S0-AIC-250

ADULT PHYSICAL CONDITIONS

Intervention Strategies for Occupational Therapy Assistants

ADULT PHYSICAL CONDITIONS

Intervention Strategies for Occupational Therapy Assistants

Amy J. Mahle, MHA, COTA/L
Founding Program Director
Occupational Therapy Assistant Program
Rowan-Cabarrus Community College
Salisbury, NC

Amber L. Ward, MS, OTR/L, BCPR, ATP/SMS
Occupational Therapy Coordinator
Neurosciences Institute Neurology-Charlotte, Carolinas Neuromuscular ALS/MDA Center
Carolinas HealthCare System, Charlotte, NC
Adjunct Instructor, Cabarrus College of Health Sciences, Concord, NC

F.A. Davis Company • Philadelphia

F. A. Davis Company
1915 Arch Street
Philadelphia, PA 19103
www.fadavis.com

Printed in the United States of America

Last digit indicates print number: 10 9 8 7 6 5 4 3 2

Senior Acquisitions Editor: Christa A. Fratantoro
Director of Content Development: George W. Lang
Developmental Editor: Jill Rembetski
Content Project Manager: Julie Chase
Art and Design Manager: Carolyn O'Brien

As new scientific information becomes available through basic and clinical research, recommended treatments and drug therapies undergo changes. The author(s) and publisher have done everything possible to make this book accurate, up to date, and in accord with accepted standards at the time of publication. The authors, editors, and publisher are not responsible for errors or omissions or for consequences from application of the book, and make no warranty, expressed or implied, in regard to the contents of the book. Any practice described in this book should be applied by the reader in accordance with professional standards of care used in regard to the unique circumstances that may apply in each situation. The reader is advised always to check product information (package inserts) for changes and new information regarding dose and contraindications before administering any drug. Caution is especially urged when using new or infrequently ordered drugs.

Library of Congress Cataloging in Publication Data

Names: Mahle, Amy J., editor. | Ward, Amber L., editor.
Title: Adult physical conditions : intervention strategies for occupational therapy assistants / [edited by] Amy J. Mahle, Amber L. Ward.
Description: First edition. | Philadelphia : F. A. Davis Company, [2019] | Includes bibliographical references and index.
Identifiers: LCCN 2018004939 | ISBN 9780803659186 (hardcover : alk. paper)
Subjects: | MESH: Occupational Therapy | Allied Health Personnel
Classification: LCC RM735.3 | NLM WB 555 | DDC 615.8/515—dc23
LC record available at https://lccn.loc.gov/2018004939

Amy's Dedication:
To my husband Scott, my endless source of steadfast love, joy, and wisdom, who with great patience endures all my pursuits and has an ear to listen. To all my family and friends, without your encouragement and support I could not have accomplished this monumental endeavor. To my son Jeremy, your contagious laughter lightens my heart. To my daughter Emily, I appreciate you sharing your gift of photography, and your love of crafting the written word inspires me. To my parents, who allowed me to be headstrong in all the right ways while growing up. To Jim and Melody, I am blessed to have always felt your love and support. To my dearest friends, many who agreed to be models for this book and all stood by me when I had little time to give. To my colleagues, who have been faithful mentors and friends. And finally, to my students, former students, and clients—you inspire me in more ways than you could imagine.

Amber's Dedication:
To my husband Bill, without whose support I would have failed miserably at this mammoth undertaking. You have bolstered me up when I have faltered, loved me unconditionally, and kept the home fires burning. To my family, who has offered unfailing encouragement and validation of my efforts, and who will have to read the book to find out what I have been up to for the past five years. To the many students and clients who inspire me daily to be a better teacher, practitioner, inventor, and mentor. To my friends and colleagues, who agreed to assist in ways large and small on this project, who have stood by me with encouragement and support, and without whose substantial efforts we would not have this book.

Dear student,
We are excited to join you along your journey into the world of occupational therapy (OT), where it may be a surprise when someone actually knows about OT. We have crafted this book, in part, based on our students' feedback on the textbooks they have used. Essentially, the feedback was that students do not read them much, if at all, and that for this to change, textbooks have to be different. You have busy lives, jobs, families, and crises, all of which do not stop just because you are in college. Our main goals for this book are to provide a high-quality and comprehensive resource, help connect both condition and intervention concepts to practice, and to make the content user-friendly. We hope that you do read it, that it helps shape you to become a compassionate and competent occupational therapy assistant (OTA), and that you do not sell it after you graduate. We know you purchased this book because it was required, but we sincerely hope it finds its way to your bookshelf, to have a place alongside other valued resources. We know the only way this will happen is if this book piques your interest, inspires you, and is a truly useful resource. We designed a few unique features and included them throughout, such as personal stories from OT practitioners and sample treatment notes and documentation, along

with critical thinking questions and real-life case studies to help make better sense of the core concepts needed to prepare you for fieldwork and entry-level practice.

As you read this book, make your notes in the margins, highlight important points, and write all over the page. Make the book yours. Use it until the pages become dog-eared. We would love that. We have been where you are and know that you have the potential to change lives through this strange and powerful concept called "occupation." We would love to hear from you regarding how the book has been helpful to you or what you suggest we do differently to improve the next edition.

Take time during your journey to study outside on a beautiful day, go for a walk, or engage in valued leisure tasks. A balance of occupations is important for your own health and wellness.

All our best,

Amy & Amber
amy.mahle.cota@gmail.com
award05otr@gmail.com

preface

As educators of occupational therapy assistant (OTA) students, we have consistently struggled to find one textbook that is specifically written for OTA students and that provides what they need to learn about occupational therapy (OT) for adults with physical conditions. We have often discussed how managing this deluge of material was both confusing and difficult. We used portions from numerous textbooks, along with other resources, to cobble together the needed content on physical conditions and interventions.

We wanted one comprehensive book that could be used throughout an OTA curriculum, contain up-to-date and relevant evidence and research, and offer students a fresh perspective. So, together, we decided we needed to write that "dream textbook." That is how this project began toward achieving our goal of having a thorough and relevant resource.

RATIONALE AND GOALS

As this project's editorial leaders, an OTA and occupational therapist, we are clinicians and educators with many years of experience, and we each brought our unique perspectives to the project. We assembled a team of 43 contributing authors, including OTAs and occupational therapists, as well as educators and/or researchers. Our shared mission has been to ensure that the textbook provides abundant evidence, the foundations of OT practice, and the practical, functional content that the OTA student craves. As editors, we have endeavored to give the chapters a consistent voice while maintaining the unique identity of the chapter authors and their expertise.

We feel strongly that textbooks, just like therapeutic interventions, need to provide the "just right challenge." With the aid of this book, the student will gain competence and confidence in addressing a variety of adult conditions and interventions.

Students often have limited time to read and may have minimal resources available to buy numerous textbooks. Many OTA students have varied life experiences, often returning to school after pursuing a different career, starting a family or upon deciding on OT as a second or third career. Thus, today's students typically have numerous other responsibilities in addition to school. To meet this challenge, this book is intended to be user-friendly and has been specifically written for the OTA, who is often a student with needs different from those of the traditional OT student. During our years of frustration with finding the right textbooks and in our focus groups with OTA students in the very beginning stages of this project, we realized that some students do not read their textbooks; and, if they do read, that task is given the least priority; or that they simply skim the pages. Our awareness emphasized the need for this book, and we knew this book must be interesting, practical, approachable, functional, and a useful resource. Our hope is that the student uses the book as the "go-to" resource through college and beyond as a new practitioner.

One option in some OTA programs is to use textbooks specifically written for the OT student. Although there is certainly crossover of content, OT and OTA programs have different needs and must meet a slightly different set of Accreditation Council for Occupational Therapy Education (ACOTE®) standards. We have worked to match the book content and features with the unique educational needs of the OTA student and to make life easier for faculty by providing a unified resource that aligns with accreditation standards at this time. Because of the requirement for the ACOTE® standards to be revised every 5 years, we specifically chose to not match chapter contents with the standards in the textbook, but added them instead to the online Instructor's Guide.

Our ultimate goal for this text is that it will help students become professional, knowledgeable, creative, and competent OTAs.

APPROACH

We have deliberately used client-first approaches throughout the book despite a trend in some groups to put the disability first. We believe that many clients are tired of being identified with their disability instead of their abilities and personhood. By using the terminology "client," rather than "patient," throughout, we align with the principles of *Occupational Therapy Practice Framework: Domain & Process, 3rd edition* (OTPF-3). We have also consciously chosen the term "occupational therapy practitioner" when a task can be completed by either the OTA or the occupational therapist and use the specific terms occupational therapist or OTA, when warranted.

We embrace the unique nature of each client and every client–practitioner interaction, and thus, the intervention portions, rather than reading as a "cookbook," present the evidence and tools to hone the clinical reasoning skills of students. The features included in each chapter were specifically created to further help students connect the concepts learned to practical applications of clinical reasoning skills.

The text contains over 300 original photos that showcase clients with disabilities as well as current equipment and technology. We worked to include a diversity of models, male and female OTAs, and individuals of different ages. Many photos capture occupations occurring in their natural environments or in specialized therapy settings. In addition to photos, the text includes a number of line art illustrations that are original and intentionally designed to demonstrate specific concepts.

ORGANIZATION OF THE TEXT

Adult Physical Conditions: Intervention Strategies for Occupational Therapy Assistants contains 37 chapters organized into four sections and has appendices and a comprehensive glossary at the end. We have integrated the guidelines of the OTPF-3, used the most up-to-date evidence, and included useful and interesting features, such as sample treatment and documentation and real-world case studies, to best illustrate chapter contents.

The chapters intentionally use cross-referencing to avoid redundancy, wherever possible. For example, the chapters on brain injury and degenerative diseases speak to those on disease-specific issues related to cognition and refer to the chapter on cognition as well. Chapter 13, Transfers Across the Continuum: Safety and Management, is intentionally comprehensive to enable readers to locate information on this topic quickly in one location. For example, this chapter includes transfers for clients with hemiplegia, severe weakness, amputations, and so on, instead of placing that content in condition-specific chapters. Our thought was that the reader would prefer to look for information on a transfer with a client with hemiplegia in one place, whatever may be the root cause of the hemiplegia. As every OT practitioner understands, tremendous differences exist among clients with the same diagnosis, and the foundational chapters will set the stage and be a reference as well.

Chapter 37, the final chapter of the book, is also a bit different. Its focus is on adult individuals with disabilities that began in childhood, such as cystic fibrosis and Duchenne muscular dystrophy, and the ways in which those conditions have affected the transition into the different stages of adulthood. This unique chapter explores how the OTA may encounter and manage clients with life-long disabilities as well as additional new conditions. This material is important in an adult-focused textbook and should not only be taught in a pediatric class, as a client with Down syndrome may have chronic diabetes, obesity, and a hip replacement, or a young adult with autism may experience ongoing sensory issues or experience a workplace brain injury.

Upon a quick glance at the table of contents, many educators may note that we have not included separate chapters on the older adult and sexual activity. Rather, we chose a different approach, weaving the topic of older adult issues and sexual activity throughout book instead of placing it in a separate chapter. The chapters include an Older Adult feature box, except in cases where it is helpful to highlight specific differences between older and younger populations. With regard to sexual activity and intimacy, we argue that discussing this subject in a separate chapter would only perpetuate the unfortunate trend of discussing sexual activity only if forced to instead of viewing it as another ADL that is part of a full and meaningful life. Sexual activity is discussed along with every other ADL in the context of every pertinent diagnosis. We hope this will lead students to genuinely connect with the importance of sexual activity and intimacy for every adult, like any other ADL, such as bathing, dressing, and self-feeding.

OVERVIEW OF CHAPTER CONTENT

Section I, *Foundations of Physical Rehabilitation, Process, and Practice,* provides to the OTA student an insight into concepts of disability, health and wellness for both the client and the OT practitioner, and the principles of teaching and learning. This section assists students to clearly understand the key elements of professionalism in OT and the expected behaviors that facilitate the transition of the student to becoming an OT practitioner. The last chapter discusses development of the occupational profile and analysis of performance skills.

Section II, *Foundations of Movement and Function,* includes essential, skill-based content, such as measuring and assessing client performance skills, all of which affect clients. Even content, such as range of motion and manual muscle testing, are holistically addressed by including not only upper and lower extremities but also intervention strategies for management. Most of the content in this section lays the foundation for subsequent chapters and is vital for the first-year student.

Section III, *Foundations of Intervention,* facilitates student understanding of all types of mobility, assistive technology, home modification, physical agent modalities, and methods of fabricating and managing orthotics. Technology, whether it is low-tech or high-tech and whether it is used at home, at work, or in the community, is an invaluable tool in the OT practitioner's kit. Driving and community mobility often mean independence for the adult and are critical issues that must be addressed even by the general OT practitioner.

Section IV, *Health Conditions and Interventions,* examines the adult physical conditions that are most commonly treated by OT practitioners and explains evidence-based intervention strategies. In addition to the conditions discussed in other textbooks, this book includes more topics in the chapters titled "Bariatric Factors and Management," "Polytrauma and Complex Multiple Conditions," "Chronic Disease Management: Utilizing a Self-Management Approach," and "The Pediatric Client—All Grown Up." Three chapters with a unique approach are "Cerebrovascular Accident: Critical Aspects and Components of Care," "Traumatic and Acquired Brain Injury: Management and Treatment," and "Spinal Cord Injury and Disease: Factors and Essential Care." The chapter on cerebrovascular accident combines the latest evidence, numerous intervention strategies, and integration with over 10 other foundational chapters. The chapter on traumatic brain injury is organized by Rancho Los Amigos Level of

Cognitive Functioning Scale with treatment interventions arranged by client symptoms. Finally, the chapter on spinal cord injury and disease includes a useful table organized by level, with skilled intervention examples, and a quick reference for chapter content presented by level of injury.

SPECIAL CHAPTER FEATURES

Each chapter contains a number of special features that will benefit students in their OT educational journey. These are as follows:

Putting It All Together: Sample Treatment and Documentation

Throughout many years of teaching, we have seen OTA students struggle to connect what they learn in the classroom and laboratory to what they will actually do in a real-life situation. Students are often confused about what to document or by the documentation process itself. A frequent comment has been: "I struggle with how to put it all together." *Putting it All Together*, included at the end of the chapters, is specifically designed to help students overcome this challenge.

This feature will help students become more prepared to use clinical reasoning and provide skilled, client-centered care. It begins with a glimpse of what an OTA might read in a client's chart—the occupational profile and basic intervention plan and goes on to illustrate the clinical reasoning process, providing a list of the tasks/activities performed in the first treatment session, corresponding goals, and rationales for selecting each task. Next is sample documentation written in the traditional SOAP note format. Finally, the student is asked to create two treatment sessions in the same format as part II (to facilitate clinical reasoning) and to write a corresponding SOAP note for each. As students practice with this format, they will build the foundation for the bridge to fieldwork and entry-level clinical practice. Because each chapter author wrote the *Putting it All Together* feature in his or her chapter, the student will see the slightly different styles of setting goals and writing SOAP notes, which is authentic to clinical practice and demonstrates that there is more than one way of "how to do it right."

Evidence-Based Practice

Although the contents of all of the chapters were written from an evidence-based perspective, this feature highlights one or more very recent research articles on a topic relevant to each chapter, with the reference(s) for accessing the resources included in the box.

OT Practitioner's Viewpoint

In this feature, each chapter author shares a personal story of first-hand experience relevant to the chapter topic. Our intention is to replicate what it would be like for the student to sit down with a seasoned practitioner and listen to a bit of wisdom or personal anecdotes.

The Older Adult

This feature highlights and examines certain aspects of the chapter content that are unique to aging and the older adult population. Not every older adult has significant health concerns, and many older adults are living long and healthy lives. Therefore, many health issues discussed will be relevant to adult clients of any age. Our goal is to help the OTA student integrate the unique concerns that affect older adults while learning the content pertinent to that function or health condition. One difference to note occurs in Chapter 33, "Cerebrovascular Accident: Critical Aspects and Components of Care," where this feature showcases "The Younger Adult," because although much of the chapter's content is about the older adult, a large number of younger adults are also experiencing strokes, and this topic may be less familiar to readers.

Communication

Timely, accurate, and clear communication is crucial to all aspects of health care, and this feature focuses on an aspect of communication unique to the chapter topic. Whether the terms and types of teamwork are interdisciplinary, multidisciplinary, or interprofessional, the bottom line is that OTAs and other healthcare professionals must communicate with each other and the client to achieve the best outcomes.

Technology and Trends

Technology advances at an exponential rate, making it challenging to pin down anything as new and innovative. Instead, the intent of this feature is to show how common technologies may be used in unique ways and to introduce technologies that are not yet commercially available.

LEARNING TOOLS

Each chapter includes a number of learning tools, which include:

- **Learning Outcomes** These serve to frame the content of the chapter and also provide a quick self-check for the reader at the completion of a chapter to ensure that the key learning objectives have been mastered.
- **Key Terms** These are listed alphabetically at the beginning of each chapter and bolded upon first use in the chapter itself. Each key term is defined in the Glossary at the end of the book.
- **Review Questions** Ten multiple-choice questions at the end of the chapters test understanding of and critical thinking about the chapter content. Since this text is designed to be used across the curriculum, the level of difficulty of the multiple-choice questions increases through the book, with the earlier chapters having more knowledge-based questions and the later chapters requiring higher critical thinking skills. Seven to eight questions in each chapter follow the traditional multiple-choice question format of four possible answers and

only one correct answer. Two to three questions follow a different format, having six options from which three correct answers are required to be selected. This aims to challenge the students to analyze multiple options; many times in OT practice, there is not just one single right answer but numerous potential solutions. Answers are provided in Appendix B.

- **Case Studies** Case studies at the end of the chapters are designed to further illustrate important learning points from the chapter. Most are real-world examples from the authors' clinical practice. The case studies are of varying lengths, and each includes questions designed to develop critical thinking skills. A few cases are formatted in a slightly different manner when they are unique to a particular condition or area of practice.

ANCILLARIES

The ancillaries include an Instructor's Guide, PowerPoint presentations and a Test Bank. These ancillaries are available at https://davisplus.fadavis.com/ to instructors who adopt and require the textbook.

The Instructor's Guide includes key documents from the book (e.g., the Putting It All Together features), which can be either printed or uploaded in a learning management system (LMS) as assignments or resources for students, such as a *Quick Reference Table to Goniometry* and a *Quick Reference Table to Manual Muscle Testing* (we strongly encourage instructors to print these tables for educational use or make available to students via the LMS). The Instructor's Guide also includes suggestions for lab activities and other valuable resources. The PowerPoint presentation for each chapter consists of basic chapter content plus key concepts designed for creative, interactive learning, and many instructors will assign them before class to spark interaction. This fresh approach is less about sitting through a lecture and more about collaborative learning and the development of critical thinking skills. These presentations are available to the educator to use "as is" or can be modified to suit individual teaching needs. Although printed in black and white in the textbook, the photos will be available in full color in the online resources in an Image Bank available to educators.

about the authors

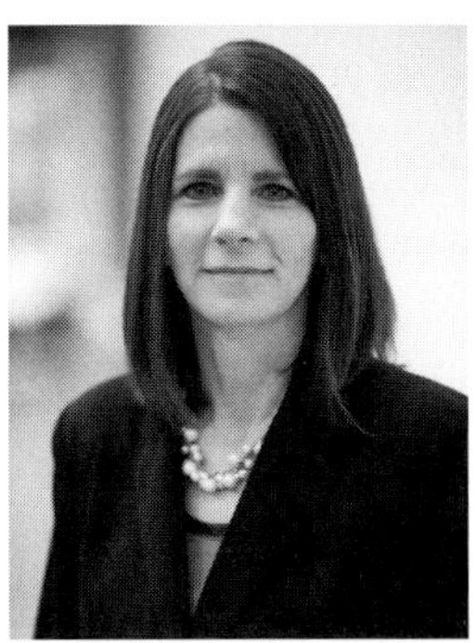

Amy J. Mahle (sounds like "mail") has been an occupational therapy assistant (OTA) for over 10 years. As many OTAs do, she found her career in occupational therapy (OT) later in life, with prior careers in social services and as a small business owner. As an OTA, she has worked in adult outpatient and acute care clinical settings and on a Brain Injury Team, and she has also assisted in the development and implementation of a Constraint-Induced Movement Therapy program. Amy enjoys creative design and problem-solving to help individuals overcome challenges, which has resulted in numerous Innovative Product Design Awards. She transitioned from clinical practice to academia on a part-time basis, eventually becoming a full-time Assistant Professor in the OTA program at Cabarrus College of Health Sciences in Concord, North Carolina where she earned the Educational Excellence Award. Most recently, she became the founding Program Director of the OTA program at Rowan-Cabarrus Community College in Salisbury, North Carolina. She regularly presents on various topics at national, state, and local levels and is especially passionate about students developing into professionals and about providing personal service to the profession and the community. She has served for several years on the board of the North Carolina Occupational Therapy Association, as Education and Research Chair, President, and most recently, Member at Large.

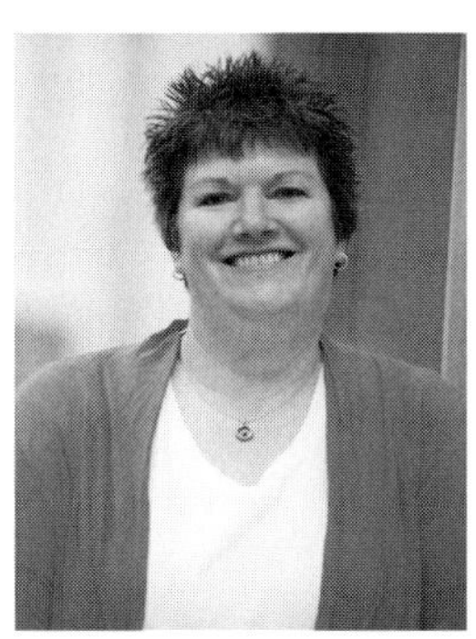

Amber L. Ward has been an occupational therapist for over 24 years—10 years in inpatient rehabilitation and more than 14 years as a full-time Occupational Therapy Coordinator, working with individuals with ALS, muscular dystrophy, and other neurological disorders. Amber has been a coordinator of a seating and wheeled mobility clinic for 12 years in addition to working in her outpatient department. She has treated a wide variety of clients of all ages and functional levels throughout her career. She has been an adjunct professor for 9 years in the OTA program at Cabarrus College of Health Sciences in Concord, North Carolina, in addition to working in the clinic. She received the RESNA Assistive Technology Professional certification in 2004, the Seating and Wheeled Mobility certification in 2014, and AOTA board certification in physical rehabilitation in 2010. Amber frequently speaks on a variety of topics at local, state, national, and international conferences. She loves to create solutions for clients with functional challenges, and she is affectionately referred to as "MacGyver" by those in her field. She has served for many years on the board of the North Carolina Occupational Therapy Association as Technology Special Interest Section Chair, Secretary, President (two terms), and, most recently, Member at Large. She has authored two journal articles about powered wheelchairs for persons with ALS and a number of other book chapters and journal articles. She is slated to receive the Roster of Fellows Award presented by the American Occupational Therapy Association just after book publication, and is proud to be added to the amazing list of professionals honored to use FAOTA in their signature.

contributors

Luis de Leon Arabit, OTD, MS, OTR/L, BCPR, C/NDT, PAM
Chapter 23
Supervisor
Department of Occupational Therapy
Adventist Health White Memorial
Los Angeles, California

Claribell Bayona, OTD, OTR/L
Chapter 24
Senior II Occupational Therapist
NYU Langone Medical Center
Manhattan, New York

Cynthia S. Bell, PhD, OTR/L, FAOTA
Chapter 6
Associate Professor and Chair of Occupational Therapy
Winston-Salem State University
Winston-Salem, North Carolina

David H. Benthall, MS, OTR/L
Chapters 25 and 26
Occupational Therapist
Durham VA Medical Center
Durham, North Carolina

Jamie Bittner, MS, OTR/L
Chapter 37
Occupational Therapist
Southeastern Cooperative Educational Programs
Norfolk, Virginia

Susan Blair, OTR/L, BCPR, BCG
Chapter 7
Clinical OT Staff Developer/Lead OT
Novant Health
Winston-Salem, North Carolina

Salvador Bondoc, OTD, OTR/L, BCPR, CHT, FAOTA
Chapter 23
Chair and Professor of Occupational Therapy
Quinnipiac University
Hamden, Connecticut

Melissa D. Brawley, MS, OTR/L
Chapter 36 and Appendix A
Home Health & Acute Care Occupational Therapist
BAYADA Home Health
Carolinas HealthCare System
Carolinas Medical Center–Main
Charlotte, North Carolina

Renee Causey-Upton, OTD, MS, OTR/L
Chapter 26
Assistant Professor
Eastern Kentucky University
Richmond, Kentucky

Megan E. Edwards Collins, PhD, OTR/L
Chapters 6 and 8
Assistant Professor
Occupational Therapy Department
Winston-Salem State University
Winston-Salem, North Carolina

Melinda Cozzolino, OTD, OTR/L, MS, CRC, BCN
Chapter 33
Associate Professor and Graduate Chair
Faculty Coordinator of Graduate Studies
Ithaca College
Ithaca, New York

Katrina Duhon Delahoussaye, MSOT/L
Chapter 17
Staff Occupational Therapist
Center for Work Rehabilitation, Inc.
Lafayette, Louisiana

Anne E. Dickerson, PhD, OTR/L, SCDCM, FAOTA
Chapter 16
Professor
East Carolina University
Greenville, North Carolina

Heather S. Dodd, MS, OTR/L
Chapter 28
Clinical Specialist
UNC Hospitals, NC Jaycee Burn Center
Chapel Hill, North Carolina

Denise K. Donica, DHSc, OTR/L, BCP, FAOTA
Chapter 37
Associate Professor
East Carolina University
Greenville, North Carolina

Joanna Edeker, PT, DPT
Chapter 29
Physical Therapist III
Carolinas HealthCare System
Carolinas Rehabilitation
Charlotte, North Carolina

Elizabeth A. Fain, EdD, OTR/L
Chapter 18
Assistant Professor
Occupational Therapy Department
Winston-Salem State University
Winston-Salem, North Carolina

Paul A. Fontana, LOTR, FAOTA
Chapter 17
Owner/Manager
Center for Work Rehabilitation, Inc.
Lafayette, Louisiana

Lori Goodnight, MS, OTR/L
Chapter 20
Subject Matter Expert
Relias Learning
Cary, North Carolina

Susan Hardesty, MS, OTR/L
Chapter 28
Occupational Therapist
Burn and Wound Therapy Co-Team Leader
Department of Rehabilitation
Eskenazi Health–Richard M. Fairbanks Burn Center
Indianapolis, Indiana

Cathrine Balentine Hatch, MS, OTR/L
Chapters 25 and 26
Lead Occupational Therapist
Piedmont Health SeniorCare
Burlington, North Carolina

Helen Houston, MS, OTR/L
Chapter 13
Occupational Therapy Clinical Specialist
Vidant Health
Greenville, North Carolina

Kelly McCoy Jones, OTR/L
Chapter 21
Occupational Therapist
NorthEast Rehabilitation
Concord, North Carolina

Brenda Kennell, BS, MA, OTR/L
Chapters 5 and 21
Program Director
Occupational Therapy Assistant Program
Central Piedmont Community College
Charlotte, North Carolina

Brittany Lorden, MHS, OTR/L, CLT
Chapter 29
Occupational Therapist III
Carolinas HealthCare System
Carolinas Rehabilitation
Charlotte, North Carolina

Amy J. Mahle, MHA, COTA/L
Chapters 1, 2, 5, 21, and 28
Program Director
Occupational Therapy Assistant Program
Rowan-Cabarrus Community College
Salisbury, North Carolina

Lisa Michaud, OTR/L
Chapter 10
Occupational Therapist
Carolinas HealthCare System
Carolinas Rehabilitation
Concord, North Carolina

Sharon D. Novalis, PhD, OTR/L
Chapter 30
Assistant Professor
Chatham University
Pittsburgh, Pennsylvania

Anna Petry, MOTR/L
Chapter 17
Occupational Therapist
The Therapy Center
Jennings, Louisiana

Lisa Pierce, COTA/L, LLCC, CEAS
Chapter 27
Certified Occupational Therapy Assistant

Jennifer C. Radloff, OTD, OTR/L, CDRS
Chapter 13
Clinical Assistant Professor, Academic Fieldwork Coordinator
Department of Occupational Therapy
East Carolina University
Greenville, North Carolina

Vivian Resnik, MHA/MBA, OTR/L
Chapter 12
Rehabilitation Director
Legacy Healthcare Services
Charlotte, North Carolina

Marjorie E. Scaffa, PhD, OTR/L, FAOTA
Chapter 4
Professor
University of South Alabama
Mobile, Alabama

Sanchala Khanolkar Sen, MSc, OTR/L, BCPR
Chapter 9
Occupational Therapist/Clinical Specialist
Novant Health Forsyth Medical Center
Adjunct Faculty
Department of Occupational Therapy
Winston-Salem State University
Winston-Salem, North Carolina

Megan McDermond Shein, OTR/L
Chapter 32
Director of Rehabilitation Services
Genesis Rehab Services
Charlotte, North Carolina

Karol Spraggs-Young, OTD, OTR/L, CHT
Chapters 19 and 22
Occupational Therapist
St. Luke's Hospital
Columbus, North Carolina
Adjunct Instructor, Cabarrus College of Health Sciences
Concord, North Carolina

LaToya Nicole Stafford, OT/L, MBA/MHA, CAPS
Chapter 3
Senior Living Program Manager II
BAYADA Home Health
Charlotte, North Carolina

Raheleh G. Tschoepe MS, OT/L
Chapter 35
Assistant Professor
Occupational Therapist
University of North Carolina–Chapel Hill
Division of Occupational Science and Occupational Therapy
Chapel Hill, North Carolina

Jordan Tucker, PT, DPT
Chapter 24
Assistant Professor
Academic Coordinator of Clinical Education
Jefferson College of Health Sciences
Physical Therapist Assistant Program
Roanoke, Virginia

Heidi A. Van Keulen, OTR/L, CBIS
Chapter 34
Occupational Therapist III
Carolinas HealthCare System
Carolinas Rehabilitation
Charlotte, North Carolina

Amber L. Ward, MS, OTR/L, BCPR, ATP/SMS
Chapters 11, 12, 14, 15, 31, and 32
Occupational Therapy Coordinator
Neurosciences Institute Neurology, Carolinas Neuromuscular ALS/MDA Center
Carolinas HealthCare System
Charlotte, North Carolina
Adjunct Instructor, Cabarrus College of Health Sciences
Concord, North Carolina

Francine Waskavitz, MS, CCC-SLP
Chapter 12
Speech-Language Pathologist
Legacy Healthcare Services
Charlotte, North Carolina

Stephanie C. Wood, OTR, CDRS
Chapter 11
Occupational Therapist, Guest Lecturer on Cognition

reviewers

We would like to thank the following reviewers for their thoughtful guidance and expertise:

Mary Kay Arvin, OTD, OTR, CHT
Assistant Professor
University of Southern Indiana
Evansville, Indiana

Janice Bacon, MEd, OTR/L
Program Director
Washburn University
Topeka, Kansas

Brandi L. Buchanan, OTD, OTR/L
Associate Professor
A.T. Still University
Mesa, Arizona

Kara Lindsay Cantoni, OTR/L
Occupational Therapist
Carolinas HealthCare System
Carolinas Rehabilitation
Charlotte, North Carolina

Michael Chan, OT
Professor
Mohawk College
Hamilton, Ontario

Megan Cook, OTR, OTR/L
Assistant Dean of OTA
Northern Virginia Community College
Springfield, Virginia

Elizabeth Joy Crawford, MSRS, OTR/L
OTA Program Coordinator
Trident Technical College
Charleston, South Carolina

LuAnn Demi, MS, OTR/L
Program Director
The Pennsylvania State University
Dubois, Pennsylvania

Dianna Fong-Lee, MA, BSc (OT)
OTA and PTA Program Coordinator and Faculty
Conestoga College
Kitchener, Ontario

Jennifer Lynn Geitner, COTA/L, BS
Academic Fieldwork Coordinator
Pueblo Community College
Pueblo, Colorado

Jennifer C. George, OTD, OTR
Instructor
Rutgers University
Scotch Plains, New Jersey

Theresa D. Gergen, EdD, OT/L
OTA Program Director
Roane State Community College
Oak Ridge, Tennessee

Laura Green, BS, MOT, OTR/L
Lead Faculty Coordinator
Kirkwood Community College
Hiawatha, Iowa

Nancy Green, MHA, OTR/L
OTA Program Chair
Cabarrus College of Health Sciences
Concord, North Carolina

Tamla Heminger, OTR, MEd
OTA Program Director
UA Cossatot
Ashdown, Arkansas

Cassady Anne Hoff, MSOT, OTR/L
OTA Program Director
Casper College
Casper, Wyoming

Lisa Ellen Hubbs, MS, OTR/L
OTA Program Coordinator
Suffolk County Community College
Brentwood, New York

Amber Jenkins, MLS, OTR/L
Coordinator
Metropolitan Community College
Kansas City, Missouri

Stephanie Johnston, MA, OTR
Professor/Fieldwork Coordinator
Lone Star College
Tomball, Texas

Amy Kampschroeder, OTR/L
Instructor
Cape Fear Community College
Wilmington, North Carolina

Linda Kelly, PhD, LOTR
Program Director
Delgado Community College
New Orleans, Louisiana

Brenda Kennell, BS, MA, OTR/L
Program Director
Central Piedmont Community College
Charlotte, North Carolina

Jeanne M. Kerschner, OT
Clinical Director and Instructor
Pennsylvania College of Technology
Williamsport, Pennsylvania

Jeanette Krajca, MS, OTR
OTA Program Director
Navarro College
Corsicana, Texas

Brenda K. Lyman, OTR/L, OTD
Professor/Associate Dean
Salt Lake Community College
West Jordan, Utah

Cynthia Lynn Meyer, MEd, MS, OTR/L, OTA
OTA Program Director and Professor
South Arkansas Community College
El Dorado, Arkansas

Mary M. Malone, MS, OTR/L
Professor
North Shore Community College
Danvers, Massachusetts

Claudia Jean Miller, OTD, OTR/L
OTA Program Chair
Cincinnati State and Technical College
Cincinnati, Ohio

Ave Marie Mitta, MS, OTR/L
Program Director
Jefferson College of Health Sciences
Roanoke, Virginia

Michelle Parolise, MBA, OTR/L
Program Coordinator
Santa Ana College
Santa Ana, California

Kimberly Renee Prevo, MS, OTR/L
Assistant Professor
Kirkwood Community College
Cedar Rapids, Iowa

Connie Rooks, MAT, COTA/L
Program Director
Western New Mexico University
Silver City, New Mexico

Jennifer J. Saylor, MEd, OT/L
Professor and Director
River Valley Community College
Claremont, New Hampshire

Karyn Shenker-Gould, OTR/L
Assistant Professor
Maria College
Albany, New York

Michelle M. Sheperd, EdD, OTR
Dean of Specialty Program
Brown Mackie College
Woodridge, Illinois

Rae Ann Smith, OTD, OTR/L
Program Director
Allegany College of Maryland
Cumberland, Maryland

Chris Sorrells, OTR/L, CHT
Instructor
Pima Medical Institute
Denver, Colorado

Amy VanCamp, OTD
Academic Fieldwork Coordinator
Clinical Assistant Professor
University of New Hampshire, College of Health and Human Services
Durham, New Hampshire

Christine Vicino, MA, OTA/L
OTA Program Director
Grossmont College
El Cajon, California

acknowledgments

We first acknowledge Christa Fratantoro, at F. A. Davis, who believed and assisted in our vision and skillfully guided us with grace and positivity to bring it to fruition. Jill Rembetski, we especially thank you for your extreme patience, careful direction, and unwavering encouragement through every stage of preparing this book for publication. You are both worthy of the title "editor extraordinaire." We also recognize others at F. A. Davis who believed in our project—George Lang, Amelia Blevins, Paul Marone, Julie Chase, Bob Butler, and many others. We are especially grateful for F. A. Davis's approach to design, which, in our visually intense environment, serves the content well.

As we embarked on this arduous, yet worthwhile and exciting journey of writing and editing a comprehensive textbook on adult conditions and OT interventions, we knew that we needed to surround ourselves with experts who were also passionate about teaching, learning, and OT. With much appreciation, we recognize all of our dedicated and talented contributing authors, who agreed to write a chapter for a textbook with two unknown main authors/editors. We are forever grateful for your contributions to the profession and, specifically, OTA education.

Throughout the project, we personally called upon several colleagues who have specialty knowledge or experience in a particular setting to help provide editorial assistance. We are incredibly grateful to Leah Holland Fisher (Chapter 11); Amy Wright (Chapter 12); Molly Shannon, Tammy Pereboom, and Amy Wright (Chapter 14); Jessica Pedersen (Chapter 15); Christa Gallie-Weiss (Chapter 33); and Kara Cantoni (Chapter 35). The collective knowledge and experience of these experts served to make this textbook even stronger in its content. We would like to acknowledge Brenda Kennell, BS, MA, OTR/L, for her expertise and considerable time in assisting us in the final stages of thoughtful editing to ensure this book is the best possible resource for instructors and students.

For the majority of the photographs, we owe special thanks to Jason Torres, who climbed up and down ladders for 4 days to get the "perfect shot." You are a master. We are grateful to Emily Rheinbolt, of Em Brooker Photography (Amy's daughter), who was ready at a moment's notice for multiple mini-photoshoots with special people and environments that we could not have otherwise captured. Many students, former students, family, friends, and clients with conditions or disabilities and their caregivers assisted with the photoshoots and generously gave of their time. Starla Daniel and Jonesha Wallace volunteered especially long hours to assist with many aspects of the main photoshoot.

We were very fortunate to have gracious hosts allow us to use their spaces and equipment. We are deeply grateful to Rowan-Cabarrus Community College and Dr. Wendy Barnhardt for permitting us to use the beautiful OTA program laboratory and North campus for the majority of the main photoshoot. We also thank Cress Goodnight and Novant Health for assistance in coordinating and hosting photoshoot locations at Novant Health–Rowan Medical Center and Novant Health Rehabilitation Center – Salisbury. We thank Diane Spicer, her therapy team, and clients at The Laurels of Salisbury. And finally, we express our appreciation of Nancy Green and Cabarrus College of Health Sciences for use of their OT laboratory and to several of their graduate OT students who were willing models.

We also want to acknowledge others who brought hard-to-find equipment and helped make these amazing photos possible—Amy Street and Steven Shope from Hanger, Inc.; Sandy Erwin from Invacare Corporation; Robert Flanagan and Worth Williams from National Seating & Mobility; Allen McKinley from Marketing Sales Logistics and his canine assistant Murphy; Regina LeFauve from Bioness; Derek Fletcher from R82; Brenda Kennell from Central Piedmont Community College; Tammy Pereboom from the North Carolina Assistive Technology Program; the Neurosciences Institute Neurology–Charlotte, North Carolina; and the loan closet and staff at the Carolinas Neuromuscular ALS/MDA Center.

contents in brief

contents

unit I

Foundations of Physical Rehabilitation, Process, and Practice

Chapter 1

Client-Centered Occupational Therapy: Disability and Participation

Amy J. Mahle, MHA, COTA/L

LEARNING OUTCOMES

After studying this chapter, the student or practitioner will be able to:

1.1 Explain the meaning of physical disability
1.2 Discuss the foundation of occupational therapy in the area of physical disability
1.3 Relate the significance of purposeful activity to an individual with a physical disability
1.4 Describe how a physical disability affects engagement in occupations
1.5 Explain common psychological and social adjustment issues associated with having a physical disability
1.6 Compare the role of the occupational therapist and occupational therapy assistant in physical disability education and treatment across the continuum of care
1.7 Summarize the role of the occupational therapy assistant on healthcare teams

KEY TERMS

Accommodation	Model of practice
Activities of daily living (ADLs)	Multidisciplinary team
Activity limitation	Participation restriction
Canadian Model of Occupational Performance and Engagement (CMOP-E)	Person-Environment-Occupation-Performance (PEOP)
Disability	Purposeful activity
Frame of reference	Short-term disability
Impairment	Theory
Inclusion	Therapeutic use of self
Instrumental activities of daily living (IADLs)	Transdisciplinary team
Interdisciplinary team	World Health Organization (WHO)
Model of Human Occupation (MOHO)	

A change in one's ability to perform meaningful, necessary, and familiar tasks, also known as occupations, can be quite a challenge to an individual and his or her loved ones—physically, emotionally, psychologically, socially, and spiritually. Occupational therapy (OT) for adults with physical conditions addresses disability in terms of the whole person, seeking to assist in returning the person to performing valued occupations through the use of techniques and tools that have been tested and proven valid. The OT practitioner partners with the client to identify meaningful occupations, create customized goals, and use intervention strategies to improve function, whether or not the person improves his or her physical condition.

PHYSICAL DISABILITY

Disability, as defined by the **World Health Organization (WHO)** and the International Classification of Functioning, Disability, and Health (ICF), is a broad term, encompassing three areas: impairments, activity limitations, and participation restrictions.[1] **Impairment** is a difficulty with a body part or parts or the way the body functions. For example, a person who has had a stroke (cerebrovascular accident [CVA]) may not be able to use one arm, and thus would be considered to have an impairment, or disability, according to the WHO and ICF. **Activity limitation** means that a person is unable to perform a meaningful task or action, such as being unable to bend over to tie one's shoes due to a severe back injury. Finally, a **participation restriction** means that a person cannot be involved in a specific life situation, for example, an individual who uses a wheelchair would not be able to perform the typical job of a police officer on patrol in the same way as someone who does not use a wheelchair.

Formerly, in the 1960s, 1970s, and earlier, disability was defined purely in physical terms, without regard to the individual and his or her complex interaction with the environment.[1] However, the new definition of "disability" is broad, and individuals who have disabilities vary greatly from those who have significant health conditions requiring extensive medical treatment to those who experience more mild forms of disability.[1] As the public becomes more aware of disability and as the perception of disability has changed over the years, the agencies that provide funding and assistance for people with disabilities have changed their objectives, too. Historically, agencies mainly provided financial assistance, but now the emphasis has altered to "supporting independence and promoting involvement in all aspects of society."[2] OT fits perfectly with the current culture of focusing on independence and engagement in society.

Consider how a physical disability affects more than just the body. A person with a disability experiences complex changes and challenges in his or her valued life roles, affecting family, friends, work, the person's many environments, and the person's psychological and emotional health. OT assists individuals with disabilities in crucial ways, including adapting the environment or task, providing rehabilitation strategies for the body, delivering education and training in adapted techniques, and promoting self-advocacy for the client with the primary goal of individuals engaging in their occupations.[3]

Prevalence of Disability

How prevalent is disability? Researchers from Cornell University discovered that in 2012, 12.1% of noninstitutionalized individuals in the United States reported living with some type of disability,[4] which is a significant portion of the population. Interestingly, the *rate* has remained almost the same since 2008, despite population growth and advances in medicine.[4] This means that the *total number* of people in the United States who are living with a disability is on the rise. The U.S. Census Bureau uses a slightly different measure of disability, because the surveys it creates use a broader definition, and reports that in the most recent census, 2010, 19% of the population (almost 1 in 5) reported living with a disability, and that more than half of those individuals were considered to have a severe disability.[2] Of further interest is that as Americans age, they become increasingly more likely to experience a severe disability. The U.S. Census Bureau reports that the possibility of an individual who is 15 to 24 years of age having a severe disability is 5%, but this increases to 25% for an individual 65 to 69 years of age.[2] The growth in the aging population due to the Baby Boomer generation may increase the total amount of people with a severe disability. When coupled with the fact that there is a 25% chance of having a severe disability after age 65, one can understand the increasing need for healthcare providers, especially OT practitioners. Figure 1-1 provides a breakdown of the U.S. Census Bureau self-reported disability data from 2010. Notice that the highest numbers of disabilities are in populations that have difficulty with ambulation, need to use assistive devices, have trouble with lifting or grasping, or have challenges performing basic **activities of daily living (ADLs)** and **instrumental activities of daily living (IADLs).** The *Occupational Therapy Practice Framework: Domain and Process, 3rd edition* (OTPF-3), a foundational document

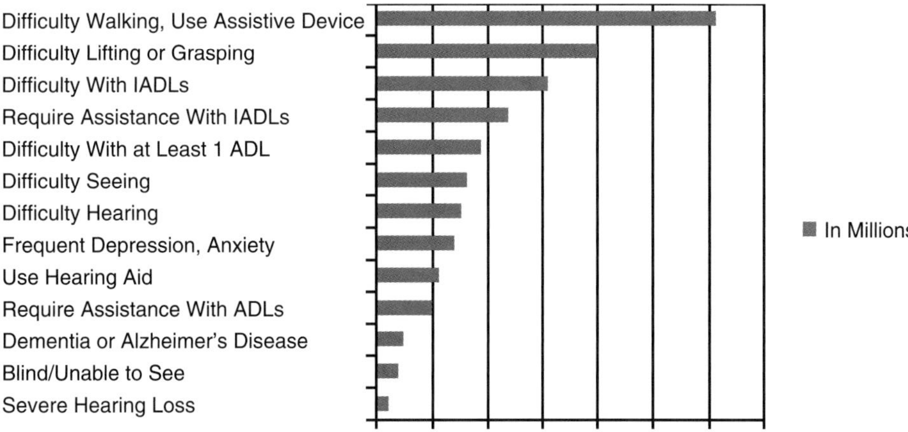

FIGURE 1-1. Types and prevalence of disability in the United States. *(Source: United States Census Bureau, 2012.)*

for the practice of OT, defines ADLs and IADLs. ADLs are tasks that one performs to take care of oneself, such as bathing, toileting, grooming, dressing, self-feeding and swallowing, moving around in one's home, and sexual activity. IADLs are tasks that are performed just beyond the scope of caring for one's own body, such as cooking, medication management, light housework, driving, grocery shopping, and taking care of children and pets.[3] Refer to the OTPF-3, available through the American Occupational Therapy Association (AOTA), for a complete list and description of ADL and IADL tasks.

Gender, Race, and Ethnicity of Disability

The U.S. Census Bureau reports on many aspects of disability, and the 2013 data from the American Community Survey (of noninstitutionalized individuals) provides detailed data regarding gender, race, and ethnicity.[5] Gender differences in the rate of disability are very small, with 12.4% male and 12.7% female rates of overall disability in the United States. When specific disabilities are presented later in this textbook, some disabilities will be noted to be more prevalent in one gender or the other.

Rates of disability are reported for the most common races and ethnicities represented in the United States. The race with the highest percentage of disability is American Indian or Native Alaskan (grouped together) at 17.1%, and the lowest is Asian at 7%. For ethnicity, the Not Latino/Not Hispanic category reports 13.8% disability, and the Hispanic/Latino (of any race) reports 8.7%.[5] Similar to gender, there are some diagnoses that are more prevalent to specific race or ethnicity. See Table 1-1 for details.

Disability Rights

In the United States, the Americans with Disabilities Act of 1990 (ADA) is a law that ensures that people with disabilities have equal access to public and commercial spaces and equal opportunities in employment, school, and transportation, as well as legal protection from discrimination.[6] The ADA defines disability broadly, and rather than compiling a list of diagnoses, states the following: "The term 'disability' means, with respect to an individual: (A) a physical or mental impairment that substantially limits one or more major life activities of such individual; (B) a record of such an impairment; or (C) being regarded as having such an impairment."[6] Before 1990, the rights of people with disabilities were not protected. For example, individuals who used a wheelchair for community mobility were denied access to public transportation because buses and airplanes were not required to be adapted for individuals with disabilities. For some, public transportation could mean the only opportunity to travel to work or medical appointments. Restaurants, stores, airports, libraries, and other public or commercial buildings and areas were not required to have barrier-free access. For example, a "handicapped accessible" toilet stall, sink, and mirror, and access to soap and towels, were not required; however, they are now all commonplace components of any public restroom.

The ADA has made a significant difference in the lives of many people with disabilities. However, despite the ADA, many physical barriers remain. For instance, some health screening equipment (mammography) is not adjustable for wheelchair users, and can only be used with people who are able to stand.[1] The ADA does not "grandfather in" (exempt them from following the law) older buildings, but instead requires existing buildings to remove barriers to access that are *readily achievable.* The ADA also states that small businesses only have to make "reasonable accommodations" for access that do not cause a financial hardship on the business. This means that the accessible entrance to a building may be in an awkward and out of the way place, rather than near the front entrance. There may be a ramp, as required by the ADA, but an automatic door opener is not a requirement, and the lack of one may cause access problems. Refer to www.ADA.gov for more detailed information.

Although the United States has made great efforts to protect the rights of individuals with disabilities, such strides do not mean that all things are actually equal. The WHO

TABLE 1-1 Race and Ethnicity of Disability

	TOTAL		WITH A DISABILITY		PERCENT WITH A DISABILITY	
SUBJECT	*ESTIMATE*	*MARGIN OF ERROR*	*ESTIMATE*	*MARGIN OF ERROR*	*ESTIMATE*	*MARGIN OF ERROR*
Gender						
Male	152,044,681	±31,462	18,912,986	71,522	12.4	±0.1
Female	159,113,423	±29,576	20,225,000	66,457	12.7	±0.1
Race and Hispanic or Latino Origin						
One Race	301,947,736	±78,375	38,110,427	±104,830	12.6%	±0.1
White alone	229,777,799	±125,936	29,948,473	±92,044	13.0%	±0.1
Black or African American alone	38,642,158	±55,396	5,392,788	±39,679	14.0%	±0.1
American Indian and Alaska Native alone	2,461,292	±28,063	420,090	±9,652	17.1%	±0.3
Asian alone	15,933,974	±35,663	1,108,627	±17,666	7.0%	±0.1
Native Hawaiian and Other Pacific Islander alone	513,332	±11,716	52,924	±3,913	10.3%	±0.8
Some other race alone	14,619,181	±129,567	1,187,525	±25,286	8.1%	±0.2
Two or more races	9,210,368	±75,419	1,027,559	±19,404	11.2%	±0.2
White alone, not Hispanic or Latino	194,651,933	±25,545	26,867,922	±86,616	13.8%	±0.1
Hispanic or Latino (of any race)	53,264,531	±12,081	4,644,799	±41,850	8.7%	±0.1

U.S. Census Bureau Data (2013), American Community Survey.[5]

identifies other factors beyond the primary physical cause that affect individuals with a disability, including unmet needs for health care, secondary conditions (such as osteoporosis, pressure injuries, increased risk for falls) that develop as a result of the primary cause, comorbid conditions, engaging in risky health behaviors, premature aging, and higher rates of premature death.[1] Healthy People 2020 is a national initiative to measure the health of the U.S. population and sets goals for the health of every American.[7] Healthy People 2020 reports specific ways that people with disabilities are disadvantaged regarding health, as shown in Box 1-1.

A subset of individuals with disability has been tracked, and through analysis, goals have been developed to address the concerns of individuals with disabilities (Box 1-2). OT is uniquely positioned to work toward helping individuals achieve goals for healthy living.

A person without a disability may have a difficult time understanding the unique needs of the disabled population and all of the challenges they face. Upon entering the profession of OT, take time to seek an understanding of these challenges. Consider how a wheelchair user accessing public transportation would perform weekly grocery shopping for the whole family. Imagine the extra time it would take to get dressed with significantly decreased range of motion (ROM) in the shoulders, or with only the use of one hand. The occupational therapy assistant (OTA) is often the change agent to help the client overcome personal and environmental concerns.

PHILOSOPHY OF OCCUPATIONAL THERAPY RELATED TO PHYSICAL DISABILITY

Formal recognition of OT as a profession began on March 15, 1917, with the founding of the National Society for the Promotion of Occupational Therapy, known today as the

BOX 1-1

Health Disparities in the Population With Disabilities[8]

Individuals with disabilities have been found to have the following health disparities in comparison with the rest of the population. They:

- Experience difficulties or delays in getting the health care they need
- Have not had an annual dental visit
- Have not had a mammogram in the past 2 years
- Have not had a Papanicolaou (Pap) test within the past 3 years
- Do not engage in fitness activities
- Use tobacco
- Are more likely to be overweight or obese
- Have high blood pressure
- Are more likely to experience symptoms of psychological distress
- Receive less social-emotional support
- Have lower employment rates

BOX 1-2

Healthy People 2020 Disability and Health Objectives[7]

Improving the conditions of daily life by:

- Encouraging communities to be accessible so all can live in, move through, and interact with their environment
- Encouraging community living
- Removing barriers in the environment using both physical universal design concepts and operational policy shifts

Addressing the inequitable distribution of resources among individuals with disabilities and those without disabilities by increasing:

- Appropriate health care for individuals with disabilities
- Education and work opportunities
- Social participation
- Access to needed technologies and assistive supports

Expanding the knowledge base and raising awareness about determinants of health for individuals with disabilities by increasing:

- The inclusion of individuals with disabilities in public health data collection efforts across the life span
- The inclusion of individuals with disabilities in health promotion activities
- The expansion of disability and health training opportunities for public health and healthcare professionals

American Occupational Therapy Association (AOTA). "Over the past century, the underlying philosophy of occupational therapy has evolved from being a diversion from illness, to treatment, to enablement through meaningful occupation."[9] OT began treating individuals with mental illness by involving them in activities and arts and crafts with an occupational focus as a diversion from their conditions, called *moral treatment*. After wounded soldiers returned from World War I, the OT field expanded to include not only clients with mental conditions but also those with physical disabilities. Part of this shift also included an effort to create vocational activities. Physical rehabilitation enabled veterans to return to productive work. Progress in the OT field has regularly centered on caring for wounded soldiers ever since.[10]

Following World War II, the Rehabilitation Movement began as an effort to move wounded veterans into job-related occupations. During this time, the OT field shifted its focus to a medical model of care and the formation of specific standards of care. This approach focused on treating the *patient's* specific illness or disorder (to relieve symptoms and compensate for disability) rather than considering the *client* as a whole person (to identify problems, set priorities, and set client-centered goals for participation in occupation). Many U.S. Department of Veterans Affairs hospitals increased in size and founded rehabilitation departments to serve wounded veterans. OT practitioners who were previously working in psychiatric hospitals were needed by the veterans, thus the OT profession shifted further away from its original roots in mental health. In addition to the effects of the war, numerous other changes to the OT field occurred during the late 1940s and into the 1950s, such as the development of thermoplastic splinting (orthotic) materials, better wheelchairs, and advanced prosthetics. OT practitioners needed advanced training in these specialized medical areas. To fill a shortage of practitioners working in psychiatric settings, the role of the OTA was developed in 1958.[11]

The OT field continued to focus on the medical model of care until debates ensued in the 1970s. Many members of the profession argued that OT had become too medically based and was lacking the "roots" of engaging clients in their occupations. Remember, the profession began as a means to engage those with mental illness in activities that would help divert the mind back to meaningful pursuits. The profession slowly began moving away from the stringent medical model, and strong proponents of the more holistic view helped refocus OT on occupation and meaning once again.[9] One such proponent was Mary Reilly, a renowned occupational therapist and theorist, who wisely summarized what she discovered as a common thread in her research of the history of the profession of OT: "That man, through the use of his hands as they are energized by mind and will, can influence the state of his own health."[12]

Purposeful Activity

The very essence of Reilly's statement describes the concept of **purposeful activity.** Think for a moment of an unpleasant task or chore. Would a person be motivated to begin,

TECHNOLOGY AND TRENDS

VETERAN AND WOUNDED WARRIOR CARE

The American Occupational Therapy Association (AOTA) has identified the veteran and wounded warrior population as an emerging niche in rehabilitation and disability due to the large number of active military personnel and the increasing number of veterans in our aging population. Of particular interest in this population is the increase in brain injuries and growing number of veterans with polytrauma (for example, one soldier who experiences an amputation, brain injury, and posttraumatic stress disorder). AOTA offers suggestions on how to become involved in working in this emerging niche, such as joining the army, serving as a civilian, or working for Veteran's Affairs.[13]

complete the task well, or even to finish it? Now consider a highly enjoyable task. Would a person be motivated to start, and give the best possible effort? During and after the preferred activity, does the person feel a sense of accomplishment, joy, or pleasure? Humans tend to spend time doing what they value when given the choice. We naturally use our minds and wills to occupy time and exert effort doing purposeful and meaningful activities.

The OTPF-3 serves as a guide for the scope of practice, areas in which OT practitioners can legally provide therapy, and the manner in which services are provided. One key term described in the OTPF-3 is "purposeful activity."[3] What makes an activity purposeful? The simple answer is an activity that the client wants to do and that has meaning for the individual. How does an OTA use activities therapeutically? OT practitioners are trained in activity analysis, which is the skill of breaking down and identifying every task into smaller parts and analyzing what is needed to perform the task or activity. When the OT practitioner works with a client, he or she understands the client's limitations in performing the activity and helps adapt the method or tools to help the client successfully complete the task. For example, Rita is a client who has difficulty grasping her favorite utensils to bring food to her mouth due to painful and progressive rheumatoid arthritis affecting her hands. The OT practitioner analyzes the task and tools and determines that even though Rita loves her utensils that she received as a wedding gift 38 years ago, they are not beneficial for her to use at this time. Because there is no cure for rheumatoid arthritis, the OT practitioner knows she must help Rita identify what changes are appropriate. The practitioner *adapts* Rita's utensils by placing a piece of cylindrical foam on their handles and also has Rita try different types of tools with built-up handles for opening containers (Fig. 1-2). Rita performs the *purposeful activity* of eating lunch with her newly adapted utensils and smiles with delight because she is no longer in pain while grasping them. She is especially thrilled that she can still use a familiar and beloved item, just with a simple modification. Purposeful activities are used as therapeutic interventions because they are motivating for the client.

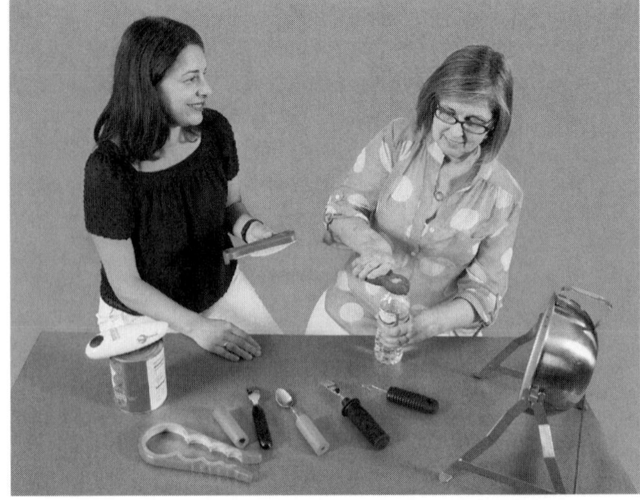

FIGURE 1-2. OTA educates client in using various adaptive equipment for the occupations of cooking and self-feeding. Shown here are various can, jar, and bottle openers, regular utensils adapted with foam tubing, utensils with built-up handles, and a bowl holder with bowl.

THEORIES, MODELS OF PRACTICE, AND FRAMES OF REFERENCE

Theories, models of practice, and frames of reference are various methods for the OT practitioner to understand the relationship between the client and what is performed in OT. They are guiding principles for providing client-centered care. Yet the terms *theory, models of practice,* and *frame of reference* and how they relate to one another are often confusing for students.

Theory

A **theory** is a broad method to understand how something works and defines the relationship between concepts. "Theories are integral to healthcare practice, promotion, and research. The choice of theory, although often unacknowledged, shapes the way practitioners and researchers collect and interpret evidence."[14] Well-known theories include Newton's law of universal gravitation (gravity) to explain why an object falls when not supported rather than float in the air. A theory is thoroughly tested and found to be true. Similarly, theories in OT help direct and guide understanding of practitioners and are foundations of models of practice. An example of an OT theory is Mary Reilly's theory of occupational behavior, in which she posited that there is a significant relationship between occupation and health.[15]

Models of Practice

Models of practice are ways of viewing the relationship of the person, the environment, occupation, and desired outcomes, and can serve to help test theories. The top three occupation-focused models included in OT programs across the United States, Canada, Australia, and the United Kingdom are the Model of Human Occupation, Person-Environment-Occupation-Performance, and the Canadian Model of Occupational Performance and Engagement.[16] Models of practice and frames of reference should be used together to inform assessment and intervention decisions. A very brief explanation is that models of practice are broad ways to understand individuals and their motivating factors for participation in occupations. Frames of reference are explanations for understanding cause and effect between individuals and their performance. The combination of the two help OT practitioners provide assessment and intervention in a client-centered manner. The next section will describe the top models of practice.

MODEL OF HUMAN OCCUPATION

The **Model of Human Occupation (MOHO)** was developed by Gary Kielhofner and has been used worldwide. MOHO focuses on "understanding and developing a person's occupational identity as well as occupational competence (the ability to participate in occupational routines and roles) in order to facilitate adaptation to the dynamic demands of the occupational life patterns."[16] The focus of intervention, then, is a client's volition (willingness to do something) and the client's habituation (how the client does things), which leads to improved competence and identity, finally leading to occupational adaptation.[17] For example, consider Rose, a client who needed to use oxygen due to a serious lung condition. She valued taking care of her flower garden, cooking meals, and playing with her grandchildren. After her lung condition worsened, she could no longer go outside to tend her garden and did not have the energy to cook the types of meals she preferred or play the same games with her grandchildren. She lost interest in all of her favorite tasks and became depressed. Using the MOHO model, an OT practitioner would determine the roles Rose valued, identify which tasks she was motivated to perform and unmotivated to perform (and why), and then implement strategies (using frames of reference) to help Rose overcome her decreased participation in meaningful occupations. The OT practitioner might change the way Rose did those tasks, the length of the tasks, the time of day, or the sequencing, to optimize her competence and identity in her valued roles and get her back to doing the things she cherishes.

PERSON-ENVIRONMENT-OCCUPATION-PERFORMANCE

The **Person-Environment-Occupation-Performance** (PEOP model; formerly the PEO model) explains the interaction between the person (intrinsic), the environment (extrinsic), the person's occupations, and the performance of those occupations in five dimensions (psychological, neurological, spiritual, physiological, and motor factors). The model centers on understanding how these dimensions interact with one another to promote well-being and quality of life. Interconnected and overlapping circles represent the model, and when one factor changes, it influences the success of occupational performance and participation.[16]

For example, consider Jason, who used to enjoy working full-time and participating in hobbies such as woodworking in his garage woodshop with friends and being a beekeeper with his wife and children. He started losing weight, feeling constantly fatigued, and having some strange sensations in his legs and feet (intrinsic–physical) to the degree that he lost the desire to work in the woodshop with his friend (extrinsic–social) or keep bees with his family (extrinsic–social). He was later diagnosed with type 2 diabetes and had a subsequent right lower extremity amputation due to uncontrolled diabetes and poor sensation (intrinsic–physical). He began to doubt his faith (intrinsic–spiritual), became depressed (intrinsic–psychological), and did little more than go to work part-time and play video games the rest of the day (decreased occupational performance and participation). Through OT, he was able to make major changes in both intrinsic and extrinsic factors, leading to increased occupational performance and participation. Several frames of reference were used to assist Jason. He gave up keeping bees because he could no longer eat honey, but started exercising and changed his diet to help control his diabetes. And after being fit with a prosthesis and obtaining an adapted bike, he began riding his bike every day (intrinsic–physical) with a friend (extrinsic–social) and cooking healthy meals with his family (intrinsic–physical and extrinsic–social). He went back to his full-time job and lived an active, healthy lifestyle.

CANADIAN MODEL OF OCCUPATIONAL PERFORMANCE AND ENGAGEMENT

The **Canadian Model of Occupational Performance and Engagement (CMOP-E)** model depicts the client at the center, with spirituality (aspects that give meaning, purpose, self-will, and determination) as the core motivating principle, which is foundational for the cognitive, affective (behavioral), and physical aspects. Surrounding this core is the individual's occupations, followed by the outermost layer, the environment.[16]

The Canadian Occupational Performance Measure (COPM) is a tool that was designed along with the CMOP-E model to be used in assessment and treatment intervention.

Frame of Reference

A **frame of reference** is a "system of compatible concepts from theory that guide a plan of action for assessment and intervention within specific occupational therapy domains."[18] More simply put, using a frame of reference helps the OT practitioner to focus specifically on addressing the underlying causes limiting occupation, whether due to activity limitation, impairment, or restriction. A frame of reference leads to practical application. Understanding the reason for the limitation the client is experiencing guides the practitioner to select a frame of reference, and by using a frame of reference, one can understand what approach to take to assist a client to meet his or her desired goals. Often an OT practitioner uses more than one frame of reference with a client. The following section is a brief overview of some of the frames of reference used in OT. In many cases, there may be specific assessments (tools to give an objective and accurate measurement) that correspond to each frame of reference. The student will have a better understanding of these frames of reference after more is learned about the conditions for which they are used.

BIOMECHANICAL

The biomechanical frame of reference applies to human movement and posture and is typically used when a client has musculoskeletal issues, hand injuries, or requires reconditioning in preparation for returning to work after an injury. Goals for the biomechanical frame of reference are for the client to gain strength, increase ROM, reduce pain or swelling, maintain joint ROM or strength, and prevent contractures (shortening of muscles and associated structures, which causes significant loss of ROM). For example, for a client who had a fracture, the muscles surrounding the bone that was fractured will become weaker and shorter without use or movement during the time the bone is healing. Once the bone is healed, typically after the removal of a cast, the muscles that are attached to the bone and cause movement to the joint can be stretched and strengthened. Examples of assessments for the biomechanical frame of reference would be a goniometer to measure joint ROM (movement) and a dynamometer and pinch gauges to measure the strength of a client's hand grasp and pinch grip (see Chapters 7 and 9).

REHABILITATION

The rehabilitation frame of reference is focused on helping a client return to the highest level of function possible, and is typically used with clients who have neurological or sensorimotor conditions, such as multiple sclerosis, spinal cord injury, CVA, or others. The goals of the rehabilitative frame of reference are to adapt the method (technique) or tools (adaptive equipment), make changes to the environment, or compensate for difficulties in performing occupations. The rehabilitative process may be long and incorporate other frames of reference. The goal is to maximize the client's participation in valued occupations. A good example is using special equipment and techniques to help with dressing and chopping/cutting food for someone who had a CVA and can functionally use only one side of his or her body.

MULTICONTEXT TREATMENT APPROACH

This approach is used with clients who have cognitive or perceptual challenges that affect the ability to engage in occupations and focuses on self-monitoring and transferring learning throughout several contexts. The approach seeks to restore cognitive and/or perceptual abilities or promote learning to adapt to compensate for decreased skills. Clients may have difficulty with any of the cognitive tasks, such as memory, problem-solving, decision-making, attention, sequencing, visual perception, and self-awareness. Using the multicontext treatment approach, clients practice skills needed in the actual context in which they occur and in varied contexts so they learn to be able to perform the task in any environment.[19]

NEUROFUNCTIONAL APPROACH

The neurofunctional approach was specifically designed for use with clients following a severe brain injury.[20] The approach recognizes that clients have decreases in some skills due to the impact of the injury, and seeks to restore skills through high-repetition, task-specific training, often in the context in which the task would normally occur. For instance, if a client had difficulty with brushing teeth, the practitioner would work on the task, such as placing the toothbrush in the mouth and initiating brushing motions (task specific) while the client is seated or standing at a sink (context).

BEHAVIORAL AND COGNITIVE BEHAVIORAL

There are multiple individual frames of reference that fall into the behavioral category. In general, this frame of reference is based on changing patterns of behavior. Conditions to which this frame of reference would apply are developmental disabilities and brain injury, and it focuses on changing objective, measurable behaviors.

COGNITIVE DISABILITY

The cognitive disability frame of reference is primarily used with clients who have experienced cognitive decline or impairment, such as following a brain injury or for a client with dementia. This frame of reference focuses on the skill of cognition and its impact on occupational performance and helps the practitioner provide activities that match the cognitive level of the client.

SENSORIMOTOR

The sensorimotor approach is used when the central nervous system has been affected, such as by a CVA or brain injury. There may be impairment in the senses, such as vision, sense of touch, or sense of movement (proprioception). Tasks are taught through repetition of movement patterns as a way of retraining the brain to gain voluntary control of movement. For example, following a CVA, a client may have decreased sensation on one side. With the sensorimotor approach, a treatment strategy may be to have the client apply lotion to the affected side and incorporate active observation and attention to the task. Eventually, the body will respond motorically to the specific sensory approach.

MOTOR LEARNING

The motor learning approach centers on the premise that movement is controlled by the neurological connections in the brain, and that those connections can be retrained to produce improved movement after a CVA, brain injury, or other condition that affects movement. A client who has had a CVA may have impaired movement (but good sensation), and this frame of reference would have the practitioner incorporate specific repetition of tasks with attention to how they are being performed and to give feedback to correct movements.

ADJUSTMENT TO DISABILITY

Imagine that a person woke up this morning suddenly paralyzed from the waist down. How would the disability change this person's routine, or roles, such as student, family member, employee, and so on? The way in which he performed his morning hygiene, prepared and ate breakfast, got dressed, and drove or walked to college? How would he carry his books? How much more time would he need to do all these tasks? If he was responsible for the care of others, would he still be able to manage that role? Whom could he rely on to help? And how would that person's roles and routines change? Would he be able to do his job? These are just several of the questions that a client with a disability faces, and for which the OTA can assist.

For the individual who did not have any prior health conditions, adjusting to a disability, even a **short-term disability** (lasting 6 months or less), can be a long, difficult process. The client may experience changes in independence, physical appearance, relationships, work status, the ability to drive, and the necessity of dealing with physical pain from the injury or illness.[21]

If the disability is caused by an injury, a tremendous amount of shock occurs in the initial days and even weeks following the injury. Life was "fine" one day, and radically different the next. The injury could be accidental, traumatic, or work related; it might occur during a leisure activity; or the client may be the victim of a crime. Each person reacts differently to injury, at times assigning blame or anger toward others, or feeling guilty for something he or she may have prevented. Nothing changes the fact that the injury is real, it will be treated and stabilized medically, and living and doing will continue. Getting through the initial stages of shock requires time. The OTA can provide honest information to the client and his or her family about the condition and also offer realistic hope. OT practitioners can help the client embrace the "new" person post-disability, listen, and provide client-centered care.

Physical Adjustment

Abundant evidence exists to support the use of OT to help clients with disabilities to improve their function in performing meaningful activities.[25] The client's acceptance of physical changes that occur with disability also depends on the critical interaction of psychosocial factors. Psychosocial means the interaction of the social aspects of the client and the psychological traits the client experiences. Clients may experience the loss of function of body parts or body systems, leaving them with a decreased ability to do the occupations they typically perform. Pain and pain management may be important considerations for the OTA to address and will be discussed in subsequent chapters.

Some ways to help clients be able to successfully transition through this process is to suggest changes to the sequence, method, or timing of tasks. For example, for a client experiencing fatigue, taking a shower every other day

COMMUNICATION

The difference between the right word and the almost right word is the difference between lightning bolt and lightning bug. —Mark Twain

Imagine for a moment that you are in the hospital, lying in a bed because you recently had a stroke. You can no longer use your dominant side and are feeling down. You hear a voice at your doorway quietly say, "I'm about to see the stroke in room 210, and I'll come chat with you afterward about the brain injury patient in room 212." In walks a smiling young woman, dressed in scrubs, stating that she is your occupational therapy assistant and is here to help you. It occurs to you that room 210 is your room. *You* are "the stroke in room 210." How would you feel? Do you want her to help you? Inaccurate and non-client-centered descriptions foster and maintain discrimination and negative attitudes toward people with disabilities.[22] People-first language (PFL) is a specific way of speaking and writing (and, ultimately, thinking), which demonstrates that the person is more important than the diagnosis. It was created with the purpose of reducing the social stigma of having a disability. To use PFL, simply state the fact about the person (client) and then follow that with the defining fact about what has affected the individual (CVA). In the example above, the individual referred to as the "stroke in room 210" would have felt more respected and valued if she had been addressed by her name and then her diagnosis stated afterward, such as "Ms. Beck, who had a CVA." Simply stated, PFL means that you put the people before the disability. People-first language describes what the person *has*, instead of who the person *is*.[23] PFL typically requires the subtle change of switching the sequence of wording, yet it can have an immense impact.

Recently, disability advocates have proposed that PFL does not always put the person first and instead propose also using identity-first language (IFL).[24] The altering viewpoint is that putting the person before the disability (i.e., person with disability) indicates, unintentionally, that having the disability is negative or shameful. Some individuals define themselves strongly with their disability and prefer "amputee" rather than "individual with an amputation." Perhaps PFL is an overcorrection in terminology?

The difference between PFL and IFL can be understood by the rationale behind each. PFL is centered on the Social Model, which represents having a disability as a trait, not something to be cured or due to a moral failure, and is intended to prevent the disability as the defining factor for the person and to reduce stigma. IFL is based on the Minority Model, sometimes called the Diversity Model, which portrays a disability as a neutral or even positive factor. IFL also stresses the group of individuals and allows for a sense of belonging to the culture of disability. IFL also acknowledges that the disability has defined the lived experience of the individual and that the person wants to use terms with which he or she self-identifies.

So what is a healthcare professional to do? Individuals with disabilities make up the largest minority in the United States. There are two seemingly opposing viewpoints on the topic.

Continued

COMMUNICATION (continued)

Some guidance can be found by considering if the language is written or spoken. For the written language, using a capital letter to indicate the group versus the individual is recommended. For example, one would write *Deaf culture* (IFL) rather than *Joanne, who is deaf* (PFL). For communicating verbally to a client it is suggested that the practitioner ask the individual how he or she wishes to be referred to, which is truly client-centered care. Overall, using both PFL and IFL is acceptable, as long as the practitioner carefully considers the audience and purpose.[24]

Examples of PFL include the following:[22]

PEOPLE-FIRST LANGUAGE:	INSTEAD OF:
Adults with disabilities	Handicapped, disabled, special needs
People without disabilities	Normal or healthy people
He has a cognitive disability.	He is mentally retarded.
She has a spinal cord injury.	She is a paraplegic.
He has Down syndrome.	He is Down's/ mongoloid.
She has a learning disability.	She is learning disabled.
He has a physical disability.	He is crippled.
She uses a wheelchair.	She is confined to a wheelchair/is wheelchair bound.
Communicates with her eyes/ device/etc.	She is nonverbal.
Congenital disability/ brain injury	Birth defect/brain damaged
Accessible parking, hotel room, etc.	Handicapped parking, hotel room, etc.

rather than every day, or using a shower seat to save energy when showering, would be helpful. For a client who experienced a CVA and now has one side of the body with limited function, the OTA might train the client to layer the underwear and pants and pull them up together on the affected side. Some clients tend to quickly learn solutions to problems and are often a great source for ideas of how to do tasks differently.

Psychological and Emotional Adjustment

Psychological and social aspects of a disability are similar to mourning the loss of a loved one.[26] The initial response is often shock, then denial, followed by anger or depression, and, finally, adjustment and acceptance. Shock is a period of physical and emotional numbness that may last from hours to days, and during which time the client may say that the events seem surreal. Denial is a coping mechanism that allows the client to gradually accept the changes that have occurred, and it may last for weeks to months. If a client gets "stuck" in denial, rehabilitation efforts and acceptance will be hindered. For example, a client with a complete spinal cord injury who thinks he will walk again may be intently focused on walking when in reality there is little or no chance of that type of recovery occurring. The client can get fixated on an unrealistic goal, and then become discouraged and depressed when the goal cannot be achieved. Anger and depression are also natural feelings of loss that are expressed as the client comes to realize the extent of a disability and begins working toward acceptance of the many changes that have occurred and still others that may occur. The last stage is adjustment and acceptance, when the client finally understands the reality of the situation, gives up false hopes, and begins to embrace new roles and routines. Acceptance does not necessarily mean the client will express joy about the condition, but instead tolerance.[26] Clients will go through the stages in their own time, and may even skip some stages. If the grief or loss is not appropriately managed, or the client becomes fixed in any stage, he or she may turn to destructive coping mechanisms, such as drug or alcohol abuse, or demonstrate depression, loss of interest in activities, fear, worry, anxiety, or irritability,[21] all of which interfere with the OT process. The OTA should remain observant of the client, watch for the stages of grief, and report to the occupational therapist any negative behaviors that may signify the client's failure to appropriately progress through the stages. Family and friends will often have their own emotional and psychological period of adjustment to a disability, and the OTA may suggest individual and/or family counseling to help facilitate healing.[21]

Social Adjustment

"People with disabilities are often socially isolated and face stigma within their very own communities. Inclusion of people with disabilities must come from the hearts and minds of everyone in a society."[27] **Accommodation** is merely making changes so an individual has the same access to work, school, and housing as individuals without a disability experience, and reasonable accommodations are mandated by the ADA. **Inclusion** goes beyond accommodation; inclusion means involving a person with a disability in all aspects of society, despite the person's disability. Law cannot mandate inclusion; instead, it must be taught. OTAs can help foster inclusion in communities by educating the public about disabilities. For example, an OTA can advocate for a summer camp experience where disabled and nondisabled teens and adults attend together. The nondisabled campers can learn firsthand that a person with a disability is the same on the inside, with the same needs and desires for friendship, fun, enjoying life, purpose, and so on.

When an individual first experiences a disability, having a support network can be crucial to successful navigation

OT Practitioner's Viewpoint

A pitfall to avoid as a student or new practitioner is the belief that you can remedy everyone who has a physical disability, that is, that every person you provide OT services to will get "better" physically. The reality of disability is that often the physical changes are permanent or degenerative. What you can do, however, is provide your absolute best for every client.

I remember early in my career being very frustrated that some clients who had excellent potential to make physical gains did not, and at the risk of overgeneralizing, I will lump them together to say *they did not want to*. They lacked the inner willpower or ability to reach out to a support system. They accepted the status quo.

Conversely, there were some clients with intense willpower who were limited by unchangeable physical conditions. No matter what evidence-based treatments and techniques I tried or how much the client worked on a task, no external physical changes occurred. Even though the actual conditions did not improve, the clients did make compensatory changes, were able to more fully engage in their meaningful occupations, and attained psychological changes. An individual's attitude is a vital element in success. Never underestimate the influence of the psyche and the effect it can have on the overall joy of occupation. ~ Amy J. Mahle, MHA, COTA/L

through the stages of adjustment. Family, friends, coworkers, neighbors, and others can visit the client, attend therapy sessions, transport the client to medical appointments, take care of cherished pets, send cards or notes of encouragement, help fundraise for medical expenses (which is becoming easier through fundraising websites and social media), provide meals, and so on. There are many meaningful ways to make a client feel appreciated or supported, and the client should be asked what would be most helpful. The client's desires may not always line up with the perceptions of well-meaning family and friends.

Coming to terms with the "new self" for the client with a disability may take some time. The client's social support system and the rehabilitation team can help the client realize that he or she is the same person, and that previously held beliefs, thoughts, and fears are most likely the same as they were before the disability. Depending on the severity and type of disability, clients may also demonstrate some personality changes. Families and close friends experience the greatest impact of any of the support systems when a client's personality changes. Many times, as in the case of brain injury, the change is permanent. The client is the same person in spirit, but may now be more impulsive, irritable, and quiet, or, conversely, more outgoing and talkative. Family and friends need to be educated on what to expect and how to respond.

Friendships that the client experiences pre-disability may drastically change post-disability. On the whole, people mean well, but sometimes they do not have the skills or maturity to cope with the "new" person post-disability. However, new friends can emerge for the client, especially if the client is surrounded by others who are also experiencing traumatic, emotional, and/or physically difficult times, which can facilitate a strong common bond.

As the client is recovering physically and still receiving OT services, the occupational therapist and OTA collaborate on steps for community reintegration, which is a more challenging social experience. If the client has noticeable physical impairments, the client should be trained how to respond to stares and questions when they occur in public. Interacting in a public setting may be a bit challenging at first both physically and socially. The client may use an assistive device for ambulation, and therefore needs to be keenly aware of environmental barriers and issues that may arise, in addition to managing any cognitive impairments or feelings of acceptance of any physical issues, such as a limp or noticeable scarring. Generally, in time, the client with a disability will find a "new normal" and be comfortable in the community (Fig. 1-3).

Some conditions are lifelong and may have actually started in childhood or in the teen years. For those individuals, growing up with a disability is their "normal" life. As those individuals move into adulthood, roles and duties often change. Chapter 37 addresses some of these transitions in more detail.

The client may find it helpful to join a local support group that can provide an additional means of social adjustment.[21] The OTA can assist the client in finding a local support group by making suggestions or, if appropriate to the client's goals, educating and training the client to perform internet searches, or contacting doctor's offices and rehabilitation centers, senior centers, or other public places. The OTA can help the client remain open to new possibilities, new friendships, and making new memories.[21]

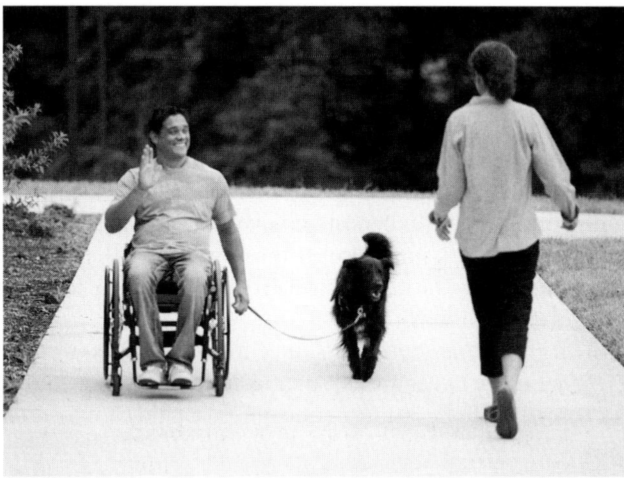

FIGURE 1-3. Individual with paraplegia and his service dog enjoying an outing in the park.

ADJUSTMENT TO CHANGES IN ROLES AND ROUTINES

As social beings, individuals fill specific roles in life, such as wife, mother, friend, uncle, teacher, civic club board member, carpool driver, choir member, volunteer fireman, and so on. Satisfaction, value, meaning, and purpose can be found in roles; they tend to define a person as an individual. The OTPF-3 defines roles as, "sets of behaviors expected by society and shaped by culture and context that may be further conceptualized and defined by the client."[3] Routines are defined as "patterns of behavior that are observable, regular, and repetitive and that provide structure for daily life."[3] Roles or routines can be either constructive or destructive. A change in physical status when an illness, injury, or disability occurs at best disrupts or changes roles, or sometimes even eliminates a valued life role.[3] Both the individual and family must learn to cope with the abrupt change in roles and routines. Expect a period of adjustment for the client and the client's family as roles shift and new routines are established. For example, the client who can no longer work the same job as before the health condition occurred may feel a keen sense of loss of the role of financial provider and also lost identity of whatever role he or she filled at that job.

Financial Adjustment

Disability has a significant impact on household income and expenses. Many families find themselves in a struggle to meet the healthcare costs for the family member with a disability. Expenses may include durable medical equipment (equipment that provides therapeutic benefit to the client, is used in the home, and is reusable, such as a wheelchair or bedside commode) not covered by insurance, prescribed medications, travel to and from specialists, deductibles and copays, and others. These expenses are in addition to the general living expenses of shelter, food, transportation, and insurance.

Depending on the client's job and potential workplace accommodations, a client may or may not need to change jobs, switch professions, or stop working altogether and apply for Social Security disability benefits. Adults age 21 to 64 with disabilities have median monthly earnings that are 28% less than adults with no disability. Furthermore, the number of adults with a disability in that same age category who are employed is only 41%, compared with 79% of the same age group of nondisabled individuals who are employed.[2] The more severe the disability, the more likely the individual will live in persistent poverty (Table 1-2). These facts are not surprising, because the more severe the disability, the less likely the individual will be able to find or perform gainful employment.

The client may need assistance from a spouse or caregiver for daily living tasks, such as toileting, self-feeding, and dressing. If the family cannot afford a paid caregiver or lacks other family support, the spouse or other family member often must stop working or take medical leave (which has time limits), and stay home to care for the individual with the disability. A parent of young or school-age children who stays at home and becomes disabled may need to hire outside help or rely on friends and family to help manage household and/or childcare responsibilities.

TABLE 1-2 Poverty and Disability (2012), United States, 15- to 64-year-olds[2]

DISABILITY STATUS	PERCENTAGE LIVING IN PERSISTENT POVERTY
No disability	3.8%
Nonsevere disability	4.9%
Severe disability	10.8%

Disability may require a client to move to a smaller house, make environmental or structural adaptations to a residence, or rent an accessible apartment. Financial issues associated with the additional cost of health care and loss of work are difficult for families, and it may be appropriate to refer them to the team social worker to assist with funding options for meeting immediate needs. Sometimes the occupational therapist or OTA may be able to help find funding sources for durable medical equipment and ramps, or locate medication programs. Any type of stress is a deterrent to healing and wellness and should be managed appropriately for best client outcomes.

ROLE OF THE OCCUPATIONAL THERAPY ASSISTANT

The roles of the occupational therapist and OTA are defined by the OTPF-3 and also by the scope of practice and laws of each state or country. The occupational therapist and OTA work collaboratively in all aspects of the OT process, but there are some specific differences in role delineation and responsibilities. The main differences are that the occupational therapist has been trained to interpret information and the OTA has not and that the occupational therapist supervises the OTA. As the supervisor, the occupational therapist is ultimately responsible for the entire process of evaluation, intervention, and outcomes review, and the OTA collaborates throughout the OT process in aspects delegated by the occupational therapist for which the OTA has gained service competency.

The evaluation process occurs at the beginning and throughout the OT process, and includes the occupational profile and analysis of occupational performance of the client. With information from the initial (and ongoing) evaluation, intervention planning (setting goals), intervention implementation, and intervention review all occur. Selecting appropriate outcomes, measuring, and applying the outcomes complete the circle of the OT process.[3] Each state has its own rules and regulations, along with supervisory

THE OLDER ADULT

With the Baby Boomer generation reaching the older adult status (65 and older) there is more opportunity for OTAs to interact with this population. Older adults desire to live at home, also called "aging in place." There are opportunities through AARP to educate clients in the HomeFit program of adapting the home for aging in place. Beyond a supportive and safe home environment, physical health and mental health are both critical to the overall health and well-being of adults aging in place. A research study has shown that older adults who participate in a written life review (writing about life chronologically and sharing how life experiences molded them), as well as an intergenerational exchange about the written life review, showed a "significant increase in sense of purpose and meaning in life," which are both determinants of preventing "cognitive decline, disability, and mortality."[28]

requirements, for occupational therapists and OTAs. OT practitioners should identify their own state-specific regulations in order to comply. In Canada, OTAs are not licensed or regulated, but are supervised by occupational therapists.

OTAs have a well-defined and significant role in treating individuals with physical conditions. The *2015 AOTA Salary and Workforce Survey* reports that 55.9% of OTAs work in long-term care or a skilled nursing facility (LTC/SNF), 11.4% in hospital settings, and 4.3% in home health, for a total of 71.6% of OTAs working in some type of physical rehabilitation capacity.[29] The OTA will likely be the healthcare provider who spends the most amount of time with the individual during skilled therapeutic intervention. Early in the process of rehabilitation, the treatment frequently occurs in sensitive situations, such as bathing, toileting, and dressing. The client relies on the OTA to be professional, reassuring, skilled, mature, and confident. But the OTA is just one member of the treatment team, and the client needs the full benefit of an interdisciplinary approach.

An interprofessional healthcare team is one that comprises various disciplines, such as OT, physical therapy, nursing, speech-language pathology, nutritional counseling, social work, and medicine, who all work together to provide the best services possible. The team is aware of the strengths of each team member and discipline, and coordinates care and communication.

The OTA can encourage the client to remain focused, positive, and realistic. Small, attainable goals will be set by the occupational therapist (the OTA may also write goals in collaboration with the occupational therapist) and when met, noted as such and new goals set. Any small sign of progress can be encouraging and motivating to the client,[21] and also to the rehabilitation team. See Box 1-3 for a list of tips and advice from the perspective of a person who experienced a disability, and what she believes will help others who are newly disabled.

BOX 1-3
Tips for the Newly Disabled[30]

The following tips are written from the perspective of a person who experienced disability and may be helpful for the OTA to share with clients. The author encourages clients to think of themselves as "Differently Able to do whatever you can Dream." The website, www.disabled-world.com, goes into further detail with an explanation about each tip, and the OTA is advised to review these for the best understanding of the author's intent.

- Expect an emotional reaction at your change in status from an "able" person to a disabled person.
- Expect others to react differently to you than they did before the onset of your disability.
- Expect changes in your energy level and the way your body and mind work together.
- Expect governmental and organizational indifference and delays, sometimes from the very medical personnel, agencies, and individuals meant to help you.
- Expect coworkers to potentially feel uncomfortable with you.
- Supplemental Security Income (SSI; the governmental Social Security disability benefit) is not a free ride.
- As a newly disabled person, you may find yourself inundated with offers for work-at-home schemes, which may or may not deal with you honestly.
- Depending on the severity of your disability, you may need a care team.
- When you are given the gift of a disability, it does not diminish you as much as you might initially think.
- Nothing is impossible.

One of the most powerful OT interventions is **therapeutic use of self,** which, in simplest terms, is how the practitioner uses herself or himself as a therapeutic tool throughout the intervention process in words and actions. Through therapeutic use of self, the practitioner builds a therapeutic relationship with the client that enables the client to achieve goals. The OTPF-3 refers to four aspects of therapeutic use of self: clinical reasoning, communication, collaboration, and empathy.[3] Empathy is the emotional component of the therapeutic relationship, which allows the practitioner to develop a healthy bond to support the client to achieve outcomes. OT practitioners must use caution when interacting emotionally with a client. Unless the OTA has been through the same situation, be cautious about using the words "I know how you feel"; false empathy may alienate the client.

Continuum of Care

All throughout the continuum of care (the places where clients receive skilled OT), OT practitioners seek to work on tasks that are client-centered and occupation-based. Jeff is a client who experienced a spinal cord injury when he was thrown from a car. Throughout his rehabilitation, occupational therapists and OTAs helped Jeff learn skills and gain independence through purposeful, client-centered activities. In the acute care hospital, an OTA provided Jeff with an adapted call bell so that he could communicate his needs to the nursing staff, and an OTA trained him how to wash his face despite his injuries. In the rehabilitation hospital, Jeff was trained by an OTA how to don (put on) a pull-over shirt (Fig. 1-4), transfer from his bed to the wheelchair, check his skin, perform pressure relief, shower using an adapted tub bench, and eat with adapted utensils.

When he left the rehabilitation hospital and went home, Jeff received OT and was able to work on transferring from his wheelchair to his own bed and maneuver his wheelchair into his own bathroom for toileting, again, with the OTA as his primary treating OT practitioner. Once he was no longer homebound, Jeff went to an outpatient rehabilitation clinic where he was ready to work on rolling in bed and lower body dressing, as well as cooking simple meals. Jeff's story provides a good example of some of the specific, occupation-based, client-centered tasks he was trained by an OTA to perform throughout the different stages of his disability experience. Remember, each client is unique.

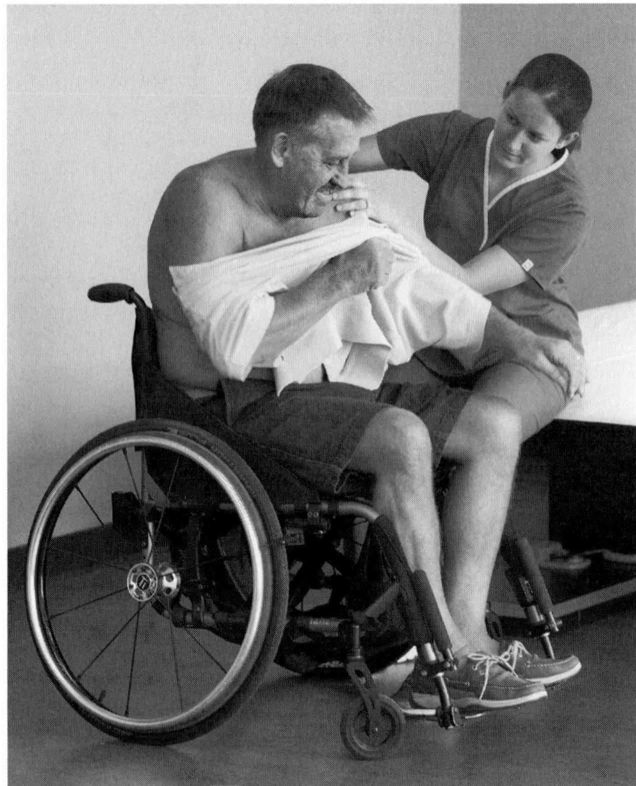

FIGURE 1-4. The OTA is training Jeff to use upper body adapted dressing techniques.

Training and Education of the Client and Family

Education and training occur in every setting of OT. The OTPF-3 provides the foundation for education and training as part of skilled OT services and also defines the client as the individual receiving OT services, plus the client's caregiver and/or family.[3] Education is defined as "imparting of knowledge and information about occupation, health, well-being, and participation that enables the client to acquire helpful behaviors, habits, and routines that may or may not require application at the time of the intervention session."[3] Training is defined by the OTPF-3 as "facilitation of the acquisition of concrete skills for meeting specific goals in a real-life, applied situation. In this case, 'skills' refers to measurable components of function that enable mastery. Training is differentiated from education by its goal of enhanced performance as opposed to enhanced understanding, although these goals often go hand in hand."[3] *Education* can be summarized as conveying information and *training* as teaching skills. OTAs will likely educate or inform the client and family on aspects of the specific disability, how it impacts function, how they can work to achieve well-being, specific strategies such as energy conservation, or other suggestions for optimal performance and function (these topics will be covered in subsequent chapters in this textbook). The education the OTA will provide can occur via verbal instruction, discussion, demonstration, and/or handouts. The OTA may refer the client to websites regarding the disability or provide information on support groups. But to

EVIDENCE-BASED PRACTICE

A recent study, "Factors Predicting Client Satisfaction in Occupational Therapy and Rehabilitation,"[31] was completed to determine the satisfaction of clients with their experience with OT in a large rehabilitation hospital. The study included 769 clients, and they were grouped into "satisfied" and "dissatisfied." The authors identified two key implications for OT practice:

- Clients highly value the ability to care for themselves. Clients who improved their functional status, especially in self-care, had higher levels of satisfaction.
- Some subsets of clients may need additional attention and/or adaptations, including those entering rehabilitation more than 15 days after the onset, those with lower abilities to function at admission or discharge, or those making limited progress.[31]

Custer, M. G., Huebner, R. A., & Howell, D. M. (2014). Factors predicting client satisfaction in occupational therapy and rehabilitation. American Journal of Occupational Therapy, *69(1), 6901290040p1-6901290040p10. doi:10.5014/ajot.2015.013094*

just educate is not enough. Suppose an OTA educates a client on ways to conserve energy or get back to gardening using adaptive equipment, but never gives the client the chance to actually practice the skills? The client will likely forget what the OTA *taught* unless he or she is *trained* to use the skills functionally (Fig. 1-5). Both education and training are important and should almost always be used to complement each other. Being observant, a keen listener, and sensitive to the client and family will help to determine what resources to provide them throughout the entire continuum of care.

Individuals learn in different ways, and there are some strategies that work best with certain types of tasks. Education and training are best used together, and the concepts should seem similar to being a student in an OTA program. Professional programs are designed to have multiple components in order to achieve the student learning outcomes, including lecture (education), laboratory work, and fieldwork (training). The training portion is when the education portion becomes more "real" to the student and is often embraced enthusiastically because it "finally makes sense." The same principle applies to the client. Chapter 5 includes more information on specific theories and methods of education and training.

Healthcare Teams

Evidence supports the idea that coordinated care provided by a team of professionals is advantageous for the client and meets best practice guidelines.[32] The client needs the specialized support and care that can only be provided by multiple types of professionals. Typically, clients who have more severe disabilities requiring extensive rehabilitation will have a greater need for more disciplines to be involved, thus the team will be larger. Team configuration and function varies historically and also in different healthcare systems and types of facilities.

Three common models of teams in treating adult physical conditions are multidisciplinary, interprofessional, and transdisciplinary. The **multidisciplinary team** consists of various professionals from different disciplines who each provide their own healthcare service to the client. A team could consist of any combination of the following: occupational therapist, OTA, physical therapist, physical therapist assistant, speech-language pathologist, dietitian, social worker, psychologist, counselor, neuropsychologist, recreational therapist, physiatrist (physician who specializes in rehabilitation), nurse, and nurse aides. Multidisciplinary teams are hierarchical in nature, and usually the highest-ranking professional member of the team is the leader.[33] Each discipline conducts its own evaluation, has separate treatment goals, and bears the responsibility for its own scope of practice and outcomes. Team members work *independently* of each other, but do have some formal communication regarding the client.[33] A challenge with a multidisciplinary team is that clients can feel overwhelmed by all the services and may even experience conflicting goals or the same goals approached differently if the team has not communicated well. Another potential issue with this type of team is that each discipline identifies and works on separate issues with the client rather than integrating care, which is shortsighted, because the client is best treated as a whole person.[33] The multidisciplinary team approach can also result in the client feeling a decreased sense of collaboration.

A more advanced multidisciplinary team will have team goals for the client that the team members decide on together (based on their individual evaluations and interpretations of the client's needs) that span the scope of all disciplines and are targeted during each individual discipline's treatment with the client. An example of an advanced multidisciplinary team is the outpatient teams created at Carolinas Rehabilitation in Charlotte, North Carolina, which are teams that are based on diagnoses, such as cerebrovascular accident and brain injury. Each team consists of one or more representatives from each discipline the client attends, including OT, physical therapy, and speech therapy. Additional team members who interact with the client, such as the vocational rehabilitation counselor, are invited to attend. The team collaborates to create multidisciplinary goals for each client, which also align with each discipline's goals. The team reviews the progress the clients have made since the last meeting and updates the team goals as needed.

In contrast, **interdisciplinary team** members work in the same setting, sharing information formally and informally, and team meetings serve as a connection point to systematically coordinate efforts and solve problems as they relate to each discipline. Many definitions have been used to describe interdisciplinary teams, but most agree that this type of team involves a variety of healthcare professionals from different disciplines who work *interdependently* on common goals for the client. In the interdisciplinary team, the lines of the professions blur and expertise overlaps based on the situation and client need.[33] The interdisciplinary approach seems to be a more integrated, collaborative approach than the multidisciplinary team, because the team

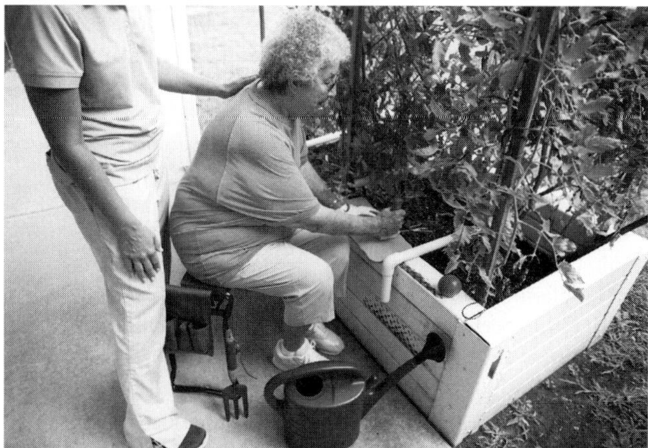

FIGURE 1-5. The client has been trained and is now able to practice gardening using a raised garden bed, garden bench for energy conservation, and adapted gardening tools to maintain proper alignment of joints.

members rely on each discipline and have common goals. One drawback of the interdisciplinary team is the logistics of meeting times. A challenge for interdisciplinary teams is that members must be willing to alter their own plans based on evidence and input from other team members.[33]

Transdisciplinary teams are primarily a type of interdisciplinary team, but interact a bit differently. Members of a transdisciplinary team often blur professional lines, believing that one professional can fill the roles of others on the team. Members train one another in aspects of their discipline and fill another's role when necessary. An example might be that a social worker may complete a client's medical intake form or an OT practitioner may record a client's social and occupational history.

Research compared the type of communication that exists between the multidisciplinary and interprofessional teams, and found that the interprofessional team used inclusive language and communicated frequently by sharing information and working collaboratively. Conversely, the multidisciplinary team members worked parallel to one another, and did share information, which may have had an effect on the interventions.[25]

Whatever type of team is experienced, the most important points to remember are that each team member needs to understand his or her own role and those of the other members, and also be able to educate team members about his or her role in client care. Although the multidisciplinary and interdisciplinary teams function differently, the OTA can participate as a member of either team, with or without the occupational therapist being present, but always in collaboration with the occupational therapist. Clear, concise, and timely communication with the occupational therapist is foundational to a good collaborative relationship. The OTA can represent the OT treatment team at larger team meetings by reporting the results of the evaluation completed by the occupational therapist, give updates on progress toward the client's goals, and report back information from the team meeting to the occupational therapist (Fig. 1-6). As the OTA becomes an experienced clinician, or takes a leadership role in the organization, the OTA may even lead interdisciplinary team meetings.

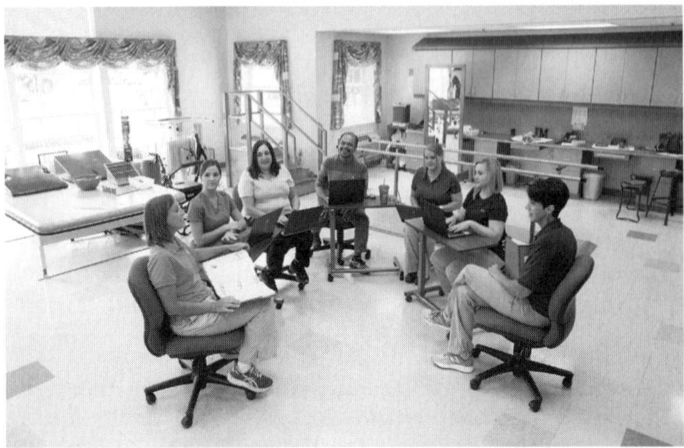

FIGURE 1-6. Team meeting led by the rehabilitation manager.

Many rehabilitation centers recruit peer counselors from the pool of clients who have successfully adjusted to disability. Although volunteers are not officially part of the healthcare team, peer counselors, also called peer mentors, can offer encouragement from a unique perspective of having gone through a similar situation. The volunteer counselors can visit with the client, meet with the family, or help run support groups. The client experiencing the disability gains a new perspective from someone who has successfully navigated the rehabilitation process, courage, and perhaps a new friend.

SUMMARY

Disability is broadly defined, affects adults of all ages, and is no respecter of persons. Individuals who are affected by disability face many challenges in overcoming and adjusting to the changes disability brings. Client-centered OT includes understanding that the client is an active part of the OT process, rather than a passive recipient. In the role of OTA, be sensitive to what the client is experiencing and the effects of disability on lifelong roles, routines, and occupations.

REVIEW QUESTIONS

1. Jason was injured while playing football. To be classified as having a disability, which three of the following are definitions of a disability?
   a. Jason must have a physical loss resulting from an injury, illness, or disease.
   b. Jason must have a physical or mental impairment.
   c. Jason must be limited in what IADL tasks he can do.
   d. Jason must have a participation restriction.
   e. Jason must have an activity limitation.
   f. Jason is restricted from participating in driving.
2. The American with Disabilities Act (ADA) would apply to which of the following situations?
   a. An individual who has a broken leg
   b. An individual who uses a wheelchair wants to access a private club
   c. An individual who complains that the local convenience store does not have an automatic door opening system
   d. An individual who needs access to the library, post office, the public bus system, and the local college
3. Occupational therapy began working with individuals with physical disabilities largely due to which of the following reasons?
   a. Physical therapy could not provide enough service to rehabilitate wounded veterans.
   b. The need to rehabilitate wounded veterans arose after each major war.
   c. There was no longer a need for occupational therapists to be involved in psychiatric care.
   d. Occupational therapists needed jobs, and working with war veterans gave them a steady income.
4. Richard experienced a CVA and as a result can only use the right side of his body. He is married, has the roles of husband, father, and grandfather, is a retired woodworker, and loves spending time with his two dogs. Which of the following is the *best* purposeful activity in OT treatment for Richard?
   a. Building a cradle for a future grandchild
   b. Brushing and playing with his dogs
   c. Taking out the trash
   d. Giving advice to his children

5. Carrie experienced an upper extremity amputation after a severe car accident. Which of the following is the *most* common challenge she faces in her experience of a physical disability that affects her engagement in occupations?
   a. Relating to other people with a changed physical appearance
   b. Becoming stuck in the stages of grief
   c. Learning to accept the physical changes that have occurred to her and persist through difficulties
   d. Not having the willpower to continue making progress
6. Carlita experienced a CVA that left her with some significant residual weakness in her right side. Due to the CVA, she has difficulty with mobility, has difficulties performing many ADLs and IADLs, and is experiencing some social adjustment issues. Which of the following is the *best* recommendation for the OT practitioner to mention to Carlita with regard to her social adjustment issues?
   a. Attend a peer support group.
   b. Only attend therapy and doctors' appointments until she feels more comfortable with her "new self."
   c. Limit social roles so the client can focus on recovery.
   d. Join a gym to improve self-image.
7. Which three of the following best depict the role of the OTA working with clients who have physical disabilities?
   a. The OTA can administer assessments and provide treatment intervention.
   b. The OTA may collaborate with the occupational therapist in all aspects of client-centered care.
   c. The OTA develops the plan of care and follows it during treatment.
   d. The OTA is solely responsible for the initial evaluation and discharge plan.
   e. The OTA is responsible to interpret results of the assessments.
   f. The OTA may collaborate with the occupational therapist to set goals.
8. An OTA is a team member on a multidisciplinary team. Which of the following tasks would the OTA *most likely* perform on the team?
   a. Schedule and run a team meeting.
   b. Set team treatment goals for the client.
   c. Report on the client's progress during a team meeting.
   d. Invite the client and family members to attend the team meeting.
9. An OTA is working with a client who has experienced a significant injury to her right upper extremity and has a very poor prognosis for regaining use of the arm. Despite being told the prognosis from her physician, she strongly believes she will recover completely. The OTA surmises that the client is *most likely:*
   a. Delusional
   b. Experiencing denial
   c. Trying to overcome the odds
   d. In a state of shock
10. The OTA uses many therapeutic interventions to affect change in James, who has been diagnosed with Parkinson's disease. The OTA works with James to help him gain skills in self-feeding. Which of the following is the best description of practicing and using actual skills?
   a. Self-advocacy
   b. Education
   c. Therapeutic use of self
   d. Training

CASE STUDY

School had just let out for the summer, and Eugene was almost finished building a tree house in the backyard for his 12-year-old son, Luke, when tragedy struck. Eugene fell 10 feet to the ground below, resulting in a spinal cord injury, a shattered ankle, and fractured tibia. He required multiple surgeries to repair his ankle and leg and to stabilize his spine. At this point he was unable to walk and used a wheelchair. Eugene spent 2 weeks in acute care and then 2 more weeks at a rehabilitation hospital. Eugene was a self-employed contractor and could no longer perform his job. Thankfully, Eugene's wife Karen was able to pick up extra hours at her part-time job to help a bit with the financial loss of income. Eugene and Karen were both worried about paying the mortgage and their health insurance premiums. Luke was supposed to go to a day summer camp with two of his friends but the family could no longer afford to send him. Karen had to take over most of the household chores and all the yard work that Eugene used to do. She did what needed to be done, but was exhausted from her job and the continual work of helping to care for her newly disabled husband. After Eugene was discharged from the rehabilitation hospital and the reality of life at home set in, he was deeply affected by the loss of his work role and most days would not get out of bed until the afternoon. Karen sensed Eugene's depression, yet felt that she could not share her own struggles and pain because she had to be the strong one.

Eugene used a manual wheelchair for mobility. His friends built him a ramp so he could enter his one-level ranch home, but unfortunately the door to the master bathroom was too narrow for a wheelchair. He was a contractor and he could not even remodel his own home. He did have a few friends who visited on occasion, but they had their own lives and troubles, and Eugene did not want to be a burden. He felt isolated, lonely, irritable, angry, and purposeless. He rarely bathed, wore the same clothes for days, and was not interested in eating much.

Luke initially felt guilty that his dad was injured while building him a tree house, but later he began to feel resentful that he could not go to summer day camp with his friends and instead had to sit home and "babysit" dad all day. He had to learn to do things to help his dad that he did not think 12-year-olds should have to do. For everyone, everything had changed in just one moment.

1. Identify the roles and routines for each member of the family before and after the accident.
2. Identify the stages of grief that Eugene experienced. Are there reasons for concern?
3. What resources could be recommended to this family?
4. What are some possible meaningful activities for Eugene? Luke?

REFERENCES

1. World Health Organization. (2015). Health information: Disabilities. Retrieved from http://www.who.int/topics/disabilities/en/
2. U.S. Census Bureau. (2012). Nearly 1 in 5 people have a disability in the U.S., Census Bureau reports. Retrieved from https://www.census.gov/newsroom/releases/archives/miscellaneous/cb12-134.html
3. American Occupational Therapy Association. (2014). Occupational therapy practice framework: Domain and process, 3rd ed. *American Journal of Occupational Therapy, 68 (Supplement 1)*, S1–S48. http://dx.doi.org/10.5014/ajot.2014.682006
4. Erickson, W., Lee, C., & von Schrader, S. (2014). *Disability statistics from the 2012 American Community Survey (ACS)*. Ithaca, NY: Cornell University Employment and Disability Institute (EDI). Retrieved from www.disabilitystatistics.org

5. Weiss, T. (2013). People with disabilities: Accommodation vs. inclusion. Retrieved from http://www.disabled-world.com/disability/accommodation-inclusion.php
6. Americans with Disabilities Act of 1990. (n.d.). Retrieved from http://www.ada.gov/pubs/adastatute08.htm#12102
7. U.S. Department of Health and Human Services. (2016). Healthy People 2020: Disability and health. Retrieved from https://www.healthypeople.gov/2020/topics-objectives/topic/disability-and-health
8. Yee, S. (2013). Health disparities research at the intersection of race, ethnicity, and disability: A national conference. [PowerPoint slides]. Retrieved from https://dredf.org/wp-content/uploads/2012/08/Yee-Intersections-Conf-disability-health-disparities-101-April-2013.pdf
9. U. S. Census Bureau, American Fact Finder. (2015). Disability characteristics, 2012 American community survey, 1-year estimates. Retrieved from http://factfinder.census.gov/faces/tableservices/jsf/pages/productview.xhtml?pid=ACS_12_1YR_S1810&prodType=table
10. Bloom Hoover, J. (1996). Diversional occupational therapy in World War I: A need for purpose in occupations. *American Journal of Occupational Therapy, 50,* 881–885. doi:10.5014/ajot.50.10.881
11. O'Brien, J., & Hussey, S. (2012). *Introduction to occupational therapy* (4th ed.). St. Louis, MO: Elsevier.
12. Reilly, M. (1961). 1961 Eleanor Clarke Slagle lecture: Occupational therapy can be one of the great ideas of 20th-century medicine. Retrieved from https://www.aota.org/-/media/Corporate/Files/Publications/AJOT/Slagle/1961.pdf
13. Wolf, T., Chuh, A., Floyd, T., McInnis, K., & Williams, E. (2014). Effectiveness of occupation-based interventions to improve areas of occupation and social participation after stroke: An evidence-based review. *American Journal of Occupational Therapy, 69*(1). doi:10.5014/ajot.2015.013409
14. Alderson, P. (1998). The importance of theories in health care. *BMJ: British Medical Journal, 317*(7164), 1007–1010.
15. Reilly, M. (1962). Occupational therapy can be one of the great ideas of the 20th century medicine. *American Journal of Occupational Therapy, 16*(1).
16. Ashby, S., & Chandler, B. (2010). An exploratory study of the occupation-focused models included in occupational therapy professional education programmes. *British Journal of Occupational Therapy, 73*(12), 616–624.
17. Kielhofner, G. (2008). *A model of human occupation: Theory and application* (4th ed.). Baltimore, MD: Lippincott Williams & Wilkins.
18. Cole, M. B., & Tufano, R. (2008). *Applied theories in occupational therapy: A practical approach.* Thorofare, NJ: SLACK Incorporated.
19. Toglia, J., Goverover, Y., Johnston, M. V., & Dain, B. (2011). Application of the multicontextual approach in promoting learning and transfer of strategy use in an individual with TBI and executive dysfunction. *OTJR: Occupation, Participation and Health, 31*(1), S53–S60. doi:10.3928/15394492-20101108-09
20. Clark-Wilson, J., Giles, G. M., & Baxter, D. M. (2014). Revisiting the neurofunctional approach: Conceptualizing the core components for the rehabilitation of everyday living skills. *Brain Injury, 28*(13–14), 1646–1656. Retrieved from http://doi.org/10.3109/02699052.2014.946449
21. Rehabilitation Institute of Chicago. (2014). Emotional adjustment to disability. Retrieved from https://lifecenter.ric.org/index.php?tray=content&tid=top262&cid=5861
22. American Occupational Therapy Association. (2015). Veteran and wounded warrior care. Retrieved from http://www.aota.org/Practice/Rehabilitation-Disability/Emerging-Niche/Veteran.aspx
23. Snow, K. (2013). A few words about people first language. Retrieved from https://www.disabilityisnatural.com/people-first-language.html
24. Dunn, D. S., & Andrews, E. E. (2015). Person-first and identity-first language: Developing psychologists' cultural competence using disability language. *The American Psychologist* (3), 255. doi:10.1037/a0038636
25. Sheehan, D., Robertson, L., & Ormond, T. (2007). Comparison of language used and patterns of communication in interprofessional and multidisciplinary teams. *Journal of Interprofessional Care, 21*(1), 17–30.
26. Taormina-Weiss, W. (2012). Psychological and social aspects of disability. Retrieved from http://www.disabled-world.com/disability/social-aspects.php
27. Snow, K. (2013). A few words about people first language. Retrieved from https://www.disabilityisnatural.com/people-first-language.html
28. American Occupational Therapy Association. (2015). Surveying the profession: The AOTA salary and workforce survey. *OT Practice, 20*(11), 7–11.
29. Chippendale, T., & Boltz, M. (2015). Living legends: Effectiveness of a program to enhance sense of purpose and meaning in life among community-dwelling older adults. *American Journal of Occupational Therapy, 69*(4), 1–11. doi:10.5014/ajot.2015.014894
30. Myers, C. (2009). Tips for the newly disabled. Retrieved from http://www.disabled-world.com/disability/newly-disabled-tips
31. Custer, M. G., Huebner, R. A., & Howell, D. M. (2014). Factors predicting client satisfaction in occupational therapy and rehabilitation. *American Journal of Occupational Therapy, 69*(1), 6901290040p1-6901290040p10. doi:10.5014/ajot.2015.013094
32. Van den Berg, J. P., Kalmijn, S., Lindeman, E., Veldink, J. H., de Visser, M., Van der Graaff, M. M., ... Van den Berg, L. H. (2005). Multidisciplinary ALS care improves quality of life in patients with ALS. *Neurology, 65*(8), 1264–1267. Retrieved from http://dx.doi.org/10.1212/01.wnl.0000180717.29273.12
33. Columbia University in the City of New York Center for Teaching and Learning. (n.d.). Postdoctoral dental education. Types of teams. Retrieved from http://ccnmtl.columbia.edu/projects/sl2/mod03_multi_1b.html

Chapter 2

Professional Considerations for Occupational Therapy Assistants

Amy J. Mahle, MHA, COTA/L

LEARNING OUTCOMES

After studying this chapter, the student or practitioner will be able to:

2.1 Identify key traits of professionalism in occupational therapy
2.2 Apply the Occupational Therapy Code of Ethics to real-world scenarios
2.3 Define advocacy as it relates to the client, community, and profession
2.4 Articulate the rationale for using evidence-based treatment
2.5 Identify suitable sources for evidence-based treatment
2.6 Describe lifelong learning
2.7 Identify a variety of methods to educate colleagues

KEY TERMS

Advocacy	Lifelong learning
Certification	Primary literature
Evidence-based practice (EBP)	Qualitative
Evidence-based treatment	Quantitative
Licensure	Secondary literature

Professionalism is a set of expected behaviors relative to a specific job or setting. General themes emerge when considering professionalism, such as self-responsibility, respect for others, integrity, maturity, maintaining a positive attitude, effective communication skills, and maintaining professional boundaries.[1] Who judges professionalism? Typically clients, peers, colleagues, or other individuals with whom the professional interacts, all of whom may judge the professional based on his or her image, communication style, competence, and demeanor.[1] In short, professionalism is often measured subjectively by the individuals involved in an interaction and healthcare providers must be keenly aware of the perceptions of all with whom they come in contact.

The general public anticipates being able to trust a healthcare provider with their health and well-being. They want to interact with someone who will listen, know the best course of action, and be able to carry it out. Healthcare providers are expected to live above reproach, to put the needs of their clients first, and to consistently act in a legal and ethical manner, both on and off the job. Additional expectations are interprofessional collaboration and effective verbal and written communication with other healthcare providers, as well as the client and family. Occupational therapy (OT) practitioners must master documentation, know the best and most current **evidence-based treatment** (OT treatments supported by the available evidence) options, embrace lifelong learning, and exhibit ethical behaviors, values, and responsibilities.[2] Professionalism is a crucial goal that must be attained and will be an interactive process of feedback, mentoring, and self-reflection.

PARADIGM SHIFT TO BEING A PROFESSIONAL

Students enter into an occupational therapy assistant (OTA) educational program with the end goal of becoming an OTA. The degree earned is quite different from other degrees one might earn in college, such as a degree in biology or welding; in the process of coursework and fieldwork students will be transformed into a *healthcare professional.*

Attitudes, thoughts, beliefs, and behaviors will morph into a new professional identity. Once the student graduates, passes the certification examination, and becomes licensed, the graduate, now practitioner, will carry new authority and responsibility. Sound daunting? It may be, but the transition starts today and will occur as long as there is an effort to do so. To begin making that paradigm shift, let's explore how being an OT professional is defined by the field of OT.

Key Traits of Professionalism

With the end goal in sight, one can begin to chart a course to becoming a professional. The American Occupational Therapy Association (AOTA) is the professional member organization and driving force behind OT in the United States. AOTA sets educational standards through the Accreditation Council for Occupational Therapy Education (ACOTE), advocates, leads and supports research, and promotes OT for practitioners and the public. AOTA also provides many resources to academic programs, such as the AOTA Level II Fieldwork Performance Evaluation (FWPE). The FWPE is an evaluation that is completed by the Fieldwork Educator at mid and end points of each Level II Fieldwork. The FWPE provides key insights into what is required to be an entry-level professional because a portion of the FWPE is dedicated to professionalism. The qualities on which every student will be evaluated are "self-responsibility, responds to feedback, work behaviors, time management, interpersonal skills, and cultural competence."[3] Let's review each of these in relation to working with adults with physical conditions; they are also summarized in Figure 2-1.

SELF-RESPONSIBILITY

Students are expected to take responsibility for their own learning. Students will be evaluated on how well they work toward service competence, which is the ethical expectation to only do what the student is trained and able to perform (and later, as an OTA professional, the definition remains the same). Each student must strive to learn as much as possible by seeking out learning opportunities from supervisors and other practitioners. Self-responsibility also means to admit when a mistake has been made and actively pursue a solution to the issue. Students can begin immediately, before ever reaching Level II Fieldwork (FW), to take education seriously and learn all that is possible from each lecture, lab, and Level I FW experience. Every assignment given is crafted to meet educational standards to prepare students for Level II FW and entry-level practice as an OTA. OTAs who demonstrate self-responsibility take every opportunity to connect what is being learned with what is already known, with the people they encounter, and with themselves. For example, if a student knows someone who has had a cerebrovascular accident (CVA) and the topic being discussed in class is CVA, seek out that person. As one relates what is being learned to what one has experienced the effectiveness of learning will increase.

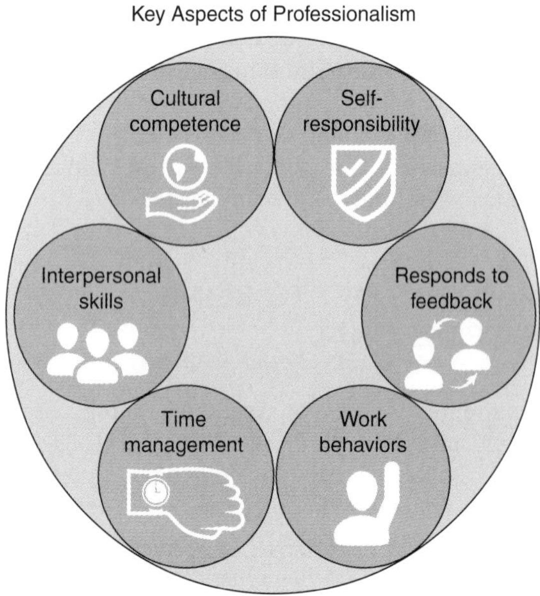

FIGURE 2-1. Professionalism.

RESPONDS TO FEEDBACK

Feedback (also called debriefing) is the written or verbal response by a peer, faculty member, or supervisor to one's actions, and can be instrumental to growth when given constructively and then reflected on. Feedback can feel uncomfortable, especially if taken as a personal assault or devaluation of self. Be assured that all students will experience varying degrees and types of feedback throughout their educational program, including the fieldwork components, in preparation for becoming a professional. The proper way to respond to feedback is to listen carefully, maintain control of emotions, and reflect on what was said or written. Refrain from automatically reacting to feedback and instead, take time to think and respond. A *reaction* is a quick reply without thought to what is being said or thought to the consequence, whereas a *response* reflects thought, time, and perspective. All OT practitioners and students should value feedback from OT colleagues who are more experienced as they can offer a unique perspective. For example, a student shared once that she valued feedback given to her by her fieldwork educator because she learned that she was using an inappropriate, childish tone with older adults. The student's background before OT had been working with children, so her natural way to respond to people she was taking care of was geared toward children, not adults. Once she was made aware of her tone through constructive feedback, she could recognize it and made efforts to change that pattern of behavior.

WORK BEHAVIORS

Supervisors, employers, and instructors all desire to have students who show initiative, are prepared, are dependable, and take care of the work or school environment. Showing initiative means to be resourceful or to look for opportunities to assist. Make sure, however, to stay within the scope of practice and defined role. For example, it would not be appropriate for a student to take the initiative to schedule his or her own fieldwork, but it may be appropriate to offer contact information for new fieldwork placements to the Academic Fieldwork Coordinator. In the classroom, an example of taking initiative would be finding a quality video on a relevant subject matter and sharing it with the instructor.

Being prepared and dependable are two traits highly sought after by employers. Being prepared means being organized, reviewing information ahead of time, bringing all items needed to class or fieldwork, and planning ahead with forethought to the situation rather than just showing up. A student may ask the following:

1. What might I need tomorrow or next week?
2. What is expected of me tomorrow or next week?
3. What tasks will need to be accomplished and do I have all the supplies, materials, and tools available and ready?
4. Have I read, studied, or practiced skills that are needed?
5. Have I communicated relevant issues/information with my professor(s), advisor, group members, or fieldwork educator(s) and in a timely manner?

Practicing those behaviors now as a student will contribute to optimal learning, decreasing stress, submitting assignments on time (or early), and overall success. Every student is relieved when he or she is placed in a group with dependable students. Be that person who can be depended on. If one adheres to one's word, meets deadlines, and arrives on time to meetings and class, that student will earn a good reputation for being dependable.

Facilities, equipment, and supplies are costly, and in the healthcare environment, one must be especially careful to take good care of the work environment to minimize the cost of upkeep or replacement. Throughout the OTA courses, students will learn how to properly care for supplies and equipment, such as hot packs and hydrocollators (the tank that heats water to the appropriate temperature to prepare and store hot packs for use with a client). Treat the educational and healthcare environments with respect and take care of the items and spaces as if they are valued personal property. Make it a habit to quickly observe any room on entering and exiting. Be the person who moves the rolling stool out of the way so a client or peer does not trip. Little things done with the right attitude and motivation make a big, positive impression on others and also help to develop one into a professional. As C. S. Lewis put it, "Integrity is doing the right thing, even when no one is watching."

Physical appearance includes clothing, hair, makeup, jewelry, shoes, and nonverbal communication. Educational programs and fieldwork sites often have a policy to follow regarding expectations for physical appearance, but broad general concepts are included here. Clothing and shoes should be appropriate, clean, and neat (no wrinkles, of the proper size and length, and not stained). Refrain from wearing scrubs or clothing that is too tight or too revealing, and remember that dressing conservatively is best. If hair is long, it should be worn away from the face to avoid contact with the client. Makeup and jewelry should be natural and at a minimum. Consider that long, dangling earrings or necklaces and most rings may become a safety risk to the wearer or the client. Fingernails should also be kept trimmed, smooth, natural, and ideally without polish. Long or jagged nails could harm a client, and artificial nails have been proven to harbor bacteria. A good safety rule for nail length is that when one looks at the volar (palm) side of the hand, nails should not extend beyond the pad of the finger. In addition, always try to be mindful of the client population and what might be offensive or dangerous to them. Scented lotions, perfumes, colognes, body sprays, hairsprays, and so on should never be worn as they may trigger an allergic reaction in a client. When working with adults, think about generational and gender differences, as well as different races and ethnic backgrounds. What may be the norm in today's society (tattoos, for example) may be offensive to the adults from a prior generation. A good general rule for professional appearance in the healthcare environment is to not wear anything that would make one noticeable—either in a positive or negative way. Nonverbal communication is also part of one's appearance, so be mindful of what one's own facial expressions and body language convey. Overall, do not allow one's physical appearance to distract the client from his or her goals.

TIME MANAGEMENT

One of the most common challenges that students struggle with is managing their time. Life is busy for all students; some have children at home, have aging parents, or may need to work part-time or full-time in addition to pursuing a degree. Just finding time to study and complete assignments is difficult.

But even beyond the juggling act of fitting in all life occupations, time management in a clinical setting poses unique challenges. One of the areas that FW educators and employers mention that students and new graduates need to work on is managing their time, including prioritizing clients and timely documentation. Exactly what does time management involve? Examine Table 2-1 to help analyze areas that may be opportunities for building these skills.[4] To complete this activity, read through and reflect on each item in the left column, then place a checkmark in column two if this is something which is a struggle. After checking all that apply, determine how the strategy can be used, and create a realistic plan to follow. For example, a person who always tends to say "yes" to everything everyone asks her to do would place a checkmark next to the strategy of "Just Say No." In the third column, "How can you use this strategy?" that person might write that saying no will enable her to devote more time to her studies. Then in the fourth column, "Create a plan," the person would state exactly how she will use this strategy. Most people are probably already aware of the situations that may arise. It might mean saying "no" to a friend's invitation to lunch and a movie because

TABLE 2-1 Self-Reflect on 10 Strategies for Time Management[4]

STRATEGIES FOR TIME MANAGEMENT	✓ IF YOU STRUGGLE	HOW CAN YOU USE THIS STRATEGY?	CREATE A PLAN TO INCORPORATE INTO PERSONAL, WORK, OR SCHOOL ENVIRONMENT
1. Set Goals			
2. Prioritize			
3. Increase Effectiveness, Reduce Urgency			
4. Delegate Effectively			
5. Manage Your Details			
6. Just Say No			
7. Control Interruptions			
8. Use New Technology			
9. Strive for Excellence, Not Perfection			
10. Control Procrastination			

that time is needed for studying or working on an assignment. In this example, saying, "I'm sorry, I can't go because I am determined to finish my assignments today, but I would love to meet you after the movie for a cup of coffee" helps preserve the time needed to finish the assignment and maintain the friendship.

INTERPERSONAL SKILLS

Interacting with others in a professional manner includes four gold standards: cooperation, flexibility, tact, and empathy.[3] Success in the OTA educational program, fieldwork, and then as a practitioner relies on successful interpersonal skills. The essence of these four gold standards of interpersonal skills is simply to put others' interests before one's own. OT is based on human relationships and using therapeutic use of self, and *cooperation* and teamwork are also integral parts of the healthcare environment. Be ready to be *flexible* if a coworker or fieldwork educator, or academic fieldwork coordinator, asks to change one's schedule. The OT field is well known for the flexibility of its practitioners, and realizing and accepting that now, as a student, will be extremely beneficial. Being *tactful* is speaking thoughtfully and diplomatically with both insight and consideration of the other person. If this skill does not come naturally, find someone who is tactful and learn skills from him or her. One tip is to always think how what is about to be said will be perceived by the other person. This requires one to be mindful of the other person and try to see an issue from his or her perspective. Finally, *empathy* is the skill of relating to individuals with compassion and caring. Clients do not want sympathy, which is commiserating, or showing pity, which is feeling sorry for someone, with the underlying belief that they are inferior. Instead, they need empathy, which is provided by a thoughtful, compassionate practitioner who will listen and respond appropriately. Consider the differences in these three statements:

1. Sympathy: "You poor thing, I can't imagine what it would be like to lose your leg."
2. Pity: "It must be just awful to only have one leg."
3. Empathy: "If I were in your position, I might feel the same way."

CULTURAL COMPETENCE

Cultural competence is defined by the FWPE as "respect for diversity factors of others including but not limited to sociocultural, socioeconomic, spiritual, and lifestyle choices."[3] Simply put, it is the ability to interact and work with people from various cultures. Cultural competence is also linked with compassion, in that the practitioner offers unbiased care and has the power to offer services to clients to improve their engagement in occupations.

Culture can be defined narrowly (for example, race, religion, gender) or broadly (grew up in the country, has a disability, prefers a certain type of music, does not eat meat or dairy products). People are different from one another in many types of ways, and everyone is a product of their own culture, which partly shapes the way individuals view others. Cultural competence is a *lifelong process* of gaining knowledge, skills, and attitudes. Cultural competence begins with cultural awareness, that is, the acknowledgment of differences between individuals and groups. Knowledge can be gained through reading, observation, and discussion. With increased knowledge, the student and practitioner can reflect on and acknowledge biases and seek to understand differences. Cultural competence requires that OT practitioners treat everyone with respect, regardless of how they arrived at their circumstance. The culturally

EVIDENCE-BASED PRACTICE

Burnout is a risk for OT practitioners due to the high levels of emotional connection with clients. A recent systematic study found that the practice of mindfulness, "the awareness that emerges through paying attention, on purpose, and nonjudgmentally to the unfolding of experience moment by moment" in healthcare professionals (including physicians, nurses, psychologists, and social workers) and teachers helped to reduce burnout in their jobs. The systematic study included eight randomized control trials. The systematic study cites from one of the research studies that participants who received mindfulness training had "decreased levels of emotional exhaustion and increased personal achievement." Another research study found that participants who wrote in a daily journal experienced "increased inner peace, calm, joy; decreased stress and anxiety, improved ability to handle stressful situations, and increased appreciation, gratitude, and compassion." Even though the research participants were not OT practitioners, the participants had similar demographic characteristics, and thus the authors state that mindfulness can likely be of benefit to OT practitioners to "monitor and maintain occupational balance and well-being."[5] Mindfulness training can occur in different structured or unstructured forms such as continuing education courses, books for self-study, and discussions with colleagues. Chapter 4 addresses burnout and stress management in further detail.

Luken, M., & Sammons, A. (2016). Systematic review of mindfulness practice for reducing job burnout. American Journal of Occupational Therapy, *70, 7002250020p1-7002250020p10. doi:10.5014/ajot.2016.016956*

competent practitioner builds trust to be able to deliver culturally sensitive care.[6] The case study at the end of this chapter further explores the issue of cultural competence.

COMMUNICATION

Communication is not specifically defined as a professional behavior on the FWPE (except in responding to feedback); however, communication is foundational to all healthcare tasks. OTA students need to learn to communicate effectively with body language (including facial expressions) and written, oral, and electronic documentation. One can convey negative body language by standing too far away from the client, avoiding touching the client, slouching while standing or sitting, crossing arms, rolling eyes, and more. Positive body language examples include nodding, good eye contact, erect posture, caring and appropriate client handling, smiling, or other facial expressions that are congruent with the situation. For example, if a client seems not to be his or her "normal self" during a therapy session (perhaps more emotional or more detached, or quiet and sad), the effective OT practitioner would communicate to the client with good eye contact, a calm voice, and perhaps a gentle hand on a shoulder or forearm, and ask the client, "You don't seem like your normal self today. Is something bothering you?" The words and tone can reflect care and concern, which are supported consistently by the eye contact, facial expression, and gentle touch.

Accurate and timely documentation is required of all OT practitioners. With the requirements of the Affordable Care Act (ACA) that healthcare providers transition to using electronic health records (EHRs), many healthcare companies have transitioned to documenting care at point of service.[7] That is, the OT practitioner is expected to be performing at least some documentation while providing client interventions. Many types of devices, software programs, and apps have been developed to help meet the documentation

COMMUNICATION

Social media use has crossed generational boundaries and is a powerful communication tool. Social media has become a context in which many students and practitioners communicate their joys, successes, frustrations, and failures, not just personally but professionally.

For communicating intraprofessionally (within the same profession) one may find closed (private) or open groups on Facebook or other social media sites dedicated to creating a forum for sharing treatment ideas, asking questions, or debating ethical scenarios. Such groups can be found for various treatment settings or populations, or may be broader. The groups can be helpful or pose issues, as the veil of social media can provide enough distance for individuals to share or say things they might not in person. Proceed with caution and use judgment when replying to posts.

With the rise of social media use, there may be some ethical dilemmas surrounding whom to connect with on social media. Does one seek or accept a client's "friend request" on Facebook or "follow" a client on Instagram? What about the request of a former client from fieldwork? Or from a professor? What are the ethical and professional boundaries that should be guarded? What if an elderly client's adult child seeks to connect via social media? Some practitioners have settled this issue by embracing the opportunity to connect in general ways with clients (cautiously and without violating HIPAA) by creating a professional Facebook, Instagram, or other type of social media account. They have wisely kept their personal and professional lives separate on social media. Ultimately, each student and practitioner must consider professional responsibilities and ethical principles as the best guides when making decisions about communicating via social media platforms.

demands, and students will most likely encounter a variety during fieldwork. One caution is to maintain as much eye contact and client-centered care as possible while using the electronic documentation devices or clients will have a difficult time developing a therapeutic bond with the practitioner. A good feature of portable devices is that the client's chart is never lost, and it is available immediately to refer to goals or see documented progress. Once the student assimilates to the point-of-service documentation, time spent documenting will be reduced and may not seem as overwhelming.

Certification and Licensure

National and state boards exist to maintain the integrity of the profession and to protect the public. To work as an OTA in the United States, one must pass the National Board of Certification in Occupational Therapy's (NBCOT®) Certified Occupational Therapy Assistant (COTA) examination, which is followed by licensure in the state where one will work as an OTA (Table 2-2). Although initial certification by NBCOT is mandatory, renewal is optional. NBCOT renewal takes place every 3 years, on proof of a specific number of professional development units (PDUs) and a renewal fee. State licensures vary, with some states having an independent board of OT, whereas the board may be combined with other types of professionals in other states. Most states require annual licensure renewal, which entails proof of a specific number of hours of continuing education (and documentation of content or skills achieved), plus a license renewal fee. Check each state board for specifics. Resources can be found on the AOTA website under the "State Policy" section.

In Canada, only occupational therapists are licensed, and not all have to pass a national certification examination to gain licensure; it varies province by province.[8] OTAs in Canada may attend a community college or gain skills through on-the-job training,[8] and they do not have to take a national certification examination.

TECHNOLOGY AND TRENDS

Continuing education is available through multiple methods: traditional face-to-face individual courses; local, regional, state, or national conferences; and online webinars, online courses, articles in *OT Practice*, in-services, journal clubs, and so on. A varied approach to continuing education is highly recommended, which would include several types of learning.

Technology has made obtaining continuing education easier to access, especially for practitioners in rural areas or those who have a difficult time attending traditional continuing education courses. Another positive aspect of online learning, especially webinars, is that one can have easier contact with presenters who live in a distant location, and who may only be available to teach their specialty area in an online format.

The sole purpose of some businesses is to deliver online continuing education, and as such, can usually offer a bundled package at a lower price than some traditional face-to-face courses purchased separately. Although the flexibility and price of purely online courses are appealing, and online courses can provide some excellent continuing education, not all companies provide the same quality. For that reason, consider asking colleagues if they have had a positive or negative experience with a specific company, and check to see if one course is available to be purchased first before agreeing to purchase a package. Also consider the course content—is it something that would be more likely to need a hands-on component? Next, think about one's learning style and which type of learning environment will be the most beneficial. Finally, attending an online course can be beneficial, but it cannot substitute for the valuable byproduct of networking with other therapy practitioners at a face-to-face course or at a conference.

Scope of Practice and Supervision

The AOTA *Scope of Practice* defines occupational therapy, OT practice components, and the scope of practice (domain and process). The document serves to highlight the distinct value of occupation and OT in contributing to client health, well-being, and participation in life occupations, and guides OT practice. The document provides guidance for the "what, how, and where" of OT, and is freely accessible to the public on the AOTA website, under "Official Documents."[9] Each state also has a state law passed by the state legislature that specifies the scope of OT in that state.

TABLE 2-2 Guide to Occupational Therapy Credentials (U.S.)*

OCCUPATIONAL THERAPIST	OCCUPATIONAL THERAPY ASSISTANT
OTS = OT student	OTAS = OTA student
OT = graduate of an accredited OT program	OTA = graduate of an accredited OTA program
OTR = an occupational therapist who passed the national board examination (NBCOT)	COTA = an OTA who passed the national board examination (NBCOT)
OTR/L = same as above, + licensed in a state	COTA/L = same as above + licensed in a state
Must maintain licensure (L)	*Must* maintain licensure (L)
Can drop the R after 3 years (not required to renew national registry)	Can drop the C after 3 years (not required to renew national certification)

*Credentials required may vary by state or country

Supervision is delineated by the AOTA document *Guidelines for Supervision, Roles, and Responsibilities During the Delivery of Occupational Therapy Services* and also at state levels.[10] This AOTA document is also available on the association website, but only to members or through access to the *American Journal of Occupational Therapy* via a library or subscription. Each state regulatory board determines the types of supervision required in its state, and they vary greatly. For example, some states have different supervision guidelines for first-year OTAs (e.g., North Carolina) whereas others do not (e.g., South Carolina). Overall, occupational therapists and OTAs work collaboratively, with the occupational therapist ultimately responsible for supervising OTAs and for the safe and appropriate treatment provided to clients (Fig. 2-2). Be sure to locate the relevant state supervision requirements.

Ethics

In the United States, the Ethics Commission, an official group that is part of the AOTA, develops the *OT Code of Ethics,* which provides core values to guide the actions of professionals and volunteers and to define the consequences of the violation of ethical principles.[11] The AOTA Ethics Commission also reviews and investigates complaints of ethical violations and takes disciplinary action with regard to membership in AOTA.

As stated earlier, OT practitioners are expected to follow personal and professional ethical principles. The terms and principles in the *OT Code of Ethics* seem rather straightforward: *beneficence* (do good), *nonmaleficence* (do no harm), *autonomy* (treat client as they wish and maintain confidentiality), *justice* (be fair and objective), *veracity* (be truthful), and *fidelity* (respect and treat all fairly).[11] However, applying these ethical principles to real-world scenarios can be challenging because sometimes the situation is unclear, or has multiple factors to consider. When facing a difficult situation and decision on the proper action to take, the first step is to read the AOTA *OT Code of Ethics* because it includes many helpful examples. Second, remember to follow the chain of command and speak directly with the supervising occupational therapist; then, if the situation is not adequately resolved, go to one's supervisor. If still confused, consider confidentially discussing the matter with a trusted OT mentor to help one see the situation from a different perspective. Ethics and adhering to ethical principles are so imperative that some state licensing boards require evidence of annual continuing education in ethics. Healthcare systems also have ethics boards that can assist in reviewing ethical situations, if needed; however, most situations can be handled with the supervising occupational therapist. Suppose an individual encounters the situation illustrated in Figure 2-3. What is the ethical violation? Is there more than one ethical principle involved? What should the OTA do?

Students will almost certainly encounter issues for which they must use the ethical principles as a guide for actions, especially during clinical and fieldwork experiences. Some examples that students have encountered in the past are "discussing clients in negative ways, stereotyping clients, referring to clients by diagnosis; failing to communicate (e.g., withholding prognostic information from clients); and breaching confidentiality (e.g., talking about clients in public)."[12] See Table 2-3 to read and consider some ethical situations. Take time to discuss which principles may be violated and the best course of action for the student or the practitioner.

The College of Occupational Therapists of Ontario suggests a step-by-step "Conscious Decision-Making Process" that is helpful to use when determining ethical scenarios:

1. Describe the situation (what are the facts, who is involved).
2. Identify the related ethical principles.
3. Identify the resources that are pertinent to the situation.
4. Determine whether further information is needed to make a decision.
5. Identify all the options.

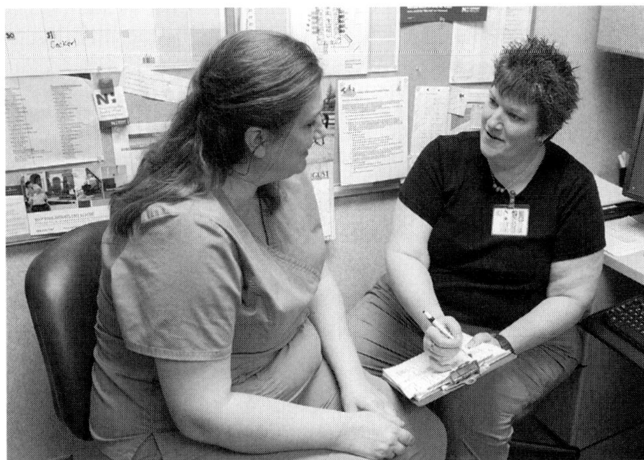

FIGURE 2-2. OTA and Occupational therapist collaborating to discuss treatment for a client.

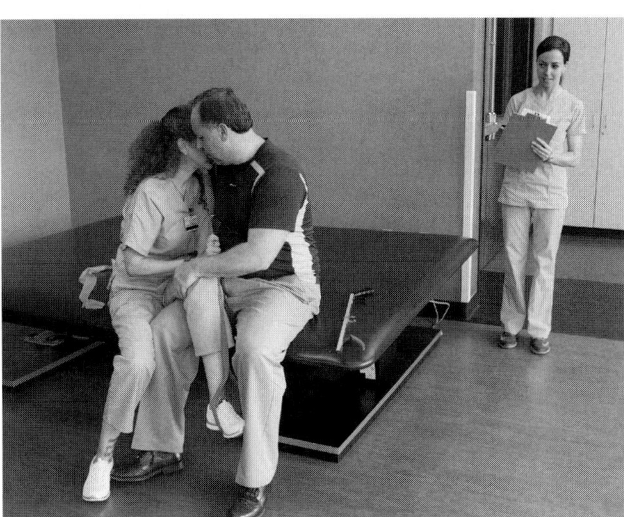

FIGURE 2-3. OTA encountering a colleague becoming physically involved with a client.

6. Select the best option.
7. Take action based on the best option.
8. Evaluate the outcome of the decision and actions taken.[6]

Try using these steps when considering the ethical situations in Table 2-3.

ADVOCACY

To be an advocate means to seek the best for another individual or group, often communicating on their behalf. **Advocacy** in the OT community must be accomplished as the profession continues to strive toward recognition of the distinct value of OT, and as the profession reaches for Vision 2025. The guiding principles that AOTA plans to attain are: "Occupational therapy maximizes health, well-being, and quality of life for all people, populations, and communities through effective solutions that facilitate participation in everyday living."[13] Every practitioner must become an advocate for the profession and for the clients served. Many physicians and other healthcare providers are still unclear on the role of OT, which presents a challenge to the OT community. OT practitioners must educate physicians, nurses, nutritionists, social workers, and other members of the healthcare team about the benefits of OT and how it both differs from and complements physical therapy and

TABLE 2-3 Ethical Scenarios

The following are scenarios based on real events. This table is meant to facilitate discussion of ethical principles and possible courses of action. Ethical scenarios can be difficult to analyze, and the course of action taken by the OTA or OTA/S may vary from person to person.

SCENARIO	WHICH ETHICAL PRINCIPLES ARE INVOLVED?	WHAT SHOULD OR COULD THE OTA OR OTA/S DO?
1. The OTA/S overheard her fieldwork (FW) educator, a COTA/L, in the hallway of the hospital talking with the physical therapist. They had all just worked with a client who was in acute care due to fracturing three lumbar vertebrae. They found out that the client (female) was injured during sexual activity and were laughing and joking about it. • What should the OTA/S do? • What principles have been violated? • Is the OTA/S at risk of violating any principles by acting or not acting?	**Beneficence** The FW educator was not acting in the best interest for the well-being of the client. **Nonmaleficence** The FW educator imposed the risk of harm by speaking openly in an unprofessional manner. **Autonomy** The FW educator did not respect the confidentiality of the client's information by speaking openly in the hallway. **Fidelity** The FW educator did not treat the client with respect, discretion, or integrity while laughing and joking in the hallway (not a private location) with another professional.	What should the OTA/S do? Options to consider: 1. Discuss the incident with her FW educator, which is following the chain of command. 2. Report the incident to the OT supervisor. 3. Report the incident to the state board that regulates OT, NBCOT, and AOTA (if the FW educator is a member). 4. Discuss the incident with the Academic Fieldwork Coordinator. Students often are hesitant to report ethical violations due to being fearful that their grade will be negatively affected. Thus the AFCW should be alerted. 5. Do nothing.
2. A new COTA/L graduate was hired to work at a long-term care facility by a contract therapy company. During her first week of work she clocked in longer on 1 day (8.75 hours) than her originally scheduled 8 hours due to a heavy client caseload, unrealistically high productivity demands (100%), and needing time to complete documentation. At the end of the week, the rehabilitation manager (an OTR/L) instructed her to alter her timesheet to reflect only working her 8 scheduled hours. This would also necessitate altering the medical record for the time she was providing	**Nonmaleficence** The OTR/L pressured the COTA/L to alter medical records and expected her to meet unrealistic productivity demands. **Justice** The COTA/L is required by this principle to report to the appropriate authorities any acts that are illegal or unethical. **Veracity** The OTR/L is requesting that the COTA/L alter documentation of a client's records and also to alter her timesheet. **Fidelity** The OTR/L is not treating the COTA/L with respect, fairness, or integrity, and is using her position as rehabilitation manager, which threatens the COTA/L's employment status if she does not comply.	What should the COTA/L do? Options to consider: 1. Refuse to change the documentation of services (alter times). 2. Refuse to alter the employee timesheet. 3. Agree to not be paid for overtime hours worked. 4. Report the actions of the OTR/L to the regional manager. 5. Report the actions of the OTR/L to the state board that regulates OT, the NBCOT, and AOTA. 6. Do nothing.

TABLE 2-3 Ethical Scenarios (continued)

SCENARIO	WHICH ETHICAL PRINCIPLES ARE INVOLVED?	WHAT SHOULD OR COULD THE OTA OR OTA/S DO?
care, because she saw the last client after the eighth hour of work, just before she left for the day. What should the COTA/L do? What principles have been violated? Is the COTA/L at risk of violating any principles by acting or not acting?		
3. The COTA/L walked into a client room at a skilled nursing facility (SNF) and found his supervising OTR/L sound asleep in the recliner, covered with a blanket. He knew that the OTR/L had been working a lot of extra hours and she also had a sick child at home. Much to his surprise, the client told him that the OTR/L fell asleep while the client was showering, and she covered her up so she could get some much needed rest. The COTA/L left the room, but later overheard that the OTR/L had billed a full treatment session and knew that it included the time she was sleeping. What should the COTA/L do? What should the OTR/L have done? What principles have been violated? Is the COTA/L at risk of violating any principles by acting or not acting?	**Nonmaleficence** The OTR/L did not remedy personal problems (lack of sleep) and the client, who needed her supervision to shower, may have been harmed. **Beneficence** The OTR/L was not demonstrating a concern for the safety and well-being of her client. **Justice** The OTR/L submitted claims for reimbursement for services not provided, which does not comply with the law.	What should the COTA/L do? Options to consider: 1. Discuss his concerns with the OTR/L about documenting and billing for services not performed. 2. Report the OTR/L's actions to the Rehabilitation Manager. 3. Report the OTR/L to the state board that regulates OT, the NBCOT, and the AOTA. 4. Do nothing.
4. The renewal period for licensure had come up quickly, and the COTA/L was waiting on the continuing education certificate to arrive from a very recent course he completed that he needed for his renewal. He was going to miss the renewal period by at least 2 days. His license was going to expire on Monday, June 30, and today was Friday, June 27th. He was scheduled to work a full week next week at the outpatient center, knew they were very busy, and did not want to have to cancel client appointments, so he went to work on Tuesday, July 1, and	**Justice** Documentation of services does not comply with laws. Practitioners must be licensed to provide OT services. **Veracity** The COTA/L represented himself as licensed when in fact he was not for 2 days. He did not report accurate records in a timely manner.	What should the COTA/L do? Options to consider: 1. Notify his supervising OT of his failure to renew his license on time. 2. Report his own actions to the state board that regulates OT for practicing OT without a license. 3. Report his own actions to NBCOT and AOTA. 4. Ensure he completes all continuing education requirements in the future well in advance of the deadline for licensure renewal. 5. Do nothing.

Continued

TABLE 2-3 Ethical Scenarios (continued)

SCENARIO	WHICH ETHICAL PRINCIPLES ARE INVOLVED?	WHAT SHOULD OR COULD THE OTA OR OTA/S DO?
worked the remainder of the week. He was able to renew his license on Thursday, July 3rd. What should he do? What should he have done? What principles have been violated? Is the COTA/L at risk of violating any additional principles by acting or not acting?		
5. A COTA/L with 5 years of experience attended a continuing education training course in kinesiotaping and has gained the skills to use kinesiotaping in the delivery of OT services. Her regular OTR/L, who is also service competent in kinesiotaping, is out on an extended maternity leave, and she is being supervised by a traveling OTR/L, who has no training or service competency in kinesiotaping. The OTR/L states to the COTA/L that she can still use kinesiotape because the COTA/L is trained, has used it in the past, and the OTR/L trusts her. What should she do? What should the OTR/L have done? What principles have been violated? Is the COTA/L at risk of violating any additional principles by acting or not acting?	Beneficence The OTR/L did not have training and therefore could not appropriately supervise the COTA/L in the delivery of services. Nonmaleficence The OTR/L may have caused harm to the client if the COTA/L made an error. The OTR/L is ultimately responsible, and if she does not have service competency, cannot supervise the COTA/L in that intervention.	What should the COTA/L do? Possible options: 1. Ask if any other OTR/Ls have service competency in kinesiotaping and ask that individual to supervise. 2. Discuss other options for client treatment interventions with the OTR/L instead of using kinesiotape. 3. Report the OTR/L to the state board of OT. 4. Wait for her full-time OTR/L to return before using kinesiotape. 5. Offer to locate a kinesiotape continuing education course for the traveling OTR/L to attend and gain service competency. 6. Proceed with using kinesiotape, per the OTR/L's instructions.

speech-language pathology. Additionally, state and federal legislators are often unaware of the role and value of OT, and efforts should be made to participate in federal or state advocacy days at the legislative buildings, such as the OTAs did in Figure 2-4.

Client

According to the *Occupational Therapy Practice Framework, 3rd edition* (OTPF-3), the term *client* includes more than just the individual receiving OT—it also comprises the family.[2] Advocating for the client may mean drafting a letter of medical necessity to the insurance company for a specific piece of equipment in collaboration with the occupational therapist. Or it could mean recognizing a change in status of the client that requires a shift in the treatment plan. It could also be helping the family to understand the unique needs of their loved one as roles may have changed. The term *client* will be used throughout this textbook in place of the older, medical model term, "patient."

Therapy Community

Advocacy within the therapy community involves collaborating with other practitioners to discuss current issues affecting the profession. Practitioners can sometimes feel isolated, especially if they are the only occupational therapist or OTA on staff, or the team is very small. Reaching out to other practitioners in the area or region is a good way to become connected with a network of therapy providers. Groups of providers tend to form naturally around a similar setting, such as geriatrics or pediatrics, and there is power

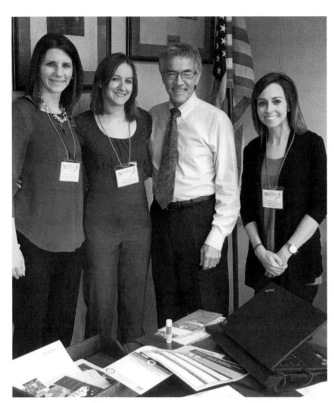

FIGURE 2-4. OTAs meeting with a member of the North Carolina State Legislature to advocate for occupational therapy.

THE OLDER ADULT

The use of technology is prevalent in current society, but older adults may not be as comfortable with using technology. A small study was conducted in which older adults were trained with an individualized home-based information communication technology program. Each participant was trained at home, using an iPad®, along key occupational areas valuable to each individual. After the training period, participants independently used the device for 3 months. At the end of that time, participants showed a significant increase in the range of activities and comfort level with technology. The study postulates that an individualized, self-paced approach in one's own context facilitated the motivation of community-dwelling older adults toward increased use of technology in leisure and social participation.[14] The additional implication is that as older adults choose to "age in place" (stay in their own home longer versus move to a facility), increasing health conditions and comorbidities may prevent social interaction, and use of technology can help the older adult with social participation.

in numbers. Practitioners can join together for continuing education, support, and advocacy for the profession and the clients served. Practitioners can meet in person or virtually to share ideas and concerns. Technology has made some methods of collaborating in the therapy community more efficient, such as using web conferencing tools. Chances are that what one practitioner may be experiencing is similar to another and the group of practitioners can begin to see patterns of concern or positive change. Scanning the current environment of what is affecting OT is a useful exercise to identify trends affecting settings in the therapy community. Once the trends are identified, they can be discussed and possible solutions brainstormed. A good way to effect change and bring attention to areas of concern is to involve the state or national professional organizations.

Professional Organizations at the State, National, and International Levels

Professional organizations spend significant time and resources lobbying and advocating for the profession, OT practitioners, and the clients served. Membership dues to professional organizations help to offset the cost of advocacy. Professional organizations may hire a lobbyist, an individual who attends legislative sessions, attends political events, and meets one-on-one with politicians to educate them regarding OT and encourage them to vote favorably on priority issues for OT. Having one or more people who can consistently represent OT to the lawmakers helps to protect the profession in services provided to citizens and jobs for licensees. When a lobbyist is not representing OT, bills can get passed that inadvertently omit it. For example, North Carolina lawmakers passed the G.S.58-50-30, "Right to choose services of certain providers," in 2001, during a time when North Carolina did not have a lobbyist for OT.[15] The general statute (G.S.), or law, ensured that clients have the right, as part of the health insurance regulations, to select their provider for many medical professions, including physicians, physical therapists, dentists, optometrists, and so on, but OT was omitted. Several years later, when the North Carolina Occupational Therapy Association (NCOTA) hired a lobbyist, the lobbyist was instrumental in communicating with lawmakers to introduce a bill, HB 208/SB 307, Occupational Therapy/Choice of Provider, to include OT. OT practitioners, students, and NCOTA board members attended an Advocacy Day in which they spoke to their individual legislators regarding the bill and educated them about OT's role in helping people. The Occupational Therapy/Choice of Provider Bill passed both the Senate and House of Representatives and was signed into law by the Governor. Without advocacy, important changes that affect the entire profession and the services that clients receive are in jeopardy. Check with state and national organizations to learn more about the current issues facing OT today.

The primary international OT organization is the World Federation of Occupational Therapy (WFOT); its mission is as follows: "WFOT promotes occupational therapy as an art and science internationally. The Federation supports the development, use and practice of occupational therapy worldwide, demonstrating its relevance and contribution to society."[16] WFOT also publishes internationally agreed on standards for the education of occupational therapists. WFOT began as an organization that only recognized occupational therapists as members, but in January 2017, WFOT began accepting OTAs as individual members. For more information, visit www.wfot.org.

EVIDENCE-BASED PRACTICE

How can an OT practitioner be sure to provide the correct intervention for the client? How does one find information on what ought to be done, especially in a rapidly changing healthcare and technological environment? What was known or used 25 years ago may or may not be the correct strategy today. OT practitioners must base interventions on the most current and reliable evidence. The AOTA reveals that **evidence-based practice (EBP)** is a blend of quality research, clinical knowledge, and input from clients regarding their values and beliefs.[17] Evidence-based practice (EBP) should be used as a clinical decision-making framework.[18] Thus EBP incorporates research and clinical expertise in a client-centered manner.

How does the new or busy OT practitioner stay current with EBP? The reality is that there are barriers associated with using EBP, such as lack of time and lack of knowledge of where to locate the EBP,[18,19] as well as lack of knowledge or training to implement interventions.[20]

Finding and Understanding Evidence-Based Practice Resources

The saying "Consider the source" holds true for evaluating scholarly work. Research is conducted in different ways and, as such, needs to be carefully evaluated. One must determine whether the results are valid, whether they are important, and whether they apply to the specific client currently being treated. The sources cited in Table 2-4 will help the OTA identify quality evidence.

Primary literature includes actual research studies conducted with research participants. The randomized control trial (RCT) is considered the most rigorous research method, in which the research subjects randomly receive the "treatment" or the "placebo" (nontreatment), and the researchers are also unaware of which subject is receiving what type of intervention or nonintervention. A controlled clinical trial is the same as an RCT, except without the randomization.[21] Although this works well in some circumstances, it is not always possible for OT research. For example, the researcher would know if a client is receiving or not receiving a specific OT intervention that is being tested, because the OT practitioner would be delivering it or not delivering it. To increase the validity of the experiment, one would need additional outside research assistants who would administer the treatment and measure outcomes, then report anonymously, which would be considered "blinding."[21]

Research can further be divided into quantitative and qualitative information (Table 2-5). **Quantitative** research deals with numbers, logic, objectivity, and finding a cause and effect. An easy method to remember this is the stem of

OT Practitioner's Viewpoint

As a student, realizing the full impact of belonging to your state and national associations is difficult. Membership may seem like just another expense and you are already spending money on tuition, fees, books, uniforms, and transportation. You may think that you'll get involved "one day." I have the privilege to travel to colleges in my state to promote the importance of advocacy and joining professional organizations. I often hear my own and other students say, "I can't afford the dues." And that may be true for some. But I would challenge you to do the math. Calculate the cost of student membership in the state and national associations and divide it by 365. The net amount is what it will cost you *per day* to advocate for OT for yourself (your future job), your clients, and the profession. Is that amount even the cost of a coffee or candy bar? State and national associations rely on membership dues to help have a daily presence interacting with legislators who make the decisions that affect our lives, jobs, and services we can provide for our clients. What are you currently doing with those dimes and quarters per day that could be better directed toward membership? If you don't advocate, who will?

Advocacy is just one of many reasons to be involved in professional associations. The obvious answer to "what's in it for me?" is the valuable resources associations provide, from discounts at conferences to discounted or free publications. Some conferences even offer specific student-only sessions custom created to meet your needs. Many states have scholarships funded by the state association. Annual scholarships are also available through the American Occupational Therapy Foundation (open to members of AOTA).

But when you dig a little deeper into professional associations, you will realize that the connections and networking are absolutely vital to your career, even as a student. You may meet your future fieldwork educator or supervisor, and have the opportunity to leave a lasting positive impression. If you haven't learned already, in this world, personal connections are fundamental. At every association conference I have attended I have made an important connection, and those connections have opened many doors that would have otherwise remained closed or even unknown.

Bottom line—get involved. Attend a State Advocacy Day or the AOTA Hill Day. Get involved in a mentor/mentee program. Apply for the Emerging Leaders Program with AOTA. Volunteer at a conference or attend just one state association conference or district meeting (at the greatly reduced student rate or perhaps at no cost) and observe and interact. Watch the networking, dialogue, learning, and advocacy. Don't be a passive student or practitioner. To be a strong, viable profession doing the most good for individuals and populations, we must unite. We must educate. We must advocate. It is your professional responsibility. ~ Amy J. Mahle, MHA, COTA/L

TABLE 2-4 Evidence-Based Practice Resource Guide

SOURCE	WHERE	WHAT
AOTA—EBP Resource Directory	www.aota.org/ebp	• Peer-reviewed journal articles • Practice guidelines • Critically appraised topics—a compilation of research answering a specific question
Cochrane	www.cochrane.org	• Systematic reviews of worldwide research that answer a specific research question • Highly authoritative
Google Scholar	http://scholar.google.com	• Search for scholarly articles
NBCOT	http://practiceblog.nbcot.org https://my.nbcot.org	• Professional blog with research topics organized categorically; summaries available to general public • Log in to MyNBCOT® to access ProQuest account for access to full articles
OT Seeker	www.otseeker.com	• Database containing abstracts of thousands of systematic reviews, randomized controlled trials, and other resources relevant to OT interventions
PubMed	www.ncbi.nlm.nih.gov/pubmed	• Citations and abstracts (some full text) for biomedical literature
OTCATS—Occupational Therapy Critically Appraised Topics	www.OTCATS.com	• Summarizes the best available research on a specific topic • Useful when a specific treatment question has been identified
Centre for Evidence-Based Medicine (Canada)	www.cebm.utoronto.ca	• Information on evidence-based medicine for a variety of health professions • Worksheets to help determine the validity and strength of a research study

TABLE 2-5 Sample Quantitative versus Qualitative Research Questions

RESEARCH QUESTION	UNIT OF MEASURE	GENERALIZE?	RESEARCH METHOD
Is constraint-induced movement therapy effective to increase independence with ADLs with clients who had a stroke?	Assessments of ADLs before and after intervention	Yes	Quantitative
What is the experience of clients who transitioned to a long-term care facility in the first month?	Nonstructured interview of clients at 1 month following admittance to a long-term care facility	No	Qualitative
What is the effect of iontophoresis on carpal tunnel syndrome?	Assess pain, numbness, and strength before and after treatment with iontophoresis (a physical agent modality)	Yes	Quantitative
For clients who have had a traumatic brain injury and are married, what is the experience of the spouse once the client returns home?	Semistructured interview	No	Qualitative

the word, "quant," similar to quantity, which is easily associated with a measurable, objective number. Quantitative research should be able to be accurately and precisely replicated, and the goal is for the results to be generalized, or applied to other similar situations.

Qualitative research aims to find answers to subjective questions, such as experiences and personal stories, which cannot be replicated. Qualitative research helps produce theories, rather than prove cause and effect.

Secondary literature is research that evaluates and sorts numerous primary research studies to identify the best overall evidence for a topic. Secondary literature can be useful to the practitioner because some analysis and evaluation has already been completed, which can save quite a bit of time. Types of secondary literature are systematic reviews, meta-analyses, EBP guidelines, and critically appraised topics (CATs). Refer again to Table 2-4, which includes some secondary literature resources. Suppose, however, that secondary literature is not available on the needed topic. One must then spend more time reviewing and evaluating research, in collaboration with the occupational therapist and perhaps even a journal club. A journal club is a group of OT practitioners who decide on an article to read, discuss, and determine its implications for practice. (More information is provided later in this chapter on Journal Clubs under Lifelong Learning). Identifying and collaborating with more knowledgeable and experienced clinicians as valuable guides for finding evidence is beneficial to any OTA student or practitioner (Fig. 2-5).[19]

Using Primary Literature for Evidence-Based Practice

The following steps are some of the ways to incorporate using EBP in everyday OT interventions.

1. *Identify clinical questions relevant to the information needed.* Formulating appropriate clinical questions requires critical thinking and a good understanding of the client. Clinical questions can be varied, such as determining the best intervention, wondering about the long-term outcomes for a client, or what common concerns the client might experience.[20]
2. *Search the literature to locate research relevant to the type of clinical question.* The research needed to answer the clinical questions largely depends on the types of questions. For example, if the question seeks to find information on concerns or experiences a client had with a particular treatment, the OTA would look for qualitative research. On the other hand, if the question were seeking which intervention had the best overall outcomes, the OTA would seek quantitative research.
3. *Critically appraise the research to determine how valid or believable it is, and to decide if the results are clinically important.* As discussed earlier, not all research has the same level of quality, and it must be carefully evaluated for research design and the number of participants to determine whether the results are statistically significant. The research article will include a section on statistical analysis and also a conclusion section, which will both give information on the ability to use the findings or not. Is the information peer reviewed?
4. *Consider how the information from the research can be applied in the clinical setting or with the client.*[20] After reviewing the literature, determine whether the results are a good fit for the client or population's context, that is, are they similar? Does the information found in the research relate well enough to the specific context of the client(s) one is working with (Box 2-1)?

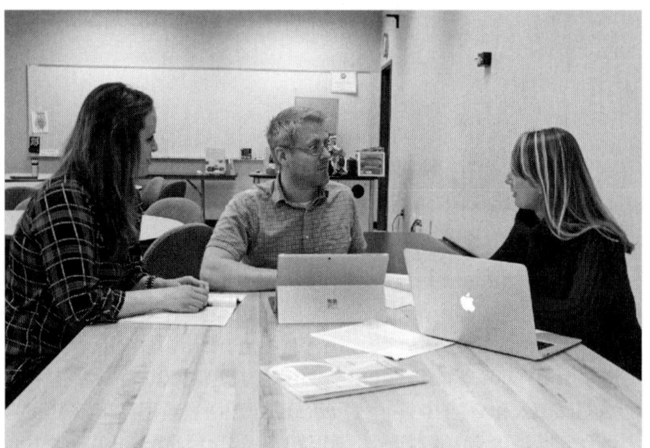

FIGURE 2-5. Students working together to find EBP.

LIFELONG LEARNING

The OT profession requires that practitioners be **lifelong learners**. In fact, the accreditation standards set by ACOTE mandate that graduates must be equipped to be lifelong learners and maintain knowledge of best practice.[22] What exactly is a lifelong learner and how does one become one? Consider the following quotes from two OTAs regarding lifelong learning: "Gaining daily insight into practice areas that will expand my understanding and provide me with new skills, education, and training to improve my professional skills in the field of occupational therapy. I attempt to accomplish it by reviewing lots of current research, networking with colleagues and other professionals in the community, attending continuing education opportunities, and fulfilling higher academic goals." Another OTA with 8 years of experience states, "Understanding I don't know everything, working to learn and try new things to improve myself as an OTA." And the following is from an occupational therapist who has over 30 years of experience: "Lifelong learning has changed for me over the years. Early on it was exploring new techniques and modalities. Then it was exploring those more deeply, looking at the nuances and how to integrate them into treatment plans. Now it's all about 'self'-discovery, work on self and just 'becoming'." The variety of perspectives on lifelong learning illustrate that the needs of the learner change over time and are unique to each learner (Fig. 2-6). Lifelong learning does not simply occur when practitioners merely fulfill their continuing education requirements; instead, the intention is to develop a natural desire to seek and discover opportunities for continual self-improvement as a practitioner and to incorporate new learning into practice.

More than Just Continuing Education Courses and Professional Development Units

At a minimum, practitioners are required to complete a specific number of hours of formal learning during a set timeframe to maintain national certification and state licensure. In the United States, the NBCOT identifies the learning as competency assessment units (CAUs) and professional development units (PDUs) and requires 36 units every 3 years after initial certification.[23] Currently, once initial certification

BOX 2-1
Practical Application of Using Primary Literature in an Evidence-Based Practice Approach

An OTA has a 49-year-old male client with a recent history of a right CVA due to an arteriovenous malformation. He has been through the continuum of care, including 5 days in the acute care hospital and a 2-week stay at the rehabilitation hospital, and has attended outpatient OT for 3 months. He has made significant progress with functional use of his left upper extremity, but he is not satisfied and wants to return to work. The OTA and occupational therapist discuss options for the client and want to determine what other evidence-based practice interventions are available to help the client make even more progress and return to work. The following are the steps in using primary literature for evidence-based practice.

1. Ask: What evidence-based treatments are available following a CVA for clients who have made some functional gains?
2. Seek: Look for literature with quantitative research (to find which specific treatments are most effective). The results found the following interventions:
   - Constraint-induced movement therapy (CIMT)
   - Bilateral upper extremity training
   - Functional electrical stimulation (FES)
   - Mirror therapy
3. Review: Carefully examine the research articles to determine their validity. Do they include a statistical analysis? Are the findings of the research statistically significant? How many participants were included in the study? Identify the top articles that meet these criteria.
   - All four therapeutic approaches have valid research. The client has already been participating in bilateral upper extremity training and FES, which has helped him make significant gains thus far.
4. Consider: Does the intervention meet the individual needs of the client? Can the client afford continued treatment? (Will insurance cover it? Is he able to pay out of pocket?) Is he able to tolerate the treatment?
   - After discussing options with the client, it was determined that CIMT was the best option for the client, due to his ability to pay out of pocket for a 2-week intensive program and results found in the research.

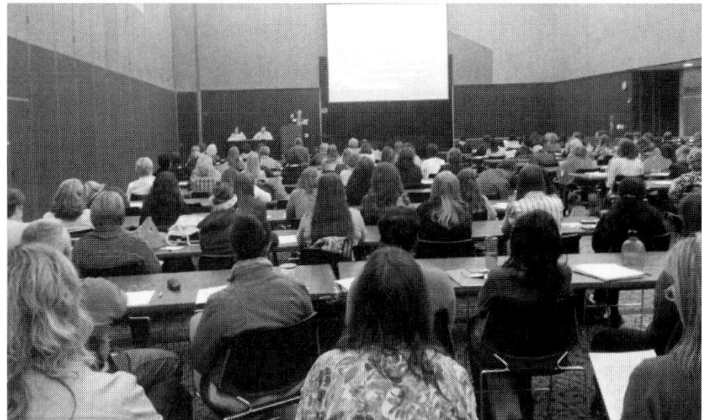

FIGURE 2-6. Lifelong learning may include attending a professional conference.

by NBCOT is obtained, a practitioner is not required to renew his or her certification. If the COTA/L allows certification to lapse, he or she may no longer use the "C" and can only legally write OTA/L for his or her credentials. Maintaining certification requires paying a fee and submitting evidence of the appropriate number and type of professional development units. OTAs should strongly consider maintaining national certification. NBCOT offers valuable online certificant-only benefits, such as basic tools to assess one's professional strengths and weaknesses to better plan for needed continuing education. NBCOT also offers to certificants the "NBCOT Navigator®," a collection of online tools to help self-reflect and further develop competencies. Furthermore, use of these and the subsequent proper documentation can be counted as CAUs for NBCOT renewal and may be counted toward a portion of continuing education requirements in some states.

Continuing education requirements vary from state to state, are managed by a state licensure board, and are sometimes called continuing competence activities (CCAs) or continuing education units (CEUs). Canadian provinces may all have slightly different requirements for occupational therapists, (many use the Annual Continuing Competence Review), but OTAs in Canada do not have continuing education requirements at this time. In the U.S., licensing boards in each state will require proof of continuing education activities, such as a certificate, handouts, notes, or other evidence of attendance and learning. Students should be familiar with the regulations and requirements in the state in which they intend to practice OT. Once initially licensed, the OTA must renew his or her license according to state requirements. Practicing without renewing a license, even for 1 day, is unethical, unlawful, and may result in disciplinary actions, such as a civil penalty, probation, or fees. Furthermore, any treatment performed by a practitioner who is not currently licensed cannot be billed for reimbursement. Each practitioner has the professional duty to renew his or her license on time and provide proof of current licensure to his or her employer. Failure to fulfill or submit proper evidence of fulfillment of continuing education requirements may also result in disciplinary actions.

Engaging Colleagues in Learning

Sharing information learned from a conference, article, or seminar is a good way to promote continued competence in the profession. Not everyone can attend the same continuing education courses, earn a certificate in a specialized field, or obtain their specialty or board certification. Nor should they. One cannot possibly afford to attend all the available conferences or continuing education events. However, when one learns information that can benefit colleagues, especially in one's practice setting, consider sharing.

When one teaches information there is a natural need to know the material well, thus sharing the information learned from a continuing education course, either formally or informally, will help to solidify one's own learning. This can be done through a "lunch and learn" in-service or just a casual conversation with colleagues. Consider preparing a simple handout with references for colleagues so they can do further reading or research on their own. When taking the time to share, colleagues can benefit from your learning, and vice versa. Employers may even be more willing to fund attendance for continuing education courses that benefit multiple employees through this type of sharing.

JOURNAL CLUBS

"The process of engaging in inquiry is as important as the result of the inquiry,"[37] and doing so with one's colleagues is even more powerful. One method to keep current with EBP is to join or even start a journal club. The club members select a peer-reviewed journal article (usually one that pertains to their practice setting), read it before the meeting, and then come together to discuss what was learned and how to incorporate the information into their practice setting. The club members can determine how frequently they meet, perhaps monthly or quarterly. A formal journal club is a powerful way to maintain dedicated time to review recent journal articles that may not otherwise be a priority amid packed work schedules and busy home lives. Some state licensing boards offer continuing competence credits toward licensure for journal clubs and require accurate documentation of the meeting and articles. OT practitioners should check with their licensing board for specific requirements. The AOTA offers journal club toolkits to assist in forming and documenting the group's activities.

PRESENTING AT LOCAL, STATE, AND NATIONAL CONFERENCES

Opportunities abound to present posters or sessions at local, state, and national conferences. A "call for proposals" is issued from the organizers of the event, which includes the types of presentation opportunities and the criteria for which the submission will be evaluated. Consider the idea of using some of the work being done in courses as a springboard for a presentation. Presenting at a local or state conference is an excellent opportunity to develop and refine important skills, including public speaking, organization, writing, and research. Consider partnering with a professor, OT practitioner, or other student(s) for the first submission. Presenting at a state conference also helps one to meet other OT practitioners in the state or region, and affords the chance to network with potential employers and future colleagues. And when working as an OTA, there may be multiple opportunities to submit a proposal to present the ways one is using evidence-based interventions, addressing ethics in a specific practice setting, interprofessional teamwork, or any other timely and important topic. Experience presenting at a professional conference looks great on a resume and will set the candidate apart from others. This can be especially helpful for new graduates or minimally experienced OTAs.

Mentorship

An excellent method of lifelong learning is to find a mentor in the profession. The mentor may or may not work in the same physical location as an OTA, but ideally the mentor should have some experience in the setting in which the OTA works. A mentor may be a supervisor, a coworker, or a more experienced OT practitioner from another area. Active involvement in the state and national association and attending local, state, or national meetings or conferences can assist in meeting a variety of individuals who may be excellent mentors. A formal mentor/mentee agreement should be established for both parties to gain maximum benefit.

At different times in the course of a lifelong career an OTA may seek a mentor. As a new graduate, a mentor can provide a good sounding board for intervention planning, finding evidence-based literature, or helping the OTA achieve balance. A seasoned mentor will have wisdom gained from experience and can offer objective advice or assist the OTA in self-reflection. A good mentor does not provide all the answers, but rather empowers the mentee and guides toward truth. An OTA who has been working for several years may find a mentor relationship helpful again when making the transition to a new place of employment, or especially when working in a different treatment setting.

In addition to the expertise and guidance a mentor may provide, activities that are well documented can be counted toward PDUs for NBCOT renewal and by some states as continuing competency activities for both the mentor and the mentee. Typically, a formal mentor/mentee relationship is well documented and should include agreed on objectives and a collaborative plan to meet the objectives, a method to log the meetings (which may be face-to-face or virtual), and then a written evaluation of the overall experience. Check the national and state boards for resources and information on documentation requirements if using toward continuing education requirements.

Other Involvement at the Local, State, National, and International Levels

Opportunities abound to become involved in OT organizations at the local, state, and national levels, beyond presenting. Organizations are dependent on volunteers. An OTA may volunteer to assist with events, host a district meeting, attend a state advocacy day or national Hill Day, serve on committees or boards, sit on a discussion panel at a college or university, or be appointed or elected to positions for the state association or the state licensing board. AOTA has a database, Coordinated Online Opportunities for Leadership (COOL), which any AOTA member may join. The database provides a pool of interested persons with various types of experience, which AOTA then uses to identify volunteers and also individuals who may be appointed to positions. For more information, visit the AOTA website and search for COOL. Entering information into COOL is an excellent way to become more involved at a national level.

For involvement internationally, consider presenting or co-presenting at a conference in another country. Also, some developing countries are good locations to volunteer time and skills on a medical mission trip and, while there, learn about another culture. Or consider volunteering with WFOT.

SUMMARY

Becoming an OT practitioner will involve a process of honest and timely feedback/debriefing and self-evaluation to obtain and demonstrate key expected professional behaviors. Students and practitioners will face ethical situations, but can be assured they have guidance from AOTA resources and should seek advice from supervisors and trusted mentors to appropriately manage the situations and maintain their own ethical behaviors. Keeping current in best practice entails locating and using evidence-based resources, maintaining licensure and certification, advocating for the profession, and pursuing desired learning rather than compensatory learning throughout one's lifetime.

REVIEW QUESTIONS

1. Juan, an OTA working in a long-term care facility, is also a fieldwork educator to Lola, an OTA/S during her Level II FW. He consistently stresses the importance to Lola of learning and growing from each interaction through self-reflection and advice he gives her. Which of the following is the professional trait to which Juan is referring?
   a. Self-responsibility
   b. Responds to feedback
   c. Work behaviors
   d. Time management
2. Taking initiative is one of the professional work behaviors valued in OT. Which of the following is the *most appropriate* way for an OTA to take initiative in her job?
   a. Sign up her supervising occupational therapist for a continuing education course.
   b. Volunteer to assist with the state association's local conference committee.
   c. Volunteer to take on extra shifts.
   d. Identify a task or process that needs to be improved, approach the occupational therapist with an idea, and gain input and permission before proceeding.
3. Jamie overheard a conversation at the nurses' station that made her think the nurses were not taking proper care of Ms. R, a client on her caseload. She knew that Ms. R. had no family or friends who ever visited and also could be very challenging to work with due to an unpleasant demeanor. Which three of the following are strategies or steps to help Jamie analyze the issues and resolve personal and organizational ethical considerations in this case?
   a. Talk to the head nurse about what she overheard.
   b. Gather all the information, describe the situation, and determine who is involved.
   c. Discuss the situation with coworkers to gain their opinions.
   d. Identify the ethical principles that apply to the situation.
   e. Determine all possible options for action.
   f. Select the option that is the easiest.
4. Seth is an OTA who works in home health with adults. He encountered a client who was in need of changes to the home environment that should have been made by the landlord. He discusses what he found with the occupational therapist, and together they decide they should:
   a. Advocate for the client by calling the landlord to discuss needed changes and the legal requirements of the Americans with Disabilities Act (ADA).
   b. Combine their resources and hire a contractor to perform the needed renovations.
   c. Notify the local county government of ADA violations.
   d. Help the client move to another house.
5. Which three of the following are the *best* examples of advocacy for the profession of occupational therapy?
   a. Write a letter of medical necessity for a client.
   b. Attend Hill Day in Washington, DC.
   c. Explain the role of OT to physicians, nurses, and other healthcare providers.
   d. Identify personal learning needs and obtain continuing education in those areas.
   e. Participate in a medical missions trip and provide OT services to underserved populations.
   f. Communicate with a state legislature about the value of OT.
6. Joanne is a COTA/L who works at an outpatient therapy clinic and is in her first year of practice. The supervising occupational therapist, Brandon, collaborates with Joanne to discuss a mutual client he just evaluated and who Joanne will treat the next day, informing her that he has not treated a client with this condition before either. What is the *best* approach for them to take?
   a. Search for peer-reviewed journal articles that are relevant to the condition.
   b. Talk to other OT practitioners in the clinic to ask for treatment ideas.
   c. Search the internet for general articles regarding the condition.
   d. Contact the referring physician for more information.
7. Blair, a COTA/L, is working at a long-term care facility. Her supervising occupational therapist has been out of school for 28 years, and admits she is "a little rusty" on finding new research. The occupational therapist asks Blair how to find evidence-based practice information. Which of the following is the *best* response to her OT supervisor?
   a. "Let's formulate a question together and search for peer-reviewed literature in a variety of scholarly databases."
   b. "Google Scholar is a good and easy source to use."
   c. "PubMed has a lot of useful information."
   d. "Summaries that can be found online contain sufficient information for practice."
8. A COTA/L wants to describe lifelong learning to his friends who are not healthcare professionals. What is the *best* description to use?
   a. Attending continuing education courses face-to-face or online to meet
   b. Attaining minimum standards of education for my license renewal
   c. Earning enough professional development units (PDUs) to renew my certification through the NBCOT every 3 years

d. Identifying my learning needs for my job and to continue to grow and develop as a COTA/L through formal and informal learning opportunities
e. Going back to school to get my master's degree in OT

9. Karina recently attended a 1-day continuing education course, and after she returned to the clinic a few coworkers were disappointed that she went and that they could not attend. What is the *best* way for Karina to respond to her coworkers?
a. Provide her coworkers with handouts from the course.
b. Share contact information for future courses on the topic.
c. Suggest her coworkers start a journal club at her facility.
d. Coordinate with the coworkers to have a "lunch and learn" session, in which she will review the key points of the course and provide handouts.

10. Jennifer, a COTA/L, has a female adult client on her caseload from a different cultural background whose husband typically also attends therapy sessions. The client seems hesitant to answer questions and waits for her husband to answer for her. Which of the following is the *best* way for Jennifer to provide culturally competent care in this situation?
a. Consider that the wife may be a victim of abuse because the husband is dominant.
b. Research the culture to learn more about communication preferences and norms.
c. Ask the husband why he will not allow his wife to answer.
d. Consult with a coworker about the client.

CASE STUDY

Jan, an OTA in a busy adult outpatient clinic situated in a large city, has worked with a variety of clients of different socioeconomic, sociocultural, spiritual, and lifestyle choice backgrounds. Lucas, a middle-aged man, came to outpatient OT after right upper extremity and left lower extremity amputations. He was unkempt with dirty, wrinkled clothing, unshaven face, unclean body, and disheveled hair. His occupational profile revealed that his living situation was uncertain. During the first treatment session Lucas shared his story. He had struggled with drug addiction most of his life, and, in fact, suffered his current injuries due to a 3-day-long drug binge that left him asleep on the train tracks. He somehow survived the accident, but had no recollection of the accident or the events preceding it due to the effects of the drugs. Eyewitnesses had related the story to him. Jan had different personal cultural experiences, but also had a relative who struggled with drug abuse, which was quite difficult for her emotionally.

1. What cultural differences might exist between Jan and Lucas?
2. Do you think Jan has any biases against Lucas? If so, what steps should she take to show impartiality toward Lucas?
3. How might Jan's personal experience of a family member with drug abuse affect her opinions of Lucas?

REFERENCES

1. Campbell, S. L., & Taylor, D. D. (n.d.). Professionalism in the workplace [PowerPoint slides]. Retrieved from http://www.umkc.edu/starr/Workplace_Professionalism.pdf
2. American Occupational Therapy Association. (2014). Occupational therapy practice framework: Domain and process (3rd ed.). *American Journal of Occupational Therapy, 68*(Suppl. 1), S1–S48. http://dx.doi.org/10.5014/ajot.2014.682006
3. American Occupational Therapy Association. (2002). *AOTA fieldwork performance evaluation for the occupational therapy assistant student.* Bethesda, MD: AOTA.
4. Thimm, R. (2010). Ten steps to better time management. *Advanced Healthcare Network for Health Information Professionals.* Retrieved from http://health-information.advanceweb.com/Student-and-New-Grad-Center/Student-Top-Story/Ten-Steps-to-Better-Time-Management.aspx
5. Luken, M., & Sammons, A. (2016). Systematic review of mindfulness practice for reducing job burnout. *American Journal of Occupational Therapy, 70,* 7002250020p1-7002250020p10. doi:10.5014/ajot.2016.016956
6. College of Occupational Therapists of Ontario. (2016). Conscious decision-making in occupational therapy practice. Retrieved from https://www.coto.org/docs/default-source/default-document-library/conscious decision making.pdf?sfvrsn=4
7. Health Information Technology. (2016). Learn EHR basics. Retrieved from https://www.healthit.gov/providers-professionals/learn-ehr-basics
8. Canadian Association of Occupational Therapists. (n.d.). Occupational therapy assistant. Retrieved from http://www.caot.ca http://www.caot.ca/default.asp?ChangeID=286&pageID=293
9. American Occupational Therapy Association. (2014). Scope of practice. *American Journal of Occupational Therapy, 68,* S34–S40. doi:10.5014/ajot.2014.686S04
10. American Occupational Therapy Association. (2014). Guidelines for supervision, roles, and responsibilities during the delivery of occupational therapy services. *American Journal of Occupational Therapy, 68,* S16–S22. doi:10.5014/ajot.2014.686S03
11. American Occupational Therapy Association. (2015). Code of ethics. Retrieved from http://www.aota.org/-/media/Corporate/Files/Practice/Ethics/Code-of-Ethics.pdf
12. Estes, J., & Brandt, L. C. (2011). Navigating fieldwork's ethical challenges: Relevant issues and appropriate resolution techniques. *OT Practice 16(7),* 7–10.
13. American Occupational Therapy Association. (2016, April 5). Academic Leadership Council meeting [PowerPoint slides].
14. Arthanat, S., & Vroman, K. (2016). A home-based information communication technology training for older adults: Effectiveness, value, and perspectives. *American Journal of Occupational Therapy, 70,* 7011520291p1. Retrieved from http://www.nbcot.org/assets/candidate-pdfs/practitioner-pdfs/renewal-handbook
15. North Carolina Legislature. (n.d.). Retrieved from http://www.ncga.state.nc.us/enactedlegislation/statutes/html/bysection/chapter58/gs_58-50-30.html
16. World Federation of Occupational Therapists. (n.d.). Fundamental beliefs, WFOT mission. Retrieved from http://www.wfot.org/AboutUs/FundamentalBeliefs.aspx
17. American Occupational Therapy Association, Inc. (n.d.). Evidence-based practice and research. Retrieved from http://www.aota.org/Practice/Researchers.aspx#sthash.ndfiOjzh.dpuf
18. OT Seeker. (n.d.). The process of implementing evidence in practice. Retrieved from http://www.otseeker.com/Resources/Implementing Evidence/TheProcess.aspx
19. Arbesman, M., Metzger, L., & Lieberman, D. (2011). Using evidence in practice: Experience from the trenches. *OT Practice* 16(7), 6–15.
20. OT Seeker. (n.d.). What is evidence-based practice? Retrieved from http://www.otseeker.com/Resources/WhatIsEvidenceBased Practice.aspx
21. University of Illinois. (n.d.). Evidence-based medicine glossary. Retrieved from http://researchguides.uic.edu/c.php?g=252338&p=1683354
22. Accreditation Council for Occupational Therapy Education. (2011). Accreditation Council for Occupational Therapy Education (ACOTE) standards and interpretive guide. Retrieved from http://www.aota.org/-/media/Corporate/Files/EducationCareers/Accredit/Standards/2011-Standards-and-Interpretive-Guide.pdf
23. National Board for the Certification of Occupational Therapy. (2016). *Certification renewal handbook.* Retrieved from http://www.nbcot.org/assets/candidate-pdfs/practitioner-pdfs/renewal-handbook

Chapter 3

The Continuum of Care and the Changing Healthcare Environment

LaToya Nicole Stafford, OT/L, MBA/MHA, CAPS

LEARNING OUTCOMES

After studying this chapter, the student or practitioner will be able to:

3.1 Describe the continuum of care
3.2 Name the various settings of the continuum of care
3.3 Develop treatment intervention plans for clients within each setting
3.4 Explain the impact the changing healthcare environment has on each setting
3.5 Explain the regulations and documentation needed to support services in each setting

KEY TERMS

Acute settings
Continuum of care
Documentation
Length of stay (LOS)
Post-acute settings
Readmissions
Reimbursement

The **continuum of care** is a concept involving a system that guides and tracks clients over time through a comprehensive array of health services spanning all levels and intensity of care.[1] As a client moves throughout the continuum of care, his or her needs may change. The occupational therapy (OT) practitioner is responsible for understanding those needs, adapting treatment strategies accordingly, and serving as a resource for discharge planning. Possessing an in-depth knowledge of what each setting offers provides a practitioner the ability to make knowledgeable discharge recommendations confidently. This chapter is particularly challenging to write, however, as health care is constantly changing as elections bring new officials into office, technology evolves, and the needs of the populace change.

As a client becomes more medically stable and functionally independent he or she moves throughout the continuum of health services. Typically, the more medically complex and fragile a client is, the more OT is needed to help identify those performance skills and client factors that may be limiting performance in his or her occupations. Figure 3-1 visually represents how the acuity level changes throughout the continuum.

In general, most settings can be grouped into one of two categories: **acute settings** and **post-acute settings.** Generally speaking, a client in an acute care setting requires daily monitoring from a physician, whereas a client receiving OT in a post-acute setting has more intermittent monitoring by a physician. Table 3-1 shows examples of both acute and post-acute settings.

Variations in research exist regarding which setting is considered acute versus post-acute.[2] Most literature categorizes inpatient rehabilitation facilities (IRFs) and long-term acute care (LTAC) facilities as post-acute settings.[2] This chapter considers these settings based on the characteristics described in Table 3-1. The description of each setting in this chapter includes details related to its client

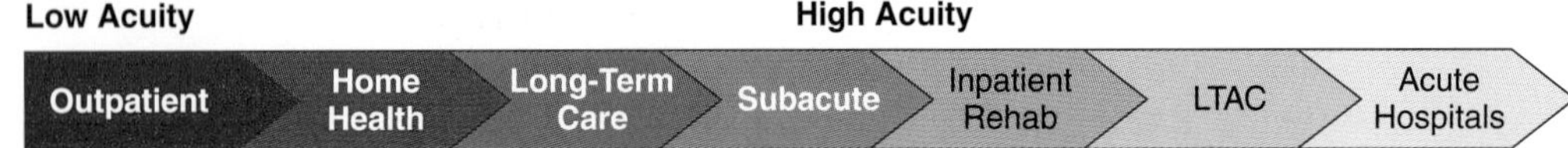

FIGURE 3-1. The level of care correlates with the setting that the client is in.

TABLE 3-1 Acute and Post-Acute Settings

ACUTE SETTINGS	POST-ACUTE SETTINGS
Acute hospital	Subacute rehabilitation Long-term care (LTC)/skilled nursing facility (SNF) Home health Outpatient services Acute rehabilitation facility/inpatient rehabilitation facility (IRF) Long-term acute care (LTAC) facility

population, the goal of OT services, treatment strategies, documentation, and reimbursement.

REIMBURSEMENT AND ITS EFFECT ON THE CONTINUUM

Before considering the unique features of each healthcare setting, it is first necessary to understand the different payers of health care. One unique connection to all of the settings is **reimbursement.** Reimbursement refers to the payment of a healthcare provider for a service. Although each setting is reimbursed for OT services in different capacities and amounts, most have the same payer sources for reimbursement. Knowing and understanding the different payer sources is beneficial for OT practitioners because it helps bridge the gap between clinical and operational expectations in each setting. The different payer sources include, but are not limited to, the Centers for Medicare and Medicaid Services (CMS), managed care, the Veterans Health Administration, workers' compensation, and private pay. Figure 3-2 gives a visual breakdown of typical healthcare expenditures of these payers. At any time in the United States, state and federal legislation can mandate changes affecting all of the reimbursement methods listed here. This is why it is very important to be a vocal advocate for the OT profession and be aware of impending legislation. The American Occupational Therapy Association (AOTA) state affairs staff monitor all bills that could potentially affect OT and provide weekly updates to state OT association presidents. There are numerous ways to get involved that will promote advocacy within each region, state, and country. One of the best ways is to join the state or national OT association to assist with time, talent, finances, and other resources.

Centers for Medicare and Medicaid Services

CMS provides several federal and state healthcare programs. Medicare is the federal health insurance program for individuals who are 65 or older, those who are younger than 65 with disabilities, and persons with end-stage renal disease (ESRD; permanent kidney failure requiring dialysis or a transplant).[3] Individuals who qualify for Medicare also have the ability to have Medicare coverage provided through a private insurance company versus the federal government. This coverage is known as Medicare Advantage or Medicare Part C. Medicare part C sometimes has drug coverage, hearing, dental, or vision services included. The only persons not allowed to transfer original Medicare to a Medicare Advantage are those with ESRD. Currently, Medicare part A covers hospital care, skilled nursing facilities, hospice, and home health services. Medicare part B covers medical costs such as ambulance services, durable medical equipment, preventive services, mental health, and limited prescription drugs. Part D is for coverage of prescription drugs. Medicare currently has dollar limits on the amount of OT services a client can receive per year.

Medicaid is a joint federal and state program that aids individuals with limited income and resources with medical expenses. Medicaid may also cover services that are not normally covered by Medicare, such as long-term supports and services and personal care services. Each state has different rules regarding Medicaid eligibility and the application process.[3] Federal and state healthcare plans are monitored and regulated very closely due to changes in federal and state spending. Many states have limits on the number of evaluations and visits Medicaid recipients may get per year, and also may have limits on durable medical equipment, which can affect clients. Medicare and Medicaid are ever-evolving as they relate to requirements for services being provided by OT practitioners.

Managed Care

Managed care insurance plans are usually offered by employers; however, individuals can purchase them independently through the healthcare marketplace. Managed care insurance plans have established agreements with select doctors, hospitals, and healthcare providers to provide care to plan members at the lowest possible cost. Many different types of managed care insurance plans are available. Among the most popular are health maintenance organizations (HMOs), preferred provider organizations (PPOs), point-of-service (POS) plans, and high deductible plans (HDPs)/consumer direct health plans (CDHPs). Managed care insurance plans usually require more frequent documentation by OT practitioners to justify services and may limit the number of visits. In many settings, managed care insurance plans usually require prior authorization before services can begin.

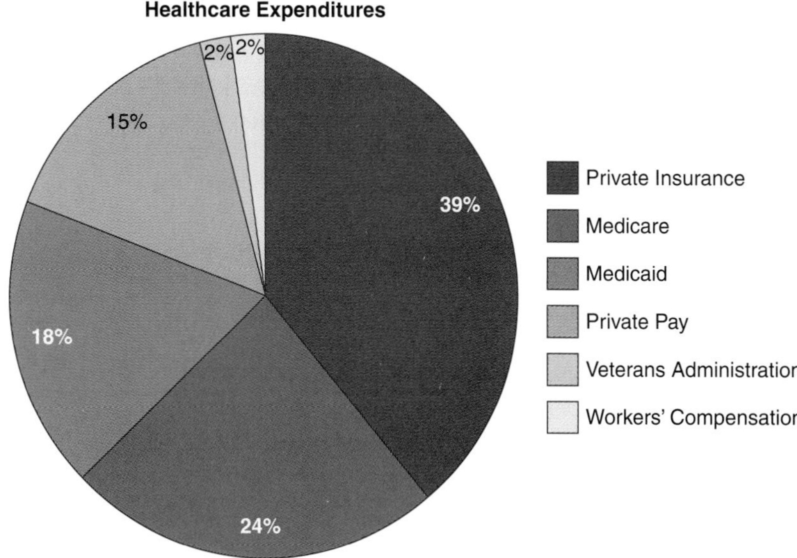

FIGURE 3-2. A breakdown of how healthcare is paid for in the United States.

Veterans Health Administration

The Veterans Health Administration (VA) provides health care for those who served in active military service and were discharged under any condition other than dishonorable. Anyone who enlisted after September 7, 1980, or entered active duty after October 16, 1981, must serve 24 continuous months or the full period for which they were called to active duty to be eligible.[4] However, there are also presumptive disability benefits, where the VA presumes that specific disabilities diagnosed in certain veterans were caused by their military service.[5] In these cases an exception is made and one does not have to serve 24 continuous months to be eligible. If a veteran served in the Vietnam War, Gulf War, or World War II, or was a former prisoner of war, and has experienced a diagnosis related to exposure of a particular element during that war, the presumptive disability benefit applies to that veteran. The presumptive disability benefit also applies to all veterans with a diagnosis of amyotrophic lateral sclerosis (ALS) who served a minimum of 90 days, or if they are diagnosed with a chronic condition such as diabetes or hypertension within 1 year of release from active duty.[5] This requirement is not true for those who enlisted before September 7, 1980. VA health care differs from Tricare, which is health insurance for all active duty service members, their families, and their survivors. OT services can occur at a VA clinic or be home based, and the services and resources available may be allotted by percentage of disability or service connectedness.

Workers' Compensation

Workers' compensation provides wage replacement and medical benefits for those individuals involved in a work-related injury. Employers in each state pay workers' compensation insurance premiums, and the employers who have jobs with a higher risk of injury pay higher premiums. The laws governing workers' compensation vary by state. Services provided by OT practitioners paid by workers' compensation are usually dictated by the workers' compensation case manager and may include individual and/or group therapy. The case manager typically dictates the frequency and duration of the OT treatment services. Authorization is usually needed after the occupational therapist completes the evaluation to continue with the recommended treatment plan.

Private Pay

Private pay refers to paying for healthcare services privately, or "out of pocket." Some settings may provide discounts to clients who pay privately, but the client typically has to ask for the discount. An additional benefit of private pay is that when clients themselves pay, they tend to have more choice in the services that they receive.

ACUTE CARE

In acute care settings, a client has more than likely experienced an acute medical episode that requires daily physician monitoring. Examples of an acute episode include an 18-year-old woman who was in a motor vehicle accident with a new diagnosis of a spinal cord injury and an 80-year-old man with a recent diagnosis of pneumonia. Each example is unique to the client; however, these clients usually present with a sudden medical change or exacerbation affecting their performance skills and likely affecting their occupations.

A client's stay in acute care tends to be short term; however, an OT practitioner can treat a client in acute care for as little as 1 day or weeks to months. The purpose of all acute care settings is to medically stabilize the client and ultimately discharge the client to the setting that will allow safe functioning with as little assistance as possible from a caregiver.

Acute Care Hospital

OT practitioners, along with physical therapy (PT) practitioners and speech-language pathologists (SLPs) in the acute care hospital, are sometimes called the "first responders" of the rehabilitation process. In this setting, OT practitioners play an important role in facilitating early mobilization, restoring function, preventing further decline, and coordinating care, including transition and discharge planning.[6] Other members within this multidisciplinary team may be a physician, nurse, dietitian, or social worker, to name a few.

When a client arrives at an acute care hospital it is often due to a sudden change in the client's medical status or an exacerbation of a chronic condition. The severity of that change varies. Five different hospital levels help delineate to which hospital a client may be taken after an event, based on the acuity or illness severity level. Table 3-2 gives a snapshot of the different levels.

CLIENT POPULATION

In an acute care hospital, one can expect to see a wide variety of client diagnoses, age groups, and acuity levels (Fig. 3-3). Table 3-2 gives an example of expected client populations and diagnoses based on the different hospital levels. The client is usually admitted to a specific specialty unit that correlates with their medical diagnosis. Examples of these specialty units include, but are not limited to, medical/surgical, neurological, orthopedic, critical care, oncology, obstetrics/gynecology, and cardiac.

GOAL OF OCCUPATIONAL THERAPY

In the acute hospital setting the occupational therapist is the first OT practitioner to have interaction with the client. The ultimate goal is preparation for the next level of care. In collaboration with the other members of the multidisciplinary team, the occupational therapist and occupational therapy assistant (OTA) are responsible for OT treatment, deciding the client's next level of care based on the current functional level, family/caregiver education and support, and insurance reimbursement issues.

OT holds a valuable and crucial role in acute care due to OT practitioners having keen activity analysis skills that enable a more accurate assessment of a client's performance skills and how the results equate to the client's discharge to the most appropriate next level of care. The evaluating occupational therapist must compare prior level of function (PLOF) to current level of function to assist with deciding the safest discharge for the client. In the event a client is not progressing as expected and the recommended discharge location is not attainable, the OTA must collaborate with the occupational therapist and case manager/discharge planner to decide what discharge location is feasible based on insurance and caregiver support. In this situation it becomes very important to use problem-solving and clinical reasoning skills to ensure that the client is discharged to a safe environment. This may mean thinking outside the box and working on tasks that would normally not be addressed in acute care such as instrumental activities of daily living (IADLs).

Another very important goal of OT in the acute care setting is to help decrease **length of stay (LOS)** by providing skilled intervention to get the client ready for the next level of care based on discharge location as quickly as possible. The LOS is the number of days a client will receive care in that setting. At admission, insurance determines an expected LOS based on a client's diagnosis and the acuity of that diagnosis. All members of the multidisciplinary team then work to get the client to the next level of care within that recommended LOS. The expected LOS is usually managed by case managers at the hospital and not by OT practitioners. Therefore open communication is expected and necessary among everyone working toward the same discharge goal.

TREATMENT STRATEGIES

Treatment strategies in this setting can vary depending on client factors, performance skills, and discharge location. A typical LOS within an acute care hospital is 3 to 5 days. Therefore purposeful and goal-directed treatment strategies in this setting become very important as clients have a shorter period of time to reach their goals. Treatment strategies in this setting can also be very challenging as one may have to manage intravenous lines (IVs), catheters, monitors, ventilators, and so on, along with working toward goals. Utilization of a rehabilitation (rehab) technician to help manage some of the external factors then becomes important. The rehab technicians in the acute care setting are trained to help manage the lines, tubes, and monitors and will work closely with OT practitioners to make sure the client is safe in all treatment sessions. Note that not all acute care hospitals have rehabilitation technicians. Also at this stage in the continuum, the client has potentially just realized that his or her functional level has changed, whether temporarily or permanently. Treatment strategies may also need to be tailored to address contextual impairments (a flight of stairs in the home of someone in a wheelchair) and performance pattern changes (such as a carpenter after the loss of an arm).

The basis of the treatment strategy should always be a direct reflection of the client's discharge location. Therefore one must always take into consideration if the client needs to be independent in a particular activity of daily living (ADL) or functional task at discharge from the hospital, or if the goal is to transfer to another setting before the client is independent in that same ADL or functional task. For example, if a client with a traumatic brain injury (TBI) is going home after discharge from the acute care hospital and the client has a tub at home for all bathing, a treatment strategy would be to focus on safety with the tub transfer. However, if another client with a TBI is going to an IRF at discharge from the hospital, treatment strategies may be related to performance skills such as balance, strength, and cognition, which may affect the client's overall occupations.

Early mobilization has also become a key initiative within this setting and thus a very important treatment strategy. Numerous studies have shown the direct correlation of early mobility and its positive impact on client outcomes. Early

TABLE 3-2 Hospital Levels

LEVEL	CHARACTERISTICS	CLIENT DIAGNOSIS EXAMPLES
I	• Comprehensive • Tertiary care • Provides prevention through rehabilitation • Specialized equipment and procedures • 24-hour in-house coverage by general surgeons and prompt availability of care in specialties • Referral resource for communities in nearby regions • Leader in prevention, public education to surrounding communities • Teaching and research to help direct new innovations in trauma care	• Spinal cord injury (SCI) • Traumatic brain injury (TBI) • Cerebrovascular accident (CVA) • Neurological-related diagnosis, e.g., multiple sclerosis (MS), amyotrophic lateral sclerosis (ALS), Guillain-Barré syndrome • Polytrauma • Severe burns • Cardiac surgeries, e.g., coronary artery bypass graft (CABG) and valve replacements • Respiratory failure • Orthopedic surgeries • Oncology • Transplant surgeries • Amputations • Myocardial infarction (MI) • General medical-surgical • Obstetrics and gynecology (OB/GYN)
II	• Able to initiate care for all injured clients • Works in collaboration with a Level I Trauma Center • Provides 24-hour accessibility to essential specialties	• CVA • TBI • Orthopedic surgeries • Oncology • Amputations • Respiratory failure • Burns • General medical-surgical • MI • OB/GYN
III	• Assessment and stabilization and emergency operations • Prompt availability of general surgeons and anesthesiologists • Transfer agreements for clients to a Level I or Level II Trauma Center	• CVA • Orthopedic surgeries • Oncology • Amputations • Respiratory failure • General medical • OB/GYN
IV	• Advanced trauma life support (ATLS) before transfer of clients to a higher-level trauma center requiring comprehensive care • Evaluation, stabilization, and diagnostic capabilities for injured clients	• Mild CVA • Pneumonia • Urinary tract infection (UTI) • Fall without injury • General medical • Chronic condition management • OB/GYN
V	• Initial evaluation and stabilization of clients for transfer to higher levels of care • Basic emergency department facilities to implement ATLS protocols	• UTI • Fall without injury • General medical clients • Chronic condition management • OB/GYN

mobilization of intensive care unit clients has been noted as one intervention to decrease the weakness and reconditioning associated with critical illness.[7] Along with PT practitioners, OT practitioners play an intricate role in helping develop early mobility protocols for the critically ill client in the hospital setting. An OT practitioner involved in an early mobility protocol would work on getting the client to sit on the edge of the bed to complete basic ADLs such as grooming and self-feeding while monitoring the client's fragile medical status. This would happen as soon as the physician feels the client is medically stable enough to get out of bed. The OT practitioner must look for many things in the client's medical chart to ensure that he or she can be mobilized, such as an order to be out of bed (OOB) by the physician, weight-bearing

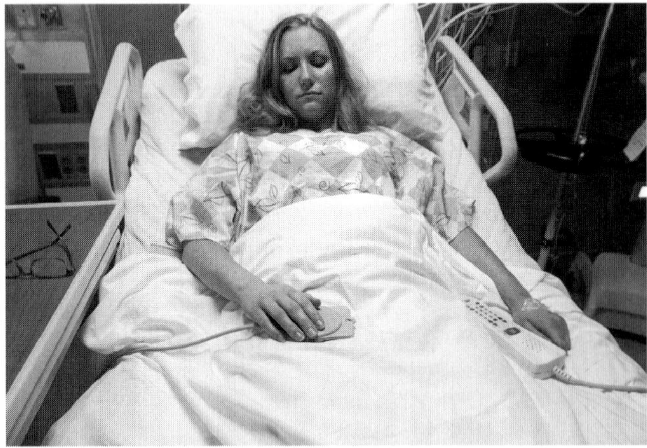

FIGURE 3-3. This is an example of what an OT practitioner might see when approaching a client in an acute care setting.

status, or even parameters for blood pressure. The OT practitioner may also work on energy conservation and activity tolerance. The one key component to consider when working with clients under an early mobility protocol is to monitor vital signs with all activity.

REIMBURSEMENT AND DOCUMENTATION

Reimbursement in the acute care setting is often determined by diagnosis-related groups (DRGs). A DRG is determined by the client's diagnosis, comorbidities (two or more chronic conditions), and the extent of the current illness (meaning if the client had any complications while hospitalized). Once a DRG is calculated, the insurance company gives the hospital a predetermined amount of money to cover all hospital expenses and any treatment needed, including OT. That DRG also helps to determine the LOS for that client.[8]

Reimbursement in the acute care hospital can get confusing as a client may not be formally admitted to the hospital, but instead placed on observation status. If under observation only, reimbursement is no longer under the DRG category, but instead OT is reimbursed from an outpatient capacity. Outpatient reimbursement is discussed later in this chapter. For clients in observation status, the hospital may incur penalties if the client returns to the hospital within 30 days of discharge.

Documentation in the acute hospital setting is critical to help case managers/discharge planners make the appropriate decision for the client's discharge. The OTA is responsible, along with other members of the multidisciplinary team, to make sure details in the documentation support the discharge location. For example, if a team member thinks a client may be appropriate for IRF, he or she should document the client's ability to tolerate 3 hours of therapy a day. If the documentation is to support discharge home with support from family, it would be important to document need for supervision.

In the acute hospital, the client's acuity level changes daily and sometimes hourly. Therefore, making sure documentation is up to date is very important. For the OT practitioner, completing reassessments is a best practice due to the sudden change in medical acuity. In such cases it becomes important for the occupational therapist and OTA to communicate with one another consistently as the client's level changes. If there is a change in medical status, the OTA is responsible to immediately contact the occupational therapist, as well as the nurse or physician, if the medical change is substantial. For example, if the client's OT evaluation states that the client can follow three-step commands and can sit up on the edge of the bed unaided, and an OTA discovers during a treatment session that the client is not oriented and requires maximal assistance to sit up on the edge of the bed, the OTA should notify the occupational therapist, nurse, and physician. One significant medical change seen is delirium, a change in mental state that can affect up to half of older adults in the hospital, and is often due to stress, pain, unfamiliar environment, lack of sleep, and medication.

POST-ACUTE SETTINGS

After a client has sustained an acute illness or injury, the client may still need further medical services to regain function before returning to the community. Post-acute care offers a range of medical care services that support the client's continued recovery from illness to wellness. Post-acute settings usually have a LOS ranging from weeks to months. The post-acute settings that we will explore directly related to OT in the U.S. are subacute rehab, long-term care, home health, and outpatient. Most clients will progress through post-acute settings back into the community, whereas other clients may remain at a post-acute setting for the remainder of their life span. Take note of the difference between an acute "setting" and "acute rehabilitation" and "long-term acute care" that are both classified as post-acute settings.

Acute Rehabilitation

An acute rehabilitation facility, also called an inpatient rehabilitation facility (IRF), provides intense, multidisciplinary rehabilitation for clients. In rehabilitation, interventions are focused on the client resuming those roles and occupations deemed important to the client's life.[9] Rehabilitation hospitals and units must, under Medicare rules, provide 24-hour, 7-day-a-week availability of physicians and nurses with specialized training or experience in medical rehabilitation. These include physicians with extensive experience in inpatient rehabilitation care and nurses with training and certification in rehabilitation nursing (certified rehabilitation registered nurse [CRRN]). Therapy includes PT, OT, SLP, therapeutic recreation, and respiratory therapy. Psychologists, social workers, vocational counselors, prosthetists and orthotists, equipment vendors, and dietitians or nutritional counselors must also be available.[10] Clients must be able to tolerate a combination of 3 hours of PT, OT, and SLP 5 days a week or 15 hours in 7 days in certain cases; some IRFs offer 4 hours for spinal cord injury, and 4.5 hours for TBI per day.

The days that the client receives therapy may vary depending on the admission day to the IRF. A client admitted on a Tuesday may have therapy services on a Saturday, or a client who misses OT on a Friday due to vomiting may have an OT session on Saturday to make up the time. Some IRFs have also decided to provide an OT or PT session on Saturday or Sunday as best practice, although that is not mandated by insurance companies. Clients admitted to an IRF usually have a definite discharge goal and discharge location.

CLIENT POPULATION

The client population in an IRF can vary. However, Medicare currently mandates a certain percentage of the facility's census to be one of the 13 following categories:

1. Cerebrovascular accident
2. Spinal cord injury
3. Congenital deformity
4. Amputation
5. Major multiple trauma
6. Fracture of femur (hip fracture)
7. Traumatic brain injury
8. Neurological disorders, including multiple sclerosis, motor neuron diseases, polyneuropathy, muscular dystrophy, and Parkinson's disease
9. Burns
10. Active polyarticular rheumatoid arthritis, psoriatic arthritis, and seronegative arthropathies
11. Systemic vasculitides with joint inflammation
12. Severe or advanced osteoarthritis (osteoarthrosis or degenerative joint disease) involving two or more weight-bearing joints (elbow, shoulders, hips, or knees but not counting a joint with a prosthesis)
13. Knee or hip joint replacement, or both with one of the following:
    - The client underwent bilateral knee or bilateral hip joint replacement surgery.
    - The client is extremely obese with a body mass index of at least 50.
    - The client is age 85 or older at the time of admission to the IRF.[10]

This list is extensive and covers many of the client populations that OT practitioners treat, but the remainder of the client populations seen at the IRF can vary. Some examples of other diagnoses might be a 70-year-old with acute respiratory failure from Guillain-Barré syndrome or a 40-year-old with a diagnosis of Hodgkin's lymphoma who is seen after chemotherapy and deconditioning. The similarity among all of the clients listed above in an IRF is that they have the potential to make substantial functional improvement in a reasonable period of time, resulting in the ability to return home or to an equivalent community setting.[11]

GOAL OF OCCUPATIONAL THERAPY

In an IRF, the ultimate goal of OT is for the client to make as much improvement in performance skills as possible in hopes of returning to the client's prior occupations. At this point the discharge location from the IRF has been decided and the OT practitioner must work toward goals associated with the client functioning in that established discharge location. All goals are centered on the client's functional potential, specifications of the discharge location, and caregiver/family support. Goals are individualized and can vary even among similar diagnoses. For example, with a 54-year-old who sustained a stroke who is functioning at a dependent level with toilet transfers and who has 24-hour family support, the goal may be for that client to perform the toilet transfer with minimal assistance from caregivers. The goal for the same client diagnosis who is functioning at moderate assist with intermittent family support may be to perform the toilet transfer with modified independence with use of assistive devices and adaptive equipment.

TREATMENT STRATEGIES

Treatment strategies in this setting can be performance skill or occupation related. Naturally, there is an emphasis on the performance skills of ADLs or IADLs as the client will be transitioning to a less restrictive environment requiring the client to be more independent. However, it is almost impossible to work on those direct occupations such as ADLs and IADLs without addressing the performance skills, such as strength, balance, cognition, and vision. Examples of such treatments could include an ADL session in the morning with a client working on showering and dressing with emphasis on following directions/sequencing, or on item retrieval for those ADL tasks with an emphasis on visual scanning. The OT practitioner may also use equipment initially for transfers while progressing a client to be more independent. Figure 3-4 shows an OTA using a mechanical lift to assist a client who is unable to stand for a transfer.

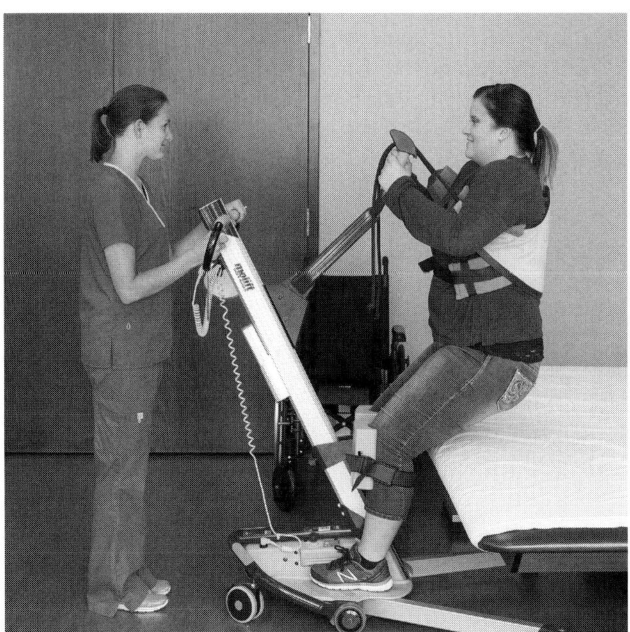

FIGURE 3-4. An example of a mechanical lift that may be used in an IRF setting to help a client transfer when unable to stand without maximal assistance.

With the goal being to discharge to an environment that will allow the client to be more independent, using simulated living environments can also be a large portion of treatment strategies in this setting. Most IRFs have a kitchen, a laundry room, and an overnight suite for family training. Some IRFs have other simulated community environments, such as a grocery store or bank. Clients are also required to bring in their own clothes (instead of wearing pajamas or scrubs) in this setting to promote returning to their routines and using objects similar to those at discharge. This is important to help the client transition back to daily activities typical before hospitalization. This also makes sure that the discharge back into the client's environment is successful.

Caregiver education and training is also a portion of treatment strategy in this setting. One of the main responsibilities in this setting is to ensure that the caregiver who will be caring for the client at discharge is safe, competent, and confident with helping the client at his or her functional level at time of discharge. This can sometimes be challenging, as a caregiver may not realize how much assistance a loved one requires until during the training, which can make the session very emotional. Therefore, the OTA may encounter psychosocial components to caregiver training as well. If this should happen, the one thing to remember is to always be compassionate and imagine how that caregiver may be feeling. It is also important to remember to put the client's needs first while providing psychosocial support to the caregiver. Social work or psychology departments may also be able to assist.

DOCUMENTATION AND REIMBURSEMENT

Reimbursement is determined in the acute rehabilitation on the initial evaluation with an assessment called an Inpatient Rehab Facility–Patient Assessment Instrument (IRF-PAI).[11] The IRF-PAI is a collective assessment of the client's physical, cognitive, functional, and psychosocial status. Once the IRF-PAI assessment has been completed, the client is placed in a Case Mix Group (CMG) that determines payment. The IRF-PAI is an assessment specifically mandated by CMS; however, many other payers also use this assessment to a certain extent for payment reimbursement.[11]

Documentation in the IRF occurs daily and many facilities use the Functional Independence Measure (FIM) assessment. There are numerous other assessments to show client progress, however, the FIM language is shared throughout the healthcare community, and it is very important for the OTA to know and understand the assessment tool to allow consistent and concise communication between the two. FIM scoring has six major categories: self-care, sphincter control, mobility, locomotion, communication, and social cognition. Each major category breaks down further into specific areas. For instance, the self-care section includes eating, grooming, bathing, upper body dressing, lower body dressing, and toileting. Seven scores within those categories correlate with the client's functional level, which is the traditional grading key used for measuring ADL status; they are dependent, maximal assistance, moderate assistance, minimal assistance, supervision, modified independent, and independent.[12] Table 3-3 gives a snapshot of the correlation between the traditional grading key and FIM scores. Some practitioners may use the term "stand-by contact-guard assistance," but to be clear, the term should be either supervision or minimal assistance. FIMs may be formally scored by the occupational therapist, but nearly all practitioners in every setting use the common FIM language of minimal, moderate, and so on to document assistance needed so that everyone is using the same terminology. (There are other formal scoring tools besides FIM that some facilities may use.) For instance, if a client requires a 25% assist by an OT practitioner to complete a transfer, the language from the FIM would dictate the level written in the note regardless of whether the OT practitioner is formally scoring or not.

Long-Term Acute Care

Long-term acute care (LTAC) settings provide post-acute care services for clients who have more medically complex conditions and require longer-term hospitalization.[13] A client who

TABLE 3-3 Functional Independence Measure (FIM) Score Correlation

A correlation between the FIM score formally used and the typical terminology used such as minimal, moderate, and maximal assistance.

GRADING KEY	FIM SCORE	CLIENT:
Dependent	1	Requires 75%–100% assistance
Maximal assistance	2	Requires 50%–74% assistance
Moderate assistance	3	Requires 25%–49% assistance
Minimal assistance	4	Requires less than 25% assistance
Supervision	5	Can physically complete task but requires supervision and/or verbal cues, no physical contact
Modified independent	6	Requires increased time or use of assistive devices or equipment
Independent	7	Can complete task without assistance from a person or from any equipment or devices

is admitted to an LTAC facility usually has an expected LOS of 25 days or longer. Most clients who are admitted to this setting are admitted directly from an acute care hospital. An LTAC setting can be seen as a cross between an acute care hospital and an IRF. LTAC facilities provide a wide variety of interdisciplinary client care services, including daily physician visits, nursing care, respiratory therapy, PT, OT, SLP, nutritional therapy, case management and social services, laboratory, radiology and pharmacy services, telemetry (machines to monitor heart rate, etc.), dialysis, pain management, and end-of-life care. OT practitioners in this setting should possess or be willing to learn a high degree of knowledge about complex medical conditions. LTAC facilities can be freestanding or be a wing or floor within a hospital. Long-term acute care hospitals have emerged as an important component in the continuum of care. Data have shown that care in an LTAC facility can result in lower costs, fewer hospital readmissions, and more successful ventilator weaning.[14]

CLIENT POPULATION

In an LTAC setting the client population and diagnoses can vary. Clients seen within the LTAC facility are similar in that they are all medically fragile, often with a primary diagnosis along with multiple active secondary diagnoses. Examples of diagnoses treated in this setting include pulmonary disease, cardiac disease, respiratory failure, pressure injuries, neuromuscular diseases, postoperative complications, and ESRD requiring dialysis. An example of someone admitted to this setting would include a client with a diagnosis of respiratory failure requiring ventilator weaning or a client with multiple wounds requiring a wound vacuum assisted closure (wound vac). A wound vac is used when a wound with depth requires assistance to heal, and it applies negative pressure to bring the edges of the wound closer to the center.[15]

GOAL OF OCCUPATIONAL THERAPY

The goal of OT in an LTAC setting is for the client to become medically stable enough to advance to the next level of care. The goal for this setting is unique, as most goals for OT in other settings are not related to medical stability because that falls within the scope of the physician. However, all members of the multidisciplinary team contribute to improving the client's medical stability in an LTAC facility.

Along with achieving medical stability, another goal of OT is to maximize the client's functional potential. With the expected LOS being 25 days or longer, the OT practitioner has an extended period of time with the client, which can make a difference in the location of the next level of care. Although there will still be clients who need to be transferred to another setting, such as a skilled nursing facility (SNF), the majority of the clients should be able to transfer to their homes from this setting.

TREATMENT STRATEGIES

Treatment strategies in the LTAC setting are centered on medically stabilizing the client in preparation for discharge to the next setting or to the home. OT practitioners will focus more on performance skills, such as activity tolerance, initially in conjunction with the other members of the multidisciplinary team. Grading activities (altering something about the activity to increase or decrease demands on the client) become very important, as the OT practitioner must change the intensity of the client's treatment session based on the client's response to treatment. To grade the activity up and/or down, the OT practitioner must have an in-depth knowledge of managing vital signs. For example, if a client is admitted with a diagnosis of a stroke and also has respiratory failure requiring intubation, the client's initial goals may be to sit on the edge of the bed unsupported for 5 minutes and comb his or her hair without a change in vital signs. Once the client meets this goal, the OT practitioner would grade up the goals. However, if the client's vitals became unstable during that treatment session, the OT practitioner would grade down the treatment by having the client sit supported for 5 minutes to complete the task. Occupational therapists and OTAs in this setting must have daily, consistent communication with each other as the client's medical status may change suddenly and require reevaluation. The client's goals may also need to be graded up or down constantly; therefore the OTA would need to communicate with the occupational therapist when a goal may need to be changed.

Treatment strategies also vary based on the client's next level of care. With the goal being to transfer to a lower level of care from the LTAC facility, discharge location plays a role in treatment strategies for the client. The majority of clients are discharged from the LTAC facility to the home, an IRF, or a SNF. Unlike some of the other settings, in an LTAC setting the client's discharge location may not be determined on admission to the facility due to the client's medical complexity. As the client progresses and starts to get stronger, it will give the OT practitioner a good idea as to which setting the client will be discharged. Once that discharge location is decided, the OTA can begin to work on specific treatment strategies related to that discharge location, especially if the discharge location is home.

DOCUMENTATION AND REIMBURSEMENT

Reimbursement in an LTAC setting is similar to that of the acute care hospital. Clients are grouped into a long-term care diagnosis-related group (LTC-DRG), which is based on the diagnosis, procedures performed, age, gender, and discharge status.[13] The LTC-DRG then determines the LOS along with the financial resources that will be provided to the hospital for the care of the client. OT treatment sessions are then reimbursed from those financial resources.

Documentation in the LTAC setting is similar to the documentation required in the acute setting in the sense that it is daily and that the client's status can change daily. One difference is that the OT practitioner will likely complete more reassessments at an LTAC facility as the client's LOS is much longer compared with an acute care hospital. If the OTA has been the primary clinician it will be important for the occupational therapist and the OTA to collaborate at least weekly to update goals. However, the collaboration between the two may be more frequent if the client's status has changed. Documentation must also include support services. Although one may not see daily progress toward meeting goals when completing documentation in this setting, the treatment notes should give specific details regarding incremental progress toward goals. For example, documenting vital signs before, during, and after a treatment session is one way to show incremental progress.

Subacute Rehabilitation

Subacute rehabilitation settings provide the tools that a client may need to help regain independence and return to the highest level of function. OT during rehabilitation in a subacute SNF is associated with a shorter LOS, as well as functional improvements for a variety of diagnoses.[16] Subacute settings provide less intense therapy and do not require 3 hours a day of participation in OT, PT, and SLP. This setting is optimal for clients who may have had a sudden debilitating illness without the stamina to tolerate the rigorous rehabilitation plan provided in an IRF. It allows for more flexibility and individuality for developing the plan of care as it relates to the amount of therapy a client receives. Clients are admitted to subacute rehab from the hospital or can be admitted from an IRF or LTAC facility as a step down before returning to the community. A client who is admitted to a subacute setting usually discharges to home or to a setting that is less restrictive. Subacute rehabilitation is often provided in a SNF. Most SNFs have a mixture of long-term care residents and residents who are there for short-term subacute rehabilitation.

CLIENT POPULATION

Clients in the subacute setting tend to be older adults admitted for medical care and rehabilitation to recover from an injury or acute illness. An OTA will likely see a large variety of physical dysfunction diagnoses in this setting, as there are no restrictions on what diagnoses can be admitted. The typical client in this setting is one who has good rehab potential but may require a longer time to reach goals compared with an IRF. On average the LOS in the subacute rehab setting is 3 to 5 weeks; however, the client can receive subacute rehabilitation for up to 30 to 100 days depending on the payer. In a subacute rehab setting there is also a requirement of a 3-night hospital admission before transfer into this setting. Therefore all clients that are seen in this setting have had a recent acute episode that required admission to an acute care hospital.

GOAL OF OCCUPATIONAL THERAPY

The goal of OT in the subacute setting, similar to the other settings, is to restore functional independence, making sure the client is ready for discharge back into the community. Subacute rehabilitation is the last step within the OT continuum that provides rehabilitation to a client in an inpatient setting. Clients are more likely to be admitted to a long-term care facility if they are unable to meet goals to return to the community. Therefore, there is a focus to get clients independent and back into the community in this setting.

TREATMENT STRATEGIES

Treatment strategies in subacute care are very similar to those of the IRF, being both performance skill based and occupation based. Although focusing on ADL tasks will be important, focusing on the performance skills to drive an increase in independence in ADLs such as balance, strength, endurance, cognition, and vision is also important. Whereas PT practitioners may work on some of the same components, OT treatment strategies focus on preparation for ADLs and other functional tasks. Balance may be worked on so that the client can safely pull up pants or endurance so that the client will be able to complete bathing and dressing without getting overly fatigued. The foundation of treatment strategies will be based on discharge location. Getting to know the client and receiving information about his or her home layout and surroundings is very important as well. The shower or tub type, toilet height, and number of levels in the house or apartment will give a good idea of how to center the treatment strategies. Similar to an IRF, the client is encouraged to get into a stable daily routine comparable to the routine at discharge. Therefore a client is encouraged to wear regular clothing within this setting and often there is a focus on IADL tasks, such as cooking and cleaning.

Caregiver training and education is also an important treatment strategy in this setting. Caregivers may have the expectation that the client will be able to function at his or her prior level at discharge, which may or may not be true. As the client transitions back into the community, the caregiver will need to understand the client's current functional level along with the amount of assistance that is needed and provide appropriate supervision and assistance.

DOCUMENTATION AND REIMBURSEMENT

Reimbursement in the subacute setting is driven by an assessment called a minimum data set (MDS). Once the MDS is completed it gives a resource utilization group (RUG), which states the financial reimbursement that the facility will receive for the client, which includes therapy. The unique thing about this setting is that therapy drives revenue. Therefore the more OT, PT, and SLP the client receives, the higher the reimbursement rate.

Because therapy services drive revenue in this setting there is a heightened awareness of documentation. Daily documentation is required in this setting with an emphasis on the treatment provided that day, and goals are updated weekly, with progress measured by the occupational therapist. Using outcome-based tools is more prominent in this setting. Many outcome tools are available for use, depending on the client's primary impairments. For example, some outcome-based tools emphasize ADLs, such as the FIM described previously; other outcome-based tools focus on balance, cognition, or endurance. It is very important for the OTA and occupational therapist to collaborate as to which outcome-based tool is the most appropriate for the client.

Long-Term Care

At times, a client is not able to transition back into the community after subacute rehabilitation due to physical and/or psychosocial factors. At that point these clients become residents of the SNF, which is then known as long-term care (LTC). LTC provides 24-hour assistance with ADLs and functional mobility and is considered the permanent residence of those who live there. The multidisciplinary team consists of but is not limited to the physician, nurse, OT, PT, SLP, dietitian, social worker, and activities coordinator. Each member of the team works to make sure that the client's quality of life remains as engaged as it would have been if living independently in the community.

CLIENT POPULATION

Most residents who live in the LTC section of the SNF are age 65 and older. However, there are also residents who may have sustained a permanent disability requiring ongoing assistance with daily activities. The resident may have been admitted to LTC directly from subacute rehabilitation or the hospital after at least a 3-day stay.

GOAL OF OCCUPATIONAL THERAPY

The goal of OT treatment in this setting is to ensure that the residents sustain their level of independence. Even though the staff at the SNF provide the residents with care needs, such as ADLs, the residents are still encouraged to be as independent as possible. Residents in this setting may have functional changes from an acute event that affects their ability to function as before with their occupations. The OT practitioners would help identify those functional changes and help the residents return to their previous functional level with that occupation.

Because the SNF is home for the residents, it is a goal of all members of the multidisciplinary team to keep the residents feeling at home. Studies have shown that the more mobile and independent the client is at the SNF, the less likely is the occurrence of an acute onset of an illness.[17] At a SNF, mobility may be via a wheelchair or with use of an assistive ambulatory device. The thing to remember is that most residents desire to be as independent as possible. The OT practitioners work to keep the residents in this setting functioning at their maximum potential to avoid acute care hospital admissions.

TREATMENT STRATEGIES

Treatment strategies can vary with the LTC resident depending on the area of functional decline. All treatment strategies will be related to restoring PLOF within the facility. For example, if a resident who normally propels her wheelchair around the facility has a functional decline, the OT practitioner may work on wheelchair propulsion. Another example would be the resident, who usually completes toileting and toilet transfer with supervision, is now functioning at a moderate assistance level due to gradual decline; the OT practitioner would work on restoring and returning the client back to that supervision level. Treatment sessions in this setting are usually 1 to 3 times per week and can vary in time, but usually last 45 to 60 minutes.

DOCUMENTATION AND REIMBURSEMENT

Reimbursement for OT services for LTC residents is through fee-for-service, which means an OT practitioner gets reimbursed for the exact services provided. All charges to the insurance provider are via the Current Procedural Terminology (CPT) codes. Common CPT codes used by OT practitioners are therapeutic activities, self-care activities, development of cognitive skills, therapeutic exercise, and so on. The CMS places a cap on how much will be paid for OT services. This cap is evaluated on a yearly basis.

Documentation for residents seen in this setting is performed at each treatment session. Due to the decreased intensity of OT services and the decrease in treatment frequency, it is imperative that each day of documentation can stand alone to support services. There is also weekly documentation for measuring goals and progress that is supported by outcome measures and tools. Medicare also mandates that an occupational therapist provides an assessment within a certain amount of visits received by an OTA. If an OTA practices in this setting it is important to check state and federal laws to ensure that regulations are met.

Home Health

Home health services are provided in the community in the client's home, which might be an apartment, a trailer, a house, or an independent or assisted living community. Requirements for receiving home health services are that the client must be under the direct care of a physician, as well as be deemed homebound, which means it must take a considerable or taxing effort to leave his or her home. A large influx in home health services provided within the United States has occurred because it has become a trend for persons with disabilities and the elderly to stay safe at home and "age in place" to reduce long-term institutionalization.[18] This is mostly due to the amount of financial resources it takes to age at home versus requiring long-term institutionalization. There has also been an increase in the acuity level of clients seen at home due to earlier discharges for home health OT.[18]

Home healthcare treatment cycles are generally billed in 60-day periods that are each called an episode. Therefore the plan of care and goals are established to be met in that time frame. The number of episodes a client can receive for home health therapy is unlimited as long as the client demonstrates progress or requires skilled treatment to prevent or slow further deterioration; the only criteria are that the client is homebound and is under the direct care of a physician. Home health is a marathon and not a sprint, compared with the other settings. Whereas OT practitioners working in other settings work toward getting the client as independent as quickly as possible, in home health care the client is already "home" so the focus is on assessing the client's need to address the tasks that will keep him or her at home as long as possible. For that reason, it is not

EVIDENCE-BASED PRACTICE

With the increased focus for all involved with health care to move toward quality-based reimbursement with prolonged outcomes, *productive aging* has become a key term. Productive aging is most widely used by OT practitioners practicing in the home health setting.[19] In 2009 close to 30% of Medicare beneficiaries over age 65 living at home reported difficulty in performing one or more ADLs, and an additional 12.7% reported difficulties with IADLs. OT practitioners are at the center of productive aging as goals for productive aging are client centered, and the framework for all OT practitioners (OTPF-3) is client-focused care. OT practitioners working within the productive aging framework focus on promoting health and quality of life, facilitating participation in meaningful daily activities, achieving positive outcomes, focusing on client-centered approaches to care for client and caregiver, and offering services that are cost-effective. The framework for productive aging as it pertains to the OT practitioner is to meet clients where they are to help them age in place, which will decrease the financial burden of the client, as well as the payer of the client's services.

American Occupational Therapy Association. (2016). Productive aging. Retrieved from http://www.aota.org/~/media/Corporate/Files/Practice/Aging/Distinct-Value-Productive-Aging.pdf

uncommon for the client to have more than one home health episode. For example, during one home health episode the focus may be getting out of bed and performing functional mobility to the bathroom safely and independently without increased fatigue. The next home health episode may focus on shower transfers and completing bathing.

CLIENT POPULATION

The clients seen in home health typically are medically stable enough to be out of a hospital but have been deemed homebound by a physician. Their homebound status can be due to their physical or cognitive limitations. If it is a considerable and/or taxing effort for them to leave the home in any capacity, they are considered homebound. Diagnoses seen in home health OT can vary. Clients admitted to home health services were likely discharged from one of the settings listed earlier. However, there is the possibility that a physician may refer a client who is already living at home for home health services without an episode at a facility if the client has sustained a functional decline. For example, a client may have sustained a fall at home without suffering any substantial injuries, but has increased back pain hindering transfers and ADLs. This client would most likely not be admitted to the hospital, but would still require some assistance from OT at home to get back to his or her PLOF.

GOAL OF OCCUPATIONAL THERAPY

The trend in describing OT's role in home health appears to be moving toward compensatory and contextual approaches that include adaptive strategies and home and environmental modifications and away from remediation, which would include strategies such as improving strength or cognition.[18] However, the ultimate goal in the home health setting for OT is safety and independence in the client's home. Some clients seen in this setting will have the capacity to regain function related to their diagnoses, whereas others will need preventive strategies put in place to avert further loss of abilities.[20] It is the responsibility of the OT practitioner and the other members of the multidisciplinary team to work together on strategies to ensure that clients can safely age in place.

TREATMENT STRATEGIES

Treatment strategies should come naturally for OT practitioners in the home health setting. After all, what better place to teach clients to be independent than their actual home? An OTA can work on bathing, dressing, meal preparation, or laundry, to name just a few functional tasks. Medication management is also a key treatment strategy that the OT practitioner can work on in this setting. Although remediation treatment strategies are not as prevalent in the home health setting, performance skills such as strength, endurance, and work simplification are still key factors to helping improve the client's overall ADL and IADL status. An OTA may work on developing a home exercise program for the client's upper extremities, which may improve the client's independence with, for example, reaching into cabinets during light meal preparation.

Getting family and caregivers involved as early as possible with treatment interventions and carryover is very important as well. For example, if a client with dementia needs to follow a home exercise program to increase strength and endurance, family/caregiver training to help carry out the plan of care would also be required. There may also be a need to educate and train family members on specific ways to give assistance with transferring a client to the toilet or how to give verbal cues to a client when performing an ADL task to promote independence.

DOCUMENTATION AND REIMBURSEMENT

Reimbursement in this setting is based on the initial assessment, called the Outcome and Assessment Information Set (OASIS). This is an assessment done by the clinician who makes the initial visit to the client, which could be a nurse, PT, or SLP. As it stands currently, per Medicare, occupational

OT Practitioner's Viewpoint

I have coined *medication management* as the unspoken IADL. As an OT practitioner I do not think we focus on medication management as much as we should, despite its inclusion under health management in the *Occupational Therapy Practice Framework, 3rd edition* (OTPF-3). Many hospitalizations could be prevented if a client managed his or her medication appropriately. Often a client will take the wrong medication, at the wrong time, in the wrong dosage. The client may have visual deficits causing an inability to see the directions correctly or a cognitive impairment that inhibits the client from filling his or her weekly pillbox appropriately. It becomes the OT practitioner's responsibility to work on compensatory techniques to help a client maximize functional independence with managing medication. We have the responsibility to our clients to keep them safe, and medication management plays an important role in that at any place on the continuum of care. ~ LaToya Nicole Stafford, OT/L, MBA/MHA, CAPS

therapists are not allowed to complete the initial assessment. After the OASIS is completed it generates a case mix score called a Home Health Resource Group (HHRG), which then determines what the lump sum financial reimbursement will be for the 60-day period to cover all services needed.

Documentation within the home health setting is completed at the time of the visit. There are also regulations surrounding how often an occupational therapist needs to complete a reassessment on the client. Because this regulation has been known to change often, it is important that all clinicians working in this setting remain current in the regulations regarding documentation. In home health care, outcome measurement tools are also important and numerous ones exist. Occupational therapist and OTA collaboration is important to determine which outcome tools are most important for each client. Due to the decreased intensity of OT treatment sessions, there is an expectation that each treatment session supports progress toward the goals set forth to be attained in the 60-day window. Community physicians have to sign the initial orders for OT and the plan of care after every 10 visits and on discharge.

Outpatient

The outpatient setting is the final step in the continuum of care. Outpatient OT services are provided in hospital-based clinics or freestanding clinics. The frequency of services provided in this setting can vary from once a month to multiple times a week, depending on the client's diagnosis and interventions being provided by the OT practitioner.

CLIENT POPULATION

A client receiving OT services in this setting lives at home or independent/assisted living but is not considered homebound. The diagnosis for which the referral has been made can be acute or chronic. The referral for this setting can come from one of the other settings discussed in this chapter or a physician's office. Diagnoses seen in this setting can vary from a client with a rotator cuff tear who lives alone to a client with multiple sclerosis having an exacerbation that changes his or her functional status.

GOAL OF OCCUPATIONAL THERAPY

The goal of OT in the outpatient setting is usually to restore function or adapt and provide compensatory training for the client. However, the goal can also be to provide services to prevent further complications related to a condition. For example, a client may be referred for pain management from a rotator cuff tear causing functional issues or be referred for strengthening and functional use of an upper extremity after a brachial plexus injury. Although the clients may have different goals, the OT practitioner still focuses on making sure both clients gain independence in their occupations of life.

TREATMENT STRATEGIES

Treatment interventions in this setting are based on the reason for the referral. For example, if a client was admitted with a flexor tendon injury, the treatment strategies would be related to restoring range of motion and strength and preventing contractures. Another example would be if a client was referred due to a visual inattention to the left side, the OTA would work on scanning and compensatory techniques related to finding and identifying objects on the left side. Treating ADL deficits in this setting can be difficult as sometimes these settings have little privacy and limited practice areas with actual tubs/showers, beds, and dressers. However, some larger or hospital-based outpatient facilities may be equipped with functioning aspects of the home, such as a sink, microwave, bed, or closet to work on occupations. If a client requires ADL-related interventions, simulation becomes key, or if available, a private room could be used for dressing skills. It also is important to utilize skills of activity analysis and work on the individual task that is difficult for carryover into ADLs. Adaptive equipment assessment, education, and training, as well as assistive technology needs, are often addressed.

Focused use of modalities and therapeutic and exercise equipment are also seen in this setting. Some examples of these are ultrasound, moist heat, and electrical stimulation. Some outpatient therapy treatment sessions are coupled with a modality to help maximize functional goals. For example, an OT practitioner may use moist heat before a joint mobilization treatment (see Chapter 18 for more details). An example of equipment one may see in this setting would be the Baltimore Therapeutic Equipment (BTE), which helps with meeting goals related to musculoskeletal impairments of the upper extremities (Fig. 3-5). Most seating and mobility and assistive technology evaluations are performed at the outpatient level. In the outpatient setting an OT practitioner may also help to introduce adaptive keyboards to assist with communication or computer access (Fig. 3-6).

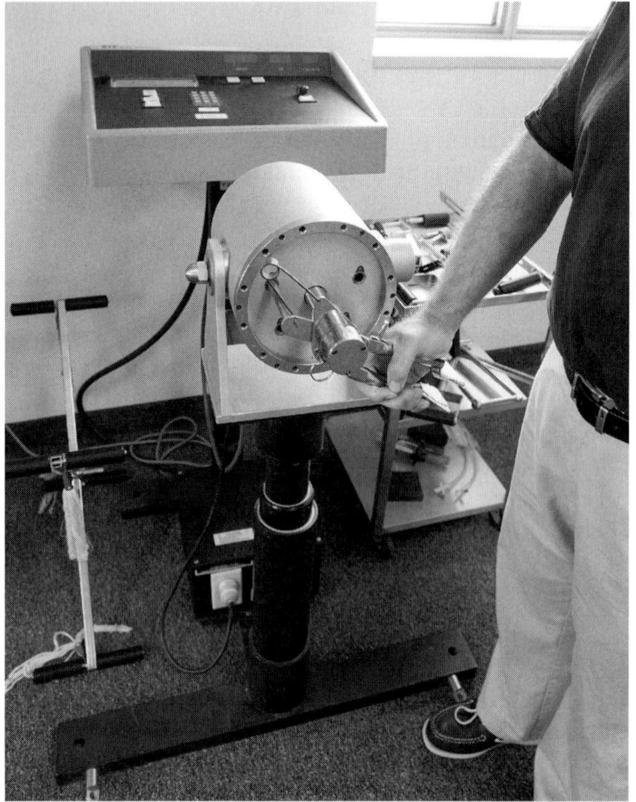

FIGURE 3-5. A BTE is a piece of equipment that is often seen in an outpatient setting that helps build upper extremity strength and range of motion.

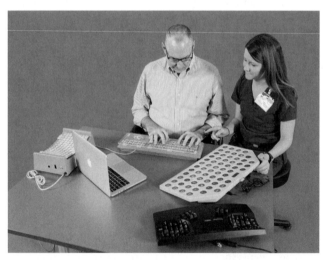

FIGURE 3-6. Adaptive keyboards are used in outpatient settings to help those who may have difficulty using a standard keyboard due to physical and/or cognitive difficulties.

DOCUMENTATION AND REIMBURSEMENT

Reimbursement in this setting is similar to that in the LTC setting. It is fee-for-service with reimbursement solely being based on the services provided through CPT codes. Medicare clients also have a cap on their OT services, which are evaluated on a yearly basis, but can be extended with proper documentation of need. Many reimbursement sources, such as Medicaid and private insurance, set limits on the number of visits allowed each year.

Documentation in the outpatient setting has to support the individual treatment session along with the client's progression toward the goals. This is another setting that uses outcome-based tools to be able to support the services being provided. Collaboration between the occupational therapist and OTA is important in this setting because rules and regulations require supervisory visits at certain points in the client's plan of care. As stated previously, regulations surrounding supervisory visits within the outpatient setting have changed over time; therefore, it is important to research the most current federal and state regulations if working in this setting.

Hospice and Palliative Care

Two additional areas that are not typically part of the continuum may be added if the need arises: palliative care and hospice. Palliative care is designed to assist in relieving symptoms of a chronic disease or disorder, focuses on quality of life, and can be added at any stage in the disease process. The basis of the palliative care team is a physician, a nurse, and a social worker. However, because palliative care can be added in any setting, the team members in that setting would also become integral members of the client's healthcare team. Palliative care can last months to years

COMMUNICATION

OT practitioners have begun to play an important role in reducing readmissions. Readmissions affect all settings and are an emerging concern for many client populations. The ultimate goal in the continuum is to progress to levels that require less medical attention and to avoid going backward. When a client is admitted back to the hospital it portrays an image that the acute care hospital did not stabilize the client well enough before discharge and/or the setting that the client was discharged to did not provide the client with the needed level of care. OT practitioners are well positioned within our scope of practice to positively affect the clinical outcomes for clients at risk for readmission back to a hospital in all practice settings. OT practitioners work to minimize the need for readmissions to the hospital while optimizing clients' abilities to interact as safely and independently as possible within their own environments, skills that are needed to stay in that setting.[21] A recent article found that "occupational therapy is the only spending category where additional spending has a statistically significant association with lower readmission rates" for the three health conditions studied: heart failure, pneumonia, and acute myocardial infarction. The authors point out that "occupational therapy places a unique and immediate focus on patients' functional and social needs, which can be important drivers of readmission if left unaddressed."[22]

and is used to support the client with pain management, personal care, and other types of care that may be difficult to manage by the outpatient or hospital-based treatment team. Hospice is a type of increased palliative care for individuals who have a life-limiting illness with a prognosis of 6 months or less to live. Under standard palliative care, an individual can continue to receive any treatment or equipment, even if it is aggressive. Under hospice, the goals switch from being restorative to providing comfort. One can receive hospice within many different settings, including the acute care hospital, SNF, and at home. Some hospice organizations also have a facility (often called a Hospice House) where a client can go for respite or to live with full care during the final stages of life. Some hospices are for profit, and some are not for profit, but all receive a lump sum for caring for the client through their insurance.

CLIENT POPULATION

All clients who receive palliative and hospice care have life-threatening diseases or disorders. Typical diagnoses seen in persons admitted to palliative and hospice services are cancer, progressive neurological disorders, end-stage dementias, and end-stage respiratory or renal disease.

GOAL OF OCCUPATIONAL THERAPY

OT practitioners play an important role in the palliative care team by identifying life roles and occupations that are meaningful to clients, and addressing barriers to performance within the context of quality of life and comfort.[23] Palliative care can be an added support system for a client in any setting; therefore the goal for palliative care will support the goal of OT within the client's setting. For hospice, however, the primary goal of OT is to help maintain the client's comfort by managing terminal symptoms and providing education and support for the family.

TREATMENT STRATEGIES

Treatment strategies would be determined by the environment or setting where the client is located. For example, if the client is receiving palliative support services in a subacute setting, the emphasis might be on safe transfers to the toilet or shoulder pain management to improve function. Hospice treatment sessions are related to the comfort of the client. Family/caregiver education is vital with hospice clients. Examples of treatment strategies are education and training on safe mobility for functional tasks, orthotic fabrication and management to maintain joint stability and to decrease pain, or even positioning recommendations for comfort.

DOCUMENTATION AND REIMBURSEMENT

Palliative care does not have a separate payment system. The reimbursement provided for the therapy services received would align with the setting in which the client resides. Reimbursement for hospice service is provided through Medicare and private insurance. OT services are contracted from the hospice provider, who takes over as the insurance.

Documentation for palliative care would follow suit with the setting in which the client is receiving services. Documentation for the hospice setting would support the client's goals, while focusing on the reason for the consultation. For example, if an OT practitioner was consulted by hospice to provide caregiver education and training on shower transfers, the practitioner would focus the sessions on training caregivers on performing shower transfers with the client.

Transitioning Between Settings

Transitioning from one setting of the continuum to another setting in the continuum can be simple and straightforward or can be complicated. Many factors determine the transition, including functional level, insurance, and family support. Figure 3-7 shows the typical transition that is seen from one setting to the next, which is a progression from high acuity to low acuity. However, a client may enter the continuum at many of the different stages. Figure 3-8 shows the array of possible discharge locations based on the admission settings.

Some of the most challenging decisions for OT practitioners to make are recommendations for what the client's next discharge location should be. Having a knowledge base of what is offered in each setting helps OT practitioners to make educated decisions and become trusted resources for case managers and discharge planners. Figure 3-9 is a decision tree to help with making recommendations for the next discharge location. However, always remember that because each client's situation is unique, a client may transition to a setting that is not considered next within the continuum.

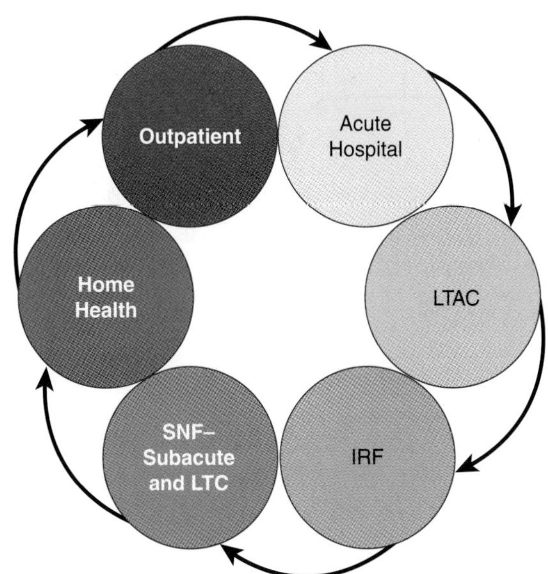

FIGURE 3-7. A representation of what the typical continuum of care for occupational therapy may look like.

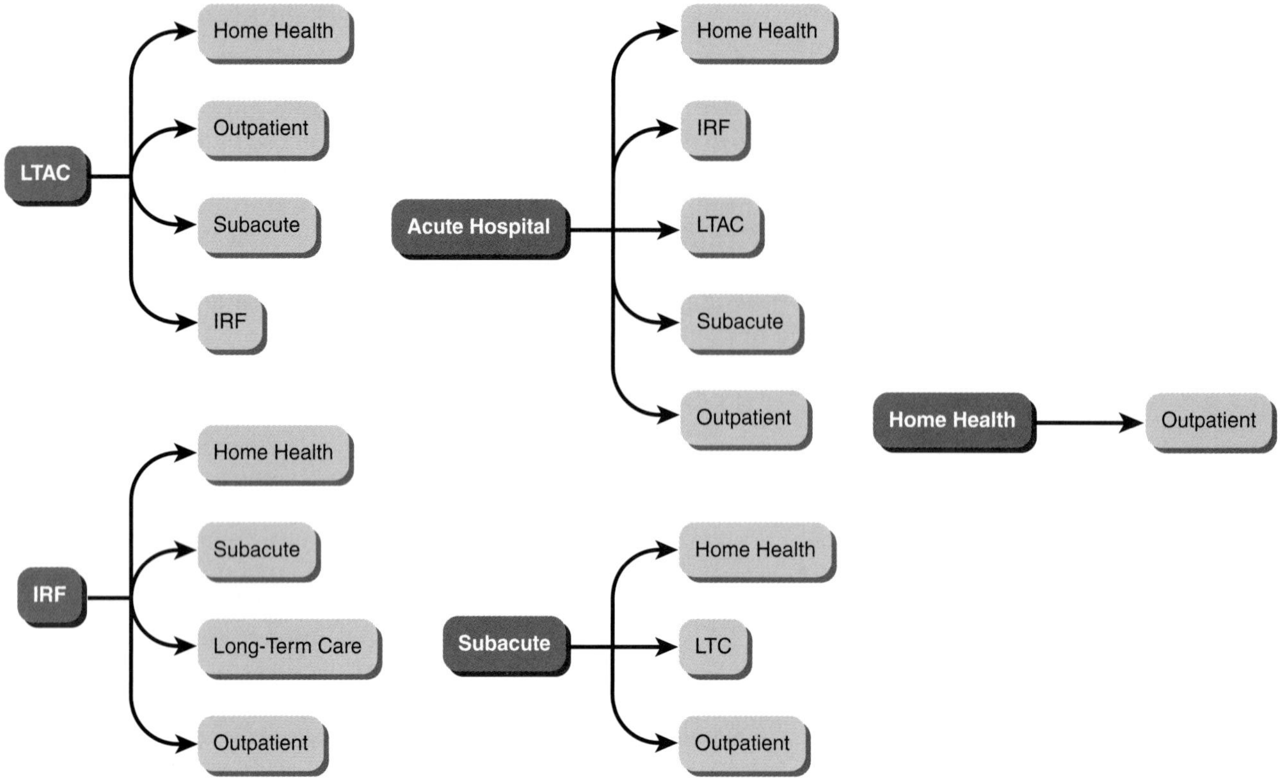

FIGURE 3-8. The typical discharge location may be based on the admission setting.

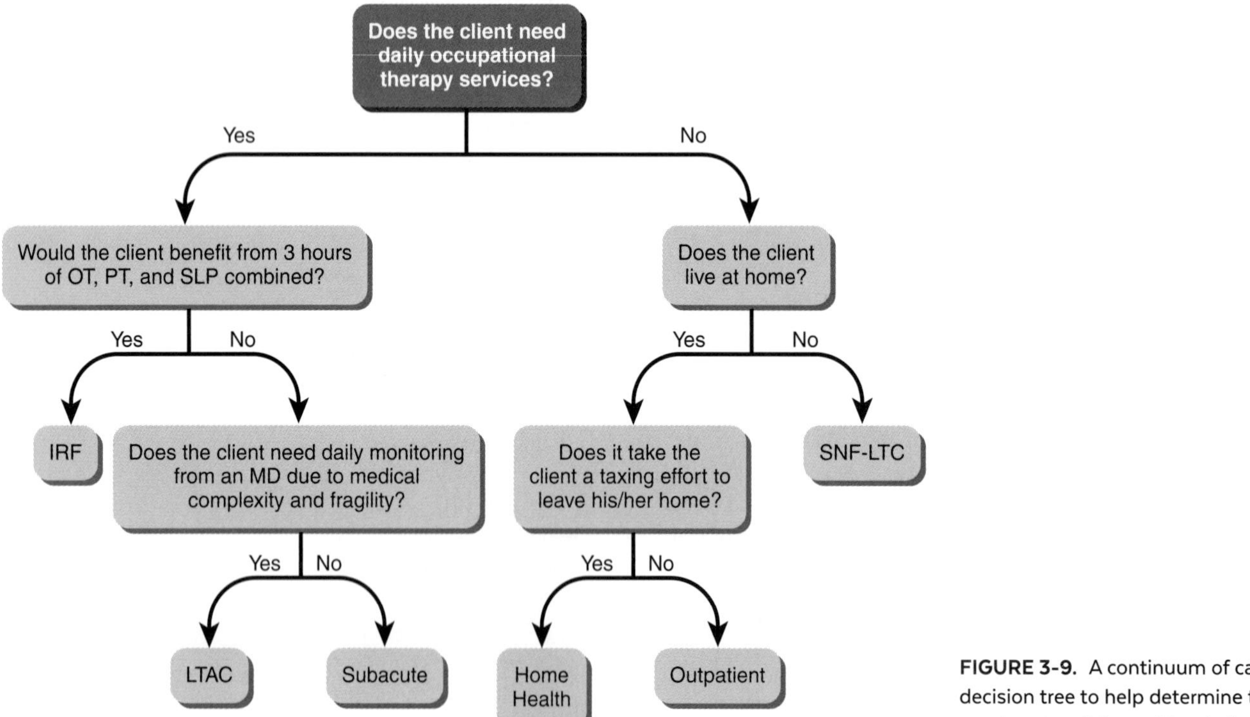

FIGURE 3-9. A continuum of care decision tree to help determine the most appropriate next level of care.

HEALTHCARE ADVANCEMENTS AND REFORMATION

Health care has evolved over the years, sometimes slowly and at times with a whirlwind pace. Recent evolution has occurred with an emphasis on preventive care along with shifting from a first curve to a second curve healthcare delivery. First curve healthcare delivery has always focused on volume-based healthcare delivery, and second curve healthcare delivery focused on value-based healthcare delivery.[24] Volume-based delivery means seeing the highest numbers of clients possible for the most numbers of sessions that are medically appropriate. Value-based delivery focuses on the quality of the care given with the amount of improvement seen. Forecasters expect that evolution to second curve delivery will start to be more aggressive in the years to come due to the Baby Boomer population aging over 65. The Baby Boomer population makes up 24.3% of the U.S. population, and 68% are still in the workforce.[25] The choices they make about whether to retire or continue to work will have profound implications for job openings and Social Security spending. Since 2011 there have been 8,000 individuals turning 65 per day, and it is estimated that by 2030, one in every five Americans will be over age 65.[25]

With a general consensus of many consumers that healthcare costs are high with disappointing outcomes, suggestions for healthcare reformation/transformation have varied.[27] The most common suggestions are single-payer systems, pay-for-performance, electronic health records, consumer-driven health plans, and value-based healthcare delivery:

- The single-payer system is one in which the government, instead of private insurers, pays for all healthcare costs.
- Pay-for-performance healthcare delivery provides an incentive bonus to providers for following processes and guidelines. As health care continues to evolve there are many forms of pay-for-performance being trialed and put into place. For instance, currently there is a negative effect on hospitals if they readmit a client within 30 days with the same diagnosis, in which reimbursement received may be cut.
- An electronic health record is the use of technology to centralize a client's medical records.
- Consumer-driven health plans require consumers to pay more of their healthcare costs from healthcare savings accounts along with high-deductible plans for catastrophic events. This allows clients to control which medical procedures and care they receive with the hopes of them becoming more responsible for their health and how healthcare dollars are spent.
- Value-based health care is defined as client health outcomes per dollars spent.[27] Therefore instead of being reimbursed for all the services provided, one would instead be reimbursed on the outcomes from the services. This is very much pertinent to OT services as our documentation with outcome-based tools could be used to determine reimbursement for services in the future more heavily.

THE OLDER ADULT

Many older adults, have multiple chronic conditions that affect their overall independence and ability to recover from an acute episode. Per the American Society of Consultant Pharmacists, almost 92% of all older adults have at least one chronic condition and 77% have at least two.[26] This means that more than likely an OTA would not just treat for the acute diagnosis but also for deficits related to any chronic conditions as well. This makes communicating and deciding the next level within the continuum imperative as chronic conditions may lead to readmissions to the hospital. The OTA must deploy critical thinking skills to help determine the reason for the many readmissions along with helping to decide the next level in the continuum. For example, if a client with congestive heart failure (CHF) and multiple readmissions to the hospital is being released to go home from an acute care hospital, an OTA may discuss with the occupational therapist the need to complete a thorough cognitive assessment to help determine whether the client can successfully manage his or her CHF medication.

Health care has also begun to switch from having a reactive approach to a more wellness and preventive approach.[28] This theory focuses on a client participating in more wellness-related activities, such as exercise classes and nutritional meal planning, to prevent health problems from developing in the future (e.g., arthritis and diabetes). As health care changes, the role that the OT practitioner plays in delivery of health care may also change. Treatment strategies can be geared toward prevention, compensation, or rehabilitation. There will always be emerging practice areas in the OT profession, encouraging continual growth of the profession alongside healthcare reformation. An example is telemedicine.

Healthcare reformation has brought discussion of how to make the continuum of care more cohesive. Historically, all settings within the continuum acted independently of each other, with nothing tying the settings together to encourage collaboration and partnership. However, due to healthcare reform many systems have been put into place to encourage collaboration. One in particular was the development of joint principles for the patient-centered medical home model (PCMH) in 2007 by the American Academy of Family Physicians (AAFP). The key principles are personal physician, physician-directed medical practice, whole-person orientation, coordinated care, and quality and safety.[30] The PCMH allows for quality and effective healthcare delivery spearheaded by a primary care physician and creates a partnership between clients and their physician. Historically, a client could have multiple physicians and healthcare providers without any cross collaboration to ensure that there was no duplication of services. The PCMH allows for a more comprehensive, personalized care delivery with

TECHNOLOGY AND TRENDS

Telehealth is a virtual healthcare delivery model where the client and the OT practitioner use technology such as a computer with a webcam or phone with a camera to communicate. This allows for increased accessibility for a client by removing all barriers to receive care, including travel. OT practitioners are using telehealth as a service delivery model to assist clients with developing skills; incorporating assistive technology and adaptive techniques; modifying work, home, or school environments; and creating health-promoting habits and routines.[29] OT practitioners develop goals that they can influence virtually. An example could be a practitioner working on time management skills with a client with a brain injury who is living at home but having a hard time transitioning back into his or her occupations due to difficulty with processing skills. Telehealth further supports the Affordable Care Act (ACA) Triple Aim. Triple Aim's goals are to improve the client's experience of care, to improve the health of populations, and to reduce the per capita cost of care per populations. When satisfaction surveys are sent out, one of the most frequent responses that link directly to client satisfaction is timeliness of care initiation and communication with the healthcare provider. Telehealth improves the client's experience of care by allowing quicker access for care management. OT practitioners' virtual role in improving the health of populations via distance education at a community support group or via a fall reduction class at a far-away setting comes as second nature as the OTPF-3 is based on identifying client factors and performance skills and patterns that may limit the health of others. An OT practitioner can also help a client establish a wellness routine virtually to assist with chronic disease management. Last, telehealth allows the OT practitioner to be fiscally responsible as it allows the practitioner to cut costs associated with traveling to see the client, as well as potential costs associated with rehospitalization through management of chronic conditions. At the time that this chapter was written, CMS has not acknowledged OT as a reimbursable telehealth service, although there is legislation in front of the U.S. Congress to do so. Therefore many practitioners are limited from being able provide care via this service delivery model.

better outcomes for the client along with a decrease in financial responsibility by insurances. However, although this model is strongly encouraged, it still remains voluntary in participation for primary care physicians.

The PCMH model bridged the gap to further reformation in the form of collaborative care via accountable care organizations (ACOs) and bundled payments. These two models have been the key to providing higher-quality and more coordinated care when a client transitions throughout the continuum.[31] An ACO consists of groups of physicians, hospitals, and other healthcare providers who have decided to voluntarily partner to give coordinated, high-quality care to their Medicare clients.[32] Although this model can be used for any population, it was designed for the chronically ill to receive the appropriate care and service by the right healthcare provider at the right time. An example of an ACO would be a hospital deciding to partner with a subacute care rehab facility and a home health agency to coordinate care for a client with congestive heart failure (CHF) who has had multiple admissions over the last several months to the hospital. Because the hospital has limited control of that client's follow-through with discharge instructions, the hospital would partner with subacute rehab or home health agency to ensure that the client continues to thrive and follow recommendations once discharged from the hospital. Many ACOs have also voluntarily decided to trial a bundled payment as well within their partnerships. A bundled payment is the concept of one lump-sum payment allotted per episode of care. Therefore, in the above example the hospital would receive one lump sum for the treatment of the client with CHF and would then have to choose how that is allocated across the continuum and with its partners.

SUMMARY

For optimal client care, collaboration between the occupational therapist and the OTA is very important regardless of the setting. Although the occupational therapist will be the one mainly conducting the evaluations, reassessments, and discharges (depending on the state) with the OTA's input within each setting, it is important for the OTA to understand each setting to be prepared to communicate with the occupational therapist regarding the client's progress. To be a resource for the multidisciplinary team, it is necessary for the OTA to understand each setting and where the client will go to next.

The continuum of care is a complicated system with many factors that determine a client's progression through it. This chapter has provided the OTA with a blueprint to help make recommendations for each setting and treatment strategies to consider. However, OTAs must look at each client case individually and establish treatment techniques based on the complex picture. Always put the client's needs first and be a support to help the transition to the level of care that is most appropriate for the client. Realize that as health care changes ever more rapidly, it is the responsibility of the OTA to be aware of changes to documentation requirements, reimbursement, coding/billing, and rules/regulations that would affect clients, as well as employers.

REVIEW QUESTIONS

1. All of the following are characteristics of the continuum of care *except:*
   a. The more medically fragile the client, the more OT is needed to return the client to his or her PLOF.
   b. The continuum of care is comprehensive.
   c. The client's needs remain the same throughout the continuum.
   d. The acuity level changes throughout the continuum.

2. An elderly client with obesity, arthritis, and osteoporosis has a fall with a hip fracture. He is transported via ambulance to the acute hospital. Due to pain and obesity, his recovery is slower than is typical, and his only available caregiver is his frail wife. Which might be his next step on the continuum?
   a. Subacute facility
   b. Home
   c. Outpatient
   d. LTAC
3. A young man with multiple sclerosis the OTA has been treating in the home for shoulder pain with decreased function is on Medicare. Which of the following is a consideration for this plan of care?
   a. That Medicare is a federally funded program
   b. That he is often seen around the neighborhood and mall in his wheelchair
   c. That Medicare does not have limits on the numbers of visits
   d. That the client is not old enough for Medicare
4. If a client just had a fracture of the spine requiring immediate surgery, what level hospital might the client be taken to?
   a. Two
   b. One
   c. Ten
   d. Three
5. An IRF and subacute rehabilitation are alike in which three of the following ways?
   a. They give 3 hours of therapy per day.
   b. The client receives multidisciplinary therapy.
   c. They are both reimbursed by RUG levels.
   d. They require a 3-night hospital stay for admission.
   e. The client may have come directly from the hospital.
   f. The client's goal is to return to his or her prior living environment.
6. Which client population would you *most likely* see at a LTAC facility?
   a. A client with acute respiratory distress requiring intubation
   b. A client with ESRD and a pressure injury requiring a wound vac
   c. A client day 2 after a subdural hematoma with unstable vitals
   d. A client with a readmission with the same diagnosis
7. LTC and outpatient facilities have which of the following in common?
   a. Both are reimbursed by CPT.
   b. Both provide 3 hours of therapy a day.
   c. Both focus on caregiver education as the primary treatment strategy.
   d. Both only accept Medicaid and private insurance.
8. After a spinal cord injury sustained during a car accident, Jean transfers to an IRF from the acute hospital. Jean is anxious to get home. The IRF multidisciplinary team is concerned that which of the following may impact her discharge directly to home health the most?
   a. The client must be deemed homebound, but loves to be outside.
   b. She only has private insurance, which will not pay for home health.
   c. The client must show daily progress.
   d. The client has a home with many steps and no plan for caregiving.
9. Palliative care and hospice have which of the following in common?
   a. They will both give excessive pain medication.
   b. They are both rehabilitative in nature.
   c. They can both be added at any stage in the disease process.
   d. They both are supportive services for life-limiting disease management.
10. When making a suggestion regarding the next level in the continuum of care, which three of the following components are the most important to consider?
   a. Prior level of independence/client's goals
   b. Discharge planner recommendations
   c. Caregiver/family support
   d. Architecture of home
   e. Family suggestions
   f. Reimbursement

CASE STUDY

Cheryl was a lively 54-year-old woman who had never been sick a day in her life. She found a lump in her left breast one day. On evaluation by a doctor, Cheryl was found to have breast cancer and would need to have surgical intervention to remove a malignant tumor and have a mastectomy. She was admitted to the hospital for surgical intervention and unfortunately had respiratory issues with respiratory failure requiring ventilation. Cheryl spent 3 weeks in the hospital, and an attempt was made to wean her from the ventilator at the hospital but was unsuccessful. Cheryl at this point had become increasingly weak and could barely tolerate sitting on the edge of the bed. Cheryl received OT within the hospital, and they focused on simple grooming while seated on the edge of the bed for endurance. Cheryl was transferred to a LTAC facility.

On arriving at the LTAC facility, the OT practitioner, along with the other members of the multidisciplinary team, focused on getting her respiratory system stronger in efforts for her to be weaned from the ventilator. Within 3 weeks Cheryl was completely weaned from the ventilator, but was not independent enough to go home as she lived with her husband who worked every day. The recommendation was made for Cheryl to be transferred to an IRF. At the IRF Cheryl made great progress. She progressed from needing moderate assistance with most ADLs to being modified independent with all ADLs. Cheryl was finally able to go home with her husband. Once she arrived home, Cheryl started receiving home health OT services as it still required an increased amount of time and taxing effort for her to leave her home. The home health OTA worked to get her modified independent in all aspects of her IADLs. Cheryl was now modified independent with all ADLs and IADLs, but still experienced some weakness and limited range of motion (ROM) in her upper extremities from her mastectomy. Cheryl then became a client at her local outpatient facility to increase her ROM in her upper extremities, and 6 months after her surgery, Cheryl returned to work.

1. What might be some treatments the OTA would have performed at each acuity level?
2. How would the OTA have assisted with the transition process?

REFERENCES

1. Health Information and Management System Society. (2014). Definition: Continuum of care. Retrieved from http://www.himss.org/definition-continuum-care
2. Long-term and post-acute care providers. (2017). American Hospital Association. Retrieved from http://www.aha.org
3. Centers for Medicare and Medicaid Services. (2014). What's Medicare? Retrieved from https://www.medicare.gov/Pubs/pdf/11306.pdf
4. Veterans Administration. (2015). Health benefits. Retrieved from http://www.va.gov/HEALTHBENEFITS/apply/veterans.asp
5. Veterans Administration. (2015). Disability compensation. Retrieved from http://www.benefits.va.gov/BENEFITS/factsheets/serviceconnected/presumption
6. American Occupational Therapy Association. (2012). Occupational therapy's role in acute care. Retrieved from http://www.aota.org/About-Occupational-Therapy/Professionals/RDP/AcuteCare.aspx
7. Lipshutz, A., & Gropper, M. (2013). Acquired neuromuscular weakness and early mobilization in the intensive care unit. *Anesthesiology, 118*, 202–215.
8. Office of Inspector General. (2001). Medicare hospital prospective payment system: How DRG rates are calculated and updated. Retrieved from http://oig.hhs.gov/oei/reports/oei-09-00-00200.pdf
9. Pendleton, H. M., & Schultz-Krohn, W. (2012). Pedretti's occupational therapy practice skills for physical dysfunction. In K. Falk (Ed.), *Practice settings for physical disabilities* (Vol. 7, pp. 43–54). St. Louis, MO: Elsevier.
10. American Academy of Physical Medicine and Rehabilitation. (2011). Standards for assessing medical appropriateness criteria for admitting patients to rehabilitation hospitals or units. Retrieved from https://www.aapmr.org/advocacy/health-policy/medical-necessity/Documents/MIRC0211.pdf
11. Centers for Medicare and Medicaid Services. (2014). Inpatient rehabilitation facility prospective payment system. Retrieved from https://www.cms.gov/Outreach-and-Education/Medicare-Learning-Network-MLN/MLNProducts/downloads/InpatRehabPaymtfctsht09-508.pdf
12. Amundson, J., Brunner, A., & Ewers, M. (2001). FIM scores as an indicator of length of stay and discharge destination in CVA patients: A retroactive outcomes study. *Journal of Undergraduate Research, 26*, 263–270.
13. American Health Lawyers Association. (2012). Overview of long term hospitals and inpatient rehabilitation facilities and their role in the post acute care continuum. Retrieved from https://www.healthlawyers.org/Events/Programs/Materials/Documents/LTC13/papers/k_marshall_yoder_yohe.pdf
14. Koranne, R. (2011). The role of the long-term acute care hospital. *Minnesota Medicine*, 38–40.
15. Wake Forest Baptist Health. (2015). Vacuum assisted closure. Retrieved from http://www.wakehealth.edu/Plastic-Surgery/Wound-Care/Vacuum-Assisted-Closure.htm#
16. Jette, D., Warren, R., & Wirtalla, C. (2005). The relation between therapy intensity and outcomes of rehabilitation in skilled nursing facilities. *Archives of Physical Medicine and Rehabilitation, 86*, 373–379.
17. Brown, C. J., Friedkin, R. J., & Inouye, S. K. (2004). Prevalence and outcomes of low mobility in hospitalized older patients. *Journal of the American Geriatrics Society, 52*, 1263–1270.
18. Craig, D. (2012). Current occupational therapy publications in home health. *American Journal of Occupational Therapy, 66*, 338–347.
19. American Occupational Therapy Association. (2016). Productive aging. Retrieved from http://www.aota.org/~/media/Corporate/Files/Practice/Aging/Distinct-Value-Productive-Aging.pdf
20. American Occupational Therapy Association. (2013). Occupational therapy's role in home health. Retrieved from http://www.aota.org/About-Occupational-Therapy/Professionals/PA/Facts/Home-Health.aspx
21. Roberts, P., &, Robinson, M. (2014). Occupational therapy's role in preventing readmissions. *American Journal of Occupational Therapy, 68*(3), 254–259.
22. Rogers, A. T., Bai, G., Lavin, R. A., & Anderson, G. F. (2016). Higher hospital spending on occupational therapy is associated with lower readmission rates. *Medical Care Research and Review*, 1–19. https://doi.org/10.1177/1077558716666981
23. American Occupational Therapy Association. (2011). The role of occupational therapy in palliative care. Retrieved from http://www.aota.org/-/media/Corporate/Files/AboutOT/Professionals/WhatIsOT/PA/Facts/FactSheet_PalliativeCare.pdf
24. Hospitals in Pursuit of Excellence. (2013). Second curve road map for health care. Retrieved from http://www.hpoe.org/Reports-HPOE/Second_Curve_RoadMap_1to4.pdf
25. Cable News Network. (2014). Baby Boomer generation fast facts. Retrieved from http://www.cnn.com/2013/11/06/us/baby-boomer-generation-fast-facts/index.html
26. American Society of Consultant Pharmacists. (2016). Senior care facts. Retrieved from https://www.ascp.com/articles/about-ascp/ascp-fact-sheet
27. Harvard Business School. (2009). Value based healthcare delivery. Retrieved from http://www.hbs.edu/centennial/businesssummit/healthcare/value-based-health-care-delivery.pdf
28. American Occupational Therapy Association. (n.d.). Wellness and prevention occupational therapy's opportunity in the era of health care reform. Retrieved from http://www.aota.org/-/media/Corporate/Files/Advocacy/Health-Care-Reform/Ad-Hoc/Wellness %20Draft%202_with %20edits-cjed.pdf
29. Cason, J. (2012). Telehealth opportunities in occupational therapy through the Affordable Care Act. *American Journal of Occupational Therapy, 66*, 131–136.
30. American Academy of Family Physicians. (2016). The patient-centered medical home. Retrieved from http://www.aafp.org/practice-management/transformation/pcmh.html
31. Centers for Medicare and Medicaid Services. (2013). Bundled payments. Retrieved from http://innovation.cms.gov/initiatives/bundled-payments/
32. Centers for Medicare and Medicaid Services. (2015). Accountable care organizations. Retrieved from https://www.cms.gov/Medicare/Medicare-Fee-for-Service-Payment/ACO/index.html?redirect=/ACO/

Chapter 4

Health Promotion and Wellness for the Client and Practitioner

Marjorie E. Scaffa, PhD, OTR/L, FAOTA

LEARNING OUTCOMES

After studying this chapter, the student or practitioner will be able to:

4.1 Describe the purpose of *Healthy People 2020*
4.2 Define health literacy and explain its impact on health
4.3 Identify occupational risk factors for health
4.4 Delineate the role of occupational therapy practitioners in health promotion
4.5 Discuss the impact of psychosocial issues on the promotion of health and adjustment to disability
4.6 Describe aspects of professional self-care

KEY TERMS

Burnout	Occupational deprivation
Chronic disease self-management	Occupational dysfunction
Compassion fatigue	Occupational imbalance
Compassion satisfaction	Occupational injustice
Ergonomics	Occupational marginalization
Health literacy	Occupational risk factors
Health promotion	Professional self-care
Health-related quality of life (HRQOL)	Resilience
Occupational alienation	Secondary traumatic stress
	Universal design (UD)
	Vicarious trauma

Within the current healthcare system, health, wellness, and preventive care present challenges to current practice and exciting new job opportunities for the occupational therapy assistant (OTA). This chapter describes the basic principles of health and wellness practice with an emphasis on promoting quality of life and the impact of health literacy on well-being. It also explores an occupational perspective on health and well-being through the identification of occupational risk and resiliency factors. Following this, the chapter discusses potential roles for the OTA in health promotion and preventive care and provides specific practice examples. The chapter concludes with a discussion of professional self-care as a means of maintaining the health and wellness of the OTA and prevention of compassion fatigue.

PRINCIPLES OF HEALTH AND WELLNESS PRACTICE

According to the World Health Organization (WHO),

> To reach a state of complete physical, mental, and social wellbeing, an individual or group must be able to identify and realize aspirations, to satisfy needs, and to change or cope with the environment. Health is, therefore, seen as a resource for everyday life, not the objective of living. Health is a positive concept emphasizing social and personal resources, as well as physical capacities. Health promotion is not just the responsibility of the health sector, but goes beyond healthy lifestyles to wellbeing.[1]

Several decades ago in the United States, the Department of Health and Human Services (DHHS) launched a national **health promotion** initiative titled *Healthy People 1990* that envisioned a future in which people live long, healthy lives. Every decade since 1990, the health status of the population has been assessed and new goals and objectives have been developed. These documents are important for occupational therapy (OT) practitioners as they provide a roadmap for OT participation in the delivery of health promotion services. The four main goals of the most recent edition, *Healthy People 2020*, are as follows:

- Attain high-quality, longer lives free of preventable disease, disability, injury, and premature death.
- Achieve health equity, eliminate disparities, and improve health of all groups.
- Create social and physical environments that promote good health for all.
- Promote quality of life, healthy development, and healthy behaviors across all life stages.[2]

In *Healthy People 2020*, health is conceptualized as being determined by the following factors: biology and genetics, individual behavior, health services, social factors, and policymaking. Although there is little that OT practitioners can do to affect biology and genetics, OT intervention certainly has opportunities to address the four other determinants of health.

Healthy People 2020 comprises 42 focus areas and more than 1,200 objectives. Focus areas that are particularly relevant for occupational therapy intervention are listed in Box 4-1. Leading Health Indicators (LHIs) are a small subset of 26 objectives from *Healthy People 2020* designed to express "high-priority" health issues and the actions that may be implemented to address them appropriately. From 2010 to 2014, progress toward achieving LHI targets was primarily positive. Some of the LHI targets in the *Healthy People 2020* initiative include access to health services; clinical preventive services; environmental quality; injury and violence; maternal, infant, and child health; mental health, nutrition, physical activity, and obesity; oral health, reproductive and sexual health; tobacco; and substance abuse. Over half (14 of 26 or 53.9%) have met their targets or at least shown improvement.[2] Some of the advancements that have occurred in the past 10 years include an increased life expectancy, as well as decreased death rates due to cerebrovascular accident (CVA) and coronary heart disease. Of course, many challenges remain in the realm of public health and health disparities. *Healthy People 2020* LHIs place a heavy emphasis on tracking progress spanning the decade as healthcare professionals work to overcome these challenges and disparities. LHIs function to assess and determine the nation's health, encourage teamwork among regions and subdivisions, and inspire positive change manifested through action at the community, state, and national levels to improve the U.S. population's health.[2]

Healthy People 2020 includes a database of evidence-based resources where individuals may look up a variety of health-related topics pertaining to current issues, events, and disorders. For example, as of May 2016 the database included 469 evidence-based resources with topics spanning fall preventions for elderly adults and immunization strategies for hepatitis B to substance abuse treatment for lesbian, gay, bisexual, and transgender individuals. The evidence is organized by the resource type and publication date. Strength of the evidence is rated on a 4-point scale, with 4 meaning the highest level of evidence.

The DHHS designed a framework, called MAP-IT, to achieve *Healthy People 2020* objectives. MAP-IT, which stands for Mobilize, Assess, Plan, Implement, and Track, assists communities with the planning and evaluation of public health interventions that lead to accomplishing the established objectives. On the *Healthy People 2020* website, links coincide with each MAP-IT step in addition to questions and resources pertaining to the step. For example, under the "Mobilize" step, some questions are, "Why do I want to bring people together? Who should be represented?" The majority of states have a *Healthy People 2020* coordinator who consistently communicates with DHHS and the Office of Disease Prevention and Health Promotion (ODPHP) as a liaison to help increase the health levels of each state's residents.[3]

QUALITY OF LIFE

One of the goals of *Healthy People 2020* is to promote quality of life. Quality of life (QoL) is also an expected outcome of OT intervention.[4] Many definitions of QoL exist, and individual perceptions will vary. The WHO defines quality of life as a "broad ranging concept affected in a complex way by the person's physical health, psychological state, personal beliefs, social relationships and their relationship to salient

BOX 4-1

***Healthy People 2020* Focus Areas Particularly Relevant for Occupational Therapy Intervention[2]**

Access to health services
Adolescent health
Arthritis, osteoporosis, and chronic back conditions
Dementias, including Alzheimer's disease
Disability and disability health
Early and middle childhood
Educational and community-based programs
Health communication and health information technology
Health-related quality of life and well-being
Injury and violence prevention
Medical product safety
Mental health and mental disorders
Nutrition and weight status
Occupational safety and health
Older adults
Physical activity
Preparedness (disaster and emergency)
Sleep health
Social determinants of health
Substance abuse
Vision

features of their environment."[5] Liddle and McKenna describe QoL as being associated with general feeling of well-being, satisfaction, and perceptions of life in relation to set goals, values, and concerns.[6]

QoL is a self-reported, subjective measure that attempts to measure the client's lived experience in the client's current stage in life, both in health and illness.[7] QoL measures can be used to assess current status, evaluate treatment efficacy, and show any progress or regression of the client's overall satisfaction with life. In addition, QoL measurements can lead to an increase in client compliance during the therapy session because QoL is relevant and is easily understood by most clients.[6] Many assessments measure QoL; some are disease specific, whereas others are generic. These assessments divide questions into several domains, including, but not limited to, social status; spiritual, psychological, and emotional well-being; community mobility; and productivity.[7,8]

Health-related quality of life (HRQOL) is a multidimensional concept that focuses on the impact of health status on QoL. It includes domains related to physical, mental, emotional, and social functioning. Venes defines *health-related quality of life* as "the measurable impact of a person's perception of his or her health and the effect that produces on satisfaction with life and wellbeing."[9] Physical disabilities can negatively affect a person's emotional and psychological well-being, producing depression and anxiety, which can decrease HRQOL.[10] Individuals with disabilities are often faced with challenges to performing essential daily living tasks and other occupations, and HRQOL may be affected by the primary disability and secondary conditions such as pressure injuries from immobility.

For example, persons with spinal cord injury exhibit a suicide rate that is two to six times greater than the general public, and fewer than 40% return to work following their injuries.[10] Individuals with traumatic brain injury may experience loss of personal control, functional limitations, limitations in work-related tasks, emotional dysregulation, and the inability to participate in previously enjoyed activities due to cognitive limitations.[8,11] These limitations can affect the person's ability to participate in all occupations, which then may affect overall QoL.

Social relationships are a key contributor to QoL. Hawton et al. determined that social isolation was negatively correlated with HRQOL.[12] Interventions are needed to promote social participation to prevent and maintain both QoL and HRQOL. Examples of interventions to promote social participation include learning how to use public transportation to attend community events and the use of social media to keep in touch with friends and relatives.

HEALTH LITERACY

Another goal of *Healthy People 2020* is to achieve health equity, eliminate disparities, and improve health of all groups. One barrier to achieving health equity and eliminating health disparities is low levels of health literacy. According to the ODPHP, **health literacy** is "the capacity to obtain, process, and understand basic health information and services needed to make appropriate health decisions."[13] Approximately 90% of adults have difficulties using the "everyday health information" that is available in retail outlets, healthcare facilities, communities, and the media in the form of signs, brochures, websites, and so on. Low health literacy is directly related to poorer health prognoses and rising healthcare costs.[14] According to DHHS, "In the only population-level study of health literacy skills conducted to date, the Department of Education's National Assessment of Adult Literacy documented that only 12 percent of US adults are proficient enough in health literacy to understand and use health information effectively."[15]

The capacity to obtain, process, and understand health information typically requires the ability to read and write and to effectively speak and listen. Living in a technological age, an individual must also be computer literate. A person must be motivated as well as socially and cognitively able to assimilate, comprehend, and use health information. OT practitioners are ethically responsible to ensure that they are providing information in a way that is appropriate for clients' individual needs, so that they can function at the highest health literacy levels possible for their abilities. According to the 2003 National Adult Literacy Survey (NALS), one in three Americans reads below a fifth-grade level, which is classified as functionally illiterate. Asking clients simple questions such as, "How confident are you in filling out medical forms?" can provide a glimpse into a person's health literacy level. Also, OT practitioners should take note of whether the client appears to read, but does not follow through with the instructions. This could denote health illiteracy as opposed to willful noncompliance.[16]

Health literacy refers to an individual's ability to understand medical language; however, it also incorporates cultural and social nuances concerning health. Health literacy goes beyond the ability to read; it is important that individuals can adequately understand health information so that they can manage their health condition. Minority groups and those with less education are not the only ones affected by low health literacy. Some individuals in the geriatric population may be experiencing changes in their vision, hearing, and cognition, which can manifest as low levels of health literacy. Compliance with medication prescriptions includes being able to count the number of pills needed daily, as well as the capacity to read and understand side effects.

OT practitioners must constantly be aware of the impact that certain factors such as diminished cognition and low vision have on health literacy. In addition, treatment interventions need to be a good fit for the health literacy level of the client. It is important to watch for clients who are embarrassed about their limited health literacy; they will sometimes disguise their inability to read by saying they prefer the healthcare practitioner to read to them or simply refuse to participate due to an inability to understand the

BOX 4-2
Warning Signs That a Client May Have Low Health Literacy[20]

Becomes angry/demanding
Is quiet and passive
Leaves registration forms incomplete
Has difficulty explaining medical concerns
Is not able to give coherent sequential history
Cannot name medications, or explain purpose, timing, or dosage of administration
Makes excuses such as "I forgot my glasses. I'll read this when I get home"
Asks no or few questions
Frequently misses appointments; skips or does not follow up on tests and referrals

directions. Some common warning signs that a client may have low health literacy are listed in Box 4-2.

Impact of Low Health Literacy

OT practitioners must be sensitive to and alert to the warning signs of low health literacy. Most health documents are written at a tenth-grade level or higher, while as previously noted, many Americans read at a much lower level. This discrepancy could cause many people to be unable to fill out their health insurance paperwork, resulting in no coverage for themselves or their families. Clients also may have trouble expressing their health history (verbally or written) while at the doctor's office or rehabilitation clinic, which could affect their treatment and outcomes as a result of potentially serious medical errors and lower-quality care. Managing a chronic disease becomes nearly impossible when individuals have insufficient health literacy. Unfortunately, individuals may be labeled as noncompliant with medications or home-based therapeutic activities when in fact they are experiencing health literacy challenges, such as having reading difficulties, lack of organization, or memory problems. Low levels of health literacy can also contribute to clients' issues with communicating with health insurance companies, overpaying for treatment and higher healthcare costs, not seeking enough treatment, having limited knowledge of their condition, and underreporting or inadequately reporting current symptoms. When OT practitioners do not communicate at the appropriate health literacy level for each client, unintended misunderstandings may occur within client interactions.[17]

Limited health literacy is also linked to less involvement in activities that foster health promotion and disease detection, riskier health choices such as engaging in drugs and alcohol, and more work-related accidents.[18] Therefore, limited health literacy can affect people's ability to find and use health information, form healthy habits, and take appropriate action in response to important public health warnings and alerts. In addition, poor health literacy affects daily tasks of living, such as purchasing healthy food and being able to follow recipes and read health labels on food containers. According to Levasseur and Carrier, "poor health literacy might be a better predictor of health status than education, socioeconomic status, employment, race or gender. The possible consequences of poor health literacy range from lower levels of empowerment and participation to situations and behaviors that could jeopardize safety and health, i.e. increase morbidity and risk of premature mortality."[19]

Integrating Health Literacy Into Occupational Therapy Practice

According to Levasseur and Carrier, there are six ways to integrate health literacy into OT practice:

1. Be aware of health literacy issues and identify health literacy problems that arise in therapy.
2. Standardize interventions to include health literacy.
3. Consider health literacy by making information accessible.
4. Strengthen interactions with clients.
5. Intervene to increase clients' health literacy.
6. Collaborate with other professionals to increase clients' health literacy.[19]

In addition, the teach-back method is a helpful strategy to help ensure that clients understand what is being asked or taught to them. With this approach, the client repeats back what the healthcare provider has said in the client's own words to demonstrate understanding.[18]

Another popular health-communication strategy is "Ask Me 3," in which clients are encouraged to ask three questions during clinical consultations. For example, clients could ask: "What is my main problem? What do I need to do? Why is it important for me to do this?" These methods promote a shame-free environment by encouraging individuals to ask questions about their health.[20]

Several tools have been created to test and measure health literacy. The most frequently used tools include the Rapid Estimate of Adult Literacy in Medicine (REALM) and the Test of Functional Health Literacy in Adults (TOFHLA). These tools test reading comprehension by assessing word recognition or by requiring the client to determine and insert the missing word into a sentence. Shortened versions of these tests also exist, and most of these tests have been validated for adults.

Adults with low literacy often experience shame, embarrassment, and discrimination, and OT practitioners can help them overcome the shame and the unfortunate stigma that many experience. A "shame-free environment" is crucial to improving health outcomes and encouraging all patients to feel comfortable disclosing when they need assistance.[20]

The following strategies are recommended to enhance understanding of health information:

- Supplement the text with pictures.
- Tailor medication schedules or health promotion activities to fit a person's daily routine, using daily events as reminders.

- Use clear captions, ample white space, and pictures or diagrams to attract the reader's attention and reinforce the message.
- Shorten sentences to 10 words or less to make written material easier to read.
- Use concepts no higher than a fifth- or sixth-grade level (see Communication for instructions on how to assess readability).
- Speak in clear, simple, culturally sensitive language to connect with patients and clients from all literacy levels.[20,21]

It is important to recognize that under duress, individuals who have excellent literacy and comprehension skills may be intimidated or challenged by the medical environment and have difficulty understanding medical information. This is especially true when such individuals are ill, anxious, in pain, or experiencing medication side effects. Under these conditions, health literacy can be challenging for anyone, regardless of an individual's reading level, socioeconomic background, or level of intelligence.[20] Enhancing health literacy will increase self-esteem and empower clients to be advocates for their own health and well-being.

COMMUNICATION

Readability measures are based primarily on factors such as the number of words in a sentence and the number of syllables in the words. A readability score indicates the reading level of the printed material. Read the following paragraph and try to guess the reading level required to understand this content accurately:

- Fennell (2003) has proposed a four-phase, interdisciplinary, team-based approach to the management of chronic disease. The phases include crisis, stabilization, resolution, and integration. Within each phase, three domains are assessed and addressed: physical/behavioral, psychological, and social/interactive. A phase model is particularly relevant because the experience of chronic illness changes over time and persons have different needs in the early phases as compared with later phases. This underscores the importance of matching interventions to the phase of illness. This approach is evidence-based and grounded in clinical practice.[22]

Two easy ways will help assess the exact reading level of this passage:

1. If using Microsoft Word: Readability statistics can be found in the Tools menu under Grammar. If the readability statistics option is checked, you will get readability statistics every time you spell check a passage.
2. If using online readability websites: Many of these are available; try this one to start: https://readability-score.com/

AN OCCUPATIONAL PERSPECTIVE ON HEALTH

A foundational premise of OT is that participation in occupation is health enhancing if the participation meets the physical, psychological, and social needs of the individual and the demands of the environment for survival and adaptation. To achieve positive health and well-being "people need what they do to offer meaning, choice, satisfaction, a sense of belonging, purpose and achievement."[23] To address occupational well-being from a population perspective, Wilcock has adopted the public health terminology of risk factors and resiliency factors.[23]

Risk Factors

Risk factors are internal or external conditions that increase a person's susceptibility to illness, disease, or disability. Many are familiar with risk factors related to health such as smoking, obesity, inactivity, and high blood pressure, for example. However, as OT practitioners, it is important to also recognize and address occupational injustice and the **occupational risk factors** that affect health and well-being. **Occupational injustice** is defined "as individuals, groups, communities, and nations experiencing a lack of meaningful occupation for its members in their daily lives."[24] Occupational injustice may manifest as the risk factors of occupational deprivation, occupational alienation, occupational imbalance, and occupational marginalization. Occupational risk factors can be considered signs of "the loss of harmony between lifestyle and the environment that humans evolved within and which ensured the healthy continuation of all capacities."[25] These occupational risk factors can result in significant health and social problems.

OCCUPATIONAL DEPRIVATION

Occupational deprivation is defined as the "deprivation of occupational choice and diversity because of circumstances beyond the control of individuals or communities."[2] Many external factors can produce occupational deprivation, some of which include technology, lack of employment opportunities, poverty, cultural values, local regulations, and limitations set by social services and education systems. Furthermore, illness and disability have social effects that can also result in occupational deprivation.[23]

Individuals with disabilities encounter occupational deprivation due to circumstances that prevent them from fully engaging in their needed and desired daily activities (Fig. 4-1). Inaccessible transportation, buildings, and community facilities are among some of the reasons why individuals with disabilities experience occupational deprivation. Unattainable social and healthcare services can also contribute to the state of occupational deprivation for individuals with disabilities.[24] Other individuals who experience occupational deprivation are caregivers, institutionalized individuals, prisoners, and persons who are

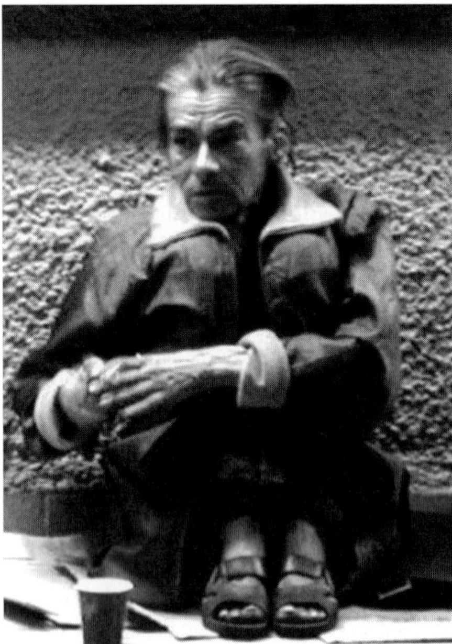

FIGURE 4-1. Occupational deprivation.

wheelchair- or bed-bound. For adults, poverty may cause occupational deprivation due to limited access to healthy foods.[24]

Occupational deprivation can produce occupational disruption and/or **occupational dysfunction.** Occupational disruption is defined as a temporary condition that transpires when an individual has an interruption in normal occupations. A disruption can be caused by an important life event, an environmental change, or a temporary illness or injury. In contrast, occupational dysfunction arises from occupational disruption that has not been resolved, occupational performance deficits, or a lengthy state of occupational deprivation. For example, prolonged bedrest due to illness or injury can result in occupational dysfunction due to loss of habits and routines. When occupational dysfunction is caused by a lengthy state of occupational deprivation, characteristics may include degeneration of an individual's natural abilities for occupations.[26]

OCCUPATIONAL ALIENATION

Occupational alienation is the "sense of isolation, powerlessness, frustration, loss of control, and estrangement from society or self as a result of engagement in occupation that does not satisfy inner needs."[23] Occupational alienation can be the result of removing individuals from their cultural occupations or by requiring people, such as the elderly or individuals with disabilities, to perform occupations that are not meaningful to them.[27] Occupational alienation is also considered "a state in which a disconnect exists between the person and his or her environment resulting in a loss of self-identity."[28] For example, individuals who are victims of human trafficking often detach or disconnect from their self-identity as a way of coping with the horrors they are experiencing; this process may result in occupational alienation. Adults who have experienced abuse and/or neglect as children are at higher risk for developing occupational alienation due to the lack of social support they received.[24]

OCCUPATIONAL IMBALANCE

Occupational imbalance is "a lack of balance or disproportion of occupation resulting in decreased wellbeing."[23] A disproportion among work, rest, and play is considered to be occupational imbalance. It occurs when an individual's occupational engagement fails to meet physical, social, mental, and rest needs. A lack of balance because of mental and social stressors of occupations can have the outcome of boredom or burnout. Students in an OTA program may have an occupational imbalance as they juggle schoolwork, families, jobs, and other responsibilities.

OCCUPATIONAL MARGINALIZATION

Occupational marginalization can be defined as "a person's occupation, although meaningful to others, lacks meaning to the individual due to underutilization of the person's full physical, social, and mental abilities."[28] Occupational marginalization is explained as an individual's inability to apply daily choices and use decision-making while engaging in occupations.[24] An example of occupational marginalization is when an individual with a disability is not included in an employment opportunity or when this individual does not even think that he or she can obtain a job.[27] Women who have been victims of domestic violence are at risk for developing occupational marginalization because fear affects their autonomy and confidence.[24]

Occupational Resiliency Factors

One approach to improving health and well-being is to reduce risk factors, including occupational risk factors. A complementary strategy is to increase protective and resiliency factors, including occupational resiliency factors.

Resilience is "a general term that signifies a person is able to endure stressful situations without suffering the physiological or psychological consequences, such as illness or disease, typically associated with such adversity."[29] Thus resiliency can be viewed as the interaction of risk factors and protective resources that produces individual variations in response to stressors.[30]

Resiliency can be promoted through risk-focused strategies, asset-focused strategies, and process-focused strategies. The emphasis of risk-focused strategies is to prevent or decrease risks and stressors to limit the impact of negative encounters. Risk-focused strategies include approaches such as parenting skills training to reduce child abuse, community policing to decrease crime and violence, and providing community recreation activities for adolescents to prevent drug and alcohol abuse. Asset-focused strategies are designed to increase available resources and access to these resources to more effectively respond to challenges and threats. Asset-focused approaches include providing tutors and other enrichment opportunities. The process-focused approach is directed toward mobilizing adaptive systems that result in influencing an individual's life. Some examples of process-focused strategies include increasing an individual's self-esteem through the successful completion of graded activities, encouraging mentoring relationships, and promoting cultural customs and spiritual practices that provide social support.[31]

Resilience is a precursor to adaptation. Persons with higher levels of resilience typically adapt more easily to changing circumstances and challenges. Positive adaptation is composed of internal and external elements. Internal adaptation is characterized as "a positive psychological adjustment as opposed to emotional distress and dysfunction."[31] External adaptation is described as "positive and effective behavioral responses to extenuating circumstances."[31] For example, individuals who have become newly disabled can value the abilities they have that remain and be grateful for the professionals and family members who are willing and able to help them (internal adaptation), and learn new strategies and skills to manage their daily living tasks (external adaptation).

THE ROLE OF OCCUPATIONAL THERAPY IN THE PROMOTION OF HEALTH AND WELL-BEING

The WHO defined **health promotion** "as a process of enabling people to increase control over and to improve their health."[1] It is the science and art of helping people change their lifestyles to move toward a state of optimal health and enhance awareness, change behavior, and create environments that support good health practices. The National Prevention Strategy, developed as a result of the Patient Protection and Affordable Care Act, identified four strategies for promoting population health:[32]

1. Healthy and safe community environments
2. Clinical and community preventive services
3. Empowered people
4. Elimination of health disparities

On an individual level, a healthy lifestyle should include the following: (1) tobacco-free living, (2) prevention of drug abuse and excessive alcohol use, (3) healthy eating, (4) active living, (5) injury- and violence-free living, (6) reproductive and sexual health, and (7) mental and emotional well-being. Through these strategies and lifestyle choices, individuals and the population as a whole can lead high-quality, longer, healthier lives and more effectively prevent and manage chronic diseases.

The profession of OT was built on the premise that engagement in purposeful and meaningful occupations can promote health and prevent disease/disability. This philosophy supports not only the use of occupation as an intervention to recover from illness, but also as a means of preventing disease and disability for persons who are generally healthy.

Through engaging in client-centered practice by having clients participate in occupations and adapt or alter their context to achieve a healthy and quality lifestyle, OT practitioners can play a role in promoting healthy lifestyles in clients' lives.[33] OT practitioners understand the interactions between people, their environments, and the activities they need to accomplish. Therefore, they can determine how these interactions benefit or hinder the individual's daily life. Some ways in which OT practitioners can promote health and wellness are as follows:

- Working with people in, or in recovery from, cancer treatment to mitigate the side effects on daily functioning
- Performing assessments for health risks, such as the potential for falls, the effect of low vision and/or cognitive issues on safety in daily tasks, and how well the home accommodates current and potential disabilities
- Teaching strategies to incorporate healthy habits and routines into daily activities for clients of all ages and abilities
- Identifying solutions to personal and environmental barriers limiting clients from engaging in healthy activities
- Providing skills training in areas such as socialization, caregiving, parenting, time management, and stress management[34]

Two official documents of the American Occupational Therapy Association (AOTA) outline the role of OT practitioners in health promotion and prevention. In the *Occupational Therapy Practice Framework: Domain and Process, 3rd edition* (OTPF-3), health promotion and disability prevention are described as approaches to intervention. The document also identifies prevention, health, quality of life, and well-being as expected outcomes of OT services. In the OTPF-3, health promotion is an approach to intervention "designed to provide enriched contextual and activity experiences that will enhance performance for all people in the natural contexts of life."[4] Disability prevention refers to the reduction of "the incidence of unhealthy conditions, risk factors, diseases, or injuries" and promoting "a healthy lifestyle at the individual, group, community, and governmental or policy level."[4]

Another AOTA (2013) official document, *Occupational Therapy in the Promotion of Health and Well-Being,* is devoted entirely to the role of OT in prevention, health promotion, and population health.[37] In it, the unique and distinct value of OT's contribution to health promotion is identified as the profession's focus on occupational engagement as a contributor to health and quality of life. Occupation-based health promotion and prevention services and programs provided by OT practitioners may address the needs of individuals, families, groups,

EVIDENCE-BASED PRACTICE

WELL ELDERLY STUDY

Dr. Florence Clark and her colleagues published a landmark study on the efficacy of a preventive OT program in the *Journal of the American Medical Association.* In this randomized, controlled trial, over 300 community-dwelling multiethnic older adults were placed into one of three groups. The control group received no intervention, the second group was engaged in a social activity program, and the third group received individual and group OT health promotion services. The OT intervention lasted 9 months and consisted of OT group services for 2 hours per week and a total of 9 hours of individual OT.

The OT intervention group participants exhibited increased vitality, physical and social functioning, life satisfaction, and general mental health. Participants also experienced a decrease in physical pain and fewer role limitations than participants in the social activity program or the control group.[35]

Even though the Clark study is older, subsequent research has demonstrated that well elderly intervention is still efficacious. In a 2016 study, a 4 month, occupation-based wellness program was completed, and the intervention group showed statistically significant improvements in general health items such as vitality and mental health, and positive trends for well-being. One of the final conclusions was that "participating in meaningful, challenging activities stimulates the occupational adaptation process"[36]; potentially, these studies are something the OTA could use to empower older persons to be active, healthy, and have a high QoL.

Azen, S. P., Zemke, R., Jackson, J., et al. (1997). Occupational therapy for independent living older adults: A randomized controlled trial. Journal of the American Medical Association, *278, 1321–1326.*

Johansson, A. & Björklund, A. (2016). The impact of occupational therapy and lifestyle interventions on older persons' health, well-being and occupational adaptation. Scandinavian Journal of Occupational Therapy, *23(3), 207–19. doi:10.3109/11038128.2015.1093544*

organizations, communities, and populations. Examples of occupation-based health promotion and prevention services include the following:

- Community-based fall prevention programs for seniors
- Workplace injury prevention and wellness programs
- Ergonomic principles applied to computer workstations in colleges and workplaces to decrease repetitive motion and musculoskeletal disorders
- Stress and anger management programs
- Parenting classes for teenage mothers, mothers in homeless shelters, or those recovering from drug dependency
- Self-management programs to enable those with chronic diseases such as diabetes, rheumatoid arthritis, and cardiac conditions to optimize health through appropriate routines (modifications when necessary) and participation in meaningful occupations
- CarFit programs for drivers to match the needs of the driver with minor adaptations to the car
- Caregiver education to prevent injury and/or burnout[34]

OT practitioners can assume any one or combination of the following roles in health promotion and prevention:

- Promote healthy lifestyles for all clients and their families regardless of disability status.
- Incorporate occupation into existing health promotion efforts developed by experts in areas such as health education, nutrition, and exercise.
- Develop and implement occupation-based health promotion programs targeting individuals, groups, organizations, and communities.[38]

TECHNOLOGY AND TRENDS

The AOTA has compiled a list of health and wellness apps that OT practitioners can use with clients. Many of these are free or low cost. Explore the possibilities. Here are a few favorites:

- Fooducate: Using your phone's camera, scan a food product's bar code to get nutritional information
- QuitStart: Developed by the National Cancer Institute, this app helps you identify smoking triggers and monitor progress toward a smoke-free lifestyle
- Calm: Meditation activities to improve mood, relax, and sleep
- Relax Me: Guided progressive muscle relaxation activity

Other health and wellness apps are readily available from other sources. Here are a few examples:

- Pillow: Measures and tracks sleep quality to identify ways to improve sleep and wake-up cycles
- Daily Yoga: Provides over 50 yoga and meditation exercises at different intensities for a variety of durations
- 7 Minute Workout: Fun exercises with no equipment needed, the challenge—7 minutes for 7 months
- Yum: Healthy and yummy recipes, shopping lists, and a digital recipe box

Health promotion programs can be provided in a variety of locations such as workplaces, college campuses, schools, community settings, health maintenance organizations, and hospitals. Stress management, weight reduction, and physical activity are a few health promotion programs in which occupational therapists and OTAs can play a role. The goal is to take action before a disease or disability occurs.

HEALTH PROMOTION PRACTICE EXAMPLES

To illustrate the role of OT, this section discusses a few health promotion and prevention practice examples in more detail; examples include weight management and obesity prevention, promotion of physical activity, chronic disease management, and enhancement of mental health and emotional well-being.

Weight Management and Obesity Prevention

The WHO classifies overweight as a body mass index (BMI) that is greater than or equal to 25, and obesity as a BMI that is greater than or equal to 30.[39] Obesity is considered to be a major public health problem in the United States. In 2014 approximately 29% of adults were obese and another 35% were classified as overweight.[40] Many of the leading causes of preventable death and morbidity are related to obesity, including heart disease, CVA, type 2 diabetes, and certain types of cancer. As BMI increases, so does the risk for these diseases. In addition to being a common comorbidity, obesity affects every aspect of health and function in an individual's life. Some of the physical effects of obesity include or lead to the following: insulin resistance, hypertension, asthma, gallbladder disease, sleep apnea, and orthopedic problems.[41] Many factors have contributed to the growing trend of obesity. On a global level, more high-fat (energy-dense) foods are available, and less physical activity is required in people's daily lives.[39] Some of the factors that contribute to the decrease of physical activity include increased modes of transportation, large increases in sedentary jobs, and increased leisure time spent watching television, playing electronic games, or surfing the Internet.

In an effort to simplify healthy eating recommendations, the U.S. Department of Agriculture (USDA) developed the MyPlate initiative. The MyPlate graphic (Fig. 4-2) is a visual representation of healthy portion sizes of fruits, grains, proteins, vegetables, and dairy.

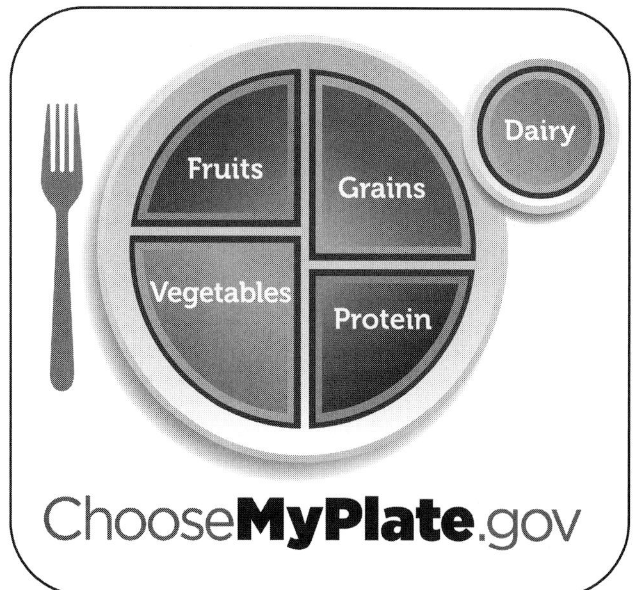

FIGURE 4-2. MyPlate.

OCCUPATIONAL THERAPY PRACTITIONER'S ROLE IN WEIGHT MANAGEMENT AND OBESITY PREVENTION

Obesity can restrict or severely limit a person's occupational performance and participation, and as a result, negatively affect their overall health and well-being. Because obesity prevents individuals from fully engaging in everyday activities, it falls within the OT domain. OT practitioners use everyday activities therapeutically to prevent the development and progression of obesity and improve their clients' health and quality of life. OT practitioners can encourage individuals to reach and maintain their healthy body weight range; facilitate weight loss; work with them to make healthier decisions through nutrition and exercise education; help them determine realistic, sustainable goals; and collaborate with them to build habits and routines that will lead them closer to their health goals (Fig. 4-3).[42]

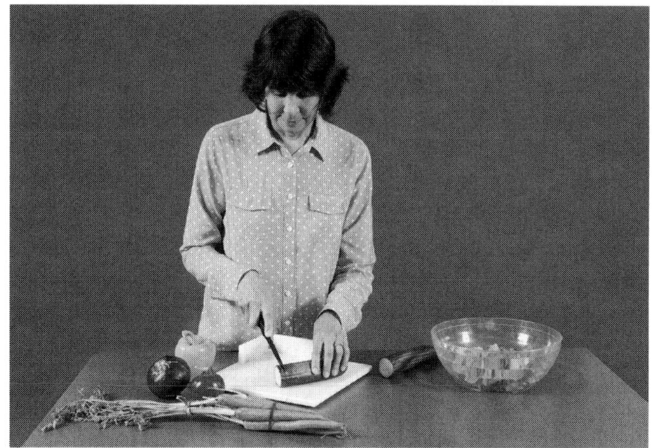

FIGURE 4-3. Preparing healthy foods is a lifestyle choice.

Promotion of Physical Activity Through Leisure

According to the WHO (2015), inadequate levels of physical activity is 1 of the 10 leading risk factors for death and is a major contributor to the rise in cardiovascular disease, diabetes, and cancer worldwide. Individuals with low levels of physical activity have a 20% to 30% higher risk of death compared with those who are adequately active.[45] In the United States, only 20% of adults meet the Centers for Disease Control and Prevention guidelines for physical activity.[46] Staying active results in many physical health benefits, including improved cardiovascular and muscular fitness; reduced risk of hypertension, diabetes, cancer, and depression; and decreased incidence of falls and fractures.[45] However, physical activity produces more than simply physical benefits, affecting QoL and psychological well-being to a large degree. The WHO defines *physical activity* as any bodily movement produced by

BOX 4-3
Lifestyle Redesign®

Lifestyle Redesign® is an evidence-based intervention approach based on the University of Southern California's Well Elderly Studies. These studies demonstrated the effectiveness of preventive occupational therapy in improving the quality of life for older adults living in the community. The Lifestyle Redesign® methodology has subsequently been applied to a variety of other populations and health conditions, such as weight management, diabetes, and chronic pain, with good results.[43] The overall goal of Lifestyle Redesign® is to enable "patients and clients to infuse sustainable, personally satisfying, health-promoting activities into daily life."[44] The key components of the Lifestyle Redesign® intervention include the following:

- Didactic presentation: Education about a topic relevant to the participants
- Peer exchange: An opportunity for participants to share information and experiences
- Direct experience: An activity or outing related to the topic designed to increase participants' self-efficacy
- Personal exploration: Time for reflection, self-appraisal, and application of what was learned to the participants' everyday lives, sometimes takes the form of "homework."[35]

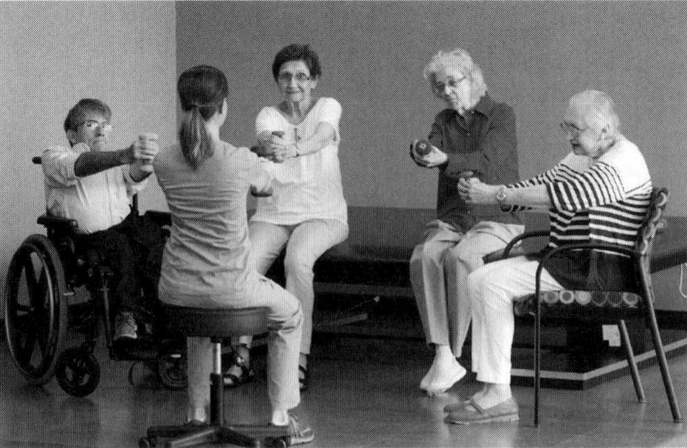

FIGURE 4-4. Physical activity group.

skeletal muscles that requires energy expenditure—including activities undertaken while working, playing, carrying out household chores, traveling, and engaging in recreational pursuits. The term "physical activity" should not be confused with "exercise," which is a subcategory of physical activity that is planned, structured, repetitive, and aims to improve or maintain one or more components of physical fitness. Beyond exercise, any other physical activity that is done during leisure time, for transport to get to and from places, or as part of a person's work, has a health benefit. Further, both moderate- and vigorous-intensity physical activity improve health.[45]

This differentiation between physical activity and exercise is very important to note. Many people often perceive physical activity as getting exercise from going to a gym or playing a sport, which may or may not have meaning for them. This perspective of physical activity as solely a strenuous or unpleasant exercise leads many to avoid even the thought of pursuing health by becoming more physically active. It should be emphasized that physical activity can be achieved in many easy and enjoyable ways (Fig. 4-4).[45]

Americans have many opportunities to be active in their everyday lives. Knowing the developmental pattern of participation in physical activity allows OT practitioners to implement plans for clients to incorporate exercise into their daily routine regardless of developmental level. Incorporating physical activity into an occupation can make it more meaningful to clients and may promote their engagement. It is important to facilitate the development of habits and routines that promote the adoption and maintenance of healthy behaviors. This can be accomplished by identifying physical activities that match a person's skills and interests, modifying the demands of the activity if necessary, and incorporating environmental supports and reducing barriers to engagement. For example, for an older adult who enjoys gardening but has arthritis, poor balance, and limited endurance, the activity could be modified by using raised flower beds and built-up handles on gardening tools, and having the person sit while working in the garden. An example of incorporating physical activity into everyday household activities is a popular program called Taskercise developed by Carolyn Barnes (Box 4-4).

Environmental factors can greatly affect a person's level of physical activity. Some factors, such as living in a place of high-density traffic, air pollution, fear of violence and crime outside of the home, or simply a lack of sidewalks, parks, and recreation facilities, may prevent people from becoming more active. It is important to consider environmental and contextual factors and provide interventions

BOX 4-4
Taskercise™

Carolyn Barnes created exercise routines that can easily be incorporated into everyday household activities. The exercises combine elements of Pilates, ballet, and isometrics and are interspersed for 30 seconds throughout normal daily tasks and chores. For example:

- Detergent bottle dumbbells
- Laundry leg lifts
- Counter push-ups
- Vacuum lunge

For more information, visit www.cleanmomma.com or read *The Clean Momma Workout* by Carolyn Barnes (2012).

that address these barriers, such as the option of virtual reality games or video workouts to allow for physical activity indoors.

In promoting an active lifestyle, the OT practitioner needs to incorporate physical activity into the client's lifestyle, work to develop sustainable habits and routines, consider the client from a holistic perspective, help the client choose desired physical activities, and incorporate evidence-based strategies that have demonstrated effectiveness. Informing clients of daily physical activity recommendations is a first step (Box 4-5).

The positive effects that physical activity has on the human body, mind, and spirit reinforce how essential it is to produce and maintain good health and well-being. Knowing the benefits of being physically active and the health risks of inactivity make choosing to be active a much easier decision. Treating from a client-centered and holistic perspective, OT practitioners can make physical activity a fun, reinforcing, and satisfying part of every person's day. Self-motivating and self-monitoring are important aspects of the process. See Box 4-6 for a simple planning and monitoring tool.

BOX 4-6
My Physical Activity Record

SUN	MON	TUES	WED	THURS	FRI	SAT

For each day, plan the activities you will do during the month. Write your goal in the box for that day.

Then throughout the month, record the activities you did for 10 minutes or more each day, the length of time you were engaged in the activity, and the intensity level.

Examples:
Walk (15 minutes, brisk/vigorous)
Gardening (30 minutes, moderate)
Swimming (60 minutes, slow)

Ergonomics and Injury Prevention

Ergonomics is "the application of human factors information to the design of tools, machines, systems, tasks, jobs, and environments for safe, comfortable and effective human use."[48] Ergonomic interventions are used in OT practice to maximize a client's occupational performance, prevent injury, and promote safety and health. OT practitioners observe client performance in a range of occupations to identify the ergonomics involved in the activity, as well as the environments in which the occupations are performed.[49] Ergonomic interventions can be provided to individuals in a variety of settings or through consultation with industry or agency personnel to develop programs and/or policies to facilitate the return to optimal function.[50]

BOX 4-5
World Health Organization Recommendations for Daily Physical Activity[46]

Adults ages 18 to 64 years: At least 150 minutes of moderate-intensity or at least 75 minutes of vigorous-intensity physical activity throughout the week, or an equivalent of both; major muscle groups should be strengthened 2 or more days a week.

Adults ages 65 and above: At least 150 minutes of moderate-intensity or at least 75 minutes of vigorous-intensity physical activity throughout the week, or an equivalent of both; for those who have poor mobility, physical activities that improve balance and help prevent falls should be done 3 or more days each week; major muscle groups should be strengthened 2 or more days a week.

OT practitioners working in industry may use ergonomic principles in the following ways:

- Conducting assessments and developing interventions for individual workers, or providing health promotion and injury prevention education programs for groups of workers
- Designing and modifying workplace tools, equipment, and behaviors to prevent injury
- Consulting with employers and insurance companies on developing programs to reduce workers' compensation costs (e.g., strategies to address the needs of aging workers)[50]

However, the workplace is not the only context in which ergonomic principles can be used. These principles and strategies can be applied to nearly any occupation in any environment. Therefore, OT practitioners in all settings must be familiar with basic ergonomic considerations, such as positioning, posture, lifting, cognitive requirements, and psychosocial factors (Fig. 4-5). Positioning and posture are important considerations for carrying out prolonged, repetitive activity safely without excessive fatigue. Good biomechanical positions are important, and no single position should be assumed for an extended period of time.[49]

Many injuries are the result of improper lifting technique and/or attempting to lift too much weight. The National Institute for Occupational Safety and Health (NIOSH) has set 51 pounds as the official lifting limit to avoid lower back pain by any single, healthy individual, for a prolonged period of time in the workplace.[54] Lifting symmetrically, without twisting the spinal column, and using large muscle groups in the legs is recommended.

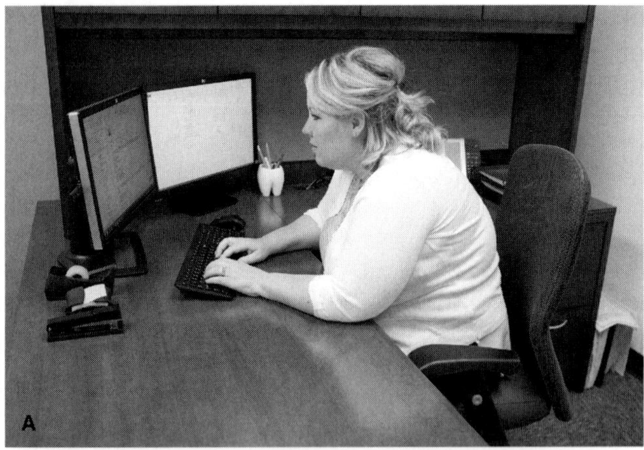

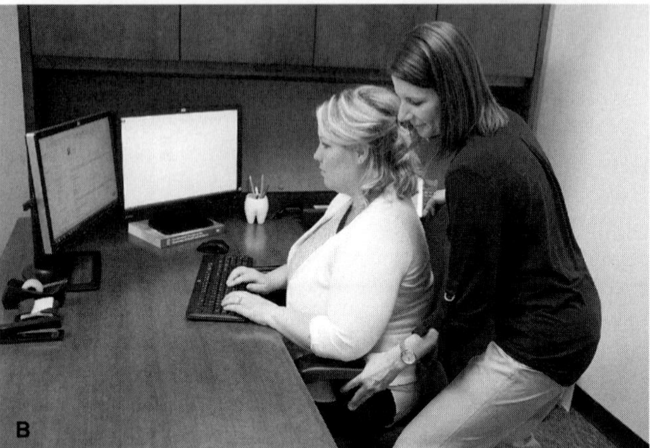

FIGURE 4-5. A. Poor office ergonomics: What can you identify as improper body mechanics in this photo? B. OTA educating the worker to make changes for improved ergonomics and the prevention of injury. Can you identify what changes were made?

THE OLDER ADULT

According to the Centers for Disease Control and Prevention, falls are the leading cause of injury and death in persons over age 65. Injuries from falls affect all areas of occupational performance.[51] Fear of falling results in a decrease in activity level with decreased endurance and strength as a consequence. So fall prevention is an important aspect of OT intervention with older adults.

One team reviewed 33 studies of fall prevention interventions.[52] Not all of the studies included OT services, but the vast majority of interventions used were within the OT scope of practice. The systematic review indicated that multifactorial interventions are strongly supported by the evidence. Multifactorial interventions combine a variety of strategies, including physical activity, home evaluation and modification, education, medication management, and assistive technology.

Home evaluation and modification are important components of a fall prevention program. Research conducted by Di Monaco et al. revealed that elderly women discharged from rehabilitation services after hip fracture can benefit from a single home visit by an occupational therapist.[53] The home visit consisted of a review of environmental hazards, performance of ADLs, and use of assistive devices. Recommendations for fall prevention were provided at the conclusion of the home visit. Risk of falling was significantly reduced in the intervention group participants, those who received the home visit, compared with those in the control group, who did not receive the home visit.

The quality of grasp of the object is another important consideration. Some objects are easily grasped (e.g., objects with handles), whereas others are more difficult (e.g., objects that are wet or slippery).

A majority of OT practitioners focus on the physical demands of tasks and work activities; however, the cognitive demands are an important ergonomic factor that can affect productivity. Cognitive workload refers to the level of mental effort or cognitive intensity needed to complete a task effectively. When cognitive demands are too low, the person may become bored. If the cognitive demands are too high, mental exhaustion, poor performance, and injuries may result.[49] Work-related and non–work-related anxiety, depression, and other forms of psychological distress are associated with increased injuries on the job, particularly upper extremity and back disorders. The association between psychosocial factors and workplace injury appears to be independent of the physical factors on the job. In addition, the impact of psychosocial factors is found in a variety of types of worksites. Therefore, psychosocial factors may be considered risk factors for the development of musculoskeletal disabilities as well.[55]

UNIVERSAL DESIGN

One strategy using ergonomic principles to improve environments for all is the universal design approach. **Universal design (UD)** is the "design of products and environments to be usable by all people, to the greatest extent possible, without the need for adaptation or specialized design."[56]

The intent of UD is to improve accessibility and usability of environments and products for persons of all ages and abilities, to enhance safety, and to prevent injury. In addition to public buildings, UD principles can be applied in a variety of settings, including education, technology, product development, worksites, home, recreational facilities, and many others. A few examples of UD are ground-level entrances without steps, lever handles for doors, ramp access in swimming pools, and signage with visual contrast.

Chronic Disease Self-Management

Chronic diseases are one of the leading causes of death and disability, and the vast majority are preventable. Chronic diseases are long-lasting conditions that can be effectively managed, but are not curable. They require ongoing medical care and/or limit ADLs.[57] According to the CDC, approximately 50% of U.S. adults have one or more chronic health conditions such as diabetes or arthritis.[58] Research has shown that **chronic disease self-management** strategies can be effective in reducing morbidity, improving QoL, and decreasing costs.[22] Self-management programs are designed to empower clients "to understand their conditions and take responsibility for their health."[59] Essentially, chronic disease self-management involves clients' active participation in the healthcare process, self-monitoring of symptoms, symptom management, making informed decisions about their health, adhering to medical recommendations, and managing the impact of the condition on their daily lives. Occupational therapists and OTAs can assist clients to manage their diseases, and engage in desired occupations in the safest and healthiest ways possible.[60]

Evidence-based self-management interventions have been developed for a number of chronic conditions, including asthma, heart disease, sleep disorders, and diabetes.[54] Of these, the most well-researched intervention is Stanford University's School of Medicine chronic disease self-management program (CDSMP).[61] The 15-hour program consists of several sessions facilitated by two trained facilitators, one a healthcare professional and the other a person with a chronic disease. The topics typically include physical activity, nutrition and meal planning, mental health issues, medication management, health literacy, social support, and evaluating new treatments and informed decision-making regarding one's health. The CDSMP has consistently demonstrated improvements in health status, healthcare utilization, self-management behaviors, and QoL. In addition, research on the CDSMP has shown that for every dollar spent on the program, 10 dollars in healthcare expenditures was saved.[61]

OT practitioners' skills in prevention, lifestyle modification, and physical and psychosocial rehabilitation are easily applicable to the management of chronic diseases.[62] OT practitioners can participate as facilitators of Stanford University's CDSMP and/or can create occupation-based chronic disease self-management programs using principles and practices from the Lifestyle Redesign® model.[43] Chronic disease self-management is explored in more depth in Chapter 25.

When working with persons with multiple chronic conditions, it is not uncommon to encounter acute emergencies. These may include hypertensive crises, seizures, hypoglycemia, sudden cardiac arrest, and choking. It is imperative for the OTA to be able to respond appropriately to these emergencies with first aid and/or cardiopulmonary resuscitation (CPR) with use of an automatic external defibrillator (AED). Box 4-7 includes brief descriptions of possible signs and symptoms of several acute emergencies and their corresponding responses. All OTAs also need to be aware of and follow any worksite, facility, or agency policies regarding emergency situations involving clients and staff.

OT Practitioner's Viewpoint

Working in home health was an eye-opener for me. I had previously worked in an inpatient rehabilitation setting in the same geographic area. Through the home health agency, I was able to provide OT services to patients discharged from the hospital. I realized that many of the occupational performance problems I was encountering with my patients (both inpatient and home health) could have been prevented. Fall prevention in the home is one obvious example. However, there are many other more subtle changes in OT interventions that could also provide impressive benefits. For example, when engaging in a cooking activity with a client, I can teach heart-healthy menu options or introduce new recipes to the person who has diabetes. I can help older adults increase their fitness levels at home by incorporating physical activities into their daily habits and routines. I can teach caregivers safe lifting techniques and energy conservation to prevent injury and fatigue. Integrating health promotion and prevention strategies into traditional OT interventions is very easy and can produce improved physical and emotional well-being for our clients and their caregivers. From this initial step, it is not difficult to imagine preventive and health promotion OT services in other arenas with a variety of populations. ~ Marjorie E. Scaffa, PhD, OTR/L, FAOTA

PSYCHOSOCIAL IMPACT

Although the focus in most adult practice settings is on improvement of physical and occupational functioning, it is critical to recognize and address psychosocial issues that affect the therapy process. Several important psychosocial considerations are discussed here, including adjustment to disability, impact of disability on the family, sexuality concerns, comorbid mental disorders, and spirituality.

Adjusting to Disability

Successful adaptation to disability requires psychological reorganization, and a four phase process of adjustment from acute injury through rehabilitation has been described.[63] The earliest phase, vigilance, occurs when the person is attempting to cope with the physiological trauma sustained from illness or injury. The person often feels detached, senses are heightened, and the cognitive demands for understanding and coping are extremely high.[63] The second phase, disruption, is characterized by disorientation, anxiety, fear of being left alone, and feelings of loss of control. Clients in this phase often perceive the environment and their caregivers as dangerous. In the third phase, enduring the self, clients become more aware of their surroundings and begin to recognize the extent of their injuries and disability. This enhanced awareness is frequently accompanied

BOX 4-7
Basic First Aid and Emergency Response

Hypertensive emergency (blood pressure [BP] exceeds 180 mm Hg systolic or 120 mm Hg diastolic)

- Possible signs and symptoms: Severe headache, shortness of breath, nosebleed, change in vision, chest pain, numbness, and weakness.
- Response: Call 911 or emergency number within your facility.

Hypotensive episode

- Possible signs and symptoms: Fainting, nausea, lightheadedness, dizziness, rapid shallow breathing.
- Response: A lower than normal BP reading is not a cause for alarm unless other symptoms are present. If other symptoms are present, consult a physician.

Seizure

- Possible signs and symptoms: Convulsions, muscle rigidity, jerking movements, brief loss of consciousness.
- Response: Stay with the person until the seizure is over, protect the person from injury, and make the person as comfortable as possible; note the length of the seizure. Do *not* restrain the person or put anything in the person's mouth. If the person is lying down, turn the person onto his or her side to prevent aspiration. If a seizure lasts 5 minutes or longer, if breathing becomes difficult, if the person appears to be choking, or if an injury has occurred, call for emergency assistance.

Hypoglycemia (low blood glucose, insulin reaction)

- Possible signs and symptoms: Shaking, sweating, chills, confusion, rapid heartbeat, impaired vision, headache, nausea, coma.
- Response: Give the person 15 to 20 grams of simple carbohydrates, for example, 2 tablespoons of raisins, one-half cup of juice or soda (not sugar free), hard candies, jellybeans, gumdrops (amounts vary). If the person becomes unresponsive, call 911.

Sudden cardiac arrest

- Possible signs and symptoms: Chest pain, shortness of breath, nausea/vomiting, racing heartbeat, dizziness, fainting, no pulse, loss of consciousness.
- Response: If trained, use an AED, begin CPR if an AED is not available; call 911.

Choking

- Possible signs and symptoms: Hands clutching the throat, inability to speak, difficulty breathing, inability to cough, skin and lips turning blue, loss of consciousness.
- Response: "5 and 5"—five sharp blows to the back between the shoulder blades with the heel of your hand, followed by five abdominal thrusts (Heimlich maneuver); call 911.

by intense psychological pain. Fostering realistic hope at this juncture is critical to the client's recovery.

The final phase, striving to regain the self, challenges the individual to merge old and new realities, both physically and psychologically. Goals in this phase are to make sense of the experience, accept the consequences, and revise and reformulate recovery expectations. This phase model provides the practitioner with a helpful framework for recognizing and anticipating the client's changing psychosocial needs during recovery and rehabilitation.[63]

Another approach to chronic disease management is a client-centered and collaborative model, focused on integration of the illness/disability into the client's life. The phases are crisis, stabilization, resolution, and integration. Within each phase, three domains are assessed and addressed: physical/behavioral, psychological, and social/interactive, which makes this model particularly relevant for OT practitioners.[64]

Phase 1, *crisis,* is characterized by shock, disbelief, and a sense of urgency. The focus is on trauma and crisis management, and the goal is stabilization. During this phase, OT practitioners can begin to establish a therapeutic relationship, offer reassurance, restructure ADLs if necessary, and provide illness education. Phase 2, *stabilization,* is characterized by low tolerance for ambiguity and a reluctance to accept the status quo. During this phase, OT practitioners can instruct clients on illness self-management (e.g., medication management), energy conservation, and work simplification techniques. Facilitation of feelings, processing grief, and the acceptance of a new normal are psychological aspects of care during this phase.[64]

Phase 3, *resolution,* is characterized by increased ability to tolerate the varying and potentially long term disease process, role and identity experimentation, and the development of a sense of meaning out of the illness experience, and the goal is the construction of a new self. During this phase, OT practitioners can facilitate the client's empowerment and self-advocacy, engage the client in life-affirming, meaningful activities, and reframe issues as challenges to be overcome. Phase 4, *integration,* is characterized by feelings of self-efficacy and acceptance, a broadened sense of meaning, reconstruction of roles and routines, and the establishment of a new normal. The focus of this phase is on the assimilation of the illness into a whole and meaningful life, and the goal is the integration of the precrisis and postcrisis self. During this phase, OT practitioners can modify and reinforce self-management strategies, and encourage and support attempts at self-advocacy. Phase 4 is often experienced transiently due to cycles of relapse and remission in many disease processes. It is not uncommon for clients to revisit previous phases multiple times.[64]

COMPLICATING FACTORS

Many factors can facilitate or hinder psychosocial adjustment to disability. Three considerations—attribution, pain, and sleep quality—are discussed here. Attribution is the process by which people make sense of their experiences. Attributions not only describe but also create reality. Some attributions are helpful to recovery, whereas others are not. Health-promoting attributions include the following:

- Faith—a belief that the illness or disability will eventually have meaning and serve a higher purpose

- Acceptance—a belief that injury, illness, and disability are part of all nature and no one is immune
- Personal responsibility—a belief that each individual bears responsibility for his or her choices and the outcome of the decision[65]

Pain is another factor that can affect adjustment to disability. Many illnesses, injuries, and disabilities have pain as a symptom. Pain perception is a personal experience and is affected not only by physiological processes, but also by psychosocial factors. Chronic pain can significantly limit occupational participation and can result in problems concentrating, altered mood, and social withdrawal. Unremitting pain, and the loss of control associated with it, can result in a sense of helplessness and hopelessness. In addition, pain often negatively affects sleep initiation, maintenance, and quality. Recognition and validation of the client's pain is a critical first step in pain management. Grading (changing the painful demands to make easier), adapting (performing a painful task in an alternate way), positioning, and emotional support are some strategies OT practitioners may use to assist clients with pain management.

Sleep is the last complicating factor to be discussed here. Recovering from illness or injury is often an exhausting process complicated by sleep problems; adequate sleep is essential for good health. Sleep deficits can result in diminished attention, memory problems, and poor emotion regulation. Immune system function can also be affected.[65]

Sleep is considered an occupation and is therefore within the OT practitioner's domain of practice to evaluate and treat. Sleep interventions typically address the sleep environment and sleep hygiene. Optimal sleep environments are "quiet, dark, cool, comfortable, clean, and safe."[65] Sleep hygiene refers to behaviors that are in harmony with the natural wake-sleep cycle. Consistent bedtimes, refraining from use of caffeine or alcohol late at night, and the use of white noise or soft music are examples of sleep-enhancing strategies.

Impact on Family

Illness, injury, and disability affect not only the individual, but the entire family. How an individual client experiences illness, injury, and disability, and how it affects the client's functioning and the effectiveness of therapy, is frequently a consequence of the person's relationships with family and significant others. Frequently, families "have tremendous expertise and knowledge related to their family members, family life, the illness or disability of their family member, and the ways in which treatment recommendations can most likely be implemented in the home."[66] As a result, families are an extremely useful resource in the therapy process.

Families are social systems, and as such when one component of the system is changed, the entire system is affected. For example, when a family member loses functional capacity, the entire family experiences grief, as well as changes in roles and routines. Therefore, adaptation to disability is a family affair; the family is forced to reorganize itself, often contrary to the desires of family members. Role renegotiation and role reorganization often result in role strain and loss or change in relationship patterns. Role strain and stress occurs when the role demands, expectations, and responsibilities in a person's life exceed the person's capabilities. For example, when a spouse who has always managed the finances, as well as cared for the home and yard, becomes seriously ill, the other spouse must learn and assume those roles, plus that of caregiver. According to Olson and Wong, "Routine relationships typically provide a sense of stability, security, and social support. As the person grieves the loss of familiar relationships and a pattern of comfortable interaction, new relationships and new patterns of interaction have not yet developed, thereby reducing support for taking on new roles."[67]

It is important to recognize that family is not simply a matter of genetics. Families come in all shapes and sizes. The critical determining factor is who the client considers to be family members.[66] OT practitioners can assist families by providing specific information about the disability, validating their feelings, fostering family inclusion in the rehabilitation process, fostering hope and effective coping, and connecting families with community resources. Some families may require a referral for family counseling.

Sexuality Concerns

Disability can also affect intimate relationships. Sexuality is an essential element of being human and is one of the ways that individuals relate to each other. The concept of sexuality does not simply refer to sexual activity, but also encompasses self-concept, sexual identity, gender roles, and sexual orientation. Chronic illness and disability can have a profound effect on relationship and sexual satisfaction and thereby affect the QoL of clients and their partners.

Disability may affect sexual desire, capacity, and performance due to reduced cardiovascular, pulmonary, and neurological function, pain, and altered body image. Medications, particularly cardiac drugs, antidepressants, hormones, and analgesics, can also impair sexual function. Sexual dysfunction associated with chronic illness may take the form of decreased sexual desire, impaired sexual arousal, inability to achieve orgasm, premature ejaculation, impotence, and painful intercourse. Sexual activity may need to be modified and/or adapted due to functional limitations imposed by illness, injury, or disability.

It is important when addressing a client's sexuality concerns to be nonjudgmental, to be sensitive to the client's sexual orientation, and to avoid sexual stereotypes.[68,69] Sexual satisfaction is an important component of well-being and should be addressed by OT practitioners. Persons with disabilities may be hesitant to engage in sexual activity for a variety of reasons, including feelings of inadequacy and undesirability, fear of rejection, and concerns about overexertion or increases in pain. Clients may need assistance to expand their concept of sexuality and to explore new means of sexual expression.

Interaction of Physical and Mental Health

Even if the client with a physical disability does not exhibit a diagnosable mental disorder, it is important for OT practitioners to facilitate optimal mental health. "Mental health is a state of well-being in which an individual realizes his or her own abilities, can cope with the normal stresses of life, can work productively and is able to make a contribution to his or her community."[70] Mentally healthy people accept their limitations, have a high level of self-awareness, effectively cope with disappointment, experience a range of emotions, establish and maintain meaningful relationships, and demonstrate the capacity for empathy and compassion toward others.[71] These are areas that can be addressed through OT intervention.

The basic principles of mental health promotion are the same as those for the promotion of physical health, and include maintaining a biopsychosocial perspective on health, promoting QoL as well as prevention of illness, intervening at a variety of levels rather than simply focusing on individual behavior, and establishing collaborative relationships with other professions. Although the research literature on mental health promotion is limited, some approaches and strategies appear promising.

An evidence-based approach to mental health promotion is described in the Positive Psychology literature as a group of strategies for promoting psychological and emotional well-being through the development of character strengths.[72] Strategies are categorized as emotion-focused, cognitive-focused, interpersonal-focused, self-focused, and coping-focused strategies. Emotion-focused strategies are designed to foster resilience, self-esteem, and emotional intelligence. Cognitive-focused strategies enhance creativity, problem-solving, and self-efficacy. Interpersonal-focused strategies encourage the development of gratitude, compassion, empathy, and altruism. Self-focused strategies cultivate humility and authenticity, and coping-focused strategies incorporate meditation, spirituality, and the pursuit of meaningfulness.[72]

Spirituality

The vast majority of models of health and wellness identify multiple dimensions of well-being, including physical, social, intellectual, emotional, environmental, and spiritual. The acknowledgment of spirituality as health-enhancing and the inclusion of spirituality in the OTPF-3 as a client factor legitimizes its incorporation in OT practice.[4]

In the OTPF-3, *spirituality* is defined as "the aspect of humanity that refers to the way individuals seek and express meaning and purpose and the way they experience their connectedness to the moment, to self, to others, to nature, and to the significant or sacred."[4] Research has demonstrated a significant relationship between spirituality and health. Numerous studies have indicated the positive influence of spirituality on mental health, physical well-being, recovery from illness, and HRQOL.[73] In addition, religious affiliation and participation has been shown to decrease all-cause mortality rates by 10% to 20%.[74] However, the mechanisms by which spirituality affects health, morbidity, and mortality remain unclear.

Persons with chronic diseases and/or disabilities face major challenges. Spirituality may provide purpose and meaning in life and provides a source of strength when coping with difficult circumstances. In addition, spirituality has an effect on the choices a person makes in life and the person's use of time.[75] Hope, coping, and resilience are resources for occupational adaptation that are often associated with spirituality. Hope is the belief in the possibility that life can be fulfilling; coping refers to the ability to effectively manage a difficult life event; and resilience is the ability to persevere despite significant obstacles.[76] A person's values, beliefs, and spirituality are important contributors to resilience. Values and beliefs such as optimism for the future, altruism, gratitude, and an appreciation for beauty contribute to resilience, whereas pessimism, fear of the future, and a sense of entitlement inhibit resilience.

Although engaging in religious and spiritual practices and rituals are obvious manifestations of meaning in a person's life, meaningful occupational participation may also include a spiritual element. Clients have reported the experience of spiritual meaning in caring for pets, caring for others, gardening, taking a walk in nature, meditating, listening to music, volunteering, and creating art through various activities. Spirituality is inherently a relationship phenomenon, a relationship with a higher power, and relationships to others. So too may the therapeutic relationship incorporate spiritual elements.[76]

One approach to understanding and incorporating a client's spiritual preferences into the therapeutic process is the use of the FICA model, which consists of four questions:

- *Faith:* What do you believe in that gives meaning to your life?
- *Importance/Influence:* How important is your faith or spirituality to you?
- *Community:* Are you part of a religious or spiritual community?
- *Address/Application:* How would you like me to address these issues in your health care?

In a survey of OT practitioners, Taylor et al.[77] found that 96% of OT practitioners agreed that spirituality influences health, yet only 37% agreed that OT should address the spiritual needs of clients. Of the OT practitioners who incorporated spirituality in the therapeutic process, 74% stated that they prayed for clients, 53% discussed with their clients how their spiritual beliefs may be helpful in their recovery, and 23% prayed with clients.[77] It is particularly important for the OT practitioner not to impose their own spiritual and/or religious beliefs on the client, nor to treat the client any differently once their beliefs are identified.

Remain respectful with the focus firmly on the occupational engagement of the client and family.

PRACTITIONER HEALTH AND WELLNESS AND PROFESSIONAL SELF-CARE

To best serve their clients, OT practitioners must attend to their own health and wellness needs. This is often referred to as **professional self-care.** In its most basic form, professional self-care means engaging in behaviors and activities that increase energy, lower stress, and contribute to health and well-being. The exact combination of behaviors and activities may vary from person to person, but there are some general principles worth following.

Interestingly, although OT practitioners often encourage their clients to focus on the basics of health maintenance, including adequate sleep, good nutrition, physical activity, and social support, there is often neglect of these aspects in the OT practitioner's life. Additional issues to consider when focused on professional self-care include injury and illness prevention through good body mechanics, infection control, stress management strategies, and the prevention of compassion fatigue.

The Basics

The basics of health promotion are restful sleep, adequate physical activity, and good nutrition. A healthy sleep-wake schedule should be composed of regularity, consistency with the body's circadian rhythm, and plenty of time for the body to have a continuous sleep. Exercising a few hours before a typical sleep time will enrich the individual's sleep. Factors such as caffeine and tobacco use have been shown to cause difficulty in falling asleep. Although alcohol is a sedative and may help a person fall asleep, it can block rapid eye movement (REM) sleep. During REM sleep, areas of the brain responsible for learning are stimulated. Another aspect of sleep is having good sleep hygiene that consists of quiet, dark, cool, comfortable, clean, and safe places to sleep.[65]

Adequate nutrition plays a pivotal role in physical and mental health. Stress can negatively affect a person's immune system and increase the body's need for specific nutrients. Healthy eating enhances focus, alertness, energy level, and overall well-being. Poor nutrition, on the other hand, can produce negative hormonal effects, weight issues, imbalances in blood sugar, immune system dysfunction, and overall poor health. Creating a reserve of healthy nutrients in the body provides protection against illness during times of excess stress.

Another health-enhancing behavior that is both simple and exceptionally effective is physical activity (Fig. 4-6). Research has shown that physical activity has many health-promoting benefits, including decreasing muscle tension, increasing release of endorphins, facilitating restful sleep, increasing oxygenation in the blood, and improving concentration.[78] Incorporating physical activity as a regular feature in one's daily routine can be extremely effective.

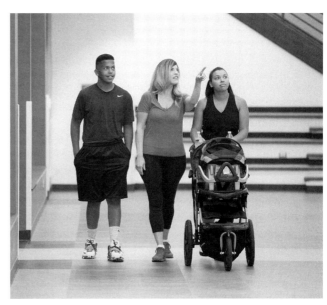

FIGURE 4-6. Physical activity and social support are important components of professional self-care.

Research indicates that social support enhances resilience and is an essential ingredient for physical and mental health.[79] Social support networks provide information, emotional encouragement, and tangible assistance when needed. A social support network comprises friends, family, neighbors, and colleagues who provide one with a sense of belonging, increased self-worth, and feelings of security. Epidemiological studies have shown that social isolation and inadequate social support are associated with increased prevalence of a variety of medical and psychiatric conditions.[79] People who have positive, fulfilling relationships live longer, healthier lives.[80]

Body Mechanics

Body mechanics is defined as "the way one moves the body, spine, and extremities during everyday activities to protect the body, especially the back, from pain and injury."[81] An OT practitioner should engage in the use of proper body mechanics when assisting clients. Proper body mechanics consist of the following techniques: keeping shoulders and hips parallel, resisting trunk rotation when lifting, maintaining feet at shoulder width apart, using larger muscle groups when lifting, bending at knees and hips while keeping back straight, and holding large items close to the body during lifts or carries.[82] OT practitioners need to know and participate in proper body mechanics to avoid any injuries. OT practitioners can apply their knowledge of proper body mechanics when performing lifts, bed mobility, and transfers with their clients.[81]

Infection Control

Infections can be spread in several different ways, including direct contact, indirect contact, droplet transmission, and airborne transmission. When an infection is spread through direct contact, the infection spreads from the infected individual straight to the other individual after an interaction. Indirect contact transmission occurs when the infected individual comes into contact with an object, such as a doorknob or another individual, who then transmits the infection to the newly affected individual. Droplet transmission occurs when infection is transmitted through respiratory droplets emitted when an infected person coughs, sneezes or talks. Airborne transmission occurs due to the airborne droplets containing an active infectious agent over a period of time and distance.[83]

Universal precautions, also known as standard precautions, are an approach to infection control created by the U.S. Occupational Safety and Health Administration (OSHA) to protect healthcare practitioners and prevent the spread of infections. Universal precautions consider all human blood and bodily fluids as if they were infectious for human immunodeficiency virus (HIV), hepatitis B virus, and other blood-borne pathogens. Healthcare practitioners should engage in thorough hand washing after any direct contact with clients (Fig. 4-7).[84] Hands should also be washed after anything has been touched that could potentially contain contaminants. Alcohol sanitizing solutions are an effective method to clean hands and prevent infection when an individual has not come into contact with any bodily fluids.[85] Additionally, healthcare practitioners need to wear disposable gloves when coming into contact with any bodily fluids and when necessary, the healthcare practitioner should wear a mask, eye shields, and a gown (Fig. 4-8). As a healthcare practitioner, one should quickly clean up bodily fluid spills with the required sanitization and protective equipment, and place harmful and sharp items in the proper waste disposals. Furthermore, healthcare practitioners should take the initiative to ensure that all wounds are properly bandaged and covered up.[84]

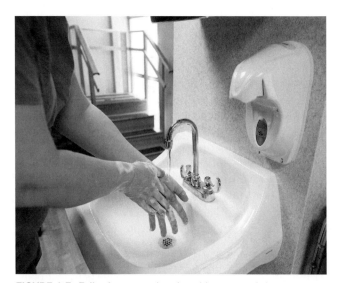

FIGURE 4-7. Following proper hand washing protocols is a requirement for all healthcare workers.

Stress Management

Stress affects everyone daily whether it is caused by environmental factors or the interaction of biological, psychological, and social (biopsychosocial) factors. Stress can be divided into three types: acute, chronic, and posttraumatic. Stress-related conditions occur when acute stress becomes episodic and then progresses into damaging chronic stress. Chronic stress has been shown to be associated with numerous mental and physical health problems, for example, depression, anxiety, heart disease, asthma, diabetes, and gastrointestinal disorders.[86] Prevention of stress-related illnesses can be challenging as people may become so accustomed to their chronic stress that it becomes accepted as a part of their daily life.

Early identification of the symptoms of chronic stress is critical to the prevention of stress-related health problems. Common symptoms include cognitive signs (memory problems, concentration problems, constant worrying), emotional signs (irritability, feeling overwhelmed, moodiness), physical signs (headaches, chest pain, lowered sexual drive), and/or behavioral (eating more or less, sleeping too much or too little, use of alcohol/cigarettes) warning signs.[86] Biofeedback therapy and relaxation strategies can assist a person to monitor physiological changes that indicate stress and take appropriate measures to reduce stress levels.[87]

Various relaxation techniques can be used for self-care by OT practitioners. Breath training focuses on addressing good breathing habits by normalizing shallow or quick breathing into deeper, diaphragmatic breathing. This slight adaptation works to provide more oxygen to the body and mind while simultaneously drastically reducing the body's waste product, carbon dioxide, which tends to build up during stressful situations when rapid breathing is most prominent. Progressive relaxation works by reducing muscle tension. Last, mindfulness practices such as sitting meditation, yoga, and tai chi are often successfully used in treating a wide range of stress-related conditions.[78] Numerous print and online resources on these practices are readily available.

Preventing Compassion Fatigue

Compassion fatigue is defined as "an emotional state with negative psychological and physical consequences that emanate from acute or prolonged caregiving of people stricken by intense trauma, suffering, or misfortune."[88] Compassion fatigue is a direct result of ignoring the symptoms of stress and inattention to personal emotions over time. One of the most insidious features of compassion fatigue is its attack on a key element of OT practice, the practitioner's empathy and the ability to show compassion.[89] The terms *burnout,*

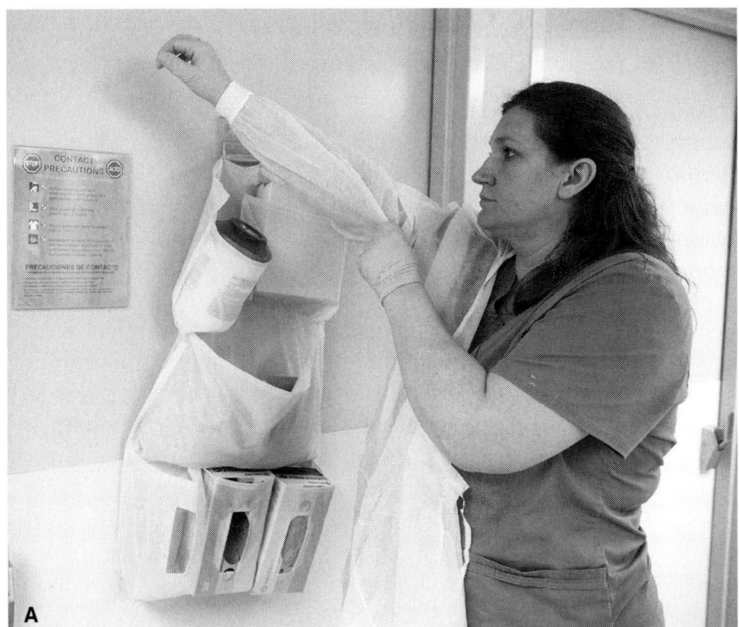
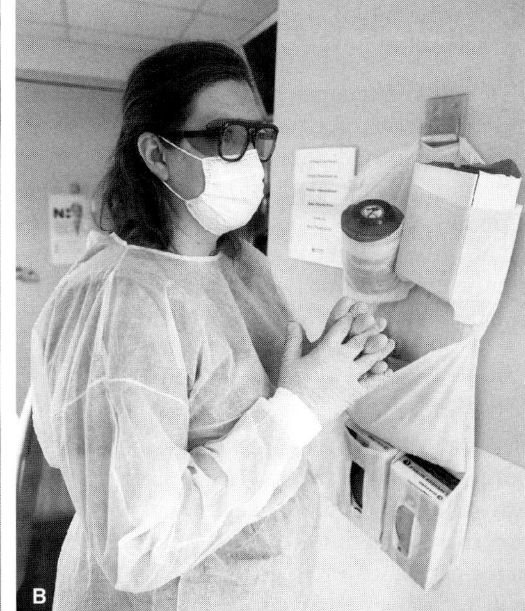

FIGURE 4-8. A. OTA applying the appropriate personal protective equipment (PPE) before entering the client's room. **B.** The OTA leaves the client's room before removing PPE.

vicarious trauma, and *secondary traumatic stress* are often associated with compassion fatigue. **Burnout** "is a psychological syndrome that involves a prolonged response to chronic interpersonal stressors on the job."[90] Burnout is described as being a chronic result of workplace stress, whereas compassion fatigue is an acute phenomenon from caring for individuals who are suffering.[91] **Vicarious trauma** "refers to the impact on a caregiver of repeated emotionally intimate contact with trauma survivors."[92] Vicarious trauma is postulated to change cognitive schemas and beliefs, which results in an interference to the practitioner's sense of meaning and worldview.[92] For example, healthcare providers experiencing vicarious trauma may question their spiritual beliefs or religious faith, feel a loss of control over their environment and a disrupted sense of safety, and experience disconnection from self and others. **Secondary traumatic stress** is closely linked to compassion fatigue and is defined as "stress resulting from knowledge about a traumatizing event experienced by another and from wanting to help the suffering person."[92] It is important to understand that compassion fatigue, vicarious trauma, and secondary posttraumatic stress are natural, unpreventable sequelae of working with traumatized, distressed clients.[88] However, the negative consequences of these conditions can be reduced, mitigated, and managed with appropriate self-care strategies.

WHO IS AT RISK?

Compassion fatigue is considered an occupational hazard, and almost everyone who works with clients or persons who have been traumatized will at some point develop a degree of compassion fatigue.[90] Caregivers who naturally demonstrate the ability to show compassion and express empathy are at the greatest risk for compassion fatigue when open to increasing grief and loss in their work.[88] Compassion fatigue is most commonly reported to be experienced by healthcare providers, from as little as one exposure to a traumatic event, but has also been reported to be experienced by family caregivers.[91] It has also been noted that "the capacity for compassion and empathy seems to be at the core of our ability to do the work and at the core of our ability to be wounded by the work."[88] Compassion fatigue not only has a negative effect on the practitioner, it also inadvertently affects client satisfaction with services. Clients have reported lower satisfaction rates from their services when a practitioner who is struggling with compassion fatigue provides care.[90]

SIGNS AND SYMPTOMS OF COMPASSION FATIGUE

Compassion fatigue presents with signs that are similar to common everyday difficulties such as stress. It is important for the practitioner to be able to recognize the following signs and symptoms:

- Trouble sleeping/exhaustion
- Amplified or exaggerated physical reflexes
- Increased emotional reactivity/hypersensitivity to emotional material
- Hypervigilance or heightened sensitivity to potential threats to self
- Diminished interest in regular activities
- Reduced ability to feel sympathy and empathy
- Anger and irritability
- Absenteeism (work, family events, social events) or poor work skills

- Difficulty separating work life from personal life
- Depersonalization
- Physical and emotional exhaustion[89]

Emotional exhaustion is known to be the primary product of compassion fatigue and can lead to difficulties with creating a genuine empathic relationship with clients, which in turn can negatively affect delivery of services.[93] Furthermore, loss of empathy can affect proper development of therapeutic relationships. These symptoms not only affect the practitioner at work, but they carry over to out-of-work contexts such as the family and home.

PREVENTING AND COPING WITH COMPASSION FATIGUE

Welsh coined the phrase "practicing responsible selfishness" when discussing ways to prevent compassion fatigue.[94] Most caregivers feel guilty for taking time out of their lives to take care of themselves, but it is important as an OT practitioner to participate in self-care activities to be an effective caregiver (Fig. 4-9). Self-care techniques include monitoring sleep patterns and physical and emotional reactivity, and participating in physical activities. Self-care methods include, but are not limited to, yoga, being with friends, laughter, engaging in light-hearted conversations not related to work, comedy, participating in hobbies, and spiritual practices.[93] Monitoring oneself for work-life balance weekly or on a regular basis is also important. If not treated, compassion fatigue can manifest in depression. It is natural for caring professionals to feel secondary effects from client trauma, but it is important to identify and treat the signs and symptoms of compassion fatigue early. If stress reduction self-care strategies are not working, it is helpful to seek professional treatment, such as counseling.[89,94]

COMPASSION SATISFACTION

Compassion satisfaction is simply defined as "the ability to receive gratification from caregiving."[95] Compassion satisfaction is the direct opposite of compassion fatigue and, in general, when levels of compassion satisfaction are higher, there is less risk of compassion fatigue.[96] OT practitioners should strive to develop a high level of compassion satisfaction within the workplace environment. Figure 4-8 depicts a simple formula to decrease the risk of developing compassion fatigue.[93] Practitioners who effectively use coping strategies to reduce stress and increase opportunities for relaxation, and at the same time remove themselves from the therapeutic setting from time to time (e.g., for vacations and holidays), are less likely to develop compassion fatigue and more likely to enhance their compassion satisfaction.

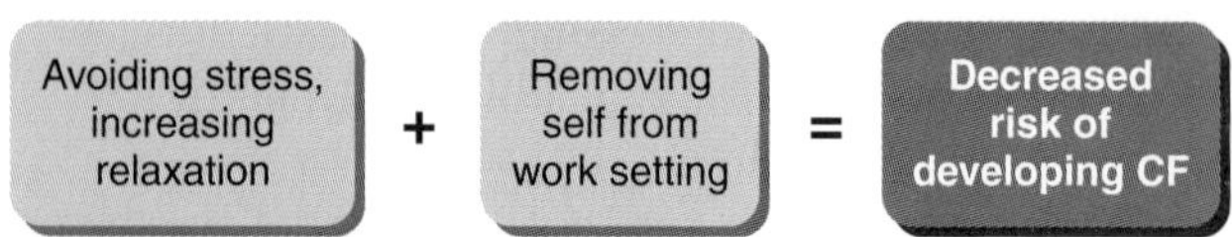

FIGURE 4-9. A formula for preventing the development of compassion fatigue (CF).

Professionals who care for their mind, body, and spirit will secondarily provide better care for clients, thereby increasing both client and practitioner satisfaction.

SUMMARY

Healthcare reform is focused on the goals of improving clients' experiences of health care, enhancing the health of populations, and reducing the per capita cost of healthcare provision. As a result, increasing emphasis is being placed on prevention, health promotion, and primary care. Health-promoting behaviors include "exercise or physical activity, nutritional strategies, lifestyle adjustment, maintaining a positive attitude, health responsibility behaviors, and seeking and receiving interpersonal support."[97] OT practitioners can make significant contributions in all of these areas for persons with and without disabilities.

Prevention and health promotion are within the domain of practice for OT practitioners and therefore are appropriate for evaluation and intervention.[4] Several accreditation standards for educational programs relate directly to prevention and health promotion and emphasize the need for skill development in these competencies.[98]

If the OT profession is to meet society's occupational needs in the future, OT educators and practitioners must develop and use innovative strategies "that facilitate the infusion of health promotion throughout occupational therapy services across the continuum of care."[99] In addition, it will become increasingly important for OT to demonstrate its effectiveness in prevention and health promotion through scientific research evidence.

REVIEW QUESTIONS

1. Jason is 55 years old and was recently diagnosed with diabetes. Both of his parents died at young ages (father at 60 and mother at 63) due to complications of poorly managed diabetes. You are concerned about his emotional reaction to the diagnosis and anticipate that Jason is likely to be experiencing which three of the following?
   a. Anger
   b. Depression
   c. Shame
   d. Guilt
   e. Anxiety
   f. Fear
2. Mr. Tillman was involved in a motor vehicle accident 2 years ago when he was 25, which resulted in a spinal cord injury (SCI) at level T3 and a mild traumatic brain injury (TBI). You and an occupational therapist have been treating him for 6 weeks in home health, and have recently noticed a decline in visitors and social support. Mr. Tillman reports that he feels worthless and that his quality of life has declined significantly. Which of the following are you most concerned about as his OTA?
   a. I am most concerned about Mr. Tillman returning to work, which previously brought him joy.
   b. I am most concerned about Mr. Tillman committing suicide due to secondary symptoms caused by his SCI and TBI.
   c. I am most concerned about social isolation and anger.
   d. I am most concerned about Mr. Tillman's difficulties with mobility and emotional dysregulation.

3. Jane has been a practicing OTA for 23 years in an acute care setting. Recently she has been experiencing increased caseloads due to company reorganization. Her supervisor notices many symptoms that suggest that Jane is experiencing compassion fatigue. Which three of the following are symptoms of compassion fatigue?
   a. Irritability
   b. Decreased emotional reactivity
   c. Diminished physical reflexes
   d. Depersonalization
   e. Reduced ability to feel empathy
   f. Over exercising
4. Cecelia has been working in an outpatient psychiatric setting for the past 10 years with adults who have experienced trauma. She feels emotionally exhausted and is having difficulty creating empathic relationships with clients. As her friend and colleague, what might you suggest to help her?
   a. Take some time off, go on vacation.
   b. See a psychiatrist for medication.
   c. Change work settings.
   d. Start a new hobby.
5. Emily is a 32-year-old single mother of three children. She has shared that she dropped out of high school when she became pregnant with her first child. She has not been taking her blood pressure medication regularly and as a result has been experiencing headaches. You suspect the cause of her nonadherence to her medication may be due to:
   a. Educational level
   b. Socioeconomic status
   c. Race/ethnicity
   d. Limited health literacy
6. Mr. Jones is a 52-year-old accountant who is depressed because he has gained 50 pounds in the past 2 years. As a result, he stays at home because he is embarrassed and self-conscious about his appearance since the weight gain. Which three of the following treatment strategies would you use to address this client's weight concerns?
   a. Help him create realistic goals for nutrition.
   b. Educate him on active leisure pursuits and help him develop a fitness plan.
   c. Tell him to change his bad habits and routines.
   d. Teach him healthy meal preparation.
   e. Encourage him to give up his friends with whom he goes out to eat.
   f. End OT treatment because he requires a psychiatrist.
7. Mrs. Porter is a 73-year-old retired nurse who likes to spend most of her time at home. Lately she has been feeling stressed out and overwhelmed by issues going on with her family. Which of the following might be the most appropriate recommendation for her to get some physical activity and relieve some of her stress?
   a. Join a weekly book club.
   b. Play computer games online.
   c. Plant some flowers in her garden.
   d. Join a local gym to work out.
8. Mr. Laramie is recovering from a CVA and is receiving OT services in a skilled nursing facility. You notice that his mood often changes abruptly with no apparent cause. Which of the following would be an appropriate intervention to address his emotional lability?
   a. Table games with other patients
   b. Meal preparation in the clinic kitchen
   c. A craft activity that requires planning and sequencing
   d. Practicing diaphragmatic breathing and guided imagery
9. Jeremy is a 25-year-old young man who has cerebral palsy. Due to his disability, he is finding the volume of work he has to complete each night challenging. The increased demands of his new job are causing him to experience significant emotional stress. Which intervention strategy would be most appropriate to use with this client?
   a. Promote his development of self-awareness and character strengths.
   b. Increase the number of coping strategies in his repertoire.
   c. Build social skills to reduce his isolation.
   d. Talk to his boss about reducing the amount of work he needs to complete.
10. Stanley recently retired from a factory job he has had for 40 years due to chronic back pain. He is not wealthy, but he has no current financial worries. Many of his friends are still working full-time. He spends most of his days watching TV and playing computer games. As a result, he has become bored and socially isolated. Stanley is experiencing an occupational risk factor known as:
    a. Occupational marginalization
    b. Occupational deprivation
    c. Occupational imbalance
    d. Occupational isolation

CASE STUDY

Robert is a 68-year-old male client diagnosed with diabetes, hypertension, obesity, and a history of heart problems. He is a retired railroad worker. He was married to his wife of 39 years and she recently passed away instantly during a motor vehicle crash. They had one son who now lives 15 hours away. The son has a wife and five children, as well as a successful, busy law career. This makes it difficult for him to visit, call, and assist his father with care. Robert's hobbies include fishing, playing cards, and watching all types of sports. Recently, he has been severely depressed due to the loss of his wife. Robert complains of numbness in his right foot and dizziness and weakness after meals. He reports that he is consuming much more than he typically would during meals, and he often snacks on large quantities of sugary foods during the day and before bedtime. Robert has been having trouble sleeping and often forgets to take his medications. Some days when he has been feeling especially depressed, he purposely is noncompliant with his medications and refuses to take them at all. He reports that he has not felt like himself lately and feels exhausted all of the time.

1. What are some of the unhealthy behaviors this client is engaged in that could be addressed by an OTA? What interventions might be used to address his unhealthy behaviors?
2. Why might Robert lack motivation to make healthy changes in his lifestyle?
3. What strategies could be used to increase his motivation?
4. How might an increase in physical activity address his health problems?

PUTTING IT ALL TOGETHER Sample Treatment and Documentation

Setting	Home health services
Client Profile	Mr. Bennett, 68 y/o, 6' 4" tall, obese male, smoker, with open, stage 2 pressure injury on buttocks due to inactivity, poor control of diabetes and inadequate medication management
Work History	Retired high school teacher
Insurance	Medicare
Psychological	Long-term history of depression, recent suicidal ideation
Social	Married 44 years, two married adult children living in other parts of the country, four grandchildren
Cognitive	Spouse expresses concern about his recent memory lapses
Motor and Manual Muscle Testing (MMT)	Deconditioned, poor endurance/activity tolerance (<10 min), participates in minimal physical activity, ambulates with cane
ADLs	Min A with lower body dressing and bathing Bathroom tub/shower combo with shower chair and hand held shower head, requires Mod A for transfers due to fall risk Standard height toilet, trouble wiping and pulling up pants
IADLs	Spouse is responsible for most IADL tasks, client no longer drives due to poor sensation in his feet
Goals	Within 4 weeks: 1. Client will be modified independent in lower body dressing and bathing with the use of adaptive equipment (AE) and techniques. 2. Client's endurance/activity tolerance for ADL performance will increase to 20 min with no complaints of fatigue. 3. Client will routinely perform pressure relief strategies to prevent future decubiti. 4. Client will adhere to medication regimen consistently with the use of a medication box and alarm system. 5. Client will engage in three physical recreational activities of choice weekly. 6. Client will demonstrate increased safety and performance of transfers for toileting and bathing.

OT TREATMENT SESSION 1

THERAPEUTIC ACTIVITY	TIME	GOAL(S) ADDRESSED	OTA RATIONALE
Educate and demonstrate to client and caregiver use of AE for lower body dressing, train and practice using reacher, dressing stick, sock aid, sock loops, long handled shoe horn, etc.	20 min	#1	*Education and Training:* Identification of most effective AE solutions for lower body dressing
Educate client and caregiver on use of raised toilet seat and handrails for safety. Practice transfers on/off toilet and use of AE to pull up pants after toileting.	20 min	#6	*Education and Training:* Enhanced safety and performance of toileting at home
Educate client and caregiver on the importance of preventing decubiti and prevention strategies, including repositioning, decreased sitting, quitting smoking, healthy nutrition, and skin care.	10 min	#3	*Education and Training:* Reduce likelihood of future development of open wounds and enhance overall health
Administer the Activity Card Sort.	10 min	#5	*Assessment:* Identification of client's interests in physical activities

SOAP note: 10/8/—, 10:00 am–11:00 am

S: Client stated that the raised toilet seat and handrails make him feel safer when transferring to commode.

O: Client was seen in home with wife present. Client reported pain (4/10) due to open injury on buttocks. Nursing staff visited yesterday to dress it, and is expected to return later today. After demonstration and practice, client preferred and was most effective using reacher, sock loops, and long-handled shoe horn for lower body dressing. However, he fatigued easily, experienced shortness of breath, and required several short rest breaks during training. With raised toilet seat and handrails, client was able to safely transfer independently, but continues to need Min A for pulling up pants. Activity Card Sort assessment indicated client interest in gardening, landscape painting, and woodworking.

PUTTING IT ALL TOGETHER Sample Treatment and Documentation (continued)

A: Transfer training and AE on commode were well received; information was provided regarding ordering equipment. Further training and practice with lower body dressing and bathing will likely increase client's ability in these ADLs. Poor endurance currently limits client participation in physical activities.

P: Continue to visit 2x per week for ADL training and introduce health management and maintenance activities, particularly medication adherence and modifying health risk behaviors. Client's readiness for change will be assessed during the next session.

Sebastian Billings, COTA/L, 10/8/—, 2:50 pm

TREATMENT SESSION 2

What could you do next with this client?

TREATMENT SESSION 3

In addition to standard OT services, what prevention and health promotion interventions might you use with this client and/or his family?

REFERENCES

1. World Health Organization. (1986). The Ottawa charter for health promotion. Retrieved from www.who.int/healthpromotion/conferences/previous/ottawa/en/
2. U.S. Department of Health and Human Services. (2015). About Healthy People. Retrieved from http://www.healthypeople.gov/2020/About-Healthy-People
3. Cohen, R. (2013). A brief introduction to the new Healthy People 2020 initiative. *Beginnings, 33*(1), 4–7.
4. American Occupational Therapy Association. (2014). Occupational therapy practice framework: Domain and process (3rd ed.). *American Journal of Occupational Therapy, 68*(Suppl. 1), S1–S48. doi:10.5014/ajot.2014.682006
5. World Health Organization. (2015). WHOQOL: Measuring quality of life: Introducing the WHOQOL instruments. Retrieved from http://www.who.int/healthinfo/survey/whoqol-qualityoflife/en/
6. Liddle, J., & McKenna, K. (2000). Quality of life: An overview of issues for use in occupational therapy outcome measurement. *Australian Occupational Therapy Journal, 47*(2), 77–85. doi:10.1046/j.1440-1630.2000.00217.x
7. Burns, T. M., Graham, C. D., Rose, M. R., & Simmons, Z. (2012). Quality of life and measures of quality of life in patients with neuromuscular disorders. *Muscle & Nerve, 46*(1), 9–25. doi:10.1002/mus.23245
8. Conneeley, A. L. (2003). Quality of life and traumatic brain injury: A one-year longitudinal qualitative study. *British Journal of Occupational Therapy, 66*(10), 440–446. doi:10.1177/030802260306601002
9. Venes, D. (Ed.). (2013). *Taber's cyclopedic medical dictionary* (22nd ed.). Philadelphia, PA: F. A. Davis.
10. Tulsky, D. S., Kisala, P. A., Victorson, D., Tate, D. G., Heinemann, A. W., Charlifue, S., ... Cella, D. (2015). Overview of the spinal cord injury–Quality of life (SCI-QOL) measurement system. *Journal of Spinal Cord Medicine, 38*(3), 257–269. doi:10.1179/2045772315Y.0000000023
11. Tomberg, T., Toomela, A., Pulver, A., & Tikk, A. (2005). Coping strategies, social support, life orientation and health-related quality of life following traumatic brain injury. *Brain Injury, 19*(14), 1181–1190. doi:10.1080/02699050500150153
12. Hawton, A., Green, C., Dicken, A. P, Richards, S. H., Taylor R. S., Edwards, R., ... Campbell, J. L. (2011). The impact of social isolation on the health status and health-related quality of life of older people. *Quality of Life Research, 20*(1), 57–67. doi:10.1007/s11136-010-9717-2
13. U.S. Department of Health and Human Services, Office of Disease Prevention and Health Promotion. (2008). Health communications activities: Health literacy improvement. Retrieved from http://health.gov/communication/literacy/#overview
14. U.S. Department of Health and Human Services. (n.d.). Quick guide to health literacy. Retrieved from http://health.gov/communication/literacy/quickguide/Quickguide.pdf
15. Koh, H. K., Berwick, D. M., Clancy, C. M., Baur, C., Brach, C., Harris, L. M., & Zerhusen, E. G. (2012). New federal policy initiatives to boost health literacy can help the nation move beyond the cycle of costly "crisis care." *Health Affairs, 31*(2), 434–443. doi:10.1377/hlthaff.2011.1169
16. Berger, S. (2014). Educating clients. In B. A. B. Schell, G. Gillen, & M. E. Scaffa (Eds.), *Willard and Spackman's occupational therapy* (12th ed., pp. 353–363). Philadelphia, PA: Lippincott Williams & Wilkins.
17. Voltz, J. (2006). Health literacy: Occupational therapists have a responsibility to communicate effectively with their clients. *ADVANCE for Occupational Therapy Practitioners, 22*(4), 54.
18. Miller-Scott, C. (2014). An evidence-based health literacy training program for occupational therapy professionals: Program development and evaluation (Capstone project). Retrieved from http://nsuworks.nova.edu/hpd_ot_student_dissertations/2/
19. Levasseur, M., & Carrier, A. (2012). Integrating health literacy in occupational therapy: Findings from a scoping review. *Scandinavian Journal of Occupational Therapy, 19*(4), 305–314. doi:10.3109/11038128.2011.588724
20. Lambert, V., & Keogh, D. (2014). Health literacy and its importance for effective communication. Part 2. *Nursing Children and Young People, 26*(4), 32–36. doi:10.7748/ncyp2014.05.26.4.32.e387
21. Scaffa, M. E. (2014). Occupational therapy interventions for organizations, communities, and populations. In B. A. B. Schell, G. Gillen, & M. E. Scaffa (Eds.), *Willard and Spackman's occupational therapy* (12th ed., pp. 342–352). Philadelphia, PA: Lippincott Williams & Wilkins.
22. Centers for Disease Control and Prevention. (2015). Preventing chronic disease: Public health research, practice, and policy. Retrieved from http://www.cdc.gov/pcd/collections/pdf/PCD_MCC_Collection_5-17-13.pdf
23. Wilcock, A. A. (2006). *An occupational perspective of health.* Thorofare, NJ: SLACK, Inc.
24. Arnold, M., & Rybski, D. (2010). Occupational justice. In M. E. Scaffa, S. M. Reitz, & M. A. Pizzi (Eds.), *Occupational therapy in the promotion of health and wellness* (pp. 135–156). Philadelphia, PA: F. A. Davis.
25. Fieldhouse, J. (2000). Occupational science and community mental health: Using occupational risk factors as a framework for exploring

chronicity. *British Journal of Occupational Therapy, 63*(5), 211–217. doi: 10.1177/030802260006300505

26. Whiteford, G. (2000). Occupational deprivation: Global challenge in the new millennium. *British Journal of Occupational Therapy, 63*(5), 200–204. doi:10.1177/030802260006300503
27. Townsend, E., & Wilcock, A. A. (2004). Occupational justice and client-centered practice: A dialogue in progress. *Canadian Journal of Occupational Therapy, 71*(2), 75–87. doi:10.1177/000841740407100203
28. Arthanat, S., Simmons, C. D., & Favreau, M. (2012). Exploring occupational justice in consumer perspectives on assistive technology. *Canadian Journal of Occupational Therapy, 79*(5), 309–319. doi:10.2182/cjot.2012.79.5.7
29. Haertl, K., & Christiansen, C. (2011). Coping skills. In C. Brown & V. C. Stoffel (Eds.), *Occupational therapy in mental health: A vision for participation* (pp. 313–329). Philadelphia, PA: F. A. Davis.
30. Rew, L., & Horner, S. D. (2003). Youth resilience framework for reducing health-risk behaviors in adolescents. *Journal of Pediatric Nursing, 18*(6), 379–388. doi:10.1016/S0882-5963(03)00162-3
31. Scaffa, M. E., Pizzi, M. A., & Chromiak, S. B. (2010). Promoting mental health and emotional wellbeing. In M. E. Scaffa, S. M. Reitz, & M. A. Pizzi (Eds.), *Occupational therapy in the promotion of health and wellness* (pp. 329–349). Philadelphia, PA: F. A. Davis.
32. Hildenbrand, W. C., & Lamb, A. J. (2013). Occupational therapy in prevention and wellness: Retaining relevance in a new health care world. *American Journal of Occupational Therapy, 67*(3), 266–271. doi:10.5014/ajot.2013.673001
33. Reitz, S. M. (2014). Health promotion theories. In B. A. B. Schell, G. Gillen, & M. E. Scaffa (Eds.), *Willard and Spackman's occupational therapy* (12th ed., pp. 574–587). Philadelphia, PA: Lippincott Williams & Wilkins.
34. American Occupational Therapy Association. (2015). The role of occupational therapy with health promotion [Fact Sheet]. *Occupational therapy: Living life to its fullest.* Retrieved from https://www.aota.org/-/media/Corporate/Files/AboutOT/Professionals/WhatIsOT/HW/Facts/FactSheet_HealthPromotion.pdf
35. Clark, F., Blanchard, J., Sleight, A., Cogan, A., Floríndez, L., Gleason, S., ... & Vigen, C. (2015). *Lifestyle Redesign®* (2nd ed.). Bethesda, MD: AOTA Press.
36. Johansson, A. & Björklund, A. (2016). The impact of occupational therapy and lifestyle interventions on older persons' health, well-being and occupational adaptation. *Scandinavian Journal of Occupational Therapy*, 23(3), 207-19. doi:10.3109/11038128.2015.1093544
37. American Occupational Therapy Association. (2013). Occupational therapy in the promotion of health and wellbeing. *American Journal of Occupational Therapy, 67*(6 Suppl.), S47–S59. doi:10.5014/ajot.2013.67S47
38. Scaffa, M. E., & Reitz, S. M. (2014). *Occupational therapy in community-based practice settings* (2nd ed.). Philadelphia, PA: F. A. Davis.
39. World Health Organization. (2015). *Obesity and overweight* [Fact sheet no. 311]. Retrieved from http://www.who.int/mediacentre/factsheets/fs311/en/
40. Centers for Disease Control and Prevention. (2014). Nutrition, physical activity and obesity: Data, trends and maps. Retrieved from https://nccd.cdc.gov/NPAO_DTM/
41. Kuczmarski, M., Reitz, S. M., & Pizzi, M. A. (2010). Weight management and obesity reduction. In M. E. Scaffa, S. M. Reitz, & M. A. Pizzi (Eds.), *Occupational therapy in the promotion of health and wellness* (pp. 253–279). Philadelphia, PA: F. A. Davis.
42. American Occupational Therapy Association. (2013). Obesity and occupational therapy. *American Journal of Occupational Therapy, 67* (6 Suppl.), S39–S46. doi:10.5014/ajot.2013.67S39
43. Dieterle, C. (2014). Lifestyle redesign programs. In M. E. Scaffa & S. M. Reitz (Eds.), *Occupational therapy in community-based practice settings* (2nd ed., pp. 377–389). Philadelphia, PA: F. A. Davis.
44. Clark, F., Azen, S. P., Zemke, R., Jackson, J., Carlson, M., Mandel, D., ... & Lipson, L. (1997). Occupational therapy for independent living older adults: A randomized controlled trial. *Journal of the American Medical Association, 278*, 1321–1326.
45. World Health Organization. (2015). *Physical activity* [Fact sheet no. 385]. Retrieved from http://www.who.int/mediacentre/factsheets/fs385/en/
46. Centers for Disease Control and Prevention. (2014). Facts about physical activity. Retrieved from http://www.cdc.gov/physicalactivity/data/facts.html
47. World Health Organization. (2016). Global recommendations on physical activity for health. Retrieved from http://www.who.int/dietphysicalactivity/factsheet_recommendations/en/
48. Chapanis, A. (1991). To communicate the human factors message, you have to know what the message is and how to communicate it. *Human Factors Society Bulletin, 34*(11), 1–4.
49. Bowman, P. (2014). Ergonomics and prevention of work-related injuries. In M. E. Scaffa & S. M. Reitz, *Occupational therapy in community-based practice settings* (2nd ed.). Philadelphia, PA: F. A. Davis.
50. American Occupational Therapy Association. (2012). Occupational therapy practitioners and ergonomics. Retrieved from http://www.aota.org/~/media/Corporate/Files/AboutOT/Professionals/WhatIsOT/WI/Facts/ergonomics.pdf
51. Centers for Disease Control and Prevention. (2016). Important facts about falls. Retrieved from http://www.cdc.gov/HomeandRecreationalSafety/Falls/adultfalls.html
52. Chase, C. A., Mann, K., Wasek, S., & Arbesman, M. (2012). Systematic review of the effect of home modification and fall prevention programs on falls and the performance of community-dwelling older adults. *American Journal of Occupational Therapy, 66*(3), 284–291.
53. Di Monaco, M., Vallero, F., De Toma, E., De Lauso, L., Tappero, R., & Cavanna, A. (2008). A single home visit by an occupational therapist reduces the risk of falling after hip fracture in elderly women: A quasi-randomized controlled trial. *Journal of Rehabilitation Medicine, 40*, 446–450. http://dx.doi.org/10.2340/16501977-0206
54. National Institute for Occupational Safety and Health. (2007). Ergonomic guidelines for manual material handling. Retrieved from https://www.cdc.gov/niosh/docs/2007-131/
55. National Institute for Occupational Safety and Health. (1997). Chapter 7: Work-related musculoskeletal disorders and psychosocial factors. Retrieved from http://www.cdc.gov/niosh/docs/97-141/pdfs/97-141g.pdf
56. Center for Universal Design. (2008). *About UD.* (para. 1). Retrieved from https://www.ncsu.edu/ncsu/design/cud/about_ud/about_ud.htm
57. U.S. Department of Health and Human Services. (2010). Multiple chronic conditions—A strategic framework: Optimum health and quality of life for individuals with multiple chronic conditions. Retrieved from http://www.hhs.gov/ash/initiatives/mcc/mcc_framework.pdf
58. Centers for Disease Control and Prevention. (2015). Chronic disease overview. Retrieved from http://www.cdc.gov/chronicdisease/overview/
59. National Institutes of Health. (2010). Fact sheet: Self-management. Retrieved from http://report.nih.gov/nihfactsheets/ViewFactSheet.aspx?csid=70
60. Chromiak, S. B., Scaffa, M. E. & Norris, S. (2014). Occupational therapy in primary health care settings. In M. E. Scaffa & S. M. Reitz (Eds.), *Occupational therapy in community-based practice settings* (2nd ed., pp. 390–408). Philadelphia, PA: F. A. Davis.
61. Stanford University. (2006). Chronic disease self-management program. Retrieved from http://patienteducation.stanford.edu/programs/cdsmp.html
62. American Occupational Therapy Association. (2015). The role of occupational therapy in chronic disease management [Fact sheet]. *Occupational therapy: Living life to its fullest.* Retrieved from http://www.aota.org/-/media/Corporate/Files/AboutOT/Professionals/WhatIsOT/HW/Facts/FactSheet_ChronicDiseaseManagement.pdf
63. Morse, J. M., & O'Brien, B. (1995). Preserving self: From victim, to patient, to disabled person. *Journal of Advanced Nursing, 21*(5), 886–896.
64. Fennell, P. A. (2003). *Managing chronic illness: Using the four-phase treatment approach.* Hoboken, NJ: John Wiley & Sons.

65. Solet, J. M. (2014). Sleep and rest. In B. A. B. Schell, G. Gillen, & M. E. Scaffa (Eds.), *Willard and Spackman's occupational therapy* (12th ed., pp.714–730). Philadelphia, PA: Lippincott Williams & Wilkins.
66. Lawlor, M. C., & Mattingly, C. (2014). Family perspectives on occupation, health and disability. In B. A. Schell, G. Gillen, & M. E. Scaffa (Eds.), *Willard and Spackman's occupational therapy* (12th ed). Philadelphia, PA: Lippincott Williams & Wilkins.
67. Olson, L., & Wong, S. J. (2015). Transition in prevention and wellness. In M. L. Orentlicher, S. Schefkind, & R. W. Gibson, *Transitions across the lifespan: An occupational therapy approach.* Bethesda, MD: AOTA Press.
68. Larsen, P. D. (2016). *Lubkin's chronic illness: Impact and intervention* (9th ed.). Burlington, MA: Jones & Bartlett.
69. McInnes, R. A. (2003). Chronic illness and sexuality. *Medical Journal of Australia, 179,* 263–266.
70. World Health Organization. (2014). Mental health: Strengthening our response [Fact Sheet No. 220]. Retrieved from http://www.who.int/mediacentre/factsheets/fs220/en/
71. National Mental Health Association. (1996). *Characteristics of mentally healthy people.* Alexandria, VA: Author.
72. Snyder, C. R., & Lopez, S. J. (Eds.). (2005). *Handbook of positive psychology.* New York, NY: Oxford University Press.
73. Tabei, S. Z., Zarei, N., & Joulaei, H. (2016). The impact of spirituality on health. *Shiraz E-Medical Journal, 17*(6), e39053. doi:10.17795/semj39053
74. Carron, R. (2016). Spirituality. In P. D. Larsen, *Lubkin's chronic illness: Impact and intervention* (9th ed.). Burlington, MA: Jones & Bartlett.
75. Radomski, M. V., & Roberts, P. (2014). Assessing context: Personal, social, cultural, and payer-reimbursement factors. In M. V. Radomski & C. A. T. Latham (Eds.), *Occupational therapy for physical dysfunction* (12th ed., pp. 50–75). Baltimore, MD: Lippincott Williams & Wilkins.
76. Humbert, T. K. (2016). *Spirituality and occupational therapy: A model for practice and research.* Bethesda, MD: AOTA Press.
77. Taylor, E., Mitchell, J. E., Kenan, S., & Tacker, R. (2000). Attitudes of occupational therapists toward spirituality in practice. *American Journal of Occupational Therapy, 54,* 421–427.
78. Davis, M., Eshelman, E. R., & McKay, M. (2008). *The relaxation and stress reduction workbook* (6th ed.). Oakland, CA: New Harbinger Publications, Inc.
79. Ozbay, F., Johnson, D. C., Dimoulas, E., Morgan, C. A., Charney, D., & Southwick, S. (2007). Social support and resilience to stress: From neurobiology to clinical practice. *Psychiatry (Edgmont), 4*(5), 35–40.
80. Seligman, M. E. (2011). *Flourish.* New York, NY: Free Press.
81. Pierce, S. L. (2014). Restoring functional and community mobility. In M. V. Radomski & C. A. T. Latham (Eds.), *Occupational therapy for physical dysfunction* (7th ed., pp. 804–843). Baltimore, MD: Lippincott Williams & Wilkins.
82. Fasoli, S. E. (2014). Restoring competence for homemaker and parent roles. In M. V. Radomski & C. A. T. Latham (Eds.), *Occupational therapy for physical dysfunction* (7th ed., pp. 844–869). Baltimore, MD: Lippincott Williams & Wilkins.
83. Siegel, J. D., Rhinehart, E., Jackson, M., & Chiarello, L. (2007). 2007 guideline for isolation precautions: Preventing transmission of infectious agents in health care settings. *American Journal of Infection Control, 35*(10 Suppl. 2), S65–S164. http://dx.doi.org/10.1016/j.ajic.2007.10.007
84. World Health Organization. (2003). Health care worker safety: Aide-memoire for a strategy to protect health workers from infection with bloodborne viruses. Retrieved from http://www.who.int/occupational_health/activities/1am_hcw.pdf
85. Snaith, L., & Rugg, S. (2006). Occupational therapists' knowledge and practice of infection control procedures: A preliminary study. *British Journal of Occupational Therapy, 69*(3), 124–129. doi:10.1177/030802260606900305
86. Sutton, A. L. (Ed.). (2011). *Stress-related disorders sourcebook: Basic consumer health information* (3rd ed.). Detroit, MI: Omnigraphics, Inc.
87. France, R. P., & DeAngelo, L. P. (2013). Biofeedback. *Magill's medical guide* (online edition). Retrieved from https://libproxy.usouthal.edu/login?url=http://search.ebscohost.com/login.aspx?direct=true&db=ers&AN=87690452&site=eds-live
88. Bush, N. J. (2009). Compassion fatigue: Are you at risk? *Oncology Nursing Forum, 36*(1), 24–28. doi:10.1188/09.ONF.24-28
89. Mathieu, F. (2007). Running on empty: Compassion fatigue in health professionals. *Rehab & Community Care Medicine.* Retrieved from http://www.compassionfatigue.org/pages/RunningOnEmpty.pdf
90. Ray, S. L., Wong, C., White, D., & Heaslip, K. (2013). Compassion satisfaction, compassion fatigue, work life conditions, and burnout among frontline mental health care professionals. *Traumatology, 19*(4), 255–267. doi:10.1177/1534765612471144.
91. Lynch, S. H., & Lobo, M. L. (2012). Compassion fatigue in family caregivers: A Wilsonian concept analysis. *Journal of Advanced Nursing, 68*(9), 2125–2134. doi:10.1111/j.1365-2648.2012.05985.x
92. Zeidner, M., Hadar, D., Matthews, G., & Roberts, R. D. (2013). Personal factors related to compassion fatigue in health professionals. *Anxiety, Stress, & Coping, 26*(6), 595–609. doi:10.1080/10615806.2013.7770
93. Negash, S., & Sahin, S. (2011). Compassion fatigue in marriage and family therapy: Implications for therapists and clients. *Journal of Marital and Family Therapy, 37*(1), 1–13. doi:10.1111/j.1752-0606.2009.00147.x
94. Welsh, D. J. (1999). Care for the caregiver: Strategies for avoiding "compassion fatigue." *Clinical Journal of Oncology Nursing, 3*(4), 183–184.
95. Simon, C. E., Pryce, J. G., Roff, L. L., & Klemmack, D. (2005). Secondary traumatic stress and oncology social work: Protecting compassion from fatigue and compromising the worker's worldview. *Journal of Psychosocial Oncology, 23*(4), 1–14. doi:10.1300/J077v23n04_01
96. Smart, D., English, A., James, J., Wilson, M., Daratha, K. B., Childers, B., & Magera, C. (2014). Compassion fatigue and satisfaction: A cross-sectional survey among US healthcare workers. *Nursing and Health Satisfaction, 16*(1), 3–10. doi:10.1111/nhs.12068
97. Pizzi, M. A. (2010). Health promotion for people with disabilities. In M. E. Scaffa, S. M. Reitz, & M. A. Pizzi (Eds.), *Occupational therapy in the promotion of health and wellness* (pp. 376–396). Philadelphia, PA: F. A. Davis.
98. Accreditation Council for Occupational Therapy Education. (2011). 2011 Accreditation Council for Occupational Therapy Education (ACOTE®) standards and interpretative guide. Retrieved from http://www.aota.org/-/media/Corporate/Files/EducationCareers/Accredit/Standards/2011-Standards-and-Interpretive-Guide.pdf
99. Campbell, R. M., Rhynders, P. A., Riley, M., Merryman, M. B., & Scaffa, M. E. (2010). Educating practitioners for health promotion practice. In M. E. Scaffa, S. M. Reitz, & M. A. Pizzi (Eds.), *Occupational therapy in the promotion of health and wellness* (pp. 512–527). Philadelphia, PA: F. A. Davis.

ACKNOWLEDGMENTS

Many thanks to the following University of South Alabama Class of 2016 master's degree occupational therapy students for their assistance in the preparation of this chapter: Taylor Anderson, Hannah Gaylord, Lori Kerr, Melinda Thornton, David J. Williams, and Montana Williams.

Chapter 5

Teaching and Learning With Clients and Community

Brenda Kennell, BS, MA, OTR/L and Amy J. Mahle, MHA, COTA/L

LEARNING OUTCOMES

After studying this chapter, the student or practitioner will:

5.1 Identify learning theories and models
5.2 Identify various learning styles and relate the appropriate teaching methods for each style
5.3 Utilize principles of health literacy
5.4 Identify important considerations for providing client-centered handouts
5.5 List factors to increase client motivation
5.6 Determine which method of teaching is appropriate given client conditions
5.7 Develop appropriate teaching plans for individuals and groups

KEY TERMS

Backward chaining
Forward chaining
Generalization
Health literacy
Identification
Integration
Self-efficacy

Occupational therapy (OT) practitioners should always be ready to explain the distinct value of the profession and educate anyone with whom they come in contact. Although the profession is becoming more well-known, many individuals still have never heard of occupational therapy or may have a limited understanding of the power and scope of practice. The role of an OT practitioner frequently includes educating and training clients and their families or caregivers, as well as colleagues and the community at-large. The focus of this chapter is on the occupational therapy assistant (OTA) as one who provides education and training to clients.

In preparing for the role of training and educating the client, the OTA first should consider that the goal of client education often aims for one or more of these three components: to change the client's method of performing a task (i.e., using adaptive equipment); to assist the client and/or caregiver to learn to perform new tasks or perform tasks in a different environment (i.e., one-handed technique); or to increase the client's understanding and acceptance of their diagnosis(es) and current abilities (i.e., spinal cord injury [SCI]). Change is the fundamental element to all listed objectives. Most humans resist change, even when change may have a potentially positive outcome. How then does the OTA become effective at educating and training, if clients are resistant to change?

At the core of most behaviors are one's beliefs and values. For example, if a student believed that studying 2 hours every day for a particular course would result in earning a passing grade, and the student valued education, then the behavior would follow the pattern of belief and the student would study for that set amount of time daily. Thus, behavior, based on one's beliefs, drives priorities and actions. The same is true for clients.

For the desired outcome to be achieved, the belief must be linked to a very likely or highly probable outcome. Sometimes the OT practitioner provides a realistic viewpoint for the client, which, although not easy, must be done. For example, if a client believed that her amputated hand would grow back spontaneously, that belief is founded on a very poor likelihood, and the belief is not helpful to the client. Unrealistic beliefs can hinder accepting a current condition and progressing toward achieving independence in meaningful, client-centered occupations. However, OT practitioners also need to be careful to not take away hope because hope is a powerful motivator. No one can predict the future, yet clients often end up proving to doctors and other medical providers that they are able to overcome seemingly impossible odds. When a client asks a question of whether he or she will be able to do a specific task again, a wise response is to state, "Every individual is unique, and therefore heals or progresses differently. Let's work on a new way to do this for now, until you see what your full recovery will be."

LEARNING THEORY AND MODELS

Several models are available that can be helpful in gaining a greater understanding of clients and the factors that influence their behaviors. The Health Belief Model (HBM), simply stated, is that a person's beliefs and perceptions affect his or her health behaviors. Those beliefs are based on four original principles: perceived seriousness, perceived susceptibility, perceived benefits, and perceived barriers. Perceived seriousness is what the individual believes about the seriousness of the disease or illness and how it may influence a person's own life. Perceived susceptibility is an individual's belief about how likely he or she is to have the disease or illness. Perceived benefits are what the individual believes are the benefits of a change in health behavior. Perceived barriers are the individual's beliefs about what would get in the way of accessing health benefits. Later additions to the model include cues to action (things that make one more likely to accept the health behavior), modifying factors (personal experiences and factors that influence behaviors), and self-efficacy (the belief that one has the power to do something).[1] A good example to illustrate the HBM is deciding whether or not to get the flu vaccine. See Table 5-1, Health Belief Model: The Flu, to help understand the model.

Albert Bandura proposed the Social Cognitive theory of human functioning, which includes self-efficacy at its core. **Self-efficacy** is an individual's self-perceptions and beliefs (and judgments) about his or her own capabilities, which have a direct effect on their actions.[2] In Bandura's theory, self-efficacy is thought to be the "foundation for human motivation, well-being, and accomplishment." Therefore, if one lacks self-efficacy, one would have a difficult time being motivated to accomplish anything or persevere in times of difficulty, because the individual believes he cannot achieve it.[2]

TABLE 5-1 Health Belief Model: The Flu

PRINCIPLES OF HBM[1]	INDIVIDUAL'S QUESTIONS/THOUGHTS	POSSIBLE OUTCOMES
Perceived seriousness–An assessment of how likely the person will be to get the illness or disease and the seriousness of the illness/disease	How serious is the flu? Will I be in the hospital? Will the flu last a long time?	The flu is not typically life threatening, so I will take my chances OR I hate to be sick, so I will get the vaccine.
Perceived susceptibility–The conclusions made that lead to a person's behavior	How likely am I to get the flu? Am I around people that would be likely to have it? Is my age a factor? How is it transmitted?	It's fairly likely that I will come in contact with someone with the flu because I work at a skilled nursing facility.
Perceived benefits–Conclusions made as to the benefits of the health behavior	If I get the flu shot, will that prevent me from getting the flu? Will that keep me from missing days from work or school?	I am going to get the shot so I do not get sick, feel miserable, and miss work.
Perceived barriers–Factors that will stop the individual from the new health behavior	Am I allergic to the components in the flu shot? How can I access it? Where is it given? Can I afford it?	My employer has a flu shot clinic on several days and also the local pharmacy is giving reduced-cost flu shots.
Cues to action–Factors that will help lead a person toward healthy behavior	There are public announcements and email reminders at work about getting the flu shot.	Because of the reminders I have seen, I am more likely to get the flu shot in a timely manner. My friend got the flu last year and was very sick. I am going to get the vaccine.
Modifying factors–Personal factors that influence whether or not to engage in the new behavior	My employer is strongly urging the flu shot. I had the flu in the past and it was miserable. I do not want to experience that again.	I might get fired if I do not take the vaccine, or at least be written up at work. I do not want to be sick. I will get the vaccine.
Self-efficacy–Personal belief that an individual can do something	I believe I am able to get the flu vaccine to avoid getting the flu.	I am going to get the flu vaccine because it will truly be to my benefit, and keep me from getting the flu.

The Locus of Control theory, by Julian Rotter, postulates that individuals have either an internal or an external locus of control. An individual with a strong internal locus of control believes he or she is largely in control of outcomes in life. Those with a strong external locus of control believe that things in life are bound to occur, and that an individual has very little, if any, control over these outcomes. Individuals who have a strong external locus of control tend to be more prone to learned helplessness and blame outside forces for their misfortunes. Learned helplessness is where an individual learns through negative experiences to feel as though they are powerless when in difficult situations, and therefore give up trying. Conversely, individuals who have a strong internal locus of control tend to accept responsibility for their actions, have a stronger sense of self-efficacy, feel confident when facing challenges, and tend to work hard for things they desire.[3] These two theories can assist the OTA to understand the client's perspective, and perhaps why one client may be more positive about being able to recover from an illness or injury, or cope with a significant disability while another client may be more pessimistic and have a more difficult time with recovery. The OTA may simply ask the client, "How do you believe change can occur in your situation?" or "What do you think will help you achieve your goals?" Analyzing the client's response will help the OTA determine the client's beliefs about the self and about change.

Another useful theory to consider is the Transactional Model of Stress and Coping, which is a framework for understanding the method in which individuals cope with stressful events.[4,5] Stress is most often a negative factor that can upset an individual's internal and/or external environments, thus affecting the physiological and psychological states for the individual who is experiencing the stress. The model proposes that an individual goes through a series of deliberations, actions, and thoughts when faced with a stressful situation:

- The individual evaluates: "Is the stress a significant event?" and "Can I control or cope with the stress?"
- The individual uses the coping mechanisms available by trying to change the stressful factors or change the way he or she feels emotionally about the situation.
- The individual may find meaningful methods to cope with the situation, which in turn perpetuate the ability to continue to cope.
- The outcomes of the coping process are directly related to the coping skills used.
- Positive outcomes are characterized by emotional well-being and positive functional status.

Coping mechanisms that are available to an individual may be influenced by an internal or external locus of control and self-efficacy. For example, if Sue, who had experienced an upper extremity amputation, had an external locus of control and poor self-efficacy, she would be less likely to cope with her condition, and the OTA would need to employ a different strategy when providing training in the use of residual limb care, strengthening, and prosthetic device use.

Another theory that is helpful to understand when working to educate and train clients is the Adult Learning Theory (also called andragogy) as proposed by Malcolm Knowles. The Adult Learning Theory has five assumptions of adult learners:

1. Self-concept: As learners mature, they move from a dependent learner to a more self-directed learner. This means that adult learners are more actively involved in the decisions that affect them and, with increasing maturity, are able to take more self-responsibility. *OT correlation: Adult clients want to be actively involved in making choices.*
2. Adult learner experience: Adult learners bring with them a wealth of personal life experience, which shapes their perceptions and learning. These personal life experiences serve as a foundation for their learning, and it is hard to separate out their experiences, as they will readily relate new information through the lens of their past knowledge and experience. Sometimes this life experience brings preconceived notions and negativity. *OT correlation: Clients have history that may be unknown to the OT practitioner, but can affect (negatively or positively) their ability and willingness to learn.*
3. Readiness to learn: As a person matures, their readiness to learn becomes more related to his or her social roles, as oftentimes an adult returns to formal education because of a change in life roles (divorce, loss of a job). Adult learners want to know why they need to know something before they learn it. *OT correlation: Explain why the client needs to do a specific task, or do it in a specific way. Connecting meaning for the client will facilitate compliance to the task.*
4. Orientation to learning: As a person matures, focus is placed more on problem-solving and learning, and readily applying this thinking to life situations. This means that adult learning should be structured around life needs rather than detached subject matter. *OT correlation: Connect therapy goals and activities to real life situations the client is experiencing.*
5. Motivation to learn: As a person matures, motivation to learn becomes increasingly internally motivated. Adult learners thrive when shown appreciation and recognition for their work (feeds self-esteem and internal motivation). *OT correlation: Use therapeutic use of self to recognize the client's hard work and motivation, but do not overdo it. Clients can spot fake enthusiasm or know when they are being flattered.*

In addition to Knowles's beliefs about the adult learner, he suggests four principles of adult learning:

1. Adults need to be involved in the planning and evaluation of their instruction.
2. Experience is the foundation for learning activities.
3. Adults learn best when the topic is of immediate value.

4. Adults are more self-directed, and prefer to learn on their own with facilitation and guidance from the instructor rather than being dependent on the instructor.[6]

The four principles of adult learning (previously stated) fit well with the tenets of how OT practitioners educate and train clients, which are:

1. Emphasize client-centered practice.
2. Build on what the client already knows.
3. Connect the task to a goal of value to the client.
4. Give guidance and support when needed and give the client space to practice skills.

LEARNING STYLES

Many practitioners have seen the quote, or something similar to it, attributed to William Glasser, in which a person learns:

- 10% of what is read
- 20% of what is heard
- 30% of what is seen
- 50% of what is seen and heard
- 70% of what is discussed
- 80% of what is experienced
- 95% of what is taught[7]

Although some say these percentages are not accurate, no one denies that people learn more when new material is presented through multisensory approaches.[8] It is important to remember this when teaching information to clients, caregivers, home health aides, and so on.

Research about "learning styles" has been around since the early 20th century. Probably everyone has taken a learning style inventory to determine personal learning style—visual, auditory, kinesthetic, and mixed. The different learning styles determine the most effective way to present new information to a learner. To determine a client's learning style, the practitioner might ask how the client learns best, or presents information in a variety of methods and observes for signs of understanding from the client. The types of learning styles include:

- Read/write–Learns best through the written word, enjoys books and other written material
- Visual–Learns best through the use of images and diagrams, not necessarily through words
- Auditory–Learns best through sound, which can include spoken words and music
- Kinesthetic–Learns best through movement, touching and manipulating things (Fig. 5-1a)
- Mixed (multimodal)–Learns best through combinations of approaches, including reading and writing

Tapscott states it is important to tailor education to the learner's style.[9] He advocates focusing on the learner, which means the "teacher" (in this case the OT practitioner) cannot deliver the same "lecture" to all learners. OT practitioners need to "step off the stage" and listen and engage in dialogue with clients and caregivers. Practitioners should also encourage learners to discover things for themselves instead of just memorizing what is told to them.[9] Multisensory approaches work well "because of the way our brain is organized."[10] Visual learning involves the occipital lobe, auditory learning involves the temporal lobes, and kinesthetic learning involves the cerebellum and motor cortex.[11] Because clients may have impairment of one or more parts of the brain, it certainly makes sense to provide client teaching in a manner that utilizes multiple brain areas (Fig. 5-1b).

Anderson also taught that even though people are born with certain tendencies toward learning styles, they are influenced by culture, personal experience, maturity level, and development. "Style can be considered a 'contextual' variable or construct because what the learner brings to the learning experience is as much a part of the context as are the important features of the experience itself."[10] *The Occupational Therapy Practice Framework, 3rd edition* (OTPF-3) defines context as "elements within and surrounding a client that are often less tangible than physical and social environments but nonetheless exert a strong influence on

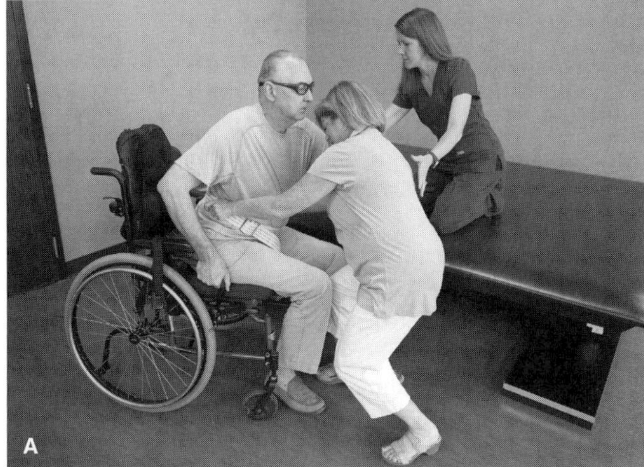

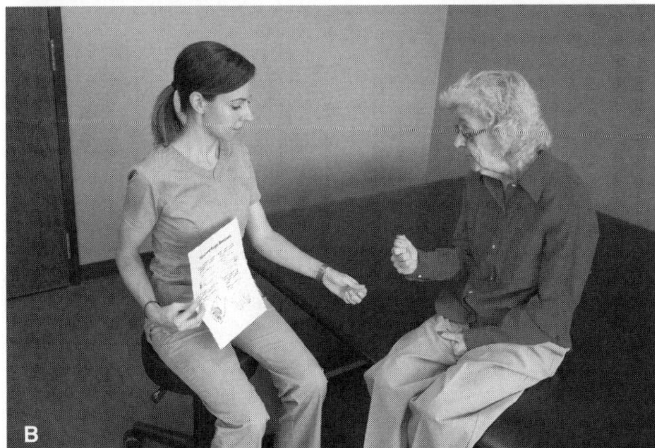

FIGURE 5-1. **A.** Training a family member to assist with transfers via kinesthetic methods is best for skills-based training. **B.** OTA using various teaching techniques, such as handouts with illustrations and clearly written directions while performing the exercise kinesthetically.

performance ... Contexts and environments affect a client's access to occupations and influence the quality of and satisfaction with performance."[12] Imagine if one day the OTA program faculty started speaking in a foreign language, holding class at 2:00 am, and making students wear flimsy pieces of material that did not cover their entire bodies. Would it affect the students' abilities to learn the material being taught? Of course it would. OT practitioners must always remember that clients are frequently in unfamiliar (and unwanted) environments and changed contexts (Fig. 5-2). They may be in pain (personal context); being treated by someone of a different gender, age group, or ethnic background (cultural context); receiving services at times of day when they are normally sleeping or working (temporal context); or being asked to read/sign forms on a tablet or computer screen (virtual context).

Strategies for Different Learning Styles

Although most of the literature about learning styles is in the academic realm, learning-style strategies can easily be applied to clients. The OT practitioner should not rely just on printed handouts or talking to a client, as the best client education incorporates all learning styles.[11,13]

- For read/write learners–Use handouts with written information clearly presented.
- For visual learners–Use charts and diagrams. Replace/complement written material with photographs or images. Highlighting certain material with different colors may help emphasize important material.
- For auditory learners–Speak to the client, but also engage the client in discussion. Having the client repeat the information or teach it to a family member may reinforce the learning. Clients may benefit from recordings of instructions that they can listen to again and again. For a client who responds well to music, it may help to set important information to a familiar melody (e.g., repeat total hip precautions to a familiar tune, such as *Twinkle, Twinkle Little Star*).
- For kinesthetic learners–Use actual adaptive equipment or practice exercises and techniques during task performance. Role-playing may be valuable. Even having clients write down information or draw diagrams for themselves can help.
- For mixed (multimodal) learners–Combine multiple techniques. Give handouts with words and pictures. Photograph and/or video the client practicing a technique (e.g., hemi-dressing/one-handed techniques, which are techniques used to dress when only one side of the body is functioning normally), and then watch it together and discuss.

Effective client teaching incorporates a variety of strategies and media. Even though a task like using a sock aid seems to be best taught kinesthetically, incorporating verbal instructions allows a learner to also process the task auditorily. Then, giving the client a handout with pictures engages visual learning, and the written instructions help the client process information in a traditional manner. With this multisensory approach, the client has the best chance of learning, remembering, and mastering the skills (Fig. 5-3). How does the OT practitioner know what teaching techniques to use and when? This will be explored further in this chapter.

LOCATING AND DEVELOPING CLIENT EDUCATION

In past years, hospitals and clinics had file drawers filled with handouts for clients and caregivers. The material may have been outdated, or may have contradicted what other disciplines were teaching, and it certainly was not personalized for the client's needs or abilities to read and understand. Some OT practitioners made their own handouts, but these were not necessarily evidence-based or even accurate.

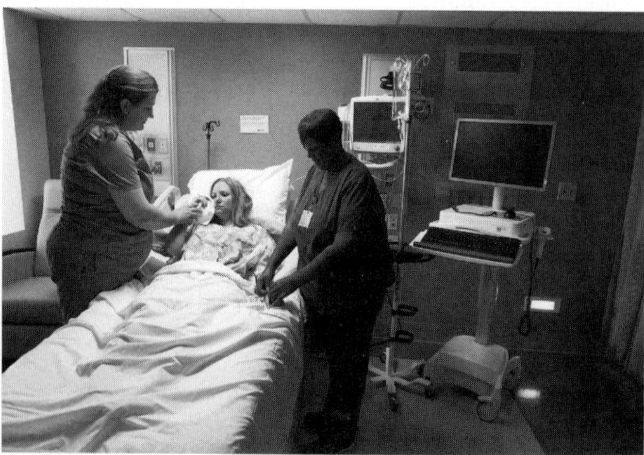

FIGURE 5-2. Client in hospital intensive care unit looks confused as a result of being in a different environment.

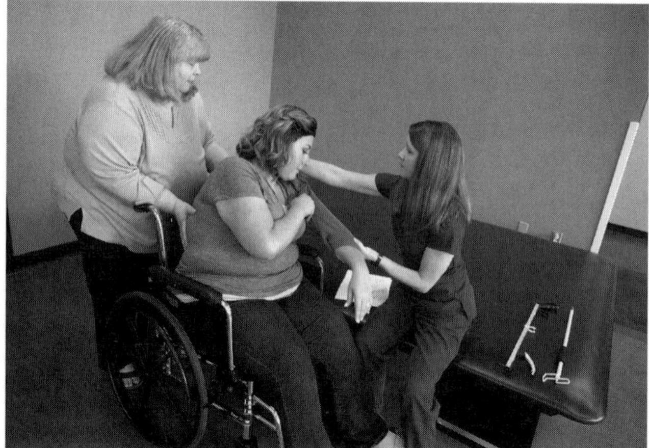

FIGURE 5-3. The OTA demonstrates using a piece of adaptive equipment through multiple learning methods, including read/write and visual (handout with directions and pictures), kinesthetic (practicing dressing), and auditory (explaining the method).

If the practitioner was a good artist, the handout might have been helpful to the client. If not, the results could have caused increased confusion, frustration, and possibly injury from doing something wrong. Sometimes OT practitioners utilized their school textbooks for resources. Depending on when the OT practitioner graduated and when the book was published, this might have resulted in more current evidence-based information. Some other resources might have been considered "OT cookbooks," with "recipes" (handouts) for different categories (diagnoses). Although a book like this might list great exercises for a total shoulder replacement, it cannot factor in whether the client might have had a previous cerebrovascular accident (CVA) and has minimal functional movement in the other arm. Although it may include handouts and illustrations for clients who have had a CVA, the handouts are generally geared toward older adults and may not be appropriate for a 27-year-old client with a CVA due to sickle-cell anemia. So how does an OTA pick quality education material that is appropriate for his or her clients?

In the 21st century, OT practitioners often obtain their client education materials electronically, either from client education software or from websites. Theoretically, this should yield more current material, as long as the OT practitioner uses respected websites or products. Using a clinical education software product allows the OT practitioner to personalize the exercises or handouts for the client. Companies such as Visual Health Information (VHI) have multiple modules, including Activities of Daily Living (ADL), Aquatic Exercise, Body Mechanics, Early Development, Lymphedema, and Neurological Rehabilitation (Fig. 5-4). An OT practitioner can put from 1 to 12 exercises or tips on a page and personalize them, directing clients on which extremity to use and how many repetitions (reps) to perform. The fewer items per page, the larger they are, so this allows the OT practitioner to adjust for the client's visual acuity. The handout can include pictures (line drawings), words, or both. An advantage to having a product like this is that the OT practitioner can save the handout, and will always have a record of what was recommended to the client, which then may be able to be added to the client's electronic health record. As always, when a client is being treated by multiple disciplines, it is important that the clinicians collaborate and do not give the client conflicting information.

Many websites include client education handouts. Students and OT practitioners need to evaluate each website for accuracy and reliability before recommending it to a client. Material produced by individuals on their personal websites may not be helpful and can indeed be harmful. Handouts from individuals or companies focusing on personal training or exercise are usually geared toward a healthy individual. Although the exercises promoted may be useful to an average, healthy adult, they could be contraindicated for someone with cardiac, pulmonary, neurological, orthopedic, or endocrine complications. Handouts that come from physical therapy practices generally are exercise-based instead of focused on occupation. For example, an OTA should not be giving a client a home exercise program (HEP) that consists solely of lower extremity and core stretches and exercises. An OT HEP should relate to the ADL, instrumental activities of daily living (IADL), work, and leisure activities that are important to the client. Yes, a client can do 20 repetitions of biceps curls and reaching toward the ceiling with a 3-pound weight; however, an OT HEP program might have the client doing a few reps with weights, and then practicing lifting three dinner dishes from the counter to the kitchen cabinet shelf and back down, carrying laundry, lifting groceries, and so on.

Some websites provide health education materials in other languages, or translate material into other languages. Some of these websites are sponsored by healthcare agencies and others by university libraries. The University of New Mexico Health Sciences Library and Informatics Center[14] has an OT resources page that includes links to Patient Education materials, which are in Spanish for Farm Worker Health, and materials for Refugee Health Information, which are available in over 50 different languages. Several websites are included in the appendix.

Health Literacy

Berkman et al. proposed a definition of **health literacy**, "The degree to which individuals can obtain, process, understand, and communicate about health-related information needed to make informed health decisions."[15] Health literacy is about much more than just the ability to read. According to the National Network of Libraries of Medicine (NNLM), "It requires a complex group of reading, listening, analytical, and decision-making skills, and the ability to apply these skills to health situations. For example, it includes the ability to understand instructions on prescription drug bottles, appointment slips, medical education brochures, doctor's directions and consent forms, and the ability to negotiate complex health care systems."[16] More recent definitions also address the importance of clear communication between healthcare providers and their clients. The U.S. Department of Health and Human Services (DHHS) has several Health Communication/Health Information Technology (HC/HIT) objectives in the Healthy People 2020 report, including one for increasing "the proportion of patients whose doctor recommends personalized health information resources to help them manage their health."[17]

The National Assessment of Health Literacy measures the health literacy of adults in the U.S. Findings show that only 12% of adults in the U.S. are at a proficient level in health literacy.[16,18] Thirty-six percent of American adults are at or below a basic level, which affects their ability to interpret information from a clearly written pamphlet or preoperative instructions sheet. Five percent of adults in the U.S. are not literate in English. The Public Health Agency of Canada reports that only 40% of Canadians and 12% of older adults are proficient at health literacy.[19] Being "health literate" involves more than just reading printed words; it includes being able to:

- Understand graphs and charts such as a height/weight chart or a medication dosage by weight chart (visual literacy).

Routine For: Client with COPD
Created By: Brenda Kennell

Sep 30, 20XX
Sample routinne for Client with COPD

STRENGTHEN - 3
Shoulder Press
(Arm / Shoulder Strength)

Using _____ lb weights, _sit_ with elbows bent and arms out from sides, palms forward. Breathe in. Raise arms above head, breathing out through pursed lips. Return slowly, breathing in.

Repeat _____ times per session.
Do _____ sessions per _day_.

Variation:
Do without weights.

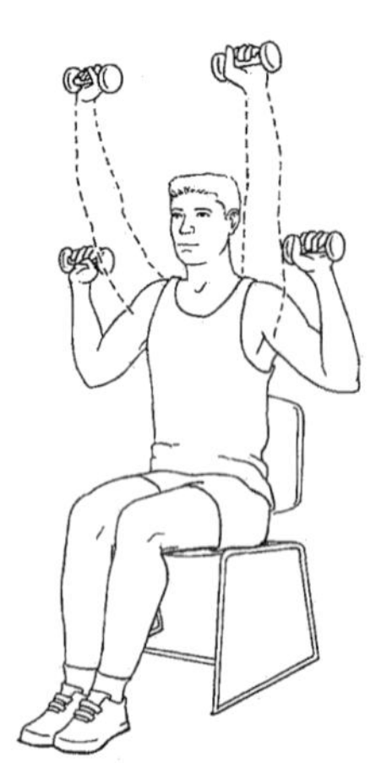

STRENGTHEN - 4
Arm Extension – Forward
(Arm / Shoulder Strength)

Using _____ lb weights, _sit_ with palms facing down at shoulder height, elbows out. Breathe in. Extend weights to front, breathing out through pursed lips. Return slowly, breathing in.

Repeat _____ times per session.
Do _____ sessions per _day_.

Variation:
Do without weights.

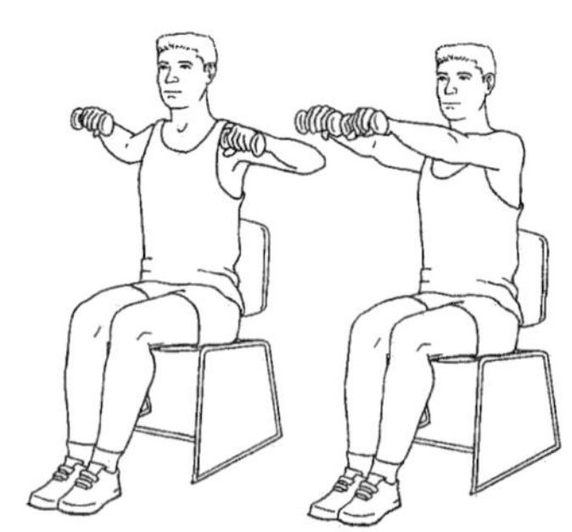

BREATHING TECHNIQUES - 1 Pursed Lip Breathing

Breathe slowly and gently in through nose and out through pursed lips (as if making a candle flame flicker, or blowing a hair off your lip).

Do not force the air out.

Breathe out for at least twice as long as you breathe in.

Repeat ______ times, times daily.

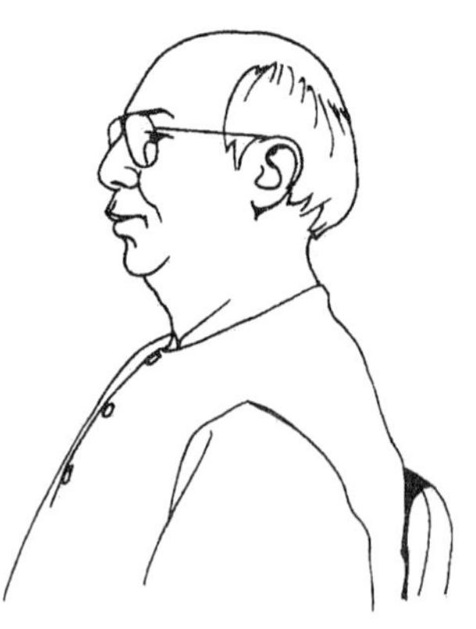

ENERGY CONSERVATION - 3
Bathing: Drying Off

Put on terry robe immediately after stepping out of shower or bath.

Sit down and pat to dry off.

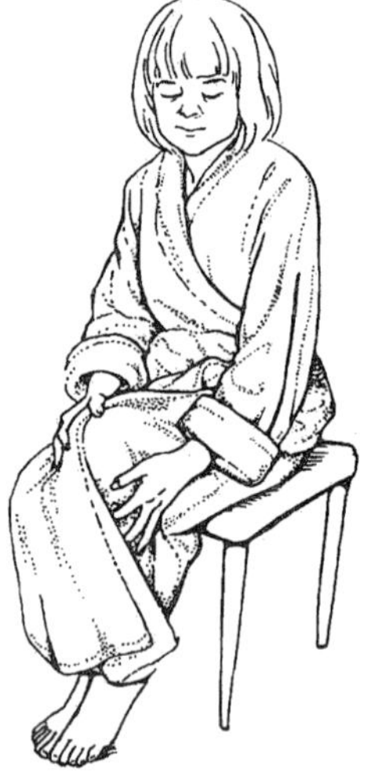

ENERGY CONSERVATION - 9 Housework: Making Bed

Bed should be placed so you can easily move around it.

Avoid heavy bedding. Use down comforter in cold weather and cotton blanket in warm weather.

Use fitted bottom sheets.

Make bed one side at a time, tucking in top sheet and blankets together.

Sit down to tuck in bedding.

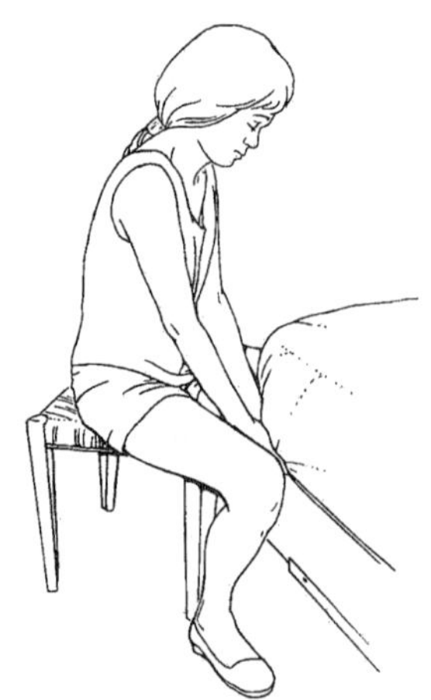

ENERGY CONSERVATION - 1
Grooming: Shaving

Sit in chair to use electric shaver.

Support arm using other hand, or rest elbow on vanity.

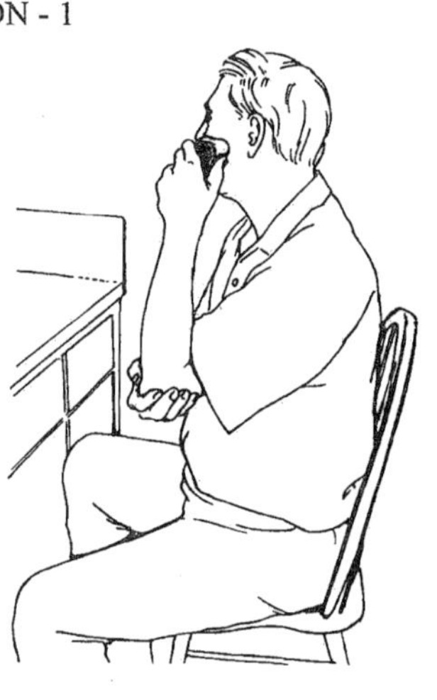

Page 1 of 1

FIGURE 5-4. Client handout - An example of a custom created handout with exercises and techniques for a client with COPD. *(Copyright © VHI. All rights reserved. www.vhikits.com. Tel: 1-800-356-0709)*

- Calculate or compute numerically such as determining the number of units of insulin to take based on blood glucose level (numerical literacy).
- Obtain and apply relevant information such as using a handout to find out which signs and symptoms necessitate an immediate trip to the Emergency Department versus a call to the physician (information literacy).
- Operate a computer, search websites, and evaluate them such as knowing which websites are reliable sources of information versus unproven or even harmful remedies (computer literacy).

People also need to have sufficient oral language skills. If a client cannot ask the right questions during a teaching session, it does not matter if the client understands the answers. Individuals need to be able to clearly articulate their confusion and/or concerns to the health professional and also to understand the responses they are receiving.

For clients who have a hearing impairment or who speak a foreign language, a healthcare facility must provide appropriate resources for the individual to understand all on which they are educated. Those resources may be a sign language interpreter or a foreign language interpreter (in person or by phone or iPad®), use of technology (applications that have translation in case of emergency or for use in home health settings), pen and paper, or some other type of electronic communication device. Any time an interpreter is used, whether for sign language or a foreign language, the OT practitioner should be aware to continue to direct conversation and body language to the client, rather than the interpreter. The interpreter is only present to assist with communication. Consistently make eye contact with the client to note a confused look and frequently ask questions to assess understanding.

Why is all of this important to OT practitioners? The OTPF-3 includes personal device care as an ADL and health management and maintenance as an IADL.[12] These include tasks that would be negatively affected by limited health literacy, such as:

- Analyzing risks and benefits to give informed consent
- Selecting the proper over-the-counter medications and the correct dosage and schedule
- Remembering the names of current and past medications
- Understanding self-management of chronic diseases, and following precautions such as hip or swallowing precautions
- Interpreting test results from healthcare providers or at-home measurements such as blood glucose level or blood pressure readings
- Evaluating the validity of advice given by (well-meaning) friends and relatives
- Following the home program proved by the occupational therapist or OTA

CREATING PRINTED CLIENT EDUCATION MATERIALS

Cognitive–When designing printed materials, it is necessary to keep the intended audience in mind. Materials should be appropriate for age and cognitive level. Line drawings are generally very simple, and they are fine to use with adults, as long as they are not too childlike. A handout for children with asthma may use red, yellow, and green like a traffic light (i.e., moving, slowing, stopping), but an adult may prefer a more specific functional analogy (i.e., if you need to take five or more breaths walking up one flight of stairs, call the doctor). Materials for clients should not use professional jargon, but rather clear, simple words. When healthcare professionals use a lot of technical words and expressions, it can negatively affect the relationship with the client who feels belittled or demeaned. This becomes complicated when there are adults who read at a lower level than expected by the health care professional. Studies have shown that the average American adult reads at a 9th grade level.[20,21] Because people generally prefer recreational reading to be 2 years below their level, many popular novels are actually written at a 7th grade level. How does an OT practitioner know what reading level is right for the client? An OT practitioner does not want to present materials that are too simplistic or too complicated. Determining the reading level of text is based in part on the ratio of syllables to words in the passage. Different text readability measures rate this paragraph from 8.7 to 11.9. This means the level a person should be reading by the 7th month of 8th grade to the 9th month of 11th grade.[22] Obviously there is a lot of variability. To play it safe, avoid long multisyllabic words when possible, and do not fill materials with extraneous words that do not add to the message. For example, it is better to list a total hip precaution as "Don't cross your leg over the other leg" instead of "Don't horizontally adduct your operative leg across midline."

Visual–Clients of any age may have visual or perceptual impairments, but the likelihood of these increases with age, after a CVA or traumatic brain injury (TBI), or with certain conditions such as diabetes. Borrowing from the principles of universal design, creation of written materials needs to be easily visually accessed by all clients. This means considering both legibility and readability. Legibility of a font refers to how easy it is for the reader to distinguish one letter from another. For example, if looking at a copy of the original Declaration of Independence, one may struggle with some words where the lowercase "s" looks like a cursive lowercase "f." Readability on the other hand refers to how easily the person can read words and blocks of text.[23] Serif fonts have little "tags" on the base and tips of letters, which increases their legibility; therefore, it is easier to distinguish the lowercase l (L) from an uppercase I in Times New Roman (serif) than the same letters "l" and "I" in Arial (sans serif). In print media, often the heading is in a sans serif font such as Arial, Calibri, or Verdana, and the body text is in a serif font such as Times New Roman, Garamond, or Courier.[24] In online media, however, sans serif fonts are typically used because of the high-resolution requirements for the serifs. Other factors also affect readability, such as when the print is crowded and too many words appear on a page. For people with certain visual-perceptual or visual contrast issues, it may be necessary to use different colored paper or overlays (Table 5-2).

Creating understandable material for healthcare consumers is so important that federal agencies are required by The Plain Writing Act of 2010 to produce clear materials that the public can understand and use.[25] The mission of the Agency for Healthcare Research and Quality (AHRQ) is to "provide Americans with health information that people can easily understand".[25] In order to comply with the Plain Writing Act, AHRQ has created a tip sheet to help determine whether a document is in "plain language." See Box 5-1 for the basic principles of plain language writing.

TABLE 5-2 Tips for Creating a Readable Client Handout

DO	DO NOT
• Use a large enough font, probably 12 to 14 point. • Set spacing between rows at least 1.15, preferably 1.5. • Have contrast between the print and the background. Sometimes this can be done with white print on a black background. • Use bullets instead of paragraphs of text. It makes it easier to see the key points. • Have at least 1-inch margins on all four sides. • Add photos or illustrations when possible.	• Use all UPPERCASE letters. It looks like you're yelling. • Use all **bold** or *italic* font. This should be reserved for emphasizing key information. • Use cartoonish drawings for adults. They may feel demeaned. • Use ambiguous photos, words, or illustrations; for example, where it is unclear which arm the person is using, or who is doing which step. • Have words overlap the pictures or graphics.

BOX 5-1
Tips for Creating Plain Language Handouts[25]

- Engage the reader.
  - Know who the reader will be.
  - Organize content for their use.
  - Write at the appropriate level.
- Write clearly and concisely.
  - Use short sentences and proper grammar.
  - Use nontechnical language.
- Display material properly.
  - Use an introduction.
  - Use short sentences and short paragraphs.
  - Use a logical and visually appealing layout that has some white space.
  - Tables help the reader see relationships more easily.
- Evaluate documents.
  - Have someone else read over to ensure plain language and readability.

THE OLDER ADULT

The U.S. Department of Health and Human Services, Centers for Medicare and Medicaid Services (DHHS, CMS) have published a "Toolkit for Making Written Material Clear and Effective," which is specifically designed to help understand changes in the older adult and to create materials that are best suited to their needs. In regard to the older adult, the toolkit states:

- Age-related changes–both physical and mental–proceed at different paces that can vary greatly from one person to the next.
- There is much diversity among older adults in terms of literacy skills.
- For any individual, literacy skills vary by context. Material is easier to read if it is familiar and harder to comprehend when worried or concerned.[26]

They state changes do occur with the normal aging process and include impaired vision, slower processing speed, less working memory (need to concentrate on one thing at a time), older adults find it harder to make conclusions from written material, and they tend to be less flexible in the way they think. The things that do not change are that they have a larger base of experience and can use that to better understand what they read, their ability to recognize and interpret pictures remains the same, and they process spoken language the same way as when younger.

Keeping the older adult in mind when creating written educational materials means following many of the same guidelines as for the general public with regard to health literacy—keep the information basic, clear, and organized and include simple, related illustrations. Two differences are to increase the font size (use approximately 12- to 14-point size, depending on the font) and ensure high contrast (very dark print on white or almost white, nonglossy paper) to help accommodate for the natural visual changes faced by older adults. Tables are not recommended for the older adult because it may be harder to compare the information presented in tables and rows and the font tends to be smaller.[26] The basic principles are easy to follow and can also be incorporated when using software programs or online sources that provide options for font size and quantity of information per page.

EDUCATION AND TRAINING METHODS

The reasons OT practitioners educate and train clients, caregivers, family, friends, and other involved people (coworkers, activity directors, nurses, certified nursing assistants, and so on) differ according to setting and population. In early intervention and pediatrics, OT practitioners may be teaching skills the client has not yet acquired, such as manipulating craft tools, self-feeding with a spoon, or gripping a pencil properly. In medical settings, OT practitioners may be helping clients relearn skills they have lost as a result of an injury or illness, such as relearning how to shave or make coffee after a traumatic brain injury.

Sometimes OT practitioners need to teach alternative or compensatory methods of performing tasks that a person was previously competent in, such as training a client in one-handed dressing techniques after a CVA. Clients may need to learn how to incorporate adaptive equipment or assistive technology into their preferred occupations, such as getting dressed while wearing an upper extremity prosthesis or preparing a meal while in a wheelchair. When a disease or disability has significantly affected performance skills, the OTA may be teaching therapeutic exercises to perform in therapy and/or at home, in order to increase strength, ROM, coordination, sensory awareness, etc. This may help the client with chronic obstructive pulmonary disease, rheumatoid arthritis, or carpal tunnel syndrome to continue participation in preferred ADLs, IADLs, work, and leisure activities. Sometimes OT practitioners need to educate clients and caregivers with important information to maintain health and safety. These may include swallowing precautions for dysphagia (difficulty swallowing), hip precautions after a total hip replacement, stress management techniques for a person with an anxiety disorder, or early signs of pressure injuries for someone with a SCI. Lastly, OT practitioners may have clients who require total care, but wish to have some level of involvement or independence. This includes educating and training individuals with debilitating conditions such as high-level SCI or amyotrophic lateral sclerosis (ALS) how to direct others to transfer them or perform their toileting program. The methods used for education and training reflect for whom, where, when, and why the education is needed.

Many different methods can be used to train a client in a task or provide information to a client. Determining which method to use depends on the client's learning style, their cognition, and the goals that need to be achieved.

Chunking

The chunking of information aids the brain to take in and organize smaller portions of data. A good example is the way phone numbers are written. When reading 9889450342 as one long chain of numbers, the brain has a hard time processing, storing, and recalling the information. In contrast, when written (988) 945-0342, the brain processes a chunk, a pause, a chunk, a pause, and then another chunk. In applying this technique to clients, present small bits of information at a time to a client. After each chunk, check with the client for recall of the information or task.

Forward and Backward Chaining

Chaining is a method of teaching skills that are performed in particular sequence. Many ADL and IADL skills are performed in a set sequence, and can be taught using either forward or backward chaining. Forward and backward chaining are commonly used in OT. A simple method to recall this method of learning is to think about the physical properties of a metal chain. One can think about a task being composed of many "links" in a chain, with the beginning of the task being the start of the chain, and the end of the task being the last link in the chain.

Activity analysis principles are necessary to understand and use forward and backward chaining. Every task is approached by thinking through all the steps required for successful performance of the task. Typically, the entire task is performed each time, but the focus point of skill acquisition differs. **Forward chaining** is used to perform a task from the very beginning of a task, step by step, adding steps as the OT practitioner progresses the client in the acquisition of skills. The OT practitioner would provide necessary assistance for step one, with the goal of less and less assistance in that first step on each successive attempt. The entire sequence is performed each time, but steps two, three, etc. are performed with assistance. The goal is for the client to eventually perform the entire task with all steps independently. **Backward chaining** occurs when the OT practitioner provides significant (or total) assistance in all steps of the sequence except the last step of the task, which the client performs. In this last step, the OT practitioner gives less and less assistance each time the task is completed, until that step can be independently performed. To progress a client in backward chaining, the OT practitioner lends less assistance in the step before the last step as the client becomes proficient, and so forth, until each step is successfully achieved. Backward chaining is implicitly rewarding because the client accomplishes the task directly after effort is given. Each time the task is completed, learning is reinforced.[27]

Let's consider the task of brushing teeth. Forward chaining would begin with the client working toward independently obtaining the toothbrush and toothpaste, but then the OT practitioner providing assistance in applying the toothpaste to the toothbrush and performing the task of brushing teeth. For the same task, backward chaining would begin with the OT practitioner providing significant assistance to the client in preparing the environment and supplies to the point where the client only has to insert the toothbrush in the mouth and brush the teeth.

How does one determine when to use forward or backward chaining? Consider using forward or backward chaining for tasks that are *sequential in nature* and when repetition of learning components is desired. One source states that little research exists for when to use which approach.[27] Another suggests these four instances where backward chaining is preferable to forward chaining:[28]

- When completion of the task provides natural reinforcement for the learner
- When "escaping" from instruction would motivate the learner
- When the learner has mastered less than half of the steps in the task chain OR when the learner is close to already having acquired the steps near the end of the chain
- When the learner is less patient or less inclined to be cooperative

Motor Learning

Motor learning refers to the acquisition (or reacquisition, as is often the case in the adult population) of skills that enable an individual to physically perform a task. A good example for most students to readily understand is learning how to type. Individuals are not born with the skill of typing/keyboarding, yet over the course of directed learning, including repetition, motivation, and outcomes, most students have learned the skill. Certainly there are different levels of proficiency, which may depend on many variables, but the goal is that the task is performed with "demonstrated consistency, flexibility, and efficiency".[29]

Inherent in motor learning is that it does not occur all at once, but rather in stages; the cognitive stage, the associative stage, and autonomous stage are the most well-known. For the OTA, being mindful of these stages can help produce optimal learning for the client.[30] Chapter 33 includes information on motor learning specific to clients following a CVA.

- The cognitive stage: The first stage, when one understands how the task is performed and what is expected. During this stage, information is gathered on how to perform the task. In the typing example, this might include becoming familiar with the keyboard, location and function of the keys, and proper hand placement.
- The associative stage: The second stage is characterized by actually performing the task and honing the skills through repetitive practice. Some of the movements may be disjointed, awkward, and inefficient. At this stage in keyboarding, typing feels awkward, and an individual is working to train fingers to make the correct movements to select the right keys. Typing is slow and mistakes are very common. Clients typically require multisensory input of tactile, visual, and auditory to learn the task. This stage is the longest.
- The autonomous stage: The final stage is when performance is almost automatic. Depending on the complexity of the task, the autonomous stage may come after years of practice or perhaps only months for a simple task. At this stage of keyboarding, the individual types without thinking about which keys to strike and is proficient and quick. To better understand the stages of motor learning, try learning the Cup Game, as explained in Box 5-2.

Many tasks that are performed by clients will require motor learning. An OT practitioner may train a client in the proper way to perform exercises with novel and/or unfamiliar items to the client, such as resistive putty or bands, or may need to train a client to perform skills in a different manner, such as utilizing proper body mechanics to lift and carry items. Perhaps even more challenging is motor learning following damage to the central nervous system (brain or spinal cord, such as after a CVA, SCI or TBI), where the client must "relearn" tasks that he or she previously performed proficiently (Fig. 5-5). The relearning is more accurately viewed physiologically and neurologically as needing to create new motor pathways for function. The client cognitively recalls how to perform the task, but because of the damage and interruption to the neurons that carry the signals to perform the task,

BOX 5-2
Try Motor Learning: The Cup Game

A fun way to understand motor learning is to try to learn a new task that has some inherent complexity. For example, "The Cup Game," if unfamiliar, is a fun multiplayer game and a good illustration of the stages of motor learning. The Cup Game requires tapping, rhythm, clapping, and moving of a cup. The game is easily found online and available with written instructions or video examples with verbal instructions. Which method would be most effective for learning a new motor game? Perhaps the whole class or a few classmates can learn this game together and apply knowledge of the three stages of motor learning. How long would it take to reach the autonomous stage? Does the rate of motor learning vary from person to person? Why or why not?

COMMUNICATION

An important part of communicating with clients during education and training is telling a client when he/she is doing a task the wrong way if it needs to be completed a particular way. Many tasks can be done in different ways with no resulting challenges or harm, such as the many ways to make a cup of tea, sweep a floor, or even don one's socks. However, some tasks must be accomplished with a high degree of specificity. For instance, to properly perform shoulder external rotation resistive exercise, one must maintain the shoulder in a slightly abducted position with the elbow flexed to properly isolate and resist the shoulder's external rotator muscles. Or, if a client has hip precautions that prevent a specific motion, the client may not be able to don socks the "normal" way and will have to learn a new method. Corrective communication may be more difficult for students, new practitioners, or those who are introverted. If the client is performing a task the wrong way, stop the client. The practitioner might use the words "Let's try that a different way" or "Let me show you the best way to (state the task and include the reason why)." Demonstrate again the proper technique with particularly clear instructions, emphasize the instructions for the part they need to improve upon, and include the reason why. If the client performs it incorrectly again, the OT practitioner may next show the client the difference between the proper and improper methods to further illustrate the point, and may also need to provide hands-on assistance to guide the client in the correct motions. The OT practitioner cannot be shy or reserved when communicating with the client, nor should the OT practitioner be harsh and punitive. Kind and encouraging words and actions offering directions for improvement are an effective communication method.

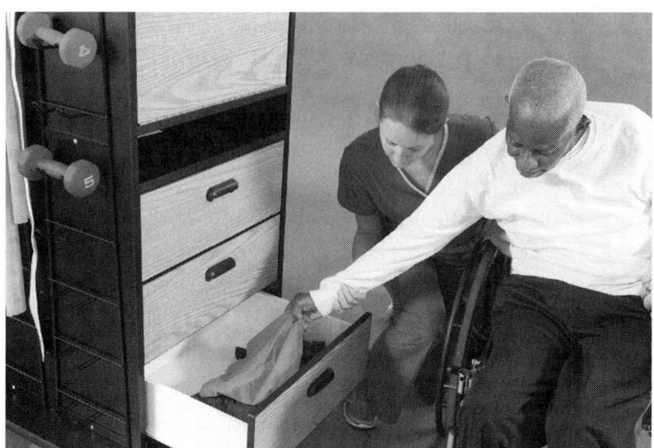

FIGURE 5-5. OTA training the client in the safe and proper positioning for obtaining items from a drawer. The client had a CVA with resulting one-sided weakness.

new neurological pathways must be created. As the client performs tasks, always keep in mind the safety of the individual. Changes in sensory or motor components may create a greater risk for falls or other injuries. Chapter 33 will discuss neuroplasticity more in depth.

According to the theory of motor learning, many systems in the body work together to accomplish a task. Researchers have been working to determine which variables in the practice environment create the best learning outcomes. A new theory of motor learning, optimizing performance through intrinsic motivation and attention for learning (OPTIMAL), suggests "motivational and attentional factors contribute to performance and learning by strengthening the coupling of goals to actions." The OPTIMAL theory explains that when a learner experiences feeling capable and competent (motivational factor), participates in a task where the learner feels in control (motivational factor), and focuses one's attention on the way the task should be performed (attentional factor), motor performance and learning is optimal.[31]

The theory fits beautifully with how OT is intended—providing the "just-right" challenge, using client-centered practice, and providing the proper environment for the client to focus on the task. The "just-right" challenge is when the OT practitioner selects a realistic yet challenging task and offers the appropriate amount of assistance, so the client can achieve success that is truly earned (Fig. 5-6). Client-centered practice takes into account the client's goals, and also acknowledges the client's strengths, abilities, and experiences as a unique individual.[12] Selecting the best environment for a task is also important. For example, selecting an environment that is not too distracting visually or auditorily will help the client focus on the task.

ADDRESSING CLIENT-CENTERED LEARNING AND OUTCOMES

Client-centered learning takes into account the learning style of the client, as described earlier, and his or her need and desire for information. But it is not just the way information is presented to the client that is important. In order for successful learning to occur, the client must have an appropriate setting and adequate time to take in the information, digest it, practice skills, and gain mastery.

- Partnership: Practitioners need to help their clients and caregivers feel like partners in the healthcare team. Clients and families do not just need to receive

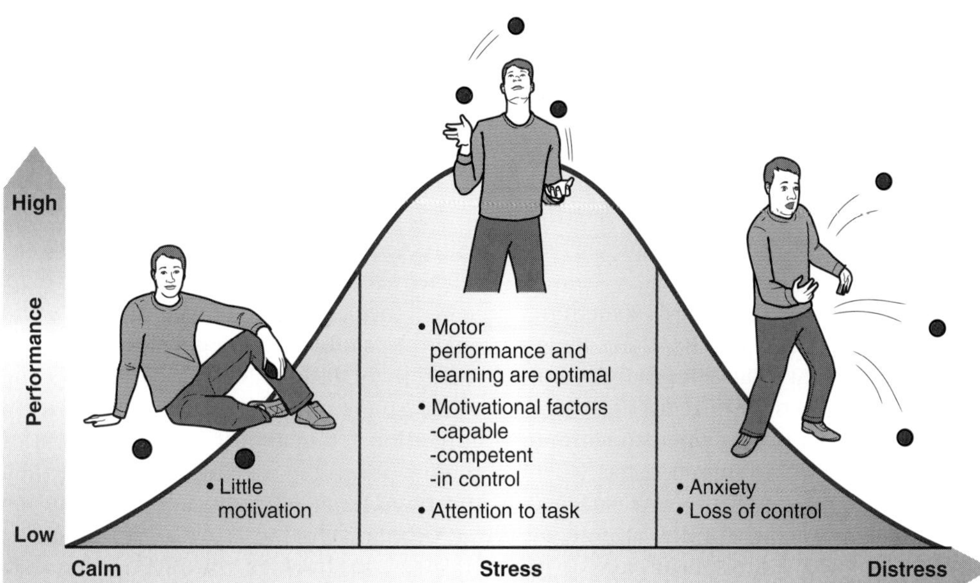

FIGURE 5-6. OPTIMAL theory. Optimal performance is achieved when just the right amount of stress motivates the learner. Too little stress yields poor performance, and too much stress impedes performance.

information, they also need to learn how to share information. The OTA can help clients learn how to ask questions and communicate clearly with their healthcare providers.[32] An example of this is educating a client on the difference between "ache" and "pain" and descriptive words for pain (e.g., stabbing, throbbing, radiating, and intermittent versus constant) so that the client can provide a clear picture of his or her feelings to the healthcare provider. To achieve positive learning outcomes, the client has to want to learn. It is critical for the occupational therapist and OTA to partner with the client and caregivers because "... collaborative communication toward defining relevant, yet feasible, rehabilitation goals (shared goal setting) can arguably increase patient's intrinsic motivation for care."[33]

- Maximize time: Teachable moments may occur outside of scheduled client education therapy sessions. The right time to provide client education is when the client and/or caregivers are available, receptive, and not distracted. It is helpful when starting out in OT to explain to the client and caregivers all that will be covered in education, and set time frames for different topics.[32] This helps people attend to what is being presented without worrying that other material will not be covered.
- Avoid overload: Material should be presented in "bite-size" portions (chunking) to avoid overwhelming the client and/or caregivers. When too much material is offered at once, a client may feel that it is impossible to learn or master it all and just give up. Obtaining mastery of certain information or a technique can help a client feel empowered and successful, and leads to intrinsic motivation for further learning.
- Return demonstration or "Show-Me" method: After demonstrating something to a client, it is not sufficient for a client to say he or she understands and can do it. The OT practitioner needs to have the client demonstrate the technique, and be able to correct any errors. For informational content, the client or caregiver can be asked to restate the taught content into their own words, or teach it to someone else.[33] If the client is unable to correctly understand or demonstrate, the OT practitioner may consider whether the correct education or training strategy was utilized.
- Practice, practice, practice: Being able to do something once does not guarantee mastery. Many times someone can do something right after being taught, but struggle the next week or even the next day. Everyone has had that experience in school when something made sense in class but was incomprehensible when trying to do homework later. To ensure success, clients need to have ample opportunities to practice skills they learn in therapy. As the client gains skills and confidence, the technique should be practiced with other items or in other settings, known as **generalization.** The client needs to be able to don different types of clothing and open different types of containers; not just the ones used in practice. The OTA should decide whether it is best for the client to practice and master one task, such as donning socks, before teaching another task. The success may help and motivate the client. However, if the topic was not of particular interest to the client, focusing on just that may actually demotivate the client. Another consideration is that if the content is difficult to master, the client may get frustrated and feel like a failure. Introducing a few things at one time and allowing the client to alternate or choose where to focus may help the client feel empowered. On the other hand, the client may not get the feeling of success because nothing is finished. There is no one right answer. The OTA must determine what is best for each client.
- Educational materials: Many sources of educational materials are available to OT practitioners. The OTA should investigate videos, handouts, brochures, and websites and determine what is appropriate for the client. A client who struggles with attention may need a printed exercise handout with only the specific exercises the client is supposed to do, not generic exercises for his or her diagnosis. A client may not benefit from watching a video of someone of different gender, age, or body size/shape doing exercises or utilizing a therapeutic technique. The client may find it helpful to watch a video of the OTA demonstrating the exercises, or a video of the OTA dressing with one-handed techniques.
- Other factors: When stress, pain, and/or fatigue are factors, the client and caregiver may exhibit a decreased learning capacity.

Utilizing Technology

To help avoid readmissions, especially in a high-risk client population, the nursing staff has begun to provide some client education materials electronically, through tablets. Clients use tablets to fill virtual pillboxes, learn about their disease, and so on. One positive effect is that the education is tied to the electronic medical record/electronic health record (EMR/EHR). However, some drawbacks exist in using technology in providing client education with tablets. Considerations involve staff development, willingness of the hospital system to invest in additional technology, the readiness of clients to use potentially unfamiliar technology, fatigue, and infection control issues.[35] Another study found that clients favored using tablet-based education for usability and the education provided to them while in the waiting room before their medical visit to a physician's office.[36]

Although the literature generally focuses on nursing staff use of technology, the OTA may also be able to provide client education materials via tablets or computers. Loading videos onto a client's or family member's tablet ensures that the resources will still be available even after discharge.

EVIDENCE-BASED PRACTICE

Because of limits on OT services imposed by insurance companies, some clients feel that they need more therapy than what is paid for by insurance. OT practitioners do their best to maximize treatment time and assist the client to reach as many goals as possible, yet for clients with a permanent life-altering diagnosis, such as SCI, the adjustment period to the change in status and community reintegration is often longer than the prescribed and allowable therapy visits. A practitioner may not be able to feel that he or she has educated and trained the client in everything they will need to know to successfully participate in social and recreational pursuits in the community. Viewed through the holistic lens, social and recreational pursuits lead to overall physical and psychological health and wellness and improved engagement in desired occupations. A recent article in *OTJR: Occupation, Participation and Health* reports on the results of a study on adult men's experiences at a wellness center for clients with SCI. The wellness center created a welcome place for those with SCI in where issues they were facing could be openly discussed and where participants felt welcome and "more than just a client." The "wellness center offered unique services designed specifically for individuals with SCI, which allowed participants to continue to improve their overall health and well-being."[34] OT practitioners should advocate for clients to use community resources that support "occupations that promote health, wellness, and civic engagement." Therefore, practitioners should be aware of available resources and be prepared to educate clients regarding those options.

Ekelman, B. A., Allison, D. L., Duvnjak, D., DiMarino, D. R., Jodzio, J., & Iannarelli, P. V. (2017). A wellness program for men with spinal cord injury: Participation and meaning. *Oxford Transitional Justice Research: Occupation, Participation and Health, 37(1), 30-39. doi:10.1177/1539449216672170*

TECHNOLOGY AND TRENDS

Clients regularly use everyday technology (ET) such as iPads®, mobile phones, and electronic household equipment, which are interwoven into everyday life. A focus study explored the perceptions of occupational therapists in regard to ETs' value, importance, and possible link to clinical practice.[37] The authors propose that the high adoption of ET doesn't necessarily mean users are competent or use the technology to its full benefit, and that OT practitioners may take for granted that their clients are adept at using ET. The takeaway points for OT practitioners are to ask clients about their ET use, determine how they are using it in their meaningful occupations, and their ability and confidence in using it. In addition, consider if the client's ET can support education (through client-centered applications, or apps, including calendars, medication reminders, and so on) and finally, be knowledgeable about modern technology to be able to train and educate clients in its use for client-centered care.

CLIENT MOTIVATION

Motivation, simply put, means to be willing to do something. A good way to begin to determine a client's motivation is to review his or her occupational profile and goals, and then ask follow-up questions while working with the client. This is part of establishing a rapport with the client and building a collaborative, therapeutic relationship.[12]

The two main types of motivation people experience are intrinsic and extrinsic. Intrinsic comes from within the client, and is the motivation to do something because of interest or meaning to the client apart from anything else.[38] It is basically doing something because the client desires to do to it and enjoys doing it. Extrinsic motivation originates from external sources to the client, such as their family, job, or OT practitioner, or even the outcome, which will come about as a result of a task performed. For example, a client may perform strengthening exercises because the outcome is to become strong enough to perform a desired occupation, but not because the client enjoys the exercise in and of itself.

Humans have an inherent need for competence and autonomy, which together lead to self-determination, the key to intrinsic motivation.[38] Being able to do a task independently and proficiently is a motivational factor for humans. Because OT goals are developed in a client-centered manner, they should be reflective of what matters most to the client, and should inherently provide a strong intrinsic motivation for clients. However, what if a client lacks the intrinsic motivation and the OT practitioner needs to help motivate them via extrinsic motivation? The practitioner could use the principles of identification and integration, as they are the methods by which extrinsic factors become more self-determined.[38] **Identification** is achieved by helping the client realize the tasks used in therapy are tied to individual client goals and have great personal value to them to achieve a desired outcome. **Integration** is the process where the individual personally values the goals and become part of his or her internal drive. They are both external motivators; clients typically achieve identification before they fully integrate a behavior.

To better understand identification and integration as motivational factors, let's consider Chuck, a client at an inpatient rehabilitation facility. He has been at the facility for 2 days and is having a difficult time being motivated to participate in therapy. He has a left transfemoral amputation (an amputation of the leg above the knee) as the result of a car accident. He is married and has two young children at home, teaches high school, and is a soccer coach for a local youth league. His OT practitioners are attempting to train and assist Chuck to transfer out of bed to a wheelchair, and then to perform residual limb care and grooming tasks. He is frustrated and just wants to be able to walk. He is worried that he will not be able to do his job as teacher or his volunteer work as a soccer coach. The OT practitioner talks with Chuck to explain that transferring to the wheelchair and achieving independence in grooming are all steps toward his goals of going home, and proper residual limb care is foundational to walking again. Chuck then identifies these tasks as very important and begins to assimilate them into personal priorities. Within a few days, Chuck has integrated the goals because he clearly connects the goals with a desired outcome, is more actively engaged in therapy, and also giving more effort to achieving independence.

Equally important to note is that intrinsic and extrinsic motivation varies among clients.[38] What may be motivating to one client, such as independently preparing a meal, may not be motivating to another. The OT practitioners must carefully consider the occupational profile (key information about the client–see Chapter 6) of the client when planning interventions. Many factors influence a client's motivation and the OT practitioner must identify those factors and attempt to mediate any that interfere with the client's progress.

Therapeutic Use of Self

Therapeutic use of self by the OT practitioner can be a powerful motivator for the client. The OTPF-3 categorizes therapeutic use of self as an intervention, and explains that it "allows occupational therapy practitioners to develop and manage their therapeutic relationship with clients by using narrative and clinical reasoning; empathy; and a client-centered, collaborative approach to service delivery."[12] The use of empathy, which is the healthy emotional connection between the OT practitioner and client in which the practitioner is able to consider things from the client's viewpoint, is a dynamic tool that helps clients communicate openly.[12] Open communication can naturally lead to fostering motivation in the client.[32] Thus, the therapeutic use of self can help motivate the client. The OTA should be a keen observer of the client's body language and what the client talks about, and also importantly, what the client does not talk about. Practitioners should pay attention to their own demeanor, body language (including eye contact), and verbal tone during the entire therapeutic process.[32] Positive body language avoids arms being crossed, hands on hips, and bored facial expressions. Instead, the OT practitioner may lean slightly forward to show he or she is listening, give intermittent head nods to show understanding while the client is speaking, and make eye contact with the client while speaking. The best healthcare professionals are those who make the client feel valued and understood, and also intentionally solely focus on the client (and caregiver, if present) for the duration of their treatment time.

CLIENT-CENTERED CARE

Part of client-centered care is helping clients find the motivation they may be lacking. Consider Jillian, who experienced a CVA; one of her goals is to prepare a simple meal for her family, based on her valued role of mom and her routine of cooking the evening meals. Currently, she only has full use of her right nondominant unaffected upper extremity and has very limited use of her dominant, affected side. The OTA is working on multiple goals simultaneously, both to restore function to the affected upper extremity (UE) and to modify tasks through compensation to allow for successful participation in functional ADL and IADL tasks. In the beginning of the treatment session, the OTA worked with Jillian to stretch her affected upper extremity and to perform small, controlled, isolated shoulder movements. Jillian became frustrated that she could not move her affected UE "normally" and questioned why the OTA was focused on "these little shoulder movements" when all she wanted to do was cook for her family. How should the OTA respond?

Frustration is a common experience for clients whose ability to perform functional tasks has been altered. Sometimes, frustration may lead to discouragement or anger. In those times, a client may think or even believe they will never "get better," or may question the methods of the OT practitioner. This has the potential to cause the client not to give his or her full effort or alternatively, to give up altogether. Part of the role of the OTA is to help the client refocus on their goals, and also to link the current activity to the stated goals (which were created in collaboration with the occupational therapist and the client).

In the case of Jillian, the OTA and Jillian reread her goals together. Next, the OTA gained agreement from Jillian that those were the goals she still desired to achieve, and then carefully explained that working with Jillian's shoulder was a method to first meet a short-term goal that was foundational to working toward restoring functional use of her entire UE. The OTA also relayed that the next task during the therapy session was to train Jillian in the use of adaptive cooking equipment. The OTA also planned with Jillian that in the following treatment session, they would work on preparing a side dish using adapted techniques and adaptive equipment. Jillian became calm, apologized for her frustration, and began working again with her affected side with renewed purpose. Reflecting on this scenario, note that the OTA patiently communicated the purpose for the treatment interventions she was performing (external motivation), and effectively refocused Jillian's mind (internal motivation) by linking the tasks to Jillian's goals, and by providing the plan for the next tasks (Fig. 5-7).

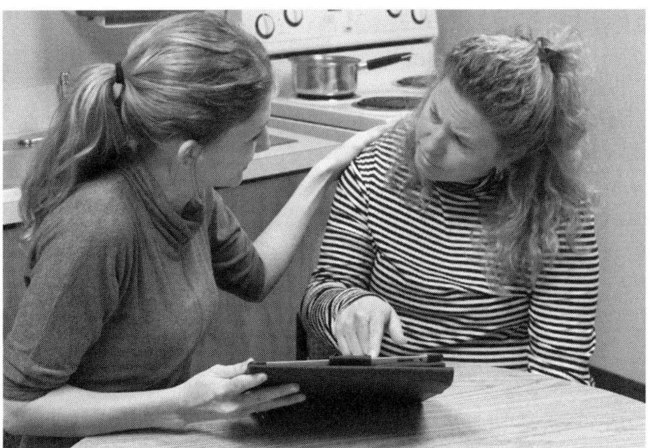

FIGURE 5-7. OTA and client, Jillian (who had a CVA), engaged in therapeutic conversation regarding her goals and the therapeutic activities that will help her succeed.

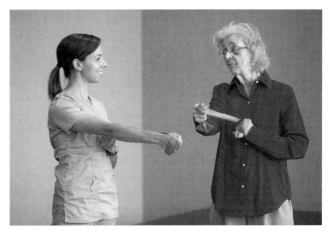

FIGURE 5-8. Demonstration of exercise with client following OTA's instruction.

ENGAGING THE CLIENT

The OTPF-3 defines the client as "persons, groups, or populations," as well as the individual and those involved in the client's care, such as family and caregivers.[12] Thus, when contemplating educating the "client," it is important to be aware of the many variations for which to be prepared to engage and educate. As an OTA, work situations will primarily be one on one with clients, but also expect to educate family, caregivers, or groups of individuals.

The Process of Client Education

Does a person become a master the first time he or she tries to ride a bicycle, crochet, or complete a tae kwon do routine? Client learning is a series of phases, with the learner gradually gaining understanding and competence. This process can end at any stage, and learners may even regress sometimes if the skills are not being used.[39]

- Acquisition phase–During this initial phase, the clinician may be identifying the right teaching style so that they client can develop strategies for successful learning. The client will be practicing and still making many errors at this stage (Fig. 5-8).
- Retention phase–At this point in the learning, the client is demonstrating recall of information when in the same or similar environment/routine. If the clinician puts the activities in a different order or starts in the middle of a routine, the client may have more difficulty.
- Generalization or transfer phase–When the client reaches this phase, he or she can spontaneously perform the task even in different settings or with different equipment. The client now can tie shoelaces on various shoes or a bow on different sized gifts. He or she can complete meal preparation in the kitchen at the rehabilitation center and at home, or can operate the washing machine in the clinic, which is coin operated (unlike the washer at home).[40]

Selecting Appropriate Materials

In order to select the most appropriate materials for the client, the OT practitioners need to have assessed the client's concerns, values, readiness to learn, barriers to learning, support systems, and learning style. Realistic learning objectives should be determined together with the client and caregivers, hereinafter referred to together as "the clients." In order to choose resources that fit the clients, the OT practitioner should determine first the clients' current level of knowledge and understanding about the condition. It is not practical to start teaching new techniques to someone who does not understand the diagnosis and prognosis. Imagine trying to teach modified grip techniques to a client with a high-level SCI if the client or the client's family does not yet realize that the condition is permanent. The OT practitioner needs to determine what the clients already know and understand, what they need to know, and what they want to know. It is also important to address any fears or concerns that the clients have that may inhibit learning the material. It can be overwhelming to present too much at one time, so the practitioner needs to be alert to signs of overload, such as confusion, frustration, or irritation.

The choice of materials may depend on the system of delivery. Is the education to be delivered one-to-one with the client, with the entire family, or in a group of people with similar needs? Does the OT practitioner expect the client and/or family to do some work on their own? Printed handouts or brochures may work well one-on-one, but not as well in a group. Demonstration may be effective when working one-on-one, but in a group setting, videos or DVDs may be preferable so that everyone in the room can see what is happening. PowerPoint™ presentations are appropriate for an inservice for other therapy department staff or when presenting to a community group, but can seem very impersonal to a client and the client's family. DVDs or YouTube™ videos may not be the best choice to teach a technique to a client and the client's family because they are not personalized, but can be great resources for them to refer back to if they forget or get confused. Another good resource for clients who have a mobile phone with a video function is to use their own mobile device to create videos during therapy sessions. The video is personalized and will allow them to have quick and easy access to the information.

The choice of who educates and trains is also important. Many clinicians are very knowledgeable about techniques, adaptive equipment, and assistive technology, but ignorant of how it feels to have a disability. Clients with permanent conditions such as SCI or amputations may respond better in some situations to trained peer educators/mentors. Since his injury in 2008, Chris Colwell (who has C5–6 quadriplegia) has made YouTube™ videos to teach people about life with a SCI. In a discussion with a class of OTA students (and one of the authors) in 2010, Chris said that he hated when OT practitioners said things such as, "Here is how *we* are going to brush *our* teeth now." According to him, he knew the OT practitioner would go home and brush teeth the normal way that night, and had no idea what it was like to not be able to do that. But he would listen if another person with C5-6 quadriplegia said, "Here is how I brush my teeth now."

When choosing education materials, it is important to review the material in advance, whether it is a printed document, a video, or a website. Be sure the material is current and accurate (look for dates and sources) and does not contradict something that another discipline taught. Accomplishing this ahead of time may be difficult when the client is also receiving physical therapy and/or speech therapy, yet there are a few methods that may work to achieve continuity. First, quickly review the client's medical record for copies of handouts or, if possible, ask other healthcare practitioners for specifics regarding the shared client. If unable to do either of those, at the beginning of the next therapy session, ask the client what he or she learned, or better yet, ask to see any handouts the client received while in physical or speech therapy.

Material must be at an appropriate educational and literacy level, and culturally appropriate. Different materials may be needed for different family members. It may be hard to find the perfect materials, but multimodal approaches are often best.[41] Lastly, remember that no printed resource can replace quality on-on-one interaction.

Maximize the Teachable Moment

Not all education takes place in planned sessions. During any OT session, the opportunity may arise to impart information to a client or the client's family. This may happen because the client or family member asks a question or struggles with a task or technique. A discussion about one-handed techniques that a client has avoided previously may now seem relevant when he is struggling to dress himself. A client who did not want to learn about adaptive equipment and says, "I am an independent person," may change her mind when she realizes she will need help with toilet hygiene. If an OT practitioner has developed rapport, gained the client's trust, and focused on the client's interests and concerns, he or she may be the logical choice when the client wants to learn or has questions.[32,42] If the OT practitioner has built trust and rapport, then the client is more likely to be at ease bringing up questions or concerns regarding sexuality. Note that the topic of sexuality will be addressed throughout this textbook in relevant locations.

Barriers

Many impediments can interfere with successful teaching and learning. These may depend on the client, the context, and/or the physical environment. Some of the barriers include cognition, education or literacy levels, communication, sensory impairments, attitudes and emotions, cultural backgrounds and expectations, environment, time constraints, pain, fatigue, stress, and sometimes medications.

COGNITIVE LEVEL

OT practitioners working with developmentally disabled adults need to have a clear understanding of their clients' levels of understanding. One study showed that generally in individuals with Down syndrome, receptive language is stronger than expressive language.[43] Just because a client cannot explain things to the OT practitioner does not mean he or she does not understand them. On the other hand, the OT practitioner is not helping the client by overestimating his or her cognitive ability and setting them up for failure. Clients with dementia or TBI will struggle with learning new information and may not remember how to perform familiar tasks. For them it will be important to keep verbal instructions short and uncluttered. The OTA will need to allow significant time for the client with cognitive deficits to process what was said before adding more instructions. It is important to determine whether a client is not learning because of a cognitive impairment or an attention deficit. Attention may improve with modifications to the environment, which is explained later in this section. Someone with significant memory or cognitive impairments who cannot remember or adhere to safety precautions must always have appropriate supervision during task performance. See Chapter 11 for more information on cognition.

EDUCATIONAL LEVEL AND LITERACY LEVEL

OT practitioners should not assume that all adults can read or understand at the same level. Clients may be functionally illiterate and unable to benefit from written client education material. They will often not reveal this information to clinicians because of embarrassment or unawareness. Furthermore, even in the current age of technology, many clients still may not own a computer, a reliable mobile or home phone, or have access to the Internet, and OT practitioners should not assume that everyone can go to a website for more information.

COMMUNICATION

The U.S. Census Bureau report from 2015 states that more than 350 languages are spoken in the home in the United States. In large cities, such as Dallas, Los Angeles, New York, Miami, and Washington DC, 30% to 50% of people ages five and older speak a language other than English in their home.[44] Although many schools, hospitals, and government agencies may have materials printed in languages such as Spanish, Chinese, Japanese, Vietnamese, Tagalog, and Arabic, it may be difficult to obtain materials or interpreters for other languages. For clients who speak English, language can become a barrier when there is neurological involvement. Receptive or expressive aphasia due to a CVA or TBI may affect the ability to understand or produce speech, respectively. Dysarthria is difficulty coordinating the muscles necessary for speech, and it may sound like the person is talking with marbles in his or her mouth. This can occur after a CVA or TBI, or with conditions such as cerebral palsy or ALS. People with injuries to the brain or certain mental health conditions may be able to speak clearly but their words are jumbled or nonsensical. Teaching and learning is affected as the clinician may have difficulty assessing understanding, and the client may not be able to ask questions. Another consideration is when a client uses a communication device, because it slows down the communication process and requires patience for both the client and the OT practitioner.

SENSORY IMPAIRMENT

Clients may have new or preexisting limitations in vision and/or hearing. A client who has always been a strong visual learner may become very frustrated when unable to read a handout because of newly developing macular degeneration or diplopia (double vision). It may be even more difficult if the client has a visual field loss after a CVA or TBI, but is unaware of it because his or her remaining vision is still clear. A preexisting hearing impairment may be present in the client, but was never addressed because the client compensated with seeing people's lips, facial expressions, and environmental context. Add in a neurological or cognitive issue and/or visual loss, and the person may no longer be able to compensate for the impairment.

Many adult clients wear glasses or contact lenses and they should have them available for use during teaching and learning. Encourage clients to maintain their glasses in good condition (clean, free of scratches) and update prescription for glasses or contact lenses. Personal device care is listed in the OTPF-3 as an ADL, so this is within the scope of practice for OT. Other clients may use hearing aids and should have them available, turned on, and certain the batteries are functioning (they must be replaced frequently). Note that in a long-term care setting, glasses and hearing aids (especially reading glasses that are taken on and off more frequently) can easily get lost in the bedding and end up missing, or clients may misplace them. The OTA may be able to assist the client in creating a safe location in the client's room for personal device storage.

ATTITUDE AND EMOTIONS

Although the OT practitioner is confident about having pertinent and valuable information to share with clients/caregivers, the clients and caregivers may not always be so convinced. Many times, especially in the acute hospital setting, people are not ready to accept what has happened. This denial and the accompanying reluctance/refusal to participate in skilled instruction from the OT practitioner may come from the client and/or the caregiver. It is a challenge for the OT practitioner when the client and family members are not "on the same page" or stage of acceptance. Emotions can also interfere with effective teaching and learning if the client and/or family members are angry, guilt-stricken, belligerent, confused, or argumentative. Outbursts can interfere with the learning of other people, so clients with behavioral issues may need to receive their education and training in quiet, isolated settings.

CULTURAL BACKGROUND AND EXPECTATIONS

When a client or family is from a cultural background different from that of the OT practitioner, it may affect the relationship with the clinician. In some cultures, women are thought to be less intelligent or less educated, so a male client will not respect information or instruction from a female clinician. Clients may not want education from a person of the opposite gender or someone much younger. Sometimes the problem is not with the practitioner but with the activity itself. Different cultures have different customs related to food, eating, bathing, toileting, and dressing. Certain cultures eat with the right hand and use the left hand for personal hygiene after toileting, so trying to teach a client with right hemiparesis (weakness in the right side of the body) how to eat with the left hand may be met with horror. The cultural mismatch can occur when trying to teach people to eat with a fork and spoon who routinely use their fingers, or trying to work on donning shoes while in their home. It is not feasible to know all the customs of every culture, but the OT practitioner needs to be alert to when an activity is offensive or uncomfortable. Asking questions or researching the client's culture can improve the relationship and lead to future success.

ENVIRONMENTAL

At some point, most students have had trouble concentrating in class because of feeling hungry, tired, or worried about something at home or had difficulty studying when someone else is talking on the phone or watching television. Some do better studying with music on, and others cannot concentrate at all unless the room is totally quiet. Think of all the environmental influences that can affect the client's learning—is the room too hot, too cold, too noisy, too crowded, too dark, too light? Are there distractions all around, or is it a blank and nonstimulating area? OT practitioners need to set up an environment that is conducive to each client's ability to attend and learn.

TIME

Sometimes teaching is not well received because of time factors. Is there insufficient time to practice? Is everyone rushed because the transportation van is here to pick up the client an hour early? Is the education and training done right before a test or procedure that is frightening or painful? Is family teaching available in the evenings or on weekends for family members who work full-time? Is the training done at the time of day when the client is most receptive? Many of us are either "morning people" or "night owls," but healthcare settings, such as hospitals and skilled nursing facilities, often do not take that into account when scheduling therapy. Also consider if the client is struggling with fatigue or lack of sleep, which can also cause a barrier in learning.

STRESS

Stress can distract clients from learning.[26] If a client seems stressed, the OT practitioner may be able to directly address the stress and help the client refocus during the session and improve learning outcomes. Sometimes listening briefly as the client identifies the stressors can be beneficial. Another strategy is to guide the client in using deep breathing techniques (take a deep breath and slowly exhale, repeat 3 to 5 times), then refocus the client back to learning.

MEDICATIONS

Sometimes medications can give clients a side effect of a mental "fog" or create a temporary altered mental status. For example, a client in the acute care setting who just had surgery to replace a hip and is receiving pain medication may be too affected by the medication to comprehend instructions for hip precautions. The OT practitioner will need to engage the client in learning at a different time.

STRATEGIES FOR GROUPS

According to Naismith and Daigle, "teaching patients in the group setting requires a clear goal and purpose with relevant and interesting topics. Through active participation and member involvement, the group develops a sense of shared responsibility for the learning."[45] The group facilitator (OT practitioner) needs to have leadership skills and knowledge of group dynamics so that he or she does not dominate the group. There are numerous group dynamic theories, but most note there is a process of how groups grow, develop, interact, and change over time. The facilitator also needs to ensure that participation of the group members is equitable, and that group members do not interfere with the learning of others. This can occur if a group member is judgmental and criticizes opinions or techniques different from his or her own. The facilitator needs to support all the group members and carefully intervene when a group member gives erroneous or potentially dangerous suggestions. The OT practitioner also must be open to suggestions from the group members, because they can contribute what actually works or does not work in their lives. Group sessions may lead to changes in attitude as well as skill and knowledge level.[45] Clients may be more receptive to "real-life" suggestions from group members or the stories from the experienced OT practitioner rather than textbook knowledge.

The group leader or facilitator must plan in advance the goals of the group and the methods that will be used to reach the goals. Each group should have an identified purpose and a targeted group member type; and the goals of the group, length, and duration would be planned in advance. For example, an OT practitioner might lead a cooking group at a senior center. Clients who would be appropriate for the group would be those with an interest and functional need to cook. The goals might be to practice skills required to prepare a hot meal with adaptive equipment or methods as needed. The group members may include those who have stopped cooking because of low energy, pain from arthritis, complications from chronic diseases, and so on.

The OT practitioner selects the leadership role most appropriate for the group and setting. There are various leadership styles depending on the type of group and clients. The styles of leadership include having complete control and directing group members in tasks, to a blend of responsibility with the group members for the group process, or being just an advisor, allowing the group to plan, execute, and self-govern. In general, more mature groups (those that have been established and functioning for some time) need less formal leadership and can function with an advisor, and the opposite is true for more basic types of groups in OT.

Each group session should be planned, at a minimum, to have an introduction, an activity (with differing levels of sharing between group members, depending on the type of group), an opportunity for sharing personal thoughts or accomplishments, and a conclusion. During the introduction the group leader facilitates general greetings and introductions of all group members and briefly communicates the purpose and plan for the group session. For most types of groups, the activity phase is the longest. Group members might be working independently, but next to another group member (parallel group) or collaboratively on a task (project group). The sharing phase, which occurs in some groups, is a time for group members to individually share their project or thoughts with the group, and then the group offers support and feedback. Peer support and feedback can be a strong influence for therapeutic change. The last phase is the summary, in which the group leader, typically the OT practitioner, gives a brief summary of the group session and may remind members of the next planned meeting. Groups and the social/shared experiences can be powerful tools for the OTA to use for educating and training. It may take practice before the OTA is comfortable not only with speaking in front of a group, but with managing and facilitating the group and the needs of individual members.

OT Practitioner's Viewpoint

Working with a therapeutic group in an outpatient setting with clients who had sustained brain injuries was one of the most challenging and rewarding parts of my job. I was the coleader of the Functional Independence Group (FIG); the purpose of the group was to help members reintegrate into the community by relearning valuable skills in social and interpersonal communication, community mobility, money management, planning, organizing, decision-making, self-reflection, and giving feedback. Group members had to meet several inclusion criteria: history of a brain injury, the ability to attend the group 3 days per week, a payer source (ranged from Workers' Compensation to Vocational Rehabilitation), and a desire to attend, make progress, and be an active participant in the group. The group leadership was interdisciplinary (the other group leader was a Speech Language Pathologist) and the style was facilitative because the group members needed some guidance to complete their tasks but also needed opportunities to try various assignments to regain independence. Each group member was responsible to identify individual goals that pertained to their own rehabilitation. As a leader, I had the task of overseeing each participant's progress (assist in setting goals, self-reflection, and progress toward goals), help the group if they came to an impasse or disagreement, and ensure everyone's safety on the outing and in the group meetings.

The group met on Mondays, Wednesdays, and Fridays. On Monday, the group members met for 2 hours and members decided together on a location they wanted to visit that week. Members each had a rotating group role, such as researching information on the Internet, making phone calls, planning the lunch location, and coordinating transportation. They had to share information and make decisions together. On Wednesday, the group took the 3-hour outing, which always included some type of activity in a public place and having lunch together at a restaurant. The group had a limited budget per person so they had to plan well and not overspend. Being in the community actually practicing the skills was incredibly beneficial for the clients and afforded many memorable experiences. One time we ate at a very nice restaurant and the members had the opportunity to practice social skills while interacting with the servers and appropriate table conversation among the group. Other trips included tours of football stadiums, local parks, gardens, a community college, using various modes of public transportation, and shopping centers. In a group of individuals with varying abilities, the members definitely had the chance to work on skills such as exhibiting patience while waiting for others to catch up or finish eating. On Fridays, the group came together for 1 hour to debrief Wednesday's trip. They reviewed the budget, evaluated and discussed their own progress toward their individual goals, and gave peer feedback. The concept of group dynamics was extraordinarily evident to me as group leader. I interacted and observed as the group members learned, worked, and supported one another in gaining their functional independence. Some members played additional roles that either supported the group goals (time keeper or organizer) or blocked them (attention-seeking roles, such as jokester or being overly emotional). I also learned how to lead more effectively in the facilitative role, determining when the members needed my assistance and when they did not. It was difficult at first to let them struggle a bit and to know the best time to step in, but with experience, facilitative leadership became more natural to me. -Amy J. Mahle, MHA, COTA/L

INTERPROFESSIONAL COMMUNICATION

Communicating with and engaging colleagues from other healthcare disciplines is integral to providing the best and most efficient client-centered care (Fig. 5-9). Each member of the healthcare team works together to provide care and education, and is aware of and respects the focus of each other's profession. However, it encompasses more than just being aware. Team members seek to support the education provided to the client by the other team members. A good example is when an OT practitioner ensures the client is using the appropriate assistive device prescribed by the physical therapist, is using it properly while working on the OT goals, and provides a brief report (typically verbal) to the physical therapist or physical therapist assistant regarding the client's performance. All healthcare providers should strive to work together in a successful team. The characteristics of an effective interprofessional team are:

- Good communication, both verbal and written, facilitated by planning meetings, client care conferences, telephone consultation, good documentation, and the willingness to go "out of the way" to make sure communication takes place
- Mutual respect among disciplines, recognizing respective areas of expertise, knowing one's limits, and teaching each other

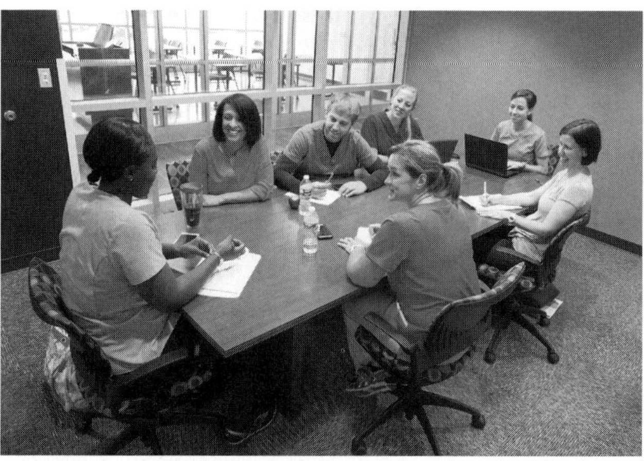

FIGURE 5-9. Team meeting of healthcare practitioners.

- A desire to work as a team and recognition of a common goal[46]

ENGAGING THE COMMUNITY

OTAs may be involved in many types of teaching in the community, such as workshops, seminars, community exercise groups, or presentations on topics of interest to a group. Audiences may include support groups, senior citizen groups, parent groups, teachers, groups of other healthcare providers, groups at homeless shelters, religious groups, free clinics, subsidized housing staff and clientele, etc. Opportunities for leading groups or providing presentations allow the OTA to promote OT to diverse groups as well as hone skills and share valuable information to the public (Fig. 5-10).

Some examples of free and powerful educational events are CarFit and the American Association of Retired Persons (AARP) HomeFit program.[47] In each of these, practitioners and students participate in training to become certified to carry out the program. The programs are community-based, free, and a powerful method to educate community members. CarFit focuses on the safe and comfortable fit of an older adult in their vehicle. CarFit events are offered nationwide. The CarFit technicians conduct a 12-point checklist to assess the community member's safe and comfortable fit in his or her car, by checking aspects of distance from the steering wheel, seat height, mirror settings to minimize blind spots, and more (Figure 5-11).[48]

The AARP HomeFit program includes a comprehensive guide that focuses on making changes in a home environment to create a safe, comfortable, and accessible fit. Booklets are available online and local AARP offices provide community trainings for HomeFit. OTAs can be involved in using the self-directed AARP booklet, on a volunteer basis, to help individuals understand and apply the information to their own home. Trainings to be qualified to use the AARP materials are held through AARP. Contact a local AARP office for additional information.

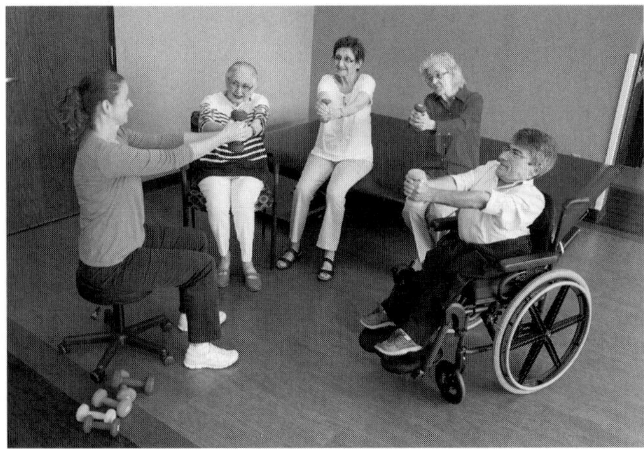

FIGURE 5-10. Teaching a group community class.

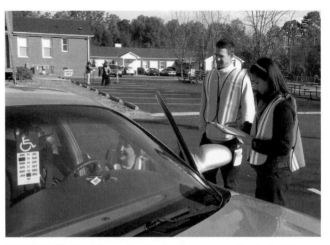

FIGURE 5-11. Providing education to the community via CarFit.

SUMMARY

Education and training are important processes occurring daily in OT in individual and group settings. To be effective in the role in educating and training clients, the OTA must understand each learner's unique life situation and conditions, preferred style of learning, and what motivates learning. Learning is affected by one's beliefs about the control he or she has to make changes (self-efficacy), the internal and external motivations for learning, and current physical and psychological conditions. Adult learners bring their experience and a desire to know why, so OT practitioners should clearly link education and training to the client's desired goals. Handouts should appeal to a broad audience and use plain language principles, include clear illustrations, be well organized, and take into account font type and size recommendations. Other types of technology also may be used for training and education and are most appropriate if customized to the client. Most often the OTA is teaching the client, including family and caregivers, but also may be providing this service to the community.

REVIEW QUESTIONS

1. Which three of the following are parts of the Health Belief Model?
   a. Perceived barriers
   b. Perceived benefits
   c. Perceived gains
   d. Perceived risks
   e. Perceived seriousness
   f. Perceived threats
2. An OTA student chooses not to study with a classmate who has a bad cold, stating, "I am afraid I might get sick." This reflects which learning theory or model?
   a. Locus of Control Theory
   b. Social Cognition Theory
   c. Health Belief Model
   d. Transactional Model of Stress and Coping
3. An elderly resident in a skilled nursing facility regularly refuses when Carl, the OTA, schedules her for shower training for her 8:00 a.m. OT session. Kathy, the certified nursing assistant

(CNA), reports no difficulty with the resident doing sponge baths in the evening. When Carl expresses frustration with the resident, the occupational therapist suggests there may be contextual variables contributing to the resident's reluctance to engage in this occupational task. After reflecting on this, which three contexts does Carl identify as the *most likely* causes?
   a. Cultural–She does not like working with a person of opposite gender.
   b. Personal–She does not like bathing.
   c. Physical–She feels more secure in her room than in the shower room.
   d. Social–She prefers to bathe alone.
   e. Temporal–She prefers bathing as part of a bedtime routine.
   f. Virtual–She does not know how to turn on the shower.
4. A client continues to have difficulty performing her home exercises. After the OTA suggests the client write down the instructions in her own words, draw diagrams, and practice, the client is much more successful. What is this client's likely preferred learning style?
   a. Visual
   b. Auditory
   c. Kinesthetic
   d. Read/write
5. The Home Health team is concerned that Mr. Smith's blood sugar is currently unstable but had been well-controlled during the 2 weeks when his daughter stayed with him. The OTA determines that although Mr. Smith has been instructed and has a handout detailing the dietary changes required, he is struggling to make sense of the information. This is an example of what component of health literacy?
   a. Functional illiteracy
   b. Informatic illiteracy
   c. Numeric illiteracy
   d. Visual illiteracy
6. Which feature is recommended for a handout on exercises for a client who has had a CVA and has a hard time processing information?
   a. Bold font to show the importance of the exercises
   b. Bulleted information instead of paragraphs
   c. Simple figures illustrating movement
   d. All uppercase letters to increase legibility
7. Leslie, an OTA, states that her client is grumpy and has said repeatedly that he wants to be independent and never have to see her again. He has almost mastered donning his lower extremity prosthesis and is eager to work on lower body dressing. Which teaching method should Leslie use with the client today?
   a. Forward chaining
   b. Backward chaining
   c. Chunking
   d. Motor learning
8. One of Jamie's long-term goals is to eat with his electronic feeder. A short-term goal is for his spouse (caregiver) to be able to set up his electronic feeder. The OTA spent two sessions with the spouse reviewing the parts of the feeder and how it works. This week's session includes the spouse practicing the set-up. She makes a few mistakes, needs several verbal cues, and refers to the written instructions a few times. The spouse is at what stage of motor learning?
   a. Associative
   b. Autonomous
   c. Cognitive
   d. Preparatory
9. Sheila is working with an 18-year-old client, Tony, after the amputation of his left leg as a result of cancer. Tony is very self-conscious about his appearance and Sheila is having a hard time motivating him to enter a driving rehabilitation program. What is the best approach for Sheila to use?
   a. Watch NASCAR races with Tony.
   b. Ask Tony if he wants to be the only 18-year-old who does not drive.
   c. Practice entering and exiting the mock car that is located in the middle of the rehabilitation gymnasium.
   d. Invite a former client, who is successfully driving after a leg amputation, to come and talk with Tony.
10. The OTA and psychologist in the rehabilitation hospital are leading a Relaxation Training and Stress Management group that meets daily for 1 week. On Monday, the group learns about the stress and relaxation responses in the body. On Tuesday, Wednesday, and Thursday, they learn and practice different techniques such as autogenic relaxation and guided imagery. On Friday, they share which techniques worked best for them and how they can incorporate them into their lives after discharge. This system illustrates which phases of group education?
    a. Acquisition, retention, generalization, and transfer phases
    b. Forming, storming, norming, and performing phases
    c. Introductory, activity, sharing, and feedback phases
    d. Planning, implementation, intervention, and outcome phases

CASE STUDY

Kim Jones is an 18-year-old male who loves to skateboard and hopes to try out for the X Games, a televised sports event, in the future. While trying to master an upside down 360-degree loop, Kim has a hard fall and fractures his cervical spine, resulting in C7 tetraplegia. The doctors try to explain what happened in Kim's spine, but his mother, Mrs. Jones, cannot stop crying or listen. Kim is frightened and not talking, but his father, Mr. Jones, listens carefully to everything the doctors say. When the surgeon comes to tell the family that Kim's surgery was successful, he draws a picture to help Mr. Jones comprehend the spinal anatomy. Mr. Jones nods in understanding, and that night at home, he goes on the Internet and reads more about cervical spine injuries. The next day he tries to explain to his wife and son how the nerves come out between the vertebrae, and why Kim will not be able to move his fingers or his legs. Mrs. Jones starts crying again, and Kim keeps asking if he can skateboard again. Kim is not receptive to the efforts of the occupational therapist, physical therapist, or nursing staff to teach him anything; repeating over and over, "I guess I'm a cripple now. No more skateboarding, no more girlfriend, no more fun. Bye, bye life." Mrs. Jones runs from the room when the registered nurse offers to show her how to catheterize Kim, saying she cannot do that. Only Mr. Jones maintains a positive attitude, telling Kim that his life still has some adventures in store for him. The night before Kim is due to transfer to a rehabilitation hospital to a spinal cord injury unit, Mr. Jones brings in a DVD for the family to watch. When Kim sees the cover of Murderball, he says, "Oh, great ... a movie about gimps in wheelchairs. Whoopee." Gradually though, Mr. Jones notices that Kim is watching, smiling, wincing, and sometimes laughing as the members of the U.S. Quad Rugby team talk, play, curse, dance, and fall out of their wheelchairs.

At the rehabilitation unit, Kim sees other people with spinal cord injuries and attends some group education sessions. After a presentation about driving rehabilitation, Kim tells his mother that he may be able to drive someday with hand controls and other modifications. Mrs. Jones does not want him to have false hope and does not share his excitement. The next day the OTA introduces the family to a man in a wheelchair, saying, "This is Mike. He is one of our peer educators." Mike tells the Jones family about his C7 spinal cord injury 10 years ago; talks about his job as a high school math teacher, and then shows them pictures of him, his wife, and their 6-year-old son skiing in Colorado. Kim is visibly relieved to hear that Mike met his wife, graduated college, got married, and had a child, all AFTER his injury. Mrs. Jones is amazed when Mike tells her that he drove to the hospital in his own car, and realizes that Kim will be able to do many things, although in a different way than before his accident.

The OTA has been trying to train Kim how to hold utensils using the tenodesis grip but her hands are different than his and he has difficulty acquiring this skill. Finally, she pulls out her tablet and searches for the Quad Smoothie video on YouTube™. In it, Chris Colwell demonstrates how he makes a smoothie, and Kim sees how Chris uses his tenodesis grip. Kim wants to practice right away at his next OT session, telling the OTA he needs to be able to hold a stylus so he can look for videos on his tablet independently. She shows him what to do, and has him demonstrate this task back to her. Over the next couple of days, Kim not only holds a fork, but also a razor, a pen, and finally a stylus. One day he calls his parents in to see a video he found of teenager Aaron Fotheringham skateboarding in his wheelchair. Something clicks and Kim is now ready to learn everything he can from the OT and physical therapy staff.

Kim asks his mother to take notes during some of his therapy sessions, so he can reread them later. He requests that the staff videotape him doing his exercises so he will remember what to do when he goes home. He gets an audiobook of *Walking Papers*, wherein Francesco Clark describes his personal journey after his spinal cord injury. Francesco started his own company, Clark's Botanicals, and became a worldwide ambassador for the Christopher Reeve Foundation. Mrs. Jones reads handouts about catheter care and verbally describes the procedure to the nurse, before practicing on an anatomic model and finally helping Kim. Mr. and Mrs. Jones read Christopher Reeve's autobiography and Mr. Jones drives to the state capitol to talk to his elected officials about sponsoring a bill for increased funding of spinal cord injury research. Mrs. Jones and Kim plan a presentation they will do for the high school students and teachers when he is ready to return to school.

A variety of teaching methods helped the Jones family as they moved through different stages of understanding and acceptance of Kim's diagnosis. By offering education in many different styles, and allowing the Jones family members to learn in the ways that worked for them, the hospital staff helped them gain confidence in critical skills. In addition, the staff gave them the means to continue learning on their own.

1. Identify multiple teaching/learning methods used by staff and the Jones family.
2. Why was Mrs. Jones able to learn catheterization later in Kim's admission? What were the barriers to her learning when the nurse first tried to teach her?
3. What was Mike's role and why was this so important?

PUTTING IT ALL TOGETHER Sample Treatment Session and Documentation

Setting	Outpatient clinic
Client Profile	48-year-old male, S/P brain injury due to a fall at home. Severe ataxia (difficulty with smooth, coordinated movements) and diplopia (double vision). Uses manual w/c for ambulation, does not self-propel. PEG tube (feeding tube in abdomen), due to be removed in approximately 3 to 4 weeks. Also receiving physical therapy and speech therapy.
Work History	Salesman, travels worldwide
Insurance	Private
Psychological	Frustrated with current need for assistance with all ADLs and IADLs
Social	Supportive spouse (primary caregiver) and two preteen children in the home; spouse attends all therapy appointments
Cognitive	Somewhat impulsive
Motor & Manual Muscle testing (MMT)	Severe ataxia affecting functional use of BUE/BLEs, trunk, speech, and swallowing MMT not tested at this point.
ADL	Max A for LB & UB dressing and UB bathing. Dependent self-feeding, LB bathing, grooming, toileting. Max A for transfers.
IADL	Dependent for all
Precautions	Needs thickened liquids. No driving.
Goals	1. Client will dress UB in a seated position with Min A within 3 weeks. 2. Client will drink with Mod I (thickened liquids) with AE in 3 weeks. 3. Client will feed himself with Mod A (puréed foods) and AE and adapted methods in 4 weeks. 4. Client will transfer from w/c to bed with Min A within 5 weeks. 5. Client will sign name on legal documents with Mod I Client will sign name with an "X" on legal documents with AE and Min A within 4 weeks.

PUTTING IT ALL TOGETHER Sample Treatment Session and Documentation (continued)

OT TREATMENT SESSION 1

THERAPEUTIC ACTIVITY	TIME	GOAL(S) ADDRESSED	OTA RATIONALE
W/C to therapy mat for transfer training with client and training of spouse. Used client's phone to video COTA/L assisting with the transfer, and then the spouse assisting with the transfer	25 min.	#4	Work on w/c to mat and mat to w/c transfers first because the bed is a softer and smaller surface. Train spouse to assist client with transfer, because she is his primary caregiver and will need to learn to help him less as he gains more skills. Have the spouse create videos of the transfer training with COTA/L for reinforcement of proper technique, and then with spouse performing transfers so she could compare techniques and observe her own body mechanics and style.
Self-feeding (drinking) with various adapted cups and stainless steel travel mugs (with and without handles)	23 min.	#2	Sample different types of cups with the client. Train client on body positioning and placement of UEs on cup for successful drinking.
Sitting balance on mat, have client retrieve clothing item	10 min.	#1	In preparation for UB dressing, work on sitting balance, stability, and retrieving items with one hand.

SOAP note: 12/30/—, 1:00 pm–1:58 pm

S: "I just want to be able to drink my morning coffee by myself."

O: Client received skilled OT for transfer training, UB dressing, and self-feeding. Client performed w/c to mat transfers x four trials. Skilled instruction provided to spouse and client on positioning of w/c to mat, placement of hands and feet, and gait belt use via demonstration with client. Client and spouse required Mod verbal cues for body mechanics and Min verbal cues for timing of transfer. Video taken with client's phone to reinforce transfer training skills, proper body mechanics, and for practice at home. While on mat, client was able to support trunk while leaning on LUE with Min A. Client required Max A for postural control while reaching for clothing items with RUE in preparation for UB seated dressing. Client seated in w/c at table with cutout for training in self-feeding (drinking) with thickened room-temperature liquid (spouse brought liquid and thickener). OTA trained client in positioning of elbows propped on cutout table, close to trunk, feet on floor, and trialed several types of cups with and without handle(s) and of various weights. Spouse took photo of positioning and cutout table to try at home with their table. Client was most successful with stainless steel travel mug without handle, firmly grasping with both hands; client was able to take five sips of thickened beverage, requiring Mod A to bring smoothly to mouth due to ataxia.

A: Client making progress toward goal of transfers and adapted self-feeding (drinking). Ataxia continues to challenge client's independence. Client and spouse responded well to training, verbalizing strategies for body mechanics and positioning. Client to work on transfers and self-feeding (drinking) at home with videos and photos as a resource.

P: Continue to work on UB dressing skills and practice donning shirt. Wait until PEG is removed for doffing shirt. Follow up with client and spouse re: transfer practice and self-feeding (drinking) at home.

Zachary Goldstein, COTA/L, 12/30/—, 4:46 pm

TREATMENT SESSION 2

What could you do next with this client?

TREATMENT SESSION 3

What could you do next with this client?

REFERENCES

1. Hayden, J. (2009). *Introduction to health behavior theory.* Burlington, MA: Jones & Barlett Publishers.
2. Pajares, F. (2009). Self-efficacy theory. Retrieved from http://www.education.com/reference/article/self-efficacy-theory/
3. Cherry, K. (2016). What is locus of control? Retrieved from https://www.verywell.com/what-is-locus-of-control-2795434
4. Park, C. L., & Folkman, S. (1997). Meaning in the context of stress and coping. *Review of General Psychology, 1*(2), 115-144. Retrieved from https://www.researchgate.net/profile/Crystal_Park/publication/232561932_Meaning_in_the_Context_of_Stress_and_Coping/links/00b4952d57e7bde419000000.pdf
5. University of Twente. (2010). Transactional model of stress and coping. Retrieved from https://www.utwente.nl/cw/theorieenoverzicht/Theory%20clusters/Health%20Communication/transactional_model_of_stress_and_coping/
6. Pappas, C. (2013). The adult learning theory–andragogy–of Malcolm Knowles. Retrieved from https://elearningindustry.com/the-adult-learning-theory-andragogy-of-malcolm-knowles
7. Think Exist. (2016). William Glasser quotes. Retrieved from http://thinkexist.com/quotes/william_glasser/
8. Thalheimer, W. (2015, March 12). Debunk this: People remember 10 percent of what they read. Retrieved from https://www.td.org/Publications/Blogs/Science-of-Learning-Blog/2015/03/Debunk-This-People-Remember-10-Percent-of-What-They-Read
9. Tapscott, D. (2009). *Grown up digital: How the net generation is changing your world,* (p. 130). New York, NY: McGraw-Hill.
10. State University of New York at Cortland. (n.d.). What are learning styles? Retrieved from http://web.cortland.edu/andersmd/learning/Introduction.htm
11. American Occupational Therapy Association. (2014). Occupational therapy practice framework: Domain and process (3rd ed.). *American Journal of Occupational Therapy, 68*(Suppl. 1).
12. Learning Styles Online. (2016). Overview of learning styles. Retrieved from http://www.learning-styles-online.com/overview/http://www.learning-styles-online.com/overview/
13. Teach.com. (2016). Learning styles. Retrieved from http://teach.com/what/teachers-teach/learning-styles
14. University of New Mexico Health Sciences Library and Informatics Center. (2016). Occupational therapy resources: Patient education. Retrieved from http://libguides.health.unm.edu/c.php?g=238055&p=1582837
15. Berkman, N. D., Davis, T. C., & McCormack, L. (2010). Health literacy: What is it? *Journal of Health Communication, 15*(Sup2), 9-19. doi:10.1080/10810730.2010.499985
16. National Network of Libraries of Medicine. (2016). Health literacy. Retrieved from http://nnlm.gov/outreach/consumer/hlthlit.html/
17. Office of Disease Prevention and Health Promotion. (2016). 2020 Topics and objectives: Health communication and health information technology. Retrieved from https://www.healthypeople.gov/2020/topics-objectives/topic/Health-Communication-and-Health-Information-Technology/objectives#4534
18. Pleasant, A., Rudd, R. E., O'Leary, C., Paasche-Orlow, M. K., Allen, M. P., Alvarado-Little, W., ... Rosen, S. (2016). Considerations for a new definition of health literacy. National Academy of Sciences. Retrieved from https://nam.edu/considerations-for-a-new-definition-of-health-literacy/
19. Public Health Agency of Canada. (2014). Health literacy. Retrieved from http://www.phac-aspc.gc.ca/cd-mc/hl-ls/index-eng.php
20. Impact Information Plain Language Services. (2013). Plain language at work newsletter: Know your readers. Retrieved from http://www.impact-information.com/impactinfo/literacy.htm
21. Institute of Education Sciences, National Center for Education Statistics. (2003). The Health Literacy of America's Adults: Results from the 2003 National Assessment of Adult Literacy. Retrieved from http://nces.ed.gov/pubsearch/pubsinfo.asp?pubid=2006483
22. Colmer, R. (2017). What is readability? Retrieved from https://readable.io/alerts/
23. Fonts.com. (n.d.). Module: Fine topography. Retrieved from https://www.fonts.com/content/learning/fontology/level-4/fine-typography/legibility
24. Wood, J. (2011). The best fonts to use in print, online, and email. *American Writers and Artists, Inc.* Retrieved from http://www.awaionline.com/2011/10/the-best-fonts-to-use-in-print-online-and-email/
25. U.S. Department of Health and Human Services, Agency for Healthcare Research and Quality. (2012). Plain language at AHRQ. Retrieved from http://www.ahrq.gov/policy/electronic/plain-writing/index.html
26. Centers for Medicare and Medicaid Services. (2012). Toolkit part 9: Material for older adults. Retrieved from https://www.cms.gov/Outreach-and-Education/Outreach/WrittenMaterialsToolkit/ToolkitPart09.html
27. Gray, C. (2016). Behavior chains and chaining. Chaining: Choosing a backward, forward or total task approach. Retrieved from http://www.cherylgray.com/cheryl/BIA2_Wk9_lecture_chaining.htm
28. Brandon, B. (2003). Last things first: The power of backward chaining. *Learning Solutions Magazine.* Retrieved from http://www.learningsolutionsmag.com/articles/325/last-things-first-the-power-of-backward-chaining
29. Muratori, L. M., Lamberg, E. M., Quinn, L., and Duff, S.V. (2013). Applying principles of motor learning and control to upper extremity rehabilitation. *Journal of Hand Therapy, 26*(2), 94-103. doi:10.1016/j.jht.2012.12.007
30. Human Kinetics. (2016). Understanding motor learning stages improves skill instruction. Retrieved from http://www.humankinetics.com/excerpts/excerpts/understanding-motor-learning-stages-improves-skill-instruction
31. Wulf, G., & Lewthwaite, R. (2016). Optimizing performance through intrinsic motivation and attention for learning: The OPTIMAL theory of motor learning. *Psychonomic Bulletin & Review, 23,* 1382. https://doi.org/10.3758/s13423-015-0999-9
32. U.S. National Library of Medicine. (2016). Maximizing your teaching moment. Retrieved from https://www.nlm.nih.gov/medlineplus/ency/patientinstructions/000460.htm
33. Jesus, T. S., & Silva, I. L. (2015). Toward an evidence-based patient-provider communication in rehabilitation: Linking communication elements to better rehabilitation outcomes. *Clinical Rehabilitation, 30*(4), 315-328. doi:10.1177/0269215515585133
34. Ekelman, B. A., Allison, D. L., Duvnjak, D., DiMarino, D. R., Jodzio, J., & Iannarelli, P. V. (2017). A wellness program for men with spinal cord injury: Participation and meaning. *Oxford Transitional Justice Research: Occupation, Participation and Health, 37*(1), 30-39. doi:10.1177/1539449216672170
35. Sawyer, T. (2016). Implementing electronic tablet-based education of acute care patients. *Critical Care Nurse, 36*(1), 60. doi:10.4037/ccn2016541
36. Stribling, J. C., & Richardson, J. E. (2016). Placing wireless tablets in clinical settings for patient education. *Journal of the Medical Library Association, 104*(2), 159-164. doi:10.3163/1536-5050.104.2.013
37. Nygård, L., & Rosenberg, L. (2016). How attention to everyday modern technology could contribute to modern occupational therapy: A focus group study. *British Journal of Occupational Therapy, 79*(8), 467-474. https://doi.org/10.1177/0308022615613354
38. Ryan, R. M., & Deci, E. L. (2001). Intrinsic and extrinsic motivations: Classic definitions and new directions. *Contemporary Educational Psychology, 25,* 54-67. doi:10.1006/ceps.1999.1020
39. EuroMed Info. (n.d.). Patient teaching into practice: Process of patient education. Retrieved from http://www.euromedinfo.eu/process-of-patient-education-introduction.html/
40. Cooper, C. (2013). *Mosby's field guide to occupational therapy for physical dysfunction.* St. Louis, MO: Elsevier Mosby.
41. U.S. National Library of Medicine. (2016). Choosing effective patient education materials. Retrieved from https://www.nlm.nih.gov/medlineplus/ency/patientinstructions/000455.htm

42. U.S. National Library of Medicine. (2016). Communicating with patients. Retrieved from https://www.nlm.nih.gov/medlineplus/ency/patientinstructions/000456.htm
43. Martin, G. E., Klusek, J., Estigarribia, B., & Roberts, J. E. (2009). Language characteristics of individuals with Down syndrome. *Topics in Language Disorders, 29*(2), 112-132. doi:10.1097/tld.0b013e3181a71fe1
44. United States Census Bureau. (2015). Census bureau reports at least 350 languages spoken in U.S. homes. Retrieved from http://www.census.gov/newsroom/press-releases/2015/cb15-185.html
45. Nasmith, L., & Daigle, N. (1996). Small-group teaching in patient education. *Medical Teacher, 18*(3), 209-211. doi:10.3109/01421599609034162
46. EuroMed Info. (n.d.). Patient teaching into practice: Interdisciplinary collaboration, patient education. Retrieved from http://www.euromedinfo.eu/interdisciplinary-collaboration-patient-education.html/
47. American Association of Retired Persons. (2014). The AARP home fit guide. Retrieved from http://www.aarp.org/content/dam/aarp/livable-communities/documents-2014/AARP-Home-Fit-Guide-2014.pdf
48. EuroMed Info. (n.d.). Patient teaching into practice: Assessing learning needs. Retrieved from http://www.euromedinfo.eu/assessing-learning-needs.html/

Chapter 6

Developing the Occupational Profile and Analyzing Occupational Performance

Cynthia S. Bell, PhD, OTR/L and Megan E. Edwards Collins, PhD, OTR/L

LEARNING OUTCOMES

After studying this chapter, the student or practitioner will be able to:

6.1 Explain the concept of an occupational profile and how to obtain the needed information for an occupational profile
6.2 Describe how to complete the Canadian Occupational Performance Measure
6.3 Demonstrate the concept of Motivational Interviewing
6.4 Identify the steps to consider when analyzing occupational performance
6.5 Discuss how to determine the activity demands associated with an occupation
6.6 Define space demands
6.7 Describe the relationship between body structures, body functions, and performance skills
6.8 Identify motor, process, and social interaction skills

KEY TERMS

Activity analysis	Grading
Activity and occupational demands	Motivational Interviewing
Adapting	Occupational performance
Canadian Occupational Performance Measure (COPM)	Occupational profile
	Performance skill

The occupational therapy (OT) profession addresses the occupations, or meaningful activities in which individuals engage, as well as utilizes occupations in practice. Two essential components of the skilled provision of OT include the practitioner's ability to develop an occupational profile and analyze the occupational performance of a client. This chapter will provide an overview of each of these concepts and highlight the role of the occupational therapy assistant (OTA). Through understanding these concepts, students and practitioners will learn how to more effectively provide OT services in a client-centered manner, using key concepts from the *Occupational Therapy Practice Framework: Domain and Process, 3rd edition* (OTPF-3) (Box 6-1).

OCCUPATIONAL PROFILE OVERVIEW

The OTA and occupational therapist should communicate and work together to establish a thorough and accurate **occupational profile,** the summary of information about the client, which includes occupational history and daily life tasks, interests, and values.[1] The occupational therapist can begin the occupational profile, and then communicate to the OTA details regarding further information that needs to be gathered and obtained. The two can collaborate and review the occupational profile to establish treatment goals and priorities. The OTA can also continue to revise and add to the occupational profile as he or she works with the client and the client progresses through the therapy process.

The occupational profile assists OT practitioners in obtaining a holistic view of the client and establishing client-centered

BOX 6-1
History of the Occupational Therapy Practice Framework[1]

The American Occupational Therapy Association (AOTA) Commission on Practice (COP) began working on the first edition of the *Occupational Therapy Practice Framework* in 1999 to develop a document that spelled out what OT involves and the process OT practitioners use with clients. The document that was developed was titled *The Occupational Therapy Practice Framework: Domain and Process* (OTPF) and was first published in 2002. The OTPF provided the basis for the profession to return to the historical roots of occupation-based practice and reinforced the need for a client-centered focus. Since the original publication of the OTPF in 2002, there have been two revisions by the COP involving feedback from AOTA members and the approval from the AOTA Representative Assembly. The second version was published in 2008, and the third and current version in 2014. The COP typically reviews official documents on a 5-year cycle.

TECHNOLOGY AND TRENDS

The occupational profile contains crucial information for the OT practitioner and healthcare team. With the increased use of electronic documentation across healthcare settings and facilities, the OT practitioner must become familiar with the layout of the documentation system their employer uses to find the most appropriate section to document information obtained from the occupational profile. There is most likely not going to be a section titled "occupational profile" for the practitioner to utilize. For example, the client's primary concerns and goals, prior level of functioning, and environmental setup may all be in different sections. Some documentation systems may have such information under a "basic information" section, or a "medical history" tab. The OTA must review the client's chart in its entirety to make sure he or she obtains all needed information.

goals. The profile explores the client's occupational history, performance patterns (e.g., routines and roles), and client factors such as their values and interests (Fig. 6-1).[1] Understanding the client's occupational history can assist the OT practitioner in becoming aware of what is meaningful and relevant to the client, including any discrepancies between the client's abilities and what he or she needs and would like to be able to do in daily life. For example, a client who has had a cerebrovascular accident (CVA) may be a grandmother who always baked cookies for her grandchildren, but can no longer do so because of decreased upper extremity range of motion and strength. While completing the occupational profile, the OT practitioner might learn that this is a role and occupation the client highly values and would like to be able to engage in again. Another client might be a rabbi who recently had a heart attack and, as a result, might report having decreased endurance and ability to participate in desired religious activities. The client and OT practitioner together can establish client-centered, occupation-based goals that help address the client's occupational needs and wants.

The OT practitioner should begin establishing the client's occupational profile when the client first begins OT. It can be completed in one session or throughout numerous sessions.[1] The OT practitioner continues to obtain new information and revise/update the occupational profile throughout the occupational process. For example, a client who has sustained a traumatic brain injury might return to work during the course of receiving OT services and encounter new challenges that need to be addressed. A client who has had a CVA might have accomplished a goal of making a simple meal like sandwiches and want to progress to making something more challenging such as lasagna. This helps ensure that the client's goals stay relevant and current, meeting her needs. Currently, for outpatient OT evaluations, Medicare requires a thorough occupational profile as part of the evaluation, and the OTA will contribute to this process as appropriate.

Information for the occupational profile can be obtained through both formal and informal conversations and interviews, and can help establish rapport with the client.[1] Obtaining such information "leads to an individualized approach in the evaluation, intervention planning, and intervention implementations stages."[1] Specific areas to address include the client's reasons for coming to OT, occupational history, values and interests, roles, current routines, and changes in their roles, routines, and occupational engagement. The OT practitioner must get a sense of the types of occupations and roles a client has, and how they have been influenced by the client's current situation (e.g., having recently had a CVA or been diagnosed with Parkinson's disease). This can assist the practitioner in determining how active the client once was and is helpful in developing meaningful, relevant, functional goals. As part of the occupational profile, clients also identify what they perceive to be their strengths and barriers, which relate to things the client feels help support occupational performance as well as things that hinder their performance. **Occupational performance** can be defined as the client's ability to desire, recall, plan, and carry out occupations based on internal desire or external stimuli and demands.[1] Looking at aspects in their physical and social environment, as well as their physical and cognitive functioning, is part of the process. For example, a client might say that he or she has learned to be extra cautious around the stove to compensate for sensory deficits, and would prefer to address how those sensory deficits are impeding the ability to safely bathe. Overall, the

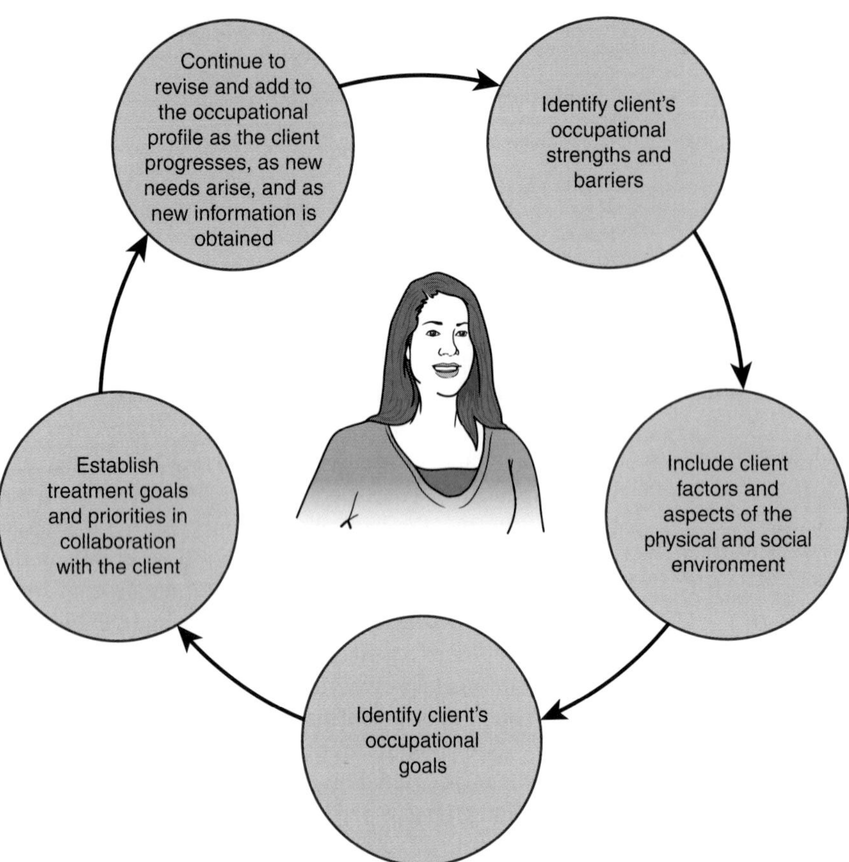

FIGURE 6-1. The Occupational Profile Process.

OT practitioner needs to explore and determine the ability of the client to perform needed and desired occupations.

The OT practitioner can utilize the occupational profile to guide intervention (including areas that might need to be evaluated further) and better understand the client's occupational needs across the OTPF-3 domains. The OT practitioner should note client strengths and how they can be utilized to enhance occupational performance. The occupational profile can be used to help determine treatment goals and priorities. Information on what the client would like to work on in OT is obtained, and his or her occupational concerns and priorities are identified. This information can be used to determine a client-centered OT intervention approach, as goals are established in collaboration with the client. These goals are all tied into functional activities and occupations, such as activities of daily living (ADL) and leisure activities. For example, a client might prefer to work on increasing his or her ability to play with children or grandchildren and rely on others' help for bathing. Another client might want to focus on leisure or work tasks, and have assistance for ADLs to conserve energy. For other clients, bathing and dressing independently may be their top priority. Every client is unique.

Sources of Information

The OT practitioner can obtain information for the occupational profile from a variety of sources. When possible, the client should be the primary source of information for the profile. As the OTPF-3 states, "by valuing and respecting clients' input, practitioners help foster their involvement and can more efficiently guide interventions."[1] This ensures that the practitioner gets the client's perspective and hears his or her goals and expectations for therapy. If the client is unable to speak or is not cognitively able to provide the needed information, the occupational profile can be created with input from family and/or caregivers. It is important to document who gave the information for the occupational profile and why it was not able to be obtained from the client. Even when the client is able to provide information, family members and caregivers can provide some additional insight and perspective to ensure that the OT practitioner gets a holistic and accurate view of the client and his or her situation and needs. For example, a client may have decreased insight and not realize that he or she is unable to fully perform self-care tasks. Other healthcare professionals working with the client might also be able to provide valuable information. This can include information on the client's functional status, strategies for working with the client, and areas to focus on during intervention. For example, a physical therapist working with a client might be able to let the OT practitioner know strategies he or she has found to be safe and effective when transferring the client or on which goals the client would like to work.

When interviewing clients, family members, and caregivers to obtain information for the occupational profile, the OT practitioner needs to be unbiased and ask open-ended questions. The practitioner needs to phrase questions in a manner that does not lead the client to answer a certain way. For example, instead of saying, "I hear you are having trouble with washing your feet. Is that right?" the practitioner can ask, "What kind of trouble, if any, are you having with bathing?" Follow-up questions can help obtain more details as needed. For example, the OT practitioner can ask if the client is able to wash his or her feet (and then other specific body parts) independently.

Cultural Awareness

The OT practitioner must take into account cultural differences when completing an occupational profile. For example, certain cultures might have dynamics where a husband or another male speaks on behalf of the wife or female, and the female is supposed to be quiet and reserved. The OT practitioner must be respectful of these differences and honor the client's cultural preferences. Regardless of the interview approach(es) taken, the OT practitioner must be culturally sensitive. This includes respecting the privacy some cultures value and maintaining an appropriate level of eye contact and personal space. For example, in Western cultures it is frequently appropriate to maintain eye contact, while in some Eastern cultures, eye contact can be seen as a lack of respect.[2] The OT practitioner must respect and respond accordingly to the client's cultural beliefs throughout the OT process. Culture may also influence the roles and occupations in which a client engages. For example, males traditionally may be more likely to engage in occupations like woodworking or working on cars, while females are more likely to engage in arts and crafts and household chores. Although cultural differences must be respected and taken into account, it is important to understand that each client is unique and the OT practitioner must not automatically stereotype a client based on his or her cultural background, religion, gender, or other factors.

COMMUNICATION

It is essential for the OT practitioner to communicate clearly, professionally, and respectfully with clients and their family members/caregivers when obtaining the occupational profile. This includes being careful with nonverbal cues, such as body language. Whether the OT practitioner is tired or having a bad day, their body language should show polite interest and engagement. Be aware of the nonverbal impact of rolled eyes, crossed arms, resting the chin on the hands, or lounging back in the chair. Sensitive topics are often brought up, and the practitioner cannot pass judgment, laugh at, criticize, or minimize what the client or others may say. This may include opinions that are significantly different than those of the OT practitioner, and may even differ from the values of the practitioner. A client may note a disdain for a certain culture or group, they might express that they are worried about sexuality issues after a severe facial burn, or that they fear their mother "taking over" their life in an attempt to assist after a spinal cord injury after an accident. Clients and caregivers often establish a level of trust and openness with the OT practitioner that is valuable and important. However the communication may occur, the OT practitioner is to be professional and respectful.

Connecting With Reserved Clients

The OT practitioner must also master the skill of how to interview and obtain information from clients who tend to be quiet and reserved, including those who might be depressed. When interviewing clients who are reserved, it is important to establish a rapport and sense of trust with the client, reinforcing the importance of collaboration and stressing the shared goal of helping him or her increase engagement in daily life by doing the things that they would like and need to do. This includes assuring the client that the OT practitioner will not judge them. It can be helpful to have the client initially complete written screens and assessments, which could be more comfortable for him or her than a face-to-face interview and also help the OT practitioner to identify key areas to address. Ensuring a quiet, private, and soothing environment might also help the client become more comfortable and open to talking with the practitioner.

Canadian Occupational Performance Measure

One way the OT practitioner can obtain information to complete the occupational profile is by using the **Canadian Occupational Performance Measure (COPM)**. Involving a semistructured interview, the COPM explores self-care, productivity, and leisure.[3] This includes looking at the things clients need, want, or are expected to do. The client identifies areas within self-care (e.g., personal care, functional mobility), productivity (e.g., paid/unpaid work, household management), and leisure (e.g., socialization, quiet/active recreation) that they may be struggling with, and rates how important the issue is to him or her on a scale of 1 to 10, with 10 being extremely important. The client then selects, at most, the five most significant problem areas for him or her. Once the top five problem areas have been identified, the client rates his or her performance abilities and performance satisfaction with each of these problem areas on a scale of 1 to 10, with 10 signifying the ability to do it well or with the highest satisfaction with performance. The OT practitioner can initially administer the COPM to assist with developing intervention strategies and goals, and use it again as desired to track changes in the client's reported performance. A literature review found that "the COPM facilitates therapists to focus on client needs, to develop meaningful intervention strategies and to demonstrate concrete and significant change scores attributable to occupational therapy practice."[4] This better enables the OT practitioner to develop and provide client-centered goals and interventions. The literature review also found that the

> **OT Practitioner's Viewpoint**
>
> I have learned so much from clients I have worked with over the years and I am always amazed at how many ways there are to complete the same task. I remember trying to work with an older gentleman who was recovering from a CVA and we were working on grooming and specifically brushing his teeth. He was very adamant that he brush all of his top teeth first, then rinse his toothbrush, reapply toothpaste, and continue brushing his bottom teeth. When I asked him why he did so, he replied, "Otherwise I am just moving the leftover food around in my mouth." He said he had learned that from his mother years ago and had always done it that way. So that is how we worked on the task. To me, this example illustrates the importance of listening to a client and asking how and why he or she typically performs a task. Listening and responding appropriately is essential and also assists to build a respectful working relationship with one another. ~ Megan E. Edwards Collins, PhD., OTR/L

COPM has "satisfactory to excellent" psychometric properties, such as validity and reliability.[4]

Motivational Interviewing

Motivational interviewing is another strategy that can be used by the OT practitioner to obtain pertinent information from a client. This approach involves demonstrating empathy and compassion toward the client while eliciting their story, and working toward enhancing the client's self-efficacy.[5,6] This can be done by asking open-ended questions, engaging in reflective listening (e.g., summarizing what the client has said), asking the client reflection questions, and identifying and reinforcing the client's strengths. Reflection questions can include looking at the client's personal goals and values and how their current actions and behaviors reinforce or are inconsistent with those goals and values.[7] The client is seen as a collaborator and partner in the process, and the motivation and ambivalence (which is recognized as being normal) toward making change is explored and addressed.[5-8] These motivational interviewing techniques require that the practitioner accept the client for who they are, including respecting autonomy and helping the client recognize strengths and how to accomplish goals.[8]

OT practitioners use the term "occupation" in a broad sense. The OTPF-3 domains include an occupation domain.[1] The occupations under the OTPF-3 domain include ADLs, instrumental activities of daily living (IADLs), rest and sleep, education, work, play, leisure, and social participation. Please see Table 6-1 for specifics. It is important that individuals have a balance between the various occupations. For example, one cannot sustain a healthy lifestyle by primarily engaging in work without participating in rest and leisure pursuits. Information on the various occupations a client engages in (including those that are needed or desired), as well as his or her overall occupational participation, should be obtained as part of the occupational profile.

TABLE 6-1 Occupations[1]

Occupation	Description
Activities of Daily Living (ADLs)	• These are basic self-care tasks such as eating, dressing, bathing, grooming, and toileting tasks.
Instrumental Activities of Daily Living (IADLs)	• These are more complex tasks than ADLs such as childrearing, pet care, cooking, cleaning, driving, money management, religious or spiritual activities, health maintenance, and shopping.
Rest and Sleep	• Getting adequate rest and sleep is essential for being able to successfully engage in other occupations. • This includes sleep preparation tasks, such as grooming and undressing before bed.
Education	• Education includes formal education environments as well as informal educational pursuits such as participating in classes or programs in a particular area.
Work	• Work includes pursuing work interests and employment opportunities, seeking employment, job-related tasks, preparing for retirement, and volunteering activities.
Play	• Play includes exploring and participating in activities that one enjoys and finds entertaining or amusing.
Leisure	• Leisure includes exploring and participating in activities that one is motivated to engage in without being required to do so.
Social Participation	• Social participation activities include engaging in activities with family, friends/peers, and community members in person or through virtual means (e.g., via the Internet, telephone, or video conferencing).

ANALYZING OCCUPATIONAL PERFORMANCE

Once an occupational profile has been gathered, the next step in the OT process is to examine how the individual performs daily tasks. This is also referred to as analyzing the occupational performance of the client. The ability to analyze occupations is fundamental to the practice of OT and is often referred to as activity analysis. **Activity analysis** is part of the OT process, allowing practitioners to understand

and address the skills and external components needed for the performance of any given activity."[9] Several components are necessary to fully analyze occupational performance. First, it is important to understand the basics of how each and every occupation is typically performed. Second, it is important to consider what actions the client uses to perform the task. In OT, this is known as analyzing the occupational demands.[1] This includes knowing the context and environment surrounding the activity, for example, the physical aspects (where the task occurs, tools and objects needed), social aspects (who is involved in the task), and temporal aspects (sequence of steps, when and how often activity occurs). Third, it is important to consider analyzing occupational performance, which is the small, observable, goal-directed actions the client uses to perform daily activities. These are referred to as the client's **performance skills,** which are learned and developed over time.[1] Analysis of performance skills allows the OT practitioner to see if the client can complete the activity in his or her current capacity and environment or whether graded or adapted means are necessary for the client to be able to engage in the activity (Fig. 6-2). **Grading** the demands of a task, by adjusting the complexity of the task, can enable or enhance functional abilities, by altering the demands or the environment, task, or assisting the client to change. An example might be a client who has had a CVA and is interested in getting back to gardening. The OT practitioner may start the client with an outside raised garden bed to grade the gardening task easier, enabling the client to perform it from her wheelchair instead of standing, squatting, or kneeling. As her strength increases, the task difficulty could increase to challenge her by grading up the task with increased difficulty in standing. **Adapting** means the practitioner would offer an alternative way to perform the task, modifying or substituting objects used in performing the activity. This might mean the client would use a large-handled trowel with a strap to keep it in her hand for easier digging. **Activity analysis** is an ongoing part of the skilled OT process used throughout every encounter with a client that requires constant examination by the OT practitioner to provide a pathway to progress toward realistic client outcomes. This part of the chapter describes the components involved in analyzing occupational performance from an activity analysis perspective.

NORMAL ANALYSIS OF AN ACTIVITY

The next step after the development of the occupational profile is to determine the typical and essential components, as well as sequence and timing that are necessary for the client to successfully complete daily tasks. For example, for the occupation of grooming and the specific task of brushing one's hair, typically the task involves an individual being able to grasp a brush or comb, move his or her upper extremity to the scalp, and move the brush or comb through the hair. The OT practitioner needs to be able to have a detailed understanding of how the aspects of a task are typically performed. Input from the occupational profile can inform this process, but it also may be necessary to ask the client for additional specifics regarding the manner in which the client engages in the task, and the frequency in which these activities are performed. Once the basic, routine information is known, the OT practitioner can move on to the next step of the specific activity and occupational demands. Remember that every individual is unique, and thus, small differences exist in how people typically perform an activity. For example, some individuals fold bath towels using a table or without a table, and some individuals fold the towels in thirds or in half. All of the examples would be considered typical ways to fold a bath towel.

Activity and Occupational Demands

According to the AOTA, "Occupational therapy practitioners analyze the demands of an activity or occupation to understand the specific body structures, body functions, performance skills, and performance patterns that are required and to determine the generic demands the activity or occupation makes on the client."[1] Another way to think about it is the specific **activity and occupational demands** are the what, where, how and when, and the who involved in a particular activity or occupation. The *what* includes any objects and their properties, tools, materials needed for the activity. The *where* includes the physical space and location, and any specific requirements of that space and location (e.g., surface, lighting, temperature). The *how and when* relates to the sequence of steps involved in the activity and whether they are fixed (have to occur in a specific sequence) or flexible (can occur in different sequences). Finally, the *who* pertains to who is involved in the activity. Is it an individual acting alone or is there more than one person involved, and is there a social aspect to the activity? Activities and occupations occur within a context (cultural, personal, temporal, or virtual) and in an environment that is physical or social.[1] For example, the task of making a sandwich is typically performed in a kitchen on a countertop (physical aspect of the environment); in addition, specific ingredients and objects are needed needed to make the sandwich: peanut butter and jelly and a knife to get the peanut butter and jelly out of their jars and spread on the bread, and a cutting board or plate, are necessary (physical aspects), and it usually does not require any assistance or communication with another (social environment). To examine this further, let's analyze the activity demands of making a peanut butter and jelly sandwich and consider all of the components involved (Fig. 6-3). An individual has a reason to make the sandwich (relevance and importance to the client); needs a plate and/or cutting board to make and serve and a knife to scoop out the peanut butter and jelly (tools); a countertop or table (equipment); peanut butter, jelly, and bread (supplies); enough room on the countertop or table (space); and performs it in a particular order, such as spreading the peanut butter and jelly before putting the two pieces of bread together (sequence). Furthermore, the individual typically uses certain actions

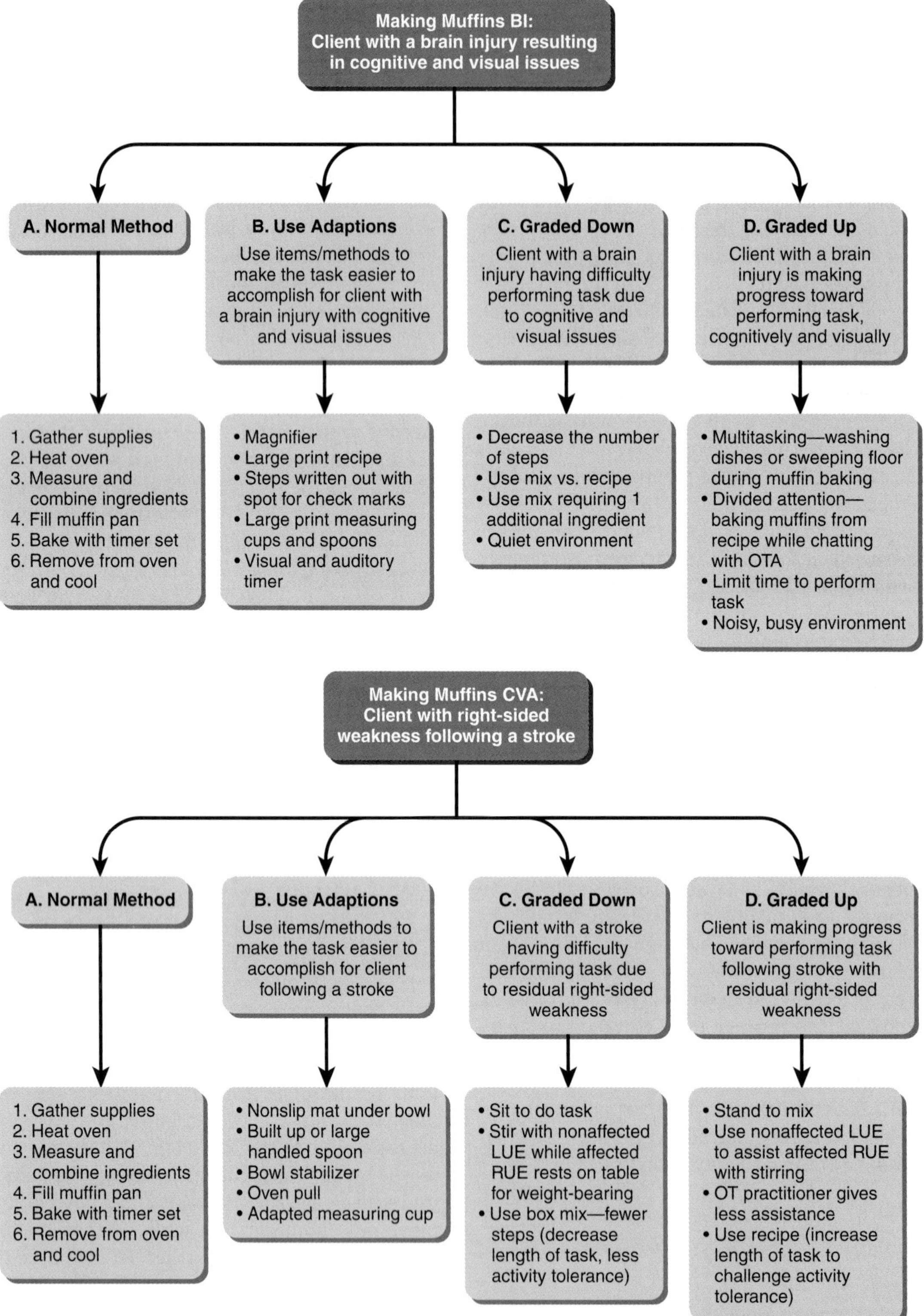

FIGURE 6-2. Each decision tree notes an example of completing a task using the normal method or adapting, grading up, or grading down.

and performance skills (moving and thinking), body functions (mobility of joints, vision), and body structures (hands, arms, eyes, etc.)

The AOTA provides a detailed description of activity and occupational demands in Table 6-2. It is important to note that a change in one aspect of an activity may alter the demands of another aspect of the activity (Fig.6-4 A & B). For example, dressing a child during the winter months may require heavier clothing and more layered items, such as a turtleneck shirt and sweater, long socks, and pants versus summer clothing that might include fewer items, such as shorts and a T-shirt, and no socks with sandals. Another

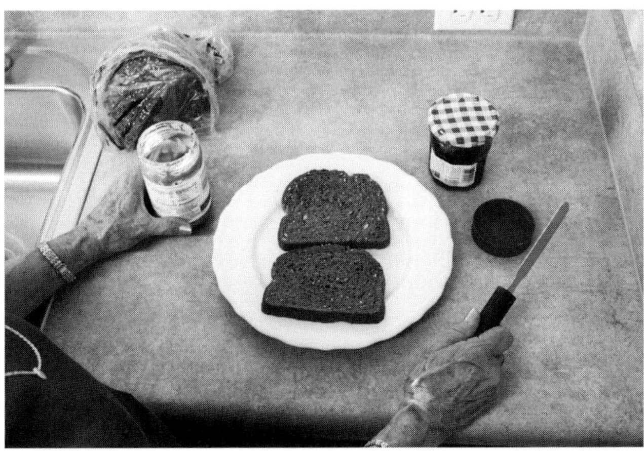

FIGURE 6-3. Preparing a peanut butter and jelly sandwich requires various activity and occupational demands.

example is baking a cake from a box mix (fewer ingredients to add) versus making a cake from scratch (more ingredients and steps to follow). An increase in the number of steps in an activity may increase the client's physical and cognitive demands necessary to complete the task. Activity and occupational demands are further described as being "barriers to or supports for participation."[1] It is up to the OT practitioner to identify when there are barriers, and make adjustments necessary that allow the client to fully participate in the occupation to the best of his or her ability. A client who has limited vision may have trouble seeing her own handwriting and the OT practitioner may recommend using a thicker, darker type of pen or pencil.

Performance Skills

To match the activity and occupational demands to a client's current cognitive, physical, and emotional functional level, the OT practitioner needs to be able to observe

TABLE 6-2 Activity and Occupational Demands[1]

Activity and occupational demands are the components of activities and occupations that occupational therapy practitioners consider during the clinical reasoning process. Depending on the context and needs of the client, these demands can be deemed barriers to or supports for participation. Specific knowledge about the demands of activities and occupations assists practitioners in selecting activities for therapeutic purposes. Demands of the activity or occupation include the relevance and importance to the client, objects used and their properties, space demands, social demands, sequencing and timing, required actions and performance skills, and required underlying body functions and body structures.

TYPE OF DEMAND	DESCRIPTION	EXAMPLES
Relevance and importance to client	Alignment with the client's goals, values, beliefs, and needs and perceived utility	• Driving a car equates with independence. • Preparing a holiday meal connects with family tradition. • Voting is a rite of passage to adulthood.
Objects used and their properties	Tools, supplies, and equipment required in the process of carrying out the activity	• Tools (e.g., scissors, dishes, shoes, volleyball) • Supplies (e.g., paints, milk, lipstick) • Equipment (e.g., workbench, stove, basketball hoop) • Inherent properties (e.g., heavy, rough, sharp, colorful, loud, bitter tasting)
Space demands (related to the physical environment)	Physical environmental requirements of the activity (e.g., size, arrangement, surface, lighting, temperature, noise, humidity, ventilation)	• Large, open space outdoors for a baseball game • Bathroom door and stall width to accommodate wheelchair • Noise, lighting, and temperature controls for a library
Social demands (related to the social environment and virtual and cultural contexts)	Elements of the social environment and virtual and cultural contexts that may be required by the activity	• Rules of the game • Expectations of other participants in the activity (e.g., sharing supplies, using language appropriate for the meeting, appropriate virtual decorum)
Sequencing and timing	Process required to carry out the activity (e.g., specific steps, sequence of steps, timing requirements)	• *Steps to make tea:* Gather cup and tea bag, heat water, pour water into cup, let steep, add sugar. • *Sequence:* Heat water before placing tea bag in water. • *Timing:* Leave tea bag to steep for 2 minutes. • *Steps to conduct a meeting:* Establish goals for meeting, arrange time and location, prepare agenda, call meeting to order. • *Sequence:* Have people introduce themselves before beginning discussion of topic. • *Timing:* Allot sufficient time for discussion of topic and determination of action items.

Continued

TABLE 6-2 Activity and Occupational Demands[1] (continued)

TYPE OF DEMAND	DESCRIPTION	EXAMPLES
Required actions and performance skills	Actions (performance skills—motor, process, and social interaction) required by the client that are an inherent part of the activity	• Feeling the heat of the stove • Gripping a handlebar • Choosing ceremonial clothes • Determining how to move limbs to control the car • Adjusting the tone of voice • Answering a question
Required body functions	"Physiological functions of body systems (including psychological functions)" (WHO, 2001, p. 10) required to support the actions used to perform the activity	• Mobility of joints • Level of consciousness • Cognitive level
Required body structures	"Anatomical parts of the body such as organs, limbs, and their components" that support body functions (WHO, 2001, p. 10) and are required to perform the activity	• Number of hands or feet • Olfactory or taste organs

Copied with permission from AOTA OTPF-3.

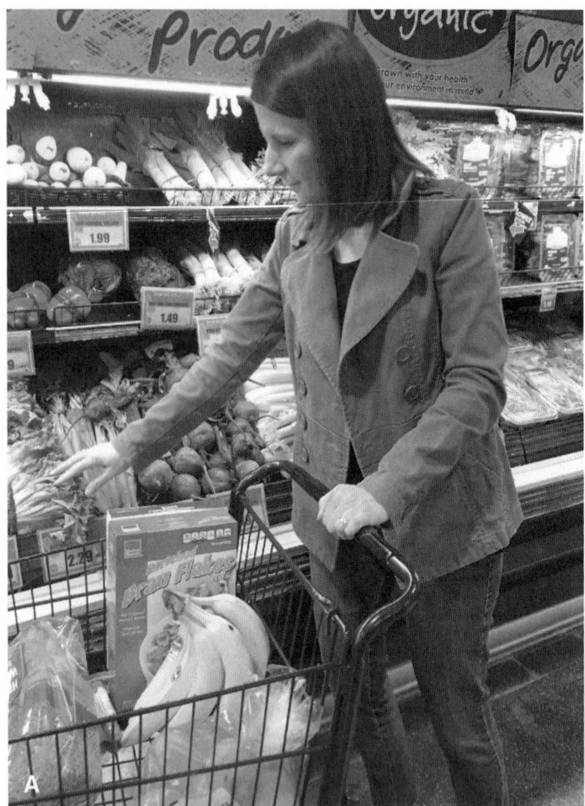

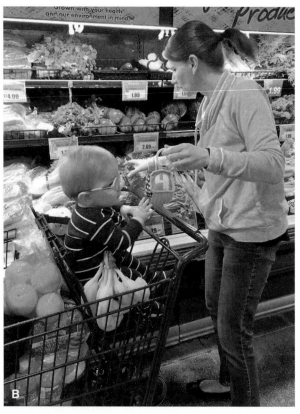

FIGURE 6-4. The aspects of a task change when activity demands are altered. **A.** Grocery shopping with the normal activity demands of remembering needing items and selecting the freshest produce. **B.** The activity demands of grocery shopping change when attention is divided between shopping and caring for a baby.

how the client's body and mind function. The AOTA OTPF-3 refers to these observable skills as *performance skills*.[1] They are organized in three categories:

- Motor skills (movement-related skills)
- Process skills (cognitive-related skills)
- Social interaction skills

A person's body functions and body structure support performance skills, and certain body structures or body functions may be required for a performance skill to be utilized. For example, tying a shoelace in a typical manner requires both hands (body structures) as well as joint range of motion (body functions). Rarely, if ever, do the performance skills categories occur in isolation to one another as overlap and combinations of the various skills are necessary to perform almost all tasks. Typically, at least the motor and process or process and social skills are used together, but some activities require skills from all categories. When a person brushes his or her hair, the person needs to *choose* the object (process skill), *grasp* the brush and *lift* it to his or her head (both of which are motor skills), and then *decide* when the hair is sufficiently brushed (terminating the task is a process skill). This activity does not involve social interaction skills. However, if an individual is fixing another person's hair, this adds social interaction skill components as well. Table 6-3 provides definitions of the most commonly used skills in each category. Figure 6-5 helps to illustrate the interaction of motor, process, and social skills. As with the activity and occupational demands, performance skills are interrelated; therefore, if one aspect of a performance skill changes, it may influence other performance skills required to complete an activity (Fig. 6-6). OT practitioners should engage in close and continual observation and analysis of performance skills to be aware of the constant interplay between the client, environment, and activity or occupation.[10,11]

TABLE 6-3 Performance Skills[1]

Performance skills are observable elements of action that have an implicit functional purpose; skills are considered a classification of actions, encompassing multiple capacities (body functions and body structures) and, when combined, underlie the ability to participate in desired occupations and activities. This list is not all-inclusive and may not include all possible skills addressed during occupational therapy interventions.

SKILL	DEFINITION
MOTOR SKILLS	"Occupational performance skills observed as the person interacts with and moves task objects and self around the task environment" (e.g., activity of daily living [ADL] motor skills, school motor skills).[10]
ALIGNS	Interacts with task objects without evidence of persistent propping or persistent leaning
STABILIZES	Moves through task environment and interacts with task objects without momentary propping or loss of balance
POSITIONS	Positions self an effective distance from task objects and without evidence of awkward body positioning
REACHES	Effectively extends the arm and, when appropriate, bends the trunk to effectively grasp or place task objects that are out of reach
BENDS	Flexes or rotates the trunk as appropriate to the task to grasp or place task objects out of reach or when sitting down
GRIPS	Effectively pinches or grasps task objects such that the objects do not slip (e.g., from the person's fingers, between teeth)
MANIPULATES	Uses dexterous finger movements, without evidence of fumbling, when manipulating task objects (e.g., manipulating buttons when buttoning)
COORDINATES	Uses two or more body parts together to manipulate, hold, and/or stabilize task objects without evidence of fumbling task objects or slipping from one's grasp
MOVES	Effectively pushes or pulls task objects along a supporting surface, pulls to open or pushes to close doors and drawers, or pushes on wheels to propel a wheelchair
LIFTS	Effectively raises or lifts task objects without evidence of increased effort
WALKS	During task performance, ambulates on level surfaces without shuffling the feet, becoming unstable, propping, or using assistive devices
TRANSPORTS	Carries task objects from one place to another while walking or moving in a wheelchair
CALIBRATES	Uses movements of appropriate force, speed, or extent when interacting with task objects (e.g., not crushing objects, pushing a door with enough force that it closes)

Continued

TABLE 6-3 Performance Skills[1] (continued)

SKILL	DEFINITION
FLOWS	Uses smooth and fluid arm and wrist movements when interacting with task objects
ENDURES	Persists and completes the task without showing obvious evidence of physical fatigue, pausing to rest, or stopping to catch one's breath
PACES	Maintains a consistent and effective rate or tempo of performance throughout the entire task
PROCESS SKILLS	"Occupational performance skills [e.g., ADL process skills, school process skills] observed as a person (1) selects, interacts with, and uses task tools and materials; (2) carries out individual actions and steps; and (3) modifies performance when problems are encountered."[10]
PACES	Maintains a consistent and effective rate or tempo of performance throughout the entire task
ATTENDS	Does not look away from what he or she is doing, interrupting the ongoing task progression
HEEDS	Carries out and completes the task originally agreed on or specified by another
CHOOSES	Selects necessary and appropriate type and number of tools and materials for the task, including the tools and materials that the person was directed to use or specified he or she would use
USES	Applies tools and materials as they are intended (e.g., uses a pencil sharpener to sharpen a pencil but not to sharpen a crayon) and in a hygienic fashion
HANDLES	Supports or stabilizes tools and materials in an appropriate manner, protecting them from being damaged, slipping, moving, and falling
INQUIRES	(1) Seeks needed verbal or written information by asking questions or reading directions or labels and (2) does not ask for information when he or she was fully oriented to the task and environment and had immediate prior awareness of the answer
INITIATES	Starts or begins the next action or step without hesitation
CONTINUES	Performs single actions or steps without interruptions such that once an action or task is initiated, the person continues without pauses or delays until the action or step is completed
SEQUENCES	Performs steps in an effective or logical order and with an absence of (1) randomness or lack of logic in the ordering and (2) inappropriate repetition of steps
TERMINATES	Brings to completion single actions or single steps without inappropriate persistence or premature cessation
SEARCHES/ LOCATES	Looks for and locates tools and materials in a logical manner, both within and beyond the immediate environment
GATHERS	Collects related tools and materials into the same work space and regathers tools or materials that have spilled, fallen, or been misplaced
ORGANIZES	Logically positions or spatially arranges tools and materials in an orderly fashion within a single work space and between multiple appropriate work spaces such that the work space is not too spread out or too crowded
RESTORES	Puts away tools and materials in appropriate places and ensures that the immediate work space is restored to its original condition
NAVIGATES	Moves the arm, body, or wheelchair without bumping into obstacles when moving in the task environment or interacting with task objects
NOTICES/ RESPONDS	Responds appropriately to (1) nonverbal task-related cues (e.g., heat, movement), (2) the spatial arrangement and alignment of task objects to one another, and (3) cupboard doors and drawers that have been left open during task performance
ADJUSTS	Effectively (1) goes to new work spaces; (2) moves tools and materials out of the current work space; and (3) adjusts knobs, dials, or water taps to overcome problems with ongoing task performance
ACCOMMODATES	Prevents ineffective task performance
BENEFITS	Prevents problems with task performance from recurring or persisting
SOCIAL INTERACTION SKILLS	"Occupational performance skills observed during the ongoing stream of a social exchange."[10]
APPROACHES/ STARTS	Approaches or initiates interaction with the social partner in a manner that is socially appropriate

TABLE 6-3 Performance Skills[1] (continued)

SKILL	DEFINITION
CONCLUDES/ DISENGAGES	Effectively terminates the conversation or social interaction, brings to closure the topic under discussion, and disengages or says good-bye
PRODUCES SPEECH	Produces spoken, signed, or augmentative (i.e., computer-generated) messages that are audible and clearly articulated
GESTICULATES	Uses socially appropriate gestures to communicate or support a message
SPEAKS FLUENTLY	Speaks in a fluent and continuous manner, with an even pace (not too fast, not too slow) and without pauses or delays during the message being sent
TURNS TOWARD	Actively positions or turns the body and face toward the social partner or person who is speaking
LOOKS	Makes eye contact with the social partner
PLACES SELF	Positions self at an appropriate distance from the social partner during the social interaction
TOUCHES	Responds to and uses touch or bodily contact with the social partner in a manner that is socially appropriate
REGULATES	Does not demonstrate irrelevant, repetitive, or impulsive behaviors that are not part of social interaction
QUESTIONS	Requests relevant facts and information and asks questions that support the intended purpose of the social interaction
REPLIES	Keeps conversation going by replying appropriately to question and comments
DISCLOSURES	Reveals opinions, feelings, and private information about self or others in a manner that is socially appropriate
EXPRESSES EMOTION	Displays affect and emotions in a way that is socially appropriate
DISAGREES	Expresses differences of opinion in a socially appropriate manner
THANKS	Uses appropriate words and gestures to acknowledge receipt of services, gifts, or compliments
TRANSITIONS	Handles transitions in the conversation smoothly or changes the topic without disrupting the ongoing conversation
TIMES RESPONSE	Replies to social messages without delay or hesitation and without interrupting the social partner
TIMES DURATION	Speaks for reasonable periods given the complexity of the message sent
TAKES TURNS	Takes his or her turn and gives the social partner the freedom to take his or her turn
MATCHES LANGUAGE	Uses a tone of voice, dialect, and level of language that are socially appropriate and matched to the social partner's abilities and level of understanding
CLARIFIES	Responds to gestures or verbal messages signaling that the social partner does not comprehend or understand a message and ensures that the social partner is following the conversation
ACKNOWLEDGES AND ENCOURAGES	Acknowledges receipt of messages, encourages the social partner to continue interaction, and encourages all social partners to participate in social interaction
EMPATHIZES	Expresses a supportive attitude toward the social partner by agreeing with, empathizing with, or expressing understanding of the social partner's feelings and experiences
HEEDS	Uses goal-directed social interactions focused on carrying out and completing the intended purpose of the social interaction
ACCOMMODATES	Prevents ineffective or socially inappropriate social interaction
BENEFITS	Prevents problems with ineffective or socially inappropriate social interaction from recurring or persisting

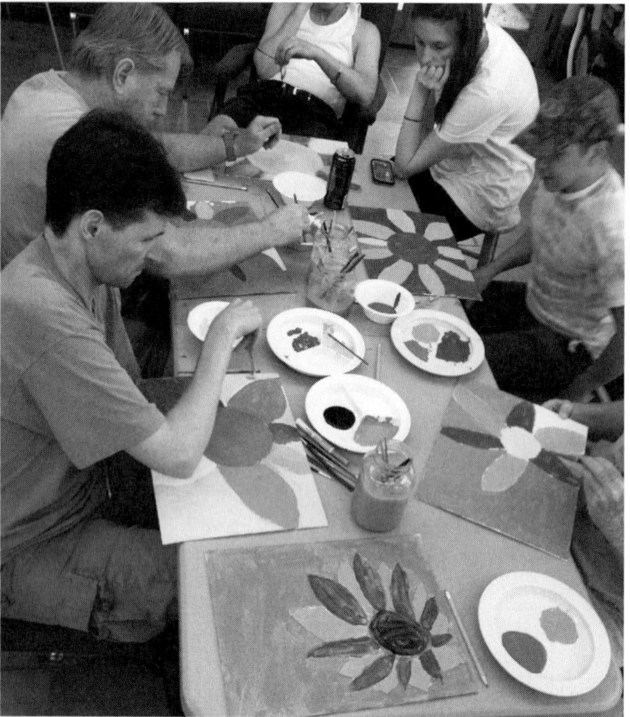

FIGURE 6-5. Motor, process, and social skills. This group craft task demonstrates the interaction of motor, process, and social skills. Note the motor skills of holding the brush, supporting the elbow on the table, and reaching for the paint. The process skills would include choosing a color, how much paint to put on the brush, and rinsing the brush between color applications. The social skills are interacting with other group members, sharing paints and brushes, encouraging others, and complimenting each other's work.

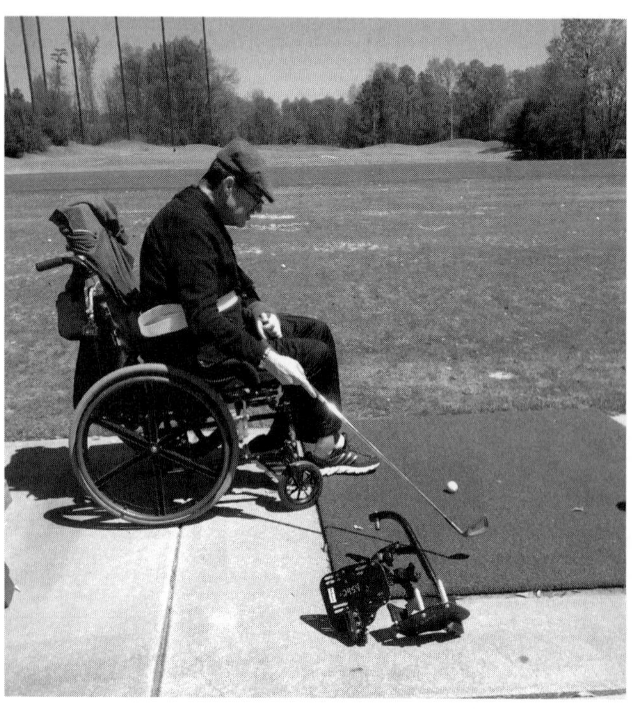

FIGURE 6-6. Client doing a task differently as a result of an injury or impairment.

CONNECTING OCCUPATIONAL PERFORMANCE AND ACTIVITY ANALYSIS TO INTERVENTION

Pulling together the client's occupational profile, occupational performance strengths and weaknesses, and the information gathered from activity analysis can be a challenging proposition for a student or practitioner. As the OTA begins to work on tasks with the client in the therapy session that were noted to be meaningful on the occupational profile, the OTA is constantly observing the client's performance and noting when the client is struggling and frustrated or when the task is too easy. This constant analysis and subsequent modification of the task being performed for that "just right" challenge is the hallmark of the therapeutic process, and one that takes time and practice to develop. An illustration of these concepts would be a treatment session with a young man with a traumatic brain injury with cognitive and behavioral deficits, where the OTA is working on money management. This client has fluctuating abilities through the day, depending on fatigue, medication levels, and alertness. The OTA spreads three quarters on the table and asks the client how much money is on the table. The client quickly notes "75 cents," and the OTA immediately grades the task with more difficulty with the addition of coins of other denominations. The OTA places three dimes, five nickels, three quarters, and two pennies on the table, and the client is directed to add up the total amount. He pauses and frowns as he tries to add up the amounts in his head. The OTA notes his confusion, and after a minute, grades down the task slightly by separating the coins into piles and asking him to count the piles separately.

Another example would be an OTA working in the home health setting in the condominium of a 75-year-old woman who fell and broke her left wrist a month ago. She has recently returned to her home with her daughter (who is staying with her temporarily) after a hospitalization and 3-week skilled nursing placement. She is quite weak from prolonged inactivity, is now in a brace instead of a cast, and is determined to get back to living independently. Many of her daily care tasks will require adaptations, such as nonslip material for the cutting board and larger handled knife for snack preparation, a buttonhook to assist with buttoning shirts, and a long-handled sponge for reaching under her right armpit and her back while bathing. Tasks that might require the OTA to observe and analyze performance would be overall endurance/fatigue with certain ADL and IADL tasks, desire and ability to perform certain tasks independently or with her daughter's assistance for energy conservation, or ability to complete a range of motion (ROM) program. The OTA may start with gentle active assistive ROM of the wrist, and then grade the ROM from session to session by providing less assistance to move through the range at the wrist as the client strengthens.

DOCUMENTATION

All OT practitioners are responsible for accurate and timely documentation of skilled services provided. Documentation becomes part of the client's legal medical record and should always be done in accordance to federal, state, and facility regulations. In legal terms, if it is not written in the note, it did not happen. Good documentation protects the OTA as well as the client. Most facilities have transitioned to the electronic health record/electronic medical record (EHR/EMR). Documentation also provides a record of the client's progress (or lack thereof), and is useful to the whole team of healthcare providers so each can review the notes of other professionals and provide optimal coordination of care.

LEVELS OF ASSISTANCE-COMMON TERMINOLOGY FOR HEALTHCARE PROFESSIONALS

The terminology used while providing healthcare services to clients is sometimes varied among practitioners and settings. Using a common language for outcomes is helpful to communicate from one setting to another and also to accurately measure and document the client's progress in therapy.

Functional Independence Measure System™

Perhaps the most commonly used outcome measure for ADLs in physical rehabilitation is the Functional Independence Measure System™ (FIM™). The FIM™ instrument measures functional outcomes in areas of ADL and is used in skilled nursing facilities, subacute facilities, long-term care hospitals, Veteran's Administration programs, and international rehabilitation hospitals.[12] The FIM™ instrument is based on language from the International Classification of Impairment, Disabilities, and Handicaps and is a licensed instrument that healthcare systems must pay to utilize. Practitioners must be trained to administer the FIM™ instrument, which is ideally scored with the consensus of the team who have been working with the client, and may take 30 to 60 minutes to fully administer.[13] The system rates a client's level of disability with regard to performing ADLs and how much assistance is needed.

The FIM™ has 18 items: 13 motor and five cognitive. Each item is rated on a scale of 1 to 7 that ranges from total assistance (complete dependence, a score of 1), to complete independence, a score of 7. FIM™ scores are often represented as a combined score, with the lowest rating at 18 and the highest at 126. The scale has had some criticism in being used as a combined number rather than reporting on each of the 18 areas individually.[14] It is important to note that for scoring, if a client requires the physical assistance of more than one person, the disability level is scored as "1," or "Dependent." Table 6-4 includes the ADL dimensions that the FIM™ measures, as well as a list and explanation of the terminology used for the client's ability to perform tasks.

The terminology portion of the FIM™ with regard to levels of disability and how much assistance is needed has been adopted, become commonplace in the rehabilitation community, and is acceptable in all adult settings.[15] Using consistent terminology across the continuum of care and in documentation benefits the client. Some refer to this as

TABLE 6-4 FIM™ Instrument-Dimensions Measured and Scoring Criteria (Levels of Disability)[13]

ADL DIMENSIONS MEASURED

PHYSICAL DIMENSIONS	*COGNITIVE DIMENSIONS*
Eating	Cognitive comprehension
Grooming	Expression
Bathing	Social interaction
Upper body dressing	Problem-solving
Lower body dressing	Memory
Toileting	
Bladder management	
Bowel management	
Bed-to-chair transfer	
Toilet transfer	
Shower transfer	
Locomotion (ambulatory or wheelchair level)	
Stairs	

SCORING CRITERIA

Independent-No Helper		
7	Complete independence (I)	Client performs all tasks without assistance and in a reasonable amount of time.
6	Modified independence (Mod I)	Client requires use of an adapted device or prosthetic, but no physical assistance. May require more than a reasonable amount of time.

Continued

TABLE 6-4 FIM™ Instrument-Dimensions Measured and Scoring Criteria (Levels of Disability)[13] (continued)

Requires Helper		
Modified Dependence-Client performs at least 50% of the task		
5	Supervision OR Setup	Client requires standby, coaxing, or cues, without any physical touch/assistance to the client. The helper sets up needed supplies or applies the client's orthoses or assistive/adaptive devices.
4	Minimal Contact Assistance (Min A)	Client can perform 75% or more of task.
3	Moderate Assistance (Mod A)	Client can perform 50% to 74% of task.
Complete Dependence-Client performs less than 50% of the task		
2	Maximal Assistance (Max A)	Client can perform 25% to 49% of task.
1	Dependent/Total Assistance (D or Dep)	Client can perform less than 25% of the task or requires more than one person to assist.

the "levels of assistance" needed as a result of the client's disability. To match FIM™ terminology, documentation should include the terminology of independent (I), modified independent (Mod I), supervision or setup (S), minimum assistance (Min A), moderate assistance (Mod A), maximum assistance (Max A), or dependent (D or Dep). See Table 6-4 for specific definitions of each. Note the FIM™ does not include contact guard assist (CGA) or stand by assist (SBA) as is noted in some sources,[16] and is not a part of the traditional FIM™ standards. Students and practitioners are cautioned to check with each facility for the specific terminology standards adopted with regard to levels of assistance. Some may use the FIM™ and some may include other terminology along with the FIM™.

SUMMARY

The essential components of the skilled provision of OT include the practitioner's ability to develop an occupational profile and analyze the occupational performance of a client. Part of this activity analysis is the ability to match the task chosen for the therapy session to the particular needs of the client and integration of all aspects highlighted in the OTPF-3. The OT profession addresses the meaningful activities in which our clients engage, and more than any other address their holistic needs. Through effectively providing OT services in a client-centered manner, OT practitioners assist in increasing quality of life, self-determination and control, role fulfillment and functional performance.

REVIEW QUESTIONS

1. Who should be the primary source of information for the occupational profile?
   a. Client
   b. Family member
   c. Physical therapist
   d. Occupational therapist
2. Which of these is the OT practitioner most likely to ask when obtaining information for the occupational profile?
   a. What did you have for breakfast today?
   b. What is your average day like?
   c. How many siblings do you have?
   d. What is the month, date, and year today?
3. Which three of the following is true regarding the occupational profile?
   a. Only the occupational therapist obtains information for the occupational profile.
   b. Information from the occupational profile includes a detailed description of the client's past medical history.
   c. It helps establish client goals.
   d. The occupational profile should be completed in one visit with the client.
   e. The occupational profile can be updated and revised as needed.
   f. It includes the client's patterns of occupational engagement.
4. Which three of the following is a key component of the COPM?
   a. Working toward enhancing the client's self-efficacy
   b. Having the client identify significant problem areas
   c. Exploring how current actions are inconsistent with the client's goals and values
   d. Asking reflection questions
   e. Conducting a semistructured interview
   f. Having the client rate the level of importance various occupations have to him or her
5. Which of the following is a key component of motivational interviewing?
   a. Looking at the client's performance satisfaction
   b. Tracking a client's progress
   c. Utilizing reflective listening techniques
   d. Asking structured questions
6. A client is having difficulty manipulating scissors to cut out paper designs. This is an indication that the client is having difficulty with which performance skill?
   a. Social interaction
   b. Endurance
   c. Fine motor
   d. Patience

7. Which of the following would be considered physical aspects of a task during activity analysis?
   a. Time of day the activity occurs
   b. Type of surface required for the task
   c. Number of people required
   d. Amount of steps to complete the activity
8. The OTA has a new client with multiple sclerosis who has difficulty with many ADL tasks because of changes in vision and cognition. When working with the client on getting dressed, which of these tasks would be considered a process skill?
   a. She tries to sequence donning her shirt before her bra.
   b. She easily lifts her leg to put it in the pant.
   c. She organizes her grooming supplies to take to the sink.
   d. She moves slowly during the ADL tasks.
9. During the OT process, analyzing a client's occupational performance occurs:
   a. Before completing an occupational profile
   b. After completing an evaluation
   c. Without the client being present
   d. After completing an occupational profile, and then throughout care
10. The OTA is working with a client with diabetes and congestive heart failure. The client is having trouble with bathing because of poor endurance. The OTA employs activity analysis to decide how to adapt the task. Activity analysis should occur:
    a. Upon initially evaluating a client
    b. Only during formal evaluation
    c. Throughout every encounter with a client
    d. Upon initial evaluation and again at discharge

CASE STUDY

Betsy Rose is a 72-year-old female and widow who lives alone in a small Pennsylvania town. Her daughter and daughter's husband live about 15 minutes away with their two young children. Betsy's daughter calls every day to check in and visits at least once a week with the children. Betsy also has a son that lives in Illinois with his family. He calls every week and visits twice a year. As a retired elementary school teacher, Betsy has many friends in the community through her years of teaching and church attendance. She loves to cook, sew, and tend to the roses in her garden. She values going to church each week and cooking meals for church and family functions. Betsy has a medical history of ovarian cancer and corrected cataracts. Betsy's daughter has noticed that she has been forgetful and has appeared confused the last few months. This includes missing church on Sunday because she did not know the correct day, forgetting recipes for her favorite dishes, leaving the stove on after cooking, and neglecting her flowers. She also volunteers at the local Senior Services Center; however, the supervisor at the center called her daughter and reported that Betsy has been forgetting to come the last few weeks. The supervisor also noted a decrease in her performance. Up until approximately 3 months ago, Betsy was independent with all ADLs and IADLs, including cooking, cleaning, and driving. An OT evaluation revealed that Betsy's upper extremity (UE) ROM is within functional limits (WFL), that her UE strength is approximately 3/5, and that she has mild neurocognitive impairment. The occupational therapist also noted that Betsy tends to have a delayed response to questions and impaired balance. Her vision is WFL with corrective lenses. Betsy's daughter made a medical appointment for Betsy and accompanied her to the appointment. Her daughter was able to share with the physician her concerns with specific examples regarding Betsy's forgetfulness, and the physician gave Betsy a diagnosis of early stage Alzheimer's disease.

1. What new questions should the OT practitioner ask Betsy and Betsy's daughter?
2. What are key elements of Betsy's occupational profile?
3. Which of Betsy's performance skills are impacted?
4. What occupations are affected by Betsy's changes in performance skills as a result of her diagnosis?

PUTTING IT ALL TOGETHER: SAMPLE TREATMENT AND DOCUMENTATION

Occupational Profile

Scott is a 55-year-old male who had a heart attack 3 weeks ago. He returned to his job as a banker last week. Since his heart attack, he has had difficulty maintaining his energy throughout the day. Although Scott reports he is able to dress and bathe himself in the morning, when he gets home from work, he requires assistance from his wife for doffing his clothes and donning pajamas. Scott is concerned about the frequent rest breaks he requires at work, how fatigued he is at night, and the assistance he needs in the evening. He states, "I can't even work on my Mustang anymore. I'm too tired. And I love to work on my Mustang."

Scott has a supportive spouse who is willing and able to assist him with ADLs and IADLs as needed. They do not have any children, and no immediate family lives in the area. He reports that his workplace is easily accessible, and that his supervisor has been understanding of his limitations and need for frequent rest breaks. Scott reports his home is not easily accessible. He lives in a second-story apartment that requires him to ambulate up 2 flights of steep stairs to enter, and he does not have any adaptive equipment to assist him with ADLs or IADLs.

Scott is very interested in Mustangs and cars in general. He enjoys cooking and listening to music. He values spending time with his wife and friends, and attending and volunteering at his church as a greeter.

Scott's daily life roles include:

- Husband
- Banker for 32 years
- Friend
- Church volunteer

Scott reports that he works 40 to 50 hours a week at the bank, with a 1-hour lunch break. He generally stays at home with his wife on weeknights. Scott will assist with dinner and household tasks in the evening, and then will work on his Mustang. He usually goes out for dinner and a movie with his wife, or shopping, on Friday or Saturday nights. Since his heart attack, Scott reports he comes home from work, eats dinner, and sleeps. He spends most of the weekend resting and watching television, only going out to attend church service.

Scott has listed these as his top priorities:

- Being independent in ADLs (especially dressing tasks)
- Increasing his endurance during the day so he requires, at most, one 30-minute break in the morning and one 15-minute break in the afternoon
- Being able to work at least 1 hour a night on his Mustang, 3 to 4 days a week
- Being able to attend church weekly, and to volunteer at church as a greeter at least two Sundays a month

Analysis of Occupational Performance

Scott's occupational profile indicates some of the activities he is having difficulty completing or keeping up with. This information, along with any medical notes and physician's orders, can provide direction on where to begin the analysis of occupational performance. After having a heart attack, his cardiovascular functions may need to be gradually improved before his endurance returns, but the OT practitioner may recommend ways to conserve what energy he does have. It would be very important to understand the specifics of the tasks he does throughout his work day as a banker and determining whether there is a better way for him to conserve his energy so that he can become more independent and engage in things he wants to in the evenings.

1. Is there a way he can sit more throughout the day and limit his walking around the bank?
2. Perhaps observing the method he is using to undress in the evenings could be important. For example, does he stand when he is undressing or could he possibly sit down? Does he have to walk far to get his pajamas? If so, could his wife possibly lay those out for him first so that he could focus solely on undressing himself?
3. As far as getting back out to the garage and working on his Mustang, what performance skills are necessary, and does he have the body functions and body structures necessary to support those skills? For example, if he is working on the engine, can he bend over for periods of time safely without his blood pressure rising? Is there heavy lifting required? Being able to analyze the various aspects of Scott's meaningful activities to understand his current capabilities, current restrictions, and what activity demands possibly could be changed, are all essential skills of an OT practitioner.

REFERENCES

1. American Occupational Therapy Association. (2014). Occupational therapy practice framework: Domain and process (3rd ed.). *American Journal of Occupational Therapy, 68*(Suppl. 1), S1-S48.
2. Akechi, H., Senju, A., Uibo, H., Kikuchi, Y., Hasegawa, T., & Hietanen, J. (2013). Attention to eye contact in the West and East: Autonomic responses and evaluative ratings. *PLoS ONE, 8*(3), e59312. doi:10.1371/journal.pone.0059312
3. Law, M., Baptiste, S., Carswell, A., McColl, M. A., Polatajko, H., & Pollock, N. (2014). *Canadian occupational performance measure* (5th ed.). Ottawa, Ontario: Canadian Association of Occupational Therapists.
4. Carswell, A., McColl, M. A., Baptiste, S., Law, M., Polatajko, H., & Pollock, N. (2004). The Canadian occupational performance measure: A research and clinical literature review. *Canadian Journal of Occupational Therapy, 71*(4), 210-222.
5. Chittenden, D. (2012). A concept analysis of motivational interviewing for the community practitioner. *Community Practitioner, 85*(10), 20-23.
6. Snyder, E., Lawrence, N., Weatherholt, T., & Nagy, P. (2012). The benefits of motivational interviewing and coaching for improving the practice of comprehensive family assessments in child welfare. *Child Welfare, 91*(5), 9-36.
7. Bohman, B., Forsberg, L., Ghaderi, A., & Rasmussen, F. (2013). An evaluation of training in motivational interviewing for nurses in child health services. *Behavioural and Cognitive Psychotherapy, 41*(3), 329-343.
8. Miller, W., & Rollnick, S. (2013). *Motivational interviewing: Helping people change* (3rd ed.). New York, NY: The Guilford Press.
9. Thomas, H. (2015). *Occupation-based activity analysis* (2nd ed.). Thorofare, NJ: Slack.
10. Chisholm, D., & Boyt Schell, B. A. (2014). Overview of the occupational therapy process and outcomes. In B. A. Boyt Schell, G. Gillen, & M. Scaffa (Eds.), *Willard and Spackman's occupational therapy* (12th ed., pp. 266–280). Philadelphia, PA: Lippincott Williams & Wilkins.
11. Hagedorn, R. (2000). *Tools for practice in occupational therapy: A structured approach to core skills and processes.* Edinburgh: Churchill Livingstone.
12. Uniform Data System. (2017). About the FIM system®. Retrieved from www.udsmr.org/Webmodules/FIM/fim_about.aspx
13. Rehab Measures. (2015). Rehab measures: FIM™ instrument. Retrieved from www.rehabmeasures.org/lists/rehabmeasures/dispform.aspx?id=889
14. Pedersen, A.R., Severinsen, K., & Nielsen, J.F. (2014). The effect of age on rehabilitation outcome after traumatic brain injury assessed by the functional independence measure (FIM). *Neurorehabilitation and Neural Repair, 29*(4), 299-307.https://doi.org/10.1177/1545968314545171
15. Centers for Medicare and Medicaid Services. (2012). Inpatient rehabilitation facility–patient assessment instrument (IRF-PAI) training manual. Retrieved from https://www.cms.gov/medicare/medicare-fee-for-service-payment/inpatientrehabfacpps/downloads/irfpai-manual-2012.pdf
16. Wayne State School of Medicine Department of Physical Medicine and Rehabilitation. (2014). Common rehab abbreviations. Retrieved from http://pmroakwood.med.wayne.edu/pdf/PMR_for_students_12-8-14.pdf

unit II

Foundations of Movement and Function

Chapter 7

Range of Motion: Assessment and Intervention

Susan Blair OTR/L, BCPR, BCG

LEARNING OUTCOMES

After studying this chapter, the student or practitioner will be able to:

7.1 Explain the various types of range of motion
7.2 List causes of range of motion loss
7.3 Describe limitations and contraindications of range of motion testing
7.4 List the steps of the range of motion procedure in correct order
7.5 Administer the range of motion assessment using given directions on a client
7.6 Describe how assessment results can be used for intervention planning

KEY TERMS

Active assistive range of motion (AAROM)
Active range of motion (AROM)
Against gravity
Axis of the body
Continuous passive motion machine (CPM)
Fulcrum
Functional range of motion (functional ROM)
Goniometer
Goniometry
Gravity eliminated
Home exercise program (HEP)
Movable arm
Passive range of motion (PROM)
Range of motion (ROM)
Screening
Self range of motion (SROM)
Stationary arm
Within normal limits (WNL)

Range of motion (ROM) is described as "the area through which a joint may normally be freely and painlessly moved."[1] Thus, ROM is the available movement a joint has, whether active or passive, measured within a specific plane.[2] When evaluating a client's ability to move his or her limbs, the occupational therapy (OT) practitioner has different methods to measure such movement. Initially, one can observe the client moving through motion while performing a functional task of everyday activities (e.g., buttoning a shirt, picking up a newspaper, or reaching up to place a bowl on a shelf) using an informal assessment such as a screening tool. If deficits in ROM are observed, then the occupational therapist or occupational therapist assistant (OTA) can use goniometry as a formal assessment. **Goniometry** is defined as the measurement of the arc of motion of a joint, and the tool used is the **goniometer**.

Joint motion is divided into multiple types: including active, active assistive, passive, self, and **functional range of motion (functional ROM). Active range of motion (AROM)** occurs when muscles act on the joint and cause voluntary movement such as bending the wrist up and down without any assistance from external forces.[2] Being able to move a body part through the ROM actively is a direct result of the client's strength, and therefore, assesses strength. **Active assistive range of motion (AAROM)** occurs when the movement of the body or any of its parts occurs partially through the individual's own efforts (or attempts at movement) and is accompanied by the aid of an individual (typically, a member of the healthcare team or a caregiver) or some device, such as an exercise machine.[1] AAROM as well as AROM is a result of the client's strength or strength limitations. A deltoid aide or a mobile arm support could be considered AAROM as well. **Passive range of motion (PROM)** refers to joint movement that only occurs when caused by an external force, such as an individual or a device, and typically has a higher degree of ROM than active movement. An example of PROM is a **continuous passive motion machine (CPM),** a motorized medical device that attaches to a limb and passively moves the joint through a set ROM as determined by medical staff.[2] Self ROM is when the client performs their own ROM, typically when the stronger limb(s) move the weaker one through movement patterns. Functional ROM is the movement required while performing aspects of self-care and everyday tasks that do not require full AROM. Functional ROM is the necessary available ROM to perform everyday tasks, but is not necessarily full ROM. An example would be reaching for a cup from a shelf just above a countertop height while standing, which requires at least 90 degrees of shoulder flexion but not necessarily full shoulder flexion of 180 degrees. **Within normal limits (WNL)** indicates that the arc of AROM is within normal acceptable guidelines (see Table 7-1). Every individual is different when it comes to ROM. People who are athletes may have greater than normal ROM because of increased flexibility and strength. Conversely, persons with arthritis may have some limitations in their ROM as a result of joint deformity or pain but not enough ROM loss to exist outside the acceptable guidelines. Some individuals have joints that are more lax (loose) than others. Remember that ROM varies from person to person, and it is wise to compare an individual's affected joint ROM with the unaffected side for comparison to his or her own body. Many factors can limit a joint's range of motion, including, but not limited to, muscle weakness, changes in muscle movement, orthopedic issues, circulation deficits, pain, swelling of the limb, structural impairments such as scar tissue, ligament injury, or tendon rupture.[3,4] These factors can affect AROM or PROM or both, depending on the condition of the client. When reaching the end of the available joint PROM, the OT practitioner will typically feel a "soft" or "hard" end feel. An example of soft end feel is full elbow flexion (the feeling that the arm could bend further if the tissue was not in the way), and hard end feel is full elbow extension, which is bone on bone. The OT practitioner should always clarify the ROM orders from the physician to establish whether there are any contraindications such as "no active ROM" with an acute proximal humeral fracture or "no abduction" with a recent rotator cuff repair.

TECHNOLOGY AND TRENDS

Robotics for improving ROM in clients with spinal cord injury (SCI) has become a frontrunner in new technological advancement efforts. Currently no cure exists for a complete spinal cord lesion, so it is crucial that ROM be maintained and that clients be able to function at the highest level of independence. The ReoGo™ device is a comprehensive therapy platform that includes a robotic guide, featuring a telescopic arm to enable high repetitions of functionally relevant UE exercises. Participants in a 2012 study used the ReoGo™ to determine whether the use of a robotic device would be beneficial as part of a comprehensive treatment approach. With today's limited resources, any intervention that can be utilized outside of therapy sessions for ongoing carryover may improve outcomes. Clients in the study demonstrated measurable improvements in active range of motion; muscle strength, as measured through manual muscle testing; perceived right UE function; and self-care performance, as measured by the functional independence measure (FIM™). The study found that although the initial results are promising and did demonstrate the efficacy of ReoGo™, more research and specific protocols that are easily reproducible with robots, such as the ReoGo™, are needed to validate this evolving treatment area.[8]

WHY IS MEASURING RANGE OF MOTION IMPORTANT?

OT is focused on a person's ability to perform tasks such as activities of daily living (ADLs) and other meaningful activities. One must have functional movement to initiate and carry through with all components of specific movements involved in such tasks. Whether reaching to empty the dishwasher, fold a basket of laundry, or feed oneself, having appropriate functional movement is an integral part of regaining independence. Assessing a client's joint ROM allows the OT practitioner to identify areas of movement impairment, develop a plan of care to address deficits, and facilitate improvement through a comprehensive therapeutic intervention program. In addition, the use of specialized therapeutic interventions, such as orthoses and positioning devices, requires formal ROM assessment to determine appropriate intervention.

HOW IS RANGE OF MOTION MEASURED?

A goniometer is a tool used to measure the arc of movement of a joint (Fig. 7-1). The word "goniometer" is derived from the Greek *gonia*, which means angle, and *metron*, which means measure.[3] Several different types of goniometers are available, from large to small, and are specific to individual joints.[5] A goniometer provides an objective measurement of ROM when properly used. Goniometers are commercially available through therapeutic equipment catalogs, and the OTA should become proficient with their use.[3,5]

A goniometer has a body axis or fulcrum, and two arms. The center point of the body has numbers and serves as the axis for measuring a joint's range of motion. The stationary

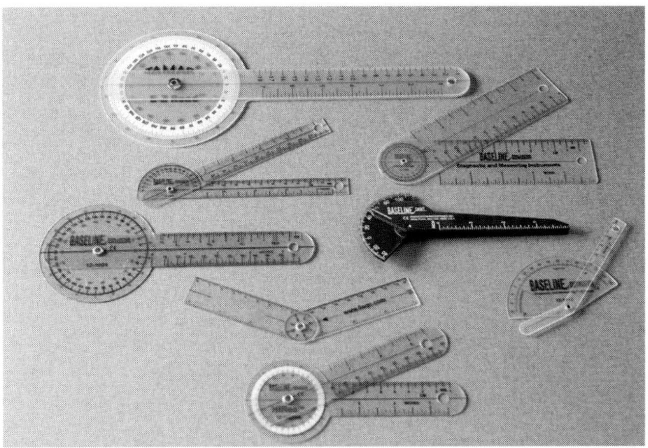

FIGURE 7-1. Goniometers of different sizes.

arm is aligned with the plane of motion proximal to the joint being measured. The moveable arm is also aligned with the plane of motion, but is distal to the joint being measured and follows the arc of movement. A plane of motion refers to the surface along which the movement is performed while the body is in the anatomical position, also known as neutral (Fig. 7-2). While in the anatomical position, the individual stands upright, legs together, knees straight, toes pointing forward, and arms by the sides with palms facing forward. The sagittal plane divides the body into left and right parts. The frontal or coronal plane divides the body into anterior and posterior parts. The transverse or horizontal plane divides the body into superior and inferior parts. Movement occurs in arcs of motion or circular motion. The vertical axis of the body runs head to feet. The frontal axis runs side to side or right to left. Finally, the anterior-posterior axis runs front to back. An OT practitioner must become proficient in the terminology that describes movement direction to ensure accurate measurement.

The planes of movement, as described, are where movement occurs and includes flexion, extension, abduction, adduction, rotation, pronation, supination, and deviation. Flexion and extension are movements that occur in the sagittal plane and refer to increasing and decreasing the angle between two body parts. Abduction and adduction are movements that occur in the frontal (also called coronal) plane, moving body parts away from (abduction) or towards (adduction) the center axis of the body. Rotation, a twisting motion, occurs in the transverse plane, which divides the body into top and bottom halves. An example is internal rotation, where the humerus in the shoulder joint and the femur in the hip joint rotates towards the center of the body. The one exception to this rule is flexion and extension of the thumb carpometacarpal (CMC) joint, which occurs in the frontal plane.

ASSESSING THE CLIENT FOR RANGE OF MOTION

How do OT practitioners actually measure ROM? Clients are rarely ever in a perfect supine (lying on the back) or prone (lying on the stomach) position on a therapy mat or hard surface. Sometimes OT practitioners have to measure a client's range of motion in different environments such as sitting on the edge of a bed, in a wheelchair, or even side-lying in a hospital bed, which can be considered a barrier to effective measurement. Another barrier can be proper alignment of the goniometer. Landmarks can be difficult to distinguish in certain conditions such as obesity, pregnancy, and advanced age. The client may be very deconditioned and unable to hold a proper position for accurate ROM assessment.

Consider several factors before beginning formal ROM measurement with a client. A thorough chart review and client interview should identify any prior AROM or PROM losses, such as a fused joint, osteoarthritis, rheumatoid arthritis, or any other limitation caused by a chronic injury. Second, identify if the client has any current joint issues such as pain, numbness, or weakness. It is a standard of care to examine a client before initiating hands-on contact to identify other limitations to joint movement, such as edema, scars, and bony protrusions.[3] To assess functional AROM, have the client move his or her extremities through a series of normal movements to determine any muscle weakness that may limit ROM. Functional ROM is less than full AROM, and there are differences within functional ROM, depending on the task (compare shoulder ROM in Fig. 7-3 and Fig. 7-4). Functional ROM instructions include directions to perform certain common tasks. To assess, the OT practitioner asks the client to perform the following motions:

- Touch the top of your head as if washing hair (shoulder flexion/abduction)
- Touch the back of your head as if washing hair (shoulder external rotation)
- Hold arms out in front as if reaching for something (elbow extension)
- Place arms behind the back as if tucking in a shirt (shoulder internal rotation)
- Touch your mouth as if self-feeding (elbow flexion)
- Bend your wrists up and down (wrist flexion and extension)
- Make a fist and then stretch out your fingers (finger flexion and extension)
- Turn your palm up and palm down, with elbows bent and arms at side (supination/pronation)

If the client is unable to perform any of these tasks, assess the need for an intervention, such as strengthening exercises with the introduction of adaptive equipment to compensate for the decreased ROM and facilitate independence to perform ADLs.

Optimally, the client will be seated, but may be supine (if unable to tolerate an upright position, such as in an intensive care unit [ICU] setting), for evaluation of ROM. During the assessment, the OT practitioner must compare each extremity and record degrees of movement. Using the goniometer and specific body landmarks, the OT practitioner can determine accurate ROM quickly and precisely. Before beginning the assessment, the OT practitioner must be aware of contraindications and precautions when measuring ROM. Contraindications may include joint

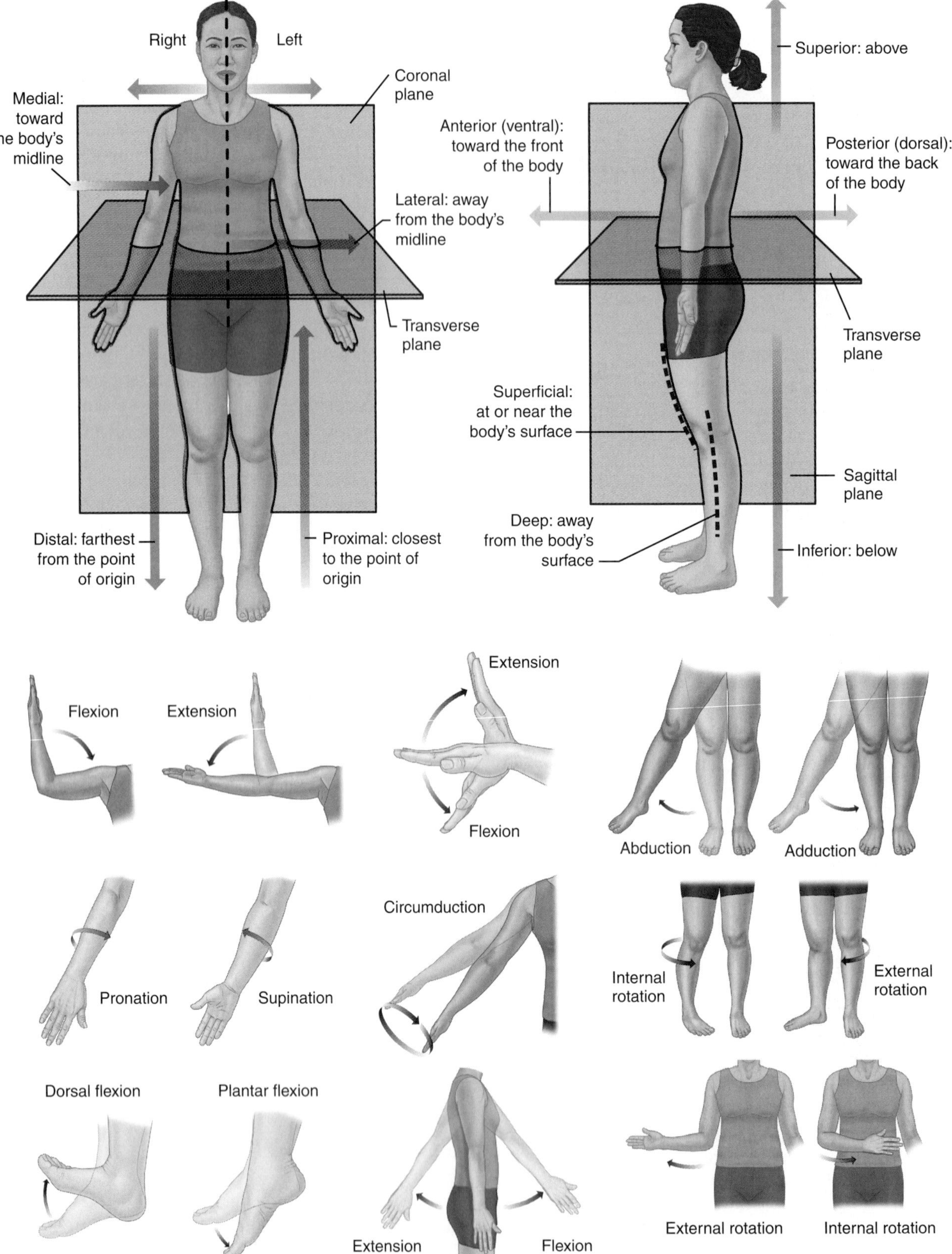

FIGURE 7-2. The basic anatomical positions and planes of ROM.

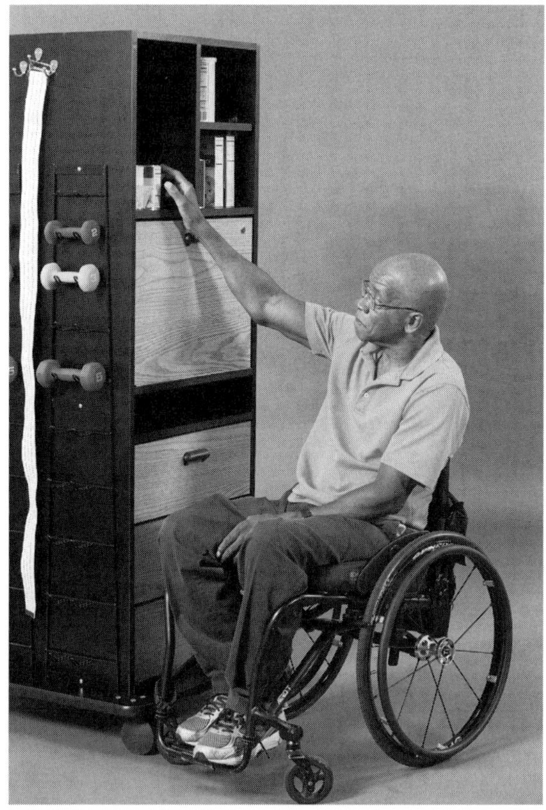

FIGURE 7-3. Client demonstrating functional ROM. He can reach to obtain an item from the shelf.

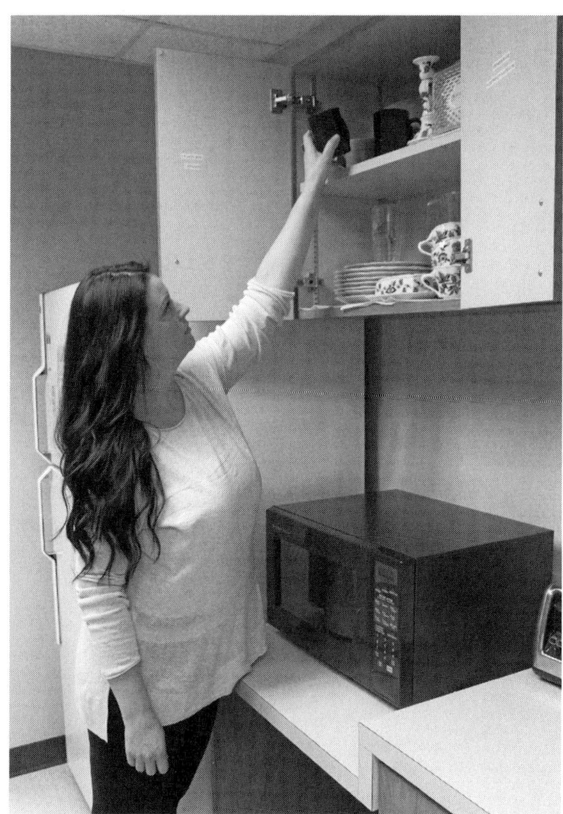

FIGURE 7-4. Client reaching overhead, requiring much more ROM, but not within WNL.

dislocation, an unhealed fracture, soft tissue damage around a joint, and myositis ossificans or heterotopic ossification, which are abnormal bone growth at the site of injury. Cognitive disorders such as dementia may limit the client's ability to follow commands for testing ROM. In this instance, the client may be observed performing functional or automatic tasks to assess ROM capabilities.[3] For clients with certain clinical conditions, use caution when measuring ROM of a client's extremities. Examples of conditions that warrant caution may include carcinoma of the bone, osteoporosis, subluxation, hypermobility of joint, newly united fracture, hemophilia, hematoma, new soft tissue injury, bony ankylosis (immobility and consolidation of a joint), or joint inflammation or infection.[3] For instance, an OTA would not want to measure shoulder external rotation in a client who has recently undergone a shoulder replacement as a result of soft tissue and muscle repair and healing. However, it is appropriate to continue to complete the remainder of the client's upper extremity (UE) ROM as indicated by the physician. Clients who are taking pain medication or muscle relaxants, or have had prolonged hospitalizations also require caution, as they may be too sedated or confused to appropriately respond to pain with ROM or overstretching.

PERFORMING RANGE OF MOTION ASSESSMENT

Before measuring a client's ROM, the OTA must understand how to use the goniometer and be familiar with medical terminology related to body position and movement. The correct process of use is:

1. Place the client in a comfortable position with the extremity to be assessed accessible to the OT practitioner.
2. Center the fulcrum (axis) of the goniometer with the center of the joint to be measured. This will be different for every joint and movement.
3. Align the stationary arm of the device with the limb being measured.
4. Hold the arms of the goniometer in place while the joint is moved through the range of motion.
5. Move the movable arm of the goniometer and line it up with the appropriate body part.
6. Read and record the numbers on the goniometer.

Two terms frequently used to define the location of an area of the body are proximal and distal. Proximal and distal are used only on the limbs, and refer to closer (proximal) or farther (distal) from the trunk. The shoulder is proximal to the hand. A point can be on the proximal third of the humerus (close to the shoulder) or distal third of the humerus (close to the elbow). During ROM measurements, goniometer placement is important because accurate results depend on proper placement of the arms and the fulcrum of the goniometer. First, an OT practitioner should stabilize or support the stationary portion of the client's body. This is the part of the body that is proximal to the joint the OTA is testing. Next, place the goniometer's stationary arm along the body part of the joint being measured. It is important that the client does not move his body in other ways while moving the joint because this leads to incorrect measurement of the movement. Review the measurement on the device before removing it from the client's body, or if it is necessary to view it closer, pinch the goniometer near the fulcrum to keep it from moving, remove from client's body, and view the measurement. Take an accurate reading of the degree of motion on the goniometer and make sure to consistently use the same stationary and movable landmarks for the joint when measuring. Be aware that baggy or loose clothing, such as a shirtsleeve, may hinder proper alignment of the goniometer. Always document the measurement. See Table 7-1 for a list of normal joint ranges.

UNDERSTANDING MOVEMENT IN PLANES

ROM must be understood in terms of the direction the movement occurs in. Flexion refers to a movement that decreases the angle between two body parts, whereas extension refers to a movement that increases the angle between two body parts. Flexion and extension are opposite motions from one another that occur in the same plane. Flexion of the elbow joint is bending the elbow, bringing the distal arm (ulna) closer to the proximal arm (humerus), and decreasing the angle. Extension of the elbow joint is increasing the angle between the ulna and the humerus, or straightening out the elbow. Another example is shoulder flexion and extension. Measuring shoulder flexion begins with the arm in the anatomical position (0 degrees of flexion) and ends with the arm reaching above the head (180 degrees of flexion). For extension, measurement begins with the client's arm in the anatomical position (0 degrees of extension), and the arm moves in the reverse direction, bringing the posterior surface away from the trunk (60 degrees of extension). Abduction and adduction are two terms that are used to describe movements away from or toward the midline of the body. Abduction is a movement away from the midline. An example is to raise the arm out to the side away from the body. Adduction is a movement toward the midline, or bringing the arm down to the side from overhead. Internal and external rotation (sometimes referred to as medial/lateral rotation) describes movement of the limbs around the long axes:

- Internal rotation is a rotating movement toward the midline. One example would be the shoulder movement when a person tucks in pants behind the back.
- External rotation is a rotating movement away from the midline. An example is the shoulder movement seen with reaching back to scratch the back of the head.

TABLE 7-1 Normal Joint Range of Motion Values[6,7]

JOINT	MOTION	RANGE
Shoulder	Flexion	0° to 180°
	Extension	0° to 60°
	Abduction	0° to 180°
	Internal rotation	0° to 70°
	External rotation	0° to 90°
	Horizontal abduction	0° to 40°
	Horizontal adduction	0° to 130°
Elbow	Flexion	0° to 150°
	Extension	0° (180°)
	Supination	0° to 80°-85°
	Pronation	0° to 70°-80°
Wrist	Extension	0° to 70°
	Flexion	0° to 75°-80°
	Ulnar deviation	0° to 30°-35°
	Radial deviation	0° to 20°
Finger	MCP flexion	0° to 90°
	MCP hyperextension	0° to 45°
	MCP abduction	0° to 25°
	PIP flexion	0° to 100°
	DIP flexion	0° to 80°
Thumb	CMC flexion	0° to 15°
	CMC extension	0° to 20°
	CMC (palmar) abduction	0° to 45°
	CMC opposition	To base of small finger; deficit is measured in cm.
	MCP flexion	0° to 50°-55°
	IP flexion	0° to 80°
Hip	Flexion	0° to 120°
	Extension	0°to 30°
	Abduction	0° to 45°
	Adduction	0° to 30°
	Internal rotation	0° to 45°
	External rotation	0° to 45°
Knee	Flexion	0° to 135°
Ankle	Dorsiflexion	0°to 20°
	Plantar flexion	0° to 50°
Ankle/Foot	Inversion	0° to 35°
	Eversion	0° to 20°

Adapted from American Academy of Orthopedic Surgeons and Eaton Hand

- Anterior: Pertaining to or toward the front plane of the body
- Posterior: Pertaining to or toward the back plane of the body
- Superior: Higher in place or position; situated above another
- Inferior: Lower in place or position; situated beneath another

Elevation and depression (of the scapula):

- Elevation refers to movement in a superior or upward direction; depression refers to movement in an inferior or downward direction.

Pronation and supination (of the forearm):

- Pronation moves the palm of the hand so that it is facing downward, like when typing on a keyboard.
- Supination moves the palm of the hand so that it is facing up, like when carrying a bowl of soup from underneath.

Dorsiflexion and plantar flexion (of the ankle):

- Dorsiflexion and plantar flexion are terms used to describe movements at the ankle. They refer to the two surfaces of the foot: the dorsum (superior surface) and the plantar surface (the bottom of the foot). Dorsiflexion refers to flexion at the ankle, so that the foot points more superiorly.
- Plantar flexion refers to extension at the ankle, so that the foot points more inferiorly.

Opposition and reposition (thumb):

- Opposition brings the pad of the thumb and the pad of any finger together, most often with the index finger.
- Reposition is a movement that places the thumb and finger away from each other.

PREPARING THE CLIENT FOR MEASUREMENT

Before initiating the ROM assessment, the OT practitioner should explain the process and accommodate any issues, such as English as a second language or other communication issues, joint limitations, or weakness. Documentation could be either via computer or a paper form based on clinic standards. The preferred client position in which to assess a client is sitting when possible. If sitting is not possible, the client may be supine or side-lying in bed or on a mat. It is rare for an OT practitioner to place a client in the prone position for measurement, and generally not in a standing position (as client may have balance problems, or may be too tall for the clinician). Also inform the client to communicate any pain experienced during joint movement. Be cautious when lining up the goniometer with the body part, especially if the clothing is loose, as the landmarks may be more difficult to distinguish.

The following are specific directions for measuring each of the joints with the most common testing position used in the majority of OT settings. Adjustments can certainly be made for the client who needs to be supine or side-lying. It is best to avoid using chairs with arms because they make it difficult to access the client and for the client to move freely through the planes of motion. However, there are times when the ideal situation is not possible, and the OT practitioner must do the best possible using these core principles of measurement.

Before measuring ROM using the goniometer, ask the client to move the body part through AROM. This helps ensure accurate communication of the movement required and is a quick way to identify any possible joint issues or weakness. Take a mental note of differences between the right and left side of the body. Also observe for any compensatory movements, such as shoulder hiking with shoulder flexion. Compensatory movements are extraneous body movements that occur as a result of the client having difficulty moving the joint through the direct line of motion. The client is often unaware of these movements because the body naturally attempts to perform the movement despite joint or strength issues.

Measuring Active Range of Motion

Note: Some of the ROM assessment photos in this chapter show the client in a standing position for photographic purposes.

CERVICAL SPINE

Motion: Flexion 0° to 40°
Use 8″ goniometer
Testing position: Seated
Fulcrum: External ear canal
Stationary arm: Perpendicular to floor
Moveable arm: Parallel to the base of nostrils
Movement: Instruct client to tuck chin to chest

Motion: Extension 0° to 50°
Use 8″ goniometer
Testing position: Seated
Fulcrum: External ear canal
Stationary arm: Perpendicular to floor
Moveable arm: Parallel to the base of nostrils
Movement: Instruct client to look up to ceiling

Motion: Lateral flexion 0° to 45°
Testing position: Seated
Fulcrum: Spinous process C7
Stationary arm: Spinous processes of thoracic vertebrae so arm is perpendicular to floor
Moveable arm: Dorsal midline of head
Movement: Instruct client to place ear to shoulder

Motion: Rotation 0° to 60°
Testing position: Seated
Fulcrum: Center of the top of the head
Stationary arm: Parallel to imaginary line between the two acromial processes
Moveable arm: In line with tip of nose
Movement: Instruct client to look toward shoulder

SHOULDER

Motion: Shoulder flexion 0° to 180° (Fig. 7-5)

Use 12″ goniometer

Testing position: Sitting in chair, feet on floor, good posture, start with arms hanging down at side

Fulcrum: 1″ below acromion process

Stationary arm: Pointed at floor

Movable arm: Along midpoint of the humerus

Movement: Instruct client to keep arm straight and raise forward and overhead as high as possible. Thumb should be pointed upward. Stationary arm stays in place, movable arm moves with humerus.

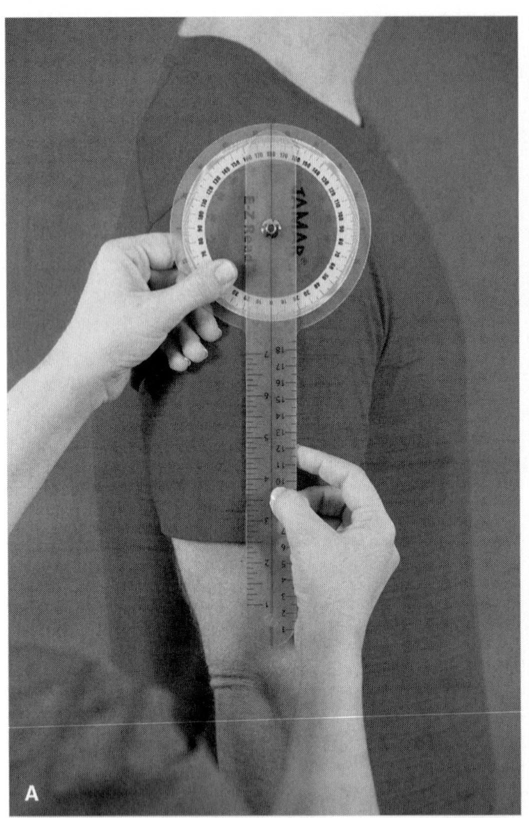

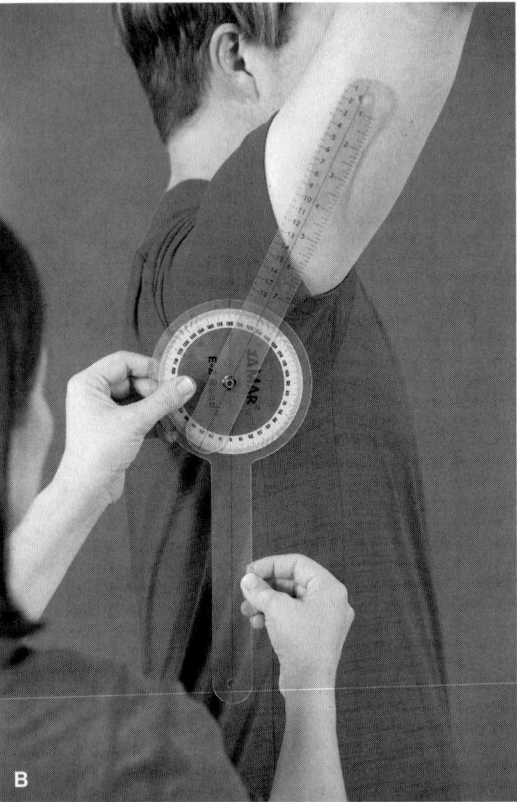

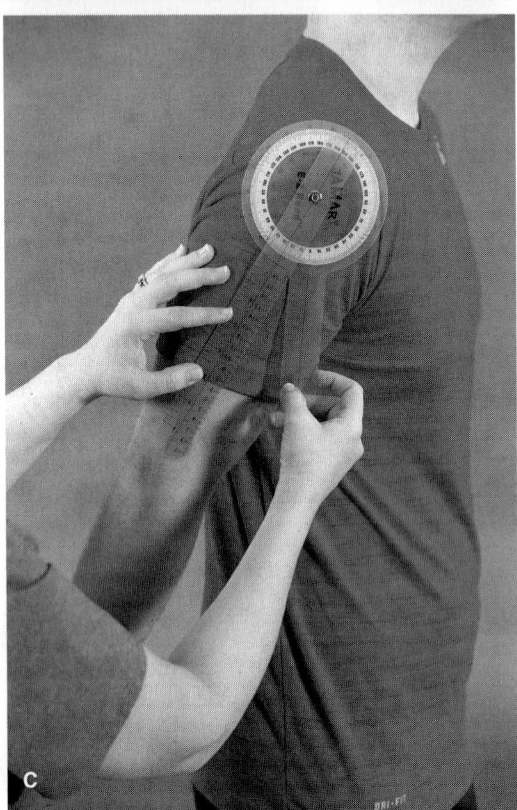

FIGURE 7-5. **A.** The start position for shoulder flexion and extension. **B.** The end position for shoulder flexion. **C.** The end position for shoulder extension.

Motion: Shoulder extension 0° to 60° (see Fig. 7-5)
Use 12″ goniometer
Testing position: Sitting in chair, feet on floor, good posture, start with arms hanging at side
Fulcrum: 1″ below acromion process
Stationary arm: Along lateral midpoint of the humerus, pointed toward floor
Movable arm: Along lateral midpoint of the humerus
Movement: Instruct client to keep arm straight and extend as far back as possible (be sure the client is not moving shoulder at an angle or rotating the shoulder). Stationary arm stays pointed to floor, in line with trunk, and movable arm moves with lateral humerus.

Motion: Shoulder abduction 0° to 180° (Fig. 7-6)
Use 12″ goniometer
Testing position: Sitting in chair, feet on floor, good posture. Measure from behind to avoid breast tissue.
Fulcrum: Posterior glenohumeral joint
Stationary arm: Along lateral midpoint of the humerus, pointed at floor
Movable arm: Along lateral midpoint of the humerus
Movement: Instruct client to abduct arm to side of body as high as allowed with palm facing forward. Stationary arm stays pointed to floor, in line with trunk, and movable arm moves with lateral humerus.

Motion: Shoulder internal rotation 0° to 70° (Fig. 7-7)
Use 12″ goniometer
Testing position: Sitting in chair, feet on floor, good posture. Humerus parallel to floor, elbow bent at a 90 degree angle
Fulcrum: Olecranon process
Stationary arm: Along middle of ulna
Movable arm: Along middle of ulna
Movement: Instruct client to keep humerus parallel to floor as the client rotates forearm down to floor. Stationary arm stays parallel to floor and movable arm moves with ulna
Alternate method: For gravity eliminated or if abduction is contraindicated, internal rotation may be measured as indicated (Fig. 7-8):
Use 12″ goniometer
Testing position: Sitting in chair, feet on floor, good posture. Humerus adducted against trunk, elbow at 90 degrees of flexion, forearm in midposition
Fulcrum: Olecranon process
Stationary arm: Parallel to floor, along ulna
Movable arm: Parallel to floor, along ulna
Movement: Instruct client to bring forearm toward trunk in motion parallel to floor without moving shoulder out of adduction. Moveable arm moves with ulna

Motion: Shoulder external rotation 0° to 90° (see Fig. 7-7)
Use 12″ goniometer
Testing position: Sitting in chair, feet on floor, good posture. Humerus parallel to floor, elbow bent at 90 degrees of flexion
Fulcrum: Olecranon process
Stationary arm: Along middle of ulna
Movable arm: Along middle of ulna

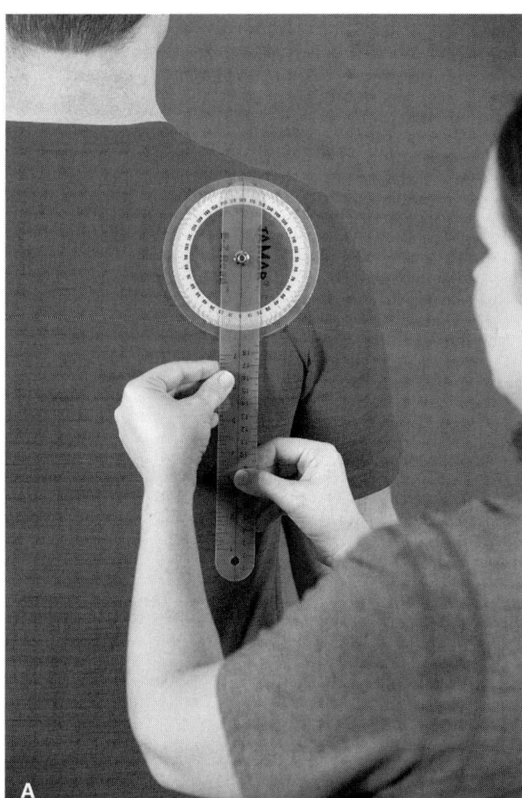

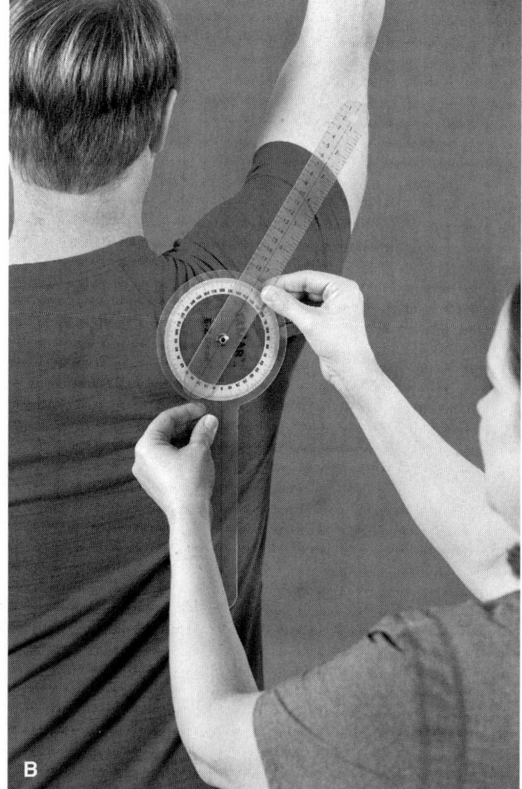

FIGURE 7-6. **A.** The start position for shoulder abduction. **B.** The end position for shoulder abduction.

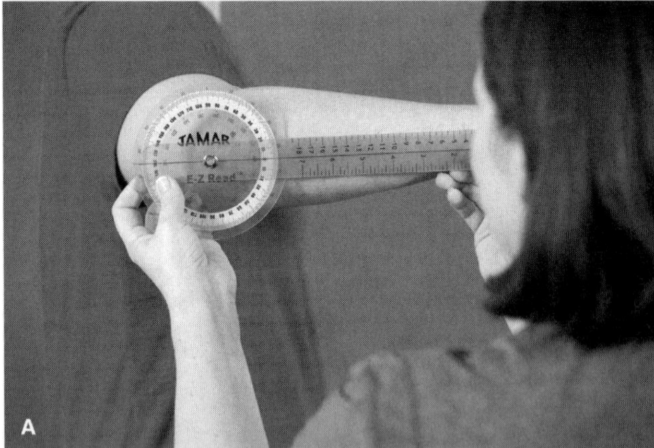

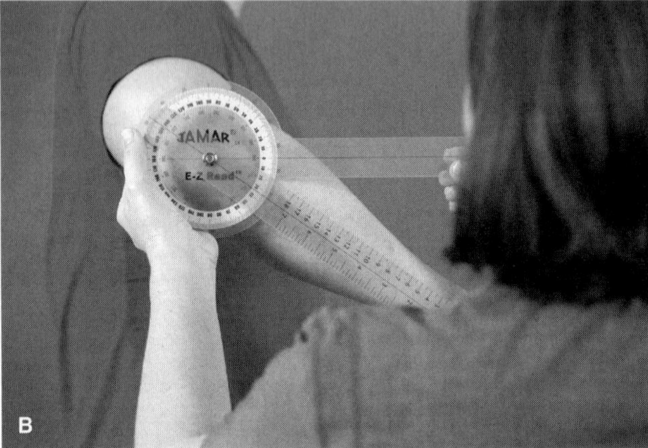

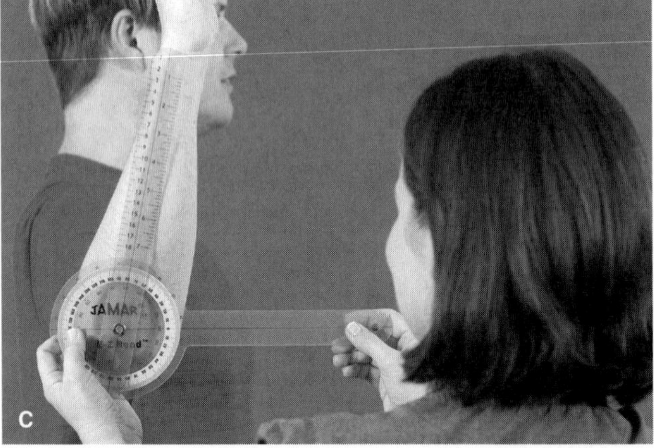

FIGURE 7-7. A. The start position for shoulder internal rotation and external rotation. **B.** The end position for shoulder internal rotation. **C.** The end position for external rotation.

Movement: Instruct client to keep humerus parallel to floor as the client rotates forearm toward ceiling. Stationary arm stays parallel to the floor and movable arm moves with ulna

Alternate method: For gravity eliminated or if abduction is contraindicated, external rotation may be measured as follows:

Use 12″ goniometer

Testing position: Sitting in chair, feet on floor, good posture. Humerus adducted against trunk, elbow at 90 degrees of flexion, forearm in midposition

Fulcrum: Olecranon process

Stationary arm: Parallel to floor, along ulna

Movable arm: Parallel to floor, along ulna

Movement: Instruct client to bring forearm away from trunk in motion parallel to floor without moving shoulder out of adduction. Moveable arm follows ulna

Motion: Shoulder horizontal abduction 0° to 40° (Fig. 7-9)

Use 8″ goniometer

Testing position: Sitting in chair, feet on floor, good posture. Arm straight out at side, parallel to body, palm facing forward

Fulcrum: Top of acromion process

Stationary arm: On top and lined up with the humerus

Movable arm: On top and lined up with the humerus

Movement: Instruct client to keep arm straight as he or she moves it parallel to floor to abduct away from the body. Stationary arm stays in starting position as movable arm travels with the humerus

Alternate method: May be measured with UE placed on top of table for gravity-eliminated position

Motion: Shoulder horizontal adduction 0° to 130° (see Fig. 7-9)

Use 8″ goniometer

Testing position: Sitting in chair, feet on floor, good posture. Arm straight out at side, parallel to body, palm facing forward

Fulcrum: Top of acromion process

Stationary arm: On top and lined up with the humerus

Movable arm: On top and lined up with the humerus

Movement: Instruct client to keep arm straight as the client moves it parallel to floor to adduct toward the body. Stationary arm stays in starting position as movable arm travels with the humerus

Alternate method: May be measured with UE placed on top of table for gravity eliminated position

COMMUNICATION

During ROM of the shoulder, it can be very easy to cause or exacerbate an impingement due to improper technique. When ranging into flexion or abduction, the client's arm should always be in anatomical position with elbow supported by the OT practitioner, forearm and wrist in neutral position, and thumb pointed up. Caregivers, family, and staff must also be trained via demonstration, written, and picture based education to protect the shoulder, not only with ROM, but also with transfers, ADLs, and bed mobility. By using the appropriate shoulder position and support in all situations, painful shoulder impingement can be prevented. Be sure to communicate this important information to your clients, caregivers, and nursing staff so they can incorporate proper alignment of the client's shoulders during all activities.

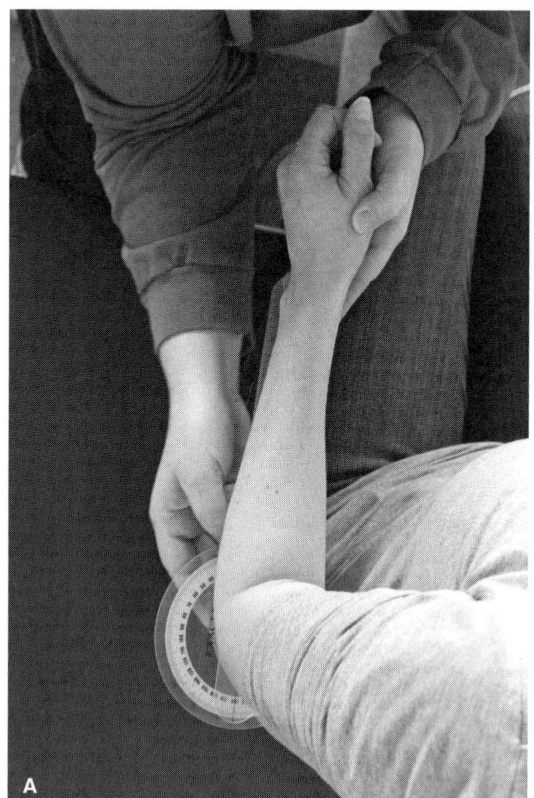

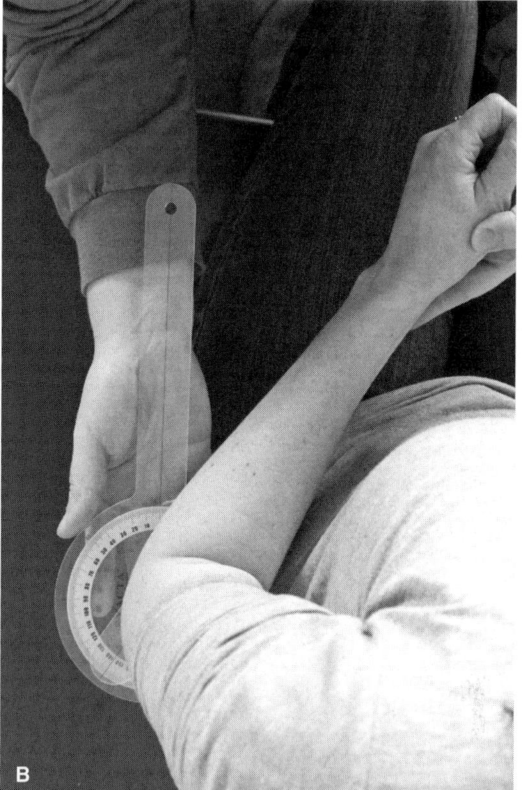

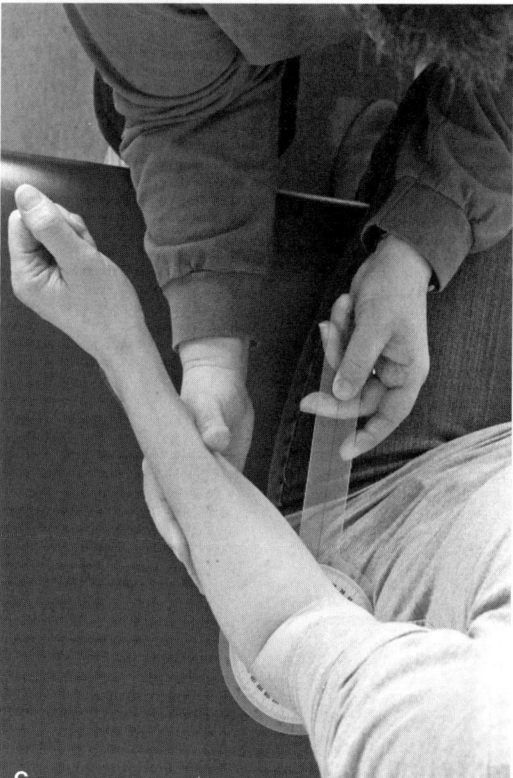

FIGURE 7-8. Alternative shoulder internal rotation if no abduction allowed or if client cannot maintain abduction. **A.** Start position. **B.** Internal rotation. **C.** External rotation.

ELBOW

Motion: Elbow extension to flexion 0° to 150° (Fig. 7-10)

Use 12″ goniometer

Testing position: Sitting in chair, feet on floor, good posture. Arm resting to side of body in anatomical position

Fulcrum: Lateral epicondyle

Stationary arm: On center of the humerus

Movable arm: On center of radius

Movement: Instruct client to flex elbow while keeping stationary arm on the humerus as movable arm moves with radius

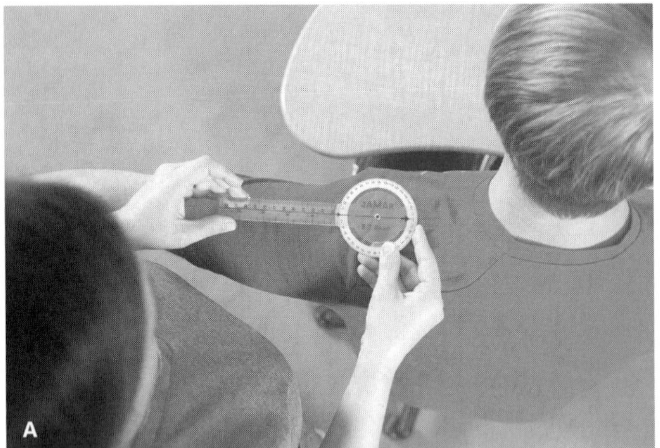

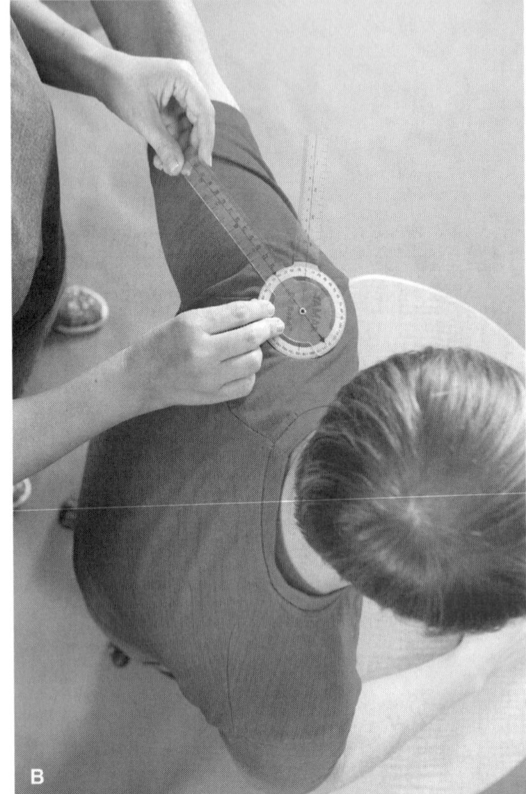

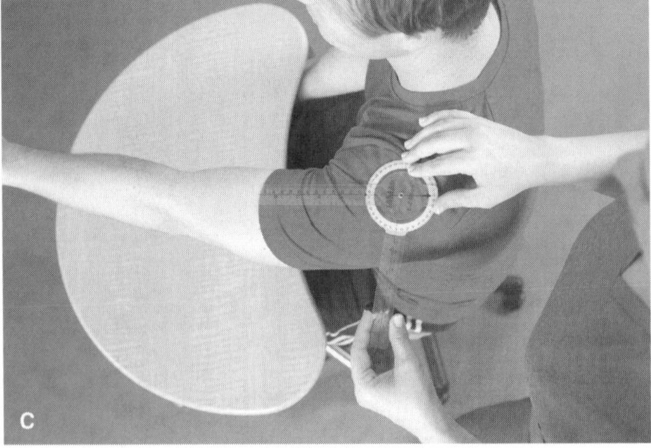

FIGURE 7-9. **A.** The start position for shoulder horizontal abduction/adduction. **B.** The end position for shoulder horizontal abduction. **C.** The end position for shoulder horizontal adduction.

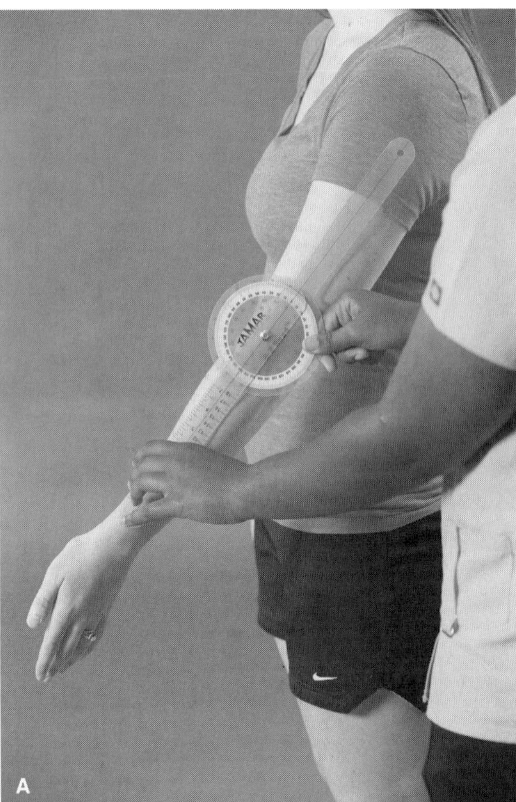

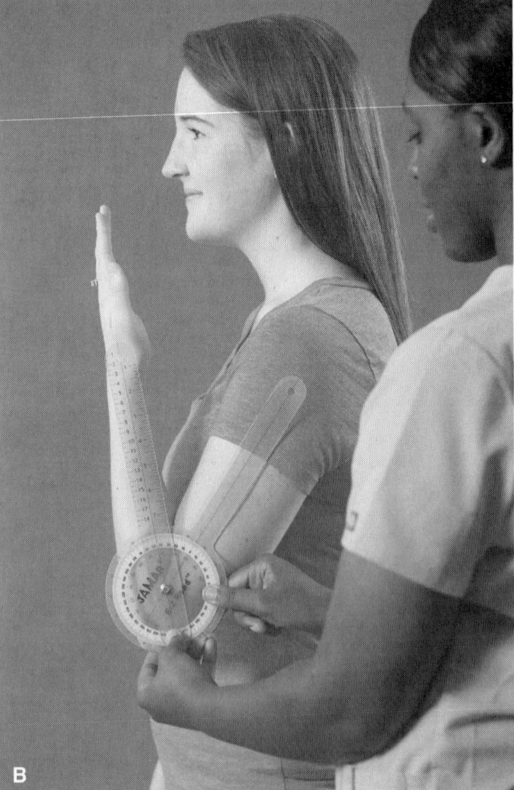

FIGURE 7-10. **A.** The start position for elbow extension and the end position for elbow flexion. **B.** The start position for elbow flexion and the end position for elbow extension.

Motion: Elbow extension 0 degrees (Fig. 7-11)
Use 12″ goniometer
Testing position: Sitting in chair, feet on floor, good posture. Arm resting to side of body in anatomical position, elbow flexed
Fulcrum: Lateral epicondyle
Stationary arm: On center of the humerus
Movable arm: On center of the radius
Movement: Instruct client to extend elbow while keeping stationary arm on the humerus as movable arm

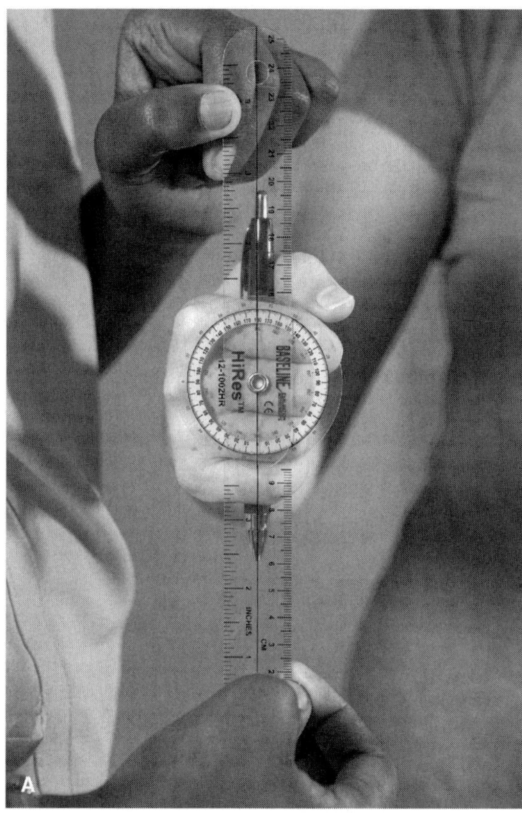

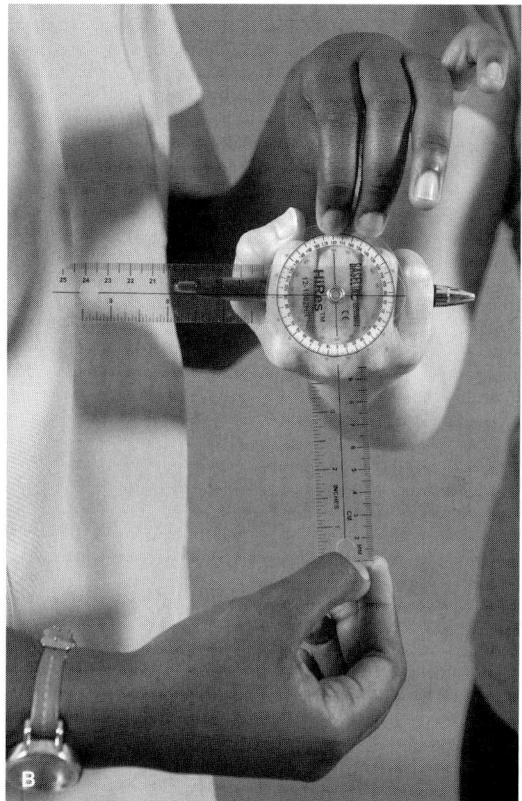

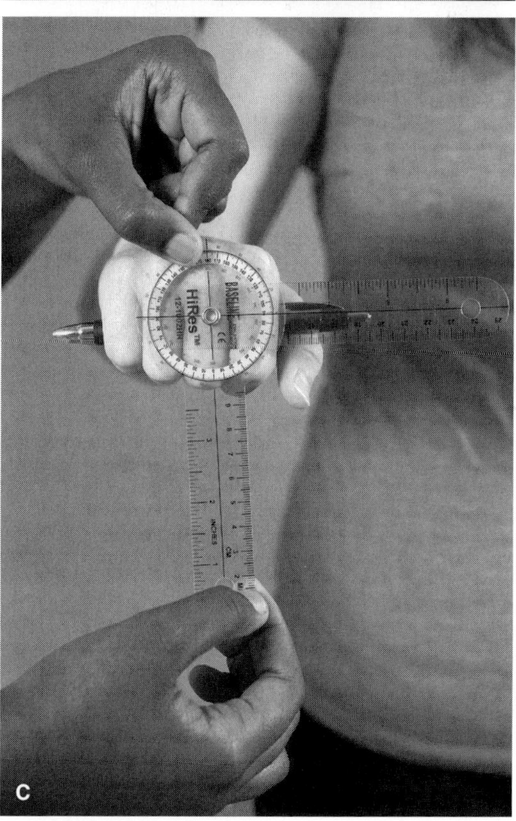

FIGURE 7-11. **A.** The start position for forearm supination and forearm pronation. **B.** The end position for forearm supination. **C.** The end position for forearm pronation.

moves with the radius. Full, normal extension is represented as 0 degrees. If the elbow does not fully extend, document this fact. For example, if the client is not able to fully extend the elbow and the measurement is noted as 10 degrees on the goniometer, then the client is lacking 10 degrees of extension, which could be documented as -10 degrees extension or as 170 degrees elbow extension. For hyperextension, document either as +10 degrees hyperextension or 190 degrees hyperextension. Follow facility protocols.

FOREARM

Motion: Forearm supination 0° to 80°-85° (see Fig. 7-11)
Use 8″ goniometer
Testing position: Start with shoulder slightly abducted and elbow at 90 degrees of flexion. Hold pencil or pen in fist
Fulcrum: Centered on 3rd proximal phalanx
Stationary arm: Pointing toward floor
Moveable arm: Pointing toward ceiling
Movement: Instruct client to supinate forearm. Moveable arm follows midpoint of pencil or pen, then take measurement. Be aware of maintaining the wrist at neutral to avoid compensation.

Motion: Forearm pronation 0° to 70°-80° (see Fig. 7-11)
Use 8″ goniometer
Testing position: Start with shoulder slightly abducted and elbow at 90 degrees of flexion. Hold pencil or pen in fist
Fulcrum: Centered on 3rd PIP joint
Stationary arm: Pointing toward floor
Moveable arm: Pointing toward ceiling
Movement: Instruct client to pronate forearm. Moveable arm follows midpoint of pencil or pen, then take measurement. Be aware of maintaining the wrist at neutral to avoid compensation.

WRIST

Motion: Wrist extension 0° to 70° (Fig. 7-12)
Use 8″ or 6″ goniometer
Testing position: Hand ulnar border down on table, thumb tucked (gravity eliminated). Allow fingers to be relaxed.
Fulcrum: Center of wrist
Stationary arm: In line with the radius
Moveable arm: In line with third metacarpal joint of index finger
Movement: Instruct client to extend wrist as far as possible and take measurement
Alternate method: May also be measured with forearm pronated on table and wrist hanging off table

Motion: Wrist flexion 0° to 75°-80° (see Fig. 7-12)
Testing position: Hand ulnar border down on the table (gravity eliminated). Allow fingers to be relaxed.
Fulcrum: Center of wrist
Stationary arm: In line with the radius
Moveable arm: In line with third metacarpal joint of index finger
Movement: Instruct client to flex wrist as far as possible and take measurement
Alternate method: May also be measured with forearm supinated on table and wrist hanging off table

Motion: Wrist ulnar deviation 0° to 30°-35° (Fig. 7-13)
Testing position: Client is seated with forearm pronated, wrist neutral, fingers in extension, and palm flat on surface
Fulcrum: Axis is the dorsum of the wrist at the base of the 3rd metacarpal
Stationary arm: Midline between the radius and ulna
Moveable arm: Dorsal midline of 3rd metacarpal
Movement: Instruct client to move wrist laterally toward ulnar direction

Motion: Wrist radial deviation 0° to 20° (see Fig. 7-13)
Testing position: Client is seated with forearm pronated, wrist neutral, fingers in extension, and palm flat on surface
Fulcrum: Axis is the dorsum of the wrist at the base of the 3rd metacarpal joint
Stationary arm: Middle of dorsum of wrist
Moveable arm: Dorsal midline of 3rd metacarpal
Movement: Instruct the client to move wrist laterally toward radial direction

DIGITS

Note: *Measurement procedures of finger ROM will vary based on the type of goniometer used.*

Motion: MCP joint flexion 0° to 90° (Fig. 7-14)
Testing position: Seated with elbow flexed, forearm in midposition, wrist neutral, forearm supported on ulnar border. If measuring from dorsum of the hand, the fulcrum is placed on the knuckle.
Stationary arm: Dorsal midline of metacarpal
Moveable arm: Dorsal midline of proximal phalanx
Movement: Instruct client to bend finger down. Focus on bending at the MCP only, not making a full fist.

Motion: MCP extension/hyperextension 0° to 45° (Fig. 7-14)
Testing position: Seated with elbow flexed, forearm in midposition, wrist neutral, forearm and hand supported on ulnar border. Depending on the goniometer, metacarpophalangeal (MCP) extension/hyperextension could be measured from the volar side. Not all clients will have MCP hyperextension.
Fulcrum: On the dorsal aspect of MCP joint of the digit being measured
Stationary arm: Volar midline of metacarpal
Moveable arm: Volar midline of proximal phalanx
Movement: Instruct client to extend finger from the MCP joint

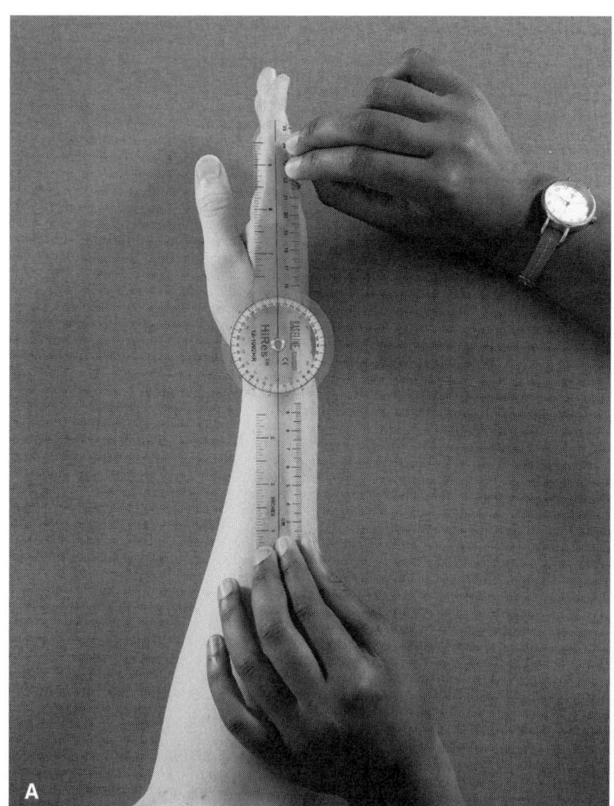

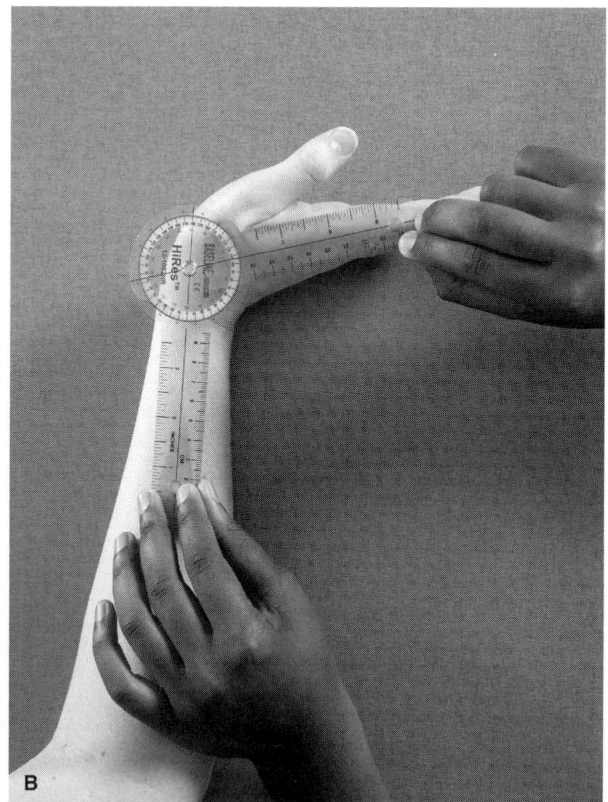

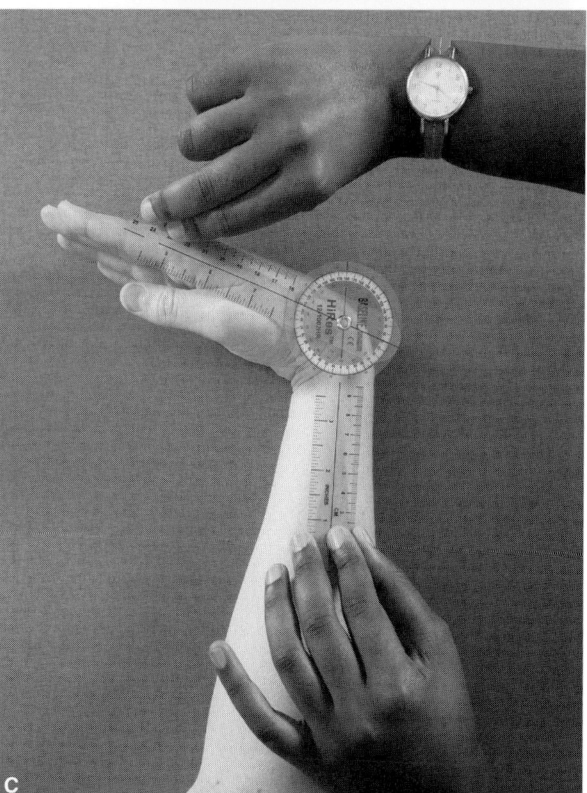

FIGURE 7-12. **A.** The start position for wrist extension and flexion. **B.** The end position for wrist extension. **C.** The end position for wrist flexion.

Motion: MCP abduction 0° to 25° (Fig. 7-15)
Testing position: Seated with forearm pronated, wrist neutral, and palm resting on table
Fulcrum: MCP joint of the digit being measured
Stationary arm: Dorsal midline of metacarpal
Moveable arm: Dorsal midline of proximal phalanx
Movement: Instruct client to spread fingers apart

Motion: PIP flexion 0° to 100° (Fig. 7-16)
Testing position: Seated with elbow flexed, forearm in midposition, wrist neutral, forearm and hand supported on ulnar border
Fulcrum: Dorsal aspect of PIP joint of the digit being measured
Stationary arm: Dorsal midline of proximal phalanx

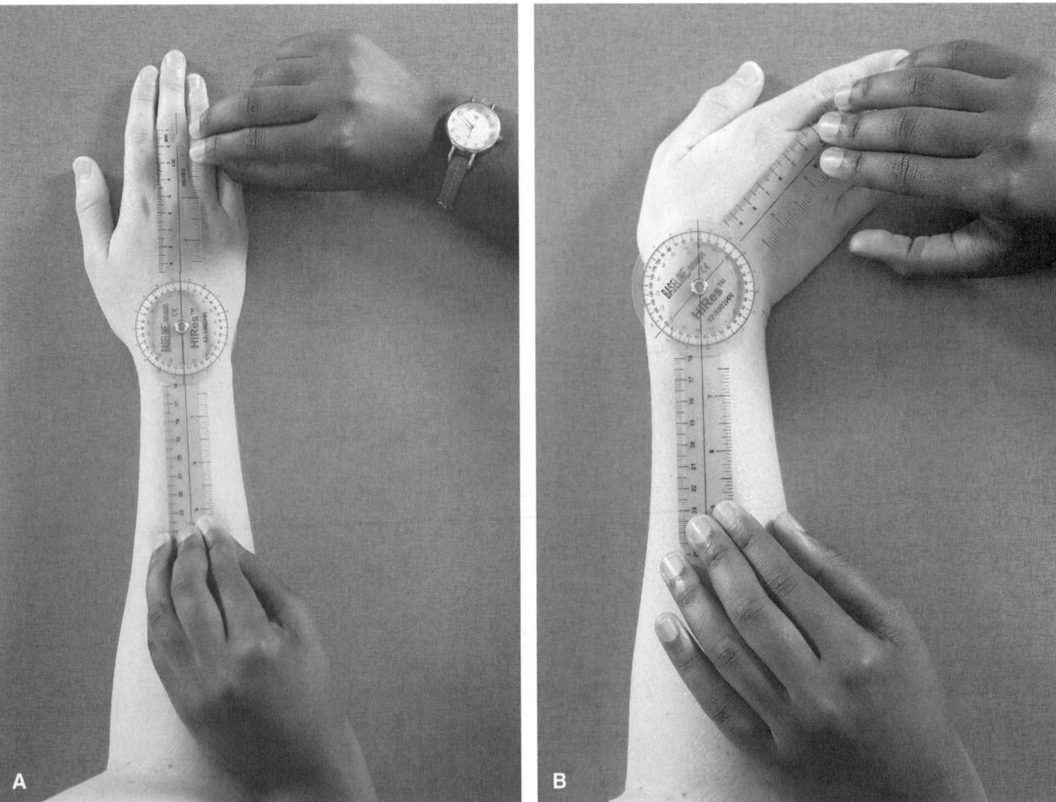

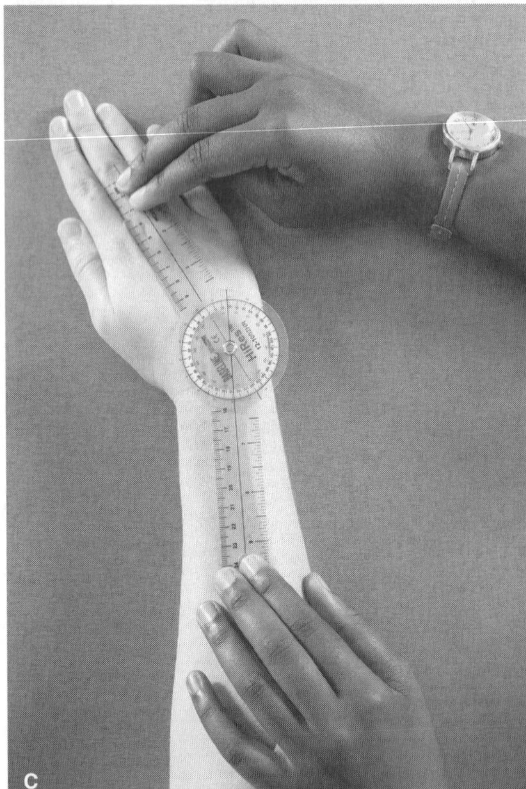

FIGURE 7-13. **A.** The start position for wrist ulnar deviation and radial deviation. **B.** The end position for wrist ulnar deviation. **C.** The end position for wrist radial deviation.

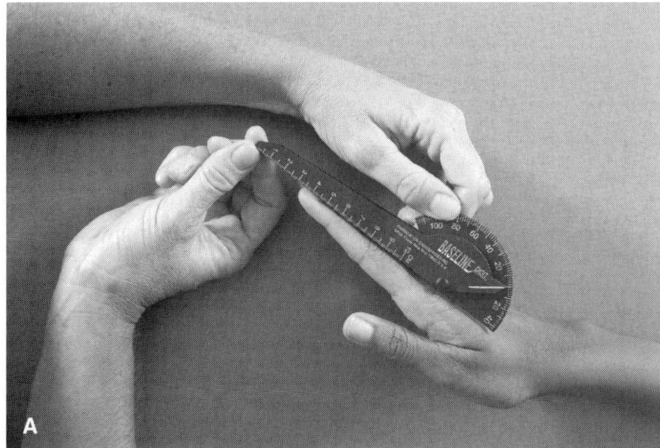

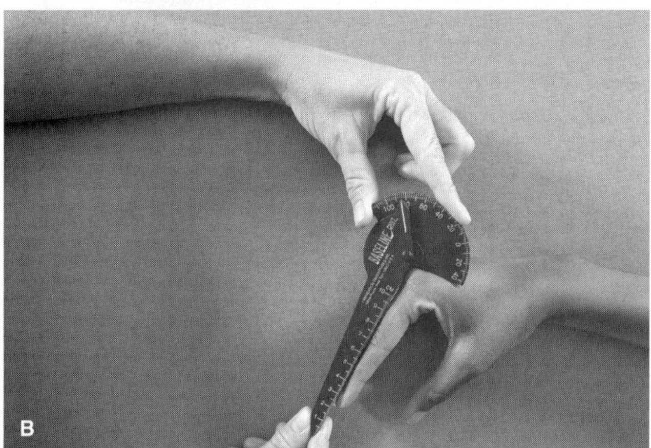

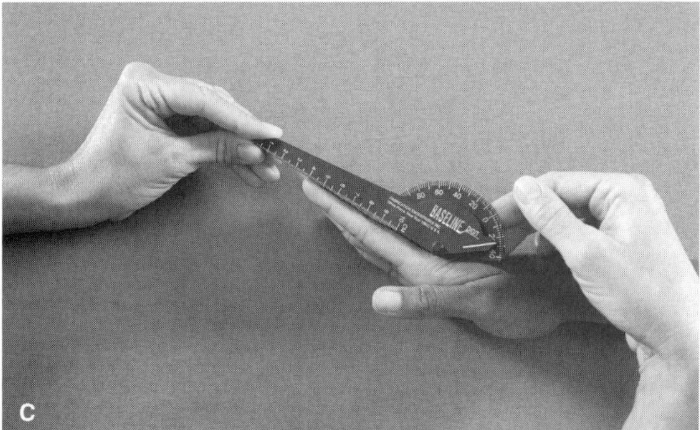

FIGURE 7-14. **A.** The start position for MCP flexion and extension. **B.** The end position for MCP flexion. **C.** The end position for MCP hyperextension.

Moveable arm: Dorsal midline of middle phalanx
Movement: Instruct client to bend finger down while maintaining MCP in neutral

Motion: Distal interphalangeal (DIP) flexion 0° to 80° (Fig. 7-17)
Testing position: Seated with elbow flexed, forearm in midposition, wrist neutral, forearm and hand supported on ulnar border
Fulcrum: Dorsal aspect of DIP joint of the digit being measured
Stationary arm: Dorsal midline of middle phalanx
Moveable arm: Dorsal midline of distal phalanx

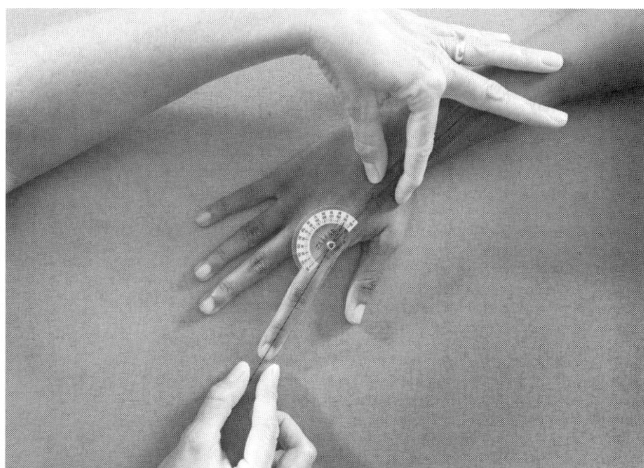

FIGURE 7-15. The end position for MCP abduction.

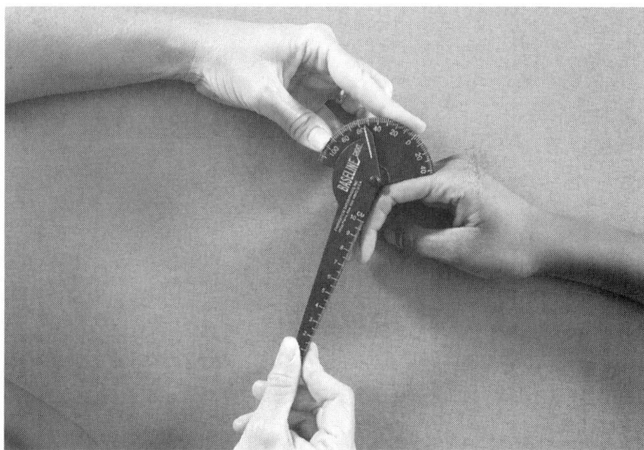

FIGURE 7-16. Measuring PIP flexion.

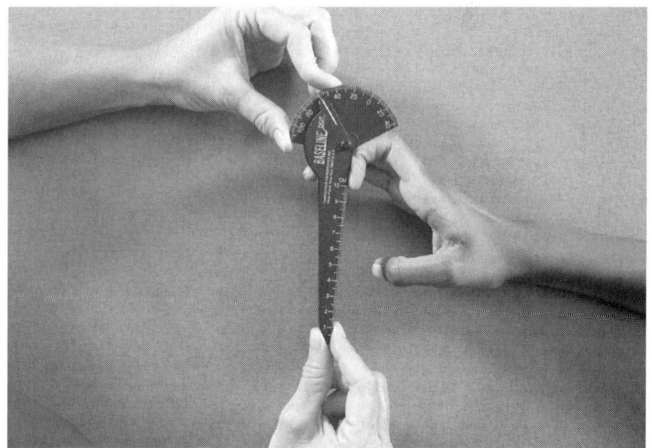

FIGURE 7-17. Measuring DIP flexion.

Movement: Instruct client to bend finger down while maintaining MCP in neutral

THUMB

Motion: CMC flexion 0° to 15° (Fig. 7-18)
Testing position: Seated with elbow flexed, forearm in supination, wrist neutral, MCP and interphalangeal (IP) joints in extension, and hand supported on hard surface

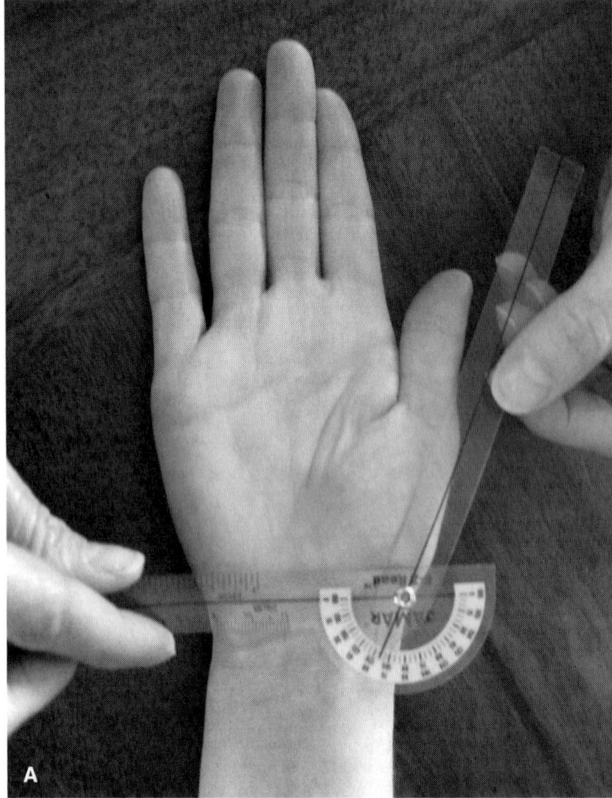

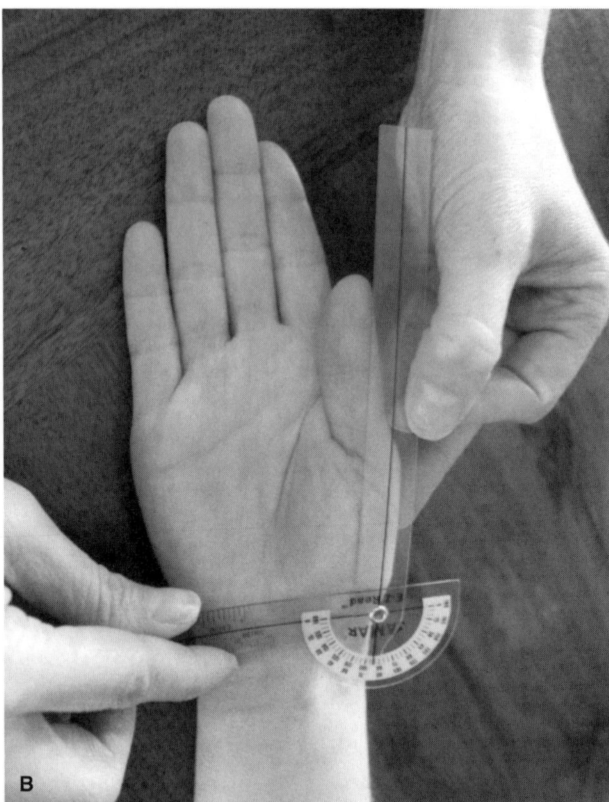

FIGURE 7-18. Measuring thumb CMC flexion at the (A) start and (B) end.

Fulcrum: Volar (forward side in anatomical position) aspect of CMC joint of the thumb
Stationary arm: Volar and perpendicular to the thumb (note the goniometer does not read 0 degrees)
Moveable arm: Volar and in line with the first metacarpal
Movement: Stabilize the wrist to prevent extra movement. Instruct client to flex the thumb toward the palm at the CMC joint. Note the difference between the degrees from the beginning of measurement to the end is the ROM

Motion: CMC extension (or radial abduction) 0° to 20° (Fig. 7-19)
Testing position: Seated with elbow flexed, forearm in pronation, wrist neutral, MCP and IP joints in extension, and hand supported on hard surface
Fulcrum: Dorsal (back side in anatomical position) aspect of CMC joint of the thumb
Proximal stationary arm: Volar midline of radius dorsal and parallel to MC
Distal moveable arm: Volar midline of 1st MC dorsal and parallel to PIP
Movement: Instruct client to bring thumb out to side, like an "L"

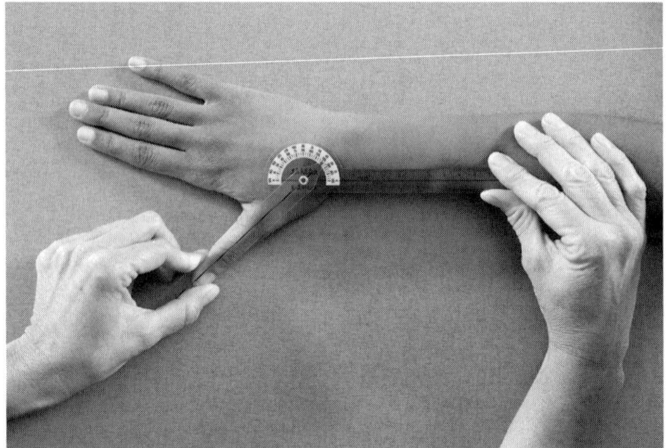

FIGURE 7-19. Endpoint for measuring thumb CMC extension (also called radial abduction).

Motion: CMC (palmar) abduction 0° to 45° (Fig. 7-20)
Testing position: Seated with elbow flexed, forearm neutral, wrist neutral, MCP and IP joints in extension, and hand supported on hard surface. Stabilize the carpals.
Fulcrum: Lateral aspect of CMC joint
Stationary arm: Lateral aspect of radius
Moveable arm: Lateral midline of 1st metacarpal
Movement: Instruct client to move thumb out away from hand

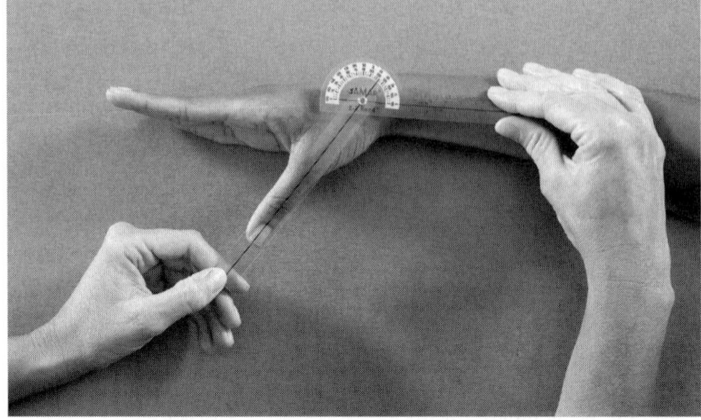

FIGURE 7-20. Measuring thumb CMC abduction (also called palmar abduction).

Motion: CMC opposition (Fig. 7-21)

Testing position: Seated with forearm in neutral midposition, wrist neutral, ulnar border of forearm and hand supported on table. Thumb rotates at right angle to palm of hand

Goniometer landmark: Tip of center of pad of thumb to pads of fingers

Movement: Instruct client to touch tip of fingers to thumb, one at a time

Measured in cm or mm from thumb pad to finger pad if not able to touch

Motion: Thumb MCP joint flexion 0° to 50°-55° (Fig. 7-22)

Testing position: Seated with elbow flexed, forearm in midposition (or full supination), wrist neutral, ulnar border of forearm and hand supported on table

Fulcrum: Dorsal aspect MCP joint

Stationary arm: Dorsal midline of 1st metacarpal

Moveable arm: Dorsal midline of proximal phalanx

Movement: Instruct client to bend thumb at MCP joint toward crease of little finger

Motion: IP flexion 0° to 80° (Fig. 7-23)

Testing position: Seated with elbow flexed, forearm in midposition (or full supination), wrist neutral, MCP and IP joints in extension, and hand supported on hard surface

Fulcrum: Dorsal aspect of IP joint of the thumb

Stationary arm: Dorsal aspect of proximal phalanx

Moveable arm: Dorsal midline of distal phalanx

Movement: Instruct the client to bend thumb at IP joint

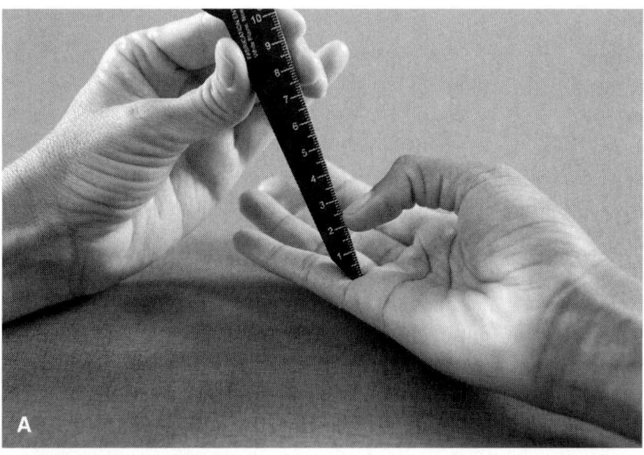

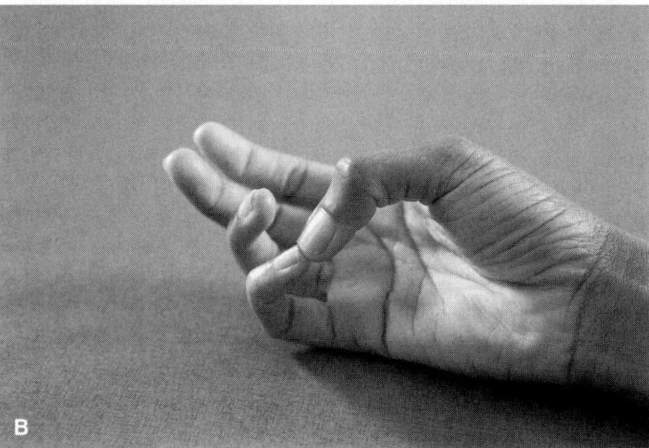

FIGURE 7-21. A. Measuring opposition when the range is limited (attempting to press pad of thumb to base of small finger). B. Client demonstrating functional opposition. Clients may perform opposition as tip to tip as the photo or pad to pad, depending on the demands of the task.

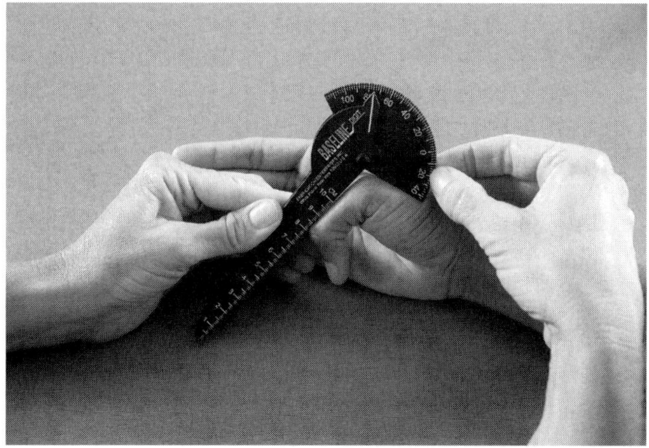

FIGURE 7-22. Measuring thumb MCP flexion.

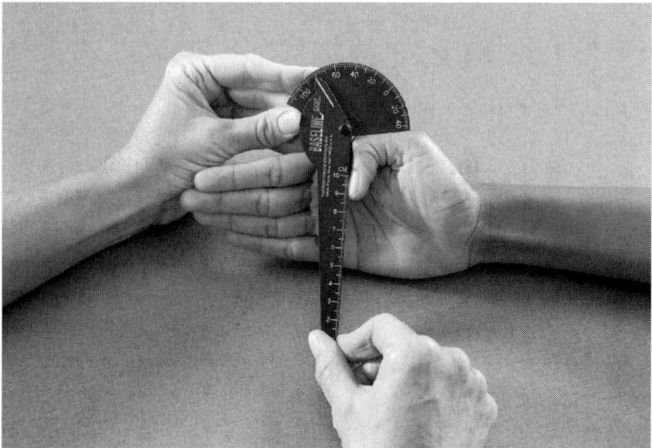

FIGURE 7-23. Measuring thumb IP flexion.

LOWER EXTREMITY

Although it may be unusual to discuss in OT textbooks, it can be important that the OT practitioner be knowledgeable in normal ROM values of the lower extremities (LEs). Loss of ROM can lead to deficits in ADLs of lower extremity dressing and bathing, limited ADL mobility, and transfer skills as well as fall risk complications. For example, a client with a total knee replacement may not possess enough functional LE ROM to access his or her feet and would benefit from education on LE adaptive equipment by the OT practitioner to maximize ADL independence.

HIP

Motion: Hip flexion 0° to 120°

Testing position: Client is supine with hip and knee in neutral extension and rotation

Fulcrum: Lateral aspect of the hip over greater trochanter

Stationary arm: Parallel to midaxillary line of the trunk

Moveable arm: Parallel to the lateral aspect of the femur

Movement: Instruct client to bend hip and move bent knee up toward chest

Motion: Hip extension 0° to 30° (hyperextension would be more than 30 degrees and is uncommon)

Testing position: Client is prone with hip and knee in neutral extension and rotation. Feet are over edge of mat

Fulcrum: Lateral aspect of the hip over greater trochanter

Stationary arm: Parallel to midaxillary line of the trunk

Moveable arm: Parallel to the lateral aspect of the femur

Movement: Instruct client to lift leg off the mat

Motion: Hip abduction 0° to 45°

Testing position: Client is supine with knees extended and hips in neutral rotation

Fulcrum: Over anterior superior iliac spine (ASIS)

Stationary arm: Horizontal, align with the femur, and remain in the starting position between both ASIS

Moveable arm: Parallel to the anterior midline of the femur, align with the femur and follow the leg through the movement

Movement: Instruct client to move leg out to the side

Motion: Hip internal rotation 0° to 45°

Testing position: Client is seated with hip in neutral rotation and 90 degree flexion. Knees flexed at 90 degrees

Fulcrum: Center of patella

Stationary arm: Perpendicular to floor

Moveable arm: Through the midshaft of the tibia

Movement: Instruct client to start with knees close together, rotate one foot away from the other out to the side and roll the knee inward

Motion: Hip external rotation 0° to 45°

Testing position: Client is seated with hip in neutral rotation and 90 degree flexion. Knees flexed at 90 degrees

Fulcrum: Center of patella

Stationary arm: Perpendicular to floor

Moveable arm: Through the midshaft of the tibia

Movement: Instruct client to rotate the foot inward as though a person might cross an ankle over the knee

KNEE

Motion: Knee extension/flexion 0° to 135°

Testing position: Client is prone with knees extended and hips in neutral rotation

Fulcrum: Lateral epicondyle of femur

Stationary arm: Parallel to lateral midline of femur

Moveable arm: Parallel to lateral midline of fibula

Movement: Instruct client to bend knee through ROM

ANKLE

Motion: Ankle dorsiflexion 0° to 20°

Testing position: Client is seated with knee flexed at least 30 degrees or supine with knees extended. Ankle in 90 degrees and foot in neutral inversion/eversion

Fulcrum: Lateral aspect of lateral malleolus

Stationary arm: Parallel to lateral midline of fibula

Moveable arm: Parallel to lateral midline of 5th metatarsal

Movement: Instruct client to point foot up

Motion: Ankle plantar flexion 0° to 50°

Testing position: Client is seated with knee flexed at least 30 degrees. Ankle at 90 degrees rotation and foot in neutral inversion/eversion

Fulcrum: Distal to lateral aspect of lateral malleolus

Stationary arm: Parallel to lateral midline of fibula

Moveable arm: Parallel to lateral midline of 5th metatarsal

Movement: Instruct client to point foot down

Motion: Ankle inversion 0° to 35°

Testing position: Client is supine with knee and hip extended and in neutral rotation, ankle 90 degrees neutral, and foot extended over edge of mat

Fulcrum: Over anterior aspect of ankle, midway between the two malleoli

Stationary arm: Parallel to anterior midline of lower leg

Moveable arm: Parallel to the anterior midline of 2nd metatarsal

Movement: Instruct client to turn the sole of the foot inward

Motion: Ankle eversion 0° to 20°

Testing position: Client is supine with knee and hip extended and in neutral rotation, ankle 90 degrees neutral, and foot extended over edge of mat

Fulcrum: Over anterior aspect of ankle, midway between the two malleoli

Stationary arm: Parallel to anterior midline of lower leg

Moveable arm: Parallel to the anterior midline of 2nd metatarsal

Movement: Instruct client to turn the sole of the foot outward

RANGE OF MOTION INTERVENTION

Individuals move through patterns of range of motion in everyday life while accomplishing functional activities. The body does not have to be perfect to complete these activities, but the movement does have to be functional, purposeful, and meaningful. Chronic or acute injury, age, gender, and other factors such as lifestyle and occupation can affect ROM.[5] In many circumstances, the loss of ROM may limit functional movement, thus causing a person's occupations to become difficult or impossible.

OT practitioners assess a client's ROM during the initial evaluation and use the results to establish an intervention plan to return that person to the highest possible state of independence. When deciding upon functional interventions to improve ROM in a client, the client's performance goals should be paramount. Certain ROM may or may not be needed by a client, depending on their desired tasks or job-related duties. ROM assessment is also used to measure progress throughout the course of treatment and again at the end of treatment to measure the outcomes of OT intervention. The first priority should be to correct ROM that limits self-care or instrumental ADLs, referred to as IADLs.[3] ROM of the elbow, wrist, and fingers is especially important in maintaining the client's ability to perform eating or grooming. Deficits of ROM at the shoulder affect the client's ability to participate in ADLs, such as donning a shirt or bathing, as well as performing high level home management tasks, such as putting away laundry or retrieving items from shelves. The OT practitioner must also always consider how each individual client's needs are different according to his or her specific occupations and environment.

The OTA must communicate with the occupational therapist to determine what category of ROM is a priority for each client. Despite deficits in PROM or AROM, a client may have enough functional ROM to perform all necessary life roles. Let's examine each category of ROM and discuss intervention strategies as they relate to life role requirements.

THE OLDER ADULT

As people age, they begin to experience functional impairments as a result of simply growing older or because of chronic comorbidities. Frailty is a result of the effects of these comorbidities on the body, which may limit a person's ability to move their joints through a purposeful and functional range. Growing old is not, in itself, a prerequisite to becoming frail. Neither does a disability, such as a loss of a limb, lead to frailty in an otherwise physically robust older person. However, there are ROM losses that can significantly impact older adults.

Loss of ROM from a fall is one of the primary reasons older adults become impaired. Hip, shoulder, wrist, and spinal compression fractures significantly affect the older adult's ability to live in their community and often result in placement into short-term rehabilitation centers, skilled nursing facilities, or assisted living centers. Each year, one out of three older adults fall. Fear of falling leads to sedentary behavior, which impairs function and creates a lower quality of life. Thus the fear leads to decreased strength and increased risk of a fall occurring. Falls are a leading cause of death as a result of unintentional injury among older adults. Deaths and injuries can be prevented by addressing risk factors.

Chronic comorbidities such as chronic obstructive pulmonary disease (COPD), arthritis, diabetes, congestive heart failure, and cardiovascular disease cause many older adults to also become sedentary, causing them to develop loss of ROM because of decreased muscle tone, an increased likelihood of pain, and a higher risk for injuries associated with disuse. Their sustained activity tolerance may be diminished, and they may no longer walk to the mailbox, walk their dog, or go to church. Their participation in life occupations diminishes and this can lead to social isolation and depression.

OT interventions designed to maximize ROM and function in older adults can help them maintain their occupational roles, participate in an active lifestyle, and reduce the risk of developing frailty, disability, and dependency.

Passive Range of Motion Intervention

PROM means that a second individual or other outside force is moving the limb through patterns of movement. PROM does not have any effect on muscle strength or muscle tone, and does not prevent atrophy; it does however, lubricate the joint and prevent stiffness. There are two approaches to intervening in this case. First, the OTA must educate the client, family, caregiver staff, and other members involved in the client's rehabilitation about positioning, protection of the limb, edema prevention, and sensory reeducation, if indicated. Positioning and edema prevention education involve placing the affected limb on a pillow or incline foam support, which reduces the risk of swelling or development of abnormal stiffness or laxity of unsupported muscles. Protection of the limb and sensory reeducation are important when sensation is impaired (see Chapter 8 for more information on sensation). A client's family members, especially those who will be physically present with the client, should be taught to perform PROM as a means to reduce the risk of contracture development, edema, or injury to the client's affected extremity.

In the case of postsurgery therapy, the OT practitioner should place special attention on the client performing the appropriate type of ROM as ordered by the physician. Initially, PROM is performed while tendons and muscles heal, which allows those structures to rest without stress and stretching. Having the client complete AROM too early can adversely affect the surgical outcome.

In performing PROM, the OTA must be positioned to support the affected limb while moving the arm through the appropriate arc of movement. The limb is supported both proximally and distally at the elbow, wrist, and hand during PROM, and the movement should be smooth and slow so as to avoid injury to joints and underlying structures such as ligaments, tendons, and soft tissue (Fig. 7-24).

Generally, the humerus moves approximately 120 degrees as the scapula rotates approximately 60 degrees, causing the ratio between the glenohumeral joint and the scapulothoracic movement to be 2:1. Because both contribute to full shoulder flexion and abduction, scapular motion will be important during all types of ROM, but especially PROM. If the scapula does not move effectively because of muscle weakness or spasticity when the arm is lifted into flexion/abduction to the full 180 degrees, the glenohumeral joint can be overstretched, and the OTA can cause long-term pain to the client as well as subluxation. Generally the OTA should move the scapula through the available range (60 degrees) of rotation with one hand as the other hand carefully lifts the arm for PROM. This would be important whether the client is in a sitting, supine, or side-lying position. The OTA can place the side of the thumb on one side of the scapula and the side of the 5th finger on the other side to assist with rotation and control. This technique of

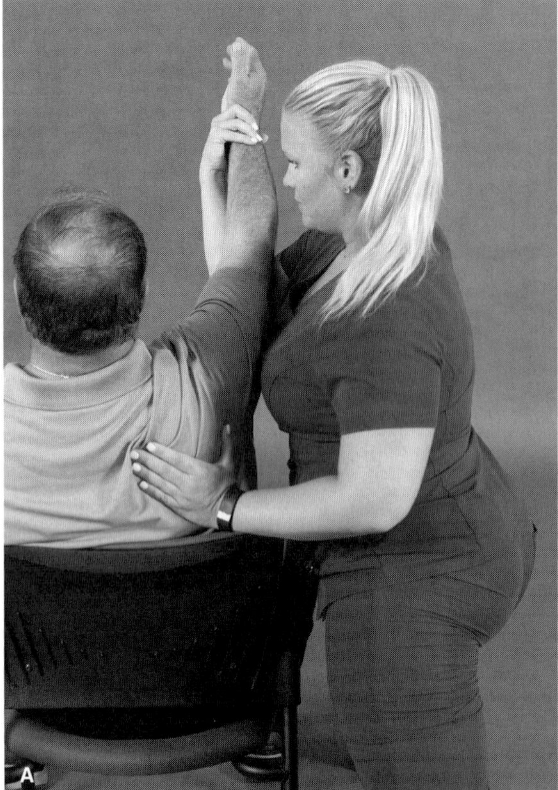

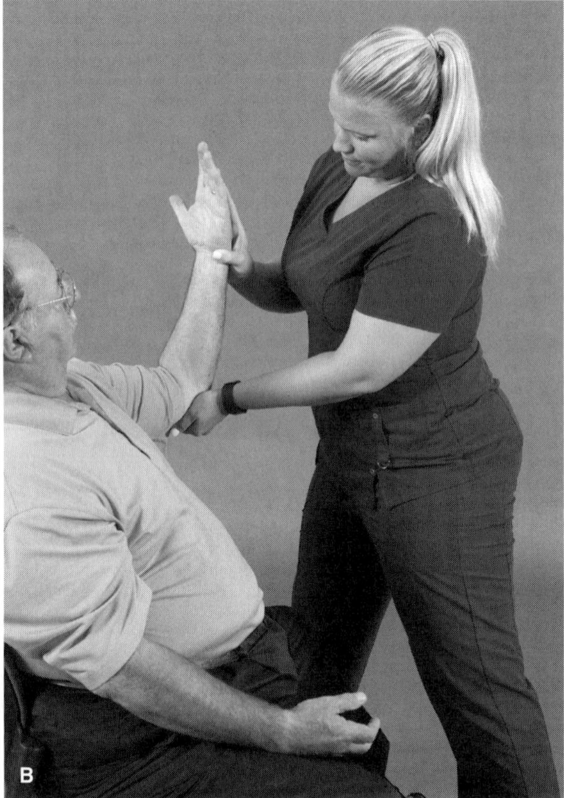

FIGURE 7-24. A. OTA performing PROM shoulder flexion. Note her hand position to guide the client's scapula and altered stance for proper body mechanics. **B.** PROM of elbow while supporting at the olecranon process.

assisted movement at the scapula should be used with shoulder flexion/extension and abduction/adduction when moving through the full ROM. With shoulder movement, much of the shoulder flexion/abduction first occurs at the glenohumeral joint (to approximately 50° to 70°) with humeral movement, and then more of the movement occurs as the scapula rotates later in the range, primarily between 90° to 120°. If the OTA is unsure of how to properly move the scapula or caregivers are unable to perform correctly, the shoulder PROM should be limited to 90° to 110° to avoid overstretching the joint capsule. For shoulder flexion, the thumb should face upward for the safest positioning through the range, and and for shoulder abduction, either palm forward or palm up.

Proper positioning for the OT practitioner and caregiver/family member is important to avoid injury and fatigue while performing PROM with the client. If the client is lying in a hospital bed, raise the bed up to a height between the practitioner's waist and elbows (be sure to lower the bed when finished). UEs that are large or have significant edema may be heavy. The OT practitioner may need to brace his or her own UEs against the trunk for stability and strength. If the client is seated, and the practitioner is tall, the practitioner may need to be seated as well. Find a position that is comfortable, maintains optimal alignment of one's own joints, and uses one's stronger joints and larger muscle groups.

For clients who have a flaccid upper extremity (no muscle tone or active movement), PROM is still an important technique to incorporate into daily activities. PROM may not necessarily be considered skilled OT and may be performed by family, rehabilitation technician, or nursing assistant. Education and training of those individuals would be considered skilled OT, as well as PROM and management of a complex, painful, and/or a subluxed joint. A flaccid joint does not necessarily need to be moved through the entire available range. It can be challenging to simultaneously maintain shoulder stability or integrity, move the scapula correctly, and hold the arm in safe positioning to full ROM. Even just halfway through the available range can be beneficial to keep the joint lubricated and to also help detect any changes in muscle tone (as often occurs after a cerebrovascular accident [CVA]). Always support a subluxed shoulder in the correct joint position during ROM, focus on scapular mobility primarily, and do not generally take the arm over 90 degrees of shoulder flexion or abduction.

Table 7-2 includes directions and illustrations for the majority of UE PROM. Take time to practice these skills with classmates and family members (seated and supine/side-lying) to gain confidence in hand placement, movements, body mechanics, and communication with the client.

TABLE 7-2 Passive Range of Motion Exercises

PROM	DIRECTIONS	
Shoulder flexion	(a) With client supine, support and hold at elbow and wrist while (b) bringing the UE into flexion. OT practitioner will need to stand-step or shift weight through motion to maintain proper body mechanics. Client may also be seated in a chair (without arms), on edge of bed, or on a mat table, but this type of client positioning will require the OT practitioner to support the weight of the limb.	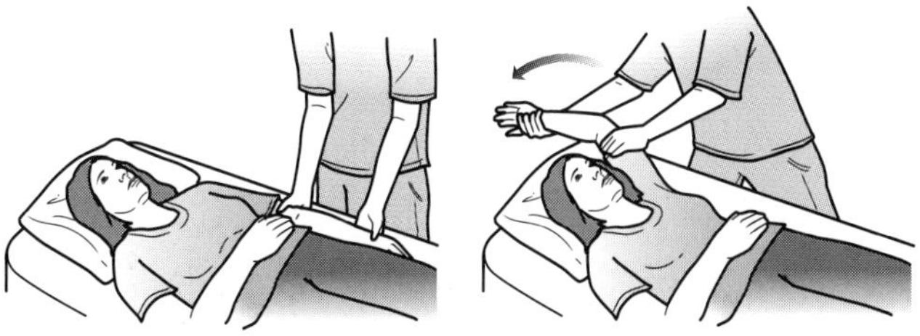 PROM shoulder flexion.
Shoulder extension	(a) Client is supine and close enough to the edge of the mat for extension to not be blocked. Practitioner stabilizes the shoulder while grasping forearm to move shoulder into extension. (b) Alternate method: Client in side-lying position, which works well for clients in a hospital bed. Be sure to support the forearm and stabilize the shoulder while guiding into extension. Client may also be seated in chair (without arms), on edge of bed, or on a mat table.	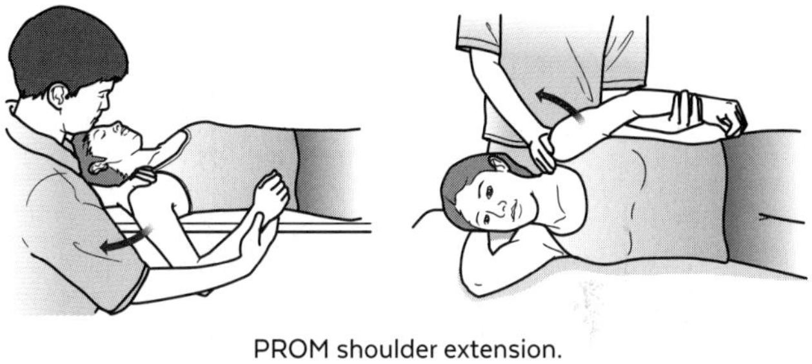 PROM shoulder extension.
Shoulder abduction	(a) With client supine, support and hold at elbow and wrist while (b) bringing the UE into abduction. OT practitioner may sit on stool or stand-step through motion to maintain proper body mechanics. Client may also be seated in a chair (without arms), on edge of bed, or on a mat table, but this type of client positioning will require the OT practitioner to support the weight of the limb.	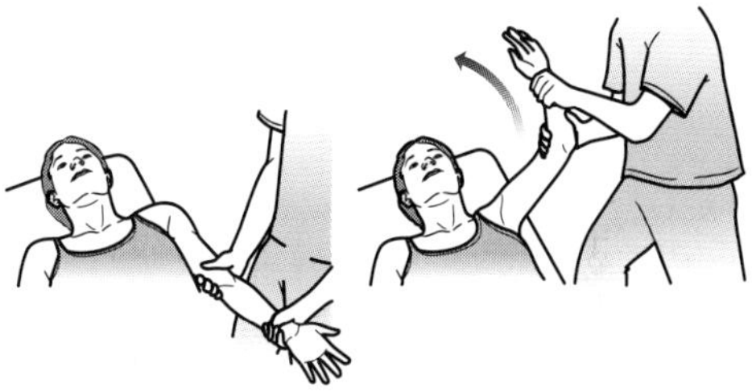 PROM shoulder abduction.
Shoulder external/ internal rotation	With client supine, support and hold at elbow and wrist while bringing the UE into external and internal rotation. Note the shoulder and elbow are both in 90° of flexion and OT practitioner supports client proximally at the elbow while directing distally at the wrist. Client may also be seated in chair (without arms), on edge of bed, or on a mat table, but this type of client positioning will require the OT practitioner to support the weight of the limb.	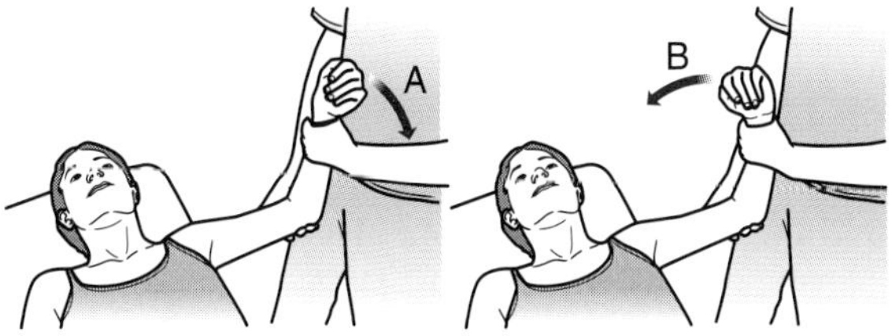 PROM shoulder external/internal rotation.

Continued

TABLE 7-2 Passive Range of Motion Exercises (continued)

PROM	DIRECTIONS	
Elbow flexion/ extension	(a) With client supine, support and hold at elbow and wrist while (b) bringing the elbow into flexion, and then back into extension. Note the OT practitioner supports the elbow proximally and directs the motion distally at the wrist. Elbow PROM may be performed with forearm pronated, supinated, and in neutral. Client may also be seated with elbow supported. For clients lacking elbow extension, it may work best for the client to lay supine on a mat. The practitioner may need to stabilize additionally at the shoulder when performing PROM elbow extension because of the tendency for compensation at the shoulder.	PROM elbow flexion and extension.
Wrist flexion/ extension and ulnar/radial deviation	Wrist PROM is performed while stabilizing just proximal to the wrist, and distally controlling the movement with opposite hand on client's hand as shown. Client may be supine or seated with elbow supported.	PROM wrist flexion/extension and wrist radial/ulnar deviation.
Finger flexion/ extension and thumb flexion/ abduction	(a) PROM fingers composite and (b) PROM for thumb opposition. PROM can be performed by individually flexing and extending each digit, each digit at each joint, or all together by wrapping the practitioner's hand around the client's fingers and flexing them into a fist (a). The thumb should be ranged separately from the fingers. For the thumb, as with the fingers, each joint can be ranged individually or all together. Grasp the thenar eminence (between the CMC and MP, near the base of the thumb) and flex (and abduct) from the CMC, rather than just the distal IP. Range all together or separately. Additionally, bring the thumb into opposition with each digit (b). Client may be supine or seated.	PROM fingers and thumb.

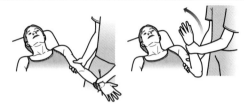

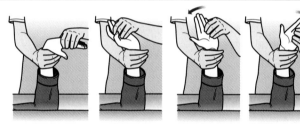

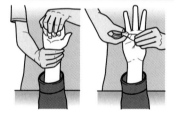

Self Range of Motion Intervention

When a client is educated on how to perform his or her own PROM, it is referred to as **self range of motion (SROM).** SROM is often difficult for individuals to perform alone, but provides focused attention on the affected UE and allows clients to be active participants in their rehabilitation. PROM and SROM are generally taught using a written or picture-based program that includes demonstration and repetition with the client and caregiver. The client performs SROM by utilizing the unaffected limb to support the affected limb. The support can be provided at the elbow by cradling the affected forearm, threading fingers together, holding the opposite wrist, or using a tabletop surface to support the limb while performing SROM (Fig. 7-25). Placing a smooth pillowcase or hand towel on the table under the UEs can assist making movements and also limits friction on skin.

OTAs can educate and train clients to perform these SROM exercises in a pain-free range:

- Shoulder flexion: Place both UEs on a tabletop. Thread fingers or grasp affected wrist with nonaffected, and slide UEs forward on the tabletop. It may be helpful to set an object on the table for the client to gently touch with clasped hands as a visual mark can be helpful to motivate. After a few repetitions, the object may be gradually moved farther away successively.
- Shoulder horizontal abduction/adduction: Place both UEs on a tabletop. Thread fingers or grasp at wrist. Use the nonaffected side to guide the affected UE in moving side to side. This may also be performed without the table.
- Alternate position for shoulder flexion: Lay supine, thread fingers or grasp wrist, carefully lift affected UE into flexion. Be careful to keep thumb pointed up to maintain shoulder in a neutral position (not internally or externally rotated) to avoid painful shoulder impingement, especially at 90 degrees and above.
- Shoulder external rotation: Sit in chair rotated 90 degrees from table. Place affected pronated forearm on tabletop, elbow at 90 degrees (try placing on top of kitchen shelf liner or a piece of Dycem). Gently and slowly lean the trunk forward, leaving UE on the table. May need assistance to maintain UE on tabletop.
- Shoulder abduction/adduction: Sit in chair or edge of therapy mat. Cradle affected UE at the elbow with the unaffected UE. Perform gentle "rocking" motions to each side.
- Elbow flexion/extension:
  - For client with weakness (or flaccidity): Place arms next to trunk, support dorsal hand/wrist with nonaffected side, bring into flexion, and then ease into extension while supported
  - For client with spasticity (stiff muscle tone): Client should be seated with legs/feet placed shoulder-width apart. Thread fingers together or grasp wrist of affected UE with unaffected side. If client has good sitting balance, have client lean slightly forward and move elbow into extension, with hands ending up between thighs. Bring back into flexion
- Supination/pronation: Grasp affected side either with threaded fingers or by the wrist/forearm, and then roll into supination, support on tabletop (on top of towel for cushioning) or in lap while seated in chair or on therapy mat. (Hint: Think of the motion used when flipping burgers or pancakes.)
- Wrist flexion/extension: Elbows bent to comfortable degree of flexion. Thread fingers together, gently push affected wrist into extension, and then bring back into flexion. Can be done on tabletop or in lap while seated in chair or on a therapy mat. (Hint: Think of the movement of windshield washers.)
- Wrist ulnar/radial deviation: Elbows bent to comfortable degree of flexion. Thread fingers together, gently move into ulnar and radial deviation. May be seated in chair or on a therapy mat. (Hint: Think of the motions of hammering a nail.)
- Fingers: Move the fingers into full flexion and extension as well as each finger into abduction and adduction. The wrist should be in neutral position.
- Thumb: Move the thumb through flexion/extension, abduction/adduction, opposition to the base of the 5th finger, and in circles in both directions.

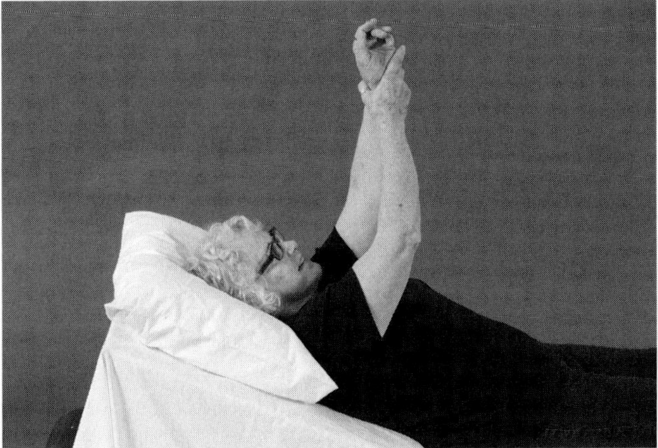

FIGURE 7-25. Client performing SROM exercises for shoulder flexion. Her stronger right hand is assisting the weaker left side.

For clients who are prescribed SROM, it is an important part of their daily routine and can be performed multiple times throughout the day. Performing SROM can empower the client to be engaged in some type of activity, even though AROM may be restricted or not possible at that time. SROM helps maintain some degree of ROM of the joint, and often clients state that it "feels good" to stretch. Clients should not perform SROM in a painful range and should stop the motion just before pain. Some practitioners may mistakenly have the client raise the affected arm through 180 degrees of shoulder SROM. This can result in significant capsular damage and pain, and should be avoided.

Active Assistive Range of Motion Intervention

AAROM is a combined effort of an outside force and the client's own muscle strength acting on the joint to create motion (Fig. 7-26). The division of effort varies according to what the client is able to do and what the OT practitioner, caregiver, or family member performs. AAROM is typically used to help the client have success in achieving ROM while the client is gaining or regaining strength. As such, the client would perform more of the motion with less assistance from the OT practitioner as he or she improves. AAROM is perhaps best used when combined with a functional task, such as self-feeding, grooming hair, brushing teeth, or reaching for an object for a purposeful and client-centered intervention.

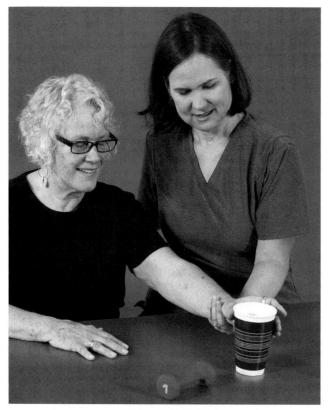

FIGURE 7-26. OT practitioner engaging the client in AAROM by supporting elbow proximally and supporting distally at the wrist to assist the client in the functional task of reaching for a cup.

Active Range of Motion Intervention

AROM is how the client moves by using his or her own muscle power. A client may have full AROM for shoulder flexion while side-lying, yet be unable to lift his or her arm into shoulder flexion against gravity to reach for objects when seated or standing. This is actually a muscle strength issue, not a range of motion issue. This difference is determined by assessing muscle strength after assessing PROM but before initiating a task (see Chapter 9 for methods to measure and improve muscle strength). AROM deficits often occur after a fracture or soft tissue injury. When a cast or orthotic (splint) is removed, the muscles and joint are tighter, which restrict motion. In this case, the OT practitioner may use therapeutic modalities such as moist heat or ice, fluidotherapy, vibration (facilitates contraction of muscle fibers), ultrasound, and electrical stimulation (stimulates muscle fibers and causes contraction or fatigue) which can be a helpful preparatory method to the program of intervention. By following the goals set by the occupational therapist, the OTA can utilize these physical agent modalities to elongate muscle fibers, facilitate prolonged stretch and muscle activation or reduce edema to allow increased ROM to be obtained. Before using any physical agent modalities, the OTA must demonstrate service competency in all methods utilized. See Chapter 18 for in-depth information on physical agent modalities.

Using the client's occupational profile, the OTA gains insight into the activities that are meaningful to the client. The OTA should always try to incorporate meaningful occupations into the AROM interventions. For example, for a client who loves to bake cookies, scooping and placing dough onto a cookie sheet at an appropriate yet challenging distance can be intrinsically motivating. Any task that is client-centered and motivating can be used in AROM such as self-feeding, games, home management tasks, or work related tasks. Just be sure to set up the task in the appropriate plane or distance to work on the specific ROM to meet the client's goal.

Home Exercise Programs

Clients who are working on PROM or AROM will benefit from a PROM/AROM daily exercise routine, called a **home exercise program (HEP).** Many resources are available to help the OTA create a customized HEP for a client, including websites, software purchased by the therapy department, or standard handouts for specific motions. Electronic versions typically have an option to print a copy for the client. Any HEP given to a client should be created to meet the client's specific goals and have clear instructions and illustrations for optimal adherence and proper performance. Be sure the client understands the HEP by educating and training the client on each exercise, because the client should be able to perform it without the OT practitioner's guidance. See Chapter 5 for methods for creating client-centered handouts.

Functional Range of Motion

Functional ROM is the primary goal of OT if the client's AROM/PROM is not normal, as it allows the client to return to his or her life occupations. An example of this occurs in older adults who experience rotator cuff tears and are unable to reach overhead. They are still able to perform all necessary self-care, drive, perform home skills, and adapt their leisure activities to compensate for their shoulder ROM loss with adaptive techniques and equipment. OT practitioners

OT Practitioner's Viewpoint

In today's rehabilitation environment, many traditional OT interventions to improve ROM focus on activities that may seem gender biased as well as age biased, such as folding laundry, kitchen tasks, reaching for beanbags, or using pegs and cones. I created a different type of table that can be used for a variety of activities that many male clients have found motivating such as taking apart a chainsaw, installing a faucet, or sanding down wood. A simple bench, accessible either by wheelchair or standing, utilizes tools, a shop vacuum, and other shop items to increase ROM through addressing a variety of IADLs. For example, supination and pronation AROM can be addressed by having a client use a screwdriver to screw items into a piece of wood. Clients can disassemble garden tools, such as leaf blowers, install faucets, and make a birdhouse or wooden box. Of course female clients may love this too! ~ Susan Blair OTR/L, BCPR, BCG

EVIDENCE-BASED PRACTICE

Functional electrical stimulation (FES) is a therapeutic method that combines the use of a physical agent modality (electrical stimulation) with performing a purposeful, functional task. OT practitioners often use FES for grasp and release patterns by enabling first wrist extension and finger flexion, then wrist flexion and finger extension. OT practitioners can use this method to increase ROM and it can also be considered a form of AAROM when instructing the client to actively engage his or her muscles, because an outside force is assisting the joint movement through electrically stimulating the muscle(s) to contract. Neuromuscular electrical stimulation (NEMS) may be accomplished through the use of a traditional NEMS device. This includes a device to deliver a specified type of electrical stimulation with programmed timing, along with wires from the device that attach to the electrodes placed on client's skin over top of the targeted muscle(s) or a neuroprosthetic, such as the H200® by Bioness. The H200® device is fit to the individual client; electrodes are embedded in the device itself, and a trained OT practitioner sets up intensity settings for the stimulation. Once the device has been fit and customized settings programed, the OT practitioner can plan functional tasks to perform while using the device. The H200® device and the traditional NEMS methods are typically used at home for high repetition of movements, which has been shown to cause changes to the neural pathways in the brain.[9]

Traditional NEMS units can be used in the same way; however, the advantages of the Bioness versus traditional NEMS units regard client follow through at home. The Bioness N200® unit is preprogramed by the OT practitioner, so the client does not need to worry about placing electrodes on the body or wires becoming tangled, thus making it simpler for clients to use on their own. Research has shown positive outcomes in "reducing impairment and maximizing function" for clients using the H200® device.[9] For more information on NEMS and other physical agent modalities, see Chapter 18.

Doucet, B. (2012). Neurorehabilitation: Are we doing all that we can? American Journal of Occupational Therapy, *66, 488-493. doi:10.5014/ajot.2012.002790*

can use creative and personalized intervention techniques based on each client's life role. For example, consider Jim, a client who loves to cook but is unable to lift his arm all the way to the top shelf. The OT practitioner can work on functional ROM by wiping off counters, stacking items in kitchen, pushing a shopping cart, and collecting items off of shelves. Education and practice with adaptive equipment such as a dressing stick, reacher, or mobile cart can be performed.

SUMMARY

The OT practitioner should be proficient in assessing and monitoring the client's ROM status. ROM impairments can be mild to severe and require a multitude of creative treatment interventions based on the underlying diagnosis. Functionally, clients can return to purposeful lives without "full or normal" ROM but the goal of the OT practitioner should be to facilitate as much functional ROM return as possible so the client can re-engage in ADLs, IADLs, work, leisure, and other life skills important to the client. The ability to engage clients in functional tasks requires only that an OT practitioner uses his or her imagination to assist a client to regain ROM and thereby regain independence. If AROM is not a feasible goal, clients and caregivers should be competent in the performance of PROM and SROM to reduce the risk of joint contractures, development of pain, and soft tissue injury.

REVIEW QUESTIONS

1. A 58-year-old male is admitted to the hospital after falling from a building scaffold. He sustains a right proximal humeral fracture and a right femur fracture. Which of the following orders would OT practitioners need to be most aware of during performance of ADLs while sitting on the edge of the bed?
   a. Weight-bearing status of RLE
   b. Low-fat diet
   c. No active ROM RUE
   d. Up to bathroom with assistance
2. An 18-year-old girl breaks her arm playing tennis and sustains a proximal radial fracture. She is casted in a long arm cast for 6 weeks and when the cast is removed, her elbow AROM is −35 degrees extension to 100 degrees flexion. What is the normal ROM for elbow extension and flexion?
   a. 0° to 125°
   b. 0° to 150°
   c. −10° to 140°
   d. −90° to 150°
3. A 40-year-old baseball player has recently undergone a rotator cuff repair of his LUE and is not allowed to abduct his L shoulder. What is an alternative method for measuring shoulder internal rotation if the client has no abduction?
   a. Side-lying on LUE
   b. Maintain shoulder adduction and 90 degrees of elbow flexion; bring forearm to torso
   c. Bend elbow and abduct shoulder
   d. Supine with UE supported on mat while in abduction
4. An OTA is working on ADLs with a 67-year-old man with a recent total knee replacement. Which of the following is the most important reason for an OTA to know how to measure LE ROM?
   a. To document knee flexion/extension and plan an AROM HEP
   b. To educate on appropriate car transfers for community reentry
   c. To provide education on LE adaptive equipment if indicated because of client's inability to reach feet
   d. To reduce the number of physical therapists needed on the orthopedic floor

5. A 48-year-old male client presents in the IP rehabilitation gym with limited RUE AROM as a result of a CVA. Which of the following interventions would be *most appropriate* to first teach the client to perform?
   a. PROM
   b. SROM
   c. AROM
   d. AAROM
6. When interviewing a client before measuring a joint, which three of the following are the most important?
   a. Discuss his or her health insurance plan.
   b. Assess his or her pain level.
   c. Discuss how the client became injured.
   d. Determine the client's prior level of function.
   e. Explain to the client what you will do.
   f. Ask the client to perform activities with resistance to measure strength.
7. How is hyperextension of the MCP measured?
   a. By bending fingers back
   b. By bending fingers down and into a fist
   c. By crossing fingers
   d. By bringing thumb to tip of index finger and measure the gap
8. Which three of the following are examples of functional ROM for shoulder internal rotation?
   a. Reaching for wallet in back pocket
   b. Putting plate on overhead shelf
   c. Washing the back of one's head
   d. Hammering a nail
   e. Placing hand in front pant's pocket
   f. Pouring water from a pitcher
9. A 35-year-old-electrician sustains an electrical burn to his dominant hand and requires multiple skin grafts from palm to forearm. At his 6-week postoperative OT appointment, he presents with a stiff edematous hand with a significant loss of passive range of motion because of which physical limitation?
   a. Swelling
   b. Tendon rupture
   c. Nonuse
   d. Muscle atrophy in forearm
10. The OTA is assessing AROM on a client who is seated in a wheelchair. To obtain the most accurate UE ROM, which of the following should the OTA do?
   a. Ask the client to be seated in a regular chair without arms.
   b. Have the client use the recline feature of the wheelchair.
   c. Request that the caregiver who accompanied the client lift and hold the client's UE while it is measured.
   d. Assist the client to transfer to the therapy mat, and ask the caregiver to provide support, if needed.

CASE STUDY

Shirley is a 67-year-old woman who recently broke her right dominant wrist while walking to her mailbox one morning. She sustained a distal radius and ulnar fracture that required casting in a long arm cast for 6 weeks. Her cast was removed, but a week later she is unable to perform ADL and leisure tasks that she could perform before the fall. She was referred to OT for right wrist therapy. Before her fall, Shirley was an active gardener, played bridge once a week, and was independent with all self-care. She lives alone with her Maltese poodle, Muffin, in a one-level home with no accessibility issues. During her initial OT evaluation, her right wrist measurements (Table 7-3) were:

The occupational therapist has identified goals to include independence with ADLs, pain free return to leisure activities, increasing grip and pinch strength by 50 percent and increasing both wrist flexion and extension to 50 degrees each.

As the OTA working with Shirley, consider the following questions:

1. What are some clinical interventions that could be used to improve Shirley's functional use of her affected hand?
2. Shirley begins to report pain with wrist extension. Her ROM has plateaued. What communication/recommendations can be made to the supervising occupational therapist?
3. Which types of adaptive equipment should be suggested for Shirley to use for ADLs until her ROM improves?
4. How can Shirley's leisure interests be incorporated into her therapy?

TABLE 7-3 Case Study ROM Measurements

MOVEMENT	AROM	PROM
Flexion	0° to 30°	0° to 55°
Extension	0° to 20°	0° to 30°
Supination	0° to 50°	0° to 60°
Pronation	0° to 50°	0° to 65°
Ulnar deviation	0° to 10°	0° to 20°
Radial deviation	0° to 10°	0° to 15°

PUTTING IT ALL TOGETHER Sample Treatment and Documentation

Setting	Outpatient, day 3 following R rotator cuff surgery
Client Profile	Mr. S, 62 y/o male, enjoys gardening and cooking
Work History	Repairs and services large industrial generators. Four years of college education, volunteers on disaster relief team across the U.S. as a chaplain, veteran
Insurance	Private
Psychological	No psychological conditions
Social	Married, lives in single-level home with one step to enter. Two grown children and four grandchildren who visit frequently.

PUTTING IT ALL TOGETHER Sample Treatment and Documentation (continued)

Cognitive	No limitations present
Motor & Manual Muscle Testing (MMT)	Client presents with normal strength in LUE as well as good postural control, RUE shoulder strength and ROM not tested because of recent surgery. • WFL AROM in LUE • WFL AROM elbow, wrist, and fingers RUE • MMT LUE: 5/5 throughout
ADL	Min A UB dressing, self-feeding with L hand at this time.
IADL	Min A with cooking as a result of wearing abduction sling.
Goals	Within 1 week: 1. Client will demonstrate Mod I for UB body dressing with AE and techniques as needed. 2. Client will demonstrate Mod I with HEP. 3. Client will demonstrate I with RUE precautions for ADLs and IADLs. 4. Client will demonstrate I to doff and don shoulder immobilizer.

OT INTERVENTION SESSION 1

THERAPEUTIC ACTIVITY	TIME	GOAL(s) ADDRESSED	OTA RATIONALE
Reviewed RUE precautions and client verbalized 100%	10 min	#3	*Education and Training:* Ensure client will be safe with postsurgical shoulder
Education and training in donning/doffing shoulder immobilizer	10 min	#4	*Education and Training:* Performance to increase independence with donning/doffing shoulder immobilizer
Distal AROM exercises 10 reps, ensure knowledge of accurately completing HEP	15 min	#2	*Preparatory Task; Education and Training:* Use energy conservation and work simplification techniques to decrease fatigue during daily occupations
Codman's exercises	5 min	#2	*Preparatory Task:* Begin gentle, nonresistive exercises postsurgery, following surgeon's protocol.
Upper body dressing techniques	8 min	#1	*Occupations:* Functional task performance to increase independence with dressing

SOAP note: 10/2/—, 9:00 am-9:48 am

S: Client stated, "It is hard to get my arm in the sleeve."

O: Seen for skilled OT to address impaired AROM/PROM RUE, impaired ADL of dressing and deficits in HEP carry through and performance for RUE. Client rated pain as 5/10 in R shoulder. Verbalized all precautions for RUE. Completed all tasks in seated position on mat. Completed doffing of sling as instructed by OTA. Stood to perform Codman's shoulder exercises using written handout as visual guide with verbal prompts for correct posture. Returned to seated position for distal AROM exercises, 10 reps of each joint exercise using HEP. Completed UB dressing task of don/doffing buttoned shirt x 1.

A: Tolerated activities well with no increase in pain during tasks. Required minimal verbal cues to don/doff sling with adjustments made for fit and function by wife, as demonstrated by OTA. Completed Codman's exercises and distal AROM exercises with moderate verbal prompts for posture and sequence. Dressed with min assist for R arm placement in sleeve.

P: Continue daily with AROM, HEP reinforcement, and adaptive ADLs.

Meredith Scott, COTA/L, 10/2/—,12:05 pm

TREATMENT SESSION 2

What could you do next with this client?

TREATMENT SESSION 3

What could you do next with this client?

REFERENCES

1. Pendleton, H. M., & Schultz-Krohn, W. (2017). *Pedretti's occupational therapy: Practice skills for physical dysfunction.* Elsevier Health Sciences.
2. Clarkson, H. M. (2000). *Musculoskeletal assessment, joint range and manual muscle testing* (2nd ed.). Philadelphia, PA: Lippincott.
3. Pedretti, L. (2012). *Occupational therapy practice skills* (7th ed.) St. Louis, MO: Mosby Elsevier.
4. Smith, H. D. (1993). Assessment and evaluation: An overview. In H.D. Smith & H.L. Hopkins (Eds.), *Willard and Spackman's occupational therapy.* Philadelphia, PA: J. B. Lippincott.
5. Norkin, C. C., & White, D. J. (2003). *Measurement of joint motion: A guide to goniometry* (3rd ed.). Philadelphia, PA: F. A. Davis.
6. American Academy of Orthopedic Surgeons. (n.d.). Retrieved from https://www.fgc.edu/wp-content/uploads/2011/12/averages-of-rom.pdf
7. Eaton, C. (n.d.). Normal range of motion reference values. Retrieved from http://www.eatonhand.com/nor/nor002.htm
8. Sledziewski, L., Schaaf, R. C., & Mount, J. (2011). Use of robotics in spinal cord injury: A case report. *American Journal of Occupational Therapy, 66*(1), 51-58. doi:10.5014/ajot.2012.000943
9. Doucet, B. (2012). Neurorehabilitation: Are we doing all that we can? *American Journal of Occupational Therapy, 66*, 488-493. doi:10.5014/ajot.2012.002790

Chapter 8

Movement, Motor Control, Sensation, Wounds, and Pain

Megan E. Edwards Collins, PhD, OTR/L

LEARNING OUTCOMES

After studying this chapter, the student or practitioner will be able to:

8.1 Describe and understand the components of normal movement
8.2 Identify the various types of coordination and how to assess
8.3 Explain how various coordination disorders impact function
8.4 Identify the various types of sensation and their impact on function
8.5 Identify the proper procedure for evaluating sensation
8.6 Identify reflexes and righting, equilibrium, and protective reactions and their impact on safety and function
8.7 Describe and understand tone and the impact abnormal tone has on function
8.8 Describe how to evaluate and address abnormal tone
8.9 Identify the causes of wounds and how to manage
8.10 Explain the importance of pain management scales and demonstrate how to administer them

KEY TERMS

Basal ganglia disorders	Maceration
Cerebellum (cerebellar) disorders	Nosocomial
Desensitization	Praxis
Flaccidity	Pressure
Graded stimuli	Primitive reflex
Homunculus	Rigidity
Hypersensitivity	Sensation
Hypertonicity	Shear
Hyposensitivity	Spasticity
Hypotonicity	Tissue necrosis
	Tone

In the absence of an illness or injury that disrupts movement, it is easy to take for granted how involved and intricate normal movement can be. Although it may seem fluid and effortless, normal movement requires a variety of complex skills and client factors. These include **praxis** (motor planning) and adequate postural control, range of motion, muscle strength and tone, and sensation. Praxis includes understanding the demands of a task and having the ability to cognitively and physically initiate and implement the necessary movements. Postural control is the ability to stabilize oneself in space and maintain balance. Range of motion (ROM) is the amount of movement an individual has in a certain joint, muscle strength is the amount of strength in a muscle, and tone is the continuous state of contraction muscles have. With these abilities in place, an individual can plan and produce the movement patterns required for functional mobility and daily occupations. Certainly, in the presence of disability, weakness, disease, or injury, these abilities can be lacking. If a client is unable to move functionally because of difficulties in any of the above areas, they are at high risk for pain and other issues, such as contractures and pressure injuries. This chapter will also address some of the complications found with lack of motor planning, adequate postural control, range of motion, muscle strength, and sensation.

COORDINATION

When a movement is coordinated, it means that it is efficient, smooth, organized, and able to result in purposeful and skilled control. The different types of coordination include gross motor, fine motor, and eye–hand coordination. Gross motor coordination is needed to perform larger movement patterns, such as coordinating arm movements to don a coat. Fine motor coordination is needed to perform smaller, more precise movement patterns, such as buttoning a dress shirt or blouse. Finally, eye–hand coordination is needed to coordinate visual input with movement of the hands, such as writing within lines.[1,2] A variety of disorders may impact a client's coordination. They are divided into **basal ganglia disorders** and **cerebellar disorders**, as both are involved in motor coordination and result in different deficits when there is a lesion.

Basal Ganglia Disorders

The basal ganglia, located in the cerebrum, are involved in regulating stereotypic motor patterns, which develop with maturation of the nervous system (an example is using a reciprocal arm swing when ambulating), and automated movements. Automated movements include walking or riding a bike, which were initially learned consciously at the cortical level but become automatic with practice. An unconscious motor system, the basal ganglia includes the caudate nucleus, putamen, and globus pallidus.[3] The caudate nucleus helps control movement, whereas the putamen and globus pallidus assist with initiating movement (Fig. 8-1). Together these structures assist an individual in performing skilled, controlled movement. Table 8-1 has examples of basal ganglia disorders.[3-5]

Cerebellar Disorders

The cerebellum is involved in the awareness of one's position in space. Information received by the cerebellum from joint and muscle receptors in the body is used to perform coordinated and controlled movements.[3] For example, an individual with a cerebellar disorder might not perceive where their hands are as they are moving them, making buttoning a shirt or reaching for a glass of water difficult. Their movements may appear jerky, segmented, awkward, and uncontrolled. Table 8-2 provides examples of cerebellar disorders, descriptions, and assessments. Standardized assessments, that could be used with these disorders, can be found in Chapter 22.

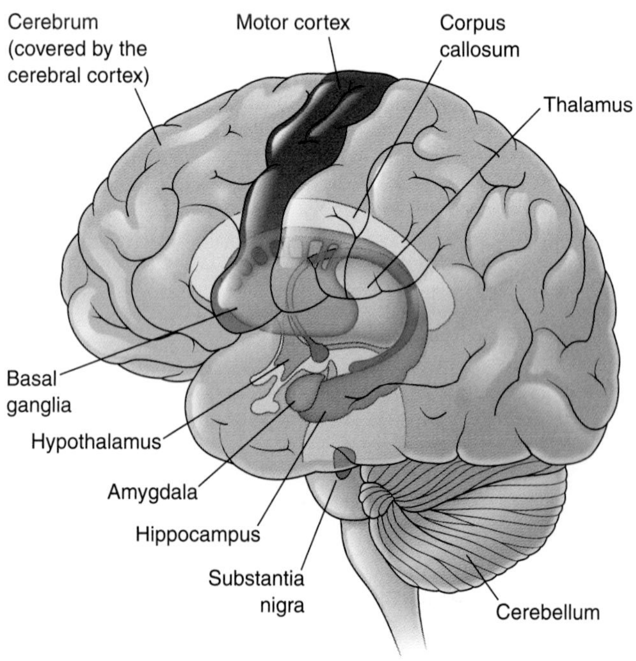

FIGURE 8-1. Basal ganglia.

Treatment of Basal Ganglia and Cerebellar Disorders

The functional impact of a coordination disorder on a client can be extensive. Decreased coordination may make it challenging for a client to feed, bathe, or dress himself or herself. Instrumental activities of daily living (IADLs), such as cooking and driving, may be extremely difficult for the client to perform. Completing basic activities of daily living (ADLs) may take extra time and fatigue the client. In addition, the social and emotional impacts of coordination disorders must be considered. A client may become depressed or frustrated that he or she is unable to complete basic ADLs, and the client may experience social stigma as a result of decreased coordination and unintentional movements.

To address the physical and cognitive effects of basal ganglia and cerebellar disorders on clients, the occupational therapy (OT) practitioner may use a variety of strategies that may include:

- Providing increased sensory input to the muscles and joints, such as exposing the client to different textures (e.g., sandpaper or felt) or by providing opportunities to bear weight through a body segment, to increase awareness of the individual's position in space.
- Utilizing compensatory strategies, such as visual or auditory cues in the environment (e.g., placing light-colored food on darker-colored plates, drawing a dark line on the edges of a sheet of paper so that the client knows where to start and end writing on a line, or having a motion sensitive sound go off when moving in a certain way) or using one hand to stabilize the other during ADLs (e.g., using holding a hairbrush in the weaker hand while the stronger hand stabilizes and moves the weaker arm and hand).
- Recommending various home and environmental adaptations for safety and ease of mobility, including removing throw rugs and other tripping hazards from the home and covering the sharper edges of furniture with foam protectors.
- Recommending adaptive equipment, such as a shower chair with suction cups on the bottom of the legs or weighted utensils, to assist with increasing occupational engagement, functioning, and safety.
- Stabilize proximally whenever possible, such as elbows on the table when eating or leaning a hip on the wall in the shower when bathing.
- Addressing muscle strength and ROM problems, including preventing contractures by splinting or providing a home exercise program that could involve ROM (passive range of motion [PROM], active assistive range of motion [AAROM], or active range of motion [AROM]) and strengthening activities.

TABLE 8-1 Basal Ganglia Disorders[3-5]

DISORDER	DESCRIPTION	DETECTED BY
Hemiballismus	Results from a lesion of the subthalamus and caudate Violent thrashing movements of the opposite extremity	Observation
Athetosis	Results from a lesion to the putamen and caudate Slow flailing of the upper and lower extremities, including continuous movements; often twisting and wormlike movements	Observation
Chorea	Results from a lesion to the caudate and putamen Sudden, involuntary jerky movements-usually of the axial and proximal limbs (e.g., shoulder shrugs, hip movements, facial grimaces, crossing and. uncrossing of the legs); movements appear dance-like	Observation
Dystonia	Sustained muscle contractions that produce repetitive twisting movements and abnormal posturing	Observation
Dyskinesia	Rhythmic repetitive movements	Observation
Tremor	Tremor: An involuntary oscillating movement caused by alternating contractions of opposing muscle groups Resting Tremor: Tremors that occur when client is at rest, diminish or disappear when movement is initiated	Observation
Tics	Repetitive, brief, involuntary purposeless movements, can involve a single or group of muscles	Observation

TABLE 8-2 Cerebellar Disorders

DISORDER	DESCRIPTION	ASSESSED BY
Tremor	Tremor: Involuntary oscillating movements caused by alternating contractions of opposing muscle groups Essential (or Intention) Tremor: Occurs when movement is initiated, tremors diminish at rest; movements often intensified toward end of movement	Observation Finger to nose assessment: Client seated, with upper extremities abducted to 90 degrees and elbows extended Client touches nose, alternating between using left and right index fingers (eyes opened initially, then switch to eyes closed) Note any tremors during task Can also have client go between his nose and practitioner's finger (which should be moved in multiple planes)[3-5]
Dyssynergia (Movement decomposition)	Movements are broken into segmented, jerky, uncoordinated movements	Finger to nose assessment Nose to OT practitioner's finger[3-5]
Dysmetria	Difficulty judging the distance needed for movement Client will overshoot (move past the needed range) or undershoot (not reach far enough)	Can observe during functional tasks or have client reach for objects[3-5]
Dysdiadochokinesia	Difficulty performing rapidly alternating movements	OT practitioner can have client alternate between forearm pronation and supination (can have client tap thighs)—if impaired, the movements will be irregular and asynchronous[3-5]
Rebound phenomenon	The opposing muscle groups are not regulated adequately	OT practitioner can have client resist pulling flexed elbow into flexion When practitioner releases client's forearm, client's arm will hit his or her torso[3-5]

Continued

TABLE 8-2 Cerebellar Disorders (continued)

DISORDER	DESCRIPTION	ASSESSED BY
Asthenia	Muscular weakness	Observed OT practitioner can have client try and maintain a fixed position (e.g., bilateral shoulder flexion) for 30 seconds[3-5]
Motor impersistence	When trying to maintain the bilateral upper extremities in a fixed position, the affected extremity will move out of position without the client noticing	OT practitioner can have client try and maintain his or her bilateral upper extremities in a fixed position for 30 seconds and observe if one side drifts[4,5]
Ataxia	Uncoordinated movement patterns impacting gait, posture, and upper extremity coordination Initiation of movement can be delayed, and the client can have errors in range and force of movement Clients frequently have a wide base of support and hold their arms away from the body in an effort to maintain their balance May have difficulty walking a straight path, tending to move toward the side of the lesion	OT practitioner can have client stand with eyes open and closed and look for any bodily sway (noting if sway increases with eyes closed)[3-5]

- Providing education on energy conservation techniques and strategies as needed, for example, taking breaks as needed, pacing oneself, and placing commonly used items within easy reach. Another strategy is for the client to do the most essential tasks earlier in the day before the client gets fatigued so he or she would have completed the most vital things first.

Interventions should usually include providing education on the functional impact of the coordination disorder, how to manage symptoms (e.g., having proximal stability and proper positioning), and a home exercise program.[6-8]

SENSATION

Sensation plays a tremendous role in everyday functioning and occupations, impacting safety and motor performance in many occupations. People receive sensory input from objects and others in the environment, as well as from their own bodies. Sensory receptors in the body react to a particular type of stimulation, such as visual input. Sensations that people receive can be tactile, auditory, visual, olfactory (smell), gustatory (taste), or vestibular (balance). The spinal cord contains ascending sensory tracts from the spinal cord to the brain. Sensory input is received by nuclei in the thalamus, which then relays it to the appropriate area in the cerebral hemispheres for interpretation. After the sensory input has been interpreted, descending motor tracts in the spinal cord relay motor responses from the brain to the body (Fig. 8-2). Normal sensation is essential for safety. For example, it is critical for clients to be able to determine the appropriate temperature of food and drinks; to feel and withdraw from sharp or painful stimuli; to smell spoiled or burning food; and to hear a smoke detector or alarm going off. It is also necessary for social interactions, such as being able to apply the appropriate amount of pressure when shaking hands with someone and to feel food on one's mouth, and for ADL performance, such as being able to determine where buttons are and manipulate them appropriately. Furthermore, through sensory input, an individual explores and learns about the environment.[4]

While conducting a sensory assessment of a client, the OT practitioner can identify sensory deficits, determine how the deficits impact the client's functioning, and establish potential treatment options. The occupational therapist may conduct sensory testing as part of his or her initial evaluation, or if service competency has been established (e.g., the occupational therapist has determined the occupational therapy assistant [OTA] can administer the assessment and obtain the same results), he or she may delegate this task to the OTA when sensory challenges are suspected. They can then discuss and interpret the findings together.

The body has various types of somatosensory receptors, which are activated by specific types of sensory input. They include mechanoreceptors, chemoreceptors, thermoreceptors, and nociceptors. Mechanoreceptors respond to tactile input, joint compression, pressure, vibration, and equilibrium changes; chemoreceptors respond to the substances released when a cell is injured or damaged as well as to particular chemicals; thermoreceptors respond to heat and cold; and nociceptors sense pain (Table 8-3).[3,5]

When considering a client's sensory abilities, it is also important to consider the **homunculus** figure (Fig. 8-3), which shows how the various areas of the body are represented in the brain. Those areas with large representation have more sensory receptors in the brain compared

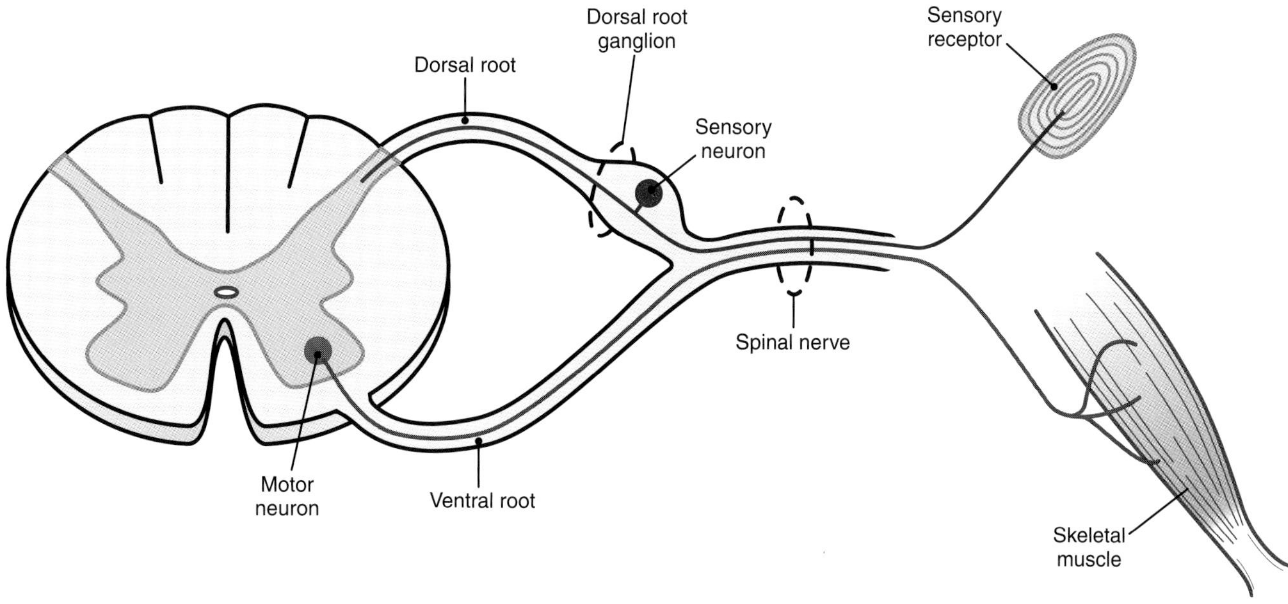

FIGURE 8-2. Sensory receptors.

TABLE 8-3 Types of Somatosensory Receptors[3-5]

Mechanoreceptors	Some skin receptors Stretch receptors in the skeletal muscles
Chemoreceptors	Olfaction and gustation
Thermoreceptors	"All over an organism's internal and external body"
Nociceptors	Mechanoreceptors, chemoreceptors, and thermoreceptors all contain nociceptors

OT Practitioner's Viewpoint

The OT practitioner should demonstrate assessments on himself or herself first so that the client knows what to expect. They should also explain to the client the purpose of each assessment, including how the area being tested can impact function and safety. The importance of this was made evident to me when a client I worked with was being, in my perception, uncooperative and slightly hostile. She refused to participate in the OT process, such as working on grooming or fine motor tasks, so I could assess her ROM and fine motor skills. After pausing for a moment and taking a deep breath, I realized she did not understand the reasoning behind what I was asking her to do. Once I took the time and effort to demonstrate, explain, and address her questions and concerns, she fully participated and engaged with me in the OT process. I simply needed to connect with her and explain what I was doing. Every client the OT practitioner works with deserves such information and respect. ~ Megan E. Edwards Collins, PhD, OTR/L

with those with smaller representation. Areas with a large amount of representation in the homunculus figure, such as the lips and hands, are more sensitive than areas with smaller representation. Such knowledge is important for the OT practitioner to know when conducting sensory testing.[5]

Sensory Testing Procedures Overview

Sensory testing should be conducted in a room with minimal distractions and noise.[4] When assessing a client's sensation, follow these steps:

- Explain to the client what is being assessed.
- Explain to the client how it will be assessed and why.
- Demonstrate the assessment on the OT practitioner's own body.
- Perform the evaluation on the client's unaffected side, requesting that the client keep his or her eyes open for practice.
- Evaluate the client's affected side with his or her eyes closed.[4]

Sensory Testing

Table 8-4 describes the various sensory tests that the OT practitioner may conduct. They include light touch (needed to detect sensation), sharp/dull (needed to detect painful stimuli), temperature (needed to detect hot and cold), stereognosis (needed to interpret tactile input through touch alone), proprioception (the ability to determine where body parts are in space without the use of vision), and vibration. It is important to note that peripheral nerve damage and injury, such as carpal tunnel syndrome, can impair the ability to receive and accurately interpret sensation.

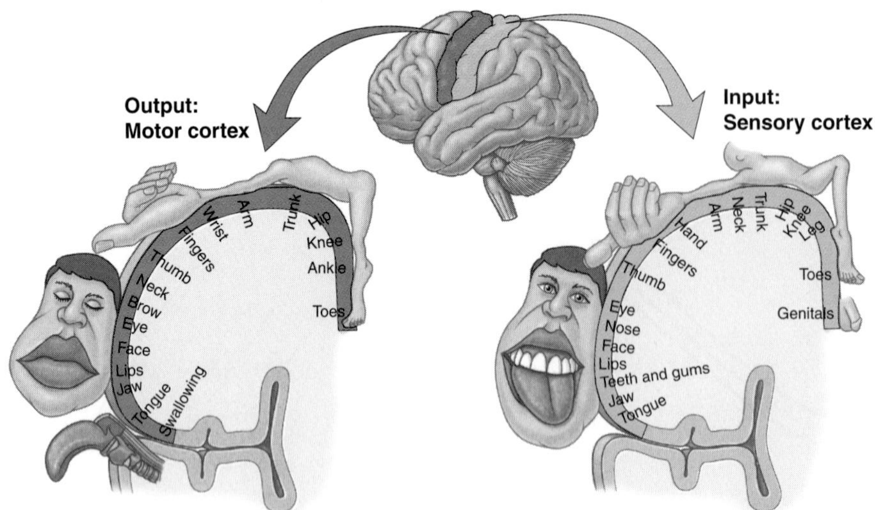

FIGURE 8-3. The homunculus figure represents how the various areas of the body are represented in the brain.

Sensory Dysfunction Treatment

Sensory dysfunction may occur for a variety of reasons, including cerebrovascular accident (CVA), spinal cord injury (SCI), peripheral nerve injury (PNI), multiple sclerosis (MS), cerebral palsy (CP), or autism spectrum disorder (ASD). **Hyposensitivity** occurs when a stimulus is applied and the client does not feel it or perceives it as less intense than it actually is.[4,5,11] For example, the client may report that he or she does not feel the object or stimulus, or that it is difficult to determine how much pressure to apply when holding an item. **Hypersensitivity** occurs when the client perceives the stimulus as being more intense than it actually is. The client might report that the stimulus is painful or irritating or react in a way that is out of proportion to the stimulus being applied. For example, the client may quickly withdraw when lightly touched with a cotton ball.[4,5,11]

Clients with either hyposensitivity or hypersensitivity will need sensory reeducation. This involves engaging the client in activities that stimulate impaired neuropathways or assist the client to work on appropriately sensing, integrating, and responding to the input.[4,5,11] The client needs to be slowly exposed to the stimulus that he or she is having trouble regulating. This will help the client learn how to appropriately regulate or perceive and react to the stimulus. Examples include touching and manipulating shaving cream, rice, or sandpaper. When a client is hypersensitive, it is usually best to start with softer textures, such as cotton balls and felt, and progress to rougher textures, such as sandpaper or steel wool. Reducing the client's response to sensory input is called **desensitization**. The process of starting with softer textures and then progressing to rougher textures can be considered **graded stimuli**.[4,5,11] However, clients who exhibit hyposensitivity might need to start with the rougher objects and as that input is integrated and interpreted more effectively and efficiently, work with softer and smoother textures. Compensatory strategies should also be used as needed to increase the client's safety and functioning.[5,11] This may include having clients utilize their vision more to account for tactile deficits, perform frequent skin inspections for any sores and redness, and learn and use safety strategies, such as using an oven mitt when taking something out of the oven or off the stove. The OT practitioner might also provide a home program to the client or his or her family.[5,11,12] This can include providing the client with a list of activities to try that involve materials with various textures, such as moleskin, felt, cotton balls, shaving cream, burlap, and sandpaper.[11] A home exercise program may also include having the caregiver, family member, or a friend place everyday items, such as a key or paperclip, in the client's hands and ask the client to identify the object with eyes closed. Alternatively, this person might ask the client to close his or her eyes, touch the client, and then ask the client to identify the area touched.

The time it takes a client to regain normal sensation will vary, depending on the specific condition and the severity and location of the lesions in the brain. In terms of nerve regrowth after a peripheral nerve injury, the average rate is around 1 mm per day, which is approximately an inch a month.[5,11] Sensory reeducation is thought to work because the sensory input and activities result in increased cortical representation and reorganization. This results in an increased ability to perceive and accurately interpret sensory input.[5,11,12]

REFLEXES, EQUILIBRIUM, AND RIGHTING REACTIONS

Reflexes are automatic movements that occur when the body is stimulated or positioned in a specific way.[3,5,13] Primitive reflexes are basic reflexes that are present during infancy or early childhood that eventually become integrated into more mature patterns.[3,5,13] Primitive reflexes are important for normal motor development and movement. With typical development, they should become integrated as movements become more controlled and no longer

TABLE 8-4 Sensory Testing

SENSE	WHEN EVALUATED	TO EVALUATE	RESULTS
Light Touch	If decreased ability to detect light touch is detected, such as in clients with Parkinson's disease or in clients who have sustained a spinal cord injury or CVA[9,10]	Using cotton ball or a Q-tip, gently apply the stimulus in random pattern on client's hand, fingers, and forearm following no particular order. Main concern is to apply the stimulus in a random pattern that the client cannot detect. Do both volar and dorsal surfaces, and apply the stimulus a total of three times to each area. Instruct the client to say "touch" or "yes" when he or she feels the stimulus.	Document the number of times the client feels the stimulus over the total number of times the stimulus was applied (e.g., 7/10). Normal is 100% accuracy.[4,5]
Sharp/Dull	If decreased sharp/dull sensation is suspected, or when concerns with safety (e.g., to sense when a sharp object has touched the skin) exist. May include clients who have had a CVA or who have Parkinson's disease[10]	Taking a safety pin that has been bent to a 90-degree angle (makes sharp/dull alternating easier) apply on client's hand, fingers, and forearm in random pattern following no particular order. Main concern is applying the sharp/dull stimulus in a random pattern client cannot detect. Do both volar and dorsal surfaces, and apply the stimulus a total of three times to each area. Instruct the client to say "sharp" when he or she feels the sharp side and "dull" when feeling the dull side.	Document the number of times the client accurately identifies the stimulus over the total number of times the stimulus was applied (e.g., 25/30). It should also be noted whether the sharp or dull stimulus was missed. Normal is 100% accuracy.[4]
Stereognosis	If decreased sensation and tactile recognition (stereognosis) are suspected, such as CVA.[9] This is important for functional tasks, such as locating an item in a purse or backpack, such as keys, without having to look at each item.	Gather a minimum of six familiar objects (e.g., paper clip, quarter, button, pen, toothbrush, and screw, with at least two of similar size and shape). Ask client to identify each item. Remember what the client calls each item. Next, have the client close eyes. Place one item in affected hand and ask client to identify it. Client should use the same name for the object as when they visually saw it. Alternatively, have two sets of each item, or pictures of each item, and have the client open their eyes after holding the item and point to the item (or picture) just held from the second set. The practitioner can help the client hold the object, if needed, and wrap the client's fingers around the object. If the client is unable to name the object, the practitioner should ask the client to identify characteristics of the item (e.g. smooth, rough, soft, hard, or round).	The client should be able to identify each object with eyes closed, using the same name to identify it as used with eyes open. A client is given credit for items he or she can describe, even if unable to identify the object. The number of items correctly identified out of the total number of item the client was presented with is documented (e.g., 5/6). Normal is 100% accuracy.[4,5]

Continued

TABLE 8-4 Sensory Testing (continued)

SENSE	WHEN EVALUATED	TO EVALUATE	RESULTS
Proprioception	If client's movements appear uncoordinated or appears to excessively rely on visual input for information on the body's position in space (proprioception), such as after a CVA.[9] Proprioception is essential for performing coordinated, controlled movements and for functionally and safely moving around the environment.	Hold the client's affected side, providing as little tactile input as possible and not crossing the joints. With the client's eyes closed, move the joint three times. Ask client to position the other extremity in the same position as the affected side. Compare the location of the unaffected arm with the affected arm.	Normal is when the client positions the unaffected arm within 15 degrees of how the affected arm is placed.[4,5]
Temperature	If client has difficulty determining and adjusting water temperature appropriately (e.g., when bathing or washing hands), such as after a CVA or brain injury.[9,10]	Use two test tubes, one with hot water and one with cold water. While client's eyes are closed, apply the hot and cold tubes, one at a time in a random pattern, to the client's arm and forearm. Apply tubes to each area three times. The client is to indicate hot when he or she feels the hot tube and cold when he or she feels the cold tube.	Document the number of accurately identified stimulus applications over the total number applied. Whether the client incorrectly identified hot or cold stimuli should be noted. Normal is 100% accuracy.[4] Hot and cold test.

TABLE 8-4 Sensory Testing (continued)

SENSE	WHEN EVALUATED	TO EVALUATE	RESULTS
Touch pressure	If decreased awareness of tactile input is suspected, such as after a brain injury.[9] Touch pressure, the ability to tell when pressure has been applied, is essential for determining when something has touched skin. Decreased touch pressure can impact safety (e.g., identifying when a noxious stimulus has touched the skin) and ADL performance (e.g., knowing that clothing is oriented correctly).[9]	Use Semmes-Weinstein monofilaments, nylon fibers of varying thickness. With the client's eyes closed, apply the 1.65 monofilament three times in a random fashion on the client's hand and fingers. Apply the monofilament with a slight bending perpendicularly to the skin, holding it for 1 to 1.5 seconds each time. The client should say "touch" when he or she feels the monofilament. If a client does not feel the stimulus, try a thicker one. Proceed in order, gradually increasing the thickness of monofilaments as needed. Only apply the larger filaments once.	1.65–2.83 is considered normal light touch. The Semmes-Weinstein Scale comes with a documentation form; use it to color pictures of the hand various colors based on the monofilament the client could feel. The thickness felt in each area of the hand should also be documented (e.g., 2.83 in the ulnar section of the hand).[4,5] **Semmes-Weinstein monofilaments.**
Simultaneous stimulation	If client may not be receiving and integrating sensory input to both sides of the body. Accurate integration of sensory input to both sides of the body is essential for ADL performance and safety.	Using the pad part of the finger, touch each of the client's arms separately (it is important for the OT practitioner to keep his or her fingernails short and not scratch the client), and then touch the left (L), right (R) or both/bilateral (B) arms together in a random pattern. The client's eyes should be closed and he or she should state whether the L, R, or both B arms have been touched.	Normal is 100% accuracy. Documentation includes recording how many times the client accurately reported whether the R, L, or B arms were touched over the total number of stimuli applied, including when no stimulus was identified (e.g., client identified with 100% accuracy when just the L or R arm was touched, but only identified both B had been stimulated 25% of the time—stating that only the R arm had been stimulated). Tactile extinction occurs if a client can identify the L and R arm correctly when done individually, but only one arm (the unaffected side) when both are touched together. In this case, input from the affected extremity is being overridden by input from the unaffected side because of a brain lesion resulting from neurological events, such as CVA or traumatic brain injury (TBI). This client may be unable to detect sensation and sensory input on one side, impacting safety and ADL performance (e.g., the client might not perceive input from one side of the body and bump into things in the environment).[4]

Continued

TABLE 8-4 Sensory Testing (continued)

SENSE	WHEN EVALUATED	TO EVALUATE	RESULTS
Tactile localization	If the client appears to have trouble identifying where an object has touched the body or is being held in the body (tactile localization). This can impact a client's safety and functional ability to hold and grasp items for ADLs.	Using finger or a small Semmes-Weinstein monofilament (the smallest one the client can feel), touch the client's forearm and hand (eyes are closed). The client then opens the eyes and touches the location where he or she believes the stimulus was applied.	Client should be able to touch where the stimulus applied within 1 cm. The OT practitioner scores this by measuring the distance between where he or she actually applied the stimulus and where the client identifies being touched.[4]
Two-point discrimination	If it is necessary to determine and document receptor density and recovery, such as following a nerve injury or repair, or after a CVA.[9] Two-point discrimination is the ability to determine whether one or two stimuli have been applied to an area of the skin. This is an important skill to have for fine motor tasks and object manipulation.	Use an esthesiometer to evaluate two-point discrimination. The device has two points, one of which can be moved along the base to increase or decrease the distance between them. Starting with the points 5 mm apart, randomly alternate between applying one or two points to the client's fingertips while his or her eyes are closed. The client is then asked to state whether one or two points were applied.	If answered correctly, the OT practitioner can decrease the distance between the points. If answered incorrectly, increase the distance between the points. Increase or decrease the distance gradually. Record the smallest distance felt accurately at least 7/10 applications. Between 1 and 5 mm is considered normal (less than 6 mm). Areas with more nerve innervation (e.g., the fingertips) will have a lower two-point discrimination than areas with less nerve innervation (e.g., the palm).[4,5] **Esthesiometer.**
Vibration	A tuning fork is used to evaluate vibration. Vibration can be essential in alerting individuals to environmental changes and dangers.	Strike a tuning fork against an object such as a table or his or her hand and then apply its stem to the joint being tested (e.g., the elbow). Strike the tuning fork again and then apply it to the same joint on the other side. Ask the client whether he or she feels the vibration, and whether it feels the same or different on both sides. The client may use words such as "It feels more or less on a side, or more intense on one side."	It should feel the same on both sides. If it does not feel the same, there could be nervous system damage. The OT practitioner should document whether or not the vibrations felt the same on both sides.[4,5]

produce automatic movement patterns.[3,5] For example, the grasp reflex includes the automatic grasping of an object placed in the hand. As infants repeatedly hold items, they will begin to have more control over their grasp and manipulation of items, and the grasp reflex will become integrated. Other reflexes emerge and are present throughout life and help provide protection and stability. For example, as individuals develop, righting reactions (desire to bring head/trunk into midline), equilibrium (a sense of being balanced), and protective reactions (using arms to stabilize the body when falling) emerge; these reactions assist with the maintenance of balance and with changing body positions, such as going from supine to sitting.[3,5]

Unintegrated primitive reflexes may impact a person's functional mobility and gross and fine motor development. When a client's primitive reflexes are not appropriately integrated or re-emerge, or when balance reactions do not emerge or are lost, such as following an insult to the brain, traumatic brain injury (TBI), or CVA, the OT practitioner must provide interventions to assist clients with their integration. Such interventions might include taking clients through developmental movement patterns or helping them regain or compensate for lost or diminished balance reactions. For example, if a client is inappropriately displaying asymmetrical tonic neck reflex (ATNR), where turning the head (the stimulus) results in extensor tone on the side the head that is turned toward and flexor tone on the opposite site, the OT practitioner would want to engage the client in tasks that involve turning the head to gradually decrease and integrate the ATNR. Table 8-5 presents primitive reflexes and how they are tested.

Primitive reflexes that are present or that re-emerge in an adult can greatly impact the adult's functional mobility and occupational performance. For example, the flexor

TABLE 8-5 Primitive Reflexes

NAME	TESTING PROCEDURE	IMPACT ON FUNCTION
Grasp reflex	An object is placed in the client's hand. A positive response is seen when the client automatically grasps the object and is unable to release it.	Can ultimately interfere with an individual's ability to hold and manipulate objects effectively (e.g., will not be able to correctly hold and manipulate a pencil or pen for writing their name), and should be integrated by 6 months of age[14]
Moro reflex	While the client is in a semi-reclined position, the head is dropped backward. A positive reaction is seen when there is a startle response such as abduction, extension or flexion, and external rotation of the arms and extension and abduction of the fingers.	Can ultimately cause an individual to have an excessive response to changes in head position, (e.g., he or she might exhibit a startle response when going to lie down in bed) and should be integrated by 4 months of age[5,15]
Flexor withdrawal	While the client is supine with legs extended and head in midposition, the sole of the foot is stimulated with a finger, feather, or other item. A positive response is exhibited by uncontrolled flexion of the stimulated leg.	Can ultimately interfere with an individual's ability to stand (e.g., whenever the leg hits the floor, the stimulation of the floor may cause the leg to immediately flex, making standing difficult or impossible), and should be integrated by 2 months of age[3,5,15]
Crossed extension	The client is initially placed in supine with one leg extended and one leg flexed and the head in midposition; The extended leg is then flexed A positive response is exhibited by extension of the leg that was initially in a flexed position.	Can ultimately interfere with an individual's ability to transfer and assume a seated position, and should be integrated by 2 months of age[3,5,15]
Asymmetrical tonic neck reflex (ATNR) *Also called *fencing reflex*	With the client supine or sitting, the client's head is turned to the side actively or passively. A positive ATNR is demonstrated when increased extensor tone is present on the extremity the client is facing while there is flexor tone in the opposite extremity.	Ultimately makes performing symmetrical movements (e.g., grasping a book or typing with two hands) difficult, and should be integrated by 6 months of age[3,5,15] **Asymmetrical tonic neck reflex.**

Continued

TABLE 8-5 Primitive Reflexes (continued)

NAME	TESTING PROCEDURE	IMPACT ON FUNCTION
Symmetrical tonic neck reflex (STNR)	With the client in quadruped, the client's head is flexed or extended. A positive STNR is indicated by flexion of the upper extremities and extension of the lower extremities when the client's head is flexed and extension of the upper extremities and flexion of the lower extremities when the head is extended.	Ultimately makes bearing weight and functional mobility tasks such as sitting up difficult, and should be integrated by 6 months of age[3,5,15] Symmetrical tonic neck reflex.
Tonic labyrinthine reflex (TLR)	The client is placed supine or prone, with the head in midposition. A positive TLR is an increase in extension tone or extension of the extremities when placed in supine position, and an increase in flexor tone or flexion of the extremities when placed in prone position.	Ultimately makes functional mobility tasks, such as rolling over, difficult and should be integrated by 4 months of age[3,5,15]
Associated reactions	The client is asked to squeeze an object. A positive reaction is seen when the client mimics squeezing the object with the other hand, or when increased tone is elsewhere in the body.	Can ultimately hinder volitional movement, and should be integrated by 8 to 9 years of age, although may be seen in healthy clients as they try to engage in strenuous movement. Clients who have had a CVA, TBI, or other neurological trauma may also exhibit associated reactions as they attempt functional tasks and movements[3,5,15]
Positive supporting reaction	With the client in a standing position, the ball of the foot is placed in contact with the floor. A positive response is exhibited by extensor tone in the legs.	Can interfere with walking and transfers, (e.g., when the foot touches the floor the increased extensor tone may make lifting the leg for transferring or walking difficult or impossible) and should be integrated by 6 months of age[3,5,15]
Righting reactions	Directing the head to maintain an upright position to maintain the normal position of head and trunk alignment, righting reactions help individuals assume a position. Often evaluated by observation during functional mobility tasks and ADLs.	Clients with impaired righting reactions may have difficulty changing and assuming positions, such as sitting up, because they are unable to keep their head and trunk appropriately aligned for functional, coordinated movements; these remain throughout life[3,5,15]
Equilibrium reactions	Considered the "first line of defense against falling," equilibrium reactions help individuals maintain a position and regain balance when the body is pushed or the center of gravity is altered (e.g., the trunk/body will curve toward the force and the extremities will extend and abduct to protect the individual from falling) Often evaluated by observation during functional mobility tasks and ADLs.	Clients with impaired equilibrium reactions may have difficulty sustaining their balance during ADLs and functional mobility tasks, leading to falls; these remain throughout life[3,5,15]

TABLE 8-5 Primitive Reflexes (continued)

NAME	TESTING PROCEDURE	IMPACT ON FUNCTION
Protective reactions	Considered the "second line of defense against falling," protective reactions protect individuals if their equilibrium reactions are insufficient to maintain balance by leading him/her to extend their arms and hands to protect the head and face. Often evaluated by observation during functional mobility tasks and ADLs.	Clients with impaired protective reactions may have frequent falls and difficulty bearing weight on their affected side when engaging in bilateral tasks; these remain throughout life[3,5,15]

withdrawal reflex, crossed extension reflex, extensor thrust reflex, and STNR can impede the ability to stand up or transfer to or off a chair. The Moro reflex can interfere with an individual's balance and coordination or increase sensitivity to sounds, light, and movement. The rooting reaction and suck–swallow reflex, when present in an adult, can make social interactions and eating challenging. The palmar grasp reflex may impair an adult's fine motor skills and coordination. Associated reactions and the asymmetrical and symmetrical tonic reflexes can decrease an individual's ability to perform controlled, volitional movements during ADLs. The OT practitioner must work with clients on integrating these reflexes by taking them through the developmental stages and addressing any safety concerns. Results from assessments the practitioner conducts aid in determining where the client is at developmentally. During interventions the client is engaged in activities that are just above his or her developmental stage to encourage skill growth.

THE OLDER ADULT

The natural aging process impacts an individual's balance, reflexes, and sensation. In general, reflexes are not as quick and efficient in older adults, placing them at a higher risk for injury. For example, if they should fall, their protective reactions might not activate in a timely manner, leading to a more severe injury. The older adult also tends to have decreased balance, which places them at an increased risk for falling. This includes trouble maintaining static balance (e.g., when sitting or standing) or dynamic balance (e.g., when walking), as well as regaining balance when starting to fall or when one's balance is disturbed (e.g., if someone bumps into them). Finally, older adults tend to have decreased sensation. This includes decreased vision, temperature discrimination, and tactile discrimination. This decreased sensation can negatively impact safety and coordination during all occupations, including leisure pursuits and activities of daily living (ADLs). Decreased reflexes, balance, and sensation perhaps play a role in the overall slower movement patterns the older adult tends to exhibit.

TONE

Muscles are in a continuous state of contraction, referred to as **tone**. An essential part of an individual's ability to stay upright and balanced, tone is also necessary for an individual to initiate functional mobility tasks and coordinated movements.[3,5] This can include movements needed for dressing, bathing, and getting in or out of bed. The OT practitioner can assess and feel tone when performing PROM on a client (described later).

Hypotonicity and Flaccidity

Hypotonicity refers to decreased muscle tone. This decreased tone is involuntary and is more than simply being weak or unfit; reflexes can also be reduced.[3,5] Hypotonicity can be the result of a lower motor lesion after a TBI, CVA, or SCI. Lower motor neurons, which are part of the peripheral nervous system, carry various messages from the brain to the skeletal muscles.[5] An individual exhibiting hypotonicity will have difficulty initiating and engaging in functional mobility tasks and ADLs, as well as picking up, using, and manipulating items. The prognosis of hypotonicity varies, depending on its underlying cause, and differs from client to client.

Flaccidity is the absence of muscle tone. An individual with flaccidity has no AROM as a result of nerve denervation (e.g., the nerve is no longer innervating the muscle), and when ranged passively the extremity will feel very heavy. Reflexes will be absent.[5] Complete SCI, cerebral damage (e.g., after a CVA or TBI), or PNI can lead to flaccidity. Although the amount of muscle tone a client gains varies, depending on the specific client and underlying cause, most clients with flaccidity develop some tone over time.[5]

Hypertonicity

Hypertonicity occurs when an individual has increased muscle tone. Reflexes may be hyperactive, and resistance to both PROM and AROM and to movement may be evident.[3,5] Hypertonicity can be the result of an upper motor neuron lesion after a TBI, CVA, or SCI, and is also seen in individuals with CP. Upper motor neurons are part of the central nervous system, and exert control over the lower motor neurons.[5] When there is an upper motor neuron lesion, the lower motor neurons are stimulated and fire, resulting in increased tone.[5] An individual exhibiting hypertonicity will have difficulty performing functional, coordinated movements for ADLs and functional mobility tasks. This can result from difficulty flexing and/or extending muscles needed to perform such occupations. Table 8-6 presents a few forms of hypertonicity. Hypertonicity is often used interchangeably with the term **spasticity**, but, technically, hypertonicity is resistance to passive movement, and spasticity is more about an increase in tone with increased velocity of movement. This means that with spasticity, the faster the passive movement, the stronger the resistance.

Evaluating Tone

Muscle tone is evaluated through passive range of motion and observation. Two common scales for rating spasticity are the Modified Ashworth Scale and the Tardieu/Modified Tardieu Scale. The Modified Ashworth Scale rates spasticity on a scale of 0 (no increased muscle tone) to 4 (rigid flexion or extension is present) after providing a quick stretch to the extremity (Table 8-7).[5,17] The Tardieu Scale rates spasticity by determining the velocity and joint angle at which the spasticity is elicited and has both slow and fast components.[5,18]

Abnormal tone can result in synergy patterns that may occur and be observed when a client tries to initiate a movement or is exposed to a stimulus. When present, the movement or stimulus will evoke a movement pattern of extension or flexion.[3,5] Synergy patterns can make ADLs, functional mobility tasks, isolated movements, and coordinated movement difficult. They can be the result of a TBI or CVA. With *flexor synergy*, muscles tend to move toward flexion and toward the body.[3,5] For example, the elbow and the knee will go into flexion, the shoulder will go into abduction and external rotation, the wrist and fingers will go into

TABLE 8-6 Hypertonicity

TYPE OF HYPERTONICITY	DEFINITION	TYPES
Rigidity	Extensors and flexors have increased tone in the same region of the body (e.g., the triceps and biceps both act antagonist muscles—to experience what this might be like, one can voluntarily flex the triceps and biceps while trying to move the elbow).	*Lead Pipe Rigidity* During PROM, constant resistance is felt throughout (can be seen in Parkinson's disease). *Cogwheel Rigidity* During PROM, resistance is felt at various points throughout the range followed by points of release/easy movement (can be seen in Parkinson's disease). *Decerebrate Rigidity* Upper and lower extremities are in extension (can occur in clients with lesions in the bilateral hemispheres of the diencephalon and midbrain). *Decorticate Rigidity* Upper extremities are flexed, lower extremities are extended (can occur in clients with bilateral cortical lesions).[3,5]

Decerebrate and decorticate rigidity.

TYPE OF HYPERTONICITY	DEFINITION	TYPES
Spasticity	Extensors or flexors have increased tone (e.g., there is increased flexor tone in the biceps; OR increased extensor tone in the triceps). It is velocity dependent.	*Clasp Knife Syndrome* After the spastic extremity is given a quick stretch, the OT practitioner will feel resistance and then the resistance will release. *Clonus* Repetitive, oscillating contractions after a quick stretch is applied to a spastic group of muscles; the number of oscillations that occur is counted and recorded.[3,5,16]

TABLE 8-7 Modified Ashworth Scale for Grading Spasticity[17]

Grade	
0	No increase in muscle tone
1	Slight increase in muscle tone, manifested by a catch and release or by minimal resistance at the end of the ROM when the affected part(s) is moved in flexion or extension
1+	Slight increase in muscle tone, manifested by a catch, followed by minimal resistance throughout the remainder (less than half) of the ROM
2	More marked increase in muscle tone through most of the ROM but affected part(s) easily moved
3	Considerable increase in muscle tone, passive movement difficulty
4	Affected part(s) rigid in flexion or extension

COMMUNICATION

When assessing muscle tone and sensation, it is extremely important for the OT practitioner to provide clear, precise directions in a manner that the client understands. Assessment results will be inaccurate if the client does not comprehend what he or she is being asked to do, and therefore does not know how to respond. It is vital to communicate with family and caregivers as well so that they manage the tone correctly. Many times, a well-meaning family member might use a light touch while massaging with lotion, which can be stimulating to an arm that has a flexor synergy and increased tone. OT practitioners can teach families techniques to inhibit or facilitate tone, as appropriate. For example, OT practitioners can explain how deep pressure can decrease tone while light touch can increase tone. Teaching ROM exercises can help address tone issues. OT practitioners can give family members activities they can do to address clients' sensory deficits, such as engaging in activities that involve various tactile sensations (e.g., playing tic-tac-toe in shaving cream). Finally, it is essential to discuss with both clients and family members how tone and sensory impairments can impact safety. This should include providing appropriate compensatory strategies, such as using a microwave for meals instead of the stove, using a thermometer to check the temperature of bathwater, and visually checking the placement of an arm when going to sit down or stand up.

flexion and adduction or ulnar deviation, and the forearm will supinate. The client will have difficulty moving out of flexion and into extension. With *extensor synergy*, muscles tend to move toward extension and away from the body.[3,5] For example, the shoulder will adduct and internally rotate, the elbow and knee will go into extension, the wrist and fingers will go into flexion, and the forearm will pronate. The client will have difficulty moving out of extension and into flexion. Figure 8-4 provides examples of flexor and extensor synergy.

STAGES OF MOTOR LEARNING AND RECOVERY

OT practitioners can describe a client's motor recovery utilizing a variety of scales and stages.

Modified Brunnstrom Stages

One common method of identifying stages of motor recovery is the use of the Modified Brunnstrom Stages of Motor Recovery (MBSMR) (Table 8-8). Frequently used to identify levels of spasticity and synergy patterns in individuals who have sustained a CVA or TBI, the MBSMR contains six stages.[5] A seventh stage, normal movement, is listed in some resources.[18] Knowing the client's stage can help the OT practitioner devise appropriate intervention activities. The practitioner can also describe the various stages to clients and family members so that they can better understand the client's progress, how his or her function may be impacted, and activities that can be used to engage the client to move forward to the next stage.

Fostering Normal Tone

The OT practitioner can take many approaches to address a client's abnormal tone. In many cases, the OT practitioner might use a combination of approaches to best meet

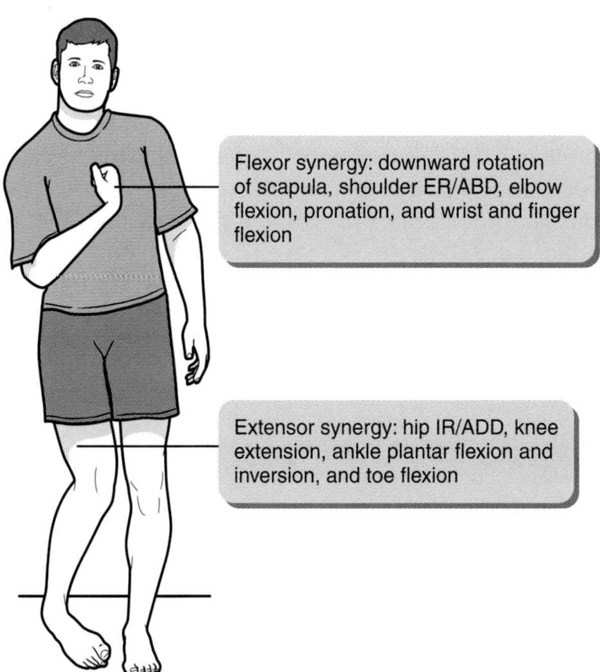

FIGURE 8-4. UE flexor synergy and LE extensor synergy. Synergies may fluctuate in the way they present through the recovery process.

TABLE 8-8 Modified Brunnstrom Stages of Motor Recovery[5,11]

STAGE	DESCRIPTION	FUNCTIONAL IMPACT
1	Flaccidity and no active movement.	The client will not be able to pick up, manipulate, or grasp any items for ADLs (e.g., a fork or toothbrush).
2	Synergy patterns (may see reflexive associated reactions) and spasticity begin to emerge.	The client might exhibit increased tone and flexor synergy patterns; the client may be able to slightly flex their finger but will not have functional controlled movements to pick up, manipulate, or grasp ADL items.
3	Spasticity is at its most severe and client can begin to use components of synergy patterns to initiate voluntary movements.	The client might be able to use a gross grasp to pick up a larger item, such as a built-up fork, with difficulty and decreased coordination; he or she may have difficulty releasing the item.
4	Spasticity is decreasing, and client can coordinate movements away from synergy patterns.	The client will have a more controlled grasp and some finger extension/thumb movement, including lateral prehension; manipulation of objects for ADLs is still very difficult and uncoordinated; Can put the hand behind the back, supinate, and pronate (with elbow flexed at 90 degrees).
5	Synergy patterns no longer dominate and spasticity continues to decrease.	The client has increased arm and hand control, enabling him or her to more functionally grasp and release objects; can bring the arm forward and overhead and pronate.
6	Client performs isolated movement easily and spasticity is minimal.	The client's arm and hand coordination and control are functional and performed with ease; decreased coordination might be the result of fatigue, or attempting to perform strenuous or quick movements.

the client's needs.[5,11] The amount of recovery and the timeline for the recovery will vary, depending on the client's specific condition and the extent of neurological damage. It is usually best to initiate treatment as soon as the client is medically stable, as the client might make the most gains shortly after the injury or illness. The overall goal is to normalize tone for maximal functioning and occupational engagement. Increased tone needs to be inhibited, whereas decreased tone requires facilitation of tone. Both tasks can be accomplished through engaging the client in specific movement patterns, placing the client in certain positions, and using a variety of sensory inputs. General interventions to work on normalizing tone are included in Table 8-9.

One intervention for tone can be weight-bearing. Weight-bearing activities are used frequently with clients who have sustained a CVA, TBI, or who have CP. Input from weight-bearing is thought to increase connections in the brain and help regulate tone. Motor neurons, which activate muscle contractions, are shown to have increased activity during weight-bearing.[19] Weight-bearing leads to stretching of muscle spindles located in the muscle. Muscle spindles carry proprioceptive input and other sensory information about the muscle's length, tension, and load. The dorsal horn of the spinal cord, containing the cell body of many spinal cord tracts, receives the proprioceptive information from the muscle spindles. Here, proprioceptive input connects to alpha motor neurons in the ventral horn. The ventral horn contains motor spinal nerve cell bodies which innervate skeletal muscles. The alpha motor neurons send messages from the central nervous system to the skeletal muscle, and this helps initiate and maintain movement. Activating the agonistic muscle (the muscle that is trying to activate) facilitates muscle movement, increasing tone. As this occurs, an alpha motor neuron inhibits movement of the antagonistic muscle. In addition, weight-bearing can be done to provide a sustained stretch, activating the Golgi Tendon organs. Located in the muscle tendons, they are proprioceptors that detect tension as the muscle is contracting. This activation causes inhibition of the agonist muscle and activation of the antagonistic muscle, temporarily decreasing tone (Box 8-1).[3]

Activities for weight-bearing can be done in the quadruped (on hands and knees) position, standing, or sitting on the edge of the bed. The OT practitioner may use his or her hands to help stabilize the client and provide further weight-bearing. These exercises can also be done during ADLs and other functional activities. For example, while the client brushes their teeth using the unaffected arm and hand, they can bear weight on the sink or bedside table with support as needed (Fig. 8-5).[5] It is important for the OT practitioner to provide education to the client and family members on how the client can incorporate weight-bearing into their daily occupations. Other weight-bearing activities can include stabilizing the client's upper extremity while he or she sits on the edge of the bed and completes grooming tasks; stabilizing

TABLE 8-9 Treatment Interventions for Tone

INTERVENTION/ APPROACH	CLIENT POPULATION	OBJECTIVES	RATIONALE	INTERVENTIONS	EXAMPLES
Neurodevelopmental Treatment Approach (NDT) *Also called *Bobath Approach*	Clients with CVA or TBI	To normalize movement patterns by normalizing muscle tone, inhibiting primitive ref exes, and facilitating normal postural reactions[5]	Weight-bearing and handling techniques on affected extremity are thought to promote proximal stability which is needed for distal mobility, and to assist with facilitating normal movement patterns and tone.[5]	Handling techniques provide increased sensory awareness and input to the client; OT practitioner may assist in facilitating normal movement patterns.[5] Weight-bearing normalizes muscle, and includes the body weight shifting over the affected stabilized arm.	Handling techniques may be used to inhibit abnormal tone or facilitate muscle contractions and normal movement patterns. Weight-bearing can be graded from having the client simply bear the weight of the arm on a table to standing and bearing weight through the arm while engaging in ADLs or a leisure activity.
Proprioceptive Neuromuscular Facilitation Approach (PNF)	Clients with CVA or TBI	To produce coordinated volitional movement by focusing on a developmental sequence of movements and the balance between agonist and antagonist movements	While an agonist muscle initiates movement, the antagonist muscle relaxes and helps control movement. [3] For example, when a client flexes the right elbow to brush teeth, the biceps are the agonist and the triceps are the antagonist. Movement is believed to develop in a proximal to distal and cephalo caudal direction (top down, from head to toe).	Mass diagonal movement patterns (frequently needed for ADL performance) are utilized in intervention to promote movement. Client may perform diagonal movement patterns to work on increasing coordination and ROM, and incorporate them into ADLs.	The D1 flexion pattern is needed when combing the opposite side of one's hair or rolling from supine to prone, the D1 extension pattern is used when opening a car door or rolling from prone to supine, the D2 flexion pattern is used when combing the same side of one's hair, and the D2 extension pattern is used when twisting to button one's pants on the opposite side. Performing such movements requires a balance of agonists and antagonists. Performing stretches that involve combinations of contracting and relaxing the agonist and/or antagonist may also assist in improving the balance between the two.[5]
Rood Approach	Clients with central nervous system (CNS) damage	Focuses on inhibiting or facilitating motor responses by applying sensory stimulation to muscles and joints.	Rood techniques often used in preparation for functional activities or in addition to other approaches for those who have abnormal tone or motor responses (e.g., after a CVA or TBI). [5,11]	Facilitatory stimulation may include tapping over a muscle belly or tendon, which can elicit a muscle contraction. Quick stretching or vibration applied to the muscle or tendon can also elicit a muscle contraction by activating the agonist muscle and inhibiting the antagonist muscle. Inhibitory stimulation includes deep pressure, slow rocking, neutral heat (hot packs, towels) and prolonged stretching.	Facilitatory stimulation: Tapping the biceps may cause elbow to extend; tapping on triceps may cause the elbow to flex. A quick stretch to the flexor carpi ulnaris can result in wrist flexion, whereas vibration to the pronator teres can cause forearm pronation. Inhibitory stimulation: prolonged stretching of the biceps can decrease extensor tone in the biceps, while prolonged stretching of the triceps can decrease flexor tone. Applying such stimulation decreases muscle activity.

BOX 8-1
Aging Issues

Stereotypes about aging adults are, for the most part, simply stereotypes. Most older adults live healthy, active lives, and incorporate any age-related changes into their lifestyles and keep going. Overall, they comprise a diverse age group that can be broken into life-stage groups, since the experiences of a 65-year-old may be very different than those of a 90-year-old. Life-stage subgroups are the young-old (approximately ages 65–74 years), the middle-old (ages 75–84 years), and the old-old (over age 85 years).[20]

Regardless of life-stage, the age-related physical changes that commonly affect older adults include hearing impairment, weakening vision, and the increasing probability of arthritis, hypertension, heart disease, diabetes, and osteoporosis.[21] Older adults of all ages may experience memory loss as the speed with which the information is received, encoded, and stored may decrease with aging.[21] Word finding ability may decline, and a general weakening of muscle strength occurs. Nine percent of those between ages 65 and 69 years need personal assistance, and up to 50% of older Americans over 85 years of age need assistance with everyday activities.[21] Older adults in lower socioeconomic situations tend to have increased chronic disease and experience the effects of older age at an earlier age.[21]

In a study on the physiological effects of aerobic exercise in older age, the researchers looked at sedentary people with a mean age of 64 years. They were split into two groups—one remained sedentary, and the physical training group received supervised aerobic exercise for three sessions per week, 1 hour each for 12 weeks. Participants' cognitive, cardiovascular fitness, and resting cerebral blood flow (CBF) were assessed at the beginning, middle, and end of the 12 weeks.[21] Physical fitness improved within the physical training group, and the researchers also found that this group significantly improved in immediate and delayed text-level memory recall relative to the control group.[21] There were also changes seen in resting regional CBF.[22] As a society, we are becoming more sedentary, and this may be changing not only our physical health, but our brain health as well.

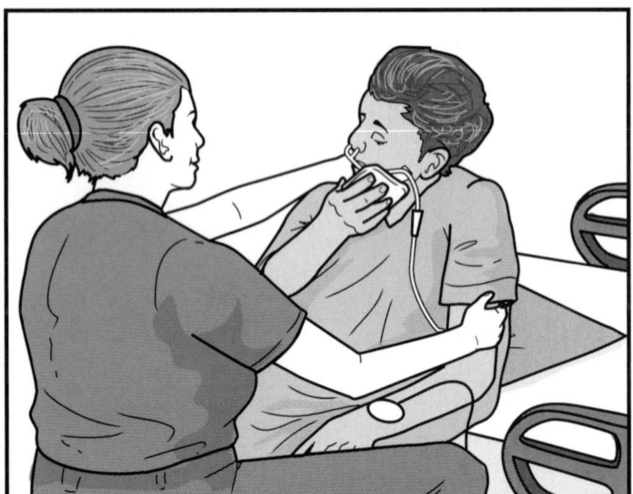
FIGURE 8-5. Upper extremity weight-bearing.

the client's upper extremity on a table as he or she stands and completes a puzzle or other meaningful task; or having the client do exercises while sitting or standing, for example, wall push-ups; the client places his or her upper extremities on the wall and leans off the wall. The practitioner should provide support and stabilization, as needed, being especially cautious to protect the shoulder and the arches of the hands.

Clients often naturally receive more weight-bearing through their lower extremities compared with their upper extremities. This is the result of functional mobility tasks, such as standing, walking, and transferring (e.g., from the bed to a wheelchair). After a neurological insult, such as a CVA, gains in ROM and control are frequently seen in the lower extremities before they are seen in the upper extremities. The increased weight-bearing in the lower extremities during functional mobility tasks may partially explain why this is the case.

Other approaches frequently used by OT practitioners are presented in Table 8-9.

It is important for the OT practitioner to understand that not all approaches work for all clients and that a combination of approaches may yield the best outcomes. This combination can be based on the client's specific needs and circumstances. Furthermore, it is important to consider what the research shows and to use evidence-based practice. Unfortunately, research has not consistently shown neurodevelopmental Treatment (NDT), proprioceptive neuromuscular facilitation (PNF), or the Rood approach to be effective.

Orthotics and casting can also be used to inhibit increased muscle tone by providing a prolonged stretch. Frequently used with clients who have neurological or orthopedic disabilities, orthotics and casting can be used to help prevent contractures, maintain or increase ROM, and/or protect joint(s).[5,11] Clients who have significant tone might require frequent orthotic adjustments as the tone decreases, or serial casting (where they are recast as the tone decreases) to slowly increase their ROM. Physical agent modalities (PAMs) are also frequently used with clients who have neurological or orthopedic disabilities. They include ultrasound, electrical stimulation, and fluidotherapy. Used to help ease pain, decrease inflammation, and improve ROM, PAMs are considered a preparatory activity and require education and practice before they are used with clients.[5,11] Finally, PROM is frequently used with clients who have neurological or orthopedic disabilities to address potential concerns and problems related to flaccidity or hypotonicity and spasticity or hypertonicity, such as contractures and adhesions.[5,11] The stretch provided during PROM can help inhibit muscle tone and keep muscles mobile and loose, helping prevent contractures and adhesions.

Addressing positioning needs is essential for numerous purposes, such as pain alleviation, safety, and joint or skin protection.[5,11] This can include providing appropriate support and cushioning to ensure proper positioning. Finally, medical interventions, such as oral baclofen (calms spasticity), an intrathecal baclofen pump (gives medicine directly into spinal cord), and botulinum toxin (Botox; blocks neurotransmitters to paralyze muscle for 3 to 6 months) can be used to decrease tone and muscle spasms.

HYPOTONICITY, FLACCIDITY, AND RELATED COMPLICATIONS

The OT practitioner can provide interventions, including home exercise and stretching programs, to address hypotonicity, flaccidity, and related complications.[3,5] In an effort to facilitate increased tone, the OT practitioner can do the following:[5,11]

- Provide a quick stretch to the hypotonic/flaccid muscles (e.g., if working on facilitating elbow extension, include a quick stretch of the triceps).
- Apply high-frequency vibration over the muscle belly to increase muscle fiber contractions.
- Tap over the muscle belly to increase muscle fiber contractions (e.g., the biceps to work on elbow flexion or the triceps to work on elbow extension).
- Provide neuromuscular electrical stimulation (NEMS) to the muscle belly to increase muscle fiber contractions.
- Engage the client in weight-bearing activities over the muscles (e.g., provide support to prevent the elbow from falling down as the client places and leans on the affected extremity while brushing teeth) to increase muscle fiber contractions.
- Ensure postural alignment (e.g., weight should be on the flaccid side the majority of the time). Working on increasing postural control (e.g., passively positioning the extremity during ADL tasks to provide sensory and proprioceptive feedback) is also essential.[5,11] Providing family education on positioning should be a part of this process. For example, the client's family can have the client place the impacted arm on the sink during grooming tasks or on the walker during ambulation.

HYPERTONICITY

With **hypertonicity**, the OT practitioner aims to inhibit muscle tone. This can include application of therapeutic ultrasound and other PAMs, such as electrical stimulation, thermotherapy (heat), or cryotherapy (cold). The device should be placed over the muscle belly. As a result of vasodilation that can occur from thermotherapy or ultrasound, muscle activity, contractions, and spasticity are decreased.[11] Vasodilation occurs when cryotherapy is applied for more than 15 minutes, temporarily reducing spasticity. When utilizing electrical stimulation, stimulating a spastic muscle is thought to fatigue the muscle and decrease spasticity, whereas stimulation applied to the antagonist muscle of a spastic muscle can help inhibit the spastic muscle.[4] Casting or the use of an orthotic, which keeps the muscle in a lengthened position, maintains pressure and provides neutral warmth, can also inhibit muscle tone.[5,11] It is also important to position and engage the hypertonic muscles in patterns that are opposite to the hypertonic or synergistic patterns.[5,11] For example, if a client is in flexion, then the OT practitioner would try and position him or her in extension. Finally, client and family member or caregiver education is essential. This can include education on positioning, orthotic wearing regimens, and home exercise programs.

WOUND DEVELOPMENT AND MANAGEMENT

Wounds are a negative outcome often seen with injuries, surgery, chronic conditions, immobility, and lack of sensation. A conservative estimate of the cost of caring for chronic wounds alone exceeds a staggering $50 billion per year.[23] Nonhealing wounds affect about 3 to 6 million people in the United States, with persons 65 years or older accounting for 85% of these events.[23] Many times, the OTA will treat a client for a wound that is the primary or secondary diagnosis, and generally, it has a significant impact on overall health, well-being, and functional abilities. Wounds can be managed in the home, hospital, or specialized wound center, and there are opportunities for health management and education on risk factor management, as well as pressure relief, positioning, nutrition, and hygiene.

Skin

Skin is an amazingly protective surface made up of the following layers[24] (Fig. 8-6):

EPIDERMIS: OUTER LAYER

- Comprised of epithelial cells
- Contains no blood vessels (avascular)
- Regenerates every 2 to 4 weeks, subject to an individual's age and friction forces applied to skin
- Receives nutrients from the dermis below
- Comprises four to five layers, depending on body location

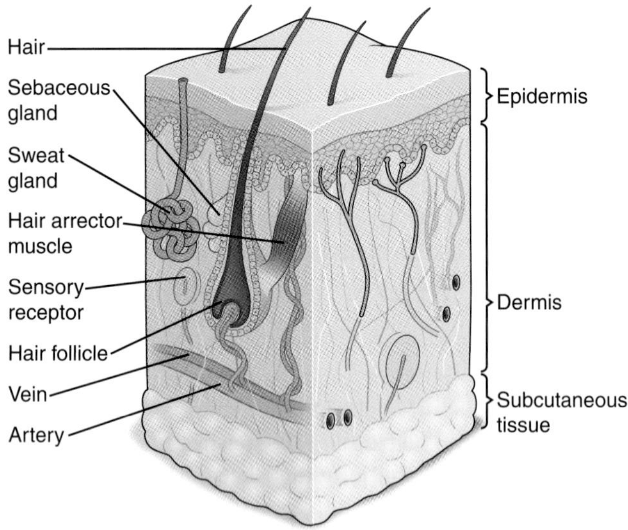

FIGURE 8-6. Layer of skin.

DERMIS: MIDDLE LAYER

- Approximately 0.5 mm thick
- Comprises two layers
- Highly vascular
- Contains nerves, connective tissue, collagen, elastin, and specialized cells, such as fibroblasts and mast cells
- Responsible for inflammatory reactions that occur in response to trauma and infection
- Contains receptors for heat, cold, pain, pressure, itch, and tickle

HYPODERMIS (SUBCUTANEOUS): INNERMOST LAYER

- Supports the dermis and the epidermis
- Varies in thickness and depth
- Comprised of adipose tissue (fat), connective tissue, and blood vessels
- Functions include storage, protection of underlying organs, insulation, and temperature regulation

Because it is exposed to the environment, skin plays an important role in protecting the body against dehydration and infections or disease. Its other functions are temperature regulation, sensation, insulation, and holding the precursor that converts to vitamin D with the assistance of sunlight. Although durable and protective, skin is fragile in some ways and can break down as a result of certain factors, such as excessive temperature, moisture, pressure, friction, and shear.

Wound Causes and Factors

Wounds can occur as a result of a multitude of reasons, which determine whether the wounds are healing or nonhealing. Examples of acute wounds are those caused by surgical procedures, trauma, abrasions, or superficial burns. Remember, every time an incision is made, a wound is created, and it must heal. Wound infections are the most expensive complications following surgery and, even after significant advancements in the healthcare field, are still a major source of bacteria that drive **nosocomial** (hospital-acquired) infection rates.[25]

Caused by surgical incisions, surgical wounds are first managed at the hospital or outpatient surgery center, and then in the home or outpatient clinic for follow-up dressing changes and wound management, as needed. Overall, infection rates of surgical sites can range from 1% to 10%, depending on the nature of the surgery.[26] The incidence of surgical site infections is related to age, and therefore is expected to continue to rise as the population ages, with a doubling of the rate in clients older than 64 years.[27] Initially after surgery, these wounds are managed with staples, stitches, drains, wound closures (glue, bandages), dressings, and wraps. In many clients, surgical wounds heal well with minimal scarring or complications. However, in clients already compromised by poor health and other factors, even a paper cut can become a significantly infected wound, or even an amputation resulting from diabetic vascular issues.

Caused by physical injury, traumatic wounds may be managed like surgical wounds to a certain extent but often involve other factors. These factors may include dirt and debris, torn and ragged edges, missing skin, and the presence of foreign objects. Wounds caused by blunt force trauma may also have excessive bleeding and bruising. Many of these factors can lead to higher infection rates and longer healing times.

Burn wounds are covered extensively in Chapter 28; such wounds can range from a simple burn resulting from touching a hot stove rack to a severe burn in multiple body areas as a result of a house fire. The different mechanisms of injury for burns include thermal, electrical, chemical, and radiation and are generally classified by the depth of the burn wound as either superficial, partial-thickness, or full-thickness wounds. Certainly, the deeper the wound, the longer and more difficult are the healing and recovery processes.

Amputation wounds can result from traumatic or chronic causes, both of which can affect the healing process differently. Important factors in healing and outcome of amputation include the client's nutritional status, age, smoking status, and the presence of coexisting diseases, such as renal failure, diabetes, and anemia. Another crucial factor is the actual amputation level because healing depends on the amount of blood flow, and in cases of peripheral vascular disease, careful selection by the surgeon is important.[28] One potential complication would be infection, and on average, clients with diabetes are approximately five times more likely to have a postsurgical wound infection compared with those without diabetes.[29] **Tissue necrosis** (death of tissue) can be another potential issue related to amputation wounds, as many amputations are performed to treat poor perfusion (blood flow and oxygenation). With amputations, the skin surrounding the suture line may also develop complications, such as edema, blistering from friction, and allergic reactions from dressings and tape. Amputation sites can develop a hematoma, a collection of blood under skin, which can attract infection, place extra pressure on the sutures and the wound, and lead to edema and necrosis.[28] Amputations are covered in-depth in Chapter 24.

Some cancers as well as cancer treatments can cause wounds. Ulcerating or fungating wounds from cancer can either be from the primary cancer site, as untreated malignant cancer infiltrates and erupts from under skin, or a secondary site after the cancer has spread. Some skin cancers, such as melanoma, can cause ulcerating wounds that may bleed, itch, ooze fluid, have a significant associated odor and pain, and be difficult to treat. Many times, the aim of treatment is symptom management more than healing. Radiation and chemotherapy can cause wounds and suppress the immune system, which deters wound healing. In addition, lymphedema after a mastectomy can cause wounds, if not treated.

Chronic wounds can be some of the most difficult to treat. Most are ulcers associated with ischemia (inadequate blood supply), diabetes mellitus, venous stasis disease (chronic leg edema from pooling fluid), or pressure.[23] Chronic wounds represent a silent epidemic that affects a large portion of the world population; they pose a major and increasing threat to the public health and economy of the United States.[25] Ischemia is often associated with peripheral artery disease and arterial insufficiency ulcers that frequently cause painful wounds on the distal leg and ankle. Diabetes is often a cause of ischemia, and frequent skin checks and close blood sugar management are important. Diabetes can also lead to neuropathy, which can cause decreased sensation in the lower limb and more advanced wounds before they are noticed. In diabetes, an elevated blood sugar level stiffens the arteries and narrows the blood vessels, which can lead to circulation problems and then can cause wounds and affect wound healing. Diabetes can also cause a decrease in immune functioning, which can lead to a higher risk for infections. Venous stasis disease can be caused by diabetes but is also seen in individuals who are obese. The primary risk factors for venous ulcer development are older age, obesity, previous leg injuries, deep venous thrombosis (blood clot), and phlebitis (inflammation of a vein).[30]

Pressure injuries, also called pressure sores or wounds, pressure ulcers, decubitus ulcers, or bedsores, are generally injuries to skin and underlying tissue resulting from prolonged pressure. The term *pressure injuries* is the preferred terminology as of 2016. When pressure is placed on a bony prominence, skin is at high risk for pressure injuries; common locations include the heels, ankles, hips, tailbone, back of the head, and areas along the spine and on the scapulae (Fig. 8-7). When pressure is combined with moisture, especially from incontinence and sweating, and shear forces to skin from transfers and moving across other surfaces it can often lead to ulceration. Clients with decreased sensation and immobility are at a higher risk for pressure injuries because either they do not feel any pain or discomfort from pressure or they are unable to move despite the feelings of discomfort. Such clients may have severe dementia, tetraplegic level spinal cord injury, or inability to communicate. Pressure injuries can develop quickly, and the skin of vulnerable individuals should be checked daily.

The National Pressure Ulcer Advisory Panel (NPUAP) redefined the definition of a pressure injury during the NPUAP 2016 Staging Consensus Conference: "A pressure injury is localized damage to the skin and underlying soft tissue usually over a bony prominence or related to a medical or other device. The injury can present as intact skin or an open ulcer and may be painful. The injury occurs as a result of intense and/or prolonged pressure or pressure in combination with shear. The tolerance of soft tissue for pressure and shear may also be affected by microclimate, poor nutrition,

EVIDENCE-BASED PRACTICE

Chronic wounds require frequent dressing changes and considerable cost in terms of time, resources, and dollars. According to Mehmood, et al., "covering an open wound with an appropriate dressing increases the healing rate, absorbs the wound exudate, and relieves pain; however, changing wound dressings hampers the process of normal wound healing and causes stress and pain to the patient."[31] These authors noted technology might assist with providing information on the proper time to change the wound dressing and report continuously on the physical environment of the wound. Ideally, sensors would note pH, temperature, humidity or moisture level, wound odor, oxygen, and bacteria, and would interface with wireless technology to convey the information to a remote location for analysis. A few such devices are already on the market, but most only track one aspect of the wound, such as moisture levels or pH. Since wound management has emerged as a major health challenge with a considerable portion of the healthcare dollars being consumed in wound care activities throughout the world, this evolving technology is important. Certainly, the cost/benefit must be weighed, but these technologies could mean faster and better wound healing in the future.

Mehmood, N., Hariz, A., Fitridge, R., & Voelcker, N. H. (2013). Applications of modern sensors and wireless technology in effective wound management. Journal of Biomedical Materials Research, 102*(4), 885–895.*

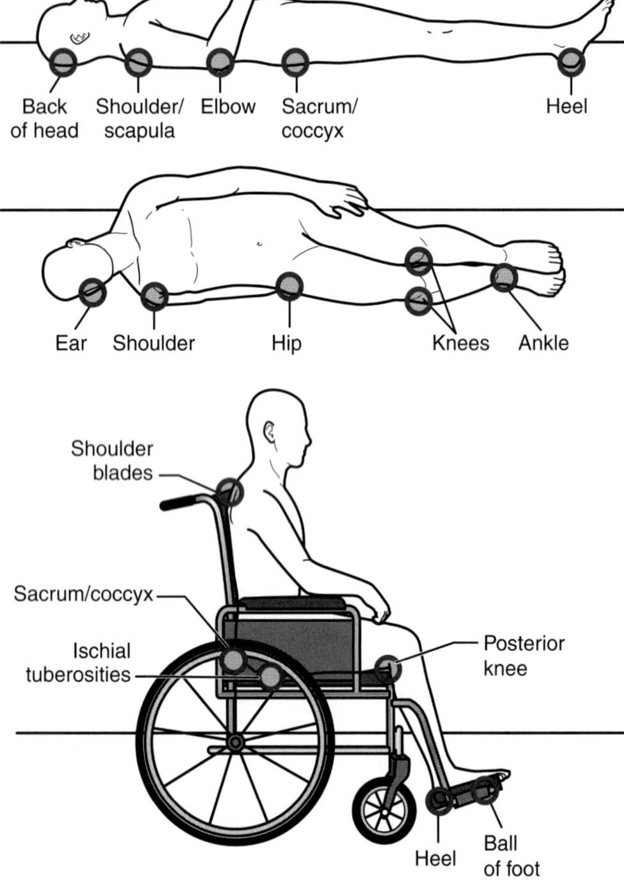

FIGURE 8-7. Bony prominences at risk for pressure injuries.

perfusion, comorbidities, and condition of the soft tissue."[32] This advisory panel also offered prevention guidelines, some of which are as follows:[33]

- Inspect skin at least daily for signs of pressure injury, especially nonblanchable redness over body points, such as the sacrum, coccyx, buttocks, heels, ischium, trochanters, scapulae, elbows, and areas beneath medical devices.
- When inspecting darkly pigmented skin, look for changes in skin tone, skin temperature, and tissue consistency compared with adjacent skin. Moistening the skin assists in identifying changes in color.
- Cleanse the skin promptly after episodes of incontinence, using skin cleansers that are pH balanced for skin.
- Use skin moisturizers daily on dry skin.
- Avoid positioning an individual on an area of erythema (reddening of the skin) or pressure injury.
- Refer to a registered dietitian all individuals at risk for pressure injury resulting from malnutrition.
- Encourage all individuals at risk for pressure injury to consume adequate fluids and a balanced diet.
- Use heel offloading devices (pressure relieving heel protectors, heel floats) for individuals at high-risk for heel ulcers.
- Use a pressure redistributing chair cushion for individuals sitting for prolonged periods in chairs or wheelchairs.
- Reposition weak or immobile individuals in chairs on an hourly basis.
- Choose a frequency for turning and repositioning based on the support surface in use, the tolerance of skin for pressure, and the individual's preferences.
- Teach the client and family about the risk for pressure injury.
- Engage the client and family in risk reduction interventions.

A pressure injury can develop in as short as 30 minutes after high pressure is exerted on a small area. Increased pressure over short periods and slight pressure for long periods have been shown to cause equal damage.

Stages of Pressure Injuries

The stages of pressure injuries were updated by the NPUAP in 2016; Table 8-10 presents the current definitions.

Note that some wounds are unstageable and their depth is unknown. The base of the pressure injury is generally covered by slough (yellow, tan, gray, green, or brown fibrinous tissue) and/or eschar (tan, brown, or black dead tissue) in the wound. Until enough slough or eschar is removed to expose the base of the pressure wound, the true depth and, therefore, the stage cannot be determined. Stable (dry, adherent, intact without erythema seen or fluid felt) eschar on the heels serves as the body's natural biological cover and should not be removed. Some wounds can be a suspected deep tissue

TECHNOLOGY AND TRENDS

Computer tablets (e.g., iPads®) can be used to evaluate and treat coordination disorders. In addition to being used for documentation, numerous applications (apps) are available that can be used to evaluate or address a wide range of concerns. Some examples include Dexteria and Cut the Buttons for fine motor skills, Dots and P.O.V. for visual perceptual skills, and iOT Session, which addresses a variety of areas, such as fine motor and visual perceptual skills. Other apps are available for work on cognition, such as BrainBaseline. Seeing the client interact with the tablet and his or her ability to touch specific areas on the tablet screen can be an engaging and functional way for the OT practitioner to observe and address motor deficits and other coordination and movement disorders. The OT practitioner can often use the results of a client's performance on an app to document progress; some apps even allow the OT practitioner to send out performance results via email. OT practitioners may also give exercises to clients who have computer tablets, and the OT practitioners can follow along with an app, such as PT and OT Helper, and other activities to do at home as part of therapy intervention.

TABLE 8-10 Stages of Wounds or Pressure Injuries[10]

STAGE	SYMPTOMS	
Stage 1 Nonblanchable erythema of intact skin	Intact skin with a localized area of nonblanchable erythema (redness), which may appear differently in darkly pigmented skin. Presence of blanchable erythema or changes in sensation, temperature, or firmness may come before visual changes.	Epidermis Dermis Fat Muscle Bone Stage I
Stage 2 Partial-thickness skin loss with exposed dermis	The wound is viable, pink or red, moist, and may also present as an intact or ruptured fluid-filled blister. Adipose (fat) is not visible and deeper tissues are not visible. Granulation tissue (tissue which fills in wounds), slough (a type of dead tissue which is usually white, gray or yellow) and eschar (dead tissue) are not present. These injuries commonly result from adverse microclimate (excess moisture) and shear in the skin over the pelvis and shear in the heel.	Epidermis Dermis Fat Muscle Bone Stage II
Stage 3 Full-thickness skin loss	Full-thickness loss of skin, in which adipose is visible in the ulcer and granulation tissue and epibole (rolled wound edges) are often present. Slough and/or eschar may be visible. Tissue depth damage varies by anatomical location; areas of significant fat tissue can develop deep wounds. Undermining (small opening for a larger wound) and tunneling (narrow passageway of dead space) may occur. Fascia, muscle, tendon, ligament, cartilage and/or bone are not exposed.	Epidermis Dermis Fat Muscle Bone Stage III
Stage 4 Full-thickness skin and tissue loss	Full-thickness skin and tissue loss with exposed or directly palpable fascia, muscle, tendon, ligament, cartilage or bone in the ulcer. Slough and/or eschar may be visible. Epibole, undermining, and/or tunneling often occur. Depth varies by location on body. If slough or eschar obscures the extent of tissue loss this is an Unstageable Pressure Injury.	Epidermis Dermis Fat Muscle Bone Stage IV

injury where the depth is unknown. In this case, one would see a purple- or maroon-colored localized area or discolored, intact skin; or a blood-filled blister caused by damage of underlying soft tissue from pressure and/or shear may be seen. The area may be covered in tissue that is painful, firm, mushy, boggy, and warmer or cooler compared with adjacent tissue.[34]

Healing

The wound healing process generally has four stages, some of which can be modified by the healing factors listed in Table 8-11, and each of these stages can be influenced by medical professionals during repair and then again by wound care after repair. Some current references use three stages of wound healing, however this textbook will use four throughout. The four stages include the following.[35]

STAGE 1: HEMOSTASIS

Immediately after injury, the tissue responds by contracting, the vessels constrict, and coagulation begins, leading to hemostasis (a stopping of blood flow). This generally lasts for about 6 hours.

STAGE 2: INFLAMMATION

Cytokines (secretions by cells in the immune system) and other chemicals are released, attracting inflammatory cells to the area, at the highest concentration at about 24 hours after the injury. Around this time, macrophages begin to migrate to the wound, peaking by day 5. These cells ingest cellular debris and also aid in activation of fibroblasts (which produce collagen) and promote collagen formation.

STAGE 3: REPLICATION AND PROLIFERATION

Simultaneously, the process of reepithelialization is occurring, and this helps sustain the growing tissue by increasing blood flow to the wound. Fibroblasts, with support from macrophages, are already forming collagen, with the process accelerated by the proliferation of new blood vessels providing oxygen and nutrients to the wound. This phase is characterized by less inflammation.

STAGE 4: TISSUE REMODELING/SYNTHESIS OR RESOLUTION

The wound then begins to contract during a process called *remodeling*, or *maturation*, which continues for several months or longer.

TABLE 8-11 Wound Healing Factors[3]

MODIFIABLE FACTORS	NONMODIFIABLE FACTORS
Stress	Oxygenation
Nutrition	Infection
Obesity	Venous insufficiency
Diabetes	Foreign substance or body
Medications, chemotherapy, steroids	Age
Alcoholism	Gender
Smoking	Immunocompromised conditions—cancer, radiation therapy, acquired immunodeficiency syndrome (AIDS)
Sex hormones	Ischemia (restriction in blood supply to tissues)
	Diseases: keloids, fibrosis, jaundice, uremia

Certainly, as part of the multidisciplinary team, the OTA would educate the client on those factors which may be modifiable, such as weight management, skin and body hygiene, diabetes management, and stress management. Wound/injury healing is a very common problem made worse by these complications. Clients may be treated for their wounds in the home setting by home health nursing and/or at a specialized wound clinic. Generally, the OTA is not cleaning and dressing the wound(s), although he or she may provide education on following precautions and on issues with bathing and toileting, to avoid making the wound worse. The client may need the OTA to advocate for setting up an evaluation for changes in mobility equipment, assistance with ordering the correct hospital bed mattress or padded commode seat, and education and training on safe transfers with a transfer board to avoid shear. The OTA can offer such options as a flexible handle inspection mirror for clients to check areas on the buttocks, feet, or back.

Some pressure injuries at stage 1 require simple moisture barrier cream and decreased pressure over the area for a day or two to heal. As the staging progresses, the injury requires a variety of plain and medicated dressings, medicated creams, and manual or surgical debridement to remove dead tissue. In more serious wounds or injuries, a skin graft may be required. A skin graft is the removal of a partial- or full-thickness segment of epidermis and dermis from its blood supply and transplanting it to another site, in this case the wound or injury site, to speed up healing and reduce the risk of infection.[34] Grafting is often done to treat burns and skin removal wounds.

Some clients with severe pressure injuries to bone, such as seen with spinal cord injury, may require flap surgery. The flap is a surgical relocation of skin and underlying muscle tissue from a nearby donor site on the client to repair a wound and is often used in stage 4 pressure injuries. The surgery involves cutting out the pressure injury (typically severe or nonhealing) and any underlying dead tissue or bone. The flap of nearby muscle helps cushion bony areas and maintain blood flow to the area.

Prevention Issues

Prevention of a wound or pressure injury long before it begins is infinitely easier than managing the painful, expensive, and extended healing process. Even long after a wound or injury has healed, the skin over the site remains more vulnerable to a recurrence compared with the skin in other areas. The OTA must collaborate with numerous team members with regard to wound and pressure injury prevention. This includes collaborating with nurses and caregivers about a rolling and turning schedule for clients who are in a bed; the wheelchair evaluator about a pressure-relieving cushion and pressure management features on the power wheelchair; the dietitian about options for increasing caloric, protein, and fluid intake for clients with swallowing issues; and caregivers about reminders for clients with memory deficits to perform pressure relief. At times, the wheelchair cushion is blamed for a pressure injury without careful observation of other places where pressure could be occurring. For example, a recliner lift chair, a hard plastic bedside commode, a shower seat, or a worn hospital bed mattress could also be contributing factors. The OTA is the perfect professional to assist with holistic management of all of these areas, with a focus on the proper equipment, education, schedule, and routine for pressure relief.

Adaptive equipment, such as a flexible mirror for skin inspection, a long-handled toe sponge for more effective cleaning between toes, a reacher or dressing stick for easier drying, and positioning boots to keep heels off the bed at night, may assist with wound prevention and management. Hospital beds can have either group 1 overlays added to the top of the standard mattress when the client is at significant risk for skin breakdown or group 2 replacement mattress systems (generally low air loss) for the client who already has two or more stage 2 injuries on the trunk or pelvis, or one or more stage 3 or stage 4 injuries on the trunk or pelvis. Group 3 air-fluidized mattresses can be used with more severe injuries as well. Medicare and insurances have specific requirements for each group. A variety of options in the type of product may be available for each grouping, so the OTA should work with an equipment supplier or manufacturer to learn about and trial options.

Chapter 15 presents many options for wheelchair cushions, many of which are effective with pressure relief. The challenge is that even with the most amazing cushioning, unrelieved pressure can still cause issues over time. When the pressure is not relieved through tilt or recline in the wheelchair, by standing or by rolling onto the side in bed, skin does not get a chance to reoxygenate at the capillary level. The pressure injury occurs when these vessels collapse under the external pressure and blood supply to the cells is cut off, limiting oxygen supply, decreasing nutrients to the cells, and decreasing removal of waste products.

Certain factors can lead to earlier and quicker development of a pressure injury if not properly managed; these may include the following:[34]

1. **Nutrition:** Inadequate nutrition is a major risk factor associated with the development of pressure injuries. Clients must receive adequate nutrients to reduce the risk of developing pressure injuries and to support healing. This may include caloric intake, fluids, and extra protein for healing. Collaboration with speech language pathologists, dietitians, nurses, and doctors may be needed. Some diseases are hypermetabolic, and the client may experience difficulty getting adequate nutrition. Swallowing, other weakness deficits, and difficulty with self-feeding can also be factors.
2. **Tissue perfusion (adequate blood flow), and oxygenation:** Tissue damage occurs when cells are deprived of oxygen and nutrients for a period. Clients must have periods of off-loading of bony prominences to keep skin healthy. A regular cycle of pressure relief is important, and alarms and other devices may be needed to establish a habit.
3. **Moisture/Maceration: Maceration** is the pronged exposure of skin to moisture, which softens the surrounding skin, causing superficial erosion of the epidermis. Primary sources of skin moisture include perspiration, urine, feces, and drainage from wounds. Encouraging clients to check all of their skin at least once a day is extremely important, especially areas with decreased or no sensation. Areas of skin folds can also be vulnerable. A focus on hygiene and a safe way for clients and caregivers to clean efficiently and effectively may be needed.
4. **Friction:** Friction is a mechanical force that occurs when two surfaces rub together, often when skin moves across a coarse surface. Generally, creating resistance between skin and the contact surface leads to friction problems. At times, this type of superficial injury is seen on bony prominences as a result of repositioning, dragging the buttocks over a wheelchair tire during a transfer, or a brace causing a blister. Removing the source of the friction is the first step, followed by problem-solving and educating all concerned about how to avoid the problem in the future.
5. **Shear:** Shear force is generated by the motion of bone and subcutaneous tissue relative to skin, which is restrained from moving because of frictional forces (e.g., when a seated client slides down a chair, when a transfer board is used, or when the head of a bed is raised by more than 30 degrees). The outer layers of skin (the epidermis and the dermis) remain stationary, whereas the deep fascia moves with the skeleton, causing a decrease in blood flow to skin and eventually leading to skin breakdown. Shear is not generally seen on the surface of skin but builds up over time as the vessels are damaged.

PAIN ASSESSMENT AND MANAGEMENT

Pain is a highly subjective, negative sensory and emotional experience, which can be the result of actual or impending damage to body structures.[36] Pain can be associated with nociceptive (sensory) and neuropathic (nerve) problems. According to the National Initiative on Pain Control (NIPC™), more than half of all Americans experience chronic or recurrent pain.[37] Understanding and assessing a client's pain is crucial to appropriate management. The presence or absence of pain must be documented for every client participating in OT.

Pain Assessment

Assessing a client's pain involves more than simply asking the client to rate his or her pain on a scale of 1 to 10. Although that method is certainly valuable, additional considerations can help the OT practitioner identify the source and cause of pain. The NIPC™ suggests using different assessment tools to determine the severity and type of pain a client experiences. The Wong-Baker FACES Pain Rating Scale is series of six faces drawn to show a happy, smiling face (1, no hurt) to the end range of a sad face with tears flowing (6, hurts worst). The client is asked to identify which face most closely relates to how he or she is feeling. The Wong-Baker scale may be used with clients aged 3 years and over and certainly may be appropriate for adults. The Numeric Rating Scale is presented visually as a horizontal line with short vertical lines for each number, 0 (no pain) through 10 (the absolute worst possible pain). The client can look at the scale and either mark a line or provide a verbal answer. The McGill Pain Questionnaire consists of a full-body, side-by-side, dorsal and volar drawing, and the client is asked to mark on the drawing exactly where he or she feels the pain, with "E" if external, "I" if internal, or "EI" if both. The Pain Quality Assessment Scale (PQAS) is a 20-item assessment that measures the quality (type) and intensity of pain with all types of pain. The PQAS uses descriptive words to identify the type of pain, including "tender, numb, electrical, tingling, radiating, throbbing, aching, shooting, cramping, and heavy."[38] The scale is a printed document with instructions to the client to rate the severity of pain and the type of pain he or she has experienced in the prior week, with each of the first 19 items using a numeric scale of 0 to 10. Item 20 includes the time component of pain, such as intermittent, variable, or stable. Even if a practitioner does not use the formal PQAS, asking the client to describe the pain in descriptive terminology helps explain the source of pain. For example, if a client feels "achy" pain in a muscle, it may have been caused by overuse, perhaps from too much exertion in their home exercise program. The practitioner can educate the client on the pain source, help alleviate fear, and re-adjust the client's activity recommendations, if needed. In addition, if a client expresses a new experience of a "sharp, stabbing pain" the OTA may need to notify the occupational therapist of the change in the client's status and together determine whether to notify the referring physician.

Pain Management

Pain management is sometimes a complicated task and, depending on the source and cause of pain, often involves additional healthcare team members, such as the physician, nurse, family member or caregiver, psychologist/psychiatrist, specialty pain clinic staff, physical therapist, and physical therapist assistant. When the client is in a hospital or inpatient rehabilitation center, there may be a standing order for medication to manage pain. The OT practitioner would be wise to coordinate therapy sessions shortly after the pain medications have been administered by the nurse. A client experiencing pain may not be able to make the best effort for performing needed therapy and thus may not progress as well toward the desired outcomes.

The American Occupational Therapy Association (AOTA) publishes a fact sheet for the OT practitioner to provide guidance on chronic pain management. Some of the educational options for the OTA that the AOTA recommends include the following:[39]

- Proactive pain control: Clients are taught to be proactive about pain management, using pain control modalities on a regular basis (e.g., heat or cold) to keep baseline pain levels lower. This allows for better participation in daily activities.
- Safe body mechanics and ergonomics: Clients are given instruction in safe body mechanics, with opportunities to practice and receive feedback. The OTA assesses and modifies any environmental factors that may be contributing to pain, such as computer monitor height in the case of neck pain. Clients learn to reduce strain and perform all occupations safely.
- Muscle tension reduction training: The OTA would educate and train the client in muscle relaxation strategies and techniques to calm the mind. This will potentially reduce pain levels.
- Communication skills training: Because chronic pain is an invisible disability, the OTA can teach assertive behavior (e.g., saying "no," explaining needs) to enable clients to manage their disability as well as appropriately communicate with the people around them.
- Proactive problem-solving: Clients can learn to anticipate potential problems with activities and plan for challenges proactively. This can increase opportunities for participating in desired activities for a client living with chronic pain.
- Pacing activities: The OTA can teach clients to pace the activities they perform routinely, for example, by taking breaks, changing the way an activity is done, or asking for help.
- A healthy lifestyle: Educate and/or train the client on physical movements, including home exercise programs, daily relaxation and medications, and health eating and weight management.

Pain management can be difficult and have a significant impact on occupational performance, and clients may have pain as a primary or a secondary diagnosis. The OTA has the opportunity to have a real impact on pain management and help clients work through their pain to maintain function.

SUMMARY

Understanding the impact that movement patterns, tone, primitive reflexes, sensation, wounds, pressure, and pain can have on a client's daily functioning and occupational engagement is essential for the OT practitioner. Immobility and the inability to effectively perform pressure relief because of these factors can cause pain as well as pressure injuries. The practitioner must address any deficits and work on integrating primitive reflexes and normalizing tone and sensation if a client exhibits dysfunction in any of these areas. Rehabilitation, if possible, along with compensation will be important, as will be educating and training the client and caregivers how to manage the consequences of each of these impairments.

REVIEW QUESTIONS

1. The client complains that she has trouble locating items in her purse without dumping everything out. Which of the following does the OTA suspect she has difficulty with?
   a. Temperature discrimination
   b. Two-point discrimination
   c. Stereognosis
   d. Proprioception
2. The client with a brain injury is exhibiting the ATNR reflex. Which of the following is the client *most likely* to experience?
   a. Trouble looking down at the sink while grooming
   b. Trouble looking ahead at obstacles in front of him with wheelchair use
   c. Trouble bringing the spoon to his mouth
   d. Trouble getting dressed
3. A client says that she tripped over a curb and injured her wrist because she put her arms out to break the fall. Which of the following did she exhibit?
   a. Equilibrium reactions
   b. Protective reactions
   c. Righting reactions
   d. Primitive reactions
4. The OTA is working with a client who has Parkinson's disease. She asks him to reach for a cup and observes that he begins to have tremors during the task. Which of the following is he exhibiting?
   a. Resting tremors
   b. Rolling tremors
   c. Intention tremors
   d. Reaching tremors

5. A client who has been attending outpatient hand therapy states she has had increasing pain in her right arm. Which three of the following options would be *most appropriate* for the OTA to do?
   a. Notify the client's physician.
   b. Discuss the client's increased pain with the occupational therapist.
   c. Use the Numeric Rating Scale to assess pain.
   d. Only tell the client that pain is expected to occur during recovery.
   e. Ask the client to describe the type and timing of pain.
   f. Ask the client to keep a pain log.
6. The OTA is assessing the client's elbow flexion strength. When he releases his hold on the client's arm, it goes back toward the client's face. Which of the following is the client exhibiting?
   a. Rebound phenomenon
   b. Tics
   c. Motor impersistence
   d. Chorea
7. The OTA is going to assess a client's sensation. Which three of the following should he or she do?
   a. Demonstrate the assessment on self.
   b. Demonstrate the assessment on the client's unaffected side with his or her eyes open.
   c. Demonstrate the assessment on the client's unaffected side with his or her eyes closed.
   d. Perform the assessment on the client's affected side with his or her eyes open.
   e. Perform the assessment on the client's affected side with his or her eyes closed.
   f. Demonstrate the assessment on the client's face first to show him or her the correct feeling.
8. The elderly client has a stage 2 pressure injury on her right buttock, a stage 1 on the back of her head, and a stage 1 on her heel. The nurse manager has asked the team to reassess the manual wheelchair for pressure relief options. What other factor is *most likely* the culprit of these three injuries?
   a. The air-fluidized bed
   b. The standard bed mattress/pillow
   c. The commode
   d. The shower chair
9. Which three of the following might the OTA use to facilitate tone in a client after a CVA?
   a. Orthotics
   b. Quick stretch
   c. Thermotherapy
   d. Weight-bearing
   e. Electrical stimulation
   f. Casting
10. The client with chronic pain cannot take any more pain medications, and she is feeling disempowered and depressed about her lack of ability to care for herself and her home because of pain. After education about the pain process and goal setting, how might the OTA assist the client with pain management?
    a. Teach how to adapt and pace activities.
    b. Teach the use of heat or cold after pain occurs.
    c. Teach an aerobic exercise program.
    d. Teach to avoid all activities that might cause pain.

CASE STUDY

Mr. Young, a 65-year-old African American male, has come to the hospital for an above-the-knee amputation as a result of complications from insulin-dependent diabetes (type 2 diabetes). He lives with his spouse, who is unable to assist with any ADLs or functional mobility tasks because of her own medical complications. Mr. Young has children who live out of state. Although his children can provide some financial assistance, they are unable to provide physical assistance. When the occupational therapist evaluates client factors, she discovers that he has peripheral neuropathy in his upper extremities (UE) and left lower extremity. He has functional UE ROM and 3+/5 BUE strength.

Mr. Young is a retired minister and hopes to return to ministry on a voluntary basis. His goals also include becoming independent with ADLs and functional mobility tasks at the wheelchair level.

1. What kind of sensory, gross or fine motor coordination, and tone assessments might the OTA conduct to determine how best to proceed with Mr. Young and to develop intervention strategies to assist him with achieving his goals?
2. How might Mr. Young's functional mobility and occupation be impacted by his amputation and diabetes?

PUTTING IT ALL TOGETHER — Sample Treatment Session and Documentation

Setting	Acute care
Client Profile	Mr. E is a 72-year-old male admitted to acute care 3 days ago for complications related to Parkinson's disease, including increased frequency of intention tremors, increasing cogwheel rigidity, and decreased balance. He was diagnosed with Parkinson's disease 15 years ago and had been independent with ADLs before admission. New stage 2 wound on right buttock from pressure and immobility, which does cause him burning pain at 4/10 level.
Work History	Mr. E is a retired naval officer and a mechanical engineer. He retired 10 years ago because of complications from Parkinson's disease.
Insurance	Medicare and Veteran's Administration Benefits
Psychological	Mild depression but overall in good spirits; exhibits a flat affect
Social	Married to a supportive spouse who is also retired. They have one daughter, who lives in town and assists client and his spouse as much as possible, and one son who is in the Navy and frequently out at sea. Spouse can provide setup and supervision for ADLs, but she is not able to provide physical assistance.

Continued

PUTTING IT ALL TOGETHER Sample Treatment Session and Documentation (continued)

Cognitive	Mild short-term memory impairment, long-term memory within functional limits
Motor & Manual Muscle Testing (MMT)	Moderate cogwheel rigidity in BUE PROM BUE is WFL RUE AROM: Shoulder flexion is 150 degrees; elbow flexion is 100 degrees; wrist flexion is 65 degrees; wrist extension is 50 degrees; finger flexion is 50 degrees; finger extension is 30 degrees LUE AROM: Shoulder flexion is 145 degrees; elbow flexion is 105 degrees; wrist flexion is 65 degrees; wrist extension is 50 degrees; finger flexion is 55 degrees; finger extension is 30 degrees MMT B Shoulders: 3+/5 MMT B Elbow Flexion: 3/5 MMT Wrist Flexion/Extension and Finger Flexion/Extension: Not tested because of tremors BLE ROM and MMT WFL: Ambulates with minimal assistance for balance and safety Client exhibits difficulty initiating and coordinating movements for functional activities Sensory evaluation revealed decreased proprioception and sharp/dull recognition
ADL	Mod A bathing while sitting on shower chair; Min A UE dressing sitting on edge of bed;, Mod A LE dressing sitting on edge of bed; difficulty manipulating buttons and zippers Setup for eating meals, including opening containers and cutting food
IADL	Not evaluated, completed by spouse before admission because of safety issues, including decreased cognition, balance, and safety awareness
Goals	Within 4 weeks: 1. Client will progress to modified independent with bathing and dressing, using adapted equipment, as needed 2. Client will increase fine motor skills for ADLs, as evidenced by being able to independently button five small buttons on a dress shirt within 30 seconds and cut soft meat with a knife 3. Client and spouse will assist client to increase AROM B shoulders to 170 degrees 4. Client and spouse will demonstrate and verbalize understanding of three strategies to assist with managing intention tremors 5. Client and spouse will demonstrate and verbalize understanding of three compensatory strategies for decreased proprioception and sensation to increase safety during ADLs and functional mobility tasks 6. Client and spouse will demonstrate and verbalize understanding of pressure relief and injury prevention and management

OT TREATMENT SESSION 1

THERAPEUTIC ACTIVITY	TIME	GOAL(S) ADDRESSED	OTA RATIONALE
UE PROM/AROM stretching	5 min	#3	*Preparatory Task; Education and Training:* Provided UE PROM and engaged client in UE AROM to loosen client's joints and muscles for ADLs and to provide suggestions on AROM exercises client can do in-between therapy sessions to increase ROM for ADLs
ADLs: Showering using hospital room's walk-in shower and shower chair; dressing sitting in wheelchair Provided education on shower chair/tub transfer bench, button hooks, long handled sponges, and reachers	45 min	#1 and #2	*Occupations; Education and Training:* Education and training for ADL Safety and on adaptive equipment
Provided client education on using weighted devices for ADLs and importance of weight-bearing activities to increase proprioceptive input	5 min	#4 and #5	*Preparatory Task; Education and Training:* Client education for strategies to increase independence and safety with ADLs

PUTTING IT ALL TOGETHER Sample Treatment Session and Documentation (continued)

SOAP note: 9/6/—, 9:00 am–9:55 am

S: "I would like to be able to dress and bathe myself—it's embarrassing having to ask for help."

O: Client performed PROM BUE exercises in all planes (10 each), PROM WFL; had client complete 10 AROM exercises each of the following to his maximal range: Shoulder flexion/extension (flexion L 155 degrees, R 145 degrees); Elbow flexion/extension (flexion R/L 100 degrees); Wrist flexion/extension (flexion R 65 degrees, L 70 degrees; extension R 50 degrees, L 50 degrees)—Education provided on doing exercises on his own one to two times a day, 10 reps each, to maintain and increase UE ROM for ADLs; Client verbalized and demonstrated understanding. Performed bathing tasks sitting on shower chair with Mod A, mostly for LE and perineal care; dressed sitting in wheelchair with Min A to don t-shirt and Mod A for donning underwear, jeans, socks, and shoes. Education provided on shower chairs/tub-transfer benches, reachers, button hooks, and long handled sponges for increased ADL safety and independence. Provided education on engaging in weight-bearing activities to increase proprioception for ADL safety and independence, including placing one hand on sink when brushing teeth, and the potential benefits of using weighted utensils and devices for ADLs to help decrease tremors during ADLs

A: Client had difficulty coordinating movements to don clothing; because of intention tremors, sensation, and decreased ROM, client is exhibiting decreased independence and safety with ADLs; would likely benefit from practice and continued education and training on adaptive equipment for ADLs and education and training on ways to increase proprioception and manage tremors.

P: Will continue to see client three to five times a week while in the hospital to work on increasing safety and independence with ADLs using adaptive equipment, as needed, pressure relief and injury management, and providing client/family education and training on ways to manage and compensate for tremors and decreased sensation; client may benefit from inpatient rehab, depending on progress

Elizabeth Jacobsen, COTA 9/6/—, 3:30 pm

TREATMENT SESSION 2

What could you do next with this client?

TREATMENT SESSION 3

What could you do next with this client?

REFERENCES

1. Neggers, S. F. W., & Bekkering, H. (2002). Coordinated control of eye and hand movements in dynamic reaching. *Human Movement Science, 21*, 349–376.
2. Pelz, J., Hayhoe, M., & Loeber, R. (2001). The coordination of eye, head, and hand movements in a natural task. *Experimental Brain Research, 139*, 266–277.
3. Gutman, S. (2017). *Quick reference neuroscience for rehabilitation professionals: The essential neurologic principles underlying rehabilitation practice* (3rd ed.). Thorofare, NJ: Slack Incorporated.
4. Gutman, S., & Schonfeld, A. (2009). *Screening adult neurological populations: A step-by-step instruction manual* (2nd ed.). Bethesda, MD: AOTA Press.
5. McHugh Pendleton, H., & Schulz-Krohn, W. (eds.). (2013). *Pedretti's occupational therapy: Practice skills for physical dysfunction* (7th ed.). St. Louis, MO: Mosby Elsevier.
6. Cloud, L. J., & Jinnah, H. A. (2010). Treatment strategies for dystonia. *Expert Opinion on Pharmacotherapy, 11*(1), 6–15. doi:10.1517/14656560903426171
7. Mainzer, K. (2012). Managing ET with occupational therapy. *International Essential Tremor Foundation.* Retrieved from www.essentialtremor.org/wp-content/uploads/2013/10/Managing-ET-with-occupational-therapy.pdf
8. Hawes, F., Billups, C., & Forwell, S. (2010). Interventions for upper-limb intention tremor in multiple sclerosis: A feasibility study. *International Journal of MS Care, 12*, 122–132.
9. Doyle S., Bennett S., Fasoli S. E., & McKenna K. T. (2010). Interventions for sensory impairment in the upper limb after stroke. *Cochrane Database of Systematic Reviews, 6*, CD006331. doi:10.1002/14651858.CD006331.pub2
10. Nolano, M., Provitera, V., Estraneo, A., Selim, M., Caporaso, G., Stancanelli, A.,... & Santorob, L. (2008). Sensory deficit in Parkinson's disease: Evidence of a cutaneous denervation. *Brain: A Journal of Neurology, 131*(7), 1903–1911. http://dx.doi.org/10.1093/brain/awn102
11. Vining Radomski, M., & Trombly Latham, C. (eds.). (2014). *Occupational therapy for physical dysfunction* (7th ed.). Baltimore, MD: Lippincott Williams & Wilkins.
12. Schabrun, S. M., & Hillier, S. (2009). Evidence for the retraining of sensation after stroke: A systematic review. *Clinical Rehabilitation, 23*, 27–39.
13. Schott, J. M., & Rossor, M. N. (2003). The grasp and other primitive reflexes. *Journal of Neurology, Neurosurgery, & Psychiatry, 74*, 558–560. doi:10.1136/jnnp.74.5.558
14. Futagi, Y., Toribe, Y., & Suzuki, Y. (2012). The grasp reflex and Moro reflex in infants: Hierarchy of primitive reflex responses. *International Journal of Pediatrics, 2012*, 191562. doi:10.1155/2012/191562.
15. Fiorentino, M. (1973). *Reflex testing methods for evaluating CNS development* (2nd ed.). Springfield, IL: Charles C. Thomas.
16. Malhotra, S., Pandyan, A. D., Day, C. R., Jones, P. W., & Hermens, H. (2009). Spasticity, an impairment that is poorly defined and poorly measured. *Clinical Rehabilitation, 23*(7), 651–658.
17. Bohannon, R. W., & Smith, M. B. (1987). Interrater reliability of a modified Ashworth scale of muscle spasticity. *Physical Therapy, 67*(2), 206–207.
18. Paulis, W., Horemans, H., Brouwer, B., & Stam, H. (2011). Excellent test–retest and inter-rater reliability for Tardieu Scale measurements with inertial sensors in elbow flexors of stroke patients. *Gait & Posture, 33*(2), 185–189. doi:10.1016/j.gaitpost.2010.10.094
19. Behrman, A. L., & Harkema, S. J. (2007). Physical rehabilitation as an agent for recovery after spinal cord injury. *Physical Medicine and Rehabilitation Clinics of North America, 18*, 183–202.
20. Lumen. (n.d.). Phases of aging: The young-old, middle-old, and old-old. Retrieved from https://lumen.instructure.com/courses/199939/pages/Section13-4?module_item_id=4575415

21. American Psychological Association. (2016). Older adults' health and age-related changes: Reality versus myth. Retrieved from www.apa.org
22. Chapman, S. B., Aslan, S., Spence, J. S., DeFina, L. F., Keebler, M. W., Didehbani, N., & Lu, H. (2013). Shorter term aerobic exercise improves brain, cognition and cardiovascular fitness in aging. *Frontiers of Aging Neuroscience.* Retrieved from https://doi.org/10.3389/fnagi.2013.00075
23. Guo, S., & DiPietro, L. A. (2010). Factors affecting wound healing. *Journal of Dental Research, 89*(3), 219–229. Retrieved from http://doi.org/10.1177/0022034509359125
24. Pressure Injury Prevention and Management. (2012). Retrieved from www.rch.org.au
25. Sen, C. K., Gordillo, G.M., Roy, S., Kirsner, R., Lambert, L., Hunt, T. K., ... & Longaker, M. T. (2009). Human skin wounds: A major and snowballing threat to public health and the economy. *Wound Repair and Regeneration, 17*(6), 763–771.
26. Posnett, J., Gottrup, F., Lundgren, H., & Saal G. (2009). The burden of chronic wounds in Europe. *Journal of Wound Care, 18*(4), 154–161.
27. Moro, M. L., Morsillo, F., Tangenti, M., Mongardi, M., Pirazzini, M. C., & Ragni, P. (2005). Rates of surgical-site infection: An international comparison. *Infection Control and Hospital Epidemiology, 26*, 442–448.
28. Harker, J. (2006). Wound healing complications associated with lower limb amputation. Retrieved from www.worldwidewounds.com
29. Ray, R. L. (2000). Complications of lower extremity amputations. *Topics in Emergency Medicine, 22*(3), 35–42.
30. Collins, L., & Seraj, S. (2010). Diagnosis and treatment of venous ulcers. *American Family Physician,* 81(8), 989-96.
31. Mehmood, N., Hariz, A., Fitridge, R., & Voelcker, N. H. (2013). Applications of modern sensors and wireless technology in effective wound management. *Journal of Biomedical Materials Research, 102*(4), 885–895.
32. NPUAP Pressure Injury Stages. (2016). Retrieved from www.npuap.org
33. Pressure Injury Prevention Points. (2016). Retrieved from www.npuap.org
34. Pressure Injury Prevention and Management. (2012). Retrieved from www.rch.org.au
35. Notley, D. A., Martin, D. R., & Hill, M. (2015). Evaluation and management of traumatic wounds. Trauma reports. Retrieved from www.ahcmedia.com
36. Fink, R. (2000). Pain assessment: The cornerstone to optimal pain management. *Proceedings (Baylor University Medical Center), 13*(3), 236–239.
37. National Initiative on Pain Control. (n.d.). Pain control initiative. Retrieved from https://www.painedu.org/nicp.asp
38. Pain Focus. (n.d.). Pain assessment scales. Retrieved from pain-focus.com/hcp/tools/pain-assessment-scales/
39. Occupational Therapy and Pain Rehabilitation. (2014). Fact sheet. American Occupational Therapy Association. Retrieved from www.aota.org

Chapter 9

Muscle Strength: Assessment and Management

Sanchala Khanolkar Sen, MSc, OTR/L, BCPR

LEARNING OUTCOMES

After studying this chapter, the student or practitioner will be able to:

9.1 List the causes of muscle weakness

9.2 Describe screening tests for muscle strength assessment

9.3 Define muscle grades by number, name, and letter

9.4 Administer manual muscle testing in various ways, depending on client needs

9.5 Describe how the assessment results can be used for intervention planning

KEY TERMS

Against gravity
Agonist
Antagonist
Concentric contraction
DeLorme's method of progressive resistive exercise (PRE)
Eccentric contraction
Gravity
Gravity-minimized (-eliminated, -lessened, -reduced)
Isometric muscle contraction
Isotonic muscle contraction
Manual muscle testing (MMT)
Muscle coordination
Muscle endurance
Muscle grade
Muscle strength
Resistance
Substitutions

The human body is able to perform tasks based on the intricate interaction of range of motion (ROM), motor control, and muscle strength. Many physical disabilities cause muscle weakness. Slight to substantial limitations of performance in occupations, such as bringing food to one's mouth, taking a bath, getting dressed, getting in and out of bed, obtaining items from a shelf or a grocery cart, and lifting a child, can result from loss of strength, depending on the degree of weakness and whether the weakness is temporary or permanent. If improvement is expected, the occupational therapy (OT) practitioner must assess the muscle weakness and plan an intervention that will increase strength and enable occupational performance.[1] Even if the weakness is permanent, knowing the strength of each muscle group will drive critical thinking about adaptations and adaptive equipment to increase functional abilities.

MANUAL MUSCLE TESTING TERMINOLOGY

Muscle strength is the maximal amount of tension or force that a muscle or muscle group can voluntarily exert in one maximal effort, when type of muscle contraction, limb velocity, and joint angle are specified.[2] In everyday language, it means the force that a muscle can produce against resistance. Types of muscle contraction include the following:

- **Isometric muscle contraction,** or static contraction, occurs when tension is developed in the muscle but no movement occurs and muscle length does not change. For example, a static contraction occurs when one squeezes a jar lid even tighter when opening it. No real motion occurs, yet one will feel the muscle contract more firmly.
- **Isotonic muscle contraction** occurs when the muscle length and the joint angle change when a muscle contracts. The muscle develops constant tension against a load or resistance. For example, when performing a bicep curl with a weight in the hand, one will feel the biceps contract and see the elbow joint

move. An isotonic contraction can be subdivided into concentric and eccentric contractions.

- **Concentric contraction** occurs when the muscles shorten and the muscle attachments (origin and insertion) move toward each other when there is joint movement. For example, picking up the weight in a biceps curl is an example of a concentric contraction of the biceps muscle. Concentric contraction is sometimes referred to as shortening contraction.
- **Eccentric contraction** occurs when there is joint motion but the muscle appears to lengthen; that is the muscle attachments (origin and insertion) move away from each other. For example, after a biceps curl, if a lifter sets the weight down slowly on the table, he or she will feel that the biceps muscle (not the triceps muscle) continues to contract, even though the joint motion is elbow extension. What is occurring is an eccentric contraction of the biceps muscle. Eccentric contraction is sometimes referred to as a lengthening contraction.[2,3]

Muscle endurance is the ability of a muscle or a muscle group to perform repeated contractions against a resistance or to maintain an isometric contraction over time.[2] This might mean the endurance to lift each brick throughout the day when building a wall or the ability to hold a sleeping child in one arm and in one position for an hour. **Muscle coordination** is the smooth rhythmic interaction of muscle function without the presence of tremors or ataxia.[2] The average person displays good muscle coordination, as indicated by not spilling when bringing soup to the mouth on a spoon or replacing the tiny screw on a pair of glasses successfully. In these examples, there is good balance between the agonist and antagonist muscles. An **agonist** is a muscle or muscle group that causes the motion and is sometimes referred to as the prime mover. An **antagonist** is a muscle that performs the opposite motion of the agonist. In the case of elbow flexion, the biceps is an agonist, and the triceps is the antagonist muscle. It has to be noted that the role of a muscle is specific to a particular joint action. In the case of elbow extension, the triceps is the agonist, and the biceps muscle is the antagonist.[3]

CAUSES OF MUSCLE WEAKNESS

Loss of muscle strength can have a multitude of causes. It could be a primary symptom or a direct result of the following diseases or injuries:

1. Lower motor neuron (LMN) diseases, such as peripheral nerve injuries, peripheral neuropathies, spinal cord injuries, Guillain-Barré syndrome, and cranial nerve dysfunction. The LMN innervates the muscle directly.
2. Primary muscle diseases, such as myasthenia gravis and muscular dystrophies
3. Neurological diseases, such as amyotrophic lateral sclerosis (ALS) or multiple sclerosis (MS)
4. Conditions in which loss of muscle strength is a result of disuse or immobilization, such as fractures, burns, amputations, hand trauma, arthritis, and a variety of other orthopedic conditions[1]

Certainly, muscle weakness can be a secondary symptom as well, with the weakness seen from immobility after a hospitalization or during and after an injury or illness. Muscle weakness can limit or prevent performance in occupations including activities of daily living (ADLs), instrumental activities of daily living (IADLs), rest and sleep, education, work, play, leisure, and social participation.[1] These limitations are assessed by the OT practitioner through observation of functional performance, screening tests, and manual muscle testing (MMT) as indicated.

SCREENING TESTS

Screening tests are useful for observing areas of muscle strength and weakness and determining whether MMT is required for certain specific areas of functioning.[2,4-6] They can help the OT practitioner avoid unnecessary testing or duplication of services. These tests are not as precise as MMT. Their purpose is to make a general assessment of muscle strength and determine areas of weakness, performance limitations, and the need for more precise testing. Screening can be accomplished by the following means:

1. Review the client's medical record for results of previous muscle test and ROM assessments by the physician or other members of the multidisciplinary team.
2. Observe the client as he or she moves about in the hospital bed, enters the inpatient rehabilitation setting or clinic, or moves around the client's home. Note any limping, difficulty with ambulation, balance deficits, holding onto walls and furniture, and near falls and how these deficits may affect independence and safety.
3. Observe the client performing functional activities, such as self-feeding, grooming, removing an article of clothing, or shaking hands with the staff.[2,4] Observing these activities will give excellent information about the strength in the limbs, functional performance, and how the client might be limited by strength issues.
4. While doing both #2 and #3, look for pain, variations in performance, or difficulty the client may have in performing these tasks.
5. Perform a quick, gross check of bilateral muscle groups where the client performs all active range of motion (AROM) of the bilateral upper extremities (BUEs) while seated or standing. Examples of these movements are as follows: reaching arms above head, touching the back of one's head and middle section of the back, touching the opposite shoulders, bending and straightening elbows, moving wrists up and down, and opening and closing hands. If the client is able to perform all these movements without significant pain or discomfort or limitations

in motion, one can assume that the AROM is within functional limits (WFL). If not, it can lead the OT practitioner to further investigate the deficits noted.

6. Perform a gross check of muscle group strength while the client is comfortably seated in a chair or wheelchair. After #5 is performed and AROM is observed, resistance (application of force) can be given to the test motions to obtain a gross estimate of muscle strength.[1] This is not a full MMT but often used to quickly screen a functional movement, such as reaching into a cupboard (shoulder flexion).

MANUAL MUSCLE TESTING

Manual muscle testing (MMT) is a means to assess muscle strength. It measures the maximal contraction of a muscle or a muscle group.[2] Criteria used to measure muscle strength include evidence of muscle contraction, amount of ROM that the joint goes through when the muscle contracts, and amount of **resistance** against which the muscle can contract. Gravity is considered a form of resistance[1,2,4] as well as other external forces that are applied and force the muscle to contract.

The purpose of MMT is to:

- Determine the amount of muscle power available
- Discern how muscle weakness is limiting functional performance
- Establish a baseline for intervention
- Determine the need for assistive devices or compensatory measures
- Aid in the selection of occupations within the client's capabilities
- Evaluate the effectiveness of intervention strategies[1]

Methods of Manual Muscle Testing

Muscle strength can be assessed in several ways. The most precise method is a test of individual muscles; in this test, called isolated MMT, a muscle is carefully isolated by proper positioning and stabilization,[7] and its strength is graded and given a number from 1 to 5.[8] Grading individual muscle strength is especially useful in hand therapy as a way to gauge return of function in individual muscles after hand surgery. Another MMT method is gross MMT, a method that is more commonly used to assess the strength of groups of muscles that perform specific motions at each joint.[4,8] This chapter will focus on gross MMT for specific motions. Muscle grading will also be discussed later in this chapter.

Contraindications and Precautions of Manual Muscle Testing

Assessment of strength using MMT is contraindicated (not recommended nor advisable) in conditions where there is inflammation or pain in the region to be tested, recent surgery, fracture or dislocation, myositis ossificans (formation of bone in a joint), bone carcinoma, or any other fragile bone condition. The OT practitioner may cause injury to the client if MMT is attempted in these cases.[2,8,9] Precautions must be taken when resisted movement could aggravate the client's condition, such as in cases of osteoporosis, subluxation or hypermobility of a joint, hemophilia (bleeding in a joint), cardiovascular risk, disease or surgery, abdominal surgery or abdominal hernia, and fatigue that exacerbate the client's condition.[2] In these cases, the amount of resistance applied may have to be carefully monitored.

Unlike the passive range of motion (PROM) assessment, MMT requires the client's complete involvement and is an active process. Therefore, the OT practitioner must be mindful of the client's understanding of the requirements of the test and willingness to expend true effort when resistance is applied and to possibly endure some discomfort during the test. The presence of cognitive deficits, language barriers, and inability to perform the motor skills required for the test may compromise the results of the MMT;[1,4] therefore, the OT practitioner should be aware of these limitations before MMT is performed. If these limitations prevent the OT practitioner from performing MMT properly, a functional or screening evaluation may have to be considered.

The knowledge and skill of the OT practitioner are of paramount importance in the validity of MMT results (both gross and isolated). Careful observation of the movement, accurate palpation, correct positioning and consistency of the procedure and experience of the practitioner are critical factors in accurate testing.[4,5,7]

To be proficient in MMT, the OT practitioner must have detailed knowledge of all aspects of muscle functions, such as origin and insertion, direction of muscle fibers, angle and line of pull on the joints, action of muscles, and possible substitutions.[4,7] They must reliably be able to test each muscle consistently and accurately over time and between individuals.

Limitations of Manual Muscle Testing

MMT cannot measure muscle endurance, muscle coordination, or motor performance capabilities of the client in functional tasks. It is not appropriate and cannot be used accurately in clients who have spasticity as a result of upper motor neuron lesions, such as cerebrovascular accidents (CVA) or cerebral palsy. In these conditions, muscles are often hypertonic, and the tone of the muscle is involuntary. Some diseases, such as Parkinson's disease, can cause muscle rigidity as well. Muscle tone and ability to perform movements can be influenced by primitive reflexes and position of head and body in space. Often, movements occur in gross synergistic or mass patterns that make it impossible for the client to isolate joint motions that are demanded in MMT procedures.[2,10-12] As spasticity wanes and synergistic patterns disappear, MMT can be used to reveal residual weakness and plan an intervention program.[1]

RELATIONSHIP BETWEEN JOINT RANGE OF MOTION AND MUSCLE STRENGTH

One of the criteria used to grade muscle strength is the ROM of the joint on which the muscle acts—that is, did the muscle move the joint through complete, partial, or no ROM? In this context, ROM is not necessarily the full average normal ROM for the given joint; rather, it is the PROM available to the individual client. When a practitioner measures joint motion, as described in an earlier chapter, it is PROM that is the measure of the range available to the client. PROM, however, is not an indication of muscle strength.[1]

When performing MMT, the practitioner must first know the client's PROM and then AROM to assign muscle grades correctly. It is possible for a client to have limited ROM at a joint but have normal muscle strength because of joint irregularities. For example, a client's AROM for elbow flexion may be limited to 0° to 120° instead of full ROM because of a previous fracture. The client may have full, normal strength within the available ROM. In such cases, the practitioner should record the specific ROM limitation along with the muscle grade.

GENERAL PRINCIPLES OF MANUAL MUSCLE TESTING

Performing MMT can involve extensive time, effort, and attention to detail to ensure that the results obtained are as accurate as possible.[13] Knowledge of the topics described below will assist the OT practitioner in making an accurate assessment.

Knowledge of Muscle Grades

MMT is a well-documented method used to evaluate muscle strength. Being aware of a client's muscle grades is crucial, as it will help the OT practitioner determine the types of therapeutic activities or exercise that can help to maintain or improve strength. Two methods of grading are commonly used to report strength testing results: number grade and letter grade. One method uses numbers 0 to 5 (0 is the weakest and 5 is the strongest) and the other uses letters, such as O = zero, T = trace, P = poor, F = fair, G = good, and N = normal. For better distinction between grades, some methods also use a "+" or "–" sign along with the number or letter grade.[3] The opposite of strength is weakness, and the scale is also used to document the degree of weakness: mild (G, 4/5), moderate (F to F+, 3/5), or severe (P to T, O, 2/5 to 0/5). Refer to Table 9-1 for an explanation of grades, and Table 9-2 for some examples of each.

Although the definitions of muscle grades are standard among healthcare professionals, assignment of muscle grade during MMT depends on the clinical judgment, knowledge, and experience of the OT practitioner, especially when slight, moderate, or maximal resistance is determined. Age, gender, body type, vocation, and leisure activities all influence the amount of resistance a particular client can take.[4,7,14]

TABLE 9-1 Muscle Grades and Definitions[5]

WORD/LETTER GRADE	NUMBER GRADE	WORD/LETTER GRADE DEFINITION
Normal (N)	5	Complete ROM against gravity, maximum resistance
Good plus (G+)	4+	Complete ROM against gravity, less than maximal resistance through full range
Good (G)	4	Complete ROM against gravity, moderate resistance
Good minus (G–)	4-	Complete ROM against gravity, minimum resistance
Fair plus (F+)	3+	Complete ROM against gravity, minimal resistance through partial ROM then breaks abruptly
Fair (F)	3	Complete ROM against gravity, no resistance
Fair minus (F–)	3-	Gradual release from test position
Poor plus (P+)	2+	Less than ½ ROM against gravity, no resistance OR in gravity-minimized plane, full ROM with minimal resistance
Poor (P)	2	Full ROM, gravity-miminized
Poor minus (P–)	2-	Partial ROM, gravity-minimized
Trace (T)	1	Palpation or observation of contraction only, no motion
Zero (O)	0	No muscle contraction observed or palpated

Normal strength of an 80-year-old female will be considerably less than that of a 25-year-old man, for example. Strength tends to decline with age, and therefore resistance applied to clients of different age groups will vary among the individual clients and needs to be considered.[2,7]

The amount of resistance that can be given also varies among muscle groups. Larger muscles with a greater cross section of fibers have greater strength and can take greater resistance. For example, the flexors of the elbow are larger, have more power, and can take more resistance than the flexors of the wrist. The OT practitioner must take this into consideration and modify the amount of resistance applied. When only one side of the body is involved in the dysfunction causing muscle weakness, the practitioner can establish the standards for strength by testing the unaffected side first.[1,2,5]

Other factors that should be considered during MMT are fatigue of weak muscles, pain, swelling, and muscle spasm. There should be no more than three repetitions of each test movement because fatigue can result in grading errors if the muscle becomes tired as a result of low endurance.[1,4] Additionally, the resistance for each muscle is generally

TABLE 9-2 Examples of Grading

SCENARIO	HOW TESTED	NAME GRADE	NUMBER GRADE
During AROM, the client cannot maintain arm fully overhead in shoulder flexion	OTA asks about pain (none), and tests PROM (within normal limits [WNL]). Since the client cannot maintain position against gravity, the grade is as noted.	Fair minus	3-/5
Client has full AROM for elbow flexion	When tested, the client can hold fairly well against resistance (moderate), although the arm moves slowly with the resistance when applied.	Good	4/5
Client cannot move wrist at all during AROM, and it is noted to be "hanging" down with ROM.	The OTA notes PROM, which is full, and tests the wrist extensors in a gravity-reduced way. The client is able to move through less than half of the ROM with gravity reduced.	Poor minus	2-/5

applied for 1 to 2 seconds, and if retesting is required, give the client a two minute break for muscle recovery.

Effect of Gravity

Gravity, the force which attracts an item to the center of the earth, occurs naturally in the environment and actually exerts a form of resistance to muscle power.[1] The effect of gravity on the client's ability to perform the movement must be considered in grading muscle strength. The **muscle grade** is based on whether a muscle can move the body part **against gravity.**[1,7] Movements against gravity occur in a vertical plane; this means they are away from the floor or toward the ceiling. Movements in the vertical plane are only appropriate for use in grades F or 3 and higher. A good starting point to understand the muscle grades is Fair or 3. If a client can move a body part completely through full ROM, against gravity and maintain it, then the MMT grade is F or 3, but may be F+ (3+), G– (4–), G (4), G+ (4+), or N (5) if they can also take resistance. To score higher than an F or 3, the client must be able to withstand manual resistance (provided by the OT practitioner) or mechanical resistance, in addition to gravity. All these movements are also performed in a vertical plane and will be graded P+ (2+) to N (5).

Tests for weaker muscles, such as 0, T (1), P (2), and P+ (2+) are often performed in a horizontal plane—that is, they are parallel to the floor to reduce the resistance of gravity on muscle power. This is because the client is not strong enough to move the body part through the full ROM against gravity. This position has been referred to as the **gravity-eliminated, gravity-minimized, gravity-reduced,** or **gravity-lessened** position.[5-7] Although gravity-eliminated is the most commonly used term, it is currently impossible to completely eliminate the effects of gravity on muscle power. Thus, the more accurate term would be gravity-minimized or gravity-lessened. The term gravity-minimized is used in this chapter.

The effect of gravity on the ability to perform movements is important in the large muscle groups of the shoulder, elbow, hip, and knee. For example, to test scapula depression in the against-gravity position, the client will have to assume an inverted position (stand on the head). Therefore, the OT practitioner may choose to do the tests for F or 3 to N or 5 in the gravity-minimized plane in these muscles. In other tests, positioning for movements in gravity-minimized or against-gravity position may not be feasible. Additionally, some clients may not be able to assume the correct position for testing for various reasons, such as confinement to bed, generalized weakness, body habitus (physique, e.g., obesity), trunk instability, medical precautions, and immobilization devices. In these cases, the OT practitioner must adapt the testing position to the client's needs and use clinical judgment to modify the grade. The practitioner should document such modifications in positioning and grading when the test results are recorded.[1]

Substitutions and Compensations

The brain thinks in terms of movement and function rather than in terms of contraction of individual muscles.[5] Thus, a muscle or muscle group may naturally attempt to compensate for the function of a weaker muscle to accomplish a movement. These movements are called compensatory movements, trick movements, or **substitutions.**[2,7] For example, to compensate for limited shoulder flexion, the client may raise up the shoulder girdle. Substitutions can occur during MMT and should be prevented. This can be achieved by giving careful instructions, correct positioning, stabilizing and palpating the muscle being tested, and ensuring correct performance of the test motion without extraneous movements or substitutions. The practitioner should palpate contractile tissue (feel by touch the muscle fibers or tendon) to detect tension in the muscle group under examination. It is only through correct palpation that the practitioner can be certain that the motion observed is not being performed by substitution.[2,5] Undetected substitutions can mask the client's problems and result in inaccurate intervention planning.[1,7]

Preparation for Testing

If several movements need to be performed at a time, testing should be organized to prevent repositioning of the client. After a chart review with notation of precautions and contraindications, the OT practitioner should ask the client about pain or other factors which would affect MMT. Then the steps would include the following:

1. Assess AROM to determine quality of movement, such as smoothness, speed and rhythm, and any other abnormal movements such as tremors.
2. Assess PROM if there is decreased AROM at a joint in order to determine available joint motion, joint integrity, and presence of tone or spasticity.
3. Decide if a full MMT is required or if the assessment will be of gross MMT only.

Correct positioning of the client and the body part is essential for effective and correct assessment. The client should be positioned comfortably on a firm surface. Bulky clothing should be removed or rearranged so that the practitioner can see the muscle or muscles being tested (for T grade). For maximum client comfort, the assessment should be administered to all muscles possible in a given position (upright, prone, supine, side-lying) before changing the client's position. If the client cannot be placed in the correct position for the test, the OT practitioner must adapt the test to the client and use clinical judgment in approximating strength grades.[6] In addition to correct positioning, test validity depends on careful stabilization, palpation of the muscles, and observation of the movements.[1,5]

Procedure for Testing

Testing should be performed according to a standard procedure to ensure accuracy and consistency. Each of the tests that follow is divided into these steps: (1) position, (2) stabilize, (3) palpate, (4) observe, (5) resist, (6) grade. Table 9-3 shows a sample form for recording muscle grades of the upper extremities. Note that the focus of this chapter is on gross MMT of movements, such as shoulder flexion or internal rotation, instead of each specific muscle, such as deltoid or brachioradialis.

The steps for the test are as follows:

POSITION

First, the client is positioned to begin the specific muscle test. The OT practitioner positions himself or herself in relation to the client. It may not be possible to achieve the optimal position, and the client may not be able to move between positions.

STABILIZE

Then, the OT practitioner stabilizes the part of the body proximal to the part being tested to eliminate extraneous movements, isolate the muscle groups, ensure the correct test motion, and eliminate substitutions. The OT practitioner then demonstrates or describes the test motion to the client and asks him or her to perform the test motion and return to the starting position. The OT practitioner makes a general observation of the form and quality of movement, looking for substitutions or difficulties that may require adjustments in positioning and stabilization.

EVIDENCE-BASED PRACTICE

"Evidence-based practice is the integration of best research evidence with clinical expertise and patient values."[1] Evidence-based rehabilitation is a subset of EBP that consists of being aware of evidence in one's field, collaboration between client and clinician, being able to apply best evidence to the client, and developing a customized interventional approach to each client.[1]

In their article titled "Effectiveness of occupation-based interventions to improve areas of occupation and social participation after stroke: An evidence-based review," Wolf et al. supported the use of occupation-based interventions to improve areas of occupation after CVA. According to their study, most of the literature targeted ADL–based interventions and collectively provided strong evidence for the use of occupation-based interventions to improve ADL performance.[15]

Studies have been performed on early mobilization in the intensive care unit (ICU) and the acute care setting and its impact on long-term function. Millions in the ICU survive critical illnesses, and the long-term consequences of these illnesses are growing concerns. These effects can be physical, cognitive, and mental health impairments. Muscle strength in healthy individuals is decreased by 1.3% to 3% per day of bed rest with no additional mitigating factors. Early intervention is the key to reducing impairments faced by these individuals. Early mobilization using an interdisciplinary approach yields the best outcomes according to the evidence. A client's participation in retraining of cognition, ROM, mobility, and functional tasks leads to shorter ICU/hospital stays, reduction in number of days spent on the ventilator, and increased savings as a result of decreased lengths of stay.[16,17]

Pedretti, L. W., Pendleton, H. M., & Schultz-Krohn, W. (2013). Pedretti's occupational therapy: Practice skills for physical dysfunction (7th ed.). St. Louis, MO: Mosby Elsevier.

Wolf, T. J., Chuh, A., Floyd, T., McInnis, K., &Williams, E. (2015). Effectiveness of occupation-based interventions to improve areas of occupation and social participation after stroke: An evidence based review. The American Journal of Occupational Therapy, 69(1), 6901180060p1-11.

Ronnebaum, J., Weir, J., & Hilsabeck, T. (2012). Early mobilization decreases the length of stay in the intensive care unit. Journal of Acute Care Physical Therapy, 3(2).

Needham, D. M. (2008). Mobilizing patients in the intensive care unit improves neuromuscular weakness and physical function. Journal of American Medical Association, 300, 1685–1690.

TABLE 9-3 Manual Muscle Testing Documentation[1]

MUSCLE EXAMINATION CHART

Client's Name:		Chart #
Date of Assessment:		
Date of Birth:		
Attending Physician:		
Date of Onset:		
Diagnoses:		

LEFT: INITIAL	LEFT: D/C		RIGHT: INITIAL	RIGHT: D/C
		NECK—Flexors		
		Extensors		
		TRUNK—Flexors		
		Extensors		
		SCAPULA—Elevators/depressors		
		Abductors		
		Adductors		
		SHOULDER—Flexors		
		Extensors		
		Abductors		
		Horizontal abductors		
		Horizontal adductors		
		External rotators		
		Internal rotators		
		ELBOW—Flexors		
		Extensors		
		FOREARM—Supinators		
		Pronators		
		WRIST—Flexors		
		Extensors		
		FINGERS—Metaphalangeal flexors		
		Proximal interphalangeal flexors		
		Distal interphalangeal flexors		
		Metaphalangeal extensors		
		Adductors		
		Abductors		
		THUMB—Metaphalangeal flexor		
		Interphalangeal flexor		
		Metaphalangeal extensor		
		Interphalangeal extensor		
		Abductors		
		Adductor pollicis		
		Opponens pollicis		

PALPATE

The OT practitioner then places his or her fingers (typically the tips of the index and middle fingers—using the thumb should be avoided because it has its own pulse) for palpation of the muscle group that is being tested and asks the client to repeat the test motion.

OBSERVE

While palpating the muscle group, the OT practitioner again observes the movement for amount of range completed and possible substitutions.

RESIST

When the client has moved the part through the available ROM, the OT practitioner asks the client to hold a position near the middle of the ROM. The OT practitioner removes the palpating fingers and uses the free hand to resist in the direction opposite that of the test position. For example, when elbow flexion is tested, the OT practitioner applies resistance in the direction of extension. The OT practitioner usually must maintain stabilization when resistance is given.

GRADE

Finally, the OT practitioner grades the muscle strength following the muscle grade chart.[1] (Refer to Table 9-1.) MMT uses the "break test" versus the "make test." In the "break test," resistance is applied after the client has reached the end of the available ROM,[1,4] whereas in the "make test," resistance is applied throughout the motion as the joint moves through the ROM. However, in the "break test," it is difficult to apply resistance at the end of the joint effectively, so in practical application, it is better to apply resistance at the midrange of the available movement for muscle testing. Midrange is the position used for most of the MMT photos and descriptions in this textbook.

Regardless of the type chosen, the client should be allowed to establish a maximal contraction before the resistance is applied. The OT practitioner applies resistance just distal to the joint on which the muscles act after preparing the client by giving the command to "hold." Resistance should be applied gradually in a direction opposite to the line of pull of the muscle or muscle group being tested.[1,4] Resistance is only applied when testing in the against-gravity positions for grades F+ (3+) and above. Resistance is not applied for tests of muscles from F (3) to 0, except for a slight resistance is sometimes applied to a muscle that has completed the full ROM in the gravity-minimized plane to determine whether the grade is P+ or 2+.[1]

Care should be taken to apply resistance just distal to the joint being tested to ensure accurate results. If the resistance is applied too distally or if it crosses a second joint, it may lead to inaccurate results. For example, in testing shoulder flexion, the resistance should be applied on the proximal humerus. If resistance is applied on the forearm, the leverage is increased and there may be an influence of the elbow joint or elbow muscles on the shoulder flexion testing.[8] Publications may differ with regard to where the stabilizing hand is placed on the body. This chapter has chosen one placement, although there may be other acceptable options. There may be differences between clients as well, as a result of pain, positioning needs, amputations, and substitutions seen, and these differences need to be taken into account. Each muscle grouping below will not note test position separately for zero (0), but will use trace position.

MANUAL MUSCLE TESTING OF THE UPPER EXTREMITY[1,8,13]

Neck Flexion

Muscles: longus capitus, longus colli, rectus capitis anterior, sternocleidomastoid, scalenus anterior
Normal (N), Good (G), Fair (F)
Position: Client is supine with shoulders abducted to 90 degrees, elbows flexed, and dorsal forearms resting on the table[13]
Stabilize: Over anterior aspect of thorax
Palpate: Over anterior aspect of neck
Observe: Ask client to tuck chin toward sternum and move neck in the direction of flexion.
Resist: Resistance is applied at the forehead in the direction of neck extension for N and G grades. Minimal resistance is applied for F+ grade, no resistance for F grade
Poor (P): Test position is side-lying. Client flexes head and neck through partial ROM
Trace (T): Test position is side-lying. No motion is seen but a palpable contraction is felt or observed, as described earlier

Neck Extension

Muscles: Erector spinae, obliquus capitus, rectus capitus posterior, splenius cervicis, semispinalis cervicis, and semispinalis capitis
Normal (N), Good (G), Fair (F)
Position: Client is prone with head in neutral rotation, shoulders abducted to 90 degrees, elbows flexed and ventral forearms resting on the table.
Stabilize: On the posterior thoracic region to avoid compensation
Palpate: Neck extensors over posterior cervical spine
Observe: Client extends head and neck through full ROM
Resist: Apply resistance over occiput in the direction of neck flexion (Fig. 9-1); Minimal resistance is applied for F+ grade, no resistance for F grade
Poor (P): Test position is side-lying. Client extends head and neck through partial ROM
Trace (T): Test position is side-lying. No motion is seen but a palpable contraction is felt or observed, as described earlier

Trunk Flexion

Muscles: Rectus abdominis
Normal (N), Good (G), Fair (F)

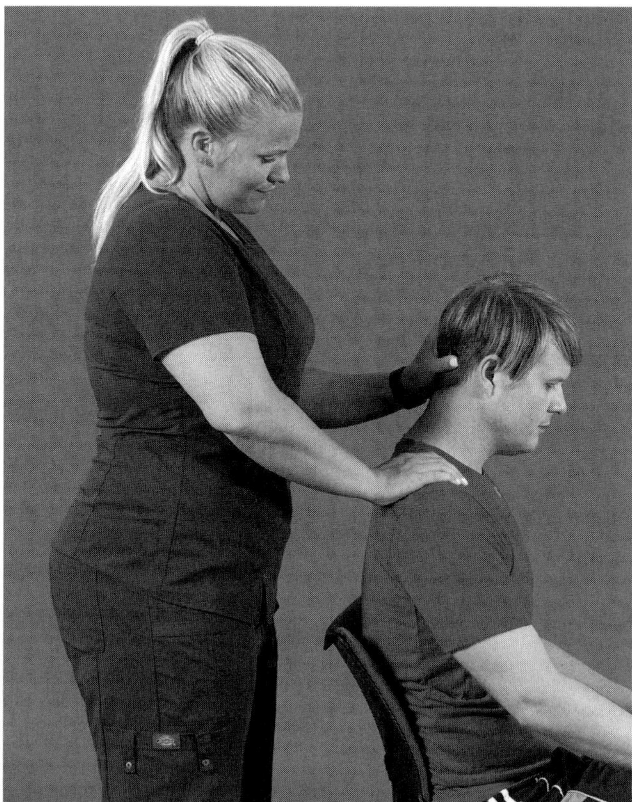

FIGURE 9-1. Cervical extension manual muscle testing.

Position: Supine with hands at sides of neck and lower extremities with slight knee flexion on a pillow for grade N, arms folded across chest for grade G and arms at sides for grade F
Stabilize: Not necessary
Palpate: Over anterior aspect just lateral to midline
Observe: Client moves in the direction of trunk flexion
Resist: Resistance is not necessary
Poor (P): Test position is side-lying. With arms at sides, client raises head and cervical spine from table, scapulae remain in contact with the surface
Trace (T): Test position is side-lying. No motion is seen but a palpable contraction is felt or observed, as described earlier

Trunk Extension

Muscles: Erector spinae, multifidus semispinalis thoracis, quadratus lumborum
Normal (N), Good (G), Fair (F)
Position: Prone with hands behind neck, pillow under abdomen, lower extremities extended for grade N, and arms folded behind back for grade G and arms at sides for grade F
Stabilize: Over posterior aspect of patient's thigh and pelvis with forearm
Palpate: Over spinous processes of lumbar and thoracic vertebrae
Observe: Client extends trunk through full ROM
Resist: Resistance is not necessary
Poor (P): Test position is side-lying. Client extends trunk through partial ROM with arms at sides
Trace (T): Test position is side-lying. No motion is seen but a palpable contraction is felt or observed, as described earlier

Scapula Elevation

Muscles: Levator scapulae and upper trapezius
Normal (N), Good (G), Fair (F)
Position: Client is sitting with both upper extremities at the side
Stabilize: Not necessary with bilateral test
Palpate: Upper trapezius just lateral to cervical spinous processes
Observe: Client moves shoulders upwards toward the ears
Resist: Over upper aspect of shoulders in an inferior direction (Fig. 9-2)
Poor (P)
Position: Client supine or prone with arms at sides, head in neutral position
Stabilize: Not necessary with bilateral test; stabilize at opposite shoulder in unilateral testing
Palpate: As in gravity-resisted test
Observe: As in gravity-resisted test
Resist: Resistance is not applied in gravity-minimized position
Trace (T): No motion is seen but a palpable contraction is felt or observed, as described earlier

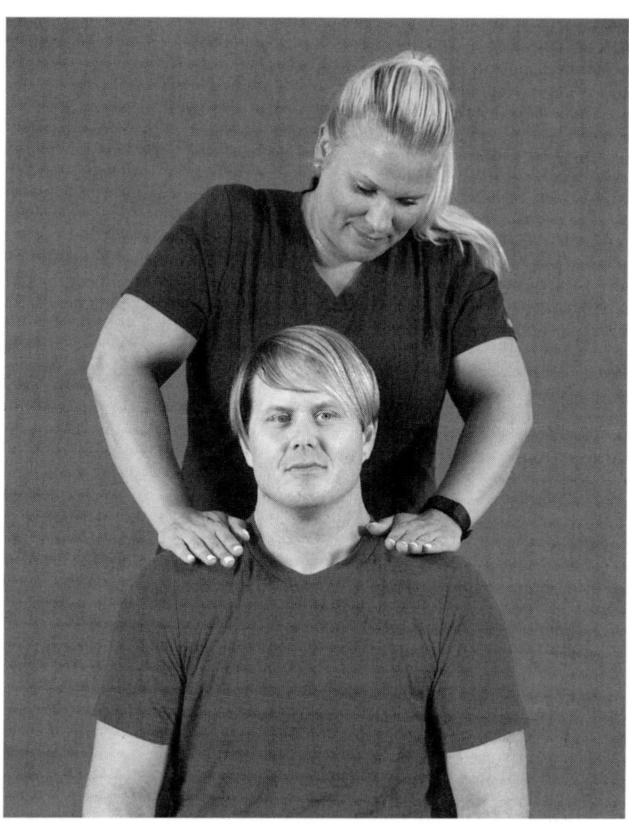

FIGURE 9-2. Both scapulae are often tested simultaneously for elevation to eliminate trunk motion.

Scapular Adduction and Depression

Muscles: Lower trapezius
Normal (N), Good (G)
Position: Client prone with arm in about 130 degrees shoulder abduction, 0 degree of elbow extension, forearm in mid position with the thumb toward the ceiling
Stabilize: With one hand over posterior aspect of opposite thorax
Palpate: At the inferior angle of the scapula
Observe: Client performs adduction and depression of scapula while elevating arm off the table to ear level (Fig. 9-3)
Resist: Over lateral aspect of scapula in direction of scapula abduction and elevation
Fair (F): Client elevates arm through full available ROM with accompanying scapular adduction and downward rotation but against no resistance (F+ minimal resistance)
Poor (P): Client elevates arm through partial ROM with no resistance
Trace (T): No motion is seen but a palpable contraction is felt or observed, as described earlier

Scapular Abduction and Upward Rotation

Muscles: Serratus anterior
Normal (N), Good (G), Fair (F)
Position: Client supine with upper extremity in 90 degrees of shoulder flexion and 0 degree elbow extension
Stabilize: Over same side of thorax to prevent trunk rotation
Palpate: Serratus anterior over lateral aspect of eighth or ninth ribs
Observe: The client reaches up toward the ceiling, abducting the scapula

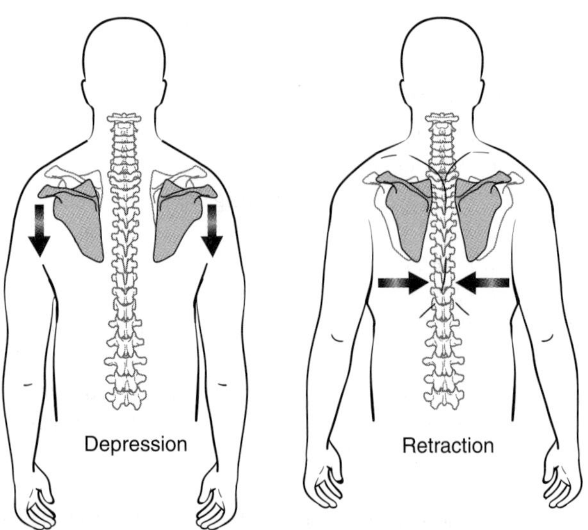

FIGURE 9-3. View of scapular movements of depression and retraction/adduction.

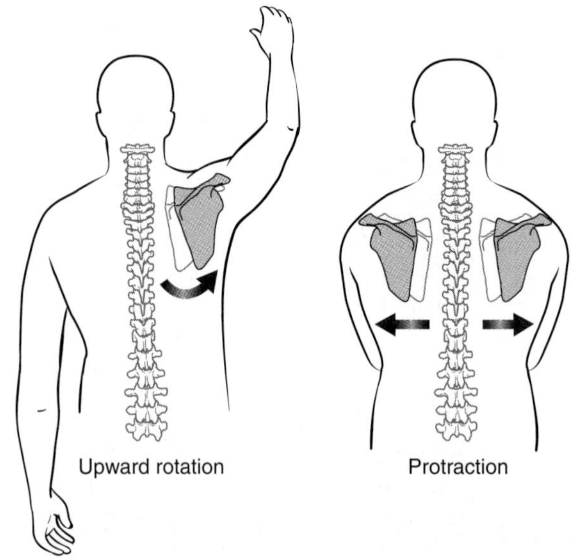

FIGURE 9-4. View of scapular movements of upward rotation and protraction/abduction.

Resist: Resistance is applied by grasping client's wrist and elbow and pushing down toward table in direction of scapular adduction
Poor (P)
Position: Client is sitting with arm supported on a table at 90 degrees of shoulder flexion and elbow extended
Stabilize: Over superior aspect of same shoulder girdle
Palpate: As in gravity resisted test
Observe: Client moves scapula by sliding arm forward on table with elbow extended (Fig. 9-4)
Resist: Resistance is not necessary in gravity-minimized plane (2+ may take minimal resistance in this position)
Trace (T): No motion is seen but a palpable contraction is felt or observed, as described earlier

Shoulder Flexion

Muscles: Anterior deltoid, coracobrachialis
Normal (N), Good (G), Fair (F)
Position: Client sitting or standing with upper extremity in 90 degrees shoulder flexion, full elbow extension, thumb upward
Stabilize: Over superior aspect of same shoulder to avoid scapular compensation
Palpate: Anterior deltoid over proximal anterior aspect of humerus
Observe: Client moves the extremity in the direction of further humeral flexion
Resist: Resistance is applied just proximal to elbow in the direction of shoulder extension (Fig. 9-5)
Poor (P)
Position: Client side-lying with arm to be tested uppermost and supported on a powder board
Stabilize: As in gravity-resisted test
Palpate: As in gravity-resisted test

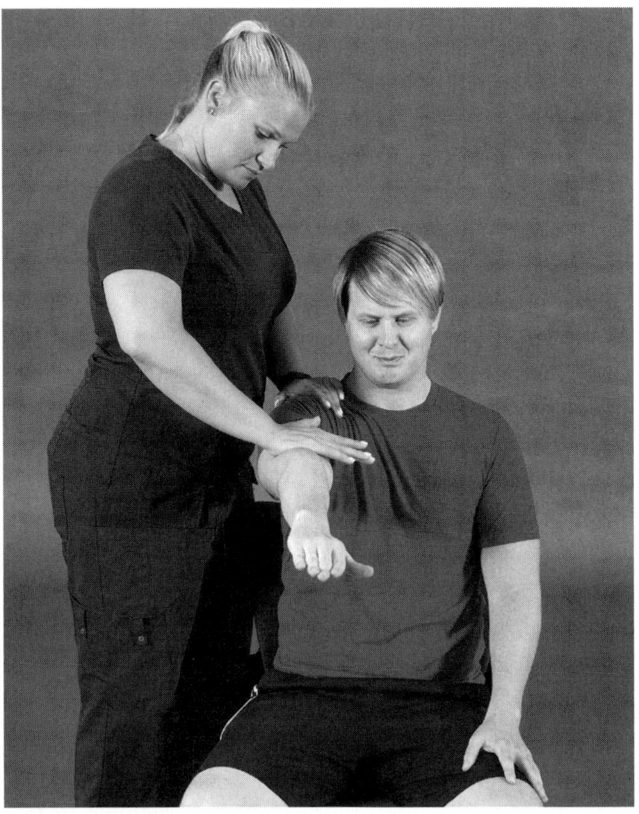

FIGURE 9-5. Shoulder flexion manual muscle testing. Note that the client can be sitting or standing for this test.

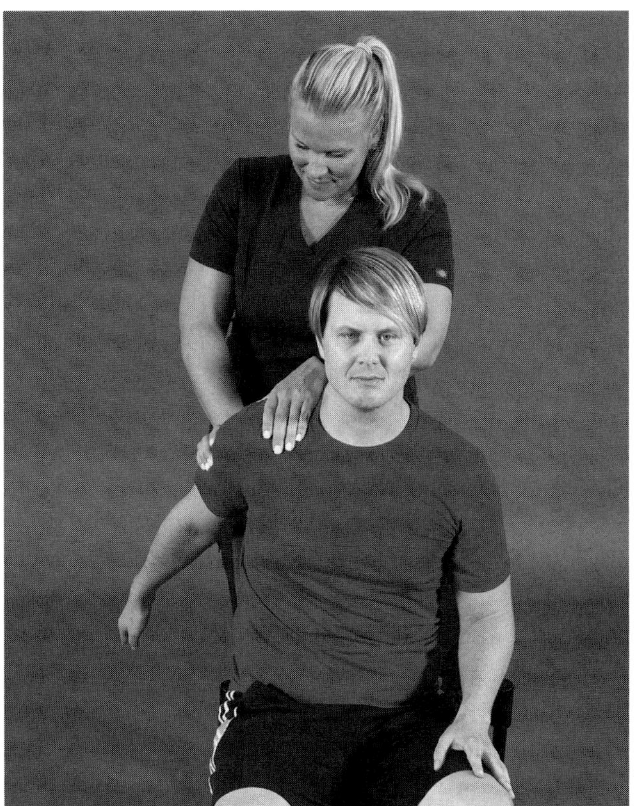

FIGURE 9-6. Shoulder extension manual muscle testing. Note that resistance is applied in direction of flexion.

Observe: Client begins motion in 0 degree shoulder flexion with palm facing trunk and attempts to move through full shoulder flexion
Resist: Not necessary in gravity-minimized position (2+ may take minimal resistance in this position)
Trace (T): No motion is seen but a palpable contraction is felt or observed, as described earlier

Shoulder Extension

Muscles: Latissimus dorsi, teres major, and posterior deltoid
Normal (N), Good (G), Fair (F)
Position: Client is prone with upper extremity at side, in full internal rotation (palm facing ceiling) and full elbow extension. (Alternatively, it can be done sitting or standing, as seen in photo but the resistance given has to be adjusted)
Stabilize: Over the scapula to avoid compensation of scapular elevation
Palpate: Latissimus dorsi along lateral side of rib cage
Observe: Client moves the arm through full range of shoulder extension while keeping shoulder adducted and internally rotated
Resist: Resistance is applied just proximal to elbow in direction of shoulder flexion (Fig. 9-6)
Poor (P)
Position: Client side-lying with arm to be tested uppermost on a powder board or supported by the practitioner
Stabilize: At the scapula to avoid compensation of scapular elevation
Palpate: As in gravity-resisted test
Observe: Client slides arm along surface through full range of shoulder extension while keeping shoulder adducted and medially rotated
Resist: Resistance is not necessary in gravity-minimized position (2+ may take minimal resistance in this position)
Trace (T): No motion is seen but a palpable contraction is felt or observed, as described earlier

Shoulder Abduction

Muscles: Middle deltoid and supraspinatus
Normal (N), Good (G), Fair (F)
Position: Client seated or standing with upper extremity to be tested in 0 degree of shoulder abduction, full elbow extension and forearm neutral
Stabilize: Over superior aspect of shoulder
Palpate: Middle deltoid over superior lateral aspect of humerus
Observe: Client moves arm into shoulder abduction
Resist: Resistance is applied just proximal to elbow in the direction of shoulder adduction (Fig. 9-7)
Poor (P)
Position: Client supine with arm to be tested in 0 degree of shoulder abduction, 180 degree elbow extension and forearm neutral

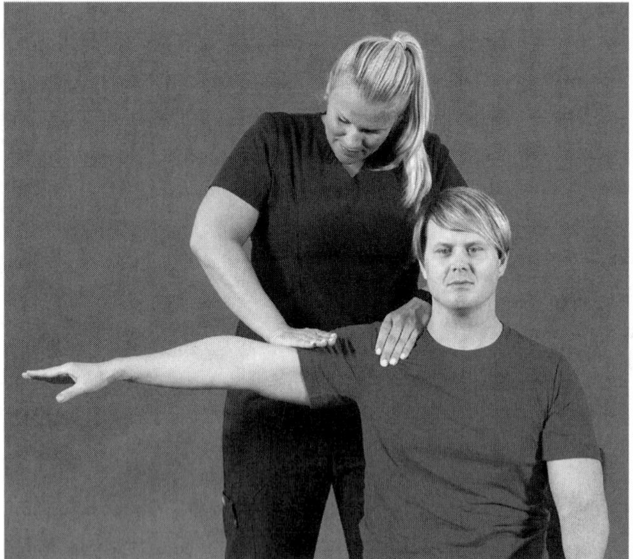

FIGURE 9-7. Shoulder abduction manual muscle testing. Note that the client can be either sitting or standing for this test.

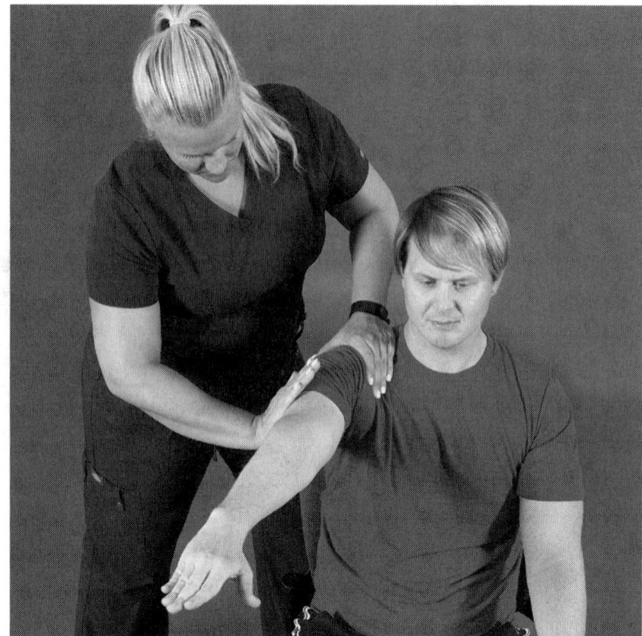

FIGURE 9-8. Shoulder horizontal abduction manual muscle testing. This test can be done in sitting or standing positions.

Stabilize: As in gravity-resisted test
Palpate: As in gravity-resisted test
Observe: Client slides arm along surface for shoulder abduction
Resist: Resistance is not necessary in gravity-minimized position (2+ may take minimal resistance in this position)
Trace (T): No motion is seen but a palpable contraction is felt or observed, as described earlier

Shoulder Horizontal Abduction

Muscles: Posterior deltoid
Normal (N), Good (G), Fair (F)
Position: Client prone with upper extremity in 90 degrees of shoulder abduction, 90 degrees of elbow flexion, and forearm hanging vertically off side of table (fingers toward the floor). Alternatively, it can be done in sitting or standing as seen in photo but the resistance given has to be adjusted)
Stabilize: Over same scapula
Palpate: Fibers of posterior deltoid over posterior superior aspect of humerus
Observe: Client moves the arm in the direction of humeral horizontal abduction
Resist: Resistance is applied over distal humerus in direction of horizontal adduction (Fig. 9-8)
Poor (P)
Position: Client seated with shoulder abducted to 90 degrees, elbow flexion to 90 degrees, humerus in neutral rotation and supported on a table or by the practitioner
Stabilize: Over superior aspect of same scapula to prevent trunk rotation
Palpate: As in gravity-resisted test
Observe: Client moves the arm in the direction of horizontal abduction
Resist: Resistance is not necessary in gravity-minimized position (2+ may take minimal resistance in this position)
Trace (T): No motion is seen but a palpable contraction is observed, as described earlier

Shoulder Horizontal Adduction

Muscles: Pectoralis major
Normal, (N), Good (G), Fair (F)
Position: Client supine with shoulder in 90 degree abduction, 90 degree elbow flexion, and forearm neutral. Alternate, as seen in photo, in sitting or standing positions.
Stabilize: Over same shoulder and upper thorax to prevent trunk rotation
Palpate: Pectoralis major on anterior border of axilla
Observe: Client horizontally adducts shoulder, bringing arm across chest keeping elbow flexed
Resist: Resistance is applied just proximal to elbow in direction of horizontal abduction (Fig. 9-9)
Poor (P)
Position: Client seated with shoulder in 90 degree abduction, elbow flexed to 90 degrees and supported on table or by the practitioner
Stabilize: Over superior aspect of same shoulder
Palpate: As in gravity-resisted test
Observe: Client adducts shoulder horizontally by sliding arm along table across chest
Resist: Resistance is not necessary in gravity-minimized plane (2+ may take minimal resistance in this position)
Trace (T): No motion is seen but a palpable contraction is observed or felt, as described earlier

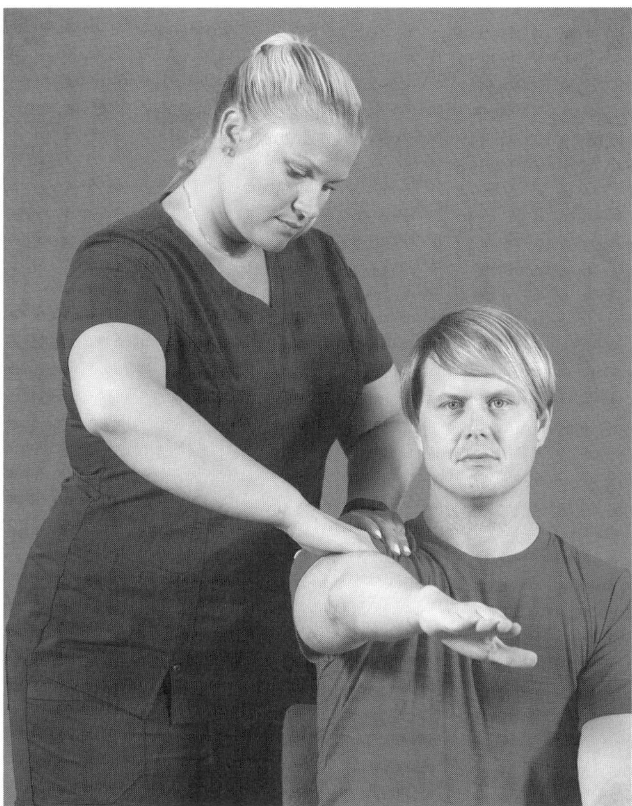

FIGURE 9-9. Horizontal adduction manual muscle testing. Stabilize at the shoulder to avoid compensation. Practitioner is using right hand to pull client's arm into abduction, resisting adduction.

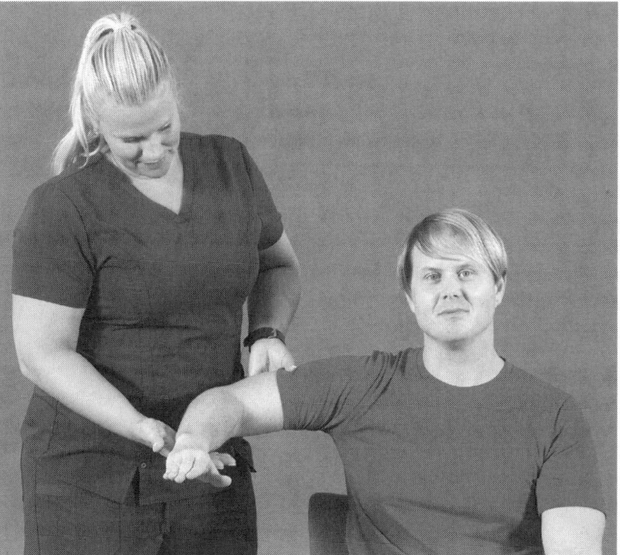

FIGURE 9-10. Shoulder internal rotation manual muscle testing. Note that this test can be done in the sitting or standing position as an alternative. Practitioner's right hand is applying resistance while left hand is supporting client.

Resist: Resistance is not necessary in gravity-minimized plane (2+ may take minimal resistance in this position)

Trace (T): No motion is seen but a palpable contraction is observed or felt, as described earlier

Common substitution: Care must be taken to see that the movement is true internal rotation and not just forearm pronation

Shoulder Internal Rotation

Muscles: Pectoralis major, latissimus dorsi, teres major, subscapularis

Normal (N), Good (G), Fair (F)

Position: Client prone with upper extremity in 90 degrees shoulder abduction, 90 degrees elbow flexion, forearm hanging vertically off side of table. A folded towel is placed under the humerus to maintain horizontal position. (Alternatively, it can be done sitting or standing, as seen in photo, or supine with the shoulder abducted to 90 degrees and elbow flexed to 90 degrees, but the resistance given will have to be adjusted)

Stabilize: At the scapula to avoid compensation

Palpate: Subscapularis deep in axilla

Observe: Client moves testing extremity in direction of humeral internal rotation

Resist: Resistance is applied just proximal to wrist in direction of humeral external rotation (Fig. 9-10)

Poor (P)

Position: Client sitting with arm at side, elbow flexed to 90 degrees, rotate the arm from neutral rotation into internal rotation

Stabilize: At the scapula

Palpate: As in gravity-resisted test

Observe: Client moves the testing extremity in the direction of humeral internal rotation

Shoulder External Rotation

Muscles: Infraspinatus, teres minor

Normal (N), Good (G), Fair (F)

Position: Client prone with upper extremity in 90 degrees shoulder abduction, 90 degrees elbow flexion, forearm hanging vertically off side of table. A folded towel is placed under the humerus to maintain horizontal position. (Alternatively, this test can be done in sitting or standing as seen in photo, or supine with the shoulder abducted to 90 degrees and elbow flexed to 90 degrees, but the resistance given has to be adjusted)

Stabilize: At the same scapula to avoid compensation (Fig. 9-11)

Palpate: Over spine of scapula

Observe: Client moves the extremity in the direction of humeral external rotation

Resist: Resistance is applied just proximal to wrist in direction of internal rotation

Poor (P)

Position: Client sitting with arm at side, elbow flexed to 90 degrees, rotate the arm from neutral rotation into external rotation

Stabilize: At the scapula

Palpate: As in gravity-resisted test

Observe: Client moves the extremity in direction of humeral external rotation[8]

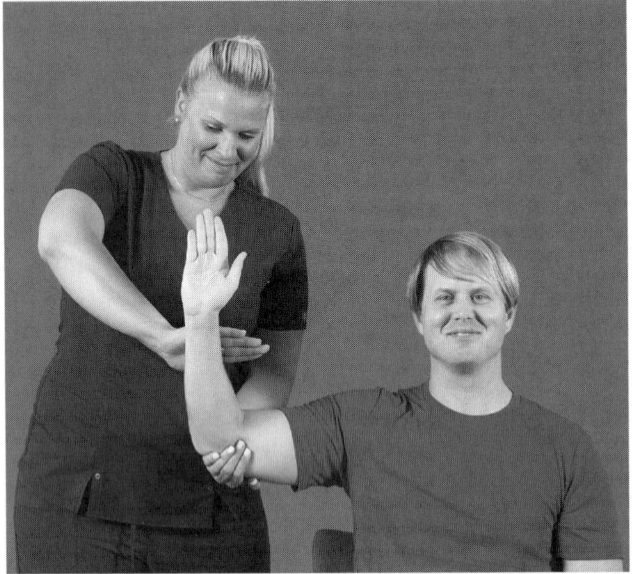

FIGURE 9-11. Shoulder external rotation manual muscle testing. This test can be done in the sitting or standing position as an alternative.

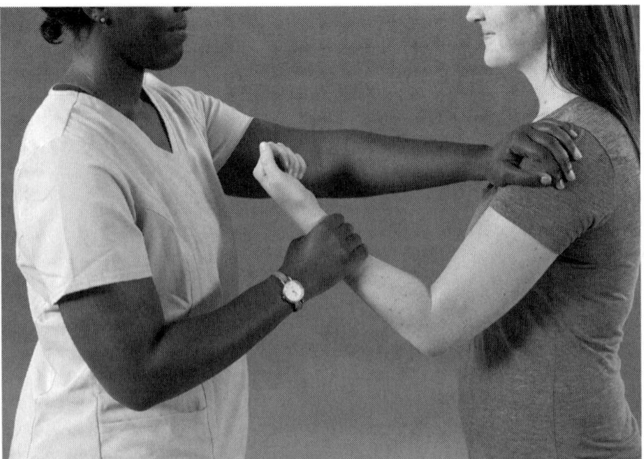

FIGURE 9-12. Elbow flexion manual muscle testing. Note that the client can be either seated or standing for this test.

Resist: Resistance is not necessary in gravity-minimized plane (2+ may take minimal resistance in this position)
Trace (T): No motion is seen but a palpable contraction is observed or felt, as described earlier
Common substitution: Care must be taken to see that the movement is true external rotation and not forearm supination

FUNCTIONAL LIMITATIONS SEEN AT THE SHOULDER

If a person has limited strength in shoulder flexors, he or she may not be able to reach overhead to comb the top of the head or reach into an overhead cabinet. Weakness in the internal rotators of the shoulders may make it difficult for a person to wash or dry the back, perform toilet hygiene, and reach into a back pocket, or for a woman to fasten her bra at the back. Weakness in the external rotators of the shoulders may make it difficult to reach behind the body or scratch the back of the head.

Elbow Flexion

Muscles: Biceps brachii, brachioradialis, brachialis
Normal (N), Good (G), Fair (F)
Position: Client seated or standing with upper extremity by the side, full elbow extension and forearm supination
Stabilize: Over anterior aspect of same humerus
Palpate: Biceps over middle third of anterior arm[13]
Observe: Client moves the extremity in the direction of full elbow flexion
Resist: Resistance is applied just proximal to wrist in direction of elbow extension (Fig. 9-12)
Poor (P)
Position: Client seated with arm supported on table, shoulder abducted to 90 degrees, elbow extended and forearm in neutral; a towel is placed under the humerus to avoid friction. (Alternatively, the arm can be supported under the forearm by the practitioner.)
Stabilize: Over anterosuperior aspect of same humerus
Palpate: As in gravity-resisted test
Observe: Client flexes elbow through full ROM by sliding forearm along table
Resist: Resistance is not necessary in gravity-minimized plane (2+ may take minimal resistance in this position)
Trace (T): No movement is seen but a palpable contraction is observed or felt, as described earlier

Elbow Extension

Muscles: Triceps brachii, anconeus
Normal (N), Good (G), Fair (F)
Position: Client supine with upper extremity in 90 degree shoulder flexion, full elbow flexion and forearm supination. (Alternative testing position is sitting or standing with full elbow flexion and about 120 degrees of shoulder flexion.)
Stabilize: Over anterior aspect of same shoulder
Palpate: Triceps over posterior surface of humerus
Observe: Client moves the extremity into elbow extension
Resist: Resistance is applied just proximal to wrist in direction of elbow flexion (flex client's elbow 45 degrees from full extension before applying resistance) (Fig. 9-13)
Poor (P)
Position: Client seated with arm supported on table, shoulder abducted to 90 degrees, elbow fully flexed; a towel is placed under the humerus to avoid friction. (Alternatively, the arm can be supported by the practitioner.)
Stabilize: Over anterior aspect of same shoulder
Palpate: As in gravity-resisted plane
Observe: Client extends elbow through full ROM
Resist: Resistance is not necessary in gravity-minimized plane (2+ may take minimal resistance in this position)

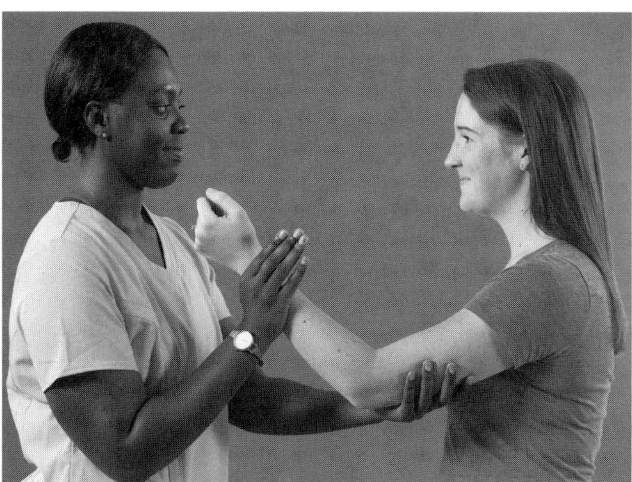

FIGURE 9-13. Elbow extension manual muscle testing. Note that the client can be sitting or standing, but substitutions have to be avoided.

Trace (T): No movement is seen but a palpable contraction is observed or felt, as described earlier

FUNCTIONAL LIMITATIONS OF ELBOW WEAKNESS

Limited elbow flexor strength will prevent bringing hand to mouth for self-feeding or grooming, as well as carrying a heavy load in the arms. Weak elbow extensors will not allow weight-bearing and pushing up from arms as to rise from chair, perform chair push-ups, or lift a heavy load onto a higher shelf.

Forearm Supination

Muscles: Supinator, biceps brachii

Normal (N), Good (G), Fair (F)

Position: Client seated with upper extremity in shoulder adduction, 90 degree elbow flexion and full forearm pronation

Stabilize: On inferolateral aspect of humerus to prevent shoulder abduction

Palpate: On anterior aspect of humerus (biceps) and posterosuperior aspect of radius (supinator)

Observe: Client moves forearm in direction of supination

Resist: Resistance is applied at the distal forearm from neutral in the direction of pronation. (Some testers prefer to use both hands to resist and stabilize across the wrist/forearm to prevent excessive wrist movement as compensation.) (Fig. 9-14)

Poor (P)

Position: Client seated with upper extremity in 90 degrees shoulder flexion, 90 degrees elbow flexion, and full forearm pronation; arm should be supported on a table with fingers pointed toward ceiling

Stabilize: Along posterior aspect of elbow

Palpate: As in gravity-resisted test

Observe: Client moves the extremity in the direction of supination

Resist: Resistance is not necessary in gravity-minimized plane (2+ may take minimal resistance in this position)

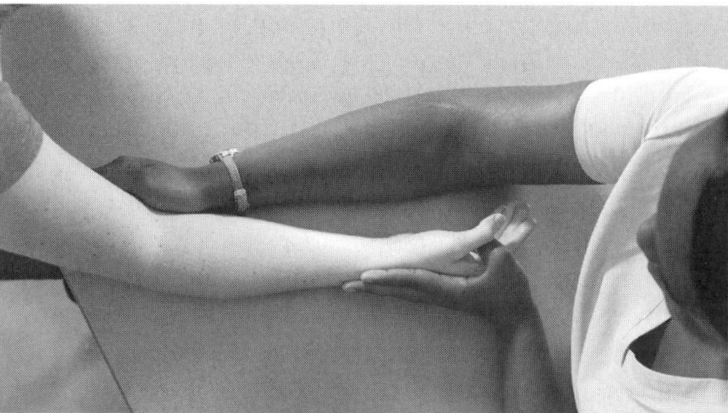

FIGURE 9-14. Forearm supination manual muscle testing. Note that the forearm should be stabilized to avoid compensation without impeding motion.

Trace (T): No movement is seen but a palpable contraction is seen or felt, as described earlier

Forearm Pronation

Muscles: Pronator quadratus, pronator teres

Normal (N), Good (G), Fair (F)

Position: Client seated with upper extremity in shoulder adduction, 90 degrees elbow flexion, full forearm supination

Stabilize: Over inferolateral aspect of humerus, preventing shoulder abduction (Fig. 9-15)

Palpate: Over anterior surface of forearm (pronator teres)

Observe: Client moves the testing extremity in the direction of forearm pronation

Resist: Resistance is applied at the distal forearm from neutral in the direction of supination (Some testers prefer to use both hands to resist and stabilize across the wrist/forearm to prevent excessive wrist movement as compensation.)

Poor (P)

Position: Client seated with upper extremity in 90 degrees shoulder flexion, 90 degrees elbow flexion, and full forearm supination; arm should be supported on a table with fingers pointed toward ceiling

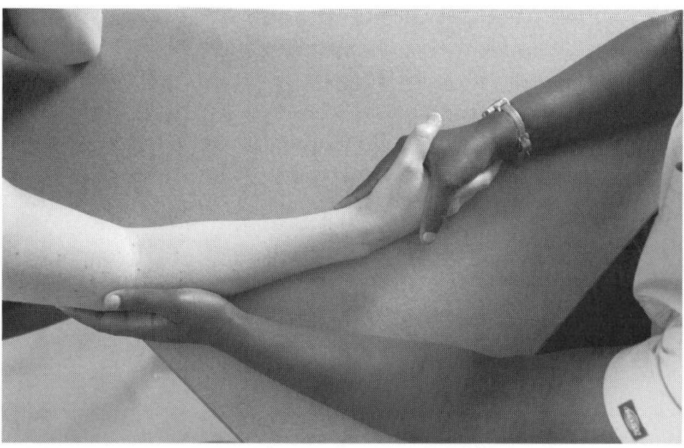

FIGURE 9-15. Forearm pronation manual muscle testing. Stabilize at the elbow to avoid compensation.

Stabilize: On anterior surface of forearm just proximal to elbow (see Fig 9.15)
Palpate: As in gravity-resisted test
Observe: Client moves the extremity in full forearm pronation
Resist: Resistance is not necessary in gravity-minimized plane (2+ may take minimal resistance in this position)
Trace (T): No motion is seen but a palpable contraction is observed or felt, as described earlier
Common substitution: Internal rotation or external rotation of shoulder may mimic forearm pronation or supination during gravity-resisted test. Care should be taken to maintain client's humerus in adduction and elbow in 90 degrees flexion during gravity-resisted test. Other compensation seen is with excessive wrist flexion or extension.

FUNCTIONAL LIMITATIONS OF WEAK PRONATORS OR SUPINATORS

Weak pronation will make it difficult to keep the spoon level during self-feeding or reaching out to pick up an item with the fingers. Weak supination will make it difficult to keep pills or coins in the palm of the hand.

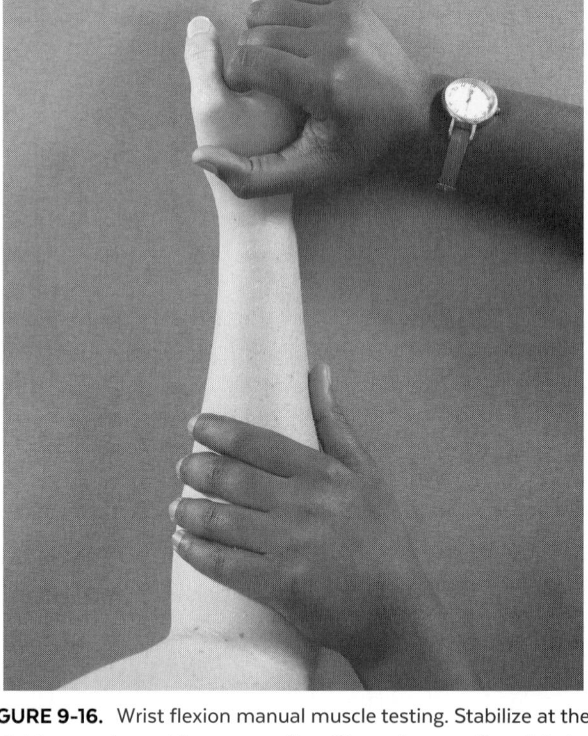

FIGURE 9-16. Wrist flexion manual muscle testing. Stabilize at the distal forearm to avoid compensation. Shown in a gravity-minimized position.

Wrist Flexion

Muscles: Flexor carpiulnaris, flexor carpiradialis, palmaris longus
Normal (N), Good (G), Fair (F)
Position: Client seated with forearm supinated on a flat surface, wrist in neutral position
Stabilize: On posterior aspect of distal forearm
Palpate: At base of second metacarpal just lateral to midline of forearm
Observe: Client moves the testing extremity in the direction of wrist flexion
Resist: Resistance is applied on the palm of the hand in the direction of wrist extension (Fig. 9-16)
Poor (P)
Position: Client seated with testing extremity on a table with forearm in neutral position (halfway between supination and pronation)
Stabilize: Along radial side of forearm
Palpate: As in gravity-resisted test
Observe: Client moves the testing extremity in the direction of wrist flexion
Resist: Resistance is not necessary in gravity-minimized position (2+ may take minimal resistance in this position)
Trace (T): No motion is seen but a palpable contracture is observed, as described earlier

Wrist Extension

Muscles: Extensor carpi radialis longus, extensor carpi radialis brevis, extensor ulnaris
Normal (N), Good (G), Fair (F)
Position: Client seated with forearm pronated and supported on a flat surface with wrist in neutral position
Stabilize: Anterior aspect of distal forearm
Palpate: Just proximal to bases of second and third metacarpals
Observe: Client moves the testing extremity in the direction of wrist extension
Resist: Resistance is applied on the dorsum of the hand in direction of wrist extension (Fig. 9-17)
Poor (P)
Position: Client seated with forearm in neutral rotation supported on a flat surface and wrist in neutral rotation
Stabilize: Along volar surface of distal forearm
Palpate: As in gravity-resisted test
Observe: Client moves the testing extremity in the direction of wrist extension[8]
Resist: Resistance is not necessary in gravity-minimized position (2+ may take minimal resistance in this position)
Trace (T): No motion is seen but a palpable contraction is observed or felt, as described earlier

FUNCTIONAL LIMITATIONS OF WEAK WRIST MUSCLES

Weak wrist extensors will cause a wrist drop putting the finger flexors at a mechanical disadvantage and giving rise to a weak grasp which will limit many ADLs. Weak wrist flexors may put finger extensors at a mechanical

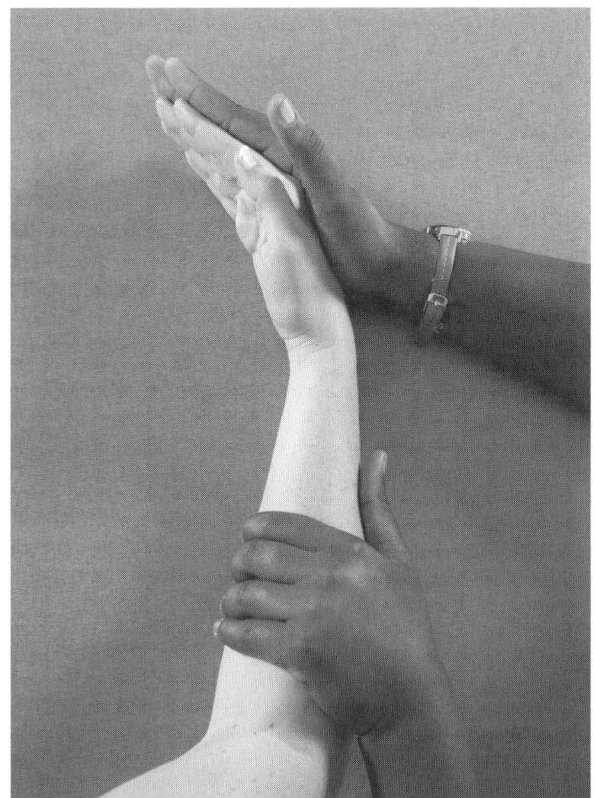

FIGURE 9-17. Wrist extension manual muscle testing. Stabilize at the distal forearm to avoid compensation. Shown in a gravity-reduced plane.

disadvantage, and may limit fine motor control and stabilization of the hand during ADL and IADL tasks.

Finger Flexion (Metacarpophalangeal [MCP])

Muscles: Lumbricals, palmar and dorsal interossei
Normal (N), Good (G), Fair (F)
Position: Client seated with forearm supinated and supported on a flat surface, wrist in neutral, fingers extended
Stabilize: Over distal dorsal surface of second through fifth metacarpals
Palpate: Is difficult but contraction may be detectable in palm
Observe: Client moves the fingers in flexion at the MCP joints while keeping IP joints extended
Resist: Resistance is applied with one or two fingers along volar surface of proximal phalanges in direction of MCP extension (Fig. 9-18)
Poor (P)
Position: Client seated with forearm in neutral rotation and supported on a flat surface, wrist in neutral position, fingers extended
Stabilize: Over dorsal surface of second through fifth metacarpals
Palpate: As in gravity-resisted test
Observe: Client flexes at the MCP joints while keeping interphalangeal (IP) joints extended

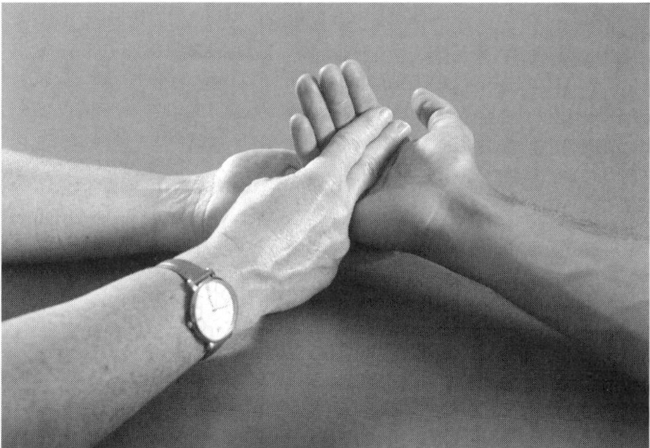

FIGURE 9-18. Metacarpophalangeal flexion manual muscle testing. Apply resistance with one or two fingers.

Resist: Not necessary in gravity-minimized plane (2+ may take minimal resistance in this position)
Trace (T): No movement is seen but a palpable contraction is observed or felt, as described earlier

Finger Flexion (Proximal Interphalangeal [PIP])

Muscles: Flexor digitorum superficialis
Normal (N), Good (G), Fair (F)
Position: Client seated with forearm supinated and supported on a flat surface, wrist in neutral position, fingers extended
Stabilize: Over palmar surface of proximal phalanges of second through fifth digits (Fig. 9-19)
Palpate: Over palmar surface of proximal phalanges
Observe: Client flexes fingers at PIP joints while keeping MCP joints extended
Resist: Resistance is applied with one finger on palmar surface of middle phalanges of second through fifth digits
Poor (P)

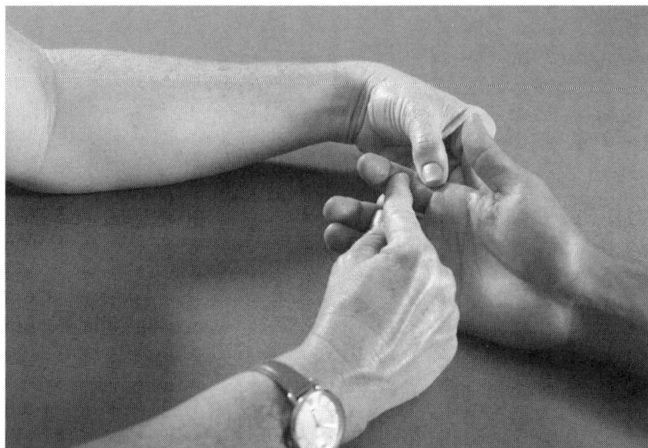

FIGURE 9-19. Proximal interphalangeal flexion manual muscle testing. Apply resistance with one or two fingers. Practitioner's left hand is blocking MCP flexion while right hand applies resistance.

Position: Client seated with forearm in neutral rotation and supported on a flat surface, wrist in neutral position, fingers extended
Stabilize: At the MCP joints
Palpate: As in gravity-resisted test
Observe: Client moves the PIP joints in flexion
Resist: Resistance is not necessary in gravity-minimized plane (2+ may take minimal resistance in this position)
Trace (T): No motion is seen but a palpable contraction is observed or felt, as described earlier

Finger Flexion (DIP)

Muscles: Flexor digitorum profundus
Normal (N), Good (N), Fair (F)
Position: Client sitting with forearm supinated and supported on a flat surface, wrist in neutral position, fingers extended
Stabilize: Over palmar surface of middle phalanges of second through fifth digits
Palpate: Over palmar surface of middle phalanges
Observe: Client moves the DIP joints in flexion
Resist: Resistance is applied with one finger on palmar surface of distal phalanges in the direction of DIP extension (Fig. 9-20)
Poor (P)
Position: Client sitting with forearm in neutral rotation and supported on a flat surface, wrist in neutral and fingers extended
Stabilize: Over middle phalanges of second through fifth digits
Palpate: As in gravity-resisted test
Observe: Client moves DIP joints in flexion
Resist: Not necessary in gravity-minimized plane (2+ may take minimal resistance in this position)
Trace (T): No motion is seen but a palpable contraction is observed or felt, as described earlier

Finger Extension (MCP)

Muscles: Extensor digitorum, extensor indicis, extensor digiti minimi
Normal (N), Good (G), Fair (F)
Position: Client seated with forearm pronated, wrist in neutral and fingers flexed
Stabilize: Proximal to the MCP joints at the metacarpals
Palpate: On the dorsum of the hand
Observe: Client moves the fingers in direction of MCP extension with IP joints flexed
Resist: Resistance is applied with fingers on the dorsal surface of proximal phalanges (Fig. 9-21)
Poor (P)
Position: Client seated with forearm in neutral rotation, wrist in neutral and fingers flexed at MCP joints
Stabilize: Over palmar aspect of second through fifth metacarpals
Palpate: As in gravity-resisted test
Observe: Client moves the fingers in direction of MCP extension with IP joints flexed
Resist: Not necessary in gravity-minimized plane
Trace (T): No motion is seen but a palpable contraction is observed or felt, as described earlier

Finger Abduction/Adduction (MCP)

Muscles: Dorsal interossei, abductor digiti minimi are MCP abductors and palmar interossei are MCP adductors
Normal (N), Good (G), Fair (F)
Position: Client sitting with forearm pronated and supported on a flat surface, wrist in neutral position and fingers extended (For MCP abduction, the digits are adducted, and for MCP adduction the digits are abducted.)
Stabilize: Over metacarpals
Palpate: Over dorso-radial aspect of second and third metacarpals, along dorso-ulnar aspect of third and

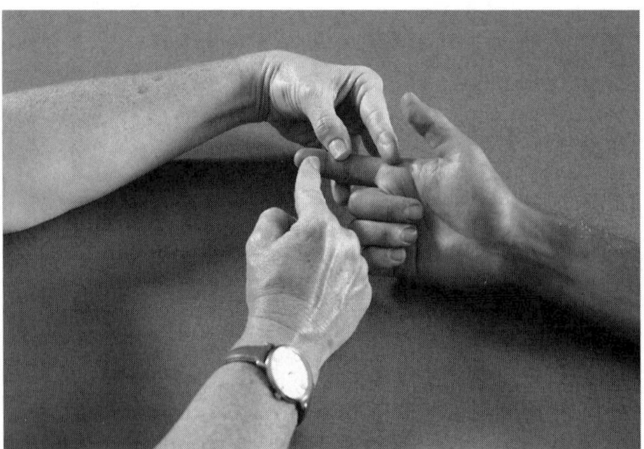

FIGURE 9-20. Distal interphalangeal flexion manual muscle testing. Apply resistance with one finger on palmar surface of distal phalanges. Practitioner's left hand blocks MCP and PIP flexion while right hand applies resistance.

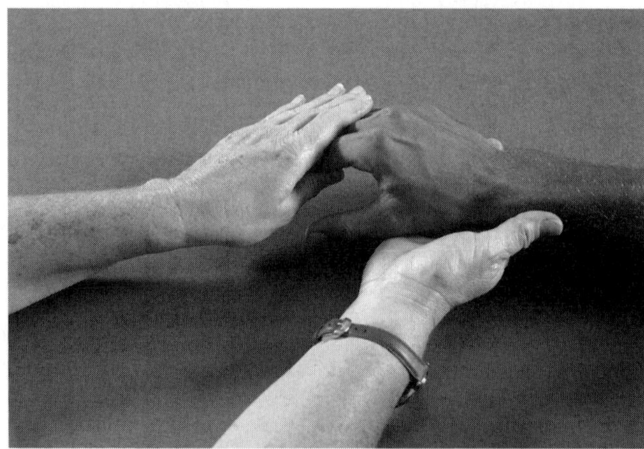

FIGURE 9-21. Finger extension manual muscle testing. Stabilize at metacarpals, and apply resistance with fingers on dorsum of proximal phalanges.

fourth metacarpals and ulnar border of fifth metacarpal (palpation is difficult)

Observe: Client moves the digits in MCP abduction or adduction depending on the test

Resist: Resistance is applied to each finger for MCP abduction in the direction of adduction and for MCP adduction in the direction of abduction. (For adduction, no resistance is applied to the third digit, but for abduction, the third digit is tested on both sides.) (Fig. 9-22)

Poor (P): Client abducts fingers through partial ROM

Trace (T): No movement is seen but a palpable contraction is observed, as described earlier

Thumb Flexion/Extension (CMC)

Muscles: CMC flexors are flexor pollicis brevis; carpometacarpal (CMC) extensors are extensor pollicis brevis and abductor pollicis longus

Normal (N), Good (G), Fair (F)

Position: Client sitting with forearm supinated and digits 2 to 5 in extension. (For CMC flexion, the thumb is in extension, and for CMC extension, the thumb is in flexion.)

Stabilize: At the wrist

Palpate: Over volar aspect of first metacarpal for flexors; palpate over dorsal aspect of first metacarpal for extensors

Observe: Client moves the thumb CMC in the direction of flexion or extension, depending on the test (Fig. 9-23)

Resist: Resistance is applied on the volar aspect of the first metacarpal with one finger in the direction of extension (for testing flexion); resistance is applied on the dorsal aspect of the first metacarpal in the direction of flexion (for testing extension). (Use one finger to provide resistance.)

Poor (P): Client flexes or extends joint through partial ROM

Trace (T): No motion is seen but a palpable contraction is observed or felt, as described earlier

Thumb Flexion/Extension (MCP)

Muscles: MCP flexor is flexor pollicis brevis; MCP extensor is extensor pollicis brevis

Normal (N), Good (G), Fair (F)

Position: Client seated with forearm supinated and supported on a flat surface with wrist in neutral position; MCP and IP joints of the thumb are extended for testing flexion and flexed for testing extension

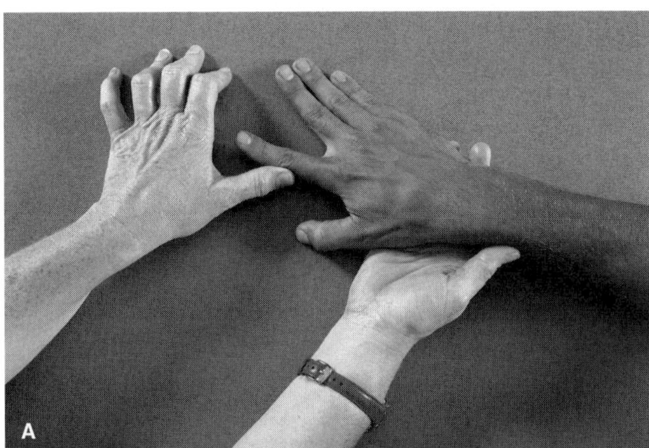

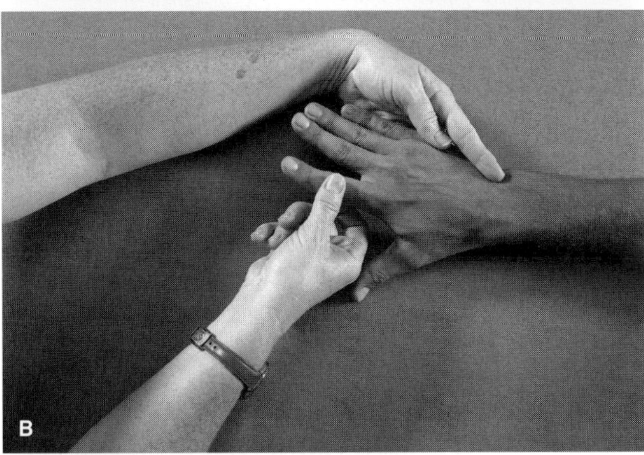

FIGURE 9-22. Finger abduction/adduction manual muscle testing. Apply resistance to each finger on both sides

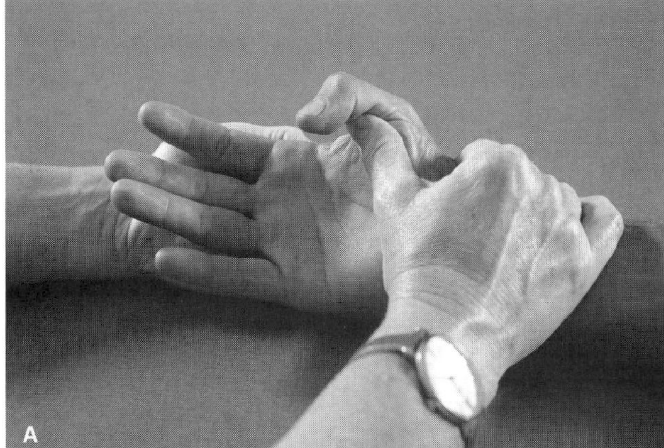

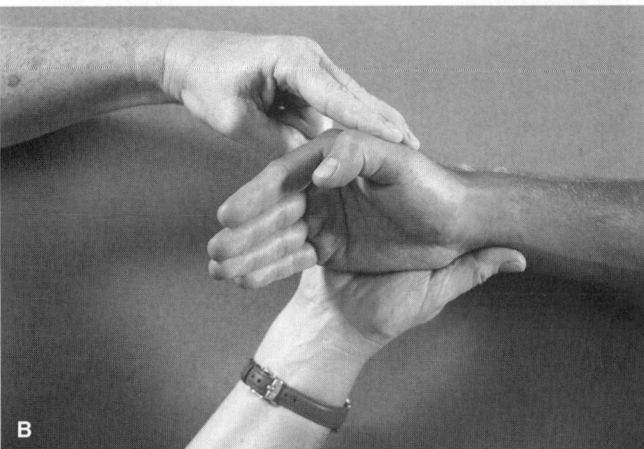

FIGURE 9-23. Thumb carpometacarpal flexion (A) and extension (B) manual muscle testing. Apply resistance on volar or dorsal aspect of thumb.

Stabilize: At the first (thumb) metacarpal
Palpate: Over volar aspect of first metacarpal for flexors; palpate over dorsal aspect of first metacarpal for extensors
Observe: Client moves the thumb MCP in the direction of flexion or extension, depending on the test
Resist: Resistance is applied along volar aspect of proximal phalanx of thumb in direction of extension (for testing flexion); resistance is applied on the dorsal aspect of proximal phalanx in direction of flexion (for testing extension). (Use one finger to provide resistance.) (Fig. 9-24)
Poor (P): Client flexes or extends joint through partial ROM
Trace (T): No motion is seen but a palpable contraction is observed or felt, as described earlier

Thumb Abduction/Adduction (CMC)

Muscles: CMC abductors are abductor pollicis longus and abductor pollicis brevis
CMC adductor is adductor pollicis
Normal (N), Good (G), Fair (F)
Position: Client seated with forearm supinated and supported on a flat surface with wrist in neutral position. (The thumb is adducted for testing CMC abduction and abducted for testing CMC adduction.)
Stabilize: At the volar surface of the wrist
Palpate: Abductors at the base and lateral aspect of thumb. Palpate adductors between first and second metacarpal bones (Fig. 9-25)
Observe: Client moves the thumb CMC joint in the direction of abduction or adduction depending on the test
Resist: Resistance is applied along lateral aspect of first metacarpal in direction of CMC adduction for testing abduction. Resist along medial surface of proximal phalanx of thumb in direction of CMC abduction for testing adduction
Poor (P): Client abducts or adducts joint through partial ROM
Trace (T): No motion is seen but a palpable contraction is observed or felt, as described earlier

Thumb Flexion/Extension (IP)

Muscles: IP flexor is flexor pollicis longus, and IP extensor is extensor pollicis longus
Normal (N), Good (G), Fair (F)
Position: Client seated with forearm in neutral rotation and supported on a flat surface and wrist in neutral

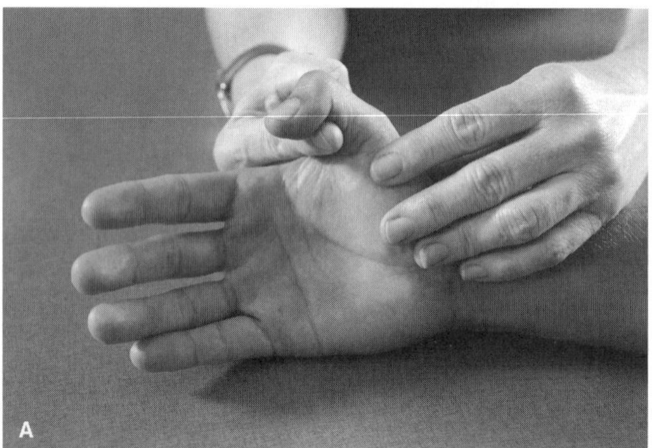

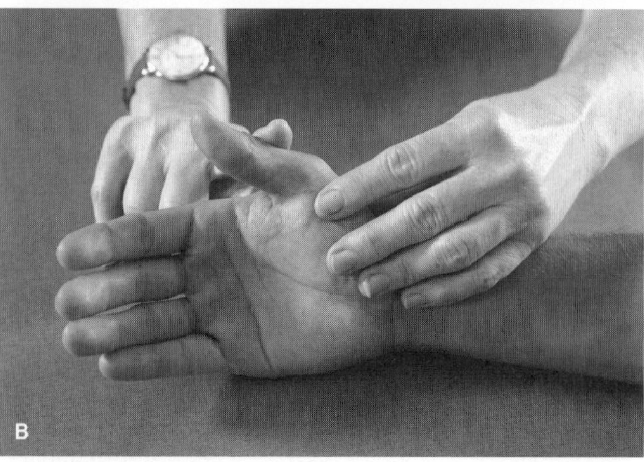

FIGURE 9-24. Thumb metacarpophalangeal flexion (A) and extension (B) manual muscle testing. Apply resistance to volar or dorsal aspect of proximal phalanx.

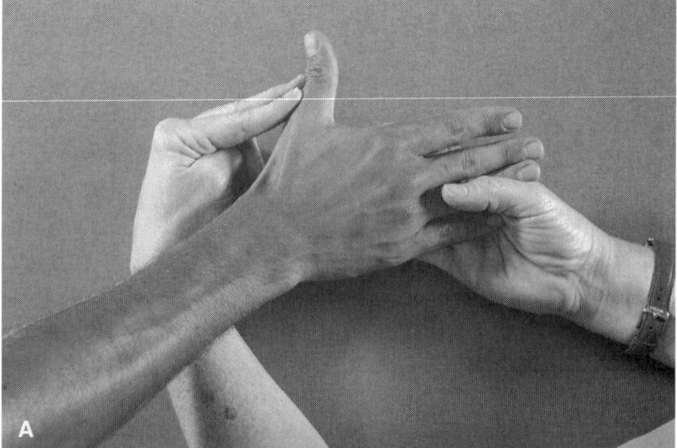

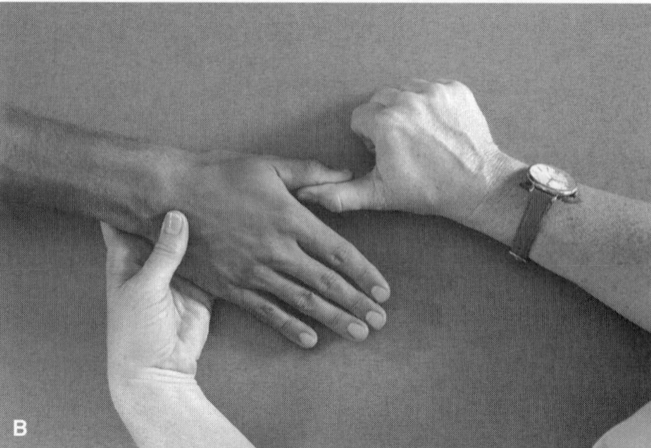

FIGURE 9-25. Thumb abduction (A) and adduction (B) manual muscle testing. Palpate adductors of thumb between first and second metacarpals.

position. (For thumb IP flexion, the joint is extended. For thumb IP extension, the joint is flexed.)
Stabilize: Sides of proximal phalanx of thumb (Fig. 9-26)
Palpate: Flexors on volar aspect of proximal phalanx of thumb; palpate extensors on the dorsal surface of proximal phalanx of thumb
Observe: Client moves the thumb IP in direction of flexion or extension depending on the test
Resist: Resistance is applied along volar aspect of distal phalanx of thumb in the direction of extension for testing flexion. (Resist along dorsal surface of distal phalanx of thumb in the direction of flexion for testing extension.)
Poor (P): Client flexes or extends IP joint through partial ROM
Trace (T): No motion is seen but a palpable contraction is observed or felt, as described earlier

Opposition of Thumb and Fifth Digit

Muscles: Opponens pollicis, opponens digiti minimi
Normal (N), Good (G), Fair (F)
Position: Client seated with forearm supinated and supported on a flat surface, wrist in neutral position and fingers extended

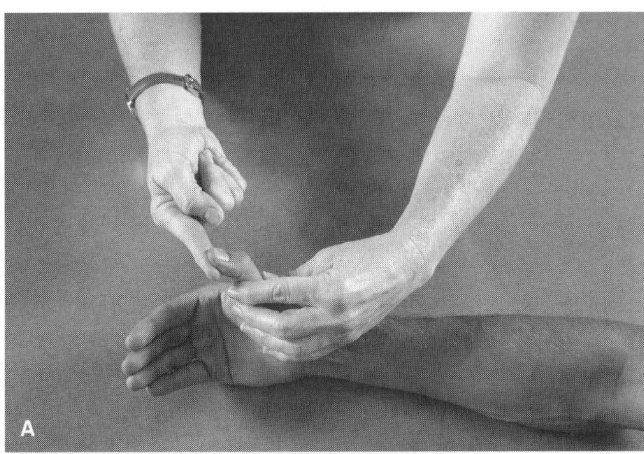

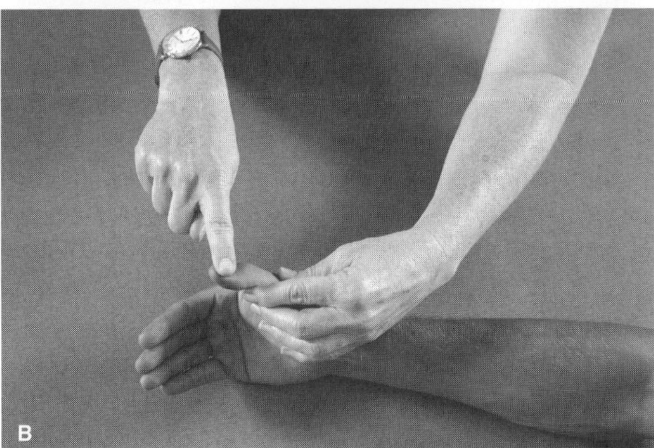

FIGURE 9-26. Thumb interphalangeal flexion (A) and extension (B) manual muscle testing. Stabilize proximal phalanx of thumb on both sides. Practitioner's left hand in A and B is blocking client's flexion, and right hand applies resistance.

Stabilize: At the wrist
Palpate: Along radial border of first metacarpal and ulnar border of fifth metacarpal
Observe: Client moves thumb and fifth finger into opposition
Resist: Resistance is applied simultaneously along volar shaft of first and fifth metacarpal bones attempting to separate first and fifth digits (Fig. 9-27)
Poor (P): Client moves joint through partial ROM
Trace (T): No motion is seen but a palpable contraction is observed or felt, as described earlier

FUNCTIONAL LIMITATIONS OF FINGER AND THUMB MUSCLES

Weakness in hand and finger muscles causes a variety of problems in hand functions. Grasp or release and opposition of thumb to fingers may hinder doing fine motor tasks like self-feeding, grooming, buttoning and tying shoe laces, writing, turning a key, opening containers, or holding on to a walker during functional ambulation.

MANUAL MUSCLE TESTING OF THE LOWER EXTREMITY

OT as a whole may not formally test the lower extremity strength as often, but it is important that there is an understanding of the testing process. The OT practitioner may want to quickly test a leg muscle before performing a functional task to assess safety. The practitioner who assesses clients for a wheelchair or mobility device will test the lower extremities each time. This section of the chapter can be a useful learning guide and a practical resource.

Hip Flexion

Muscles: Iliopsoas, sartorius, tensor fascia latae, rectus femoris
Normal (N), Good (G), Fair (F)

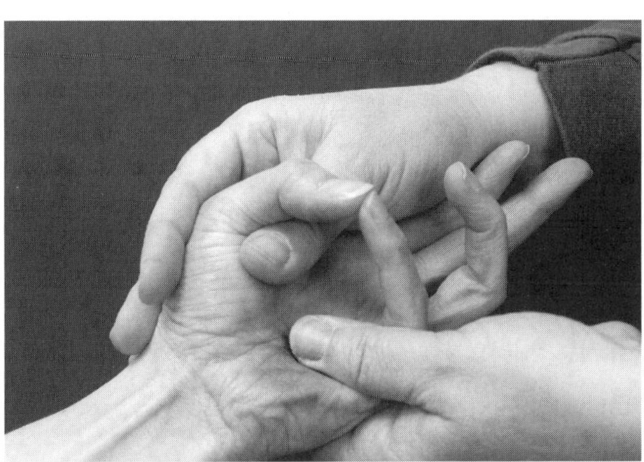

FIGURE 9-27. Thumb opposition. Apply resistance at both the first and fifth metacarpal bones away from opposition.

Position: Client seated at edge of table with knee at 90 degrees and foot unsupported, holding onto table edge with hands
Stabilize: At the contralateral iliac crest of the pelvis
Palpate: Distal to anterior superior iliac spine
Observe: Client moves the testing extremity in direction of hip flexion
Resist: Resistance is applied over anterior aspect of thigh proximal to the knee in direction of hip extension for Normal and Good strengths (No resistance is applied when testing Fair strength.)
Poor (P)
Position: Client is lying on non-test side holding this extremity in hip extension and knee flexion
Stabilize: The side-lying position and the pelvis while supporting the testing extremity
Palpate: As in gravity-resisted test
Observe: Client moves the testing extremity into maximal hip flexion
Resist: Not necessary in gravity-minimized position (2+ may take minimal resistance in this position)
Trace (T): No motion is seen but a palpable contraction is felt or observed, as described earlier

Hip Extension

Muscles: Gluteus maximus, semitendinosus, semimembranosus, biceps femoris
Normal (N), Good (G), Fair (F)
Position: Client in prone with lower extremities extended
Stabilize: At the pelvis
Palpate: Over buttock and upper thigh posteriorly
Observe: Client moves the testing extremity in the direction of hip extension while keeping the knee extended (if knee flexed, only testing gluteus maximus)
Resist: Resistance is applied over posterior aspect of the thigh proximal to the knee in the direction of hip flexion for Normal and Good strengths. (No resistance is applied for Fair strength.)
Poor (P)
Position: Client is lying on the non-test side holding this extremity in hip and minimal knee flexion
Stabilize: The side-lying position and the pelvis while supporting the testing extremity
Palpate: As in gravity-resisted test
Observe: Client moves the testing extremity into maximal hip extension
Resist: Resistance is not necessary in gravity-minimized position (2+ may take minimal resistance in this position)
Trace (T): No motion is seen but a palpable contraction is felt or observed, as described earlier

Hip Abduction

Muscles: Gluteus medius, gluteus minimus
Normal (N), Good (G), Fair (F)
Position: Client is in side-lying on non-test side holding this extremity in hip neutral and knee extension (client may require non-test hip/knee flexed for balance)
Stabilize: At the pelvis
Palpate: Above greater trochanter on lateral side of pelvis
Observe: Client moves the testing extremity in the direction of maximal hip abduction
Resist: Resistance is applied over the lateral aspect of the thigh proximal to the knee in the direction of hip adduction when testing Normal or Good strengths. (No resistance is applied when testing Fair strength.)
Poor (P)
Position: Client is supine with hips fully adducted and knees extended
Stabilize: The pelvis
Palpate: As in gravity-resisted test
Observe: Client moves the testing extremity into maximal hip abduction
Resist: Resistance is not necessary in gravity-minimized position (2+ may take minimal resistance in this position)
Trace (T): No movement is seen but a palpable contraction is felt, as described earlier

Hip Adduction

Muscles: Adductor magnus, adductor longus, adductor brevis, pectineus, gracilis
Normal (N), Good (G), Fair (F)
Position: Client is in side-lying on test side with hip in neutral and knee extended on testing surface (Non-test extremity is in abduction with knee extended, held up by tester.)
Stabilize: Support the non-test extremity in abduction
Palpate: On medial aspect of thigh
Observe: Client moves the testing extremity in the direction of hip adduction toward the non-test extremity
Resist: Resistance is applied over the medial aspect of distal thigh in direction of hip abduction for Normal and Good strengths (No resistance is applied when testing Fair strength.)
Poor (P)
Position: Client is supine with hip in neutral and full abduction and knee extended
Stabilize: At the pelvis
Palpate: As in gravity-resisted test
Observe: Client moves the extremity into maximal hip adduction
Resist: Resistance is not necessary in gravity-eliminated position (2+ may take minimal resistance in this position)
Trace (T): No movement is seen but a palpable contraction is felt or observed, as described earlier

Hip External Rotation

Muscles: Piriformis, quadratus femoris, gemellus superior and inferior, obturator internus and externus
Normal (N), Good (G), Fair (F)

Position: Client seated with legs off side of table with testing hip in 90 degrees flexion and knee flexed
Stabilize: At the anterolateral aspect of the distal thigh
Palpate: On posterior aspect of pelvis between sacrum and greater trochanter (external rotators are deep and hard to palpate)
Observe: Client moves the testing extremity into maximal hip external rotation
Resist: Resistance is applied over the medial aspect of the lower leg proximal to the ankle in the direction of internal rotation for testing Normal and Good strengths. (No resistance is applied when testing Fair strength.)
Poor (P)
Position: Client is supine with testing hip in internal rotation and knee extension
Stabilize: At the pelvis
Palpate: As in gravity-resisted test
Observe: Client moves the testing hip into maximal external rotation
Resist: Resistance is not necessary in gravity-minimized position (2+ may take minimal resistance in this position)
Trace (T): No movement is seen but a palpable contraction is seen or felt, as described earlier

Hip Internal Rotation

Muscles: Gluteus medius, gluteus minimus, tensor fascia latae
Normal (N), Good (G), Fair (F)
Position: Client seated with legs off side of table with testing hip in 90 degrees flexion and knee flexed
Stabilize: At the medial aspect of the distal thigh
Palpate: On anterolateral aspect of pelvis
Observe: Client moves the testing extremity into maximal hip internal rotation
Resist: Resistance is applied over the lateral aspect of the lower leg proximal to the ankle in the direction of external rotation for testing Normal and Good strengths. (No resistance is applied when testing Fair strength.)
Poor (P)
Position: Client is supine with testing hip in external rotation and knee extension
Stabilize: At the pelvis
Palpate: As in gravity-resisted test
Observe: Client moves the testing hip into maximal internal rotation
Resist: Resistance is not necessary in gravity-minimized position (2+ may take minimal resistance in this position)
Trace (T): No motion is seen but a palpable contraction is observed or felt, as described earlier

FUNCTIONAL LIMITATIONS OF WEAK HIP MUSCLES

Full flexion and extension of the hip are required for many ADLs and IADLs. Weak hip muscles may make standing difficult. Squatting, bending to tie a shoelace with the foot on the ground, and toenail care all require full or nearly full hip flexion. Sitting on and rising from a chair, ascending or descending stairs, bathing feet in a bathtub, and crossing of legs to access feet for washing or dressing lower body are other activities that require moderate to full flexion and extension.[1]

Knee Flexion

Muscles: Biceps femoris, semitendinosus, semimembranosus
Normal (N), Good (G), Fair (F)
Position: Client is prone with lower extremities extended
Stabilize: Over posterior aspect of pelvis
Palpate: On lateral aspect of posterior thigh
Observe: Client moves the knee into 90 degrees of flexion
Resist: Resistance is applied over posterior aspect of leg proximal to the ankle in the direction of knee extension for testing Normal and Good strengths (No resistance is applied when testing Fair strength.)
Poor (P)
Position: Client side-lying on non-test side with hip and knee extended
Stabilize: The testing thigh and support the testing extremity to minimize gravity without assisting the motion
Palpate: As in gravity-resisted test
Observe: Client moves the testing extremity into knee flexion
Resist: Resistance is not necessary in gravity-minimized position (2+ may take minimal resistance in this position)
Trace (T): No motion is seen but a palpable contraction is observed or felt, as described earlier

Knee Extension

Muscles: Quadriceps femoris
Normal (N), Good (G), Fair (F)
Position: Client seated with legs off side of table with a folded towel under distal thigh of testing extremity
Stabilize: The testing thigh
Palpate: Over anterior aspect of testing thigh
Observe: Client moves the testing extremity into knee extension
Resist: Resistance is applied over anterior aspect of distal lower extremity in the direction of knee flexion for testing Normal and Good strengths. (No resistance is applied when testing Fair strength.)
Poor (P)
Position: Client is side-lying on non-test side with hip extended and knee flexed.
Stabilize: The testing thigh and support the testing extremity to minimize gravity without assisting the motion
Palpate: As in gravity-resisted test

Observe: Client moves the testing extremity into knee extension
Resist: Resistance is not necessary in gravity-minimized position (2+ may take minimal resistance in this position)
Trace (T): No motion is seen but a palpable contraction is observed or felt, as described earlier

FUNCTIONAL LIMITATIONS

Knee weakness will make standing and walking difficult increasing the risk of falls as a result of buckling. ADLs that require moderate to full range of knee flexion and extension are lower body self-care tasks, such as donning pants and socks, squatting to lift an object from the floor, crossing legs and sitting down, and rising from a chair or commode.[1]

Ankle Plantar Flexion

Muscles: Gastrocnemius, soleus
Position: Client prone with knee extended and testing foot over edge of table, ankle in neutral position. (Alternate position may be in sitting with leg suspended.)
Stabilize: The lower extremity proximal to the ankle
Palpate: On posterior aspect of leg
Observe: Client moves the testing ankle into plantar flexion with toes relaxed
Resist: Resistance is applied on the posterior aspect of the calcaneus in the direction of dorsiflexion for testing Normal and Good strengths (No resistance is applied when testing Fair strength.)
Poor (P)
Position: Client side-lying on test side with testing extremity extended at hip and knee, ankle in neutral position
Stabilize: The lower extremity proximal to the ankle
Palpate: As in gravity-resisted test
Observe: Client moves the testing ankle into plantar flexion
Resist: Resistance is not necessary in gravity-minimized position (2+ may take minimal resistance in this position)
Trace (T): No motion is seen but a palpable contraction is observed or felt, as described earlier

Ankle Dorsiflexion

Muscles: Tibialis anterior
Normal (N), Good (G), Fair (F)
Position: Client seated with legs off table, testing ankle in neutral position
Stabilize: The lower extremity proximal to the ankle
Palpate: Over anterolateral aspect of tibia
Observe: Client moves the testing extremity into ankle dorsiflexion
Resist: Resistance is applied over dorsal surface of medial side of foot in the direction of plantar flexion for testing Normal and Good strengths. (No resistance is applied when testing Fair strength.)
Poor (P)
Position: Client side-lying on test side with testing extremity extended at hip and knee, ankle in neutral position
Stabilize: The lower extremity proximal to the ankle
Palpate: As in gravity-resisted test
Observe: Client moves the testing ankle into dorsiflexion
Resist: Resistance is not necessary in gravity-minimized position
Trace (T): No motion is seen but a palpable contraction is observed or felt, as described earlier

Foot Inversion

Muscles: Tibialis posterior
Normal (N), Good (G), Fair (F)
Position: Client sitting with lower leg and foot off table, ankle and foot in neutral position
Stabilize: The lower leg proximal to the ankle
Palpate: Over anteromedial aspect of tibia
Observe: Client moves the foot in inversion
Resist: Resistance is applied on the medial aspect of the foot in the direction of eversion for testing
Poor (P)
Position: Client supine with knee in extension, foot and ankle in neutral position
Stabilize: The lower leg proximal to the ankle
Palpate: As in gravity-resisted test
Observe: Client moves the foot in inversion
Resist: Resistance is not necessary in gravity-minimized position (2+ may take minimal resistance in this position)
Trace (T): No motion is seen but a palpable contraction is observed or felt, as described earlier

Foot Eversion

Muscles: Peroneus longus, peroneus brevis
Position: Client sitting with lower leg and foot off table, ankle and foot in neutral position
Stabilize: The lower leg proximal to the ankle
Palpate: Posterior to lateral malleolus
Observe: Client moves the foot in eversion
Resist: Resistance is applied on the lateral aspect of the foot in the direction of inversion for testing Normal and Good strengths. (No resistance is applied when testing Fair strength.)
Poor (P)
Position: Client supine with knee in extension, foot and ankle in neutral position
Stabilize: The lower leg proximal to the ankle
Palpate: As in gravity-resisted test
Observe: Client moves the foot in eversion
Resist: Resistance is not necessary in gravity-minimized position (2+ may take minimal resistance in this position)
Trace (T): No motion is seen but a palpable contraction is observed or felt, as described earlier

FUNCTIONAL LIMITATIONS WITH ANKLE MUSCLE WEAKNESS

Ankle weakness will cause instability with balance deficits and make a person more prone to sprains or fractures of the ankles. It will also increase the risk of falls, which may limit mobility and increase pain. ADLs and IADLs that require some ankle movement are donning socks, depressing the accelerator on an automobile, tying shoelaces, and walking on uneven ground.[1]

GRIP AND PINCH STRENGTH

Grip strength of the hand (gross grip) can be tested using a standard adjustable-handle dynamometer (Fig. 9-28). Testing position has been researched and must be followed to correctly assess grip strength[1]. The subject should be seated, with the shoulder slightly abducted and neutrally rotated and 0 degrees of shoulder flexion, the elbow flexed at 90 degrees, forearm in neutral position, and wrist between 0 and 30 degrees of extension. Observe the client for attempts to compensate by holding the shoulder in a tightly adducted position, flexing the shoulder, or extending the elbow. The dynamometer handle is generally set at the standard second position (the handle can be set at three different positions, depending on the size of the hand), and three trials are done for each hand. The examiner should stabilize the dynamometer lightly to prevent accidental dropping of the device, but be aware of the client pushing into the hand of the assessor for increased force or leverage. The practitioner may want to remove the client's rings for more comfortable testing, and alert the client that there may be no feeling of movement in the dynamometer, whatever the strength exerted. An average of the three trials should be documented. Both hands should be tested, either for evaluative information or so that the "normal" or non-affected hand can be used for comparison. Normative data may be used to compare strength scores.[1] Variables, such as age, vocation, prior injuries, pain, and disease process, may affect the strength measurements. There may be a variation of sides because of right or left hand dominance (dominant hand may be as much as 5-20 pounds stronger), which is typical. Refer to Table 9-4 for normative data of grip strength.

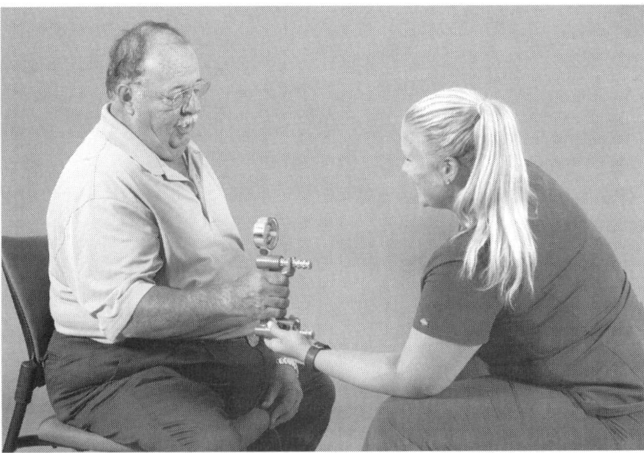

FIGURE 9-28. A hand-held dynamometer in a testing position.

Pinch strength should also be tested, using a pinch gauge or a pinch meter (Fig. 9-29). A variety of prehension patterns of pinch can be tested with the pinch gauge. Two-point pinch (thumb tip to index fingertip), lateral or key pinch (thumb pulp to lateral aspect of the middle phalanx of the index finger), and three-point pinch or the three jaw chuck (thumb tip to tips of index and middle fingers) should be assessed. As with the grip dynamometer, three successive trials should be performed, the average documented, and then compared bilaterally.[1] The practitioner should also hold the device to keep it from being dropped because weakness and oils on the skin of the client can make the fingers slide off the device during testing. Compensation efforts may include pushing the pinch gauge into the examiner's hand, the table, or the lap for more force.

Maximal voluntary effort during grip, pinch, or muscle testing may be affected by pain in the hand or extremity. The OT practitioner should note if the client's ability to exert full force is limited by subjective complaints of and presence of pain.[1] Consistency in noting pain with the use of a pain

TABLE 9-4 Average Grip Strength Versus Age (Pounds)

		MALES		*FEMALES*	
AGE	**HAND**	**MEAN**	**SD**	**MEAN**	**SD**
20-24	R	121.0	20.6	70.4	14.5
	L	104.5	21.8	61.0	13.1
25-29	R	120.8	23.0	74.5	13.9
	L	110.5	16.2	63.5	12.2
30-34	R	121.8	22.4	78.7	19.2
	L	110.4	21.7	68.0	17.7
35-39	R	119.7	24.0	74.1	10.8
	L	112.9	21.7	66.3	11.7
40-44	R	116.8	20.7	70.4	13.5
	L	112.8	18.7	62.3	13.8
45-49	R	109.9	23.0	62.2	15.1
	L	100.8	22.8	56.0	12.7
50-54	R	113.6	18.1	65.8	11.6
	L	101.9	17.0	57.3	10.7
55-59	R	101.1	26.7	57.3	12.5
	L	83.2	23.4	47.3	11.9
60-64	R	89.7	20.4	55.1	10.1
	L	76.8	20.3	45.7	10.1
65-69	R	91.1	20.6	49.6	9.7
	L	76.8	19.8	41.0	8.2
70-74	R	75.3	21.5	49.6	11.7
	L	64.8	18.1	41.5	10.2
75+	R	65.7	21.0	42.6	11.0
	L	55.0	17.0	37.6	8.9

Adapted from the User's Manual of Lafayette Instruments, with permission.

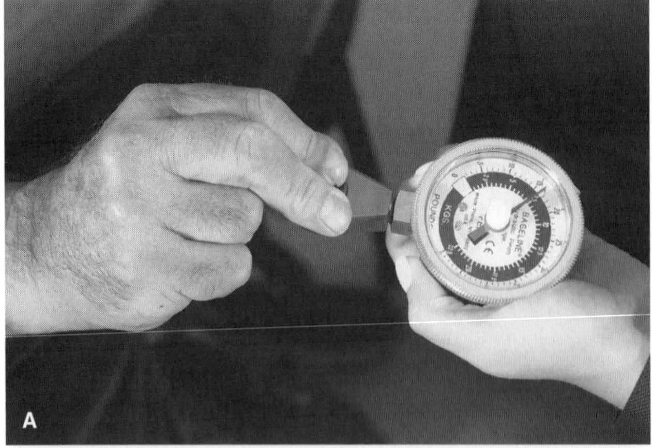

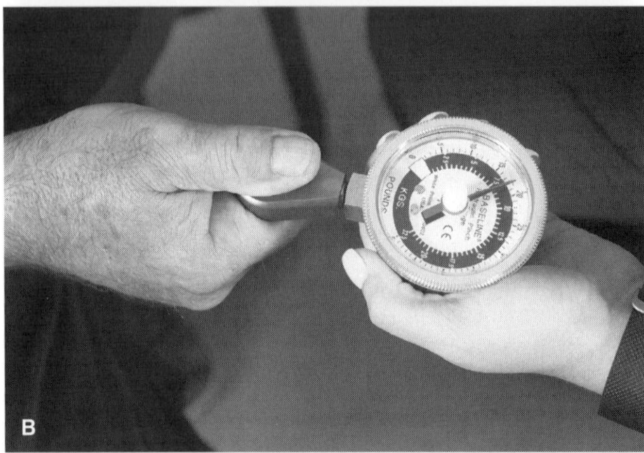

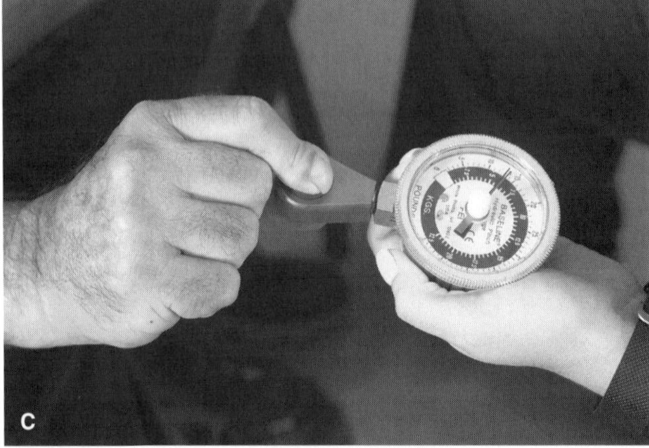

FIGURE 9-29. Assessing client's most common pinch strengths with a pinch gauge. **A.** Three jaw chuck. **B.** Lateral pinch. **C.** Two-point pinch.

scale and localization of the pain symptoms will help the clinician assess the role that pain is playing in the client's recovery process.

In a recent comparative study of millennials' grip and lateral pinch strength by Fain and Weatherford,[18] the authors concluded that there was a significant decrease in both strengths for the millennial population compared with older norms. This was noted in the study as resulting from a change in societal occupations and increase in use of technology, such as cellular phones, specifically by the millennial generation. Certainly, society as a whole is more sedentary than in the past, and this may affect strength in many muscle groups.

TECHNOLOGY AND TRENDS

MMT is the most traditional method to test muscle strength. Although it is inexpensive, readily available, and valid in assessment of lower grades, it is not so sensitive to gradations of strength above grade 4. A standard adjustable handle dynamometer is recommended for assessing grip strength. Pinch strength can be accurately tested using a pinch gauge.[13] The advent of technology and the need for more objective measures of human performance has led to the development of various devices to measure force created by human segments, primarily during isometric conditions.[13]

Hand-held dynamometry (HHD) is developing as an important part of science as applied to practice. The data have relevance for determining patient function before, during, or as the result of intervention. Instruments have been developed to objectively measure isometric forces. Recording is usually done via manual resistance at the place where the resistance hand would generally be placed for MMT. Studies have established a high reliability of the measures within tester and within session.[13] Nuclear Magnetic Resonance Imaging scans are used to assess the cross-sectional area of muscles to estimate the muscle volume and detect atrophy in muscles in research and outcome studies. Electromyography (EMG) assessment of muscle activity can be done with surface electrodes or percutaneously with needle electrodes. This can assist the physician to detect abnormal activity in a muscle and help in treatment planning.[13,24]

BASIC INTERVENTION STRATEGIES FOR IMPROVING MUSCLE STRENGTH

Preparatory methods and tasks may be used as a preliminary to occupations and activities and generally involve strengthening, decreasing pain, or increasing function of the muscle groups. When used by the OT practitioner, they are meant to prepare the client for occupational performance. Examples of these are therapeutic exercise, orthotics, assistive technology, physical agent modalities, and simulated activities or components of occupation. Therapeutic exercise and activities are described in this chapter, assistive technology in chapter 14, physical agent modalities in chapter 18, and orthotics in chapter 19.

Results of Assessment

During intervention planning for improvement or maintenance of muscle strength, the OT practitioner must consider several factors in the clinical reasoning process, including the following:

- What is the degree of weakness?
- Is the weakness generalized or specific to one or more muscle groups?

COMMUNICATION

Good and timely communication between the occupational therapist and the OTA is paramount for a successful outcome for the client. In muscle strength assessment and intervention, the contraindications and precautions need to be clearly mentioned in the initial evaluation by the occupational therapist and thereafter revisited by the OTA regularly as the condition warrants. In clients with osteoporosis, resistance applied during assessment or resistive activity used for intervention could aggravate the condition. In a very frail person, the OT practitioner's excessive enthusiasm could cause considerable damage in the form of torn muscles or fractures. Certain cardiovascular conditions, abdominal surgeries, or hernias also may have strict precautions for movement and resistance, and these have to be communicated clearly during the intervention process. For example, a client with recent coronary artery bypass surgery and a sternal incision may suffer a wound dehiscence (rupture along the surgical incision) as a result of resistive exercises prescribed by the occupational therapist. This could result in serious consequences for the client in terms of resuturing of the wound, loss of function and increased lengths of stay.

- Is there a significant imbalance between the agonist (muscle movement/direction desired) and the antagonist (muscle movement resisting/slowing the movement)?
- How are the client's occupations affected by this weakness or imbalance?
- Is an orthosis needed to protect or support the weak muscles?

When substantial imbalance between opposing groups of muscles is noted, intervention goals may be directed toward strengthening the weaker muscle group while maintaining the strength of the stronger group. Muscle imbalance may also suggest the need for an orthosis to protect the weaker muscle from overstretching while recovery is in progress. Examples of such orthoses are the ankle foot orthoses for nighttime used to prevent overstretching of the weakened ankle dorsiflexors, and the wrist cock-up orthosis, which is used to prevent overstretching of the weakened wrist extensors in radial nerve palsy.[1]

Muscle grades will suggest the level of therapeutic activities or exercises that can help maintain or improve strength. Is the weakness mild (G or 4 range), moderate (F to F+ or 3 to 3+ range), or severe (P to 0 or 2 to 0 range)?[9] If the client has mild weakness, the activities will involve strengthening exercises and performance of ADL/IADL tasks to increase strength and endurance. Muscles graded F+, for example, can be strengthened without added resistance, but with increased repetitions while lifting the weight of the arm and ADL/IADL tasks with light activity against gravity. Likewise, muscles graded P may require exercise or activity in the gravity-minimized plane, or by active assisted exercise, where the occupational therapy assistant (OTA) provides assistance with moving through the ROM with little or no resistance to increase strength.[1]

Endurance of the muscles—that is, the number of repetitions of the muscle contraction possible before fatigue sets in—is an important consideration in intervention planning. A frequent goal of the therapeutic activity program is to increase endurance as well as muscle strength. Since MMT does not measure endurance, the OT practitioner must assess endurance by engaging the client in periods of exercise or activity graded in length to determine the length of time that the muscle group can be used in sustained activity. A correlation between strength and endurance should be noted. Muscle endurance must be assessed after the muscle strength has been tested. Weaker muscles tend to fatigue faster than stronger ones. When selecting intervention modalities for increasing endurance or tolerance to sustained activity, it is better to emphasize repetitive action of muscles at a submaximal contraction and not tax the muscle to its maximal ability.[1,9]

Sensory loss, which often accompanies muscle weakness, complicates the client's ability to perform an activity or exercise program. For example, impaired tactile or proprioceptive sense may make the muscle appear weaker and ineffective even when strength is adequate for performance of a specific activity.[1]

Other considerations in the OT practitioner's clinical reasoning include the diagnosis and expected outcome of the disease, length of the recovery period, effect of exercise on muscle function, and any precautions or contraindications to exercise. A client with ALS may not be able to recover any lost strength because of the fast progression of the disease, and the focus would be on compensatory adaptations and equipment. Clients with MS may have the ability to strengthen muscles that have been weakened after an exacerbation of the disease but also are severely affected by overheating, and therefore caution must be taken during exercise and activity.

The OT practitioner should assess the effect of muscle weakness on the client's ability to perform ADLs and other occupations; this can be observed during various assessments. Which tasks are more difficult to perform because of muscle weakness? How does the client compensate for the weakness? Which tasks are most important and meaningful for the client to perform? Is special equipment necessary or desirable for the performance of some occupations? For example, in clients with weakness of the shoulder and elbow, the use of suspension slings or a mobile arm support could be beneficial to increase independence in self-feeding and increase sense of self-worth. For a client with difficulty lifting the leg against gravity, a sock aid to don the socks without crossing the leg over or a stool to place the foot on may be effective.

Roles of the Occupational Therapy Assistant and Occupational Therapist and Common Goals for Clients

For the occupational therapist and the OTA to work together effectively, understanding of roles and good communication between the two practitioners is of utmost

OT Practitioner's Viewpoint

In today's fast-paced rehabilitation environment, the push is to do "more" and "do it faster." New practitioners and students may feel the need to rush to meet a facility's productivity rules. As a result, therapies may not be as client centered or functional. My experience as an occupational therapist for over 30 years in almost all settings has given me some perspective. Listening to clients "tell their story" during the initial assessment has been an important step in building rapport with them and has made the subsequent intervention sessions much easier for both of us. So, do take the few minutes initially to hear them out.

It is very easy and tempting to use gadgets and equipment as a means of performing strengthening exercises. Often, these are meaningless and out of context for the clients. Stacking cones, lifting a dowel rod, and using the arm ergometer may be a quick warm up to a functional task but should not be the treatment in its entirety. If you must use these items, do so judiciously, and always explain the rationale behind your decision to your clients in simple layperson's terms. Clients are bound to be more compliant and engaged in the task if they understand the meaning and value behind it. Do not underestimate the value of occupations. Use of upper extremities for simple self-care tasks, even in very early stages of rehabilitation, has a lasting effect on function and self-esteem. Studies have shown that early mobilization in the form of exercises or activity decreases the length of stay for clients in intensive care units.[25]

Education of client and his or her family needs to start early and continue throughout the client's stay in the setting. If the client agrees, take the time and opportunity to teach whoever is present with the client during your session with them. I have had great results with compliance of exercises or continuation of ADLs when I have taken the time to review them with multiple family members or friends. So, in the end, it has been a win-win situation. ~ Sanchala Khanolkar Sen MSc, OTR/L, BCPR

importance. A successful occupational therapist–OTA relationship, in which the two practitioners complement each other, is beneficial both to the client and the facility. They work together to achieve the common goals of maximizing client's' independence.

OTAs can administer MMT after they have demonstrated service competency in the United States, and with supervision by the occupational therapist in Canada. The OTA can collaborate with the occupational therapist and the client to develop portions of the intervention plan (e.g., planning for dressing training).[20] As determined by the occupational therapist, an OTA can also implement interventions (where competence has been demonstrated) related to client factors of strength or ROM. Implementation of daily exercise or activity programs, upgrading or downgrading the activity according to the demands of the task and the tolerance of the client, progressing the client through daily participation in occupations, and contributing to documentation, education, and training of the client and family regarding home exercise program and equipment needs can be done by the OTA under the supervision of the occupational therapist.[1]

Common Intervention Approaches for Increasing Muscle Strength

The biomechanical approach to intervention is likely to be used in conditions where improvements in strength, ROM, and muscle endurance are the goals of OT. The understanding of kinematics (movement of objects) and kinesiology (human body movement) serves as the foundation for the biomechanical frame of reference. The OT practitioner views the limitations in occupational performance from a biomechanical perspective, analyzing the movement required to engage in the occupation.[1] The OT practitioner should use a variety of therapeutic exercises and functional activities to promote client engagement and function. The OT practitioner should use caution with simply performing exercises with weights or machines, as the hallmark of what distinguishes OT from physical therapy (PT) is the focus on function and occupation. Clients should clearly be able to distinguish OT from PT, even though both may be working on strengthening. The days of the OT practitioner working only on the arms and the PT practitioner on the legs should be gone if the OTA maintains a holistic and occupation-based focus.

PURPOSES OF THERAPEUTIC EXERCISE AND THERAPEUTIC ACTIVITY

The general purposes of therapeutic exercise, as with therapeutic activity, are to:

- Develop awareness of normal movement patterns.
- Aid in overcoming ROM deficits.
- Develop strength and endurance to perform tasks in a functional way.

Strengthening may be graded by an increase or decrease in resistance. Methods include changing the plane of movement from gravity-minimized to against-gravity, adding weights to the equipment or to the client, and using tools of increasing weight.[1]

Endurance may be graded for "just the right challenge" by moving from light to heavy work and increasing the duration of the work period. For example, folding napkins or sorting kitchen utensils can be done at first in supported sitting (chair level), then unsupported sitting (edge of bed or mat), and then progressed to standing and organizing household items onto shelves.[1]

In degenerative conditions, such as muscular dystrophy, MS, or ALS, the OT practitioner must take care to accommodate the client's diminishing endurance and grade the activity accordingly. In certain situations, adding exercise to muscles fatigued by the daily routine can lead to decreased functional performance and to safety risks. An example might be the client using a squeeze ball 50 times and then not having the strength in the hand to button a shirt.

Preparatory tasks and methods may be used as a preliminary to activities, which prepare the client for improved occupational performance. An exercise program for muscle strengthening is considered an example of a preparatory method because if the client has increased strength, he or she is able to increase occupational performance.[20] A muscle must contract at or near its maximal capacity and for enough repetitions and time to increase strength. Active-assisted, active, and resistive isotonic exercises and isometric exercises are used to increase strength.

ACTIVE-ASSISTED EXERCISE

In active-assisted exercise, the client moves the joint through partial ROM or gives some assistance throughout the range, using isotonic muscle contraction, and the OT practitioner or a mechanical device completes the range (Fig. 9-30). Slings, pulleys, weights, springs, or elastic bands may be used to provide mechanical assistance.[21]The goal of active-assisted exercise is to increase strength of trace (T), poor minus (P–), and fair minus (F–) muscles while maintaining ROM and performing functional tasks. In the case of trace muscles, the client may contract the muscles with the practitioner's encouragement, while the practitioner completes the entire ROM. The exercise is graded by decreasing the amount of assistance until the client can perform active exercises independently.[22,23] Active-assisted exercise completed in a functional way could be hand-over-hand self-feeding or assisting to push a weaker arm forward into a shirt. This type of active-assisted exercise can be very motivating to clients, can be easily graded for changing needs over time, and involves the client in their own care.

ACTIVE EXERCISE

Isotonic muscle contraction is used in active exercise, but eccentric contraction may also be used. With active exercise, the client moves the joint through its available ROM independently against no outside resistance (Fig. 9-31). The goal of active exercise is to increase strength of poor to fair muscles while maintaining ROM. It may be used with higher muscle grades for the maintenance of strength and ROM when resistance is contraindicated. If exercise is performed in a gravity-minimized plane, a powdered surface or board may be used to decrease resistance produced by friction. Using a pillowcase between the body part and the surface may also help decrease friction. The exercise is graded by a change to resistive exercise as strength improves.[22,23]

RESISTIVE EXERCISE

Resistive exercises use isotonic muscle contraction against a specific amount of weight to move the load through a certain ROM.[22-24] It is also possible to use eccentric contraction against resistance. Resistive exercise is used primarily for an increase in the strength of F+ to normal muscles. It may also be useful for producing relaxation of the antagonists to the contracting muscles if increased range is desired for stretching or relaxing hypertonic antagonists. An example is performing a resistive triceps exercise such as pressing up on the armrests from the wheelchair seat to decrease hypertonicity in biceps.

The client performs muscle contraction against resistance and moves the part through the available ROM (Fig. 9-32). The resistance applied should be the maximum against which the muscle is capable of contracting for the desired repetitions. Resistance may be applied manually or by weights, springs, elastic bands, sandbags, or special

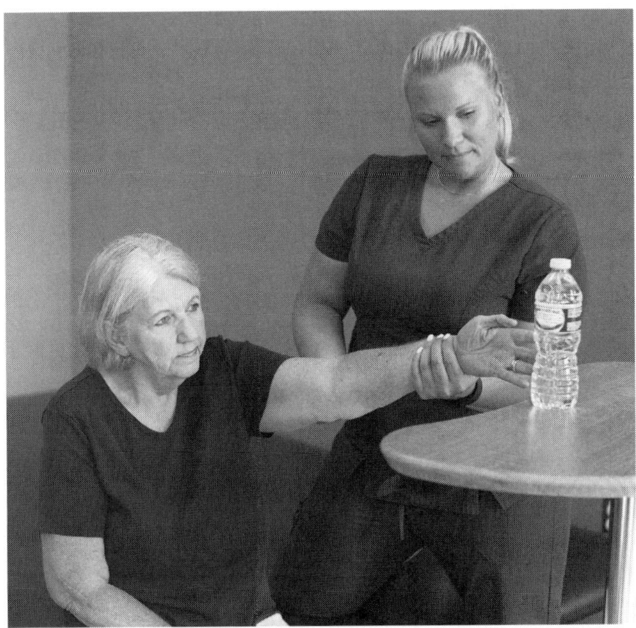

FIGURE 9-30. OTA assists client in reaching for a beverage as functional active-assisted exercise.

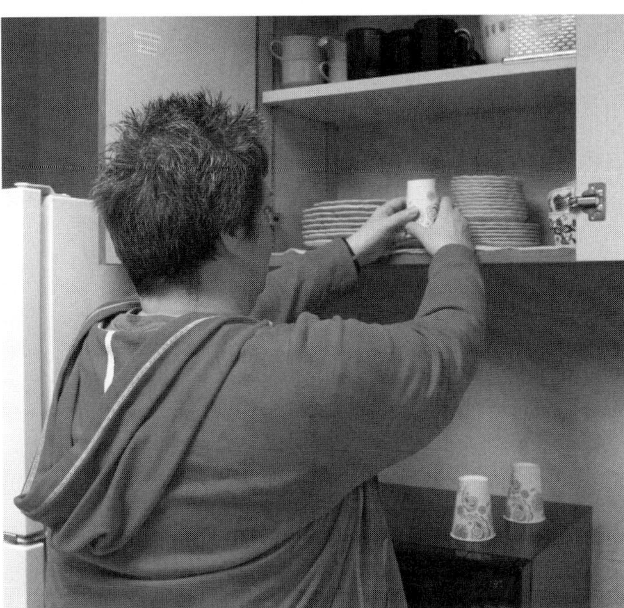

FIGURE 9-31. Client performing functional task of placing lightweight paper cups as simple active exercise.

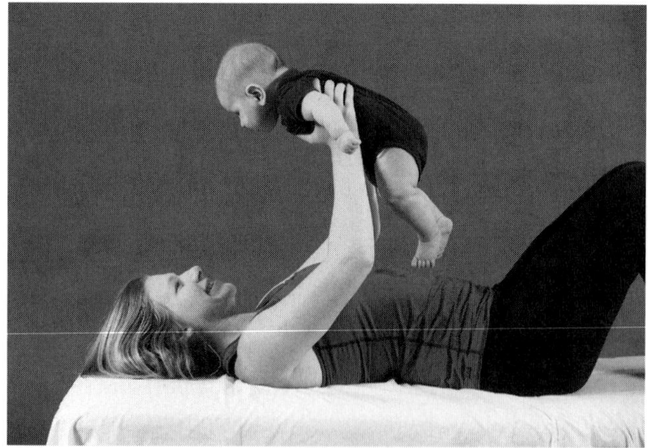

FIGURE 9-32. Client performs meaningful resistive exercise lifting her baby.

devices. The resistance is graded progressively with an increasing amount of resistance and the number of repetitions depends on the client's general endurance and the endurance of the specific muscle.[22-24]

Progressive Resistive Exercise One specialized type of resistive exercise is the **DeLorme's method of progressive resistive exercise (PRE).**[21,25] PRE is based on the overload principle. During the exercise procedure, small loads are used initially and increased gradually after each set of 10 repetitions (Fig. 9-33). It consists of three sets of 10 repetitions each, with resistance applied as follows: first set, 10 repetitions of 50% of maximal resistance; second set, 10 repetitions of 75% of maximal resistance; third set, 10 repetitions at maximal resistance.[21,24,25]

An example of a PRE for strengthening a biceps muscle, which can withstand a maximum of 12 pounds of resistance, is as follows: Flex the elbow first against 6 pounds for 10 repetitions, then against 9 pounds for 10 repetitions, and the final 10 repetitions against 12 pounds.

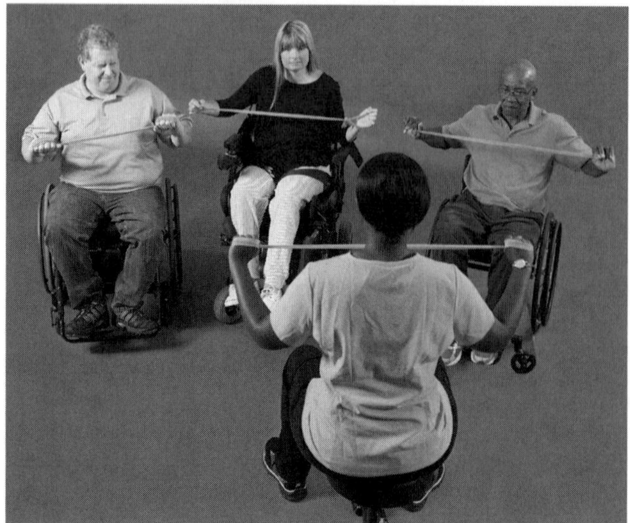

FIGURE 9-33. Performing resistive exercises with resistive bands; stronger bands can be used as clients gain strength.

ISOMETRIC EXERCISE

Isometric exercise uses isometric contractions of a specific muscle or muscle groups. In isometric exercises, a muscle or a group of muscles is actively contracted and relaxed without producing motion of the joint that it ordinarily moves. The purpose of this type of exercise is to maintain muscle strength when active motion is not possible or is contraindicated. It may be used with any muscle grade above trace. It is especially useful for clients in casts, after surgery, and with arthritis or burns.[24] It can be done with or without resistance.

The client is taught to set or contract the muscles voluntarily and to hold the contraction for 5 to 10 seconds. The OT practitioner can assist to set the muscles by providing a kinesthetic touch with fingers without offering resistance. If passive motion is allowed, the OT practitioner may move the joint to the desired point in the ROM and ask the client to hold the position. This is isometric exercise without resistance.[1]

Isometric exercise with resistance uses isometric muscle contractions performed against some outside resistance, for example manual resistance, weights, or an outside surface. Its purpose is to increase muscle strength in muscles graded fair or 3, to normal or 5. A small weight held in the hand while the wrist is stabilized at neutral requires

THE OLDER ADULT

As global population ages, research into the causes and characteristics of aging has grown dramatically. OT practitioners need to be aware of the evidence supporting theories of aging so that they are able to distinguish normal aging from aging caused by disease. Aging is caused by the passage of time. Biological theories have determined that aging is highly influenced by damage caused to cells as a result of wear and tear. Lifestyle choices, such as poor diet, smoking, a sedentary lifestyle, and lack of exercise, have been correlated with earlier aging and increased susceptibility to disease.[26]

Sarcopenia or age-related muscle loss occurs when there is no intentional effort or intervention to prevent decline. It can also occur as a result of some diseases and their effects, such as prolonged immobilization. According to Carmeli et al, 20% or more of skeletal muscle mass is lost by age 80.[27] This can give rise to decreases in muscle tone, strength, and endurance, resulting in falls and other complications. OT practitioners can help older clients establish occupational habits and routines to maintain their health and delay the progression of disease. OT interventions in older adults can provide education on the importance of daily exercise. Developing a daily routine of exercises or activities to build into client's schedule, such as walking for 30 minutes before breakfast, climbing up or down stairs while doing laundry in the basement, gardening, and so on can go a long way in establishing a healthy lifestyle. Although age causes loss of muscle mass, strength, and maximum ROM, a motivated, well older adult is able to maintain the functional ROM and strength needed for daily tasks.[26,28]

isometric contraction of the wrist flexors and extensors.[1] Isometric exercise should be used with caution as it affects the cardiovascular system in some clients and conditions (e.g., a recent myocardial infarction or heart attack). It may cause a rapid and sudden increase in heart rate and blood pressure, depending on the client's age, intensity of contraction, and the muscle mass being contracted.[23] Therefore, cardiovascular precautions are particularly important and must be taken into consideration with this type of exercise. All types of exercise can have an effect on the heart rate, blood pressure, and oxygen saturation of the client, and it is very important for the OT practitioner to note precautions from the chart and monitor vitals as needed.

SUMMARY

Muscle weakness may be the result of many diseases and injuries. Screening tests can be used to assess the general level of strength available for the client to engage in the occupations of ADLs, IADLs, rest and sleep, education, work, play, leisure, and social participation. These tests can determine which clients and which muscle groups may need MMT.[1] MMT assesses the level of strength in a muscle or muscle groups. It does not measure muscle endurance or coordination and cannot be used accurately when spasticity is present in a muscle group. Accurate assessment of muscle strength depends on the knowledge, skill, and experience of the OT practitioner. Although there are standard definitions of muscle grades, clinical judgment is important for an accurate assessment.

Muscle test results are used to plan intervention strategies to increase strength, compensate for muscle weakness, and improve occupational performance. Results can also be used to track the progression and expected course of some diseases, which, in turn, can assist the OT practitioner to choose appropriate intervention modalities and strategies.[1]

Engagement in occupation is the primary goal and objective of OT practice. OT practitioners can use therapeutic exercises and activities to help clients meet their physical and personal goals. Be wary of performing exercises exclusively without a functional approach, as purposeful, occupation-based activity is the core of OT practice.[1] A client could unload a dishwasher or lift canned goods to strengthen in a functional way instead of sitting at a weight machine. Appropriate therapeutic exercise and activity are individualized and designed to be purposeful, goal directed, meaningful, and interesting to the client while meeting therapeutic objectives. It can be adapted and graded to meet the special needs of clients or the environment.

REVIEW QUESTIONS

1. Screening tests for muscles are useful in which three of the following?
   a. Observing areas of strength and weakness
   b. Reducing pain
   c. Determining which areas require specific MMT
   d. Assessing sensory impairments
   e. Testing specific muscles in isolation
   f. Evaluation of performance limitations
2. You are an OTA student in inpatient rehabilitation. In your second week, your supervisor asks you to perform MMT on Mr. Roberts, who is supine in his hospital bed. How should you position your client for MMT of shoulder flexion against gravity?
   a. Prone
   b. Supine
   c. Sitting
   d. Side-lying
3. How should you position your client for MMT of horizontal adduction against gravity?
   a. Prone
   b. Supine
   c. Sitting
   d. Side-lying
4. Your supervisor tells you to perform MMT on your client without getting her out of bed. How would you position your client for MMT shoulder extension, gravity-minimized?
   a. Prone
   b. Supine
   c. Hook-lying
   d. Side-lying
5. Some limitations of MMT are listed below. Which three of the following are correct?
   a. It cannot measure muscle endurance.
   b. It discerns how muscle weakness is limiting performance in function.
   c. It cannot accurately measure strength in spastic muscles.
   d. It cannot measure muscle coordination.
   e. It is a means of evaluating muscle strength.
   f. It determines the amount of muscle power available.
6. Before performing manual muscle testing, the OT practitioner must measure the client's _______ to assign muscle grades correctly.
   a. Sensation
   b. PROM
   c. Isolated joint motion
   d. Muscle endurance
7. Mary is a 60-year-old woman who had a left CVA and is attending outpatient OT services. During functional muscle testing of her right arm, the OTA notices that the client can raise her arm all the way up but that it falls down immediately. What muscle grade is the client exhibiting?
   a. 2+
   b. 3
   c. 3+
   d. 5
8. John is recovering from Guillain-Barré syndrome. While checking his muscle strength in his R wrist extensors, the OTA notices that the muscle contracts but the joint does not move. What muscle grade should be assigned to the client's wrist extensors?
   a. 0
   b. 1
   c. 2
   d. 4
9. You ask your client to raise her arm in the air in front of her. She is unable to lift it. In a gravity-minimized position, she has some ROM, but it is less than full. What MMT grade would you assign her?
   a. 2
   b. 1
   c. 2−
   d. 3

10. Your supervisor at the outpatient clinic asks you to complete a sensory assessment on a client. She tells you that your client has good (4/5) muscle strength in his upper extremities (UEs). Which one of the following answers will you choose for his muscle strength?
    a. Full ROM in the gravity-minimized plane
    b. Partial ROM against gravity
    c. Full ROM against gravity with moderate resistance
    d. Partial ROM against gravity with minimum resistance

CASE STUDY

Lydia is a 35-year-old school teacher who was very active, worked full time, exercised, and took care of her 2-year-old daughter. She woke up one morning and experienced tingling and numbness starting from her feet and ascending upward. By that evening, she had increasing numbness and weakness in her extremities with shortness of breath. She was admitted to an intensive care unit and intubated because of worsening respiratory distress. In addition, she complained of pain and tenderness in her muscles, decreased sensory processing, and difficulty swallowing, and she was very agitated and fearful. She was diagnosed with acute Guillain-Barré syndrome and was placed on a ventilator.

The OT practitioner fitted her with resting/positional orthotics to support her hands and reduce her muscle belly tenderness. In addition, a communication system was devised with the help of her husband. Lydia would blink her eyelids at the correct letters on a board to make a word and thus try to make her needs known. Daily PROM exercises were taught to the nursing staff and family to prevent contractures of her extremities as she had very minimal active movement of her joints.

When Lydia was moved out of the intensive care unit as her condition began to improve, the OT practitioner was able to reduce her fears by adapting a system that gave her more control of her environmental context, allowing her to operate her call button, room lights, bed, and television.[1] After a few weeks on the general floor, Lydia was transferred to the inpatient rehabilitation unit and eventually discharged home with her husband and 2-year-old daughter in a one-story house. Her mother and sister live nearby and are willing to assist her, as needed. Her husband works full time in a bank and is very supportive. Before onset of her disease, Lydia was very active, worked out at a gym three times a week, and enjoyed an active social life. She was a regular volunteer at the local soup kitchen.

Six months later, Lydia is now participating in OT in an outpatient setting. Guillain-Barré syndrome is in the recovery phase, with remyelination resulting in a generalized increase in muscle strength. Lydia continues to be unable to fully engage in occupations that are meaningful to her, primarily because of residual weakness in her distal extremities and moderate limitation in endurance. She uses a walker at home but needs a wheelchair for long-distance mobility. A home health aide comes in the morning to assist her with bathing and personal grooming and to drive her to her outpatient appointments. Her mother and sister help care for her daughter. Lydia states, "Although I can do things for myself, it takes so long that I end up getting exhausted and need a lot of rest breaks to complete the task. I need help to safely shave my armpits and legs. Blow drying and curling my hair can be daunting tasks."[1]

Lydia has also indicated that she cannot complete home management tasks, such as meal preparation, grocery shopping, and laundry, without assistance. She is unable to provide care to her daughter, which greatly concerns and saddens her. She is limited in her ability to participate in outdoor and community occupations, which used to give her a great deal of satisfaction. She has been able to take family leave from her job but hopes and wants to return to work as soon as she can. She has indicated that with all the progress she has made, she and her husband are trying to be realistic but are more and more hopeful about her making a full recovery.

In reviewing the above occupational profile, the OT practitioner must focus on those client factors that are interfering with body function, namely, decreased muscle strength and endurance. Maintaining the arms at or above shoulder level without taking several rest breaks when brushing the teeth or hair remains a problem for Lydia. Another problem is applying enough force to open jars or chop foodstuff during meal preparation. These deficits are prohibiting the client from fully engaging in occupations for participation in the physical, social, personal, cultural, and spiritual contexts that bring meaning to her life.[1]

1. At what stage in this client's recovery should the OT practitioner first administer a muscle strength assessment?
2. What are some other methods to assess muscle strength? What information regarding the client's status can be gained from each of these methods?
3. How can the above information be used to develop an intervention plan for this client?

PUTTING IT ALL TOGETHER — Sample Treatment and Documentation

Setting	Inpatient rehabilitation center
Client Profile	Ms. J is a 60-year-old female admitted to acute care 2 weeks ago for pneumonia with congestive heart failure and COPD. She was initially in the ICU and then in acute care. Now she is transferred to inpatient rehabilitation for further therapy. Before this episode, Ms. J was independent in ADLs and IADLs. She lives in a one-level house with no steps, has a standard toilet, tub/shower with glass doors, and no DME.
Work History	Ms. J works part time as a secretary in a large firm.
Insurance	Blue Cross Blue Shield
Psychological	Mild anxiety over her situation at times, but overall in good spirits
Social	Married to a supportive spouse who also works. They have one daughter who lives in town and two grandkids, who they love spending time with. Ms. J also loves to paint and dance.
Cognitive	Intact

PUTTING IT ALL TOGETHER Sample Treatment and Documentation (continued)

Motor & Manual Muscle Testing (MMT)	Dominance—R hand dominant PROM—intact all four extremities AROM—about 50% to 75% through ROM at all UE joints MMT—shoulders: 3-/5; elbows: 3-/5; wrists: 3-/5; and 30 pounds grip in right hand, 27 pounds grip left hand, 12 pounds lateral pinch in both hands Sensation—intact
ADL	Feeding—Min A with AE (builtup utensils) Grooming—Mod A Bathing—Max A UB dressing—Min A LB dressing—Max A Toileting—Mod A to bedside commode
IADL	Not appropriate at the present time
Goals	1. Client will feed self all 3 meals with setup using adaptive equipment prn—1 week 2. Client will groom self with setup at sink level in sitting—1 week 3. Client will tolerate 1 hr of OT session with one to three rest breaks in gym area—2 weeks 4. Client will complete bathing tasks with Min A in supported sitting—3 weeks

OT TREATMENT SESSION 1

THERAPEUTIC ACTIVITY	TIME	GOAL(s) ADDRESSED	OTA RATIONALE
Teach use of AE during self-feeding and grooming	30 min	#1 and #2	*Education and Training; Occupations:* Education and training in use of builtup handles on feeding and grooming utensils during morning ADL session, correct technique with rest breaks for energy conservation
Training and practice of strengthening exercises/trunk control to increase muscle strength and endurance	30 min	#3 and #4	*Preparatory Tasks:* For bathing use graded upper extremity strength exercises at chair, mat level in sitting with rest breaks to increase strength, trunk control for ADLs

SOAP note: 9/6/—, 9:00 am-10:00 am

S: "I need to rest and take my time while eating."

O: Client participated in skilled OT intervention in room and gym area for morning tasks of self-feeding and grooming. Client was educated and trained in use of adapted utensils to feed self and groom with builtup handles on hair brush and comb. Client needed Min A with 3 rest breaks to complete tasks. Client also completed bilateral UE strength and trunk control exercises sitting at edge of mat with frequent rest breaks because of decreased activity tolerance.

A: Client tolerated activities well, with no pain reported during tasks. Required rest breaks due to fatigue and minimal SOB, was able to feed self with setup and groom with Min A. Client is very motivated and tries hard. Client has great potential to increase independence in ADLs.

P: Will continue to see client 5 times a week while in inpatient rehabilitation to work on increasing strength, endurance, and independence with ADLs with the use of adaptive equipment, as needed, and providing client/family education.

Elizabeth Jacobsen, COTA/L 9/6/—, 3:30 pm

TREATMENT SESSION 2

What could you do next with this client?

TREATMENT SESSION 3

What could you do next with this client?

REFERENCES

1. Pedretti, L. W., Pendleton, H. M., & Schultz-Krohn, W. (2013). *Pedretti's occupational therapy: Practice skills for physical dysfunction* (7th ed.). St. Louis, MO: Mosby Elsevier.
2. Clarkson, H. M. (2000). *Musculoskeletal assessment: Joint motion and muscle testing* (2nd ed.). Philadelphia, PA: Wolters Kluwer/Lippincott Williams & Wilkins Health.
3. Lippert, L., & Lippert, L. (2006). *Clinical kinesiology and anatomy* (4th ed.). Philadelphia, PA: F. A. Davis.
4. Hislop H. J., & Montgomery, J. (1995). *Daniels and Worthington's muscle testing* (6th ed.). Philadelphia, PA: W. B. Saunders.
5. Daniels, L., & Worthington C. (1986). *Muscular testing* (5th ed.). Philadelphia, PA: W. B. Saunders.
6. Pact, V., Sirotkin-Roses, M., & Beatus, J. (1984). *The muscle testing handbook.* Boston, MA: Little, Brown.
7. Kendall, F. P., & McCreary, E. K. (1983). *Muscles, testing and function: With posture and pain* (2nd ed.). Baltimore, MD: Williams & Wilkins.
8. Latella, D., & Meriano, C. (2003). *Occupational therapy manual for evaluation of range of motion and muscle strength.* Clifton Park, NY: Thomson/Delmar Learning.
9. Killingsworth, A. (1987). *Basic physical disability procedures.* San Jose, CA: Maple Press.
10. Bobath, B. (1978). *Adult hemiplegia: Evaluation and treatment* (2nd ed.). London, UK: Heinemann Medical Books.
11. Brunnstrom, S. (1970). *Movement therapy in hemiplegia: A neurophysiological approach.* New York, NY: Harper & Row.
12. Landen, B., &Amizich, A. (1963). Functional muscle examination and gait analysis. *Journal of American Physical Therapy Association, 43,* 39–44.
13. Reese, N. B. (2005). *Muscle and sensory testing* (2nd ed.). Philadelphia, PA: W. B. Saunders.
14. Crepeau, E. B., Cohn, E. S., & Schell, B. A. (2009). *Willard & Spackman's occupational therapy* (11th ed.). Philadelphia, PA: Lippincott Williams and Wilkins.
15. Wolf, T. J., Chuh, A., Floyd, T., McInnis, K., &Williams, E. (2015). Effectiveness of occupation-based interventions to improve areas of occupation and social participation after stroke: An evidence-based review. *The American Journal of Occupational Therapy, 69*(1), 6901180060p1-11.
16. Ronnebaum, J., Weir, J., & Hilsabeck, T. (2012). Early mobilization decreases the length of stay in the intensive care unit. *Journal of Acute Care Physical Therapy, 3*(2), 204–210.
17. Needham, D. M. (2008). Mobilizing patients in the intensive care unit improves neuromuscular weakness and physical function. *Journal of American Medical Association, 300,* 1685–1690.
18. Fain, E., & Weatherford, C. (2016). Comparative study of millennials' (age 20-34 years) grip and lateral pinch with the norms. *Journal of Hand Therapy, 29*(4), 483–488.
19. Silva-Cuto, M. A., Prado-Medeiros, C. L., Oliveira, A. B., Alcantara, C. C., Guimaraes, A. T., Salvini, T. F., ... & Russo, T. L. (2014). Muscle atrophy, voluntary activation disturbances, and low serum concentrations of IGF-1 and IGFBP-3 are associated with weakness in people with chronic stroke. *Physical Therapy Journal, 94*(7), 957–967.
20. American Occupational Therapy Association. AOTA standards of practice for occupational therapy. (2010). *American Journal of Occupational Therapy, 64,* 106th ser.
21. Schram, D. A. (1984). Resistance exercise. In J. V. Basmajian (Ed.). *Therapeutic exercise* (4th ed.). Baltimore, MD: Williams and Wilkins.
22. Huddleston, O. L. (1961). *Therapeutic exercise.* Philadelphia, PA: F. A. Davis.
23. Kraus, H. (1963). *Therapeutic exercise.* Springfield, IL: Charles C. Thomas.
24. Ciccone, C. D., & Alexander J. (1988). Physiology and therapeutics of exercise. In J. Goodgold (Ed). *Rehabilitation medicine.* St. Louis, MO: Mosby.
25. DeLateur B. J., & Lehmann J. (1982). Therapeutic exercise to develop strength and endurance. In F. J. Kottke & G. K. Stillwell (Eds.). *Krusen's handbook of physical medicine and rehabilitation,* Philadelphia, PA: W. B. Saunders.
26. Coppola, S., Elliot, S., & Toto P. (2008). *Strategies to advance gerontology excellence—promoting best practice in occupational therapy.* Bethesda, MD: AOTA Press.
27. Carmeli, E., Coleman, R., & Reznick, A.Z. (2002). The biochemistry of aging muscle. *Experimental Gerontology, 37*(4), 477–489.
28. Liebesman, J. L., & Cafarelli, E. (1994). Physiology of range of motion in human joints: A critical review. *Critical Reviews in Physical and Rehabilitation Medicine,* 6(20), 131–160.

Chapter 10

Vision and Visual Perception

Lisa Michaud, OTR/L

LEARNING OUTCOMES

After studying this chapter, the student or practitioner will be able to:

10.1 Describe the visual system and how it relates to vision deficits

10.2 Identify vision conditions related to neurological impairment and their functional effects

10.3 Describe low vision conditions and their functional effects

10.4 Develop treatment intervention plans for clients with vision impairment

10.5 Discuss the psychosocial impact of vision impairment as it relates to the client and the client's family

KEY TERMS

- Agnosia
- Central Vision
- Compensatory strategies
- Contrast
- Convergence
- Cranial nerve palsy
- Diplopia
- Hemianopsia
- Hemi-inattention
- Hemi-neglect
- Legal blindness
- Oculomotor control
- Perceptual completion
- Peripheral vision
- Scotoma
- Visual attention
- Visual field deficit
- Visual fields
- Visual scanning

When hearing the word "vision," most people think of going to the eye doctor every year to get an eye examination, hoping to avoid glasses. But vision is actually a complex neurological system, comprised not only of the eyes, but the brain as well. The eyes obtain the visual information from the environment by controlling the muscles that look for and find a target. The brain then receives and interprets this information, allowing for an action to be taken. "A primary mission of vision in the human organism is the organization and manipulation of space."[1]

Vision (sight) is one of the five senses, and is the most primary sense. Humans will always try to use it and will rely upon it, no matter how impaired it may be. To quote Oscar Wilde, "It is in the brain that the poppy is red, the apple is odorous and the skylark sings."

All people rely on vision to obtain information about the environment, such as:

Are there obstacles I need to walk around?
Do I recognize the people in the room I just entered?
Do my clothes match?

Without this visual information, reactions to others and responses to the environment will be affected. If there is a reception of incorrect visual information, then the processing of this information does not happen accurately. This chapter will discuss the most common vision impairments occupational therapy (OT) practitioners address and treatment ideas and resources for clients. The goals of the occupational therapy assistant (OTA) who is working with someone with vision impairment are to improve the client's safety and independence in his or her home, community, and work environment and to improve quality of life to meet the client's individual goals.

TREATMENT TEAM

The concept of a treatment team is imperative when discussing treatment of vision impairment. OT is well suited to address vision impairments because of its focus on increasing clients' independence in home and community, via modified environments, compensatory strategies, and use of adaptive equipment. OT practitioners also have the training to manage medical conditions that some clients have when experiencing vision deficits, such as cognitive impairments, impaired sensation related to diabetes, and balance deficits related to neurological conditions. OT practitioners may earn specialty certification in low vision (SCLV or SCLV-A for the OTA) through the American Occupational Therapy Association (AOTA).

In addition to OT practitioners, the treatment team is comprised of other healthcare professionals who address different components of the client's visual needs. It is important for the client with vision impairment to have an accurate medical diagnosis and receive appropriate medical intervention when the team initiates therapeutic interventions.

Ophthalmologist

An ophthalmologist is a medical doctor (M.D.) who specializes in eye care. An ophthalmologist attends 4 years of undergraduate education, 4 years of medical school, 1 year of internship, and 3 years of residency. An ophthalmologist's primary role is diagnosing conditions that cause vision loss and medical management of these conditions. Ophthalmologists can also complete further training in neuro-ophthalmology, specializing in vision deficits related to a neurological deficit.

Optometrist

An optometrist receives a doctor of optometry (O.D.) degree, after successful completion of 4 years of undergraduate education and followed by 4 years of optometry school. An optometrist is not licensed to practice medicine. Optometrists perform eye examinations to assess general eye health and the need for corrective lenses, and prescribe certain medications for eye diseases. Optometrists may also receive training in vision therapy (exercises designed to help improve visual skills). Optometrists can further their education in vision therapy and vision rehabilitation, which may result in achieving a board certification as a Fellow of the College of Optometrists in Vision Development (FCOVD). They may also be known as neuro-optometrists or behavioral optometrists.

> **COMMUNICATION**
>
> Vision impairment can be a very overwhelming topic to explain to families, especially when their acuity is "normal" but functionally their vision has limitations. Remember the results of the evaluation and stick with the facts of the evaluation. Use handouts and diagrams, such as the vision hierarchy, to assist with the explanation. For example, the OTA might say, "I know John's near vision tested at 20/20 but he presents with limited range of motion in his eyes to the left, making it difficult for him to move his eyes to see the left side of the paragraph. This makes it difficult for him to keep his place when reading." The client and family will need continued reinforcement of the purpose of the OT intervention to improve functional performance and independence, not necessarily to restore vision.

Physiatrist

Also known as a physical medicine and rehabilitation doctor, a physiatrist completes 4 years of undergraduate education followed by medical school, a residency, and board certification in physical medicine and rehabilitation. Physiatrists are the physicians who care for clients after cerebrovascular accident (CVA) or brain injury and who work closely with the OT practitioner in treatment planning. The physiatrist, as well as any physician, can refer the client to the optometrist or ophthalmologist when vision impairments are present.

Certified Low Vision Therapist

A certified low vision therapist (CLVT) works with clients with visual impairment to improve their functioning with daily skills, using remaining vision and adaptive devices. These skills may include computer use, communication skills such as reading and writing Braille, and home management. CLVTs must obtain at least a bachelor's degree in a low vision area, complete at least 350 hours of internship under the supervision of a CLVT, and pass an examination to receive certification. A CLVT may also be an OT practitioner, nurse, doctor, or other healthcare professional.

Certified Vision Rehabilitation Therapist

A certified vision rehabilitation therapist (CVRT) works with clients to increase their independence with adaptive living skills, including home management and outside employment. There are master degree programs in CVRT, and a practitioner must at a minimum have a bachelor's degree with an emphasis on vision rehabilitation therapy, with a 350-hour internship to be eligible to sit for the examination.

Certified Orientation and Mobility Specialist

A certified orientation and mobility specialist (COMS) completes 2 years of graduate-level education following a bachelor's degree. COMS specialize in teaching clients travel and mobility skills. This may include using a sighted cane or white cane, used to locate obstacles that may be in the way of mobility, and preparing to utilize a guide dog. The COMS also addresses community mobility, such as public transportation and managing cross walks. The goal of the COMS is to increase a client's independence with mobility in the community. Sometimes OT practitioners will receive this certification to complement their treatments with low vision clients.

THE VISUAL SYSTEM

The visual system consists of the eye as well as structures in the brain. Visual input is received through the eye and then transmitted via an impulse to the optic nerve that then reaches the visual cortex of the brain, located in the occipital lobe. Given that these impulses are traveling from the eyes to the back of the brain, many areas within the brain are vulnerable to an injury that could lead to visual impairment. Let's focus on the areas of the eye that bring the information into the system to be processed. Review Figure 10-1, which

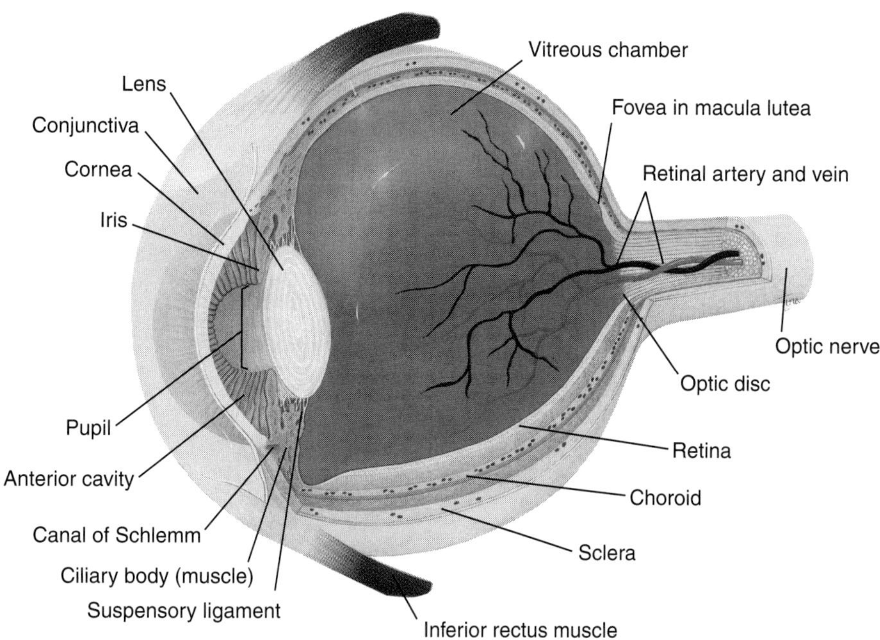

FIGURE 10-1. The eyeball.

presents the structures of the eye, and Table 10-1, which describes the physiology of these structures and how they work together to transmit information to the brain.

The Eye

The eye is a complex bit of anatomy with many vital pieces in a very small object. The lens, cornea, pupil, and vitreous body all work together to bring light into the eye. The macula and fovea make these images clear and focused. The retina and optic nerve allow the image to be transmitted to the brain. All these areas work together, allowing the brain to perceive accurately what is in the environment.[2]

MUSCLES OF THE EYE

The eye has seven muscles that work in conjunction to allow full range of motion for scanning the environment to bring information to the brain (Fig. 10-2).[2] If one of these muscles is impaired, or if the muscle is not receiving the message from the brain because of a nerve injury, this will affect the eye's range of motion (Table 10-2). For example, if the lateral rectus is impaired, the eye will not move out to the side. Some of the muscles have more than one function, such as the superior rectus. If this muscle is affected, you may see weakness with adduction of the eye but that movement is the primary function of medial rectus so that

TABLE 10-1 Features of the Eye and Their Functions[3]

ANATOMICAL FEATURE OF THE EYEBALL	FUNCTION
Lens	Focuses light rays onto the retina
Cornea	Clear part covering the pupil and iris; lets light into the eye
Pupil	Dark, round center of the eye; opens and closes to regulate the amount of light the retina receives
Iris	Colored part of the eye
Vitreous Body	Lies between the lens and the retina and holds these structures in place. Contains a clear jelly, called vitreous humor, which assists with transmitting light
Optic Nerve	Nerve that carries impulses from the eye to the visual cortex to the brain
Fovea	Located in the retina, provides the most acute vision
Macula	Located near the middle of the retina. Enables visualization of objects with great detail
Retina	Sensory membrane that lines the eye. Receives images from the lens and converts them into signals that reach the brain via the optic nerve
Choroid	Layer of blood vessel; provides nourishment to the back of the eye
Sclera	White portion of the eye

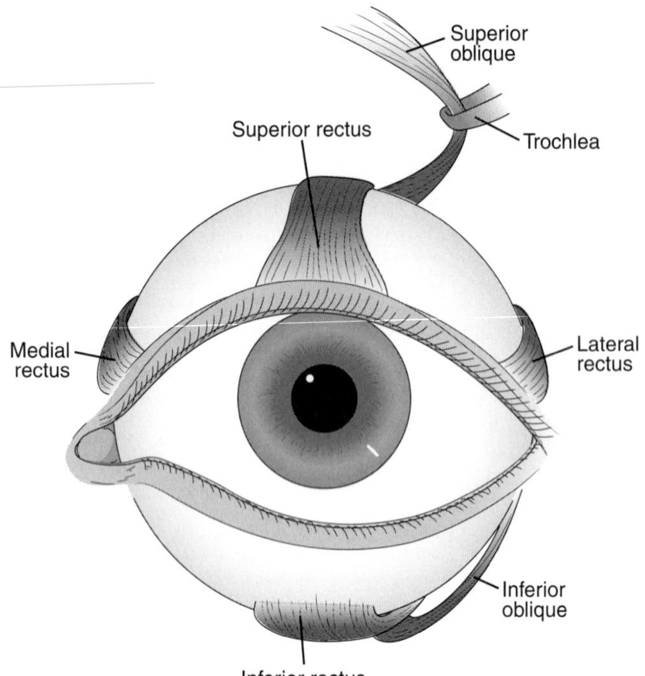

FIGURE 10-2. Muscles of the eye.

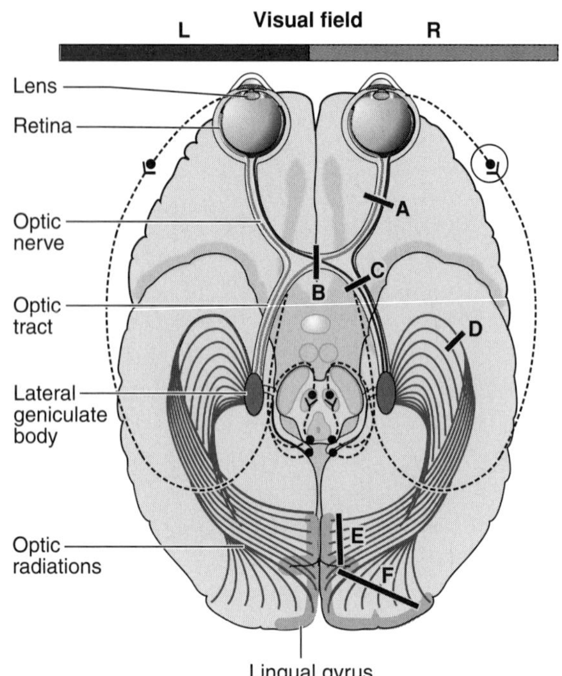

FIGURE 10-3. The visual pathway.

movement may be preserved. If the lateral rectus is affected, it is most likely that abduction will be affected because that is the primary function of that muscle, but the superior rectus will assist with abduction.

Visual Pathway

The visual pathway brings information from the eye to the areas of the brain for processing. As demonstrated in Figure 10-3, this is a complex system but also vulnerable to injury, given the number of areas located throughout the brain. The following is a brief review of these structures.

The optic chiasm is where the two optic nerves intersect at the brain, forming the optic tract. This is where the fibers cross to the contralateral side of the brain.[4] A lesion anterior to the optic chiasm will affect only one eye. A lesion posterior to the optic chiasm will affect both eyes.

The lateral geniculate nucleus is located in the posteroinferior nucleus of the thalamus. It serves as a processing center in the pathway from the retina to the visual cortex, via the optic radiations. Optic radiations are nerve fibers ending in the primary visual cortex of the occipital lobe.[5] Finally, the visual cortex receives and interprets the visual input into information the brain can understand.

Cranial Nerves

The cranial nerves (CN) are another important aspect of the nervous system and are necessary for communication to and from the visual systems.[2] The cranial nerves provide motor and sensory information throughout the head and neck. The cranial nerves begin in the midbrain and run to their dedicated areas. There are 12 cranial nerves; four cranial nerves, II, III, IV and VI, are dedicated to vision (Fig. 10-4 and Table 10-3).

Damage to cranial nerves II, III, IV or VI may result in different outcomes depending on which nerve or combination is affected. For example, damage to the anterior to

TABLE 10-2 Muscles of the Eye and Their Functions[3]

MUSCLES OF THE EYE	FUNCTION
Superior rectus	Elevates the eye (primary function), rotates top of eye toward the nose (secondary), adducts the eye (tertiary)
Lateral rectus	Abducts the eye
Inferior oblique	Rotates top of eye away from the nose (primary), elevates the eye (secondary), abducts the eye (tertiary)
Inferior rectus	Downward gaze (primary), rotates top of eye away from nose (secondary), adducts eye (tertiary)
Medial rectus	Adducts the eye
Superior oblique	Rotates top of eye toward nose (primary), depresses eye (secondary), abducts eye (tertiary)
Levator palpebrae	Works with the superior rectus to elevate the eyelid

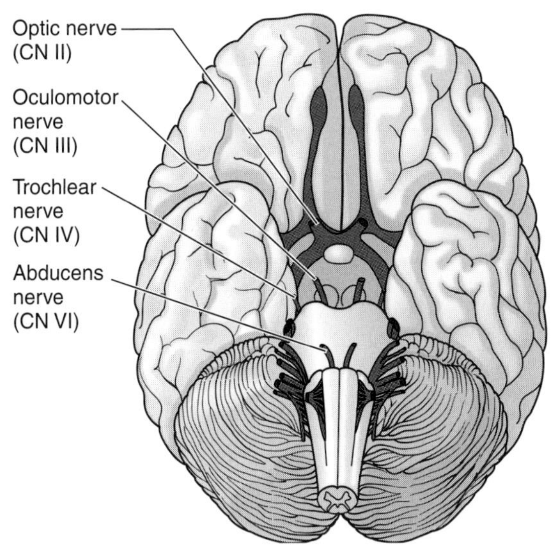

FIGURE 10-4. The four cranial nerves dedicated to vision are II, III, IV and VI.

the optic chiasm of CN II will result in blindness. Damage posterior to the optic chiasm of CN II will lead to various visual field impairments, which will be discussed later in the chapter. Damage to CN III, IV, or VI will lead to weakness or paralysis of the eye muscles. These are known as **cranial nerve palsy**. Damage to CN II is usually not referred to as palsy (Table 10-4).

The initial medical treatment for cranial nerve palsy is to see if it will resolve on its own; the ophthalmologist will usually wait 6 months before implementing any medical intervention, which may include surgery. This is where OT plays a significant role, in assisting the client with ways to manage the effects of the palsy to maintain independence. The treatment will be symptom-specific. These are discussed later in the chapter with other interventions.

Healthcare professionals also frequently use the terms "anterior visual system" and "posterior visual system." For example, a practitioner might refer to "a meningioma of the anterior visual system." The anterior visual system refers to structures anterior to the lateral geniculate nucleus. Posterior visual system refers to the structures posterior to the lateral geniculate nucleus (Fig. 10-5).

VISION CONDITIONS RELATED TO NEUROLOGICAL IMPAIRMENTS

As the preceding figures have demonstrated, vision areas are found throughout the brain. CVA, traumatic brain injury (TBI), and tumors frequently cause vision impairment. As many as 50% of clients with neurological impairments have vision deficits.[6] This demonstrates the importance of performing visual screening when a client is diagnosed with these conditions.

TABLE 10-3 Cranial Nerves Dedicated to Vision[2]

NERVE	NAME	FUNCTION
Cranial Nerve II (CN II)	Optic nerve	Carries impulses from the retina to the brain (vision)
Cranial Nerve III (CN III)	Oculomotor nerve	Moves all extraocular muscles, except the superior oblique and lateral rectus. Also controls the size of the pupil and elevating the eyelid
Cranial Nerve IV (CN IV)	Trochlear nerve	Motor control of the superior oblique muscle
Cranial Nerve VI (CN VI)	Abducens nerve	Motor control of the lateral rectus muscle

TABLE 10-4 Types of Cranial Nerve Palsies[3]

NAME	PRESENTATION	CLINICAL IMPLICATIONS
CN III palsy	Eye turns down and out, eyelid droops (ptosis), dilated pupils	Diplopia (double vision), difficulty with depth perception, difficulty with reading, convergence insufficiency
CN IV palsy	Outward rotation of the upper portion of the eye	Vertical diplopia, difficulty with reading, computer work, and walking down steps. Client may turn his or her head down and out to compensate

Continued

TABLE 10-4 Types of Cranial Nerve Palsies[3] (continued)

NAME	PRESENTATION	CLINICAL IMPLICATIONS	
CN VI palsy	Eye drifts in toward the nose	Diplopia; client may turn head to the side to compensate	

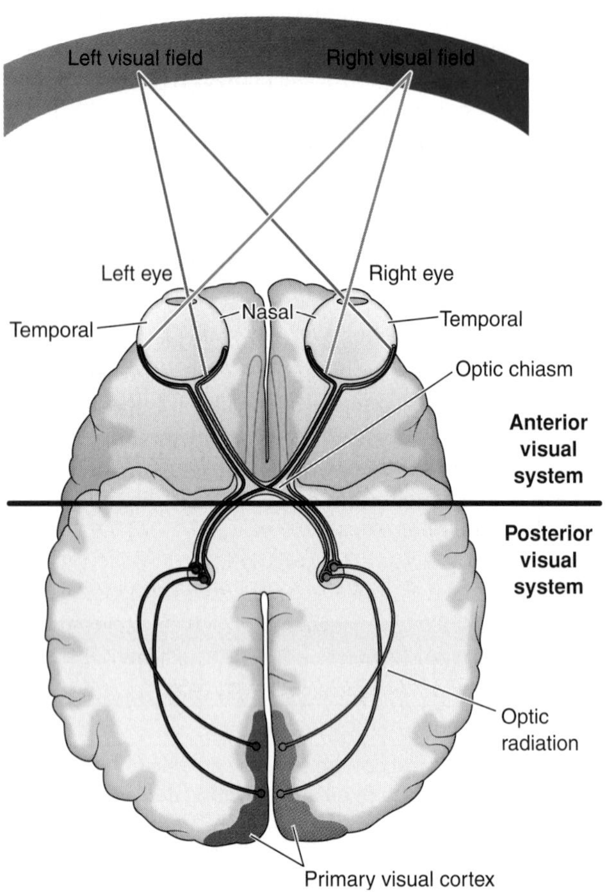

FIGURE 10-5. The anterior and posterior visual system.

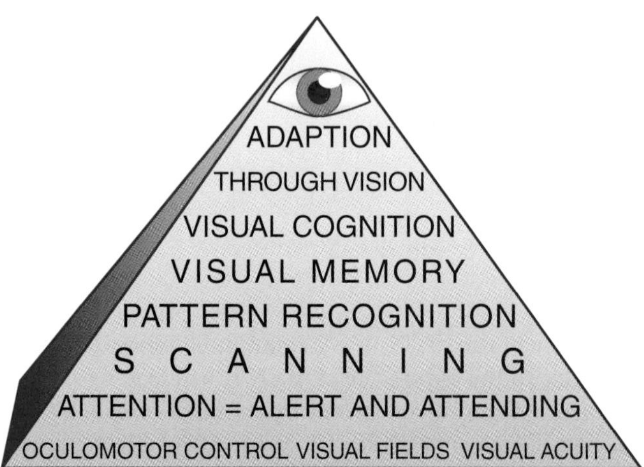

FIGURE 10-6. The visual hierarchy.

Understanding the different functions of the visual system will make it easier to address each deficit and understand how one deficit will affect other areas and overall function. Mary Warren, an occupational therapist who pioneered and expanded the role of OT in vision rehabilitation, describes this in her Hierarchical Model (Fig. 10-6).[7] The premise of the model is that each skill is dependent on the one before it, and a deficit in that skill will affect the next skill on the hierarchy. For example, visual cognition cannot be intact if there are deficits in visual scanning and visual memory. The most basic visual skills are acuity, **visual fields** (total area where objects can be seen), and **oculomotor control** (control of eye movements). These are the functions that allow us to take visual information in correctly. Deficits in these areas need to be addressed before moving up the hierarchy to address the higher levels. If deficits persist in the lower levels (acuity, visual fields, and oculomotor control) the other (higher) levels cannot be adequately addressed, as they rely on the information being accurate as it is coming to the brain to be processed.

Acuity

Acuity is typically defined as sharpness of vision. A person with blurry vision is having difficulty with acuity. If the visual information that is being taken in is not clear, then the client may not be seeing the information accurately, which means the information may not be processed accurately. For example, if impaired acuity affects the client's ability to read medication instructions, then the client may not take the medication correctly. When working with clients who are having difficulty with visual acuity, it is important to have them perform all visual tasks with the best corrected acuity, meaning with their glasses on if they are updated. If the client does not have an updated prescription, enlarging print will be helpful until the new glasses are available.

ACUITY INTERVENTION

Although the OT practitioner can assess a client's visual acuity to check for deficit, treatment is managed by the optometrist or ophthalmologist, usually through a prescription for new glasses or contacts. Functionally, this deficit can be addressed temporarily by managing the font size to accommodate the client's impaired acuity. Improved lighting and increased contrasts may assist, and the client may also use a magnifying glass, their smartphone camera or zoom functions in electronics.

Visual Fields

Visual fields refer to the extent of visual space that is visible to an eye in any given position; it is approximately 65 degrees upward, 75 degrees downward, and 95 degrees outward.[3] Functionally, the visual field is the area that can be seen when eye is looking straight ahead—about 180 degrees horizontally and 125 degrees vertically (Fig. 10-7).

Each eye can be divided into superior and inferior halves, and right and left halves. These can be subdivided into quadrants. These terms are related to where the vision loss is noted as well as its extent. Full access to each visual field ensures that the visual information the client is processing is complete. If a client is not receiving the full information from the environment, his or her ability to process that information will be compromised.

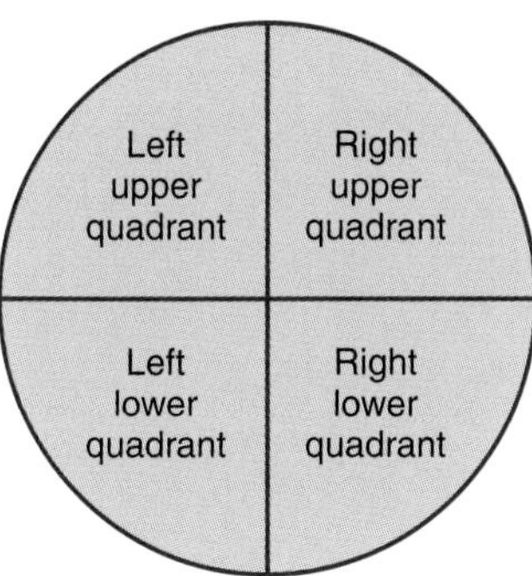

FIGURE 10-7. The visual fields.

VISUAL FIELD DEFICITS

Visual field deficits (VFDs) refer to blind spots in a portion of the visual field. These may occur based on the location of the injury in the brain (Table 10-5 and Fig. 10-8).

Reviewing the illustrations shown in Table 10-5 and Figure 10-8 will help clarify the location of each type of deficit. A right **hemianopsia** in the right eye is a blind spot on the lateral side of the right eye, the right outside vision. A right upper quadrantopsia is a field deficit in the upper right corner of the left eye, toward the nose. A left homonymous hemianopsia is a blind spot on the left side of both eyes, so toward the nose in the right eye and the outside vision on the left side. Many variations of field impairments are possible; therefore, knowing the terminology can help the OT practitioner determine the location of the field impairment. When describing a field impairment, it is always described from the client's point of view, which of the client's visual fields are impaired. A client may have full eye movement and still have a visual field impairment; the two are not related. A full visual examination is key to determining the specific visual impairment.

Common observations of clients with VFDs include bumping into objects on one side, turning the head away from the affected side, tripping over objects, reading difficulty because of missing words, and/or driving accidents. With a more severe deficit, clients may not shave their entire faces or brush all their hair because they do not see that side.

The most important aspect of treating a VFD is the client's awareness of the deficit. A client who is aware a visual deficit is present can carry over the treatment techniques and will be more successful than a client with poor awareness, impaired memory, or hemiparesis (weakness on one side of the

TABLE 10-5 Types of Visual Field Deficits (VFDs)

Hemianopsia	Vision loss in one half of the visual field in one eye	Right hemianopsia of the right eye (L, R)
Homonymous hemianopsia	Vision loss in one half of the visual field on the same side of both eyes	Right homonymous hemianopsia (L, R)
Quadrantopsia	Vision loss in one quarter of the visual field	Right upper quadrantopsia of the left eye (L, R)

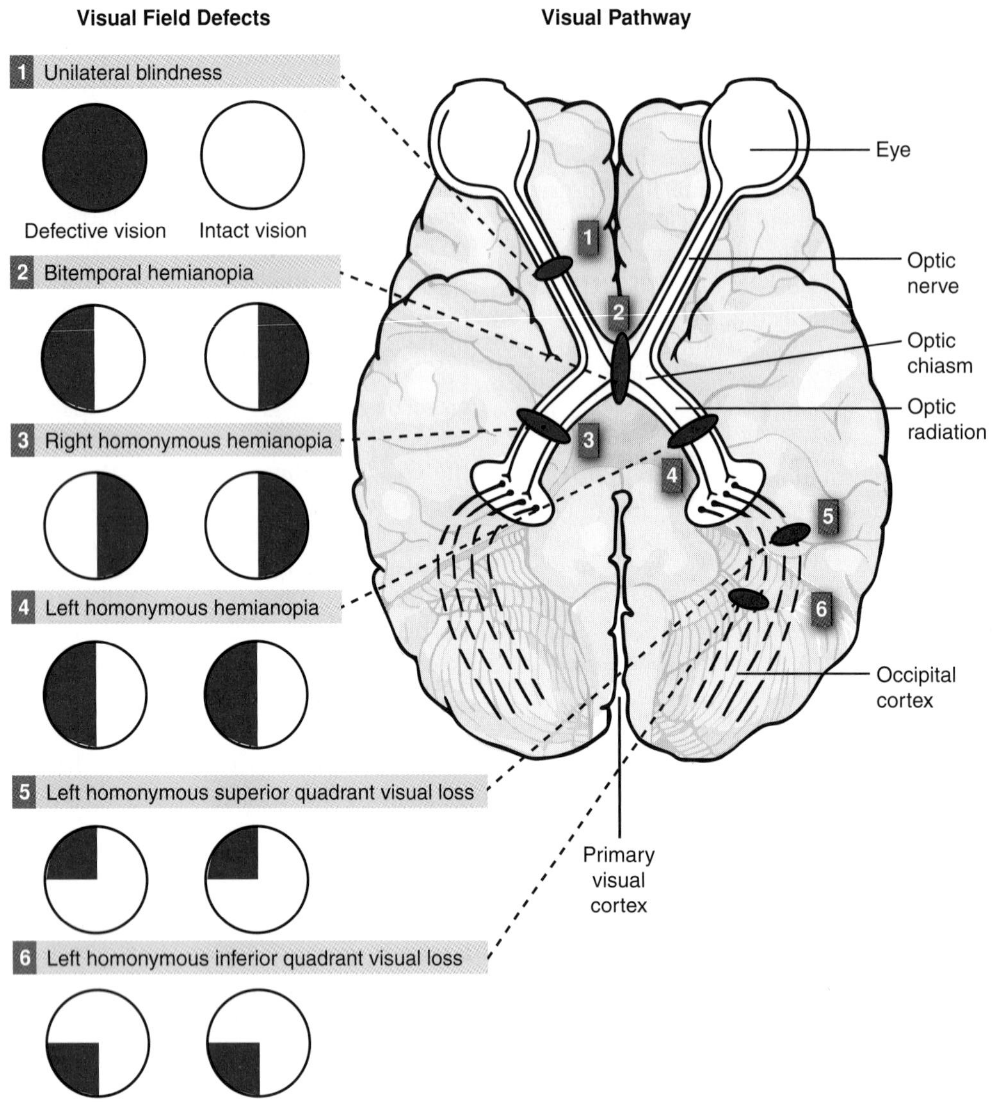

FIGURE 10-8. Visual field deficits.

body) with impaired proprioception (the ability to know where our body parts are in relation to the rest of our body). Providing a client with objective information may help the client realize that his or her vision is impaired. The OT practitioner can perform an objective assessment by providing the client with reading and writing tasks, or a letter cancellation task where the client might cross out all the H's on lines full of random letters. However, some clients will demonstrate poor insight into their vision impairments because of the cognitive deficits related to their injury or CVA. The functional prognosis for these clients is not as good, as they will not understand the importance of implementing the treatment techniques or may have difficulty recalling them. Fifty percent of clients will have some natural recovery within the first month of the neurological insult. Little recovery occurs after 6 months,[8] and full recovery of visual field impairment rarely occurs.[8]

When a client is dealing with a sudden loss of vision, such as a visual field impairment related to CVA or TBI, they may experience **perceptual completion**. Sometimes the brain cannot process that there is a partial vision loss and it will "fill in" the blind spots with what it thinks should be there. When a client is looking at another person, they may not be seeing the person's entire body, but the brain will fill in the information based on what information it is receiving. This can be confusing for the client, as they may think what they are seeing is accurate. Perceptual completion can be a safety issue, especially with mobility and driving, because what the client is "seeing" may not be accurate but only an optical illusion.

INTERVENTIONS FOR VISUAL FIELD DEFICITS

OT interventions for VFD often include **compensatory strategies**. These usually begin with having the client turn his or her head toward the impaired visual field to bring the areas they are missing into view. Then the strategy would progress to having the client keep the head still and moving only the eyes toward the impaired visual field. This strategy is helpful with all functional tasks and is a building block for future tasks, as the client is learning they will need to be in the habit of moving the blind spot out of the way when performing all functional tasks.

READING WITH A VISUAL FIELD DEFICIT

Clients with peripheral field loss will have the most difficulty with locating the beginning of a line and/or knowing when the sentence or line ends. A finger or line guide may be helpful, as well. A finger guide refers to using a finger to keep the reader's place in the text. A line guide is something that is placed under the line that is being read (an index card of contrasting color works well). Using anchor lines, which are lines drawn in a contrasting color on either side of the page to provide visual cues for the beginning and ending of the line, is also very helpful. When beginning training with a client, start with a short sentence or paragraph and progress to longer text and different page layouts. Instruct clients that sometimes moving the page around but keeping the eyes in one spot is helpful. Use task lighting and good contrast with the print. It is important for clients with neurological visual field impairment to keep items, such as reading materials and dishes when eating, in midline to encourage them to attend to the deficit side.

Paper-and-pencil tasks such as letter cancellation, mazes, and connect-the-dots are good starting points to begin to get the client into the habit of scanning to the affected side. After these beginning treatments, the OTA can then progress the client to self-care and home management tasks. Incorporating reading bills and recipes, or making sure the entire carpet is vacuumed, are great ways to incorporate functional tasks into therapeutic interventions.

Another potential treatment in this area is visually scanning while mobilizing (either ambulating or self-wheelchair propulsion) (Fig. 10-9). Scanning while moving is often more functional than sitting still and will improve awareness of environment. Treatment can include having the client mobilize with the OT practitioner (either wheelchair or ambulating) to retrieve items that will be used in the therapy session. Having the client locate and retrieve specific clothing items in the closet and grooming items on the sink

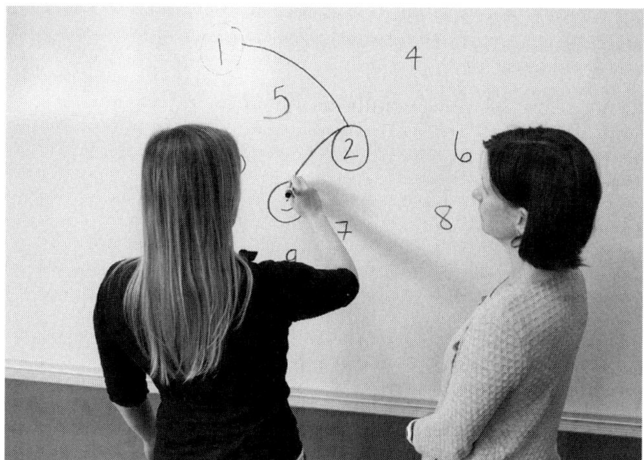

FIGURE 10-9. Scanning treatment.

needed for ADLs would be an option. Progress to visually scanning in the community, such as locating items in a grocery store. The client should be fairly comfortable managing the home and other small familiar places before attempting larger, more unfamiliar surroundings.

Oculomotor Control

Oculomotor control refers to control of the eye muscles and ensures that eye movements are accurate and efficient. Just like a person will need good control of the arm and leg muscles to function efficiently, the same is true of the eye muscles. Oculomotor control allows for binocular (both eyes) vision and is what stabilizes images on the retina and fovea.

CONVERGENCE

Convergence means moving both eyes symmetrically toward midline to focus on a single point. Convergence insufficiency refers to the eyes not moving normally toward midline, and often leads to reading difficulties or diplopia (double vision).

SACCADES

Saccades refers to small rapid eye movement between two points of fixation. The act of reading uses saccades, moving from letter to letter or word to word. Driving is another example of using saccades because it requires looking from the dashboard to the mirrors to the road and back.

FIXATION

Fixation is keeping the eyes on one object to obtain information about it for the brain to process. This is accomplished by using the eye's fovea. Fixation can be limited at times by decreased attention, as the client may not attend to the object long enough for the brain to process the information.

OCULOMOTOR IMPAIRMENTS

Deficits with oculomotor control commonly occur when a cranial nerve is injured or are due to weak muscles on the hemiparetic (weaker or affected) side. This means that the eye may not move in all directions (impaired range of motion) or the eye movements may not be coordinated with each other. A client with impaired oculomotor control may have difficulty moving his or her eyes to the information needed to see. Common clinical observations with impaired oculomotor control include the client's:

- Inability to read, with head turning or tilting
- Difficulty locating items in a closet or drawer
- Decreased safety with ambulation and driving
- Convergence insufficiency
- Diplopia (double vision)

INTERVENTIONS FOR OCULOMOTOR IMPAIRMENTS

Warren's prereading and writing exercises were developed to improve oculomotor control as well as attention to the affected side. These exercises are designed to progress the client from easy to more difficult scanning tasks to prepare the client for reading text and scanning the environment.[9]

Diplopia

Although humans have two eyes, they only see one image. In normal vision the eyes work together to make one image or to converge. Diplopia is caused by the two eyes not working together because of muscle or nerve weakness (convergence insufficiency). Diplopia often results in the client keeping one eye closed. The clinician may also observe a disconjugate gaze, meaning that the client's eyes are not lined up.

INTERVENTIONS FOR DIPLOPIA

One intervention for diplopia is the use of a translucent patch that is worn as needed by the client for relief of symptoms of diplopia. It can be worn on whichever eye the client prefers. The client may prefer to wear the patch over the nondominant eye. To assess a client's eye dominance, roll an 8.5" x 11" paper into a tube and hand it to the client. When the client is asked to look through it, he or she will bring the paper tube to the dominant eye.

Another treatment for diplopia is partial occlusion (Fig. 10-10). This is the preferred method of managing diplopia, as it tends to be less disruptive to balance and orientation. The client must have glasses for partial occlusion; however, they can be clear lens glasses if the client does not require prescription glasses. To create partial occlusion, the OT practitioner places a strip of transparent material (3M Transpore™ surgical tape is one brand of transparent tape) over the full lens of the nondominant eye. As the client focuses on a target, the OT practitioner removes one small strip of tape at a time, starting at the outside of the lens, until the client begins to report diplopia. At this point, the OT practitioner replaces the last strip of tape removed. Every few days (or at each visit), assess if client can tolerate removal of a small portion of tape, until tape is eventually no longer needed. This process may take days, weeks, or months and is different with every person. The tape performs the same function as the translucent patch but also allows the client to use the affected eye more, allowing for muscle strengthening (Fig. 10-11).

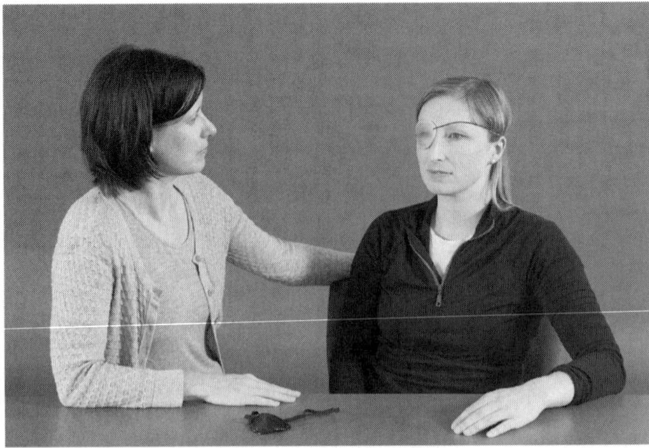

FIGURE 10-11. Client with translucent patch. Black patch is also featured.

Although using a black patch is no longer considered best practice, it is still commonly used. The black patch is worn as needed for relief of symptoms of diplopia in the same way the translucent patch would be. It must be alternated from eye to eye frequently (typically every 2 hours) to minimize the risk of muscle atrophy of the eye. The OT practitioner may initiate this, or depending on practice location, a physician order for a black patch may be necessary.

Physician Guided Treatment for Diplopia A physician may be called upon for treatment of diplopia. One medical treatment option is a prism, which is a device either placed on the lens of the glasses or made directly into the lens of the glasses, which helps redirect the line of sight into one image. The prism is used only until the diplopia is resolved. Surgery is often performed only as a last resort, when all other options have been attempted and unsuccessful, and at least 6 months post injury or illness. The surgery is usually performed by realigning the eye muscles for improved alignment.

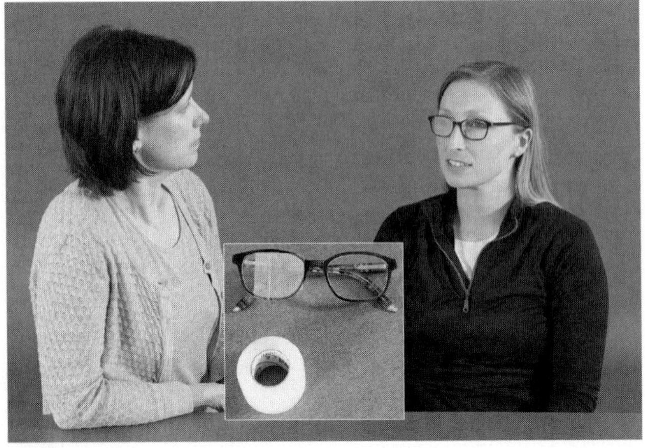

FIGURE 10-10. Client with partial occlusion.

OT Practitioner's Viewpoint

In my treatment session, I may begin with a simple vision-only task for a few minutes, to warm up the eyes. Then I will progress to incorporating more body movements, balance, and functional tasks. For example, the client will transition to sitting on balance foam while performing the same visual scanning task for improved proprioception and trunk control. I may also have clients perform visual scanning while standing in the kitchen, retrieving specific items from the cabinets, and then returning them back to where they found them, to incorporate memory, if appropriate. Multitasking during a treatment session is vital when treatment time may be limited and is also more true to "real life." ~ Lisa Michaud, OTR/L

Visual Attention

Visual attention is the ability of the visual system to attend to visual information in the environment, as well as to determine what information is relevant and irrelevant to a situation. This is a cognitive ability that allows individuals to determine which information is important to the task at hand. For example, when a client is reading a bill, he or she will use visual attention to determine which important areas of the bill to attend to for efficient task completion. A client with impaired visual attention may require increased time to locate the important information, and therefore be less efficient with task completion.

INTERVENTIONS FOR IMPAIRED VISUAL ATTENTION

To improve a client's attention to a task, begin by removing all distractions. Look at the environment where the treatment is taking place. Is the television or music turned off? Can the treatment occur in an environment without other people, or where the client is not distracted by looking out a window? Begin in these quieter environments and as the client becomes more successful with performing the tasks, begin to add small distractions. For example, when a client is dressing, turn on music. Try having the client perform his or her exercises in front of the window, or where other people are exercising, to integrate the attention component.

Visual Scanning

Visual scanning (sometimes called smooth pursuits) refers to how the eyes move to obtain information. The normal scanning pattern is left to right, top to bottom, in the alphabets of English and French (Canada). A client with an impaired scanning pattern may have difficulty with reading, as they may not be able to stay on the line. Visual scanning may be impacted by impaired oculomotor control, impaired visual attention, or both.

When reading, clients may have difficulty staying on the line or may completely lose their place. When paying bills, clients may have difficulty locating where the amount or date due is located on the bill. When functionally ambulating, clients may not be able to locate specific items in the environment that the OTA is asking them to find. It is important to determine the cause of these issues before determining the best course of treatment.

INTERVENTIONS FOR IMPAIRED VISUAL SCANNING

As normal scanning patterns are left to right and top to bottom, the OTA would begin treatment with tabletop scanning in these directions in an organized manner. As the client progresses, begin to utilize a more disorganized pattern and then progress to incorporating this into a functional task, such as scanning for items in the kitchen of the therapy clinic, or in another distracting environment. Always be mindful of the role attention to task has in completion of these functional activities.

These previous areas (acuity, visual fields, oculomotor control, attention, and scanning) describe how information is brought into our visual system. The next areas refer to how the brain processes the information that is brought in. Keep in mind that vision is a "system," meaning that one part of the system relies on the other parts of the system to work effectively. If any of the areas that bring information into the brain continue to demonstrate deficits, the information will not be processed correctly.

Pattern Recognition

Pattern recognition is the ability to identify details of objects to determine what the objects are. Pattern recognition is knowing the difference between a fork and a spoon by looking at them, because of knowing the fork has tines to pierce food and a spoon has a rounded bowl-like shape.

INTERVENTIONS FOR PATTERN RECOGNITION

Deficits with pattern recognition are managed by utilizing compensatory strategies by teaching clients different ways to determine what they are seeing. If a client is having difficulty distinguishing the right shoe from the left shoe, teach them to look at the shoes' features to see the differences. For example, the flatter side of the shoe goes on the outside of the foot. When differentiating between a pencil and a pen, the pencil usually has an orange or pink top (the eraser). Grooming items or utensils may also be marked differently, such as with colored duct tape. The OTA may even write the object's name on a piece of tape and attach it to the object.

Visual Memory

Visual memory is remembering what is seen. If the information that is being seen is interpreted incorrectly, this will lead to inaccurate visual memory. If the client's ability to visually recall information is impaired, difficulty recalling information just read or looked at will result. Examples of visual memory include remembering a few items from a shopping list, signs while driving, directions for taking medications, or parts of an address or phone number.

INTERVENTIONS FOR VISUAL MEMORY

When visual memory is impaired, compensatory strategies include writing down what needs to be remembered or writing the specific features of an item to assist with recall of the features of that specific item. Treatment may need to begin with basic tabletop tasks. For example, present one photo or object for five seconds, remove it from view, and ask the client to immediately choose the object from two or three choices. As the client progresses, increase the number of objects. Allowing the client to verbally describe the object to himself or herself may assist with immediate recall as well. Visual memory can have a significant impact on the ability to read and recall the information, and the ability to follow written directions, such as a recipe. Progress to these types of functional activities as the client tolerates.

Visual Cognition

Visual cognition is using all of the information obtained from the lower areas of Mary Warren's hierarchy to make decisions regarding the information the brain is receiving and processing. If the client has mastered the lower areas of the hierarchy and continues to demonstrate difficulty with the cognitive aspects of functional tasks, it may be time to focus more on cognition instead of vision. Chapter 11 will focus on cognitive issues and management.

This section has been focusing on visual tasks, but the visual system does not work in isolation. The performance of everyday tasks utilizes all the senses together to obtain information. One option is to progress the client from performing visual tasks while sitting then standing and progressing to stand on a balance disc or while functionally ambulating (be mindful of the risk involved with these balance activities). Remember that, with all treatments, vision does not work by itself but with proprioception, balance, touch, and other senses. Making treatments multisensory, such as incorporating balance and mobility, makes them more functional. Have clients stand on a balance board while performing scanning tasks. When performing reaching tasks, provide proprioceptive input to the opposite hand, such as by leaning or using a surface for weight-bearing.

VISUAL PERCEPTION

As previously discussed, the visual system is focused on the structures that obtain visual stimulation and move it to the brain for the information to be processed. As defined by Bouska, Kauffman, and Marcus, perception involves "...the dynamic process of receiving the environment through sensory impulses and translating those impulses into meaning based on previously developed understanding of that environment."[10] Sensory impulses refer to all five senses: vision, hearing and equilibrium, taste, touch, and smell. For the purposes of this chapter, the content will be focusing on visual perception. Simply put, visual perception is how the human brain understands what the eyes see.

Perception is variable from person to person, and after an injury or event, visual perceptual deficits may be present. Differences in perceptions may exist even without a specific deficit, based on a person's previous life and visual experiences (Fig. 10-12). In average everyday lives, these differences can cause arguments about what tie matches the chosen shirt, or what is actually seen in a photo. Certainly, when a deficit in perception is present, the client will have an even larger disconnect. When the client experiences a sudden change in how his or her brain perceives an environment, it can be upsetting and confusing. The client may verbalize that something is "off" but may not understand what it is. These deficits can lead to impairments with independence in home and community because the client may be seeing images or the surroundings differently than he or she is used to. For instance, an older woman may insist someone is coming in and washing her walls and floors when she is away because they seem so clean. Meanwhile, the woman's daughter visits and notices the dirt in the corners, and hand prints near the light switch.

TECHNOLOGY AND TRENDS

Therapeutic technology devices for vision come in varying sizes, and many address visual tasks utilizing touch screens. The Dynavision D2™ visual-motor training system is a 48-inch by 48-inch wall- or mobile-stand mounted board with multiple small lights in linear and circular patterns, which have touch control. The Dynavision D2™ has multiple functions, but at its most basic level, the client is instructed to touch the light as it turns on. A screen located in the center of the board can be used to challenge visual and cognitive skills, including speed of recognition, visual discrimination, divided attention, and information processing. Programmable software facilitates individualized training programs for clients of various ages, abilities, and conditions. Each hit of the target provides automatic multisensory feedback to reinforce learning. Raised buttons offer tactile input, while an audible beep indicates a successful hit. If the OTA wants to simply address attention to one side, it can be programmed to have more of the lights activate on that specific side. When the goal of the session is to incorporate vision with balance, the tasks can be performed standing.

Bioness Integrated Therapy System (BITS®) comes with a portable stand and screen sizes in 48 inches or 55 inches. BITS® comes with 24 customizable programs to address visual areas such as visual motor skills, visual field loss, visual neglect, and contrast sensitivity. These tasks can be performed in sitting and standing positions to incorporate balance.

Vision Coach™, developed by Perceptual Training Inc., is a programmable, interactive light board that can be used to address visual skills such as dynamic acuity, saccades, fixation, tracking, reaction time, and depth perception. The Vision Coach™ is 50 inches by 34 inches and is Wi-Fi compatible. It is height adjustable, so it can be used in sitting or standing positions.

Disorders of Perception

Perception is a complex area and each person will present differently with his or her deficit, and each client's particular needs will vary. Understanding visual and perceptual deficits can be very difficult for the client and family because they are not always immediately obvious. Client and caregiver education throughout the rehabilitation process and beyond is extremely important. Symptoms of visual perceptual deficits may include:[3]

- Using other senses to interpret visual information
- Confusing right and left
- Giving poor attention to visual tasks
- Missing visual details of tasks
- Demonstrating impaired handwriting
- Demonstrating slow task performance

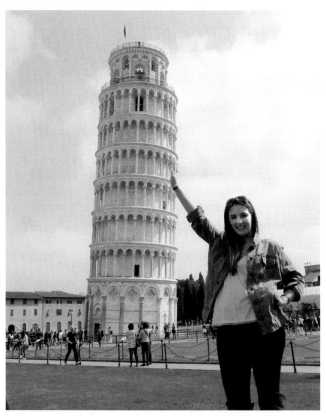

FIGURE 10-12. The Leaning Tower of Pisa. The client's interpretation of this photo will be based on how one's brain perceives the information and previous visual experiences.

Interventions for Spatial Relations

Utilizing functional tasks is a great way to address spatial relations (Table 10-6). Examples of functional tasks might include having the client place laundry into the washing machine, with the focus being on the "into" aspect of the command. Placing the plates on top of one another and putting the toothpaste cap back onto the toothpaste are also great ways to utilize functional tasks for treatment. Also, try to incorporate the client's environment as the "space" to which they are relating. Ask clients to place objects around the therapy space or their own kitchen and request that they recall where they placed those items and retrieve them. Decreasing environmental clutter will also increase the client's success with these tasks, as there are fewer items they need to scan through.

Interventions for Form Discrimination

Initiate treatment for form discrimination with an activity that has the client sort two different types of similar objects, such as utensils (forks from spoons) or clothing (shirts from pants). As the client progresses, increase the number of types of objects to be sorted. Minimizing clutter is helpful, as well as organizing the storage space of items, allowing objects to be presented in a manner where the objects can be viewed individually.

Interventions for Figure Ground

If the client is in the hospital, the meal trays are a great option to utilize in treatment for figure ground, such as having the client locate specific items on the tray. This task can be graded based on the number of items that are on the tray. Other options are sorting a food pantry or a clothing drawer to locate specific items or sorting by color or size. Utilizing contrasting colors can also help the client with locating or identifying specific items for increased independence.

Interventions for Visual Closure

Interventions for visual closure may need to begin with basic tabletop activities before progressing to a more complex functional task, such as reading or managing money. These tasks should be mostly visual, and minimize the motor component, to truly focus on the visual aspects of the task. Begin with matching a complete picture with a partial picture of

TABLE 10-6 Visual Perception

PERCEPTUAL SKILL	DEFINITION	EXAMPLE
Spatial relations	Knowing where an object is in relation to self and others	Knowing that a glass is sitting in front of a person and on top of the table, while the table is under the tablecloth
Form discrimination	Discriminating the important features of different objects such as shapes, colors, and letters	Knowing the difference between the number six and the number nine, between a square and a rectangle
Figure ground	Distinguishing objects from surrounding objects	Locating a specific pair of socks in the drawer
Visual closure	Perceiving the whole picture when only pieces are available for visual interpretation	Being able to identify a tree when only branches are presented
Depth perception	Knowing how far away an object is	Being able to reach for an object without overshooting or undershooting, navigating steps without over or under stepping

letters or simple pictures of objects, and progress to simple words and a slightly more complex picture. As the client becomes proficient with these tasks, then they may be ready to progress to a more complex task such as reading.

Interventions for Impaired Depth Perception

The cause of the depth perception impairment should be addressed first; it is usually an oculomotor issue. However, for the safety of the client, compensatory strategies should be introduced while treatment is ongoing. This may include educating the client and his or her caregivers on the deficits and their safety implications, such as falling, bumping into objects, or spilling things. When ambulating in an unfamiliar environment, the client may need assistance to manage curbs. When the client is reaching for objects on the table, gently moving the client's hand on the table until he or she reaches the object will reduce the chance the client will knock something over, perhaps causing a spill.

Hemi-Inattention and Hemi-Neglect

The parietal lobe of the brain is responsible for integrating visual input received through the eyes. Damage to the right side may produce **inattention** or **neglect**. The terms "neglect" and "inattention" are often used interchangeably and can be difficult to differentiate. The following discussion will explore their differences.

Hemi-inattention is decreased awareness of one side of the body and/or the environment. This more commonly occurs to the left side of the body when there is an injury to the right side of the brain. Impaired sensation may occur on the affected side with visual acuity and visual fields are intact. Impaired sensation with visual field and/or acuity changes may also occur. A client with this deficit will require cues to attend to the affected side when performing self-care tasks and with mobility, especially in distracting environments. Clients with visual inattention will bump into objects or miss items on the affected side. Clients with hemi-inattention are often able to recall that they have this deficit and its functional implications. However, there are also deficits related to task attention, and this leads to decreased carryover of the treatment techniques, making this a very difficult diagnosis to treat (Box 10-1).

BOX 10-1
Visual Attention Versus Hemi-Inattention

Although the words are similar, the meaning is very different. Visual attention refers to attention of the entire environment and how the visual system brings in all information. Hemi-inattention refers to lack of attention to one side. Documenting these accurately is very important to minimize confusion among the team as well as those auditing the documentation.

The treatment for visual inattention is to provide environmental adaptations to increase stimuli to the affected side. For example, stand by the client's affected side during conversation, ensuring the client is looking at who is talking. Another option is to place stimuli to the affected side during functional tasks to increase attention to that side. Interventions may include reorganizing the client's room to ensure more visual input is coming to the affected side, including from the entry door or television. Also making sure functional items are placed to the affected side will encourage the client to attend to that side. For safety, keep the phone or hospital call bell where the client can see it, in case of emergency. Family education is vital to ensure carryover of techniques outside of the clinical environment, as the client will have difficulty with carryover of these techniques. Mirrors are extremely useful to provide visual feedback. Place a piece of colored tape vertically down the midline of the mirror and also on the client's shirt in midline, and assist the client in lining up his or her body with the midline pieces of tape.

Weight-bearing through the affected side will also provide proprioceptive input to the muscles for improved awareness of the affected side. This is effective for both midline awareness and improving attention to the affected side. This can be completed standing or sitting for lower body input. If standing, position the affected upper extremity on a table while performing a simple reaching task with the unaffected side, toward the affected side. The same can be done sitting, placing the affected side on the mat or chair next to the client. Complete these tasks with a full length mirror placed in front of client for added visual feedback, if tolerated.

Hemi-neglect, also called unilateral neglect, is a severe form of hemi-inattention that refers to no awareness of the left side of the body and/or environment. At times, a left homonymous hemianopsia (refer to Table 10-5) is present. Usually the client is unaware of a deficit; therefore, poor functional outcomes are typically found with unilateral neglect. Unilateral neglect may also be related to impaired task attention, so addressing attention to task is crucial.[11] Caregiver education is vital to ensure carryover of techniques outside of the clinical environment.

Treatment techniques are similar to those used for a homonymous hemianopsia, including tactile cues if sensation is intact, and use of mirrors to increase visual cues of left side. For example, the OTA can use a handheld mirror, moving it to the client's left side while encouraging the client to follow with their eyes. Encourage clients to maintain eye contact with the person to whom they are speaking. Using daily tasks such as bathing and dressing, writing, knitting, and washing a car, are wonderful ways to encourage task completion.

Determining Deficits

During the occupation therapy evaluation, the occupational therapist should determine whether the client has a deficit related to visual field, hemi-inattention, or neglect

(Table 10-7). If this was not assessed initially and there is a suspicion of a vision deficit, the OTA should discuss this with the occupational therapist. During the treatment session, a client with only a visual field deficit may be aware that something is wrong with his or her vision, but may not know quite what it is. Sometimes clients think they are blind in one eye when they actually have a homonymous hemianopsia. These clients will bump into walls or people on their affected side, or they may miss text on the affected side when reading. In general, these clients will be able to learn to compensate for their deficits, and they will utilize compensatory strategies well.

Conversely, clients with a hemi-inattention may be unaware that they do not pay full attention to one side. Their visual fields will be intact; however, they simply do not notice certain parts of their environment. They will often be impulsive and unorganized when completing functional tasks and mobility. Clients with hemi-inattention often do not utilize compensatory strategies well. This can make their prognosis worse than having a visual field deficit alone.

Finally, a client with neglect will demonstrate very poor awareness of their affected side, at times even exhibiting decreased awareness of their own body. Usually a visual field impairment will also be present. These clients will only scan to their unaffected side and may have difficulty even coming to midline with their eyes. These clients generally have no awareness of these deficits, therefore, make no attempts to compensate. The prognosis is very poor for clients that neglect to recover these skills.

AGNOSIA

Visual agnosia is the inability to recognize an object by sight despite adequate cognition, normal language skills, normal visual acuity, and intact visual fields.[13] Functionally this may be evident when clients are unable to identify common objects such as a shoe or a pen. They may not recognize a family member who walks into a room until they hear his or her voice. They may not be able to identify objects in pictures. Agnosia can be difficult to diagnose, as all these examples may be related to other vision impairments or a language impairment. Keep in mind that visual acuity and visual fields are all intact with agnosia, and that full cognition may or may not be intact. Types of agnosia include:

- Prosopagnosia: Inability to recognize a familiar face
- Simultagnosia: Inability to perceive entire picture or integrate its parts
- Tactile agnosia: Inability to recognize objects by tactile inspection alone (also known as astereognosis)
- Auditory agnosia: Inability to recognize familiar sounds
- Object agnosia: Difficulty with recognizing familiar objects

Treatment for agnosia is compensatory. Although there may be some spontaneous recovery, no cure exists. Education of the client and caregivers is key, as there is frequently a denial of the deficit or poor awareness of it. If the client is not aware of the deficit, it is very difficult to implement compensatory strategies. Utilizing the client's other senses to compensate for the vision impairment can assist, such as providing tactile cues to identify the features of an object for correct identification, or smelling food items to identify.[14] Consistency and organization of the environment is very important, as clients may be unable to rely on their vision for accurate feedback. Knowing that the toothpaste or other item is always in the same place can increase independence. Organizing clothing by color for improved accuracy may also assist. Keeping containers of items that are used together, such as bowls and spoons, can significantly reduce a person's stress and reliance on others.

LOW VISION

According to the National Eye Institute, low vision is a visual impairment that cannot be corrected by medical or surgical intervention and is severe enough to interfere with the performance of activities of daily living, but allows some usable vision.[15] Low vision is typically caused by diseases of the eye itself and does not involve the brain.

A person with low vision is not blind. Being blind means a lack of light perception and usable vision. A client with

TABLE 10-7 Visual Field Deficit Versus Hemi-Inattention Versus Neglect[12]

VISUAL FIELD DEFICIT	HEMI-INATTENTION	NEGLECT
Visual deficit	Cognitive deficit	Cognitive deficit
Organized scanning pattern	Disorganized scanning pattern	Disorganized scanning pattern
Will attend to the affected side but not completely	Will scan only in unaffected side	Will only scan in unaffected side
Not impulsive and will double check work for errors	Impulsive and will not double check work	Impulsive, poor attention to task, may not complete task
Blind spot present	Blind spot not present	Blind spot may be present
Will verbalize awareness of deficit	Variable awareness of deficit	No awareness of deficit
Respond quickly to compensatory strategies	Minimal attempts to utilize compensatory strategies	No attempt to utilize compensatory strategies

low vision does have vision that can be used for functional tasks, but may need to learn to use their vision differently or need adaptive devices to assist with independence.

Another low vision term, **legal blindness**, can be confusing as well. This is a term used by the government to determine whether a client qualifies for government services and benefits. Legal blindness means that the acuity is no better than 20/200 with best correction in the better-seeing eye (glasses or after surgery) or only 20 degrees of total visual field or less in the better-seeing eye. This is still very usable vision. A client with 20/800 acuity still has usable vision for ADLs.[16]

Low Vision Lesions and Damage

Anton-Babinski syndrome is a rare form of cortical blindness caused by bilateral occipital lobe lesions. Individuals with this syndrome are unable to visually recognize objects. Because of poor awareness of their deficits, they often confabulate, or make-up, stories of what they see.[17] Both CVA and TBI can lead to this syndrome, although it is more common post CVA. **Cortical blindness** can also occur where the individual does have awareness of their total or partial vision loss. Recovery of vision is possible over time but, in some cases, not all.

Charles Bonnet syndrome (CBS) results in pseudovisual hallucinations or phantom visions and occurs in individuals who have suffered notable visual impairment as a result of damage to the visual regions of the brain or eye diseases such as macular degeneration. False images such as faces, lights, and shapes can be superimposed on the environment. An example of this is a client who saw a horse's head everywhere she looked in her visual environment. Individuals who experience this syndrome are aware the images are not real but often are afraid to share this information with their doctors because of fear they will be viewed as crazy. Research has shown that approximately 75% of individuals living with CBS continue to experience symptoms for 5 years or more.[18]

THE OLDER ADULT

When dealing with any diagnosis in an older adult, there are always some considerations that are different than in a younger population. At this time in a client's life, he or she is often looking forward to, or enjoying, the freedom that comes with retirement and having the children finally out of the house. There can be a difficult adjustment to a diagnosis that will lead to loss of vision, as that will be perceived as a loss of freedom and quality of life. Other considerations may be that the client was a caregiver for a spouse, or perhaps an aging parent. A large concern for these clients may not be only a loss of their independence but their ability to be a caregiver. With their grown children working and dealing with their own families, there may need to be changes made to the entire family dynamic, as those not used to being a caregiver may need to step up and deal with a change of roles. The OT practitioner can assist the client with regaining or maintaining independence, but also assisting the client in the adjustment of possibly having to give up some roles that may become too difficult. The OT practitioner is well suited to address these areas with the holistic approach that is the hallmark of the profession of OT.

Symptoms of Low Vision

The symptoms of the diseases that cause low vision may have a gradual onset, so clients may not notice a change in their vision immediately. This is why regular eye examinations are so important. Symptoms can include difficulties with daily skills such as reading or driving, decreased participation in leisure or social activities, difficulty identifying faces, difficulty with writing, bumping into objects with mobility, holding reading materials at an odd angle or close to the face, or mealtime challenges. Even going to the store can be stressful because it may be difficult for the person with low vision to recognize someone who greets him or her. Managing finances will be difficult for the client who cannot see the lines on the checks or cannot stay on the line when writing. A client who is an avid reader may no longer be able to read standard-size print.

Many different conditions cause low vision. This chapter will focus on the conditions that affect adults who are most likely to receive OT services: age-related macular degeneration (ARMD, sometimes seen as AMD), diabetic retinopathy (DR), and glaucoma.

Age-Related Macular Degeneration

The macula is part of the retina, in the posterior portion of the eye (refer to Fig. 10-1). The macula is responsible for **central vision**, which is the most acute and clear vision. Central vision is necessary for reading, facial identification, and object identification. Clients with ARMD lose their central vision but keep their **peripheral vision**. Peripheral vision is commonly known as side vision but also includes upper and lower vision and enables the effective navigation of the environment and anticipation of surrounding objects. Clients with ARMD can be fairly independent with mobility because their peripheral vision is intact. Clients with ARMD experience significant impairment with reading, writing, and identifying objects. Functional examples include reading words on prescription bottles, seeing the controls on the stove or microwave, or looking at photographs.

The two types of ARMD are wet and dry. Wet ARMD is characterized by the formation of new leaky blood vessels in the retina. When the blood leaks, it damages the macula, which leads to impaired central vision. Dry ARMD is characterized by atrophy of the macula because of lack of oxygen. This lack of oxygen causes small yellow spots (drusen) to form on the macula.[16] Clients can begin with the dry form, and then develop the wet form. Ten to 15 percent of clients with dry ARMD will develop wet ARMD.[16] Clients may have dry ARMD on one eye and wet ARMD in the other. Wet ARMD progresses more quickly than dry ARMD. A client with wet ARMD may notice changes in a day or a week, whereas a client with dry ARMD may not notice changes for months or years. The rate of progress will vary from person to person and can differ in each eye. It is difficult to predict how quickly it will progress.

The central blind spot that occurs with ARMD is also known as a **scotoma.** It is important that the location of the scotoma is identified during the initial eye examination, as this will affect treatment techniques. Knowing the location of the scotoma will determine how the client needs to move his or her eyes and utilize remaining vision effectively. This will be discussed in detail in the next sections.

MEDICAL MANAGEMENT

Macular degeneration is not reversible, and the medical treatments are meant to preserve vision and prevent future vision loss. Medical management of AMRD includes:

- Medication injected directly into the eye to stop blood leaking and the development of new abnormal blood vessels
- Laser treatment to destroy new abnormal blood vessels or to destroy the drusen related to dry ARMD
- Photodynamic laser therapy that injects medication to be absorbed by the abnormal blood vessels, followed by a cold laser to activate the medication to destroy the abnormal blood vessels
- Diet to slow the progress of ARMD. The National Eye Institute published a study in 2013 determining that high doses of vitamin C and E, beta-carotene, and the minerals zinc and copper can slow the progress of ARMD.[15] This is important information for OT practitioners to be able to educate their clients, when discussing disease management and how to slow progression. This is known as the AREDS2 (age-related eye disease study) formula and supplements are labeled this way for over-the-counter purchase. The OT practitioner can also provide education regarding an eye-healthy diet. This includes utilizing foods with a low glycemic index; increasing intake of dark, leafy greens, fish, fruits, and nuts; and managing cholesterol and blood pressure.[19]
- Simple lifestyle changes to help prevent or slow the progression of ARMD. These include stopping smoking, regular exercise, wearing sunglasses outdoors to block UV light, and having regular eye examinations.[19]

OTHER TREATMENT FOR MACULAR DEGENERATION

A relatively new implantable miniature telescope for ARMD is a treatment option. The implantation of the telescope is an outpatient surgical procedure where the lens of the eye is removed and replaced by the telescope. The telescope projects images from the field of view to the healthy retina, the area typically used for peripheral vision. Criteria for the procedure is that the client must be at least 65 years old, have advanced but stable macular degeneration, need cataract repair, and demonstrate improved acuity by three lines on the eye chart with an external telescope. The procedure is performed only on one eye. The operated eye becomes the eye used for central vision and the nonoperated eye is used for peripheral vision. The OT practitioner is involved after this procedure to provide the client with training on using the telescope for the most effective use of vision. The implant can typically be used 4 to 6 weeks post-surgery. After the procedure, clients will continue to require glasses and handheld magnifiers. Functionally, clients reported they were less dependent on others, less worried about their vision, and had improved recognition of facial expressions and reactions.[20]

Diabetic Retinopathy

Diabetic retinopathy (DR) affects clients with both type 1 and type 2 diabetes. DR affects the blood vessels of the entire retina, causing decreased circulation and hemorrhages that will lead to varying levels of vision loss (blind spots). This vision loss can also be variable from day to day or week to week, as new hemorrhages are created and heal and as blood sugar levels fluctuate. Diabetic retinopathy is a leading cause of vision loss in American adults, where ARMD is the leading cause of vision loss in Canadian adults. DR is sometimes referred to as "Swiss cheese vision," because of the variability of blind spots. These clients typically have good visual acuity, but are limited functionally by these variable blind spots. Managing blood sugar levels will decrease these daily vision changes, and educating clients about how to locate their most useful vision each day will increase their successes with daily tasks. This will be discussed further in the treatment section.

A team approach is very important for a client with diabetes. DR is preventable with the proper management. If a client effectively manages blood sugar, the likelihood of developing the disease decreases. If a client has not already seen a Certified Diabetes Educator (CDE), it is imperative that is set up. The CDE educates clients about how to effectively manage the disease, its complications, and prevent complications. The OT practitioner plays a crucial role in working with the CDE to reinforce their education and assist with incorporating this education with daily tasks. OT practitioners who work in low vision sometimes become CDEs as well. In this case, the client can then do "one-stop shopping," receiving OT services and diabetes education in the same treatment session. This also allows the OT practitioner to ensure clients are adequately managing their disease from multiple aspects.

MEDICAL MANAGEMENT

Ophthalmologists manage DR with medicated eye drops and laser treatments. Managing a client's blood sugar levels is important to prevent future damage.

Glaucoma

Glaucoma is caused by increased pressure within the eye itself. In this condition the eye does not drain fluid as it should, and this buildup causes permanent damage to the optic nerve. Glaucoma leads to decreased peripheral vision. If untreated, the loss of peripheral vision can be severe, leading to "tunnel vision" or complete loss of vision. These clients typically have good visual acuity because central vision is intact, but limited mobility because of decreased peripheral vision.

MEDICAL MANAGEMENT

Prevention is key, and regular eye examinations must include monitoring the pressure in the eye, which is sometimes the first sign of a problem as glaucoma can have no symptoms. Once glaucoma is diagnosed, ophthalmologists manage it with medicated eye drops, oral medication, and laser treatments.

Low Vision Occupational Therapy Treatment

Before beginning treatment with clients with low vision, it is important to understand the emotional aspects of these diagnoses. These clients may not fully accept the functional implications of their diagnoses or understand the progression and permanence of their conditions. They also may not understand that they will have usable vision and will not be completely blind. The OT practitioner's role is not only to increase their clients' independence, but also to provide education and emotional support, as clients deal with this life-changing diagnosis. OTAs should educate clients about the goals of OT treatment to ensure that clients understand that treatment will not improve their vision to the same level as it was previously. Instead, the OTA can provide education and tools to help clients use their usable vision more effectively for increased safety and independence. When the client fully understands the purpose of low vision treatment, it will be easier for him or her to establish appropriate goals for their treatment, thus guiding the treatment plan.

Some of the treatments an OTA may provide for clients with low vision may include environmental adaptations, which means making changes to the environment for increased function. Examples of environmental adaptations are removing a door that is in the way or adding a lamp to a dark spot in a room. Another example is reducing clutter, removing objects that are tripping hazards, and removing unnecessary items from counters and tables. Removing throw rugs and managing electronic cords to reduce the tripping hazard are also important. The OTA should also consider visual clutter and minimize objects in the client's visual field to what is necessary to avoid object confusion and decrease effort spent on tasks. Examples of reducing visual clutter include removing all but a few necessary items from the bathroom counter to more easily locate the toothbrush and toothpaste.

Contrast refers to the ability to distinguish between similar shades of light and dark, or the color contrast between an object and its background. For example, a black pen on a white piece of paper has good contrast, but a yellow pen on a white piece of paper has poor contrast. Without contrast, objects may disappear visually to the client. Some examples of high contrast include pouring coffee in a white cup, using blue gel toothpaste on the toothbrush so it can be seen on the typically light-colored bristles, using solid colored plates instead of plates with designs to allow the food to be distinguished more easily, using one color fitted sheet and another color for the top sheet, outlining door frames with contrasting color paint or placing contrasting color duct tape on the edge of stairs for safer mobility, using contrasting colors on furniture such as a throw on the couch or a coffee table book on the edge of the coffee table to help with identifying the edge.

Using tactile cues can help compensate for impaired vision as well. Placing rubber bands on objects is one way to do this, such as placing one band on a shampoo bottle to help distinguish it from the conditioner. Some clients also will vary the number of rubber bands used, to distinguish between different items, such as one rubber band on blood pressure medicine and two rubber bands for arthritis medicine. Placing raised dots or pieces of hook Velcro® on the most commonly used stove or microwave controls assists with this as well.

Lighting has many aspects that require consideration because adequate lighting is important for clients to be able to utilize vision effectively. Overhead lighting is important for safety, and lighting throughout a room will help decrease shadows. However, task lighting may be necessary for performing specific activities, such as reading, knitting, or even working on a car. Task lighting may be a desk lamp or a floor lamp with a shade and a gooseneck so the light can be directed toward a specific task. When possible, the task lighting should come from behind and over the shoulder, positioned as close to the work surface as possible, with even illumination on the task items. Placing the light on the opposite side of the hand being used for the task may help to decrease shadows. Demonstrating these different types of lighting to the client may assist with increasing awareness of the importance of adequate lighting. The types of light bulbs used are also important.[21] Because everyone experiences low vision differently, it is important to experiment with different types of lamps and bulbs to see what is most comfortable for the client.

Fluorescent bulbs work well for general tasks for extended periods and usually provide good color and contrast. Incandescent bulbs work well for up-close tasks and are inexpensive to purchase, but they produce heat and are more expensive to use. Incandescent bulbs do not work well for general room lighting because of producing shadows and glare. Light emitting diode (LED) bulbs are designed for reading lamps. They are more energy efficient and are not as hot as incandescent lights. They work well in task lighting with low vision.

In addition to choosing the correct light bulb, lumens are important as well. Lumens refer to the brightness of the bulb. The higher the number of lumens, the brighter the bulb; however, high lumens may increase the glare. Using coated bulbs may help with decreasing glare. Because glare is a normal reflection of light, glare can become uncomfortable for clients with low vision and affect their ability to perform functional tasks. This is an area that is important for the OT practitioner to address. The client will have to think about whether to sit near a window, and consider the glare from a glass-topped table. Besides awareness, this can be accomplished with different devices such as coated glasses, coated light bulbs, or different window coverings.

Low Vision Aids

Low Vision aids are pieces of adaptive equipment used to assist clients with visual tasks. Examples include magnifiers, writing aids, kitchen aids, medical aids, and computer aids. Magnifiers will make the print larger, but will not make it clearer (Fig. 10-13). They also decrease the field of view, providing fewer letters at a time. Types of magnifiers include handheld, stand-mounted, and lighted, as well as microscopes and telescopes that are mounted onto glasses. All magnifiers can be purchased without the input of a medical professional, but a magnifier prescribed by a low vision physician will best meet the client's needs. Clients need to understand that the magnifier will not provide "normal" vision. Proper training by a low vision professional in the use of magnifiers is extremely important. Many times clients will state that their magnifier does not work. This is usually due to not having the correct magnifier for their impairment or not knowing how to use it correctly.

Writing aids may assist clients with increasing independence with writing tasks. Many items are available online, including paper with raised lines to help readers keep their places, which also comes in yellow to decrease glare. Another example of a writing aid is a plastic template to help clients keep their places when writing checks or signing their names on documents. Most banks also offer large checks, large checks with raised lines, and large check registers, upon request. Some OT practitioners trained as low vision specialists only use these guides as a last resort, as many of the training compensations will assist clients to adapt without external guides. For increased safety and independence, many types of adaptive equipment are available for use in the kitchen (Fig. 10-14). Examples of kitchen aids include talking food scales and talking food thermometers. Liquid level indicators can be placed on the edge of a glass or mug and chime when it is three-fourths full. Other examples are large print measuring cups and spoons and finger guards to protect fingers when cutting up foods.

EVIDENCE-BASED PRACTICE

Evidence-based practice (EBP) refers to integrating individual clinical expertise and the best external evidence. Although each OTA presumes to know what works best for clients, research is needed to convince those paying for the services that these practices are necessary and effective. These are some examples of EBP related to vision.

An article by Lamoureux et al. discusses research in how effective low vision rehabilitation is in a client's participation in daily living and quality of life.[22] This study included 192 participants, most with age-related macular degeneration. The rehabilitation interventions included the optometrist, orthoptist, occupational therapist, and an orientation and mobility specialist. The participants' rehabilitation programs were tailored to their specific needs and goals, and services were deemed complete when the goals were met or the participant was unable to identify further needs. The overall results of the study demonstrated improvements with emotional well-being, reading, and accessing information.[22] Mobility and independence were only improved for those participants who received OT, orientation and mobility services.

Mohler et al. investigated the factors affecting readiness for low-vision interventions in older adults.[23] The study used the Transtheoretical Model (TTM) to address the client's readiness for change; change specifically in this study included utilizing low-vision interventions. The study's goal was to determine "what factors facilitate or inhibit change in the way older adults with low vision perform valued activities."[23] The TTM describes the client's' willingness to accept change with these six stages: precontemplation, contemplation, preparation to make change, action, maintenance of behavior change, and termination (the change in behavior is complete). The study utilized 10 participants with various low vision diagnoses. The study concluded three areas related to positive change, including the desire to maintain or regain independence, positive attitude, and the presence of a formal social support system (professionals, support groups). Factors that inhibited readiness for change were a limited knowledge of options and the activity was not a priority. This study demonstrated the importance of utilizing a client-centered approach to address the areas that are important for the client as well as understanding where the client is in the process of understanding and accepting his or her diagnosis.[23] EBP appears to be more relevant in the area of low vision than with a diagnosis of vision deficits related to a neurological-based diagnosis. Perhaps this is an area for future research to demonstrate the effectiveness of OT with these clients.

Lamoureux, E. L., Pallant, J. F., Pesudovs, K., Rees, G., Hassel, J. B., & Keefe, J. E. (2007). The effectiveness of low-vision rehabilitation on participation in daily living and quality of life. Investigative Ophthalmology and Visual Science, 48, *1476-1482.*

Mohler, A. J., Neufeld, P., & Perlmutter, M. S. (2015). Factors affecting readiness for low vision interventions in older adults. American Journal of Occupational Therapy, 69, *6904270020. doi:10.5014/ajot.2015.014241*

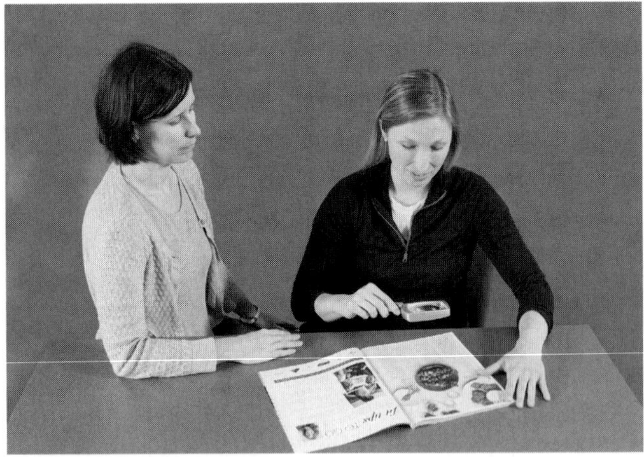

FIGURE 10-13. Hand held magnifier.

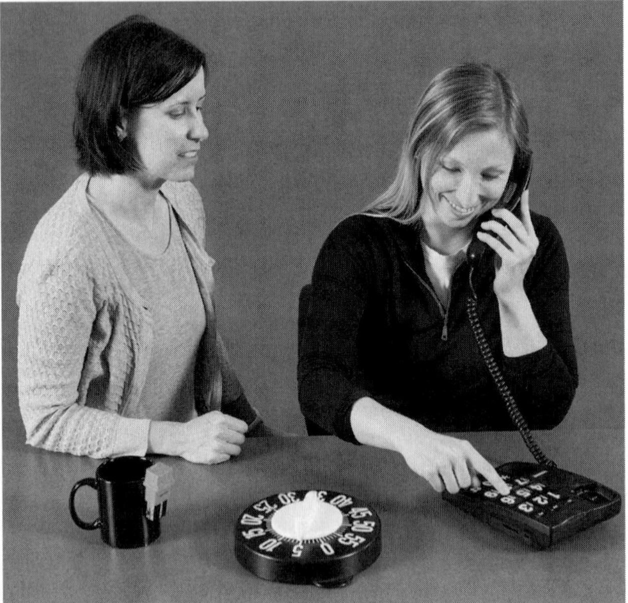

FIGURE 10-14. Kitchen aids. *From left:* Liquid level indicator makes a sound when the liquid hits the sensor, a large-print kitchen timer, and a large numbered phone.

Other aids increase a client's independence with managing medical conditions. These include large print pill boxes, talking blood pressure machines, and talking glucose monitors. Large size numbers on an adapted phone will assist with dialing correctly as well.

Some basic computer aids within the control panel of all computers include the brightness and contrast controls on computer screens and the ability to resize fonts. Also available are large print keyboards and devices that decrease the glare on the keyboards or screen. E-readers, such as a Kindle™, have changed the landscape for clients with low vision as well. It is quite easy to change the font and contrast on most devices, and many also have an audio option that allows clients with low vision to continue to enjoy their books by listening to them.

Many electronic devices also include adaptations to facilitate their use by clients with low vision. Most smartphones have the options of various settings to help with low vision. Increasing text size to allow for easier reading, and there are often options for making the print bold and increasing the contrast. Some devices may have a built in magnifier or one can be added as an app. Inverting the colors, making the background black and the text white, also increases the contrast and makes it easier to read for some clients. Voice options are useful as well. Smartphones can be set to read texts and voicemail, as well as set up for voice commands. All devices are set up differently; please refer to the instructions for the specific devices.

Reading with Low Vision

Learning to read with low vision can be frustrating but ultimately rewarding. Reading techniques will vary based on a client's diagnosis and field of view; the techniques are also different for peripheral field loss and central field loss. With reading, glare can be an issue. Using matte paper instead of glossy paper can help. The OTA may also encourage clients to use finger guiding, placing their fingers on the text and moving along with the words to help them keep their places. Anchor lines on the sides are also very helpful. When beginning reading training with a client, start with an easy sentence or paragraph and progress to longer text and different page layouts. Make sure task lighting is utilized as well as good contrast with the print. If the client is dealing with a scotoma or tunnel vision, font size does not necessarily need to be increased. Making the font larger may bring the words more into the blind spot, making the task more difficult.

READING WITH CENTRAL FIELD LOSS

Eccentric viewing is a technique that moves the scotoma, related to central vision loss, out of the way.[16] This is known as locating the preferred retinal locus (PRL). The client's PRL is typically located during the initial OT low vision assessment, before a treatment session. Scotoma awareness and PRL training are essential for treatment to be effective. Eccentric viewing involves looking to the left, right, above, or below the target. When a client is using eccentric viewing, his or her eyes do not seem as though they are looking at the intended target. Because these clients are unable to use central vision effectively, they learn to use the healthier part of their retina in a different way. Instruction in this technique is essential, as this is not a natural technique. The client begins with scrolling one line of text, keeping eyes in one spot, and then progresses to longer text.

Vision Changes Related to Aging

With aging, many changes naturally occur in the body that are not related to a disease process. For example, the eye muscles that control the pupil lose strength, leading to decreased ability to respond to changes in lighting. This means a person may need more lighting than he or she did at age 25. Decreased tear production may also cause dry eyes (artificial tears will help with this). Peripheral vision also naturally decreases with individuals losing up to 30 degrees of peripheral vision by age 80.[24] Perhaps the most well-known age-related vision change is presbyopia. This occurs when the lens loses flexibility, making it difficult to focus on near tasks. The easiest treatment for this is reading glasses.

PSYCHOSOCIAL IMPACT OF VISUAL DEFICITS

A new diagnosis of a condition that has led to vision deficits or will lead to vision loss can be devastating for the client. Often times these clients will experience depression related to their loss of function and independence.[25] Depression itself may cause clients to be less compliant with the treatment recommended by their physicians or OT practitioners, as they may not see the purpose in the treatment. Clients experiencing new vision loss may also experience anxiety. Clients may not be able to perform their job as they used to, and unemployment is twice as likely among people with visual impairment compared with fully sighted people.[25] They may no longer be able to drive safely or navigate in the community, safely complete IADLs or perform leisure tasks they once enjoyed, and may feel a loss of roles, routines, and habits. Clients may also experience anxiety related to anticipating future vision loss (such as with ARMD) and anticipated loss of function.

The role of the OTA includes providing the emotional support to the client and the family to allow for adjustment to a "new normal." Providing information for local support groups or individual counseling may assist with the process. Understanding and addressing the emotional impact this has on the client, as well as the family, will make the education and treatment sessions more effective for both.

Leisure

Participation in leisure activities and the psychosocial impact of vision loss seem to go hand in hand. Someone dealing with anxiety and depression related to a new vision deficit may be more socially isolated and, therefore, may have less participation in the social activities that were previously enjoyed. The OT practitioner can play a large role in assisting the client in identifying and locating resources for leisure activities. These may be activities specifically designed for clients with a vision impairment. The OT practitioner also may utilize an OT session to find ways to modify an activity the client previously enjoyed for increased independence and social satisfaction. If the client enjoys crafts, educating in correct lighting and increasing contrast will increase the client's success with this task. Adaptive equipment for low vision, such as large playing cards or bingo cards, is available as well as modified board games. Educating clients about how to access audio books can allow them to continue their joy of reading. Participation in social activities can have a positive influence on managing depression and lead to improved management of anxiety. Small support groups can provide social support and provide the increased confidence needed to promote continued participation in the leisure activities of the client's choosing.

SUMMARY

The visual system is important in functional and daily living tasks and is quite complex. It is an integration of many areas of the brain as well as structures of the eyes themselves. Numerous impairments can arise that affect vision, visual-perception, and the client's ability to maintain independence. With all vision impairment, the level of cognitive impairment will affect functional outcomes. A client who is not aware of the presence of a visual impairment will not have motivation to utilize the treatment techniques or compensatory strategies necessary for functional independence. A client with memory impairment may be aware that a deficit exists yet be unable to carry over the treatment techniques because of decreased recall. This chapter has explored numerous visual deficits as well as the treatment and compensatory options for management. The OTA will find that visual deficits will affect every aspect of a client's occupational performance, and with hope, this chapter has prepared the new practitioner to tackle these.

REVIEW QUESTIONS

1. John has been diagnosed with oculomotor impairment. Which three of the following ways might this present functionally?
   a. He will have difficulty reading because of losing his place.
   b. He will have difficulty locating items in his closet because of an impaired scanning pattern.
   c. He will demonstrate hemi-inattention.
   d. He will report diplopia.
   e. He will have difficulty orienting his clothing front to back and left to right.
   f. He will have difficulty using his toothbrush and combing his hair correctly.
2. A client with left homonymous hemianopsia demonstrates poor awareness of her left side. Where should treatment begin?
   a. Scanning tasks to increase attention to the left
   b. Educating the client's family on how to carry over compensatory strategies
   c. Training the client how to utilize tactile cues
   d. Increasing contrast on the left side
3. Jennifer is a client you have been working with in the hospital. She was admitted with a new diagnosis of CVA. She has just begun to be able to participate more in therapy and you note that she is not paying attention to her left side as much. Which of the following is the next course of action?
   a. Continue with the current treatment plan.
   b. Begin to address this inattention by bringing visual stimuli from the left side and initiate education.
   c. Discuss this new finding with the occupational therapist to determine whether a new treatment plan needs to be implemented.
   d. Discuss with Jennifer's mother about possibly needing glasses.

4. Your client is reporting double vision during your first session. This is not mentioned in the notes you received from the occupational therapist. You should:
   a. Give the client a patch because you know it will probably be needed.
   b. Tell the client not to worry about it, as diplopia usually resolves on its own.
   c. Make the print larger on their home exercise program so the client can see it better.
   d. Discuss the client's report with the occupational therapist and refer to a neuro-optometrist or neuro-ophthalmologist.
5. Your client has been successful with simple organized visual scanning tasks to address oculomotor control. Which three of the following should they progress to next?
   a. Reading a paragraph with a line guide
   b. Reading a paragraph in a book
   c. Working on a more disorganized scanning task, possibly including standing or ambulation
   d. Scanning tasks with less lighting to increase muscle strength
   e. Scanning tasks with one eye occluded to increase muscle strength
   f. Reading a recipe
6. It is your first visit with a client with age-related macular degeneration. You begin with:
   a. Providing education on the client's PRL
   b. Reviewing goals and ensuring the client understands the diagnosis
   c. Addressing magnification needs
   d. Providing education on increasing contrast in the home
7. Bob is demonstrating difficulty with self-feeding, specifically with using the correct utensil. Treatment will include:
   a. Educating the family to give Bob the utensil he will need at the proper times
   b. Only providing Bob with a spoon
   c. Educating Bob on the difference in the utensils and what each is used for
   d. Utilizing plastic utensils for safety, when he chooses the wrong utensil
8. A client is being seen for the first OT session after a new left below-knee amputation related to an infected wound. The client has begun to report intermittent blind spots at various times of the day. What may be the cause?
   a. Hemianopsia
   b. Diabetic retinopathy
   c. Agnosia
   d. CVA
9. A new client is requiring significant education regarding the new diagnosis of low vision. Which of the following are appropriate points of education to be addressed?
   a. Therapy tasks will improve vision if they are performed every day.
   b. Therapy will include education in the use of proper lighting and contrast.
   c. Therapy will progress the client from mobility devices.
   d. Therapy will allow the client to stop using their magnifiers.
10. Your highly motivated client with diabetic retinopathy states he continues to have difficulty with functional tasks at home. He is successful with you during treatment sessions, is demonstrating carryover of treatment techniques, and completing his home program. You think he is close to discharge from outpatient OT. What would *most likely* cause this discrepancy?
    a. The lighting is different at home.
    b. The client is not utilizing low-vision techniques at home.
    c. The client does not want to stop therapy.
    d. The client is using the wrong magnifier.

CASE STUDY

RW is a 59-year-old right-handed male diagnosed with cerebrovascular accident. The client reports that he stood from the toilet at home and fell to the floor, and was unable to get up. He also experienced dizziness and slurred speech. In the emergency department, a computerized tomography (CT) scan of the head showed a 5.7 cm x 2 cm right basal ganglia intracerebral hemorrhage with compression of right lateral ventricle, with a 7-mm midline shift from right to left. His intracerebral hemorrhage was managed nonoperatively. RW's previous medical history includes hypertension, alcoholism, and tobacco abuse. He lives alone and works full time. He does not have medical insurance.

After 7 days in acute care, client was transferred to inpatient rehabilitation, where he received OT services. The OT evaluation was completed on day 2 of his rehabilitation stay. Client presented with 0/5 strength in left upper and lower extremity, impaired sensation left side. He also presented with a right gaze preference. Functionally, the client presented as follows:

Feeding: Required set up, including opening packages and cutting food. Verbal and tactile cues to attend to left side

Grooming: Completed 50% of tasks without assistance. Assistance to brush hair on left side of head, set up to wash face. Overall total assistance to shave because of impaired attention to task, impaired safety, and left inattention

Bathing: Client washed his abdomen, chest, left arm, perineal area, and right thigh. Assistance required with remaining areas because of left hemiplegia, left inattention, and overall impaired attention to task. Bathing was completed at bed level as a result of impaired activity tolerance and safety.

Upper body dressing: Client required 75% assistance to don a pullover shirt. He required total assistance to thread left upper extremity and incidental assistance to thread right upper extremity. He was able to don over his head with verbal cues for technique.

Lower body dressing: Completed while supine in bed due to impaired balance. Client threaded right lower extremity but was dependent for remainder of task due to left hemiplegia. Client dependent to roll to don clothing over hips

Toileting: Required total assistance for clothing management and hygiene

Toilet transfer: Unsafe to perform because of impaired mobility and balance

Shower/tub transfer: Unsafe to perform because of impaired mobility and balance

In addition, client presented with moderate deficits with verbal expression, problem-solving, and memory.

The OT treatment plan consisted of addressing sitting balance, standing balance, neuromuscular reeducation, positioning, range of motion, safety education, ADL retraining, family education, and wheelchair mobility. A vision evaluation, performed by an OT practitioner, was also ordered by the physician. The focus of this case study will be the vision rehabilitation he received during his rehabilitation stay.

The OT vision evaluation was performed on day 7 of his rehabilitation stay. Client presented with these on the vision evaluation:

Acuity: Distance 20/20, near 20/30, completed with reading glasses for near assessment
Extraocular ROM: Unable to move either eye laterally to the left
Fixation: Impaired with horizontal movement
Convergence: Impaired right eye
Visual fields: Left homonymous hemianopsia per confrontation field testing
Reading: Assessment completed with large print paragraph. He was dependent due to the inability to scan to the left and locate the next line. Client with impaired awareness of difficulty with reading
Scanning: Significantly impaired per letter cancellation test. The occupational therapist provided interventions at this time to initiate education on compensatory strategies, including turning head, anchor line, and finger guiding.

Cross Out the H

Visual scanning before treatment.

Cross Out the H

Visual scanning after treatment.

At completion of assessment, the OT practitioner educated the client on the results of homonymous hemianopsia, combined with decreased oculomotor control, the typical prognosis with this condition and the treatment plan. Client did verbally demonstrate understanding of the results of the assessment.

As the client's vision impairment was obvious from admission, he was placed in a room that was set up to promote attention to left side. When the client was sitting in his wheelchair or in bed, the door was on his left, to provide stimulation to that side both with hallway traffic and people entering his room. The television was midline. Initially his call bell was placed to his right side for safety, as he needed to be able to easily assess this to address his basic needs. The OTA educated the client's family, when they were present, to place the call bell on his left so they could encourage him to scan in that direction. The OTA provided a written handout for the family and educated his sister to minimize stimulation to his right side in order to promote attention to his left side, such as being on his left side during conversation. As the client progressed with attention to his left side, call bell was placed more frequently to his left.

A portion of each OT session was spent directly addressing visual scanning, oculomotor control, and attention to left side. This was achieved via paper-and-pencil tasks, simple ocular exercises to address range of motion, and tabletop reaching tasks with right upper extremity with focus on reaching toward left side, usually to locate a specific target. In a specific visual scanning task, the OTA placed playing cards in front of client, and asked client to read the cards from right to left. As the client progressed, the OTA either placed more cards or increased the distance between the cards to increase distance of scanning. To further progress the client, the OTA provided gentle tactile cues to the client's head to minimize his head movement to encourage eye movement. A large rolling mirror placed across the table was also used as a reference to ensure quality and efficiency of visual scanning.

The OTA also utilized bathing and dressing sessions as an opportunity to address attention and scanning to the left side. Initially during his rehabilitation stay, the OTA placed items in midline for the client to locate, to draw attention away from his right side. As he progressed, the location of grooming supplies on the sink, or where he needed to look for his clothing when getting ready to dress, made their way toward the left. Meal times were also a great way to address attention and scanning to the left. Before beginning to self-feed, the OTA had the client identify items on the tray. He initially required significant prompting to attend to the left. During the first session, the client ate all items on the right side of the plate and stated he was done. The OTA then prompted him that there was more food on the left side of the plate, but he continued to state he was finished. When the OTA turned the plate so the food was then in his right visual field, client again began self feeding and progressed to finish the remainder of the meal. In subsequent sessions, the OTA would provide cues such as, "There are two items to the left of the plate" or asked client to locate a specific item that was placed on the left. As the client progressed with his meal, he would require cues to recall and attend to the left, but the cues became less frequent.

When the OTA was addressing other aspects of his treatment plan, such as facilitation techniques for his left extremities or sitting and standing balance, tasks were always geared to address attention and scanning to his left side. Specifically, when neuromuscular electrical stimulation was placed on his left upper extremity, he was instructed to visually attend to this side and to attempt to actively engage these muscles. This provided both visual and tactile stimulation.

Fourteen days into his rehabilitation stay, the client demonstrated improving ocular ROM to his left side, but not full ROM. He continued to demonstrate impaired fixation.

Knowing the client would have difficulty with carrying over these treatment techniques, family education was essential. Although education with the client's sister addressed the physical aspects of his care, a significant amount of time was spent reviewing how the OT practitioner was addressing his vision needs and how she could carry this over at home. This included education handouts as well as her observing our therapy sessions and followed this up with the sister returning demonstration of these techniques.

After 28 days in rehabilitation, the client was discharged to his sister's home, as he continued to require physical and cognitive assistance.

Functionally, the client required 25% to 50% physical assistance with self-care tasks and functional mobility. He was functioning at a wheelchair level. The client continued to be limited by left hemiplegia and cognitive impairments. The team recommended follow-up with neuro-optometrist to address left homonymous hemianopsia, as well as outpatient OT to follow up with therapy techniques initiated in rehabilitation.

1. Where do you think RW will be functionally 1 year from discharge from inpatient rehabilitation?
2. Because RW did not have medical insurance, how much follow-up therapy did he receive specifically related to his vision impairments?
3. How did RW's vision impairment affect his performance with ADLs?
4. Did RW's impaired sensation affect his performance with visual tasks?

PUTTING IT ALL TOGETHER — Sample Treatment & Documentation

Setting	Inpatient rehabilitation
Client Profile	30 y/o female s/p second CVA with hx of CVA
Work History	Cashier at a franchised food establishment
Insurance	Medicaid
Psychological	Immature affect
Social	Lives with parents and 5-year-old child
Cognitive	Impaired insight into deficits
Vision	Impaired oculomotor control related to this, as well as previous CVA, difficulty scanning, decreased figure ground, and decreased depth perception
ADL	Assist required due to impaired balance, impaired upper body motor control, vision impairments
Instrumental Activities of Daily Living (IADLs)	Impaired reading, impaired financial management, impaired ability to perform child care
Goals (related to vision)	1. Client will read four lines of continuous text without error and demonstrate full comprehension within 2 weeks. 2. Client will perform simple food prep with supervision by discharge. 3. Client will safely complete basic ADL tasks at a Mod I level within 2 weeks.

OT TREATMENT SESSION 1

THERAPEUTIC ACTIVITY	TIME	GOAL(S) ADDRESSED	OTA RATIONALE
Utilizing visual scanning skills with kitchen tasks. Made a cheese sandwich after gathering all ingredients and tools	30 min	#2	*Occupations and Activities:* Increased independence with child care tasks, as well as simple snack prep for herself and her child
Grooming task at sink to find items required and maintain balance in standing while performing	20 min	#3	*Occupations and Activities:* Addressed both visual scanning and figure ground to find grooming items as well as balance and motor control in standing

PUTTING IT ALL TOGETHER Sample Treatment & Documentation (continued)

SOAP note: 3/12/—, 10:00 am–10:50 am

S: "I need to be able to make a school lunch every day."

O: Client ambulated in the therapy kitchen with Min A for balance, without an assistive device to address visual scanning. She retrieved items from cabinets and drawers with verbal cues to incorporate scanning strategies to locate specific items needed to make a sandwich. Once all items were on the counter, in a visually uncluttered environment, she was able to organize task and complete making the sandwich without assistance. OTA educated client in her improved performance with an uncluttered environment and recommended she incorporate this into her home environment. OTA recommended when client is at home, she sit on a stool at the counter or sit at the table to complete task, for safety with her balance. Client verbalized understanding. Client also performed grooming task at sink with minimal cues and assist to find items at side of sink and Min A for standing balance.

A: Client progressing toward goal of modified independence with simple food prep and toward ADL goal. She does display decreased safety awareness, which may be a combination of visual and balance issues.

P: Continue to incorporate visual scanning skills into functional tasks. Incorporate balance tasks into ADL and visual scanning tasks. Initiate family education to ensure safety and carry over of therapeutic techniques into IADLs at home.

Javier Bloom, COTA/L 3/12/—, 10:45 am

TREATMENT SESSION 2

What could you do next with this client?

TREATMENT SESSION 3

What could you do next with this client?"

REFERENCES

1. Suchoff, I. (1981). Visual-spatial development in the child: An optometric theoretical and clinical approach. New York, NY: State University of New York.
2. Wilson-Pauwels, L., Stewart, P. A., Akesson, E. J., & Spacey, S. D. (2010). *Cranial nerves: Anatomy and clinical comments.* Shelton, CT: People's Medical Publishing House.
3. Scheiman, M. (2002). Understanding and managing vision deficits: A guide for occupational therapists, (2nd ed.). Thorofare, NJ: Slack, Incorporated.
4. Miller-Keane encyclopedia and dictionary of medicine, nursing, and allied health, 7th edition. (2003). Retrieved from http://medical-dictionary.the free dictionary.com/optic+chiasm
5. Millodot, M. (2009). Dictionary of optometry and visual science, 7th edition. Butterworth-Heineman. Retrieved from http://medical-dictionary.thefreedictionary.com/optic+radiations
6. Applebaum, S. (2004). Head injury and stroke vision rehabilitation. Retrieved from www.visionhelp.com
7. Warren, M. (1993). A hierarchical model for evaluation and treatment of visual perceptual dysfunction in adult acquired brain injury, Part I. *The American Journal of Occupational Therapy, 47* (1), 42-54.
8. Zhang, X., Keder, S., Lynn, M., Newman, N., & Biousse, V. (2006). Natural history of homonymous hemianopsia. *Neurology, 66*, 901-905.
9. Warren, M. (2016). Pre-reading and writing exercises. Retrieved from http://visabilities.com
10. Bouska, M. J., Kauffman, N. A., & Marcus, S. E. (1990). Disorders of the visual perceptual system. In D. A. Umphred (Ed.), *Neurological rehabilitation*, St. Louis, MO: Mosby.
11. Kaldenburg, J., & Smallfield, S. (2013). *Occupational therapy practice guidelines for older adults with low vision.* Bethesda, MD: AOTA Press.
12. Zoltan, B. (2007). *Vision, perception, and cognition: A manual for the evaluation and treatment of the adult with acquired brain injury* (4th ed.). Thorofare, NJ: Slack, Incorporated.
13. Berryman, A., Rasavage, K., & Politzer, T. (2010). Practical clinical treatment strategies for evaluation and treatment of visual field loss and visual inattention. *NeuroRehabilitation, 27*, 261-268.
14. Burns, M. S. (2015, Mar 3). Update on neuroscience: Disorders of perception [Webinar]. Joint appointment professor. Northwestern University.
15. AREDS2 Research Group. (2013). Lutein/Zeaxanthin and omega 3 fatty acids for age-related macular degeneration: The Age Related Eye Disease Study 2 (AREDS2) randomized clinical trial. *JAMA*, 309(19): 2005-2015. doi:10.1001/jama.2013.4997
16. Mogk, L., & Mogk, M. (2003). *Macular degeneration: The complete guide to saving and maximizing your sight.* New York, NY: Random House Publishing.
17. Overview of cerebral function. (n.d.). Retrieved from http://www.merckmanuals.com/professional/neurological-disorders/
18. Misconceptions. (n.d.). Retrieved from http://www.charlesbonnet syndrome.org/
19. Knobbe, C. A. (2016). Macular degeneration prevention. Retrieved from http://www.allaboutvision.com
20. VisionCare and Ophthalmic Technologies, Inc. (2015). Implantable Miniature Telescope. Retrieved from http://www.centrasight.com
21. Warren, M. (Ed). (2000). Low vision: Occupational therapy intervention with the older adult: Lesson 1. A self-paced course from the American Occupational Therapy Association.
22. Lamoureux, E. L., Pallant, J. F., Pesudovs, K., Rees, G., Hassel, J. B., & Keefe, J. E. (2007). The effectiveness of low-vision rehabilitation on participation in daily living and quality of life. *Investigative Ophthalmology and Visual Science, 48*, 1476-1482.
23. Mohler, A. J., Neufeld, P., & Perlmutter, M. S. (2015). Factors affecting readiness for low vision interventions in older adults. *American Journal of Occupational Therapy, 69*, 6904270020. doi:10.5014/ajot.2015.014241
24. Segre, L. (2015). Vision over 60. Retrieved from http://www.all aboutvision.com
25. Shahid, K. S. (2012).Visual impairment: Understanding the psychosocial impact. Retrieved from Medscape.com

Chapter 11

Cognition

Stephanie C. Wood, OTR, CDRS and Amber L. Ward, MS, OTR/L, BCPR, ATP/SMS

LEARNING OUTCOMES

After studying this chapter, the student or practitioner will be able to:

11.1 Identify common acute and degenerative conditions that lead to cognitive deficits

11.2 Recognize the characteristics and symptoms of various cognitive deficits

11.3 Identify treatment options for common cognitive deficits and how to provide effective occupational therapy services for clients with cognitive changes

11.4 Describe how to correctly utilize group therapy models for treatment

11.5 Recognize the importance of generalizing cognitive skills addressed in the therapy clinic to "real-life" activities outside of the therapy clinic

KEY TERMS

Acalculia
Agnosia
Agraphia
Alexia without agraphia
Alternating attention
Anosognosia
Anterograde amnesia
Anticipatory awareness
Aphasia
Attention process training (APT)
Cerebral akinetopsia
Chaining technique
Chunking
Cognitive rehabilitation therapy (CRT)
Constructional apraxia
Divided attention
Emergent awareness
Episodic memory
Errorless learning technique
Executive functions
Explicit/declarative memory
Focused attention
Generalization
Global amnesia
Implicit/procedural memory
Initiation
Intellectual awareness
Long-term memory
Phasic alertness
Post-traumatic amnesia
Response inhibition
Retrograde amnesia
Selective attention
Semantic memory
Sensory memory
Short-term memory
Spaced retrieval technique
Sustained attention
Topographical orientation
Vascular dementia
Working memory

As occupational therapy (OT) practitioners, one of the most interesting and complicated areas of practice involves addressing cognitive impairment. What is cognition? **Cognition** is "the mental action or process of acquiring knowledge and understanding through thought, experience, and the senses."[1] Cognition becomes easily impaired when the brain no longer functions like it should as a result of acute, chronic, or degenerative neurological conditions. In fact, cognitive impairment is one of the most devastating long-term consequences of brain injury.[2] According to the Centers for Disease Control and Prevention (CDC), more than 16 million people in the United States are living with cognitive impairment.[3]

All occupations have a cognitive component, no matter how basic. It is through task analysis that the attention, executive function, memory, and behavioral components of tasks can be identified by the occupational therapy assistant (OTA). Cognitive capacities, such as attention and judgment, affect a client's process performance skills and ability to organize actions in a timely and safe manner.[4] As humans, the skill set needed for each daily task completed is taken for granted. Most of these activities are very routine, automatic, and overlearned. Completion of most daily tasks is done without thinking about or processing the activity. Imagine if the ability to concentrate, problem solve, organize, or remember was lost. Even the most simplistic tasks would no longer be easy to complete. This is what clients who have cognitive impairments struggle with on a daily basis.

The brain is truly the most complex machine ever created. According to Stephen Smith, a professor of molecular and cellular physiology at the Stanford University School of Medicine, "a single human brain has more switches than all the computers and routers and Internet connections on Earth."[5]

The reality of the brain's complexity is best summed up by this quote by Emerson M. Pugh: "If the human brain were so simple that we could understand it, we would be so simple that we couldn't."[6] Every year new research is published regarding information not previously known about the brain. With this research comes new evidence as to what techniques and strategies lead to the best therapeutic outcomes for individuals with cognitive impairment. Resources like the American Congress of Rehabilitation Medicine's Cognitive Rehabilitation Manual: Translating Evidence-Based Recommendations into Practice are critical to keeping up to date on the best practices in cognitive rehabilitation and should be sought out by OT practitioners working in this area.[7]

NEUROANATOMY OF COGNITION AND FUNCTIONAL LIMITATIONS ASSOCIATED WITH DAMAGE TO EACH LOBE

In order to provide the best quality therapy, an OT practitioner must first understand how the different areas of the brain control function. On average, the human brain has 86 billion neurons.[9] The cerebral cortex is a thin layer of brain tissue that covers the cerebrum as well as most structures in the brain (Fig. 11-1). It is made up of "gray matter," consisting of mostly nerve cell bodies. It is the largest part of the human brain and is the most highly specialized in cognitive function including language, thinking, and perceiving.[10] The "white matter," consisting of mostly myelinated axons, sits below the gray matter. The white matter connects areas of gray matter and carries nerve impulses between the neurons.

The cerebral cortex is divided into four lobes: frontal, temporal, parietal, and occipital. Each lobe has distinct roles that contribute to the overall function of the human body and more specifically cognition (Fig. 11-1). In addition, the brain is divided into two hemispheres (Fig. 11-2). The corpus callosum connects the right and left hemispheres, and is made up of more than 200 million nerve fibers.[11] Each hemisphere has specialized functions, including the control of the opposite side of the body. More specifically, the left hemisphere is often described as being verbal and analytical. The right hemisphere is thought to control spatial tasks, art and music, creativity, imagination, intuition, body awareness and control, and emotions.[12]

No one area of the brain is more important than the others. Together, the lobes make up a complex superhighway of information processing. Damage to any one area of the brain significantly disrupts this processing of information and can result in mild to severe functional impairments.

EVIDENCE-BASED PRACTICE

OT practitioners have traditionally focused on cognitive rehabilitation and compensation to increase occupational performance after an injury or disease process that causes cognitive deficits. With the profession's focus on evidence to drive effective treatment, a systematic review was recently published that noted the effectiveness of various interventions to address cognitive impairments and improve occupational performance. In the article by Radomski et al. in 2016, strong evidence was found to support use of:

1. Direct attention training: An intensive drill approach to improving attention using simple to more complex mental tasks
2. Attention process training: An attention-training method using the types of attention as a hierarchy
3. Dual-task training: Two tasks performed simultaneously, such as walking and talking
4. Executive function training: Strategies to improve organization and regulation
5. Encoding techniques for memory: Strategies to assist with recall and retention of memories
6. Compensatory strategy training for memory: Internal (e.g., mnemonics, imagery, association) and external (e.g., memory aids, PDAs, calendars) strategies
7. Cognitive assistive technology: Low and high level technology to assist with cognitive abilities and compensation[8]

Although each of these techniques improves a client's abilities in the specific domain, much less evidence was found to tie the techniques to short- and long-term influences on occupational performance. Particularly strong evidence was found involving cognitive assistive technology, and this may be because of its relevance to OT practice in the ways that low- and high-tech options are put in place for rehabilitation and compensation by the OT practitioner. The OTA could use low-tech strategies, such as pictures, to describe the steps for grooming, or color-coded shirts and pants for coordinated dressing. High-tech options could be used such as a smart phone calendar with alerts or a speech-to-text program for getting thoughts on paper. OTAs should frequently check the evidence in their practice area to foster lifelong learning with a focus on effective treatment strategies. Many cognitive interventions may help clients, especially when "provided by OT practitioners who have the knowledge and skills to tether client-centered, occupation-oriented approaches to cognitive interventions supported by evidence."

Radomski, M. V., Anheluk, M., Bartzen, M. P., & Zola, J. (2016). Effectiveness of interventions to address cognitive impairments and improve occupational performance after traumatic brain injury: A systematic review. The American Journal of Occupational Therapy, *70(3), 1-17A. doi:http://dx.doi.org/10.5014/ajot.2016.020776*

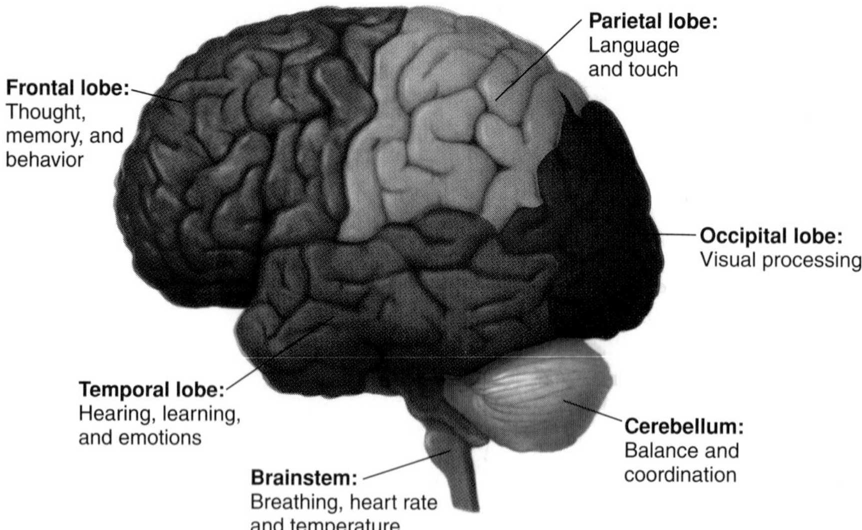

FIGURE 11-1. Lobes of the cerebral cortex.

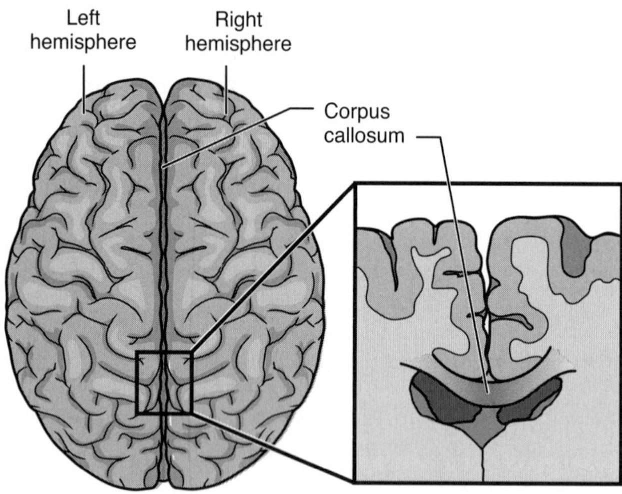

FIGURE 11-2. The two hemispheres of the cerebral cortex are connected by the corpus callosum.

Frontal Lobes

The frontal lobes are large and are positioned at the front of the cranium. These physical characteristics paired with their proximity to the sphenoid wing make them very vulnerable to injury.[13]. The frontal lobes are best known for their role in carrying out executive functions. These **executive functions** help individuals to be organized, make decisions, problem solve, and regulate behavior in a way that allows for independence and safety in managing daily activities. To have optimal executive function and self-regulation skills, good working memory, mental flexibility, and self-control are needed.[14] Without optimal executive function and self-regulation skills, tasks involving planning, focusing, remembering, and multitasking cannot be completed with success.[14] This can negatively impact an individual at home, school, work, in the community, and with driving. Frontal lobe impairments can also alter personality and change the way in which people and problems are approached. Negative behaviors such as anger, low frustration tolerance, impulsivity (acting without thinking), disinhibition (a lack of restraint), apathy, poor **initiation** (inability to begin a task), decreased motivation, or inattentiveness can stress any relationship and affect job performance. Families who experience loved ones with frontal lobe impairment may find it challenging to relate to the person their loved one has become. Individuals experiencing frontal lobe impairment may find that relationships with family, friends, and coworkers become difficult to successfully maintain.

Temporal Lobes

The temporal lobes play a critical role in organizing sensory input. They participate in auditory sensation and perception, selective attention of auditory and visual input, visual perception, organization and categorization of verbal material, language comprehension, long-term memory, personality and affective behavior, and sexual behavior.[15,16] Individuals with right temporal lobe lesions (injury or damage) can experience difficulty with making sense of nonverbal auditory stimuli such as music, whereas left temporal lobe lesions can result in significant difficulties with language. Specific areas of impairment can include recognition, memory, and formation of language.[17]

Parietal Lobes

The parietal lobes are responsible for sensation, perception, and integrating sensory input, especially visual input. Damage to the left parietal lobe can cause a variety of impairments including right-left confusion and **aphasia** (a disorder involving impaired expressive and/or receptive language). It can also cause **agraphia** (impaired ability to write), **acalculia** (impaired ability to calculate numbers), and **agnosia** (impaired ability to recognize common objects).[18] Damage to the right parietal lobe can result in neglect of body parts or space on the left side of the body, known as left neglect or hemi-inattention. This can have a significant impact on self-care and overall independence for the client with these deficits. In addition, right parietal damage can cause difficulty drawing, **constructional apraxia** (difficulty putting things together), and **anosognosia** (denial of impairments).[18]

Occipital Lobes

The occipital lobes are the visual processing center and are made up of the primary visual cortex and visual association areas. They are the smallest of the lobes and are located at the back of the brain. The occipital lobes receive and interpret visual input from the retina. Damage to this area of the brain can result in a variety of visual disorders involving partial to complete vision loss and visual hallucinations. The right occipital lobe controls vision to the left half of each eye and the left occipital lobe controls vision to the right half of each eye.

ACUTE AND DEGENERATIVE CONDITIONS THAT CAN LEAD TO COGNITIVE DECLINE

A variety of conditions can lead to cognitive decline. Some of these conditions are due to acute neurological changes from a single event. These include traumatic brain injury (TBI), acquired brain injury (ABI), cerebrovascular accident (CVA), aneurysm rupture, or an arteriovenous malformation (AVM) bleed. Other conditions causing cognitive decline can be chronic, degenerative conditions such as Parkinson's disease (PD), multiple sclerosis (MS), amyotrophic lateral sclerosis (ALS), dementia (including Alzheimer's disease [AD]), and Huntington's disease (HD). In addition, brain tumors, autism, specific genetic and chromosomal abnormalities, and other developmental impairments can impair cognition.

Traumatic and Acquired Brain Injury

According to the Brain Injury Association of America, "Traumatic brain injury (TBI) is an injury to the brain caused by an external force after birth. Common causes of a traumatic brain injury include gunshot wounds, motor vehicle crashes, assaults, or falling and striking your head." They define an ABI as including "all types of traumatic brain injuries and also brain injuries caused after birth by cerebral vascular accidents (commonly known as stroke), and loss of oxygen to the brain (hypoxic brain injury)."[19] There is a debate in the brain injury field as to what to call traumatic injuries, but this book will use the term TBI for traumatic injuries, CVA for strokes, and ABI for all other types of brain injuries. Brain injury almost always causes cognitive deficits and can affect every area of cognition. There is often a direct impact injury from force, as well as further injury from the brain moving inside the skull, causing other nondirect injuries. Cognitive impairment can present itself with deficits in attention, concentration, memory, executive function, behavior, and awareness. Although each type of brain impairment results in different types of cognitive difficulties, this list of common cognitive impairments typically occurs after experiencing a TBI:

- Difficulty problem-solving and reasoning through daily tasks and dilemmas
- Saying and doing things that are out of character
- Reacting to situations impulsively
- Repeating words or stories
- Talking incessantly and providing too much detail
- Sharing inappropriate information or doing inappropriate things
- Drifting off-topic during conversation
- Forgetting names and details, both new and old
- Difficulty remembering how to do common daily activities
- Difficulty concentrating and screening distractions
- Difficulty attending to more than one thing at a time
- Difficulty generating words or comprehending conversation
- Inability to identify impairments and how these impact daily life
- Defensiveness when impairments are discussed[20]

Cerebrovascular Accident

A CVA, or stroke, occurs when nutrients and oxygen being carried in the blood through an artery to the brain are blocked. This can occur because of a blood clot or rupture of an artery, and leads to brain cell death.[21] A CVA can cause many types of cognitive and physical impairments, depending on the location of injury in the brain. Left hemisphere CVAs can result in deficits on the right side of the body as well as:

- Receptive aphasia: Difficulty understanding speech
- Expressive aphasia: Difficulty with speaking
- Decreased initiation, slowness of thought
- Personality and behavioral changes
- Increased frustration
- Memory impairment[22]

Right hemisphere CVAs can result in deficits on the left side of the body as well as:

- Left-sided inattention to body and space
- Decreased concentration
- Problem-solving difficulties
- Distractibility
- Decreased insight into deficits
- Impulsive behavior
- Short-term memory loss[22]

Aneurysm

A brain aneurysm or cerebral aneurysm is caused by a bulging or weak area in an artery supplying blood to the brain. Typically this abnormality goes unnoticed but on rare occasions can rupture and cause a type of CVA called a subarachnoid hemorrhage. The severity of the hemorrhage determines whether brain damage or death occurs. Deficits common after aneurysm include:

- Visual and verbal memory impairments
- Significant fatigue
- Changes in language skills
- Executive function changes
- Anxiety and depression
- Sleep disturbances and changes in sleep patterns[23]

Arteriovenous Malformation

A brain AVM is a tangle of abnormal blood vessels in the brain that connect arteries and veins, which can lead to symptoms over time or a rupture.[24] The AVM disrupts the vital process that arteries and veins do to circulate oxygen-rich blood from the heart to the brain and back to the heart and lungs. Cognitive and other related deficits common after an AVM rupture include:

- Ataxia: Loss of coordinated and controlled movements
- Apraxia: Loss of motor planning of skilled movements
- Memory impairments
- Slight confusion to full dementia
- Hallucinations
- Sensory changes[25]

THE OLDER ADULT

Cognitive impairment can be seen in older adults for a variety of reasons. This population experiences a variety of neurological impairments such as Parkinson's disease, CVAs, Alzheimer's disease and other types of dementias at a more significant rate than younger age groups. In addition, age itself can gradually decline cognition. Working with older adults with cognitive impairment can be extremely rewarding but challenging, too. These individuals can be challenged physically and cognitively, not to mention with their hearing and vision. Also, they are many times used to certain routines and may have trouble adjusting to change. Whereas younger clients many times embrace technology as a way to overcome certain impairments, older adults may not have experiences using technology that will allow them to rely on it as a strategy. Creativity is critical in identifying the best ways to assist older adults in overcoming cognitive change. In addition, those with degenerative conditions may need to be monitored over time so that adjustments in the strategies used to enhance their independence can be modified as their cognition declines. Never judge a client's ability based on age alone. Some 65 year olds may appear more impaired than 85 year olds. Be open minded and do not judge a book by its cover. Treat the individual, no matter the age, and tailor the treatments to their current ability, past interests, and desire for independence.

Parkinson's Disease

PD is a motor system disorder caused by a loss of brain cells responsible for producing dopamine. Most people recognize the motor impairments common to Parkinson's, but the cognitive deficits seen with the disease can be subtle and become progressively worse as the disease progresses. Researchers estimate that at least 50% of individuals with PD have mild cognitive impairments with as many as 20% to 40% showing more severe impairment or dementia.[26] As resourced from the Parkinson's (disease) Foundation website, "Many people with Parkinson's are surprised to find that they feel distracted or disorganized, or have difficulty planning and carrying through tasks. It may be harder to focus in situations that divide their attention, like a group conversation. When facing a task or situation on their own, a person with PD may feel overwhelmed by having to make choices. They may also have difficulty remembering information, or have trouble finding the right words when speaking. For some people these changes are merely annoying, for others they interfere with work or with managing household affairs."[27] Cognitive deficits common with PD include:

- Bradyphrenia: Slowness of processing information
- Multitasking and concentration deficits
- Problem-solving deficits
- Decreased memory and recall
- Visual-spatial deficits[28,29]

Multiple Sclerosis

MS occurs when there is damage to the myelin coating around the nerve fibers in the central nervous system that causes a disruption in the nerve signals sent throughout the body. It is considered to be a chronic, progressive autoimmune disorder. The cognitive symptoms seen with MS can vary widely both in type and severity. According to the National Multiple Sclerosis Society, only 5% to 10% of individuals with MS develop severe cognitive impairments that significantly affect everyday activities, yet more mild cognitive impairment is common and occurs in 50% of all cases.[30] Common cognitive deficits seen with MS include:

- Memory and concentration deficits
- Decreased attention
- Decreased initiation and motivation
- Poor mental acuity, processing delays, slowness of thought
- Difficulty making decisions
- Impulsivity
- Distractibility
- Difficulty staying on task
- Planning or organizational deficits
- Executive function changes
- Problems understanding what is read or heard
- Perseveration: Getting stuck on one thought
- Decreased self awareness, especially of deficits
- Spatial orientation challenges: Getting lost
- Decreased selective attention[31]

Amyotrophic Lateral Sclerosis

ALS is a progressive neurodegenerative disease affecting the brain and spinal cord and results in the wasting away of muscles as a result of motor neuron involvement. Through the years it has also been referred to as Lou Gehrig's disease, named for the American baseball great who was afflicted with the disorder, and in many countries, it is known as motor neuron disease. What some people do not know is that up to 50% of individuals with ALS experience cognitive and behavioral changes.[32] Up to 25% of those with ALS will develop dementia.[32] The cognitive and behavioral changes, provided by the ALS Association, that can occur in individuals with ALS are:

- Behavior changes
- Disinhibition: Lack of restraint to follow social norms
- Decreased attention to hygiene
- Decreased judgment for decision making
- Lack of concern for self and others, future
- Inability to concentrate
- Perseveration/fixation: Response or thought repetition
- Increased aggression
- Difficulty with expression in writing and speech
- Loss of spelling
- Difficulty following and recalling instructions
- Decreased memory[32]

Dementia

Experts in health care agree, dementia is not a specific disease yet rather a broad term used to describe a significant decline in mental function capable of interfering with daily activities. According to the Alzheimer's Association, 60% to 80% of individuals with dementia have AD.[33] The second leading cause of dementia is **vascular dementia** caused by CVA, or series of CVAs, or other vascular changes. At least two of these cognitive functions must be significantly impaired for a diagnosis of dementia to be considered:[34]

- Impaired memory
- Attention deficits
- Communication and language deficits
- Visual perceptual deficits
- Decreased reasoning and judgment

Huntington's Disease

HD is a rare, inherited disease that causes the progressive breakdown (degeneration) of nerve cells in the brain. HD has a broad impact on a person's functional abilities and usually results in movement, cognitive, and psychiatric disorders.[28] According to the Huntington's Disease Society of America, the symptoms that occur with this disorder are:[35]

- Personality changes
- Decreased judgment
- Depression and mood swings
- Forgetfulness

Temporary Cognitive Changes

There are times when cognitive changes can be temporary, such as with a medication side effect, urinary tract infection, deficiencies in certain vitamins and other nutritional issues, insomnia and sleep issues, and many cancer and chemotherapy treatments. For some clients, simply being out of their familiar environment can cause increased confusion. A term called hospital delirium, which may affect clients who are frail and mildly demented, is caused by the combined impact of medications, dehydration, infection, and many times surgery, and the after effects of sedation. For most, once the contributing factors are resolved, so does the cognitive change.

COGNITIVE REHABILITATION THERAPY

Without appropriate therapeutic intervention, individuals with any type of cognitive impairment can have difficulty carrying out their daily routine. This in turn can lead to an overall reduction in independence and safety. Activities that were once automatic can now require a great deal of effort or become impossible to complete and may require **Cognitive Rehabilitation Therapy (CRT)**. CRT has many definitions; according to the Brain Injury Interdisciplinary Special Interest Group (BI-ISIG) of the American Congress of Rehabilitation Medicine, "cognitive rehabilitation is a systematic, functionally oriented service of therapeutic cognitive activities, based on an assessment and understanding of the person's brain-behavior deficits. Services are directed to achieve functional changes by (1) reinforcing, strengthening, or reestablishing previously learned patterns of behavior, or (2) establishing new patterns of cognitive activity or compensatory mechanisms for impaired neurological systems."[29,36] The Society for Cognitive Rehabilitation offers this definition: "...CRT is the process of relearning cognitive skills that have been lost or altered as a result of damage to brain cells/chemistry."[2] They identify that CRT has these four components:

1. Increasing an individual's awareness of deficits by identifying cognitive strengths and weaknesses through education.
2. Problem resolution by retraining impaired cognitive skills.
3. Compensation for impaired cognitive skills through implementation of internal, external, and environmental strategies.
4. Generalization of learned skills into real-life environments by implementing the first three components of CRT.

It is estimated that 95% of rehabilitation facilities treating individuals with TBI and ABI offer cognitive rehabilitation through individual, group, and community-based interventions.[37] In addition, a recent study concluded that "participants receiving intensive cognitive rehabilitation programs (ICRP) showed significantly greater improvements in community integration than participants receiving standard rehabilitations. Although both groups improved, the participants receiving ICRP were over twice as likely to show clinically significant improvement in community integration as those receiving standard rehabilitation programs (SRP)." These same individuals showed significant improvement in attention, processing speed, and immediate-memory recall.[38]

The Role of Occupational Therapy in Cognitive Rehabilitation Therapy

Published in the *American Journal of Occupational Therapy* in 2013, "the American Occupational Therapy Association (AOTA) asserts that occupational therapists and occupational therapy assistants, through the use of occupations and activities, facilitate individuals' cognitive functioning to enhance occupational performance, self-efficacy, participation, and perceived quality of life. Cognition is integral to effective performance across the broad range of daily occupations such as work, educational pursuits, home management, play, and leisure. Cognition also plays an integral role in human development and in the ability to learn, retain, and use new information in response to changes in everyday life."[39] The Accreditation Council for Occupational Therapy Education (ACOTE) in 2012 stated, "occupational therapy practitioners are well-qualified to assess and address cognitive performance issues affecting daily activity performance because of their education and training in cognitive functioning, task analysis, learning, diagnostic conditions, and a holistic understanding of the wide range of factors and contexts that affect performance."[39]

Numerous cognitive assessments can be used by OT practitioners as well as other members of the multidisciplinary team. The OTA should have familiarity with the types of assessments that are commonly used as well as what the results of the tests may mean for functional treatment. Although the neuropsychologist is viewed as the expert on analyzing cognitive function through the administration and interpretation of neuropsychological tests, OT practitioners also have access to cognitive assessments. These tools are designed for the OT practitioner to use in order to collect data regarding their clients' cognitive function. Some of these tools look at cognitive function in multiple areas and others are more specific to a cognitive domain such as attention or memory. Table 11-1 shows a listing of the cognitive assessments commonly used by OT practitioners and which cognitive domain(s) are being tested.

Many newer OT practitioners are unsure how their approach to cognitive deficits would differ from other teammates, especially the speech-language pathologist (SLP). The OT practitioner addresses cognitive performance as it relates to occupational performance, functional abilities, and task completion. OT practitioners are taught to focus on functional activities and the skills necessary to complete them, and to recognize that health is supported and maintained when clients are able to engage in home, school, workplace, and community life.[4] The SLP addresses the same components of cognition, particularly as they relate to communication, and the physical therapist addresses cognition from a motor and safety perspective.

More specifically, the OTA should work with a client on the cognitive issues that particularly interfere with their ability to complete daily tasks at home, school, and work, in the community, and with driving. For example, if a client is experiencing difficulty remembering to take their medications on time because of attention and memory impairments, an OTA may implement a reminder system to address these cognitive impairments and effects on the client's independence. Treatment sessions would involve creating a written or electronic schedule for medication management, implementing auditory cues (e.g., alarms) or visual cues (e.g., pill organizer, paper schedule, etc.) to ensure the client follows through, practicing the process in therapy and at home, and making adjustments as needed to ensure success. Involving family in the process will also assist with follow through outside of the therapy clinic. The SLP, on the other hand, may also address this client's memory and attention impairments but provide these interventions through memory and attention-specific tasks and strategies to enhance the individual's overall cognitive-communication abilities.

A Multidisciplinary Approach to Cognitive Rehabilitation

Cognitive rehabilitation is extremely beneficial when approached from a multidisciplinary perspective so that the cognitive components that affect each skill area are not overlooked. According to the Society for Cognitive Rehabilitation, "CRT cannot be seen as a 'stand alone' therapy, but must form part of the multidisciplinary approach."[2] In the multidisciplinary setting, many professionals will address cognition. Each discipline addresses cognition differently and is integral to achieving a positive functional outcome. A multidisciplinary team includes OT, SLP, physical therapy, neuropsychology, physicians, and nurses. In some instances, therapeutic recreation, music therapists, behavioral specialists, and social workers may also be part of the team.

The role of the neuropsychologist is critical in order for the OT practitioner to best understand what cognitive abilities have been impaired by the neurological condition. Neuropsychological testing is a tool they use to identify specific cognitive impairments. This information can help guide the entire therapy team in choosing appropriate interventions for the client as well as identifying potential for recovery.

Variables That Affect Cognitive Rehabilitation

Many variables affect cognitive treatment, and include the severity and range of impairment, the degree of unawareness, emotional reactions, premorbid psychiatric issues, and family factors.[7] In addition, client factors, including premorbid

TABLE 11-1 Abbreviated List of Cognitive Assessments Used in the Occupational Therapy Setting[40-44]

TEST	CHARACTERISTICS	ORIENTATION	MEMORY	ATTENTION/ CONCENTRATION	EXECUTIVE FUNCTIONS/ THINKING OPERATIONS	VISUAL & SPATIAL PERCEPTION	VISUOMOTOR ORGANIZATION	CALCULATIONS
Mini Mental State Examination (MMSE)	30 questions 5-10 minutes Used often in dementia	X	X	X	X			X
Lowenstein Occupational Therapy Cognitive Assessment (LOTCA)	21 subtests in 4 areas, 30-45 minutes to administer, adaptations for communication deficits, 20 up to 70 years of age	X			X	X	X	
Lowenstein Occupational Therapy Cognitive Assessment-Geriatric (LOTCA-G)	71-90 years of age, 23 subtests in 7 cognitive areas 15-30 minutes	X	X		X	X	X	
Montreal Cognitive Assessment (MoCA)	Distinguishing clients with mild cognitive impairment from normal elderly clients 10-15 minutes	X	X	X	X	X		X
Allen Cognitive Level Screen (ACLS)	Performance of three visual motor tasks of increasing complexity. Uses leather lacing tools/stitches		X	X	X			

Continued

TABLE 11-1 Abbreviated List of Cognitive Assessments Used in the Occupational Therapy Setting[40-44] (continued)

TEST	CHARACTERISTICS	ORIENTATION	MEMORY	ATTENTION/ CONCENTRATION	EXECUTIVE FUNCTIONS/ THINKING OPERATIONS	VISUAL & SPATIAL PERCEPTION	VISUOMOTOR ORGANIZATION	CALCULATIONS
Short Blessed Test	Detects early cognitive changes 5 minutes or less	X	X	X				
Test of Everyday Attention (TEA)	15-80 years, 45-60 minutes; test comprises 8 subsets that represent everyday tasks			X				
D2 Test of Attention	10 minutes to administer Selective/sustained attention, scanning			X				
Contextual Memory Test (CMT)	5-10 minutes to administer Uses familiar objects as the items to be remembered		X					
Rivermead Behavioral Memory Test (RBMT)	Ages 16-96, 20-30 min visual and verbal recall, recognition, memory Acquired brain damage		X					
Neurobehavioral Cognitive Status Screening Examination (COGNISTAT)	Adults, elderly, 15-20 min to administer	X	X	X	X			X

COMMUNICATION

Communication is a significant issue that is addressed in many ways with those who are cognitively impaired. For example, it may be addressed by assisting an individual with expressive language impairment in communicating while out in the community during a grocery shopping errand or with buying a ticket and popcorn at the movie theater. Communication is integral to any activity involving the interaction of two or more people. The appropriateness of communication may also need to be addressed as part of the therapeutic process. Negative and awkward behaviors are common among those who have cognitive impairments. OT practitioners should not shy away from confronting these behaviors head-on as part of the communication process. An example of this is when a client who was college-aged with a brain injury pulled down her shorts in a private therapy room during her first introduction with the occupational therapist who was getting ready to begin the in-clinic portion of her driving evaluation. The client shared she was putting a special lotion on her thighs to keep her shorts from rubbing her skin. In response, the occupational therapist casually but matter-of-factly confronted the individual about the awkwardness of the interaction. The issue of behaving this way, both in general, and when meeting a new practitioner, had to be addressed. "Confronting with compassion" should be the approach used by OT practitioners to assist individuals in overcoming behaviors that negatively affect communication. If OT practitioners do not take the time to do this, who will? The longevity of a client's relationship with family and friends depends on it. It is the connection felt with those who are close that keeps individuals invested and engaged in those relationships. Nothing kills those connections more than awkward, negative behaviors.

values, beliefs, and spirituality, influence participation in all life activities[4].

Even clients with mild cognitive impairments can have significant difficulty adjusting to their deficits. When individuals have strong educational backgrounds and are successful in high-level work positions (i.e., business executives, dentists, lawyers, doctors, principals, etc.), they can become hyperaware of even the smallest changes in function. These clients are used to relying on their advanced memory, attention, problem-solving, and multitasking skills to complete their jobs. Even small changes in function can feel monumental when trying to complete high-level cognitive tasks. This can result in difficulty adjusting to previous routines and activities despite being capable of resuming independence with these tasks. Other clients may be less aware of deficits until they begin to impact their functional performance. Clients may try to explain away problems with memory or confusion as being tired or stressed. Many individuals who experience a neurological change can also experience a personal loss related to their loss of function. This in turn can lead to an emotional reaction such as depression and other negative psychological issues.[45]

INTERNAL AND EXTERNAL COGNITIVE STRATEGIES

The ways in which cognitive impairments are addressed in therapy are through the use of strategies. Strategies are tools used to compensate for cognitive deficits. These strategies can be internal or external. An internal strategy represents a type of thought process or behavior that is not written down but instead memorized and accessed as needed. For example, categorizing and visualizing information to remember details are types of internal memory strategies. Other examples of internal strategies used to address attention and memory deficits include working slowly, double-checking work, and using acronyms and word associations to remember things. These strategies are introduced to the client by the OT practitioner. Training is provided to the client during therapeutic tasks until the client is able to self-monitor and apply these internal strategies on his or her own. Greater cognitive ability is required to carry out internal strategies versus external strategies because the strategy itself has to be remembered and implemented at the very time the individual begins to struggle with a task.[2] According to the Society for Cognitive Rehabilitation, "strategy training should be matched to the level of awareness shown by the person with brain injury. As awareness increases, different strategy training should be incorporated."[2] Internal strategies are more difficult to use than external strategies and should be reserved for individuals with more mild cognitive impairment. Therefore, the more impaired the client, the less able they will be to utilize internal memory strategies successfully.

For those clients who are moderately to severely impaired, the use of external memory strategies will be critical to their success with rehabilitation and their ability to return to independence with daily tasks. External strategies represent tools that are external to the client. These include orientation and memory notebooks, notes and labels, smart phones, alarms, and electronic and paper calendars. Not only should the strategies chosen match the level of awareness of the individual, they should also match the client's premorbid learning styles and interests. If an external strategy, such as an electronic device, will add more confusion to a person's daily life, it should be replaced with a simpler tool. Depending on an individual's progress in therapy or lack thereof, the strategies used during the rehabilitation process may need to be adjusted to allow the individual to gain the highest level of independence possible.

ATTENTION AND CONCENTRATION IMPAIRMENTS

Attention is a complex cognitive function that is essential for human behavior.[46] It serves as a foundational skill for all other cognitive processes. Without the ability to sustain attention, new memories cannot be encoded, problem-solving and judgment can become altered, and behavior impairments can occur.

Many areas of the brain play a role in attention, making it a very common problem after a brain injury. Even subtle impairments can significantly impair a client's ability to complete daily tasks independently and safely.[7] For example, if a person loses focus and wanders away from the cooktop during a meal preparation task, a safety issue—as minor as a pot boiling over or as major as a fire—could ensue.

Attention can be directed voluntarily or automatically. For instance, if an individual is looking for a park bench to sit and rest on, that would be an example of voluntary attention. On the other hand, when one hears a gunshot or thunder, attention shifts automatically. The ability to process internal and external stimuli depends on maintaining a certain level of awareness of the environment. It is normal for attention to fluctuate throughout the day. A person's ability to pay attention and concentrate depends on many factors such as stress, disruptive thoughts, background noise, and level of fatigue. Most brain activities require a lot of attention, whether it is to memorize information, understand a text, or find an item.[47] Without attention to external stimuli, new learning simply does not happen, which in turn affects memory. As might be expected, adequate attention is needed to successfully complete many daily tasks. Difficult tasks such as driving in an unfamiliar city require more focused attention versus an automatic task such as brushing teeth, which requires less.[48] To sustain attention there also needs to be motivation from the client to do so and cognitive processing to juggle competing information and stimuli.[49]

Types of Attention

Phasic alertness is an individual's momentary, rapidly occurring (within milliseconds) readiness to respond, such as to a reaction time test or when awoken abruptly from a nap. Phasic alertness is a short lived attentional effect, often related to focused attention as one orients to the sound of a baby crying or the smell of gas in the house.

Response inhibition is the ability to inhibit the inclination to direct attention toward something distracting.[50] The ability to maintain attention means a person has good response inhibition. Examples of this are when an individual is not distracted during a conversation with someone even though another person in the room is talking loudly on their phone or when a person is able to stay focused on conversation even though a person's hairstyle or clothes are distracting. Generally, the longer attention is sustained, the degree of response inhibition decreases. This, in turn, can lead to the person attending to stressors and distractions. For example, during a long meeting, an individual may start to focus more on the sore bottom they have developed from sitting rather than listening to the speaker.

Focused attention is thought to be the most basic level of attention. This type of attention allows for the identification of specific sensory information. For example, it is focused attention that allows a person to orient to sounds, smells, and tactile stimuli during the daily routine.

Sustained attention is the ability to remain focused and on task for an extended period of time.[51] Sustained attention is often called vigilance or tonic alertness,[49] and is the readiness to respond over longer time intervals, generally over 10 minutes. It is also known as intrinsic alertness, or the internal control of attention in the absence of cues.[52] This might involve attending to a speaker during a long class or focusing on a game of Solitaire. It is at this level of attention that working memory occurs, which allows an individual to hold information in mind while mentally manipulating it in some way.[53]

Selective attention enables a person to focus on one item while mentally identifying and distinguishing the nonrelevant information.[54] This skill gives the ability to filter out extraneous information coming into a person's sensory system. It is this type of attention that allows for picking out an individual's face in a crowd or locating a certain name on a list of names. The brain does not focus on every face or name, but scans for particular features or letters. Significant amounts of information come into sensory systems throughout the day, and no one could possibly focus on all of it at the same time. Things which are selectively attended to include a person's name being called, the smell of dinner, noticing the toy on the floor which must be stepped over, as well as hundreds of other pieces of information. Among all this information, selective attention prioritizes information according to the situation at hand.

Alternating attention allows for shifting focus between two tasks or activities, each which require thought, such as taking notes in class while listening to the lecture. Another example might be helping a child with homework while cooking on the stovetop. Stepping away from stirring a pot of soup to check on a child sitting at the kitchen table completing a math worksheet, and then returning to meal prep demonstrates how attention can shift back and forth between two activities all the time in one's daily life.

Divided attention allows for simultaneously attending to multiple stimuli. Many situations require a person to attend in two directions at once, such as listening for a child playing in the living room while noticing that the vegetables are browning in a pan during dinner preparation. One of the tasks is generally more automatic and requires less focus than the other, such as brushing hair while listening to the news. The ability to split attention is an essential skill that allows one to multitask in even the most basic ways. Having a conversation with a family member while dusting the living room demonstrates divided attention. Humans live in a world today that expects a high level of multitasking. Technology keeps the connection at all hours of the day and in all environments, whether it is desired or not. No matter where a person goes, the impact of this is seen, while people drive and talk on the phone and text during their kids' sporting events. Like it or not, multitasking has become a way of life.

TECHNOLOGY AND TRENDS

Cell phones, smartphones, and tablets have become the new way of managing our calendar, schedule, and life, and they can be invaluable for those with a cognitive deficit. Both voice-to-text and text-to-voice programs exist that can make communicating easier both by text, email, and in person. Alerts and alarms can be set for medication reminders and appointments. Note pages can be used to write down information the client does not want to forget, and photos of medication bottles texted by family at certain times can remind the client to take those medications. Photos can also be used to document the client's life as it happens and can be reviewed at the end of the day or the next day. Also, photos can be used to remember what to buy at the grocery store or at Target. Global positioning system (GPS) devices can assist with finding the way, whether driving or on foot. Many applications, or "apps," can assist with reading, learning a new skill, simple cooking strategies, memory games, and so much more. Technology can be a burden at times, but can be a lifesaver for a client with a cognitive deficit.

Specific Treatment Interventions

The focus now will shift from attention as a condition, to treatment strategies that the OTA can employ to compensate or rehabilitate for attention deficits.

GENERAL ATTENTION STRATEGIES

In everyday life, strategies are employed to enhance attention without realizing it. Some of the techniques that are used automatically become difficult to implement when a neurological injury or condition occurs. Therefore, OT practitioners will need to reintroduce these strategies to their clients. These are general ways to enhance attention:[55]

- Alter the environment to eliminate noise and distractions.
- If a noisy environment cannot be altered, ear plugs can be worn.
- When fatigue sets in, take a break.
- Do not complete complex tasks when tired.
- Work slowly and focus on details.
- Double check work for errors.
- If lost in conversation, ask for clarification.
- If unable to write down information fast enough, request that information be repeated.
- Get a good night's sleep.
- Stick to routines.

ATTENTION PROCESS TRAINING

Sohlberg and Mateer have done much work in the area of attention and have developed an attention training method for those with neurological impairment called **Attention Process Training (APT)**.[54] Their framework for addressing attention is based on the hierarchical model that places focused attention as the most basic level of attention and divided attention is the most complex. If thought of as a pyramid, focused attention would be on the bottom with sustained attention next, then selective attention, alternating attention, and lastly divided attention on top. Therefore, the more impaired an individual is cognitively, the more difficulty they will have utilizing higher-level attention skills[7] (Fig. 11-3). The use of the APT approach entails both quantitative and qualitative measures and does require a specialized set of materials and techniques outlined in the APT manual. Research has shown that it is an effective method for addressing attention impairments. As part of the APT program, generalization of attention skills is incorporated into treatment so that "real-world" tasks requiring different levels of attention are specifically addressed.[56]

ATTENTION TREATMENT ACTIVITIES

At the end of this paragraph, therapeutic activities that can be used to generalize attention skills are listed under the type of attention each one addresses. Once an individual can focus their attention and sustain it for a period of time, activities can be introduced to address selective, alternating and divided attention by adding in more distractions. Any activity can be used to address attention by modifying it appropriately for the level of function of the client. Ultimately, training of attention skills needs to be tied back into functional activities that relate to the individual's daily routine at home, in the community, and at work or school.

Sustained attention includes:

- Self-care tasks, such as bathing or dressing
- Household management tasks, such as cooking or cleaning
- Work or school-based tasks, such as answering phone calls, using the computer, taking notes, and making calculations
- Community-based tasks, such as banking or grocery shopping

Selective attention includes:

- Self-care or household management activities while the TV or music is on

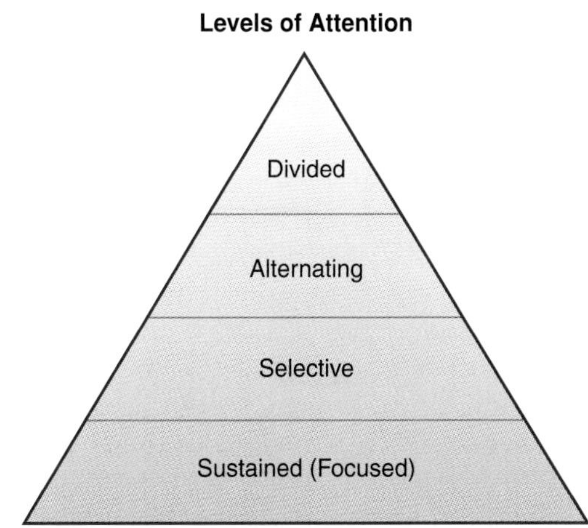

FIGURE 11-3. Pyramid of attention concepts.

- Completion of a puzzle or craft with noise or conversation in the room
- Ordering a meal at a noisy restaurant
- Reading a book or newspaper with the TV or music on

Alternating attention includes:

- Completing household chores with occasional phone interruptions
- Watching the news in the living room and walking to the dryer in the laundry room to check clothes as needed
- Cooking a meal in one room, and then walking to another room to check on kids
- Checking an item off a grocery list after finding it on the shelf
- Completing work or school tasks with frequent interruptions
- Reading the newspaper while stopping to highlight each time a certain word is used in an article
- Alternating between two activities, e.g., folding one shirt, then completing a crossword answer, alternating between the tasks

Divided attention includes:

- Cleaning the kitchen while talking on the phone
- Cooking while listening to the news
- Having a conversation while eating a meal
- Putting the dishes away while discussing current events with a loved one

Importance of Attention as a Foundational Skill for All Other Cognitive Abilities

Attention is the beginning and end for all other cognitive abilities. It is a foundational skill that underlies and supports all cognitive functions.[7] For example, attention is a necessary prerequisite for memory. New memories cannot be made if the information to be remembered has not been encoded properly. If an individual cannot attend to information coming from the environment, then the individual will not remember what was heard, seen, touched, smelled, or tasted; be able to process this information; or make good decisions regarding safety, including moving away from something dangerous. This impaired ability to process new information then leads to a decreased ability to encode details. This, in turn, leads to an inability to form new memories. If highly distracted, an individual can have difficulty retrieving old memories, too. Without the ability to attend, learn, or retain information, most functional tasks become extremely difficult. For example, even the simplicity of carrying out a morning routine involving self-care activities can be extremely difficult when individuals cannot sustain, alternate, or divide their attention effectively enough to complete multistep tasks. Strategies to enhance independence at home that incorporate attention and memory skills, such as a morning checklist, may be necessary to keep the individual focused on the tasks to be completed. This type of checklist might need to be posted in the bathroom for the severely impaired, with assistance from a caregiver to carry through with each task. For less impaired individuals who still need assistance to attend to each detail, a checklist could be housed on an electronic device with assistance as needed to carry through with each step. Time should be spent practicing these strategies both in the clinic and in the home if possible. Caregivers would need appropriate training to know what the expectation is for using this technique.

MEMORY IMPAIRMENTS

Memory impairments can be functionally devastating for the person with acquired neurological deficits, as remembering even the most basic details of what is needed to do or where to go may be compromised. Often what is thought of as "memory" is long-term memory because that type of memory holds the details of the past, which is so important in defining who individuals are, through facts and events as well as the mental map for how to do daily routines. However, there is also short-term and sensory memory. Memory function is not localized to one specific brain region; therefore, memory impairment is common with any type of neurological insult (Fig. 11-4).

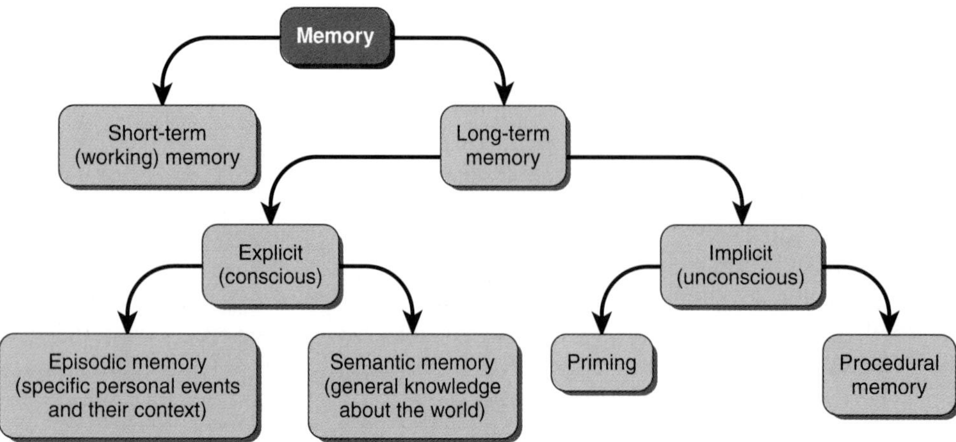

FIGURE 11-4. Types of memory.

Types of Memory

Sensory memory is often linked with perception, but is actually a form of unconscious memory. An individual's senses are constantly taking in information. Some is ignored, and some is put into sensory memory for perception by the brain. The information is used and stored for less than 1 second, and then is gone. Sensory memory is used to be able to look at something for a split second, and to be able to describe it. Another example is the momentary notice of a bad smell coming from someone passing in a crowd at a festival. These memories are used by the brain to move through and interact with the world, but are not retained.

Short-term memory is referred to as the brain's "Post-it" note, and will retain about seven items for about 10 seconds to 1 minute.[57] It can be thought of as the ability to remember and process at the same time. Examples of this are when one speaker remembers the argument of the other speaker until it is his or her turn to talk, or when an individual remembers a phone number long enough to dial it without writing it down. When information is held in the mind and is manipulated, it is referred to as **working memory**. This information will quickly disappear if not consciously retained by rehearsing it, associating it with other information already in long-term memory storage, or by giving it meaning (something of strong interest to the individual). The prefrontal cortex is the area of the brain that when damaged causes difficulty with short-term memory (see Fig. 11-1). Short-term memory has limited capacity, but there are certain ways to increase the time these memories can be used. One way is through the use of strategies such as categorizing information by type. Rehearsing out loud can also help with short-term memory. Often new information will push out older information, and certainly distractions will interfere with short-term memory. Imagine the significance of severe short-term memory impairment. Day-to-day details that give lives structure, order, and meaning would no longer be encoded successfully. There would be a sense of emptiness when it came to recalling dates, appointments, schedules, and memories of events that occurred that day.

Long-term memory is for the storage of information and memories over a long period of time. Although some things seem forgotten, the capacity for long-term memories in a healthy person is unlimited, and does not degrade much at all over time. Long-term memory encodes memories semantically or by meaning and association versus sound or visual information, as with short-term memory.[57] When there is trouble recalling information from long-term memory, it may be that a neural connection has degraded or another memory of close association has laid down on top of it, confusing the issue. Long-term memory is stored throughout the brain, although most long-term memories go through the hippocampus for consolidation on the way to storage. Because long-term memories are stored in so many places, memory impairment is common with many neurological disorders.

Long-term memory is often divided into two further main types: **explicit** (or **declarative**) **memory** and **implicit** (or **procedural**) **memory.**[58] Explicit/declarative memory is the memory of facts and events. These memories can be consciously recalled, such as the memory of a friend dancing on the table at a Christmas party 3 years ago. Explicit/declarative memory can be further broken down into episodic and semantic memory. **Episodic memory** is responsible for storing information about events (i.e., episodes) that were experienced. An example would be a memory of the first day at school.[59] **Semantic memory** is responsible for storing information about the world. This includes knowledge about the meaning of words, as well as general knowledge.[59] Examples of this would include knowing the names of the state capitals, how a car generally works, or the definition of hypermetabolic.

All explicit/declarative memories require conscious thought to recall and use. Procedural/implicit memory is more about remembering how to perform tasks, such as riding a bicycle or playing the piano, and is automatic, without conscious thought. Even individuals with amnesia generally have procedural memory that remains intact. Deficits in procedural memory are typically seen with degenerative neurological conditions such as dementia, as the severity of the impairment increases. Initially, procedural memory can be a very helpful learning tool for individuals with significant declarative memory loss. By repeating the same procedures over and over again in therapy, an individual can start to make new memories that can enhance independence with daily routines. Individuals who experience both declarative and procedural memory impairments over time are limited in the ability to benefit from traditional cognitive rehabilitation techniques.

Amnesias

Post-traumatic amnesia (PTA) is the period of confusion immediately after a TBI when the individual is unable to make new memories. During this state, clients can be disoriented to person, place, and time. They may demonstrate distractibility, agitation, anger, fear, emotional lability, impulsiveness, confabulation (the combination of imagination and memory), and disinhibition.[60] Rehabilitation techniques used during this period need to be modified in order for the client to benefit. The length of PTA is viewed as one of the best indicators of the severity of brain injury and long-term functional outcome. Therapy during PTA should focus on orientation, self-care, and motor and mobility activities that require limited attention. Repetition of familiar routines is critical because encoding of new memories is absent. Orientation protocols involving reviewing personal information and place and time both verbally and with visual cues are necessary. Brief activities and frequent breaks support the severely impaired attention span seen in individuals with PTA. Depending on the severity of the brain injury, PTA may persist beyond inpatient rehabilitation into the outpatient rehabilitation setting.

Retrograde amnesia is the loss of memory of events and information that occurred before the brain injury or condition. **Anterograde amnesia** is the inability to make new memories after a neurological event. These individuals can usually recall information before the onset of their condition. This type of amnesia can be extremely debilitating and permanent. Both retrograde and anterograde amnesia can be present in an individual, which results in a **global amnesia** (almost total disruption in memory).

Specific Treatment Interventions

Internal memory strategies are tools that should be used for clients with mild cognitive impairment only. The success of these strategies relies on the client's ability to learn, remember, and apply these strategies as needed to assist with encoding and recalling information during daily tasks. Individuals with more significant cognitive impairment will not be able to utilize these strategies on their own with success. In addition, individuals without a cognitive impairment, and who are in school or training and attempting to recall numerous facts, will also use these techniques with success. They include:

- **Visualization:** Making a mental picture of information
- **Verbalization:** Repeating information over and over verbally
- **Storytelling:** Linking items together by telling a story about them
- **Association:** Mentally associating new information with something familiar
- **Organization:** Organizing items to remember them in meaningful ways
- **Categorization:** Organizing long lists by putting items in categories
- **Acronyms:** Using or creating acronyms (an abbreviation formed from the initial letters of other words and pronounced as a word) to assist with memory
- **Chunking:** Breaking down information into small chunks, such as when we group a long phone number into three groups (area code, first three numbers, and then the last four numbers)
- **Humor:** Creating a thought that is funny or humorous to assist with remembering
- **Rhyming:** Using rhymes to remember items

External memory strategies are tools that are necessary for individuals with more severe memory impairments (Fig. 11-5). Just as it sounds, these strategies are external to the client and do not rely on the individual applying internal concepts to situations to encode and recall information. Tools such as these are often called cognitive assistive technology, and may include low- and high-tech options such as:

- Orientation notebook with autobiographical orientation page
- Memory notebook with daily schedule, memory log, and a "things to do" section

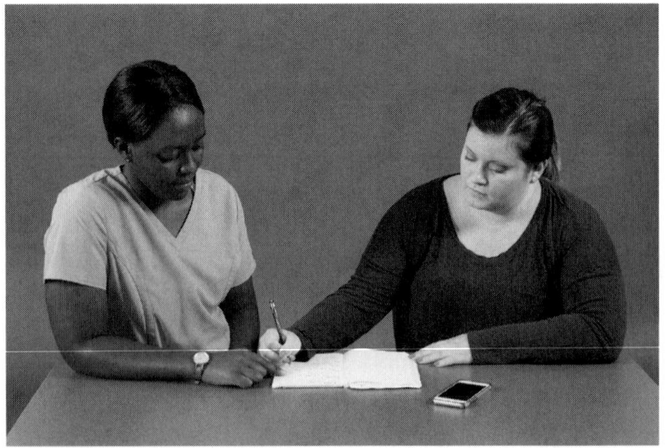

FIGURE 11-5. Client using external memory strategies, including a notebook and smartphone.

- Electronic devices such as cell phones, pagers, alarms, and voice recorders
- Signs, labels, checklists, and pocket notebooks

The decision to implement a memory notebook versus an orientation notebook depends on the severity of the memory deficits. Memory notebooks are appropriate for clients with mild to moderate memory impairments who are aware they are having difficulty remembering. They generally consist of a daily schedule, memory log, and a "things to do" section.[46] Orientation notebooks, on the other hand, should be used with individuals with severe memory impairment or persisting PTA. They generally only have two parts, including an autobiographical orientation page and an additional orientation information page.[7] The ACRM Cognitive Rehabilitation Manual gives very specific guidelines on how to implement and train individuals in the use of orientation and memory notebooks. They do recommend several training strategies for individuals with severe memory impairments. These include:[7]

- **Errorless learning technique:** A tool for presenting important information to a client in a way that eliminates trial and error and guess work. When a client does not learn information correctly, they may think and worry about it. By taking out the "guess work," the individual is not allowed to make a mistake when learning information. This is especially important when clients are relearning orientation information, such as name and age. The client is presented with the information, and then immediately asked to repeat it. For example, "Your name is Sam. What is your name?"
- **Spaced retrieval technique:** The exact same technique as errorless learning, yet the client is asked to remember the information for increasingly longer periods of time. For example, the client is told, "Your name is Sam. What is your name?" Then after a 15 second delay, the question "What is your name?" is asked again and if the client is accurate, the question is asked again at a 30-second delay, and so on.[61]

- **Chaining technique:** A tool for breaking down functional tasks into steps, and then chaining them together one by one as the client learns each step. Instead of looking at a task as a whole function, the task is viewed in parts, starting with the first and progressing to the last as each are learned successfully. Backward chaining can also be used and involves teaching the steps of the task from the last to the first, such as buttons before donning a shirt.

Other helpful strategies for working with the memory impaired include the following:

- Keep distractions (e.g., music, noise) to a minimum and have client focus on one task at a time.
- Have the client keep to routines.
- Use a self-care checklist or household management checklist.
- Keep household objects in the same place.
- Use labels or notes for safety reminders, e.g., "Don't turn on stove."
- Use the same route to walk to the mailbox or bus stop. If getting lost is a problem, the OT practitioner can label doors or color code doors inside the house or hang arrows to indicate directions. When going out, the client should be accompanied initially to ensure the route is understood. A simple map can be sketched from the bus stop to the house, and the client must always carry a personal address book and emergency phone numbers.[62]

Importance of Memory for Learning and Generalizing Strategies

Memory can be affected by numerous factors that influence the making of new memories as well as the retrieval of long-term memories. Whether a client has a short-term memory deficit, a long-term memory deficit or both, the effects can lead to significant disability. Impairments in short-term memory make new learning challenging because when information is not encoded properly, difficulties occur with retrieval of this information. The more significant the memory impairment, the more structured the strategies have to be to assist with independence in this area. The more structured the tools used to track new and old information, the less ability the client will have in generalizing these strategies to all daily activities without assistance.

EXECUTIVE FUNCTION IMPAIRMENTS

Executive functions are self-regulating and control functions that direct and organize cognition and behavior. Executive functions include planning, initiation, decision making, directed goal selection, flexible problem-solving, self-awareness, self-inhibition, self-monitoring, and self-evaluation (see Fig. 11-3).[63] Because these skills integrate information at higher levels across cognitive domains, damage to the executive system typically involves a cluster of deficiencies, not just one ability. The loss of that "administrative" control affects the ability to organize and regulate multiple types of information and, therefore, behaviors.[63] The frontal lobe is best known for its role in carrying out executive functions. Damage to this area of the brain can lead to a multitude of cognitive and behavioral impairments, leaving individuals ill-equipped to successfully negotiate a very complex world. Without these executive functions helping individuals organize, make decisions, problem solve, and regulate behavior, a client may begin to experience breakdowns in the ability to independently and safely manage their daily routine. Tasks involving planning, focusing, remembering, and multitasking cannot be completed with success.[14] In order to have optimal executive function and self-regulation skills, good working memory is needed as well as mental flexibility and self control.[14] Executive functions help an individual to:

- Manage time
- Pay attention
- Switch focus
- Plan and organize
- Remember details
- Avoid saying or doing the wrong thing
- Anticipate and do things based on experiences[64]

Damage to the executive system can lead to:

- Inappropriate behavior involving disinhibition
- Mood swings
- Decreased awareness of impairments
- Impaired ability to anticipate problems and analyze situations
- Poor ability to apply consequences from the past to current situations
- Difficulty interpreting abstract concepts
- Difficulty planning and initiating the steps needed to successfully execute a task
- Difficulty with verbal fluency
- Impaired ability to multitask
- Difficulty processing, storing, and/or retrieving information
- Lack of concern toward others, including animals
- Loss of interest in previous activities
- Difficulties making plans for the future[63]

Types of Executive Function

Executive function can be divided into two groups: **organization**, which is gathering information and preparing it for evaluation, and **regulation**, which is taking stock of the surroundings and changing behavior in response to it. For example, seeing a piece of pumpkin pie at the Thanksgiving table may be tempting. That is where executive function can step in. The organizational part reminds an individual that the slice of pie is likely to have hundreds of calories. Regulation tells an individual that eating the pie conflicts with goals that they may have, such as eating less sugar or losing weight.[64]

Organization includes skills such as attention, working memory, planning, sequencing (breaking down complex actions and prioritizing), problem-solving, abstract thinking (high level or symbolic thinking), cognitive flexibility (ability to use different strategies in different situations), and rule acquisition (learning and using the rules that apply to situations).[63] For example, a client may display difficulty with performing a cooking task if there is an ingredient missing, and would not be able to figure out a substitution or backup plan to have the recipe work out. In an emergency, the client may not be able to determine what to do first. Another client might have difficulty deciding what to do if a store does not have the item that he or she came to purchase or if the item has been moved to another part of the store.

Regulation includes skills such as initiation, emotional regulation, monitoring internal and external stimuli, moral reasoning, decision making, and self-control.[63] An example of regulation difficulties might be angry outbursts over small problems, or having excessive difficulty making a simple decision such as whether to get up from a seat and get a drink of water or not.

Specific Treatment Interventions

In order to enhance success, treatment intervention goals for executive function impairments should:[7,65]

1. Enhance a client's awareness of deficits.
2. Assist the client in anticipating and planning for difficulties related to impairments.
3. Address the client's ability to execute the task at hand and self-monitor all of the steps involved, making adjustments as needed.
4. Assist the client in evaluating how well the task was completed.

These techniques can be used to accomplish the aforementioned goals:[7]

- **Self-talk:** Research shows that teaching clients to talk through the steps of a task can be beneficial.[51,66] For example, if a client is preparing a recipe, each step can be spoken aloud while completing the activity. As an individual progresses with this skill, talking aloud can be reduced to a whisper and eventually the client can silently process the steps to themselves.
- **Goal-plan-do-review (GPDR):** This technique involves the client writing down the goal, identifying the plan for accomplishing the goal, completing the task, and then reviewing successes and failures after the task is completed.[65] The ACRM Cognitive Rehabilitation Manual offers a detailed form and a short form for GPDR, either of which can be completed by OT practitioners working with clients with executive dysfunction.[7]
- **Predict-perform:** Due to the degree of unawareness that can be present in individuals with executive function impairment, a simple technique of having the client predict how he or she will do on a certain task and then analyze success once the task is completed can be very beneficial. It can be executed as simply as having clients give a percentage of how they think they will do on a task, e.g., a check-writing task. Clients with executive function impairment often minimize their difficulties and predict they will complete a task with 100 percent success even though they may only execute the task with 50 percent accuracy. This tool can help them see the discrepancy between their prediction and their performance. The OTA should be prepared for clients to experience more emotional reactions (e.g., sadness or frustration) to their performance as awareness increases.

Additional executive function strategies offered by Geffner include:

- Alter the workspace to allow for movement.
- Limit distractions.
- Work away from doors that are open.
- Break down large projects into smaller steps.
- Allow for breaks.
- Keep a notepad and pen handy.
- Prioritize tasks.[67]

The OTA can put in place the structure clients are often missing with executive function impairment by teaching them how to use external strategies for assistance. An example would include using a smartphone for note taking and tracking appointments with calendar functions. In addition, the volume can be muted for less distraction. Alarms and watches can assist with time management, including teaching a client to start early enough to manage ADL tasks in a timely fashion. The OTA can work with the client on socially appropriate behavior both by modeling as well as role-playing and providing education on how to interact in certain situations (Fig. 11-6). In order to enhance problem-solving and overall focus, the client can work with the OTA on simplifying and organizing the steps required to complete challenging tasks using strategies that include GPDR and self-talk. By adding in the predict-perform technique, a client can start to see the degree of difficulty being experienced and thus improve overall awareness of their impairments.

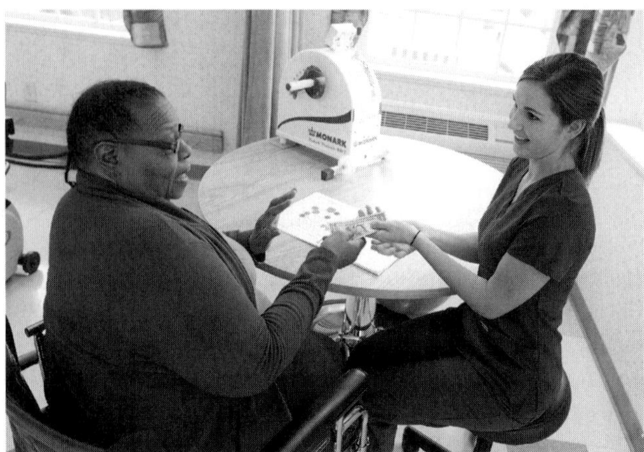

FIGURE 11-6. Cognitive treatment for money management.

COPING STRATEGIES FOR ADULTS WITH EXECUTIVE FUNCTION IMPAIRMENT

Living with executive function impairments can be frustrating and overwhelming at times. These coping strategies are recommended to assist individuals who have executive function impairments lead happy, productive lives:

- Use external structure; make notes and lists to plan and keep organized.
- Acknowledge limitations.
- Gather information about this type of disability.
- Have a coach to assist with planning, organizing, and problem-solving.
- Join or start a support group.
- Think positively and try to decrease negative thoughts.[67]

Importance of Reasoning and Problem-Solving on Overall Independence

When there are deficits in executive functioning skills such as reasoning and problem-solving, the effects can be far reaching in terms of functional independence. If a client cannot reason through how to solve a problem with a bill or determine whether food is spoiled, then the ability to live at home and be independent will suffer. When difficulties with problem-solving are present, the OTA might see a client become paralyzed with indecision when faced with the simple problem of whether to take a shower before or after self-eating, or what to do if an ingredient is missing when making muffins. The types of difficulties one might see when a client cannot plan and organize or manage time effectively might include being continuously late for meetings and events, not checking to see whether there is soap before starting a load of laundry, or often wandering around the grocery store without a list.

BEHAVIORAL IMPAIRMENTS

Behavior goes hand in hand with cognition. Socially unacceptable behavior is a significant impairment when it comes to forming and maintaining interpersonal relationships and holding a job. It can be one of the most difficult skills to manage as well. The person with behavioral deficits may talk a mile a minute, stand too close to someone they are talking to, or have difficulty initiating a response to a question in a timely manner. Individuals may be extremely focused on themselves and can be very emotional. Clients may say and do things they never would have done in the past, which can be extremely disturbing to family and friends. Another possible behavioral/emotional impairment is flat affect, a lack of emotions shown on the face, unchanging expression of emotions in response to various situations, as well as a potential emotional disconnect from others.[49] Behavioral difficulties and changes are common with neurological impairment.

OT Practitioner's Viewpoint

After years of working with clients who have a brain injury, I thought nothing could surprise me. I was working with Albert, a young man who was impulsive and easy to agitate. We were in the bathroom of his room at the rehabilitation center, and he was seated in his manual wheelchair to work on grooming. He was fairly good at automatic tasks, but any tasks that required attention or problem-solving were frustrating to him. The face washing went fairly well, and then we moved on to tooth brushing. He at first thought the toothbrush was a hair brush, and I stopped him from brushing his hair with it. I rinsed it off, added a bit of toothpaste, and gently moved the toothbrush in his hand toward his mouth. I said, "Brush your teeth Albert." Instead of brushing his teeth, he threw the toothbrush across the bathroom. It landed in the toilet like a basketball in a hoop, and he said, "You are the worst therapist I have ever seen in this bathroom!" When I stopped giggling to myself and got a new toothbrush, we began the process again. It is never dull when you work with clients with cognitive deficits, and often times quite humorous. Appreciating the humor can give you the energy you need to work with such significant, serious, life-changing impairments that otherwise could be overwhelming, not only for the client but also for you, the practitioner. ~ Amber L. Ward, MS, OTR/L, BCPR, ATP/SMS

Types of Behaviors With Definitions

A large collection of behaviors are considered to be socially acceptable by society. It is when these behaviors start to interfere with the ability to carry out daily activities as well as lead to extremely awkward interactions and alienation of family and friends that they are deemed inappropriate. Table 11-2 provides a list of maladaptive behaviors that can be experienced by individuals with cognitive impairment.

Specific Behavioral Treatment Interventions

Successful reintegration into the community and return to previous activities is often dependent on the individual's ability to modify maladaptive behaviors that may result from injury or illness.[68] Client factors such as specific mental functions, global mental functions, and body functions will also be factors in reintegration.[4] The most important issue to address in order for an individual to begin to modify these negative behaviors is to make sure the client is aware of them. Initially, awkward behaviors are easily overlooked by family and friends because no one wants to make the individual feel uncomfortable by drawing attention to these issues. The truth is that behaviors an individual is unaware of cannot be modified. Many times instead of addressing these issues head-on, they are danced around until friends and sometimes even family start to drift away and spend less time with the individual because the interactions are too uncomfortable. This is where the OT practitioner must step in to educate both the client and family and offer strategies

TABLE 11-2 Types of Maladaptive Behaviors and Intervention Strategies

	MALADAPTIVE BEHAVIOR	OT INTERVENTION STRATEGY
Hyperverbosity	Talking continuously, and not necessarily with clear thoughts	Redirect clients as needed to keep them focused on the task at hand.
Tangentiality	Difficulty staying on topic and sharing information and stories unrelated to the main topic	Refocus clients to the original topic as often as needed.
Overinclusiveness	Sharing too much detail in conversation and not recognizing when to stop talking, even when the person being spoken to loses interest	A discussion with clients regarding the amount of detail they have given or the length of time they have been talking will assist them in gaining awareness of this problem. Educate clients on signs that their audience has lost interest, e.g., decreased eye contact or walking away.
Confabulation	Sharing stories that are a mix of memories and imagination that clients believe to be true. For example, a client shared that his foot was impaired because he had a palm tree that grew out his toe that had to be removed.	Reorienting clients to the facts is imperative.
Perseveration	Saying or doing the same thing over and over again	Drawing clients' attention to the number of times they have physically or verbally repeated themselves will help boost their awareness.
Impulsivity	Acting before thinking, leading to rushed and inappropriate actions	Teaching clients to think and slow down before acting
Hyperactivity	Increased movement, high energy, impulsive decisions, short attention span, and distractibility	Educating clients regarding their symptoms of hyperactivity will heighten their awareness.
Decreased initiation	Slowness of movement and/or slowness in speech and thought	Verbal cues to increase the pace of participation may be helpful to improve speed of performance. Give time for clients to process requests and begin movements.
Egocentric behavior	A focus on one's self that may cause a lack of empathy for others. This can lead to having difficulty seeing situations through someone else's eyes. The result can be thoughtless or hurtful remarks or unreasonable, demanding requests.	This behavior stems from a lack of abstract thinking. Providing clients with clear examples of their self-centeredness will be necessary to heighten their awareness.[62]
Aggression	Angry and hostile behavior	As long as safety is not an issue, try to ignore the behavior or agree with them if possible to help diffuse the situation. Focusing on the root of the anger can help clients regain a sense of control.
Emotional volatility	Uncontrollable and inappropriate angry outbursts or uncontrollable laughing and crying, which can fluctuate depending on the situation	Remain calm, and try to focus on the fact that the behavior is unintentional. Remember clients have decreased control over their emotions. Focus on times when they are able to maintain control and implement strategies as appropriate.
Flat affect	Lack of emotion; sometimes a client will not show regular emotions such as laughing, crying, or anger when faced with certain situations.	Remember clients are not doing this on purpose and may not realize what is going on. Encourage the client to notice if someone is smiling or crying, and to provide the appropriate response.
Disinhibition/ sexual inappropriateness	Saying or doing inappropriate things because of a distinct lack of control over thoughts that are spoken out loud as well as actions; can include those sexual in nature. In general, there is an impaired filter for all thoughts and feelings, and for behaviors that are typically suppressed as a result of social and societal restraints. This can get the person into trouble with others and the judicial system as they act on impulses. It can be especially shocking to family and friends when coming from a client who before their neurological impairment would never have behaved in this way.	When inappropriate interactions do occur, stay calm and do not react emotionally to these comments or behaviors. Give clients feedback regarding their inappropriateness, but know that until their brain starts to recover and their awareness starts to improve, these inappropriate interactions may continue and are not intentional.

to manage these behaviors. Some of the treatment strategies for the OTA to offer clients and family members when working with someone with a behavior problem might include:

- Enlisting a family and friend support network: Have clients with the behavioral problems confide in their support network about their difficulties, and enlist their support to understand triggers and to learn how to avoid them. Teach clients to walk away if they feel an emotional outburst could happen.[69] Likewise, family members need to be able to share with others their emotions regarding the challenges of living with a loved one with these difficulties.
- Get regular exercise: Not only is it good for the body, but exercise can calm the mind.
- Relaxation/meditation: These practices can assist with calming an outburst or avoiding one in the first place. The OTA can train the client in these techniques, and have them use the techniques to avoid a problem. Regular sleep cycles can be disrupted with cognitive changes, and relaxation or meditation before bed may assist with sleep.
- Social skills training: The OTA can both model appropriate social skills as well as train clients through role-playing to be aware of the social cues they may encounter. For example, helping a client understand the importance of eye contact, how close to stand to another person while talking, or what clothing is appropriate to wear in public may be necessary.
- Anger management: Some clients with cognitive/behavioral changes will require anger management classes, training, or techniques to understand their triggers and how to cope with them.
- Behavior checklists: Clients benefit from education about their negative behaviors by receiving clear feedback from practitioners, peers, and family. This can be provided through structured feedback forms used to monitor negative behaviors in the therapy clinic and at home. An example of how this is used effectively is for the OTA to help identify any inappropriate behaviors and list them on a chart. This chart can be housed in a memory notebook that the client takes from interaction to interaction. When negative behaviors in the categories listed occur, the practitioner in each session can mark the chart and a count can be kept on a daily basis of the incidence of each behavior. Education should be provided to the client regarding how often these behaviors are occurring (Fig. 11-7).
- Videotaping: By video recording interactions during functional tasks, clients can see first-hand the negative behaviors that they have been told about but have previously minimized or not recognized.
- Treatment groups: When a client receives direct feedback from peers in a group setting under the direction of a neuropsychologist or OT practitioner regarding negative behaviors, this can be many times more beneficial than receiving similar feedback from practitioners or family outside of the group setting.

Self-monitoring Behavior Checklist for John Smith Date:________

Behavior		No Problem				Severe Problem
Did I listen and let others talk?	Self-rating	1	2	3	4	5
	Other rating	1	2	3	4	5
Did I stick to one topic at a time?	Self-rating	1	2	3	4	5
	Other rating	1	2	3	4	5
Did I limit answers to 1–2 sentences?	Self-rating	1	2	3	4	5
	Other rating	1	2	3	4	5
Did I get my facts straight?	Self-rating	1	2	3	4	5
	Other rating	1	2	3	4	5

FIGURE 11-7. Behavioral checklist. The "other" rater could be anyone who observes the behavior, including a family member, friend, or caregiver.

- Neuropsychological intervention: Counseling is extremely beneficial for all clients with cognitive and behavioral impairments negatively affecting their everyday life.

Impact of Behavior on Social Relationships and Sexuality

Behavioral changes can be even harder for family and friends to manage than cognitive changes. Often the behavior is hurtful and angry, and it can be difficult to remember that the person cannot always control or manage it. Also, some behaviors make it so that no one wants to be around the person, and finding caregivers who will stay on or friends who will visit can be very difficult. Children may not understand why their parent is mad all the time, and may think it is their fault. The behavioral changes may get the person in trouble with the law or may cause separation or divorce from a spouse. Some behavioral changes lead to hypersexuality, which can lead to adultery, accessing prostitutes, sexually transmitted diseases, and behaviors that are out of character and may result in broken relationships. Sexual relationships can be difficult with either cognitive or behavioral challenges, as the person with the changes may want a sexual relationship more or less than their partner does. Also, the caregiver may be too tired or stressed from caregiving and managing the behaviors to even think about a sexual relationship. In addition, individuals with behavioral challenges may act in ways that are a turnoff to their partner and these behaviors may include anger/aggressiveness, child-like acts, irritability, sadness, nervousness, or self-centered actions. Other difficulties can also affect social and sexual functioning, such as with these examples:

- Attention: Paying attention to other people walking by instead of a date
- Memory: Forgetting what a partner likes and does not like during sex
- Communication: Pouting or getting angry instead of talking about a problem
- Planning ahead: Calling for a reservation or thinking about the need to bring a condom

- Reasoning: Thinking through why a partner may be upset
- Imagining: Putting themselves in another's shoes[70]

Activity and occupational demands are specific to each activity, and simple affection such as a kiss may have very different demands behaviorally and cognitively than sexual intercourse and safe sexual behavior.[4] It is important for the OTA to address all occupations which are affected by deficits, including sexuality.

THE COGNITION IN VISION

When an individual thinks of vision, the most immediate thought is of the eyes themselves. Although damage to the eyes can cause a variety of visual symptoms, damage to the brain can also have a devastating impact on vision. The ability to pay attention to both the right and left side of the visual environment, visually recognize objects and patterns, and remember what is seen are skills controlled by the brain. Brain impairment can negatively influence visual attention, visual perception, and visual memory. Many visual disorders and details about the visual system are found in Chapter 10. In addition, there are a variety of lesser-seen disorders of complex visual processing that have increased cognitive components and affect independence and safety with daily occupations. These are complex disorders that may cross between vision and cognition (only key terms appear in bold font here):[71]

- **Alexia without agraphia:** Inability to read letters, words, or sentences, yet ability to write
- Disorders of topographic orientation: Topographical orientation gives a mental map as to where things are located in both public and personal spaces and assists in interpreting landmarks to find the way. Difficulties with this skill impair the ability to negotiate the community on foot or in a motor vehicle as a result of an inability to recognize public places. This can also affect the ability to find rooms in a home.
- Constructional ability disturbances: Difficulty constructing a copy of an object or model by drawing or using blocks
- Achromatopsia: A disorder of color processing in which there is partial or complete loss of color vision
- **Cerebral akinetopsia:** An inability to perceive movement of objects, such as a ball.

OT practitioners provide valuable compensatory strategies for deficits in visual memory, visual perception, and visual attention. Internal and external memory strategies already mentioned can assist with visual memory as well. Similarly, inattention to visual input such as from one side can be addressed with attention strategies noted earlier. See Chapter 10 for specific visual information and treatment strategies. All adaptive and retraining options may be affected by cognitive impairments; however, the OTA will need to take into account the best learning and retention strategies in this area.

AWARENESS

Anosognosia is the inability to identify impairments in one's self. This is a common problem with moderate to severe brain impairment. Self-awareness requires complex brain processes that the person may no longer possess, either temporarily or permanently. The client's impaired self-reasoning and abstraction skills lead to an inability to generalize appropriate thoughts and behaviors from one situation to the next. For example, the client might lack the ability to identify, "This is a bad idea" or "I need to keep my shirt on even though it's really hot in the restaurant." Many people with cognitive and behavioral challenges with unawareness think they are perfectly fine. They have difficulty understanding why they have been told they cannot drive or why they have had other medical restrictions imposed on them such as being told they should not have a drink with their friends because of the detrimental affect this could have on their brain recovery. This can be an amazingly difficult challenge for caregivers who are trying to provide supervision and assistance to someone who is not self-aware of their deficits. According to a study done by Sherer et al., 76% to 97% of clients with a TBI in the post-acute phase of rehabilitation experienced some degree of unawareness.[72]

Types of Awareness

According to Crosson et al., there are three types of awareness that occur in a hierarchy.[73] The most basic level is **intellectual awareness**. This allows a client to identify that impairments do exist. When asked, clients would be able to verbalize some or all of their impairments. The next level is **emergent awareness**. This type of awareness allows the client to identify the impairment as it is occurring. For example, a client might say, "I can't remember what you said to do first. Maybe I should write it down because my memory is impaired." The highest level of awareness is **anticipatory awareness**. This type of awareness allows the client to anticipate the effects of the impairment before it actually occurs. For example, clients might identify they need to write out a grocery list before going to the store because they are aware they will forget what needs to be purchased if they do not have a list.[74]

Significance of Awareness to Success in Rehabilitation

An ongoing lack of awareness is a predictor of poor functional outcomes in individuals with any sort of brain injury. Clients cannot fix problems they do not know they have. In order for strategies to be effective, a client needs to understand why they are important as well as how and when to use them. If an individual does not recognize his or her impairments, this cannot effectively happen and independence and safety issues will persist. Ways to enhance an individual's awareness of their impairments include educating the client through discussion in therapy sessions, videotaping performance and discussing problems seen, implementing a behavioral checklist to track negative behaviors and pointing out the frequency of occurrence, and implementing strategies such as "predict-perform" to compare the client's perception of how he or she is performing with the reality of their performance.

COGNITIVE REHABILITATION WITH DEGENERATIVE CONDITIONS

Cognitive rehabilitation for someone with an acute condition such as a brain injury or CVA who may improve is very different than for a client with a progressive condition such as PD or AD. Much of the "rehabilitation" for the progressive population is actually accommodation for the cognitive problems or adaptation of the environment and regulation of the amount of supervision. Initially the individual might need only a few strategies to maintain independence but over time progress to needing more strategies to maintain only partial independence. For example, when a client with dementia has mild memory deficits that may involve losing the car keys regularly, the adaptation might be a digital noisemaker attached to the keys. When the memory impairment worsens, and the client gets lost driving the car, driving might need to be stopped entirely. As the condition worsens, the family may have to provide supervision for safety with tasks such as cooking because of forgetfulness with turning off the stove or with household management as a result of forgetting to lock the door at night. The changes are continuous, and so must be the solutions. Many OTAs provide short-term therapy in these cases, where the OTA may see a client in the home to problem solve safety issues and provide education for a few weeks, and then the occupational therapist will discharge the individual. The client may need to be seen again in 6 months to a year when new cognitive changes and problems have occurred that affect function and home safety. Some clients will not be able to stay in their homes alone after a worsening of cognitive function, and must move in with family, to a memory care facility, or to a long term care facility. OTAs work in these specialized centers to keep the residents functioning at the highest level possible despite significant cognitive deficits. See Chapter 32 for further information and treatment strategies for clients with dementia.

COGNITIVE REHABILITATION IN VARIOUS SETTINGS

The OTA may see clients with cognitive deficits in every setting and with every type of disease or disorder. In the acute setting, a variety of cognitive impairments are seen in individuals with TBI, CVA, infections, and other neurological conditions. Inpatient rehabilitation centers often have specialized units for clients who have had a TBI, CVA, or other condition that causes cognitive impairment. Intensive rehabilitation is offered to these individuals with a team approach to care involving multiple disciplines.

Some outpatient therapy clinics are highly specialized brain injury facilities providing a holistic approach to care for all types of cognitive impairment. It is in these facilities that both individual and group treatments may be offered and where the end goal is community reintegration. In a traditional outpatient setting, OT practitioners also can see individuals with a primary diagnosis of TBI or CVA but may also see cognitive deficits as a secondary diagnosis in individuals with degenerative conditions. For example, individuals with ALS or PD who might be referred for treatment to work on transfers or independence with self-care activities might also begin to work on cognitive strategies as the OT practitioner or caregiver identifies this as an issue. Skilled nursing facility OTA staff will often see clients with more significant cognitive deficits, as many times these individuals cannot remain at home with age-related dementias, AD, or other neurological disorders. Home health OTAs often come across clients who are at risk for safety issues or being able to remain in their home because of cognitive concerns. Also, these OT practitioners may see clients with physical deficits from a CVA and discover they have cognitive issues, too.

INDIVIDUAL VERSUS GROUP TREATMENT

OTAs providing cognitive rehabilitation in an outpatient setting may choose to provide some treatments in individual sessions and some treatments in a group setting. There are benefits to both. In terms of individual sessions, choices must be made as to where the individual session takes place. Although room options in some therapy departments may be limited, providing cognitive rehabilitation in a noisy therapy gym is usually not ideal. If that is the only choice, choosing a quiet corner away from the hustle and bustle is necessary. Given that many cognitively impaired clients have difficulty concentrating and screening distractions, quiet environments, such as a private room where the door can be closed, are beneficial. If a client is specifically working on divided attention and screening distractions, then a noisy environment may be of benefit to accomplish this goal. Besides assisting the client in concentrating, therapy in a quiet, private room may allow a client to feel more comfortable with sharing emotions regarding task performance and discussing impairments. This type of environment also allows the OT practitioner to give direct feedback regarding difficulties in a very private, personal way.

Providing group therapy can be beneficial for clients with cognitive impairment. It can feel extremely overwhelming for clients to not be able to think through and do things that were once automatic. Therefore, interacting with others with similar difficulties can provide a level of comfort and hope that OT practitioners cannot always provide on their own. Many clients have said through the years that "There is comfort in knowing I'm not alone." Imagine feeling like the only one experiencing certain deficits and therefore, feeling completely misunderstood and alone; how miserable this would be. Part of accepting a disability is recognizing that everyone has strengths and weaknesses. It is an amazing experience when clients' awareness improves to allow them to recognize that they may have a significant impairment in one area of function but at the same time can identify other things they do well. An example of this is when a client is able to identify that although they have paralysis on one side of the body and memory difficulties, at least speech is intact. By interacting closely with fellow clients in a group setting, this enhanced self-awareness of deficits is possible. In addition, the ability to get to know others with disabilities and see them progress can be very encouraging. Sharing experiences and ideas not only provides emotional support but also stimulates new ideas and strategies among clients. When it comes to negative behaviors, feedback from peers can often be more meaningful than from therapy practitioners.

Group therapy can be provided to address most any aspect of cognition (Fig. 11-8). Memory skills group, problem-solving group, ADL group, and community reintegration group are all examples of groups that have been successfully implemented in therapeutic settings to address cognition at both foundational and functional levels. For example, a community reintegration group might perform a grocery-shopping task in the community to work on money management, problem-solving, social awareness, attention, and memory. Generally, Medicare and Medicaid do not fund long-term outpatient groups. Some private insurance companies will pay to certain limits, but many longer-term groups and day treatment programs are funded by the families of the person with cognitive deficits or through private grants. State and federal funds are also available for some aspects of treatment through Vocational Rehabilitation services (VR) for individuals who are eligible based on their disability and long-term goal of returning to work.

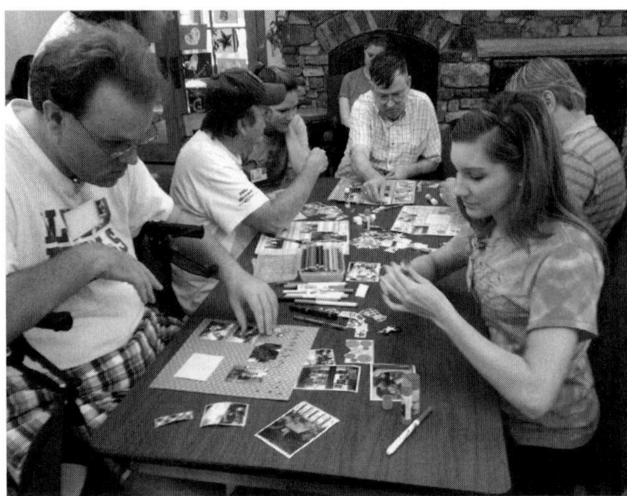

FIGURE 11-8. Cognitive group therapy.

IMPORTANCE OF FAMILY INVOLVEMENT

Families play a critical role in the rehabilitation process. Out of concern and need, families are there from the start to assist with an individual's care. Just like the client, they, too, grieve the loss of function a disability can cause. This loss of function can dramatically impact family dynamics and roles. In turn, significant stress can occur for those family members who are serving as caregivers. The physical, emotional, and financial demands can be overwhelming.

Family involvement is important for multiple reasons. When an individual is cognitively impaired, having an advocate in the healthcare environment is helpful. The nature of the cognitive disability often results in clients being unable to independently manage their own care. Families bridge this gap initially by stepping in to make appropriate decisions regarding the individual's medical care and to educate the rehabilitation and hospital staff as to who the client was before impairment. The information that is shared regarding the client's personality, interests, learning styles, and coping mechanisms can be critical in developing realistic, appropriate goals for the client. Families also play a critical role in encouraging the client. "Families who inspire hope can help the individual to adjust and become more confident in his or her own abilities."[75] This is extremely important, given that self-esteem and self-image problems can present themselves in individuals with a disability. Clients need acceptance for who they are, not what they can do, and families can provide this.

Helpful ways to offer support to families during the rehabilitation process include:

- **Decrease anxiety with education.** Families need appropriate education as to what medical issues have led to their loved one's cognitive impairment as well as what to expect functionally. The best way for families to overcome their fears and lessen their apprehensions is to provide them with knowledge. This in turn assists them in the coping process.
- **Always provide honest, thoughtful answers to questions.** Families rely on healthcare providers for medical information and therapy expectations. It is common for families to ask therapy practitioners about recovery. When a client's prognosis is uncertain, an OT practitioner must walk a fine line between sharing realistic expectations and making certain not to remove hope that recovery is possible. Sharing what research suggests or patterns of recovery seen in the clinic with other clients with similar impairments can be helpful, yet always remember there will be clients whose recovery proves everyone wrong. Acknowledge that each client will heal differently and that the effect of rehabilitation on recovery is not an exact science.
- **Families need encouragement too.** Spouses, children, and other family members can experience intense grief, frustration, and sadness in response to their loved one's cognitive impairments. Without

support, more significant issues, including anger and depression, can occur. As a therapy practitioner, just being available to listen to concerns and answer questions goes a long way to providing support and encouragement to the family. Acknowledging their emotions and praising their efforts to be good caregivers is often what a family needs to get through such a difficult situation.

- **Factor in family dynamics.** Every family is different. Personalities, education, and coping styles make for different experiences when facing adversities, such as cognitive impairment in loved ones. Respect these differences and adjust therapeutic interactions as needed to best meet the needs of each individual family unit.
- **Help families identify needs that must be managed.** Becoming a caregiver overnight can be very overwhelming. With that comes many details and needs that have to be addressed. These may include keeping track of therapy schedules, funding sources, and locating support groups. The OT practitioner can be a great resource to the family.
- **Give families permission to step back as the client progresses.** It is natural for families to manage each and every detail of an individual's care initially when a disability occurs. Over time as a client progresses in independence, it is important for the individual to take more ownership of life and the rehabilitation process, and for families to relinquish some control. This can be painful and challenging for some caregivers and they may require extra encouragement and support to do this.

IMPORTANCE OF THE THERAPEUTIC RELATIONSHIP IN ACHIEVING GOALS

Through the years there have been many names for a positive therapeutic relationship with a client. These include therapeutic use of self, conscious use of self, client-centered therapy, rapport, and therapeutic alliance. Currently, the *Occupational Therapy Practice Framework: Domain and Process, 3rd edition* (OTPF-3) designates the term "therapeutic use of self" to describe the process of establishing a good working relationship with a client, which, in turn, is integral to achieving a good therapeutic outcome.[4] Regardless of the term, the client's relationship with the OT practitioner is necessary for success in achieving therapeutic goals. Clients can be very defensive regarding cognitive and behavioral issues. This can be due to impaired awareness as well as premorbid coping strategies. Without a good working relationship, a practitioner's ability to shape cognitive skills and behaviors is often limited. When an individual does not feel understood, it is difficult to receive critical feedback regarding issues that need to improve. Imagine not feeling emotionally connected to a practitioner and then being told by that individual that there are problems with talking too much, not staying on topic, poor organization, and the need for a memory notebook to recall information. For many clients, this could be a tough realization and could lead to a wall building up between the OTA and the client. In turn, progress could be inhibited.

To establish a therapeutic relationship with a client, an OT practitioner must first start by getting to know the individual. This includes identifying who the individual was before the cognitive impairment with respect to roles, habits, and routines as well as who the individual is now with performance skill impairments. Although the occupational therapist will perform a thorough evaluation, the OTA should also assimilate information regarding the client's injury or medical condition, and how this is negatively impacting the client's awareness, cognitive abilities, behaviors, and life skills. Family can provide critical information as to the client's premorbid educational level, personality, and coping style. Sometimes clients react to their disability in unexpected ways. Understanding their styles before their disability may help make sense of this.

A psychologist by the name of Malcolm L. Meltzer, Ph.D. experienced significant memory impairment as a result of anoxia after a cardiac arrest at the age of 44. He was able to put into words the importance of the therapeutic relationships based on his own personal experiences during his 2-year rehabilitation. "Realize that the patient may feel alone and incompetent, and more important than the rehabilitation techniques used is the relationship with you—somebody who is interested and cares."[40]

To establish a good working rapport with the client, there must be a relationship based on trust and respect. Suggestions as to how to accomplish this include:

- Avoid judging behaviors and demonstrate understanding and respect.
- When addressing impairments, point out strengths before deficits, and be encouraging.
- Engage clients in discussions regarding their difficulties and attempt to get clients to acknowledge differences in their abilities now instead of before their cognitive impairment.
- Establish treatment ideas and strategies *with* the client, not *for* the client. Individuals must "buy in" to the treatment strategies being presented in order for them to initiate their use.
- Always follow-up on issues important to the client. This helps the individual develop trust with the OT practitioner and feel cared for.

Additional ways to provide support and encouragement to the client include:

- Do not be afraid of clients feeling down about their current situations. Tears and other expressions of sadness, frustration, or anger are normal and should be expected.
- Never pretend to know exactly what a client is feeling. Every client and his or her circumstances are different. Respect that! Offer encouraging words such as, "I don't know what it is like first hand to be going

through your situation, but I can only imagine how difficult it must be and what you might be feeling."

- Do not "over talk" during treatment sessions. Periods of silence are acceptable and can be very contemplative for both the OT practitioner and the client.
- Do not feel there has to be completion of a specific activity during the treatment session if a client is struggling emotionally. Only a part of a functional activity may be completed before needing to discuss the client's performance or reaction to the task. Time to process feelings and issues is extremely therapeutic and necessary during some treatment sessions. Documentation about cognitive tasks as a whole can be difficult, especially when emotional issues play a role in the treatment session, and OTAs should refer to the policies of their specific site for guidance.

IMPORTANCE OF GENERALIZING SKILLS INTO "REAL-LIFE" ENVIRONMENTS

What does "generalization" of skills mean? **Generalization** is the ability to apply learned skills to both predictable and unpredictable environments. Neurological impairment can have a significant impact on the ability of an individual to take what has been practiced in the therapy clinic and apply it to "real-life" situations. OT practitioners are trained to bridge this gap by addressing life skills in a variety of environments, including home, community, work, school, and driving. By addressing an individual's occupations during therapy, the client can experience firsthand how to incorporate strategies directly into their daily routine (Fig. 11-9). According to the Society for Cognitive Rehabilitation, "All cognitive rehabilitation tasks should focus on improving real life functioning."[2]

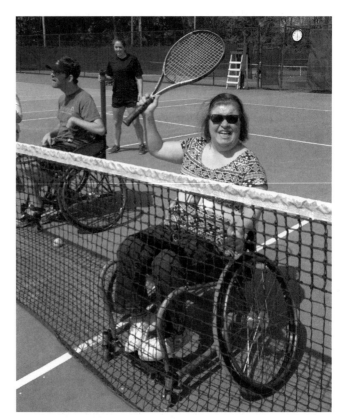

FIGURE 11-9. Adapted tennis.

It is very common for cognitive impairments that were not evident in the therapy clinic to show up in these "real-life" environments. When considering these environments in rehabilitation, OT practitioners should be concerned with how clients constructed their occupations in their lives to fulfill their perceived roles and identity and whether they will be able to do so in the future.[4] There will always be a place for some clinic-based pencil-and-paper cognitive tasks in OT, but if there is no attempt to assist the client in generalizing the strategies learned during these activities to other environments, then as OT practitioners, there is only completion of half of the job.

OT should never be thought of as a routine, "one-size fits all" approach but, instead, as a well thought-out, individualized plan of care. The degree of cognitive impairment paired with the client's premorbid lifestyle, interests, activities, and abilities sets the tone for the daily life skills chosen to be addressed by the OT practitioner. Daily activities that would not have been completed before the client's cognitive impairment should not be prioritized during treatment sessions. For example, if a client's husband has always been responsible for all aspects of household financial management, time should not be spent addressing this with the client. Basic skills of money management, including money counting, check writing, and credit card use necessary for community independence would be a better use of time. Likewise, if an older client is only accustomed to using the microwave to heat up meals, time should not be spent addressing more complex meal preparation with the oven and stove. A better use of therapy time would be to address microwave meal preparation and review general safety guidelines for stove and oven use. Collaborating with the client to identify which cognitive strategies work best for that individual for each task is imperative to success. There will always be some degree of trial and error necessary when choosing the most effective strategies.

If possible, OTAs should accompany their clients into a variety of environments to work on generalization. Some OT departments provide opportunities for practitioners to transport clients in company-owned vehicles. When this is not possible, some therapy departments allow practitioners to meet clients and their families in their homes, communities, workplaces, and schools. Even walking from the rehabilitation setting to a nearby store or gas station can provide a physically and cognitively challenging outing.

The types of activities addressed in the home environment may include self-care, child-care, pet care, cleaning, meal preparation, financial management, and lawn care. Again, OT practitioners should not use a "cookbook approach" to rehabilitation. Time only should be spent addressing those activities that are integral to the client's resuming independence. An exception to this rule is in regard to role changes caused by a disability. If a client is unable to work and will need to take over household responsibilities because a spouse will be returning to work, then all aspects of household management will need to be addressed during OT sessions in the home or clinic.

The type of activities addressed in the community may include shopping at grocery, drug, and department stores and specialty stores in malls; banking inside banks and at bank machines; utilizing a gas pump for putting gas in a vehicle and for payment; and participating in leisure activities, including libraries, museums, sports, movie theaters, and restaurants. Taking time to identify a client's previous responsibilities in the community as well as leisure interests will help narrow down the activities that should be addressed. Working on cognition in the form of community reintegration can be fun and challenging. Always expect the unexpected. Depending on the mobility needs of a client, even tasks such as accessing public restrooms can be challenging and should be addressed. Bathrooms come in all shapes, sizes, and configurations. Some are easier to negotiate with mobility aids and wheelchairs than others. Also, the distance needed to travel to locate a restroom in public can be physically challenging and may require proper planning. Clients with impairments in initiation, planning, and problem-solving may be very challenged with this type of task.

Unfortunately, not all therapy departments and clinics are able to provide these opportunities for OT practitioners and their clients to go into the client's home and community. In these situations, OT practitioners must be flexible and creative in providing generalization opportunities that do not involve leaving the facility or accompanying the client to different environments. Ways in which this can be done include using available resources. Examples of this include:

- Provide outings to the hospital cafeteria to address strategies needed to be successful with making choices, food ordering, money management, and appropriate socialization skills.
- Provide outings to the gift shop in the hospital to address strategies needed to be successful with shopping, including locating items and money management.
- Use the hospital map and signage to locate restrooms, chapel, cafeteria, gift shop, and other areas. This would be similar to using maps at museums, malls, and other places.
- Locate the bank machine in the hospital or facility and review proper procedures for use.
- Use a building directory, if available, to locate offices in the facility.
- Work with the client to successfully negotiate crossing streets with and without stoplights outside of the hospital or clinic.
- Practice a variety of appropriate socialization skills necessary for success outside of the clinic.
- Give family homework assignments to do with the client in the community and ask them to report back on the individual's performance.

SUMMARY

Cognitive challenges can affect every part of a client's life. These impairments can be devastating to the client's work, family, home, and social roles, and can disrupt the performance of all tasks in the daily routine. The costs associated with cognitive impairment are also substantial in terms of lost wages, increased healthcare costs, as well as lost productivity in society. Many disorders result in some degree of cognitive impairment, and millions of clients and their families are affected every day by the impact of these cognitive issues on independence and safety. The OTA has an important role with assisting individuals in the rehabilitation of their cognitive deficits as well as in the long-term management for those with intractable or progressive disorders affecting cognition. It is through OT that long-term success can be achieved in resuming independence with daily tasks at home, in the community, at school, at work, and with driving for individuals with cognitive impairment.

REVIEW QUESTIONS

1. You would like to take your client who has attention and judgment issues on an outing to the main hospital gift shop to work on following directions and attention to task when making a purchase. You know that the client will try to buy candy even though the client has diabetes, and you would like to prevent that before it happens. The actions you take before the outing are:
   a. Call the gift shop to put away the candy.
   b. Practice in the therapy gym to make careful choices when offered a variety of tempting items.
   c. Write a list of approved items to buy.
   d. Take the client to the park instead of the gift shop for less temptation.
2. A client is impaired in his ability to complete self-care and household tasks, yet his wife handles all the cleaning and cooking at home. The issues that need to be addressed are sequencing, following directions, memory, and safety awareness. A cooking task meets all of these needs. What should the OTA do?
   a. Perform a cooking task to "surprise" his wife with a meal.
   b. Only perform woodworking tasks that he enjoys.
   c. Only perform exercise tasks.
   d. Perform a shaving task that can also work on these cognitive issues.
3. You are covering a relatively new client for a coworker who neglected to tell you anything about the client except that she had a CVA. After talking with her, she appears to have impaired speech, impulsiveness, and impaired problem-solving ability. Where might her CVA have been located?
   a. Left hemisphere
   b. Brainstem
   c. Right hemisphere
   d. White matter
4. Which brain lobe participates in auditory sensation and perception, selective attention of auditory and visual input, visual perception, organization and categorization of verbal material, language comprehension, long-term memory, personality and affective behavior, and sexual behavior?
   a. Cerebellum
   b. Frontal lobe
   c. Parietal lobe
   d. Temporal lobe

5. Attention can be directed voluntarily or automatically. An example of automatic attention would be:
   a. Turning the head to a gunshot sound
   b. Scanning the ball field for a certain player
   c. Noting where you parked in the parking deck
   d. Tuning out conversations around you at a coffee shop
6. Which three of the following include ways to increase short-term memory?
   a. Clunking
   b. Chunking
   c. Use of aides, such as lists
   d. Distractions
   e. Rehearse out loud
   f. Push out older information with newer information
7. You have an adult with a TBI as an outpatient, and he is determined to get back to work. You offer coping strategies for his executive function impairment, one of which would be:
   a. Knowing and accepting limitations
   b. Rehearsing information out loud
   c. Telling coworkers about all personal issues
   d. Starting a TBI support group at work
8. Sometimes a person with cognitive problems will not show the regular emotions such as laughing, crying, or anger when faced with certain situations. This is called:
   a. Emotional volatility
   b. Flat affect
   c. Lack of judgment
   d. Protective behavior
9. Which three of the following are tools used to compensate for cognitive deficits?
   a. Using a smartphone calendar
   b. Viewing pictures in the bathroom of the steps for grooming
   c. Logging in to Facebook or social media
   d. Working in the noisy gym to challenge the client
   e. Putting on noise-canceling headphones while working
   f. Relying on information from the Internet
10. You have an elderly client who has had MS for 25 years. He is having difficulty taking the skills you are teaching him and applying them to real-life situations at home and in the community. As an OTA, you know that all clinical skills must be:
    a. Generalizable
    b. Repeatable
    c. Interesting
    d. Effective

CASE STUDY

M.B. is a 52-year-old, left-handed male who suffered a TBI in a motor vehicle accident. Frontal lobe impairment is present as well as a right hemisphere ischemic CVA caused by a left carotid dissection, which occurred from seatbelt trauma to the neck. According to the neuropsychologist, he is exhibiting left-sided weakness; general attention impairments in the areas of selective, alternating, and divided attention; slowed information processing, mild-to-moderate memory impairment; and severe executive function impairment with all aspects of awareness, reasoning, problem-solving, and organization as well as behavioral regulation. M.B. is impulsive and disinhibited with his actions, often saying and doing things completely out of character, and is overinclusive with his speech, sharing way too much detail. In addition, he is struggling with poor frustration tolerance and bouts of anger. In general, he is lacking safety awareness and he is struggling with multistep tasks, new and old.

Before the accident he was in sales for an office supply company and relied heavily on his friendly personality, sense of organization, and management of details to be successful. He is a married father of three children, ages 21, 16, and 11. He and his wife have always had a strong relationship but she is struggling with the personality changes that have occurred with his brain injury. His children have all been active in sports and he was currently coaching his 11-year-old son's baseball team at the time of his injury. M.B. is an active member of his church and has a strong social circle. At home, he is primarily responsible for financial management and yard work but also enjoys cooking with his wife.

1. Identify at least four maladaptive behaviors that will need to be addressed in treatment.
2. Identify and explain the use of two tools/techniques that could be used to heighten the client's awareness regarding his cognitive and behavioral impairments.
3. Outline two activities for residential, vocational, and community that are appropriate for the client to complete during therapy sessions in each of the impaired areas of attention.
4. Identify how a memory notebook could be of use to this client and what sections would be appropriate. Explain how this could be incorporated into treatment sessions.
5. Identify two internal memory strategies and two external memory strategies, other than the memory notebook, that might assist this client and explain how to implement them into functional tasks during your treatment sessions. Use a different activity for each strategy.
6. Explain how an OT practitioner would handle questions from the client's wife regarding projected cognitive, behavioral, and physical outcomes. She is hoping that her husband will have a full recovery with no residual impairments; however, the OT practitioner knows some residual impairment is most likely.
7. Develop a home program of two community-based tasks that family could complete with M.B. outside of the therapy clinic with specific guidelines for completion.

PUTTING IT ALL TOGETHER Sample Treatment and Documentation

Setting	Inpatient rehabilitation, referred from acute hospital, where client spent 4 weeks
Client Profile	Mr. M, 25 y/o, experienced a TBI 4 weeks ago, resulting in mild L-sided weakness, poor balance, and numerous cognitive and behavioral deficits
Work History	In college, master's level in business administration
Insurance	Insurance through Blue Cross
Psychological	Easily agitated, impulsive, often swears, refuses treatment at times
Social	Single, lives in apartment with three other guys near campus, 2nd floor apartment
Cognitive	Short-term memory impairment, impulsivity, and attention and executive function deficits
Motor & Manual Muscle Testing (MMT)	Client presents with mild weakness in his LUE • WFL AROM in BUEs • MMT RUE: 5/5 throughout • MMT LUE: Shoulder 3+/5, elbow 4/5, wrist 4/5, hand 4/5 • Grip R 135#, L 67# • Ambulates with supervision to Min A for balance
ADL	Min A bathing, supervision to Min A LB dressing, supervision UB dressing, supervision grooming
IADL	Max A with all because of decreased safety awareness and cognitive deficits
Goals	Within 4 weeks: 1. Client will require Mod I for bathing and dressing with the use of appropriate AE and techniques 2. Client will increase strength in LUE to 4+/5 at shoulder to increase ability to perform functional ADL tasks 3. Client will prepare a simple microwave meal with Mod I for safety and adapted techniques 4. Client will prepare a daily schedule and follow it with Mod I and adaptive strategies

OT TREATMENT SESSION 1

THERAPEUTIC ACTIVITY	TIME	GOAL(S) ADDRESSED	OTA RATIONALE
Bathing on shower seat in shower area in room, handheld shower	15 min	#1	*Occupations:* Performance, cognitive retraining, and safety awareness
Upper and lower body dressing, grooming	15 min	#1	*Occupations:* Functional task performance, cognitive retraining
Perform shoulder AROM exercises with demonstration and hand over hand as required, in standing near mat. Shoulder flexion, shoulder abduction, protraction/retraction, and elevation	10 min	#2	*Preparatory Task; Education and Training:* Strengthening and exercise to increase active control over LUE, memory and recall of exercises, balance
Prepare microwave popcorn, working on following directions, and safety precautions	15 min	#2 and #3	*Occupations:* Functional task performance, cognitive retraining, sequencing, attention, following directions, IADL performance, safety

SOAP note: 10/3/—, 7:00 am–7:58 am

S: Client states, "Do I smell?" when asked to take a shower. Mother present for treatment session.

O: Client participated in inpatient therapy session to address ADL, IADL performance, cognition, and strengthening of LUE. No c/o pain. Client was able to ambulate to bathroom with Min A, although required repetition of directions to start the shower process and sit on the shower seat. He required Min A for thorough bathing and drying after shower. He was able to complete UB/LB dressing with moderate cues and occasional Min A from OTA for clothing orientation and safety. Client performed UE exercises in all planes with min hand over hand and moderate cues to attend to task. Client worked on IADL task in kitchen, and did require cues for impulsivity, safety and attention as well as Min A for balance.

A: Client did not become agitated this session, and was able to complete ADL, IADL, and exercise tasks with multiple cues. He is noted to have cognitive deficits which affect his functional performance. Client will benefit from continued ADL/IADL program & support from mother for HEP due to short term memory and attentional issues.

P: Continue to work on ADL/IADL tasks, cognitive retraining, functional use of LUE, & follow up on HEP.

Jane Brooker, COTA/L, 10/3/—, 5:15 pm

TREATMENT SESSION 2

What could you do next with this client?

TREATMENT SESSION 3

What could you do next with this client?

REFERENCES

1. Oxford Dictionaries. Dictionary, thesaurus, & grammar. (n.d.). Retrieved from http://www.oxforddictionaries.com
2. Best Practice Recommendations. (2004). Retrieved from http://www.societyforcognitiverehab.org/
3. Centers for Disease Control. Cognitive impairment: A call for action, now! (2015). Retrieved from http://www.cdc.gov/
4. American Occupational Therapy Association. (2014). Occupational therapy practice framework: Domain and process (3rd ed.). *American Journal of Occupational Therapy, 68*(Suppl. 1). http://dx.doi.org/10.5014/ajot.2014.682006
5. Moore, E. A. (2010). Human brain has more switches than all computers on Earth. Retrieved from http://www.cnet.com/
6. Pugh, E. M. (n.d.). Quote. Retrieved from http://www.goodreads.com/quotes/123391
7. Haskins, E. C. (2012). Cognitive rehabilitation manual, translating evidence-based recommendations into practice. American Congress of Rehabilitation Medicine.
8. Radomski, M. V., Anheluk, M., Bartzen, M. P., & Zola, J. (2016). Effectiveness of interventions to address cognitive impairments and improve occupational performance after traumatic brain injury: A systematic review. *American Journal of Occupational Therapy, 70*(3), 1-17A. http://dx.doi.org/10.5014/ajot.2016.020776
9. Herculano-Houzel, S. (2012). How many neurons make a human brain? Billions fewer than we thought. Retrieved from http://www.theguardian.com/science/blog/2012/feb/28/
10. Cerebral cortex. (n.d.). Retrieved from http://biology.about.com/
11. What is the corpus callosum? (n.d.). Retrieved from http://nodcc.org/
12. Right brain hemisphere. (n.d.). Retrieved from http://psychology.jrank.org/
13. Frontal lobes. (n.d.). Retrieved from http://neuroskills.com/brain-injury/frontal-lobes.php
14. Executive function & self-regulation. (n.d.). Retrieved from http://developingchild.harvard.edu/
15. Kolb, B., & Whishaw, I. (1990). *Fundamentals of human neuropsychology*. New York, NY: W.H. Freeman and Co.
16. Temporal lobes. (n.d.). Retrieved from http://neuroskills.com/braininjury/
17. Overview of cerebral function. (n.d.). Retrieved from http://www.merckmanuals.com/professional/neurological-disorders/
18. Parietal lobes. (n.d.). Retrieved from http://neuroskills.com/braininjury/
19. What is the difference between an acquired brain injury and a traumatic brain injury? (2015). Retrieved from http://www.biausa.org/
20. Neumann, D., & Lequerica, A. (2009). Cognitive problems after TBI. Retrieved from http://uwmsktc.washington.edu
21. Ischemic strokes (clots). (n.d.). Retrieved from http://www.strokeassociation.org/
22. Effects of a stroke. (2012). Retrieved from www.strokeassociation.org/strokeorg/about
23. al-Khindi, T., Macdonald, R. L., & Schweitzer, T. A. (2010). Cognitive and functional outcome after aneurysmal subarachnoid hemorrhage. *Stroke*, 41, e519-e536. Retrieved from http://stroke.ahajournals.org/content/41/8/e519.full
24. Overview: Brain AVM. (n.d.). Retrieved from www.mayoclinic.org/diseases-conditions/brain-AVM/home/omc-20129992
25. Arteriovenous malformations (and other vascular lesions of the central nervous system). (2014). Retrieved from www.medicinenet.com/
26. Davis, C. P. (2015). Parkinson's disease dementia. Retrieved from www.emedicinehealth.com/
27. Cognitive impairment. (n.d.). Retrieved from http://www.pdf.org/en/cognitive_impairment_pd
28. Mayo Clinic Staff. (n.d.). Huntington's disease definition. Retrieved from http://www.mayoclinic.org/
29. Harley, J. P., Allen, C., Braciszewski, T. L., Cicerone, K. D., Dahlberg, C., Evans, S., ... Smigelski, J. S. (1992). Guidelines for cognitive rehabilitation. *NeuroRehabilitation 2*, 62-67.
30. Cognitive changes. (n.d.). Retrieved from http://www.nationalmssociety.org/Symptoms-Diagnosis/MS-Symptoms/Cognitive-Changes
31. Lou, J. Q., Tischenkel, C., & DeLange, L. (2009). Cognitive deficits in MS. Retrieved from http://www.msfocus.org/
32. Rush, B. K. (2014). Cognitive and behavioral changes in ALS: A guide for people with ALS and their families. Retrieved from http://www.alsa.org/
33. Alzheimer's Association. (2015). 2015 Alzheimer's disease facts and figures. *Alzheimer's and Dementia, 11*(3), 332-84.
34. What is dementia? (n.d.). Retrieved from http://alz.org/
35. What is Huntington's disease? (n.d.). Retrieved from http://hdsa.org/what-is-hd/
36. Koehler, R., Wilhelm, E., & Shoulson, I. (Eds.). (2011). Defining cognitive rehabilitation therapy for traumatic brain injury: Evaluating the evidence. Committee on Cognitive Rehabilitation Therapy for Traumatic Brain Injury; Board on the Health of Select Populations; Institute of Medicine. doi:10.17226/13220
37. Mazmanian P. E., Kreutzer J. S., Devany C. W., & Martin K. O. (1993). A survey of accredited and other rehabilitation facilities: Education, training and cognitive rehabilitation in brain-injury programmes. *Brain Injury, 7*, 319-331.
38. Cicerone K. D., Mott T., Azulay J., & Friel J. C. (2004). Community integration and satisfaction with functioning after intensive cognitive rehabilitation for traumatic brain injury. *Archives of Physical Medicine and Rehabilitation, 85*, 943-50.
39. Giles, G. M., Radomski, M. V., Champagne, T., Corcoran, M. A., Gillen, G., Kuhaneck, H. M., Wolf, T.J. (2013). Cognition, cognitive rehabilitation and occupational performance. *American Journal of Occupational Therapy, 67*(Suppl.), S9-S31.
40. OT assessment index. (n.d.). Retrieved from http://mh4ot.com/resources/ot-assessment-index/
41. Groves, D., Coggles, L., Hinrichs, J., Berndt, S., & Bright, L. (2010). An innovative algorithm for cognitive assessments. *Occupational Therapy Now, 2*, 20-23.
42. Asher, I. (2007). *Occupational therapy assessment tools: An annotated index*. Bethesda, MD: AOTA Press.
43. Itzkovich, M., Averbuch, S., Elazar, B., & Katz, N. (2000). Lowenstein occupational therapy cognitive assessment (LOTCA) battery (2nd ed.). Pequannock, NJ: Maddak.
44. Allen, C. K., Austin, S. L., David, S. K., Earhart, C. A., McCraith, D. B., & Riska Williams, L. (2007). *Manual for the Allen cognitive level screen-5 (ACLS-5) and large Allen cognitive level screen-5 (ACLS-5)*. Camarillo, CA: ACLS and LACLS Committee.
45. Mateer, C. A., Sira C. S., & O'Connell, M. E. (2005). Putting humpty dumpty together again: The importance of integrating cognitive and emotional interventions. *Journal of Head Trauma Rehabilitation. 20*(1), 62-75.
46. Donaghy, S., & Williams, W. (1998). A new protocol for training severely impaired patients in usage of memory journals. *Brain Injury, 12*, 1061-1076.
47. Attention. (2016). Retrieved from http://www.happy-neuron.com/brain-and-training/attention
48. Sladyk K., Jacobs K., & MacRae N. (Eds.). (2014). *Occupational therapy essentials for clinical competence (2nd ed.)*. Thorofare, NJ: SLACK Incorporated.
49. Oken B. S., Salinsky M. C., & Elsas, S. M. (2006). Vigilance, alertness or sustained attention: Physiological basis and measurement. *Clinical Neurophysiology, 117*(9), 1885-1901.
50. C8 Sciences. (n.d.). Sustained attention. *Cognitive Skills: The 8 Core Cognitive Capacities*. Retrieved from http://www.c8sciences.com/about/8ccc/
51. Cicerone, K. D., & Giacino, J. T. (1992). Remediation of executive function deficits after traumatic brain injury. *NeuroRehabilitation, 2*(3), 12-22.
52. Weinbach, N., & Henik, A. (2012). Temporal orienting and alerting–The same or different? *Frontiers in Psychology, 3*, 236. http://doi.org/10.3389/fpsyg.2012.00236

53. NINDS cerebral aneurysms information page. (2015). Retrieved from http://www.ninds.nih.gov/
54. Sohlberg, M. M., & Mateer, C. A. (1987). Effectiveness of an attention-training program. *Journal of Clinical Experimental Neuropsychology, 9*(2), 117-130.
55. Attention and brain injury. (n.d.). Retrieved from http://www.brainline.org/article/attention-and-brain-injury.html
56. Sohlberg, M., Johnson, L., Paule, L., Raskin, S., & Mateer C. (2001). Attention process training II: A program to address attentional deficits for persons with mild cognitive dysfunction. Puyallup, WA: Lash & Associates Publishing/Training Inc.
57. Mastin, L. (2010) Short term (working) memory. Retrieved from http://www.human-memory.net/types_short.html
58. Mastin, L. (2010). Declarative (explicit) & procedural (implicit) memory. Retrieved from http://www.human-memory.net/types_declarative.html
59. McLeod, S. (2010). Long term memory. Retrieved from http://www.simplypsychology.org/long-term-memory.html
60. Post-traumatic amnesia (PTA) & brain injury. (n.d.). Retrieved from www.synapse.org.au/information-services/post-traumatic-amnesia-(pta).aspx,
61. Brush, J., & Camp, C. (1998). *A therapy technique for improving memory: Spaced Retrieval.* Beachwood, OH: Menorah Park Center for Senior Living.
62. Family Caregiver Alliance. (1996). Coping and behavior problems after head injury. Retrieved from https://caregiver.org/coping-behavior-problems-after-head-injury
63. Executive functions. (n.d.). Retrieved from http://memory.ucsf.edu/ftd/overview/biology/executive/single
64. What is executive function? (n.d.). Retrieved from http://www.webmd.com/add-adhd/guide/executive-function
65. Ylvisaker, M., & Feeney, T. (1998). *Collaborative brain injury intervention: positive everyday routines* (1st ed.). San Diego, CA: Singular.
66. Cicerone, K. D., & Wood, J. C. (1987). Planning disorder after closed head injury: A case study. *Archives of Physical Medicine and Rehabilitation, 68*(2), 111–115.
67. Geffner, D. (2007). Managing executive function disorders. ASHA Convention, St. John's University, NY.
68. Beatty, C. (n.d.). Interventions for behavioral problems after brain injury. Retrieved from http://www.brainline.org
69. Behavioral & emotional symptoms. (n.d.). Retrieved from http://www.brainline.org/
70. Sander, A. M., & Maestas, K. (2014). Sexuality after traumatic brain injury. *Archives of Physical Medicine and Rehabilitation,* 95,1801-1802.
71. Mesulam, M. (2000). *Principles of behavioral and cognitive neurology* (2nd ed.). New York, NY: Oxford University Press.
72. Goverover, Y., Johnston, M., Toglia, J., & DeLuca, J. (2007). Treatment to improve self awareness in persons with acquired brain injury. *Brain Injury, 21,* 913-923.
73. Crosson, B., Barco, P. P., Velozo, C. A., Bolesta, M. M., Cooper, P. V., Werts, D., & Brobeck T. C. (1989). Awareness and compensation in postacute head injury rehabilitation. *Journal of Head Trauma Rehabilitation, 4,* 46-54.
74. Fleming, J. (2010). Self-Awareness. In J. H. Stone & M. Blouin (Eds.). *International encyclopedia of rehabilitation.* Buffalo, NY: Center for International Rehabilitation Research Information Exchange (CIRRIE). REHABDATA Accession Number 020715.
75. Effects of rehabilitation on the family. (n.d.). Retrieved from http://www.hopkinsmedicine.org/

Chapter 12

Self-Feeding, Swallowing, and Communication

Amber L. Ward, MS, OTR/L, BCPR, ATP/SMS, Vivian Resnik, MHA/MBA, OTR/L, and Francine Waskavitz, MS, CCC–SLP

LEARNING OUTCOMES

After studying this chapter, the student or practitioner will be able to:

12.1 Discuss the social impact of self-feeding, swallowing, and communication impairments

12.2 Explain typical self-feeding, swallowing, and communication patterns

12.3 Describe the anatomy and physiology of the swallowing mechanism

12.4 Identify modified diet textures and liquid consistencies

12.5 Explain and implement the use of adaptive equipment and assistive technology for self-feeding and communication

12.6 Describe the roles of the interdisciplinary team in regards to self-feeding, swallowing, and communication

KEY TERMS

Airway obstruction	Object permanence
Aphasia	Paralinguistic communication
Apraxia	Penetration
Aspiration	Phasic bite
Augmentative and alternative communication (AAC)	Pragmatic communication
Bolus	Presbyphagia
Bruxism	Receptive communication
Dysarthria	Sialorrhea
Dysphagia	Swallowing
Expressive communication	Tongue thrust
Feeding	Viscosity

Imagine, it is Thanksgiving Day, the turkey is roasting, the cider is warming, and pumpkin pie is baking in the oven. The home is full of delicious aromas as family and friends gather around the table to enjoy a holiday meal in good company. Everyone is waiting, watching the stove and the oven patiently, taking in the sights, sounds, and smells of the holiday and dreaming of dinner time. Now imagine this same holiday gathering while being dependent on someone else to eat. Imagine the embarrassment and frustration if unable to enjoy the same foods as those dining nearby. Longing to say thank you, attempting to join in on conversation as thoughts race through, and yet no sounds emerge.

It is important to imagine the challenges clients will encounter day to day with self-feeding, eating, and communication. After reading this chapter, the student will understand the role of occupational therapy (OT) for individuals with impairments affecting self-feeding, swallowing, and communication. Occupational therapy assistants (OTAs) are an integral part of the interdisciplinary team and therefore must be able to recognize the roles of other disciplines as well as their own. In some settings, the speech language pathologist (SLP) works on deficits in eating and swallowing, but according to the American Occupational Therapy Association (AOTA), "feeding, eating, and swallowing are within the domain and scope of practice for occupational therapy. Occupational therapists and OTAs have the knowledge and skills necessary to take a lead role in the evaluation and intervention of feeding, eating, and swallowing problems."[1] Furthermore, at times, the SLP may take the lead role in the treatment of communication and language deficits, but as noted in the *Occupational Therapy Practice Framework: Domain and Process, 3rd edition* (OTPF-3), the OT practitioner manages the occupation of communication management, the client factors of voice and speech, the performance skills related to producing speech and speaking fluently, and the social skills related to language, to name a few.[2] To provide client-centered care and follow best practices, all disciplines must integrate to create a holistic approach to each client. Each discipline brings unique strengths to the treatment team, and the OTA, who focuses on occupation and function, is a valued member. Providing daily treatment, following the established plan of care, and communicating progress and setbacks to the supervising occupational therapist all contribute to the interdisciplinary approach.

THE SOCIAL IMPACT OF SELF-FEEDING

Mealtime is an integral part of daily life. It is often a part of social events and gatherings and is shared as quality time with family and friends. During a meal, one must be able to demonstrate effective communication and social interaction skills in addition to self-feeding. Cultural and societal norms also play a role in mealtime etiquette. A person's difficulties with self-feeding, swallowing, or communication greatly impact his or her mealtime experiences. People with difficulties in one or more of these areas often experience significant distress, which can lead to isolation and reduced quality of life.

SELF-FEEDING AND EATING

Changes in eating and food preparation can be caused by deteriorating health, reduced mobility, and routines becoming controlled by dietary requirements or medication regimens.[3] This is especially true for those clients with chronic conditions and for the older adult. Many reasons can cause functional deficits in the occupation of self-feeding and may include client factors as well as performance patterns.[2] Whether it is a movement function or a process skill that may be causing functional difficulties, the role of the OT practitioner is to empower a person to be as independent as possible to facilitate the highest level of quality of life.

The Basic Principles of Feeding

The ability to feed oneself allows a person to regulate the amount of food and liquid taken in for adequate nutrition and hydration. Being able to consume food and liquids is essential for muscle use, as well as brain and organ function. The action of **feeding** oneself includes getting the food or drink and bringing it to the mouth. Although this may seem to be a simple task, it is actually a highly complex process.

The physical process of self-feeding has three main parts; (1) scooping the food, (2) managing the food on the utensil, and (3) bringing the food to the mouth. A person must be able to manage the food, by using his or her hands, by scooping with a spoon, or by piercing with a fork. This requires hand grasp, gross and fine motor coordination, hand–eye coordination, arm and hand strength, and range of motion (ROM) at the shoulder, elbow, wrist, and hand.

Beyond the physical requirements of self-feeding, an individual also requires visual–perceptual, cognitive, and social skills. A person needs to be able to locate items needed for self-feeding—the food on the plate, as well as utensils, condiments, and beverages. Cognitively, feeding incorporates sequencing, problem-solving, attention, and sorting. The social aspects of self-feeding can range from individual interaction to that in a large group setting, each with its own obstacles to navigate.

Typical Feeding Patterns

To complete the process of self-feeding, every individual integrates multiple systems, including physical, visual–perceptual, cognitive, and social aspects involved in this activity of daily living (ADL). Before determining the best course of rehabilitation, an OT practitioner must understand the typical patterns for self-feeding. There are multiple ways to bring food and drink to one's mouth. Commonly, a person uses both hands to manipulate utensils. Some cultures use the dominant hand to cut with the knife, with the fork in the nondominant hand. Later, the knife is placed on the plate, and the fork is placed in the dominant hand to use for scooping or piercing bites of food. Other cultures choose not to switch hands, keeping the fork in the nondominant hand for scooping or piercing. Still other cultures use breads and other foods to scoop and transport the food to the mouth and use fingers instead of utensils. Finger foods, such as sandwiches, French fries, and many fruits, eliminate the need for utensils altogether. As the food reaches the mouth, a number of processes occur, including jaw protrusion toward the food, lip stabilization around the food, and jaw and lip closure to keep the food in the mouth. Any of these processes can be interrupted with weakness or other deficits and will lead to food or drink falling out of the mouth or inability to pull food from the fingers or utensil.

Typical patterns for liquid intake are less varied compared with patterns used for food. For adults, the typical pattern is to directly drink from a cup or drink through a straw held in the hand. This is deceptively simple, as there are many different types of cups, glasses, goblets, and mugs that require different grasp patterns needed for safe manipulation. Typical patterns include a power grasp for a simple cup or glass. Some people utilize a lateral pinch grasp or a three-jaw-chuck grasp for stemmed glasses. Holding a mug allows for several options of grasp that require isolated or combined finger, hand, and wrist movements. Drinking liquid from the cupped hand assumes that the client can pull the hand and fingers into that position and keep the hand level as it reaches the mouth. Drinking from a cup can be affected by decreased lip and jaw strength as well as decreased tongue movement. Difficulty drinking from a straw can be attributed to decreased lip closure, decreased ability to make a seal, or decreased diaphragmatic control.

SELF-FEEDING IMPAIRMENTS

Because self-feeding patterns can differ among cultures, there may be a wide variance in how deficits in sensation, vision, strength, and motor control affect self-feeding. The OTA will observe performance skills in this area and assist to increase the client to effectively get the food and drink to the mouth.

Factors Impacting Feeding Abilities

Impairments that impact self-feeding can range from mild to profound, and an OT practitioner provides skilled intervention for all. The first task is to determine when to focus on rehabilitation versus compensation for optimal independence. A rehabilitative stance focuses on a return to typical patterns, whereas a compensatory stance focuses on teaching new patterns and the use of equipment to compensate for the loss of function.

PHYSICAL

Physical impairments that may affect self-feeding can range from mild muscle weakness, decreased ROM, and incoordination to more severe deficits, including contractures, tremors, spasticity, hemiplegia, and tetraplegia. Skilled interventions for OT practitioners involve determining the root cause of the client's feeding difficulties and initiating the use of either rehabilitation or compensatory strategies, including adaptive equipment. For example, if a client is unable to lift the arm to bring food to the mouth, what is the root cause? Is it weakness of the arm, which potentially can be strengthened, or a limitation in scapular ROM, which decreases available shoulder flexion for the arm to reach the mouth? It is important for the OTA to understand the complex nature of self-feeding to be able to carry out the treatment plan prescribed by the evaluating occupational therapist.

Posture and positioning play a significant role in self-feeding and should be the first priority when determining how to increase a client's independence and safety with this ADL. Typically, to eat at the table, people sit in chairs with postural alignment of the hips, knees, and ankles to achieve an upright position (Fig. 12-1). The inability to get into or maintain this upright position can interfere with self-feeding. Abdominal muscle weakness, hip instability, and even decreased sensation in the lower extremities can make sitting upright more difficult. The preferred table height is one that allows a person to keep the shoulders in neutral alignment and rest the hands comfortably on the table with elbows bent at a 90-degree angle. A table that is too high or too low may interfere with the ability to self-feed effectively. Some clients prefer to eat from a recliner or a bed; however, lack of adequate support or a table surface can limit functional abilities. When working with a client in a hospital bed, always have them sit up as much as is possible, even at the edge of the bed, as this can safely increase the client's ability to self-feed and drink. Clients with trunk weakness may eat more easily seated in a wheelchair with proper support. Some cultures eat from low tables, sitting on the floor on cushions or pillows, but this can be difficult to manage if there is decreased trunk or arm strength and difficulty getting off the floor and may need to be limited at first.

For a client with muscle weakness and decreased active range of motion (AROM), treatment interventions may focus on strengthening the muscles of the trunk and upper extremities as well as increasing the client's activity tolerance. Stretching exercises can increase ROM and flexibility of the bilateral upper extremities. Some clients have progressive weakness or are unable to perform strengthening tasks and will require compensatory equipment and techniques. Self-feeding effectively requires movement and control at the hand for grasp and utensil manipulation, as well as angle, wrist flexion/extension/ulnar and radial deviation, forearm movement for supination/pronation, and elbow flexion/extension. Despite the root cause of the weakness, the use of lightweight utensils and cups can facilitate a client's ability to bring food to the mouth. Utensils with builtup, elongated, or specially curved handles can also minimize the effort required to scoop food and assist those with decreased ROM or strength. Plates and bowls with suction bases or the use of nonskid mats stabilize dishes on the table. Plate guards and scoop dishes provide

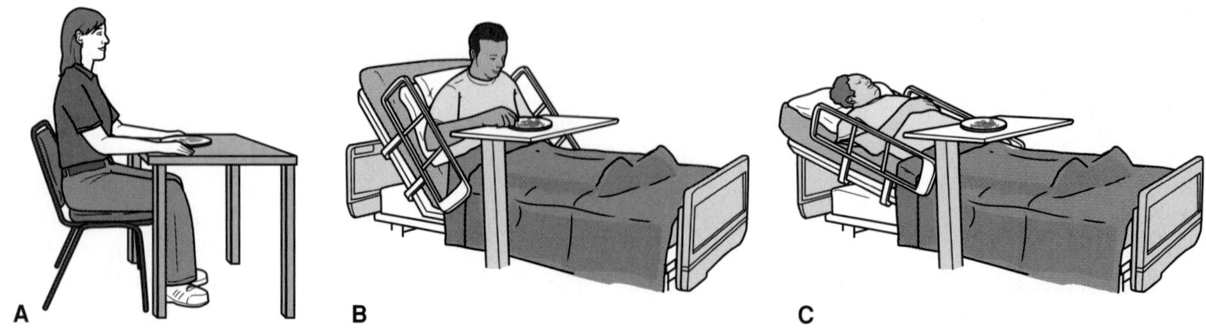

FIGURE 12-1. Note the differences between the drawings, and imagine the difficulties with eating/swallowing when reclined back.

a vertical edge to ease scooping of food and prevent it from sliding off the plate. For drinking liquids, providing extra-long straws with a straw clip will position the straw for the client, eliminating the need to grasp the straw with the hand for support. Straws with one-way valves and varied lengths and diameters may also be helpful. Plastic cups with covers, spouts, and handles will decrease the risk of spilling or breaking a grasp if the client is unable to maintain the grasp on the cup. At times, more severe arm weakness will require an elevating mobile arm support to provide mechanical advantage for self-feeding. The mobile arm support attaches to the wheelchair or table and uses rubber bands to lift the weight of the client's arm in a supported way (Fig. 12-2). A pivot point at the forearm assist allows the elbow to drop to bring the hand to the mouth. Careful setup and adjustment are often required for best control. For another reduced-gravity option, the plate and the client's elbow can be placed on books or boxes to raise the height of both, and bring the plate and the elbow closer to the mouth. This means the client can scoop the food at the mouth height instead of scooping it at a lower level at the plate and then bringing it up to the mouth.

Clients with decreased sensation as a result of a cerebrovascular accident (CVA) or numbness from neuropathy may experience difficulty holding onto utensils and cups or bringing the items to the mouth accurately. If the decreased sensation is in the face or lips, the client may have difficulty with pulling food from the utensil or keeping it in the mouth effectively. They may lose food from the mouth when chewing and drinking.

FIGURE 12-2. Client using a table mount mobile arm support, utensil in universal cuff, and scoop plate.

Rehabilitation or compensation of the movements involved in holding the utensil may include grasp and release, as well as pinch. Some clients are able to work on strengthening of the hand and wrist, but others need adaptive equipment and techniques to manage the utensil. Cylindrical foam can be placed over the utensil handle to create a larger-diameter grip; many caregivers create customized options, such as adding a piece of tubular pipe insulation to a handle or wrapping it with a washcloth that is then secured with tape. Various cuffs and attachments are available to keep a utensil in the hand, including those that are only hand-based and those that also stabilize the wrist (Fig. 12-3). The utensil generally slides into the cuff that is attached to the hand. The cuff compensates for the inability to hold onto the utensil because of weakness. When using a cuff or gross grasp, the fork or spoon may need to have a bent handle and a curve toward the mouth to keep the food from falling off and to reach the mouth at the proper angle. Creating a longer handle on a fork or spoon may allow clients with decreased ROM or strength to more easily bring the utensil to the mouth.

Clients with incoordination and tremor often have difficulty with self-feeding and drinking. Generally, this population requires compensation and adaptive techniques. Getting as much of the client's upper extremity supported on a firm surface, such as a table, will avoid multiple joints moving at once. One of the options may be a raised table with risers under each leg or some height adjustability. Some clients will benefit from weights on the wrists and weighted utensils, although for some, the weight only increases the movement seen. In an article that tested the use of weighted cuffs in persons with tremors resulting from static brain lesions, McGruder et al. found that "the application of weight to the wrist of a person with upper-extremity tremor is accompanied by some functional improvement

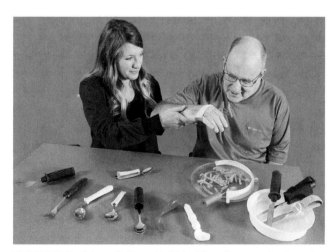

FIGURE 12-3. Adapted plate with high sides, plate guard, adapted utensils and a universal cuff with utensil on the client's hand.

in self-feeding for some individuals. The size of benefit seems to be sensitive to the amount of weight used."[4] A randomized controlled trial of persons with Parkinson's disease using weights noted no support for this recommendation,[5] and in a resource for essential tremors, it was seen that in a small proportion of clients, tremors could be dampened down to improve function with weights on the wrists.[6] Despite the current evidence, the OTA may find many OT practitioners continuing to use the technique of adding weight to offset the effects of the tremors during functional tasks.Using a fork or spoon with a built-in gyroscope, such as Liftware Steady™, will assist many clients with tremor with bringing the food to the mouth. Keeping a drink on the table and using a lid and a straw will assist clients with getting the liquid in with less spilling. Most of the time, a mobile arm support will only exacerbate the problem because it actually increases available motion. Timing the administration of medications for movement disorders around mealtimes may also make self-feeding less messy for some clients.

Clients with spasticity and motor control issues will often have difficulty with hand-to-mouth movement and often overshoot or undershoot the mouth, tip the spoon or fork, and lose the food. ROM and contractures can also be a concern with this population. Attaching the utensils to the hand may assist clients with steadying the utensil, and often a deeper spoon or one with an edge can help keep the food in the spoon. Generally, a cup with a lid and a straw or spout will assist with minimizing spillage. Educating the client to mix foods, such as peas in mashed potatoes, or crackers to thicken soup, may be helpful as well. Some clients may benefit from an automatic power feeding machine that will scoop and bring the spoon to the mouth. The power feeder may also be used with clients with severe weakness, tremor, spasticity, or other control issues, and may have a substantial cost associated with purchase.

VISION AND VISUAL-PERCEPTUAL SKILLS

A variety of vision and visual–perceptual impairments can impede a person's ability to self-feed. During self-feeding, vision and visual–perceptual skills play as important a role as physical skills. A significant part of self-feeding involves visually perceiving what is in front of oneself at the table. This includes the food and liquids one intends to consume, the utensils required, and the condiments on the table, as well as other people's items. Low vision is a broad term that covers a wide range of visual impairments that can affect this ADL. The term refers to more than simply requiring glasses to comfortably see what is in front of oneself, and all OT practitioners need to understand the differences between these conditions to provide best practice. Table 12-1 provides a quick reference chart regarding common vision conditions and their effects that may impact self-feeding. Refer to Chapter 10 for further information on vision.

In addition to their effect on vision, which include depth perception, scanning, visual fields, figure ground, and object permanence, visual–perceptual skills can also have a significant effect on functional skills. Depth perception allows a person to determine how close or far an item is from him or her. This is essential to facilitate retrieving a glass, scooping food, or grasping a napkin or other item. Depth perception is also utilized when returning items to the table, passing items to another person at the table, or even communicating with others. The OTA could assist a client with depth perception deficits during self-feeding by using weighted cups that will not tip over if bumped, training the

TABLE 12-1 Visual Conditions, Effects, and Strategies[7]

CONDITION	EFFECT ON VISION	OT STRATEGIES FOR SELF-FEEDING
Cataracts	Clouding of the lens of the eye can affect one or both eyes Increased glare from lights	Lower bright lights Higher contrast between plate and food
Diabetic retinopathy	Directly caused by diabetes damage to blood vessels in the retina Usually affects both eyes Blood vessel leakage causes "blind spots" and blurred vision	Turn head to avoid blind spots while eating Higher-contrast plate, cup, and napkin
Glaucoma	Tunnel vision May eventually lead to complete vision loss in one or both eyes	Teach client to put same type of food in same place on plate, utensils and cup in same place Turn head to compensate for tunnel vision
Legal blindness	Central visual acuity 20/200 or less in the "better" eye with the best possible correction Visual field of 20 degrees or less	Teach the clock method with the client and caregiver to describe which food is on the plate by position on a clock Teach client to put same type of food in same place on plate, utensils and cup in same place
Macular degeneration	Sharp, central vision is damaged first Common complaints of "blank spots"	Turn head to compensate for blank spots High-contrast plate and napkin

client to compensate by assigning specific places for all items on the table, as well as training the client to note size differences to identify items that are farther from or closer to them.

Scanning is the ability to attend from one visual field to another; this allows a person to identify all items on a table and to locate items that are shared among others sitting at the table. Typically, a person is able to scan horizontally, vertically, and diagonally and to utilize peripheral vision in addition to direct, focused sight. The client must scan to locate not only the food on the plate but also their drink, condiments, napkin, and others around the table. Turning the head from side to side or using touch can help compensate if the eyes are less able to scan the full environment. Many clients who have very low vision or are blind are able to learn compensatory strategies for independent self-feeding, such as using divided plates, always putting the same types of foods in the same location, using touch, and using alerts on cups indicating when nearly full.

Figure ground and object permanence play important roles in locating and identifying objects on the table. Figure ground is the ability to recognize objects as being different from the background. For example, a person is able to identify light-colored food items on a white plate, or see silverware (figures) on the table (background). Without the ability to differentiate objects from the background, locating food and bringing it to one's mouth becomes a much more difficult task. A compensatory option that the OTA can offer a client is the use of high-contrast plates, cups, and napkins to distinguish them from the food and the tablecloth. A black or red placemat could be placed under a lighter-colored plate, for example.

Both inattention and neglect of one side of the body or one visual field can affect a client's ability to self-feed. Often, inattention can be compensated for with scanning techniques and reminders. For example, placing a bright-colored strip of tape on the side less attended to or asking the client to look for a certain target on that side can direct the client to look to that side. Neglect is more substantial than inattention and occurs when the visual field simply does not exist for the client; it is very difficult to change. In cases of neglect, the OTA should move the client's plate, food, and drink to the side that the client attends to or does not neglect. When assisting the client with inattention or neglect with self-feeding, the OT practitioner can sit either on the client's affected side or on the unaffected side, depending on the severity of the problem. If the OTA is sitting on the affected side, the client would be forced to attend to that direction. However, with severe neglect, the OTA may simply not exist to the client when sitting on the affected side. In rehabilitation situations, the OTA may want to challenge the client by having him or her gradually attend to the entire plate or items on the affected side with cues and assist. In a compensation situation, the OTA may ask caregivers to place all food and drink items on the unaffected side to increase independence with the self-feeding task.

Visual field cuts can also affect a person's ability to self-feed. A person with a visual field cut is not able to see anything in the impaired area and may include any portion of the eye or the entire eye, affecting all or part of the vision of that eye.[8] Visual field cuts can present separately or exist in combination with inattention or neglect. When field cut is not accompanied by neglect, the client can often learn to scan to compensate for the lost visual field. Cues to find certain food items by turning the head can also help compensate. If the client has difficulty with compensation, the OTA should help by placing items on the table within the unaffected visual fields. The individual will be able to see items required during meals by using these new consistent routines, and eventually habits will form. Alternatively, turning a client's plate after everything in the available visual field has been consumed will assist as well.

Another issue that is typically thought of as a cognitive aspect and has roots in the visual areas as well is called **object permanence.** Object permanence ensures that despite an object being outside of the visual field, the person is still able to recognize that the item is available and present. This relates to remembering the napkin on the lap and other people at the table who may have left the table temporarily. With severe neglect, the items on the affected side simply do not exist for the client and may lose object permanence. Other clients with severe short-term memory deficits may lose this skill as well. Frequent scanning and establishing routines may be helpful.

COGNITIVE

Cognitive aspects of self-feeding include sequencing, attention, memory, and executive functions. A person sequences the steps for self-feeding by first scooping food before bringing the utensil toward the mouth. Sequencing also occurs when a person takes a bite of food to his or her mouth and determines when to open the mouth, insert the food, and close the mouth. More severe sequencing impairments can affect a person's safety, from eating or drinking something that is too hot to attempting to take another bite before swallowing. Compensation for sequencing deficits would be rehearsal of the steps required, a written home or maintenance program that includes the cuing needed for independence, or providing picture sequences for caregivers or family members to follow.

Attention can be broken down into four types—sustained, selective, alternating, and divided—and all four have a role in self-feeding. Sustained attention is the ability to maintain the focus on the meal and eating with external stimuli. Selective attention is the ability to maintain focus on one stimulus when multiple stimuli are occurring—for example, the bite of food being too hot when the client is tasting it, moving the utensil, looking at a partner, and many other stimuli. Sustained attention and selective attention are used to focus on an individual task, whereas alternating attention and divided attention are used to attend to multiple stimuli. Alternating attention is the ability to switch the focus back and forth between tasks during self-feeding.[9] This might be seen when the client has to attend to cutting food and then look at a partner for conversation. Divided attention is the ability to process two or more responses or demands at the same time.[9] This might be the ability to talk to a partner while bringing a fully loaded spoon to the mouth without spilling. During self-feeding, there is a need to focus on an individual task when scooping food, bringing food to one's mouth, and identifying food and drink to consume. Alternating attention and divided attention are called upon when a person needs to interact with others during a meal or to attend to multiple items in front of them. The OTA can assist with attention issues by noting the environment for the meal and reducing distractions as well as talking while eating. Cues for attention as well as offering only one food at a time may be necessary.

Mealtime, as well as the time outside meals, can be affected by a person's memory. Remembering the last time one ate or drank as well as what was consumed is essential, not only for satisfying the needs of hunger and thirst but also for nutrition and hydration tracking. It is also important to remember the amounts consumed in conjunction with medications to minimize the potential negative effects of any medication. Memory is divided into short-term and long-term memories, and both have roles to play in self-feeding. Short-term memory with regard to self-feeding, incorporates remembering when food has been scooped onto a utensil, recall of what was ordered (e.g., in a restaurant), and how much of the meal has been consumed. A client who does not recall how much she has eaten can overeat or undereat, impacting nutrition and hydration. If unable to recall whether or not she has scooped food onto a utensil, the client may bring an empty utensil to her mouth, which exerts unnecessary energy that may not be expendable. Portion sizes, as well as taking a photo of the plate before eating, can help the client track consumption. Recording the food and drink consumed may also be helpful.

Long-term memory is any information that is no longer stored in short-term memory and has been placed beyond conscious awareness. Long-term memory impairments resulting from dementia or visual deficits, such as visual agnosia (impairment of recognition of objects), may impede an individual from remembering how to use utensils, how to differentiate utensils from each other, or even what a utensil is. Increased severity of long-term memory impairments can include forgetting how to coordinate bringing food to one's mouth, chewing, or even swallowing. Procedural memory is specifically linked to self-feeding, as once routines are learned, they can be performed without conscious thought.[10] Motor, cognitive, and perceptual skills associated with the learning of movement-based information make up procedural memory, with such tasks as brushing teeth, tying shoe laces, and self-feeding.[10] Procedural memories can often be tapped into for the performance routine tasks, such as self-feeding, in the case of persons with dementia. Many times, just placing a plate in front of the person and handing them a utensil (or pre-loaded utensil) will initiate self-feeding.

Executive functions related to self-feeding include problem-solving, planning, and self-regulation. A person subconsciously solves problems during mealtime with each bite. Determining the appropriate-sized bite to scoop, cut, and pierce needs to be assessed each time a person brings food to the mouth. Problem-solving impairments may include simply being unable to decide whether to use a fork or a spoon, if a bite is the right size or not, or even whether another bite is wanted. Problem-solving can also affect meal preparation and choices, shopping for food, and following multistep directions in a recipe. The OTA can assist with practice with problem-solving as well as cuing during the meal and during meal preparation. Planning deficits may impact the ability to determine the timing of meals, impact getting adequate nutrition, and performance of simple tasks, such as setting the table with a spoon instead of a fork to eat soup. Meal preparation as well as self-feeding and drinking can have multiple steps that require organization and planning.[11] Self-regulation plays a significant role in whether to continue eating or not, which impacts nutrition and hydration directly and can also have negative impacts on one's health as a result of stomach discomfort and bowel and bladder irregularity. The social aspects of self-feeding, including interactions with others, use of condiments (e.g., salt and pepper on food), and communication with others present during mealtime also relates to self-regulation.

SOCIAL

Self-feeding and mealtime are social events, involving family, friends, and sometimes strangers. Interactions with familiar people are generally easier, but a person may also need to interact with strangers. At a restaurant, for example, a person has to be able to communicate wants and needs throughout the meal to those they are dining with and also to wait staff serving them. Verbal communication plays an essential role during mealtime. Other social aspects of mealtime include observing manners and customs. Each culture has various social norms that must be adhered to for a successful mealtime interaction—customs ranging from what utensils are used, if utensils are used; eye contact and conversation during meals; and even obtaining various items from the table. Cultural sensitivity plays a large role in the success of OT interventions. The OT practitioner should be familiar with common cultural norms beyond his or her own to facilitate successful intervention.

Pragmatics is an area of social language skills that can have a role with the social aspects of self-feeding and mealtime. Clients with pragmatic deficits may have difficulties with taking turns (when reaching for food), body language (if a guest dislikes a served food), asking for help when needed (to cut food), speaking too loudly (intonation of voice), and speaking with the mouth full. Treatment for these deficits may involve modeling desired behavior, practicing specific scenarios, role-playing, and offering visual cues through the use of pictures or cue cards.

Social impairments can manifest as social anxiety, inappropriate behaviors, or communication barriers. Social anxiety may stem from communication, physical, neurological, visual–perceptual impairments or a combination of any of these. For example, a person who is unsure of his or her ability to speak may choose to remain silent, which limits the ability to communicate wants and needs, interact with others at the table, or communicate with a caregiver who is assisting with self-feeding. A person with social anxiety may limit his or her intake during self-feeding because of difficulty with managing food or utensils. Persons with mild cognitive deficits are often anxious as they know they have difficulties with memory and judgment and are afraid to make a social mistake. Many times, the OTA can offer increased practice with repetition, safe exploration, role-playing, and gradually increased demands to overcome these social impairments.

Inappropriate behaviors can be aggressive or passive. Striking a caregiver, grabbing for food items not belonging to oneself, or even throwing unwanted food are examples of aggressive physical behaviors. Passive behaviors are also known as *avoidance behaviors*. Examples can include ignoring others who are attempting to communicate or turning one's head away from a utensil brought to the mouth. Often, clients with brain injury will display inappropriate behaviors during mealtimes, such as impulsively reaching for a food item, talking with the mouth full, and stuffing more food in the mouth than can be chewed. The client with aggressive behaviors may need to be isolated for a time at meals for the protection of other clients, with application of behavioral strategies and ongoing therapy to manage these behaviors.

Communication barriers may range from not hearing what is being said to not understanding for any reason. Those clients with hearing loss may hear during the meal more easily in a quiet environment with fewer people and background noises. If a person's memory is impaired, he or she may not recall donning hearing aids or replacing batteries, making communication increasingly difficult. Clients with dysarthric (garbled) or quiet speech can be easily frustrated in a noisy environment as well.

Other parts of the environment can play a role in the functioning of the client during self-feeding as well. The color of the room, tablecloth, or dishes, as well as the presentation of the food, may enhance or diminish appetite. Red and yellow are colors that tend to increase appetite. Blue and green tend to be calming. Music can assist with the rhythm of swallowing and intake and introduce a relaxing or stimulating mood.

MALNUTRITION AND DEHYDRATION ISSUES

Some clients who are able to bring food and drink easily to the mouth still are malnourished and dehydrated. The reasons for this include lack of appetite, inability to get easily or safely to the toilet, reduced mobility or strength to retrieve food and drink, difficulty with food preparation, and difficulty with getting to the store to buy food and drink. Many persons with disabilities face one or more of these challenges. Lack of appetite occurs fairly frequently in older adults because as their taste buds undergo age-related change, food does not taste as good. Refer to the feature, "The Older Adult," to learn about some other issues that may impair an older adult's ability to self-feed. Depression and medications can also cause lack of appetite. If a client does not have a dependable way to perform toileting, he or she may voluntarily withhold food and/or drink to avoid needing to urinate or defecate while their caregiver is away from the home. This may be especially true for women who cannot easily use a urinal and have to pull down clothing to urinate. A new product on the market is called PureWick®, which is a female external catheter that hooks to a standard suction machine to wick away the urine into the collection canister. Food and drink retrieval and preparation from a walker or wheelchair can be difficult; and pain, decreased balance, fatigue, and other factors may hinder these tasks as well. The OTA has a strong role in adapting and modifying the environment, as well as offering adaptive equipment and techniques for management. A tray for carrying items on the walker and adaptive clothing or a reacher to retrieve items from the refrigerator could be useful. Although services for food and drink delivery, such as "Meals on Wheels" are available, many clients with disabilities struggle to get other supplies from the store. Even with delivered food, the client may be unable to open the wrapper on a sandwich, cut up an apple, peel an orange, or open a small packet of pepper. Certainly, adaptive techniques and equipment, such as a self-opening scissors to cut the package, an adapted cutting board and knife, and a spring-loaded needle nose pliers to assist with the packet of pepper, could assist with these tasks. Mobility, reaching, endurance, and transportation issues can limit abilities to procure, retrieve, and prepare food. The OTA may work with the client on a management plan to include caregivers (paid and unpaid) and community resources, such as a church group or volunteer groups. More grocery delivery options as well as online shopping and home delivery are now becoming increasingly available.

CAREGIVER EDUCATION AND TRAINING

Functional recovery and therapy sessions are not only limited to one-on-one interaction between the OTA and the client. Education and training of caregivers is essential for follow-through outside of therapy sessions and to optimize quality of life after discharge from skilled therapy. It is the responsibility of the OT practitioner to educate and train not only the client but also any caregivers who may be responsible for assistance with self-feeding. Thorough education involves the use of handouts, trials, hands-on learning, and examples and is part of skilled treatment as a billable education session. Presentation of education using multiple methods may assist with learning. For example, during the first part of the meal, the OTA may demonstrate to the caregiver the adaptive techniques for the client with arm weakness and a visual field cut. The next step for skilled

THE OLDER ADULT

The United States National Institute of Aging describes "failure to thrive" (FTT) as a "syndrome of weight loss, decreased appetite and poor nutrition, and inactivity, often accompanied by dehydration, depressive symptoms, impaired immune function, and low cholesterol."[12] FTT has been found to be associated with increased admission rates to the hospital, low level of independence in all activities of daily living (ADLs), and cognitive impairment.[13] The four chief characteristics of geriatric failure to thrive are impaired physical function, malnutrition, depression, and cognitive impairment.[14] Clients hospitalized with this diagnosis often have underlying health issues as well as acute needs, and it can be a warning sign for more serious concerns.[15] For clients with FTT, the OTA may address self-feeding and eating, as well as other areas of occupation, ROM and contracture management, assistive device needs, mobility and positioning in mobility devices, strengthening, balance activities, and pain management. The OT practitioner will also address safe preparation of simple, yet nutritious meals, and work with caregivers to increase overall nutrition. Adaptive strategies for cognitive changes that affect ADLs and IADLs will be needed, as will working with caregivers and community resources on a plan for increased socialization and options to increase activity level.

OT intervention can often be training the caregiver for the second half of the meal. The OTA will supportively observe and cue the caregiver, as needed, with regard to ensuring safety with swallowing and the optimal setup for promoting the client's independence in self-feeding. A follow-up after the meal may be a handout with the techniques listed or even a video of the techniques. The OTA can train caregivers how to position a client for best self-feeding or swallowing, adapt for various weaknesses, and even the proper way to dependently feed a client. When feeding another person, it is important to make eye contact to determine whether he or she is ready for a bite of food or a swallow of liquid. Bite and sip amounts and the rhythm and pace of feeding are also important when feeding someone else to avoid causing choking. To know the wants and needs of the client, effective communication plays an important role in caregiver-assisted feeding. It is important to remember that caregivers may not have the specialized education of an OT practitioner, and care must be taken to determine that the education and training have been successful and that caregivers are competent to continue providing care without the supervision of an OT practitioner.

SWALLOWING

Swallowing plays a pivotal role in an individual's ability to adequately gain and maintain nutrition and hydration to sustain life. Although there are options for nutrition and hydration that do not involve swallowing, such as a feeding tube, the inability to safely swallow even saliva can result in choking, aspiration, pneumonia, and death. The OT practitioner will often collaborate with other team members, such as the dietitian and the SLP, so that the entire team is working toward the goals, including safe swallowing.

Basic Principles of Swallowing

The process of swallowing involves four phases—the oral preparatory, the oral transit, the pharyngeal, and the esophageal. Each phase of the swallow plays a key role in safely transporting nutrients from the mouth into the stomach. The phases of swallowing function will be explored later in the chapter.

ANATOMY AND PHYSIOLOGY OF THE SWALLOWING MECHANISM

Swallowing is a complex process involving the mouth, pharynx, larynx, and esophagus. These systems work together to form the swallowing mechanism and are responsible for transporting foods and liquids from the mouth into the stomach for digestion. See Figure 12-4 for an anatomical view of the body structures involved in the swallowing process.

SWALLOWING IMPAIRMENTS

Although most people swallow without difficulty, numerous impairments, diseases, and disorders can cause one or more parts of the process to break down. Without complete coordination of the four phases of the swallow, clients will have swallowing impairments.

Dysphagia

Many diseases and impairments can impact the ability to swallow; these impairments in feeding and swallowing functions are referred to as **dysphagia**. Some causes of dysphagia in adults are CVA, brain injury, spinal cord injury, Parkinson's disease, amyotrophic lateral sclerosis (ALS), multiple sclerosis (MS), muscular dystrophy, cerebral palsy, and dementia. Swallowing can also be impacted by poor dentition; cancer in the mouth, neck, or throat; and/or injury from surgery to the head or neck. General signs or symptoms of dysphagia include, but are not limited to, laborious effort in moving food from a utensil into the mouth, difficulty or prolonged chewing or swallowing of food, leakage of food or liquids from the mouth, coughing during or following intake, choking on solid foods, a wet and gurgly vocal quality following intake, nasal drainage, and/or watering eyes. Recurrent pneumonia, weight loss, and dehydration are also possible signs and symptoms of dysphagia. These signs and symptoms of dysphagia are listed in Table 12-2.[16] Individuals with dysphagia are inadvertently at risk for serious medical conditions, including

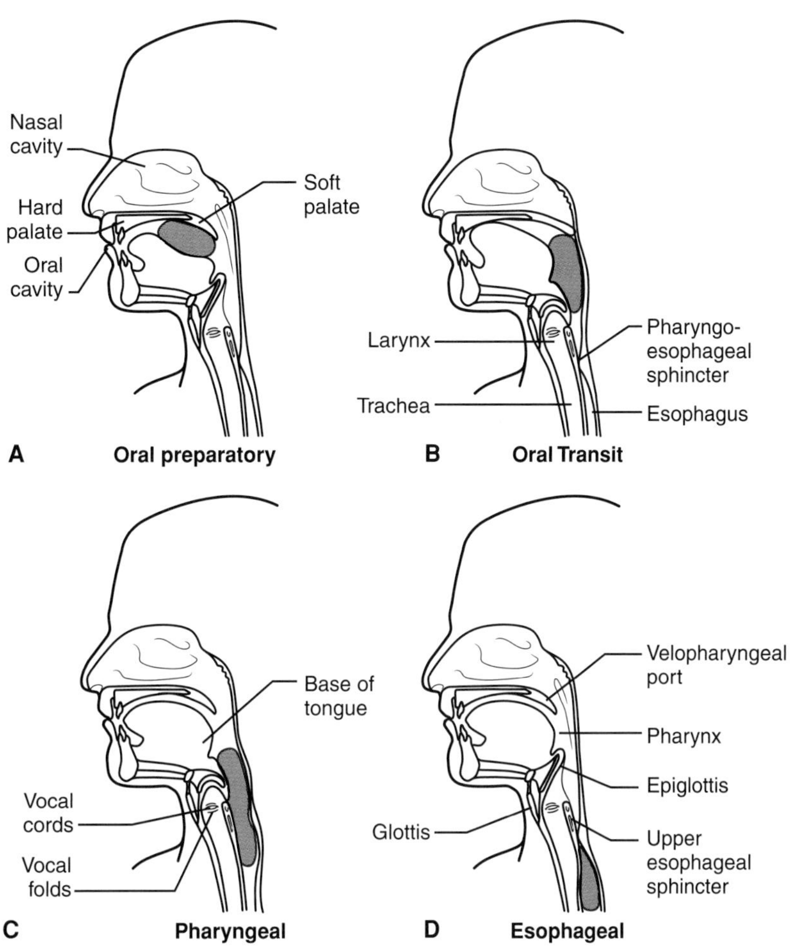

FIGURE 12-4. Structures of swallowing mechanism.

TABLE 12-2 Signs and Symptoms of Dysphagia[16]

PHASE	SIGNS AND SYMPTOMS OF DYSPHAGIA
Oral or pharyngeal dysphagia	Difficulty with or prolonged chewing Leakage of food or liquids from the mouth Drooling Coughing Choking Delayed swallow initiation Weight loss Change in dietary habits Nasal drainage Watering eyes Wet, gurgly vocal quality Penetration and/or aspiration Aspiration pneumonia
Esophageal dysphagia	Regurgitation Sensation of food "sticking" in the chest Unexplained weight loss Recurrent pneumonia

airway obstruction and/or aspiration pneumonia, as a result of swallowing impairments. **Airway obstruction** is a blocking of the airway as a result of choking on foods, which impedes normal breathing. Materials that bypass the airway protection during swallowing into the laryngeal region but do not make it past the vocal folds into the trachea are considered to cause **penetration**. Penetration of materials into the upper airway increases an individual's risk for aspiration. **Aspiration** occurs when any substance actually enters the airway or trachea and can lead to pneumonia. In a normal swallow function, when penetration has occurred, one will experience a cough response to discharge the material from the airway. However, many people with dysphagia exhibit what is known as *silent aspiration*, in which materials enter the airway because of the absence of an overt cough response to clear the material.

The Phases of Swallowing

Each phase of the swallowing process plays a key role in safely transmitting nutrients from the mouth into the stomach (Table 12-3). Dysphagia can occur in one or more phases of the swallow. This section explores the phases of swallowing in normal functioning adults and how dysphagia impacts the swallowing process.

The purpose of the oral preparatory phase is to prepare food to be swallowed. Sensory recognition for taste, touch, and temperature are required for an individual to form an appropriate and safely sized bolus. A **bolus** is an assemblage of solids and liquids that will be swallowed and is created as one chews this mixture of materials into a cohesive unit. As

TABLE 12-3 Phases of Swallowing[17]

PHASE	PROBLEMS MAY BE CAUSED BY:	OTA TREATMENT
Oral preparatory	Poor dentition Fatigue during chewing Behavioral feeding deficits Decreased sensation in the oral cavity Weakness or atrophy of lingual or labial muscles	Recommendation for dental visit Rest breaks, as needed Smaller bites Softer consistency foods for less chewing
Oral transit phase	Velopharyngeal insufficiency Decreased anterior to posterior transfer Lingual incoordination or weakness Delayed activation of the pharyngeal muscles One-sided weakness	Extra time given for each bite/sip Food directed to stronger side with tongue or spoon Softer consistencies, thicker liquids Smaller bites/sips
Pharyngeal phase	Decreased or absent laryngeal elevation One-sided weakness Decreased tongue base retraction Decreased epiglottic inversion Poor airway coverage Residue pooling in the pyriform sinuses and valleculae	Chin tuck Multiple swallows per bite/sip Smaller bites/sips Care with straws (may get too fast or too much)
Esophageal phase	Decreased upper esophageal sphincter (UES) opening GERD Decreased peristalsis Strictures, narrowing, spasms, tumors, etc.	Consultation with MD about medications for GERD Avoiding spicy and acidic foods Sitting up during and after eating

food enters the mouth (oral cavity), during this phase, several processes begin to prepare its breakdown. First, sensory recognition of food or drink approaching the mouth cues saliva production. Saliva assists in the breakdown of food particles and allows for the formation of a cohesive bolus. As the food or drink approaches the oral cavity, saliva production continues while the tongue, lips, and teeth prepare to remove the bolus from the utensil. Upon introduction of the food into the mouth, saliva begins the process of breaking down the food and assists the tongue, teeth, and palate in the creation of a cohesive bolus. During the oral preparatory phase, adequate mastication (chewing) is required to prepare the bolus for safe swallowing. Mastication and bolus manipulation can be greatly impacted by poor dentition and/or fatigue during mastication caused by generalized weakness and changes in endurance. Lingual strength—that is, tongue strength and coordination—also plays a large role in swallowing function for manipulation and propulsion of the bolus to the pharynx. At the conclusion of the oral preparatory phase, the bolus is positioned on the tongue for transport into the pharynx.

The next phase is the oral transit phase, during which the bolus is passed from the back of the mouth into the throat. This process is called anterior-to-posterior propulsion of the bolus. During propulsion, the soft palate closes to form a barrier between the mouth and the nasal cavity. This closure prevents foods and liquids from entering the nasal cavity during the swallow.

As the bolus is propelled posteriorly, the muscles for the pharyngeal swallow are activated, and so begins the pharyngeal phase. During this phase, the laryngeal framework elevates and moves forward while the epiglottis inverts to protect the airway. Epiglottic inversion forms a barrier, acting as the primary defense against penetration into the airway. Within the larynx, the vocal folds close tightly as a secondary defense to materials entering the trachea, thereby preventing aspiration. At this time, the base of the tongue contacts the pharyngeal wall, and the bolus moves around the epiglottis and through to the upper esophageal sphincter (UES), where the final phase of the swallow begins. Figure 12-5 shows an abnormal swallow with penetration into the airway and aspiration.

The final phase of the swallow is the esophageal phase, in which the bolus travels down the esophagus and into the

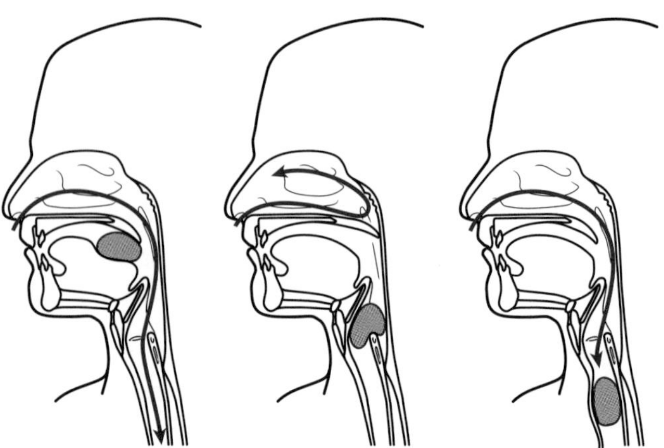

FIGURE 12-5. Abnormal swallow with penetration and aspiration.

stomach. Once the bolus reaches the UES and is accepted into the esophagus, a process known as *peristalsis*, in which muscle contractions transport the bolus inferiorly, pairs with gravity to assist the movement of the bolus into the stomach for the process of digestion. The swallowing process has been completed once the bolus reaches the stomach and digestion begins.

Esophageal dysphagia causes difficulty with the final phase of the swallow. Strictures (narrowing from scar tissue due to irritants), spasms, tumors, and/or the absence or weakening of the peristalsis function may characterize these impairments. Esophageal disorders are typically diagnosed and treated by a gastroenterologist with medications or surgical procedures. Gastroesophageal reflux disease (GERD) can also play a role in aspiration or penetration at the pharyngeal level from acid reflux propelling substances up through the UES and into the airway. GERD is typically managed with medications, restrictive diets to reduce acidic intake, and positioning recommendations to reduce the risk of reflux caused aspiration.

Evaluation of Dysphagia

Dysphagia affects more than just one's ability to swallow and often impacts a person's mental, physical, and social integrity. These factors play a large role in evaluation and treatment considerations. To evaluate for dysphagia, an OT practitioner or SLP specializing in swallowing disorders will complete a comprehensive chart review and client and/or caregiver interview, followed by a bedside swallow examination (BSSE). For assessment, practitioners may also utilize instrumental examinations, such as fiberoptic endoscopic evaluation of swallowing (FEES) and/or the videofluroscopic swallowing study (VFSS), which is also commonly known as the modified barium swallow study (MBSS).

A BSSE begins with a comprehensive chart review for medical history and will be completed with the client as the initial mode of assessment. During a BSSE, the practitioner assesses the client's oral motor function and swallowing mechanism for strength and coordination. Following the oral motor examination, the practitioner assesses the integrity of the client's laryngeal elevation and completes a diet texture analysis. A diet texture analysis begins with "by mouth" or PO (PO from the Latin, *per os*) trials of different solid and liquid consistencies to determine the least restrictive, yet safest, diet. The practitioner will also utilize this time to determine the appropriate compensatory strategies to maximize safety in oral intake. Following a BSSE, an instrumental examination may be necessary to gain more information on the pharyngeal and esophageal phases of the swallow, as they cannot be observed superficially.

Instrumental examinations allow a practitioner to observe the swallowing process with the use of cameras, videos, and x-rays. The FEES utilizes a flexible tube equipped with a small camera and light that are connected to a video monitoring system. The tube, or endoscope, is gently inserted through the client's nose and down into the throat and allows the practitioner to view the pharyngeal phase of the swallow on the video monitoring system. During the assessment, the client will be instructed to eat or drink different solid and liquid consistencies to complete a thorough examination for the least restrictive, yet safest, diet recommendation. The device for FEES is often portable and allows for assessment of the client in various positions. Ear, nose, and throat specialists (ENTs) often assist or complete the FEES as well.

VFSS/MBSS is utilized to assess dysphagia. An OT practitioner will complete a VFSS in a radiology unit or department in conjunction with a radiologist. During a VFSS, the client will sit or stand in front of an x-ray machine and be asked to swallow different solid and liquid consistencies that have been mixed with barium, which makes it possible to view the entire swallowing process. Throughout these trials PO, the client is instructed on different compensatory strategies and positions to determine which ones are most appropriate for reducing the risk of aspiration or penetration during intake. The VFSS also allows for a view of the esophageal phase of the swallow for further assessment of esophageal dysphagia.

Dysphagia impacts a client's mental, physical, and social well-being. As such, OT practitioners are faced with using their best clinical judgment to determine which assessments are the most appropriate on an individual case basis. Some factors that may impact the determination for the most appropriate assessment include the client's cultural background and beliefs, medical diagnoses and condition, ability to follow instructions, and ambulation ability to receive assessment; the payer source or facility resources are also a consideration.

Presbyphagia

Presbyphagia refers to characteristic age-related changes in the swallowing mechanism of otherwise healthy older adults.[18] Although the swallowing mechanism is not inherently impaired in older adults, they certainly can be at higher risk for dysphagia as a result of an acute illness, surgery, multiple medications, and age-related conditions.

A person with presbyphagia may, along with these other factors, exhibit signs of weakening muscles interfering with eating, which may be consistent with signs of dysphagia, such as coughing and choking. A study on swallowing in both younger and older women found that swallowing function is influenced by both age and bolus size.[19] As muscles weaken, the airway becomes more susceptible to penetration, and the risk for aspiration increases. Because of these factors, while eating, the person may experience discomfort, such as coughing and a feeling of choking, and is at risk for weight loss, dehydration, malnutrition, and/or aspiration pneumonia.[20]

DIET MODIFICATIONS

In the treatment of dysphagia, an obligation exists to minimize the client's risk for aspiration or penetration while maximizing the client's safety with the least restrictive diet. The term *least restrictive diet* refers to the highest level of diet that a client can safely eat or drink without a high risk of choking or aspiration. Some important considerations regarding diet habits and modifications include the client's quality of life, cultural background, food and drink preferences, prognosis, and/or the etiology of dysphagia.

Table 12-4 shows the hierarchy of diet texture levels to maximize and maintain safety with oral intake. This hierarchy begins with regular solids, which include all foods without texture-based restriction. Next is a regular chopped diet, in which foods must be chopped into smaller pieces. Regular chopped diets still require a client to demonstrate adequate chewing, bolus formation, and manipulation. Mechanical soft consistencies are a step down from chopped diets and consist of foods that are ground, moist, and semisolid. At this level, foods require less chewing, and the risk of choking is reduced. Pureed solids are the final diet texture in the hierarchy, in which foods are altered to be pudding-like and require very little to no chewing.

Sometimes, a client will require a modified solid diet, such as mechanical soft foods, because of poor dentition. Dentures can be challenging to manage in the best of cases, and well-fitting dentures can be financially out of reach for some. Tooth and mouth pain can also be issues for managing foods that are harder to chew. A blender will transform food from a chopped diet to mechanical soft consistency; generally, meats are cooked well and then ground, as needed, for consistency and moistness. Vegetables are cooked very soft and then ground, and fruits are generally served already ground, such as with applesauce, or blended, such as with canned peaches. To puree, food items should be ground in a blender with additional liquid, such as adding broth or gravy to meats and vegetables and adding juices to blended fruits, to get a more pudding-like texture.

Liquid consistencies also have a hierarchy of modifications based on viscosity as follows:

Thin liquids → Nectar Thick Liquids → Honey Thick Liquids → Pudding Thick Liquids.

TABLE 12-4 Examples of Modified Solid Diet Levels

SOLIDS	EXAMPLES
Regular solids	All foods without texture restriction
Regular chopped solids	Meats chopped into small, bite sized pieces—for example, chicken cut into small cubes, sausage chopped into small bites, etc.
Mechanical soft solids	Ground, moist, semi-soft texture—for example, ground beef or ground turkey moistened with sauce or gravy
Puree solids	Altered to be pudding-like—some naturally occurring examples of puree solids include pudding, applesauce, mashed potatoes, etc.

Viscosity refers to a liquid's thickness or resistance to flow. Liquid consistencies utilized for clients with dysphagia include thin (regular) liquids, followed by nectar-thick liquids, honey-thick liquids, and finally pudding-thick (spoon-thick) liquids. Modifications to liquids are recommended when the client has a delay in the swallowing process, resulting in liquids reaching the back of the throat before the swallowing process has been initiated. As a result, the client will be at a higher risk for aspiration, penetration, and/or pneumonia. Modifications in the liquid consistencies to increase the viscosity allow for improved control of the liquids and decrease the client's risk of aspiration. Thickening agents are commercially sold and are generally available in a tasteless powdered form to add to liquids. Nectar-thick liquid is what might be found in a can of peaches in heavy syrup. Generally, the more the thickening powder added, the thicker the liquid becomes. For most powders, the longer the liquid sits, the thicker it gets, and the OTA should carefully follow package directions.

Mixed consistencies are a final consideration for diet textures. This term refers to foods that contain both solid and liquid components. These foods can occur naturally and/or be created. For example, some naturally occurring mixed consistencies include fruits, which require adequate chewing to safely swallow but also contain a liquid component. Other examples of mixed consistencies include chunky soups, sauces, or cereals with milk. Foods that melt are also mixed consistencies. Ice cream, gelatin, milkshakes, and so on may appear to be pureed at first; however, they melt to a thin liquid. For individuals with dysphagia, these consistencies can be especially difficult to swallow safely.

The following recommendations for eating and drinking are useful to clients with dysphagia:[21]

1. Eat slowly.
2. Avoid eating or drinking when rushed or tired.
3. Consume small amounts of food or liquid at a time.
4. Eliminate distractions, and concentrate on eating.
5. Avoid mixing food and liquid in the same mouthful.
6. Place the food on the stronger side of the mouth if weakness exists on one side.

In some cases, when an individual has severe dysphagia or is at risk for nutritional decline because of decreased alertness impacting oral intake or infection from intake following a surgical procedure, a client will be deemed NPO. The term NPO stands for the Latin term *nil per os*, which means "nothing by mouth." NPO serves as a medical instruction for a person who is not able to safely ingest foods, liquids, or medications PO and must receive alternative forms nutrition. When NPO status is related to severe risk for aspiration pneumonia, the therapy team works with the client's physician to make the final decision. The client's physician will ultimately decide on feeding tube placement and feeding protocol from that point on. Important considerations for NPO status include the client's and family's wishes and cultural beliefs, as well as the client's prognosis and mental status. NPO status can be permanent or temporary and may include all foods and drinks, including ice chips. Caution should be taken when performing oral hygiene, as a client could aspirate on toothpaste or water when rinsing. The OTA must be able to recognize when an individual is NPO and maintain compliance to best meet his or her needs.

CHOKING

Sometimes a client will choke despite diet modifications, NPO status, or training because of severe weakness, weak coughing reflex, or other reasons. The OTA must be familiar with cardiopulmonary resuscitation (CPR) protocols for clearing the throat of a person who is choking and also know the facility's emergency medical procedures. Despite learning CPR using a mannequin on the floor or a table, it can be an entirely different experience to have a client in a wheelchair with multiple medical issues who is choking. A client may not be actually choking but may be merely having a very hard time coughing something up because of a weak cough reflex or the presence of thick mucus. This type of client may require an assisted cough, and information and an illustration can be found in Chapter 35.

DROOLING

Some clients will have not only difficulty with liquids and foods, but their own saliva. Drooling can be a very challenging and embarrassing symptom of dysphagia for the adult client. Some clients completely stop leaving the house when drooling begins in the course of their progressive disorder. The OT practitioner can provide bibs and other options to collect or manage the drool and certain medications that have a side effect of dry mouth can be helpful. Often, physicians have a difficult time regulating between drooling and severe dry mouth. Botulinum toxin (Botox®) can be injected periodically by a physician into the salivary gland, which can assist to limit drooling, but there are other potential risks. It is important for the client to stay hydrated, so any saliva left does not turn into thick mucus.

FEEDING TUBES

When the client is completely unable to swallow in the short term after an incident, such as a CVA, the physicians may decide to feed the client through a nasogastric (NG) tube, which goes through the nose to the stomach. If the swallowing problems are long term or permanent, a percutaneous endogastric (PEG) tube, commonly called a feeding tube, may be surgically placed through the abdominal wall to the stomach. The PEG tube allows formula, medications, and water to go through the tube for nutrition and medical management. Some clients with PEG tubes learn to care for the tube and manage all feedings independently, in which case the OTA may work with the dietitian and the client on strategies to open cans and water bottles, crush medications, and reach all supplies. Often, food is poured in the tube, and then the client or the caregiver raises the tube so that gravity assists with propelling the liquid through it. Clients who cannot reach up because of weakness may need an adapted tool to assist. Some clients and caregivers are concerned about chemicals and artificial ingredients and will inquire about blending their own foods into a formula. However, this can be difficult, and the dietitian can assist with determining the proper amounts of calories and nutrients. In some clients, swallowing may improve over time, and eventually the tube may be removed and the hole will close easily. It is not unheard of for the tube to be pulled out by an OT practitioner accidently during a transfer or treatment session; therefore, care must be taken to ensure that gait belts, clothing, and other items do not pull on the tube. If the tube does become dislodged, it must quickly be replaced, as the hole can close within 30 minutes. Nursing staff must be immediately notified if they are available on site, or the physician's office must be notified if a feeding tube gets pulled out during a home visit. This may mean a trip to the emergency room if the client is at home and the tube cannot be put back in quickly.

Client's quality of life, cultural background, food and drink preferences, prognosis, and/or the nature of one's dysphagia are just some of the factors that are considered before and during diet modifications. As OTAs, it is crucial to be able to recognize modified diets to maintain dietary compliance during therapy for self-feeding. These diet modifications may also play a role in feeding recommendations. OT practitioners and SLPs work together to maximize safety with feeding and swallowing.

COMPENSATORY STRATEGIES AND PRECAUTIONS

Compensatory strategies are techniques or modifications to behaviors and environments to compensate for an impairment affecting function. With regard to dysphagia, compensatory strategies are utilized to maximize safety with the least restrictive diet. The interdisciplinary team's job is to ensure that clients and/or their caregivers understand the risks of aspiration and the associated medical concerns and to educate and train each client on the importance of consistent strategy use.

The type of strategy or precautions recommended are dependent on the nature of the client's dysphagia, willingness or ability to modify mealtime behaviors, cognitive status, and mental alertness, as well as the client's potential to self-monitor. Common strategies for clients with dysphagia to improve safety and attention during mealtimes include environmental modifications. These modifications are used to reduce distractions in the mealtime environment—for example, turning off the television, positioning the client facing a wall or empty space versus a busy dining area, and/or simplifying the place setting to only the necessary utensils. Appetite and attention to the task of feeding can also be increased through client-centered selection of music and television shows. The color of the room in which clients are fed or self-feeding is also an important consideration. The color orange increases appetite and alertness. Caregivers may bring in photos of the client's home setup to assist the OTA to offer options for environmental modifications.

Positioning recommendations may be provided as a precaution. Common positioning recommendations include having the client sit upright at or as close to 90 degrees as possible to reduce the risk of aspiration. For individuals with esophageal dysphagia or acid reflux, positioning recommendations to remain upright for 30 to 60 minutes after the meal are common. A physician's prescription often indicates how long a client with a traumatic brain injury, cardiac condition, dysphagia, or post-thyroid surgery status need to stay in a supported upright sitting position following a meal. Upright positioning allows for gravity to continue to assist in the process of esophageal transit and reduces the risk of materials flowing upward into the pharynx. The OT practitioner should educate the caregiver that the hospital bed allows for seating the client at about 30 degrees (or less if the client has slid down in the bed). Meals may be better completed in a wheelchair or a more upright chair if 90-degree positioning is required.

No matter the solid consistency, the recommendation may be slowing down eating to allow enough time for adequate chewing. Further recommendations may include the use of different temperatures to increase awareness of the bolus, taking smaller bites and smaller sips, and alternating liquids and solids to reduce the amount of *stasis*, or residue, remaining in the mouth. Some clients may become agitated by constant cues given by caregivers with regard to these recommendations. One strategy is to only offer small amounts of food on the plate at one time and a smaller spoon or fork to slow down the eating. Clients with decreased bolus manipulation, coordination, or propulsion may exhibit larger amounts of residue remaining in the mouth or pharynx following the swallow. For this reason, the recommendation is multiple swallows to safely clear all materials before continuing with a meal.

Some clients with primitive oral motor chewing patterns and reflexes, such as **tongue thrust**, **phasic bite,** and gag will also require these strategies and diet consistency modifications. These holdover reflexes can cause **sialorrhea** (drooling), **bruxism** (grinding of teeth), and difficulty swallowing and chewing. Tongue thrust is often referred to as reverse swallow and is seen when the tongue pushes forward during the attempt to chew and swallow. A phasic bite, in which the jaws move up and down with no lateral movement, is generally ineffective for chewing. The gag reflex can be very strong in some individuals and may hinder swallowing. Many of these patterns and reflexes are seen in adults with cerebral palsy and severe and profound developmental disabilities.

For pharyngeal dysphagia, recommendations vary more and tend to require more training. Some common recommendations include utilizing an effortful swallow, avoiding the use of large straws with liquids, completing multiple swallows, or utilizing more technical strategies to improve the elevation of the larynx, sensation of the pharynx, and protection of the airway. These classic strategies and treatment methods, such as the chin tuck method, may assist in airway protection. In the chin tuck method, the client puts the chin down toward the chest and holds it there during the entire bite/sip and swallow. More research is recommending a neutral head position versus a chin tuck position, unless a MBSS has shown it to be effective for the client with dysphagia. Using a "nosey cup" that has a cut-out for the nose to allow a chin tuck or a small straw with the cup held lower will help clients tuck their chins while swallowing (Fig. 12-6). Recognizing and encouraging continued use of all recommended compensatory strategies by the client and the caregiver to maximize safety is an important skill for OTAs.

A final and imperative consideration in dysphagia is oral hygiene, or the practice of keeping the mouth clean. Compared with oral care in normal-functioning adults, oral care in individuals with dysphagia can be more challenging because of increased residue and decreased oral clearance during the swallowing process. Oral hygiene is a strong predictor of aspiration pneumonia; however, not all individuals who experience aspiration will acquire aspiration pneumonia. Aspiration of bacteria that develops in the oral cavity increases the risk of infections, such as aspiration pneumonia.[22,23] In individuals with NPO status, oral hygiene is of utmost concern because bacteria can form more rapidly in the absence of any food or liquids entering and clearing the mouth. OTAs often assist with ADLs, such as brushing teeth and completing hygiene routines, and it is imperative for them to recognize the importance of oral hygiene, especially in clients who present with dysphagia. For individuals who have swallowing precautions, brushing teeth with toothpaste may present a safety issue; in these cases, using a toothbrush or Toothette® oral swab that is dipped in mouthwash and then shaken or squeezed will provide a pleasant taste without the risks. For individuals on respiratory devices and suction machines, to manage secretions, a special toothbrush can be hooked to the suction machine to prevent fluids going down the airway during brushing.

Dysphagia Treatments

Although treatment for dysphagia is often compensatory and exercise based, other strategies are available for OT practitioners to employ with clients. The first is neuromuscular electrical stimulation (NMES), which involves the placement

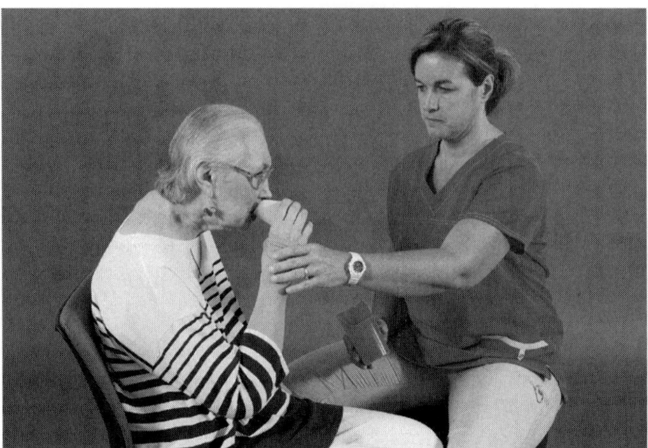

FIGURE 12-6. A nosey cup with chin tuck.

of electrode on the front of the neck, causing a muscle contraction from an electrical current.[16] The research results regarding the effectiveness of NMES are mixed, with some studies showing significant improvement and others modest to no improvement. One study noted that a combination of NMES and exercises may produce the best results.[24] Ice massage and tactile thermal stimulation are often performed to initiate a pharyngeal swallow, with varied results, although some studies showed more improvement with ice massage than with tactile thermal stimulation.[16] Some OT practitioners will use lip, lingual, and/or tongue strengthening exercises, with lingual and tongue strengthening exercises reported in the literature showing improvement in strength[16] but not assisting in functional swallowing.[25] The McNeill Dysphagia Therapy Program focuses on progressive strengthening and coordination of the swallow in the context of functional swallowing activities. A study of this method versus traditional therapy found superior outcomes with the program.[26]

One less-considered aspect of dysphagia is the client's feelings about a feeding tube as far as body image, sexuality, and ability to complete desired occupations, such as swimming laps in the pool or in the ocean. Having a tube protruding from the belly is hardly anyone's definition of sexy, and when inserted long term, can have significant effects on relationships, how a client perceives themselves, and their self confidence. The feeding tube site is also not supposed to be submerged underwater unless completely protected, and coverings can be bulky and difficult to make securely waterproof.

Although the management of dysphagia is mostly addressed by OT practitioners and SLPs, carryover of recommended compensatory strategies, oral hygiene routines, and diet compliance methods can only be achieved with a strong team approach. All therapy professionals rely on each other, clients, staff members, and caregivers to implement the recommendations from all disciplines to maximize function and safety for the client.

COMMUNICATION

Human beings rely on communication every day. There is communication at school, at work, at home, on the road, and at the store. Communication can be with peers, coworkers, family members, teachers, employers, and friends. In each of these interactions, communication methods or devices may be used, including speech, email, telephones, gestures, writing, signals, pictures, texting, and so on, with the ultimate goal of conveying a message.

Modes of Communication

The term communication refers to the sending and receiving of messages between and among individuals. The multiple modes of communication include verbal, nonverbal, and written communication. It is important to understand the benefits and usage of each mode to provide the best client-centered care to each client. Verbal communication defined is as simple as it sounds—speaking and vocalizing meaningful content, such as words, phrases, questions, and directions. Nonverbal communication includes facial expressions and hand expressions, or gesturing. This includes informal gestures, such as pointing, and formal versions of standardized communication, such as American Sign Language. Written communication involves handwriting or typing letters, words, diagrams, shapes, and objects. OTAs need to be able to recognize and/or utilize all modes of communication to effectively provide client-centered care to a wide range of individuals.

Language for Communication

Although communication is more than just spoken language, the ability to speak and be understood as well as to understand language is extremely important. Many individuals take these skills for granted until a challenge occurs. Simple examples are difficulty in understanding what a family member is saying because of a bad cell phone signal or trying to get a point across to someone who does not speak English. Imagine the stress and fear experienced after waking up from a CVA when everything that is said sounds like gibberish. Language has four parts; each will be covered in the following section.

RECEPTIVE COMMUNICATION

Receptive communication is the comprehension, or ability, to understand, language. Receptive communication plays a large role in communication competence, as one must be able to receive, process, and comprehend information to effectively communicate with a partner. For example, in an interaction involving two people sharing a meal, if one says, "Pass the salt, please," the recipient must be able to receptively process the request, understand the action requested, locate and discriminate the salt from the pepper and other items on the table, and complete the action of passing the item to the individual who requested it. Receptive communication is the basis of effectively completing a communication exchange, as one must understand the topic, request, or statement presented to respond appropriately. When the client has receptive communication deficits, the OTA may see the client experiencing difficulty understanding verbal directions. Using gestures, facial expressions, and other nonverbal communication strategies may assist with understanding. Caregivers should be educated to remain patient and to resist the temptation to speak louder to be understood.

EXPRESSIVE COMMUNICATION

Expressive communication refers to interconnecting thoughts, questions, ideas, and concerns with those of the intended recipient(s). Speaking, writing, and gesturing, or any combination of the three, are forms of expressive communication. Using the last example of two people sharing a meal, one individual used expressive communication to request the salt. From an expressive language standpoint, the individual requesting the salt must be able to verbally or gesturally request what is needed or to convey the request through a form of written communication. The individual must also direct this communication to the correct person, assess the outcome of the interaction, and complete the action of accepting the item that was passed. Expressive communication is essential to meeting the wants and needs of each individual as well as for social interaction. Deficits with expressive communication will cause individuals to have significant difficulty making their needs known. The OTA may see frustration in these clients, and they may be upset for no clear reason. Some clients will restate a single word over and over with varying inflection and expression or simply utter nonsensical phrases. See Chapter 33 for further information on these communication deficits.

PARALINGUISTIC COMMUNICATION

Paralinguistic communication refers to the nonverbal parts of communication, such as gasps, sighs, and/or facial expressions. These accessories assist in conveying meaning and emotion during a communication interaction. For example, the facial expressions of an individual who is excited will likely reflect that excitement in a smile, a higher pitch and volume of tone, and an exclamation of his or her elation, resulting in the communication partner understanding the individual's enthusiasm.

To effectively convey the significance of the expressive content, one's paralinguistic actions must be compatible with the verbal or written expression communicated. For instance, an individual who is smiling and appears excited and yet is verbally expressing sadness will cause confusion in his or her communication partner, or the mismatched behaviors may be interpreted as sarcasm. Clients with severe facial weakness, such as those with ALS, may be very happy and amused, but their facial expression remains flat as their muscles can no longer move well. This makes it seem like they are always angry or unhappy, which may not be the case. A client with flat affect from a brain insult or injury may have similar issues. Paralinguistic properties play an important role in effective communication.

PRAGMATIC COMMUNICATION

Pragmatic communication is utilized to explain the verbal and nonverbal rules that govern social communication. These rules include the use of language for different purposes, such as greeting, informing, and requesting. Pragmatics also involve modifying language to meet the needs of the communication partner, such as different ways of speaking at work and on a date; addressing a child and an adult differently; and following rules of conversation, such as taking turns, appropriate eye contact, topic maintenance, and/or repairing communication breakdowns if and when they occur. Pragmatic communication is essential in social interactions to maintain communication competence. In the adult population, pragmatic impairments can occur from CVA, traumatic brain injury, and other neurological deficits. The OTA can often use modeling and role-playing with the client or in a treatment group to address deficits with pragmatics and to bring increased awareness to deficits.

COMMUNICATION IMPAIRMENTS

As discussed, communication is the sending and receiving of messages that can carry ideas, facts, opinions, attitudes, directions, and emotions. Communication plays a vital role in a person's life impacting emotional, physical, and mental well-being. Impairments in communication can be developmental or acquired as a result of CVA, brain injury, tumors, and/or degenerative diseases. Communication impairment is defined as a breakdown in one's ability to receive, send, process, and comprehend information.[27] These impairments can present in the processes of hearing, language, speech, or any combination of the three.

A hearing disorder, such as deafness or hearing difficulty, is the result of an impaired auditory system. Age-related hearing loss is referred to as presbycusis. Impairment in the process of hearing can result in a decrease in one's ability to comprehend information or can reduce the ability for production of clear speech. People with hearing impairments may see an audiologist for a full hearing assessment to correct or compensate for the problem. Other individuals may rely on alternative methods of communication, such as reading/writing and using gestures or sign language. Many adults have some amount of hearing loss, and it is important for the OTA to accommodate their pitch, tone of voice, volume, and speed to be clearly understood. Many times, to be clearly heard, the OT practitioner will not need to increase his or her volume but instead deepen the tone. Hearing aids may not be covered by an individual's insurance or may not work effectively, and often, clients are socially isolated because of their hearing deficit.

An impairment in language may impact one's ability to comprehend and/or express information. Language impairments can affect a person's auditory comprehension, verbal expression, reading, and writing, thereby impacting functional communication. A speech disorder is an impairment in the areas of articulation, fluency, and/or voice. The term articulation refers to the physical production of speech sounds. Fluency means the flow of speech sounds, syllables, words, and sentences and is characterized by a speaker's rate and rhythm during presentation of spoken information. Voice is characterized by vocal quality, loudness, resonance, and pitch. Speech disorders can have a strong impact on an individual's intelligibility, or ability to be understood, in verbal communication exchanges or the presentation of information.

As previously stated, communication plays a vital role in everyone's life. OT practitioners use communication to direct clients in therapeutic activities, to relay information to other health care professionals, and to educate caregivers with strategies and home exercise programs. An important skill for the OTA is having knowledge of different communication disorders and their nature to be able to provide the best client-centered care to those individuals who present with these deficits.

Aphasia

Aphasia is a communication impairment affecting receptive and/or expressive language abilities. Clients can present with mild aphasia, with only minimal word finding deficits, or aphasia that is severe enough to make any communication a challenge. Aphasia is most often the result of a CVA with insult to the left hemisphere of the brain, or the language hemisphere. However, it can also be the result of tumors, brain injury, or neurological disease.

The severity of aphasia varies, depending on the location and impact of insult to the brain. Some of the more common types of aphasia include Broca's aphasia, Wernicke's aphasia, and global aphasia. Broca's aphasia occurs as a result of damage impacting the left frontal area of the brain. This region of the brain is responsible for expressive language abilities, allowing the use of words together to form sentences to communicate. Individuals with Broca's aphasia will present with difficulty with expressive language characterized by placing words together without function words, such as "is," "and," or "the," and/or difficulty with word finding, which is also known as *anomia*. Anomia is the loss of the ability to name, recognize, or recall objects or names; it can be receptive or expressive; can be present at the word level, the phrase level, the sentence level, or the conversation level; and can make communication very frustrating. Imagine yourself with the feeling of having words at the tip of your tongue but being unable to speak them out; individuals with Broca's aphasia face that same feeling daily when trying to communicate simple wants and needs.

Wernicke's aphasia occurs from damage to the posterior portion of the left hemisphere of the brain, impacting comprehension of information. A person with Wernicke's aphasia will present with deficits characterized by a poor understanding of information and the production of sentences that have the correct structure but contain nonsensical words and phrases. Because of this disconnect of comprehension, those with Wernicke's aphasia often will not be able to recognize or understand that their communication is impaired. These individuals can often produce fluent sentences; however, the sentences do not necessarily contain meaningful communication.

Global aphasia occurs when a catastrophic event inflicts extensive insult on the left hemisphere of the brain in multiple areas. Individuals with global aphasia will present with impairments that impact both receptive and expressive language abilities, thereby affecting comprehension as well as expressive communication. Clients with this severe type of aphasia will have a combination of the many deficits in Broca's and Wernicke's aphasia, including difficulty understanding words, phrases, and sentences; difficulty forming words and sentences; disfluencies; use of nonsensical words and utterances; and the inability to recognize or understand that their communication is impaired. Global aphasia is the most severe because it affects more avenues utilized to compensate for impaired communication.

Aphasia may strain or limit one's ability to speak, read, write, and/or comprehend, and this will, as a result, make communication difficult. Although individuals may present with difficulty understanding information and/or expressing themselves, it is crucial to remember that aphasia is an impairment of language and not intellect. In addition, the OTA must remember that clients with impairments in spoken language often will have impairments extending to other modes of communication as well, including reading and writing. These impairments may require OT practitioners to think outside the box, utilize alternative methods of communication, or go above and beyond to communicate with these individuals to provide the best possible therapy (Table 12-5).

Dysarthria

Dysarthria is a motor speech impairment caused by damage to the brain. Some causes of dysarthria include traumatic brain injury, CVA, tumors, and/or progressive neurological diseases, such as Parkinson's disease, Huntington's disease, ALS, or MS. A motor speech disorder, such as dysarthria, results from impaired movement of the muscular structures involved in speech production, including the lips, tongue, vocal folds, and diaphragm, causing muscle weakness that affects speech production. These impairments in movement are a result of damage to areas of the brain responsible for the motor planning, execution, and regulation of the muscles.

A person with dysarthria may experience challenges related to volume, coordination of breathing during speech, tone of voice, vocal quality, timing of muscle movement for articulation, vocal strength, ROM, and speed. The type and severity of a client's dysarthria determines the challenges a client will experience as well as the abnormality or intelligibility of his or her speech. The OTA must be able recognize the presence of a speech impairment to be able to apply appropriate methods of communication during a session. The client with dysarthria may need to write, type on a device, or use gestures to communicate. Many clients will continue to try to talk in spite of their dysarthria, and although familiar listeners, such as caregivers, may understand them, the OTA may need to ask for permission to use an alternative method. Dysarthria may or may not come with any cognitive deficits, so the OTA must not assume a decrease in speech to mean difficulties with thinking.

Apraxia

Apraxia of speech is also a motor speech disorder. It is caused by damage to the area of the brain that is responsible for coordinated and controlled muscle movement; it can be a comorbidity to aphasia or dysarthria. Some causes of apraxia include traumatic brain injury, CVA, tumors,

TABLE 12-5 Suggestions to Improve Effective Communication With a Person With Aphasia

TYPE OF APHASIA	IMPAIRMENTS	STRATEGIES TO INCREASE EFFECTIVE COMMUNICATION
Expressive	Deficits impacting communication of thoughts, emotions and/or ideas	• Encourage the client to utilize gestures and pictures to assist in communication. • Allow additional time for the client to communicate thoughts and ideas. • Offer writing as an alternative or supplement to speaking. • Refer to the SLP for treatment and/or training with a communication aid.
Receptive	Deficits impacting comprehension of information, instructions and/or questions	• Use demonstration paired with written and verbal instructions to direct the client in therapeutic tasks. • Provide a model of exercises. • Use hand-over-hand and tactile assistance to guide a task or exercise. • Break down verbalizations. • Use gestures in addition to verbalizations. • Simplify directions to one at a time. Once each step is mastered, continue to build the task to multistep.
Mixed	Deficits impacting both incoming and outgoing information and/or messages	• Use a combination of some or all the above recommendations. • Be sure to always allow more time for processing information.

and/or progressive neurological disease. In individuals with apraxia, the messages from the brain to the mouth are disrupted—that is, the person trying to communicate cannot move the lips or tongue to the right place to articulate sounds correctly, even though the muscles involved are not weak.[27] A person with apraxia will present with inconsistent speech errors, including difficulty producing speech sounds; repeating words or sounds; speech errors characterized by changing, substituting, or leaving out sounds; and/or a slow speech rate and impaired rhythm and intonation of speech. Individuals with apraxia will often demonstrate groping, or appear to be blindly searching, for the tongue and lips to produce speech sounds or to correct errors. Apraxia, as with other communication disorders, can vary in nature and severity on a case-by-case basis.

Communication disorders come in all shapes, sizes, and severities, and it can often be difficult for an OT practitioner to distinguish one from another. It is important to work together with other disciplines to support clients requiring various compensatory methods for communication. A team approach is always the key to improving the client's overall function and generalization of the trained skills and strategies.

COMPENSATORY STRATEGIES FOR COMMUNICATION

Compensatory strategies for communication serve as a supplement to existing or unaffected communication skills to improve a client's receptive and expressive language abilities. These techniques may involve altering the environment or client behaviors to improve reciprocal communication. During a treatment session, it is imperative to provide an environment that facilitates success because environmental considerations can greatly impact the treatment outcome. Some methods for improving the environment include modifications, such as reducing background noise and distractions by turning off music or the television, removing the client from a noisy or crowded room, and/or reducing clutter in the client's visual field. Removing distracting items from sight, or seating the client facing a less distracting space during therapy, can make the environment more conducive to reciprocal communication. For example, during a therapy session scheduled in the busy gym, it may be beneficial to move the client to the therapy kitchen or outdoors for a quieter environment.

Strategies to maximize effective conversation with an individual who presents with a communication impairment can include using environmental techniques in conjunction with providing face-to-face communication, simplifying instructions and statements to only a few content words, using yes/no questions, or using simple closed-ended questions while providing a field of choices. For example, to simplify instructions, one could say, "use this spoon" while holding up the correct spoon instead of "use the spoon to the right of your plate." To provide a field of options during a simple closed-ended question, one could say, "Do you want these black pants or your blue jeans?" while holding up both options to eliminate distraction. When offering choices or providing simple one- to two-word explanations, holding the objects up to the client, such as holding the food item close to the mouth, will increase his or her understanding and conceptual development. In addition, using multimodal approaches to communicate, such as speaking in conjunction with writing and gesturing, may be effective. For example, writing "stand up" on a whiteboard while modeling and verbalizing the request may be needed to communicate with some clients. It is important to pause between questions, instructions, and statements to allow the individual enough time to process and communicate. The amount of time required to process and respond to conversation or instructions will vary with each individual.

Augmentative and Alternative Communication

Augmentative and alternative communication (AAC) is a term used for all forms of communication other than speaking; this form of communication is utilized to communicate wants, needs, and ideas. The purpose of AAC is to restore an individual's ability to effectively communicate in all aspects of daily life. Individuals with communication impairments can utilize AAC by supplementing intact expressive language or speech abilities or by replacing speech or language with a compensatory AAC system. Systems to replace verbal communication with AAC can include the use of symbols, pictures, and/or written communication and can be simple and low-tech or complex, depending on the needs of the client. A low-tech option might include a pen and a notebook, laser pointer on a wall-mounted letter board, or finger-pointing to pictures or a dry-erase board. High-tech options might be a complex communication device that allows the client to access letters and words by scanning with a toe switch or to type by hovering over a letter and using word prediction with a camera trained at the client's eyes.

It is important for an OTA working with adults with communication impairments to have knowledge of AAC systems to be able to use them to communicate effectively with these clients. For example, writing to communicate with a client via a portable whiteboard or sheet of paper is utilizing AAC. Simple communication boards containing a field of words, such as yes, no, food, drink, and so on, may be used to prompt a client to say a word to communicate a basic need. To help the client express basic needs, the OT practitioner can create a simple communication board using general pictures of items or actual photographs of the client's personal items, such as hair brush, bed, phone, and cup (Fig. 12-7). The more the items on a communication board, the more complex it becomes. Some clients will function better with only a few items on a page whereas others may be able to use boards containing the alphabet, 10 or 15 pictures or words, and/or pain scales.

The growth of technology has led to many easy-to-access forms of AAC. Touch screen cell phones and tablets can be transformed into communication devices with the use of applications created to supplement or replace

OT Practitioner's Viewpoint

I worked with Frances, a client with a diagnosis of dementia, who resided at a skilled nursing facility; she was referred to OT for decreased self-feeding ability. The initial evaluation revealed some discoordination of gross motor skills, but Frances demonstrated good trunk control and no limitations in ROM in any joint. The biggest area of deficit for Frances was found in her cognition and communication. She was often frustrated if her meal was too hot or cold, not cut in the right-sized pieces, or if there was too much noise in the lunchroom. She displayed her frustration by wildly waving her hands for a caregiver's attention, and refusing to eat. The treatment focused on functional communication, including verbal expression of needs via a picture board made specifically for mealtime and education of caregivers on how to best interact with Frances at meals. She was not easy to understand, and the pictures made it quicker for both Frances and the caregivers. The interventions also focused on hand-to-mouth coordination and cutting of food. I practiced with Frances at snack and mealtimes to get her food the size she liked and implemented the use of a large handled, utensil bent towards her mouth as well as a plate guard. As a result of the treatments and the education of Frances and the staff, she became less frustrated and began to complete her meals in a timely fashion. ~ Vivian Resnik, MHA/MBA, OTR/L

COMMUNICATION

The ability to communicate is crucial for relationships, making needs known, and quality of life. Many clients who are unable to speak or be understood note difficulties with communication despite the advances in communication device technology, apps, or other resources. Many times, it is not so much about the ability to communicate simple wants and desires as it is about vocal inflection and meaning, conversational flow with one person or a group, timing of responses and jokes, and overall speed. The average person talks at 110 to 160 words per minute, and the average person types at 40 words per minute. Some clients with AAC devices type on a keyboard, but many use scanning, onscreen keyboards, picture based icons, and other much slower options. Even for those who type, hand weakness and fatigue can slow typing rate even further. A client who uses an AAC device may feel left out of conversations or be embarrassed that the conversation comes to a halt while the group waits for the comment. Sometimes the conversational flow has moved on while the client is still typing the original thought. This can be frustrating, and often the client will avoid social situations he or she used to enjoy.

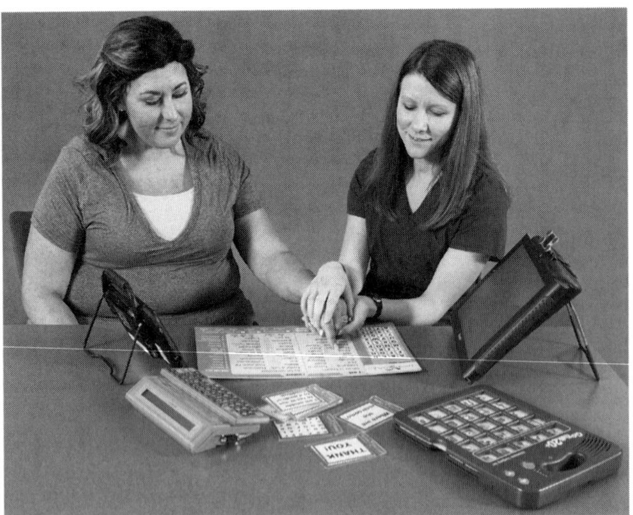

FIGURE 12-7. Simple and complex communication boards.

verbal communication. Phone and tablet devices can carry applications that can be tailored to meet the client's specific needs by creating a general or comprehensive communication board. These communication boards can become interactive with a simple touch of the screen to verbalize a word, phrase, or sentence for the individual. These devices can also be utilized to type out words or sentences or draw pictures to communicate.

Other devices are specifically devoted to running a communication system. These devices can often be customized for individuals with weakness or paralysis, visual impairments, and/or hearing impairments by capitalizing on the client's strengths. For example, a client with ALS may be fitted for an eye gaze communication device. Such a device can be controlled entirely with a camera that notes the position of the client's eyes (retina), enabling him or her to communicate. The access method for a communication device could be typing, touching a switch (technology access method), tapping a touch screen, using eye gaze technology, moving a mouse, or utilizing a head mouse (a camera that reads a reflective dot on the forehead or glasses as the head moves). It is important to note that the average person types at 40 words per minute, whereas the average AAC user is getting out about 8 to 10 words per minute, and this can go up to 12 to 15 words per minute with rate enhancement strategies, such as word prediction.[28] The average English speaker uses 110 to 160 words per minute. This means that no matter how proficient the user of AAC is, social communication abilities will be seriously compromised. See Chapter 14 for further details on devices, switches, and technology.

A specially trained professional, beyond the services of a general practitioner, will complete client evaluation, education, and implementation. The OTA will assist in carrying out the strategies and techniques established by this professional during skilled intervention. This may involve assisting various caregivers to access the device with the client during toileting or bathing and problem-solving how and where to place the device on the table during a meal. The use of alternative communication allows for improved expression in the absence of normal-functioning speech abilities. Gaining familiarity and practice with these alternative methods will improve the OTA's skills when working with diverse client populations.

EVIDENCE-BASED PRACTICE

Pullin and Hennig published an article entitled "17 Ways to Say Yes: Toward Nuanced Tone of Voice in AAC and Speech Technology" in 2015.[29] This article discusses that all AAC devices speak in a monotone, and clients lose all nuances of speech, such as tone of voice, emotion, and expressiveness, affecting intent. Think for a moment about the numerous ways an English speaker can say the word "really." It can be a question, a statement of disbelief, a note of excitement, or a sarcastic comment. As a person with amyotrophic lateral sclerosis (ALS) who used a speech-generating device (SGD) as part of communication, Colin Portnuff described his need for more expressive tone of voice: "I want to be able to sound sensitive or arrogant, assertive or humble, angry or happy, sarcastic or sincere, matter of fact or suggestive and sexy."[30] Pullin and Hennig noted that part of the reason for the lack of tone of voice is the incredible complexity of adding it to AAC devices, when combined with issues of culture and native language, gender, speech patterns, and emotions ranging from boredom to hatred or happiness. Technology exists that uses the client's own voice (called voice banking). The client speaks numerous phrases into a database which tries to harvest sounds, words, speech patterns and other individual aspects of speech. The difficulty often lies in that clients are already losing intelligibility by the time they seek voice banking. Other clients simply record phrases such as " I love you" in their own voice to add to the ACC device at a later point. The article also discussed the need for open dialogues and forums, as well as research into the ability to initially assign a tone of voice to a statement and later to have it naturally occur in the output from an AAC device.

Pullin, G., & Hennig, S. (2015). 17 Ways to say yes: Toward nuanced tone of voice in AAC and speech technology. Augmentative and Alternative Communication, *31(2), 170–180. http://doi.org/10.3109/07434618.2015.1037930;*

Portnuff C. (2006). Augmentative and alternative communication: A user's perspective. *Lecture delivered at the Oregon Health and Science University. Retrieved from http://aac-rerc.psu.edu/index-8121.php.html*

TECHNOLOGY AND TRENDS

Some clients with severe disorders, such as amyotrophic lateral sclerosis (ALS) use communication devices after they lose their voice. They may start with typing with both hands, but as the disease progresses, they may have to use one finger, head pointing, scanning with a switch, or eye gaze. Depending on the progression, having a consistent muscle movement to press a switch becomes nearly impossible. A newer switch called an *EMG switch* uses minute electrical impulses from muscle contractions and turns that impulse into switch control. The input to the EMG switch comes from electrodes placed on the skin, and the EMG switch continuously monitors the signal under the electrodes. When the signal level exceeds an adjustable threshold (as when the muscle twitches as the client attempts to contract it), it provides the switch action. Almost any controllable single muscle on the body can be used to control the EMG Switch, such as pectoral muscles, brow muscles, jaw muscles, cheek muscles, and others. Many severely impaired clients can still communicate for much longer with the aid of this technology.

IMPLEMENTATION OF STRATEGIES DURING OCCUPATIONS

As a member of the larger team, following through with the recommendations and suggestions from other team members is essential to best serve clients. Incorporating strategies from other disciplines can progress the goals set by the supervising occupational therapist for the betterment of the client. For example, assume that an SLP determines that a diet modification from regular solids to a mechanical soft diet should be made for a client with difficulty swallowing. Based on the diet modifications, the OT plan will change as well. Cutting is no longer required for self-feeding tasks, and there may be increased use of a spoon versus a fork for bringing food to the mouth. Work, leisure, social, and sexuality issues in addition to ADL and IADL tasks may need to be addressed for the client who drools, has a feeding tube, or who has communication difficulties. A client who has dysarthria and drives must plan ahead for a traffic stop so an officer does not think the client is drunk due to garbled speech. A young mother with ALS may look for strategies for drooling management before meeting her child's kindergarten teacher for the first time. Many clients with language and communication deficits as client factors will experience difficulties with performance skills in relation to occupations as well. These deficits may include an impact on simple tasks, such as asking for a drink of water or expressing the need to use the toilet, to complex tasks, such as banking, map reading, and following verbal or written directions for cooking or setting up a new computer. These difficulties with occupations may mean that despite their excellent physical skills, some clients cannot resume role participation or full independence after an injury or event. It is important to consider the client holistically, and see beyond the disability to the impact the change has on all aspects of life.

SUMMARY

When entering the field of OT, an understanding of impairments and treatments for individuals with self-feeding, swallowing, and communication deficits is essential. These skills play a large role in the client's social interaction, function, and quality of life and are a priority for providing client-centered treatment. Self-feeding, swallowing, and communication are multisensory tasks and require a holistic approach to improve function and achieve goals.

Back to the original scene. Thanksgiving Day, surrounded by family and friends, mouthwatering food abounds at the table. This time, however, the client is not isolated. Family and loved ones understand the person's needs for self-feeding, swallowing, and communication, assimilating and accommodating these needs at the table. The table bears a plate full of the favorite foods of the correct consistency and a cup with a lid and a straw; the hostess has turned down the background music for easier communication. It is important for the OTA to recognize the larger impact each treatment session will have on a client's life, and to always be working toward the client's goals.

REVIEW QUESTIONS

1. While working with a client on feeding skills during a meal, the client presents with a severe cough accompanied by a wet, gurgly vocal quality. It is likely that this client has dysphagia that is:
   a. Pharyngeal
   b. Abdominal
   c. Epiglottal
   d. Nasal
2. During a feeding session, you are working with a client on a diet of pureed solids and nectar-thick liquids. Which of the following would be appropriate to provide?
   a. Cold cereal with milk
   b. Ice cream
   c. Pudding
   d. Bacon and eggs
3. A client who presents with a communication impairment characterized by difficulty articulating messages correctly in the absence of muscle weakness likely has:
   a. Dysphagia
   b. Apraxia
   c. Dysarthria
   d. Aphasia
4. When focusing on self-feeding skills with a client with tremors, which of the following pieces of adaptive equipment is not recommended?
   a. Plastic cup with lid and spout
   b. Scoop plate
   c. Mobile arm support
   d. Weighted utensils
5. Which of the following is an example of utilizing a multimodal approach to communication during a session?
   a. Modeling an exercise in a group setting
   b. Verbalizing instructions in a quiet environment
   c. Providing written instructions in conjunction with verbal instructions and further supplementing with a demonstration of the task
   d. Providing tactile cues during an exercise using weights

6. James has Parkinson's disease and is referred to OT services in his nursing home for assistance with self-feeding breakfast while still reclined in bed. Nursing says he makes a mess and often tires partway through the meal. What might be the first option the OTA would try the next morning?
   a. Get James sitting more upright, either in the bed or in the wheelchair.
   b. Use a Liftware Steady™ spoon.
   c. Decrease the distractions by turning off the TV during the meal.
   d. Alert nursing that James requires to be fed.
7. When substances enter the airway below the level of the vocal folds, it is referred to as:
   a. Penetration
   b. Aspiration
   c. Dysphagia
   d. Apraxia
8. A client with MS has severe dysarthria and mild cognitive deficits. The family has noted the client has difficulty spelling words with the communication device that utilizes a keyboard. Which three of the following might be included as the next options for this client?
   a. Picture-based board using familiar items
   b. Eye gaze communication
   c. Text to speech on her phone
   d. Board with common words and phrases
   e. Word prediction on current device
   f. Adapted stylus for using tablet based communication
9. Mrs. Cannon has moderate dysphagia with difficulty swallowing thin liquids. She also has some weakness in her dominant UE. The preferred positioning for her to self-feed is:
   a. Side-lying with a pillow between the knees only
   b. Reclined to a 120-degree seat to back angle in wheelchair
   c. Seated with hips, knees, and ankles in 90-degree angles with table height promoting elbow flexion at 90 degrees
   d. Seated in a soft chair with deep cushions
10. John is a 56-year-old gentleman with a recent diagnosis of CVA. He has dominant right-sided weakness, with decreased hand grip, right visual inattention, and receptive language deficits. Which three of the following might be strategies the OTA could employ at the first self-feeding session?
   a. Sitting back and observing John at the meal
   b. Setting the table with a large-handled spoon and U-cuff
   c. Setting the table with the plate in midline
   d. Setting the table with the plate completely on the left side
   e. Giving multiple verbal directions to assist John during the meal
   f. Using gestures and few words during the self-feeding session

CASE STUDY

Phyllis is a 79-year-old female who resides in an assisted living facility. She was diagnosed with Parkinson's disease (PD) approximately 20 years ago, and as her disease progressed, she required more assistance, resulting in a move from her daughter's home with family assistance to an assisted living facility. Before the onset of PD, Phyllis worked as an art and theater instructor at a local college. She was often involved in creating props for theatrical events, instructing students in role play, and leading musical arrangements. According to her daughter, Phyllis always prided herself on her social and acting skills; however, because of the changes in her physical status with the disease progression and the change in her environment, she has had to modify her favorite activities. At this time, Phyllis' favorite hobbies at the facility include spending time in the gardens, joining the chorus club, and attending meals with friends in the dining room.

Phyllis recently noticed a significant increase in right hand weakness and difficulty swallowing. Nursing staff also reported decreased safety with her power mobility device. Because of her increasing difficulties, Phyllis has had consultations for skilled occupational and speech therapy. An occupational therapist has completed her evaluation, and an OTA is scheduled to work with her in her next therapy session.

While preparing for the session and reviewing her goals, one goal noted by the OTA is for Phyllis to address self-feeding. Phyllis is on a modified diet of mechanical solids and nectar-thick liquids.

1. What might the OTA work on with this client?
2. What types of adaptive equipment would be helpful?

PUTTING IT ALL TOGETHER Sample Treatment and Documentation

Setting	An assisted living facility
Client Profile	Ms. M., 66 y/o female presents with decreased ability for self-feeding, as reported by caregivers in dining room. The registered dietitian assessed weight loss during recent visit and expressed concerns regarding the client's intake of liquids and solids. The client was discharged from speech therapy services approximately 1 month ago, and is currently on a mechanical soft diet with thin liquids.
Work History	Retired for approximately 10 years from job as purchasing agent
Insurance	Medicare part B primary (covers 80% of therapy costs); AARP private insurance secondary (covers remaining 20%—client has already met deductible for this plan)
Psychological	No DSM-IV diagnosis. Multiple caregivers report increased "outbursts" during meals. Decreased attention, increased agitation, inappropriate behaviors
Social	The client has 2 adult children living locally. They visit often.
Cognitive	Alzheimer's disease. A & O x 1

PUTTING IT ALL TOGETHER Sample Treatment and Documentation (continued)

Motor & Manual Muscle Testing (MMT)	BUE AROM 100% of normal range MMT BUE: 4-/5 R hand dominant Gross motor coordination intact Fine motor coordination minimally impaired Sensation grossly intact BUE Tone normal BUE Moderate impairments with motor planning
ADL	Max A for ADLs; supervision to Min A for transfers; Min A holding her hand for all functional mobility
IADL	The client enjoys watching TV. Leisure activities significantly limited due to severely impaired cognition
Goals	In 30 days: 1. The client will increase fine motor coordination of BUE to 100% accuracy in order to complete self-care tasks. 2. The client will effectively use least restrictive assistive device to feed self 100% of meal increasing to Mod A requiring 75% verbal instruction/cues. 3. The client will verbalize wants and needs during meals 3/5 times and 75% verbal instruction/cues. 4. The client will demonstrate adequate sustained and divided attention for self-feeding with Mod A for 50% of meal.

OT TREATMENT SESSION 1

THERAPEUTIC ACTIVITY	TIME	GOAL(S) ADDRESSED	OTA RATIONALE
Limitation of items presented visually during meal to one dish at a time for decreased divided attention and problem-solving needs	5 min	#2, #3, and #4	*Preparatory Task; Education and Training:* Decreased number of items on table limits need for divided attention. The client is better able to attend to what is in front of them and more successfully self-feed.
Education provided to caregivers in dining room regarding decreased field of choices at mealtime	10 min	#2, #3, and #4	*Education and Training:* Education of caregivers promotes unified front to provide best practice to the client. This also facilitates increased carryover of strategies taught during skilled intervention, as the client is unable to recall new information due to progression of Alzheimer's dementia.
Fine motor coordination utilizing various grasp patterns for items presented during meal	45 min	#1 and #2	*Occupations:* Determination of functional grasp patterns that are most habituated for client with plans to compensate mealtime needs as client is able

SOAP note: 10/7/—, 12:00 pm–1:00 pm

S: "I like pickles. I don't like when people rush me."

O: Client participated in skilled OT in community dining room for lunch meal this date. Seated at "assistance table" with caregiver to provide feeding assistance. Client's lunch arrived with three items on plate. OTA removed sandwich and placed on small plate, with original plate removed from client's visual field. Client was able to grasp sandwich and coordinate sequence to bring to mouth with no cues. Following completion of sandwich, plate with other items placed in front of client for continued completion of lunch meal. Able to sequence scooping with spoon for remainder of meal 8/11 attempts. Integration of eating and drinking during meal noted with min cuing.

A: Client required 75% initial verbal cues for attention during self-feeding, progressing to 50% verbal cues as meal progressed. Limitation of items present provides increased ability for sustained attention by the client this date. Finger foods are successful for the resident with 100% accuracy. Fine motor coordination becomes increasingly impaired as the client fatigues. The client will benefit from continued skilled OT to increase fine motor coordination, grasp strength, and cognitive skills for increased independence with self-feeding.

P: Continue with established intervention plan. Next visit with focus on functional grasp patterns for increased manipulation of utensils and other items at meals. Follow-up with supervising occupational therapist regarding need for formal education with dining room staff to implement compensatory strategies.

Evelyn Planer, COTA/L, 10/7/—, 1:10 pm

TREATMENT SESSION 2:

What could you do next with this client?

TREATMENT SESSION 3:

What could you do next with this client?

REFERENCES

1. Clark, G. F., Avery-Smith, W., Wold, L. S., Anthony, P., Holm, S. E. (2007). Specialized knowledge and skills in feeding, eating, and swallowing for occupational therapy practice. *American Journal of Occupational Therapy, 61*(6), 686–700.
2. American Occupational Therapy Association. (2014). Occupational therapy practice framework: Domain and process (3rd ed.). *American Journal of Occupational Therapy, 68*(Suppl. 1).
3. Plastow, N. A., Atwal, A., & Gilhooly, M. (2015). Food activities and identity maintenance among community-living older adults: A grounded theory study. *American Journal of Occupational Therapy, (69)*6, 6906260010p1-6906260010p10.
4. McGruder, J., Cors, D., Tiernan, A. M., & Tomlin, G. (2003). Weighted wrist cuffs for tremor reduction during eating in adults with static brain lesions. *American Journal of Occupational Therapy, 57*, 507–516.
5. Meshack, R. P., & Norman, K. E. (2002). A randomized controlled trial of the effects of weights on amplitude and frequency of postural hand tremor in people with Parkinson's disease. *Clinical Rehabilitation, 16*(5), 481–492.
6. What is essential tremor? (n.d.). Retrieved from www.hopkins medicine.org.
7. Eye Health Topics. (n.d.). Retrieved from https://nei.nih.gov/health.
8. Warren, M. (2009). Pilot study on activities of daily living limitations in adults with hemianopsia. *American Journal of Occupational Therapy, 63*(5), 626–633.
9. Types of attention. (n.d.). Retrieved from http://thepeakperformance center.com.
10. Lewis, S. C. (2003). *Elder care in occupational therapy*. Thorofare, NJ: SLACK Incorporated.
11. Cattie, J. E., Doyle, K., Weber, E., Grant, I., Woods, S. P., & The HIV Neurobehavioral Research Program (HNRP) Group. (2012). Planning deficits in HIV-associated neurocognitive disorders: Component processes, cognitive correlates, and implications for everyday functioning. *Journal of Clinical and Experimental Neuropsychology, 34*(9), 906–918.
12. Aguilera, A., Pi-Fiquews, M., Arellano, M., Torres, R. M., García-Caselles, M. P., Robles, M. J., ... & Cervera A. M. (2009). Previous cognitive impairment and failure to thrive syndrome in patients who died in a geriatric convalescence hospitalization unit. *Archives of Gerontology and Geriatrics Suppl, 9*, 7–11.
13. Verdery, R. B. (1997). Clinical evaluation of failure to thrive in older people. *Clinics in Geriatric Medicine, 13*(4), 769–778.
14. Robertson, R. G., & Montagnini, M. (2004). Geriatric failure to thrive. *American Family Physician, 70*(2), 343–350.
15. Kumeliauskas, L., Fruetel, K., & Holroyd-Leduc, J. M. (2013). Evaluation of older adults hospitalized with a diagnosis of failure to thrive. *Canadian Geriatrics Journal, 16*(2), 49–53.
16. Vose, A., Nonnenmacher, J., Singer, M., & Gonzalez-Fernandez, M. (2014). Dysphagia management in acute and sub-acute stroke. *Current Physical Medicine and Rehabilitation Reports, 2*(4), 197–206.
17. Matsuo, K. & Palmer, J. B. (2008). Anatomy and physiology of feeding and swallowing–Normal and abnormal. *Physical Medicine Rehabilitation Clinicians of North America, 19*(4), 691–707.
18. Humbert, I. A., & Robbins, J. (2008). Dysphagia in the elderly. *Physical Medicine Rehabilitation Clinicians of North America, 19*(4), 853.
19. Higashijima, M. (2010). Influence of age and bolus size on swallowing function: Basic data and assessment method for care and preventive rehabilitation. *American Journal of Occupational Therapy, 64*, 88–94.
20. Hansen, T., Lambert, H. C., & Faber, J. (2012). Ingestive skill difficulties are frequent among acutely-hospitalized frail elderly clients, and predict hospital outcomes. *Physical & Occupational Therapy in Geriatrics, 30*(4), 271–287.
21. Ney, D. M., Weiss, J. M., Kind, A. J., & Robbins, J. (2009). Senescent swallowing: Impact, strategies and interventions. *Nutrition Clinical Practice, 24*, 395–413.
22. Coker, E., Ploeg, J., Kaasalainen, S., & Fisher, A. (2013). A concept analysis of oral hygiene care in dependent older adults. *Journal of Advanced Nursing, 69*(10), 2360–2371.
23. Yoon, M. N., & Steele, C. M. (2013). Monitoring oral colonization as a risk for pneumonia in complex continuing care: Lessons learned from a pilot study. *Canadian Journal of Speech-Language Pathology & Audiology, 37*(2), 134–145.
24. Miller, S., Jungheim, M., Kuhn, D., & Ptok, M. (2013). Electrical stimulation in treatment of pharyngolaryngeal dysfunctions. *Folia Phoniatrica et Logopaedica, 65*, 154–168.
25. Di Pede, C., Mantovani, M. E., Del Felice, A., & Masiero, S. (2016). Dysphagia in the elderly: Focus on rehabilitation strategies. *Aging Clinical and Experimental Research, 28*(4), 607–617.
26. Carnaby-Mann, G. D., & Crary, M. A. (2010). McNeill dysphagia therapy program: A case-control study. *Archives of Physical Medicine and Rehabilitation, 91*, 743–749.
27. American Speech-Language-Hearing Association. (1993). Definitions of communication disorders and variations [Relevant Paper]. Retrieved from www.asha.org/policy.
28. Higginbotham, D. J., Shane, H., Russell, S., & Caves, K. (2007). Access to AAC: Present, past, and future. *Augmentative and Alternative Communication, 23*(3), 243–257.
29. Pullin, G., & Hennig, S. (2015). 17 Ways to say yes: Toward nuanced tone of voice in AAC and speech technology. *Augmentative and Alternative Communication, 31*(2), 170–180.
30. Portnuff, C. (2006). Augmentative and alternative communication: A user's perspective. Lecture delivered at the Oregon Health and Science University. Retrieved from http://aac-rerc.psu.edu/index-8121.php.html

ACKNOWLEDGMENTS

I would like to thank Dr. Kelli Fellows from Pfeiffer University for assisting with editing and bringing a non-healthcare professional's perspective to the information.

Chapter 13

Transfers Across the Continuum: Safety and Management

Jennifer C. Radloff, OTD, OTR/L, CDRS and Helen Houston, MS, OTR/L

LEARNING OUTCOMES

After studying this chapter, the student or practitioner will be able to:

13.1 Demonstrate basic principles of body mechanics for transferring clients safely

13.2 Explain the importance of back injury prevention principles in relationship to transfers

13.3 Describe the multiple factors that help determine the type of transfer to use with a client

13.4 Discuss the steps needed to complete traditional transfers to a variety of surfaces

13.5 Explain the different lift systems that are used for clients who require significant assistance

13.6 Discuss modifications to traditional transfers to accommodate for unique needs of clients with specific diagnoses

KEY TERMS

Assistive devices	Side-scoot transfer
Body mechanics	Squat-pivot transfer
Injury prevention	Standing lift
Orthostatic hypotension	Stand-pivot transfer
Pressure injuries	Stand-step transfer
Safe-patient-handling (SPH) equipment	Transfer
Shearing forces	Transfer belts
	Transfer boards

The ability to move in one's environment equates to independence in many of an individual's desired occupations. When considering an average day, a person will **transfer** (move from one site to another) out of the bed in the morning, transfer to the commode for toileting, transfer into the shower or bathtub for bathing, transfer to furniture in the living room and dining room, and transfer in and out of a vehicle to access the community to participate in work, school, shopping, and socializing, which also contains various types of transfers. When experiencing an illness or injury, this will often result in the need for assistance with transfers. The occupational therapy assistant (OTA), along with most medical professionals, will need to assist clients with transferring from one surface to another. This chapter will provide education on reducing risk of injury during transfers, use of good body mechanics, factors to consider before assisting with a transfer, appropriate methods and techniques used to perform transfers, determining which transfer to use, and proper use and positioning of assistive devices.

INJURY PREVENTION

Healthcare workers have one of the highest incidence rates of nonfatal work-related injuries among all U.S. workers; many of these injuries are attributed to transferring clients.[1] What constitutes many of the work-related injuries are higher-risk client-handling activities, including repositioning clients in bed and transferring clients to a variety of surfaces.[2] Researchers have found that occupational therapy (OT) practitioners have an annual injury incidence rate of 16.5 injured per 100 full-time workers and found that practitioners are poor self-reporters of injuries.[3] Training on proper body mechanics that should be used when transferring clients is one step toward reducing potential for work-related injuries. When working with clients who require significant assistance or are dependent, severely debilitated, or bariatric, practitioners should use **safe-patient-handling (SPH) equipment**. Examples of SPH equipment include manual and electric portable lifts, overhead track lifts, and standing-aid lifts. Use of this equipment has been found to reduce work-related injuries.[4] This chapter will provide information on manual (traditional) transfers as well as dependent transfers using SPH equipment.

Body Mechanics

Body mechanics is a term that conveys the concept of how to best position the body in space and has foundational principles in anatomy and kinesiology. This is one reason OT practitioners have core classes in these areas as part of their academic preparation. Having this foundational understanding promotes increased efficiency of movement and reduces the possibility of injury.[5] When transferring a client, the practitioner should always follow primary guidelines for proper body mechanics (Table 13-1).

Gaining an understanding of and being able to consistently use good body mechanics is very important, but it is not the only factor that ensures a safe transfer. The OTA should also become skilled at practicing the different types of transfers, problem-solving different scenarios that they might encounter when transferring clients, and using the best methods for educating and training clients and caregivers about proper body mechanics, safe transfers, and fall prevention. By gaining and implementing these skills, practitioners will be prepared for different scenarios that they may face and will ultimately prevent injuring themselves.

Educating and Training Clients and Caregivers

Clients who have disorders or diseases that result in disability may need assistance with transferring or may have a modified method for completing transfers independently. It is important for the practitioner to educate clients and caregivers about proper body mechanics to reduce their risk of injury. Many times, clients and caregivers will opt for efficiency in transfers; however, the long-term consequence for both clients and their caregivers may be wear and tear on joints and muscles, resulting in the need for therapeutic intervention, medications, or surgery to repair preventable damage to the body. Therefore, the OTA has a responsibility not only to train the client and the caregiver how to perform a safe transfer but also to explain why the methods that the client and caregiver have been taught can prevent future injuries. Fall prevention information should also be provided to clients and caregivers with the goal of reducing potential injuries. Last, the clients and caregivers may encounter situations, typically environmental, in which they are unable to perform the transfer steps exactly as taught. After learning about good body mechanics, the client and the caregiver will be more equipped to problem-solve in the situation and make the safest decision to protect their bodies from injury.

PREPARING FOR TRANSFERS

Before beginning any transfer, the OTA should consider his or her own physical abilities, client factors, optimal body positioning for the practitioner and the client, the environment, type of transfer belt, assistive devices, and the goal of the transfer, all of which impact the success of the transfer. The supervising occupational therapist should provide direction and guidance in deciding which type of transfer to use. Additionally, when decisions need to be made with

TABLE 13-1 Primary Guidelines for Proper Body Mechanics

GUIDELINE	POSITIONING	RATIONALE
Position self close to the client while maintaining normal spinal alignment.	Flex at hips, knees, and ankles with the head/neck in slight flexion.	Maintains center of gravity
	Scoot client to the front edge of the surface that he or she is sitting on and ensure that the hips, knees, and ankles are flexed.	Maintains the client's center of gravity and positions him or her closer to you in preparation for the transfer
Ensure a good base of support (pelvis and lower extremities).	Stagger the feet, one more forward than the other, and about shoulder width apart.	Allows for weight shifting between the lower extremities during the transfer
Use knee(s) to block client's knee(s).	Use either inside and/or outside of the knee to block opposing side of client's knee.	Provides support to weaker lower extremity(ies) to prevent buckling of client's knee(s)
Avoid twisting of the trunk.	Isometrically contract trunk muscles.	Reduces chance of twisting at the trunk
Do not use arms to lift the client.	Ensure shoulders are in no greater than 45 degrees of flexion, elbows are flexed and in locked position, and wrists are in neutral position.	Prevents injuries to the upper extremities
Weight shift in unison with the client.	Perform small rocking motions to promote weight shifting.	Produces counterbalancing of load between practitioner and client

regard to selection of assistive mobility devices, assistive transferring devices, and durable medical equipment (DME), the supervising occupational therapist must be consulted to ensure agreement with the intervention plan.

Client Factors and Performance Skills

When preparing to transfer a client, the practitioner must consider various *client factors* and *performance skills* that can directly impact the success and safety of the transfer. *The Occupational Therapy Practice Framework: Domain and Process, 3rd edition* (OTPF-3), identifies client factors as mental, sensory, motor, cardiovascular, respiratory, and skin functions.[6] Performance skills categories include motor skills, process skills, and social interaction skills.[6]

Mental functions include sustained attention, memory, sequencing, alertness, orientation, and accurate perception of sensory information. Examples of process skills include pacing, initiating, continuing, and terminating. Unanticipated limitations, such as decreased alertness, inability to initiate a task, or inability to follow directions by a client during a transfer, could lead to increased risk of injury.[3]

Sensory functions include vision, hearing, vestibular system, touch, pain, pressure, and proprioception. Motor functions include joint mobility and stability, muscle power and tone, and reflexes and voluntary control of movement. Examples of motor skills are bending, coordinating, and calibrating. An older client who has sustained a cerebrovascular accident (CVA) and has a history of diabetes could have reduced proprioception (sense of position in space) as a result of neuropathy, reduced joint mobility, and limited ability to calibrate movements because of neurological changes. The OT practitioner has to take all of these factors into account when considering the best method for safely transferring the client.

Cardiovascular functions (blood pressure, heart rate, and rhythm) and respiratory functions (rate, rhythm, and depth) work in tandem for physical endurance. Skin functions include consideration of skin integrity and prevention of wounds. During transfers, friction and **shearing forces** (e.g., pushing skin one direction and bone/muscle in another) are likely to occur on the client's skin. This typically happens along the buttocks, specifically to the skin over the ischial tuberosities when the client slides forward or backward along the bed, wheelchair seat, or when inaccurately using a transfer board (e.g., client should not slide). The soft tissues of the scapulae, elbows, and heels are also common areas that receive significant shearing forces when the client is lying or repositioning in bed and when transferring onto or out of a bed.

Social interaction skills, such as producing speech, questioning, or replying, improve communication between the client and the practitioner when conducting transfers. The more information the OTA can glean about specific client factors and performance skills deficits, the better the OTA will be able to predict the level of assistance the client will require and how best to educate the client or caregiver.

Occupational Therapy Assistant's Physical Abilities

Reflecting on the client factors and performance skills listed above, the OT practitioner must be aware of his or her own strengths and limitations in each of these areas. When deciding between a manual transfer and use of SPH equipment, OTAs should consider:

- Their own height and weight in comparison to the height and weight of the client
- The amount of physical assistance level required by the client
- The ability of the client to actively participate in the transfer
- The best form of communication with the client, the caregiver(s), and other medical professionals to ensure success of the transfer

Body Positioning

Before beginning any transfer, consider the best use of body mechanics, the assistance level of the client, and the surface to which the client is being transferred. In many surface-to-surface transfers, the practitioner may choose to position himself or herself in the front of the client at midline for best mechanical advantage when dealing with clients who need a significant amount of physical assistance. When using assistive mobility devices, such as a walker, the OTA may choose to position himself or herself to the side of the client for best use of proper body mechanics.

When considering body positioning, the OTA should determine the goal of the transfer. If the goal is to enable the client to eventually transfer independently or to participate as much as possible in the transfer, then every attempt should be made to position the client to where the client can assist with the transfer. In certain situations, the goal may be for the caregiver to transfer the client; this requires careful consideration of best body positioning to promote the safety of both the caregiver and the client. An additional consideration is that if the client has any type of restrictions (e.g., weight-bearing precautions), body positioning of the practitioner or the caregiver and of the client will need to be adjusted to promote adherence to these restrictions.

Preparing Environment for Transfer

Consideration of the environment is very important when preparing for a transfer. The environment includes furniture (e.g., bed, chair, tables), lighting (e.g., overhead, lamp, incandescent), assistive devices (e.g., mobility devices and DME), flooring surfaces (e.g., smooth versus textured), medical equipment (e.g., oxygen lines, intravenous lines, and catheter tubing), and obstacles (e.g., clutter, throw rugs). When transferring from one surface to another, it is optimal to have transfer surfaces that are equal in height, nonmoving, firm, and close in proximity. However, this is not always possible, depending on the environment, client factors, and other variables.

Before a transfer, hospital bed wheels should be placed in the locked position. Wheelchair locks should be fully engaged and accessories, such as arm or leg rests, should be moved out of the path of movement. All medical equipment (e.g., intravenous lines and catheter tubing) should be positioned before moving the client so that there is no tugging or pulling on the lines during the transfer. Always consider the ending position when clearing lines and leads. When transferring to surfaces in the bathroom, the use of DME (e.g. raised toilet seats, tub benches) should be considered if its use would promote the client's independence and increase his or her safety. Assistive mobility devices, such as walkers or canes, should be placed such that they support the client and do not hinder the safety of the transfer. To reduce the risk of falls, it is important to ensure that the immediate environment is free of clutter and that the client is wearing proper footwear (e.g., shoes or anti-slip socks).

Transfer Belt Application

Most institutions require the application of **transfer belts,** also referred to as *gait belts*, when transferring or mobilizing a client to decrease the risk of falls or injury during a transfer. Transfer belts should be positioned low on the client's waist (just above the iliac crests) and snug to prevent slipping along the abdomen and trunk. The transfer belt may need to be tightened when the client comes to the standing position from the seated position and may need to be loosened when returning to the seated position.

Special consideration of transfer belt placement should be given if a gastrointestinal tube, colostomy bag, chest tube, or other medical devices are present along the client's abdomen, back, or sides of the trunk. The transfer belt should never be placed over any medical device. In these situations, the transfer belt is placed around the client's upper chest, just underneath the axillae, or low on the hips to avoid riding up and pulling tubes. When working with bariatric clients, if a single transfer belt will not fit the client's waist, two buckle-style transfer belts can be joined to increase the overall length allowing for a transfer belt to be used. Longer transfer belts can be obtained for long-term use for these clients.

Several types of transfer belts are available (Fig. 13-1). They are available in different widths, lengths, and fabrics, such as those that are washable, antimicrobial, or disposable; they can have plastic or metal buckles, or Velcro® closures. Some transfer belts have integrated handles to keep the wrists in neutral and to facilitate ease of grasp for care providers.

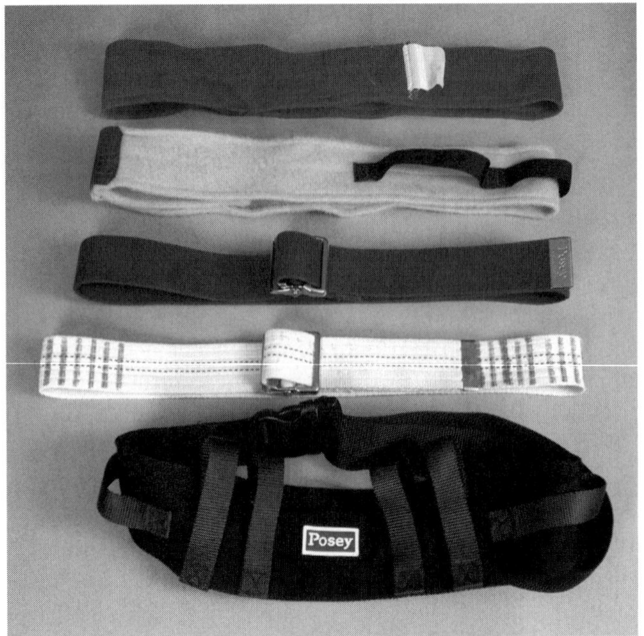

FIGURE 13-1. Types of transfer belts.

Assistive Devices

Some clients will be unable to transfer to the standing position. The reason may be neurological impairment, weakness, weight-bearing limitations, or cognitive impairment; these clients will require an adaptive way of transferring between surfaces. An adaptive way of transferring simply means a side-scoot, partial-stand, or squat-pivot transfer between surfaces. These will be described in detail later. Some clients may require additional assistive devices, such as transfer boards, to increase the safety of the transfer. Assistive devices can help compensate for client weakness and/or increased distance or height difference between surfaces.

Transfer boards are flat, smooth boards made of wood or plastic and vary in length, weight-bearing capacity, weight, shape, and function (Fig. 13-2A). Certain types of transfer boards have an additional feature to reduce friction and to facilitate glide by incorporating a dynamic component that moves with the client, a decreased friction cloth feature, or by adding rollers within the board itself.[7] Push-up blocks are an assistive device that the client can use to increase the mechanical advantage of the upper extremities for providing weight shifting off of the buttocks (see Fig. 13-2B). Pivot discs can be used with clients who are able to bear weight through the lower extremities but are unable to easily move their lower extremities and buttocks while in the sitting position (see Fig. 13-2C). The pivot disc allows a caregiver to rotate the client from one surface to another without the need to move the client's feet. When nonmovable surfaces are farther apart, a transfer platform device may be used for a client who has challenges with moving lower extremities when in a weight-bearing position (see Fig. 13-2D). However, with this device, the client should be able to assist with the transfer while transitioning from sitting to standing.

Decision Making

To ascertain which type of transfer to use with a client, it is necessary to consider the following factors in addition to those already discussed. The overriding principle is ensuring the safety for all concerned; it is imperative to not cause harm to clients, practitioners, or caregivers. The "just right

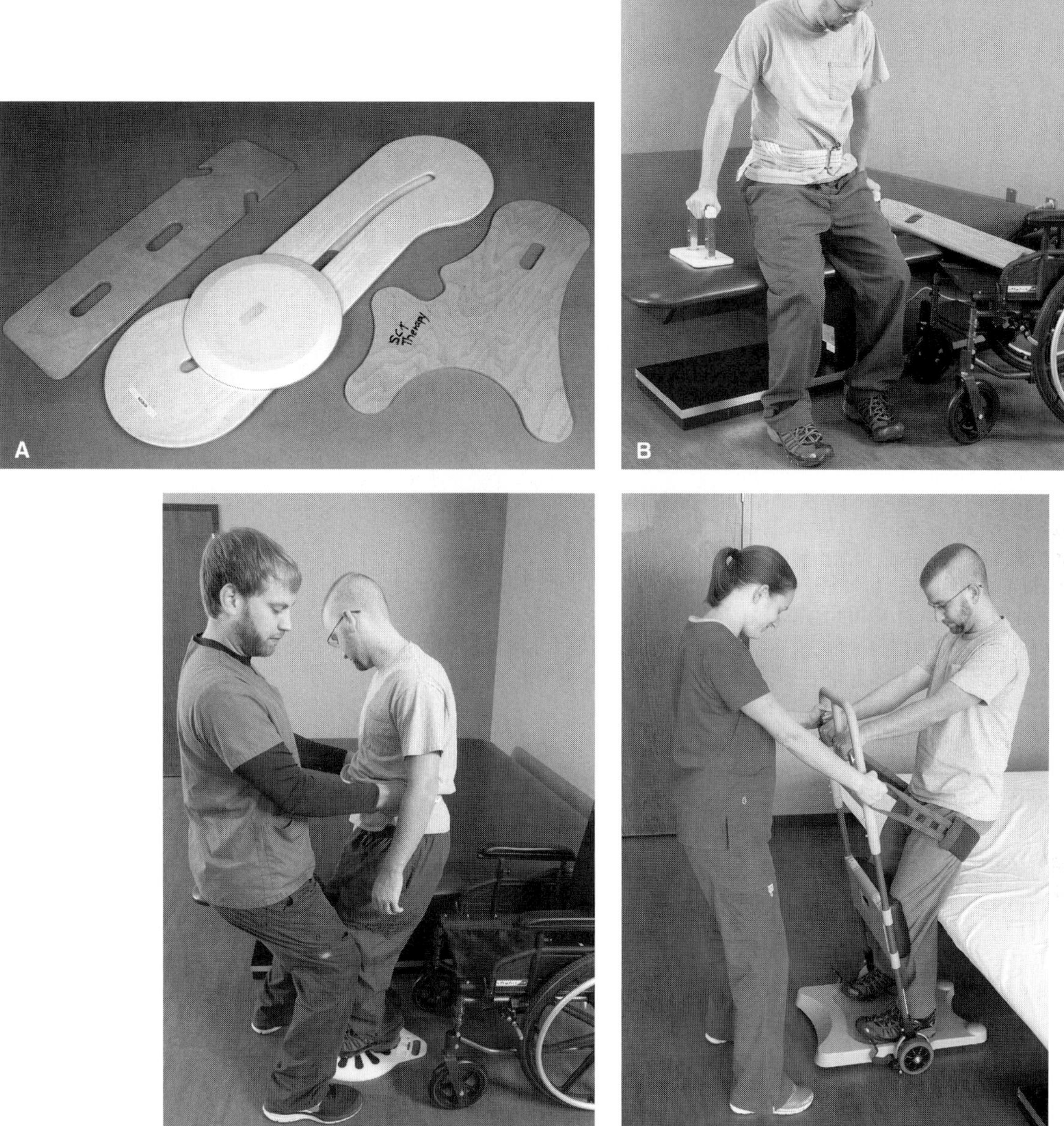

FIGURE 13-2. Examples of assistive devices: **A.** Transfer boards. **B.** Push up blocks. **C.** Pivot disc, placed under lower extremities to assist with transfer. **D.** Transfer platform device; Etac Molift Raiser™.

challenge," is when the practitioner selects the type of transfer based on the client's current abilities while considering limitations or restrictions for the purpose of optimizing functional independence. The OTA should encourage the client to participate in a transfer that facilitates the client to be as independent as possible while reducing the burden of care. As one example of decision making, the practitioner selects specific transfers that reinforce motor learning while increasing strength and activity tolerance for a client who has sustained a CVA. As a second example, the supervising occupational therapist and the OTA collaborate and select transfers that incorporate DME to reduce fatigue and facilitate energy conservation for a client who has multiple sclerosis.

Taking developmental levels of functional mobility into consideration can be useful to the practitioner and help decide on the appropriate transfer. For example, if a client is unable to actively participate in bed mobility, he or she is unlikely to be able to sit on the edge of the bed (unassisted) and therefore may need to use SPH equipment to transfer out of bed. If unable to sit without assistance, the client is unlikely to be capable of standing, and therefore ambulation without significant assistance is improbable. Although a seemingly basic concept, developmental levels can be very useful to the

THE OLDER ADULT

It is important to consider comorbidities that can be associated with aging, such as reduced visual skills, reduced bone density, reduced muscle strength and coordination, reduced skin integrity, and longer healing times, if injured. These comorbidities can impact the selection of a transfer method for the client to ensure safety during transfers, especially when the client is returning home. An additional consideration is the aging caregiver. When providing education and training on transfers to caregivers, the practitioner should determine the capabilities of the caregiver to ensure selection of the best transfer method that meets the safety and needs of both the client and the caregiver. Therefore, the same comorbidities mentioned above apply not only to the client but also to the caregiver when determining the safest transfer methods.

An example is as follows: After a cerebrovascular accident, the client is demonstrating increased independence with a squat-pivot transfer. The client's wife attends the therapy session, and the OTA determines that the wife has compromised strength and is at risk of falling or injuring herself if she assists the client with this transfer method. The OTA communicates this to the supervising occupational therapist, and as a team, they decide that it is best to use a transfer board or side-scoot transfer. This decision is made because the client demonstrates the greatest potential to be safe with the wife, only needing to provide supervision while using these two types of transfers to various surfaces.

COMMUNICATION

In many practice settings, it can be challenging for the supervising occupational therapist and OTA to communicate. However, when considering the individuality of each client and his or her associated deficits, environmental differences, variety of assistive devices, and safe-patient-handling (SPH) equipment on the market, it is imperative that the two practitioners communicate consistently to ensure that the most appropriate options for the client are being selected and implemented into treatment.

The following is an example of lack of communication impacting the care of a client. The client has a tub with overhead shower at home and needs Mod A with transferring, so the OTA recommends a hard plastic tub bench. However, the OTA did not communicate with the supervising occupational therapist before making the recommendation to the wife; the wife went out and purchased the tub bench in preparation for the client's return home. The supervising occupational therapist read the OTA's documentation note regarding the recommendation and knew that the recommendation was not best for the client's home environment. The supervising occupational therapist knew this because she had spoken with the client's daughter and found out that the doorway into the bathroom was too narrow to accommodate a wheelchair; this eliminated the bathroom as a viable option for the client's use while he was wheelchair bound. Both practitioners were at fault; the supervising occupational therapist should have discussed the piece of environmental information that he had learned with the OTA, and the OTA should have discussed the recommendation for the assistive device with the supervising occupational therapist before making it to the wife.

practitioner to determine which transfer type to attempt with the client. If the next developmental level of transfer is to be attempted, it is recommended that a second care provider assist the practitioner with the transfer to prevent injury or that an alternative method be selected if a second care provider is not available.

TRADITIONAL TRANSFERS

The transfers discussed below can be used by any care provider to assist the client with safe transfers. However, the majority of transfers covered in this section are primarily utilized by therapy practitioners in a variety of settings. These transfers are designed to support clients throughout the transfer while providing best positioning in which clients can use their own abilities to participate in the transfer. For all transfers, there are initial considerations and steps that should always be followed before beginning any transfer (Table 13-2).

Bed Mobility

Bed mobility includes moving up and down in the bed, rolling from side to side, transitioning from supine to sitting and sitting to supine, and optimal positioning in preparation to transfer out of the bed. When working in practice settings, including hospitals, home health, skilled nursing facilities, and long-term care facilities, the OT session will frequently be initiated at the client's bedside. The OTA needs to consider how much the client might be able to participate in the bed mobility process as an aspect of OT care and should encourage the client to assist as much as the client is capable.

MOVING UP IN BED

For moving a client up in bed, two care providers are required, and they use a draw sheet (a smaller sheet positioned underneath the client's trunk and thighs) that is on top of the fitted mattress sheet. The V-method can be used to move a client toward the head of the bed.

1. Both practitioners stand at a corner at the head of the client's bed.
2. With legs positioned shoulder width apart, each practitioner grasps a corner of the draw sheet with both hands.
3. On the count of three, each practitioner transfers the weight from the front foot (closest to the client's feet)

TABLE 13-2 Initial Considerations and Steps Before Any Transfer

DID I:	EXAMPLES:
Set up the environment to ensure safety during the transfer?	Position the wheelchair, lock the wheels, and remove the leg rests.
Get all the assistive devices needed for the transfer?	Use transfer board or walker; bathtub bench.
Inform the client what is about to happen?	"I'm going to help you get out of bed."
Tell or show the client where they are transferring to?	"I am going to help you move from your bed to the wheelchair."
Tell the client how to assist during the transfer?	"I need you to push off the armrests with both hands and use both your legs to stand up."
Position the client's body for optimal mechanical advantage to assist with the transfer?	Move client to the edge of the seating surface before transferring to another surface.
Position all the medical lines to prevent pulling or disconnection?	Position catheter bag, intravenous line(s), and ventilator tubing.
Apply a transfer belt to client?	For movements other than bed mobility, apply a transfer belt.
Determine who is providing the directions during the transfer if another care provider is assisting with the transfer?	Discuss who will provide the directions to the client during the transfer.

and transition to bear weight on the back foot (closest to the client's head) (Fig. 13-3). In this way the practitioners' trunks are not twisted, and they use the large muscles of the hip girdle and legs instead of the back muscles, which can frequently be injured during client repositioning.

4. The transfer is completed by straightening the sheets, adjusting the pillow, and ensuring that the client is comfortable.

Some clients will require significant assistance because of their complete dependence, sedation, or physical size. In these cases, it may be deemed unsafe to manually move the client through the techniques listed above, and SPH equipment should be utilized. The SPH equipment allows the client to be moved up in bed without increased risk of injury to care providers. The types of SPH equipment, as well as how and when to use them, will be discussed later in the chapter.

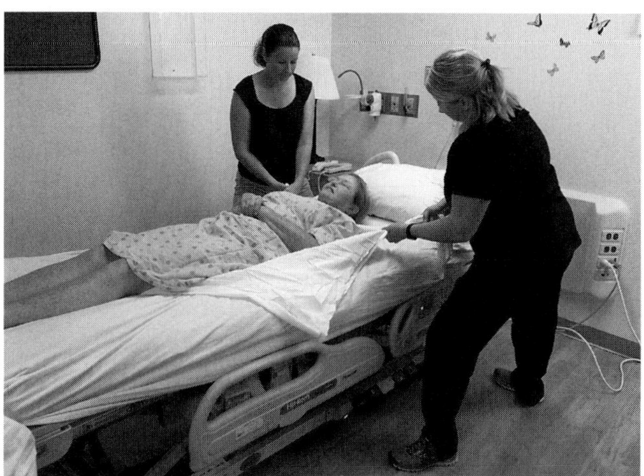

FIGURE 13-3. Using the V-method to slide a client up in bed.

USE OF EQUIPMENT FOR BED MOBILITY

Mechanical beds (electronic or manually adjusted), referred to as hospital beds, can be useful in assisting the client to increase participation with bed mobility. In many settings, the practitioner can encourage the client with initial use of a trapeze bar (triangular overhead bar) if available, elevate the head of the bed, and utilize bed rails to facilitate mobility, increase upper body strength, and encourage client participation in pressure-relief techniques to promote skin integrity. The OTA should also consider environmental adaptations that the client will need to make after discharge from therapy and discourage reliance on these bed modifications if the client will not have them available at home.

Trapeze bars can be very useful with weaker clients to let them assist with the bed mobility process and give them a measure of independence. However, they can limit relearning of bed mobility techniques, such as rolling in bed, as they only provide movement in one plane and may limit the client's ability to transition from supine to sitting for this reason. Elevating the head of the bed can assist with supine to sitting transfers as well as with swallowing and breathing. However, this position can frequently result in clients migrating toward the foot of the bed. This makes it necessary to move the client up toward the head of the bed for comfort, to achieve optimal feeding position, and to meet respiratory needs.

Mechanical beds can be used to assist with repositioning by temporarily placing the bed flat or in the Trendelenburg position (the head of the client is between 15 to 30 degrees lower than the feet). Either of these positions allows the client and care providers to more easily move the client toward the head of the bed for improved bed positioning.

Note of caution, laying the bed flat or using the Trendelenburg position may be contraindicated for clients with certain restrictions (e.g., nasogastric tubes, intracranial pressure monitors). The medical chart should always be checked to ensure that there are no contraindications before placing the client in either of these positions.

Rolling a client from side to side can frequently be performed by one practitioner with the use of a draw sheet that is positioned lengthwise underneath the client's body (Fig. 13-4). With clients who are obese or others who require total assistance, rolling in bed may require two care providers or more and/or the use of equipment. An air-assisted mat can be used for clients who are unable to assist sufficiently. This involves the use of a nylon mat placed under the client and then inflated with the use of an electric pump, thereby reducing friction and burden of care, as well as the risk of skin breakdown as a result of shear forces. Another useful assistive device to reduce shearing/friction and reduce the forces required to facilitate movement is a transfer sheet, which is used to reposition a client in bed. A transfer sheet is made of continuous nylon loop fabric that helps caregivers glide the client in all directions (Fig. 13-5).

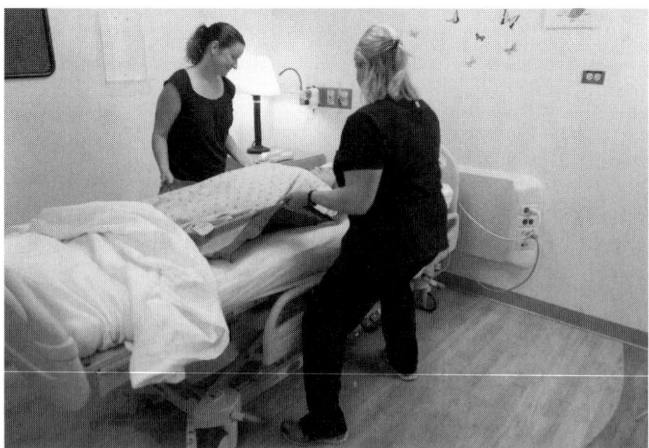

FIGURE 13-5. A transfer sheet may be used to glide a client in all directions.

BED MOBILITY WITHOUT EQUIPMENT

To move the client up in bed, the following steps are used when the client is able to assist with bed mobility, and the goal is for the client to be independent in bed mobility without the use of equipment. Encourage clients to engage their core muscles (abdomen and back) as well as all four extremities as they are able.

1. Instruct the client to roll toward one side and push up with both upper extremities in order to prop upper body onto the elbow and forearm (Fig. 13-6A). The OTA can assist by providing support along the client's shoulders to facilitate rolling and positioning of the client's arms.
2. When the client is rolling back toward midline, instruct the client to bend the opposing elbow in order to prop the upper body onto both elbows and forearms.
3. Instruct the client to bend both knees bringing both feet flat onto the bed.
4. When the client is engaging all four extremities, instruct the client to *bridge* by lifting the back and buttocks off of bed and shifting weight in the direction of the head of the bed. The OTA can provide assistance by helping the client lift the hips off the bed with hand placement along the low back and the hip to promote engagement for bridging. The OTA must also shift his or her own weight between the lower extremities (see Fig. 13-6B).
5. If client still needs to move higher up in the bed, instruct the client to reposition the upper and lower extremities and shift weight again until reaching desired position in bed.
6. End the transfer by having the client return the extremities to a comfortable position.

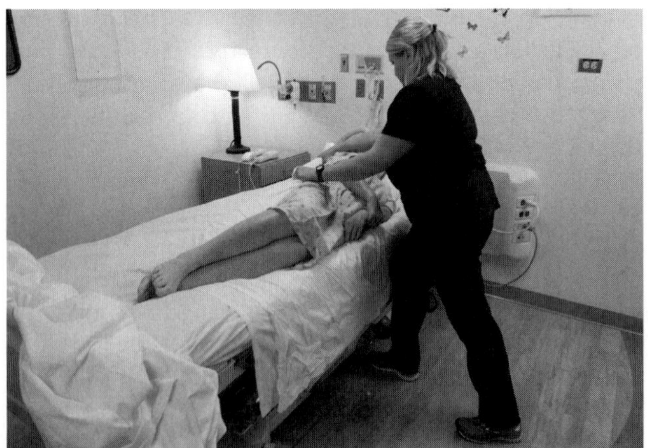

FIGURE 13-4. An individual OT practitioner can use a draw sheet to roll a client from side to side.

Supine to and From Sitting on Edge of Bed Transfers

1. Select a side to roll toward. For the purposes of conveying instructions, these steps will have the client rolling onto the left side of the body.
2. Remove any barriers, such as the right lower half of bed railing, if using a hospital bed.
3. Instruct the client to bend the right knee and place right foot flat on the bed. While the client is pushing off with the right foot, instruct the client to reach to the left for the upper bed railing with the right hand (or edge of the bed) to roll onto the left side. The OTA should stand facing the client's upper body. Placing the right hand on the client's right scapula and the left hand on the client's right hip, the OTA should provide assistance, as needed, while the client rolls onto the left side (Fig. 13-7A).
4. Instruct the client to bring the legs off the side of the bed. The OTA places his or her left hand along the

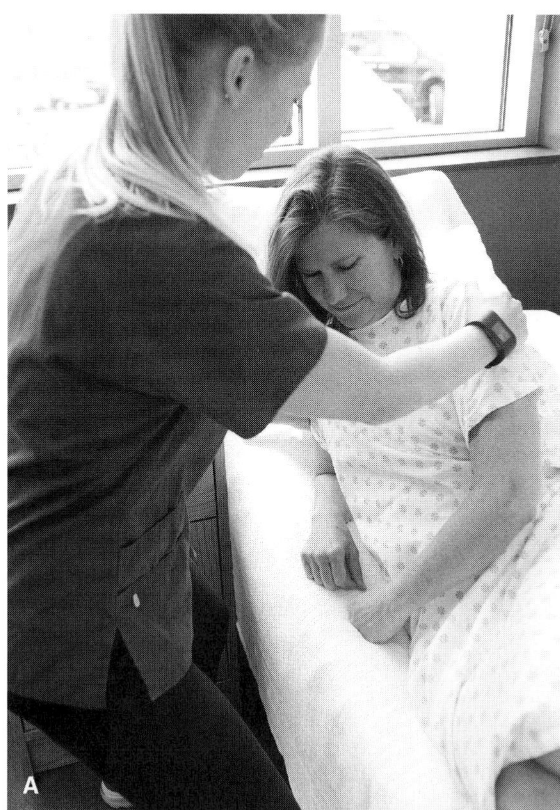
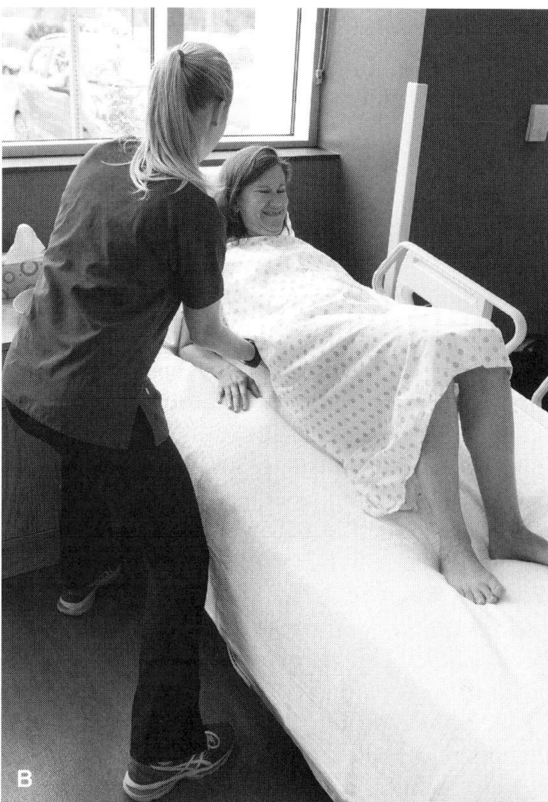

FIGURE 13-6. A. The client rolls to one side and begins propping up on elbow and forearm. B. Bridging buttocks, using all four extremities to move up in bed.

client's posterior right hip (or along the back of the client's legs), assisting, as needed, until the client's lower legs are off the side of the bed.

5. Instruct the client to use both upper extremities to push off the mattress (or bed rail) and get into the sitting position. The OTA should place his or her right hand on the outside of the client's left shoulder and the left hand along the client's right hip and assist the client into the sitting position. During this movement, the OTA should shift weight from the right foot to the left foot (see Figs. 13-7B and 13-7C).
6. End the transfer with the client's feet touching the floor, trunk in midline, and upper extremities placed on mattress next to thighs.

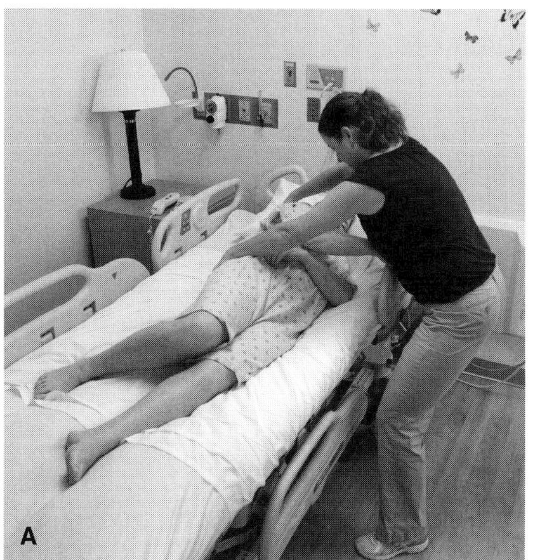
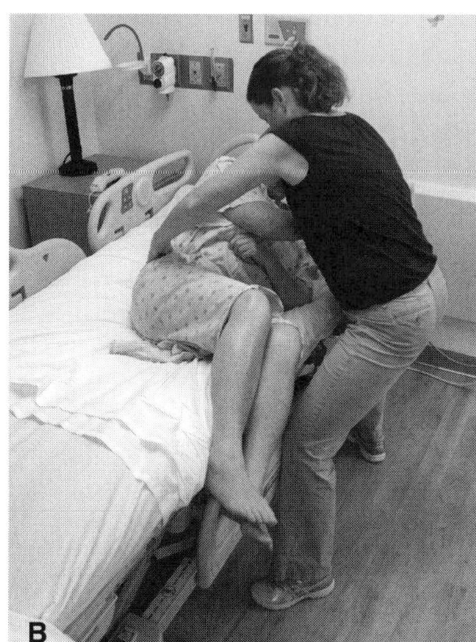
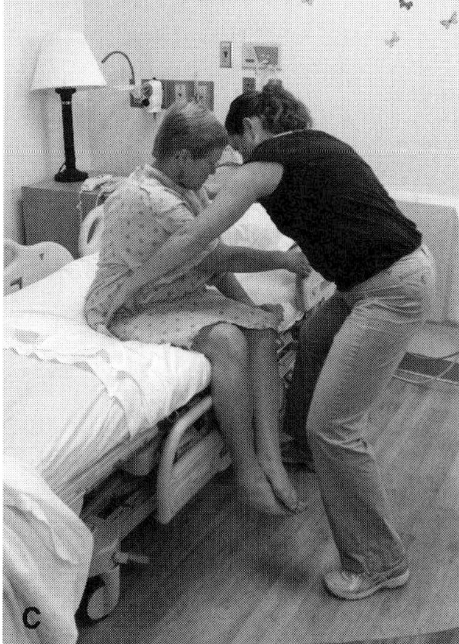

FIGURE 13-7. A. The OTA assists the client to roll onto her right side. B. The OTA places her left hand on the client's posterior hip. C. The OTA assists the client into the sitting position.

Stand-Step Transfers: Wheelchair to Other Surfaces

This transfer is used with a client who requires less assistance and is able to step with lower extremities when in the standing position. The instructions for this transfer begin with the client sitting in a wheelchair and do not incorporate use of adaptive equipment beyond the wheelchair to simplify the steps. The basic concepts of the transfer can be applied to a variety of surfaces, such as a bed, toilet, bath bench, or chair.

1. Swing away or remove both leg rests.
2. Position wheelchair parallel, or at a slight angle to the surface to which the client is being transferred.
3. Fully engage the wheelchair locks.
4. Place the transfer belt on the client.
5. Instruct the client to scoot to the front edge of the wheelchair. The OTA may need to assist by either helping the client weight shift from side to side while scooting the hips forward or instruct the client to lean back into the backrest and slide the hips forward. The latter option should only be used if there are no skin integrity issues on the buttocks (Fig. 13-8A).
6. The client's feet should be positioned flat on the floor and shoulder width apart.
7. Instruct the client to place hands on the wheelchair armrests.
8. The OTA should align his or her body directly in front of the client and place the arms along the sides of the client's trunk, with both hands on the transfer belt to ensure readiness to assist with the transfer, as needed.
9. Instruct the client to shift weight anteriorly onto the arms and legs and come to the standing position (see Fig. 13-8B).
10. Instruct the client to take step(s) toward the surface being transferred to. The OTA should realign himself or herself, as needed, to ensure that alignment with the client is maintained for the best counterbalancing of weight. The client should be encouraged to not hold onto the practitioner; however, clients will often need to do this to increase their balance or feeling of security. If this is necessary, have the client place his or her hands on the practitioner's forearm or elbow, which limits any risk to the practitioner. The client should never place the upper extremities around the neck of the practitioner.
11. Once the posterior side of the client's legs are touching the surface being transferred to, instruct the client to reach back with the upper extremities and place the hands on the surface being transferred to while slowly lowering the hips and buttocks onto the new surface (see Fig. 13-8C).
12. End the transfer with the client's feet touching the floor, trunk in midline, and upper extremities positioned comfortably. If client has decreased trunk balance or weakness, the OTA must ensure support to the trunk before releasing the transfer belt.

A

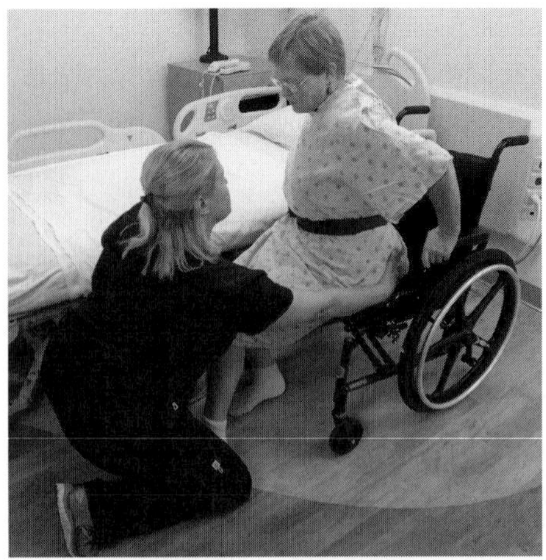

B

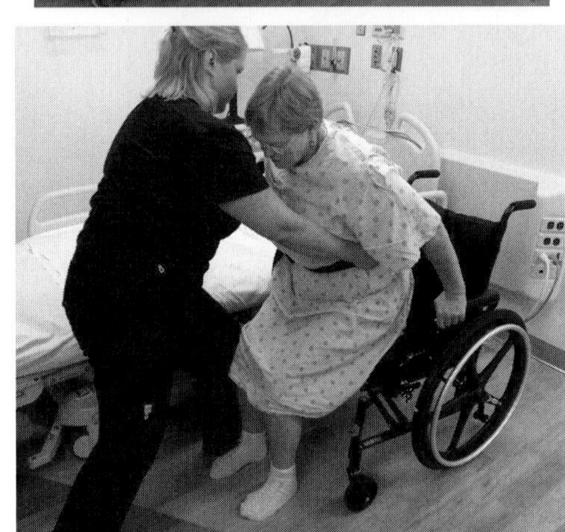

C

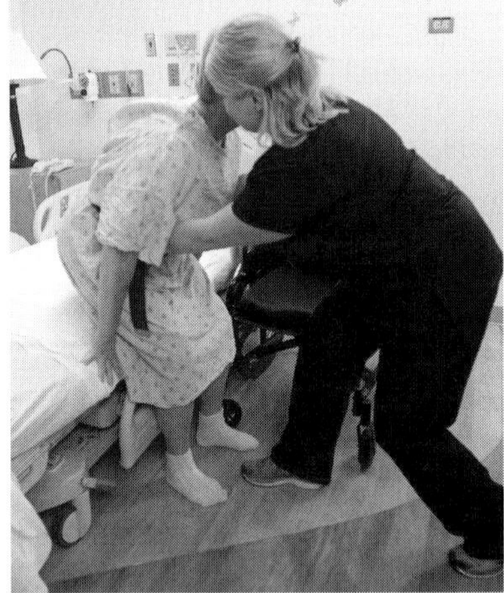

FIGURE 13-8. **A.** The OTA helps the client to scoot to the front edge of the wheelchair. **B.** The OTA instructs the client to shift weight anteriorly onto her arms and legs and come to the standing position. **C.** The OTA instructs the client to reach back and place hands on the surface being transferred to while slowly lowering hips and buttocks onto the bed.

Stand-Pivot Transfers: Wheelchair to Other Surfaces

The stand-pivot transfer is primarily used with a client who needs less assistance but is unable to step with the lower extremities when in the standing position. This transfer is also utilized when the space to complete the transfer is very confined. As with the previous transfer, the instructions begin with the client in the wheelchair, but the concepts can be utilized when transferring from other surfaces.

1. Swing away or remove both leg rests.
2. Position wheelchair at an approximately 45-degree angle to the surface being transferred to (front closer, back farther away) This angle places the buttocks closer to the surface being transferred to once the client scoots forward in the wheelchair.
3. Fully engage the wheelchair locks.
4. Place the transfer belt on the client.
5. Instruct the client to scoot to the front edge of the wheelchair. The OTA may need to assist by either helping the client weight shift from side to side while scooting the hips forward or instruct the client to lean back into the backrest and slide the hips forward. The latter option should only be used if there are no skin integrity issues on the buttocks.
6. The client's feet should be positioned flat on the floor, shoulder width apart, with heels turned slightly toward surface being transferred to and the foot closest to new surface should be slightly forward of the other.
7. Instruct the client to place both hands on the armrests.
8. The OTA should align his or her body directly in front of the client and place the arms along the sides of the client's trunk, with both hands on the transfer belt to ensure readiness to assist with the transfer as needed.
9. Instruct the client to shift weight anteriorly onto the arms and legs to come to the standing position (Fig. 13-9A).
10. Have the client pivot on the balls of the feet so that both heels shift toward the surface being transferred to. The OTA should maintain grip on the transfer belt and assist with weight shifting while pivoting on his or her feet (be alert to not twist the back) (see Fig. 13-9B).
11. Once the posterior side of the client's legs are touching the surface being transferred to, instruct the client to reach back with his or her upper extremities and place the hands on the surface being transferred to and slowly lower the hips and buttocks onto the new surface (see Fig. 13-9C).
12. End the transfer with feet touching floor, trunk in midline, and upper extremities positioned comfortably. If client has decreased trunk balance or weakness, the OTA must ensure support to the trunk before releasing the transfer belt.

Squat-Pivot Transfers: Wheelchair to Other Surfaces

Squat-pivot transfers are typically used with a client who needs greater-than-minimal assistance or is unable to come to the standing position. Steps for this transfer begin with the client in the wheelchair; however, the concepts can be modified for transferring from different surfaces.

1. Swing away or remove both leg rests.
2. Position wheelchair at a 45-degree angle to the surface being transferred to.

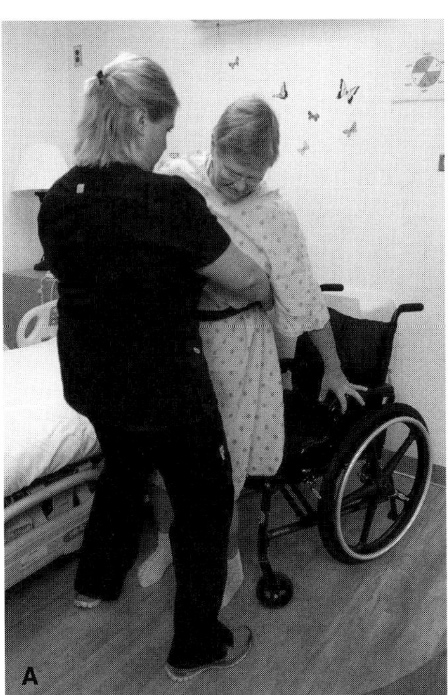

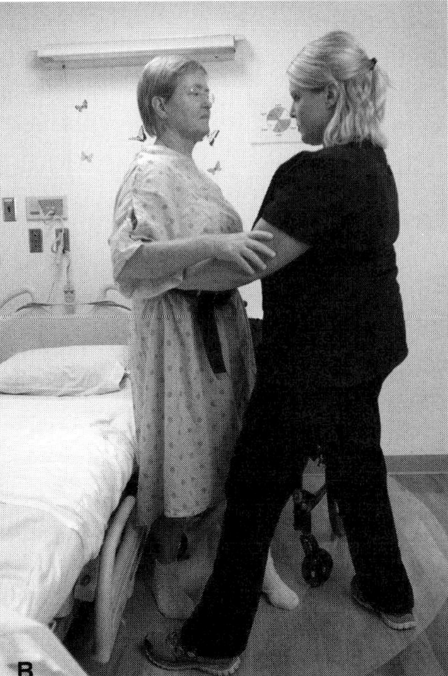

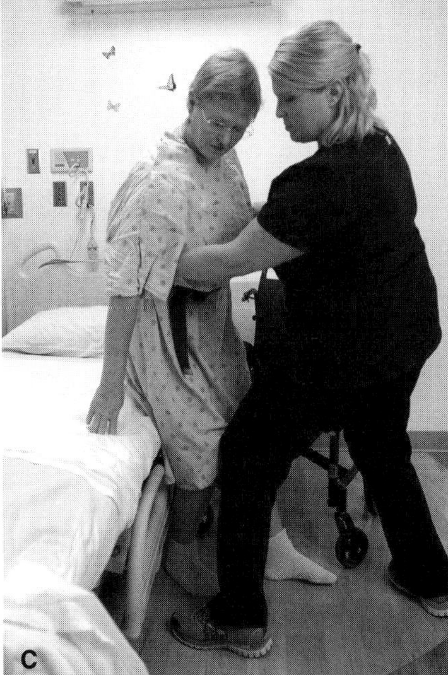

FIGURE 13-9. A. The OTA instructs the client to shift weight anteriorly onto the arms and legs to come to the standing position. B. The OTA maintains a grip on the transfer belt and assists with weight shifting while pivoting on her feet and not twisting her back. C. When the posterior side of the client's legs touches the bed, the OTA instructs the client to place her hands on the bed and slowly lower her hips and buttocks.

3. Swing away or remove the armrest closest to the surface being transferred to because this will prevent the hips and buttocks from striking the armrest during the transfer.
4. Fully engage the wheelchair locks.
5. Place the transfer belt on the client.
6. Instruct the client to scoot to the front edge of the wheelchair. The OTA may need to assist by either helping the client shift weight from side to side while scooting the hips forward, or instruct the client to lean back into the backrest and slide the hips forward. The latter option should only be used if there are no skin integrity issues on the buttocks.
7. The client's feet should be positioned flat on the floor, shoulder width apart, with heels turned slightly toward the surface being transferred to, and the foot closest to new surface should be slightly forward of the other.
8. The OTA should align his or her body directly in front of the client and place the arms along the sides of the client's trunk, with both hands on the transfer belt to ensure readiness to assist with the transfer, as needed. Additionally, the OTA may block the client's weaker lower extremity to prevent knee buckling of knees during the transfer (Fig. 13-10).
9. Instruct the client to shift weight anteriorly into his or her arms and legs to remove weight from the hips and buttocks. Have the client pivot on the balls of the feet and swing the hips to the surface being transferred to. The OTA should maintain grip on the transfer belt and assist with weight shifting while pivoting on the feet (be alert to not twist the back).
10. End the transfer with the client sitting upright with feet touching the floor, trunk in midline, and upper extremities positioned comfortably. If client has decreased trunk balance or weakness, the OTA must ensure support to the trunk before releasing the transfer belt.

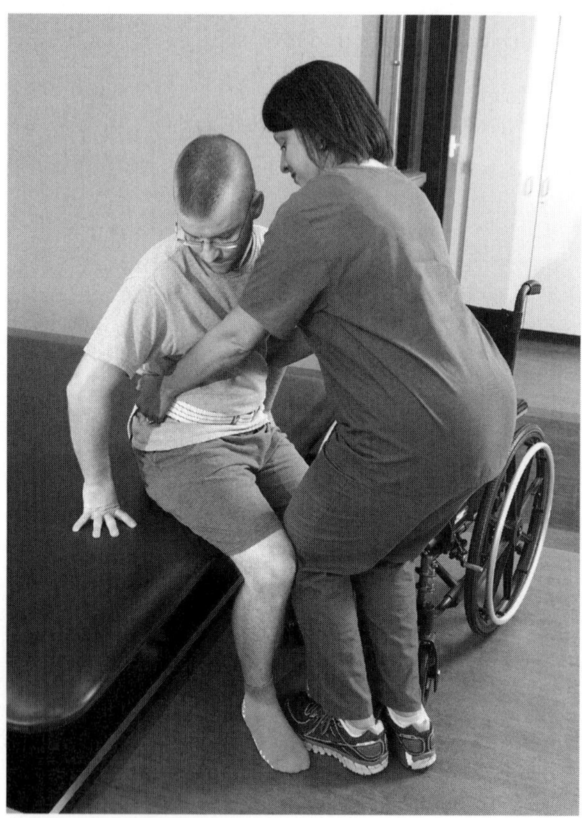

FIGURE 13-10. The OT practitioner blocks the client's weaker lower extremity to prevent knee buckling.

Side-Scoot Transfers

This type of transfer is typically used for a client who has greater weakness of the lower extremities and has adequate strength of the upper extremities to assist with lifting buttocks off of a seated surface and when pivoting on the feet is not ideal or possible.

1. Surface heights must be equal in height and in very close proximity.
2. Swing away or remove both leg rests.
3. Swing away or remove the armrest closest to the surface being transferred to because this will prevent the hips and buttocks from striking the armrest during the transfer.
4. Fully engage the wheelchair locks.
5. Place the transfer belt on the client.
6. Instruct the client to scoot to the front edge of the wheelchair. The OTA may need to assist by either helping the client weight shift from side to side while scooting the hips forward, or instruct the client to lean back into the backrest and slide the hips forward. The latter option should only be used if there are no skin integrity issues on the buttocks.
7. The client's feet should be positioned flat on the floor, shoulder width apart.
8. Instruct the client to place one hand on the wheelchair armrest and the other hand on the surface being transferred to.
9. The OTA should align his or her body directly in front of the client and place the arms along the sides of the client's trunk, with both hands on the transfer belt to ensure readiness to assist with the transfer, as needed.
10. Instruct the client to use both upper extremities in an extension/depression pattern while leaning the trunk anteriorly, lifting the buttocks off of the surface, bearing weight into the knees and feet, and performing a small sideways motion toward the new surface. The client repeats this motion until fully seated on the new surface. The OTA should maintain grip on the transfer belt and assist with weight shifting (be alert to maintain good spinal alignment) (Fig. 13-11).
11. End the transfer with the client sitting upright with feet touching the floor, trunk in midline, and upper extremities positioned comfortably. If the client has

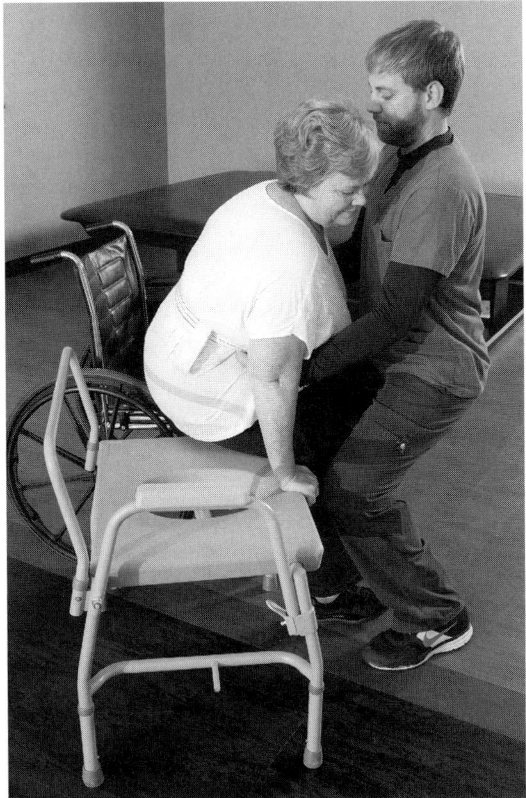

FIGURE 13-11. During the side-scoot, the OTA maintains his grip on the transfer belt and assists with weight shifting, keeping his spine in alignment.

decreased trunk balance or weakness, the OTA must ensure support to the trunk before releasing the transfer belt.

Transfer Board Transfers

Transfer boards have been referred to as *sliding boards*, but use of this terminology should be discouraged because clients should not slide across the transfer board; sliding can result in increased friction to the skin along the buttocks. The overall steps for transferring with a transfer board is similar to those for the side-scoot transfer. The transfer board is used when surface heights are not even, there is a large gap between the surfaces, there is arm weakness, there is disparity in the sizes of the caregiver and the client, or the client is unable to bear the full weight of the body through the upper extremities.

1. Start with the client in the seated position.
2. Place the transfer belt on the client.
3. The client leans away from the direction of the transfer, while the OTA places the transfer board between the ischial tuberosity of the hip and knee (e.g., mid-thigh) and with one-third of the board beneath the thigh. The OTA may need to assist with leaning safely to the side while positioning the transfer board. Ultimately, the client should be taught to independently place the transfer board (Fig. 13-12A).
4. The client then returns to the upright sitting posture.
5. The OTA should align his or her body directly in front of the client and place the arms along the sides of the client's trunk, with both hands on the transfer belt to ensure readiness to assist with the transfer, as needed.
6. The client leans anteriorly, reducing weight off the hips and increasing the load-bearing of the foot/feet and hands and performs small side-scoot motions toward the surface he or she is transferring to by lifting the buttocks and shifting the hips. To reduce skin integrity concerns, the client does not slide along the board but partially lifts the buttocks off the board in small increments, using the board like a bridge to span the distance between the two surfaces. The OTA assists, as needed, with weight shifting and ensuring that the buttocks come off the board. If a second care provider is needed, this provider should be behind the client (see Fig. 13-12B).
7. This motion is repeated until the client is fully seated on the new surface.
8. Have the client lean away from the transfer board while the OTA removes the transfer board. At times, a second care provider may be needed to ensure safety (see Fig. 13-12C). With time, the client should be taught to independently remove the transfer board.

Throughout the transfer, the OTA will assist through verbal directions and by promoting accurate weight shifting. If use of the transfer belt is insufficient for weight shifting, a draw sheet (e.g., sheet folded lengthwise) can be placed under the client's buttocks and can be used to facilitate this weight shift if the client is unable to provide sufficient power alone, or for education purposes.

Clients who are unable to shift weight off of their buttocks or have skin integrity issues can utilize a transfer board that has a dynamic seat component (e.g., Beasy® board). This type of transfer board is placed in a similar manner with the dynamic component underneath the buttocks (Fig. 13-13). The client does not perform the side-scoot motions, but instead, the OTA assists in leaning the client anteriorly and guiding the client's hips to engage the dynamic movement of the sliding surface component.[7]

Two-Person Transfer

If the OTA is unable to safely transfer a client alone, a second practitioner may be involved. The two practitioners can position themselves in front of and behind the client during a seated or standing transfer, or they can position themselves side by side, as in a two-hand-hold transfer (frequently used for clients who have cognitive deficits and are unable to use an assistive device). In either configuration, communication among the practitioners and the client is essential to ensure that they all work together as a team. The practitioner most familiar with the client should be the facilitator and most frequently is positioned in front of the client so that he or she can have eye contact with the client.

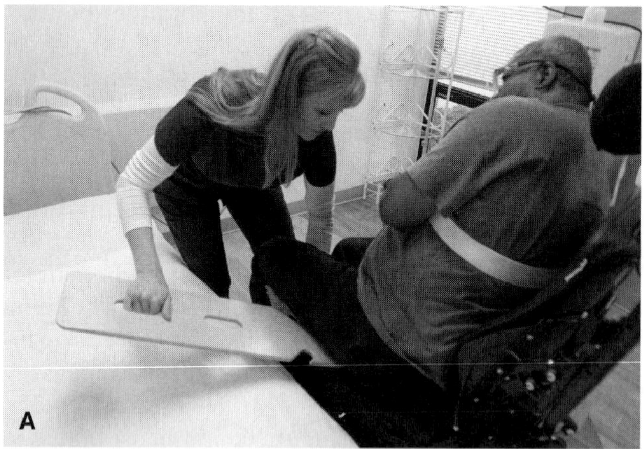

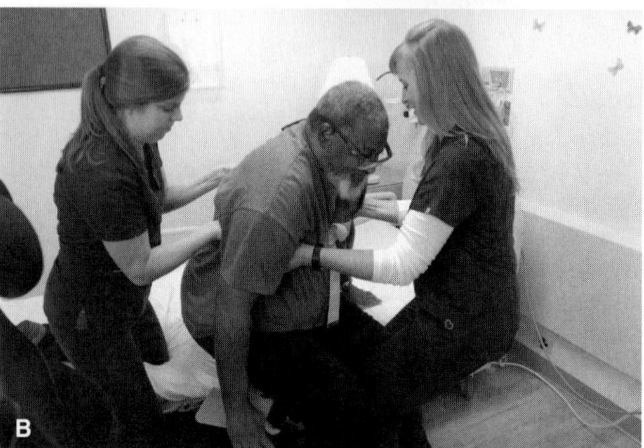

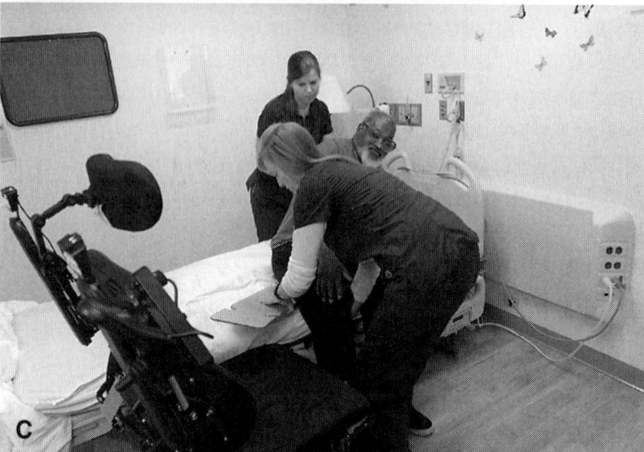

FIGURE 13-12. A. The OTA places the transfer board between the ischial tuberosity of the hip and knee. B. The client partially lifts his buttocks off the board in small increments, using the board like a bridge to span the distance between the two surfaces. C. The OTA removes the transfer board.

A transfer plan must be established and communicated clearly so that both the practitioners and the client are clear about their respective roles during the transfer. Agreeing on a number to count to for initiating the movement component of the transfer can unify effort and ensure that the client and the practitioners are all putting forth effort at the same time during the transfer. The use of SPH equipment will be discussed later in the chapter.

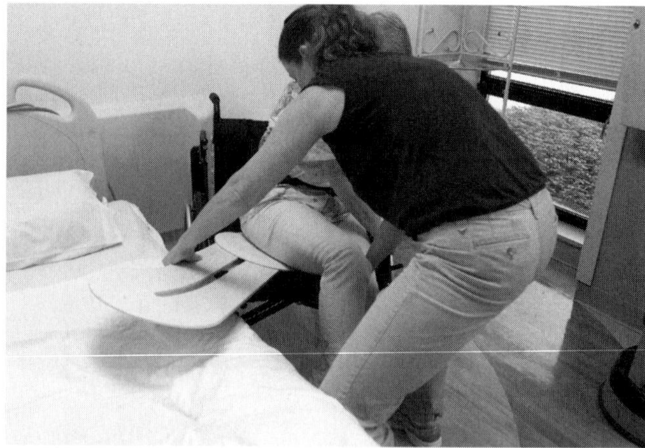

FIGURE 13-13. Place the dynamic component of the transfer board underneath the client's buttocks.

Toilet Transfers

Transfers to and from the toilet may sometimes be challenging because of limited space around the toilet. Standard toilet seat heights are between 14 and 16 inches as will be found in most clients' homes. The 2010 Americans with Disabilities Act (ADA) Standards for Accessible Design requires toilet seat height be a minimum of 17 inches and maximum of 19 inches.[8] Therefore, if working in an ADA-compliant practice setting, the OTA can expect the toilet height to be within these ranges or know what recommendations to make to clients regarding home modifications. The OTA will need to determine the best method of transferring based on consideration of the environment (e.g., toilet height, space around the toilet), mobility equipment (e.g., wheelchair, walker), transfer assistance level of the client, and body positioning for both the client and the practitioner. Additional consideration of DME, such as elevated toilet bases, elevated toilet seats, toilet safety frames, wall-mounted grab rails, or 3-in-1 commodes, can be used in conjunction with the toilet to improve the success of the transfer.

If unable to access the toilet, a 3-in-1 commode can be used in a more open space to allow easier access. A 3-in-1 commode can be ordered with additional features, such as drop-arms to allow for unobstructed access (e.g., side-scoot transfer or use of a transfer board) on one side while providing an armrest on the opposing side. All DME has weight limitations; therefore, the OT practitioner must make sure to use equipment that is rated appropriately for each client, especially when working with bariatric clients.

Clients who have decreased strength in their lower extremities may use their assistive mobility device (e.g., cane or walker) as a stabilizer when lowering themselves to or rising from the toilet. However, this should be discouraged because it increases the risk for falling. Therefore, the practitioner will need to ensure that the client can safely lower himself or herself to and rise from the toilet without using the assistive mobility device. Clients who are unable to do this independently should use DME (e.g., an elevated toilet seat, toilet safety frame, or grab rail). For transferring the client, the OTA should ensure that the client has on a transfer belt, and the OTA should place himself or herself at the best mechanical advantage to assist the client in the given space. The best position for mechanical advantage might be in front of the client while holding onto each side of the transfer belt, or to the side of the client while holding onto the posterior and side (closest to the practitioner) of the transfer belt (Box 13-1).

With clients who are using a wheelchair, the OTA will need to determine how the wheelchair can be placed (parallel, perpendicular, or head-on position). Consideration is then given to the amount of assistance needed, if the client can come to the standing position (stand-step), if the client will need to pivot (standing or squatting), or if a transfer board will be needed. The OTA will need to predetermine whether any DME is needed for improving the success and safety of the transfer. Last, the OTA must be able to maintain safe body mechanics throughout the transfer given the environment restrictions. The transfer steps used for stand-step, stand-pivot, squat-pivot, side-scoot, or transfer board transfers can be slightly altered to accommodate transferring between the wheelchair and the toilet (Box 13-2 and Box 13-3).

Bathtub and Shower Transfers

If the information was not available during the initial evaluation, the OTA needs to inquire how the client was bathing before needing OT services. Gaining insight into the type of bathroom fixtures (e.g., bathtub or shower stall) and the prior bathing method used (e.g., sitting in bathtub or standing to shower) will enable the OTA to make the safest decisions when determining the type of transfer to use and if DME is available or will be needed. At times, this decision making will need to occur with the supervising occupational therapist based on the experience level of the OTA.

If the client desires to stand for showering and has the strength and endurance to stand, then the OTA will need to teach the client how to use the upper extremities to brace against the shower walls for added stability while stepping over the shower curb or the side of the tub. For best safety considerations, the installation of wall-mounted grab rails into load-bearing studs or heavy duty suction cup grab rails along the shower wall should be recommended. The client should be instructed not to use towel racks, wall-mounted soap dishes, shower doors, or shower curtain rods for support because these items are not properly anchored to support

BOX 13-1
Toilet Transfers

Look closely at this figure. The client uses a rolling walker because of decreased balance and decreased strength following a traumatic head injury. The OT practitioner is addressing the occupation of toileting and therefore needs to ensure that the client can safely transfer on and off the toilet. Because of the use of the rolling walker, the practitioner has used clinical reasoning to position herself at the side of the client, demonstrating best mechanical advantage to assist the client while ensuring proper body mechanics. Additionally, the OT practitioner will instruct the client to transition his hands from the walker to the grab rails before lowering himself onto the toilet. Note the client's right hand on the grab rail; the next step would be for the client to move his left hand to the grab rail before lowering himself to the toilet.

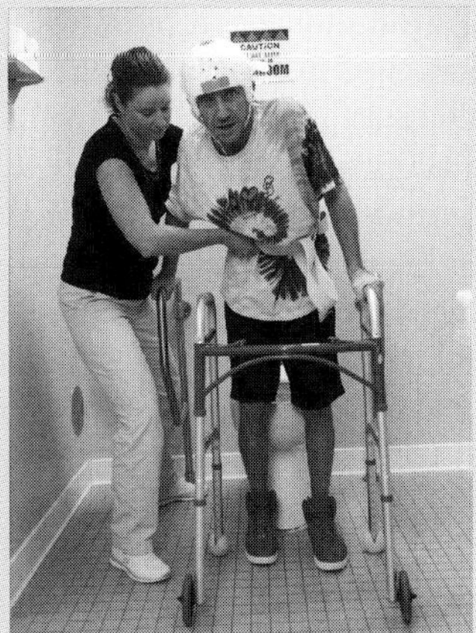

Toilet transfer safety rails at toilet.

BOX 13-2
Toilet Transfers From a Wheelchair

Look closely at this figure. The client uses a power wheelchair because of an incomplete spinal cord injury in the cervical region. The OT practitioner has taken note of the layout of the bathroom and the positioning of the toilet in relationship to the sink and wall. Knowing the physical deficits of the client, she has clinically reasoned to use a heavy-duty 3-in-1 commode with a drop-arm feature in conjunction with a transfer board. The wheelchair has been positioned closely to the toilet with the armrest swung out of the way. She has adjusted the height of the 3-in-1 commode to assure equal heights between the toilet seat and the wheelchair seat. Last, she has positioned herself in front of the client for best mechanical advantage to assist the client with weight shifting while ensuring proper body mechanics.

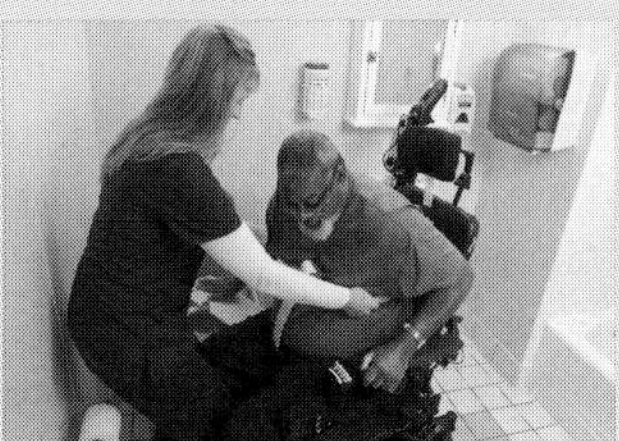

Toilet transfer board.

BOX 13-3
Sexual Activity

An individual's ability to perform bed mobility transfers more independently is connected to more than just moving around in the bed but to also be able to position oneself for engaging in sexual activity. Clients and caregivers can be educated on how the client can position himself or herself in the easiest manner without a significant amount of assistance so that bed mobility challenges do not interfere with participation in this valued occupation. Many times, OT practitioners are so focused on helping the caregiver be able to transfer the client that they forget it is important that the relationship between the client and his or her significant other need not always be based on a mindset of "patient and caregiver." Instead, OT practitioners need to be sensitive to the fact that intimacy between the client and his or her significant other needs to be encouraged and determine the transfers and occupations that allow for autonomy.

The following is an example of decision making that alters the caregiver role while taking care to support intimacy. Through therapeutic intervention, T. B. has regained her independence with the hygiene aspect of toileting and can now complete transfers to/from a bedside commode with modified independence; however, this requires her significant other to empty the commode several times throughout the day and a commode has to be present in their bedroom, which impacts their intimacy. The practitioner has also worked with T. B. on transferring to/from the commode in the bathroom, but she needs minimal assistance with the transfer only because of the environmental layout of their bathroom. The practitioner discusses the situation with T. B. and her significant other, and together they determine that the significant other will assist T. B. with transferring to the commode in the bathroom versus keeping a bedside commode in their bedroom.

the weight of the client. If the client is able to safely step over the side of the tub but does not have the endurance to stand for an entire shower, then the recommendation of a shower chair can be made.

The following is an example of a shower stall transfer with an ambulatory client. The practitioner has set up the area to simulate the client's home environment, which requires the client to step over the shower curb, and to incorporate the recommended use of installed grab bars and a shower seat because of the client's decreased standing balance.

1. Client has transitioned his hands from the rolling walker to the grab rails installed along the walls and aligned his body to face the shower entrance.
2. Using grab rails, client steps over the small curb. The practitioner assists, as needed, for balance and safety, ensuring use of good body mechanics (Fig. 13-14A).
3. The client continues to take small steps to align the back of his lower extremities with the front edge of the shower seat, using grab rails for balance and support.
4. The client is instructed to reach his hands back to the shower seat and begin lowering his hips toward the seat (see Fig. 13-14B).
5. Final positioning is buttocks on seat with feet flat on the floor.

A client who needs assistance for transferring in or out of a bathtub (either with or without an overhead shower) should use a tub transfer bench. The tub transfer bench allows for safe transferring over the side of a tub from the seated position to reduce the risk of falling. If the client requires the use of a wheelchair, the practitioner will determine the best positioning of the wheelchair based on the environmental setup of the bathroom (toilet, sink, walls), similar to the considerations mentioned in the toilet transfer section.

One example of a tub bench transfer is as follows:

1. Position the wheelchair close to the tub bench.
2. Use a squat-pivot transfer to transition the client from the wheelchair to the outer portion of the tub bench (Fig. 13-15A).
3. Have the client pivot his or her hips while moving the legs toward the side of the tub.
4. Have the client lift one leg over the side of the tub. The OT practitioner assists with lifting the leg, as needed, while incorporating good body mechanics.
5. The client scoots the buttocks further into tub area along the tub bench and then lifts the second leg over the side of the tub (see Fig. 13-15B).

An additional example of transferring to the tub bench for a person using a stand-step transfer method and a rolling walker can be viewed in the Paraplegia and Tetraplegia section of this chapter.

A variety of tub transfer benches are available on the market to accommodate a variety of specific client needs. Therefore, the OTA should confer with the supervising occupational therapist until a strong knowledge base of all the features and rationale for selection has been gained. Similar to the toilet transfer, decision making regarding the safest type of transfer to use is determined by the space available, the assistance level of the client, the type of assistive devices being used, selection of DME, and the best body positioning of the client and the practitioner. At any time, if the OTA is unsure about decision making, he or she should discuss the issue with the supervising occupational therapist.

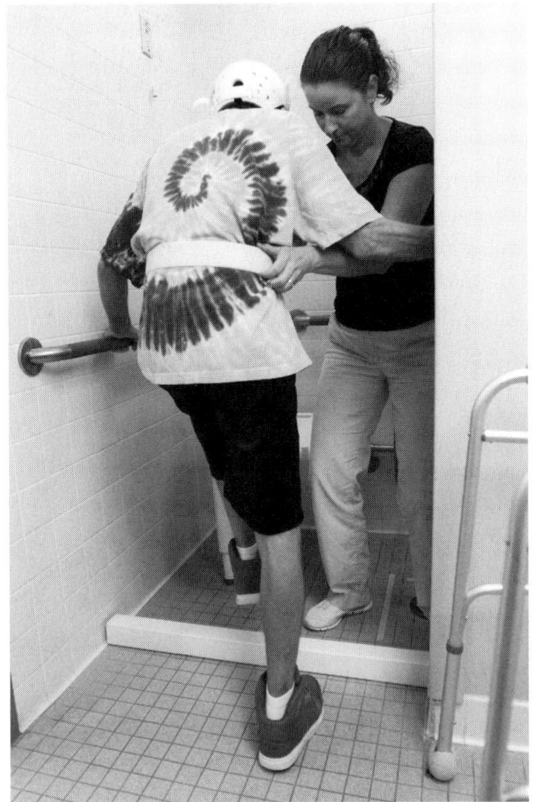

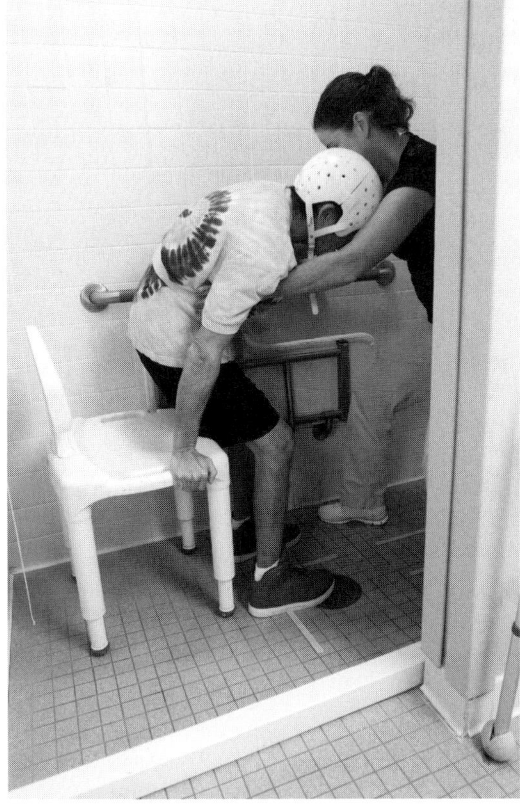

FIGURE 13-14. **A.** The OTA assists client to step over shower curbing. **B.** The OTA instructs client to reach hands back to shower seat and begin lowering hips toward seat.

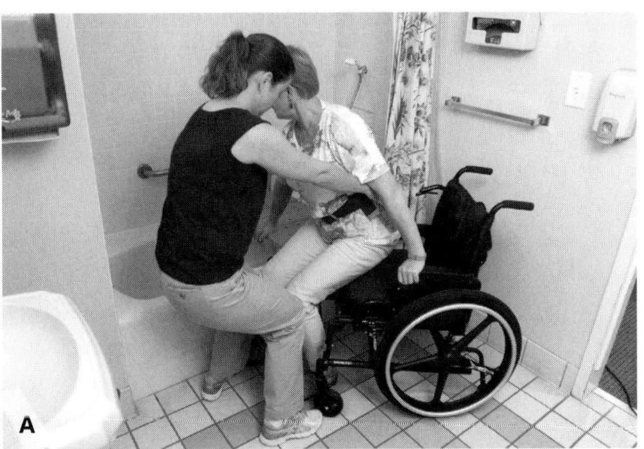

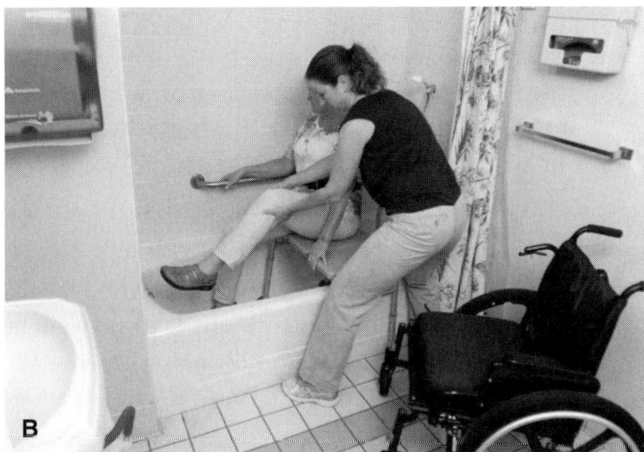

FIGURE 13-15. **A.** Using a squat pivot transfer to transition the client from the wheelchair to the outer portion of the tub bench. **B.** After scooting her buttocks further into tub area, the client lifts her second leg over the side of the tub.

Transferring With Assistive Ambulatory Devices

Assistive ambulatory devices, such as walkers and canes, are used by some clients to increase independence and safety with mobility. The selection of these devices is typically determined by the physical therapy (PT) practitioner. The OTA needs to ensure that the assistive ambulatory device is safely incorporated into the transfer. Consider an example of a client who is using a standard walker to increase stability when ambulating.

When coming to the standing position from a seated surface (e.g., bed, chair, or toilet), the following must be done:

1. Position the walker directly in front of the client.
2. The OT practitioner should be positioned to the side of the client, with one hand on the posterior aspect of the transfer belt and the other hand on the side of the transfer belt, ensuring that the OT practitioner's arms will not impede the transitional movement of the client's arms from the seated surface to the walker (Fig. 13-16A). When determining which side to

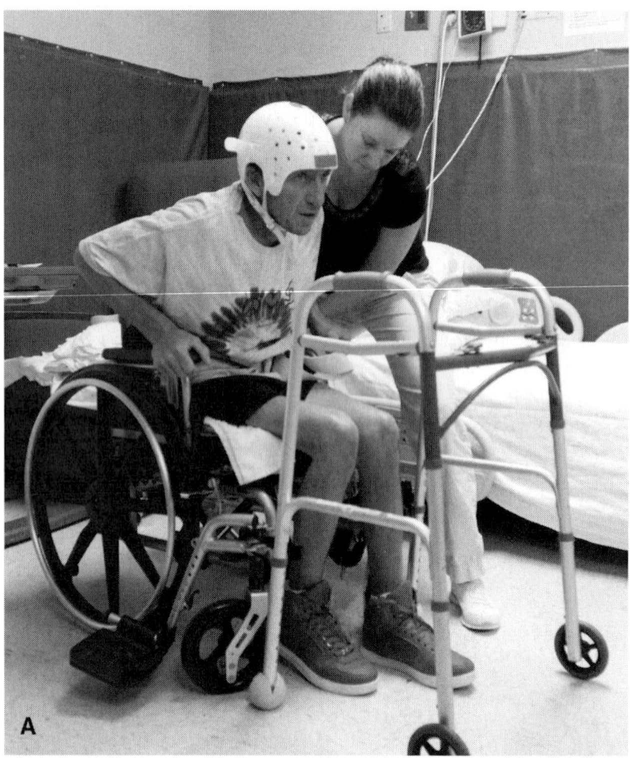

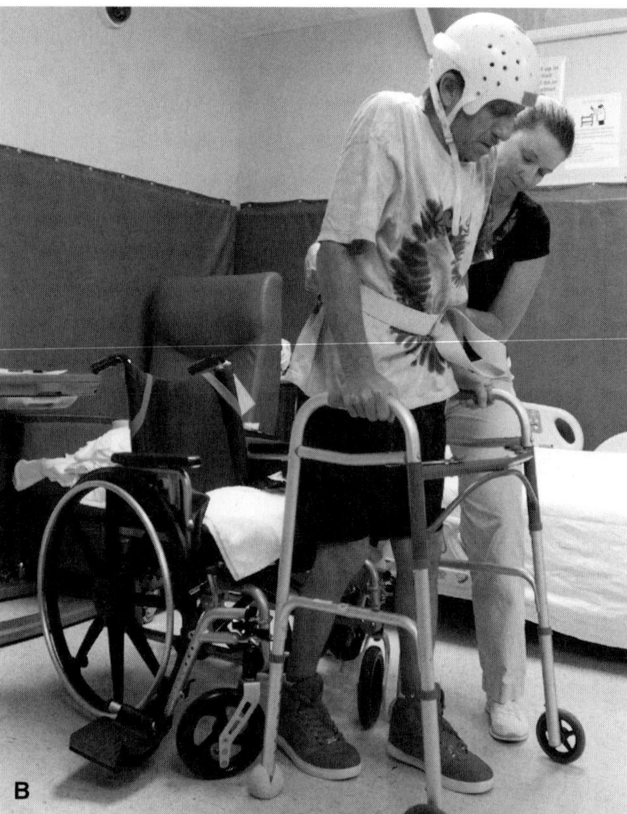

FIGURE 13-16. A. OT practitioner positions herself to the side of the client, with one hand on the posterior aspect of the transfer belt and the other hand on the side of the transfer belt. B. Proceeding with ambulation once client has gained balance.

stand on, the OTA could choose to be positioned on the client's weaker side or the side that is least confined by the environment or out of the path of upcoming mobility.

3. Instruct the client to use the upper extremities to push up from the seated surface, or armrests, while shifting weight anteriorly to engage the lower extremities to come to the standing position. The tendency will be for the client to pull himself or herself up by using the walker; however, this should be discouraged because the walker will not provide stability.
4. During this weight-shift transition, instruct the client to reach up for the walker.
5. Ensure that the client has gained balance before proceeding with ambulation (see Fig. 13-16B).

With clients utilizing a cane, the cane should be placed on the side where the cane will be used. The cane is typically used on the weaker lower extremity side; however, the physical therapist will make this determination on the basis of several factors, and the OTA should follow-through with the physical therapist's recommendations.

1. Have the client place the cane handle leaning securely against the seated surface.
2. Typically, the OTA will be positioned on the side opposite to the cane; one hand should be on the posterior aspect of the transfer belt and one hand on the side or anterior aspect of the transfer belt.
3. Instruct the client to use both upper extremities to push up from the seated surface, or armrests, while shifting weight anteriorly to engage the lower extremities to come to the standing position (Fig. 13-17).
4. Upon achieving standing balance, the client can reach back for the handle of the cane.

Transfers From the Floor

Despite the best efforts of OT practitioners, clients do occasionally fall or have to be lowered to the floor. The decision to lower a client to the floor is made when there is a greater risk of injury to the client or the practitioner while attempting to maintain an upright position. It is important for clients and their caregivers to practice this transfer to reduce the risk of injury and to learn how to get up safely if this occurs.

To practice transferring from the floor, the practitioner must demonstrate and assist the client to lower himself or herself to the floor. This is usually done on a padded surface (typically carpeting or thin portable therapy mats) to prevent injury. A variety of methods can be used to transfer up from the floor, and the method used will depend on the strength and agility of the client and the caregiver, as well as the equipment that they have available.

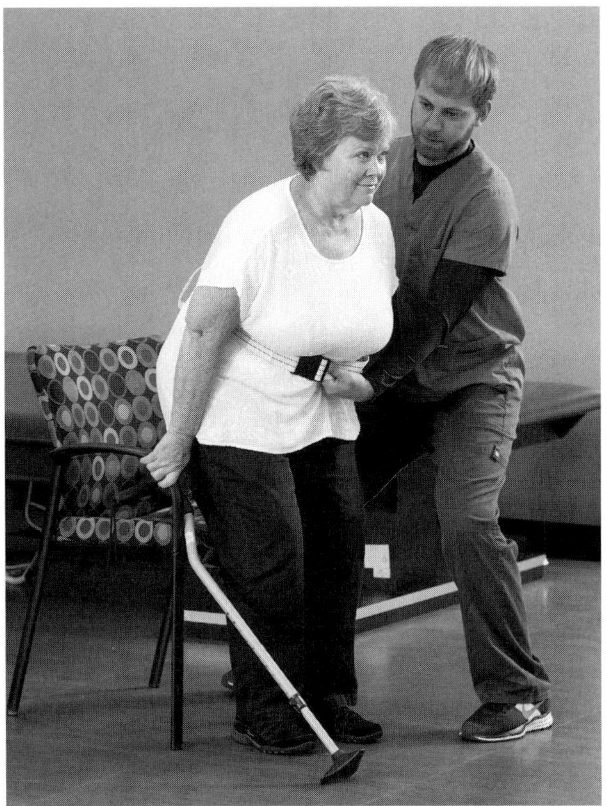

FIGURE 13-17. Preparing to stand and placement of cane.

For a client who needs total assistance, the best method is to use SPH equipment (discussed in the next section). If this equipment is not available (e.g., in the home), then emergency services (e.g., 911) may need to be called to prevent further injury to the client or the caregiver.

Clients with good trunk and upper-body strength can be taught to maneuver themselves from the floor back into the seat of a wheelchair, chair, or firm couch. A sequential series of steps can be used or created by placing sturdy objects that are progressively taller next to each other to form a "staircase," and the client can be assisted to transfer from one level to the next until reaching the chair (Fig. 13-18).

Some clients are able to learn to transfer directly from the floor to a firm couch, chair, wheelchair, or bed by placing their hands on the seat surface (Fig. 13-19A), pushing the lower body into partial kneeling (see Fig. 13-19B), swinging their hips onto the couch (see Fig. 13-19C), and then repositioning self, as needed, on the couch. Ambulatory clients are often able to transfer themselves off the floor by using a sturdy piece of furniture, such as a chair, couch, or chest of drawers, to pull themselves upright, "walking" their lower extremities underneath them into a more vertical position.

FALL PREVENTION

As a healthcare provider, an OT practitioner needs to ensure the safety of clients by preventing falls. In hospital settings, 84% of all adverse events are associated with falls,[9] with

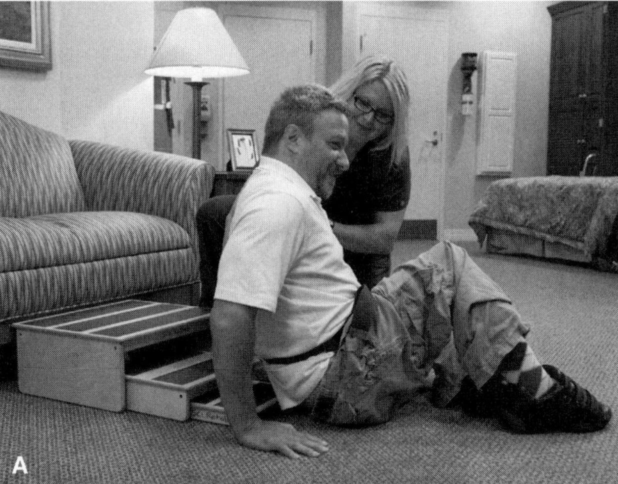

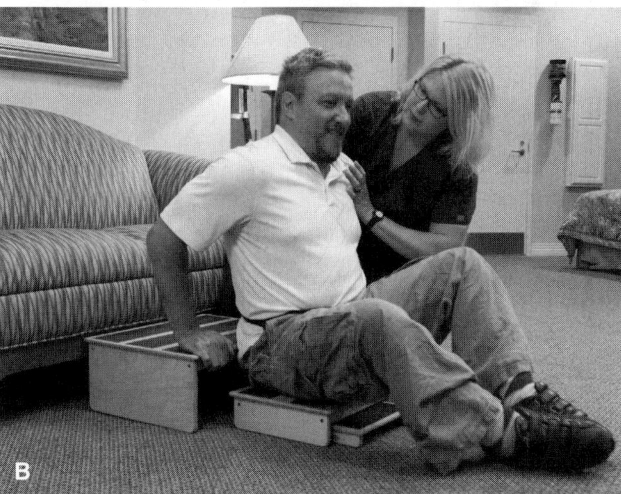

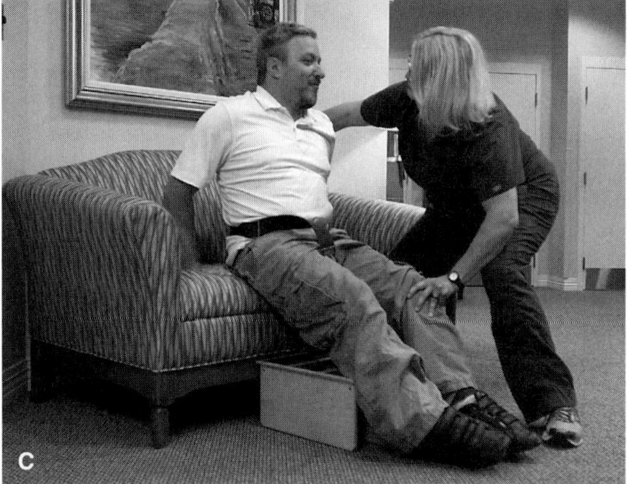

FIGURE 13-18. A client with good trunk and upper-body strength can learn to maneuver himself from the floor back into the seat of a wheelchair, chair, or firm couch. **A.** Client prepares to lift lower body onto first raised surface **B.** Practitioner spots client as he lifts himself level by level. **C.** Client lifts onto the couch with OTA guiding and assisting as needed.

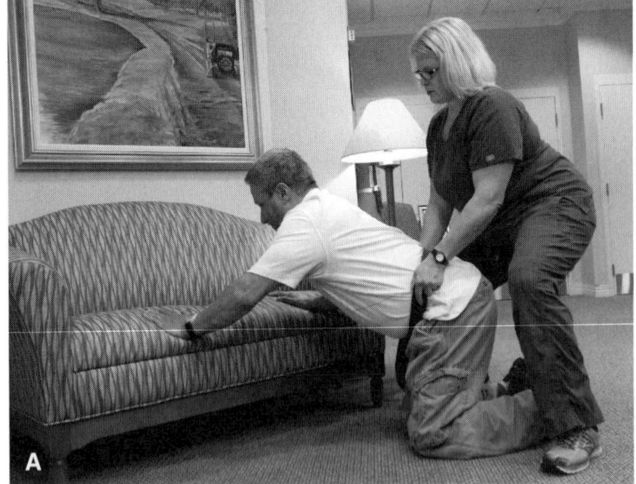

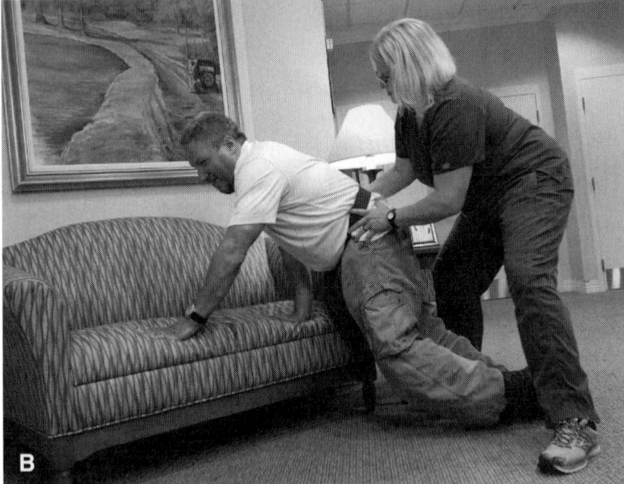

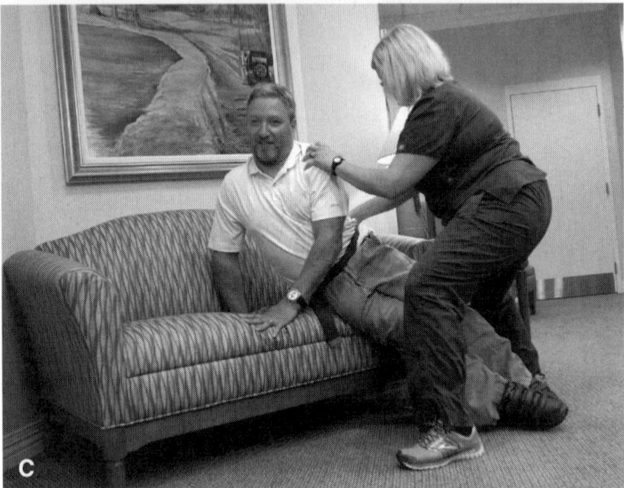

FIGURE 13-19. A client transferring directly from the floor to a firm couch. **A.** OTA holds to belt, and assists client to knees. **B.** Client begins to pivot around, while OTA guides legs and spots him. **C.** Client rotates to sit on couch, while OTA makes sure he is on enough to not slide off.

approximately 33% of falls resulting in injury.[10] Falls are linked to longer hospital stays and an increase of hospital discharges to nursing centers.[11] The Centers for Medicare and Medicaid Services[12] will not pay for costs associated with injuries from falls if deemed a preventable error. Approximately one third of community-dwelling people age 65 years and older experience accidental falls annually,[13] similar to nonambulatory nursing home residents in this same age group reporting at least one fall annually.[14] Medical conditions, such as amputations, CVA, and cognitive impairments, alter a person's center of gravity, thus reducing stability, putting the individual at a greater risk for falls.[15] The above evidence supports the necessity for all practitioners to address fall prevention and education as an aspect of intervention for clients and their caregivers.

One aspect of fall prevention is being aware of the risk factors and being alert to these when reviewing a client's medical history. Risk factors include advanced age; previous falls; decreased balance/gait; visual, cognitive, and auditory impairments; musculoskeletal deficits; comorbidities (two or more chronic conditions); side effects of medications; and environmental factors.[16] A component of OT services is to address the above-mentioned deficits and impairments. By ensuring that these deficits are addressed within occupations, the OT practitioner is helping clients learn effective problem-solving skills and reduce their risk of falling in the future. At times, OT intervention cannot improve the client's deficits or impairments, and therefore the OT practitioner will need to make environmental modifications and change the selection of transfers to reduce the risk of falling.

Another aspect of fall prevention is providing education in conjunction with addressing environmental factors, such as proper selection and installation of DME, increased lighting, and appropriate footwear.[16] A recommendation to reduce clutter and ensure a clear path of travel in and around the environment (home, hospital, or long-term care home, etc.) can be made to reduce the risk of falling. As the OTA practices transfers with a client, he or she needs to reinforce the rationale for and proper use of ambulation devices[17]; ensuring wheelchair locks are engaged; surfaces, such as beds, chairs, and couches are stabilized; and DME (e.g., tub benches, 3-in-1 commodes) is appropriate to the client's needs and installed correctly. The OT practitioner should ensure that lighting around the home is sufficient, especially in darker areas of the homes, such as hallways and stairwells. Education should be provided to the client stressing the importance of wearing proper footwear and use of lighting in the overnight hours when there is a greater risk for falls when transitioning between the bedroom and bathroom for toileting. If bowel or bladder urgency is an ongoing concern, then the suggestion of a bedside commode or the use of urinals/bed pans should be encouraged to reduce the risk of falling. Last, when providing home safety recommendations for the home, clients should be encouraged to keep a cordless or mobile telephone on their person at all times or to use a medical alert system such as a necklace or wrist-watch attachment that can be activated to summon immediate assistance from family or emergency response teams, if needed.

SAFE PATIENT-HANDLING EQUIPMENT

A variety of products on the market can fall under the category of SPH equipment. In this chapter, the term *SPH equipment* refers to lift systems that are used for assisting clients with safe transfers. Typically, SPH equipment is used when a client requires complete assistance or significant assistance to transfer. As part of the lift system, the OT practitioner must also select the most appropriate type of sling based on the client's needs. The next section will first discuss the types of slings and steps to apply a sling under the client in preparation for the transfer. This is followed by a discussion of the three most common types of lift systems and includes steps for performing a transfer with a lift system. Although the content that follows provides examples on the use of lifts, all practitioners should be trained on the proper use of the SPH equipment that is available in their practice setting before using it with a client.

Sling Selection and Application

When using a lift system, a sling that supports the client's weight is required. A variety of slings can be used with lift systems. The following is a list of the most common sling types and a brief rationale for each sling to assist the practitioner in the decision making process for selecting a sling type that aligns with the needs for transferring the client.

- A *full-length body sling* extends from the head or shoulders to behind the client's knees. It is an older style of sling and is used for clients that need full support. It can only be positioned when the client is supine; therefore, the client will have to remain sitting on the sling when transferred to seating surface (e.g., wheelchair) and increases the risk of skin breakdown if the client is in the seated position for long periods.
- A *divided-leg sling* is recommended for transferring clients between supine and sitting positions and for most other transfers. The leg straps are positioned between the client's legs, reducing the likelihood of the client's buttocks sliding forward out of the sling. This sling can be positioned when the client is either in the supine or sitting position. It is a preferred sling to use if the client will remain sitting for long periods. This sling type has several variations (e.g., addition of head/neck support).
- *Toileting slings* have a circular cut-out, which is positioned below the client's buttocks and perineal area. This sling can be used for bathing as well.
- A *standing sling* is used in conjunction with a standing-aid lift. This sling supports the torso and thus avoids interfering with hip movement when transitioning between sitting and standing positions.

To apply a sling, the client can be in either the sitting or the supine position. Make sure to have the sling in the correct orientation, the top versus the bottom of the sling. See Figure 13-20 for an example of correct orientation of a divided leg sling.

The steps to apply a sling when the client is in the seated position (typically in a wheelchair) are as follows:

1. Assist the client with leaning the upper body forward by placing hands behind the client's shoulders. Do not pull on client's arms, but provide support, as needed. While the client is leaning forward, the care provider slides the sling behind the client's back to the seated surface (Fig. 13-21A).
2. If using a divided leg sling, move the client's lower extremities, as necessary, to bring both leg straps to the inside of the thighs in preparation to attach the sling to the lift (see Figs. 13-21B and 13-21C). If using a toileting or other sling, lean the client side to side to work the sling under the buttocks.

For a client who is in bed, use the following steps:

1. Assist the client with rolling onto the side by placing a hand behind the client's shoulder and hip girdle. The sling is rolled vertically halfway and placed underneath the client until it reaches the vertical midline of the client (Fig. 13-22A).
2. Roll the client toward the opposite side in a similar manner and then unroll the sling to a flattened

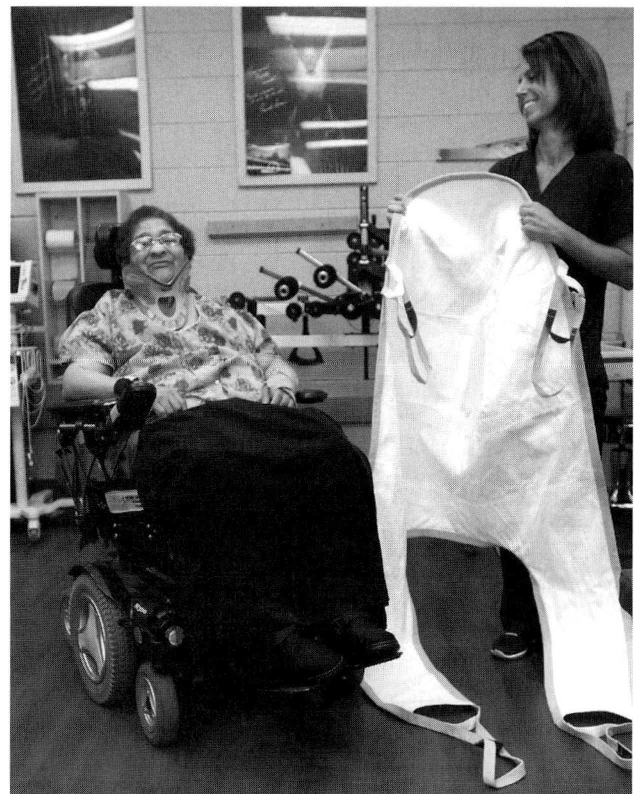

FIGURE 13-20. Divided leg sling in the correct orientation.

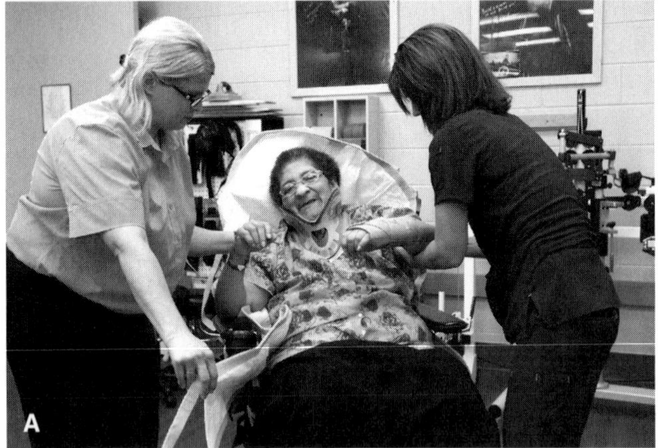

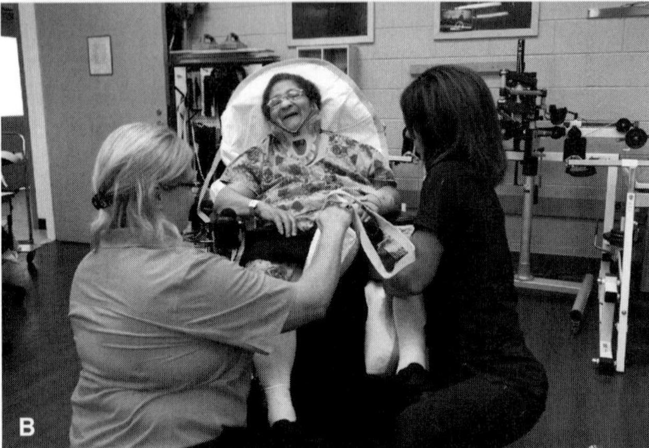

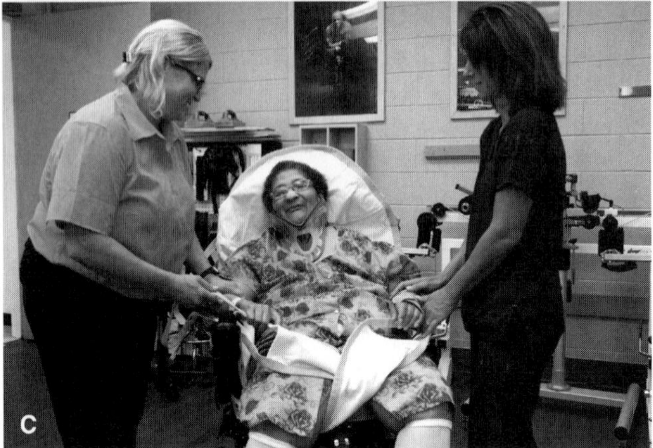

FIGURE 13-21. Applying a divided leg sling: A. First slide behind back all the way to seat surface, and bring side wings along outside of thighs. B. Slide side wings under each leg from the outside to the inside, just above the knee. C. Shows crossing straps, but can leave uncrossed, as desired.

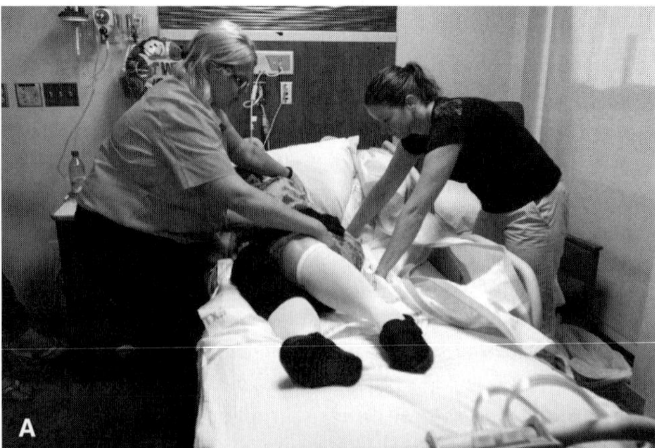

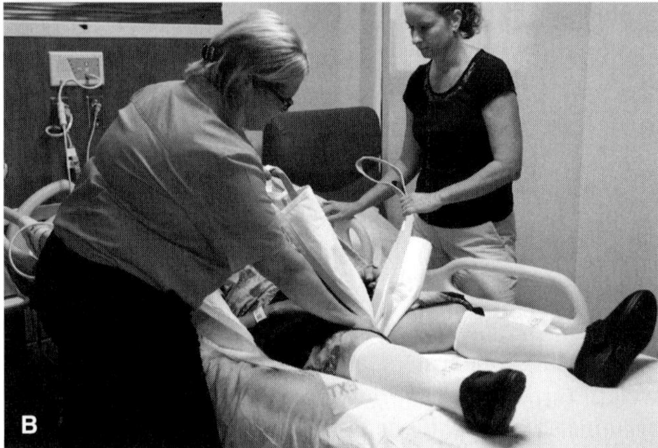

FIGURE 13-22. Applying a sling to a client in bed. A. Roll client, and slide half of sling under body. Roll back slightly to other side, and pull out sling until fully under client. B. Bring side straps from outside of thighs to inside at lower thighs above knees. Cross or not as desired.

position that spans the client's shoulder to the hip girdle.

3. Assist the client with rolling back into supine. If using a divided leg sling, move the lower extremities, as necessary, to bring both leg straps to the inside of the thighs in preparation to attach the sling to the lift (see Fig. 13-22B).

The above steps can be performed when only one practitioner is involved. For clients who are unable to assist, have significant cognitive impairment, or are overweight, it is best to have a care provider assist the OT practitioner for additional safety, as demonstrated in the figures. To remove the sling, the above steps are performed in the opposing direction. It is important that slings be removed upon completion of the transfer to reduce the risk of skin irritation.[18]

Portable Lifts

The first type of SPH equipment we will discuss is a portable lift. Depending on the vendor, portable lifts are also referred to as *floor lifts*; the common term "Hoyer lift" is one of many available brands. Portable lifts are either manual (mechanical) or electric (powered). Manual portable lifts require the care provider to manually pump a lever arm that uses hydraulics to lift the client off of a surface. Electric portable lifts are operated by pushing a button on the control panel to activate the hydraulic system for lifting the client off of a surface.

Portable lifts are the most common type of SPH equipment and can be found in a variety of settings, including hospitals, skilled nursing facilities, nursing homes, school systems, and private homes. Portable lifts are affordable and enable the care provider to transfer the client safely between two surfaces (e.g., bed to the wheelchair). This type of lift

EVIDENCE-BASED PRACTICE

OT practitioners are taught to have hands on the client to influence his or her functional outcome. Some practitioners have taken this general concept and applied it to educating clients on transfers; the result is that lift systems are not used therapeutically. However, the implementation of SPH protocols across facilities are changing the way practitioners are incorporating the use of lift systems into the therapeutic process.

Darragh et al.[19] found that practitioners using lift systems reported an increase in treatment options and an increase in client participation. The availability of lift systems in facilities allows practitioners to incorporate SPH equipment into the therapeutic process. Additionally, there is an increasing variety of options for lift systems over the past few years, allowing for the use of lift systems in a variety of settings and situations (e.g., ceiling lifts versus a portable lift that takes up significant floor space in the therapy gym). The choice to use a lift system can increase the comfort levels of some clients who are fearful of a practitioner transferring them because of the client's reduced ability to assist with the transfer, and conversely, some clients are very fearful of being suspended in the air by the lift.[19]

Practitioners have reported that the use of lift systems assist with mobilizing clients earlier in the therapeutic process, allowing for the ability to get more dependent clients out of bed easily.[19] The use of lift systems allow more time during intervention sessions to address other areas of occupations versus a considerable amount of time being spent on transferring the client before and at the end of the session. Last, practitioners have reported that the use of lift systems reduces the risk of injuries by increasing safety for practitioners as well as clients who require a considerable amount of assistance to transfer.[19]

Darragh, A. R., Campo, M. A., Frost, L., Miller, M., Pentico, M., & Margulis, H. (2013). Safe-patient-handling equipment in therapy practice: Implications for rehabilitation. American Journal of Occupational Therapy, 67, 45–53. *http://dx.doi.org/10.5014/ajot.2013.005389*

system is advantageous to medical facilities because one portable lift can be used for several clients on a hospital floor or residents living in a long-term care facility. Another advantage of the portable lift is that it can be used to transfer a person from one room to another room (e.g., bed to the toilet). A limitation of the portable lift is that it requires a large footprint, thus needing open floor space to be used between the two surfaces.

The following is one example of using a portable lift to transfer a client. Note that all OT practitioners should be trained by the facility on the proper use of portable lifts before use with a client. The instructions for this transfer begin with the client sitting in a wheelchair and assume that the divided leg sling has already been placed properly (use sling application steps in previous section). The basic concepts of this transfer can be applied to a variety of surfaces, such as a bed, toilet, bath bench, or other supportive surface. Before beginning the transfer, the process should be explained to the client to decrease potential anxiety about the transfer.

1. The two surfaces (e.g., wheelchair and bed) should be placed optimally so that the OTA can achieve a triangular steering pattern (e.g., lifting the client from the wheelchair, backing the lift away from the wheelchair, and steering the lift toward the bed).
2. Remove any obstacles between the path of the transfer so that the client can be transferred smoothly once suspended in the sling. *Note:* leaving the client hanging for an extended period can cause anxiety and discomfort.
3. Fully engage the wheelchair locks.
4. Align the lift to the client.
5. Lower the cradle and attach sling straps (Fig. 13-23A).
6. Lock the wheels of the lift; raise the cradle lifting the client off of the seated surface, only need to raise high enough for the buttocks to clear both surfaces (see Fig. 13-23B).
7. Unlock the wheels of the lift, and maneuver the lift until the client is aligned over the new surface.
8. Lock the wheels of the lift; slowly lower the cradle while providing guidance to the sling to ensure the best positioning of the client on the new surface; at times, a second care provider may be needed to assist with positioning. Note: make sure attention is paid to the cradle position as it approaches the client's head (as they lower fully to the seat) to avoid injury.
9. Once the client is fully supported by the new surface, remove the sling straps.
10. Raise the cradle, unlock the wheels on the lift, and move the lift out of the way.
11. Remove the sling from underneath the client.

Overhead Track Lifts

An overhead track lift is a second type of SPH equipment that combines an electric lift with a railing system that is suspended from overhead. Overhead track lifts can be freestanding or mounted to the ceiling. Although not portable, an overhead track lift does not require a large amount of floor space, and this can be very helpful in small spaces. This type of lift has become more common in rehabilitation settings, where they are installed in therapy gyms and client rooms.

The advantage of this lift system is that it can be set up in a single room or the ceiling-mounted railing can transition throughout an entire house, although it is often cost-prohibitive to do so.

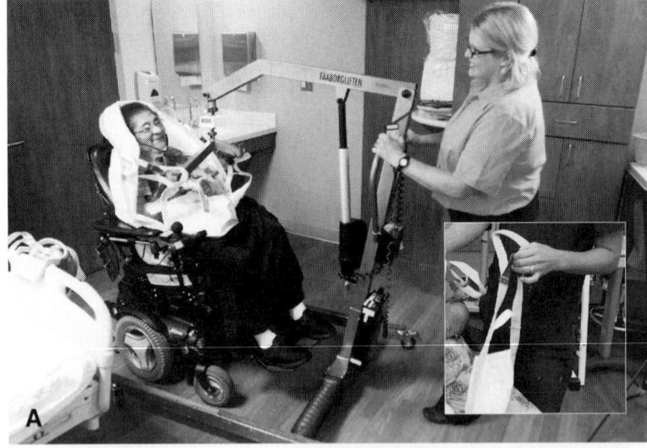

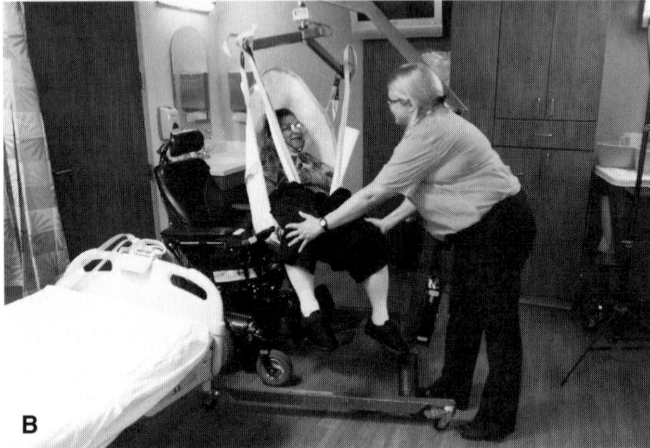

FIGURE 13-23. Using a portable lift to transfer a client. A. Hook straps onto lift cradle (see inset for detail). B. Roll lift over to chair and carefully lower client; make sure bottom is fully on seat before unstrapping.

Practitioners should be trained by the facility on the proper use of the overhead lift system before use with a client. The instructions for this transfer begin with the client sitting in a wheelchair and assume that the divided leg sling has already been placed properly (use sling application steps in previous section). The basic concepts of this transfer can be applied to a variety of surfaces, such as a bed, toilet, bath bench, or other supportive surface. Before beginning the transfer, the process should be explained to the client to decrease potential anxiety about the transfer.

1. Align the overhead lift to the client.
2. Lower the cradle, and attach the sling straps (Fig. 13-24A).
3. Using the control panel, raise the cradle lifting the client off of the seated surface; it only needs to be raised high enough for the buttocks to clear both surfaces.
4. While the client is suspended, provide guidance to the sling/client to maneuver the lift toward the new surface.
5. Ensure best positioning of client over the new surface, and slowly lower the cradle while providing guidance to the sling/client, as needed; at times, a second care provider may be needed to assist with positioning. Note: make sure attention is paid to the cradle position as it approaches the client's head (as they lower fully to the seat) to avoid injury.
6. Once the client is fully supported by the new surface, remove the sling straps.
7. Raise the cradle, and move the lift out of the way.
8. Remove the sling from underneath the client.

Standing-Aid Lifts

Standing-aid lifts are used to assist persons who have the ability to bear weight in their lower extremities but need a significant amount of assistance to transfer from the sitting position to the standing position. Similar to the portable lifts described above, standing-aid lifts are portable and operate on either manual or electric hydraulics. This lift is exceptionally useful to facilitate toilet transfers; the client's lower body clothing can easily be accessed and removed to encourage use of a commode. This upright position improves bowel and bladder functions and allows the client to use upper-body muscles more independently.

The following instructions describe how to use a standing-aid lift. The client should wear nonskid footwear (preferably shoes). Before beginning the transfer, the process should be explained to the client to decrease potential anxiety about the transfer.

1. Begin the transfer with the client in the seated position.
2. Assist the client with leaning forward by placing the sling around the client's waist and attaching the sling

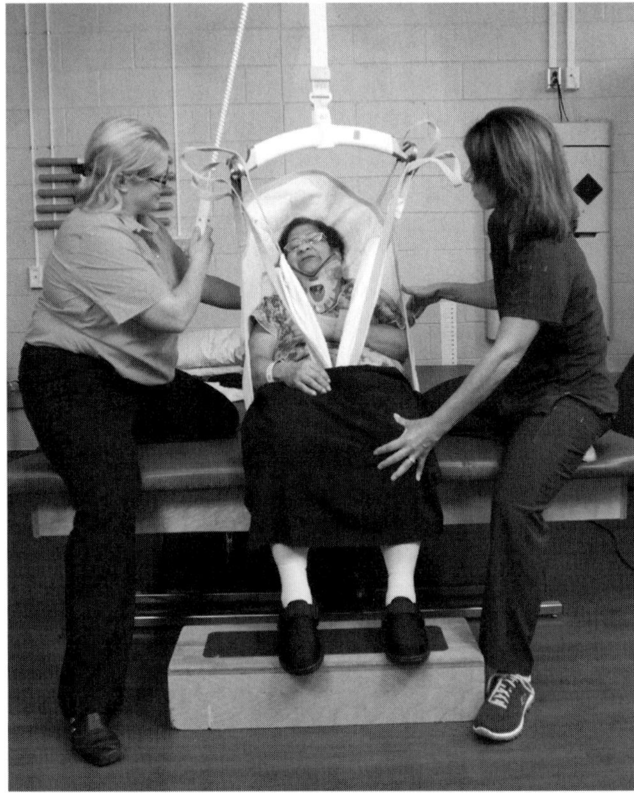

FIGURE 13-24. Transferring a client using an overhead track lift.

TECHNOLOGY AND TRENDS

New technology in transfers is combining the concept of overhead track systems with the capability of being portable. These overhead portable lift systems can be set up in a variety of settings—from therapy settings to home settings. Many times, the lifts sit on two or four legs and are braced against the wall, with the lift suspended from an overhead horizontal beam(s) connecting and stabilizing the product. This allows for use in facilities or home environments that have limited floor space, places where overhead ceiling tracking cannot be installed, or places where the flexibility for the lifts to be used in more than one space is required. Some of these lifts can be disassembled to be accommodated in a large/long duffle bag for travel. As with other lift systems, the use of lifts can decrease worker or caregiver injuries and increase safety for clients.

to fit snugly between the client's iliac crest and rib cage over the soft tissue of the client's torso. *Note:* if this strap is not sufficiently tight, the sling can slide up the trunk causing an unsafe and unstable position during transfers.

3. Align the lift to the client.
4. Place the client's feet on lift platform, with client's knees positioned against knee pads to prevent excessive knee flexion.
5. Attach the sling straps to the lever arms, and lock the wheels of the lift.
6. Encourage the client to hold onto the handles during the transfer while raising the lever arms to lift the client off of the seated surface into the standing position.
7. When ready to return the client to the seated position, lower the lever arms until the client is fully supported by the new surface.
8. Remove the sling straps, and move the lift out of the way.
9. Remove the sling from around the client.

Note that clients should not use a standing-aid lift if they have weight-bearing precautions in the lower extremities or if they have had a lower extremity amputation that prevents equal weight-bearing through both lower extremities. Clients with significant weakness in the trunk or neck, or with back pain may be unable to use this type of lift.

TRANSFERS FOR POSTSURGICAL RESTRICTIONS

Immediately after surgery and at times for several weeks to months afterward, physicians will give medical orders to restrict certain movements in an attempt to allow the site of surgery or other medical intervention to heal. These are called *postsurgical restrictions;* some practice settings also use the term *precautions.* It is important that the supervising occupational therapist and the OTA discuss how the restrictions or precautions will impact the client's treatment plan. The medical chart should be consulted before beginning any treatment to determine whether restrictions are the same or if they have changed. The OTA will need to alter transfer techniques, under the advisement of the supervising occupational therapist, to allow for or to teach clients to incorporate these restrictions or precautions into their daily transfers.

Orthopedic Restrictions

Clients who have recently undergone orthopedic procedures, such as hip pinning, total hip replacement, partial hip replacement, or total knee replacement surgeries, are likely to have movement restrictions and weight-bearing restrictions. The OTA must be familiar with the movement restrictions and weight-bearing restrictions and adapt transfers accordingly. Clients with lower extremity joint replacements will be utilizing a walker postoperatively; therefore, a stand-step transfer or stand-hop transfer between surfaces will be used, with the practitioner standing on the surgical side of the client to provide assistance throughout the transfer. Stand-step transfers should be used with clients who can follow partial to full weight-bearing restrictions. Stand-hop transfers should be used with toe-touch to non–weight-bearing restrictions. With movement restrictions, that is, not flexing the hip more than 90 degrees, the client will need to slide out to the edge of the seated surface and will extend the surgical leg, increasing the hip angle to allow for slight trunk flexion when using arms to push up from the seated position. This same attention to detail should be given when preparing to seat the client. The client should place the surgical leg anteriorly to increase hip angle while the nonsurgical leg bears the majority of the weight to slowly descend to the seating surface.

Sternal Restrictions

Clients who underwent cardiac surgery have medical orders for sternal restrictions. Additionally, these clients will have limited activity tolerance and strength. The following are common sternal restrictions and are typically maintained until 8 weeks after surgery. Note that it is important for the OT practitioner to consult the cardiac physician and medical chart orders about restrictions specific to each client.

- No pulling or pushing with arms
- No lifting more than 10 pounds
- No reaching past midline

Implementation of sternal restrictions makes it necessary for the client to learn to perform transfers without pushing up using the arms. The OTA must instruct the client to place his or her hands in the lap or hug a pillow, to prevent weight-bearing through the upper extremities because this could cause displacement of the midline incision and result in nonhealing of the bones. For bed mobility, the OTA needs to teach the client with sternal restrictions to roll in bed by using the lower extremities because the client is not allowed to pull on the bed rails using the upper extremities. When transferring from sitting to standing, a client should be taught to rock anteriorly several times to increase weight shift from the buttocks onto the feet. Environmental modifications, such as raising the heights of seating surfaces, may be needed if these clients are unable to regain sufficient strength to perform transfers from siting to standing without the use of their upper extremities. Education regarding pulse monitoring will need to be taught so that these clients do not overexert themselves. Clients may use ambulatory assistive devices, such as a walker or cane, as long as they are not putting their entire body weight onto this device during functional mobility.

Pacemaker Restrictions

Restrictions for clients who have pacemakers implanted are very similar to sternal restrictions, except that they typically only apply to the arm on the side of the pacemaker placement (frequently the left arm); and in most cases, clients only have to adhere to the pacemaker restrictions for 2 weeks after surgery. For each client, the OTA must read the medical orders and educate the client on the client's specific restrictions ordered by the physician with regard to transfers and participation in daily occupations.

Spinal Restrictions

Clients who have had spinal surgery have spinal restrictions that they are to follow until the physician changes or discontinues the restrictions. Spinal restrictions are usually maintained 3 months after surgery. Typical spinal restrictions include the following:

- No bending (the area of the spine involved)
- No lifting more than 10 pounds
- No twisting (the area of the spine involved)
- No straining (e.g., Valsalva maneuver)

Clients who undergo neck or back surgery may or may not have to wear spinal orthotics in the form of cervical collars, thoracic-sacral orthoses, and lower-back braces. Some of these can be donned sitting on the edge of the bed, but many clients have to perform upper-body bathing and dressing in the supine position. The client will then don the orthosis with assistance and then sit on the edge of the bed to complete activities of daily living.

OTAs need to modify instruction for these clients ensuring that they perform bed mobility by "log-rolling," keeping the entire spine in alignment, rather than moving segmentally. The practitioner must educate these clients and their caregivers about donning of orthoses. Cervical collars must be donned in the supine position, keeping the head in alignment with the body, without a pillow under the head, with a caregiver stabilizing the neck while the anterior and posterior sections of the collar are placed individually, one at a time. Thoracic lumbar sacral orthosis (TLSO) braces are typically donned over a thin shirt while the client is in bed. The OT practitioner will use a log-rolling technique while a caregiver positions the anterior and posterior sections of the TLSO separately before the head of the bed is raised past 30-degree flexion.

Lower-back braces or corsets are often donned while seated on the edge of the bed, but care must be taken to ensure spinal alignment when transitioning clients from supine to sitting. OTAs may need to obtain clarification from the physician or the orthotist about showering with the orthosis—including scheduling time to allow the orthosis to dry completely. Clients with spinal precautions are often not allowed to have the head of the bed raised beyond 30 degrees without their spinal orthosis in place. Because of the motion limitations imposed by the orthoses, OTAs may need to provide additional assistance, especially when clients transition from supine to sitting on the edge of the bed.

TRANSFERS FOR SPECIFIC DEFICITS

The traditional transfers discussed earlier in the chapter are primarily utilized with clients who have use or some use of all four of their extremities. Modifications will need to be made to these transfers when the client has a diagnosis that results in specific associated deficits. This next section considers transfer modifications for persons with hemiparesis, paraplegia, tetraplegia, or lower extremity amputation.

Clients who have one or more of the above deficits will have associated complications that the practitioner must be knowledgeable about to be prepared to address them when performing transfers. **Orthostatic hypotension** is common in clients who have been bedbound primarily in the supine position for extended periods (e.g., because of medically induced comas or prolonged recovery from surgery) or have had blood loss or dehydration. Symptoms include dizziness or lightheadedness, fainting, nausea, blurry vision, weakness, and confusion from a sudden drop in blood pressure. Clients may experience orthostatic hypotension when transitioning from supine to sitting on the edge of a bed or when transitioning from sitting to standing. Therefore, a second care provider may be required to assist when first initiating transfers because the client may experience a drop in blood pressure and become unresponsive. Should a client experience orthostatic hypotension, he or she can be placed in the Trendelenburg position. In the Trendelenburg position, the client is positioned supine with the feet positioned higher than the head by 15 to 30 degrees, to manage the drop in blood pressure. This position can easily be achieved with the use of a hospital bed or power wheelchair with a tilt-in-space function, or even in a manual wheelchair tipped backwards with the brakes locked.

Pressure injuries may also be an associated complication that must be considered when preparing to transfer a client. See Chapter 8 for information. The National Pressure Ulcer Advisory Panel defines a pressure injury as "an area of unrelieved pressure over a defined area, usually over a bony prominence, resulting in ischemia, cell death, and tissue necrosis."[20] Additionally, pressure injuries can be initiated or healing can be prolonged as a result of shearing forces occurring during transfer between surfaces. Persons with hemiparesis, paraplegia, tetraplegia, or lower extremity amputation are at risk for pressure injury development because of prolonged supine or sitting positions or shearing forces. Prolonged positioning causes more than 32 mm Hg forces (sufficient to decrease blood supply to the tissues involved) to be exerted, causing deep tissue injury and pressure injuries.[21] Therefore, OTAs play an important role in educating clients and caregivers about reducing shearing forces during a transfer, proper positioning after transfer to a new surface, and application of pressure relief techniques to reduce the risk of development of pressure injuries.

Hemiparesis

Hemiparesis is weakness on one side of the body affecting the function of the upper and lower extremities. Deciding between transferring toward the hemiparetic side versus the nonhemiparetic side involves consideration of client factors, the environment, and the purpose for the transfer. Client factors to consider are strength and movement of the hemiparetic side, assistance level, visual–perceptual deficits (e.g., hemianopsia or neglect), and cognitive deficits (e.g., ability to follow directions).

When unfamiliar with the client, the OTA should attempt to transfer the client toward the nonhemiparetic side as the client will have a greater sense of security and generally be able to assist more with the transfer. The use of a squat-pivot or stand-pivot transfer is suggested in combination with transferring toward the nonhemiparetic side because less movement of the hemiparetic upper and lower extremities is required. With increased familiarity with the client and as the client progresses toward discharge, the OTA must work with the client and the caregiver on transferring in both directions to ensure safety. Some environmental situations require the client to be able to transfer in both directions, for example, transfers to and from the toilet or a motor vehicle because these are fixed surfaces.

OT Practitioner's Viewpoint

I find that my clients make faster progress in transfer status when the OT and PT practitioners regularly discuss how we are going to help the client progress in becoming more independent with his or her own transfers. Furthermore, once the decisions are made, I take the time to discuss the type of transfer and reasoning for the transfer selection with the nursing staff. Taking this time with the nursing staff tends to improve follow-through by the nursing staff to reinforce and ultimately increase the client's transfer performance. The caregivers and/or families are also more comfortable with transferring the client because they are seeing consistency among healthcare professionals in transfer methods. ~Dr. Jennifer C. Radloff, OTD, OTR/L, CDRS

BED MOBILITY

At the beginning of bed mobility training with the client, the client may be more dependent on assistive devices, such as bed railings and trapeze bar, but he or she should be encouraged to rely less and less on such equipment as improvements in mobility are made. For moving up in the bed, the OTA must consider the assistance level of the client. In some circumstances, the OTA should request the assistance of a second care provider to avoid injury (refer to two-person bed mobility transfer for steps). For the client who requires minimal assistance and has some return of function on the hemiparetic side, a modified transfer for moving up in bed can be used. For direct application of steps, we will assume that the client has left-side hemiparesis.

1. Position the bed completely flat. Ensure that the trapeze bar is within comfortable reach of the right upper extremity.
2. Stand on the client's hemiparetic (left) side, facing the bed.
3. Instruct the client to place the left upper extremity across the abdomen with the assistance of the right upper extremity, as needed.
4. Instruct the client to bend the right knee, with the right foot placed flat on the bed.
5. Instruct the client to assist with bending the left knee to place the left foot flat on the bed. Place the client's right hand underneath the knee to provide physical assistance to bend the knee while the client's left hand is placed around the left ankle providing assistance to place the foot flat on the bed.
6. The OTA should place the right hand under the client's left posterior hip and the left hand on the anterior aspect of the client's left knee.
7. Instruct the client to reach up for the trapeze bar with the right upper extremity and lift the upper body while using the right lower extremity to lift the buttocks off the bed; assist with bridging the left hip, and encourage use of the left lower extremity to assist with bridging to scoot up in the bed.
8. Repeat the previous step until the desired upward position is reached.

A modification to moving up in bed is to have the client roll onto his or her side and push up into sitting on the edge of the bed. Have the client place both feet on the floor and perform side-scoot movements by using the nonhemiparetic hand, bending the trunk anteriorly to bear weight on both legs to lift the buttocks off of the bed while performing small "hops" toward the head of the bed. When reaching the top one third of the bed, the client transfers from sitting on the side of the bed to the supine position. The practitioner assists, as needed, throughout this transfer to ensure safety.

SUPINE TO AND FROM SITTING ON EDGE OF BED

For transitioning from supine to sitting on the side of the bed, the practitioner should stand on the side of the bed that the client is rolling toward. In some situations, the OTA will provide a combination of verbal instructions and physical assistance, as needed. If the client has receptive aphasia or cognitive processing deficits, it is recommended that very little verbal directions be used and more tactile cueing be used instead.

For direct application of steps, we will assume that the client has left hemiparesis. In addition, the client has been making progress and therefore the OT practitioner has decided to have the client learn to transfer toward the hemiparetic side; therefore, the client will be rolling onto his or her left side.

1. Stand on the left side of the bed facing the client.
2. Instruct the client to bend his or her right knee, placing the right foot flat onto the bed.
3. Instruct the client to reach for the left hand with the right hand and either interlace the fingers or hold onto the left wrist. Instruct the client to "reach toward the ceiling" to promote scapular protraction and approximately 90 degrees of shoulder flexion.
4. The OTA should place the left hand on the client's right hip and the right hand on the superior/posterior aspect of the client's right shoulder to assist with rolling the client.
5. Instruct the client to turn the head to the left while moving the arms to the left and pushing off with the right foot to log-roll toward the left side (Fig. 13-25A).
6. Instruct the client to place the right hand on the mattress or the upper bed rail in front of the torso to provide support while lying on the left side.
7. Instruct client to hook the right ankle/foot behind the left lower leg to assist with moving both lower extremities off the side of the bed. Assist the client, as needed, with placement of the right lower extremity and movement of both lower extremities with the left hand to perform the sweeping motion of moving the lower extremities off the bed.
8. Instruct the client to use the right hand to push off the mattress or the upper handrail to lift the upper body off the mattress to come into the sitting position. Facilitate this movement by placing the right hand underneath the client's left shoulder and the left hand at the superior aspect of the client's right hip along the side of the trunk and assist the client into the sitting position. During this movement, the OTA should weight shift from the right foot to the left foot (see Fig. 13-25B).
9. End the transfer with the client's feet touching the floor, trunk in midline, and upper extremities placed in a position to support sitting balance (see Fig. 13-25C).

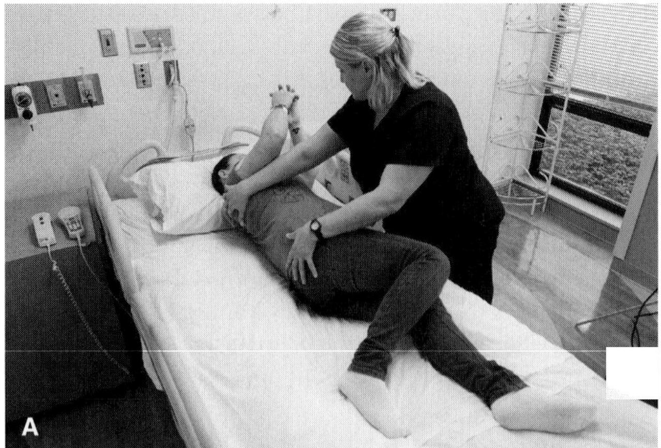

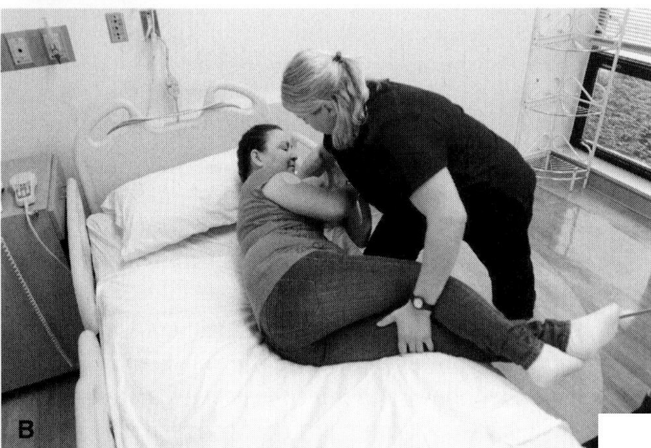

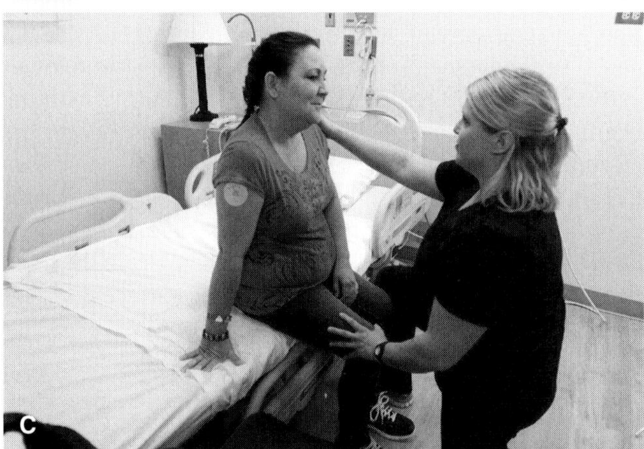

FIGURE 13-25. Assisting the client with left hemiparesis from the supine position to sitting on the edge of the bed. **A.** Assist to begin rolling. **B.** Moving from side lying to begin sitting up. **C.** Stabilize in sitting.

WHEELCHAIR TO AND FROM OTHER SURFACES

As with all other transfers, the OT practitioner should consider the environmental setup and select the type of transfer on the basis of the client's assistance level and progress. For direct application of steps, we will assume the client has left-side hemiparesis. The client has stated the importance of being able to self-transfer to a couch upon discharge; because this is the first time practicing this transfer, the OT practitioner has decided that it is safest to transfer toward the nonhemiparetic side (i.e., right side) and will use a stand-pivot transfer.

1. The OT practitioner should be positioned facing the client in midline, with one hand on each side of the transfer belt. Note that if the hemiparetic

upper extremity cannot assist in the transfer, then the OTA can encompass the client's arm inside the OTA's own arm and then hold onto the transfer belt.

2. Instruct the client to push off the armrest with the right (nonhemiparetic) hand while leaning anteriorly to bear weight into the lower extremities. The OTA should block the client's left (hemiparetic) knee with the OTA's right lower extremity to prevent buckling of knee when the client transitions to the standing position (Fig. 13-26).
3. Assist the client with pivoting of the feet and movement of the body toward the new surface. During this motion, the OTA should shift weight from an anterior position to a posterior position in space to counterbalance the weight of the client.
4. Instruct the client to reach toward the new surface with the right (nonhemiparetic) hand and slowly lower himself or herself onto the new surface. The practitioner should provide support to the client's left (hemiparetic) knee on the descent to ensure a smooth transition.

As with all transfers, modifications can be made to this transfer to best match the environment, client factors, assistance level, and assistive devices. The type of transfer is likely to change throughout the therapeutic process as the client gains more return of function on the hemiparetic side.

Tetraplegia and Paraplegia

Depending on level of spinal cord injury (SCI), whether the lesion is complete or incomplete, the American Spinal Injury Association (ASIA) impairment scale (AIS) (motor versus sensory impairments), and the presence of additional comorbidities or dual-diagnoses, the type of transfer that clients are able to perform and the amount of assistance that they need will vary immensely. Individuals with a complete SCI (AIS A) will have no motor or sensory responses at and below the level of injury, whereas an individual with an incomplete SCI (AIS B, C, or D) may have either motor or sensory responses. Individuals with an incomplete injury may also have spasticity, increased tone, or fluctuating tone—often flaccidity and spasticity simultaneously, which may impede function. The proper transfer technique will be one that compensates for and addresses these fluctuations.

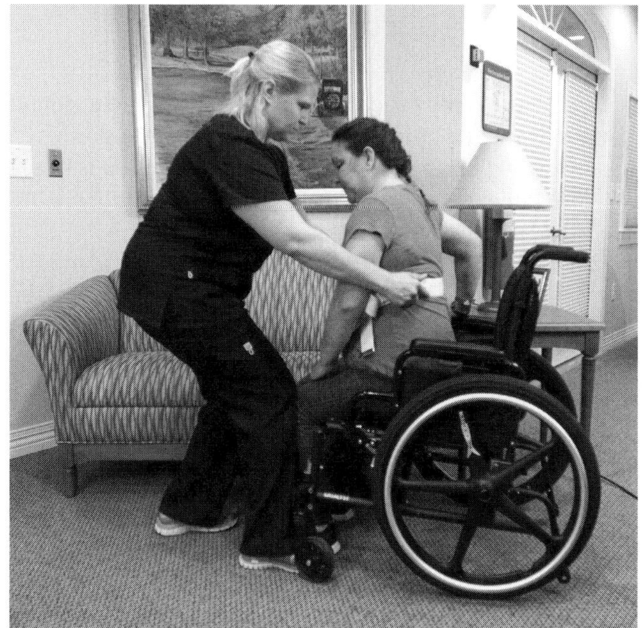

FIGURE 13-26. Assisting the client with left hemiparesis from the wheelchair to the couch.

For the purpose of this chapter, we will address modified transfer techniques and the expected levels of assistance that will be required for clients with SCI and no additional comorbidities. Clients with high-level tetraplegia (C5 and higher) will require total assistance of one or two caregivers and therefore will primarily use SPH equipment for most transfers. Clients with lower level tetraplegia (C6 to T2) will probably only require the assistance of one caregiver, and clients with paraplegia (T3 and below with no upper extremity involvement) may often transfer independently with modified techniques and assistive devices. To be able to address the varying types of transfers, we will divide each type of transfer into the following classifications: high-level tetraplegic (C5 and higher), low-level tetraplegic (C6 to T2), and paraplegic: (T3 and below). Note that individuals with SCI are more likely to have incidences of orthostatic hypotension, especially early on in the recovery phase, and are at an increased risk of developing pressure injuries throughout the remainder of their life. In addition, during the first year following the injury, the client will likely need the most assistance, and some clients classified with C5 or lower, especially those with incomplete injuries, may need less assistance with transfers than in the beginning. Refer to Chapter 35, Spinal Cord Injury and Disease: Factors and Essential Care for more specifics on clients with SCI.

BED MOBILITY

The practitioner should refer to some of the previous sections—Assistive Devices, Use of Equipment for Bed Mobility, and SPH Equipment—because the interventions and skills discussed there can be implemented to assist clients with SCI with bed mobility. Additional considerations and techniques specific to the different levels of SCI are discussed below.

High-Level Tetraplegia (C5 and Higher): People with high-level tetraplegia, AIS A, require total assistance for bed mobility. Therefore, the use of SPH equipment, such as nylon mat, air-assisted mat, or lift systems, are recommended. In addition to providing this information, the OTA can educate the client to participate actively in the transfers by learning how to instruct caregivers on how to roll, scoot toward the head of the bed, and position the client. Encouraging clients to be self-advocates is important, as few caregivers or family members have experience with assisting people with this level of impairment.

Techniques to consider with bed mobility transfers for persons with high-level tetraplegia are as follows:

- Place a hand behind the scapula when rolling a client toward the OTA, as opposed to pulling on an arm; this can prevent subluxation and associated pain and deformity.
- Use of leverage, such as flexing the knee of the client when rolling, is an effective technique despite the lack of innervation to the lower extremities.
- Avoid shear forces by using low-friction surfaces, such as nylon sheets or an air-assisted mattress.
- Use the Trendelenburg position to move the client toward the head of the bed.

Low-Level Tetraplegia (C6 to T2): Clients with lower-level tetraplegia are able to assist with bed mobility primarily by using their upper extremities along with assistive devices (e.g., trapeze bar or bed rails). Techniques listed in the section "High-Level Tetraplegia (C5 and Higher)" should be used to reduce injury; however, the client should be encouraged to use the available upper extremity function to assist with bed mobility. A client with a SCI, AIS A, at C6 is able to perform wrist extension (tenodesis technique) and use the bicep/deltoid, although has no elbow extension. These individuals can use these movements as a modified technique in conjunction with a bed rail to assist with rolling into the side-lying position. Individuals with C7–T2 can also use a trapeze bar to move the upper-body to assist with repositioning toward the head of the bed or use the bed rails to roll from side to side.

Paraplegia (T3 and Below): Individuals with innervation at or below T3 are able to use their upper extremities to perform rolling over in bed and for moving upward toward the head of the bed. Many are able to perform these tasks independently once educated by the OTA.

Techniques to consider with bed mobility transfers for persons with paraplegia are as follows:

- Use of a leg lifter or thigh straps to flex the knee or grasping behind the knee can be taught for repositioning the lower extremity. By flexing the knee, the added weight of the flexed knee can be used as leverage to roll from supine to side lying.
- Strengthening of elbow and shoulder extensor muscles is valuable to facilitate training the client to move the body toward the head of the bed by propping on the elbows and then extending the elbows with shoulder depression.
- Incorporation of assistive devices (e.g., trapeze bar, bed rails, or bed ladder), as needed, to assist with bed mobility.

The OTA may initially need to assist with these movements and should use the techniques described in the paragraphs above, but as the client's strength, range of motion, and technique improve, the OTA may decrease the amount of assistance so that clients are able to do as much as possible for themselves.

SUPINE TO AND FROM SITTING ON EDGE OF BED

The practitioner should refer to some of the previous sections—Assistive Devices, Traditional Transfers–Supine to/from Sitting on Edge of Bed, and SPH Equipment—because the interventions and skills discussed there can be implemented, with slight modifications, to assist clients with SCI. Additional considerations and modified techniques specific to the different levels of SCI are discussed below.

High-Level Tetraplegia (C5 and Higher): Clients with this level of injury, AIS A, have little, if any, innervation of the trunk musculature, which makes sitting unsupported on the edge of the bed a dangerous position. The OTA must train these clients to attempt to reposition, or influence the position of their body, by movements of the head and neck. Total assistance is required to transfer these clients from supine to sitting on the edge of the bed.

The use of a lift system is strongly recommended for this transfer because it reduces the risk of injury to both the caregiver and the client. As a general "rule," if two caregivers are required, a lift system should be used to perform this transfer. Note that individuals with higher-level tetraplegia, AIS A, will be unable to maintain their legs in adduction and their legs may tend to "splay" when positioned in the sling. If using a divided leg sling, it is advisable to cross the straps so that the strap under the right leg is attached to the lower hook on the left side, and vice versa. This should bring the lower extremities into a more adducted position, which can be maintained with positioning pads in the wheelchair to keep the legs parallel.

If a lift system is unavailable or not working, a two-person supine to sitting on edge of bed transfer can be performed. Note that if the client is required to wear a torso or cervical orthosis, it should be donned before the transfer is initiated. For direct application of steps, the client will be rolling onto his or her left side to transition from supine to sitting on the side of the bed.

1. The OTA is positioned on the side of the bed that the client will be rolled toward and is facing the client. The second practitioner is on the opposite side of the bed, facing the client. The height of the bed is raised to prevent low back strain for both practitioners. All bed rails are lowered.
2. A pillow is placed between the client's legs, and the right leg is flexed at the knee and is used to roll the client toward the OTA. The use of a pillow reduces stress to the spinal column when transitioning to side lying.
3. The client is assisted, as needed, with positioning the left arm by abducting the left shoulder by approximately 25 degrees so that this arm does not become trapped under the client's trunk while rolling onto the side.
4. The practitioners should provide support at the client's shoulders, right hip, and right upper leg. Working as a team to assist the client with rolling onto the left side, the client is log-rolled toward the OTA

maintaining spinal alignment (the head, shoulder, and hip girdle in line with one another) (Fig. 13-27A).

5. Each of the practitioners place one of their hands underneath the client's left shoulder while using their opposing hands to slide the client's lower extremities off the bed (see Fig. 13-27B).
6. As a team, the practitioners transition the client from side lying to sitting on the edge of the bed.
7. The practitioner behind the client will be needed to maintain sitting balance once the client is fully upright, and the OTA in front must block the knees of the client to ensure that the pelvic girdle does not slide anteriorly off the edge of the bed (see Fig. 13-27C).
8. Using one hand, the OTA can lower the bed and then reposition the client's lower extremities to ensure that both feet are on the ground to provide additional support.

Low-Level Tetraplegia (C6 to T2): Clients with a lower-level tetraplegia will have varying function of the upper extremities (e.g., elbow flexion and extension, wrist extension, and possibly hand function spared). The role of the OTA is to train the client to perform the supine to sitting on the edge of bed transfer by using a combination of the muscles available to use and assistive devices (e.g., a bed ladder, trapeze bar, or a powered bed) to assist with these movements. Although the use of a lift system is often the transfer method of choice, these clients can frequently participate more during this transfer and therefore alternative methods may be possible. Transfer steps for the OTA are essentially the same as those described for providing assistance to individuals with high-level tetraplegia, but the client should be able to physically assist more with the transfer and should be encouraged to do so. In the early stages of recovery, the use of a lift system is the safest transfer method for all concerned; however, maximal use of all available muscle groups should be encouraged.

Paraplegia (T3 and Below): With therapeutic intervention, individuals with paraplegia (AIS A) are likely to be able to perform supine to sitting on the edge of the bed transfer with modified independence (using assistive devices and additional time) before they are discharged from the hospital setting. Essentially, the same transfer steps are used as with persons who have tetraplegia; however, the client will have use of the upper extremities to assist in the transfer. Clients who have greater use of their upper extremities, including increased strength, may only need one practitioner to assist with the transfer when beginning therapeutic intervention.

In the early stages of recovery, clients with paraplegia may be wearing a TLSO brace (typically 3 months after surgery) and may need additional assistance. The brace should be donned before the transfer is initiated. The following are steps for direct application; the client will be rolling onto the left side to transition from supine to sitting on the side of the bed with the assistance of only one practitioner.

1. The OTA is positioned on the side of the bed that the client will be rolled toward and is facing the client. The height of the bed is raised to prevent the risk of low back strain for the practitioner. The upper bed rails are left in upright locked position because they will be used by the client to assist with the transfer.

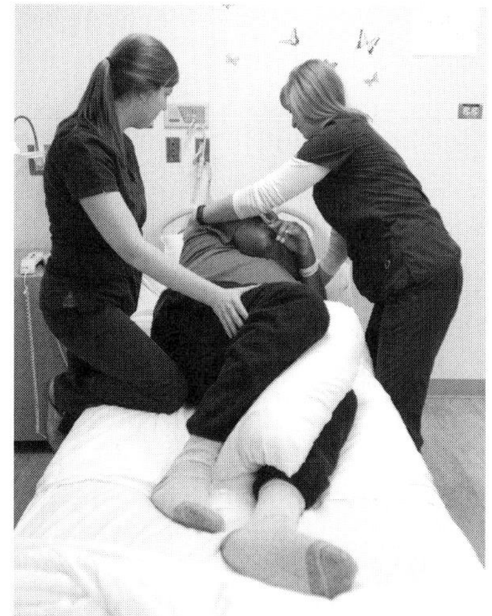
A

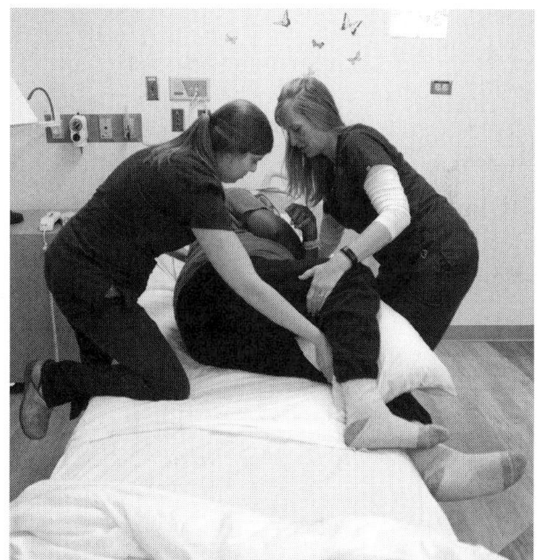
B

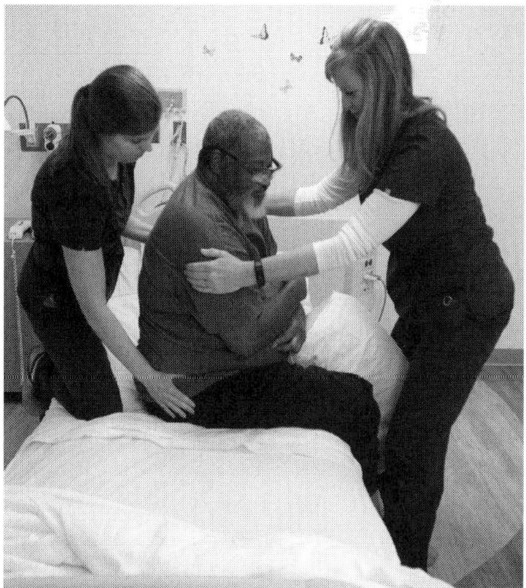
C

FIGURE 13-27. Performing a two-person transfer from supine to sitting on edge of bed for a client with high-level tetraplegia. **A.** Rolling to side. **B.** Assistance to move from side-lying to begin to sit. **C.** Bring upright and support sitting.

2. A pillow is placed between the client's legs, and the right leg is flexed at the knee and is used to roll the client toward the OTA. The use of a pillow reduces stress to the spinal column when transitioning to side lying.
3. The practitioner places his or her right hand on the client's right scapula and the left hand on the client's right hip. While encouraging the client to use both upper extremities as much as possible to assist with the transfer, the practitioner assists the client with rolling onto the left side, and the client is log-rolled toward the OTA maintaining spinal alignment (the head, shoulder, and hip girdle in line with one another) (Fig. 13-28).
4. The practitioner repositions his or her right hand to underneath the client's left shoulder while using the left hand to slide the client's lower extremities off the bed. The client is instructed to use the upper extremities (left elbow pushing into the mattress and the right hand pushing off the mattress or rail) as much as possible to transition from side lying to sitting on the edge of the bed.
5. The OTA should maintain one hand on the client's upper shoulder while blocking the knees of the client to ensure that the pelvic girdle does not slide anteriorly off the edge of the bed.

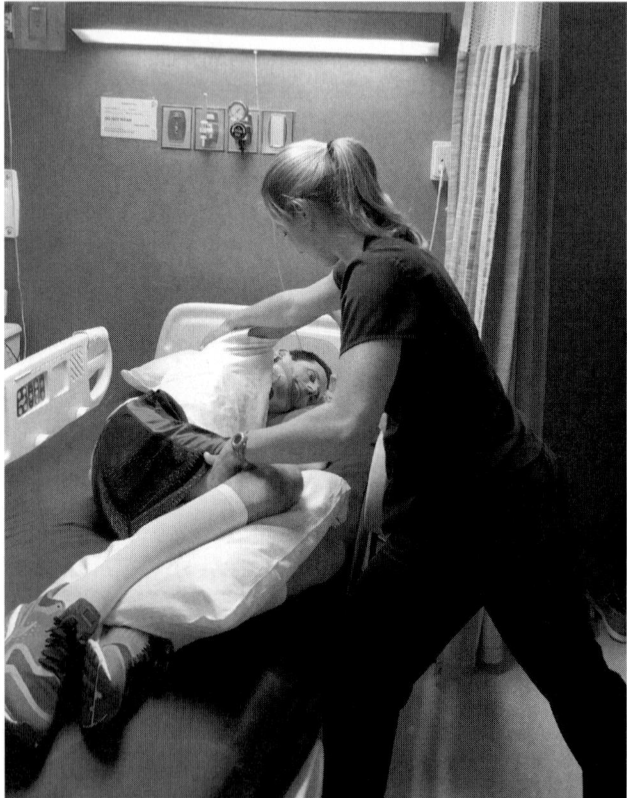

FIGURE 13-28. Performing a transfer from supine to sitting on the edge of the bed for a client who has paraplegia.

6. Using the opposing hand, the OTA can lower the bed and then reposition the client's lower extremities to ensure that both feet are on the ground to provide additional support.

WHEELCHAIR TO AND FROM OTHER SURFACES

Most individuals with SCI will spend a large percentage of their days in a wheelchair. It is important to educate the client and the caregiver(s) on how to transfer to various surfaces, such as a toilet, tub bench, and chair or couch. It is important for the OTA and the supervising occupational therapist to discuss recommendations for the most appropriate SPH equipment and assistive devices based on the client's level of function and the environments the client will encounter upon discharge from OT services. Environments can differ greatly, requiring an individualized treatment approach to ensure increased independence and autonomy for each client.

High-Level Tetraplegia (C5 and Higher): Most clients with this level of injury will require the use of a lift system for transfers and power wheelchairs as their primary mobility device because of the tilt-in-space features, power steering options, and optimal seating positioning availability. Power chairs tend to be bulky, and it may be difficult to approximate the height of the surfaces or get the wheelchair close enough for transferring between some surfaces. In most hospital settings or extended care facilities, portable lift systems can be used for transfers to/from the bathroom. However, because of the large footprint of the portable lift systems, these types of lifts are not conducive for many home bathroom environments unless significant home renovations are done. Therefore, bowel care and bathing may be provided in the bed by caregivers, or a bedside commode can be used in the bedroom. If a portable lift can fit into a bathroom area, the client can only be transferred onto the edge of a tub bench versus fully into the tub because of the design of portable lifts. A tub transfer bench with sliding seat could be used to transfer clients with high-level tetraplegia into the tub without sliding or shear forces (the seat itself slides on the bench into the tub). An alternative, but more expensive, home modification is the installation of an overhead lift/ceiling track system that extends into different rooms within the home. This allows clients to be transferred between various surfaces. Refer to the SPH equipment section of this chapter for transfers using a lift system.

For clients with incomplete high-level tetraplegia who are able to transfer without a lift system, modifications to traditional transfers listed earlier in the chapter can be used to transfer between the wheelchair and other surfaces. For direct application of steps, here is an example of a client who has incomplete high-level tetraplegia: The practitioner is assisting the client with transferring from a power wheelchair to a standard tub bench. The practitioner determined that it was necessary to involve a second practitioner for added safety. Next, the practitioner selected a stand-step transfer with the use of a platform walker. These decisions were made on the basis of the client's current level of function.

1. Position the wheelchair parallel to the tub, allowing enough transitioning space for the client, practitioner, tub bench, and assistive mobility device.
2. Place the walker (this example is using a platform walker) in front of the client; because of the environment, the practitioners position themselves on either side of the client with hands on the transfer belt. An alternative hand position (shown in Fig. 13-29A) is to have one hand on the transfer belt and one hand on the front of the shoulder to provide additional trunk support.
3. Instruct the client to lean forward and use the legs to assist with transitioning from sitting to standing.
4. Once the client is standing, the primary practitioner supports the client with both hands when the client is taking a step but then transitions one hand to the walker to assist with moving the walker (see Fig. 13-29B); then the practitioner returns the hand back to the transfer belt when the client takes the next step. The second practitioner provides support, as needed (e.g., on the transfer belt or at the anterior shoulder, or assisting the client's lower extremity with stepping or positioning).
5. Continue to have the client take steps until the back of the client's legs are touching the outside of the tub bench.
6. Because of the environment, the primary practitioner has moved to the front of the client with both hands on the transfer belt while the second practitioner is standing in the tub with hands positioned on the client's hips. The client is instructed to slowly lower onto the edge of the tub transfer bench while the practitioners assist, as needed.
7. Train the client on how a leg lifter can be used to assist with lifting one leg at a time into the shower. One practitioner demonstrates the use of the leg lifter while the second practitioner provides sitting balance support (see Fig. 13-29C).
8. Perform small side-scoot motions, as needed, to move client's buttocks along the tub bench until the full body is inside the tub. Side-scoot can be done by one practitioner positioned in front of client by standing in tub, using both hands on transfer belt, and assisting the client with lifting the buttocks off of tub bench (reducing shearing forces to buttocks).

Low-Level Tetraplegia (C6 to T2): As with high-level tetraplegia, clients with low-level tetraplegia will most likely utilize lift systems in the early stages of recovery and may continue use of lift systems depending on the return of function in the client. For clients with this level of SCI, transfer boards can be used with assistance; however, the dynamic transfer board is recommended for transfers in which the surfaces are close in height. By using a dynamic transfer board, shearing forces to the buttocks are reduced. Refer to the section on transfer board transfers for instructions.

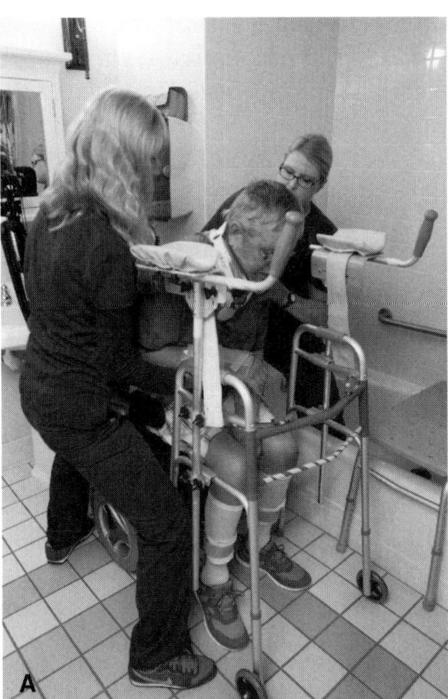

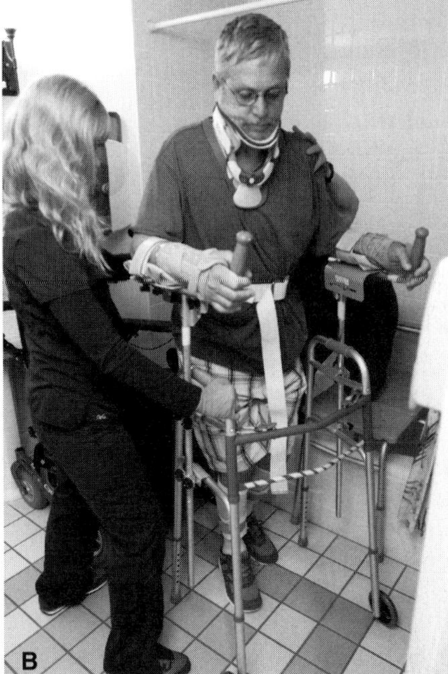

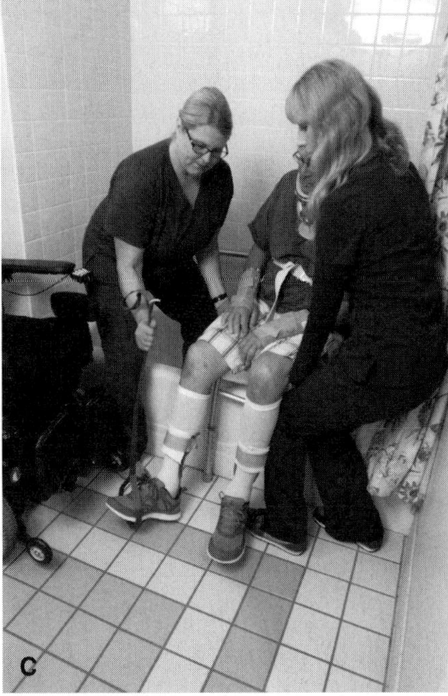

FIGURE 13-29. Assisting a client who has incomplete high-level tetraplegia with transferring from a power wheelchair to a standard tub bench. A. Both practitioners assist client to move forward on the seat and prepare to stand. B. Once standing, practitioners assist client to put arms on troughs of walker, and gain stability to pivot. C. Client sits on tub bench, and OTA assists with the leg lifter so client can move his leg into the tub.

Additional techniques in doing the transfer board transfer with this level of injury are as follows:

- Ensure that the upper body is always supported.
- Ensure that the client's lower extremities remain in a weight-bearing position throughout the transfer.
- The practitioner's knees should be blocking the client's knees to provide support.

If surfaces vary too much in height to use a transfer board, a traditional transfer (e.g., squat-pivot) may be used with assistance.

For tub bench transfers, a transfer board can be used. An alternative method is the use of a hand-towel or alternative material placed under the buttocks and upper thighs of the client to facilitate this transfer—especially when transferring out of the tub when the client is damp and fatigued.

Another alternative method is the incorporation of transfer blocks or modified transfer blocks to increase the arm leverage so that clients can achieve a greater lifting capacity. Depending on return of function, some clients will not require a transfer board as their upper body becomes stronger and they become more skilled in performing this transfer (Box 13-4).

Clients with some trunk stability can use a standing lift versus a portable full support lift (see SPH equipment section for transfer instructions), which can be very useful to transfer to any seating surface. Toileting with the assistance of gravity in the seated position, on a commode, bedside commode, or drop-arm commode is optimal for bowel and bladder needs. Therefore, it is important to work toward individuals with low-level tetraplegia transferring to a commode versus having bowel movements in bed.

Paraplegia (T3 and Below): Lift systems are generally unnecessary for clients with paraplegia because of the preservation of upper extremity function. With functional upper body strength, the OTA can train the client on how to perform transfers from the wheelchair to another seating surface, with or without the use of a transfer board. Level surfaces, with no gap between them can frequently be spanned by a client with paraplegia without a transfer board; however, increased distances between surfaces or transferring up an incline may require the use of a transfer board to bridge the gap.

Environmental modifications or assistive devices that allow the majority of transfers to be made to level surfaces will lessen the wear and tear on the shoulder joints of the client and are useful for energy conservation purposes. The frequent use of transfer boards can lead to compromise of skin integrity. The OTA should instruct the client to lift the buttocks off the board as much as possible and not slide along the transfer board, to reduce shear forces. To preserve good skin integrity, it is essential to ensure that the client's skin remains dry and that the transfer board is dried before transferring from a wet surface. Once a client has an area of ulceration, the client may need to use a lift, regardless of level of assistance needed, to preserve skin integrity.

Trunk stability is less of a concern with clients who have paraplegia. However, it is still important for the practitioner to remain alert during the transfer and provide support, as needed. As with clients with tetraplegia, the practitioner should make sure that the lower extremities maintain a weight-bearing position, when possible, and provide blocking support at the client's knees when assisting the client in a transfer. Clonus, which are brisk or sustained involuntary muscle contractions, can be dangerous for both the client and the OTA as sudden onset may impact the client's ability to transfer or maintain stability within the transfer.

Clients with paraplegia should be encouraged to complete bowel movements over a commode as gravity assists with evacuation of bowels; assistive devices may be needed to ensure safety and modified independence with the transfer. A tub transfer bench can be utilized for transferring into a tub for bathing, and the client may or may not need a leg lifter and additional grab rails for increased independence. Last, it is important to train clients on how to transfer to other surfaces around the home, including floor transfers, to ensure that the client can perform transfers without assistance.

BOX 13-4
Leisure

The pursuit of leisure interests takes various forms for different individuals. The ability to transfer out of a bed and into a wheelchair or transfer out of a chair and ambulate with prosthetics allows greater possibilities to pursue leisure interests both inside and outside of the home. Several areas of leisure require an individual to be transferred into a wheelchair or other seats to open the door of possibilities. For example, a client who sustains a lower-level spinal cord injury can learn to transfer onto an adapted ski and resume their interests in skiing. A client who is dependent with transfers can be transferred by using a lift system into a power wheelchair to go to the zoo or explore a museum with their family.

Lower Extremity Amputation

Persons who have had lower extremity amputation(s) will need to learn many new ways of moving from surface to surface. Initially, the practitioner should educate the client to transfer without a prosthesis while the residual limb is healing, and then if the client receives a prosthesis, he or she should be trained on how to transfer with the prosthesis. After becoming a prosthetic user, persons with amputations may on occasion choose or need to transfer without the prosthesis (e.g., to get into a tub/shower), and different methods may be used as people age. It is beneficial to learn several different transfer methods that can be selected, as needed, depending on environmental challenges.

To conserve energy and protect the joints of individuals with amputations and their caregivers, it is important to realize that the more similar the heights of the two surfaces involved in the transfers, the more independent the client will be, and less effort will be needed from all concerned. Strengthening upper extremities, abdominal and trunk muscles, and residual limbs as much as possible will help compensate for the absence of the part of the lower extremity that has been amputated. As with all transfers, the proximity of the surfaces, the firmness of the surfaces, fewer obstacles, and a feeling of security in the client will all strongly influence the ease of the transfer. Communication between the person performing the transfer and the OTA assisting with the transfer is essential to ensure that all parties are working together as a team. Initially, clients who have had a recent amputation may need assistance for all mobility and transfers, but with training of the person and the caregiver, environmental modifications, and strengthening, the majority of individuals should be able to learn to transfer by themselves.

BED MOBILITY

In the hospital setting, the OT practitioner will begin with the powered bed in the flattened position and can incorporate bed rails, trapeze bars, or other modifications, as needed. As the client gains greater independence, these modifications can be removed. In the case of a unilateral lower extremity amputation, the client should be trained on incorporation of bilateral upper extremities and the full lower extremity limb and on using the three extremities for bridging the trunk and buttocks off of the bed to move up in the bed, similar to the steps listed in the section on traditional transfers. If the client has had bilateral lower extremity amputations, he or she will need to use the upper extremities and trunk muscles with the practitioner providing assistance, as needed. Additionally, SPH handling equipment, such as a nylon sheet, can be used to assist with moving up in bed and reducing shear forces until the client is able to successfully incorporate the upper extremities.

Rolling from side to side and being able to maintain the side-lying position is important for completing hygiene and lower body dressing following a recent amputation. The more proximal the lower extremity amputation, the more trunk and upper extremity strength is needed for bed mobility. Disassociation of the shoulder and hip girdles is necessary to allow one area of the body to stabilize while the rest of the body is moving. Clients with a leg amputation should also be trained on rolling into the prone position (or as close to this position as is tolerated) as the prone position assists with reducing hip flexion contractures.

SUPINE TO AND FROM SITTING ON THE EDGE OF BED

Train individuals with unilateral lower extremity amputation or bilateral below-knee amputations on how to safely transition to sitting on the edge of the bed. However, individuals with bilateral above-knee amputations, who are sitting up without their prosthesis, should not be encouraged to sit on the edge of the bed because of balance concerns but, rather, to sit up in the center of the bed. Transitioning from supine to sitting on the edge of the bed may require some environmental modifications for clients who have had an amputation.

Use of a powered bed (elevating the head of the bed), the use of bed rails, and physical assistance from the OTA may be needed. When providing assistance, the client must be encouraged to independently perform as much of the movement as he or she can, in whatever manner works best, as long as the method is safe. Some clients may use a trapeze bar to lift the upper body from the supine position, although this method does not always allow for completion of the entire transition. A bed ladder, either commercially obtained or created by the OTA by tying knots progressively in a sheet or rope attached to the foot of the bed, may be more useful. The client can progressively move his or her hands further and further toward the foot of the bed by reaching for knots/rungs farther and farther away.

If facilitation is needed, the OTA can have the client roll toward the OTA and then bring the leg toward the OTA and over the edge of the bed, to gain a mechanical advantage. To transition into the sitting position from the side-lying position, the practitioner can assist by placing a hand under the scapula or behind the shoulder and encouraging the client to push up through the upper extremities into the seated position.

WHEELCHAIR TO AND FROM OTHER SURFACES

Many persons with a unilateral lower extremity amputation can perform transfers by using traditional transfer methods, with or without assistive devices, and their upper extremities to compensate for the amputated leg. It is best to begin with transfers that keep the buttocks low to the surfaces being transferred to (e.g., side-scoot or squat-pivot) to reduce the risk of falling. Once balance has improved, clients not using a prosthesis may be able to transition to using a stand-pivot transfer and some may be able to perform a stand-hop method in conjunction with a walker.

Individuals with bilateral lower extremity amputations (at least one amputation is below the knee) should begin with using a transfer board or side-scoot transfer incorporating the use of both upper extremities. Push-up blocks can greatly improve the success of lifting the buttocks off surfaces until increased upper body strength has been achieved. At times, a person with bilateral lower extremity amputations may only wear one prosthetic. It is important to train the client on additional transfer methods, such as a squat-pivot or stand-pivot, in conjunction with a walker, thus offering more options of transfer methods to increase independence and safety with regard to any type of surface they might encounter.

For individuals with bilateral above-knee amputations, a modified method is used to transfer in and out of the wheelchair to increase safety. To transition from sitting in the center of the bed to the wheelchair, the OTA should have the client face the opposite direction of the wheelchair and move the hips posteriorly into the wheelchair (Fig. 13-30). If there is a gap between the wheelchair seat and the edge of the bed, a small blanket can be rolled and wedged in-between to reduce the gap.

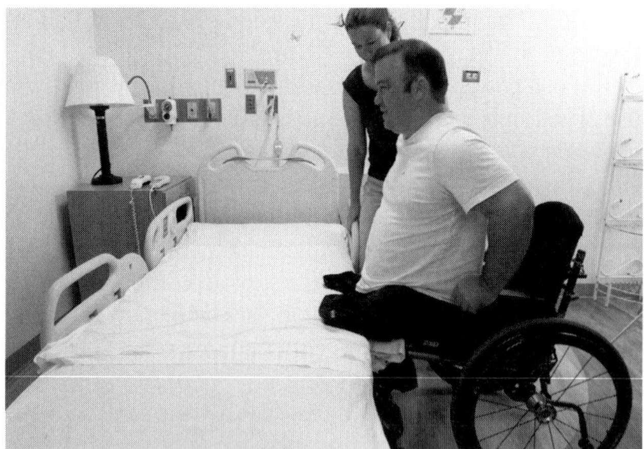

FIGURE 13-30. A client with a bilateral above-knee amputation transfers from the wheelchair to the bed.

When transferring from a wheelchair to a commode, the importance of equal surface heights is even more important, as there is less surface area for support. Toilet surfaces can be raised by using handicapped-height commodes, elevated toilet seats, or by placing a 3-in-1 or drop-arm commode over a standard height commode for energy conservation and safety purposes. Clients with bilateral above-knee amputations should be encouraged to position the wheelchair directly in front of the commode and to transfer onto the commode by using an anterior approach (Fig. 13-31). All other individuals with lower extremity amputations can use a transfer board to perform a side-scoot transfer, or they may be able to perform a squat-pivot transfer with the wheelchair placed at 45 degrees to the commode. By using a walker or crutches, many individuals with unilateral amputation or those using prostheses can ambulate into the bathroom or perform a stand-step transfer.

When clients with an amputation take a bath, they have to remove their prosthesis, so many will sit on a chair or tub bench while showering. The safest way for a client to transfer is by using a tub bench placed over the edge of the tub or the edge of a walk-in shower so that they can sit and then scoot sideways into the tub or shower. Many individuals with amputations are able to walk into the bathroom wearing their prosthesis, sit down on the bench/chair, remove the prosthesis, and leave it outside the tub or shower. Clients with bilateral above-knee amputations might prefer the anterior–posterior method when transferring to/from the tub bench from a wheelchair, as this requires less balance and affords more support throughout the transfer, thus increasing overall safety.

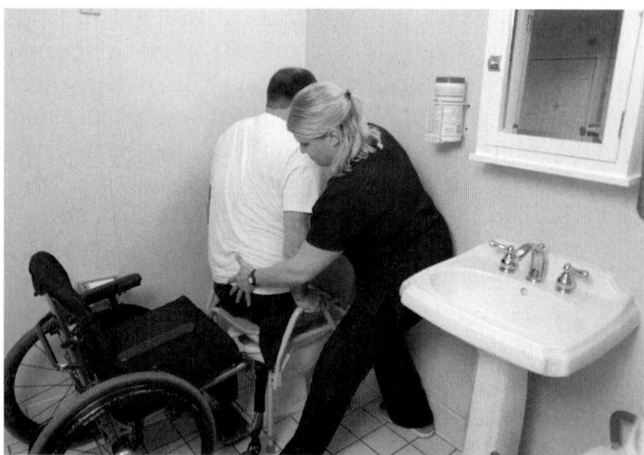

FIGURE 13-31. A client with a bilateral above-knee amputation transfers from the wheelchair to the commode.

If residual limb pain or phantom limb pain is of concern, padded tub benches can be used, although these benches typically require increased vertical lift (onto the tub bench) and are not as durable as hard plastic tub benches. Placement of a hand towel on the bench will reduce the risk of slipping when the client is wet and soapy and can facilitate a side-scoot transfer if physical assistance is needed when getting into or out of the tub or shower. It is possible for individuals to transfer from the edge of a tub, down into a tub, but it requires significant upper body strength and agility.

TRANSFERS INTO MOTOR VEHICLES

An area of occupation that should be addressed during OT practice is how a client accesses the community. Some clients may have driven vehicles previously but are currently not driving because of a recent change in medical status or only travel as a passenger (Box 13-5). These clients will need to be trained on transferring in and out of the passenger area of a vehicle. If it is determined that the client will return to driving, then it is important to ensure that the client can safely transfer in and out of the driver's side of the vehicle. Many of the transfer principles that have been discussed in this chapter thus far will be applicable to transferring in and out of a motor vehicle.

The OT practitioner will need to ask the client what type of vehicle he or she will be primarily using to be able to gain insight into the height of the seating and options for stowing mobility devices. If access to the vehicle is not possible, the OTA can ask the caregiver to measure the height between the ground and the vehicle seat, and this would help the OTA decide to use an adjustable mat inside the therapy setting to practice transferring to/from this seat height, if this mat is available. The optimal practice situation is to use the actual vehicle and train with both the client and the caregiver to ensure success of the transfer and the safety of the client and the caregiver. An additional step to vehicle transfers is to ensure that the client or the caregiver is able to stow the needed mobility device (e.g., cane, walker, or wheelchair) in the vehicle independently.

General Weakness

Clients who are able to use all four extremities but have generalized weakness may need a compensatory strategy to get in and out of vehicles that sit lower to the ground. The following steps apply to the client who is ambulatory with or

BOX 13-5

Psychological Impact Following a Medical Status Change

The psychosocial impact to an individual following a medical status change can have consequences to their ability to participate in therapy. This applies to participation in transferring between surfaces. A client may require significant encouragement because of feelings of loss, and therefore, selection of a transfer method in which the client can be encouraged to participate more and see greater accomplishment during that session builds therapeutic rapport. For an individual who may be very angry or confused, a method of transfer that helps maintain the highest level of safety for both the client and the practitioner should be selected. The sense of accomplishment of needing less assistance from the care provider can be a great boost to self-efficacy, especially if the medical change has stripped the individual of his or her autonomy.

Here is an example of how much increased independence in a "simple transfer" can change a client's outlook on life. J. T. was hospitalized for 6 weeks following an acquired brain injury caused by a motor vehicle accident. His family never thought he would live, much less regain the ability to participate in daily occupations. One of his last treatment sessions was to practice motor vehicle transfers. That day, he was able to independently transfer into the passenger seat of a car, telling his OT practitioner that he finally felt like himself again because he could get out and go again and not be trapped in his home.

without a device or to a wheelchair user who can transition from sitting to standing and pivot on the feet without steadying assistance and has no weight-bearing restrictions for the arms or legs.

ENTERING THE VEHICLE

1. With the passenger door open, place the client in the standing position or have the client come to the standing position and turn in space until the back is positioned toward the seat. OT practitioner facilitates the transfer through verbal directions, standing next to the client while maintaining at least one hand on the transfer belt for guidance and safety.
2. The client positions the left arm on the passenger door armrest and the right hand on the outer side of the seat back and slowly lower the buttocks to the seat by bending forward at the waist while the OT practitioner provides assistance, as needed.
3. The client moves the left hand behind the body to the front of the seat (or dashboard), brace the right forearm along outer side of seat back, and lifts the left leg into the vehicle while slightly spinning in seat. Assist with lifting the leg, as needed, or incorporate the use of a leg lifter.
4. The client is instructed to lean the trunk against the seat back, lift the right leg into the vehicle, and spin slightly in the seat to align self properly in the passenger seat. Assist with lifting the leg, as needed, or incorporate the use of a leg lifter.

EXITING THE VEHICLE

1. Have the client place the left hand either on the raised center console or the front of seat and use it as leverage to spin the legs toward the door. Have the client lift the right leg out of the car.
2. Have the client continue to spin until able to bring the left leg out of the car; it might be helpful for the client to lean posteriorly in the seat.
3. When both legs are now outside of the car, instruct the client to use the trunk muscles and push off with the left hand to flex at the waist so that the client is sitting upright on the edge of the seat facing the door. The OT practitioner should assist by placing the left hand along the client's scapula and the right hand on the transfer belt.
4. Instruct the client to place his or her right hand either on the seat or the outer side of seat back or to use elbow/upper arm on outside of car and flex at the waist while the left hand pushes down on the passenger door armrest or along the frame of the car (Fig. 13-32) to come to the standing position or pivot off the feet and swing the buttocks into the wheelchair seat. Note that the client should not perform a pulling motion on the armrest because this can cause the passenger door to move inward and potentially injure the client. The OT practitioner should position the hands on the transfer belt, and assist, as needed.

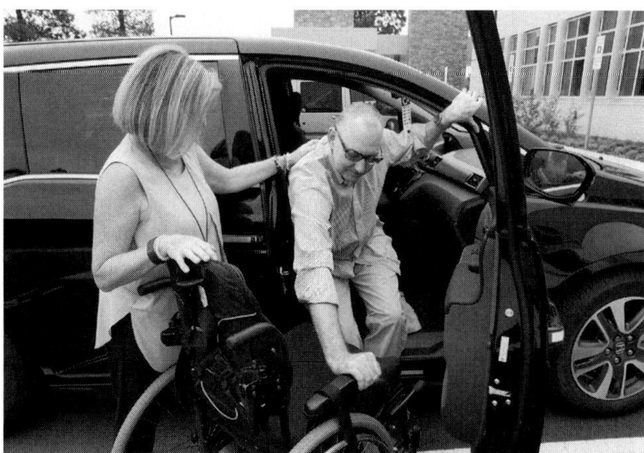

FIGURE 13-32. Client demonstrating the method for exiting a vehicle with caregiver assist. The method is utilized for general weakness or other conditions.

If the client struggles when using arms for assistance, an adaptation called the Handybar® can provide additional leverage and handhold placement for the right hand for lowering into the vehicle or pushing up to exit the vehicle. For the client who has difficulty spinning on the seat, placement of an unfolded kitchen trash bag underneath fully clothed buttocks or use of a swivel seat can reduce friction. Should a client use any of these assistive devices, the devices must be removed for safety purposes before operating the vehicle.

If the client requires the assistance of a caregiver for this transfer, the caregiver should stand just off center to the client's right-hand side and assist by slowly lowering the client onto the seat by using the transfer belt for entering the vehicle or assisting the client to shift weight forward for exiting the vehicle. The caregiver should be trained to avoid pulling or holding onto the client's arms and instead use a transfer belt.

Postsurgical

Depending on the type of surgery, physicians may recommend that a client not operate a motor vehicle for a certain period. For clients who have sternal precautions, the physician may advise the client to limit riding as a passenger because of the positioning of the seat belt across the chest; as well, if a motor vehicle accident should occur, the engagement of the seat belt, along with the release of the airbag, could cause serious injury to the chest that is still healing. The OTA should educate and train the client with sternal precautions to adhere to the recommendations of not pulling with the arms and instead using the legs when entering and exiting the vehicle. For the client who has a pacemaker, the seatbelt should not cross over the incision site, and the client should not use the upper extremity to push or pull when entering or exiting the vehicle.

Clients who undergo spinal surgeries need to be mindful of all of their restrictions or precautions, which may include transferring in and out of a vehicle. The OTA should educate and train clients not to twist their bodies, but to perform small scoots on their buttocks to ensure straight alignment of the spine. The client who has a restriction on bending will need to be educated and trained on how to keep the spine straight, not bending anteriorly while flexing the hips and knees to sit on the vehicle seat.

Hemiparesis

For clients who have pronounced hemiparesis and require assistance to transfer, the OTA should consider the type of transfer being utilized to other surfaces. For example, the client who is able to complete a stand-pivot transfer with equal or less than minimal assistance, the OTA could use a modified version of the steps listed in the section on hemiparesis in this chapter. The client would be encouraged to use the nonaffected side as able and to incorporate the affected side as able to promote use and independence. Assistance from the OTA or caregiver will mostly occur with slowly lowering the client into the vehicle or rising from the vehicle seat, ensuring flexion at the waist to avoid bumping the head, shifting of hips in the seat, and lifting the hemiparetic leg in and out of the vehicle. An adaptation would be to recline the seat back slightly or move the base of the seat back to create additional room for maneuvering.

A client who can perform a squat-pivot transfer from the wheelchair, with equal or less than minimal assistance, may be successful in transferring into the vehicle. The following are the transfer steps for an individual with hemiparesis:

1. Remove the wheelchair leg rests, and swing away the armrest closest to the passenger seat.
2. Propel the wheelchair forward into the area between the seat and the open vehicle door.
3. Engage wheelchair locks, and have client scoot to the edge of the wheelchair seat.
4. Practitioner will be positioned in front of the client, slightly to the right side of the client, with both hands on the transfer belt.
5. Have the client use the nonaffected arm and place his or her hand on the wheelchair armrest.
6. Instruct the client to shift weight into the unaffected arm and legs to remove weight from the hips and buttocks. The client should pivot on the balls of feet while swinging the hips to the vehicle seat.
7. Once the client is securely seated, instruct the client to lean the trunk against the seat back, lift one leg at a time into the vehicle, alternating with spinning the buttocks in the seat to align self properly in the passenger seat. Assist with lower extremities, as needed, or incorporate the use of a leg lifter.

The assistive devices mentioned above can be used if the client has difficulty spinning the buttocks in the seat; however, the devices must be removed before the vehicle is operated.

An additional adaptive transfer would be to incorporate the use of a transfer board between the seat of the wheelchair and the vehicle seat. Educating and training the client on the use of a transfer board could reduce the need for physical assistance and thus potential injuries to both the client and the caregiver. Although it is possible to transfer a client who needs greater levels of assistance, vehicle transfers place the caregiver at a mechanical disadvantage to assist and may result in injury. Therefore, the OTA will need to consider alternative options, such as special vehicle seating or adaptive vehicles, for the client who requires moderate to full assistance over the long term. The OTA should have a discussion with his or her supervising occupational therapist about referral of the client to a driving rehabilitation specialist and adaptive mobility vendor for vehicle seating options or about the possibility of the client's has the potential to resume driving.

Paraplegia and Tetraplegia

In the initial stages of recovery, clients with paraplegia or tetraplegia will need a greater level of assistance with transfers and will most likely utilize alternative transportation options, such as adaptive vans or buses, to access the community. As the client regains function, vehicle transfers will need to be addressed. The client who has paraplegia and demonstrates greater independence in transferring will most likely be able to either transfer in and out of a lower-sitting vehicle (e.g., car) with an adapted side-pivot, side-scoot or use a transfer board independently. Clients who do not regain adequate upper body strength or those who had sustained a higher level of injury will need to be educated about special vehicle seating or adaptive vehicles in which to ride in their wheelchair. The OTA should have a discussion with his or her supervising occupational therapist about referral of the client to a driving rehabilitation specialist and adaptive mobility vendor to ensure that mobility needs to access the community are met.

Amputation

The OTA should consider the type of transfer the client has been using for most other surfaces as the steps of the transfer will be familiar to the client, leading to greater success. Clients with a lower extremity amputation not wearing a prosthesis can transfer into a car by using stand-pivot, squat-pivot, side-scoot, or a transfer board, depending on the level of assistance needed. The client wearing the prosthetic limb will most likely use a stand-step transfer. For the client who has bilateral lower extremity amputations and not wearing prostheses, a side-scoot or transfer using the transfer board is appropriate. If the client is wearing both prostheses, then he or she will most likely perform a stand-step transfer. Clients are not allowed to operate the gas or brake pedal with a prosthetic limb; therefore, it is important to refer the client to a driving rehabilitation specialist if the client has a right lower extremity amputation because many driving adaptations with proper fitting and training are available. For further information, see Chapter 16, which focuses on driving and driving adaptations.

SUMMARY

Transfers are an integral part of participation in everyday occupations. Clients and their caregivers should be educated and trained on transfers to as many different surfaces as possible so that when they encounter a new environment, they have the ability and confidence to problem-solve and to determine the safest method of transferring. It is important for the OTA to discuss with the supervising occupational therapist the environmental challenges that the client is facing so that as a team they can determine the best and the safest transfer solutions, which could include recommendations of SPH equipment and assistive devices, for each individual client and the client's family.

REVIEW QUESTIONS

1. C. E. is a 26-year-old male who has been diagnosed with C4 AIS A tetraplegia. One of his goals is to be able to be transfer to the commode for his bowel movement; to the roll-in shower for bathing; and to the recliner in his enclosed patio to rest in the afternoons. What transfer device would you recommend?
   a. A ceiling lift
   b. A standing lift
   c. A free-standing mechanical powered lift
   d. A platform rolling walker
2. J. W. is a 52-year-old female who underwent a coronary artery bypass graft (CABG) and has sternal precautions. She has general weakness in her lower extremities from lack of activity in the past several months. What type of transfer would be *most appropriate* for her?
   a. Transfer board with push-up blocks
   b. Modified stand-pivot transfer
   c. Traditional squat-pivot transfer
   d. Manual mechanical lift transfer
3. D. D. is a 59-year-old male who has been diagnosed with Guillain-Barré syndrome, which is characterized by progressive weakening from distal to proximal, followed by progressive strengthening of muscles from proximal to distal. He is currently in the progressive stage, wherein he is regaining his strength. He would like to be able to transfer to a bedside commode for his toileting instead of using a bedpan; however, he continues to need maximum assistance for stand-pivot transfers and total assistance (two caregivers) for toileting—one to help him stand and the other to perform hygiene and manage the pants. His wife would like to be able to take him home, but she is the only caregiver. What device would you recommend to maximize his independence so that he and his wife can manage at home?
   a. A transfer board with a sliding seat
   b. A manual lift with a full-body sling
   c. No device, to encourage him to use his own strength
   d. A powered lift with a divided leg sling
4. L. P. is a 53-year-old male with type 2 diabetes. He has recently had both his legs amputated above the knee. He is afraid of falling and has decided not to get prostheses, but to use a power wheelchair instead, for mobility. His power wheelchair will not be able to get through his bathroom door at home because the door is too narrow. Which transfer method would you recommend that would make him feel secure while transferring onto a 3-in-1 commode placed next to his bed?
   a. A squat-turn transfer
   b. An anterior–posterior transfer
   c. A side-scoot transfer
   d. A transfer board with toilet seat cut-out type of transfer
5. B. K. is a 68-year-old client who had a fall at home and sustained compression fractures to her lumbar spine. She underwent spinal surgery and has to put on a thoracic-lumbar-sacral orthosis (TLSO) when upright. You note the client required max A × 1 during the initial evaluation. It is your first treatment session and the first time transferring the client in the therapy gym. Which transfer would you select?
   a. A transfer board transfer
   b. A squat-pivot transfer
   c. A stand-pivot transfer
   d. A stand-step transfer
6. A. D. is a 34-year-old male who underwent a gastric bypass surgery that resulted in medical complications. He has been in the acute care setting for 3 weeks and has become debilitated. He currently weighs 450 lb (204 kg). He needs to be moved up in bed frequently. The primary nurse consults with the OTA assigned to A. D. regarding the best transfer method to use. How would you recommend that the nurses move him up toward the head of the bed to reduce the risk of injury to the staff?
   a. A draw-sheet placed vertically, and two staff members performing the transfer
   b. A nylon sheet, and two staff members performing the transfer

c. An air-assisted mat, and two staff members performing the transfer
d. Assisting the client with rolling side to side until he works himself up in the bed

7. F. Z., a 68-year-old female, will be discharged from the hospital tomorrow. She had been admitted to acute care after a motor vehicle collision. She is continuing to experience severe vertigo and is unable to maintain her static balance when seated on the edge of the bed. The medical chart has her weight at 350 lb (113 kg). What transfer method would you recommend to her family to assist her with transferring from the bed to her wheelchair?
   a. A stand-step transfer using a large-based quad cane
   b. A mechanical lift transfer using a sling with divided legs and a head support
   c. A bariatric transfer board as it would have a larger transfer surface area
   d. A squat-pivot transfer using a transfer belt
8. G. G. sustained a T10 complete spinal cord injury (SCI) 4 weeks ago and has been making steady progress but still needs Mod A × 1 with most of her basic transfers. The occupational therapist recommends that the OTA work on motor vehicle transfers to the passenger seat in preparation for discharge to home in the next week. Which transfer would it be safest to attempt for the first-time car transfer?
   a. Squat-pivot from the wheelchair, with OTA in front
   b. Side-scoot from the wheelchair, with OTA on right side
   c. Transfer board from the wheelchair, with OTA on right side
   d. Transfer board from the wheelchair, with OTA in front
9. S. B. is an 82-year-old female who was recently admitted to the memory care unit in a skilled nursing facility because of the progression of Alzheimer's disease. The OT evaluation stated that the client required Mod A × 1 once the transfer was initiated, required Max A with activities of daily living (ADLs), and had deficits with regard to following verbal directions. The physical therapist reported Mod A with ambulation because of decreased standing balance. The OTA plans to work on grooming with the client at the sink and therefore needs to transfer the client from the bed to a wheelchair. Which three of the following transfer methods would be the safest while encouraging client participation aligning with her current abilities?
   a. Use of a stand-step transfer method
   b. Use of a standing lift to transfer
   c. Use of a stand-pivot transfer method
   d. Use of a side scoot transfer method with transfer board
   e. Use of a pivot disk to transfer
   f. Use of a squat-pivot transfer method
10. V. H. sustained a CVA 2 weeks ago and needs minimal assistance with most of his transfers and continues to fatigue easily. The OTA learns that V. H.'s bathroom at home has a tub with an overhead shower and a standard-height toilet seat. When making decisions regarding transfers for bathing, which of the following three durable medical options would ensure safety and completion of ADLs?
   a. Shower chair with a hand held shower for showering in the seated position
   b. Tub transfer bench with a hand held shower for showering in the seated position
   c. Tub transfer bench with grab rails for showering in the standing position
   d. Shower chair with grab rails for showering in the standing position
   e. Elevated toilet seat
   f. Toilet safety frame

CASE STUDY

M. W. is a 74-year-old woman who was recently diagnosed with leiomyosarcoma (a soft tissue sarcoma or cancer). She has been told that her tumor is progressive and untreatable surgically, and her oncologist estimates that she has less than a year to live. M. W. has agreed to receive palliative chemotherapy to manage her symptoms and pain. She has no children, but her friends and neighbors (all approximately her age) are willing to provide assistance around the clock so that she is able to spend the remainder of her life at home and not in a nursing facility.

The home health OTA has been asked to recommend the best transfer methods for fall prevention and caregiver education and training on safety for assisting client with transfers, including potential assistive device needs that the caregivers are likely to need as her condition worsens and she becomes weaker. M. W. is currently able to perform functional mobility using a single-point cane, although her ambulation has become slower and more unsteady, and she recently fell in the bathroom in her home.

1. Considering the deterioration likely with M. W.'s condition, identify the assistive devices related to transfers that the client might need.
2. Identify the types of transfers that the OT practitioner would recommend as the client's condition worsens, providing connection to assistive devices that have been considered in the first question.
3. Identify a few important points related to transfers on which the OTA should educate and train the caregivers regarding care of this individual.

PUTTING IT ALL TOGETHER — Treatment Session and Documentation

Setting	Inpatient rehab, referred from acute care where the client spent 1 week
Client Profile	K. J. is a 32 y/o female that was diagnosed with MS, relapse-remitting type, 2 years ago. She had an exacerbation 1 week ago and was admitted to the hospital with left side weakness and mild left hemianopsia. She is married with 2 children (7 y/o and 9 y/o).
Work History	She is college educated. She is a baker and has a small catering business that she runs in her home.
Insurance	Private (husband's employer); limited to 30 visits

PUTTING IT ALL TOGETHER Treatment Session and Documentation (continued)

Psychological	When initially diagnosed with MS, she struggled with minor depression and continues to take medication, which she reports has significantly helped. Additionally, she reports her husband, extended family, and church family are a major support system for her.
Social	She and her family are very active in their church participating in Bible study groups as well as weekly church services. Their children are active in Boy Scouts, and the family loves to hike and go camping.
Cognitive	Mild deficits with sustained attention/concentration
Motor and Manual Muscle Testing (MMT)	RUE • AROM is WNL • MMT 4+/5 overall, grip strength 45# LUE • Decreased gross and fine motor coordination • Tone between Brunnstrom stage 5 and 6 • AROM: Sh flex 100, sh abd 85; elbow, wrist, hand WNL • MMT: Shoulder not tested due to limited ROM; elbow 4−/5, wrist 4−/5, grip strength 30# Trunk is weaker on left side but able to sustain dynamic sitting balance; Min A with bed mobility, Mod A with transferring to/from bed, toilet, tub bench, and chair/couch. She is ambulating with Min A using a rolling walker.
ADL	Mod A with grooming, bathing, and dressing
IADL	Mod A with simple meal prep, Mod A with laundry
Goals	(Emphasis on connection between transfers, adaptive equipment, and occupation) Within 3 weeks (d/c): 1. Client will require Mod I with bed mobility for participation in sleeping/resting. 2. Client will require Mod I with transfers to/from bed for participation in sleeping/resting. 3. Client will require Mod I with toilet transfers, including toileting hygiene and clothing management with the use of AE as needed. 4. Client will require Mod I with tub bench transfer for participation in bathing. 5. Client will require Mod I with transfers as an aspect of participation in IADLs (simple meal prep and laundry) demonstrating energy conservation techniques and use of AE as needed.

OT TREATMENT SESSION 1

THERAPEUTIC ACTIVITY	TIME	GOAL(S) ADDRESSED	OTA RATIONALE
Assessment of medical devices attached to client and environment, determination, selection, and placement of AE (e.g., rolling walker, toilet safety frame), removal of obstacles in environment	5 min	Indirectly #1, #2, and #3	*Preparatory Tasks:* Explain to client the plan for session, placement of AE in preparation for transfers, clear environment of hazards, check medical equipment lines in preparation for transfers.
Client education and training on proper body mechanics and best use of current ROM/strength to transfer between supine and sitting edge of bed	12 min	#1 and indirectly #2	*Occupations; Education and Training; Preparatory Tasks:* Verbalize proper body mechanics, determine current ROM/strength for transferring safely and how much assistance OTA will have to provide
Client education and training on proper body mechanics and best use of current ROM/strength to transfer between sitting and standing at edge of bed; safety considerations with incorporation of rolling walker	10 min	#2 and indirectly #3, #4, and #5	*Preparatory Tasks; Education and Training:* Verbalize and demonstrate proper body mechanics, determine current ROM/strength for transferring safely and how much assistance OTA will have to provide, purpose and application of transfer belt, transition safety with rolling walker to reduce risk of falling.
Ambulating with rolling walker from bedroom to bathroom for participation in toileting	3 min	#3 and indirectly #4 and #5	*Occupations; Education and Training; Preparatory Tasks:* Determine current ROM/strength for ambulating safely and how much assistance OTA will have to provide, safety with rolling walker to reduce risk of falling.

Continued

PUTTING IT ALL TOGETHER Treatment Session and Documentation (continued)

THERAPEUTIC ACTIVITY	TIME	GOAL(S) ADDRESSED	OTA RATIONALE
Client education and training on proper body mechanics and best use of current ROM/strength to transfer between standing and sitting on toilet; safety considerations with incorporation of toilet safety frame and rolling walker	10 min	#3 and indirectly #4 and #5	*Occupations; Education and Training; Preparatory Tasks:* Verbalize and demonstrate proper body mechanics, determine current ROM/strength for transferring safely and how much assistance OTA will have to provide, transition safety with rolling walker and toilet safety frame to reduce risk of falling.
Client education and training on clothing management and toilet hygiene in relationship to transferring (safety to reduce fall risk)	6 min	#3 and indirectly #4 and #5	*Occupations; Education and Training:* Verbalize and demonstrate proper body mechanics, determine current ROM/strength for safety and how much assistance OTA will have to provide, transition of clothing and hygiene management to reduce risk of falling.
Ambulation from bathroom to bedroom; sitting in bedside chair	3 min	#3 and indirectly #4 and #5	*Occupations; Education and Training:* Determine current ROM/strength for ambulating safely and how much assistance OTA will have to provide, safety with rolling walker to reduce risk of falling.
Verbal review of transfers, including techniques, body mechanics, best body positioning, incorporation of AE and overall safety to prevent falls	8 min	#1, #2, and #3; indirectly #4 and #5	*Education and Training:* Review concepts taught today for reinforcement of concepts and answer questions.

SOAP note: 07/09/—, 8:30 am–9:27 am

S: Client stated "I am still feeling very tired but I am ready to do therapy because I need to be as independent as possible to return home quickly to my family."

O: Client willing participant in OT tx session to address transfer safety for participation in occupations. Client provided with education and training for bed mobility to promote independence for self-positioning in preparation to sleep/rest and to get in/out of bed. She required Mod A for bed mobility and transferring from supine to sitting edge of bed with Max v/c's. Needed cueing for proper hand placement to push off of bed then reach up for rolling walker when transitioning from sit to stand; required only Min v/c's for same procedure when transitioning stand to and from sit to toilet using toilet safety frame. Required Mod v/c's and Mod A for maintaining dynamic balance for clothing management and toilet hygiene, otherwise able to pull clothing up/down and wipe peri-area without assistance. Ambulation to return to bedroom and to sit in bedside chair required Mod A (dynamic balance) and Min v/c's to remind ct. about hand placement transitions. Reviewed best body mechanics and safety for transfers determining verbal recall of steps, needing Min v/c's. Will need to reinforce transition positioning of UEs to increase safety with rolling walker and AE in bathroom.

A: Throughout entire treatment session, client was very willing participant and demonstrated good effort into all activities. Overall required Mod A for bed mobility, supine to sitting EOB, ambulation to/from bathroom, toileting transfers due to weakness and fatigue. Noted instability with dynamic standing balance (fair +) due to weakness. Noted some carry-over of skills from beginning of session to latter aspect of session when transferring off of toilet and returning to bedside chair by less v/c's being required for body positioning and safety.

P: Continue to address goals and review of body positioning for safety with transfers to increase independence with desired occupations for return home.

Paula Ricco, COTA/L, 07/09/—, 9:40 am

TREATMENT SESSION 2

What could you do next with this client?

TREATMENT SESSION 3

What could you do next with this client? Are there other goals to address?

REFERENCES

1. U.S. Bureau of Labor Statistics. (Dec 2014). Employer-reported workplace injuries and illnesses-2013. Retrieved from http://www.bls.gov/news.release/archives/osh_12042014.pdf
2. Hodder, J. N., MacKinnon, S. N., Ralhan, A., & Keir, P. J. (2010). Effects of training and experience on patient transfer biomechanics. *International Journal of Industrial Ergonomics, 40,* 282–288. doi:10.1016/j.ergon.2010.01.007
3. Darragh, A., Huddleston, W., & King, P. (2009). Work-related musculoskeletal disorders and injuries: Differences among older and younger occupational and physical therapists. *Journal of Occupational Rehabilitation, 19*(3), 274–283.
4. Thomas, D. R. & Thomas, Y. L. N. (2014). Interventions to reduce injuries when transferring patients: A critical appraisal of reviews and a realist synthesis. *International Journal of Nursing Studies, 51,* 1381–1394. doi:10.1016/j.ijnurstu.2014.03.007
5. Johansson, C. & Chinworth, S. A. (2012). *Mobility in context: Principles of patient care skills.* Philadelphia, PA: F. A. Davis.
6. American Occupational Therapy Association. (2014). Occupational therapy practice framework: Domain and process (3rd ed.). *American Journal of Occupational Therapy, 68*(Suppl. 1), S1–S48. http://dx.doi.org/10.5014/ajot.2014.682006
7. BeasyTrans Systems, Inc. (2012). Beasy premium transfer boards: Instruction guide (pp. 1–23). Retrieved from http://beasyboards.com/pdfs/BeasyInstructionBrochureFINAL2012.pdf
8. Department of Justice. (2010). 2010 ADA Standards for Accessible Design. Retrieved from http://www.ada.gov/regs2010/2010ADAStandards/2010ADAstandards.htm#c6
9. Gallardo, M., Asencio, J., Sanchez, J., Banderas, A., & Suarez, A. (2012). Instruments for assessing the risk of falls in acute hospitalized patients: A systematic review protocol. *Journal of Advanced Nursing, 69*(1), 185–193.
10. Choi, Y., Lawler, E., Boenecke, A., Ponatoski, E. R., & Zimring, C. M. (2011). Developing a multi-systematic fall prevention model, incorporating the physical environment, the care process and technology: A systematic review. *Journal of Advanced Nursing, 67*(12), 2501–2524.
11. Miake-Lye, M. I., Hempel, S., Ganz, D. A., & Shekelle, P. G. (2013). Inpatient fall prevention programs as a patient safety strategy: A systematic review. *Annals of Internal Medicine, 158*(5), 390–396.
12. Centers for Medicare and Medicaid Services. (2012). *Hospital-acquired conditions.* Retrieved from http://www.cms.hhs.gov/HosptialAcqCond
13. Jensen, L. E., & Padilla, R. (2011). Effectiveness of interventions to prevent falls in people with Alzheimer's disease and related dementias. *American Journal of Occupational Therapy, 65,* 532–540. doi:10.5014/ajot.2011.002626
14. Rice, L. A., Ousley, C., & Sosnoff, J. J. (2015). A systematic review of risk factors associated with accidental falls, outcome measures and interventions to manage fall risk in non-ambulatory adults. *Disability and Rehabilitation, 37*(19), 1697–1705. doi:10.3109/09638288.2014.976718
15. Vieira, E. R., Freund-Heritage, R., & da Costa, B. R. (2011). Risk factors for geriatric patient falls in rehabilitation hospital settings: A systematic review. *Clinical Rehabilitation, 25*(9), 788–799. doi:10.1177/0269215511400639
16. Spoelstra, S. L., Given, B. A., & Given, C.W. (2012). Fall prevention in hospitals: An integrative review. *Clinical Nursing Research, 21*(1), 92–112.
17. Letts, L., Moreland, J., Richardson, J., Coman, L., Edwards, M., Ginis, K. M., ... & Wishart, L. (2010). The physical environment as a fall risk factor in older adults: Systematic review and meta-analysis of cross-sectional and cohort studies. *Australian Occupational Therapy Journal, 57,* 51–64. doi:10.1111/j.1440-1630.2009.00787.x
18. Brienza, D. D. (2015, March). National Pressure Ulcer Advisory Panel. Retrieved from http://www.npuap.org/wp-content/uploads/2012/01/NPUAP-Lift-Sling-White-Paper-March-2015.pdf
19. Darragh, A. R., Campo, M. A., Frost, L., Miller, M., Pentico, M., & Margulis, H. (2013). Safe-patient-handling equipment in therapy practice: Implications for rehabilitation. *American Journal of Occupational Therapy, 67,* 45–53.
20. Haesler, E. (2014). National Pressure Ulcer Advisory Panel (p. 12). Retrieved from http://www.npuap.org/wp-content/uploads/2014/08/Updated-10-16-14-Quick-Reference-Guide-DIGITAL-NPUAP-EPUAP-PPPIA-16Oct2014.pdf
21. Graff, M. B. (2000, Nov 6). Preventing heel breakdown. Retrieved from http://www.nurses.com/doc/preventing-heel-breakdown-0001

ACKNOWLEDGMENTS

The authors would like to recognize Grace Ferrell, MS, OTR/L, for her contributions to the spinal cord injury section; Megan Inman, MLIS, at East Carolina University Laupus Library, for her assistance in locating research literature to support the evidence discussed in the chapter; and Rachel Gartz, graduate OT student at East Carolina University, for the literature review for the fall prevention section. We would also like to thank the patient volunteers and occupational therapy practitioners from Vidant Medical Center, Greenville, NC, who assisted us with the majority of photographs used in this chapter.

unit III

Foundations of Intervention

Chapter 14

Assistive Technology and Home Modifications

Amber L. Ward, MS, OTR/L, BCPR, ATP/SMS

LEARNING OUTCOMES

After studying this chapter, the student or practitioner will be able to:

14.1 Define the occupational therapy assistant role with assistive technology

14.2 Explain the differences between low- and high-tech assistive technology

14.3 Identify assistive technology items required for activities of daily living, instrumental activities of daily living, leisure, and work

14.4 Determine the types of assistive technology required for various disabilities

14.5 Identify funding sources and options for assistive technology

14.6 Identify home modifications that can be performed to adapt for disability

KEY TERMS

Adaptive equipment (AE)
Assistive technology (AT)
Electronic aids to daily living (EADLs)

Assistive technology (AT) is an umbrella term that includes assistive, adaptive, and rehabilitative devices for people with disabilities and also includes the process used in selecting, locating, and using them.[1] Most individuals, regardless of disability, use AT. It might be a rubber jar opener, reading glasses, or a remote start for the car. AT can be anything from a simple (low-tech) device, such as a magnifying glass, to a complex (high-tech) device, such as a computerized communication system. It can be big—an automated van lift for a wheelchair—or small—a grip attached with Velcro® to a pen or fork. AT can also be a substitute, such as an augmentative communication device that provides vocal output for an adult who cannot communicate with the voice.[2] Assistive technologies enhance the ability of a person with a disability to participate in major life activities and to perform tasks that would be otherwise difficult or impossible for the individual to carry out. The principle of enhanced ability includes an increased level of independent action, a reduction of time spent in activities of daily living (ADLs), more choice of activities, and greater satisfaction in participating in activities.[3] AT can also specifically be **adaptive equipment (AE)** that is used to enhance occupational performance, such as a device to assist with buttons or a larger-handled fork.

According to the United States Assistive Technology Act of 2004, AT refers to "any item, piece of equipment, or product system, whether acquired commercially, modified, or customized, that is used to increase, maintain, or improve functional capabilities of individuals with disabilities."[4] Occupational therapy assistants (OTAs) are one of the prime inventors, creators, educators, matchers, and finders of AE and AT equipment and devices for their clients, and must be fully aware and up to date on options. The OTA must realize that training (to use any AT device) and providing ongoing technical assistance is necessary not only for the client, but also for family members, caregivers, service providers, and other people who are significantly involved in a client's life. It is also important to integrate and coordinate any AT with other therapies, interventions, or services.[2]

Every state is mandated to have a federally funded AT program in at least one location in the state. Often a state will have multiple locations, each with a fully functional office, loan closet, training and education center, and staff who can see the clients in the center or at home. Any professional, including occupational therapists or OTAs can refer to an AT Center, and the clients can also self-refer. The AT Center often will present at local and regional conferences, as well as provide education for local students of all ages. OTAs can find their program by state at assistivetech.net—the national public website on assistive technology.

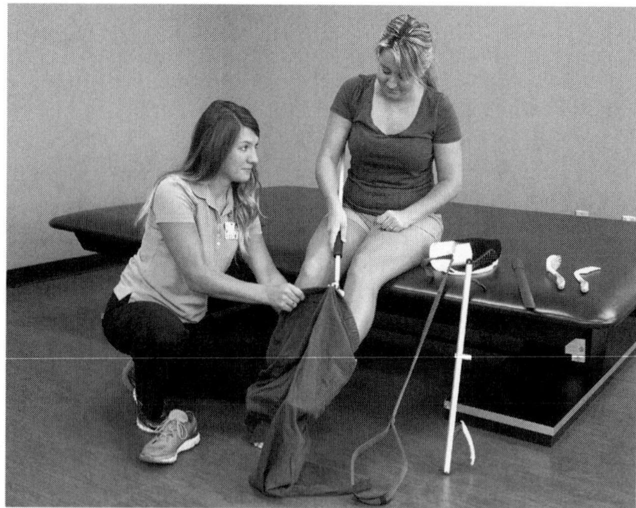

FIGURE 14-1. Various AT items for dressing. The client and OTA are using a dressing stick with a leg lifter. A reacher, long-handled shoehorn, long-handled brush, and comb are sitting nearby.

ACTIVITIES OF DAILY LIVING

ADLs are some of the prime tasks for which OTAs and their clients use AT. Many clients focus on improving or maintaining independence for as long as possible and are willing to accept small pieces of equipment or an adaptive technique to continue with their occupational tasks and roles in the home, community, and workplace.

Dressing

For dressing tasks, OTAs select tools based on the particular strengths and weaknesses of the client. The client who has difficulty buttoning a shirt could use a buttonhook or replace the buttons with Velcro®. The cuff and collar buttons can have an elastic band/button combination to avoid the need to unbutton them. A dressing stick can be used to push up a bra strap, pull up a pair of pants, pull a sweater down off a shelf, don a jacket, or open a drawer. Clients may use a reacher tool not only to pick up dropped items but to grab the waistband of the pants to begin donning them over the feet or to pull a shoe nearer. A long-handled shoehorn assists with donning shoes, and elastic or magnetic shoelaces in place of standard laces avoid the tying difficulty (Fig. 14-1). Other ways to avoid tying shoes include Velcro® closures, numerous other shoelace types, and adaptive tying methods—including one-handed tying. If the pants fall down as the client stands from the toilet, he or she might use a pant clip or suspenders (Fig. 14-2).

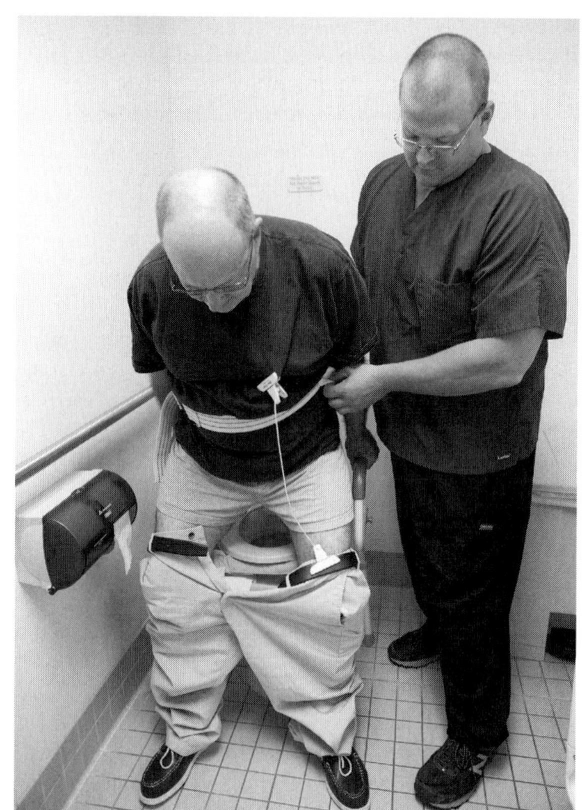

FIGURE 14-2. A pant clip can be used to keep the client's pants from falling to the floor when two hands are needed to come to a standing position.

Zippers that are difficult to pull up and down can be easily adapted by attaching a commercially available zipper pull or any empty key ring, fishing line, or ribbon. Anything that makes a loop large enough for the client to put a finger in can be inserted through the zipper hole to assist with moving the zipper up or down. A sock aid assists clients who cannot either bend down or reach their feet to don a pair of socks or stockings. The sock is loaded onto this device, heel down, and with the straps, the user gets the sock aid near the foot, pushing the foot through the sock, as the sock aid is pulled onto the foot (Fig. 14-3). Compression stockings can be particularly challenging because they are tight fitting, and there are specific tools and techniques for clients to manage them. Bras are often difficult, and a front-opening style bra with Velcro® might be easier than one that fastens in the back. One technique is to fasten a back-opening style bra in the front where it is easier to see and reach and spin it around or to replace the clasps with Velcro® to assist. Many women choose to use a sports bra in a slightly larger size or a camisole with a shelf to make donning overhead easier, or to wear no bra for an easier dressing experience.

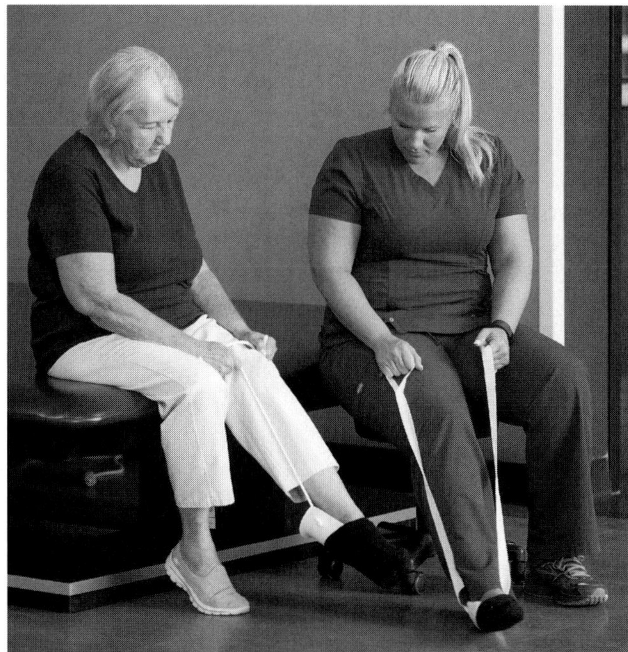

FIGURE 14-3. OTA training a client to use a sock aid.

Bathing

Bathing can be a particularly dangerous occupation when the client has a disability of any sort. Certainly one-sided weakness can make it unsafe to access the tub, decreased balance may lead to a fall, shoulder weakness may cause difficulty washing hair, or decreased sensation may make it difficult to assess water temperature. The next section is subdivided into bathing equipment for access and seating, and equipment for actual washing and drying.

THE OLDER ADULT

Many younger OT practitioners may assume that their older clients loathe to use and integrate technology. This is not necessarily true, but many of the "Silent Generation" born before 1946 are slow to change to newer or more efficient ways of doing things, especially those involving electronics. They can be very independent, and often will not readily accept assistance, such as adaptive equipment. Because they were born around the Depression era, they may not spend money to purchase a gadget or device that the OTA recommends from a catalog unless they have actually tried it and see its value. When working with these clients, the OTA may have better luck connecting with a loaner closet or manufacturer to trial and borrow needed equipment, such as a transfer tub bench or bedside commode, if not covered by insurance. This-era client may not want to change their home to accommodate a new disability or hire assistance to help with tasks such as mowing the lawn or cleaning the gutters. Because this generation is generally hard working, they will often embrace technology if they see in a practical way how it will assist them, but may require additional training with unfamiliar technology. An example might be a grandmother who uses FaceTime to talk with grandchildren who live across the country, a retiree who spends the day on the computer searching the Internet, or an automatic food/water dispenser for a beloved pet.

BATHING EQUIPMENT

Bathing equipment is often required in the tub or shower because of poor balance, weakness, or endurance. In such cases, shower seats, transfer tub benches, rolling shower chairs, and other equipment options can assist. A small shower seat can have a back or be just a stool, and typically has height-adjustable leg rests and slip-resistant rubber feet to safely fit in a tub or shower stall. If space is particularly tight, the small shower seat or corner shower seat may be chosen without a backrest. If sitting balance is an issue or may become an issue, then a seat with a back and even handles may be required. They come in many sizes, shapes and materials, such as wood/teak, plastic, and padding covered in vinyl. There are seats with a commode cutout, seats with padding, and seats of varying sizes, including bariatric seats for those clients who are over 250 pounds. The choice of which seat to use may depend on the bathroom decor, the need for pressure relief or padding, the client's strengths, or the seat's functional use. If the client is particularly tall or has difficulty with sitting to standing, then an extra tall shower seat with handles can be purchased. Shower seats are not typically covered by any insurance.

Transfer tub benches are longer seats with two feet that sit in the tub and have either a clamp on the side of the tub or two feet that sit outside of the tub (Fig. 14-4). They allow a client to slide into the tub versus stepping into it. Transfer tub benches work best with a shower curtain, which can tuck in to avoid water leaking on the floor versus a shower door. Tub benches can have a commode cutout for the tub portion, as well as a sliding seat. The sliding seat starts on the portion of the bench outside the tub, and after the user sits on the seat, a latch can be opened, and the whole seat

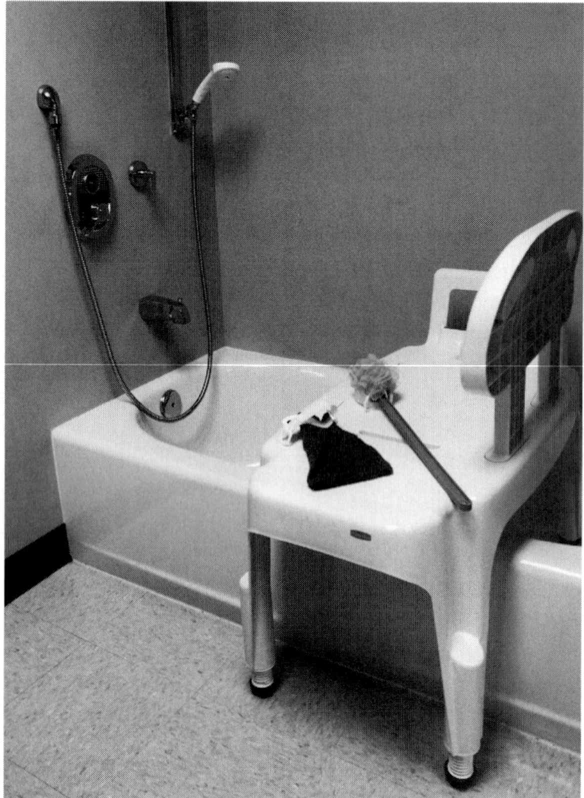

FIGURE 14-4. A transfer tub bench, long handled sponge, wash mitt, and handheld shower.

slides into the tub. With standard tub benches, the user must slide or be moved along the bench, which can be challenging if weakness is substantial. Clients may sit on a hand towel or sheet to allow caregivers to assist with sliding and to decrease friction and shear. Padded seats with commode cutouts or solid seats are also available for those with risk of skin breakdown or pain. A leg lifter will assist with putting the client's leg into the tub (and can also be used for the car and bed) (Fig. 14-5).

Rolling shower chairs typically are also commode seats, and can be used for toileting as well as bathing. They are usually aluminum chairs on wheels, and will roll into an open and accessible shower area. The user can use a commode bucket with the rolling seat by the bedside as well. Some rolling shower chairs are made of PVC materials, which make them much larger than the aluminum ones, but are much less expensive. Rolling shower commode chairs can have the option of tilt (seat tips backward to help with balance and head control) (Fig. 14-6) and recline (backrest lays backward) with padded seats, headrests, and other supportive items such as lateral pads for trunk stability and seatbelts. Some rolling shower chairs will slide into the tub or small shower stall to avoid an expensive renovation. In the case of the slider, a frame stays in the tub or shower, a rolling shower chair locks into the frame, and then the seat slides across into the tub or shower stall, as seen in the photo in Figure 14-7. There are companies that sell shower floor inserts to build up the inside of the shower to the shower lip height, and then a small ramp is added to the outside of the shower. This allows the rolling shower commode chair to be used without a major renovation in a standard shower.

Portable showers are another bathing option that allows the client to shower in the kitchen or garage—wherever there is a water supply and drain. Although expensive, they can avoid a more costly renovation, and allow flexibility for bathing. Portable showers hook to the water supply, and have a pump to push the water back into the drain. Whenever a seat for bathing is used, a handheld shower hose can assist with getting the water where it is needed, and often these long shower heads will have handles, hooks to attach

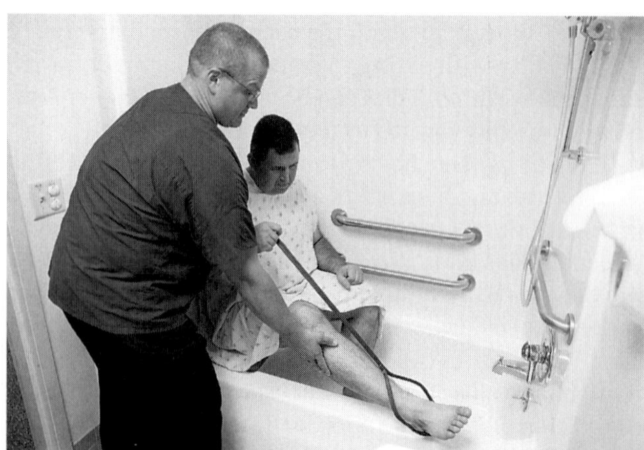

FIGURE 14-5. Training a client to use a leg lifter to lift the client's leg into the tub.

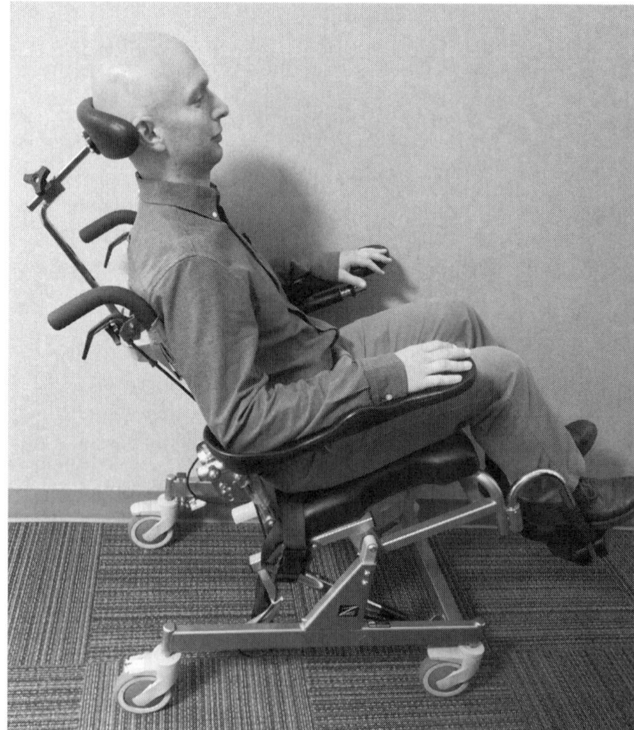

FIGURE 14-6. A rolling shower commode chair with tilt and supportive features. Many of this type of chair can roll first over the toilet and then into an accessible shower, to save multiple transfers and conserve energy for caregiver and client. Some are height-adjustable for easier transfers, have a padded cut-out seat, and other features can be added if a client's condition progresses.

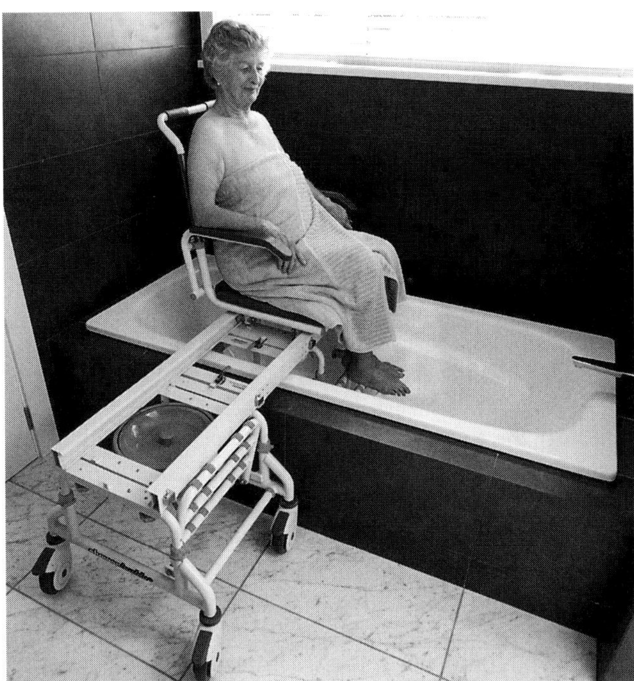

FIGURE 14-7. A tub slider. A frame stays in the tub and there is a rolling shower chair. The chair meets up with the frame, and the seat itself slides over into the tub. *(Courtesy of Shower Buddy, LLC, www.myshowerbuddy.com)*

on the wall, or a shower bench holder and shut off valves to temporarily turn off the water as needed. Always test the water temperature coming from the handheld shower before directing it on the client. Being able to direct the water can keep ventilators and feeding tubes dry as well as keep water out of the client's face and keep the caregiver drier. These hoses are available from local hardware or home improvement stores, are easy to install, and not typically covered by insurance. Power body dryers can be added if using a towel is difficult. These are a less common item, but are installed in the shower stall, typically in the corner away from the water supply. The jets of air are turned on, and the dryer works like a vertical row of hand dryers, such as those found in a public bathroom.

OTHER BATHROOM EQUIPMENT

OTAs may obtain various other types of easy-to-find assistive equipment to aid clients in the bathroom. Empty pump bottles that are sold at many drug stores or battery-powered automatic dispensers can assist with dispensing liquid soap and shampoo. As a note, many brands of soaps come in liquid form, and may be easier to manage than the bar. Wash mitts where the whole hand slides into the folded and sewn washcloth, or poofs with string handles can assist with easier holding of the washcloth. The client may be able to find a "soap on a rope" or create their own with a drill and soft rope. Long-handled and bendable sponges and brushes can assist with washing the feet and back. If the client has shoulder weakness, then the bendable brush should be chosen for easier reaching. Specific foot-washing devices that suction to the tub or shower floor are also available. Towels with loops can make for holding onto the towel better for easier drying, and is an easy sewing project. Loops made of 1-inch soft cotton belt webbing can be sewn on each side of the narrow ends of the towel to wrap around the person. Experiment with the size of towel and the size of the loops for the particular client's needs. A terrycloth robe can dry the client without effort once donned, or the client could try a chamois. Rubber mats may be needed on the shower floor to avoid slipping, or water/beach shoes may be purchased for less sliding. A small 4- to 6-inch lip on the shower may seem like a mile high for a client with leg weakness, therefore, a grab bar installed in a strategic location near the shower entrance and one inside the shower may assist with balance and safety (Fig. 14-8). A word of caution about suction cup grab bars: although they can be invaluable for travel, they may not hold a person's full body weight, and can dry out behind the suction cups, causing them to fall off the wall. If suction grab bars are used, they need to be checked frequently, and kept slightly moist in the suction cup. A grab bar fully mounted into a stud is always a safer option, and are recommended to be installed by a professional, especially if the studs are behind tile.

Toileting

Toileting and toilet hygiene are ADLs that can be very difficult for the user to complete safely and thoroughly, and the OTA will often assist with modifications of all kinds. The client may have the bathroom and toilet safely and functionally set up at

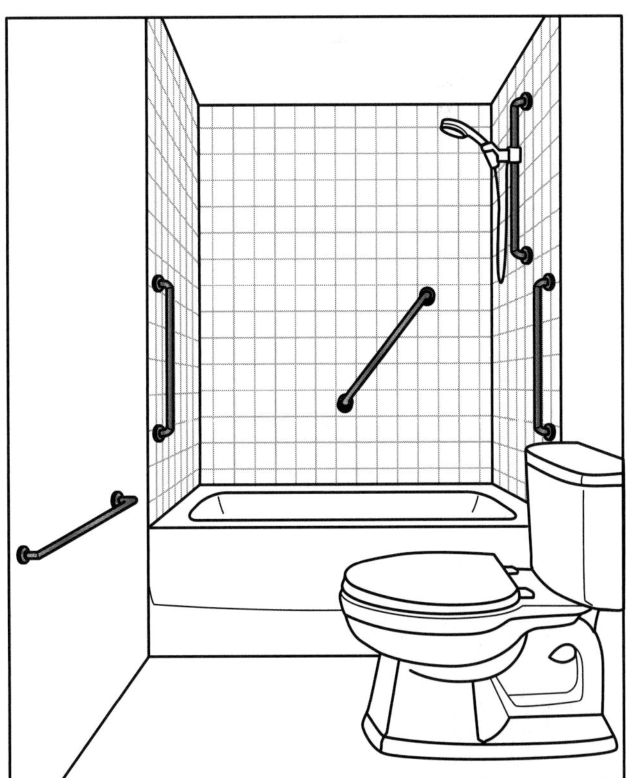

FIGURE 14-8. The OTA can offer many options for installation of grab bars, but final placement selection may depend on the strengths and weaknesses of the client and logistics of the space. A few options are shown.

home, but be foiled by a public bathroom. A caregiver of the opposite sex, use of mobility equipment in small bathrooms, toilet seats that are too low even in handicapped stalls and grab bars in the wrong location can all be issues in public bathrooms. Some users will have a portable raised toilet seat in a duffel bag to take along with them into public bathrooms or for travel, or a suction grab bar to temporarily mount to the wall. Many clients will have difficulty with clothing management to use the toilet, whether from the button or zipper, pulling up the pants, or managing a difficult transfer while also managing clothing. Women often have a more difficult time than men, as they cannot use a urinal or other collection devices, and often need to get onto the toilet, commode, or bedpan each time. Adapted clothing can include Velcro® instead of buttons and zippers, suspenders to assist with pulling up pants (put arms in suspenders while sitting on toilet to shoulders, and stand up), pants with Velcro® or snaps in the inseam or side seams, and "buttless" pants. These pants are commercially available from adapted clothing online stores, and have a flap instead of a bottom seat on the pants for easier toileting access (Fig. 14-9). Women can use wrap around skirts; they would fully open the skirt, leave it in the chair, and transfer to the toilet (no underwear).

Adaptations to the actual toilet can include a riser underneath or above the toilet to raise the height. The riser underneath the toilet, called the Toilevator®, raises the toilet 3.5 inches, which is of benefit to very tall clients, as they could have both the riser underneath and one on top of the toilet seat. It is also very stable because it mounts under the toilet with longer screws provided to become one unit, is less visible, and easier to clean. The riser for on top of the toilet typically clamps on or sits on the toilet, and may or may not have handles (Fig. 14-10). This type tends to be less stable, but can remove for travel and other toilet users in the home. A toilet safety frame does not have a seat, but simply consists of handles that attach into the screws that secure the toilet seat and lid. They can assist a user to get to their feet. A 3-in-1 or bedside commode may be covered by insurance, and has the option of being used by the bedside with the bucket, or over the toilet without the bucket. They have rubber feet and height adjustable legs. They can also come in a wider size for easier wiping or for bariatric clients over 250 pounds. If used by the bedside, easier clean up can be achieved with small trash bags or even kitty litter in the bottom of the pail. If needed, padding generally can be added in the form of a Velcro® on foam, gel, or air seat, which would be purchased separately. Additionally, the legs in the front and back may be adjusted to different heights to fit the client's needs. For example, adjusting the rear legs slightly higher than the front legs can assist a client to stand up. The OTA would use clinical reasoning to make such adjustments and consult with the occupational therapist as needed.

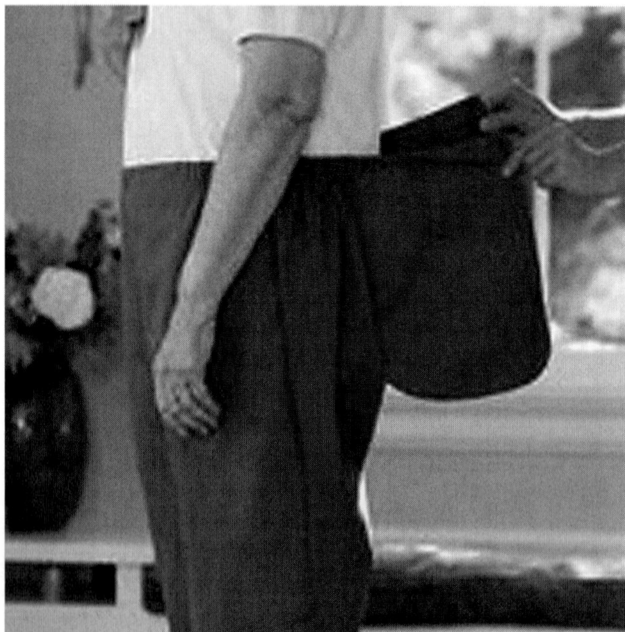

FIGURE 14-9. "Buttless" pants with flap. The client goes without underwear, and the flap covers the buttocks. When the client is seated on the toilet, the opening is large enough for toileting, and this avoids clothing removal. *(Courtesy of Buck & Buck, Seattle)*

For toilet hygiene, a bottom wiper is about as low-tech as it gets, but can maintain independence with a task which is very important to many people. The toilet tissue or wet wipe attaches temporarily to the wiper, and is easily removed once wiping is completed. Wipers have a variety of handles and ways to hold the paper for people with various weaknesses (Fig. 14-11). The highest tech AT option for toileting is the bidet seat, which is a seat and lid that attaches to the toilet (in place of the regular seat) and provides a warm water wash and warm air dry at the touch of a button. A bidet can also be an entirely separate toilet, but these may be low to the ground. Portable bidet options that hook into the water supply in the hotel bathroom are available for traveling. Many clients who are bed bound use a bedpan for toileting, but this is not ideal because of discomfort and difficulty with eliminating when in supine. External catheters can assist men with collecting urine into a bag, and temporarily attach on the outside of the penis with a collection bag. The collection bags can be smaller for

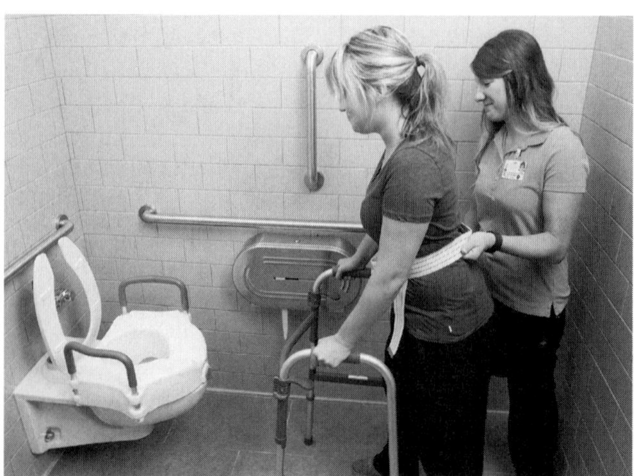

FIGURE 14-10. Portable raised toilet seat with handles, placed and clamped onto the toilet.

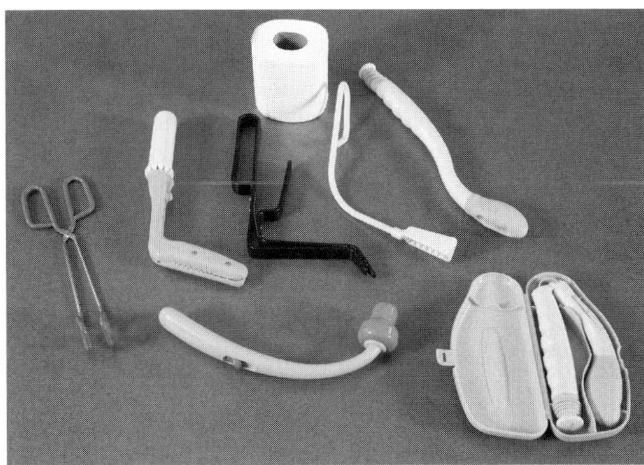

FIGURE 14-11. Multiple bottom wipers. For all, the toilet paper or wet wipe wrap around to allow the client easier reaching for toilet hygiene. Some require hand strength for the button to release the paper.

attaching to the leg under clothing or larger for overnight or hooked onto the wheelchair. The external catheter attaches with a glue substance to the penis, and then a tube goes from the catheter to the collection bag. Standard urinals can be of assistance for men, and spill-proof models exist as well. The OTA may recommend other empty bottles or containers, such as from juice, that fit the situation and may have a more reliable lid or cap than a standard urinal. Women have to use collection devices, such as specialty urinals, with different ends for the shape of women's bodies. Another option for a woman is a portable urine management item, typically used for camping or traveling, to direct urine in standing or sitting toward the toilet (Fig. 14-12). A new product on the market is called PureWick®, which is a female external catheter that hooks to a standard suction machine to wick away the urine into the collection canister. Women may require adaptations with orthotics or holding devices for inserting or retrieving tampons when they have weak fingers, or they can use pads.

Self-Feeding and Drinking

Many utensils to keep a person eating are available, including those that are large-handled, weighted, lightweight, curved, flexible, clip-on, and adjustable. Many of these utensils can be purchased by the client, but are not covered by insurance.

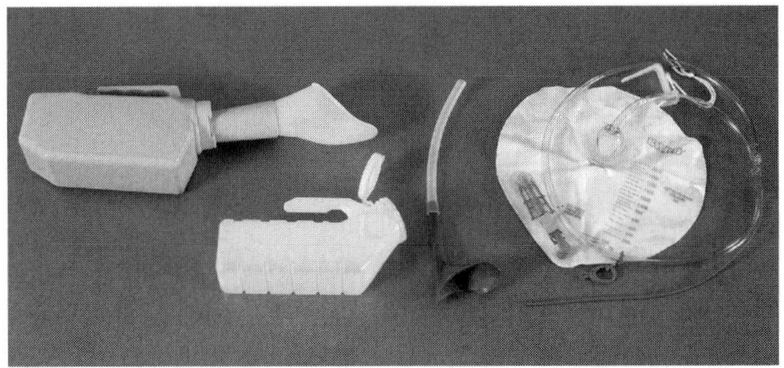

FIGURE 14-12. *From left:* A spill-proof urinal with female attachment, a standard urinal, a Whiz® Freedom urine device for women (stand to urinate), and an internal catheter system with collection bag used for either sex.

A universal cuff or economy wrist-forearm orthosis (a universal cuff that also supports the wrist) can go around the hand, and allow the utensil to be attached to the hand when the client has hand and/or wrist weakness (Fig. 14-13). Generally, when the hand is weak enough to require these items for support, the utensil has to be bent to allow the food to stay on the spoon or fork, and to be at the right angle when approaching the mouth. Another option is to use very inexpensive silverware that bends easily to the correct position, often just with the hands. Many adaptations for plates and bowls exist; some have higher sides or one side higher for easier scooping, and plate guards can be added to any plate to make a high side. A divided plate will separate food into sections, and plates and bowls with suction will keep them from moving. Dycem® (a nonslip material) or inexpensive rubber shelf liner can also keep the plate and bowl from moving as much. When the client's arm is weak, a mobile arm support can attach to the table or wheelchair for self-feeding, grooming, and other uses. It can lift the arm into the air with rubber bands and a support, and has a pivot point at the elbow for self-feeding. High-tech feeding devices in which a user presses a button and the spoon comes to the mouth are available, but these can be very expensive. For persons with tremors, a spoon called Liftware Steady™, which has a built-in gyroscope, minimizes tremors resulting in increased independence for self-feeding. The Liftware Level™ is a utensil with leveling technology to maintain the utensil level regardless of how a client's hand or arm moves.

A rocker knife or alternatively shaped knife handle can assist with cutting. The rocker knife allows the client to roll the knife back and forth for easier cutting, or a sharp pizza cutter can work as well for less friction. Alternatively shaped knives have the grip either at a 90-degree angle to the knife blade, or in a pistol grip for easier holding, because of the particular hand position needed for maximal force. The knife may be permanently attached at the tip of the blade to the cutting board for increased safety (Fig. 14-14). Sometimes a very sharp knife will actually cut better than a steak knife, which requires more force and sawing. When

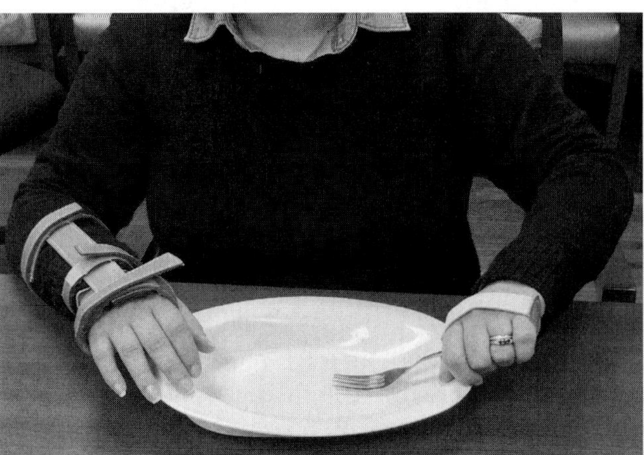

FIGURE 14-13. Universal cuff with wrist support *(left)* and universal cuff *(right)* for self-feeding.

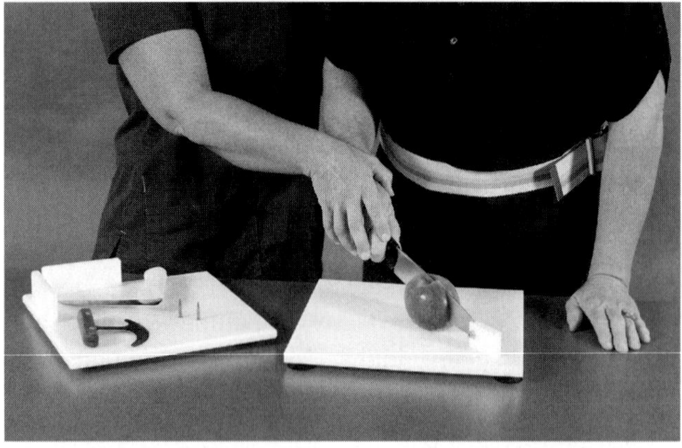

FIGURE 14-14. *From left:* Adapted cutting board, adapted knives, and cutting board with knife blade attached to the board.

at a restaurant, a client can request the food to be cut into bite-sized pieces in the kitchen so that there is no struggle to cut the food at the table. Cylindrical foam can be put over a utensil to make it easier to hold. Foam comes in different sizes and densities for use with different types of utensils and different amounts of hand weakness. The foam should be removed before placing utensils in dishwasher or be hand washed only. In a pinch, pipe insulation can serve as an inexpensive foam covering as can masking tape or plastic cable ties over a piece of washcloth or foam to build up the handle of the utensil.

For drinking, cups with ridges on the sides, a series of rubber bands applied (to keep cup from sliding out of the hand), handles, sippy lids, long straws, or one-way valve straws can assist with drinking when the hand or arm is weak. The one-way valve straws have a ball bearing in the bottom, and once the liquid is slurped to the top, it stays at the top. This makes it easier for people with poor diaphragmatic control or mild lip weakness to still drink from a straw. Clients can put their fingers through a handle of a cup so that the weight of the cup is on the side of the hand instead of the weaker finger grip. Sometimes lightweight coffee travel mugs are ideal for many clients as the mugs often have a lid and handle. Clients who are supposed to tuck their chin for safer swallowing often have difficulty drinking from a cup, and should generally not use a straw because of potentially larger amounts of liquids ingested at a time. A nosey cup has a cut out for the nose that allows the chin to stay more tucked. Long straws can be up to two feet long, but beware of the diameter. It is nearly impossible to suck a beverage up 2 feet long, large diameter straw, even without lip or diaphragm weakness. Many cup holders will attach the cup or a beverage holder with Velcro® or more permanently with screws to the wheelchair or walker, and some even have flexible gooseneck arms to keep the drink straw right where it is needed.

For those who have tube feeding through a feeding tube, but want to perform this task independently, a tool to pop the tab on the can of formula or Dycem® to open the bottle may be required. Sometimes pliers come in handy to pinch open the plug on the end of the tube. If clients have a gravity drip, then they need to raise the syringe and tube up high so the tube is straight, and the liquid flows downhill. If they have weak shoulders, a homemade tube lifter or holder may be necessary. The client stands to fill the syringe with food, then sits with the syringe in the holder to allow the tube to be lower and use gravity assist to drip the food through the tube (Fig. 14-15). Water bottles to flush the tube can be opened with Dycem® or a commercially available bottle opener tool.

Grooming and Personal Hygiene

An electric shaver, electric toothbrush, and power flosser are about as high-tech as grooming gets most of the time. An electric shaver may be heavier, so a cuff or interlocking loops of Velcro® can keep it in the hand. Some clients will even shave while lying in the bed for an easier time. If they need a regular razor, a piece of cylindrical foam can make the razor easier to grab, or the client could use a wider women's razor. Online vendors sell razors on long arms for reaching more difficult areas. An electric toothbrush can be a little bit heavy because of the batteries, but once turned on, can make brushing much easier. Propping the arms on the sink or table will take the weight from the razor or brush. Many clients will use cylindrical foam over their make-up brushes as well. An angled mirror can be used for all grooming tasks set up at the kitchen table or bar with a spit cup and water. Sitting at the table and resting the elbows on the table can be much easier for the client with weak legs or poor balance for standing, or who has weaker arms with difficulty reaching. A variety of pump bottles and alternative toothpaste options make lotions, soaps, and toothpaste easier to manage. Toothpaste comes in pumps and different size tubes, or the client's caregiver may want to empty all the toothpaste into a container that is easier to use. Denture brushes suction to the counter for one-handed cleaning or for those with weakness. A hair dryer holder can hold the hair dryer in the correct position for a one-handed user, clients with upper body weakness, or decreased shoulder active range of motion (AROM) to manage. Long-handled brushes and combs can also assist with reaching the back of the head and sides for brushing or combing. Large-handled grooming supplies such as nail clippers and files can be found at most drug stores for easier holding. A manicure or pedicure is a possibility when nail clipping is more difficult. Suction cup nail clippers can attach to the sink or counter for easier management for clients with poor grip or difficulty with coordination, and one-handed clippers are available as well. There are also clippers with a magnifying glass attached. A device does not yet exist for inserting and removing contacts, although the OTA may assist with minor adaptations, and some clients have a caregiver assist or wear glasses.

Personal hygiene can be difficult for clients with a disability, and the opening/donning of deodorant, reaching the head to comb, shaving, and tooth brushing can be

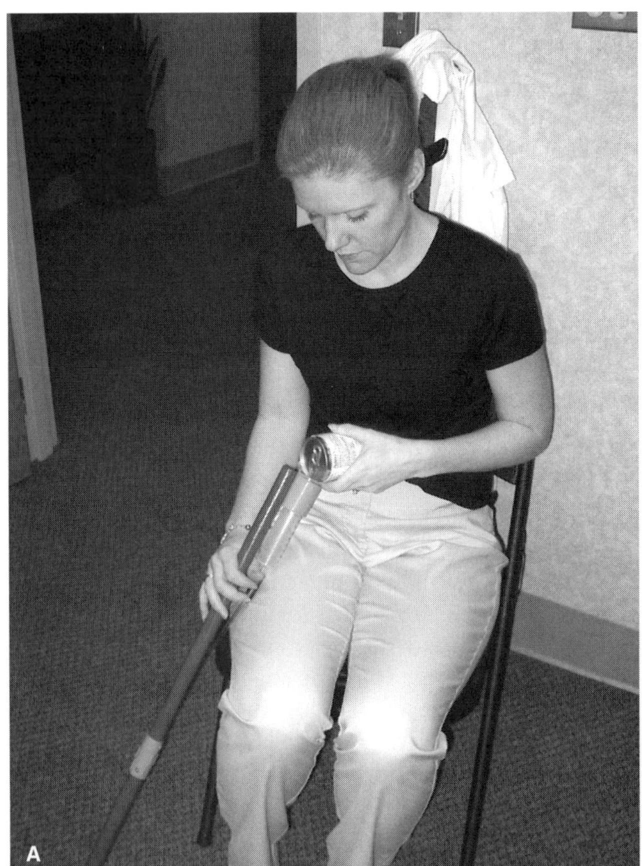

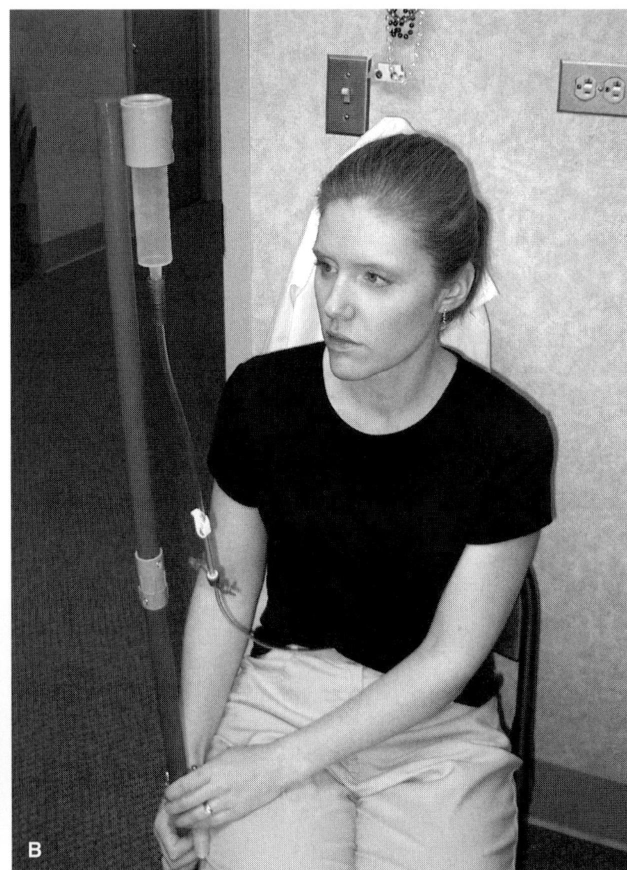

FIGURE 14-15. Homemade tube lifter or holder. **A.** The client lowers the dowel to fill the syringe, and **B.** walks the dowel upwards with the hands to allow the liquid to gravity drip into the stomach. This is often used when the client is not strong enough in the shoulders to lift the tube or syringe in the air for a gravity drip.

difficult. Also, some clients may not realize they have a problem with odor, and it will be the OTA's job to assist with awareness and management of these hygiene tasks. A salon can assist with short- or long-term hair removal if this is an issue for the client.

Sexual Activity

Sexual activity is an ADL that the OTA needs to quickly become comfortable talking about with clients. OT practitioners are the front-line professionals when it comes to discussing sex and intimacy and, often, because a trust is built during treatment sessions, the client will feel comfortable talking with the OTA. Adaptive equipment may need to be fabricated to hold onto dildos and vibrators, or for holding the fingers, hand, or wrist steady for pleasuring a partner or themselves. OTAs can direct clients to stores that sell a variety of aids that are commercially available, and assist with adapted and safe positions for sexual encounters. Patient lifts (commonly called Hoyer lifts) with divided leg slings can assist with positioning for the partner with disabilities as well. A variety of supportive seats, wedges, and chairs meant to assist with disability positioning and movement during sex are commercially available, such as Intimate Rider® (Fig. 14-16).

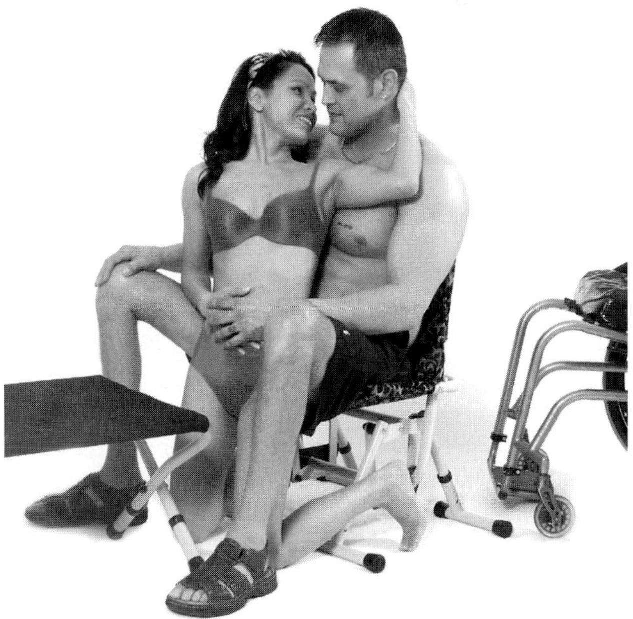

FIGURE 14-16. Intimate Rider®. The male client with leg weakness, such as from paraplegia, sits on the chair, in which it glides forward and backward. Generally, the partner leans over the other supportive seat for full access. There are many varieties of adaptive devices on the market for specific disabilities. *(Courtesy of Health Postures)*

INSTRUMENTAL ACTIVITIES OF DAILY LIVING

Sometimes OT practitioners are so concerned about basic ADLs, that they do not spend adequate time on instrumental activities of daily living (IADLs), which can sometimes be the deciding factor in whether a client stays at home or goes to a facility. In many apartments and townhomes, the laundry is not on the main floor, so it is out of reach for a person who uses a wheelchair or cannot carry a laundry basket and manage stairs at the same time. The IADL of cooking can be difficult because of heavy pots and pans, opening jars and cans, and reaching/pressing microwave buttons. IADLs can take a tremendous amount of resources and energy, and so this section on the use of AT for IADLs can be particularly important.

Health Management and Maintenance: Medication Management

Many adaptations for medication management are readily available to the general public. When asked, the pharmacist will put medications in easy-to-open bottles. Pill holders organized by the day, week, or month can assist to keep the client safe and organized. Pill holders are also available with timers. Many phones have alerts that can be set for medication reminders, and some power wheelchair joysticks have this capacity as well. Sometimes if the client already has an emergency alerting system, it can be set so that the company calls at certain times of the day to remind about medication. The OTA may to color-code bottles or put in groupings in bins to allow the client to keep medicines that are taken at certain times of the day or night together. Easy-to-read charts with names and medication pictures placed in a central location may also assist with reminders and keeping medicines straight. For the client with swallowing difficulties, pill splitters and pill crushers are commercially available. When the person with a feeding tube takes pills, generally the pills must be finely crushed. Eye drop assists that direct medicated or lubricating drops into the eye more easily also are available.

Home Management: Laundry and Cleaning

A reacher or dressing stick can assist to get items out of the washer or dryer. A front loading, stacked, or top loading machine may need to be considered depending on the needs of the client. A laundry bag can be used instead of a basket if one arm is weak, or the basket can go on the walker seat. There are even laundry bins on wheels. Another adaptation is to attach a strap to each side of the laundry basket, then to put the strap over the head. This works like a vendor selling drinks at a sporting event, and allows the stronger back muscles to stabilize the basket if one side or both arms are weak. It also allows a hand to be free to hold onto the rail when navigating the stairs. Smaller bottles of detergent or pods can be easier to hold and manage than large ones, or a caregiver can put detergent into empty small water or other small bottles for easier handling. A pump bottle for stain remover and bleach may be easier than opening the bottles and sticks. Soaking stains before washing may help a client who is weaker to avoid scrubbing on them. Tools to assist with turning washer knobs can help the client with weaker pinch. A long-handled dustpan can accompany a broom, and long-handled scrubbing sponges and long-handled toilet brushes work well to reach without stooping. Lightweight vacuums and mops may be less fatiguing, and cleaning products that can soak on and involve less scrubbing are easier to use as well. If funding resources are available, a cleaning service may be appropriate.

Meal Preparation

Large-handled stirring spoons, cheese slicers, and peelers can make those tasks easier with less effort, especially for those with a weak grip or arthritis. A Y-shaped peeler keeps the wrist in neutral for an improved ergonomic grasp. For clients with low vision, a talking measuring cup, one with large print, or a large print cookbook can assist. Book stands can hold heavy cookbooks, and some clients simply load recipes onto phones and tablets. A cutting board with nails driven through the back side so that they stick up 1 inch on the top side can hold an apple or potato for peeling and cutting (refer to Fig. 14-14). Some cutting boards have one side with edges built up for holding bread for one-handed spreading. Sharp knives are easier to cut with than dull ones, and a sharp pizza cutter can have less friction as well. A folding, rolling cart can be a lifesaver in the kitchen, for setting the table, transporting hot pans to the table, and carrying heavier items. If sitting to cook at the stove, a special steam-resistant, angled mirror mounted over the stove will help the user see into the pots, but cannot be used in conjunction with a range hood because it would block the air flow. Stove knobs on the front of the stove make it more convenient and safe for cooking (Fig. 14-17). Items are available to hold a gallon or half gallon of milk or other beverage for pouring, or for working with one hand, such as for stirring a pot or mixing a batch of cookies. These tools hold the pot handle from spinning when stirring with one hand (see Fig. 14-17), and a special suction bowl to keep it from spinning and moving when stirring with one hand use. Many caregivers will transfer gallons of milk and juice into smaller containers, such as empty water or juice bottles, after grocery shopping, to avoid the client having to lift the heavy containers. Automatic jar openers and can openers are appliances that can sit on the counter and make those tasks less strenuous, although jar pops, rubber, and other handheld jar openers are low-tech options that can also assist. One-handed and power can openers are available, as well as openers that open the lid with no sharp edges for those with numbness. Picture cookbooks can be easier to follow and recipe websites and videos can assist with following a recipe for those

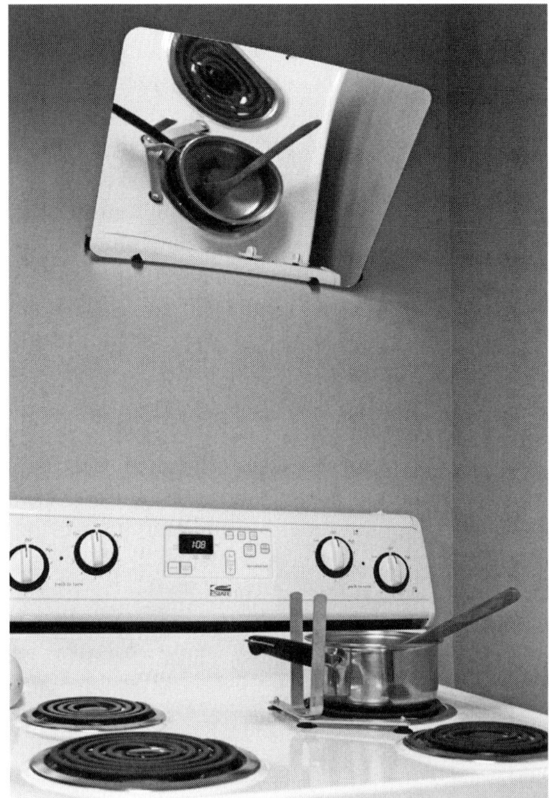

FIGURE 14-17. Stove with angled mirror so the client can see in the contents of the pot on the stovetop while seated and a pot handle holder when stirring with only one strong hand to keep the pot from spinning.

with decreased attention or ability to follow directions. Self-opening scissors, standard scissors, or a commercial bag opener can get open cereal and chip bags more easily. Simple spring-loaded needle nose pliers can assist with opening ketchup packets or resealable or zip-top bags when the thumb is weaker than the grip.

Shopping

Shopping can be a particular challenge for clients with disabilities, from driving, parking, getting into and out of the store, navigating the store, reaching and carrying items, and carrying and unloading items to and from the home. Many times, clients will arrange for friends or family who are going to the store to shop for needed things. Organization can assist with activity tolerance management by navigating the store in an efficient manner, and a power cart may assist as well. Having a list that follows the order of the store will help make sure nothing is forgotten, as well as keep the client organized. The standard shopping cart can assist with balance, and is a place to store a cane. Plastic bag holders with large grips are available to keep the heavy bags from digging into arthritic joints, and asking the bags to be packed lighter may assist. Using cloth bags with shoulder straps may make carrying easier as well. Some stores have services where the client orders online, the store employees shop for them, and the store either delivers the items or someone drives to the store for pick up, where the groceries are loaded into the car. Some clients choose to order all grocery items online for home delivery.

Care of Pets and Child Rearing

Pet leashes and harnesses that keep the family dogs from pulling a client off their feet are available, and many people will attach the leash to their waist or the wheelchair. The client will have to watch the dog to avoid getting tangled. Many pet feeders and waterers allow the client or caregiver to load a week's worth of food at one time or automatic feeders dispense a certain amount at a certain time of day. Ball throwing machines and tools can assist for those high-energy dogs for those clients with weak arms. Horse curry combs have straps, which actually can also be used for dogs, or the OTA may adapt dog or cat brushes and combs for easier use. Companies can be hired for everything from occasional fish tank cleaning to daily walks with the dog. Consider the size of the pet and the long-term care needs before bringing them into the home.

The OTA can help create or recommend child changing areas that are wheelchair accessible for the home, and many diapers and wipes can be pulled and managed with one hand. Some clients will need to move baby-changing areas to a bed or the floor for ease of reaching or to prevent rolling off or other safety issues. Baby and toddler carriers can assist with carrying the child around the home or when out in the community, and a pillow can position the child for effective nursing or bottle feeding. A specifically designed carrier for holding babies securely (with no hand use) when the client is seated is called LapBaby®, and is available online. A piece of Dycem® or thick woven shelf liner can help hold the bottle or bowl steady while placing on the top or stirring. Change those tiny snaps, zippers, and buttons to Velcro® when possible. The "leashes" for toddlers are not ideal, but can keep a toddler from running off from a parent with a disability. A useful resource for parents with disabilities or those who wish to be is www.disabledparenting.com, and the OTA can use this resource to guide clients as well.

Home Management: Yardwork

Garden kneelers allow clients who are weaker to have handles to push on to get off the ground, a padded place to kneel, and when flipped over, a seat to sit on while gardening. Long and lighter weight garden tools can assist as well as those with extra grips and assists to manage (Fig. 14-18). Smaller scale pots on the porch may be more manageable than using shovels and rakes in the acreage out back. Power or riding mowers can assist with lawn mowing. Yard tools that are electric may be easier to start, lighter to carry, and require less maintenance than gas tools. Garden beds can be raised to a height that a wheelchair will fit underneath the edge for easy access to plant, weed, water, and harvest. Plans and photos can be found online.

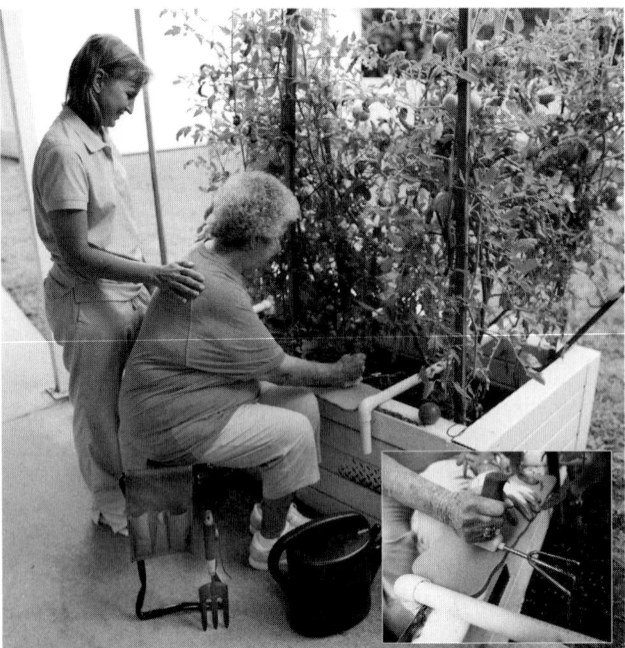

FIGURE 14-18. Gardening items. Large handled watering can, garden kneeler stool which can be flipped over when kneeling on the ground for handles to assist with getting up, and a raised garden bed. *Inset:* Adapted garden tool.

EDUCATION AND WORK

Some clients with disabilities may not be encouraged to continue with higher education because of the perception that they are not capable of all the occupations involved, but the OTA can often make enough adaptations and offer resources to make this dream a reality. A wheelchair, scooter, or power wheelchair may be required to conserve energy, and increase safety and the ability to get across campus. Transportation may also be wheelchair accessible to also get across campus. The OTA can advise on packs and bags that attach to wheelchairs, either under the seat, by the feet, or on the backrest. Adaptations for taking notes, including recording them and using a computer or iPad®, may be possible. Clients may use large-sized pens or add cylindrical foam to a pen or pencil to increase the grip, or the OTA may need to custom fabricate a writing device for the client's specific needs. When the ability to press down is weak, ball point pens are less easy to write with when the ability to press is weak than slim markers or gel/roller ball style pens. Signature stamps can be created by stationary stores or online if the client has to sign frequently. Adaptations may be required to stay organized with the class and homework/test schedule, and planners, phone applications, and charts may be needed. The adult student should contact the disability services office at the school for required accommodations, such as making class resources available before class for easier note taking, having increased time for test taking, or having a classmate take notes.

Many adult clients have been in the work world for years before an injury or disease process makes it difficult to continue working, and others have had a life-long disability and would like to enter their chosen field. The OT practitioner can certainly assist in a multitude of ways, including adaptation of work tasks or environment, functional mobility and safety within a building or from and to parking, education and training of the client, supervisor, or coworkers, use of AE and technology, and workplace assessments. Some adaptations for getting from the parking into the building and back would be mobility devices such as a scooter or power wheelchair, wheelchair transportation, and a handicapped parking tag to park closer. Employees and students can advocate for a power opening door at the entrance of the building and for bathroom accessibility. Adaptations for keyboards, mouse access, and phone access would be similar to ideas offered in other parts of this chapter. Ergonomics would be important, as well as building in rest breaks and potentially a couch or surface to lay flat to rest. At times, work tasks may involve reaching and carrying papers, folders, and books which may be too heavy or difficult for the client. A reacher, rolling cart, shoulder bag, or alternative storage of items may be needed. Employers must provide reasonable accommodations for qualified employees per the ADA to allow them to work despite a disability if it does not cause the business "undue hardship." There is a lot of gray area with this issue, as some employers claim hardship to put up a grab bar in the bathroom, and others are willing to extensively renovate to accommodate a client with a disability. Some employees may require an assistant to fully manage all the physical tasks required of the job, or may not be able to return to paid employment in any fashion due to difficulties with balance, fatigue, or strength.

Volunteerism, categorized under the occupation of work in the *Occupational Therapy Practice Framework: Domain and Process, 3rd edition (OTPF-3)*, can be an effective boost to quality of life, and the OTAs may have to adapt the project, tools, or items for the client to have success with the group or charity of their choice. Clients may be able to volunteer to make calls or stuff envelopes from their own homes, or use the volunteering to get out of the house for social interactions. Some clients participate in peer mentoring programs where they volunteer to talk to newly injured or diagnosed clients with that same disability. This process can be very rewarding for the client as a volunteer opportunity.

COMMUNICATION

Although communication is addressed thoroughly in Chapter 12, a review of low- and high-tech AT devices is found here. Because communication is so inherent to quality of life and functional performance, the OTA will inevitably work with the rest of the team and the client/caregivers on procurement, functional use, and training.

Low Technology for Communication

Communication is a vital skill, and a tool as simple as a picture board with yes or no options and pictures and letters to point to can be effective. A laser light attached to a hat or headband can point to letters on a board on the wall. A clear plexiglass letter board allows the client and caregiver to communicate letter choices by matching eye contact through the board (Fig. 14-19). Some clients and families have boards memorized where the client blinks or nods when the row number or letter is reached to choose letters to spell words. Simple recorders can play back a desired phrase when a certain switch is hit, or merely record thoughts to assist with memory. For people who speak softly, an amplifier can make the difference in being understood, especially in a crowded room. For writing, there are larger pens, ones with various grips, and ways to attach the pen to the client's hand (Fig. 14-20). Typing or using text on the phone, iPad®, or tablet to communicate may be easier than writing for some people.

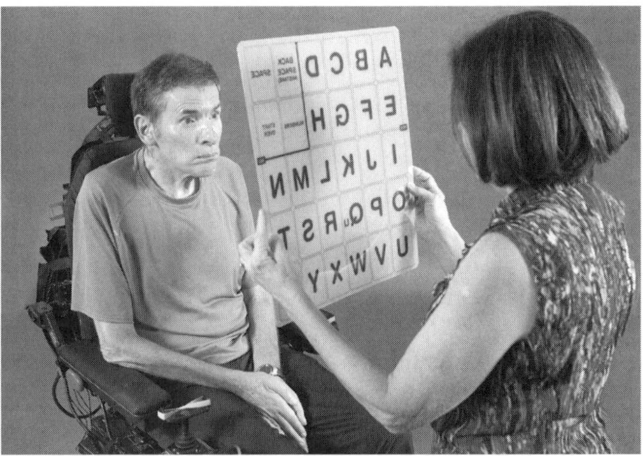

FIGURE 14-19. Clear letterboard being used between client and caregiver.

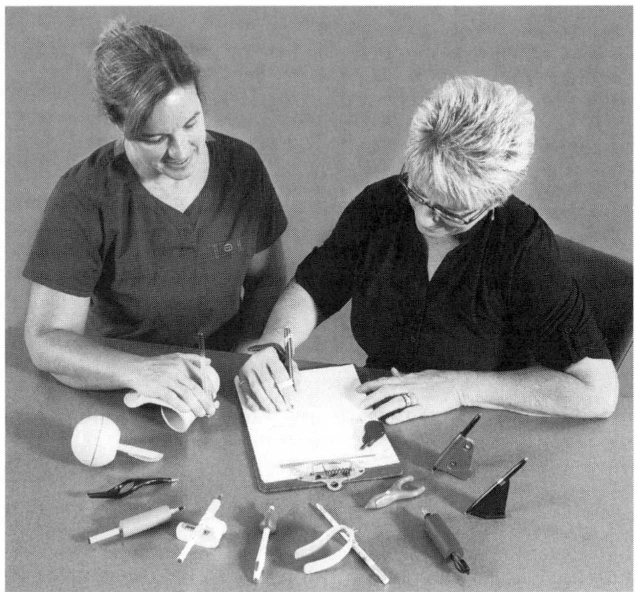

FIGURE 14-20. Various adapted writing options to trial and test with larger handles, alternate grips, and some which hold a pen stable for the client. The client in the photo is using a Wanchik's Writer®.

High Technology for Communication

Although texting and e-mailing are frequently the preferred methods of communication for younger adults, adults of all ages are becoming more comfortable with using their phones for more than just dialing. Many smart phones have hands-free, voice-activated dialing and answering capabilities that go beyond a speaker phone.

Communication devices are often computer-based and can be very complex. Access of the device by use of the hand is generally with a mouse, a touch screen, or keyboard. Many are compatible with multiple methods of access, including manual/touch, head-pointing, eye-tracking, Bluetooth via power wheelchair controls, and switch/scanning via any number of different switches. When accessed with a switch, a button is plugged into the device that, when activated, causes an action to happen. For instance, if a client is able to activate a foot switch by pressing it with their big toe, it may choose a word that was highlighted to speak. Switches can be activated by any part of the body where the client has consistent, volitional control. They come in many sizes and require different amounts of force or pressure for activation (Fig. 14-21). Some do not even require force, such as proximity switches, where activation occurs when the client gets close to the switch or fiber optic switches that activate when a beam of light is broken. An electromyography (EMG) switch is activated by an electrode sensor that detects very small amounts of muscle movement for those with very limited mobility (Fig. 14-22). It is also possible to change repeat and delay rates within the "ease of access center", "accessibility" or "system preferences" (depending on computer type) to avoid hitting multiple letters at once or repeating keys. A head mouse is a camera device that tracks a reflective dot worn typically on the forehead or bridge of glasses, and allows individuals to control the mouse via head movement (Fig. 14-23). This may be used

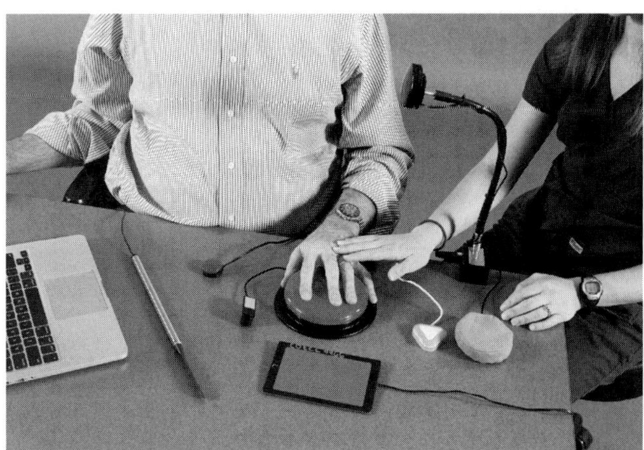

FIGURE 14-21. Numerous switches. *From left:* Leaf switch; small buddy button; microlite; large buddy button (round); pressure switch (rectangular); proximity switch, which doesn't involve direct contact (triangle); pillow switch; and buddy button on a gooseneck clamp for moveable positioning.

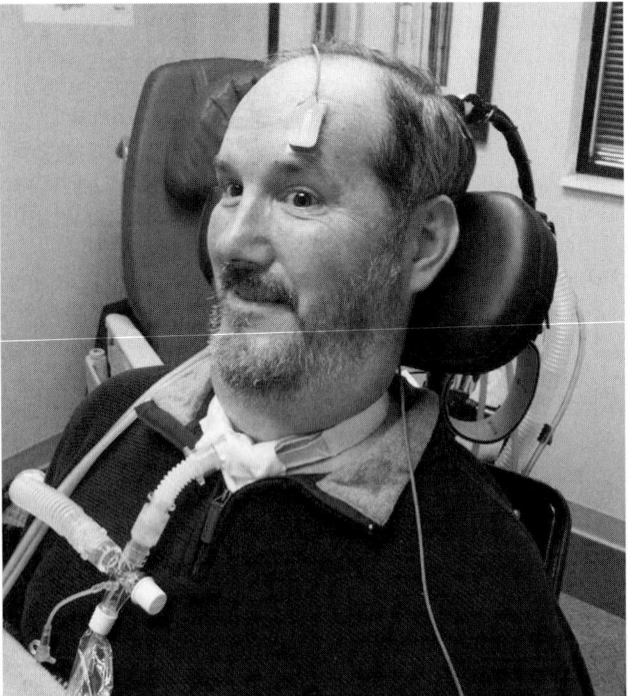

FIGURE 14-22. A wired EMG switch to activate the client's communication device with forehead muscle activation.

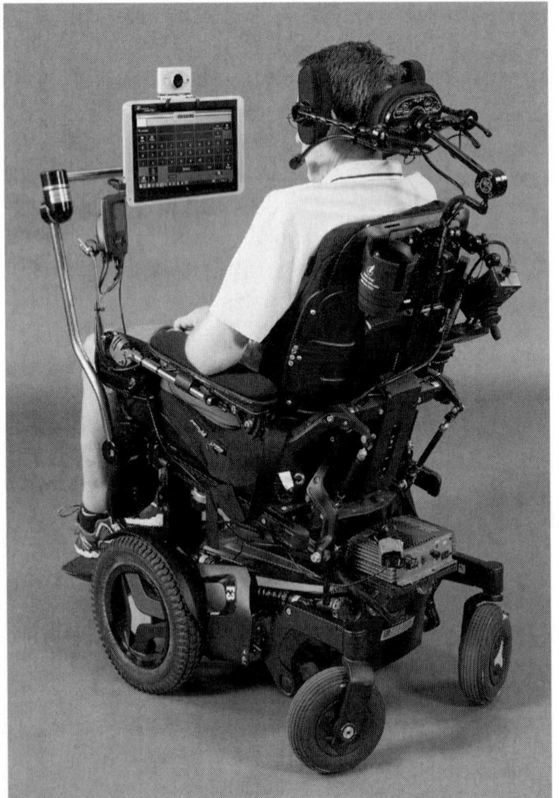

FIGURE 14-23. This client is accessing his communication device while mounted to his power wheelchair. He chooses the letters and words on the screen via a camera mounted to his computer (head mouse), which reads the position of a reflective dot worn on his forehead. As he moves his head, the camera reads the dot's position, and when he hovers over a choice for a preset amount of time (dwell), the device then makes that choice.

when the hands/feet are weak, but the neck is relatively strong, and is often easier to transition to than eye gaze and it does not require such fine control. The eye gaze access option uses a camera to track cornea and pupil reflections. Eye tracking devices are calibrated by following users' eye movements. Successful calibration and selection accuracy are dependent on maintaining optimal positioning. If the arms or hands are weak, mouse clicks can be performed by blinking, hitting a switch with another part of the body, or using mouse-click emulation software ("dwell click") that clicks automatically after a set length of time. Some programs are beginning to use web cameras as a lower-cost mouse option via facial recognition software. Brain-computer interface is a newer access method designed for those with little to no observable volitional muscle control. The user wears a cap (like a tight swim cap) with sensors that read EMG signals from the scalp. These signals are analyzed by the device for certain specific features, which then translates the features into actions. The action might be a yes/no option or to choose a certain letter on a screen. It is a slow, emerging technology, but has good promise for the future. Some communication devices are icon- or picture-based, and some are letter-based. The icon user can still communicate in full sentences/paragraphs when combining icons as needed, or quickly get a one-word thought across. The number of buttons or keys on a dynamic display device can be customized. There can be many choices or as few as two, depending on communication needs and cognitive status. They often include preloaded phrases or pictures and are capable of storing jokes, speeches, voice recordings, and other personal messages. Many text-based communication devices have word prediction to increase the speed of communication. Applications are available to assist with picture-based communication as well as text-to-speech output for communication via smart phone, tablet, or iPad®. Numerous mounting systems are available to attach a communication device, tablet, or phone to the wheelchair. The OTA may fabricate a custom mount from a clamp, gooseneck, Velcro® or thermoplastic splinting material, and there are online sites that sell gooseneck pieces and clamps for AT uses (Box 14-1).

VISION

While vision is covered thoroughly in Chapter 10, some specific AT and adaptations are presented here. Magnifiers and glasses can assist with decreased acuity, as can brighter lights and bright paint and tapes on the edge of each step of stairs, shower edges, or cupboard corners. An audio labeler can assist with finding items in the cupboard; when the item label is scanned, the device audibly identifies the item. With low vision, home organization is key and always putting items in the same locations will help. Screen readers are devices that can offer increased access to the text on the computer, by loading the reading application, positioning the

EVIDENCE-BASED PRACTICE

In the 2016 article, *Meanings and Experiences of Assistive Technologies in Everyday Lives of Older Citizens: A Metainterpretive Review*, authors performed a literature review on articles involving older adults and technologies of varying sorts. One reviewed article noted that many older adults are conflicted about technology, and although they see the potential value (especially for others), they did not necessarily want it in their home.[5] They found that older people in general have a positive attitude toward technologies and recognize the potential of technology in a wide range of areas.[5] Sometimes, the need for technology was an admission of an increasing disability, and many elders note they have a hard time keeping up with the changes in technology. Skymne et al. found that a prerequisite to become a user of technologies "is that you have trust in the experts, that you have the right information, and that you have confidence in yourselves."[6] This places a large burden on the OTA who assesses for, prescribes, educates on, trains, and uses assistive technology with this population to provide information in a way that inspires trust and self-confidence. For many active, independent, and self-sufficient older adults, "not being a burden" is the motivational factor for using AT.[5] In a study of elderly cerebrovascular accident (CVA) survivors, Barker et al. found different categories of acceptance of wheelchairs as technology: "Reluctant acceptance is when the wheelchair is seen as a necessity, grateful acceptance is when the wheelchair is experienced as a great asset, and internal acceptance is when the wheelchair is experienced as 'a part of me.'"[7] Many times, clients may be extremely reluctant to consider a technology, and then find it life changing once it is adapted into their paradigm. The notion that clients must be dependent on technology to be independent in their interactions with others puts AT in an uncomfortable spot for many users.

Dahler, A. M., Rasmussen, D. M., & Andersen, P. T. (2016). Meanings and experiences of assistive technologies in everyday lives of older citizens: A meta-interpretive review. Disability and Rehabilitation: Assistive Technology, *11,8.*

Skymne, C., Dahlin-Ivanoff, S., Claesson, L., & Eklund, K. (2012). Getting used to assistive devices: Ambivalent experiences by frail elderly persons. Scandinavian Journal of Occupational Therapy, *19(2), 194–203.*

Barker, D. J., Reid, D., & Cott, C. (2004). Acceptance and meanings of wheelchair use in senior stroke survivors. American Journal of Occupational Therapy, *58,221-230.*

BOX 14-1
Details of Mounting Options

Many times it is the responsibility of the OTA to devise an option to allow a device to attach closely and securely enough that the client will have full access at whatever height, angle, and location is required. Some devices, such as eye-gaze access, require the device to be at eye level and very stable, yet easily removable for transfers. It might be necessary to Velcro® a smartphone to the thigh, opposite wrist, or wheelchair armrest for easy access. The phone or tablet can mount to the armrest, seat rail, or joystick with permanent, removable, or swing away mounts as well. The tablet may require a stand on the lap, a flexible mount, or moveable system so if the client is reading or typing, the access and location can change. If a flexible or gooseneck option is required, then a website such as www.modularhose.com has many AT options with clamps, plates, and other mounting options. It is the responsibility of the OTA to be familiar with the options available and how to procure these devices.

mouse over the beginning of the text, and clicking the mouse to start and stop reading. They can also be accessed through headings using keyboard shortcuts. Screen readers will also read the icons verbally on the screen. Video magnifiers take an image on a piece of paper and enlarge sections to the desired size on a screen. They come in portable or desktop versions, and can magnify other items besides an image on paper, including a medication bottle, needlepoint, or a food label. One could also use a larger movie screen to see the computer or TV screen. Textures and raised bumps/dots on items can determine colors of clothing in the closet or the flour container versus the sugar. These raised dots are from one-quarter to 1 inch in diameter, made of plastic or felt, sticky on one side, and are generally found in a hardware store to protect a table or floor from a scratching item. The dots could be used to tell the position of the dial on a stove or washer, or the sizes of a measuring cup (e.g., two dots for one-half a cup, and three dots for three-quarters a cup). They also come in bright colors for those with low vision. Applications are now available on the phone to assist with color, item, and money identification for the client with low vision. The camera on a smart phone can be used to take a photo of a label in small print and enlarge it with the zoom feature directly on the phone. Guide sticks, long white canes, talking GPS, and guide dogs can assist someone who is completely blind to navigate the environment, and there are agencies in most large cities to assist with information and training.

HEARING

The standard device for a client who is hearing impaired is a hearing aid, but many people cannot afford them and require other options such as a personal amplifier or FM (frequency modulation, similar to radios) system. A personal amplifier can be used to amplify conversation when a person who is hearing impaired cannot see the speaker's lips for lip reading, such as in the car. Organizations such as churches often use FM systems, where the sermon is amplified in the room only for those wearing a certain device. FM systems can be less expensive than hearing aids. Hearing aids now have many options for programming, with use of Bluetooth to stream the phone or TV directly into the aids. Phone apps can often change programming on the hearing aids without having to go back to the audiologist's office. Many phones have not only volume controls but amplifiers, too. For the person who is hearing impaired, a light can be set-up to flash in the home for the doorbell or phone. Lights can also come on to wake up the person, or a device can go under the mattress to have the bed shake to wake them up. Telecommunications-relay services exist where the client types in words, and an operator types what the person on the other end is saying. It is also available to communicate with someone who uses sign language, where the operator speaks to the verbal person, then signs to the deaf person. Video phones are used for sign language users as well as video phone chats for FaceTime and other systems. Closed caption TV is an option for the text to appear on the TV screen for the deaf and hard of hearing.

COMPUTER, IPAD®, TABLET, AND PHONE ACCESS

Technology access can be varied, and numerous shapes, sizes, and types of input options are available for device access. Every computer has accessibility settings in the control panel or system preferences for items such as contrast, size of the type, and color scheme. Just as with communication devices, clients can use a computer with hand, foot, head, switch, or eye movement for full control. A person who is using their eyes to move the mouse will either hover over an icon for a determined amount of time, blink, or activate a switch for the clicks. All computer functions can be performed with a single access point. For example, if a person can only access a mouse, an onscreen keyboard will allow them to input text. An onscreen keyboard is available on every computer or can be downloaded, and takes up the bottom portion of the screen with the keyboard. The onscreen keyboard can be sized so the user can see it well, and are available in various keyboard styles such as ABC, frequency, and QWERTY formats. Mouse options can be varied depending on the strength and mobility of the limb using the control (Fig. 14-24). Clients who have weaker hands may use a mouse with the feet, and these come in many sizes. Keyboard options are just as varied, depending on whether the client only uses one hand or prefers a different order of the keys, has ataxia, and needs the keys protected and separated, or prefers smaller/larger keyboards (Fig. 14-25). The wheelchair joystick or control on complex rehabilitation power wheelchairs for clients with significant disabilities can serve as the mouse via Bluetooth access. The client can press

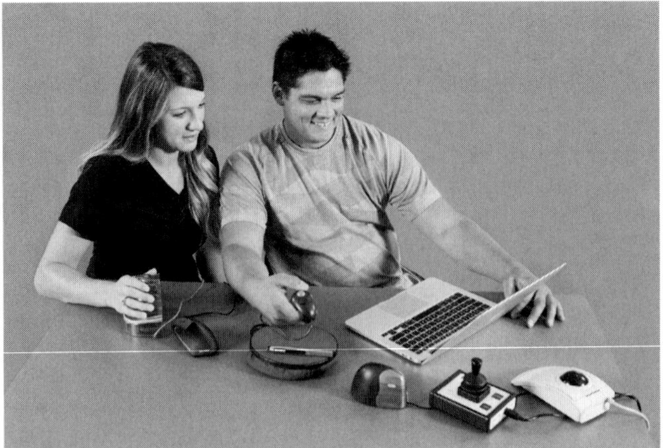

FIGURE 14-24. *From left:* Mouse options: vertical mouse, standard mouse, handheld mouse, beanbag mouse pad (to sit on leg), a different vertical mouse, a joystick mouse, and a track ball.

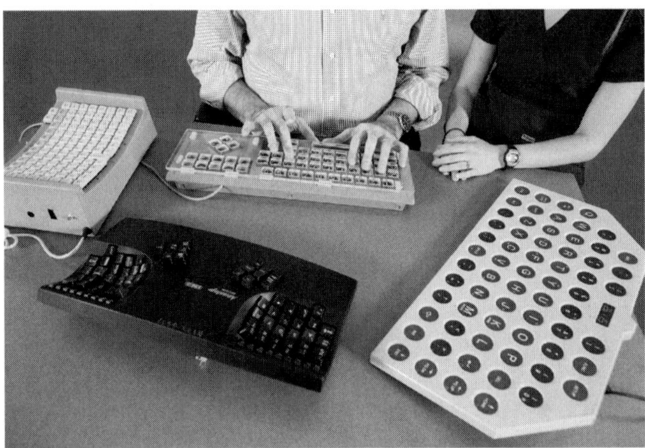

FIGURE 14-25. Keyboard options. *Clockwise from top left:* Curved keyboard, large keyboard with key guard for clients with ataxia, large colored/inset keyboard, and Kinesis™ Advantage split ergonomic keyboard.

switches or keys on the joystick for mouse clicks or simply dwell for selection. A touch screen with a conductive stylus or finger provides access to cell phones, iPads®, and tablets. These devices can also be accessed with a Bluetooth switch or using head movement as the switch. Figure 14-26 shows many options for differently shaped styluses and typing aids for control. A fabricated or commercially available adapted stylus can make access easier for those with hand weakness, or the OTA may need to fabricate a finger orthotic to maintain strong pointing when the finger wants to flex. Power wheelchair control is also available to use with most smart phones and tablet computers through Bluetooth technology. A headset or speakerphone can provide hands-free access to a cell phone or landline for those unable to lift or grasp the phone. A large button landline phone can be useful for decreased vision or limited finger dexterity. Various holders and mounts can attach the computer or cell phone to the wheelchair or a stand for access. Switches can assist when the person is using scanning on the computer for mouse clicks or with a switch interface

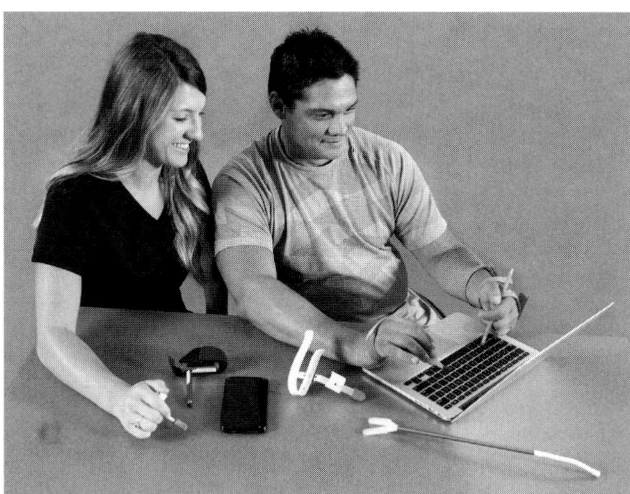

FIGURE 14-26. Stylus and pointer options for computer access. *From left:* T handle stylus, stylus with cuff, MaxiAids typing aid, mouthstick, standard typing aid, and economy wrist support holding pencil-eraser end down to hit keys.

and, as noted earlier, can be found in all shapes, sizes, and types for various needs (refer to Fig. 14-21). Many clients who do a lot of typing at home or work prefer to dictate their words into text, and Dragon®, Apple products, and Windows speech recognition software can assist. The accuracy is improving all the time, and the programs can be trained to a specific voice. The mobile arm support mentioned for self-feeding is very useful for computer, iPad®/tablet, and phone use when mounted to the wheelchair for use at home and the community.

TECHNOLOGY AND TRENDS

One of the most exciting technological trends is the advent of the Kinova® Jaco robotic arm, which can be controlled and integrated into complex power wheelchair controls. The robotic arm has multiple joints, as well as two fingers and a thumb on the hand for grasp and release. It mounts to the side rail of the power wheelchair, and however the client is controlling the chair, such as with joystick, foot, lip, or single switch, is also how the robotic arm is controlled. The robotic arm removes easily as needed. There are also memory functions that allow the arm to move to a preset place, such as for shaving, and the user only presses one button. These robotic arms are expensive, but may be well worth getting through insurance, fundraising, or finding other funding sources if it means increasing independence.

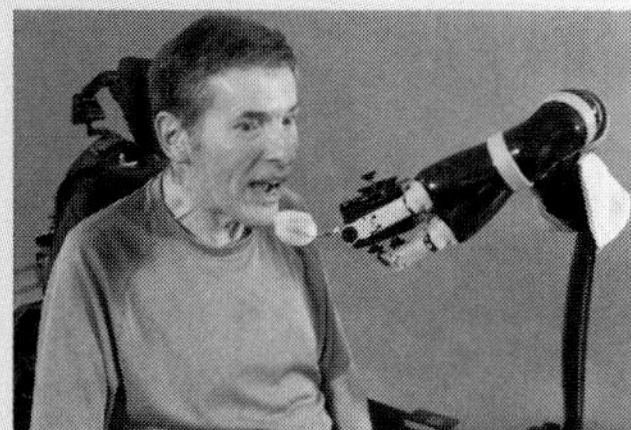

Client using robotic arm to self-feed.

DOOR OPTIONS, ALERTING, AND ELECTRONIC ACTIVITIES OF DAILY LIVING

Home access can be a significant limitation in many ways for clients with disabilities. With smaller doors, swing-clear or off-set hinges can replace standard hinges to get the door farther out of the way to increase the usable space (Fig. 14-27). A power door opener or automatic lock can get the client in or out of the house without the need to manage the lock or knob physically. A lever door handle versus a round knob can be easier to get open without requiring grip strength. A rope or string tied to the door handle can assist to get the door pulled open or shut when using a wheelchair or walker. A dressing stick, mouthstick or dowel rod could be used to push elevator buttons and doorbells. A wireless doorbell can be used to alert a caregiver that the client needs help, and can also be switch-adapted. The doorbell pressing portion could be attached to Velcro® on the wheelchair, a wrist strap, or bed rail. Louder alarms are available as well for a hard of hearing caregiver. These alerts can be hooked in through the home alarm system or computer system. Lights and appliances

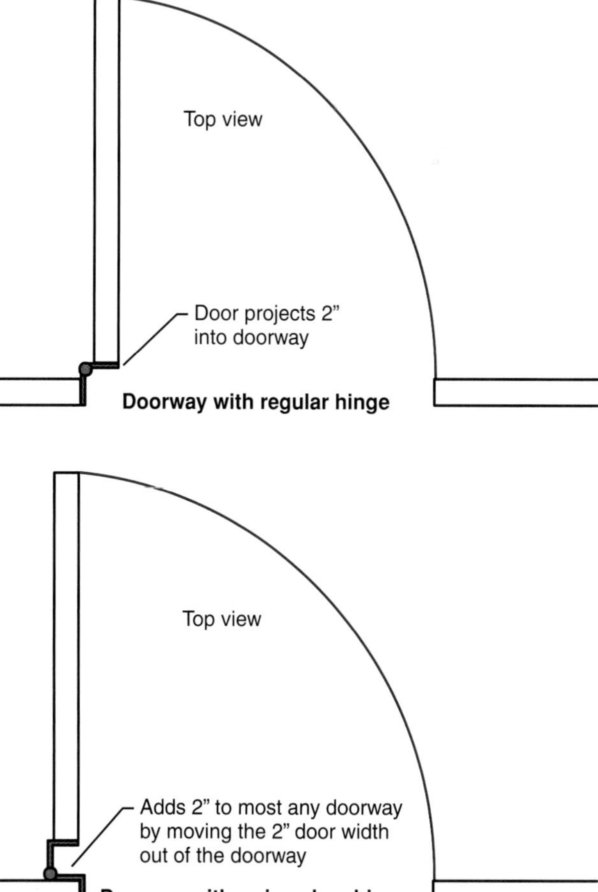

FIGURE 14-27. Swing clear hinges. Note the extra room in the available door opening with the swing clear hinges.

can be made to turn on through motion, timers, remotes, switches, or home automation. **Electronic aids to daily living (EADLs),** also known as environmental control units (ECUs), allow a client with a disability to interact and manipulate television, lights, telephone, drapery controls, doors, appliances, and bed controls from a wheelchair, phone, computer, tablet, or a remote and potentially can be set up by the OTA. The client can use an X-10 device or power link, into which lights or other appliances are plugged. Clients keep the remote/phone/activation option, and when they want light "A" to turn on, they press that button, and light "A," which is plugged into slot A, turns on. The potential is unlimited, and they can work via infrared, radio waves, and Bluetooth as well. Many smartphone systems are now linking to electronic devices in the home via Wi-Fi, so that the client could say "goodnight" via voice control, and a preset group of items could react, such as the door locking, lights turning off inside, and the thermostat changing. Many options for voice control for clients who cannot talk exist within smart phone and communication device technology. If the OTA has interest in assisting clients with setting up this sort of home automation, further study with the state AT program staff or online resources may be required. The OTA may also want to pursue a certification as an assistive technology professional (ATP) via the Rehabilitation Engineering Society of North America (RESNA).

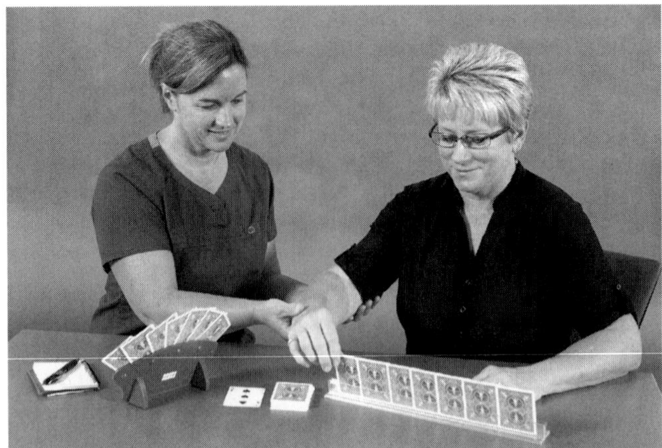

FIGURE 14-28. Playing card holders. A very low-tech option is to use a board game (lid on) flipped over, and cards can be held in the space.

LEISURE

Quality of life is important for all clients at any stage, and leisure is a large part of that. Quality of life is not necessarily tied to physical functioning status, and the OTA can adapt and introduce leisure activities throughout the lifespan. Crossword puzzles, Sudoku, Solitaire, and games of all sorts can be found on computers, tablets, iPads®, and pen/paper. Card holders can assist to hold playing cards, and an automatic shuffler can shuffle the cards (Fig. 14-28). A board game box flipped over intact has a nice space to line cards up in for an inexpensive card holder. Crafts can be adapted with items for holding a crochet hook or yarn more easily, gloves for quilting or sewing, which are rubberized to hold the fabric steady, or pliers for beading jewelry. Books can be held securely with a book holder or a clipboard with a chip clip or rubber band on the other end to hold the book securely to the clip board. The clip board then leans on a pillow to get the angle needed. A Kindle® or e-reader may be easier to hold, lean against a pillow, or to turn pages than a book. Large print books can also be found in libraries and bookstores, and the font on e-readers can be enlarged. Books on CD, apps, phones, e-readers, or MP3 players can be listened to if reading is difficult. Each state has a library for the blind and physically disabled to provide physical access to books, magazines, and newspapers, where the items can be checked out for free, and often mailed to the home and shipped back for free. Libraries also have many books available for free download in multiple formats.

Golf, fishing, and other sports have numerous adaptations available. Golfing adaptations include gloves to help hold the club, straps that attach the person to the golf cart to assist with balance, special seats to sit while hitting the ball, and longer and shorter clubs. A ride in the golf cart may be an option to spend time with friends and be outside if physically playing is not an option. Fishing adaptations include power casters and reelers, as well as pole holders for a belt and the wheelchair. Swimming pools can be adapted to have seats to lower the person in the pool as well as supportive straps and seats for in the pool, and many public or YMCA pools are already outfitted with these devices or have zero entry. Many public pools have shower seats and adapted locker rooms for clients with disabilities. Beaches often rent beach wheelchairs for getting to the water because most wheelchairs are not designed to move on top of sand (Fig. 14-29).

Travel can be very enjoyable, and there are many travel websites and agencies that specialize in adapted travel. Many state and national parks have accessible trails and access points. Hotels generally have a limited number of adapted rooms but calling ahead is useful to make sure the client's specific needs are met. Airlines require at least 48 hours' notice for clients with disabilities, and the client/caregiver may want to call multiple times to alert airport staff, especially for a client with significant disabilities. Take the client's own wheelchair all the way to the gate, and have the chair "gate-checked" under the plane. Then, the chair will be brought up at the arrival gate in the destination city. The client generally has to be transferred into a very small wheelchair designed to go down airplane aisles, and this can be challenging for a client who has significant weakness. Leave plenty of time for connecting flights. The airline should be able to accommodate ventilators, oxygen, bilevel positive airway pressure (BiPAP), and other medical devices, but a letter from the doctor may be required. Power wheelchair batteries currently are safe for travel and do not need to be removed or disconnected. Since the wheelchair or walker is stored under the plane with the luggage, damage can be a very real possibility. Remove anything which might fall off or which is very fragile

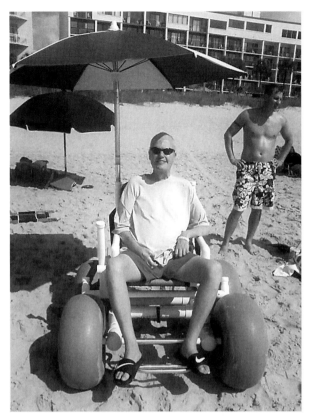

FIGURE 14-29. Client in a beach wheelchair. Large tires provide easy access.

and place in a carry-on at the gate. Accessible cruises, train travel, RV rentals, van rentals, and scooter/wheelchair rentals can be found as well. Careful pre-planning can make a dream trip a reality.

Some communities have adapted sports programs where people with all kinds of disabilities can learn basketball, snow skiing, water skiing, tennis, cycling, rugby, baseball, and many other opportunities. Horseback riding can be adapted to be therapeutic as well as fun.

SERVICE ANIMALS

Although many types of animals can be part of the family, a service dog is a working dog, not a pet, and is specifically trained to assist a person with a disability. The ADA recognizes service dogs and grants rights to the dogs and their human handlers access to anywhere the public is generally allowed to go.[8] The service dogs may assist a client with disabilities in many ways, including assisting a client with navigating streets, retrieving dropped items, pulling a wheelchair up a hill, or calming a client who has post-traumatic stress disorder (PTSD) and is having an anxiety attack.

Emotional support animals, comfort animals, and therapy dogs are not service animals under the ADA, and other species of animals, whether wild or domestic, trained or untrained, are not considered service animals either.[8] It does not matter if a client has a note from a doctor that states the person has a disability and needs to have the animal for emotional support. These support animals provide companionship, relieve loneliness, and sometimes help with depression, anxiety, and certain phobias, but do not have special training to perform tasks that assist people with disabilities.[8]

If the OTA has a client who requires a service dog for particular tasks and needs related to the disability, there are lists of groups that train service dogs. Often a client can start by working with local or national organizations related to the disability (e.g., Multiple Sclerosis Society). The wait lists can be long, but may be well worth it.

CREATING CUSTOM ASSISTIVE TECHNOLOGY DEVICES

One of the most enjoyable parts of an OTA's role may be creating custom AT devices to meet client needs. What if the client cannot push the remote control with their hand but have foot motion? Create a toe orthotic to hit the TV remote keys. What if the client cannot reach the back knobs on a stove? Create a tool to attach to a reacher to turn the knobs. The sky is the limit, and many practitioners keep Velcro®, extra splinting material, elastic, duct tape, foam, gooseneck, PVC pipe, glues, and other working tools for creating what clients need. Often the OTA can be an inspiration for a caregiver, friend, or family member to assist the client as well. Offering a riser option for raising the couch so the client can get out of it may mean that the family builds a platform for the recliner and other chairs as well. If a raised toilet seat is not tall enough, the OTA can educate the family to raise up each leg on sections of wood with holes drilled in for the legs. Dycem® or rubber shelf liners can have a multitude of uses from holding a communication device on a tray and a plate steady to turning a car key. Give your clients the building blocks for adaptation and creation of their own AT devices (Box 14-2).

BOX 14-2
Tablet Holder

A female client with a speech deficit as her only weakness was becoming frustrated with trying to type with one hand on her tablet with keyboard while she was up and walking. She was a fast typist, and was trying to keep up with the flow of the conversation. The OT practitioner working with her devised a holder for the tablet. It was made from a large piece of thermoplastic splinting material that was bent in an L shape. One part of the L held the tablet, and the other leaned against the client's abdomen to make a shelf for the tablet to sit on. A Velcro® strap around her neck held the shelf close so she could use two hands to type freely. A piece of Dycem® kept the holder/tablet from rotating forward as it leaned against her. Very inexpensive, very practical, and it did not exist commercially.

OT Practitioner's Viewpoint

I think the creativity and creative process are the most rewarding and exciting parts of my job. To make something from scrap or from wandering around the hardware store is so amazing and often meets a very unique need. One of the strangest and most simple devices was a U-bolt with extra nuts on the ends of the U-shape to make the device heavier. This simple device allowed a woman with multiple sclerosis who had only the use of one hand to be able to hit Ctrl/Alt/Delete keys all at the same time to log into her computer. Her technology department could get rid of this log-in requirement at all times except for the first log in, and the client did not like asking other staff to log her in, as she was the boss. The weighted U-bolt sat upright pressing down the Ctrl and Alt keys, and then she pressed the Delete key with her functioning hand. She uses the tool for about three seconds a day, but what a difference it made for her. ~Amber L. Ward, MS, OTR/L, BCPR, ATP/SMS

COMMUNICATION

Consideration of AT by the whole team working with the client can be important and difficult as well, at times, and communication among all team members is vital. For example, a client with amyotrophic lateral sclerosis (ALS) who attends a multidisciplinary clinic in another state from his home, might have an occupational therapist, physical therapist, speech language pathologist (SLP), respiratory therapist, dietitian, neurologist, pulmonologist, gastroenterologist, and equipment vendor representative on his team. The client may also have a home care team with nursing aides and OT or physical therapy practitioners, as well as a team of friends and family. The client may also have a palliative care team and a primary care doctor. All of these people may be affected by how the eye-gaze communication device mounts to the power wheelchair and whether there is a rolling mount for the hospital bed. How easily it goes into the correct place each time and yet removes by a variety of people for toileting transfers will be vital. Also important is how stable the device is on the chair, and whether it makes the chair too wide to go through the home's doorways. The training of all these people as well as communication with others who are not as familiar with the technology is also important, and communication can quickly breakdown.

CHOOSING CORRECTLY

Choosing AT may be a decision that the OTA makes alone, and sometimes together with a team of professionals and consultants as well as the occupational therapist, client, and family. An AT team may include family physicians, regular and special education teachers, speech-language pathologists, rehabilitation engineers, occupational therapists, physical therapists, physical therapist assistants, and other specialists, including consulting representatives from companies that manufacture devices.[9] To determine the AT needs of a person with a disability, an AT assessment should be conducted. Many AT professionals use the SETT framework for the AT process from start to finish. SETT is an acronym for Student, Environment, Tasks, and Tools. The SETT framework is a model intended to promote collaborative decision-making in all phases of AT service design and delivery from consideration through implementation and evaluation of effectiveness[10]. The result of an assessment is a recommendation for specific devices and services. Once it is agreed that AT would benefit a person, issues related to design and selection of the device, as well as maintenance, repair, and replacement of devices should be considered by the team before ordering.[2]

DEVICE USE AND ABANDONMENT

Many times, a well-meaning practitioner will issue or recommend an AT device, and then clients will refuse to use it or say they will use it, take it home, and then abandon it. Was there a clear dialogue between the client, family, and practitioner, and were all the needs and environments taken into consideration? Issues of design, consumer preference, cost, and policy can influence the use, disuse, or abandonment of AT, and the assessment process can be complicated. For example, if the wheelchair is too large to get through the doorways in the home, the wheelchair will not be used. If the client is not comfortable in the new wheelchair, they may just continue to use the older one. Multiple factors are related to the abandonment of AT devices, including failure by providers to take the client's, family's, and caregiver's opinions into account, lack of easy device attainment, poor AT device performance, and changes in client needs or priorities.[3] If the OTA is cautious from the beginning to really listen to the client, carefully train to use the product, and provide the necessary support and follow-up when things go wrong, then the user-technology match will be greater and the overall effectiveness higher. Certainly, clients evolve over time as their condition changes and they age, so the AT may need to modify over time as well. A client with a progressive disorder may begin by eating with foam attached onto a utensil, then progress to a feeding cuff to hold the spoon, then a mobile arm support, and then an automatic feeder.

WHO PAYS?

AT can be very inexpensive, such as a pair of elastic shoelaces ($3), or as expensive as a standing power wheelchair ($60,000). At times, the client's insurance will assist with the cost of the items, but often they will not, and the client is left scrambling. The next section lists some of the many payer options:

- Government programs (whether Medicare, Veteran's benefits, or Medicaid agencies) pay for certain AT if it is prescribed by a doctor as a necessary medical device. This generally does not include small gadgets, but instead items such as communication devices, patient lifters, wheelchairs, and bedside commodes. At times the items will be rented for 13 months instead of outright purchased by certain agencies.
- Private health insurance (as determined by the plan) pays for certain AT if it is prescribed by a doctor as a necessary medical device or is used for rehabilitation.
- Vocational rehabilitation and job training programs, whether funded by government or private agencies, may pay for AT and training to help clients get a job or function in college/technical school.
- Employers may pay for AT that is determined to be a reasonable accommodation, so an employee can perform essential job tasks.
- Private funding options such as grants, charities, fundraising, and gifts
- Self-pay

Other sources of funds may be available in a state or community, including private foundations, charities, and civic organizations. The Assistive Technology Industry Association (ATIA) has developed a Funding Resources Guide to offer sources and resources to investigate and explore as prospective funding options.[11] The state AT program may have ideas on funding as well. Some states offer a program with low interest rates for purchasing AT, and other states offer a "reuse" program to allow people to buy, sell, donate, and trade used AT items.

In addition, almost all companies that sell AT can provide more specific answers about funding opportunities for their products and may help the OT practitioner find financial support from these or other funding sources. Sometimes clients and families have to use their own money for the AT they think is important. An example of this might be a seat elevator on a power wheelchair which raises the seat straight up, so clients can reach in cupboards as well as stand to their feet for transfers. This is not typically covered by funding agencies, but often paid for out of pocket by families who feel that it is important for function and safety. But remember that persistence pays off. Funding availability has changed over the years, and some technology that was not covered only a few years ago is now funded. Find the appropriate technology first, and then look for the money.

ASSISTIVE TECHNOLOGY RESEARCH

With the introduction of AT, some people with disabilities found that they were able to perform many occupations without the help of family members or paid assistants. For example, some individuals were able to participate in parenting, improve work productivity, and join in active recreational activities. Others were able to avoid being institutionalized. However, although many clients with disabilities report that the use of AT has greatly improved their quality of life, measurement of changes in their satisfaction, self-esteem, adaptability, safety, and competence have been rarely studied. This has prompted the development of several means for objectively evaluating the benefits of AT.

The Quebec User Evaluation of Satisfaction with Assistive Technology (QUEST) collects information about the benefits of AT and attempts to measure individuals' satisfaction with their devices. QUEST uses different types of variables to measure user satisfaction, including those that take into account the environment, pertinent features of the person's attitudes, expectations, and perceptions, as well as the characteristics of the AT itself.[12] QUEST allows the user to determine the relative importance of each of the satisfaction variables. The Psychosocial Impact of Assistive Devices Scale (PIADS) is a questionnaire that provides a measure of user perception and other psychological factors associated with AT devices. The three main components of PIADS are adaptability, competence, and self-esteem. PIADS has been applied to the measurement of outcomes with a variety of AT devices, from wheelchairs and eyeglasses to EADLs.[13] PIADS and QUEST provide reliable measures of the consumer perspective and often are considered in conjunction with assessments of functional status. It is the responsibility of all practitioners to contribute to the body of knowledge about AT and OT. This is important so that AT and OT services continue or improve with reimbursement. Take courses or continuing education on research, and consider writing a case study for a journal or OT news magazine about an interesting client solution or adaptation.

RESOURCES: REHABILITATION ENGINEERING SOCIETY OF NORTH AMERICA, STATE AGENCIES, AND THE INTERNET

As previously noted, every state has a government-funded AT program that offers device demonstrations and loans as well as training and information for both clients and families as well as practitioners. A listing of these programs can be found at the Association of Assistive Technology Act Programs website (www.ataporg.org). Another great resource is the RESNA, which trains and certifies ATPs as well as Seating and Mobility Specialists (SMS) and also publishes a journal, sponsors research, and writes position papers (www.resna.org). ATIA, is another good resource that offers training through conferences and webinars as well as an informative website for consumers and professionals. The Internet is a wealth of information and resources for locating options, creative solutions, and the AT that the client requires to manage mobility, ADL, IADL, work, and leisure skills.

HOME MODIFICATIONS FOR DISABILITY

Even minimal disabilities can require the need for home modification or adaptation. When the client has visual disabilities, home organization can be vital so the client can confidently navigate through the home. When one leg has weakness, the client may not be able to get into a standard tub or shower, and a renovated space may be required. When a new power or manual wheelchair is added into the mix, the need to organize and modify the space for use of the wheelchair is a vital strategy to enhance mobility within the home environment.[14] One of the key concerns with use of power wheelchairs indoors is the extent of damage caused to property because of problems with drivability and restricted space.[14] Time, effort, and financial and family/community resources are often required to make large and small home modifications. For a wheelchair, a 36-inch wide door works best for most users' access, but depending on the size of the chair, may need to be widened even more. For the bariatric client, a significantly wider or double door may allow access. Most disability design specifications note a 5-foot turning radius is generally sufficient for a manual wheelchair or power wheelchair, but again, individual needs may differ. Options are available for modification of steps, including a ramp, porch lift (lifts the chair and client straight up), stair glide lift (chair glides along the stairs to upper floor), or elevator.

Universal Design

The universal design (UD) concept, developed in 1997, has seven guiding principles that allow for a goal of any home or business space to be accessed, understood, and used in the widest possible extent, for all people at any age and with any disability without extra adaptations[14]. These concepts include:[15]

- Equitable use: Provides the same means of use, either identical or equivalent
- Flexibility in use: Accommodates a wide range of abilities and preferences
- Simple and intuitive use: Avoid unnecessary complexity and allow to be easily understood
- Perceptible information: Allows for adequate contrast, size, legibility, and various modes of delivering information
- Tolerance for error: Design minimizes hazards
- Low physical effort: Minimizes fatigue, strain, and energy expenditure
- Size and space for approach and use: Allows for adequate access, no matter the client's disability, size, or shape

OT practitioners are increasingly involved in advocating for, designing and consulting on environments which facilitate and promote participation. This is becoming more common as clients with disabilities and older adults are committed to living in their homes and not in facilities, and as the "baby boomer" population of active older adults demands full access to the world. Part of what UD accomplishes is access for all, in a way that is seamlessly integrated and does not draw attention to the client's particular disability. An example would include a newly built home with a built-up lawn and concrete sidewalk to move directly into the home without steps, in comparison to a home with a large ramp out front. Both provide access, but the concrete path allows for access without drawing attention to the need for accommodations. Other examples might include a master bedroom and bathroom on the main floor instead of upstairs, a stove with the controls in the front, larger print in an instruction guide, motion sensitive lights in a hallway or room, or 36 inch wide doorways.

Home Access

ADA ramp requirements note that 12 inches of length is needed for every 1 inch of rise for commercial buildings, but some private residences are not able to achieve that standard because of financial or space constraints, and must make shorter and steeper ramps (Fig. 14-30).[16] Material selection is important so that the material is weather and slip resistant. Clients and their families can put up grab bars in hallways and bathrooms for increased safety with transfers and ambulation, and there are many types of rails discussed earlier made for the toilet, tub, and shower. Some grab bars attach to the wall with a flip back portion to allow closer access to the toilet when not in use. Another type of bar/pole can clamp vertically between the floor and ceiling so it can be placed almost anywhere for firm support. Floor selection is important, as carpet is often difficult to roll or walk over. The transition between different floor materials should be as smooth as possible. Transitions can be difficult for those with mobility, visual, or perceptual disabilities, and may need to be brightly marked. Small ramps may be needed for one-half inch or higher transitions, especially for the entry door.

The OTA may complete an informal home assessment during the home health therapy process, which can be a simple safety checklist with recommendations about doorway widths, lighting, and throw rugs, or can participate in a more formalized process with the occupational therapist with a significant evaluation and follow-up report. Numerous home assessment checklists exist (many free or low cost); some have the client performing certain functional tasks, some focus on the environment and structure of the home and yard, and some are more interview based. This excerpt from Rebuilding Together's Safe At Home Checklist is one small subset on exterior entrances and exits to highlight the detail in the average home safety assessment and includes:[17]

- Note condition of walk and drive surface; existence of curb cuts

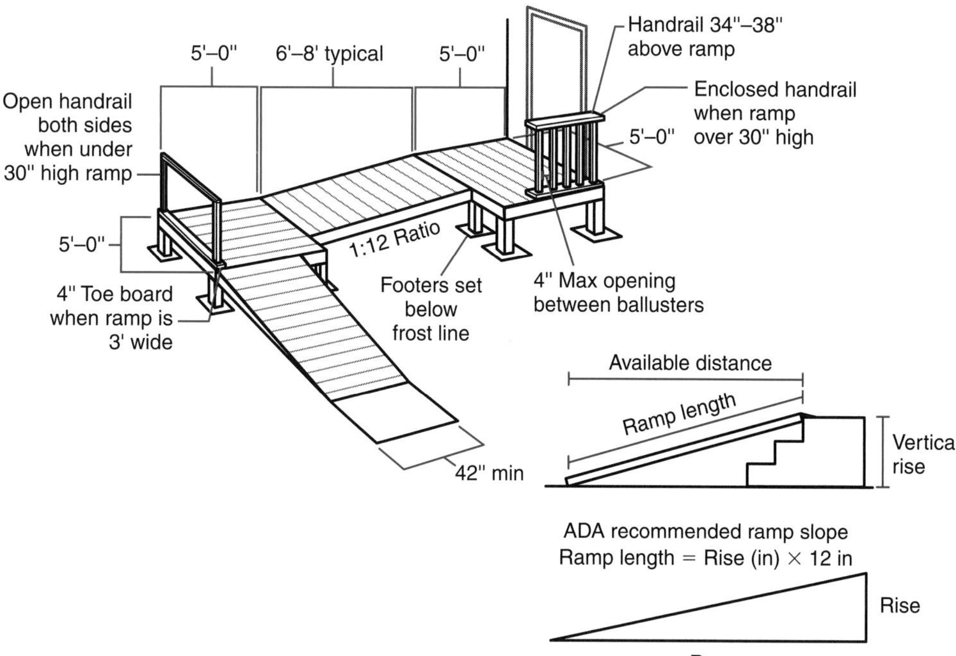

FIGURE 14-30. ADA ramp design and recommended ramp slope.

- Note handrail condition, right and left sides
- Note light level for driveway, walk, porch
- Check door threshold height
- Note ability to use knob, lock, key, mailbox, peephole, and package shelf
- Do door and window locks work easily?
- Are the house numbers visible from the street?
- Are bushes and shrubs trimmed to allow safe access?
- Is there a working doorbell?

Generally, the final report will have notations of potential problem areas, with suggestions to increase safety and make changes. Sometimes the recommended changes will be outside of the financial means of the client, and the OTA will be able to assist with lower cost changes. For example, the OTA could offer options, outside of widening a doorway, that include swing-clear or offset hinges or temporary door/facing removal with a shower curtain on a tension rod to block the view in the doorway. Another option might be a kitchen reorganization to avoid a step-stool or use of a reacher to clean items off the floor in the traffic paths.

SUMMARY

The rationale for how to choose the "right" AT option for the client is an art and a science for the OTA. The art is considering the esthetics and appearance of the choice as it fits into the client's life, and the science is the features and types of AT devices available as well as the financial, space, and other constraints. A good rule of thumb when trying to make a decision between options is often what is the easiest, cheapest, and simplest is best. The greater number of moving or computerized parts, the higher the chance for breakdown and expense. The OTA can be the creative professional who thinks outside the box to maximize the client's occupational performance: "To invent, all you need is imagination and a pile of junk." ~Thomas Edison

REVIEW QUESTIONS

1. A young adult client who has C5 complete tetraplegia will need to access his environment from his power wheelchair at home, at college, and with friends. Which is important to consider *first* when choosing assistive technology for this client?
   a. Client's needs in all environments
   b. Cost
   c. Bulkiness
   d. User abandonment
2. Mrs. B is a 48-year-old woman with facioscapulohumeral muscular dystrophy, resulting in shoulder and elbow weakness. She struggles in the morning to get ready in time for work. Which three of the following tasks could Mrs. B use a dressing stick for?
   a. Pushing up a bra strap
   b. Picking a pen up off the floor
   c. Donning a shirt
   d. Pushing off socks
   e. Retrieving glassware from the cupboard
   f. Scratching the middle of the back
3. A married, 65-year-old client has had a CVA resulting in mild right-sided weakness. He can ambulate with a walker with supervision. He and his spouse live in an older home with four steps to enter, a small bathroom with tub/shower combination, a sunken living room, and a four-poster high bed. Which three of the following home modifications might the OTA suggest be completed before discharge?
   a. Renovate the bathroom to be a roll-in shower
   b. Bring the living room to the height of the rest of the home
   c. Widen bathroom door to accommodate the walker
   d. Ramp for the four-step entrance
   e. Remove the box springs to lower the bed height
   f. Install a rail for the hallway

4. What might be appropriate piece(s) of adaptive equipment for a person who works in an office who has weak hands and low vision?
   a. A reacher
   b. Computer with large print and a dictation program for typing
   c. Books on CD
   d. A buttonhook and a zipper pull
5. What is required by the ADA for the height-length ratio of a ramp?
   a. 1:15
   b. 2:12
   c. 1:20
   d. 1:12
6. The OTA has three clients on caseload who are potential candidates for considering options for computer access. What characteristics of the client would require a computer accessed with eye gaze technology?
   a. When the client's hands are weak
   b. When the client's upper extremities, body, and neck are weak
   c. When the client's legs are severely weak
   d. When the client cannot speak clearly
7. A client with amyotrophic lateral sclerosis (ALS) is living at home and is having difficulty accessing many electronic items without assistance. Some of the items that can be controlled by an EADL unit would be:
   a. A power wheelchair and hospital bed
   b. A communication device
   c. A washing machine and dishwasher
   d. Lights, TV, and power door
8. A client has no use of her arms whatsoever, but has fairly strong legs, and wants to press the TV remote herself. What easy and practical way could the OTA suggest to meet this need?
   a. A toe splint with a pointer attached to it, to press the buttons with foot
   b. A large button TV remote to press with nose
   c. An environmental control unit for the TV, controlled with eye gaze
   d. A mobile arm support attached to the recliner
9. Which item would NOT be considered assistive technology?
   a. Garden kneeler
   b. Large-sized pen
   c. Velcro®
   d. Elastic shoelaces
10. The 28-year-old client the OTA is treating in the outpatient AT clinic for a new communication device has cerebral palsy, uses his current 7-year-old communication device mounted to his wheelchair, and lives alone in an accessible apartment. He has personal assistants coming into his home two times a day. He uses an outdated access style and the OTA knows there are many easier options currently. The OTA is also aware that he has a very small window of available control and functional independence. What is the best strategy to discuss the recommended product ?
    a. Insist that he order the newest product.
    b. Order the same product he has been using for 7 years.
    c. Show product/access options and let him decide how to proceed.
    d. Change his access method because it will be easier for him.

CASE STUDY

Kara is a 24-year-old who has Charcot-Marie-Tooth disease, which causes her to have hand pain and weakness, ankle weakness, and pain with use of ankle-foot orthotics (AFOs). She has fair balance in standing and difficulty performing her work tasks as an administrative assistant at a large law firm. The master bedroom with a tub/shower combination is upstairs in her townhouse and she has no bedroom and only a half bath downstairs. She works the day shift, and has two young children, ages 1 and 3. Her spouse is a truck driver, but is local and is usually home by 7 pm at night. She is having difficulty with many ADL and IADL tasks, including laundry, cleaning, childcare, cooking, and food preparation. She enjoys shopping and reading. Problem solve a list of tasks that probably require assistive technology, and think of potential solutions the OTA might need to make, such as:

Bathing and dressing, balance, clothing retrieval, drying, opening and squeezing shampoo, holding soap, buttons, zippers, socks, tying shoes
Toileting, wiping, getting off low toilet
Laundry, carrying and folding
Cleaning
Cutting food, holding utensil, holding heavy cup
Food preparation, cutting/chopping, making lunches, making bottles, cooking, transporting groceries
Child care, fasteners, diapers, bath time
Work tasks, typing, writing, transcribing, phones, emails, carrying, filing
Transportation, safe driving, turning key, getting in and out of car, getting kids in and out of car seats

Look through the chapter and also think of creative solutions for these problems.

1. Most will be low-tech solutions, but are there high-tech solutions that might help as well?
2. What unique equipment or gadgets would help her?
3. How will she pay for everything you recommend, and are there less costly alternatives to those you recommend?

PUTTING IT ALL TOGETHER Sample Treatment Session and Documentation

Setting	Client's home
Client Profile	Mrs. S is a 43-year-old woman with a 3-year diagnosis of multiple sclerosis. She is married with 3 boys, ages 5, 9, and 13. She is a stay-at-home mom who is active at her son's schools.
Work History	Stay-at-home mom
Insurance	Blue Cross Blue Shield from husband's job
Psychological	Client reports short-term memory issues.

PUTTING IT ALL TOGETHER Sample Treatment Session and Documentation (continued)

Social	Mrs. S enjoys time with her family and friends. The children are very active in sports and activities, and she spends significant time in the car. Hobbies include exercise, book club, and crafting.
Cognitive	Mild deficits noted in short-term memory.
Motor & Manual Muscle Testing (MMT)	UE Testing: • WNL ROM in BUE's • 4+/5 shoulder strength/elbow, 4/5 wrist • 25 pounds grip on left, 20 on right, 5 pounds lateral pinch on left, 2 pounds on right LE Testing: • WNL AROM in BLE's • 5/5 - bilateral hip/knee/ankle strength: No functional deficits noted. She notes significant fatigue with daily routine; takes occasional naps or rests in the middle of the day
Sensory	Vision: Wears contacts for distance Hearing: WNL Touch: Reports mild numbness and tingling in hands bilaterally
ADL	Mrs. S reports independence in performance of all ADLs in the home; however, further assessment results revealed that performance of ADL tasks are noted to be frustrating, with increased time required and occasional assistance for items such as necklace clasps, small buttons, shoe tying, bra fastening, and many other parts of her daily routine.
IADL	Mrs. S has difficulty with IADL tasks such as making the children's lunches, cooking, cleaning, and other tasks.
Functional Mobility	Mrs. S has no difficulty with functional mobility, and no balance deficits noted.
Goals	Within 3 weeks: 1. Mrs. S will perform morning ADL routine with modified independence, utilizing adaptive equipment and adaptive techniques. 2. Mrs. S will utilize memory compensation strategies with modified independence for management of her daily routine. 3. Mrs. S will verbalize and demonstrate use of adaptive equipment and strategies with modified independence for cooking and kitchen tasks. 4. Mrs. S. will verbalize and demonstrate use of adaptive equipment and strategies with modified independence for home management tasks. 5. Mrs. S will independently verbalize 5 energy conservation strategies she can incorporate into her daily routine.

OT TREATMENT SESSION 1

THERAPEUTIC ACTIVITY	TIME	GOAL(S) ADDRESSED	OTA RATIONALE
Client education and training on adaptive equipment and techniques for morning bathing, dressing, and grooming routine	20 min	#1	*Occupations; Education and Training:* Demonstrated use of adaptive equipment and techniques as well as energy conservation.
Set up of smart phone with memory compensation strategies	10 min	#2	*Occupations; Education and Training:* OTA demonstrated how to utilize smart phone options.
Completion of kitchen meal prep task, including training in use of adaptive equipment/compensatory techniques	25 min	#3 and #5	*Occupations; Education and Training:* Trained and educated on AE options/compensatory strategies as well as energy conservation for meal prep task in kitchen.

SOAP note: 10/5/—, 9:00 am–9:55 am

S: At OTA arrival, Mrs. S was noted to be well-groomed and dressed, but said, "I'm exhausted today; just getting ready and getting the kids out the door is a chore."

O: Client participated in skilled OT in home to address ADL, IADL, memory, and energy conservation tasks. OTA demonstrated use of AE including reacher, button hook, elastic shoelaces, and dressing stick for dressing tasks, and client returned demonstration with supervision and min cues. Education was provided today on strategies to use such as a shower seat for bathing, sitting to don clothing and other energy conservation tasks. Client demonstrated proficiency at Mod I level with use of calendar, alerts, and notes for memory enhancement once trained by OTA. OTA and client worked on simple meal prep task in kitchen involving use of knives and other tools, opening packages and bottles and item retrieval. Client required supervision to Min A to manage many of the tools, and frequently dropped items. Client was educated and trained on various AE and adaptive techniques to increase performance with meal prep as well as energy conservation during these tasks.

Continued

PUTTING IT ALL TOGETHER Sample Treatment Session and Documentation (continued)

A: Client did understand use of AE for ADL and IADL tasks, although had difficulty incorporating use effectively into task performance due to hand weakness and numbness. Client plans to begin incorporation of memory strategies on smart phone into daily routine immediately. Client is an excellent candidate for further work to address ADL/IADL performance and energy conservation due to motivation and willingness to work on occupational performance. Client would benefit from continued skilled OT services to maximize understanding of energy conservation principles and reinforce teaching of adaptive equipment/compensatory strategies for ADL/IADL tasks.

P: OTA to see client 2x/week for 3 weeks for 50–60 minutes to address personal and home management as well as energy conservation. OTA will continue plan of care with progression of home and self-management instruction, including further exploration and education and training with strategies for independent performance of ADL and IADL tasks with AE and adaptive techniques. Considerations to explore include use of a stool or chair in the kitchen, jar and bottle opener, needle nose pliers for pinching packages and Ziploc bags, and which techniques and equipment will assist most for ADL tasks.

Ethan Staver, OTA/L 10/5/—, 2:32 pm

TREATMENT SESSION 2

What could you do next with this client?

TREATMENT SESSION 3

What could you do next with this client?

REFERENCES

1. Assistive Technology Act of 1998. (1998). Retrieved from https://www.section508.gov/assistive-technology-act-1998
2. Assistive Technology Fact Sheet. (2015). In *Center on Technology and Disability*. Retrieved from http://ctdinstitute.org/library/2014-10-13/fact-sheet-assistive-technology-101
3. Assistive technology. (2015). In *Encyclopædia Britannica*. Retrieved from http://www.britannica.com/topic/assistive-technology
4. Assistive Technology Act of 2004. (2004). Retrieved from http://www.gpo.gov/fdsys/pkg/BILLS-108hr4278enr/pdf/BILLS-108hr4278enr.pdf
5. Dahler, A. M., Rasmussen, D. M., & Andersen, P. T. (2016). Meanings and experiences of assistive technologies in everyday lives of older citizens: A meta-interpretive review. *Disability and Rehabilitation: Assistive Technology, 11*(8), 619-29.
6. Skymne, C., Dahlin-Ivanoff, S., Claesson, L., & Eklund, K. (2012). Getting used to assistive devices: Ambivalent experiences by frail elderly persons. *Scandinavian Journal of Occupational Therapy*. 19(2), 194–203.
7. Barker, D. J., Reid, D., & Cott, C. (2004). Acceptance and meanings of wheelchair use in senior stroke survivors. *American Journal of Occupational Therapy*. 58, 221-230.
8. Brennan, J., & Nguyen, V. (2014). Service animals and emotional support animals: Where are they allowed and under what conditions? ADA National Network. Retrieved from https://adata.org/publication/service-animals-booklet
9. What is assistive technology? (2015). Assistive Technology Industry Association. Retrieved from http://www.atia.org/i4a/pages/index.cfm?pageid=3859
10. Zabala, J. S. (1999). Get SETT for successful inclusion and transition. Retrieved from http://www.ldonline.org/article/6399/
11. ATIA funding resources guide. (2015). Assistive Technology Industry Association. Retrieved from http://www.atia.org/i4a/pages/index.cfm?pageid=4219
12. Demers, L., Weiss-Lambrou, R., & Ska, B. (1996). Development of the Quebec User Evaluation of Satisfaction with Assistive Technology (QUEST). *Assistive Technology, 8*(1), 3-13.
13. Day, H., Jutai, J., & Campbell, K. A. (2002). Development of a scale to measure the psychosocial impact of assistive devices: Lessons learned and the road ahead. *Disability and Rehabilitation, 24*(1-3), 31-7.
14. Arthanat, S., Nochajski, S. M., Lenker, J. A., Bauer, S. M., & Wu, Y. B. (2009). Measuring usability of assistive technology from multi-contextual perspective: The case of power wheelchairs. *The American Journal of Occupational Therapy, 63*, 751-64.
15. What is universal design: The 7 principles. (2014). Retrieved from http://universaldesign.ie/What-is-Universal-Design/The-7-Principles/
16. ADA standards for accessible design. (2010). Information and Technical Assistance on the Americans with Disabilities Act. Retrieved from http://www.ada.gov/2010ADAstandards_index.htm
17. Safe at Home Checklist. (n.d.). Rebuilding Together. Retrieved from http://www.aota.org/practice/productive-aging/home-mods/rebuilding-together/assessments.aspx

Chapter 15

Seating and Wheeled Mobility

Amber L. Ward, MS, OTR/L, BCPR, ATP/SMS

LEARNING OUTCOMES

After studying this chapter, the student or practitioner will be able to:

15.1 Identify the differences between the types of manual and power mobility devices
15.2 Identify when a client should go to a seating clinic specialist
15.3 Identify the differences between cushion material types
15.4 Describe accessories that can be used on a wheelchair
15.5 Identify the characteristics between power wheelchair drive control styles

KEY TERMS

Complex rehabilitation technology (CRT)
Drive lockout
Joystick throw
Manual wheelchair
Mobility-related activities of daily living (MRADLs)
Power wheelchair
Scooter
Tilt-in-space manual wheelchair
Tremor dampening
Wheeled mobility

Wheeled mobility, whether from a walker, manual wheelchair, power wheelchair, scooter, or motor vehicle, has a vital contribution to the well-being, quality of life, and independence of the client. It is imperative for the occupational therapy assistant (OTA) to be involved in the therapeutic process as it relates to the functional needs of the client, assisting in determining the appropriate level of technology, and integrating the mobility device fully into the client's life. This chapter will address the realm of wheelchair mobility needs—from simple to complex—to give the OTA a working knowledge of the many options for daily use by clients. We will also discuss the issues around a poor mobility choice, including pain, fatigue, pressure injuries, and loss of function. The goal of this text is that the student reading this chapter will acquire an appreciation for how and when to intervene as a generalist with the client with mobility needs or know whether it is necessary to refer the client to a seating clinic specialist (Box 15-1).

At times, a doctor or another team member might prescribe or recommend a wheelchair for a client without the full understanding of what the evaluation, documentation, delivery/fitting, and training process entails. The wrong mobility device can be uncomfortable, unsafe, or even deadly, as in the case of a pressure injury or device without the proper support. Complications of a poorly configured wheelchair and seating system may include:

- Pressure injuries
- Shoulder dysfunction
- Progressive scoliosis/kyphosis or other progressive positioning problems
- Pain
- Hip dislocation
- Decreased respiratory function
- Decreased ability to propel the wheelchair
- Decreased ability to function in the environment.[1]

Because sitting is not a normative position for movement, but instead a transitional phase or position of rest, it can be difficult for the seated client to be comfortable for 12 to 18 hours at a time, which is the duration they might typically be in their wheelchair.[2] Besides the potential for harm to the client, the wrong device is also a waste of the client's insurance or grant money, and they are often stuck with the device for a number of years. Unfortunately, some stakeholders involved in selling wheelchairs either do not have enough education to understand the potential for harm to vulnerable consumers, or are more motivated by sales than by best practice or best outcomes.[1] The OTA can have a pivotal role on the team working with the client and assist to integrate the technology into their lives successfully.

BOX 15-1
Functional Ambulation

In this chapter on wheeled mobility, a moment must be taken to discuss ambulation and specifically functional ambulation and mobility. Many times in the career of an OTA, he or she might hear something such as, "I don't want to work on getting dressed. I just want to walk again." A nonverbalized thought may be "What? Are you going to walk around dirty and naked?" The ability to walk is extremely important to most individuals and society as a whole, and often getting a wheelchair or losing/not regaining the ability to ambulate is seen as a therapy "failure," both by clients and practitioners. Although physical therapy (PT) partners may focus on the ambulation process, the OTA must also focus on function. Sometimes, the ambulation efforts take so much energy, risk falls, or cause so much pain/debility that use of a mobility device would be more functional. If the client used the device to get where they were going and then stood up, they may not be too fatigued to then perform the task. Clients with progressive disorders often say, "I am not giving in to the disease by getting a wheelchair." Meanwhile, they fall frequently, have muscle pain and cramping from overuse, and give up many desired activities outside or at a distance, such as going to the mailbox or across their yard because of decreased mobility.

A paradigm shift is required to see the mobility device as a tool to be functional, and not a statement about the self-worth of the client, a lack of success/abilities, or a failure with "giving up." How is it that a pair of glasses as a tool to see better or a handrail added to outside steps to assist does not have nearly the emotional connection or the angst as a wheelchair?

As the OTA, assisting clients to assimilate change and assistive devices into their lives is often the focus of the therapy process. The OTA can certainly acknowledge the desire to walk with a statement such as, "I hear what you are saying. Let's focus on what will get you home the soonest," or "Let's stand at the sink while you brush your teeth to work on those muscles." Ultimately, the client makes the decisions, but the OTA can guide the client toward the options that will make life easier, safer, and more functional for the client, be it reacher, elastic shoelaces, or a power wheelchair.

DECISION TREE FOR WHEELCHAIRS

The wheelchair service provision process is not simply assessment followed by delivery. Providing a client with an appropriate wheelchair requires a full spectrum of services by a variety of providers.[3] This can include the client and family/caregivers, physician, occupational therapist or OTA, or physical therapist or physical therapist assistant (PTA), supplier or vendor (who sells the wheelchair), and assistive technology professional (ATP). The ATP designation is a certification from Rehabilitation Engineering Society of North America (RESNA), and an individual with this certification is recognized by Medicare and other insurances as a necessary team member and mandatory for the supplier who provides complex rehabilitation technology. **Complex rehabilitation technology (CRT)** products and associated services, including devices that require a specialty process (evaluation, fitting, programming, and training) to meet the specific needs of clients with congenital, progressive, or degenerative neuromuscular disorders as the primary diagnosis[3]. An example of CRT would be a power wheelchair for a client with advanced multiple sclerosis or Parkinson's disease, but not a basic power wheelchair for a client with diabetes and arthritis. The OTA and other professionals can study and work toward the ATP certification to increase competency and for professional development, but Medicare currently only requires the supplier representative have this designation when working with CRT seating and wheelchairs.

The purpose of a decision tree for wheelchairs is to visually assist the OTA with deciding what type of mobility system the client may require, and how to direct him or her to the correct place for assessment and procurement of the device (Fig. 15-1). An ultra lightweight or positioning **manual wheelchair** and complex rehabilitation **power wheelchair** evaluation should automatically require a seating specialist and a supplier with an ATP designation, but there are some gray areas with more basic or simple systems. Some suppliers simply sell scooters or basic wheelchairs over the phone, and they are dropped off at the client's home. Many reputable suppliers prefer to take their scooter and basic power wheelchair evaluations to a seating specialist for the expert advice and evaluation, documentation, and additional justification options for insurance. This process not only determines which seating option is ideal (it may not be a basic chair), but also offers the client increased choices, assurance of the correct product to match his or her needs, and increased accountability.

SEATING EVALUATION

A seating evaluation can be performed by an occupational or physical therapist, and is typically conducted at a hospital-based or freestanding outpatient clinic with demonstration products to trial during the process. The OTA could also be involved in many parts of this process, as will be noted in the later sections. The evaluation can be performed in the client's home by a home health occupational or physical therapist as well, and the supplier would bring product to the home to try. The overarching goals of the positioning and wheelchair seating evaluation and product selection would be[3]:

- Adequate support for orthopedic alignment for comfort and function (type of cushion, angle of backrest)

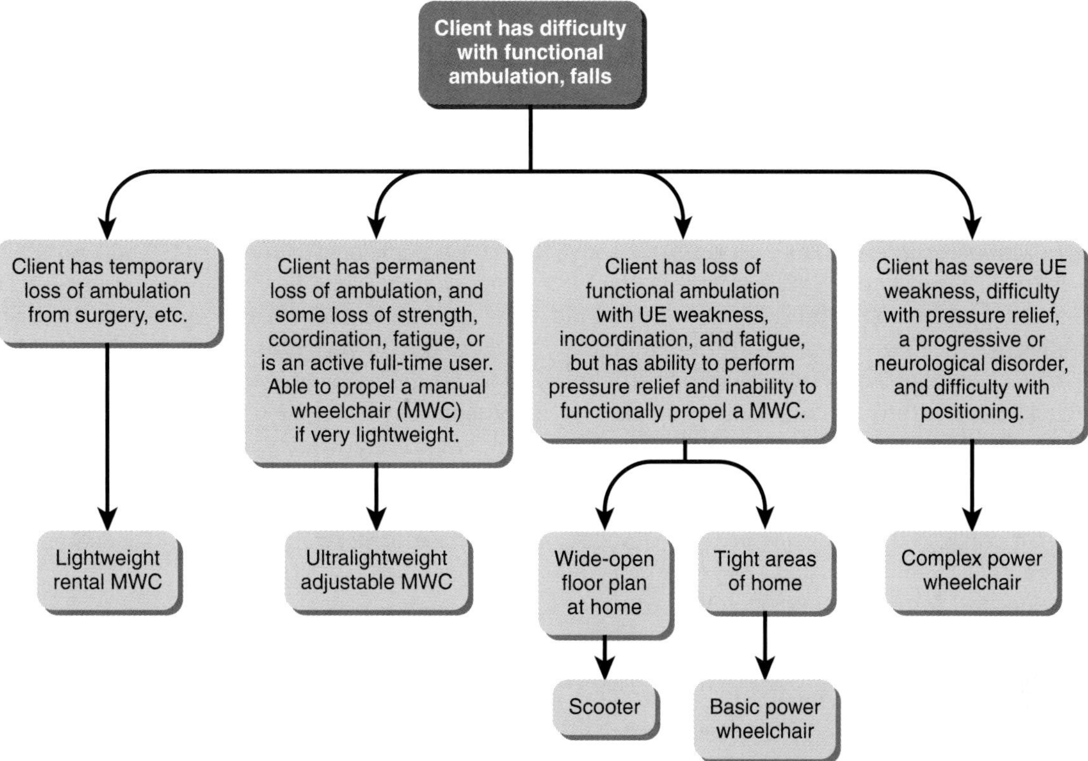

FIGURE 15-1. The decision tree can assist the OTA to decide how best to proceed when a mobility device is required.

- Accommodation of fixed asymmetries (scoliosis, pelvic position, leg length differences)
- Adequate stability and mobility to enhance function
- Adequate pressure distribution and comfort to increase sitting tolerance
- Integration of the device into **mobility-related activities of daily living (MRADLs)** (any activity of daily living [ADL] for which the mobility device would be used)

The seating evaluation should typically consist of numerous parts, each of which will be discussed next (as adapted from the *RESNA Wheelchair Service Provision Guide*).

Referral

The referral for a new product is generally physician-based and determined by a medical need. According to RESNA, "both the therapist and the supplier should be skilled, qualified professionals with specific training and experience in seating and mobility. The participation of both the therapist and the supplier is critical, as they possess different and complementary skill sets."[3] The referral leads to the set-up of an appointment for the evaluation.

Evaluation

The evaluation is multipart and will determine the needs of the client, including for environment of use, tolerance of technology, body function and structures, activity demands, and participation. Typically, it is performed by the occupational or physical therapist, although the OTA or PTA may contribute. For example, the OTA could take the history and perform specific assessments for which competency has been established. For the rest of the chapter, it will be assumed that the occupational therapist and OTA are completing the assessment for the mobility device, and further detail on the specifics of the evaluation will be discussed later in the chapter.

Equipment Recommendation and Selection

The occupational therapist or OTA and supplier match the equipment selection and the needs of the client, caregivers, and environment. According to RESNA, "the recommendation, trial and selection process should be an educational experience for the client/caregiver(s) to assist them in making informed decisions. The process should include a discussion of options, including the range of products available to meet the client/caregivers' specific needs and goal(s). The results of the evaluations should be used to establish priorities based on the client's needs, goals and activities."[3] Equipment may not be available from just one manufacturer, and may come from many different manufacturers to meet the client's needs. Generally, product trial and mock-up is done with attention to whether specific off-the-shelf products can be used, or whether the client requires something more custom. Sometimes this particular step will take more than one evaluation session if the client's needs are particularly complex.

Funding and Procurement

The occupational therapist, OTA, and supplier must discuss coverage criteria, benefit requirements and limitations, and limitations of the desired mobility equipment with the client and caregiver(s). If resources or sufficient coverage are not available, then the team needs to discuss the client's personal resources, such as fundraising, nonprofit or community organizations, grants, or loaner programs. It is important to assist the client to prioritize/compromise based on options available; education and equipment trials will assist with informed decision making. Documentation is also an important component, with medical and functional justification addressed with recommendations and rationale, as well as why a less expensive option will not work. The occupational therapy (OT) practitioner writes both the evaluation and a letter of medical necessity, justifying each part on the chair and why it is medically necessary. All the documentation goes to the prescribing physician for approval and signature. Also in this period, most insurance companies require a face-to-face visit by the client with the physician, where a discussion about the mobility device needs and justification are documented[3].

Product Preparation

According to RESNA, "the supplier should submit the specific documentation to meet all funding source requirements in order to maximize the likelihood of obtaining authorization. When there is a funding source limitation on the wheelchair or components, any exclusions or restrictions should be discussed with the client. Any adverse decision made by the funding source should be discussed with the client and an appeal strategy should be developed."[3] The supplier also orders the product and assembles the product to the measurements and specifications before the fitting.

Fitting

The fitting process determines whether the product chosen by the client/caregiver, supplier, and OT practitioner is going to ultimately be the correct option for comfort and function. Generally, at this time, the client is transferred into the wheelchair, modifications are made for fit and postural support, education and training are performed, and the client test-drives the chair (if power mobility). Programming modifications for power mobility, such as turning speed and acceleration, may be done at this time, and the chair is tested by the client in both slow speeds in tight quarters, and in fast speeds outdoors. Modifications to ultralightweight manual wheelchairs may include backrest position and axle placement for optimal propulsion. Adjustments to mechanical components on the wheelchair and initial seated adjustments to tolerance are made. At times because of the complexity of the chair, multiple fitting appointments may be required as the client adjusts to the seating system. Sometimes the items initially chosen may ultimately not work for the client, and others will have to be ordered and put on the chair. This might be a cushion that is uncomfortable or a thigh support that is too short. It is important that the whole team remain involved in this process for the best outcome.

Training

Training the client on how to use the device can be performed by the occupational therapist or OTA and/or supplier, and can happen at the clinic, the home, community, or all three. Both the client and caregivers will require education to understand how to use the device, its seating and positioning considerations, as well as maintenance, follow-up, and repair. Multiple sessions may be required for safety and functional performance as well as integration into the client's daily routine. The occupational therapist or OTA may begin the training in an outpatient setting, and then have the client transition to home health for further training in the home setting.

Delivery

The product is taken to the client's home if he or she does not have a method of transporting it, or, if the client has an adapted vehicle, the chair is loaded into the vehicle/lift. The client takes final possession of the chair and the responsibility that goes along with it.

Follow-Up Maintenance and Repair

Maintenance and repair of the device is an ongoing process where the team follows the client to monitor and reassess his or her body structures and function, activities and participation, and the environment, as needed.[3] Changes such as a spinal rod surgery for scoliosis or weight gain/loss can substantially change how the chair fits and functions, and a new visit to the seating specialist or team may be required. Repairs are initially under warranty, and then typically covered by the funding source, and completed by the supplier's repair team. Significant changes in medical condition may require a new visit with the seating specialist to make changes to the chair.

Outcome Measurement

Outcome tools exist that can allow the team to quantify the client's performance before and after obtaining the correct seating and wheeled mobility product. This assists with future decision making, adds to the body of evidence, and allows the team to assess performance and decisions made. According the RESNA, "professionals involved in the provision of wheelchairs should apply outcome measures to raise the standard of practice, to support evidence-based practice, and to improve the level of accountability."[3]

Assessment

Even though the OTA will not complete the evaluation for the seating and wheeled mobility system, he or she can play a vital role in the process. Because the process has so many parts, there is an ample place for all team members. The

OTA may take the medical history, perform range of motion (ROM) measurement, assist with the mat evaluation, discuss current technology and the environment, test drive chairs with the client, and have many other roles. It is extremely important that the OT practitioner self-assess and receive training in the assessment process for the mobility product so they do no harm. Because there is currently a shortage of qualified seating professionals, some practitioners may be asked to perform a seating assessment when they are unskilled in this particular practice area. This has significant ethical implications as an unskilled practitioner might end up relying on the supplier for all information or may chose incorrectly for the client's needs.

The evaluation includes the following parts:[3]

- Medical status and history
- Determination of current technology and mobility products and the environments of use as well as satisfaction, age, and repair needs
- Environments of use at home, school, and community and how the client functions in those environments with the technology, including barriers to use. This includes reaching, functional activities, controlling, maneuvering, and transfers into and out of the system.
- Client's support system that is in place to manage all aspects of owning the equipment and tolerance for technology
- Current and desired levels of performance of MRADLs and instrumental activities of daily living (IADLs) using the product. Functional needs for wheelchair design and components are also discussed.
- Body systems and structures including ROM, strength/weakness, tone issues, motor planning, contractures, pain, gross and fine motor control, balance in sitting and standing, former and current skin integrity, and skeletal deformities. Much of this information will be found during the comprehensive mat evaluation, which is typically performed by the occupational therapist or physical therapist, and requires extra training (Table 15-1 and Fig. 15-2).
- Skills and function with current seating and wheelchair components and future needs from the new product
- Product trials for determining preferences, what meets client's needs, methods of access, and capabilities for using the products safely

As is evident, the seating and wheelchair mobility process and procurement is complicated and time consuming, but extremely rewarding and can change the client's life for the better. OTAs should play a role whenever they have a client who has or requires a mobility device, even if just to give information to the seating specialist and perform training with the new device. Many times the seating clinic will be a long distance from the client's home, and after the fitting and delivery, much of the training for safety and functional use will be completed in the home by the home health practitioner. It is important that the OTA familiarize themselves with seating and wheeled mobility products and how they are used to maximize independence and function as well as safety and control.

BALANCE TESTS

Often, the seating evaluation will include standing balance assessment to assist with determinations of mobility needs. One test is the Timed Up and Go (TUG) assessment, which is a commonly used screening tool to assist practitioners to identify clients at risk of falling. To perform the TUG, time clients from when they rise from an armchair, walk at a comfortable and safe pace to a line on the floor three meters (approximately 10 feet) away, and turn and walk back to the chair and sit down again.[6] The client wears his or her regular footwear and uses the customary walking aid (cane or walker) if necessary.[7] A faster time indicates a better functional performance, and a score of more than

EVIDENCE-BASED PRACTICE

Because of the aging population and many other factors, OT and physical therapy practitioners are not being trained in seating and wheeled mobility in large enough numbers to meet the public need. With that in mind, researchers and clinicians are looking toward creative alternatives. One of these is telerehabilitation, where the experienced seating and mobility clinician may be hundreds of miles away from the client and the generalist practitioner is performing the hands-on portions and product trial. Robert Schein et al. have published numerous articles in this topic area, showing that the long-distance consultation does work to get clients the products they require without driving hundreds of miles or even to another state. In their study from 2011 that looked at 50 in-person evaluations and 48 via telerehabilitation in remotely located clinics, they noted equally effective results from both types. Study findings were based on the level of function the participants showed with their new wheeled mobility and seating devices as measured by using the Functioning Everyday with a Wheelchair (FEW) outcome tool.[4] This tool was designed as a self-report questionnaire to be administered over time to clients with wheeled mobility and seating technology as an indicator of perceived user function related to wheelchair/scooter use.[5] Telerehabilitation is becoming more prevalent and will continue to grow in the area of seating and wheeled mobility as technology continues to improve.

Schein, R. M., Schmeler, M. R., Holm, M. B., Saptono, A., & Brienza, D. M. (2010). Telerehabilitation wheeled mobility and seating assessments compared with in person. Archives of Physical Medicine and Rehabilitation, *91(6), 874-878.*

Holm, M., Mills, T., Schmeler, M. R., & Trefler, E. (n.d.). The functioning everyday with a wheelchair (FEW) seating-mobility outcomes measure. Retrieved from http://www.few.pitt.edu/

TABLE 15-1 Parts of the Mat Evaluation[3]

Sitting posture and postural tendencies	Determine whether fixed or flexible, in seated and supine positions: • Posterior pelvic tilt • Anterior pelvic tilt • Pelvic obliquity • Pelvic rotation • Kyphosis • Lordosis • Scoliosis • Windswept deformity
Range of motion in relation to sitting	Hamstring range with knee extension, hip flexion All joint ROM from neck to ankle, effects on ROM-tone, contracture, pain
Muscle strength	Manual muscle testing
Skin integrity	Skin inspection for skin issues, suspected or confirmed
Tone	Hypotonicity, spasticity, rigidity
Balance	Sitting balance and standing balance, if applicable, along with balance tests
Endurance	Tolerance for sitting with and without support and for how long
Support required for function	Possible trunk and/or pelvic support, other areas

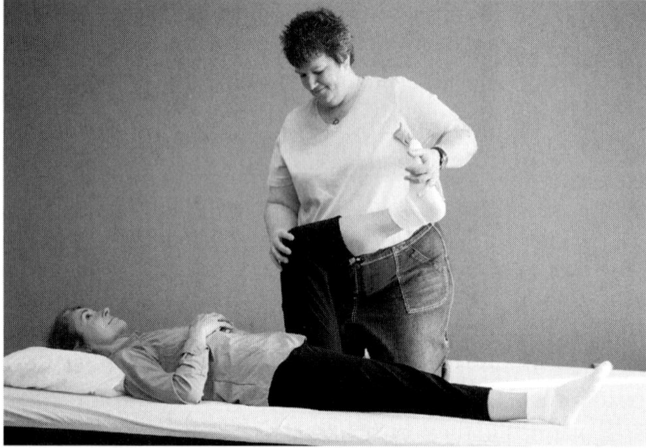

FIGURE 15-2. Mat evaluation. The OT practitioner is assessing hip range of motion.

or equal to 13.5 seconds is used to identify those at increased risk of falls.

Another common test is the Berg Balance Scale to assess static balance and fall risk in adults. It is a 14-item list with each item ranging from 0 to 4, with 0 indicating the lowest level of function and 4 the highest level of function. A score of 56 indicates functional balance, while a score of less than 45 indicates individuals may be at greater risk of falling.[8] The tasks include:[8]

Sitting to standing
Standing unsupported
Sitting unsupported
Standing to sitting
Transfers
Standing with eyes closed
Standing with feet together
Reaching forward with outstretched arm
Retrieving object from floor
Turning to look behind
Turning 360 degrees
Placing alternate foot on stool
Standing with one foot in front
Standing on one foot

Each task has specific scoring and directions, such as:[8]

Sitting to standing:
INSTRUCTIONS: Please stand up. Try not to use your hand for support.
4: Able to stand without using hands and stabilize independently
3: Able to stand independently using hands
2: Able to stand using hands after several tries
1: Needs minimal aid to stand or stabilize
0: Needs moderate or maximal assist to stand

The test is available free online and from numerous sources.

COMMUNICATION

Communication is very important to consider when prescribing a power or manual wheelchair. There must be interaction between the treating OTA, the evaluating occupational therapist, caregivers and family, the physician and nurse, the supplier, the manufacturer of the wheelchair, the insurance company, and of course the client. How the client uses the chair functionally in all situations must meld with the physical and support needs to maintain a proper body alignment and provide positioning and pressure relief. For example, the caregiver may want ankle supports to keep the client's feet on the footplates, but the client does not want to be restricted. In another situation, the OTA working in home care sees how little the client touches the backrest and does not use the footrests at home, but the client uses all items in front of the physician and evaluating occupational therapist. Other times, the client wants a chair exactly how the last one was, even though the client's condition and body needs have changed. Without good communication, there will be technology abandonment or poor outcomes. The client is ultimately in control if competent to make decisions, even if the decisions are—in the rest of the team's estimation—a bad idea.

MANUAL WHEELCHAIRS

Manual wheelchairs are often perceived as the most simple and direct of the pieces of mobility equipment to prescribe, but this is not often the case. A multitude of types, features, and support systems for positioning and pressure relief as well as weight are available. The OTA should consider the current physical status of the client, as well as future needs, as many insurance companies are expecting 5 to 7 years of use or more from any mobility device. Many insurance companies primarily focus on "in the home" use, and although the client can take the device out of the home, it must be able to be used in the home effectively and safely for completion of functional activities or self-care.

Rental and Basic Manual Wheelchairs

The most basic wheelchair is a transport chair, which is a simple folding wheelchair with 4 small wheels, limited sizes, and no or limited armrest removal or adjustment. The cost of the transport chair is generally under one hundred dollars. A simple, standard, or lightweight manual wheelchair rental from a wheelchair equipment supplier could suffice for a client with a wheelchair need of 6 months or less or for the client with a basic and straightforward need (Fig. 15-3). The client might have a recent broken leg or a hip fracture. Most clients can go directly to the wheelchair supplier of their choice with a prescription from their physician for rental. Most insurance companies will rent a lightweight manual wheelchair for 13 months, and at the end of the rental period, the chair belongs to the client. If the client goes to the hospital or to a nursing facility before the 13 months is over (these locations are responsible for providing a wheelchair), or no longer needs the chair because of improvement, then the wheelchair goes back to the supplier. These basic manual wheelchairs offer limited sizes and features, and their weight is commonly 33 pounds at the lightest. They could have basic swing-away legrests or manual elevating swing-away legrests for leg elevation, a basic cushion, a straight up or reclining backrest, and anti-tippers on the back (to avoid accidental tipping over), as required. Basic manual wheelchairs tend to have cloth or leatherette seats, a backrest at 90 degrees, and have little to no adjustability. Sling fabric or leatherette seats, although lighter, provide little pressure relief, tend to hammock downward over time, and lead to hip adduction and internal rotation for the client. Some clients will need to propel the manual wheelchair with only one arm and one leg or two legs. These clients will need attention to the overall height of the seat with cushion to the floor so their feet touch the floor securely. If the seat is too high, it will cause the client to potentially scoot forward in an unsafe manner to reach the floor. These chairs with a lower height are often called "hemi-height" manual wheelchairs.

However, if the need is over 6 months, the client may consider a lighter weight manual wheelchair with positioning and pressure relieving components, as they are presumably using the wheelchair throughout the day and throughout their life. The OTA could assist with this decision making process of choosing a simple rental versus a more complex manual wheelchair, and also assist the client to find a qualified seating specialist. If the client answers "yes" to the following questions, then the rental or simple manual wheelchair would be the correct answer in the decision process:

1. Will the client use the manual wheelchair only part time, for longer distances only, or for a short period of time?
2. Does the client have someone to propel him or her and load/unload the chair from the vehicle?

Ultralightweight Custom Rigid and Folding Manual Wheelchairs

There are times when the client has a longer-term need for a manual wheelchair, usually due to weakness, poor balance, ataxia, incoordination, shoulder pain or potential/risk for shoulder pain, fatigue or decreased sensation, or when a standard lightweight wheelchair may not suffice functionally. The next step for these clients would be a custom ultra lightweight manual wheelchair, which would be in the 12- to 20-pound range with accessories, for a full-time and active user (Fig. 15-4). These wheelchairs have fully adjustable (e.g., vertical and horizontal) rear wheel axles that enable reducing or elongating the overall chair length/height and subsequently wheelbase length and seat height.

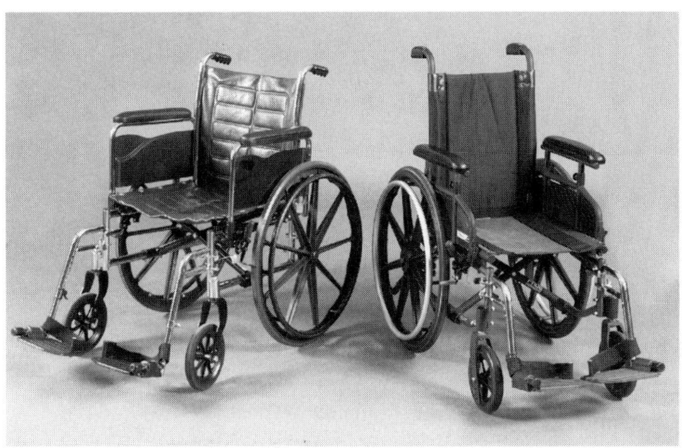

FIGURE 15-3. Both of these wheelchairs are basic, folding, rental options.

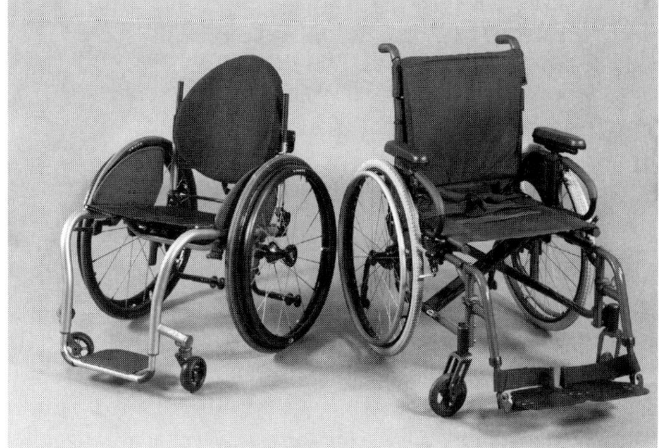

FIGURE 15-4. Ultra lightweight chairs can be rigid *(left)* or folding *(right)* and have more customizability with less weight.

When the rear wheels are moved forward on the frame, it can enhance maneuverability in tight quarters,[9] but may increase the potential to tip over backward. A longer wheelbase will increase stability, but may put the wheel out of reach for efficient propulsion. The axle height and frame position have a direct effect on efficiency of movement and propulsion for the client. For a properly fitted adult chair, the elbow angle when the hand is at the top of the wheel should be 110 to 120 degrees, and when fully extended, the finger tips should touch the middle of the wheel.[10] The adjustable axle plate assists to put the wheel in the correct position. These manual wheelchairs can be as light as 12 pounds without the wheels/armrests/footrests, and can be more efficient for clients to propel and easier to transport. In a 2011 study by Oyster et al., participants who used ultra lightweight manual wheelchairs accumulated significantly more minutes of propulsion time per day compared with those who used just lightweight (standard) manual wheelchairs, thus making higher quality wheelchairs a potential factor related to mobility.[11] This means that because the clients with the higher quality and lighter weight chairs used their chairs more, these chairs may affect their mobility in that they may get less fatigued or have more efficient mobility.

The frames of ultra lightweight manual chairs can be rigid or folding, and both have advantages and disadvantages. Rigid frames allow the majority of the propulsion energy to go into movement, whereas the folding frame chair flexes more at the folding mechanisms, and this flex can consume some of the propulsion energy. The rigid frame generally has a fold-down or removable backrest, and the wheels can come off, leaving the rigid frame in an L-shape for transport. The folding frame wheelchair folds by pulling up on the seat fabric and the two wheels come together and can be removed as needed. Rigid chairs typically have a solid one-piece footplate and legrests to offer more stability and rigidity, and some have a footplate that will flip back. The folding frame chairs typically have swing-away legrests with flip up footplates. The armrest choices vary with each chair, but are typically flipped back or swung away and are height adjustable. Many custom manual wheelchairs will have a supportive backrest and a pressure relieving and/or positioning cushion. These options will be discussed later in the chapter. A client who might use an ultra lightweight manual wheelchair might have paraplegia, spina bifida, or slowly progressing multiple sclerosis.

Standing, Power Assist, and One-Arm Drive Wheelchairs

Manual wheelchairs may have additional options, such as the ability for the seat to raise to stand the client, the ability to add power-assist wheels, or a one-arm drive feature. The standing feature is typically a manual hydraulic lever, and often the chair is not able to roll when the person is standing. The standing feature offers pressure relief and weight-bearing through the hips and legs. Standing has other physiological benefits as well, including increased bowel/bladder efficiency, bone density, circulation, hip, knee and ankle range of motion, and decreased edema.[12] Clients could use the standing feature to more effectively reach items at home and work, perform toileting, make a meal, see over crowds, and have eye-to-eye contact with other individuals (Fig. 15-5). The power-assist wheels have small battery-operated motors that go in place of the standard wheels or are integrated into the frame, and allow the client to push on the wheels and have an exaggerated response. With one push, a client could go 20 to 30 feet because of the push assist versus 1 to 2 feet with a standard push on the wheels. It is also helpful for hills and ramps, as it allows for more effective propulsion with much less effort. By lowering the stress and energy needed to accomplish MRADLs, power-assist wheels should enable participation in a range of activities that might otherwise be impractical.[13] These might include increased access to diverse terrain, such as gravel, grass, and inclines such as ramps, to novel and social activities, and for increased freedom. The power assist may ultimately decrease pain and stress on the shoulders, wrists, and hands of an active user. The power-assist wheels do add weight to the chair, so this must be taken into account when independently loading/unloading the chair; some clients have both power-assist wheels and standard wheels for various circumstances and environments.

The one-arm drive is for clients with one-sided weakness or one upper extremity amputation, who may have only

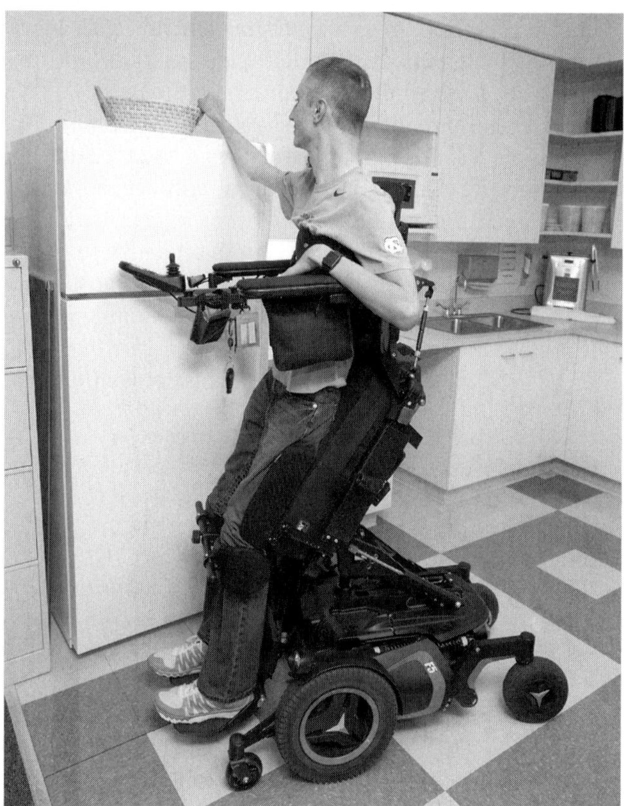

FIGURE 15-5. The ability to stand for a wheelchair user can be important for function as well as for reaching, pressure relief, and many other reasons. The standing feature can be found on manual as well as power wheelchairs.

one functional arm with which to propel the manual wheelchair. There are two types available. Lever drive one-arm drive systems are a lever mounted to the front caster area of the wheelchair with linkages back to the rear wheel. The lever drive has a forward, neutral, and reverse setting, and when the lever is "pumped" forward and back while in gear, the chair moves in the direction chosen. The other type is a double hand rim one-arm drive. It has two hand rims on the same side of the wheelchair that control the rear wheels on both sides. The outer (larger) hand rim controls the wheel on the same side of the wheelchair and the inner (smaller) hand rim controls the wheel on the opposite side of the wheelchair. It can be difficult to get insurance companies to cover these features at times, but for the clients who have them or are seeking them, they can be worth the fight.

Dependent Manual Wheelchairs

Another option for a manual wheelchair is one where the client is unable to physically propel the chair, and may be cognitively, physically, or visually unable to use a power wheelchair. A dependent manual wheelchair typically has four smaller wheels, and is usually pushed by a caregiver (Fig. 15-6). This type of wheelchair can have manual tilt typically controlled by the caregiver, and some brands can add manual recline as well. This type of manual chair is often known as a **tilt-in-space manual wheelchair**. Tilt is when the whole seat tips backward on the base, offering rest, pressure relief, and repositioning without changing the seat/hip angle. Recline is when the backrest alone leans backward for positioning and pressure relief, and goes into a more lying down position. Most of the time, the tilting/reclining manual wheelchair will have extensive positioning, pressure relieving, and support items on the chair to assist with safe use. The client who may be appropriate for this type of chair could be one with advanced Parkinson's disease, severe and profound developmental disabilities, dementia, later-stage multiple sclerosis, and significant issues with motor control, vision or cognition. Those support items will be described at length later in the chapter. Typically, there are swing away legrests, and they may elevate for positioning assistance as well. It is possible to have full size back wheels for some propulsion by the client and still have manual or power tilt. These manual wheelchairs can be heavy however, and the tilt mechanism differs as the seat tilts back and downward so the client does not lose contact with the wheels. At times, the chair can be configured so the client can also foot-propel the chair. There is a handle for clients to tilt themselves with hydraulic assist or power assist or a trigger for the caregiver to tilt the client. The client who might benefit from this variety of tilt-in-space chair is one who has dementia and needs to independently move in space to calm agitation, but still needs the pressure relief and positioning throughout the day.

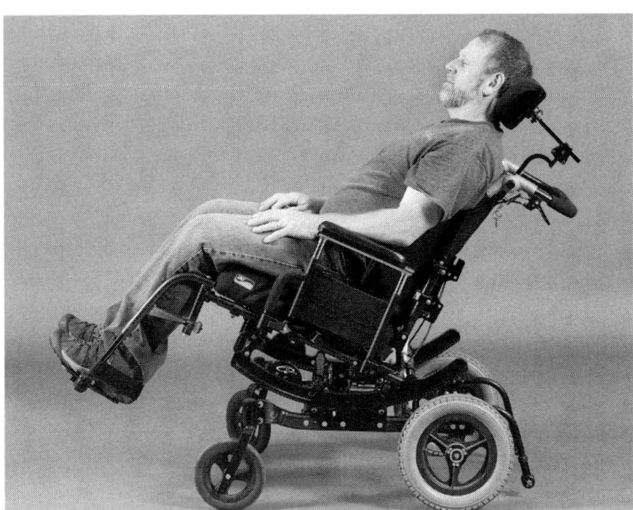

FIGURE 15-6. Note the ability to change position and offer pressure relief in the tilt position in a manual wheelchair.

SCOOTERS

Scooters are often difficult to get insurance to pay for because they tend to be better used outside of the home, and many insurances require "in-the-home" use for the mobility device. Scooters also tend to be longer than they are wide, and can at times be more unstable or tippy side to side when going over uneven ground. The longer length also makes the base less maneuverable in the home. Scooters do have their place, however, and many clients appreciate the ease of taking apart the mobility device and of the caregiver or the client putting it in the car trunk, as well as the lightweight mobility option. There are three-wheeled and four-wheeled scooters. The three-wheeled scooters are more maneuverable in general, and the four-wheeled variety tend to be more stable. The seat on the scooter is generally one size fits all; however, bariatric (for larger clients) scooter options are also available. The seats generally swivel for safer transfers. The client using the scooter must have gross and fine motor strength, as the scooter turns with a tiller (central post in front of the seat for turning), and has bilateral thumb switches for forward and reverse. In addition, the key must be turned for on/off and removed at times. In order to qualify for a scooter under most insurances, the client must be unable to effectively use an optimally configured manual wheelchair, and as mentioned, the client must require the use of the scooter in the home (Fig. 15-7). Some clients want a scooter because of portability or the perception that they look "less disabled" to the general public. The OTA should counsel the client who has a more significant disability, very tight spaces in the home, a progressive condition, and trouble standing from a standard height seat to consider a power wheelchair instead.

POWER WHEELCHAIRS

Power wheelchairs are mobility devices that are the next level up from a scooter, and have a variety of configurations and options. Clients using power wheelchairs make up a

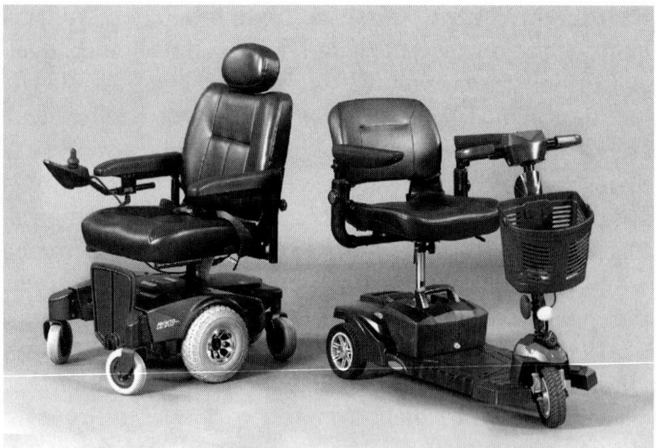

FIGURE 15-7. The basic power wheelchair *(left)* and scooter *(right)* are viable options for clients with less significant disabilities.

highly heterogeneous population with wide-ranging mobility-related impairments and activity needs within the settings of home, workplace, school and/or community.[14] A client may use a power wheelchair for certain occupations and mobility in the home and community, or use the chair full time, specifically using it for all mobility, home and community based occupations, as well as potentially for napping and/or sleeping. The next sections will outline the wide variety of options available to meet various medical and functional needs of a client related to power wheelchairs.

THE OLDER ADULT

Many frail older adults live with mobility challenges in skilled nursing facilities. Medicare and many insurance providers may not pay for wheelchairs or scooters (even repairs) while the client is in the facility because Medicare/insurance pays the facility to care for all the needs of the client. It is left to the administrators of the mostly for-profit facilities to provide the expensive equipment, in combination with OT and PT staff who often are not trained in seating and wheeled mobility issues. This can be a recipe for disaster, with the potential consequences of pain, pressure injuries, increasing contractures and deformities, decreased safety, and behavioral challenges; however, there are solutions to this pervasive problem. Many reputable suppliers are willing to provide education and training to practitioners for little to no cost on options to assist their clients. These experienced ATPs can assist with product selection and problem-solving to meet client needs. Even though the medically necessary and correct product may be expensive, the cost savings in decreased wounds, pain, deformity, infection, and staffing should be tempting for any administrator. It is often up to the allied health staff of the facility to initiate the necessary steps to facilitate improving the lives of the residents they work with, by increasing their education, and researching the ways to meet both the fiscal needs of the facility and the quality of life of their clients.

Basic Power Wheelchairs

Basic power wheelchairs are generally a captain's or van style leatherette seat on a power wheelchair base. The basic power wheelchairs are usually driven with a standard joystick with an on/off button or switch and a speed control. They have some range of seat size options, such as 18 × 18 inches or 16 × 16 inches, but very little ability to change the seating. The armrests generally will flip back, and the single footplate flips up as well for transfers. The client can order swing-away legrests instead of the single foot platform, or swing-away legrests that manually elevate upwards. Some basic power wheelchairs will have the ability for the seat to swivel for easier transfers. Most backrests have a lever for slight recline, and the backrest can fold forward for transport as well. These chairs are maneuverable in tight spaces, but may get stuck in rough terrain outdoors and at slow speeds over some thresholds and carpets because of their potentially smaller motors and wheels. The battery range is typically 8 to 10 miles, and there is a charger. Most clients go under a mile a day around the home and yard, but some clients use their wheelchairs as full transportation devices to reach a store or the mall many miles away. Generally, to get a basic power wheelchair, a client needs a nonprogressive, nonneurological diagnosis or diagnoses, which lead to difficulty with ambulation as well as difficulty propelling an optimally configured manual wheelchair or using the tiller of a scooter. Sample diagnoses might be a client with arthritis, spinal stenosis, obesity, congestive heart failure, chronic pain, degenerative joint disease, or chronic obstructive pulmonary disease (COPD). A client with a progressive or changing condition needs to think twice about a basic power wheelchair because of the inability to make changes or have flexibility with this chair. Similar to the scooter, some clients want this type of chair versus a more complex power wheelchair due to the perception that the basic chair makes them appear less disabled or that the basic power wheelchair is smaller. Actually, most basic power wheelchairs have similar lengths/widths to many more complex power wheelchairs. Most insurance requires 5 to 7 years of use from a mobility device, and clients with a progressive disorder may not find the basic chair suitable for long-term use. A pressure relieving or positioning cushion, power tilt, power seat elevate, and manual or power elevating legrests can in some circumstances be put on a basic chair for the client who does not have a qualifying diagnosis for a more substantial power wheelchair but still has significant medical needs. However, the payment by insurance providers for these chairs is generally too low for many suppliers to be willing to add numerous expensive features.

Complex Power Wheelchairs

Complex power wheelchairs (also known as CRT) are another step up in long-term function, comfort, pressure relief, positioning, and flexibility for certain qualifying clients (Fig. 15-8). The diagnosis must typically be neurologically significant (congenital, progressive/degenerative, injury/trauma) and serious, causing disability in the short

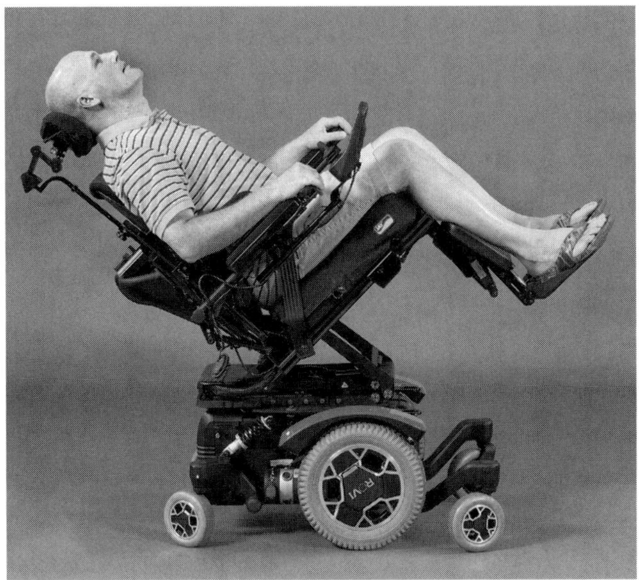

FIGURE 15-8. Complex power wheelchairs offer significant flexibility for short- and long-term needs. Note the tilt used in this chair for pressure relief and repositioning.

and long term. Deciding on the perfect complex power mobility device can be a challenge for the client, the caregiver, and the team; ideally, the equipment should address not only the client's physical needs, but his or her safety, lifestyle, and budgetary limitations as well.[15] These chairs have the flexibility to change their seated position into power tilt, recline, seat elevate (when the seat raises straight up 8 to 14 inches), and leg elevation/articulation (when the legrests raise up and articulate out to straighten the legs), as well as the drive control style from driving with a standard joystick with the hand to driving with the head, chin, foot, or finger. The cushion is simply attached with Velcro®, so hundreds of cushion options with either positioning, pressure relieving, or both properties can be chosen to meet the client's medical needs. These power chairs typically come with a plush headrest that is removable and has flexibility in positioning. Many additional supports at the trunk, head/neck, chest, shoulders, pelvis, hips, thighs, and knees may be added as required by the client's condition. These power wheelchairs often have to meet the needs of clients with complex body shapes, scoliosis, progressive disorders with constantly changing needs, increased or decreased muscle tone, contractures, as well as motor control problems. One can see how the complexity of the chair would increase quickly. If the mobility device is ill-fitting and/or wrong for the client's needs, the client may have little recourse for a proper device because many insurance providers will not cover another chair for 5 to 7 years unless a new diagnosis or significant change in condition occurs. It is extremely important for a qualified seating specialist be involved in the case to achieve the best outcome for the client.

The entire process timeline can vary, depending on the efficiency of the seating practitioner, physician, and supplier in generating and completing paperwork, and the insurance company in generating the approval. The chair process can take increased time if any parts on the chair are not approved initially and must be appealed, or are custom built. The wheelchair process from evaluation to delivery in the United States can be anywhere from 2 weeks to 6 months or more. The average seems to be 6 weeks to 3 months. The costs to the client can vary dramatically, depending on copays, deductibles, co-insurance, and other variables. For instance, a client with only Medicare (pays 80%) requiring a complex power wheelchair could owe multiple thousands of dollars because a complex power wheelchair could cost $15,000 to $50,000 retail or more. In many countries the process for wheelchair procurement can be quite different.

DRIVE WHEEL CONFIGURATION

One important factor to consider with a power wheelchair is the drive wheel configuration between front wheel drive, center, or mid wheel drive, and rear wheel drive. Each drive style has its pros and cons, and will be discussed in Table 15-2.

TABLE 15-2 Drive Configuration Options[9]

WHEELCHAIR TYPE	TURNING	OBSTACLES/TRANSITIONS	STABILITY	FASTER SPEEDS
Front wheel drive	Great 90° turns, good turning radius	Generally drive easily over small obstacles, good over transitions and rougher terrain	Some brands are likely to tip forward down severe inclines, forward anti-tippers often used	Can require reduced speeds for full control, although technology is much improved
Mid wheel drive	Excellent turning radius	Can high center mid wheel (power wheel loses contact with ground due to terrain), can turn going over threshold if not hit squarely, climbs small obstacles	Some tipping onto casters on severe inclines, up or down	Good control, responsive to turns
Rear wheel drive	Poor turning radius, especially turns from hallway to room	More easily stuck over transitions because power is in back	Likely to tip back going up steep hills/over inclines, rear anti-tippers	Good control

According to Koontz et al., mid wheel drive power wheelchairs required significantly less space to perform a full 360-degree turn in place compared with front wheel drive and rear wheel drive models because equal portions of the frame pivot about the center point of the wheelchair.[9] These authors also found that front and mid wheel drive wheelchairs are better than rear wheel drive wheelchairs for maneuvering in confined spaces.[9] The front wheel drive chair allows a better 90-degree turn into a room, where the rear wheel drive has to swing wider to get into the room. Front wheel drive chairs could be considered some of the best over more varied terrain, and the rear wheel drive at the highest speeds for tracking straight, but as technology continues to improve, all the chair drive styles are meeting more of the needs of consumers.

POWER FEATURE OPTIONS

The power tilting feature on the power wheelchair is when the whole seat tips backward up to 55 degrees on the wheelchair base, maintaining the seated position (see Fig. 15-8). Benefits to the client include pressure relief, capillary refill in the skin of the bottom, repositioning, especially scooting back in the chair, rest, and pain relief.[16] Some clients use some degree of tilt all the time when driving the chair for increased stability and balance in sitting, head/neck control, and for less slumping forward. This can be especially useful when going downhill or down ramps. Power recline is when the backrest itself lays backward, allowing the client to move into a lying down position when used in combination with elevating/articulating legrests (Fig. 15-9). Recline is used to open up the hip angle for clothing management, toileting and urinal use, repositioning, pressure relief, tone management, and pain management, especially in the back and hips. Power center mount or swing-away elevating legrests allow the legs to elevate and articulate up to a fully extended knee position. Leg elevation provides stretching, tone/spasticity management, ROM, edema management, and pain relief, and when positioned down in a flexed position, allow the chair to turn in tighter spaces. A combination of tilt, recline, and leg elevation can get the hip angle opened to a wider degree and the feet higher than the heart, which can assist with edema management. The seat elevate allows the entire seat to move upward 8 to 14 inches, allowing the client to reach cupboards, stovetops, and closets, perform safer transfers, see over crowds, and be in a socially advantageous position (Fig. 15-10). Many chairs will allow driving in an elevated position to allow moving from refrigerator to counter in the kitchen or closet to bed in the bedroom. Some even have the stability to drive up to 3.5 miles an hour in an elevated position. Many other custom and specialty power features are also available on power chairs that may not be covered by some insurance providers. A few examples include power: standing, tilting to the sides laterally (where the whole seat leans side to side), anterior recline (backrest closes tighter than 90 degrees), and anterior tilt (to tip the seat and backrest forward to assist with transfers and reaching), power headrest positioning, power armrest movement to assist with transfers, power legrest/footplate movement down to the floor or out of the way, and a power seat where the whole seat comes forward and down to the floor for a client with difficulty getting into a standard height seat. The power standing feature typically requires a sturdy base with altered suspension to allow the client to safely drive in standing. There are blocks at the knees and across the chest for support. The chair can stand directly from a seated position, or stand from a lying down position, and can stop at any

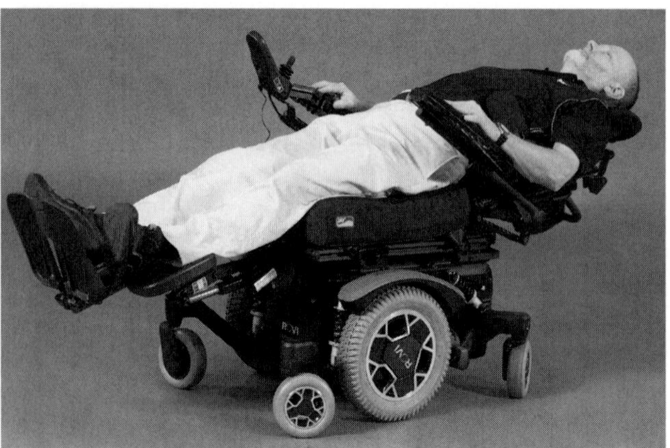

FIGURE 15-9. The client can use the power features for pressure relief, repositioning, head control, rest, and many other functions. As seen in this picture, both recline and an elevating foot platform are required to get into a fully supine position.

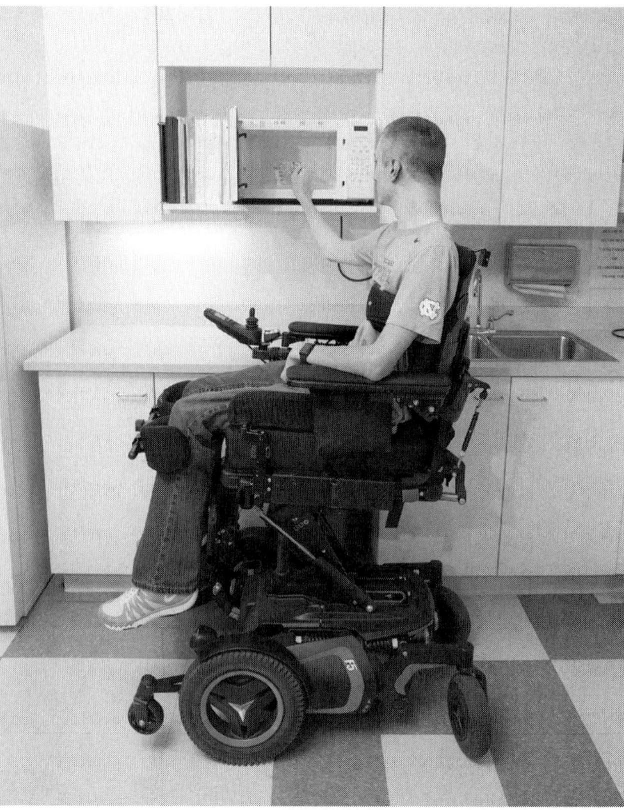

FIGURE 15-10. Seat elevate currently is not a covered feature by many payer sources, but is extremely functional for the client.

point along the way if the client cannot tolerate fully upright. See Figure 15-5 for a standing power wheelchair.

CUSHIONS

A multitude of cushion choices are available for the client, but cushion types fall into a few categories: foam, gel, air, and hybrids (Fig. 15-11 and 15-12). See Table 15-3 for details of the cushion materials, properties, and specifics.

The cushions all have insurance codes, and generally the cushion is categorized as general use, positioning, skin protection, or both positioning and skin protection. The client's diagnosis will determine the cushion category for which the client qualifies, and the client's specific positioning needs (pelvic positioning, scoliosis) and history of skin breakdown will be taken into account by the practitioner. During the evaluation, the client should try as many cushions in the qualifying category as possible, for as long as possible. Some seating specialists will modify the off-the-shelf cushions with wedges and cut cushions for leg length discrepancies. Most cushion manufacturers will make custom sizes and shapes for the client's particular needs. A pressure mapping system can be used to see which cushion style is best for that consumer by offering a look at the pressure distribution under the bony prominences. Pressure mapping will be explained in further detail later in this chapter. Most cushions will have a cover which can be removed for washing, and education and training must be provided on putting not only the cover back on correctly, but the cushion back in the chair in the correct orientation. Vulnerable clients can quickly develop a pressure injury from sitting on a cushion backwards. Some cushions are available with internal liners to protect the cushion from urine and other fluids. The OT practitioner should warn clients and caregivers about multiple layers between the client and the cushion, such as absorbent pads, towels, slings, and heavy clothing, as these may decrease the effectiveness of the cushion and its pressure relieving properties. Not only do these layers not allow the bony prominences to immerse into the pressure relieving layers, but also can cause increased moisture and pressure from wrinkles.

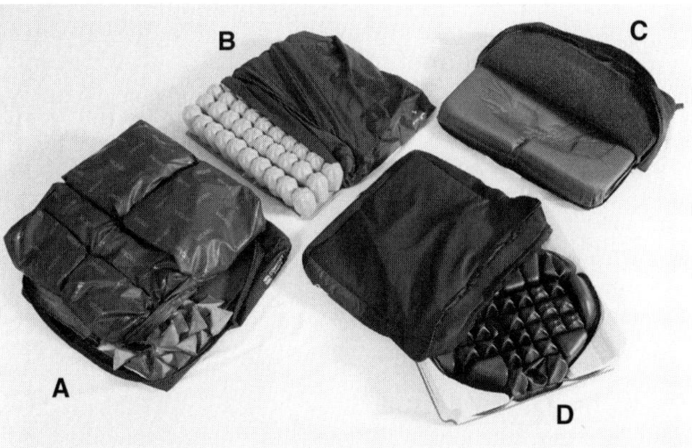

FIGURE 15-11. Air can be very effective for pressure relief, but can be difficult to maintain at times. Cushions are: **A.** Comfort Company Vicare® with individual air packets, **B.** Star Cushion with adjustable air cells, **C.** Varilite Evolution™ that is foam over an adjustable air bladder, and **D.** Roho® Hybrid Elite SR® with adjustable air cells in the back and foam in the front.

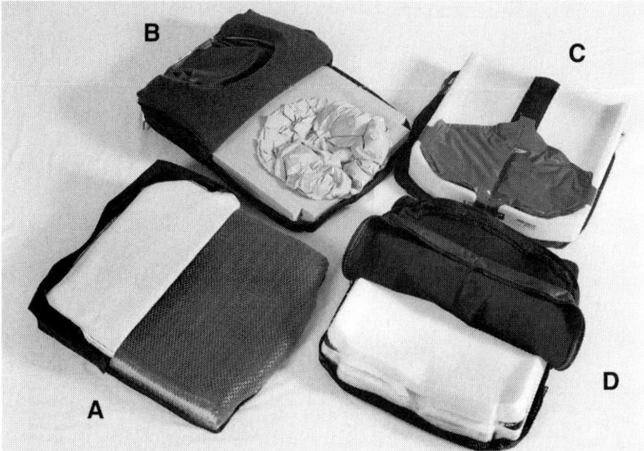

FIGURE 15-12. Cushions can be made from a variety of materials. **A.** Supracore's Stimulite® Contoured XS honeycomb style thermoplastic cushion. **B.** Jay J3® gel cushion with a gel pack in the back and foam in the front. **C.** Invacare Matrx Libra®, which is a fluid pack over foam. **D.** Jay Union®, which is a gel pack between foam layers.

Most insurance companies cover only one cushion every 2 to 3 years. Give careful thought to the cushion choice for a client with a progressive disorder or who has fluctuations in ability to stand for pressure relief from day to day. For example, a basic foam cushion may be fine for the client who can stand to relieve pressure, but not necessarily for someone who sits all day. Cushion coverage is generally diagnosis driven, and so if the client has a pressure injury or a certain diagnosis at risk for skin issues, the option is available for a pressure-relieving cushion. When there is a scoliosis or other positioning diagnosis, a positioning cushion can be ordered. Clients with complex needs may require cushions with both properties. At times, the cushion chosen for initial comfort for the short time at the evaluation may not be the best long term choice, and practitioners should assure that clients are educated on options.

BACKRESTS

Backrests come in many shapes and styles with air, gel, foam, and combinations, as well as positioning components (Fig. 15-13). Sling backs, which are typically found on basic manual wheelchairs, are the lightest-weight option but can lead to a kyphotic posture over time as the material stretches and ages. An adjustable tension type fabric backrest with horizontal Velcro® straps allows for some adjustability as the back straps can be tightened to provide a mild contour and provide more support over the life of the product. Off-the-shelf backrests have generic contours and are available at various heights and depths of contoured support. Lower heights allow more functional trunk and scapular movement and do not interfere as much with access to the wheels for propelling a manual wheelchair. Higher backrests provide increased posterior support for weakness or tone and can have built-in contour or swing away lateral trunk

TABLE 15-3 Wheelchair Cushion Types

TYPE OF MATERIAL	WEIGHT	HEAT	MAINTENANCE	IMPACT ABSORPTION	ENVELOPMENT
Foam	Can be light or heavy	Can be hot	Damaged by moisture and light Not easily cleaned	Good	Good at first, poor as cushion ages
Air	Lightest	Coolest	Can be punctured Easily cleaned	Excellent	Excellent, if inflated correctly
Gel	Heaviest	Cold in winter, cool in summer	Can be punctured Easily cleaned	Fair	Fair, gel can migrate out from under the bony prominences
Combo: Foam and gel	Heavy	Midrange	Combo of characteristics	Fair to good	Good
Combo: Foam and air	Light	Midrange	Combo of characteristics	Good to excellent	Good

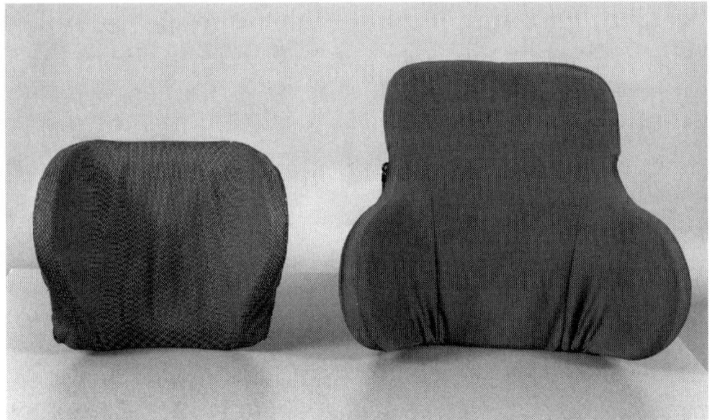

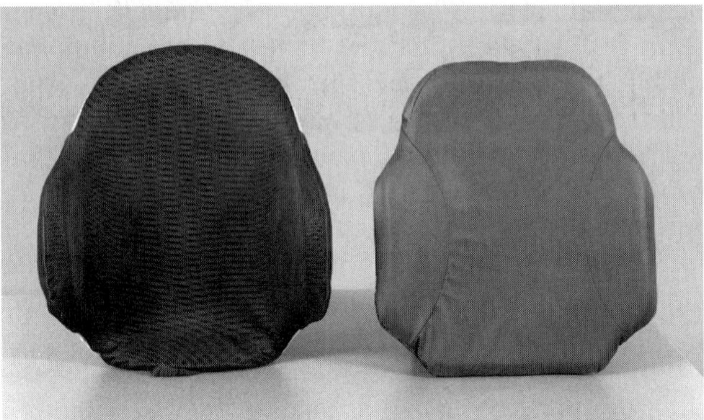

FIGURE 15-13. Backrests can be mounted onto almost any chair and can have different contours, materials, height and widths, and levels of support. Many off-the-shelf backrests can be customized for particular client needs, including inserting air or gel areas behind bony prominences. increasing lateral support, or making accommodations for mild kyphosis or lordosis.

supports. Off-the-shelf backrests can mount to the back panel or back canes of a manual or power wheelchair when the standard backrest does not have the positioning or pressure relieving properties required for the client. Most have hardware that allows for movement in all directions to accommodate for pelvic positioning or spinal scoliosis needs. Some solid backrests have adjustable vertical metal stays or horizontal wires, which can also assist with positioning a client who has kyphosis, lordosis, or scoliosis. Backrests with air support generally are either all air cells, or have the adjustable air cells along the spine and lateral areas.

Some clients have very significant contractures and asymmetries that cannot tolerate an off-the-shelf product and require a custom molded seat (back rest, seat cushion, or both) (Fig. 15-14). Generally, a mock-up of the mold is created, and then either the mold is poured as liquid foam that hardens, or a plaster mold or a digitized picture is sent to the manufacturer for creation. Because these seats are

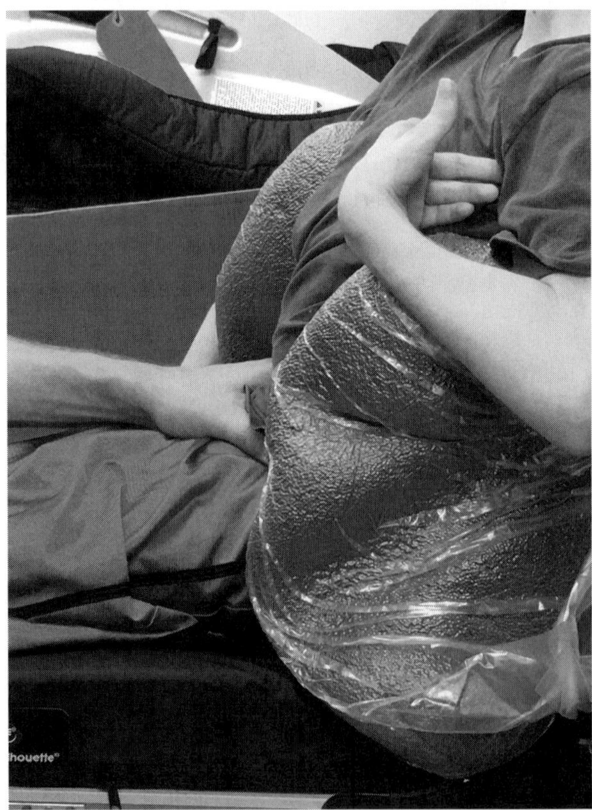

FIGURE 15-14. A molded seat can accommodate an unusual body that cannot be effectively supported with an off-the-shelf product. This is a picture of a mold in process. The molded shape from the evaluation is sent to the manufacturer to be made either from a plaster mold or a digitized file.

built for the individual, many custom curves can be created, but the chair generally can only have the tilt feature for positioning and pressure relief. Recline can change the position of the client's body against the backrest, causing the molded position to shift, while tilt keeps the mold in a stable position relative to the client. Molded seats provide maximum pressure distribution, and provide maximum support and stability when required but do not accommodate growth, weight changes, or other seating changes.

ELECTRONICS

Scooter and basic power wheelchairs generally have an on/off switch or button and some speed control as the only electronic options. For complex power mobility, the upgraded electronics in the joystick (or other control method) are programmable and adjustable. The supplier or wheelchair evaluator can place a handheld, in-line, or computer programmer to adjust the control method and change parameters such as turning speed, acceleration, and deceleration speeds as well as the **joystick throw** (how far the joystick is pushed before something happens). **Tremor dampening** is a programming feature that can be used for clients with a tremor or less controlled movements, as it keeps the chair moving straight despite extraneous movements. Switches can be added for control of on/off and mode to move through the power features and be placed where necessary for a client who cannot reach the standard controls. This type of programmability, control options, and flexibility is not possible in the more basic chairs.

At times during the evaluation, the client may demonstrate the inability to use the joystick for control due to weakness, contracture, tone abnormalities, or tremors. Alternative drive controls may also be assessed at that time to maximize full control over the chair. Any time there is an alternative drive control, the standard joystick can be replaced by a separate control display screen, which allows the client to know what speed, mode, or drive the wheelchair is in. Numerous options exist for full control, such as a foot controlled joystick that mounts one of the footplates, switches to perform various chair tasks, or a head-controlled option called head array where sensors are built into the headrest pads (Fig. 15-15 and 15-16).

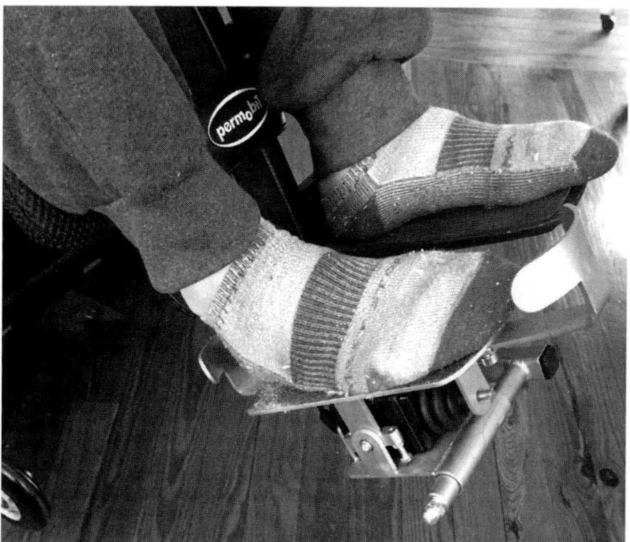

FIGURE 15-15. The actual (black) joystick is positioned under the footplate and is connected to the footplate. As the client moves his or her foot, it operates the joystick for full proportional control.

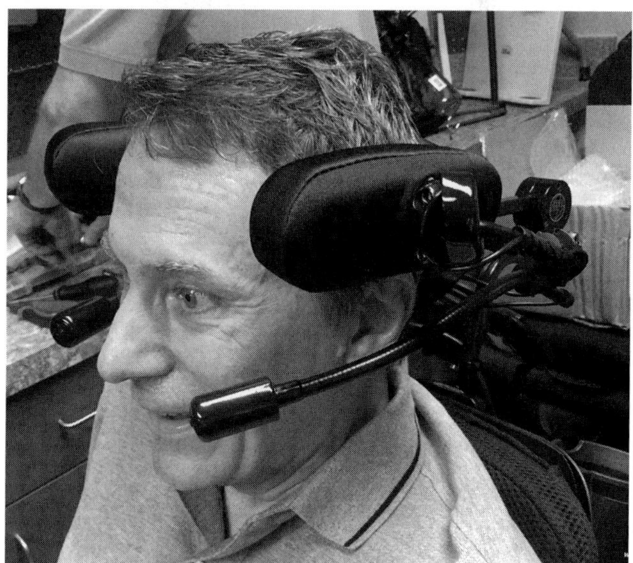

FIGURE 15-16. This client is using sensors in the headrest pads (head array) to control the chair movement, as well as switches near his chin for on/off and mode (power feature and other function) control.

A number of companies have created sensor options for the headrest or headband that allow control with very little movement. A client may use sip and puff technology that uses breath/lip control into a straw for chair control. Generally the client sucks on the straw (sip) either softly or firmly, or puffs/pushes air into the straw (puff) softly or firmly and these air movements are translated into drive controls. The client may use a soft puff for forward, a hard sip for reverse, or many other options, depending on the client's needs. A client could drive with a miniature joystick using one finger or even with the miniature joystick positioned at the lower lip (Fig. 15-17).

Options are also available to place various types of switches in locations where the client has controlled movement, such that one switch might be forward, one reverse, one right and one left around a thumb, both thighs, or on a tray. Switches are powered through the chair and can require force to activate or simply require the client to get near them (proximity switches) without touch required to activate. Switches can be as tiny as breaking a beam of light to operate, known as fiber optics (Fig. 15-18), or as large and force tolerant as needed for a client with ataxia. If a client has very few useful movements with consistent control, the numbers of switches can be lowered to even just one switch for full chair control. In this case, the client would activate the switch to go forward, then the chair would stop when body part is removed or comes away from the switch. At that point via scanning on their display, the client would hit the switch again to make a choice to select right, stop, forward, and so on. Each directional choice is maintained only while the body

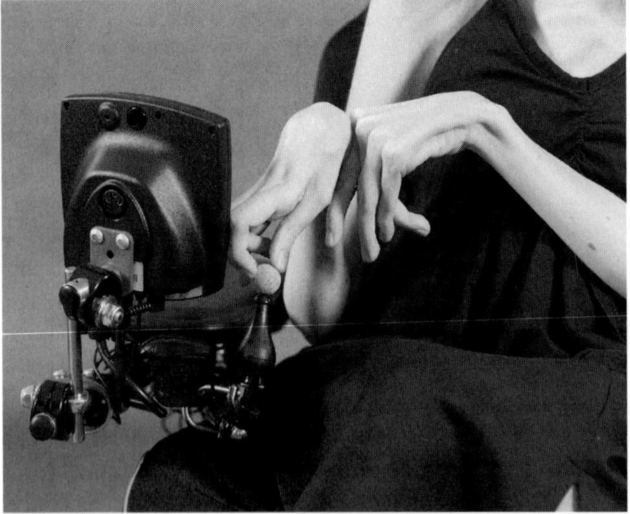

FIGURE 15-17. The miniature joystick requires less force to move and is often a good option for clients with significant hand weakness or contracture.

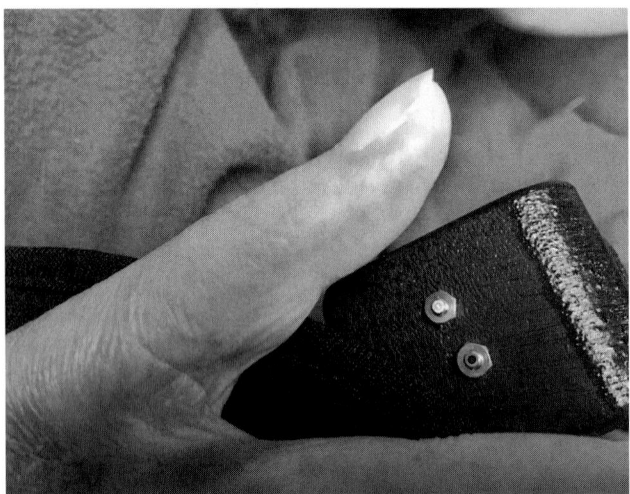

FIGURE 15-18. Fiber optics chair control. The client is using her thumb to cross a beam of light coming through a wire. This client has the control configured so the left switch turns left, the right switch turns right, and when both are covered it moves forward.

part maintains activation of the switch. Although cumbersome, many clients rely on this option for driving as well as power seating control. Generally, the client also has a secondary joystick on the back of the wheelchair for caregiver control over the chair, which is called an attendant control. The attendant control is typically not covered by insurance until an alternative drive control is used. The attendant control has full capability to control the chair for driving as well as power features for positioning/pressure relief.

ACCESSORIES

Accessories required for a client's wheelchair can vary dramatically, depending on the client's functional and positional needs. Many clients can maintain trunk and pelvic positioning simply via the backrest and seat, but clients with increased weakness, abnormal tone or asymmetries may require lateral trunk support pads, often on swing-away hardware for full trunk control. It can be difficult at times to get the lateral pads positioned so they support the client fully for function, yet do not interfere with movement or cause pain/pressure. Anterior supports include support at the trunk and hips, and can include shoulder straps, shoulder retractors (firmly keep shoulders back), chest straps (horizontal strap across chest), and vests (a larger 4-point anterior support). A chest strap or vest keeps a client with poor trunk balance from falling forward in the chair over rough or varied terrain or during transportation and promotes trunk extension and scapular retraction.

A variety of anterior pelvic supports, such as pelvic positioning belts with various buckles and straps, and solid anterior pelvic supports called subasis bars are available. Subasis bars control the pelvis at the anterior superior iliac spine. Lateral hip and lateral thigh supports can be added at the side of the hips and/or outside the lower thigh or the knee for leg and pelvic control. This can be necessary when in full tilt/recline/leg elevation when gravity and weakness may make the knees fall to the side and therefore the feet to fall off the legrests. Other clients have very wide-spread leg positioning, and may require the lateral leg support to fit through doorways and decrease pain at the hips. Medial support to keep the knees apart is also possible through a medial pommel. Most of the time, these supports are removable or flip down for transfers. If the foot falls off the legrest or requires positioning, a toe strap or shoe/ankle huggers attached to the footplate can assist. See Figure 15-19 for many of these options. Gel or air pads can be placed almost anywhere on the chair for better pressure relief of bony prominences, and typical spots are on the footplate, armrests, laterals, and head supports. These may not be covered by insurance, and some caregivers and clients have their own pads sewn or created.

Armrest supports can vary in length and height, and can have straps and built up sides to keep weak arms from

TECHNOLOGY AND TRENDS

Students, clients, caregivers, and the public often ask why power wheelchairs do not have the ability to be controlled by the eyes or the voice for people with severe disabilities. Although these technologies do exist, they have not become readily available. There are a few significant safety issues to consider. If there is a camera or tablet reading the client's eye position, would it be in the way of the client seeing where they are going? How would the camera account for eye fatigue, bright sunlight, dark hallways, bumps, and jostling, which are a part of normal use of a power wheelchair? Would the chair turn toward whatever the client happens to glance at? As far as controlling the power wheelchair with a voice command, it is very difficult to filter out loud talking or noises in public places and make the user safe. Technology is amazing, and it is with hope that someday the regular consumer will be able to use products such as these to increase function and mobility.

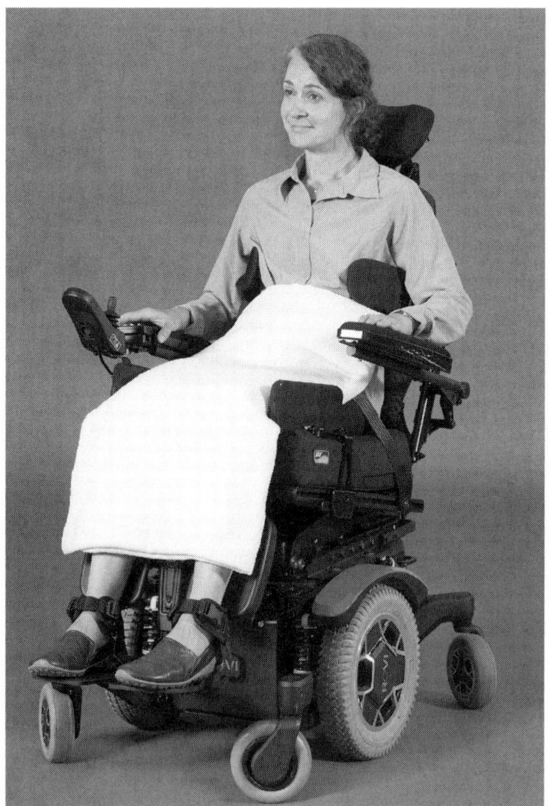

FIGURE 15-19. Most positioning components are adjustable as well, and will move out of the way for transfers. This client is using lateral pads at the trunk, thigh guides for the outside of the legs, and ankle huggers to maintain her feet on the footplates.

falling off. Elbow blocks and contoured armrests keep the arms from sliding backward while the chair is in full tilt, which could cause injury (Fig. 15-20). Headrest supports can be a standard plush 10-inch cushion with adjustable and removable hardware, or they can be a wider or longer headrest with more support laterally or along the occiput. Lateral facial pads can attach to the headrest and offer side support for the head when needed for neck weakness, and dynamic head straps attach to the headrest for when the head would fall forward without support (Fig. 15-21). Generally, sitting back in some tilt whenever in the chair will assist to keep the head erect and posture straighter for someone with weakness. This position can also be useful when going down hills and ramps to decrease fear or actual risk of falling forward.

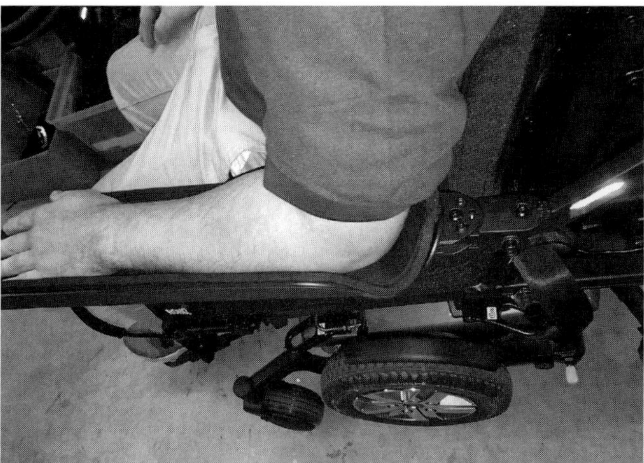

FIGURE 15-20. Arm troughs can assist with keeping the weakened arm from falling off the armrest or backward when using tilt and recline.

PRESSURE RELIEF AND WOUNDS

Pressure relief over the bony prominences is a major issue for clients who are very weak, have poor nutrition, fragile skin, and require wheelchairs a significant portion of the day. Pressure injuries can be a constant battle to prevent, even if the client has full sensation and the ability to perform pressure relief, because of the cumulative effect of sitting for hours, days, months, and years. The cushion, backrest, armrest, legrest, and headrest choices are all important considerations in maintaining adequate pressure relief. Although the head is not usually considered a weight-bearing surface, pressure injuries to the back of the head and the ears are not uncommon. Many times, the bony aspects of the spine and scapula are danger points, and of course the seated surfaces of the ischial tuberosities and the sacrum (coccyx, trochanters) are also vulnerable. Seating clinics and specialists often have a pressure mapping system that can demonstrate the pressure or pressure relief of various cushion options to choose from in the wheelchair prescription process. The mapping system is a thin pad with sensors that goes between the client and the

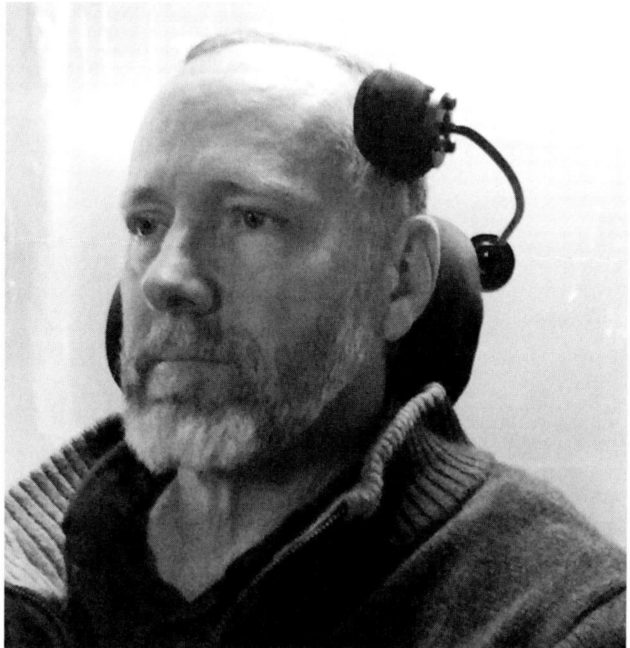

FIGURE 15-21. Numerous options for head control exist, but these lateral facial pads are multiadjustable and will swing out of the way for transfers.

seated surface, and provides a color picture of the amount of pressure and distribution in each area (Fig. 15-22). It will show which cushion or surface distributes the pressure the best or what happens when the client leans forward or to the side. Also, pressure mapping can be used as an educational and training tool for biofeedback with visual impact for clients who are fearful or neglectful of performing frequent pressure relief.

Pressure injuries are categorized by stages, and can be as simple as a reddened area and as deep as to the bone itself. The best management is prevention, but at times the pressure or shear factors are too great, and a wound appears. Certainly, other factors can influence skin integrity besides just pressure, and those factors are skin health in general, nutrition, moisture from urine or sweating and heat, shear (sideways movement of layers of skin across another such as from a slide board), and sensation (or lack of).[17] Some clients never really perform any pressure relief, sit on a basic cushion, and still never get a pressure injury, while others sit on a flat air cushion for 30 minutes and develop an injury. Pressure injuries tend to be round and those from shear more irregular or oblong. See the wound section of Chapter 8 for more information.

If the client is uncomfortable, or the caregiver notes the beginnings of a pressure injury, then a visit to the seating specialist is needed. The seating specialist can help determine the origin of the injury and suggest alternative products and solutions. Although at times the seating system is the suspected culprit, pressure points from the bed or shower/toilet chair, shear from transfers, and rubbing over the wheel of the chair or on the sling during transfers may also be the cause.

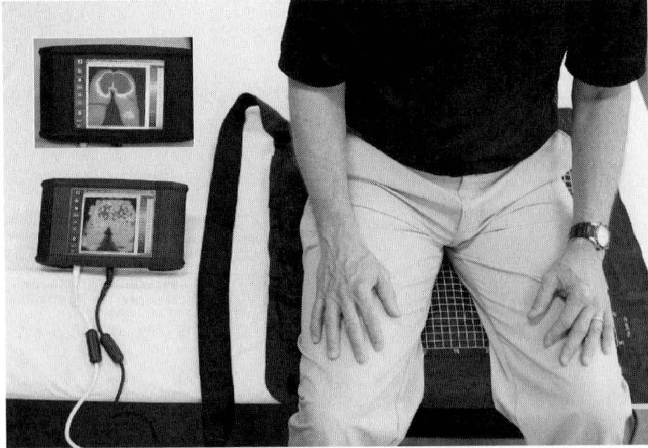

FIGURE 15-22. The pressure mapping pad and sensor system go between the client's bottom and the cushion surface, and show the pressure distribution in a color gradient on the screen. The picture on the top *(inset)* shows the pressure from sitting on the firm therapy mat table, and picture of the tablet wired to pad shows the pressure more evenly distributed with a pressure relieving cushion. There are still some darker spots on this cushion, and others would need to be trialed as well.

PRESSURE RELIEF OPTIONS AND TRAINING

Even if a client uses a well-fitting and supportive wheelchair, an ideal cushion for their needs, and have ideal posture, they still may have pressure related issues, and need to perform pressure relief. Pressure relief allows oxygenation and blood flow to the tissues under the bony prominences and can assist to keep those tissues healthy. A variety of methods are available to perform pressure relief, depending on the client's strength, mobility, and pain issues. No matter the method, the evidence notes that pressure injury risk is highly varied, and there are no consistent guidelines for pressure relief procedures in the literature based on a 2015 systematic review.[17] Some standards suggest to relieve pressure every 30 minutes for 5 minutes, while others note every 15 to 20 minutes for 1 to 2 minutes. Certainly, some clients will have a difficult time with this frequency of pressure relief, but these seem to be the most common recommendations. Clients who are new to pressure relief or have new pressure issues may require an alarm or alert on their phones or watches to remind them of pressure relief times. Technology also exists that allows the OT practitioner to monitor the frequency of pressure relief, degrees of tilt and recline, and length of time that the client performs the task. This information can be uploaded as a teaching tool, equipment justification, or method for determining reasons for new pressure areas. The OTA can provide education on various pressure relief options, which are appropriate to the situation and condition of the client. The specific technique depends on the type of wheelchair, type and level of injury, and the functional abilities of the client. The options include:

1. Power wheelchair positioning: Certainly the best option for effective pressure relief is a combination of tilt and recline, specifically combining 25 to 45 degrees of tilt with 110 to 150 degrees of recline to maximize pressure relief.[16,17] Standing wheelchairs (manual and power) are also exceptionally effective for pressure relief in the standing position.
2. Lean side to side: The client should lean far enough to the side to unweight one ischial tuberosity on one side, accounting for balance challenges by hooking an arm over the armrest, backrest or push handle, or leaning over a table or counter. The client should lean at least 1 minute on each side.
3. Lean forward: The client should ensure he or she is all the way back in the seat, and then lean as far forward as possible to unweight both sides of the buttocks. Care should be taken for balance deficits, and some clients could lean toward a couch or low table and keep the seatbelt on for increased safety.
4. Independent push-ups: The client uses both arms on the wheels or armrests to lift the body so the buttocks have no weight on them. Although the quickest and

easiest method for many clients, this method does put extra strain on the shoulders, so should be limited in favor of the earlier options for many clients.[17] Note: pictures of the pressure relief styles can be found in Figure 35-16.

TRAINING ON WHEELED MOBILITY

Training the client for community mobility will initially be done by the seating team of which the OTA may be a part, and the client may also require further training in the environment at home or a facility that the OTA may perform. At times, the client may have obtained the chair from a supplier who just dropped it off, and did not perform any real training besides how to charge the battery. The seating specialist may often be based in the clinic, and require assistance from a home health practitioner to continue the training in the home environment with its specific challenges. Increasing the amount of wheelchair skills training provided to the client may also increase social and community participation by increasing comfort with the chair.[18] A wheelchair or scooter of any sort can be a dangerous piece of machinery in the wrong hands or without proper training. Some clients are good and careful users from the first moment they get into the chairs, and some clients require significant training and safety awareness education to be independent with their devices. The seating specialist may arrange for an OT practitioner to visit the residence to train the client further on the mobility device. Training may include safe ways to store the device, transfers on and off, integration into the daily routine, entering and leaving the house over thresholds and ramps, independent and assisted transportation options, and how to use the mobility aid for outside use over varied terrain and transitions. OTAs who work with clients who are poor or unsafe wheelchair or scooter users should speak to the occupational therapist about including a safety goal in the plan of care. In a suburban environment, lawn chairs set up in the driveway can be a great start to learn obstacle avoidance and stopping distance awareness. In more urban settings, a lobby of a hotel, a mall, or quiet sidewalk can be options for training, but with close supervision. Clients with cognitive disabilities may potentially be able to control the wheelchair, but require some extra training and supervision to be safe in all areas and terrain. This list provides some thoughts about education, training, and safety that the OTA can use.[19]

1. Always watch the terrain as one or both front caster or drive wheels can suddenly be turned sharply by encountering a crack in the pavement, rock, bump, threshold, drop-off, or sideways incline.
2. Always steer straight up or straight down an incline. Never travel across an incline because the wheelchair is more likely to fall over sideways on steep grades. For wheelchairs with casters in front, avoid areas in the pavement or path that tilt to one side to avoid having the wheelchair roll off the path.
3. Work with clients to understand stopping and reacting quickly with their particular mobility device. Clients with power wheelchairs must understand that increased stopping distance is generally required with increased speed. All clients must be able to stop and react quickly as needed and understand principles of turning with their specific type of wheelchair.
4. Fully charge batteries before leaving home. It is dangerous to be stranded outdoors in a power wheelchair with a dead battery.
5. Avoid rain and snow if possible, which are especially hazardous to clients with power wheelchairs and to the expensive equipment. Try to stay out of falling rain or snow; try to stay off wet, slippery surfaces coated with rain or snow because of the risk of sliding or getting stuck. Ramps can be treacherous and slippery with rain, ice, and snow.
6. Turning in tight spaces will be approached and managed differently with every chair configuration, size, and type. The practitioner should work with the client and caregiver on moving furniture, clutter, and other obstacles as well as how to safely approach the turns within space constraints.
7. Assist the client to recognize potential safety hazards, such as attempting to go off a full curb, driving through a deep puddle, deep water channels at the end of some driveways at the street, ditches, deep gravel/sand, and others. Use activity analysis skills to analyze the environment and identify potential hazards.

OT Practitioner's Viewpoint

I have performed seating evaluations for the past 12 years, and love the challenge it can bring. One type of client I really enjoy working with is the young adult with Duchenne muscular dystrophy. As the disease progresses, the clients will typically drive with a joystick until they absolutely cannot manage to control the chair. They often have a difficult time changing to a new drive control on the chair, especially when it is all they have ever known. A miniature joystick is often a very good joystick to switch to, because it takes very small amounts of motion, is very sensitive, and young men with Duchenne often retain finger/thumb control the longest. It can be mounted in a tray or off the end of the armrest in almost any angle and configuration. When the drive control is ordered and being delivered at the seating clinic, there is nervous laughter and outright stress about making a change. When the chair is transitioned over to the miniature joystick and the client trials it for the first time, they are usually amazed and happy. It takes so much less effort, and they retain independent and full control over the chair and the power features. It makes the job worthwhile, and has the client set for many more years. ~Amber L. Ward, MS, OTR/L, BCPR, ATP/SMS

COMMON REPAIRS AND CHANGES

Ensuring a client is comfortable in a seated position for long periods of time involves certain principles of seating. Although the OTA may not perform a full seating evaluation, he or she still has ways to make clients more comfortable in the chair. The OT practitioner can request a prescription for changes or repairs and refer back to the seating clinic as needed. If the client is a resident in a skilled nursing facility or other care center, most insurance providers generally require the facility to pay for any repairs or a new chair. The difficulty is that most facilities will not buy a client batteries, much less a new chair, and clients may need to turn to loaner closets or self-pay options to stay independently mobile. Most chair repairs (as needed) will be performed by the supplier who sold the chair or the seating specialist, but there are a few small and common things that the handy OTA may be able to adjust or fix without a special visit.

Sliding Out of the Chair

In cases where a client is sliding out of the chair, the first step is to understand whether the client has a neutral or posteriorly tilted pelvis (Fig. 15-23). Posterior tilt of the pelvis is when the top of the pelvis is tilted backward, comes with slouched sitting, and can be flexible, preferred, or fixed in that position. Often with a posterior tilt comes hamstring tightness on the back of the knees, which means, at times, the legs will not stretch out to fit on the legrest angle without pulling the hips forward. Also, with a fixed posterior tilt, the client may not be able to tolerate sitting in a fully upright position, and if seated in that sort of chair, will slide forward out of the chair to raise the head and keep the eyes level. Many times, some recline in the backrest will assist with positioning with posterior pelvic tilt or kyphosis as well as some tilt to keep the client firmly back in the chair. Also, noting the legrest position and moving the footplates back may assist to increase foot contact. Some clients slide out trying to find a more comfortable spot, and the OTA may want to look for a more pressure relieving cushion, as well as institute a pressure relief schedule. A visit to a seating specialist may be warranted as well.

Legrest or Foot Platform Length

Many manual and power wheelchairs have adjustments that can be made for leg length. Ideally the client should have equal weight distribution through the entire length of the femur and foot. If the legrests are too high, all the weight goes into the ischial tuberosities and coccyx/sacrum, often causing tailbone pain and instability. If the legrests are too low, the seating stability can be compromised, as well as unequal weight distributed through the back of the thigh. Low legrests can also pull a person out of the seat as they attempt to stabilize on the footplates. Most legrests and foot platforms adjust with an Allen wrench or socket wrench, and if the OTA runs across these repairs frequently, a set may be worth purchasing.

Legs Falling Out to Sides

Many clients with leg weakness may require support on their outer thigh because of the leg falling out to the side, including a thigh guide mounted to the side rail of the seat or a knee guide mounted to the legrest. If the client does not have thigh or knee guides on their chair, and their legs are falling, a visit from the supplier or to the seating clinic to assess may be warranted. Many guides remove or flip out of the way for transfers and are multipositional. A temporary or emergency measure might be a gait belt or Velcro® wrapped around the lower thighs if the client is in danger of running over their feet as the legs fall to the side and cause the feet to fall off the legrests. This use of a strap can cause pressure areas, so is a temporary/emergency option only. Repositioning and moving the thigh or hip guides, either along the track forward and back or as they touch the client, typically requires the use of Allen wrenches.

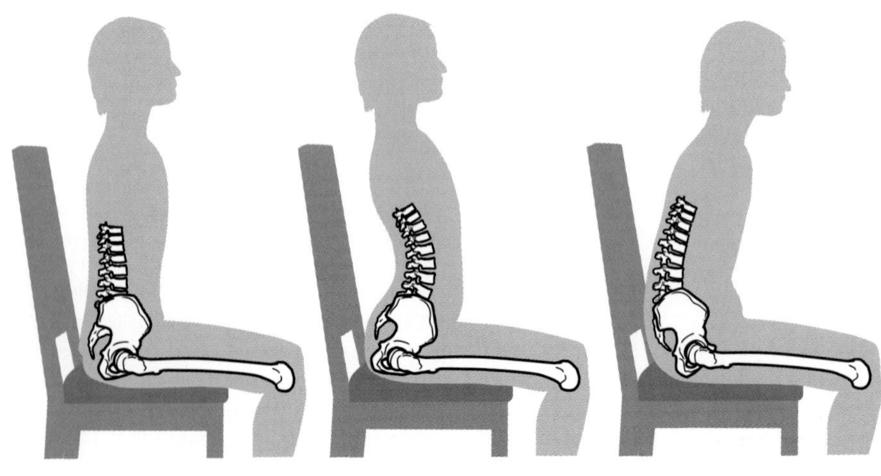

FIGURE 15-23. Note the differences with pelvic positioning as labeled and think about what each position will mean for function.

Leaning to the Side

Some clients have progressive trunk weakness and may start leaning to the side in the chair, some to the point of falling out of the chair. Generally, this indicates the client needs lateral support in the chair. Lateral support cannot be added to a basic manual or power chair, so if the client is in a basic chair, a visit to a seating clinic to explore options for a more flexible and complex chair will be needed. A temporary measure might be a pillow between the body and armrest, a wedge under the bottom or cushion or a strap around the trunk, but this is not appropriate long term, and may cause pressure issues and create more positioning problems. Some facilities may also consider a strap as a restraint.

Headrests

The headrest is the most frequently adjusted item on the complex power chair. When the client tilts back, the headrest generally stays in position with relation to the body, but with recline, the headrest tends to move upward in relation to the client. Try to use the Allen wrenches to move the headrest to a comfortable midway point where the client spends the most time or needs the most support. If the head falls sideways or forward, additional supports may be required. An emergency support for head positioning might be soft Velcro® added to the headrest and across the client's forehead, but this can be a safety issue if it slides down, and the client should not be alone or on transport with this sort of strap.

Joystick Position

Usually, a thumbscrew, knob, or bolt holds the joystick in place, which keeps the joystick from turning or moving while driving. The whole joystick can be rotated slightly to give a client a mechanical advantage inward or outward for full joystick control, or it can be moved closer or farther from the client. The joystick can also be moved to the other side if needed because of increased weakness.

Power Wheelchair Will Not Drive

If the power wheelchair turns on but will not drive, check two things. Note that the chair was not accidently taken out of gear by a lever near each motor of the chair. Also, check that if they have power features, that the chair is not in drive lock out. **Drive lockout** is a safety feature, and if the chair is tilted or reclined too much for safe driving, the chair simply will not move. The solution is to bring the chair into a more upright position. The supplier can adjust the drive lockout if needed for ramps and hills for a comfortable seated position. Another culprit may be low or dead batteries, and the client may require replacement of the batteries or charger.

Power Wheelchair Is Driving Slowly

If the power wheelchair is driving slowly, the batteries may require replacing, or the chair may be slow because of positioning of the seat. In seat elevate, and in some chairs with the legrests brought fully into the base, the chair will be automatically slowed down. Look for a turtle or a yellow "caution" light on the display screen to indicate the slow mode; the speed adjust knob may be turned all the way to the slowest level.

TRANSPORTATION FOR WHEELED MOBILITY

When using a manual wheelchair that folds, the client may carry the chair in a vehicle's trunk or behind the seat; the folding type can be difficult to self-load if the client has weakness. For a rigid manual wheelchair, the back folds, cushion, and wheels come off, and the remaining L-shaped frame generally fits into the trunk or back seat, or the client can disassemble and independently load into the passenger seat by bringing the pieces across the body. The driver's seat generally needs to be somewhat reclined and back all the way to accomplish this and does take practice. Some tilting/reclining manual wheelchairs will fold to a certain extent, although many clients are transported in their mobility device. Although chairs are crash tested, riding in them while in the vehicle is generally not considered safe, although with both the chair and client restrained by both a seatbelt on the chair and a shoulder restraint from the vehicle, it may be safer than a very weak client in a standard car seat. Scooters have the advantage of disassembling into three to four pieces, which still can be heavy, but more easily transported in a standard vehicle. Some basic power wheelchairs allow the seat to remove, but the base still can be over 100 pounds.

Many clients receive a power mobility device and have no way to transport it. Some large communities with a bus system have transportation options for clients with mobility devices, and taxi and accessible vans for hire may be options although can be expensive. Some consumers will put a wheelchair or scooter lift on the back or inside of their vehicles, but they must consider the weight of the mobility device as well as the weight of the lift on the vehicle frame and hitch. The chair must be safely restrained with these options. Some complex power chairs can weigh over 400 pounds, and cannot be put on the back of many vehicles. Some SUVs and minivans can be retrofitted with an arm lift that puts the chair inside the vehicle, although those typically work best with scooters and small basic power wheelchairs. A small trailer can hold the weight of the power wheelchair more easily for a smaller vehicle, or a hitch lift can be added to a larger vehicle. Chair restraints can either be ratchet straps attached onto official tie-down spots, or a bolt mounted under the chair that then locks into a device on the van or trailer floor. The best option, although more expensive, is a vehicle that has been modified with a raised roof or lowered floor, and a ramp or lift to accommodate the client riding in a wheelchair inside the vehicle. The ramped vehicles (generally a minivan) can have a power or manual ramp, which come off the side or rear of the van. Full-sized vans typically have a vertical lift that puts the chair and client in the vehicle. Once the client and the chair are in the vehicle, both must be restrained for the ride. The chair gets tied down with ratchet straps/hooks or a locking system, and ideally the client transfers to a regular car seat. If the client must ride in the chair, the client must have a seatbelt and shoulder harness that is hooked to the vehicle. As with manual wheelchairs, the wheelchair seat belt alone is not enough to restrain the client sitting in the power wheelchair while in the vehicle. Some chairs are crash tested but some brands may not be. Many clients drive the vehicle themselves, either from the standard driver's seat, or with the driver's seat removed, and the locking station placed so the client drives from the wheelchair. Generally, clients with power wheelchairs require specialized designed vans, minivans, or SUVs if they intend to drive from the wheelchair. Because it often takes weeks or months to acquire and adapt vehicles, it is best practice to immediately bring in the driver rehabilitation specialist to consult with the client and family.[20] This saves money because family members may unknowingly replace a small vehicle with a particular vehicle that cannot be adapted or is not designed to carry a power wheelchair. For example, this could occur when the client's spinal cord injury happens in a vehicular accident and the vehicle needs to be replaced by the family. Many used vans that are already adapted are available for purchase from either a dealer or an individual.

INTEGRATION OF MOBILITY DEVICES AND OTHER TECHNOLOGY

Many times the client with the manual or power wheelchair will need to have other items integrate with that device. Something as simple as the weight of a backpack for college hanging on it can affect how a manual wheelchair moves and reacts. Where does the person store his or her phone, keys, drink, and personal items on the mobility device? The OTA can assist with designing and finding bags, holders, and attachments of all sorts. Something as simple as a fanny pack can buckle onto the armrest of a chair, or a pocket could be sewn into the front of the wheelchair cushion. More complex items must also integrate with the wheelchairs, such as a mobile arm support, and require decisions about how it will attach to the wheelchair for self-feeding, grooming, and computer use. Many clients have communication devices, laptops, tablets, e-readers, and phones that need to be in the correct position for access. Various mounts can be added to the side rails, posts, and tubing of the chairs and are multipositional. Mounts generally must lift off for transfers, but some can be moved in and out independently by the client. Some power wheelchairs will have a display attached to the power wheelchair when the client uses an alternative drive control. Many practitioners and clients do not realize that this control often has infrared control, and can control the client's TV through the chair control. Manufacturers also have added in Bluetooth that allows the client to control the mouse of their computer through the chair's drive controls. The same control can be achieved with a smart phone of any type so the phone is controlled through the chair control. Many home automation options use Bluetooth as well. There are complex power wheelchair additions, which will send smart phone reminders to tilt back and perform pressure relief, as well as store the information on how often and for how many degrees the client moved in a day. This information can then be uploaded by the OT practitioner and used for educational and research purposes. A power inverter can be added to the power wheelchair batteries and allow the ventilator, bilevel positive airway pressure (BiPAP), or other devices to run off those batteries. The ventilator, suction, oxygen, and other items must have a secure way to mount or hang from the wheelchair through trays, supports, hooks, or push handles. A device exists that plugs into the wheelchair charger port that has a USB connection. It allows any device to be charged from the wheelchair batteries. One client took their power wheelchair to a car stereo shop and had undercarriage lights put on the power wheelchair, which pulsed to music played through stereo speakers mounted to the chair, while the music was controlled through the client's phone. Many power wheelchair manufacturers offer light packages as well. The integration of all the needed and desired items on the chair can be complex. Most of these accessories are not covered by insurance, but are options for clients to pursue as needed or desired.

SUMMARY

Working with clients and their seating and mobility needs can be a challenging, yet very rewarding opportunity. The incorrect piece of equipment can mean pain, pressure injuries, deformities, dependence, lack of support, and decreased function, while the correct equipment can provide independence, comfort, and function, as well as positioning and pressure relief. Results from a study of clients with amyotrophic lateral sclerosis (ALS) by Ward et al. showed power wheelchairs can also affect aspects such as quality of life and sense of control for the user.[21] Mobility-related ADLs are vital to the client with a mobility disability, and the device they use can affect task performance to a significant degree. The correct device may mean the client can attend college, stay in the home instead of a facility, live pain free, and have safe mobility in all areas of life. It is the responsibility of the OTA to self-assess his or her skills in this area before working with clients on their mobility needs. The OTA should seek continuing education or practical knowledge from seating specialists, suppliers, and/or manufacturers if assisting clients with their mobility needs or if he or she is interested in working in this exciting and fulfilling practice area.

REVIEW QUESTIONS

1. Although outcomes and benefits will vary, the overall goal of every seating intervention is to:
   a. Maximize the individual's function.
   b. Maintain midline alignment in the chair.
   c. Reduce contractures.
   d. Obtain the best cushion possible to minimize the risk of developing pressure ulcers.

2. To achieve distal mobility and function, a client being evaluated for seating and positioning must have:
   a. Good visual acuity
   b. Kinesthetic awareness
   c. Proximal stability
   d. Adequate room for movement
3. A client, who uses a power wheelchair, lives in a trailer that has a tight hallway with a sharp 90-degree turn into the bathroom. Which drive wheel configuration would *best* suit the client's needs?
   a. Rear wheel drive
   b. Mid wheel drive
   c. Front wheel drive
   d. All terrain drive
4. A client reports a sore bottom after sitting upright on a 3-year-old cushion for 2 hours. The pain is said to go away when the client returns to bed. What should be the OTA's *first* response?
   a. Ask the client to go back to the seating specialist for pressure mapping and a new cushion order.
   b. Research all cushion choices for the client.
   c. Ask the nurses to put the client back to bed after 2 hours.
   d. Refer the client to a wound clinic.
5. The OTA has a client who tends to be hot natured and sweaty in the summer, has paraplegia at the T12 level, and has no sensation below the level of injury. The client wants a lightweight cushion with excellent pressure relief for their manual wheelchair. Which type of cushion should the OTA trial *first?*
   a. Memory foam
   b. Gel
   c. Air
   d. Combination of foam and gel
6. When would a scooter be an appropriate choice for clients with a progressive disorder?
   a. It is always appropriate for this type of client.
   b. When the client is progressing slowly and still walking functionally most days
   c. When the client has amyotrophic lateral sclerosis (ALS)
   d. When the client has poor sitting balance
7. Mrs. Staver has poor sitting balance with a lean to the right in sitting, severe leg weakness, and decreased sensation in her lower legs from multiple sclerosis and diabetes. She has a complex power wheelchair with a fairly basic cushion and backrest on it. Which three of the following should be added to her chair for full support?
   a. Hip guides and toe straps
   b. Gel footplate pads
   c. Thigh guides
   d. A contoured backrest with lumbar support plus lateral pads
   e. A foam seat cushion
   f. Arm troughs
8. The OTA at a skilled nursing facility is asked to manage the manual wheelchair of a client who keeps sliding out of her chair and find a solution. The OTA has limited experience with seating and positioning, and worries about adequate skills in this area. What would be the *first* step toward finding a solution?
   a. Tell the OT supervisor of the refusal to work on the wheelchair.
   b. Check the client's hamstring length and hip ROM.
   c. Take online classes about seating and positioning.
   d. Put a stronger seatbelt on the client.
9. An OTA works with an occupational therapist who dabbles in seating evaluations, but never performs a mat evaluation, saying it is not necessary for a good result. The OTA remembers learning that the mat evaluation was part of a good outcome. What should the OTA say to the occupational therapist?
   a. "You are doing a great job, and your chairs always seem to work out well."
   b. "You are not doing what is best practice."
   c. "I am worried we do not do mat evaluations here. Can you look over this RESNA position paper about the wheelchair evaluation process so we can talk about it?"
   d. "I will perform the mat evaluation from now on."
10. Three complications of a poorly fit wheelchair can include:
   a. Loss of function
   b. Independent ADL performance
   c. Functional mobility
   d. Pressure injuries
   e. Pain
   f. Independent control over the power features

CASE STUDY

Georgia is a 55-year-old woman who has had Parkinson's disease for 20 years. She lives at home alone, has 24/7 paid caregivers, and has a sister who lives 4 hours away and is involved. Georgia is coming into the seating clinic today for a power wheelchair. She is unable to stand or ambulate, and generally sits in her recliner chair or in a transport chair. She spends her days watching television, having visitors, and reading. She has poor sitting balance, her legs have rigidity and fall to the right, and she is noted to lean heavily to the right in her transport chair when coming into the clinic room. Georgia's sister has already talked with the OT practitioner over the phone, and is excited about getting Georgia something comfortable she can tilt/recline back in and also have increased support and functional mobility. Georgia has mild cognitive deficits, very quiet and mumbled speech, and more rigidity than tremors. Georgia soon makes it clear that she only wants a very small, take-apart, basic power wheelchair, and is not interested in a complex power wheelchair. The OT practitioner is worried about Georgia falling out of a basic chair to the right unless strapped into the chair in some way. Georgia and her sister have an angry discussion in the office, and Georgia seems unwilling to change her mind despite her sister's protests.

1. How might the OT practitioner convince Georgia that a complex chair would be medically and functionally better for her?
2. How might a trial of each type of wheelchair be useful?
3. Would the OT practitioner have the supplier take both to the home?
4. If the OT practitioner cannot convince her, should he or she order what Georgia wants?
5. What are the ethical issues surrounding client choice when the OT practitioner believes that it is a bad choice?

PUTTING IT ALL TOGETHER — Sample Treatment Session and Documentation

Setting	Home health, referred from neurologist who treats client for multiple sclerosis, based on seating clinic recommendations
Client Profile	Mr. T, 55 y/o, had a basic power wheelchair for 6 years and recently got a complex power wheelchair with tilt, recline, elevating leg platform, and seat elevate to manage his medical changes
Work History	Currently on disability, was a small business owner
Insurance	Medicare, Medicaid
Psychological	Well-adjusted to use of the basic power wheelchair for nearly all mobility
Social	Married, two grown children, lives in a home with ramp, which is accessible to his current power wheelchair
Cognitive	Within normal limits
Motor & Manual Muscle Testing (MMT)	Client presents with weakness in bilateral upper and lower extremities • WFL AROM in BUEs • MMT LUE: 4/5 throughout • MMT RUE: Shoulder 3+/5, elbow 4/5, wrist 3/5, hand 3/5 • MMT LLE: 3-/5 hip, 3/5 knee, 3/5 ankle • MMT RLE: 2/5 hip, 3-/5 knee, 2/5 ankle with AFO • Grip R 23#, L 45# • Unable to ambulate, squat pivot transfers with Min-Mod A
ADL	Min A bathing from tub bench, Min-Mod A LB dressing, Min A UB dressing, Mod I grooming, Min A toileting with raised seat, all from power wheelchair
IADL	Mod I to Min A for all from power wheelchair
Goals	Within 3 weeks: 1. Client will require Mod I for safe use of power wheelchair in home for MRADLs. 2. Client will perform full tilt every hour for 2 minutes with smart phone reminders while in the chair with no other cues for pressure relief. 3. Client will use full recline, full leg platform elevation, and 25-degrees of tilt for 30 minutes every 3 hours with minimal cues for edema management. 4. Client will perform maneuvering of power wheelchair with Mod I for in and out of home, including managing door and safety. 5. Client will use seat elevate to increase level of independence with transfers to Min A.

OT TREATMENT SESSION 1

THERAPEUTIC ACTIVITY	TIME	GOAL(S) ADDRESSED	OTA RATIONALE
Maneuvering new power wheelchair in and out of all rooms in home, getting in correct position near toilet and tub bench for safe transfers	10 min	#1	*Occupations; Education and Training:* Functional task performance, mobility, mobility retraining as it pertains to ADLs, safety awareness
Practice using the power features, including tilt/recline/legs for pressure relief, repositioning and edema management.	15 min	#2 and #3	*Education and Training:* Functional task performance, power feature use training
Work on pulling open the outside door and maneuvering power wheelchair to get out the door, over threshold, and down the ramp safely.	10 min	#4	*Occupations; Education and Training:* Functional task performance, safety awareness
Practice the use of seat elevate for transfers to bed, toilet, and tub bench.	20 min	#5	*Occupations; Education and Training:* Functional task performance, ADL performance, safe mobility and transfers

SOAP note: 5/5/—, 10:00 am–10:58 am

S: Client states, "This chair is much bigger" when asked about functional use since delivery of the new power wheelchair.

O: Client participated in home health therapy session to address functional mobility, ADL and IADL performance, and home safety. No c/o pain. Client was able to drive the power wheelchair to bathroom with Mod I, although required min cues to maneuver to a safe position for toilet and tub bench transfer. He required Min-Mod A for transfer to both toilet and tub bench with use of seat elevate. He was able to complete full tilt with some recline position with moderate cues for pressure relief, and

PUTTING IT ALL TOGETHER Sample Treatment Session and Documentation (continued)

correct recline/leg elevation and tilt position for edema management with Min cues. Client performed outside door opening with Min A and addition of a pull rope and dressing stick. Client worked on safely maneuvering the larger power wheelchair through the home, required Min cues for centering in the doorway openings, and did not hit any walls or door jambs.

A: Client began to work on transfers and use of power wheelchair in a safe manner for MRADL tasks. His new chair is slightly larger in length and width, which affects his functional performance. Client demonstrated good safety awareness with thresholds and ramp, although did require cues for correct positions for pressure relief, repositioning, and edema management. Client will benefit from continued work on functional and safe use of power wheelchair in the home.

P: Continue to work on MRADL tasks, functional mobility, home safety, and safe use of power features for medical management.

Maxine Austin, COTA/L, 5/5/—, 7:30 pm

TREATMENT SESSION 2

What could you do next with this client?

TREATMENT SESSION 3

What could you do next with this client?

REFERENCES

1. Walls, G. (2011). Reaching for best practice. A focus on power wheelchair seating and mobility protocols. *Rehab Management, 24*(1), 14-17.
2. Hastings, J. D., Fanucchi, E. R., & Burns, S. P. (2003). Wheelchair configuration and postural alignment in persons with spinal cord injury. *Archives of Physical Medicine and Rehabilitation, 84*, 528-534.
3. Shea, M., Arledge, S., Armstrong, W., Babinec, M., Dicianno, B., Digiovine, C., ...Stogner, J. (2011). RESNA Wheelchair service provision guide. Retrieved from www.resna.org.
4. Schein, R. M., Schmeler, M. R., Holm, M. B., Saptono, A., & Brienza, D. M. (2010). Telerehabilitation wheeled mobility and seating assessments compared with in person. *Archives of Physical Medicine and Rehabilitation, 91*(6), 874-878.
5. Holm, M., Mills, T., Schmeler, M. R., & Trefler, E. (n.d.). The functioning everyday with a wheelchair (FEW) seating-mobility outcomes measure. Retrieved from http://www.few.pitt.edu/.
6. Barry, E., Galvin, R., Keogh, C., Horgan, F., & Fahey, T. (2014). Is the timed up and go test a useful predictor of risk of falls in community dwelling older adults: A systematic review and meta-analysis. *Bio-med Central Geriatrics, 14*, 14.
7. Podsiadlo, D. & Richardson, S. (1991). The timed "up & go": A test of basic functional mobility for frail elderly persons. *Journal of American Geriatric Society, 39*(2), 142-148.
8. Berg, K., Wood-Dauphinee, S., Williams, J. I., & Maki, B. (1992). Measuring balance in the elderly: Validation of an instrument. *Canadian Journal of Public Health, 2*, S7-S11.
9. Koontz, A. M., Brindle, E. D., Kankipati, P., & Feathers, D. (2010). Design features that affect the maneuverability of wheelchairs and scooters. *Archives of Physical Medicine and Rehabilitation, 91*, 759-764.
10. Guthrie, M. (n.d.). Basic wheelchair biomechanics. Retrieved from https://courses.washington.edu/anatomy/KinesiologySyllabus/WHEELCHAIR.pdf
11. Oyster, M. L., Karmarkar, A. M., Patrick, M., Read, M. S., Nicolini, L., & Boninger, M. L. (2011). Investigation of factors associated with manual wheelchair mobility in persons with spinal cord injury. *Archives of Physical Medicine and Rehabilitation, 92*, 484-490.
12. Arva, J., Paleg, G., Lange, M., Lieberman, J., Schmeler, M., Diciano, B., Babinec, M. (2007). RESNA position on the application of wheelchair standing devices. *Rehabilitation Engineering & Assistive Technology Society of North America*, 1-17.
13. Levy, C. E., Buman, M. P., Chow, J. W., Tillman, M. D., Fournier, K. A., & Gaicobbi Jr., P. (2010). Use of power assist wheelchair results in increased distance traveled compared to conventional manual wheeling. *American Journal of Physical Medicine and Rehabilitation, 89*(8), 625-634.
14. Arthanat, S., Nochajski, S. M., Lenker, J. A., Bauer, S. M., & Wu, Y. B. (2009). Measuring usability of assistive technology from multicontextual perspective: The case of power wheelchairs. *The American Journal of Occupational Therapy, 63*, 751-764.
15. Petito, C. (2010). Customizing power. A holistic approach to complex power wheelchair and seating systems. *Rehab Management*, 10-13.
16. Dicianno, B. E., Arva, J., Lieberman, J. M., Schmeler, M. R., Souza, A., Phillips, K., ...& Betz, K. L. (2015). RESNA position on the application of tilt, recline, and elevating legrests for wheelchairs literature update. *Assistive Technology, 27*(3), 193-198.
17. Groah, S. L., Schladen, M., Pineda, C. G., & Hsieh, C. H. (2015). Prevention of pressure ulcers among people with spinal cord injury: A systematic review. *Physical Medicine and Rehabilitation, 7*(6), 613-636.
18. Smith, E. M., Sakakibara, B. M., & Miller, W. C. (2014). A review of factors influencing participation in social and community activities for wheelchair clients. *Disability and Rehabilitation, Assistive Technology, 11*(5), 361-374. doi:10.3109/17483107.2014.989420
19. Mobility Training for Client and Public Safety. (2004). National Institute of Rehabilitation Engineering. Retrieved from http://www.agis.com/SqlFileResource.axd?id=438&resource=pdf
20. Stressel, D., Hegberg, A., & Dickerson, A. E. (2014). Driving for adults with acquired physical disabilities. *Occupational Therapy in Health Care, 28*, 148-153.
21. Ward, A. L., Hammond, S., Holsten, S., Bravver, E., & Brooks, B. R. (2015). Power wheelchair use in persons with amyotrophic lateral sclerosis: Changes over time. *Assistive Technology, 27*(4), 238-224. doi:10.1080/10400435.2015.1040896

Chapter 16

Driving and Community Mobility

Anne E. Dickerson, PhD, OTR/L, SCDCM, FAOTA

LEARNING OUTCOMES

After studying this chapter, the student or practitioner will be able to:

16.1 Describe the unique contributions of occupational therapy practitioners with expertise in driving and community mobility.

16.2 Discuss the roles of occupational therapy practitioners when addressing the instrumental activity of daily living of driving and community mobility.

16.3 Appreciate the complexity and meaningfulness of the occupation of driving for the older adult and the adult with disabilities.

16.4 Describe the adaptive options for driving as well as alternative transportation options for clients with a disability.

KEY TERMS

Alternative transportation	Interactive driving simulator
Baby Boomers	Medically at-risk drivers
Comprehensive driving evaluation	National Highway Traffic Safety Administration (NHTSA)
Driver rehabilitation specialist (DRS)	Older drivers
Fitness to drive	Vehicle modification

Except for a few major cities, most people use their personal vehicles to get to where they need and want to go. Even most people who use the subway, train, or bus to get to work depend on their personal vehicles to travel to events and places outside the range of public transportation. In fact, driving is the most accepted form of community mobility in the United States.[1] Because community mobility is recognized as the means to participate in other occupations, it is considered an occupation enabler.[2] Thus, persons who do not or cannot drive face consequences that affect their abilities to participate in some aspects of life.[1]

Driving is one of the most valued instrumental activities of daily living (IADL).[3] This is highlighted by the change in the revised *Occupational Therapy Practice Framework: Process and Domain, 3rd edition* (OTPF-3),[4] with driving and community mobility as an identified IADL, rather than just community mobility. The definition of this IADL remains the same; driving is one means of community mobility along with walking, biking, as well as other transportation systems. However, identifying driving as part of the IADL reflects the importance of driving to our clients and the recognition that the majority of adults use their own personal motor vehicle as their means of community mobility and will continue to do so in the foreseeable future.[5]

BABY BOOMERS WILL CHANGE OCCUPATIONAL THERAPY PRACTICE

The generation born between 1945 and 1964 is known as **Baby Boomers**. The proportion of the U.S. population aged 65 years and older will increase from one in eight in 2010 to one in five by 2030.[6] In 2021, the oldest of this generation will be turning 75, the age at which fragility issues will begin to affect this generation in greater ways.[6] It is critical to understand the effect of these numbers on occupational therapy (OT) practice. In addition to the obvious increase in client numbers, Baby Boomers are a unique group of individuals who, for example, will insist on adaptive equipment that is both useful and attractive. Their work ethic will demand that OT practitioners find better ways to adapt work environments, modify home environments, and address the occupations beyond those of dressing, self-feeding, and bathing. Most importantly, Baby Boomers will expect to remain independent and live at home. For this generation, nothing means independence more than their having their car ready to go when and where they want and need to go.

It is essential to recognize that the Baby Boomer generation grew up with the development of motor vehicles. In the 1940s and 1950s, the "car" was the status symbol of independence, the method of interacting with others, and provided the means to engage in occupations. Many teenagers, particularly those who lived in suburban areas, counted the days to get their driver's licenses because having and driving a car was the social network of this generation. In other words, the car was the equivalent to the newest smartphone today! Consider driving down Main Street as comparable to posting the latest on Facebook or Twitter–making sure friends are aware of who is a companion, and what is most valuable. Although phones were used to communicate, the most popular method of socialization was driving to the local gathering places whether it was a high school sports game, ice cream shop, concert, or swimming pool. Additionally, with the expansion of the interstate highway system during this period, families increasingly lived and worked well beyond their immediate communities. Activities such as going for a Sunday drive or watching a movie at the drive-in theater were popular activities for many families of this generation. Thus, driving, for Baby Boomers, is not just about community mobility and getting to where they want and need to go, but also about the occupation of driving. Regardless of whether **alternative transportation** (any other form of transport besides driving, such as biking or public transportation) is available or not, when an older adult is at risk of losing his or her ability to drive, OT practitioners must understand and consider that for these individual clients, it may not be just about losing an option of community mobility, but losing their valued occupation of driving their car. Furthermore, it is recognized that driving is crucial to engaging in other occupations.

COMMUNICATION

Most OT practitioners, especially those living in suburbia and rural areas, depend on driving to get to where one needs and wants to go. This is also true for older adults. However, driving is not just about transportation for Baby Boomers. As addressed in this section, driving is also an occupation! Many older adults like to drive–just like the younger generation enjoys computer games or keeping in touch with Twitter, driving was what Baby Boomers did for "fun" and entertainment. Driving is their connection to the world and why they consider it important for independence. Therefore, it is important to communicate the understanding of the loss when a client is told they cannot drive for even a short time and why it is devastating when told they can never drive again. Do not jump in with options of real-time ridesharing or why family members can drive them, without first listening to their loss. It is not just about getting to the doctor, grocery store, or bank. For some, it is another loss because of aging and they feel it will change their life–and it will! Be mindful of this loss and communicate understanding in anticipation of the time they will be able to work on methods of maintaining their community mobility.

Finally, it is important to recognize that older adults are generally safe drivers, overall having the lowest risk of collisions compared with other age groups. This is partly due to lower exposure to the risk factors of being on the road during rush hour, night driving, and avoidance of high-speed interstates. Additionally, research has clearly demonstrated that it is not "age" that leads to declines in driving, but instead the functional impairments associated with medical conditions that put **older drivers** at risk.[5] With normal aging, a person has slower information processing and motor responses. As with most activities, older adults compensate for this by driving more slowly and conservatively. It is not until drivers are over the age of 70 years that crash risk increases when, for example, intersections require quick information processing and immediate decisions (e.g., yield signs, flashing signals).[7] Moreover, the frailty and fragility of some older adults puts them more at risk to die of a crash than younger or middle-aged adults,[8] which is why driver safety is so important. The issue to understand about age and driving is that the number and implications of medical conditions increase as one ages.[9] Thus, the older adults who are at risk are typically clients who have medical conditions with functional impairments that will affect driving skills. However, it is important to also understand that drivers of any age who have a disability may benefit from the skilled services of OT practitioners who will address each individual's unique needs, thus promoting engagement in the occupation of driving and community mobility.

OCCUPATIONAL THERAPY ROLES IN ADULT REHABILITATION

As addressed in other chapters of this text, the role of the occupational therapy assistant (OTA) in intervention with adults differs by setting and disability. Typically, after a medical event, the client is seen by the OT practitioner in acute care, where he or she is concerned with assessment of performance skills to prevent further deterioration and/or enhance recovery from functional disabilities. Moving quickly into the subacute and/or rehabilitation phase, the OTA works in collaboration with the occupational therapist on intervention strategies and contributing to the process of ongoing evaluation. It is the role of these OT practitioners to address each occupation, as identified by the OTPF-3. What is not always clear to practitioners is that the occupation of driving and community mobility is related directly or indirectly to all other occupations (Table 16-1). Consequently, it is critical that practitioners consider driving and community mobility in their intervention plan and not assume it will addressed later in the therapeutic process.

Although the value of occupations is different for each individual, in the therapeutic process, interventions generally start with basic activities of daily living (ADLs) to ensure the individual is able to perform their daily tasks of self-care. As the client improves, attention can be addressed in areas

TABLE 16-1 Linkage Between Occupations and the Instrumental Activity of Daily Living of Driving and Community Mobility

OCCUPATIONS: IDENTIFIED BY THE OTPF-3[4]	CONSIDERATIONS WHEN PLANNING INTERVENTIONS AND DISCHARGE FOR DRIVING AND COMMUNITY MOBILITY
Activities of Daily Living Bathing/showering, toileting and toilet hygiene, dressing, swallowing/eating, feeding, functional mobility, personal device care, personal hygiene and grooming, sexual activity.	• Management of incontinence to use transportation • Securing mobility devices in vehicle • Ingress and egress from a motor vehicle • Storage of wheelchair or scooter
Instrumental Activities of Daily Living Care of others, care of pets, childrearing, communication management, driving and community mobility, financial management, health management and maintenance, home establishment and management, meal preparation and clean up, religious and spiritual activities and expression, safety and emergency maintenance, shopping.	• Transporting family members who do not drive (e.g., spouse, grandchildren, parents) • Transportation to physician office, pharmacy, and clinical therapy appointments, grocery stores, and/or restaurants, bank, post office, social activities • Religious activities • Traveling to vacation home
Rest and Sleep Sleep preparation, sleep participation, rest.	• Fatigue increases crash risk
Education Formal education participation, informal personal education needs or interests exploration, informal personal education participation.	• Attending community college classes (e.g., computer skills, retirement planning, estate planning) • Attending community recreational activities such as senior sports, painting, quilting, playing cards
Work Employment interests and pursuits, employment seeking and acquisition, job performance, retirement preparation and adjustment, volunteer exploration and participation.	• Employment outside the home requires a form of transportation • Volunteer in community (older adults are the largest age group of volunteers)
Play or Leisure Exploration and participation.	• Access to play or leisure when desired, any day or time • Sports, fishing, golf, yard sales, boating, walking, hiking
Social Participation Community, family, peer/friend	• Visiting friends, family, colleagues • Social events like graduations, movies, concerts, birthday parties, reunions, and other celebrations • Vacations with family or friends

of instrumental activities of daily living (IADLs) (e.g., meal preparation, medication management, shopping). Because OT practitioners have limited time in present day health care systems, they must work with their clients, caregivers, and team to address essential unmet goals with appropriate discharge planning. Driving and community mobility will likely be an area that is not directly addressed during initial services. However, it will be essential to the recovery of function and quality of life for clients. Practitioners must understand that many of the ADLs and most of the IADLs are affected by whether someone is able to be mobile in his or her community. Thus, practitioners must ensure that clients and families have the information to address these IADLs in the future as they recover at home and want to participate in more complex occupations, such as driving.

During the rehabilitation process, when the question of driving arises from the client or family, the OT practitioner must acknowledge and respond to this critical IADL without hesitation. That does not mean the practitioner is making a decision about the licensure to drive. Because of their role in intervention (i.e., direct interaction with clients) in ADLs and IADLs, OTAs may actually have the best perspective in terms of the client's true functional abilities and deficits. The OTA observes performance and can identify whether there are functional deficits that will affect the activity of driving. Identifying potential risk for clients when considering driving is not significantly different from identifying risk with other complex tasks. If a client has difficulty independently organizing a meal, determining how to put on garments, or managing the household budget, the OTA informs the occupational therapist of their observation. If the client is at risk for safety with other complex IADLs, there is real potential for risk with the IADL of driving and community mobility.

Consider that, with driving, the identification process is not more complex, but it is more complicated. This is because the potential risk is not just about the client and caregivers, but potentially affects the public if a driving outcome proves negative (a crash). Unfortunately, the fear of making a decision about driving is often the reason OT practitioners do not have the confidence to address driving.[10] However, driving and community mobility is within the scope of OT practice. In fact, it is the ethical obligation of the practitioner to identify risk.[1,11]

The reality is that OT practitioners do not make decisions about driver licensing–only the state licensing agencies do. However, because OT practitioners observe functional performance and identify risk, they have been identified as the "go to" profession for driver evaluation and rehabilitation.[12] Furthermore, unless all OT practitioners step up to address this IADL with all clients, it will be a practice area lost to other less qualified service providers (without medical training or education) who are already devising certificate programs that purport to be able to evaluate adults with disabilities and older adults effectively.[10,13]

Unlike a normal aging individual, a **medically at-risk driver** (Box 16-1) may have specific visual, perceptual, motor, and cognitive issues that are best addressed by professionals with medical training.[1] Without that expertise, the medically compromised driver may not be accurately assessed, offered inappropriate advice on vehicle adaptations, or told driving is no longer an option when that may not be true. To preserve this critical IADL and foster quality of life, every possibility to return to the client's favored method of community mobility (in most cases driving) must be pursued by those who understand activity analysis and the occupation of driving. Thus, the goals of this chapter are to assist the OTA in 1) understanding the IADL of driving and community mobility, 2) assisting in identifying risk, and 3) addressing this IADL through appropriate interventions.

OT Practitioner's Viewpoint

As an expert and researcher in driving, I attend several national conferences related to transportation and gerontology. As one of the few occupational therapists at these conferences, it is always exciting to see how other professionals attending these conferences value OT practitioners who practice in the area of driving and community mobility. In fact, 80 percent of DRSs (an interdisciplinary field) are occupational therapists. At this time, this is a practice area in which we do not have threats from physical therapy, speech therapy, or nursing taking over the assessment/intervention of this IADL. However, we soon will–unless we step up to meet the need! Baby Boomers want to remain independent and want to continue to drive. As OT practitioners, generalists and specialists, we must address this IADL or we will lose this practice area to some other group. We absolutely have the skill set to be able to address driving as an IADL–as outlined in this chapter–and we should make sure we do not lose this to another less skilled group or worse yet, no one deals with driving and our clients either become at risk or lose their ability to be mobile in their community. ~Anne E. Dickerson, PhD, OTR/L, SCDCM, FAOTA

BOX 16-1
Medically At Risk Definition

The Medically At-Risk Driving Centre of the University of Alberta defines a *medically at-risk driver* as:

A person who, regardless of age, has a medical condition or conditions that could affect driving performance, but further assessment or testing is needed to determine whether the medical condition(s) has made the person be unsafe to drive (e.g., some drivers with diabetes are safe to drive, others are not).[14]

THE PROFESSION OF DRIVER REHABILITATION

The profession of driver rehabilitation is a multidisciplinary field that plans, develops, and implements driver rehabilitation services for individuals with disabilities. The **driver rehabilitation specialist (DRS)** field encompasses a diverse group of providers (e.g., engineers, driving instructors, health care professionals) who specialize in driving rehabilitation, with requirements for certification and education that vary from state to state. The driver rehabilitation field developed in the 1950s, soon after the proliferation of the automobile when occupational therapists, driver educators, and engineers collaborated to provide driver rehabilitation based on medical and vocational rehabilitation service models.[1] The focus was rehabilitation through **vehicle modification** and adaptive equipment for individuals with physical impairments (e.g., spinal cord, amputation, dwarfism). Only recently have programs been expanding to include older adults with physical and cognitive disorders because of the increasing numbers of older adults (i.e., Baby Boomers) living longer with chronic conditions who want to maintain their independence through driving. In fact, the first **National Highway Traffic Safety Administration (NHTSA)** collaborative agreement with the American Occupational Therapy Association (AOTA) was initiated in 2003 with the recognition that expansion of driver rehabilitation service programs, policies, and strategies was required to meet the need for services.

From this historical perspective, the diverse roles of the DRS functioned well. Because it was often a matter of determining fit of hand controls to drive or teaching an individual with a spinal cord injury (SCI) on their use, a DRS with an engineering or driver instructor background was practical (Table 16-2). However, because of the medical complications of cerebrovascular accident (CVA), traumatic brain injury (TBI), or Parkinson's disease, the medical background of a

EVIDENCE-BASED PRACTICE

One of the most exciting studies for OT practitioners is one that was not done by OT practitioners–but by researchers in business and public health. The study by Rogers, Bai, Levin, and Anderson found that "occupational therapy is the only spending category where additional hospital spending has a statistically significant association with lower readmission rates" for the three health conditions studied: heart failure, pneumonia, and acute myocardial infarction.[15] What does that mean for OT as a profession? It is quite significant. It shows the OT intervention made a difference–that when the hospital spent more money to provide OT services, the clients stayed out of the hospital. Other services were also evaluated (including physical therapy and speech therapy), but these did not make a difference. The researchers indicated they believe the results show that OT is important because OT practitioners focus on issues important to readmission–how to discharge the client to be safe in his or her environment. The authors specifically mentioned 1) providing recommendations and training for caregivers; 2) determining whether the person can live independently or requires further rehabilitation or nursing care; 3) training in use of assistive devices for activities of daily living (e.g., using the bathroom, bathing, getting dressed, making a meal); 4) doing home safety assessments and suggesting modifications; 5) assessing the ability to do IADLs, such as manipulating items (e.g., medication containers) and provide training when necessary; and 6) working with physical therapists to increase the intensity of inpatient rehabilitation. So, how is this related to driving and community mobility? Although this study does not mention it, it is one of the valued IADLs of clients. If OT practitioners can address this IADL as well as the others mentioned in this study, OT will be known as the profession that keeps the client out of the hospital and doing the activities they need and want to do!

Rogers, A. T., Bai, G., Lavin, R. A., & Anderson, G. F. (2016). Higher hospital spending on occupational therapy is associated with lower readmission rates. Medical Care Research and Review, *1–19. https://doi.org/10.1177/1077558716666981*

health professional becomes essential. Thus, determining who has the essential qualifications to become a DRS becomes much more complicated. Individuals with DRS credentials can be as diverse as the practice areas of OT (e.g., school-based practitioners, mental health practice, and long-term care practitioners). Unlike OT however, DRSs may include individuals with an educational background that did not address medical conditions. Furthermore, the terminology of driver rehabilitation has become complicated and clarification is recognized as a goal for researchers, stakeholders, and practitioners in the larger arena of transportation.[16] Table 16-2 provides definitions for important terms in driver rehabilitation as defined by leaders in the transportation field.[17] Although not officially established yet, the table offers a reflection of current driver rehabilitation terms and definitions.

THE DRIVER REHABILITATION SPECIALIST/OCCUPATIONAL THERAPY PRACTITIONER

A DRS who is also an occupational therapist typically performs a **comprehensive driving evaluation** to determine an individual's driving knowledge, skills, and abilities. The comprehensive driving evaluation is defined as "a complete assessment of an individual's driving knowledge, skills, and abilities by a healthcare professional that includes: 1) medical and driving history, 2) clinical assessment of physical, cognitive, vision, and/or perception abilities, 3) on road assessment, as appropriate, 4) an outcome summary, and 5) goals and recommendations for inclusive mobility plan including transportation options."[18] Potential outcomes of the evaluation might be findings of decreased vision or attention to traffic, or ankle weakness with decreased reaction time. Specifically for adults with new or ongoing medical conditions, the individualized plans may include recommendations for rehabilitation of skills (e.g., increase scanning skills through designed intervention), compensation through training (e.g., learn to drive a roundabout, learn to use hand controls), compensation through adaptation of the vehicle (e.g., using a steering knob for one-handed turning), cessation of driving, or a combination.

Because of the advances in technology, a wide range of options and innovations are available to compensate for physical disabilities. For example, bioptic telescope systems for individuals with low vision, hand controls for individuals with lower limb amputations, a left foot accelerator for a missing or impaired right leg or foot, or joystick steering for the individual with high level SCI are all technological advances that make driving possible (Fig. 16-1). However, although rehabilitation or compensation through training or adaptation is the ideal goal, the individual must have the capacities for new learning and skill development. Technological advances are not yet able to compensate for deficits in executive functioning, a key determinate of driver strategies, tactics, and safety.[16] Furthermore, individuals with decreased insight[19] or poor cognitive abilities[20] in addition to their physical impairment, may no longer have the ability to voluntarily limit or adapt their behaviors to be deemed fit to drive. This is where the OTA may be extremely helpful in the identification process. As the OTA is working with a client and observes that new learning is difficult, or conversely, the individual is able to learn new skills, the OTA

TABLE 16-2 Definitions for Select Commonly Used Terms in Driver Rehabilitation

Term	Definition
Fitness to drive	A driver characteristic, defined by the absence (or the extent to which) of any functional (sensory, perceptual, cognitive or psychomotor) deficit or medical condition that significantly impairs an individual's ability to competently operate the vehicle while conforming to the rules of the road and/or that significantly increases crash risk.
Driving competency	The demonstration of fitness to drive that meets criteria recognized by a body responsible for driver licensing.
Driving skill	The demonstration of vehicle control decisions at operational and tactical levels in a range of traffic and environmental conditions a driver may be exposed to in everyday experience.
Driving ability	The necessary sensory, perceptual, cognitive, or psychomotor skills needed to control a motor vehicle for a designated range of traffic and environmental conditions, plus a knowledge of the rules of the road that meets jurisdiction requirements.
Clinical driving evaluation	A healthcare professional obtaining, interpreting, and documenting data to determine fitness to drive through assessment of sensory, perceptual, cognitive, or psychomotor abilities using specific tools or instruments.
On-road assessment	A driving evaluation in a motor vehicle to examine a person's driving abilities and skills in the operational, tactical, and strategic levels using a method of scoring or determining attainment levels.
Comprehensive driving evaluation	A complete assessment of an individual's driving knowledge, skills, and abilities by a healthcare professional that includes: 1) medical and driving history, 2) clinical assessment of sensory, perceptual, cognitive, or psychomotor abilities, 2) on-road assessment, as appropriate, 3) an outcome summary, and 4) goals and recommendations for inclusive mobility plan, including transportation options.
Behind the wheel	Performing driving maneuvers using a vehicle or simulated vehicle for purposes of instruction/training on public roads or off-road settings.
On road	Driving on roadways that are private or on public roadways, streets, or highways.
Driving test	An examination of driving maneuvers and knowledge of the rules of the road performed in a motor vehicle on a public highway or street.
Off road	A component of the on-road assessment that is conducted on roadways or areas that are not publicly managed as roadways (e.g., private road, parking lot, closed course). It should be noted that in some areas or disciplines, this refers to the clinical assessment done before the on-road assessment.
Closed course	A driving venue separate from publicly traveled roadways, with known and controlled driving parameters that is used for evaluation of skills or abilities, or practice of driving maneuvers.
Naturalistic driving (study or assessment)	A methodology to monitor or evaluate driving behavior, using instruments installed unobtrusively in a driver's own car, that 1) provides an objective driver identification number and driving data for each trip, and 2) requires no interaction from the driver.
Standardized road test	A road test with specific components always performed (e.g., right turns, highway, intersections) to establish a score on a scale with at least interval data properties that is comparable across individuals.

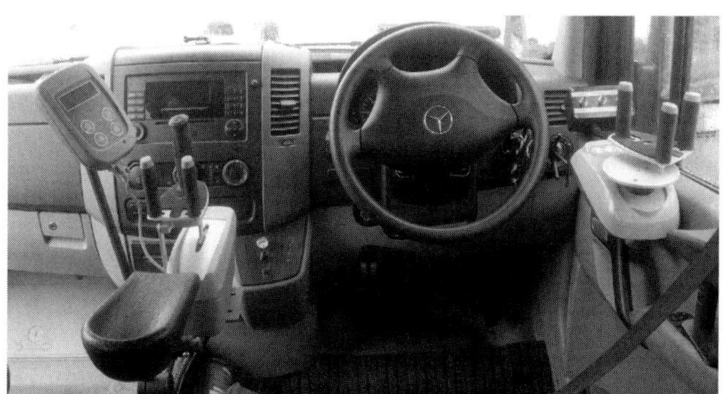

FIGURE 16-1. Joystick drive control. *(Photo courtesy of www.tetraplegicliving.com)*

should consider driving and the learning abilities needed and inform team members about the client's observed potential or risk.

LEVELS OF SERVICE FOR DRIVING

As described, the profession of driver rehabilitation is evolving with the changing needs of clients, state licensing authorities, and technology. To complicate matters, physicians are frequently asked about driving by their clients and/or family members and may not know about the services of driver rehabilitation or the role OT has in driving and community mobility. Understandably, consumers are also confused by the concept of or complain about cost of a medically based comprehensive driving evaluation because they do not understand the level of service that is needed for completing one. Consumers (e.g., clients, caregivers, family members) may not understand why the licensing authorities may simply withdraw a license based on a diagnosis and where to go for help if that happens.

In an effort to clarify services, the two professional associations most closely related with driver rehabilitation, the Association for Driver Rehabilitation Specialists (ADED), and the AOTA, created and adopted a document describing the range and diversity of driver services.[21] The development of this seminal document was completed over an 18-month period through funding by NHTSA, and it is the first time the diverse types of services related to driving have been described and differentiated.[21]

The *Spectrum of Driver Services* has two sections. The first section illustrates the range of available services from community awareness to specific services of driver rehabilitation (Table 16-3). The second section breaks driver rehabilitation programs into three general groupings according the levels and complexity of services (Table 16-4). The significant features of Table 16-3 include:

1. The differentiation between community-based education; medically based assessment, education, and referral; and specialized evaluation and training with driver rehabilitation programs.
2. Under each of five different program types (driver safety programs, driving schools, driver screening, clinical IADL Evaluations, and driver rehabilitation [DR] programs), the typical providers are described with their credentials. This will assist in determining which programs use providers with a medical background.
3. Under each program type (as listed previously), the required providers' knowledge and typical services will assist the reader in being able to differentiate preventative services (i.e., updating driving skills or acquiring a driver's license) from medically based assessment. These sections also articulate the differences in the screening at a physician's office, a clinical (or IADL) assessment that might be done by a generalist occupational therapist, and the specialized services provided by the DRS.
4. The outcome of each program type is clearly stated. Because driver safety programs provide education and awareness and driving schools enhance skills for healthy drivers, these two categories should not be the intervention resource for those with medical conditions. The medically based assessment, education, and referral programs that indicate risk or the need for referral to the specialized programs are the appropriate programs for these individuals.

Table 16-4 illustrates the different levels of driver rehabilitation programs. The significance is that all healthcare providers referring to driving programs (e.g., physicians, neuropsychologists, medical licensing boards, and OT practitioners) should understand that not all driver programs are the same. Specifically for clients with physical impairments, the differentiation may be critical. For example, if the client has any upper or lower extremity paresis, he or she should be referred to a low tech program because adaptive equipment may be needed to compensate for operation of primary or secondary controls of the vehicles. A basic program would not be appropriate because the typical evaluation vehicle does not have any modification and, therefore, the most effective and efficient evaluation could not be completed.

SCREENING AND EVALUATION PROCESS FOR DRIVING AND COMMUNITY MOBILITY

Using standardized assessment tools or tools based on research evidence is critical to obtaining reliable information for justifying services.[22] However, one of the issues with evaluation of a dynamic and complex activity such as driving is that, based on present research, there is not one single assessment tool to comprehensively evaluate **fitness to drive** (meeting necessary mental or physical requirements to drive) or driving performance.[23,24] Groups of tools are being analyzed together to capture some of the skills and abilities needed (e.g., vision, cognition, perception, and motor function).[25-28] Studies have focused on assessments that increase predictive validity for fitness to drive in older adults[29] while others have examined tools in samples with specific medical (or clinical) conditions.[30] The point is that the activity of driving, as a complex IADL, needs to be considered within a performance based context, not according to the scores of a computer-based or pencil-and-paper test. This is where the OTA's role is valuable. The observations of performance during daily tasks are essential contributions to the tasks of determining risk by the OT practitioner.

Although all DRS use an array of assessment tools, it is the data gathered in the behind-the-wheel (BTW) or on-road assessment that is primarily considered when making a recommendation of fitness to drive.[31] However, not all clients need the BTW component. When the individual does not meet the minimum capacities to be able to safely operate a motor vehicle (e.g., significant visual deficit, moderate or severe dementia), there is no justification for a specialist's referral. Thus, the OTA who sees that the client has difficulty managing his adaptive equipment for dressing or does not recognize the left visual field, it is not a leap of faith to make the connection to driving performance. The OTA already familiar from observing and working with their clients should recognize that when a client struggles with other complex IADLs, the OTA can collaborate with the occupational therapist to make a driving recommendation with confidence because the same abilities and skills the client needs to perform most complex IADLs are the same

TABLE 16-3 The American Occupational Therapy Association and Association for Driver Rehabilitation Specialists' Document Showing the Spectrum of Driver Services, Used With Permission.

SPECTRUM OF DRIVER SERVICES: RIGHT SERVICES FOR THE RIGHT PEOPLE AT THE RIGHT TIME

	Community-Based Education		*Medically Based Assessment, Education, & Referral*		*Specialized Evaluation and Training*
PROGRAM TYPE	**DRIVER SAFETY PROGRAMS**	**DRIVING SCHOOL**	**DRIVER SCREEN**	**CLINICAL IADL EVALUATION**	**DRIVER REHABILITATION PROGRAMS (*INCLUDES DRIVER EVALUATION*)**
TYPICAL PROVIDERS AND CREDENTIALS	Program-specific credentials (e.g., AARP and AAA Driver Improvement Program)	Licensed driving instructor (LDI), certified by state licensing agency or Dept. of Education	Health care professional (e.g., physician, social worker, neuropsychologist)	Occupational therapy practitioner (generalist or driver rehabilitation specialist#) Other health professional degree with expertise in instrumental activities of daily living (IADL)	Driver rehabilitation specialist#, certified driver rehabilitation specialist*, occupational therapist with specialty certification in driving and community mobility+
REQUIRED PROVIDER'S KNOWLEDGE	Program specific knowledge. Trained in course content and delivery	Instructs novice or relocated drivers, excluding medical or aging conditions that might interfere with driving, for purposes of teaching/training/refreshing/updating driving skills.	Knowledge of relevant medical conditions, assessment, referral, and/or intervention processes. Understand the limits and value of assessment tools, including simulation, as a measurement of fitness to drive.	Knowledge of medical conditions and the implication for community mobility including driving. Assess the cognitive, visual, perceptual, behavioral, and physical limitations that may impact driving performance. Knowledge of available services. Understands the limits and value of assessment tools, including simulation, as a measurement of fitness to drive.	Applies knowledge of medical conditions with implications to driving. Assesses the cognitive, visual, perceptual, behavioral, and physical limitations that may impact driving performance. Integrates the clinical findings with assessment of **on-road** performance. Synthesizes client and caregiver needs, assist in decisions about equipment and vehicle modification options available. Coordinates multidisciplinary providers and resources, including driver education, healthcare team, vehicle choice and modifications, community services, funding/payers, driver licensing agencies, training and education, and caregiver support.
TYPICAL SERVICES PROVIDED	1. Classroom- or computer-based refresher for licensed drivers: Review of rules of the road, driving techniques, driving	1. Enhance driving performance. 2. Acquire driver permit or license. 3. Counsel with family members for student driver skill development. 4. Recommend continued training	1. Counsel on risks associated with specific conditions (e.g., medications, fractures, postsurgery). 2. Investigate driving risk associated with changes in vision, cognition, and	1. Evaluate and interpret risks associated with changes in vision, cognition, and sensory-motor functions due to acute or chronic conditions. 2. Facilitate remediation of deficits to advance client readiness for driver rehabilitation services.	Programs are distinguished by complexity of evaluations, types of equipment, vehicles, and expertise of provider. 1. Navigate driver license compliance and basic eligibility through intake of driving and medical history. 2. Evaluate and interpret risks associated with changes in vision, cognition, and sensory-motor functions in the driving context by the medically trained provider.

Continued

TABLE 16-3 The American Occupational Therapy Association and Association for Driver Rehabilitation Specialists' Document Showing the Spectrum of Driver Services, Used With Permission. (continued)

PROGRAM TYPE	DRIVER SAFETY PROGRAMS	DRIVING SCHOOL	DRIVER SCREEN	CLINICAL IADL EVALUATION	DRIVER REHABILITATION PROGRAMS (*INCLUDES DRIVER EVALUATION*)
	strategies, state laws, etc. 2. Enhanced self-awareness, choices, and capability to self-limit.	and/or undergoing licensing test. 5. Remedial Programs (e.g., license reinstatement course for teens/adults, license point reduction courses).	sensory-motor function. 3. Determine actions for the at-risk driver: • Refer to IADL evaluation, driver rehabilitation program, and/or other services • Discuss driving cessation; provide access to counseling and education for alternative transportation options 4. Follow reporting/referral structure for licensing recommendations	3. Develop an individualized transportation plan, considering client diagnosis and risks, family, caregiver, environmental, and community options and limitations: • Discuss resources for vehicle adaptations (e.g., scooter lift) 4. Facilitate client training on community transportation options (e.g., mobility managers, dementia-friendly transportation) • Discuss driving cessation. For clients with poor self-awareness, collaborate with caregivers on cessation strategies • Refer to driver rehabilitation program 5. Document driver safety risk and recommended intervention plan to guide further action. 6. Follow professional ethics on referrals to the driver licensing authority.	3. Perform a comprehensive driving evaluation (clinical & on-road). 4. Advises client and caregivers about evaluation results, and provides resources, counseling, education, and/or intervention plan. 5. Intervention may include training with compensatory strategies, skills, and vehicle adaptations or modifications for drivers and passengers. 6. Advocates for clients in access to funding resources and/or reimbursement. 7. Provide documentation about fitness to drive to the physician and/or driver-licensing agency in compliance with regulations. 8. Prescribe equipment in compliance with state regulations and collaborate with Mobility Equipment Dealer^ for fitting and training. 9. Present resources and options for continued community mobility if recommending driving cessation or transition from driving. Recommendations may include (but not restricted to): 1) drive unrestricted; 2) drive with restrictions; 3) cessation of driving pending rehabilitation or training; 4) planned reevaluation for progressive disorders; 5) driving cessation; 6) referral to another program.
OUTCOME	Provides education and awareness.	Enhances skills for healthy drivers.	Indicates risk or need for follow-up for medically at-risk drivers.		Determines fitness to drive and provides rehabilitative services.

#DRS-Health professional degree with specialty training in driver evaluation and rehabilitation, **CDRS*-Certified Driver Rehabilitation Specialist-Credentialed by ADED (Association for Driver Rehabilitation Specialists), +*SCDCM-Specialty Certified in Driving and Community Mobility* by AOTA (American Occupational Therapy Association), ^Quality Approved Provider by NMEDA (National Mobility Equipment Dealers Association).

TABLE 16-4 The American Occupational Therapy Association and Association for Driver Rehabilitation Specialists' Document Showing the Range of Driver Rehabilitation Programs, Used With Permission.

SPECTRUM OF DRIVER REHABILITATION PROGRAM SERVICES

PROGRAM TYPE	DRIVER REHABILITATION PROGRAMS		
	Administer comprehensive driving evaluation to determine fitness to drive, and/or provide rehabilitative services.		
LEVELS OF PROGRAM AND TYPICAL PROVIDER CREDENTIALS	**BASIC**	**LOW TECH**	**HIGH TECH**
	Provider is a driver rehabilitation specialist (DRS)# with professional background in OT, other allied health field, driver education, or a professional team of CDRS or SCDCM with LDI**.	DRS#, certified DRS*, occupational therapist with specialty certification in driving and community mobility+, or in combination with LDI. *Certification in driver rehabilitation is recommended as the provider for comprehensive driving evaluation and training.*	DRS#, certified DRS*, occupational therapist with specialty certification in driving and community mobility+. *Certification in driver rehabilitation is recommended as the provider for comprehensive driving evaluation and training with advanced skills and expertise to complete complex client and vehicle evaluation and training.*
PROGRAM SERVICE	Offers comprehensive driving evaluation, training and education. May include use of adaptive driving aids that do not affect operation of primary or secondary controls (e.g., seat cushions or additional mirrors). May include transportation planning (transition and options), cessation planning, and recommendations for clients as passengers.	Offers comprehensive driving evaluation, training and education, with or without adaptive driving aids that affect the operation of primary or secondary controls, vehicle ingress/egress, and mobility device storage/securement. May include use of adaptive driving aids, such as seat cushions or additional mirrors. At the low tech level, adaptive equipment for primary control is typically mechanical. Secondary controls may include wireless or remote access. May include transportation planning (transition and options), cessation planning, and recommendations for clients as passengers.	Offers a wide variety of adaptive equipment and vehicle options for comprehensive driving evaluation, training and education, including all services available in Low Tech and Basic programs. At this level, providers have the ability to alter positioning of primary and secondary controls based on client's need or ability level. High tech adaptive equipment for primary and secondary controls includes devices that meet the following conditions: 1. Capable of controlling vehicle functions or driving controls, and 2. Consists of a programmable computerized system that interfaces/integrates with an electronic system in the vehicle.
ACCESS TO DRIVER'S POSITION	Requires independent transfer into OEM^ driver's seat in vehicle.	Addresses transfers, seating and position into OEM^ driver's seat. May make recommendations for assistive devices to access driver's seat, improved positioning, wheelchair securement systems, and/or mechanical wheelchair loading devices.	Access to the vehicle typically requires ramp or lift and may require adaptation to OEM driver's seat. Access to driver position may be dependent on use of a transfer seat base, or clients may drive from their wheelchair. Provider evaluates and recommends vehicle structural modifications to accommodate products such as ramps, lifts, wheelchair and scooter hoists, transfer seat bases, wheelchairs suitable to utilize as a driver seat, and/or wheelchair securement systems.

Continued

TABLE 16-4 The American Occupational Therapy Association and Association for Driver Rehabilitation Specialists' Document Showing the Range of Driver Rehabilitation Programs, Used With Permission. (continued)

LEVELS OF PROGRAM AND TYPICAL PROVIDER CREDENTIALS	BASIC	LOW TECH	HIGH TECH
TYPICAL VEHICLE MODIFICATION: PRIMARY CONTROLS: GAS, BRAKE, STEERING	Uses OEM^ controls.	Primary driving control examples: A) mechanical gas/brake hand control; B) left foot accelerator pedal; C) pedal extensions; D) park brake lever or electronic park brake; E) steering device (spinner knob, tri-pin, C-cuff).	Primary driving control examples (in addition to low tech options): A) powered gas/brake systems; B) power park brake integrated with a powered gas/brake system; C) variable effort steering systems; D) reduced diameter steering wheel, horizontal steering, steering wheel extension, joystick controls; E) reduced effort brake systems.
TYPICAL VEHICLE MODIFICATION: SECONDARY CONTROLS	Uses OEM^ controls.	Secondary driving control examples: A) remote horn button; B) turn signal modification (remote, crossover lever); C) remote wiper controls; D) gear selector modification; E) key/ignition adaptions.	Electronic systems to access secondary and accessory controls. Secondary driving control examples (in addition to low tech options): A) remote panels, touch pads, or switch arrays that interface with OEM* electronics; B) wiring extension for OEM^ electronics; C) powered transmission shifter.

DRS-Health professional degree with specialty training in driver evaluation and rehabilitation, **CDRS*-Certified Driver Rehabilitation Specialist-Credentialed by ADED (Association for Driver Rehabilitation Specialists), +*SCDCM-Specialty Certified in Driving and Community Mobility* by AOTA (American Occupational Therapy Association), ^OEM-Original Equipment installed by Manufacturer. Reference: NMEDA Guidelines http://www.nmeda.com.
**LDI-licensed driving instructor

as with driving. The recommendation "to refrain from driving at this point in the recovery process" can be stated with confidence, without a referral to a DRS.

WHEN TO REFER TO A DRIVER REHABILITATION SPECIALIST

When a client tells the OTA "I want to drive when I am discharged," it becomes a responsibility of the OTA to respond appropriately. Figure 16-2 may assist both the OTA and the supervising occupational therapist to make appropriate plans for the client; this graphic is based on the image of a stoplight, which goes from green (go) to yellow (caution), to red (stop). It is a matter of considering the evidence from evaluation results, intervention with the ADL/IADL skills, using clinical judgment, and the risks involved with driving. The client with significant impairments in all areas of function (e.g., cognition, vision, motor) represents the individuals who are in the "higher risk" area of Figure 16-2. When the generalist OT practitioner recognizes that the client with severe or multiple impairments exceed the thresholds in one or more areas, it means that driving is a high-risk activity. Therefore, informing the client, family, and rehabilitation team is appropriate. Sending the client to a DRS is unwarranted in terms of cost for a specialized evaluation or the emotional turmoil of a negative outcome. That is not to say the client will never drive again. In fact, like all other valued occupations, practitioners can use this desire to return as motivation to work toward improvement. Importantly, driving and community mobility should be part of the overall goal-setting and intervention plan to preserve mobility by planning for supportive transportation until a final driving decision might be made.

Conversely, clients who recover quickly from their medical event and demonstrate no impairment with other complex IADL skills likely have no need to see a DRS either. If there are no indications or "red flags," driving may not be a concern. However, this does not mean the OT practitioner is saying, "The client is a safe driver." The client may actually be a poor driver because of bad habits; however, the evaluation results do not warrant further investigation. For the older adult, it is also a good time to share information about changes associated with aging and encourage the older adult to maximize skills to maintain driving skills and abilities.

The middle group on Figure 16-2 refers to individuals in this area, as those drivers in the "gray" area. These clients are recovering from their condition, demonstrating gains in the functional areas of cognition, motor, vision, and perception. They will likely return to many previous roles and functional abilities. This group may also include clients with degenerative disorders who are losing strengths and skills. These clients

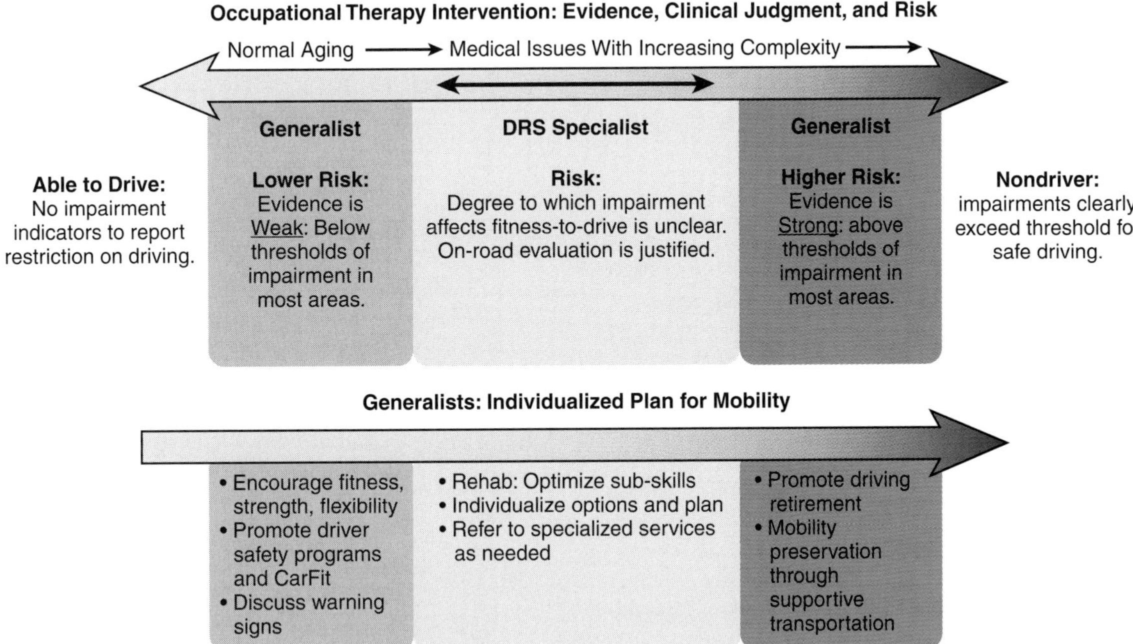

FIGURE 16-2. Decision making graphic. The original graphic used green/yellow/red colors to represent levels of risk, which in this graphic are in more muted colors. *From left:* Lower risk (green-go), risk (yellow-caution), and high risk (red-stop), to guide the OT practitioner in decision making.

"in the gray area" are the ones in which the general practitioner cannot definitively make the decision about fitness to drive and thus need to refer on to a specialist. Research has shown that an outcome of assessment of IADLs validity predicts how someone might do on a driving evaluation.[1] Specifically, using the Assessment of Motor and Process Skills (AMPS)[18] differentiated between drivers who passed and drivers who failed a driving evaluation. This research supports the general OT practitioner's roles in contributing critical information to the specialist. Thus, general OT practitioners should develop referral pathways to the specialist by providing valuable referral information, specifically including results of assessment tools or evaluation outcomes that allows the specialist to specifically target the questionable areas rather than having the client undergo a lengthy, broad-based evaluation, duplicating services and evaluations already completed and paid for by the client or third party payers.

It has been argued that there are not nearly enough DRSs in the United States to provide comprehensive driving evaluations for each client who wants and needs to resume driving.[1,32] This is true in some areas of the country, but the focus needs to be on increasing capacity of DRSs and OT generalists who collaboratively work together to meet the needs. In fact, the goal of the Gaps and Pathways Project–a joint collaboration of NHTSA and AOTA–is to build and expand the pathways or referral links between the OT generalists and driver rehabilitation specialists.[13] Similarly, in Canada, the Canadian Association of Occupational Therapists works closely with ADED, collaborating via joint conferences, education, and services. The general OT practitioner has the skills, knowledge, and abilities to observe and describe their client's functional performance and prepare the client for referral when appropriate.

CLINICAL OBSERVATIONS OF FUNCTIONAL PERFORMANCE

OT practitioners observe, analyze, and describe functional performance using clinical reasoning. Recently, Dickerson and Bédard[33] developed a decision tool for clients with medical issues, specifically a generalist's framework for identifying driving risk as well as the potential to return to driving. The framework is based on Michon's three levels of driving behaviors: strategic, tactical, and operational.[34] The strategic or highest level is the decision-making process of planning trip goals and mode of transport (e.g., vehicle, walking, biking) to get to the destination. Strategic planning is also needed when a driver comes upon an accident and has to make the decision of whether to find an alternative route.[35]

The second level consists of tactical behaviors, the behaviors related to decisions made during driving maneuvers such as slowing for weather, when to pass a vehicle, making a turn, using a turn signal, and other maneuvers. The lowest level, operational behaviors, is the overlearned human-machine interactions necessary to control the vehicle. These include using the brake, turning the steering wheel, and pressing the accelerator. There are the skills one does automatically; for example, driving a familiar route every morning so that memory of driving the actual route is forgotten.

Dickerson and Bédard[33] described and linked person factors needed for safe driving (i.e., physical/sensory, cognitive, emotional regulation, insight) under each of the three levels of driving behaviors (Table 16-5). Using examples of clinical observation questions for each level of behavior (Table 16-6), the OTA can use these questions to complete the designed checklist (Fig. 16-3). The decision tool

TABLE 16-5 Occupational Therapy—Performance Appraisal for Driving (OT-PAD)[33]

Purpose: Driving is a complex instrumental activity of daily living (IADL). Consequently, using clinical reasoning based on evaluation results, knowledge of the client, and observation of clients performing other complex tasks, OT practitioners can make recommendations about the activity of driving. The OT-PAD has been designed as a clinical tool to assist practitioners in making the link between their knowledge and the activity of driving as well and considerations for supports or requirements for community mobility options.

The person factors that are most likely to affect driving include: *physical/sensory, cognitive, emotional regulation,* and *insight.* Questions are separated into three sections, based on Michon's three levels of Driving Behaviors.

WHEN RELATED TO DRIVING, THESE ARE DEFINED AS:	
***Strategic** level: Decision-making process, affecting all levels of driving*	• Determining trip goals and mode of transport (e.g., bike, drive, walk) • Navigating how to get there as well as being able to modify or change "plans," both in anticipation of trip and while on the road
***Tactical** level: Decisions/maneuvers made during driving maneuvers*	• Slowing down due to weather • Knowing if it is safe to make a left turn • Deciding whether to pass a slower vehicle
***Operational** level: Human-machine interaction used to control the vehicle*	• Steering, pushing brake pedal, using turn signal • Having the physical skills to carry out the tactical maneuvers • Possessing the overlearned skills developed through driving experience
EXAMPLES OF IADL APPLICATIONS FOR EACH OF THE THREE LEVELS.	**CLIENT NOTES:**
Strategic: *Does the client have the cognitive ability to make decisions at the strategic level?*	
• Does the client know whether he or she has the information to make an appropriate decision? Does the client initiate seeking additional or clarifying information?	
• If the client were to make a meal, would he or she be able to plan it correctly (with similar competence to prior his or her medical condition)?	
• Can the client recognize, organize, reorder from pharmacy, and remember to take medication accurately and safely?	
• Can the client plan a meeting with a friend or family member or make an appointment and appropriately follow through without instructions from others?	
• Is the client able to calm down and perform tasks after being surprised, flustered, or annoyed by any incidents or other people?	
• Does the client plan how to manage his or her physical mobility within the immediate environment without significant assistance (i.e., how to plan to get his or her wheelchair in and out of a vehicle as well as in and out of the home)?	
Tactical: *Does the client have the performance skills to perform actions at this level?*	
• Does the client immediately slow down when there is a wet floor or pavement?	
• Does the client acknowledge others passing by in the hallway or on the sidewalk to say hello in recognition?	
• Does the client adjust or accommodate immediately and appropriately when problems occur, such as being disconnected on a phone call, when coffee is spilled, a pet jumps up and down, a family member doesn't show up, a household item breaks, or food burns on the stove?	
• Is the client able to multitask (i.e., one task being automatic), like walk and talk, read and drink, wash dishes and talk on the phone, tell a story and exercise, give instructions and make coffee?	

TABLE 16-5 Occupational Therapy—Performance Appraisal for Driving (OT-PAD)[33] (continued)

EXAMPLES OF IADL APPLICATIONS FOR EACH OF THE THREE LEVELS.	CLIENT NOTES:
Operational: *Does the client have the performance skills to perform actions at this level?*	
• Does the client perform normal daily tasks efficiently and automatically without cues (e.g., brushing teeth, self-feeding, dressing)?	
• Does the client have difficulty manipulating tools like cutlery?	
• Does the client bump into doorways or walls?	
• If the client loses balance, is his or her recovery effective?	
• How does the client react to environmental changes?	
• How fast does the client recognize change in the environment? For example:	
• Does the client immediately see when someone enters the room?	
• Does the client recognize sounds and the sources of the sound?	

TABLE 16-6 Degree of Impairment[33]

The OT-PAD facilitates the *link* between daily tasks and driving. Using clinical reasoning based on evaluation results, knowledge of the client, and clinical observations, indicate the degree of impairment for each *person factor* under each *level of driving behavior.*

LEVELS	*DESCRIPTORS OF HOW TO CONSIDER EACH FACTOR UNDER EACH LEVEL: PHYSICAL/SENSORY, COGNITIVE, EMOTIONAL REGULATION, AND INSIGHT*	DEGREE OF IMPAIRMENT			
		None	*Mild*	*Moderate*	*Severe*
Strategic: *Does the client have the cognitive ability to make decisions?*	**Physical/sensory**–Aware of physical limitations and is able to plan for successful compensation (e.g., if in a wheelchair, demonstrates ability to plan time and/or assistance for transfer).				
	Cognitive–Demonstrates ability to plan in advance using appropriate decisions to meet the goals of the task; self-regulates with insight into decisions; organizes steps to complete task.				
	Emotional regulation–Can plan with appreciation of the emotional state (e.g., Does not drive if experiencing excessive, anxiety, depression, or anger).				
	Insight–Has accurate awareness of the skills and abilities he or she possesses to meet the demands of the task (e.g., to clean the windows, skills/abilities to use a ladder safety? Can make modified decisions based on driving experience and/or training.)				
Tactical: *Does the client have performance skills to perform actions at this level?*	**Physical/sensory**–Is aware of his or her physical limitation and adjusts as required (e.g., if floors are wet, walks more slowly).				
	Cognitive–Can evaluate a complex, dynamic context and adjust or accommodate through appropriate actions.				
	Emotional regulation–Can recognize and manage emotions that arise in challenging situations.				
	Insight–Can accurately gauge the risk and skills/abilities needed to meet the demands of a task requiring immediate decisions.				
Operational: *Does the client have performance skills to perform actions at this level?*	**Physical/sensory**–Meets the minimum requirements (e.g., vision) or is able to compensate for limitation (e.g., with training, will be able to use hand controls to compensate a lower extremity amputation)				
	Cognitive–Awareness and flexibility to use the appropriate actions to achieve desired results.				
	Emotional regulation–Emotional state does not negatively affect performance of automatic tasks.				
	Insight –Not applicable.				

		None	Mild	Moderate	Severe
Strategic	Physical/Sensory				
	Cognitive				
	Emotional				
	Insight				
Tactical	Physical/Sensory				
	Cognitive				
	Emotional				
	Insight				
Operational	Physical/Sensory				
	Cognitive				
	Emotional				
	Insight				

FIGURE 16-3. Sample write-up form.

was designed to assist practitioners with extrapolating from the client's performance of tasks identifying fitness to drive.[33] In other words, this decision tool will help the OTA to identify risk and identify the degree of impairment (i.e., none, mild, moderate, severe). Because this is a new tool, there is no research to identify how many "flags" warrant a recommendation, but it can be used as a tool for the OTA to discuss issues of concern with the supervising occupational therapist. This discussion may lead to 1) further evaluation, 2) changes in intervention to addresses performance underlying driving and community mobility, or 3) a referral to a DRS as discussed previously.

INTERVENTIONS TO FACILITATE RETURNING TO DRIVING

Because driving is so important to clients, they may not ask about driving to avoid the answer "You cannot drive." Families or caregivers may not recognize driving as an issue or may want to avoid the responsibility of a spouse, parent, or sibling who will need assistance with transportation. Because of these possibilities, it is important for the OT practitioner to bring up the issue of mobility with the client as well as the primary caregiver. This is especially true as the client is recovering function and is gaining independence or losing function as with a progressive disorder. As an occupation, community mobility is essential to maintain connections to community and quality of life and, therefore, is a part of the OT practitioner's ethical obligation.[1]

If the client does ask about returning to driving, the obvious question becomes what exercises or therapies improve function in the areas needed for driving. Because driving is a complex task that requires the integration of sensory, motor, visual, and perceptual skills with good executive functioning, it is not a simple answer with cookbook specific activities to practice. Doing exercises on paper to improve scanning skills, block sorting for facilitating perceptual skills, or computer rehabilitation may improve discrete skill sets, but using actual complex activities are necessary to challenge the integration of the neurological system and facilitate the reorganization process.

Other chapters in this book will expand on many of these processes and specific therapeutic interventions. The main point here is that the occupation of driving uses all the same underlying processes used in other complex IADLs. Therefore, therapeutic interventions to assist the client in regaining driving skills and abilities are not any different from other ADL or IADL tasks. As a client makes a meal in the kitchen, he or she is using the same component skill set for driving, including vision, coordination, problem-solving, attention, and many others. The key to success is using all the therapeutic interventions possible to ensure the client has recovered functionally and has the potential to pass the on-road assessment before sending the client for a comprehensive driving evaluation or driving test. That said, there is one possible exception of a therapeutic activity that might be contextually unique for driving, the interactive driving simulator.

INTERACTIVE DRIVING SIMULATORS

An **interactive driving simulator** is defined as a computer-controlled environment that represents selected aspects of the driving experience considered to be representational of real-world driving. It allows objective measurements of clients' responses to designated driving tasks and scenarios and how the responses influence subsequent events within the limits of the parameters of the simulation program through accelerator, brake, and steering components (Fig. 16-4). There is a wide range of simulators, from desktop computer programs with one screen to total immersion, where one sits in a motor vehicle and views a wide screen projection of a driving scene. However, for OT providers, there are a handful of models that have been designed and developed specifically for clinical use. Furthermore, there is beginning evidence for the efficacy of using driving simulators for both assessment and intervention in driver rehabilitation.[1,36] In a study with clients who were 6-month post-CVA the researchers found that performance on the on-road test improved significantly more in the simulator group than in the cognitive tasks group, supporting the argument that "rehabilitation of driving skills after CVA should focus on direct training of functional skills rather than its component parts."[37] These results also support other studies that suggest driving simulator skills can be generalized to real-world driving.[38–40]

These results have two major implications for OT practice. First, the studies support the concept that performing occupation-based activities provide greater rehabilitation potential. That is not to say that component-based therapy is not useful, but the integration and use of functional tasks at the right level of challenge will improve function over component-based exercise. The second implication is the recognition of recovery of function often occurs over time. It is therefore important to make sure clients have adequate resources and information for pursuing driver evaluation and rehabilitation beyond the short time they are in rehabilitation services.

A barrier to the use of driver simulators is simulator adaptation syndrome or simulator sickness. Simulator sickness is similar to motion sickness,[41] a physical discomfort experienced when driving a simulated vehicle because of the incompatible sensations of visual, auditory, and motions systems. Symptoms include dizziness, restlessness, cold sweats, nausea, and vomiting. Clients are more susceptible if they are over 70 years of age and female. The contextual and environment design of the scenarios (e.g., curves and turns), duration, simulator configuration, and calibration of the brake and accelerator also contribute. However, mitigation strategies can be effective and include diet (not an empty stomach but not full, and water and/or crackers can settle the stomach), room temperature and airflow (cooler works better, and a fan may help), and keeping turns to a minimum.[36,42] The other barrier to driving simulators is training. Driving simulators are deceptively easy to use. Regardless, using a driving simulator is a complex tool and the OT practitioner wanting to use it "needs to seek and obtain the appropriate education and training to use this tool effectively, appropriately, and with the knowledge to minimize simulator sickness."[36]

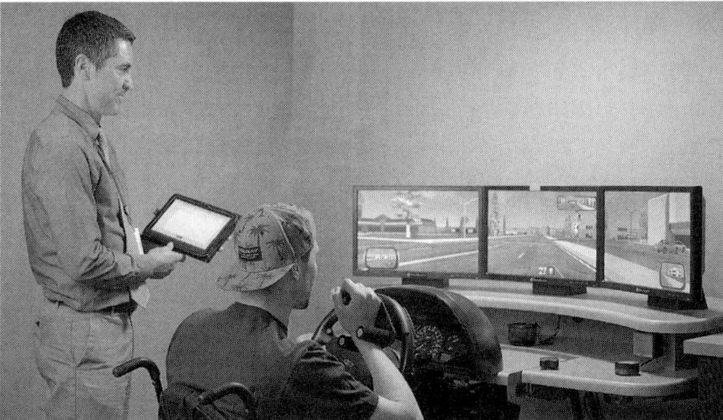

FIGURE 16-4. A client learns to use adaptive equipment on a DriveSafety CDS-200 driving simulator. The driving simulator provides a wide range of driving scenes for the client to experience before driving on the road. *(Courtesy DriveSafety, Inc.)*

ADAPTIVE EQUIPMENT AND VEHICLE MODIFICATION FOR DRIVING

For OT practitioners working with adults, adaptive equipment, demonstration, and practice for the transferring in and out of a vehicle should be a priority for all clients who are returning home. The client and family will be in all likelihood returning to their home via a motor vehicle and will have follow-up medical appointments, including therapy. Techniques of transfers do not necessarily differ from other types of transfers, but tools such as the HandyBar® that provides a portable support on either side of the vehicle or a car caddie attaches to the frame of a vehicle and can be used to offer balancing support (Fig. 16-5). A padded swivel seat might be used to allow more lateral and rotational

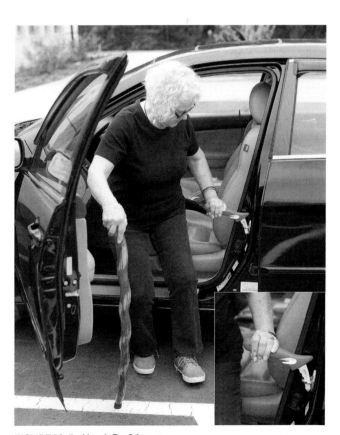

FIGURE 16-5. HandyBar® in use.

movement. However, motor vehicles seats are designed to prevent injuries during a crash and any change to the design, like adding a cushion, changes the dynamics of the vehicle protection, so this should be avoided unless absolutely necessary.

With some conditions, such as CVA, there is impairment that requires the use of adaptive equipment that will change the functioning of the primary or secondary functions of the motor vehicle. If these are needed, the specialized training and/or experience of the DRS is needed as identified in Box 16-2. Thus, if the client needs adaptive equipment, a referral to a DRS is necessary. Based on Box 16-2, the practitioner needs to decide the level of program complexity required by the client. For those adaptations that require some modification of a vehicle, the DRS's low tech level will meet these needs. When the client may not be able to transfer or has significant disabilities, such as a C5 SCI, a high tech referral would be best. Table 16-7 describes some common types of adaptations, so the OTA understands what options are available for the client. It is important for the OTA to be aware of the range of possibilities for adaptation to vehicles so that physical limitations do not prevent returning to driving, but also understanding the driver-vehicle interaction is complex and needs the appropriate level of expertise to prescribe, fit to the vehicle, and to train. Young adults with life-long disabilities such as muscular dystrophy or cerebral palsy generally will require specialized evaluation, equipment, and training by a DRS to be able to drive. These clients may need adapted driver's education, may drive with joystick and computerized controls, and will have very specific and individualized options designed for them. Some disabilities, unfortunately, will preclude ever driving in a safe and controlled manner, and the OTA can address alternative transportation options.

BOX 16-2

Adaptive Equipment for Vehicles: When Is it Appropriate to Refer to a Driver Rehabilitation Specialist?

- When the client has the potential to drive with specialized equipment in their vehicles
- If the client will need a new vehicle to accommodate a motorized wheelchair. If a client was in a motor vehicle accident and will need a wheelchair, often the family replaces the damaged vehicle without realizing the need for a specialized vehicle. In these cases, an early referral is important to have the best information for purchasing a vehicle that meets the needs of the family
- To determine whether the installation of the equipment meets the client's needs (e.g., a check to see if the adaptive equipment is functional for the client)
- To assist to train the client to use any type of specialized equipment
- To offer opportunities to "try out" different types of equipment (e.g., models of hand controls are varied)

VEHICLE OPTIONS

For the client who uses a wheelchair, especially a power wheelchair, transportation can be an issue. Complex power wheelchairs can weigh over 400 pounds, and certainly do not disassemble to go into a vehicle. Even a small scooter can have the heaviest part at 35 pounds, which may be unreasonable for a caregiver to manage. Lifts can be added externally in the hitch or internally to a vehicle to allow these

TABLE 16-7 Common Adaptive Equipment for Personal Motor Vehicles

Steering wheel additions	If a client has an amputation, weakness in grip, or a nonfunctional arm, there may be limitations on the ability to steer the motor vehicle, and a steering wheel attachment could be installed to use for steering. It would also be used with hand controls for increased control over the wheel. There are different types, sizes, and positions of the mount, depending on the client's specific deficits. Some hold the hand attached safely to the wheel when the client has decreased grip strength.	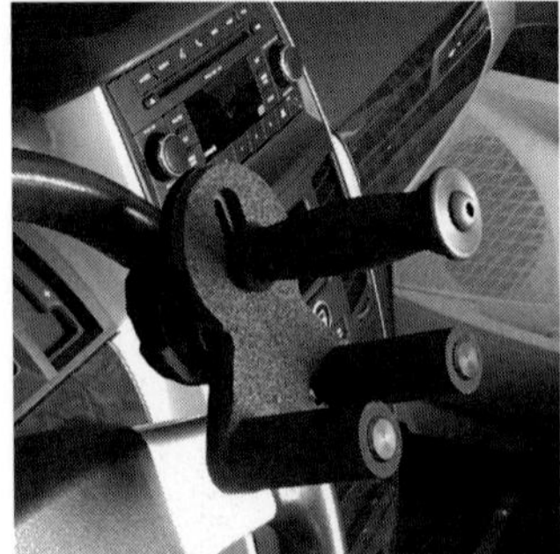 Tri-pin on steering wheel. *(Courtesy of Veigel North America-www.veigel-na.com.)*
Secondary control extensions	To drive safely, one hand must always be on the steering wheel. Therefore, turn signal extensions as well as other extensions for wipers, cruise control, gear selector, or headlights can be installed to facilitate the use of the controls of the vehicle without taking one hand from the wheel. These are designed differently, depending on the unique needs of the client and the vehicle.	

TABLE 16-7 Common Adaptive Equipment for Personal Motor Vehicles (continued)

Left foot accelerator	When the client does not have full functioning of the right leg, then the person may require a left foot gas pedal. This will allow the client to use both accelerator and brake with the left unaffected limb. The alternative is hand controls. It is always important to get an evaluation for determining which is best for the client.	
Hand controls	These are often used when the driver has mild to severe leg weakness and cannot use the right or left foot accelerator and brake. The client holds a lever off the left side of the steering column, and one direction is gas and one is brake. Typically used with a steering wheel adaptation to allow for easy turning with one hand.	Hand controls mounted in a car.
Panoramic mirrors	Special mirrors can be used when neck range of motion is limited or to increase visual awareness to the rear, sides, and blind spots. It is important to note that these mirrors do not compensate for field cut deficits. The client with a field cut should see a rehabilitation optometrist as well as a DRS. Some states have certain restrictions, so visual acuity, contrast sensitivity, and field cut should be measured precisely.	
Adapted seats	Vehicles can be adapted with special seats, either in the driver's or passenger's position. The seats, with power, can rotate and move in multiple directions, and even lower outside the vehicle for a safer transfer.	
Safety restraints	All wheelchairs must be securely tied down or attached in the vehicle to avoid being a projectile out of the vehicle in an accident. Most chairs have specific tie down spots designated or recommended for securement. The client can use four ratchet straps, or there are automatic securement systems such as EZ Lock Wheelchair Docking Systems™ or Q-Straint®. These systems have a V-shaped metal piece attached in the floor of the vehicle and a bolt attached under the wheelchair. The client simply drives the bolt into the slot, and the whole chair bolts to the vehicle. It releases with a remote button push.	

Elements of this chapter are the result of working with Elin Schold Davis, Project Coordinator of the Older Driver Initiative at the American Occupational Therapy Association, on the *Gaps and Pathways Project* funded by the National Highway Traffic Safety Administration.

important mobility devices to be taken to destinations with access, thus providing the client with more flexibility in mobility than with a cane or walker (Fig. 16-6). If the mobility device is carried externally, the weight of the device on the frame of the car must be considered. Hitch lifts can have a ramp that folds out to load the mobility device or a battery-operated, height adjustable platform. Certainly loading and unloading as well as carrying the device in the rain and weather is a consideration as well as transferring the potentially dependent client into a vehicle seat. A small trailer may allow a smaller vehicle to carry the weight of a heavier chair, and a grill cover tied down over the chair can keep off the rain.

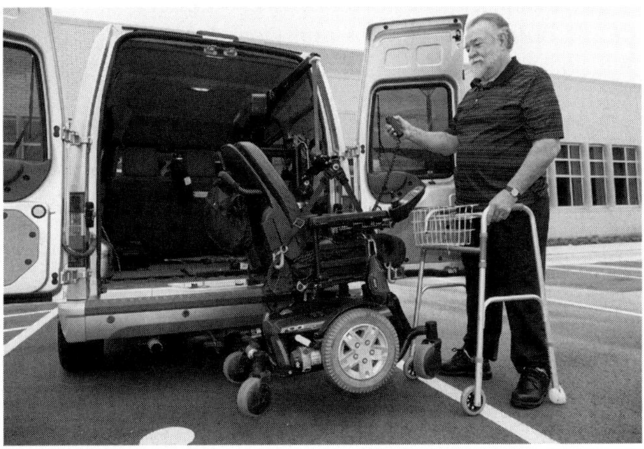

FIGURE 16-6. Loading a power wheelchair into the back of a van with a power lift system.

Another option can be a vehicle that is modified to carry a wheelchair inside it during transport. This is generally a minivan or full-sized van, which has been modified with a raised roof and/or lowered floor for increased headroom so clients can enter the van sitting in their mobility device. Either a ramp will fold out of the back or side, or a lift will raise and lower to allow this (Fig. 16-6 and Fig. 16-7). Once inside, the client can transfer to the driver's or passenger's seat (preferable), or stay in the wheelchair (if it is designed/tested for this purpose). Either way, the wheelchair must be secured, and the person must be secured as well, not only by the wheelchair seat belt, but a safety shoulder harness and belt attached in the vehicle.

Accessible vehicles can be rented by the day, week, or month as required for a specific need if the client does not

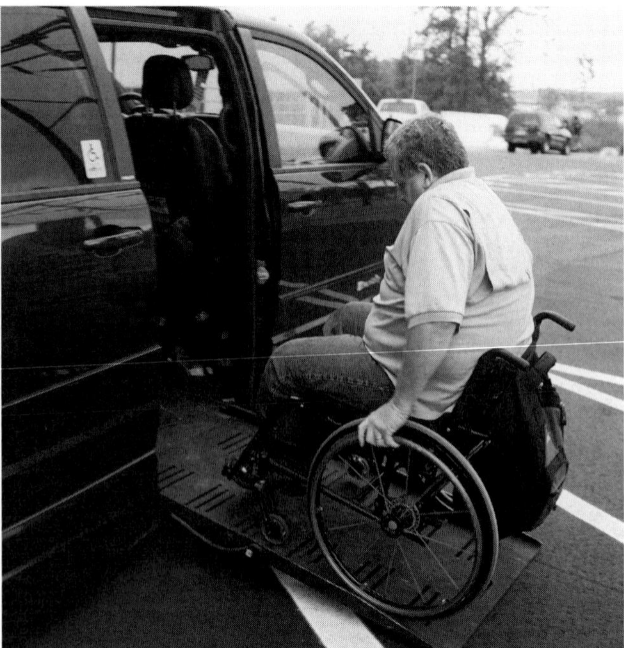

FIGURE 16-7. Manual wheelchair going into an accessible van.

have the resources to outright purchase an accessible vehicle. There are also wheelchair transport companies that will offer rides for a fee, and accessible taxi services. Vocational Rehabilitation and Worker's compensation, as well as private fundraising and grants, may assist to purchase a vehicle.

ALTERNATIVE TRANSPORTATION OPTIONS

The reality is that for some adult clients, there will not be enough functional recovery to learn to drive or return to driving, usually as a result of significant deficits in physical, perceptual, or cognitive functions. This is often very difficult for the client to accept,[1] and in fact, many individuals continue to drive regardless of the medical recommendation.[5,43] The loss of a driver's license can change a person's life dramatically. The client may no longer be able to live alone and will need to depend on others for transportation. If there are no family members or friends available, the client will be further isolated because if driving is not possible due to medical impairments, it is possible that any sort of public transportation will not be an option for those same reasons. This will further eliminate many social activities that are important for maintaining contact with others. Although taxis, ridesharing services, and wheelchair transport options may be seen as expensive, one strategy is to work out a budget with the client to show that this sort of transportation may be cheaper than owning a car and paying for maintenance, gas, parking, and insurance.

OT practitioners need to make sure clients have community mobility through transportation planning and by providing the client and family with information and resources. Working through the client's actual transportation needs on paper as well as with family and friends, who might provide assistance, may alleviate the anxiety of not being able to get to where the person needs and wants to go. As with any client who needs to retire from driving, the OT practitioner needs to address the client's community mobility needs. Because each community is unique, practitioners should build relationships and work with local agencies (e.g., local councils on aging, Area Agencies for Aging, public transport), national agencies (e.g., American Association of Retired Persons (AARP), Veteran's Administration) as well as disease/disability specific organizations (Muscular Dystrophy Association, Multiple Sclerosis Society) to develop a specific list to guide clients and caregivers.

For adults with disabilities that would preclude them from driving, the OTA can assist with planning how to get around the community and to the places the individual needs and wants to go. This may include:

- Educating and training the family, extended family, or friends on how to appropriately transfer the client in and out of vehicles

TECHNOLOGY AND TRENDS

With technology growing exponentially, it is often heard in social media that self-driving cars will be the answer in the next 5 years. Individuals who are blind or have cognitive deficits will be able to get into a vehicle and tell it where to go. More than likely, however, the population is years from having self-driving cars for all individuals who may need it. Why? Although advancements such as the advance crash warnings that work well on highways or city traffic to inform the driver if the vehicle ahead makes a sudden stop or is slowing down, they are not able to replace the driver entirely. What these warnings not been perfected to do is to see a deer or pedestrian that comes, not from the front, but an odd angle that is not within the "range" of the sensor. The second major issue is liability. If there is a crash because of the technology, who is at fault? The driver? He or she was dependent on the car to "self-drive." The car dealership or manufacturer? Imagine how that can possibly happen. The problem is that technology breaks down. Humans "take over" when cruise control turns off. If Mr. Smith has dementia and is using a self-driving car that has a problem—is he capable of "taking over?" OT practitioners struggle with deciding how impaired someone has to be retiring from driving. With the self-driving car, it is the same questions-how impaired can a person be to use a high tech car so that the person is "safe" if it fails? The last major issue is the environment. Self-driving cars use environmental technology to get to their destinations. This can be done in many ways, but most envision sensors in the roadways to track and monitor the car to get to the destination. In one city alone, how will this technology be able to be incorporated into the environment without being cost prohibitive? So, either way, OTAs working in driving and community mobility will be needed long into the future, and actually will be able to make a significant contribution to keep clients as independent as possible.

- Assisting the client and family to explore other types of personal transportation options, such as purchasing a used adapted van
- Assisting the client and family to find private medical transportation, such as local companies who have accessible vans
- Training in the use of public transportation (e.g., buses, subways, trains) in order for the client to get to where he or she wants and/or needs to go
- Training the client to access and read public transportation schedules, plan routes, and assess the cost and method(s) of payment
- Contacting the client's community's public transportation to determine how to access Americans with Disabilities Act (ADA)-required public transportation
- Assisting with potential volunteer transportation programs, taxi services, or new services such as ride sharing or apps, especially if finances are an issue
- Discussing safety concerns of using public transportation
- Helping establish new routines for family/caregivers if they need to provide transportation for the client (for example, providing transportation for a college student who needs to attend classes at the local university but still lives at home)
- Training and educating wheelchair users who live in urban areas to navigate the challenges of traffic, pedestrians, weather, and also safety concerns

Finally, as described in the beginning of this chapter, driving is a valued occupation, especially for older adults who grew up with the "car." The occupation of driving is and will continue to be an activity that defines adults of all ages in terms of success and independence. Sometimes it is not just about getting where they need and want to go–but the feeling of being independent, able to do what they want to do when they want to do it. Some older adults do not need to drive, but they like seeing the vehicle there–"just in case." It is important to respect that losing the ability to drive is a loss for any adult–just like losing a pet or loved one, losing walking ability, or losing one's home or independence. The OTA does not always need to find the answer, but respect the client's feelings and demonstrate understanding and empathy.

Because driving and community mobility is such a major issue for Baby Boomers, there has been an explosion of websites and resources developed to address this issue. Although many of these websites have good information, there are often competing agendas and opinions, and just because it is on the Internet–does not make it true! It is critical to be informed and make sure the most evidenced-based information is available. Thus, it is important to use resources and websites that are driven by medically based or research-based information without trying to "sell" something. One such website is the new Clearinghouse for Older Road Users (ChORUS), funded by the U.S. Department of Transportation's Federal Highway Administration (FHWA) and the NHTSA. This site serves as a centralized, user-friendly, and dynamic source of information pertaining to highway safety for aging drivers, passengers, pedestrians, and cyclists. Built as a comprehensive resource, it covers all three major components of highway safety: safe roadways, safe road users, and safe vehicles. A board of subject matter experts approve what is put on the website to ensure the information is accurate, up-to-date, and focused on providing the best information.

SUMMARY

This chapter discusses driving and community mobility with the emphasis on why and how the OTA should address this valued and important IADL. Community mobility, regardless of the method (e.g., walking, biking, driving, public transit) is critical to our medically impaired clients. The skilled observation of performance is the key for identifying risk, making appropriate referrals to driver rehabilitation specialists, as well as receiving additional intervention to assist with community mobility options. Additionally, when informing someone of a recommendation for cessation of driving, the client and caregiver may not be emotionally ready to receive additional referral information, if even available. A pathway between generalist and specialist can work both ways; if the client fails evaluations to be able to drive a vehicle, then they could be referred back to the general OT practitioner to work on community mobility through alternative transportation.

Although driving is a privilege granted by the state or province, community mobility is a right for everyone. As OTAs work with adult clients, there is an obligation to take on the challenge of addressing driving and community mobility. One of the most important takeaways from this chapter is the ability for the OTA to understand that it is important to address driving and community mobility as an IADL. It is vital to consider how the OTA can assist a client with his/her mobility needs, and when it is necessary to refer to a driver rehabilitation specialist. Collaborating with the specialists in the community and region will mean that OTAs are able to serve the functional needs and occupations of their clients. OT has an opportunity to be the nationally recognized profession meeting the needs of driving–one of the most valued functional activities for young and older adults.

REVIEW QUESTIONS

1. A client has had a mild CVA, but still has mild right-sided weakness and inattention to the right. The OTA knows the client drove to their outpatient appointment, and when asked, the client says it was fine to drive. What is the *first* step the OTA should take?
   a. Call the client's family.
   b. Call the client's medical doctor.
   c. Ask the occupational therapist to assess the client further.
   d. Refer the client to a driving evaluator.
2. The OTA is observing a client having difficulty with making a sandwich for lunch. The client planned to use ham but instead made a peanut butter and jelly sandwich when he saw the jar of jelly. The client then comments his wife is happy he is being discharged because she does not like to drive and he will take

over driving again when he is discharged tomorrow. Which three of the following should the OTA do?
  a. Talk to his wife about not allowing him to drive.
  b. Investigate whether cognitive impairment has been identified with the client.
  c. Ignore the comment, as the OTA was not asked to evaluate his driving ability.
  d. Document the observations.
  e. Speak with the supervising occupational therapist or team member about the observations.
  f. Remind him about his desire for ham on his sandwich.
3. The hospital is considering getting a driving simulator. The occupational therapist asks the OTA to read up on how to use the simulator for intervention. Which three things should the OTA do?
  a. Practice on the driving simulator.
  b. Seek training for use of the driving simulator through continuing education or mentorship.
  c. Call AOTA about how to charge for services on the driving simulator.
  d. Find a document to show that using a driving simulator is not appropriate for the OTA.
  e. Investigate the types of simulators available on the Internet.
  f. Call a colleague who uses simulation.
4. The client has recovered fairly well from his CVA. He really wants to return to driving, but has some physical and visual impairments that may affect driving. A referral to a driver rehabilitation specialist is appropriate at which level?
  a. Basic
  b. Low tech
  c. High tech
  d. A referral is not appropriate
5. The client has progressive dementia. Both he and his spouse understand it is safer for him to cease driving, but the wife has done virtually no driving for the past ten years. Which three of the following are the *most appropriate* recommendations?
  a. Encourage him to continue to drive, as long as the wife is able to be a passenger and direct him.
  b. Encourage the wife to see a driving instructor to brush up on her driving abilities and skills.
  c. Encourage the wife to see a driver rehabilitation specialist for a comprehensive driving evaluation.
  d. Encourage the client to see a driver rehabilitation specialist for a comprehensive driving evaluation so he can continue to drive.
  e. Speak with the occupational therapist and/or the team about alternative methods of transportation for the couple.
  f. Offer resources about driving safety to both the client and his spouse.
6. For a client with a permanent disability, such as a SCI, when would be the ideal time to bring in the driver rehabilitation specialist?
  a. Soon, in the beginning of the rehabilitation process
  b. After the client has completed inpatient rehabilitation
  c. After the client has completed all hospital-based rehabilitation
  d. When the client is optimally recovered and ready to drive
7. The client with vascular dementia has a significant cognitive impairment that will prevent her from returning to independent driving. What would be the next intervention for the OT practitioner to do?
  a. Discuss options for using public transportation because the client lives near a bus line.
  b. Work with the family on options for maximizing the client's mobility with a transportation plan.
  c. Discuss options for learning to use a taxi or ride sharing service.
  d. Give a list of potential volunteer driving programs.
8. A typical OT practitioner who specializes in driver rehabilitation provides:
  a. Comprehensive driving evaluations, training, and recommendations for modifications of vehicles
  b. Driving education, comprehensive driving evaluations, training, and recommendations for modifications of vehicles
  c. Comprehensive driving evaluations, training, recommendations for modifications of vehicles, and alternative transportation education
  d. Driving safety education, driver training, comprehensive driving evaluations, training, recommendations for modifications of vehicles, and alternative transportation education
9. The client is an 80-year-old man who had a mild CVA and is recovering quickly. During ADLs and IADLs, the OTA observes that his cognitive abilities do not appear to be impaired. However, his son and daughter come to the OTA and ask to tell him he should not drive anymore because of this CVA. The OTA should:
  a. Refer the family to the physician to speak about driving.
  b. Discuss observations about his cognitive abilities and assure them he is likely safe to drive.
  c. Refer the family to the occupational therapist to consider screening tests for driving.
  d. Tell the family to make an appointment for a comprehensive driving evaluation.
10. A client with a TBI has been using the driving simulator to regain skills necessary for driving. He continues to improve on the simulator to where he does well on all of the scenarios. What is the next step?
  a. Allow him to try driving in the parking lot in his family's car.
  b. Refer him for a comprehensive driving evaluation.
  c. Discuss his progress with the occupational therapist to consider other driving evaluations.
  d. Continue with the simulator scenarios, adding difficulty with multitasking activities while driving.

CASE STUDY

Sam is a 22-year-old male with a diagnosis of autism spectrum disorder. Although high functioning, his parents identified that he has significant issues with motor planning, multitasking, following two-step directions, and anxiety. They also identified some problems with focus and attention. Sam lives part-time with his mother, stepfather, and younger half-brother, and part-time with his father. Sam has a learner's permit, but both parents were concerned about his driving safety. Sam shows little interest in driving because he does not feel the need to drive (parents are available to drive him) and he has anxiety about crashing.

Sam's mother signed him up to participate in the East Carolina University's Department of Occupational Therapy's Driving and Community Bootcamp with the goal of increasing independence and determine whether independent driving is a safe option. The Bootcamp included multiple interventions, but for Sam, the simulator was the primary focus of his participation. Each simulator intervention session was approximately 45 minutes. There were pre- and post-testing on the simulators, using the exact same drives. Sam was enthusiastic about training on the driving simulators, stating, "This is really cool. I can't wait to drive in it!"

First session: The focus of the driving sessions was on regulatory signs and signals (e.g., stop signs, traffic lights). As an orientation, the simulated drive first only included stop signs to practice judging distances when stopping, coming to a complete stop at the stop line, and looking in each direction for traffic before proceeding. Sam showed good awareness of all stop signs during the drives, but demonstrated some difficulty with judging when to begin braking. The OTA verbally prompted Sam to press the brake when approaching a stop sign for each stop sign. During subsequent trials, Sam showed improvement in this area, braking for a stop sign appropriately at 5/8 stop signs. Sam demonstrated good awareness and perception of the environment, looking in each direction at the stop sign before safely proceeding 100 percent of the time.

Second Session: While Sam demonstrated appropriate understanding of traffic lights changes, he was initially unable to apply this understanding to traffic situations when the light was green. Sam slowed for yellow and stopped for red, but also stopped for green lights. When the OTA asked why, he stated, "to ensure that there is no traffic coming." The OTA agreed that it is a good practice to always look both ways before crossing an intersection, but it is important to continue through at a green light, as traffic behind expects a driver to continue through and stopping at the intersection would be an unsafe practice. In subsequent trials, Sam stopped at green light intersections 2/8 times and slowed at these intersections 6/8 times. Specific drives for traffic lights will be utilized at the next session to allow Sam additional trials to continue practicing appropriate responses based on the traffic light.

Third Session: Sam drove the same drives and showed marked improvement. He stopped appropriately at stop signs and assessed for traffic before safely proceeding 4/4 times. However, he still demonstrated some difficulty managing green traffic lights.

Fourth Session: This session focused on turning appropriately. The OTA verbally prompted Sam through various scenarios of turning left and right, and lane changes for these turns. Sam verbally expressed understanding, but required verbal prompting 75 percent of the time to remember lane changes before a turn. Sam required no verbal cuing to turn into the appropriate lane when multiple lanes existed. When the OTA asked, Sam was able to accurately verbalize strengths and weaknesses, demonstrating improved self-awareness.

Fifth Session: As Sam became more comfortable with turning, the OTA noticed Sam's speed increased during turns, causing the turns to become unsafe. The OTA then verbally prompted Sam to slow before a turn, to which he responded appropriately. Sam managed stop signs and traffic lights in the turning drives appropriately 7/8 times, showing improvement in this driving skill.

Sixth Session: The OTA discussed speed maintenance and lane maintenance before starting. Sam was prompted to follow the speed limit when safe, but to slow in certain situations. Sam demonstrated good speed maintenance and demonstrated 90 percent competency with all lane changes and stop signs.

Seventh Session: Sam wanted to work on lane maintenance in turns. Turns were accurate and there was 100 percent appropriate use of turn signals. Sam practiced turns on a four-lane road to learn differences in road lines and when to change lanes when turning. Sam verbalized understanding the difference. Sam used mirrors to change lanes 90 percent of the time.

1. Should the OTA prompt the correct maneuvers or allow the client to "crash" and recognize his or her own errors?
2. How can one grade an activity to make it harder when using the same scenario on a simulator?
3. What are some other activities the OTA can use with Sam other than the driving simulator to increase his community mobility skills?

PUTTING IT ALL TOGETHER — Sample Treatment and Documentation: Using the OT-PAD for Decision Making

Mrs. Doris Dobson is a 76-year-old widower with osteoarthritis who is recovering from total hip replacement surgery on her right side. She has been referred to OT for evaluation of ADL and IADL. Mrs. Dobson has high blood pressure and her hospital stay after surgery was extended because her blood pressure was uncontrolled after the surgery. The occupational therapist performed her initial evaluation and found that Mrs. Dobson was mildly confused, but the nurse indicated this was new and likely because of medication changes. Mrs. Dobson has functional range of motion, low stamina, and needed moderate assistance with all ADL activities. Carolyn, the OTA assigned, was asked to address Mrs. Dobson's ADLs (dressing and bathing) in the morning and assist her with making a sandwich or other easy meals in the kitchen in the afternoon, with the goal to teach her precautions for total hip replacements.

Mrs. Dobson was a pleasant woman who welcomed Carolyn and appeared delighted to work on getting dressed independently. Carolyn reviewed the precautions about total hip replacements before starting the bathing, toileting, and dressing. Although Mrs. Dobson indicated she understood, Carolyn had to intervene two times during the 30-minute process to stop Mrs. Dobson from bending over too much. Mrs. Dobson asked why there was a raised toilet seat on her toilet and only understood after Carolyn again explained it in relation to her recent surgery.

Mrs. Dobson came to the OT clinic later that afternoon. She was anxious to perform well in the clinic, as her doctor informed her that once she was independent in her ADLs/IADLs, she would be able to go home. She was chatting about wanting to return home soon, as she missed her grandchildren whom she was "in charge of" after school. Mrs. Dobson informed Carolyn that once she recovers, she would return to picking up the grandchildren after school. As a widower, she loved that she could help her daughter and son-in-law and feel useful.

Carolyn asked Mrs. Dobson what kind of sandwich she would like to make. With the choices, Mrs. Dobson decided on a tuna sandwich with chopped celery and mayonnaise, and a cup of green tea. After orienting her to the clinic's kitchen, Carolyn watched Mrs. Dobson as she used her walker about the kitchen to make the sandwich and tea. Mrs. Dobson started the hot water for tea first, and then went to retrieve the materials for the sandwich. Mrs. Dobson opened a can of chicken, chopped some onion and

Continued

PUTTING IT ALL TOGETHER Sample Treatment and Documentation: Using the OT-PAD for Decision Making (continued)

celery, and used the salad dressing in the mix. Instead of using the wheat bread she initially requested, Mrs. Dobson instead took used white bread that was already opened. She completed the sandwich and finished by making instant coffee, but forgot to turn off the burner of the stove. Mrs. Dobson moved slowly about the kitchen and seemed to get slower as time passed, needing to stop to rest before finishing the kitchen task. She had to ask Carolyn where the cups and milk were for the coffee, even though she was oriented to both those items earlier.

After sitting down to eat the sandwich and drink the coffee, Mrs. Dobson asked Carolyn when she thought she could go home. Carolyn replied that Mrs. Dobson appeared to need to increase her strength and independence. She would give her report to the occupational therapist and the rest of the team, including her physician, and the team would decide the best for her. Mrs. Dobson again remarked that it was important for her to get home so she could help her daughter with the grandchildren.

Carolyn was concerned about Mrs. Dobson returning to home too soon and caring for her grandchildren. It was evident from the performance of making a light lunch that Mrs. Dobson had some cognitive impairment. Although Carolyn could not determine whether it was temporary because of medication or not, it was concerning for her to return to home independently. Carolyn noted this in her documentation and was going to speak to her supervising occupational therapist about observations.

Although she did not ask about driving, Carolyn was wondering if "going home" also implied that Mrs. Dobson was ready to return to the more complex IADL of driving and community mobility. In preparation for reporting to her supervisor and team, Carolyn completed the Occupational Therapy Performance Appraisal for Driving (OT-PAD) (refer to Table 16-5) to address the issue of driving in case driving was not addressed by other team members. From the OT-PAD, Carolyn was able to describe that once Mrs. Dobson recovered from the hip replacement, she may be able to drive at the operational level (the overlearned tasks), but might have difficulties at the tactical and especially the strategic level, where decision making and fast processing were necessary. Carolyn suggested that a comprehensive driving evaluation might be warranted if Mrs. Dobson's confusion or cognitive impairment did not improve.

Documentation

LEVELS	DESCRIPTORS OF HOW TO CONSIDER EACH FACTOR UNDER EACH LEVEL	DEGREE OF IMPAIRMENT			
		None	*Mild*	*Moderate*	*Severe*
Strategic: *Does the client have the cognitive ability to make decisions?*	**Physical/sensory**-Aware of physical limitations and is able to plan for successful compensation (e.g., if in a wheelchair, demonstrates ability to plan time and/or assistance for transfer)			X	
	Cognitive-Demonstrates ability to plan in advance using appropriate decisions to meet the goals of the task; self-regulates with insight into decisions; organizes steps to complete task			X	
	Emotional regulation-Can plan with appreciation of the emotional state (e.g., Does not drive if experiencing excessive, anxiety, depression, or anger)	X			
	Insight-Has accurate awareness of the skills and abilities he or she possesses to meet the demands of the task (e.g., to clean the windows, skills/abilities to use a ladder safety? Can make modified decisions based on driving experience and/or training)			X	
Tactical: *Does the client have performance skills to perform actions at this level?*	**Physical/sensory**-Is aware of his or her physical limitation and adjusts as required (e.g., if floors are wet, walks more slowly)		X		
	Cognitive-Can evaluate a complex, dynamic context and adjust or accommodate through appropriate actions			X	
	Emotional regulation-Can recognize and manage emotions that arise in challenging situations	X			
	Insight-Can accurately gauge the risk and skills/abilities needed to meet the demands of a task requiring immediate decisions			X	

PUTTING IT ALL TOGETHER Sample Treatment and Documentation: Using the OT-PAD for Decision Making (continued)

Documentation (continued)

LEVELS	DESCRIPTORS OF HOW TO CONSIDER EACH FACTOR UNDER EACH LEVEL	DEGREE OF IMPAIRMENT			
		None	*Mild*	*Moderate*	*Severe*
Operational: *Does the client have performance skills to perform actions at this level?*	**Physical/sensory**-Meets the minimum requirements (e.g., vision) or is able to compensate for limitation (e.g., with training, will be able to use hand controls to compensate a lower extremity amputation)	X			
	Cognitive-Awareness and flexibility to use the appropriate actions to achieve desired results		X		
	Emotional regulation-Emotional state does not negatively affect performance of automatic tasks	X			
	Insight -Not applicable				

REFERENCES

1. McGuire, M. J. & Schold-Davis, E. (Eds.). (2012). *Driving and community mobility: Occupational therapy strategies across the lifespan*. Bethesda, MD: AOTA Press.
2. Stav, W. B., & Lieberman, D. (2008). From the desk of the editor. *The American Journal of Occupational Therapy, 62*(2),127-129.
3. Dickerson, A. E., Reistetter, T., & Gaudy, J. R. (2013). The perception of meaningfulness and performance of instrumental activities of daily living from the perspectives of the medically at-risk older adults and their caregivers. *Journal of Applied Gerontology, 32*(6), 749-764.
4. American Occupational Therapy Association. (2008). Occupational therapy practice framework: Domain and process (3rd ed.). *American Journal of Occupational Therapy, 68,* S1-S48. doi:10.5014/ajot.2014.68006.
5. Coughlin, J. F., & D'Ambrosio, L. A. (Eds.). (2012). *Aging America and transportation: Personal choices and public policy*. New York, NY: Springer Publishing Company.
6. Federal interagency forum on aging-related statistics. (2008). *Older Americans 2008: Key indicators of well-being.* Washington D.C: US Government Printing Office.
7. Dickerson, A. E., Molnar, L. J., Eby, D. W., Adler, G., Bedard, M., Berg-Weger, M., ... & Trujillo, L. (2007). Transportation and aging: A research agenda for advancing safe mobility. *The Gerontologist, 47*(5), 578-590.
8. Sifrit, K. J., Stutts, J., Staplin, L., & Martell, C. (2010). Intersection crashes among drivers in their 60s, 70s and 80s. *Proceedings of the Human Factors and Ergonomics Society Annual Meeting, 54*(24), 2057-2061.
9. Kent, R. (2010). The biomechanics of aging. *NTSB Forum on Safety, Mobility, and Aging Drivers.* Washington, DC: Transportation Research Board.
10. Carr, D. B., Schwartzberg, J. G., Manning, L., & Sempek, J. (2010). *Physician's guide to assessing and counseling older drivers* (2nd ed.). Washington, DC: National Highway Traffic Safety Administration.
11. Dickerson, A. E., Schold Davis, E., & Chew, F. (2011). *Driving as an instrumental activity of daily living in the medical setting: A model for intervention and referral.* Presentation at the Transportation Research Board: Emerging Issues in Safe and Sustainable Mobility for Older People. Washington, DC.
12. Slater, D. Y. (2014). Consensus statements on occupational therapy ethics related to driving. *Occupational Therapy in Health Care, 28*(2), 163-168.
13. Dickerson, A. E. (2014). Driving with dementia: Evaluation, referral, and resources. *Occupational Therapy in Health Care, 28*(1), 62-76.
14. What is a medically at-risk driver? (2011). The Medically At-Risk Driving Centre of the University of Alberta. Retrieved from http://www.mard.ualberta.ca/FrequentlyAskedQuestions.aspx
15. Rogers, A. T., Bai, G., Lavin, R. A., & Anderson, G. F. (2016). Higher hospital spending on occupational therapy is associated with lower readmission rates. *Medical Care Research and Review,* 1–19. https://doi.org/10.1177/1077558716666981
16. Dickerson, A. E., Davis, E. S., & Staplin, L. (2014). Can clinicians, researchers, and driver licensing officials build a shared vocabulary? *Occupational Therapy in Health Care, 28*(2), 188-193.
17. Pellerito, J. M. (2006). Pioneers in driving rehabilitation. In J. M. Pellerito (Ed.), *Driver rehabilitation and community mobility: Principles and practice* (pp. 32-34). St. Louis, MO: Elsevier Mosby.
18. Dickerson, A. E., Reistetter, T., Davis, E. S., & Monahan, M. (2011). Evaluating driving as a valued instrumental activity of daily living. *American Journal of Occupational Therapy, 65*(1), 64-75.
19. Rizzo, M. & Kellison, I. L. (2010). The brain on the road. In T.D. Marcotte & I. Grant (Eds.), *Neuropsychology of everyday functioning* (pp. 168-208). New York, NY: The Guilford Press.
20. Anstey, K. J., Wood, J., Lord, S., & Walker, J. G. (2005). Cognitive, sensory and physical factors enabling driving safety in older adults. *Clinical Psychology Review, 25*(1), 45-65.
21. Carr, D. B., Duchek, J. M., Meuser, T. M., & Morris, J. C. (2006). Older adult drivers with cognitive impairment. *American Family Physician, 73*(6), 1029-1034.
22. Lane, A., Green, E., Dickerson, A. E., Davis, E. S., Rolland, B., & Stohler, J. T. (2014). Driver rehabilitation programs: Defining program models, services, and expertise. *Occupational Therapy in Health Care, 28*(2), 177-187.
23. Doucet, B. M., & Gutman, S. A. (2013). Quantifying function: The rest of the measurement story. *The American Journal of Occupational Therapy, 67*(1), 7.
24. Dickerson, A. E., Meuel, D. B., Ridenour, C. D., & Cooper, K. (2014). Assessment tools predicting fitness to drive in older adults: A systematic review. *American Journal of Occupational Therapy, 68*(6), 670-680.
25. Bedard, M., Weaver, B., Dārzin, P., & Porter, M. M. (2008). Predicting driving performance in older adults: We are not there yet! *Traffic Injury Prevention, 9*(4), 336-341.
26. Barrash, J., Stillman, A., Anderson, S. W., Uc, E. Y., Dawson, J. D., & Rizzo, M. (2010). Prediction of driving ability with neuropsychological tests: Demographic adjustments diminish accuracy. *Journal of the International Neuropsychological Society, 16*(04), 679-686.
27. Classen, S., Witter, D. P., Lanford, D. N., Okun, M. S., Rodriguez, R. L., Romrell, J., ... & Fernandez, H. H. (2011). Usefulness of screening tools

for predicting driving performance in people with Parkinson's disease. *American Journal of Occupational Therapy, 65*(5), 579-588.

28. Molnar, F. J., Marshall, S. C., Man-Son-Hing, M., Wilson, K. G., Byszewski, A. M., & Stiell, I. (2007). Acceptability and concurrent validity of measures to predict older driver involvement in motor vehicle crashes: An emergency department pilot case–control study. *Accident Analysis & Prevention, 39*(5), 1056-1063.
29. Zook, N. A., Bennett, T. L., & Lane, M. (2009). Identifying at-risk older adult community-dwelling drivers through neuropsychological evaluation. *Applied Neuropsychology, 16*(4), 281-287.
30. Crizzle, A. M., Classen, S., & Uc, E. Y. (2012). Parkinson disease and driving: An evidence-based review. *Neurology, 79*(20), 2067-2074.
31. Dickerson, A. E. (2013). Driving assessment tools used by driver rehabilitation specialists: Survey of use and implications for practice. *American Journal of Occupational Therapy, 67*(5), 564-573.
32. Fisher, A. G. (2006). *Assessment of motor and process skills: Volume I and II* (6th ed.). Fort Collins, CO: Three Star Press.
33. Dickerson, A. E., & Schold Davis, E. (2014). Driving experts address expanding access through pathways to older driver rehabilitation services: Expert meeting results. *Occupational Therapy in Health Care, 28*(2), 122-126.
34. Dickerson, A. E., & Bédard, M. (2014). Decision tool for clients with medical issues: A framework for identifying driving risk and potential to return to driving. *Occupational Therapy in Health Care, 28*(2), 194-202.
35. Michon, J. A. (1985). A critical view of driver behavior models: What do we know, what should we do? In L. Evans & R. Schwing (Eds.), *Human behavior and traffic safety* (pp. 485-524). New York, NY: Plenum Press.
36. Bedard, M. B., Parkkari, M., Weaver, B., Riendeau, J., & Dahlquist, M. (2010). Assessment of driving performance using a simulator protocol: Validity and reproducibility. *The American Journal of Occupational Therapy, 64*(2), 336-340.
37. Classen, S., & Brooks, J. (2014). Driving simulators for occupational therapy screening, assessment, and intervention. *Occupational Therapy in Health Care, 28*(2), 154-162.
38. Devos, H., Akinwuntan, A. E., Nieuwboer, A., Tant, M., Truijen, S., De Wit, L., ... & De Weerdt, W. (2009). Comparison of the effect of two driving retraining programs on on-road performance after stroke. *Neurorehabilitation and Neural Repair, 23*(7), 699-705.
39. Akinwuntan, A. E., Wachtel, J., & Rosen, P. N. (2012). Driving simulation for evaluation and rehabilitation of driving after stroke. *Journal of Stroke and Cerebrovascular Diseases, 21*(6), 478-486.
40. Kewman, D. G., Seigerman, C., Kintner, H., Chu, S., Henson, D., & Reeder, C. (1985). Simulation training of psychomotor skills: Teaching the brain-injured to drive. *Rehabilitation Psychology, 30*(1), 11.
41. Lundqvist, A., Gerdle, B., & Ronnberg, J. (2000). Neuropsychological aspects of driving after a stroke—in the simulator and on the road. *Applied Cognitive Psychology, 14*(2), 135-150.
42. Hettinger, L. J., Berbaum, K. S., Kennedy, R. S., Dunlap, W. P., & Nolan, M. D. (1990). Vection and simulator sickness. *Military Psychology, 2*(3), 171.
42. Patomella, A. H., Johansson, K., & Tham, K. (2009). Lived experience of driving ability following stroke. *Disability & Rehabilitation, 31*(9), 726-733.

Chapter 17

Work Rehabilitation and Retraining

Paul A. Fontana, LOTR, FAOTA, Katrina Duhon Delahoussaye, MSOT/L, and Anna Petry, MOTR/L

LEARNING OUTCOMES

After studying this chapter, the student or practitioner will be able to:

17.1 Define and differentiate between work conditioning and work hardening

17.2 Explain the unique role of the occupational therapy practitioner in the industrial setting

17.3 Demonstrate how to properly administer and score specific assessments to identify the presence of symptom magnification

17.4 Explain the importance of addressing psychosocial factors to increase the client's compliance/success and quality of life

17.5 Define the purpose of functional capacity evaluations in relation to facilitating return to work

17.6 Identify the components of a functional capacity evaluation and why it is important to see the client for multiple days in succession to ensure a defensible result

KEY TERMS

Functional capacity evaluation (FCE)
Functional capacity report (FCR)
Maximum medical improvement (MMI)
Physical job description
Symptom magnification
Work capacity evaluation (WCE)
Work conditioning
Work hardening

Occupational therapy (OT) has an important role to play in work and industry, including injury prevention programs as well as return to work (RTW) programs. Within the realm of injury prevention, the OT practitioner will incorporate onsite analysis of the job and development of physical job descriptions, perform post-hire assessments of the newly hired employees, and provide onsite ergonomics education and training.

The RTW programs will include the following aspects, which will be covered in this chapter:

- Work conditioning
- Work hardening
- Functional capacity evaluations (FCEs)

Following an injury, the injured employee will undergo medical treatments in an attempt to resolve the injury. This may include surgery, injections, medications, and possibly a variety of therapies (OT, physical therapy [PT], chiropractic). Once the client reaches **maximum medical improvement (MMI),** the individual will often require one of the industrial OT programs mentioned above to ensure readiness to reenter the workforce. An individual is considered to have reached MMI when either additional medical interventions or traditional therapy interventions are no longer of benefit to the client. When this occurs, the goal changes from attempting to resolve the medical issues or pain complaints the client may have to improving the individual's function within his or her pain tolerance.

Work conditioning and work hardening programs are designed to improve a client's strength, endurance, and ability to tolerate more extensive activities so that the person can return to competitive employment. **Work conditioning** will focus on specific physiological issues (flexibility, strength, and endurance) that prohibit the client from participating in more work-related activities, whereas **work hardening** uses the client's participation in real work activities to improve his or her functional improvement. Through active participation in these types of programs, the psychosocial issues that developed as a result of being in the injury management system for extended periods will also often be resolved.

The use of real work activities in an injured client's rehabilitation has its roots in OT from the profession's inception. When an injured employee has been in the injury management system for a prolonged period, he or she will benefit from a work conditioning program designed to improve the physical ability to tolerate work. As this individual is able to tolerate 8-hour workdays, the employee will progress to work hardening, which uses real work activities to "harden" or strengthen him or her to improved tolerance for work. Both work conditioning and work hardening will conclude with a **functional capacity evaluation (FCE)** that identifies the client's real abilities and/or limitations to perform sustained work. At times, the FCE will also be used alone to determine disability and provide a one-time assessment.

Workers' compensation insurance is the payer source for the vast majority of medical claims for injuries occurring on the job and also for the cost of the RTW programs (reimbursement for OT and related disciplines). Workers' compensation specifics vary from state to state and from country to country. Generally, injured workers are paid a portion of their salary while out of work, undergoing medical care, and attending work conditioning and/or work hardening programs.

Within the *Occupational Therapy Practice Framework, 3rd edition* (OTPF-3), work is defined as "labor or exertion, to make, construct, manufacture, form, fashion or shape objects, to organize, plan or evaluate services or processes of living or governing, committed occupations that are performed with or without financial reward."[1] For OT practitioners working in an industrial rehabilitation setting, working with an employee who is attempting to RTW from either a work-related injury or non–work-related injury or illness, job performance is a particular consideration. The client must be able to perform the essential functions of the job, including those involving work skills and patterns, before returning to work in the same capacity as before the illness or injury. The OT practitioner can assist clients who are unable to perform essential functions or are otherwise unable to return to their previous jobs with exploring other employment interests and pursuits and assist them in seeking and acquiring employment. By identifying the client's abilities and limitations in performing work activities, the OT practitioner provides the vocational counselor and the client with the appropriate physical parameters in the search for a new occupation. This may also include teaching clients to advocate for themselves in the job market or identifying the jobs that are best suited to them as determined by their physical capabilities and personal interests.

COMMUNICATION IN WORK REHABILITATION

Communication, both verbal and written, is always an important part of any OT process, but there are some specific areas, which need to be addressed in the work rehabilitation setting. Essential to a good work conditioning program, work hardening program, or FCE is good communication between the occupational therapist and the occupational therapy assistant (OTA) and between the OT practitioners and the client. It is imperative that the client relays to the OT practitioner how he or she is tolerating a task. It is equally important that the OTA relays to the occupational therapist what the OTA has observed from the client's participation in the activities—thus adding that objective piece

EVIDENCE-BASED PRACTICE

A recent article from the *American Journal of Occupational Therapy* presented 9 years of data from a facility providing occupational rehabilitation. The two research questions the authors studied related to "whether a set of client factors previously reported in the literature would significantly predict successful program outcome and whether the presence of interventions in the area of occupations and activities via simulated work tasks would be associated with successful outcomes."[2] The success of the program was determined when, at discharge, clients met one or more of the following criteria: They returned to work at any job; clients were cleared by a physician to return to work and initiated a job search process; or they progressed to a vocational rehabilitation plan meant to support obtaining employment.[2] This study noted that therapeutic intensity was a predictor of success because clients who could tolerate increasing time in the program tended to do better compared with those who could not. The other important predictor of success was participation in occupation-based activities.[2] Specifically, participating in work simulation activities increased the odds of success by more than six times.[2] The authors noted that "given the centrality of the occupation of work as a life role and its contribution to people's purpose and sense of meaning, occupational (i.e., work) rehabilitation is a natural match for occupational therapy practitioners."[2] A focus on activities of daily living is often the norm in physical rehabilitation, and the generalist OTA may want to consider the use of work-related, occupation-based activities, even if the OT practitioners do not work in the work hardening field specifically.

Hardison, M. E., & Roll, S. C. (2016). *Factors associated with success in an occupational rehabilitation program for work-related musculoskeletal disorders.* American Journal of Occupational Therapy, *71(1), 7101190030p1-7101190030p6.*

of information to the client's subjective complaints. Some further information would include:

1. The documentation needs to be thorough, complete, and timely. Documentation must accurately describe all observations or professional opinions (pain posturing).
2. Documentation needs to be in complete sentences, using correct grammar.
3. Documentation needs to be such that if the OT practitioner is called upon in 2 to 4 years to respond in a deposition, the OT practitioner is able to describe exactly what occurred in the clinic accurately and with confidence.
4. Progress notes for work conditioning and work hardening need to be documented at least weekly with a complete reevaluation performed every ten visits. The weekly documentation should be short and to the point, without extraneous sentences that do not reflect what occurred in the clinic that week. Documentation is addressed to the physician, with copies sent to everyone on the chart: attorney(s), medical case manager, rehabilitation nurse, vocational counselor, insurance provider, and so on. Documentation should include:
   - How many visits have been attended/how many missed and reasons
   - Cooperation and attitude of the client
   - Overall goals/objectives being worked on and the activities used to reach these
   - Summary of pain complaints over the week
   - Problems or concerns that have come up
   - Plans for the future—this can include the following:
     - The date for which the reevaluation is scheduled
     - Pain complaints that are causing concerns and any questions that need to be addressed
     - Plans for the future
5. Reevaluation format: A full reevaluation should occur at least every ten visits and include all areas that were not within normal limits (WNL) during the baseline evaluation. The reevaluation format recommendation has three columns. The first column lists the activity; the second column lists how the client performed on the baseline assessment; and the third column lists how the employee performed on the day of the reevaluation. Documenting the reevaluation in this manner helps even a nonmedical person (e.g., a claims adjuster) to see and understand the necessity for continued therapy or see that the client's condition has plateaued and the client needs to be discharged.
   - *Reevaluation Format Sample:*

Activity:	Baseline:	Reevaluation:
Fl-W Lifting	Jan 2, 20XX—15 lbs	Jan 12, 20XX—25 lb

6. Discharge note: This note will summarize what happened in the weeks of work conditioning or work hardening. The work conditioning discharge note will conclude with the recommendation for future therapy—generally to include a work hardening program or an FCE. The work hardening discharge report will include the results of the discharge FCE.
7. Other documentation: There needs to be a place to document any and all phone contacts with anyone involved in the case: client, physician, attorney(s), employer, vocational counselor, medical case manager, and insurance company. This documentation is useful to ensure that an accurate log remains to explain any issues regarding scheduling, transportation issues, and so on. Anytime there is a phone contact or in-person contact of significance, the OT practitioner should write a summary letter to all involved, updating each on the conversation and the plans for the future. If the therapy department is having a difficult time getting approval for the request for work conditioning, work hardening, or the FCE, scheduling for the client, or the client is not attending as directed, the OT practitioner must write a letter summarizing the issues and the plans for follow-up. The letter is addressed to whomever referred the client for the industrial program, with copies to all those on the file. When having difficulty contacting the client to schedule an evaluation or work conditioning/work hardening program, the letter should be addressed to the client and sent by registered mail, with a request for return receipt. Copies should be forwarded to all parties listed on the intake sheet.

OCCUPATIONAL THERAPY ASSISTANT'S ROLE

The OTA plays an important role in industrial OT programs. After completing training and gaining service competencies on each component of the initial baseline assessment and musculoskeletal assessment, the OTA is able to complete these areas of the assessment. "The occupational therapy assistant contributes to the evaluation process by implementing delegated assessments and by providing verbal and written reports of observations, assessments, and client capacities to the occupational therapist."[3]

COMMUNICATION

Communication between the occupational therapist and the OTA must be open, honest, and frequent to ensure that a client's activity programs are adjusted on the basis of the client's progress or lack thereof. Because the client's participation, especially during the early stages of the work conditioning and work hardening programs, can change significantly from day to day or from morning to afternoon, the occupational therapist must be readily available to consult with the OTA or reassess the client to ensure a timely change in activities as the client's participation warrants.

By working closely with the occupational therapist, the OTA is able to point out any areas where the client's performance is not WNL so that the occupational therapist or the OTA is then able to retest and confirm these findings, if needed.[4] For example, the OTA may take repeated volumetric or circumferential measurements or repeat grip testing and distraction grip testing (test in various ways and with distractions to decrease cheating) with a client, all of which will help document the client's performance.

To be an effective team member during the work conditioning and work hardening programs or during functional capacity testing, it is imperative that the OTA be knowledgeable about the results of the baseline evaluation results, including the physical problems that were identified during the assessment and that the client will be working to resolve in the rehabilitation programs. Often, a client's prior OT or PT program has focused solely on resolving the problems associated with the injured body part, such as a knee, shoulder, or hand, for example. The work capacity assessment looks not only at the injured area, but also identifies abilities and problems that prohibit the client from wholly engaging in a full RTW program. By understanding the client's OT goals as developed by the occupational therapist, the OTA will be able to effectively collaborate with the occupational therapist and the client in selecting appropriate client-centered functional activities and exercises that will be motivational to the client and facilitate a resolution of the client's physical problems. The OTA will assist with the implementation as well as the modifications of activities and intervention techniques based on the client's performance.[3]

Furthermore, the OTA's role is also to ensure that the client remains on task and to document vital signs and pain complaints during activities. By providing good observations of the client's performance and discussing with the occupational therapist any problems and issues observed, the OTA is instrumental in helping to identify the client's true abilities and limitations. Through close and continual observation, the OT staff is able to put an objective component to a subjective complaint. This gives the OT practitioner insight as to whether indications of self-limiting or symptom magnification may exist. An example of this would be when the client is rating his or her pain as an 8/10, where 10 equates to maximal intense pain requiring hospitalization, yet the OT practitioner documents, when distracted, the client is able to actively engage in normal conversation and laughter with the OT staff and other clients. Another example is a client reports a maximal intensity of leg pain or total numbness in the leg, yet the OT staff observe that the client limps during certain activities and walks normally in others.

The OTA can also assist with distracting the client during activities. Some clients will stop performing an activity after a few minutes, not necessarily because they cannot continue due to pain or fatigue, but rather out of boredom. Other clients will behave differently when the OT practitioner is working with or observing them than they will behave when they are with other staff members. If the client performs at a significantly higher level during distraction testing than without the distraction, it is a sign of symptom magnification. For instance, a client stops a walking activity after 5 minutes, reporting that he or she is in too much pain to continue. Yet later in the day, when distracted by conversation with the OTA or other staff members, the client demonstrates the ability to walk for an hour without any outward sign of difficulty.

The role of the OTA in the documentation of the weekly progress notes and regular reevaluation notes is also critically important. He or she works closely with the occupational therapist to ensure that all pertinent information data about the client's active participation (or lack thereof), progress or regression, issues and concerns, and so on are clearly raised, discussed, and documented. The documentation of the objective observations of both the OTA and the occupational therapist is critical in ensuring defensibility of all of these programs.

WORK CONDITIONING PROGRAMS

Unfortunately, traditional medical treatments following a major injury or illness generally focus solely on the injured body part. For instance, the client participating in a rehabilitation program following a knee injury will perform specific knee exercises until the range of motion (ROM) and strength of the affected knee are equal to or as close as expected to those of the unaffected knee. Or if an individual is in rehabilitation following a serious hand injury, he or she will participate in therapy until the affected hand is as close as possible to the unaffected hand with regard to ROM, function, and strength.

Although the affected extremity may be strong (or as strong as possible) following the rehabilitation program, without active participation in continual aerobic and strength building activities, the individual will show a continual decline in his or her ability to function at a preinjury state over time. Even healthy, noninjured individuals will have a significant decrease in cardiopulmonary function as well as strength, endurance, and flexibility when they become relatively inactive for a period. Muscle strength and the function of the cardiopulmonary system start to decline almost immediately following inactivity. Studies show that strength will decrease by 4% per day during the first week of inactivity. After 12 weeks of inactivity, the client will lose 68% of the strength. In the first 3 weeks of inactivity, maximum oxygen intake declines by 27% and cardiac stroke volume and output decrease by 25%.[5,6] An article published in *Spine Journal* reported that individuals with low dynamic trunk muscle endurance and low aerobic endurance simultaneously had an increased risk of incidence of low back pain (LBP).[7] Thus, it is no wonder that following a 3- to 6-month recovery period from a back, shoulder, knee, or hand injury, the individual is unable to RTW safely without restrictions or modifications, at least initially, once he or she has reached MMI.

As early as World War II, reconditioning programs were set up within Veterans' Administration hospitals to reduce the effects of prolonged hospitalizations of injured veterans by "increasing muscle tone and work tolerances, reestablishing work habits, and promoting mental alertness."[8] This was accomplished by the OT practitioner assigning these long-term clients to work in the hospital's industrial workshop or giving them work assignments in the hospital's landscaping or office areas.[8] The concept of "work conditioning" first came into existence in the late 1970s and early 1980s and aimed to reduce the "economic and human costs of work-related injuries."[9] Work conditioning, as described in the literature, is intertwined with work hardening. Today, work conditioning programs are commonly defined as individualized and structured treatment programs designed to restore and improve the specific work performance skills of individuals recovering from long-term illness or injury.[9-12] This type of treatment program focuses on restoration of the worker's cardiovascular and musculoskeletal systems, specifically strength, endurance, flexibility, motor control, and cardiopulmonary functions.[11,13] A work conditioning program is initiated after the client has completed basic rehabilitation treatment but is unable to tolerate an 8-hour-per-day job or a work hardening program. A client who is beginning a work conditioning program has reached MMI. This does not mean that the individual is necessarily cured or pain free but, rather, that the medical profession has no further treatments to offer to the client. The goal of the work conditioning program is to help improve the client's function.

THE OLDER ADULT

As the population ages, many adults are working longer and longer before retiring, and it is becoming increasingly more difficult to retire comfortably. Some adults retire from a long-term career and after a few years of retirement, go back to part-time or full-time work either to get out of the house or for additional income. Others delay retirement for increased social security benefits or to retain insurance benefits. By 2019, over 40% of Americans 55+ years of age will be employed, making up over 25% of the U.S. labor force.[14] Employers often rate older workers high on characteristics, such as judgment, commitment to quality, attendance, and punctuality.[14] Certainly, older adult workers make up a significant portion of the workforce and may be seen in a work hardening program or a situation where the OTA may assist with modification or adaptation of work tasks. This might include adapting the keyboard for someone with a hand that is weak or painful or using a voice-to-text mode to avoid significant typing. It also may mean a focus on body mechanics and other factors that may have led to an issue with work performance. The older adult may take longer to rehabilitate or have more physical conditions that impact work performance, but they are certainly a vital part of the workforce.

Work conditioning programs consist of 4 hours of progressive, aggressive therapy per day, 5 days per week, for upward of 4 to 6 weeks, depending on the client's tolerance level. When the individual is able to return to a modified form of real work for 2 days a week, the treatment may then be a combination of work and 3 days of work conditioning. OT treatment sessions consist of both passive and active–assisted stretching to help improve the client's flexibility and mobility, along with exercises and functional activities designed to improve both strength and aerobic fitness. Intensive education regarding a tailored home exercise program, back education, and biomechanical training for proper material handling and lifting techniques, and safety training are incorporated (Fig. 17-1). This, along with limited use of passive physical agent modalities for symptom control, will assist in resolving the associated issues that come with deconditioning.

Initial Evaluations

The comprehensive evaluation that precedes the work conditioning program or the work hardening program is called **work capacity evaluation (WCE).** This assessment, as

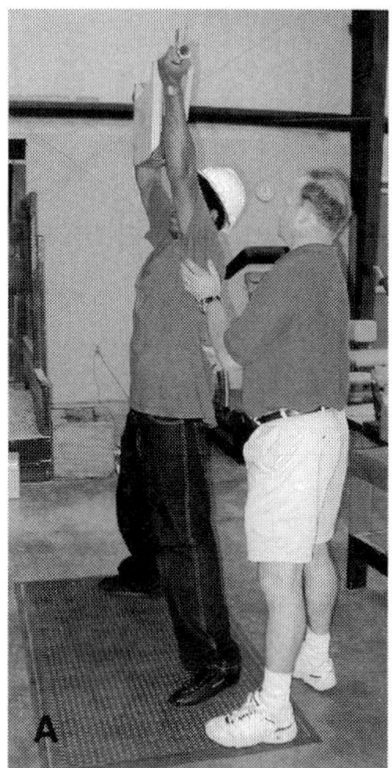
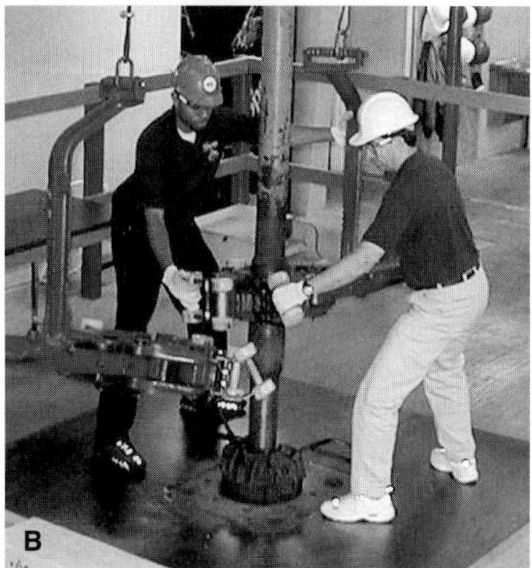

FIGURE 17-1. A. Lifting heavy object overhead while learning to maintain proper alignment of back. B. Using proper body mechanics for a two person simulated drill floor (oil rig).

will be described in detail later, not only covers the client's musculoskeletal abilities but also includes the ability to perform work-related functions. The purpose of the WCE is to assess the function of the client's injured body part (knee, hand, etc.) as well as the pertinence of that body part to performance of work.

Both the occupational therapist and OTA have a role in performing the client's baseline WCE. Although the occupational therapist typically performs the WCE, the OTA is able to assist with each aspect of the evaluation in which he or she has been assessed and noted to have competency by the occupational therapist. The occupational therapist and the OTA are able to work together to assess the client, performing the initial interview as well as each aspect of the musculoskeletal assessment along with the assessment of critical work-related functional tasks.

The initial (baseline) WCE for work conditioning and work hardening or for FCE will all have very similar components. This baseline assessment provides a snapshot of the client's status at the onset of whichever program he or she is beginning. The major areas of each assessment will include an initial interview, a musculoskeletal (full body) assessment, and job-specific functional activities.

INITIAL INTERVIEW

The initial interview includes the following:

- Previous medical and rehabilitation history
- Job description: General physical requirements
- Current prescription medication, along with any side effects reported by the client

The client should be asked to bring his or her medications to the appointment in the original prescription containers so the occupational therapist or OTA is able to make a determination if the client is taking the medications as prescribed. The OT practitioner should read the label to find out when the prescription was last filled and how many tablets were included. The number of pills still in the bottle should be counted, adding to it the number of pills the client should have consumed since it was last filled to determine if the numbers add up. If it is determined that the client is abusing medications by consuming them at a faster rate than prescribed or if taking them at a slower rate than prescribed, the OT should inform the physician who prescribed the medication. A follow-up documentation of this discussion in the client's medical records should be included, with copies to all parties affiliated with the case. The following should be documented:

- Any predetermined limitations or restrictions placed on the client by the physician, either temporary or permanent restrictions. Typical restrictions include the following:
  - Medium work level on clients who undergo a lumbar fusion
  - No bending, stretching, or extended reaching during first 6 weeks to 3 months following implementation of a dorsal column stimulator.
  - Limited lifting of weight for a relatively recent shoulder repair.
- Client's understanding of the diagnosis, perception of his or her current abilities and limitations pertaining to self-care, physical daily living, work, leisure activities, and previous OT, PT, and chiropractic care.

Written restrictions placed on the client by the treating physician are not to be exceeded without express written approval by the treating physician and surgeon. Often, the treating physician will place temporary restrictions or guidelines that the client must follow when he or she is at home. However, when in doubt, it is wise to always get the restrictions or updated restrictions in writing from the treating physician before exceeding them. The FCE that occurs at the conclusion of the work conditioning (or work hardening) program will establish the true restrictions that the physician should consider.

Questioning the client about his or her previous medical care, along with prior OT, PT, or chiropractic care, helps the OT practitioner make a determination as to whether or not the client has had the benefit of good progressive therapy or not. Previous medical care may include physician services, surgeries, and/or injections. Keep in mind that this is subjective information from the client and may not be a true and accurate picture of the therapy received. This consideration becomes important as the occupational therapist attempts to make a determination as to whether the client may be able to make further functional improvements with proper rehabilitation. When the client relates that he or she has participated in an OT, PT, or chiropractic therapy program that has been primarily based on passive modalities, the occupational therapist may reasonably predict that with appropriate care the client may expect to function at a higher level, which may result in a possible referral to a work conditioning or work hardening program. The OT practitioner must know all about the client's medical history to ensure that the activities the practitioner is going to request of the client will not put the client at risk of being reinjured.

It is important for OT practitioners to gain a clear understanding of a client's perception of pain before they participate in any physical activities. Having the client document the pain location, description, and intensity rating before attempting any activity will give the OT practitioner a baseline for comparison once activities are initiated. Having the client rate his or her pain at its worst over the past month and what activities the client was performing when the pain reached that level also gives the OT practitioner much valuable insight as to what to expect from the client during the FCE or WCE. Before participating in any functional activities, if the client reports that "while at home doing very little or not even anything, my pain was very intense," it would indicate to the OT practitioner that the pain was worse at home before the evaluation. In other words, the client may report experiencing significant increases in pain at home without having participated in any activities or after having participated in only minimal activities. This indicates to the OT practitioner that the client's pain may reach these levels at home and that it is not necessarily related specifically to the activities performed during the evaluation. This information can be useful in the defense of the practitioner if a claim is made that the assessment worsened the client's pain.

Note the client's description of pain complaints over the previous month and at the time of the evaluation, including what alleviates the pain and what makes it worse. When a client states that nothing can alleviate the pain, this statement provides a clue that making this individual feel better is going to be a difficult task.

MUSCULOSKELETAL ASSESSMENT (FULL BODY ASSESSMENT)

The musculoskeletal assessment component of a WCE must be performed on the client's whole body because the purpose is to identify issues with regard to readiness to RTW. With individuals who are relatively pain free and ready to RTW, the assessment can take 20 to 30 minutes, whereas with an individual who has been in the injury management system for a long time (greater than 6 months) and still reporting a fair amount of pain, the assessment can take 60 to 90 minutes to complete. The components of the assessment include the following:

- Baseline resting heart rate and blood pressure
- Height and weight
- Sub-maximal aerobic fitness: Assessment compared with age and gender norms
- Grip strength: Compared with age and gender norms
- ROM: Includes cervical and trunk ROM, as well as upper-extremity (UE) and lower extremity (LE) ROM. All limitations are clearly identified, along with any objective observations made by the OT practitioner. A goniometer is required to ensure accuracy of the observation of limitations. In addition to accurate measuring of active range of motion (AROM) and passive range of motion (PROM), the OTA must consider the client's reports of pain with these movements, paying particular attention to the client's reports of pain once ROM is stopped. For example, if a client reports an increased pulling pain at end range, but no pain (or significantly reduced pain) once the muscle is taken off tension, this denotes muscle tightness. This directly relates to the treatment protocol for this issue. (Similar documentation would occur for the muscle length/flexibility assessment.)
- Manual muscle testing (MMT): Includes all major muscle groups for the UE/LE
- Muscle length and flexibility: Primarily for individuals with low back or hip issues because this will help the OT practitioner determine which areas to concentrate on when stretching the client
- UE coordination: For a client who has had a hand or shoulder injury, standardized coordination testing will be appropriate. Otherwise, gross functional finger dexterity or coordination is assessed to screen for other potential issues that may affect the RTW potential.
- LE gross coordination: Screening for potential issues that may affect the RTW potential for any client.
- Proprioception: Gross proprioception screening: for UE, fingers to nose with eyes closed; for LE, box step with eyes closed.
- Balance: Unilateral static balance as well as dynamic balance will be assessed. Dynamic balance will be assessed in the client's ability to independently transition to and from the floor, the ability to squat (partial or fully), kneel, bend, or assume a variety of postures and positions required on the job.
- Stereognosis: Screening for all clients; have the client close the eyes and identify a common object placed in his or her hand only by touching it.
- Sharp/dull discrimination: For clients with UE and LE neurological issues.
- Provocative tests: Tests that are designed to purposefully elicit positive signs of medical issues. The client will be using his or her entire body to perform the work that they will return to. Because most acute therapies are limited to the injured body part, the baseline assessment should include various provocative tests that might identify other issues that can put the individual at risk of further injury should he or she participate in a variety of activities and can affect the RTW decision. Provocative testing can include a variety of shoulder stability tests, such as the "empty can test" for shoulder impingement issues, deep palpation over the lateral epicondyle to test for tendonitis, Tinel's and Phalen's signs for identifying carpal tunnel syndrome, or the Finkelstein test for de Quervain's. These assessments are performed quickly and easily without increasing the cost or time of evaluation and can elicit valuable information about the individual's status that can help prevent injuries. Many of these assessments are described in detail in Chapters 22 and 23.
- Screen for neurological issues: Neurological assessments are recommended to be included in the work capacity baseline testing for any type of client. These assessments are performed quickly and easily without increasing the cost or time of evaluation. They also allow the OT practitioner to eliminate neurological issues that may not be considered by other disciplines who focus their evaluation only on the injured body part.
  - Straight leg raise (SLR): Recommended for use with every client because it is a quick and easy way to assess whether the client has radicular pain. For clients with low back injury the angle of the supine SLR versus the seated SLR can be compared to check for consistency or inconsistency of effort and possible symptom magnification.
  - Slump test: Another quick and easy check for neurological symptoms. This will also put the dura on

stretch and reproduce radicular pain. By having the client bend his or her trunk forward while forward flexing the neck and coming to standing on the heels, the OT practitioner is tightening up the dura and putting the client's sciatic nerve on stretch. If the client is displaying positive neurological signs, he or she will experience a "shocking" sensation down the leg, similar to what one feels when hitting the lateral epicondyle, producing pain throughout the UE as a result of irritation of the ulnar nerve.

- Toe rise: Performed by having the client come up on the toes with equal effort, without rolling out to the lateral aspect of the foot; this tests for L5/S1 nerve dysfunction.

- Other assessments specific to different types of issues will also be performed.
  - For injuries where edema is a concern, circumferential or volumetric measurements are performed before and at the conclusion of activities on bilateral extremities (hand, foot, ankle, etc.); permits comparison of the nonaffected extremity (the client's normal fluid exchange) with the affected extremity. Chapter 22 contains more detailed information regarding edema management.
  - B200 isoinertial back assessments for lumbar back injuries (evaluates for strength, power, and range of motion)
  - Standardized coordination testing for UE injuries
  - Shoulder or knee stability test for shoulder or knee injuries

Job-Specific Functional Activities

Because one of the purposes of the WCE is to identify any problem areas that prevent an individual from returning to competitive employment, the assessment must include the client's participation in a variety of functional and work-related tasks. These include prolonged standing, walking, lifting, carrying, pushing, pulling, stair and ladder climbing, and so on. Depending on job requirements, the evaluation can include crawling, transitioning to or from the floor, swinging sledge hammers, torquing on wrenches, walking on uneven surfaces, and so on. Some of the functional tasks assessed include the following:

- Prolonged walking
- Climbing stairs and ladders (Fig. 17-2)
- Back education
- Body mechanics and proper lifting
- Material handling training
- Job-specific lifting and carrying:
  - Floor: Overhead
  - Floor: Shoulder
  - Floor: Waist
  - Carry: Including up/down stairs

The work conditioning baseline assessment identifies problems that will interfere with the client's ability to participate in 8 hours/day of simulated work activities. After the baseline assessment, if it is determined that the client is able to consistently and actively participate in 8 hours/day of simulated activities, 5 days a week, then the client is not appropriate for work conditioning but, rather, is ready for work hardening. Work hardening will be discussed in the next section.

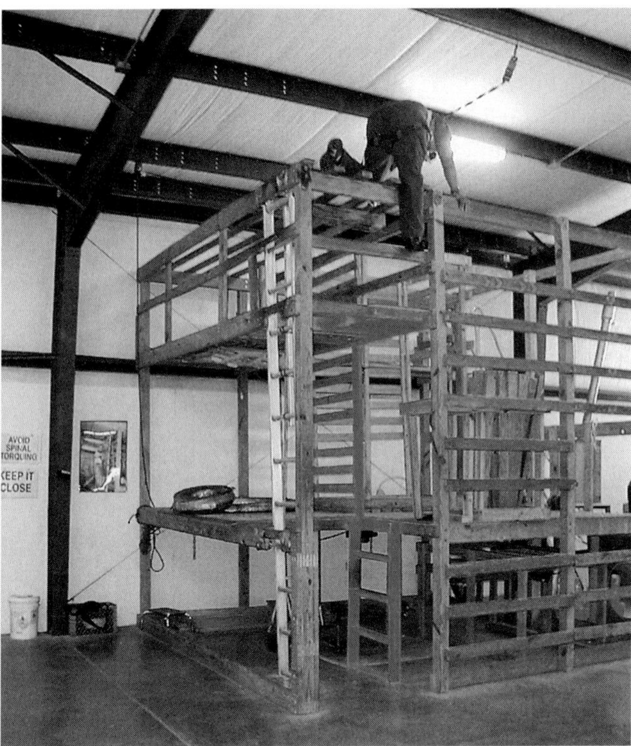

FIGURE 17-2. Worker climbing ladder (wearing a safety harness).

Program Development

The occupational therapist, with input from the OTA, will design an activity program for the client. The program goals initially are not necessarily job related but, rather, are intended to resolve problems that have been identified in the initial baseline assessment and that are preventing the client from RTW at this time. An example of a problem list would be similar to the following:

1. Very tight craniosacral or back muscles, including back extensors, hip flexors, quads, piriformis, hip extensors, hip internal, and hip external rotators, with resulting LBP complaints; or very tight shoulder/rotator cuff muscles, resulting in UE pain complaints or limitations
2. Poor aerobic fitness compared with other men or women of the client's age and gender
3. Poor muscle strength/endurance and ROM
4. Decreased tolerance to prolonged standing, walking, or sitting
5. Decreased ability to climb stairs and ladders
6. Decreased grip strength and power/endurance
7. Decreased ability to lift or carry weights or push and pull forces

On the basis of this type of problem list, the occupational therapist identifies and establishes a series of short-term and long-term goals in collaboration with the client and input from the OTA. A daily activity program can be developed from this list of goals to resolve the problems. The 4 hours of work conditioning activities will consist of a series of exercises and stretching in conjunction with the client's participation in progressive functional activities. The exercises can include the client's participation in the following:

- Structured circuit weight training
- Progressive functional lifting/carrying/squatting activities
- Monitored and OT practitioner-directed aquatic therapy
- Progressive, OT practitioner-directed stretching twice during the 4-hour session

The OTA is responsible for having the client carry out these activities, for documentation, and for informing the occupational therapist when the client is not progressing as expected, when the activities are not sufficiently challenging, or when the client is not participating actively.

Progress Notes and Reevaluation Notes

Proper documentation of a client's progress and reevaluations are essential to ensure accountability. It is imperative to document the client's weekly progress, or lack thereof, in the work conditioning program. Unlike other settings, the weekly progress notes and reevaluation notes are directed to the referring physician. These notes, in a letter format, are completed every Friday and cover the previous week's sessions; they should cover the following areas:

- Number of work conditioning sessions completed—including any absences and the reasons for these
- Statement regarding the client's attendance, promptness, and whether the client is participating actively in the rehabilitation program, as described
- Summary of the activities the client is participating in and the general goals being worked on or completed
- Summary of the client's pain complaints
- Issues, problems, or questions for the physician
- Plans for the future including progression toward discharge

Figure 17-3 shows an example of a progress note, which should be printed on the rehabilitation center's letterhead. The OTA's role in the development of the weekly progress notes and the regular reevaluation notes is critically important. The OTA will work closely with the occupational therapist to ensure that all pertinent information about the client's active participation or lack thereof, progress or regression, issues, and concerns, are clearly documented. Documentation of the objective observations of both the OTA and the occupational therapist is critical for ensuring the defensibility of the work conditioning program.

Accountability is of utmost importance in sustaining a work conditioning program. To aid those involved in determining whether the work conditioning program should be continued or discontinued, it is important to document the initial status and the current status in all the appropriate areas side by side so that all interested parties can make a comparison easily. The progress note for a particular week summarizes what the reevaluation note quantifies.

WORK HARDENING PROGRAMS

Work hardening programs were developed in the early 1980s to fulfill a need in the transition of injured workers returning to work at some capacity. Before this, in the 1960s and 1970s, many OT practitioners had "dropped out of work programs for the industrially injured" because of the shift in focus toward the medical model in the OT profession and the "pressure to develop a scientific rationale for its practice."[8] When this occurred, vocational evaluators assumed the roles vacated by OT. The vocational rehabilitation programs were able to find the "best vocational direction for the individual, given his or her interests, aptitudes, general physical abilities, skills, worker traits, and the local labor market."[8] However, these programs did not adequately address or physically prepare an individual to RTW through exercise and realistic job simulation activities.[8]

Leonard Matheson and Linda Ogden at Rancho Los Amigos in Southern California developed a unique partnership that incorporated the client's participation in real work activities as a means to assess the client's ability to RTW in a safe manner. The Matheson and Ogden WCE model considered work tolerance and employment feasibility as primary evaluation factors, or the frames of reference, for the evaluation. This evaluation became a multiweek process wherein injured workers would gain improved physical work tolerance through conditioning, learn pain management techniques, gain increased confidence in their abilities, and demonstrate an improved attitude, all through the structured use of real work and functional activities as the therapeutic medium. Over time, this process evolved into a "separate intervention service for the industrial injured," and the term work hardening evolved.[8] Injured workers would be "hardened" back to work.

Work hardening programs are the last step in the treatment plan before the client is discharged to a functional work level. Work hardening is defined as:

> "a highly structured, goal oriented, individualized treatment program designed to maximize the individual's ability to return to work. Work hardening programs, which are interdisciplinary in nature, use real or simulated work activities in conjunction with conditioning tasks that are graded to progressively improve the biomechanical, neuromuscular, cardiovascular/metabolic, and psychosocial functions of the individual. Work hardening provides a transition between acute care and return to work while addressing the issues of productivity, safety, physical tolerances, and worker behaviors."[8]

Work hardening guidelines indicate that work hardening programs are up to 6 weeks in length. When assessing whether the client is ready to transition from work

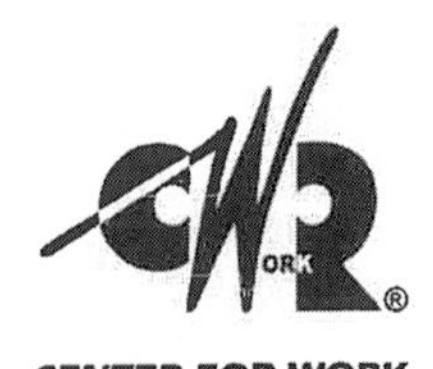

CENTER FOR WORK REHABILITATION, INC.®

Ergonomic Consultation

Functional Capacity Evaluation

Work Hardening

Occupational Therapy

Back Education Programs

On-Site Job Analysis

Job Description Development

Post-Offer Testing

ADA Consultation

FITNESS AND HEALTH

Private and Group Swim Lessons

Fitness Memberships

Aquatic Programs

Aerobics & Zumba

Yoga & Pilates

Weight Training

Personal Training

Massage Therapy

Silver Sneakers

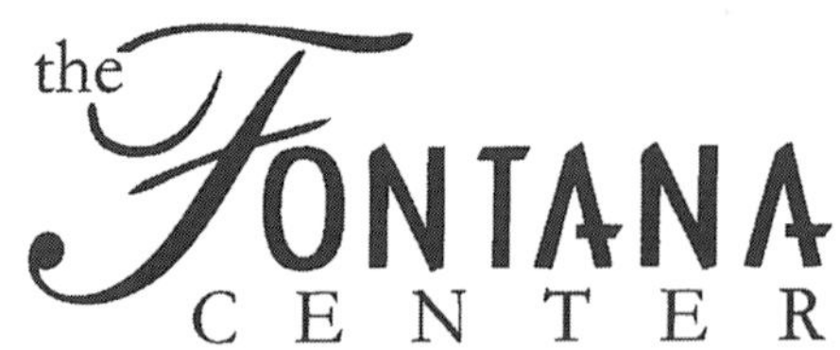

Feb 1, 2016

Dr Bob Jones
1234 Any Avenue
Suite 2500 D
New Orleans, LA 70777

RE: Work Conditioning Program for Mable Carter

Dear Dr Jones,

This is to follow up on Ms Mable Carter's work conditioning program that was initiated on January 14, 2016. She has attended 11 sessions thus far, only missing Monday of this week due to personal reasons. She has reported that she has been actively engaging in the home stretching program.

Ms Carter has been participating in activities and exercises designed to strengthen/condition her tolerance to participation in functional and work tasks. This includes:

- ❑ Therapist directed progressive/aggressive stretching of hamstrings, piriformis, and quadriceps, as well as implementing the Mckenzie techniques.
- ❑ Body mechanic training and implementation of safe material handling process including participation in a gentle warm up stretching program.
- ❑ Progressive holistic strengthening/conditioning program designed to strengthen/condition her for standing, walking, squatting, and other functional activities.
- ❑ Trigger point techniques to Bilateral Upper Traps/right IT band

	Week 1	Week 3
MAX. LIFTING CAPACITY		
Overhead	10 lbs Waist-OH	15 lbs Knee-OH
Shoulder	15 lbs Waist-S	20 lbs Knee-S
Waist		25 lbs Knee-W
Bench to bench carry	15 lbs	25 lbs
Repetitive lift/carry	5 lbs W-OH 10 lbs W-S	10 lbs K-OH 15 lbs K-S 20 lbs K-W
Treadmill	15 minutes at 2.0 mph	30 minutes at 2.5 mph

She experiences essentially the same pain, reporting a dull aching pain in center of her lower back, right buttocks, as well as across the right upper trap, and it ranges from 30—70 (Decreased from last week 40—80) out of 100 where 100 equates to hospitalization pain. She continues to respond well with hamstring stretches and prolonged lumbar extension.

Ms Carter has had a significant/positive change in her attitude towards the program, walking around much more cheerfully and making comments like "I can tell how much this is helping already; I need to keep going". We will continue the program as described this week and look to re-assess how she is doing each day, adjusting activities as she tolerates. Ms Carter is being daily encouraged to continue to walk, stretch, and stay active at home.

Thank you once again for the referral. Please contact us at the Center for Work Rehabilitation Inc. with any questions or concerns.

Sincerely,

Paul A. Fontana, OTR, FAOTA
Occupational Therapist
Fellow, American Occupational Therapy Association

Katrina Duhon Delahoussaye, MOTR/L
Occupational Therapist

cc: Sara Jones, Adjuster

709 Kaliste Saloom Rd.
Lafayette, LA 70508
337-234-7018 *fax* 337-232-3891
www.fontanacenter.com

FIGURE 17-3. Weekly progress note sent to the referring physician.

conditioning into the work hardening program, the OT practitioner should evaluate the client to ensure that:

1. The client is able to sustain a level of function 8 hours per day, 5 days per week.
2. The 6-week period will enable the client to make sufficient progress to either RTW or plateau at the highest work level reasonably projected by the OT practitioner.

If the physician has not approved a work hardening order before the date projected for the transition, then the occupational therapist should make a formal written request at a minimum of 1 to 2 weeks before the period that the occupational therapist would like the work hardening program to commence. This will give sufficient time for the physician to respond and for the carrier to approve the work hardening program so that no lapse in rehabilitation occurs when the work conditioning program ends and before the work hardening program begins.

A client is eligible for a work hardening program once he or she has reached MMI and is expected to reach his or her functional goals and limits or is able to return to his or her former job, within 4 to 6 weeks of work hardening. The client is *not* considered a candidate for work hardening and should begin in the work conditioning phase when:

- It is believed that the client will not be able to tolerate a minimum of at least 6 hours of physical activities per day, 5 days a week.
- Within the 6-week period for a work hardening program, the client will not reach maximum functional level or job goal requirements (should this be the case, the client should be placed in a work conditioning program).

A critical component to any work hardening program is the ability to provide the client with realistic or simulated work-related activities (Fig. 17-4). Through performance in graded functional work tasks, the client will not only improve his or her physical abilities to perform work but also improve from a psychosocial standpoint, gaining confidence in the ability to tolerate the demands of the work to which he or she will be returning. In the initial stage of a work hardening program, the OT practitioner may continue with some of the strengthening, conditioning and stretching components used in the work conditioning program. However, to be considered work hardening, the program must have the ability to simulate real work or the critical components of real work activities. As the client progresses in the work hardening program, the use of circuit weight training and treadmill, elliptical, or upper body ergometer (UBE) type of exercise equipment will be replaced by only simulated work-type activities throughout the 8-hour days.

Work hardening programs will improve the client's ability to sit, stand, lift, carry, climb, sustain a variety of postures and positions, and handle other unique stresses required for a specific job. These might include the ability to

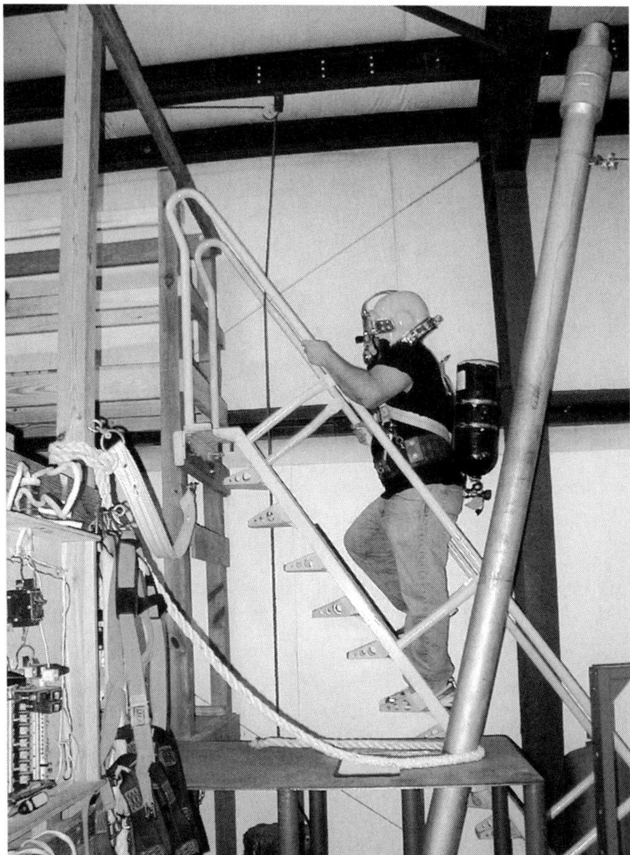

FIGURE 17-4. Firefighter climbing stairs with breathing apparatus.

cope with vibrations when swinging a sledge hammer, to swing on a swing rope or climb a ladder repeatedly throughout the day, or to stand and walk on nonlevel surfaces while wearing steel-toed boots throughout the 8-hour work day. Increasing the client's productivity and safety through proper body mechanics will be carried over from the work conditioning program, where appropriate, or will be introduced if the client did not begin with participating in a work conditioning program.

Initial Evaluations

The initial evaluation for a work hardening program is very similar to that of a work conditioning program in that it also includes an initial interview and a musculoskeletal assessment. However, understanding the description of the job to which the injured worker is going to be returning is more important at this stage than when the client was in the work conditioning phase. The RTW option may be the job the client was performing at the time of the injury. When it is believed that the previous job is not a viable option any more, a vocational counselor may become involved. A vocational counselor is trained in performing an inventory of various interests and an aptitude test, assessing the client's vocational interests and identifying potential career prospects that meet a client's needs. The vocational counselor will require the results of the FCE or WCE or a projected functional work level by the OT practitioner to properly assist the client in identifying potential

OT Practitioner's Viewpoint

Julia Child was quoted as saying: "If you can find your niche, I think you could find your life."[15] Finding your niche in OT will allow you to bring passion to your work; that will culminate in the richness of your work and will fuel you throughout your work lifetime. As an occupational therapist, I have found that working with industrial customers, analyzing jobs, identifying those critical work demands that present problems for his or her ability to return to competitive employment, and then following up with a meaningful program that will improve the client's functional abilities so that he is able to regain his life brings to me the fulfillment that I did not find in other areas of practice. You will have more opportunities to use clinical reasoning and your creative intellect in this area of practice than in any that I am aware of. As the client begins to make incremental improvements in his or her functional abilities, I see great gains in the client's psychosocial state. Having an individual go from believing that he or she will never be able to return to competitive work or possibly even be able to pick up their children or play with them, to the point where he is able to work full 8-hour work days in competitive employment, gives me the satisfaction that I have made a positive difference in a person's life.

A wonderful example of this is given in the sections on work conditioning and work hardening. A young man was in pain management following a "successful" lumbar fusion; he was using narcotic pain medication every day and believed that he was going to be a "patient" for the rest of his life. He was depressed—as can be expected of someone only 42 years old and had permanent restrictions limiting his ability to even pick up his children, let alone ever return to work. It was truly amazing to watch his attitude change almost daily, as he began making progress in his therapy. He was so excited when he came in and told us that he had not taken any pain medication in a week and was still relatively pain-free. Talk about helping folks "live life to the fullest!" ~Paul Fontana, LOTR, FAOTA

jobs. The vocational counselor may identify another reasonable and feasible option that is based on the client's intellect, schooling, interests, and job availability within 50 miles of the client's home. However, this planning requires the input from the OT practitioner as to a reasonable work level the client will be able to attain following a work hardening program. In many cases, no projected job options are considered until a realistic functional work level is delineated.

The results of the WCE or FCE will help the OT practitioner to:

- Determine appropriateness of care—whether the client is appropriate for a work conditioning program or a work hardening program.
- Establish a baseline for quantifying progress.
- Provide for realistic cross checks to determine the client's validity or consistency of effort and possible symptom magnification behaviors (Box 17-1).
- Identify problem areas that must be resolved if the client is going to be able to improve functionally and RTW.
- Estimate a discharge work level so that a realistic RTW scenario can be established.
- Develop the plan of care—that is, the activity program designed by the OT practitioner to resolve the identified problems and return the individual to his maximum level of function.

Physical Job Description

A **physical job description** is imperative for determining a work hardening program. To be effective, the job description should identify the physical requirements necessary to perform the job's essential functions. When these physical requirements are identified in quantifiable, measureable terms, the simulated work tasks and abilities can be used in the rehabilitation process. If the specifics of the job are not known and those functions cannot be simulated closely, the OT practitioner cannot, in good faith, release

BOX 17-1
Assessments Help Identify Issues

The Center for Work Rehabilitation, Inc. (CWR) at the Fontana Center in Lafayette, LA, was asked to perform a baseline assessment on an individual who was thought to be a "malingerer" by the company because the client had made no progress in spite of a year of physical therapy. The orthopedic surgeon who evaluated the client could not find anything that would "cause" the pain complaints expressed by the client. "Malingerer" is a medical-legal term, which means that the individual has no pain and is making up pain complaints. There is no way to objectively measure pain, so the OT practitioners at the CWR do not use the term *malingerer* to describe any client but, rather, use the term *symptom magnifier*, which was proposed by Dr. Leonard Matheson, to describe individuals who magnify their pain behaviors, either consciously or unconsciously, for secondary gain.

Following an 8-hour baseline assessment and a B200 isoinertial back evaluation, which showed no inconsistencies or nonphysiological behaviors, it was the opinion of the occupational therapist at the CWR that the individual not only gave a valid and consistent effort but also demonstrated that he had significant low back muscle weakness and muscle tightness. The year of physical therapy did not address any of the client's physical problems but, rather, consisted of passive modalities. After 3 weeks of work hardening, which included progressive, aggressive stretching by the occupational therapist and the OTA, along with daily B200 back rehabilitation, the client was released without restrictions back to full duty at his job as a fisherman.

BOX 17-1
Assessments Help Identify Issues (continued)

OOC Evaluation Results for 26-JUL-00

Demographic Data

		Resistance Settings
Age: 31	Sex: M	Rotation 25%: 17 lb-ft
Height: 5 ft 09 in	Weight: 180 lbs	Rotation 50%: 34 lb-ft
		Flex/Ext 25%: 25 lb-ft
Diagnosis: Lumbar Strain		Flex/Ext 50%: 50 lb-ft
Surgical Category: Non-Surgical		Lat Flex 25%: 23 lb-ft
Activity Level Category: Very Heavy Work		Lat Flex 50%: 46 lb-ft

Abnormal Indicators 3

	Rotation 25%	Rotation 50%	Flex/Ext 25%	Flex/Ext 50%	Lat Flex 25%	Lat Flex 50%
Isometric Max Torque						
Max Velocity		↓	↓	↓		
Rotation Sec Max Torque						
Flex/Ext Sec Max Torque						
Lat Flex Sec Max Torque						

Non-Physiological Indicators 1

1) not observed
2) max velocity 50% greater than or equal 25%, seq 2: L F
3) not observed
4) not observed
5) not observed
6) not observed

Baseline Rehabilitation Data

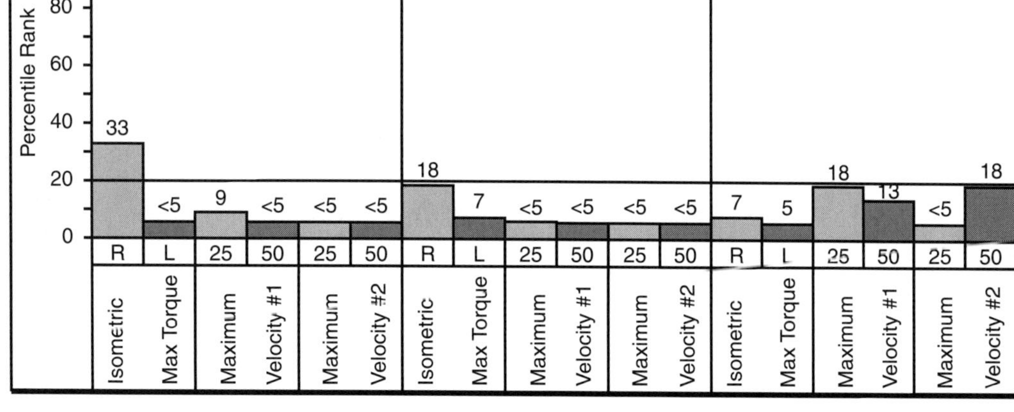

Test Administered By: Signed: ______________ Date: ________

Physiological Test but demonstrates current back dysfunction and not recommended for hire.

Continued

BOX 17-1
Assessments Help Identify Issues (continued)

OOC Evaluation Results for 10-May-00

Demographic Data

Age: 36 Sex: M
Height: 5 ft 04 in Weight: 196 lbs

Diagnosis: Non-Symptomatic
Surgical Category: Non-Surgical
Activity Level Category: Heavy work

Resistance Settings

Rotation 25%: 30 lbs-ft
Rotation 50%: 60 lbs-ft
Flex/Ext 25%: 33 lbs-ft
Flex/Ext 50%: 71 lbs-ft
Lat Flex 25%: 38 lb-ft
Lat Flex 50%: 63 lb-ft

Abnormal Indicators 8

	Rotation 25%	Rotation 50%	Flex/Ext 25%	Flex/Ext 50%	Lat Flex 25%	Lat Flex 50%
Isometric Max Torque	↑					
Max Velocity						
Rotation Sec Max Torque			↑			
Flex/Ext Sec Max Torque						
Lat Flex Sec Max Torque			↑			

Non-Physiological Indicators 1

1) not observed
2) max velocity 50% greater than or equal 25%, seq 2: F/E
3) not observed
4) not observed
5) not observed
6) not observed

Baseline Rehabilitation Data

Percentile Rank (0–100)

	Isometric (R)	Max Torque (L)	Maximum (25)	Velocity #1 (50)	Maximum (25)	Velocity #2 (50)
Rotation	95	79	84	79	34	37
Flexion/Extension	58	25	60	79	37	58
Lateral Flexion	81	75	83	89	76	94

Test Administered By: Signed: ______________________ Date: __________

Physiological Test with no signs of any weakness or dysfunction

the client back to work. Without this knowledge, the OT practitioner has to speculate as to whether the individual will be able to meet the critical job demands; this would place clients at an increased risk of injury by returning them to jobs that they may not be able to perform safely. It also can deny employment to an individual who really would be able to RTW. Without a valid physical job description that quantifies in measurable terms the physical requirements needed to perform the work safely, the OT practitioner will not be able to develop an effective work hardening program where the client performs these critical job demands.

A valid job description allows the client to gain valuable knowledge about his or her ability to perform a task that he or she may be fearful of performing, as well as learn, practice, and become proficient in performing a task correctly thereby decreasing the risk of injury. Many job descriptions provided for clients in work hardening programs may convey how much weight needs to be lifted in very general terms (occasionally lift 50 lb or frequently lift 25 lb), but very few quantify what the term "frequent" or "occasional" mean. When this is the case and the OT practitioner is unable to perform an onsite job analysis, it is imperative to ask the necessary questions so that the OT practitioner understands the critical components of the job as it affects the client and can properly simulate those tasks in the program. This will be covered more extensively in the section on FCE.

Program Development

The baseline WCE identifies problems that will interfere with the client's ability to return to his or her previous work level (or job). When the return to a former job is an unrealistic expectation, the goal of the work hardening program is to promote the client's maximal level of function. Furthermore, the baseline WCE provides the OT practitioner with the information he or she needs to project what functional level the client should be able to realistically achieve following the work hardening program. The OT practitioner will develop a program, including exercises, functional work activities, and training designed to:

1. Resolve or ameliorate the problems identified on the baseline assessment.
2. Simulate real work activities or the critical components of real work requirements so that the client can:
   - Develop the strength/endurance to safely perform the task as required on the job.
   - Learn the correct posture/position or technique to safely perform the task.
   - Develop the confidence to safely perform the task.

It is important to educate the client on the "why" behind job simulation activities that have a revised technique—that is, the client has to understand the reason behind the revision and simulation—and generally, if the client fully understands the reasoning, this results in increased client compliance.

If it is determined that the client will be unable to reach his or her previous work level, the program will focus on improving the client's functional abilities, reducing the client's physical restrictions or limitations, and reducing his or her pain complaints. The program will conclude when the client's improvement or ability to sustain an increase in physical activity reaches a plateau. For example, if a client is only able to perform a quarter partial squat because of permanent limited ROM and pain, the program will have the client perform quarter or partial squatting with a gradual increase in frequency or the weights lifted as the client tolerates. An initial work hardening activity program may include the activities listed in Figure 17-5.

A valuable component of a work hardening program is improvement in clients' psychosocial attitudes and opinions of themselves as productive members of their families and society. Often, when clients have been out of work or in constant pain and unable to fulfill their usual roles in life for an extended period, it takes a toll on their self-perception as a productive member of society and therefore can influence their recovery process. It is not uncommon that the work hardening program is the place where the client has the time to develop a rapport with the OT practitioner and is able to confront some of these psychosocial issues with the assistance of a trained and educated professional. Depression is a normal response when a 42-year-old man or a 35-year-old woman is unable to take care of the family and is confronted by the possibility of never being able to RTW. As the client makes progress toward his or her previous functional abilities through the work hardening program, the resolution of these issues becomes a real possibility, and the client's attitude and perspective on life will improve.

Clients can be medically mismanaged by not getting the appropriate therapy or surgery or the correct follow-up therapy in a timely manner. Many clients are never properly educated about their injuries, actual diagnosis, or realistic outcomes with the right medical treatment approach. Some do not clearly understand their injuries or have been told something false (by friends, attorneys, or even medical practitioners) and will refuse to participate in different activities out of fear of further damaging the injury or because it may cause pain. In other cases, clients may have healed properly from surgery or their injuries; however, they may still have some form of muscular dysfunction surrounding the injured area as a result of scar tissue, tight muscles, or poor strength recovery. This can be a significant cause of pain. When this occurs, it is the responsibility of the OT practitioner to provide education to the client about the anatomy and physiology of the spine, muscles, and joints. This allows the individual to understand the cause, the possible "cure," and how active participation in the work hardening program will resolve those issues. For example, a client who equates pain with further damage to an injured site may be more willing to work actively with the OT practitioner if he or she (and significant others) understands that muscle fatigue and/or muscle tightness may be the cause of the pain and that the pain experienced while participating in certain activities could be the result of this. When clients are properly educated on their injuries and the recovery process, they feel more empowered to take control of their recovery and, in turn, are more compliant and dedicated to the process.

It is not always possible for a client to make a full "pain-free" recovery. Often, if resolving the client's pain was a realistic goal, it would have been accomplished before the client reached the work hardening program. With such

Work Hardening Program Example: Job: Bridge Tender for Railroad Co.

Target Heart Rate:________/________ BP:________/________

5 minutes	Debrief with therapist/pain sheet
15 minutes	Warm up stretches
20 minutes	Bike at 2.5–3.0 mph (5 minute intervals)
20 minutes	Arm bike: switching direction every 60 seconds
60 minutes	Repetitive lifting: 1. Squat lift 40 lbs from the floor, carry 25 feet to OH height then carry back 1 x 60 seconds for 20 minutes 2. 5 minutes standing: push/pull BTE lever with 200 lbs of force with both hands x 10, then 140 lbs of force 1 x 5 seconds for 5 minutes. 3. Squat lift 50 lbs from the floor, carry 25 feet to waist height then carry back 1 x 60 seconds for 20 minutes 4. 3 minutes kneeling push/pull BTE lever with 120 lbs of force directly in front of him, like cranking a jack. 5. Climb stairs carrying 40 lbs, repeat x 10 once each minute switching hands
10 minutes	Break
10 minutes	Lifting assessment: 1. Floor–OH 40 lbs x 2 2. Floor–W 50 lbs x 2 3. B-B carry 50 lbs x 2 4. Swing 16 lbs sledge hammer x 15, rest 1 minute and repeat.
60 minutes	Treadmill at 3.5 mph Reassess grip strength: R _____ _____ _____ _____ _____ L _____ _____ _____ _____ _____
20 minutes	BTE ladder pull/push: Resistance 350 in lbs standing 1 minute in each direction. Use a small block to put one foot on while standing
20 minutes	Brick shelving unit. Place 15 lbs object from the Floor–Waist–Shoulder–Overhead (all positions) within one minute. Repeat for 20 minutes.
30 minutes	Lunch
15 minutes	Warm up stretches
15 minutes	Crawl under 4' high structure, begin threading chain with rope at eye level for 10 minutes (squatting/kneeling/sitting on heels), every 2 minutes, lift and hold 5 lbs object at eye level for 10 seconds x 2, climb out and perform 2 back extensions. Lift and carry 15 lbs tools up/down 3 flights of stairs.
20 minutes	Squat lift 40 lbs from the floor, carry 25 feet to OH height then carry back 1 x 60 seconds for 20 minutes
20 minutes	Seated ladder pull with 350 lbs 1 minute in each direction (place one foot on 6" block)
10 minutes	Break
20 minutes	Push/Pull sled with 120 lbs force for 10 feet 1 x 60 seconds
30 minutes	Squat lift 50 lbs from the floor, carry 25 feet to waist then carry back 1 x 60 seconds for 20 minutes. Then perform BTE seated with R hand 120 lbs 1 x 5 seconds for 5 minutes, then repeat with L hand.
15 minutes	Standing: Push/Pull BTE lever with 200 lbs force with both hands x 10
20 minutes	Multi assembly working from floor to overhead.
20 minutes	P/P sled with 120 lbs force 1 x 60 seconds
10 minutes	Standing: P/P BTE lever with 200 lbs force (position 4) with both hands x 10, then 140 lbs (560 in lbs on pos. 4) of force 1 x 5 seconds for 2 minutes. Then kneeling P/P BTE lever with 120 lbs of force directly in front of him, like cranking a jack for 3 minutes. Then performing light hand activity on bus bench at floor level for 5 minutes (kneeling/squatting/sitting on his heels)
15 minutes	Cool down stretches/pain sheet BP:________/________

FIGURE 17-5. Sample work hardening program plan.

clients, at some point in time, pain resolution is no longer the goal of rehabilitation. Rather, improving the individual's level of functioning within his or her pain tolerance is a viable goal. Most people, in general, are not pain free, but they are able to continue to function well in society and within their jobs within their pain tolerance. Where possible, the OT practitioner's role is to identify the source of the client's pain and work to resolve it. Often, when the pain, such as LBP, is the result of tight craniosacral muscles or scar tissue, participation in progressive and aggressive stretching and strengthening exercises and activities often reduces or possibly resolves it. If the client still experiences pain, the goal is to maximize function within his or her pain tolerance. Improving a client's function often will increase the ability to return to competitive employment. For example, standing tolerance may be increased, and the client may be able to perform jobs at work; squatting tolerance may be increased, and the client is able to lift safely; or sitting tolerance may be increased, and the client is able to return to driving a truck at work. This improved function will also enhance clients' lives outside of work. Along with being able to return to competitive work; being able to take care of the home; playing with one's children; and being able to stand long enough to play golf, go hiking, or work in the yard will go a long way to improving one's quality of life.

Another important aspect of a successful work hardening program is using an interdisciplinary approach. It is important that all those involved in the client's RTW issues be actively engaged in and knowledgeable about the client's status and situation. This includes the client's physician, significant others (spouse, children, etc.), attorney, medical case manager, rehabilitation nurse, vocational counselor, insurance provider, employer or potential employer (when known), along with any other integral professional, such as spinal cord stimulator representative, prosthetic representative, and so on. By working closely with this team, the OT practitioner is helping the client have the best chance at succeeding in their RTW program. This can include speaking with the physician regarding a change or possible increase of the client's medication (for pain, sleep) at the onset of the program, requesting transportation for the client to and from the clinic each day, or having the spinal cord stimulator or prosthetic representative attend several sessions to help minimize pain or optimize function. When a rehabilitation nurse, medical case manager, or vocational counselor is assigned to work with the client, having this professional attend regular meetings with the OT practitioner and the client will ensure that each understands the problems being encountered, assistance that is needed, and what the realistic goals are and when they may be achieved. Every member of the interdisciplinary team should understand and be aligned with the plan of care and know what role he or she needs to play for the client to have the best chance for success.

Progress Notes and Reevaluation Notes

It is imperative to document the weekly progress, or lack thereof, that the client is making in the work hardening program. The notes contain the same type of information as was previously discussed in the work conditioning section.These notes are to be completed every Friday and cover the previous week's sessions. Reevaluations are to be completed every 2 weeks (10 sessions). Clients in work hardening programs need to have a reevaluation covering any problem areas that were identified during the initial baseline assessment. All documentation is to be sent to the treating physician, the insurance carrier, or whoever is paying for the work hardening program, the medical case manager, rehabilitation nurse or vocational counselor who is assigned to the case, and any attorneys who may be involved.

A complete reevaluation covers all the problem areas that were identified in the baseline evaluation. It will be performed every 10 sessions to determine whether the OT goals are still appropriate and also to document the progress the client has made since the initial evaluation. The same format that was described in the work conditioning session will be used here. The subsequent weekly progress note will summarize the findings of the reevaluation along with outlining the plan for the future (Fig. 17-6).

TECHNOLOGY AND TRENDS

Computerized programs are available on the market for completing a FCE and may help reduce the time involved in paperwork. However, this type of software may inhibit the OT practitioner's ability to accurately document what actually occurred in the clinic as he or she is looking at the computer screen and not the client. If that is the case, then this type of documentation system is not a valuable addition to documentation in the clinic. Technological advances can certainly provide some exciting new additions to the ability of the practitioner to simulate work activities. However, it is important not to "get hung up on the bells and whistles." If the individual has to lift 100-lb sacks, then they should be made to lift 100-lb sacks in the program. If they have to repetitively swing a 16- or 20-lb sledgehammer, then they must repetitively swing a 16- or 20-lb sledgehammer in the program. It is the job of the occupational therapist or the OTA to simulate the work activityor the critical demands of the work activity that is of particular concern to the client with regard to his or her ability to return to work (RTW). The closer the simulation is to the actual job, the easier it is to defend the results. Furthermore, the OT practitioner must be able to come up with activities that do not require him or her to speculate as to whether the client will be successful in his RTW situation. For instance, lifting a milk crate with handles is not the same as handling the same weight on an item that does not have handles. Static strength tests do not correlate to what a person is able to lift dynamically.

Discharge

Discharge criteria are met when:

1. The client has demonstrated that he or she is able to RTW without restrictions.
2. The client has demonstrated that he or she is able to RTW with restrictions as identified by the potential employer as reasonable.
3. The client has plateaued in his or her progress and thus has reached his or her maximum functional improvement.

When the decision is made that the client has achieved one of the discharge criteria, a detailed FCE will be provided. The discharge note to the physician will include the following:

- Summary of the number of days in the work hardening program, along with a statement regarding the client's participation, cooperativeness, and attitude
- Discharge functional work level along with a statement that the report has been reviewed verbally word for word with the client who is in agreement with the report and if the physician also is in agreement there is a place for his signature at the end of the attached functional capacity report (FCR)

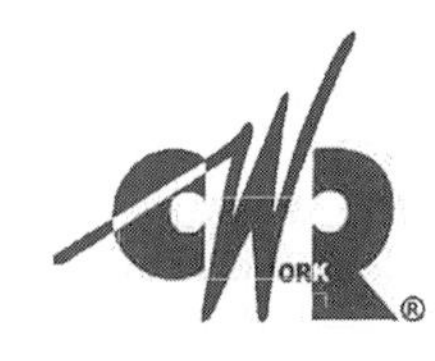

CENTER FOR WORK REHABILITATION, INC.®

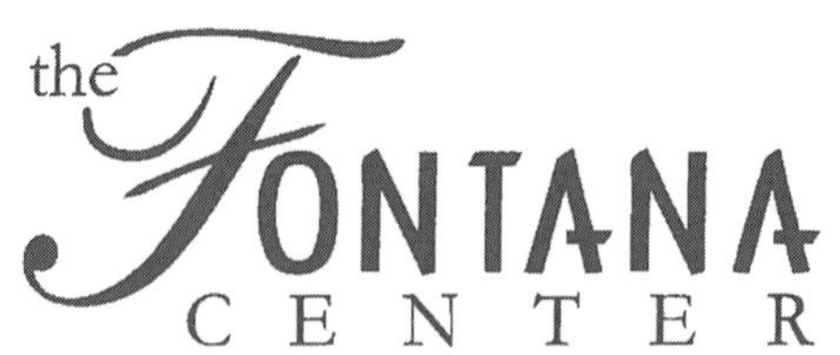

Ergonomic Consultation

Functional Capacity Evaluation

Work Hardening

Occupational Therapy

Back Education Programs

On-Site Job Analysis

Job Description Development

Post-Offer Testing

ADA Consultation

FITNESS AND HEALTH

Private and Group Swim Lessons

Fitness Memberships

Aquatic Programs

Aerobics & Zumba

Yoga & Pilates

Weight Training

Personal Training

Massage Therapy

Silver Sneakers

April 8, 2015

Dr Bruce Miller
1234 Jones Street
Lafayette, LA 70508

RE: Work Hardening program with Joe Smith

Dear Dr. Miller:

This is to follow up on Mr Joe Smith's Work Hardening program. He has completed 4 sessions of work conditioning and 7 sessions of work hardening (6 hours). Mr Smith is cooperative and is actively participating in all that we have requested of him. Mr Smith is participating in activities and exercises designed to strengthen/condition his tolerance for participation in functional and work tasks.

	INITIAL EVALUATION DATE: 3 / 22 / 15 Week 1	**RE-EVALUATION DATE: 4 / 1 / 15 Week 3**
MAX. LIFTING CAPACITY		
Overhead (OH)	15 lbs	30 lbs
Shoulder (S) from knee height	20 lbs	50 lbs from floor
Waist (W) from knee height	20 lbs	60 lbs from floor
Repetitive lift / carry	10 lbs Floor - OH	20 lbs Floor - OH
	20 lbs Knee - S	30 lbs Floor - S
	30 lbs Knee - W	40 lbs Floor - W
Treadmill	20 minutes at 1.5 MPH	30 minutes at 2.0 MPH
Stairs	5 (1 x 60 seconds for 5 min)	20 (1 x 60 sec for 20 minutes)
Push / pull	30 lbs force	70 lbs force

Mr Smith continues to report a dull aching pain across the center of his low back and a burning pain over bilateral lateral thighs (SLR is negative bilaterally) and rates it a 40 to 50/100 throughout the day. Although he is reporting the same amounts of pain as he has previously, he has improved the amount of work and functional activities he is able to tolerate significantly.

Mr Smith has completed 6 hour sessions all week and tolerated them well. We will transition his progress to 8 hour sessions each day next week, re-assessing his tolerance to activities and adjusting activities as he tolerates. Mr Smith is being encouraged daily to continue to walk, stretch, and stay active at home.

We would like to thank you again for this referral. Should you have any questions regarding this correspondence, please feel free to contact us here at the Center for Work Rehabilitation Inc.

Sincerely,

Paul A. Fontana, OTR, FAOTA
Occupational Therapist
Fellow, American Occupational Therapy Association

Katrina Duhon Delahoussaye, MOTR/L
Occupational Therapist

Enclosure

cc: Sara Jones, Claims Adjuster
Mary Williams, Case Manager
Bruce Davis, Attorney

709 Kaliste Saloom Rd.
Lafayette, LA 70508
337-234-7018 *fax* 337-232-3891
www.fontanacenter.com

FIGURE 17-6. Reevaluation note to physician.

- A statement regarding any special tests that were performed, such as volumetric measurements, circumferential measurements, repeated grip test, isoinertial back evaluation, and a summary of the results
- If there is a job description available for the expected RTW position, a statement regarding the client's ability to RTW without restrictions or with restrictions would be included.

At the time of discharge following participation in a work hardening program, the client does not have to undergo another WCE. The OT practitioner has seen the client actively participate 8 hours per day for multiple days in succession at the discharge work level, so he or she is able to develop an FCE report based on the observations as well as objective testing. No additional testing or charges should be added to the client's program.

FUNCTIONAL CAPACITY EVALUATION

A FCE is an objective and comprehensive assessment of a person's demonstrated ability to sustain work in a competitive job market. It's not simply a musculoskeletal assessment and lifting assessment, neither is it what a person may be asked to be conditioned to but, rather, what an employer can expect from the client the next day. The FCE will include a summation of the individual's current abilities and limitations, ideally compared with his or her previous job or, when no job description is available for comparison, simply a listing of the individual's current abilities and limitations within his or her pain tolerance.

History of the Functional Capacity Evaluation

The FCE has evolved over the past 45 years since its inception in the early 1970s. Through work at Rancho Los Amigos Hospital in Downey, California, initially with cardiac clients, the client's participation in real work tasks was implemented and graded to identify safe work levels for these individuals. By having the clients use hammers and saws, carry items up and down stairs, push and pull on wrenches, shovel gravel, and carry toolboxes and sacks, all the while being monitored with electrocardiography equipment, the staff was able to specify those activities that the client was safe to handle and those that were resulting in an unsafe physiological response of their cardiac system. If healthcare professionals discharge individuals to perform levels of work that are too stressful or difficult for them, then these cardiac clients could potentially experience another cardiac event. The FCR helped both the client and his or her doctors establish the safe work level for the client. The client would then be able to return to full duty without restrictions or to a modified work capacity, or the person would know that he or she would not be able to return to that type of work and would need to explore alternative employment.[16]

Matheson and Ogden, through their work in this area, saw the value in the medical team being able to quantify specifically a person's demonstrated ability to safely perform tasks as a means of helping individuals return to meaningful work. Because back-related issues were costing business and industry the most in terms of dollars and the clients in terms of loss of function, the team at Rancho Los Amigos quickly realized the need to expand its program beyond cardiac issues and incorporate all work-related injuries and illnesses. Matheson, in his role as a scientist, helped build the framework of terminology that we use today to clarify the components of this aspect of industrial rehabilitation—namely, work conditioning, work hardening, and FCE.[16] In addition, he developed and defined the term symptom magnification and helped OT practitioners understand how to both identify and work with individuals who were magnifying their pain behaviors in either a conscious or unconscious manner for secondary gain or to control their environment.[17]

PITFALLS OF THE MODERN FUNCTIONAL CAPACITY EVALUATION

FCE, as first described and taught by Matheson, was best conducted over five consecutive 8-hour workdays because this was what individuals are expected to do once they complete the assessment process. What has happened over the years, however, is insurance companies do not want to pay for this extensive evaluation. As the rate they reimburse providers has decreased, providers (primarily OT and PT) have looked for ways to provide the results of a 5-day, 8-hour FCE in much less time and with less involvement on the part of the OT practitioner. This explains the evolution of the 2- to 4-hour, computer-based FCE. The problem with these less personalized, "cookbook" types of assessments will be discussed further in this section.[16]

In one of his earlier publications on this subject, Matheson quoted Ralph Waldo Emerson in his preface to what was called back then, *work capacity evaluations*:

"As to methods there may be a million and then some, but principles are few. The man, who tries methods, ignoring principles, is sure to have trouble."[16]

This section on FCE is not intended to be a description of a step-by-step cookbook approach to performing FCEs. To identify whether a person can safely lift, carry, and otherwise handle a 100-lb sack on his job, the OT practitioner has to have him lift a 100-lb sack in the clinic in the same manner as he would on the job. If the job requires him to repeat this 50 times in a day, then he has to do it 50 times a day in the clinic. The OT practitioner cannot determine whether an individual can stand or walk for 2 hours by having him walk 100 feet and repeat it three times, looking at the coefficient of variation, as some computerized assessments claim. At a training conference that Matheson was teaching, when asked about how to develop an FCE, he said (paraphrased), "You're an occupational therapist. You know how to do this. You know how to perform a thorough musculoskeletal assessment. You know what normal behavior is and how to identify nonphysiological behaviors. And you understand how to do an activity analysis. What you need to do is incorporate the use of real work, functional activities and tasks that relate to the client's job or the critical components of the job so that you can assess his abilities to safely perform the work."[18]

Components of a Functional Capacity Evaluation

This section does not aim to provide a step-by-step instruction manual to performing FCEs but, rather, help to illustrate the principles involved so that the OTA and the occupational therapist can use their training in OT to develop an assessment tool that is ethical and one where their professional opinions can be defended.

The results of the FCE, a **functional capacity report (FCR)**, is a definitive statement of what the employer can reasonably expect from the client the next day and continually thereafter. Areas that will be included in the FCR include the individual's ability to sit, stand, stoop, squat, bend, walk, climb (both ladders and stairs), lift and carry (including up and down stairs), push and pull (both while walking as well as stationary unilaterally), and work in a variety of postures and positions within their pain tolerance.

It is critically important that the results are objective and that the OT practitioner does not speculate as to the individual's abilities or limitations. To ensure defensibility it is imperative that the assessment include:

- On site interaction/supervision by professional therapy personnel
- Multiple 8-hour days in succession and not rely on a client's ability to perform a task one or two times to determine whether he is able to safely perform the task day in and day out
- Use of real work activities and or simulations of the critical components of tasks the individual may have difficulty with

Under most state Practice Acts, FCEs or assessments are performed by occupational or physical therapists with many of the daily interventions performed by the OTA or physical therapist assistant. According to some state Practice Acts, occupational and physical therapists cannot delegate this supervision to athletic trainers or other semiprofessionals but must provide onsite supervision of the daily activities in FCEs.

Every FCE, regardless of the diagnosis, should incorporate, at a minimum, all of the following components:

- Initial interview
- Job analysis, where applicable
- Extensive, full body musculoskeletal assessment
- Education regarding anatomy and physiology of the spine, disc pressures associated with everyday activities, and instruction in proper biomechanics for lifting and material handling
- Job-specific or client-specific dynamic lifting assessment
- Realistic simulated work activities
- 8 hours/day for multiple days in succession
- Distraction testing

INITIAL INTERVIEW

The initial interview will be the same process as previously discussed.

JOB ANALYSIS

As previously discussed, having a good written physical job description that clearly identifies the physical requirements necessary to perform the essential job functions in measurable terms is vital to aiding the OT practitioner in developing real work scenarios for the client to participate in.[19] Ideally, the OT practitioner, with his or her expertise in activity analysis, should travel to the work site and conduct a thorough job analysis and develop a reliable physical job description that quantifies the physical requirements needed to do this job in measurable terms. Quite often, the job descriptions provided to the OT practitioner list the physical requirements of the job in generic, nonmeasurable terms (Fig. 17-7). The problems come when trying to quantify the occasional or frequent postures and positions or lifting scenarios in a meaningful way. The Department of Labor quantifies the frequencies of an activity or posture in very generic terms:

- Occasional: Zero to one-third of a work day
- Frequently: One- to two-thirds of a work day
- Constantly: Greater than two-thirds of a work day[19]

What constitutes "frequent" lifting at one company or to one individual may not constitute "frequent" lifting to another. Thus, it is left up to the OT practitioner to determine how often "occasional" or "frequent" lifting, bending, squatting, or stair climbing, is (whether frequent lifting is 1×/hour throughout the day or 1×/10 minutes throughout the day). This decision will determine whether a client is able to RTW or not and cannot be left to the practitioner's unjustified guesswork.

When the job description uses these generic terms to describe the job and when the OT practitioner is not able to go on site, it is then necessary to analyze the job and develop a written and quantifiable physical job description. It is critically important that the OT practitioner question the client extensively so as to gain a good understanding of at least the client's description of the job. When looking to identify the weights of items lifted and carried along with their frequency, it is useful to have the client state the name of the item and his or her best guess as to its weight. Remember this is the client's description of the job. The OT practitioner may then use this information in his or her discussion with the company's representative to confirm the weights used on the job. When possible, the OT practitioner should also contact the employer and question a representative about the physical requirements for the position while remembering that this is the employer's perception of the job requirements. It is important to document the name and title of the employer's representative. In some cases, a written physical job description that identifies the job's physical requirements does not exist, and the client and the company's verbal descriptions of the job vary greatly. When this occurs, the OT practitioner must document what both the client and the employer state about the job's physical requirements. The OT practitioner must furthermore indicate which requirements he or she is using as the basis for his or her professional opinion, along with a clarifying statement

Employer Name: ____________________

Job Title/Classification: Mechanical Tech

JOB REQUIREMENTS AND PHYSICAL DEMANDS CHECKLIST

DESCRIPTION OF JOB RESPONSIBILITIES (LIST OR DESCRIBE ESSENTIAL JOB FUNCTIONS):
MECH TECH:

1. WALK DOWN PROJECT DRAWINGS FOR ACCURACY
2. OVERSEE FLUSHING AND LEAK TESTING ACTIVITIES OF PROJECT PIPING AND MECHANICAL SYSTEMS
3. VERIFY ALIGNMENTS OF SHAFT AND BELT DRIVEN EQUIPMENT SUCH AS: PUMPS, FANS, GENERATORS, COMPRESSORS, ETC.
4. ASSIST IN RUNNING EQUIPMENT TO PROVE SYSTEMS FUNCTION AS PER PROJECT DESIGN BASIS
5. COMPLETE PROJECT DOCUMENTATION THAT ENSURES EQUIPMENT QUALITY CHECKS HAVE BEEN PERFORMED PER SPECS.

Using the following definitions, please identify the extent to which each required activity is present during the workday:

N–*NEVER*: not required or not a significant component of the work
O–*OCCASIONAL*: activity or condition exists up to 1/3 of the workday (or, 1x–4x per hour)
F–*FREQUENT*: activity or condition exists from 1/3 to 2/3 of the workday (or, 5x–24x per hour)
C–*CONSTANT*: activity or condition exists 2/3 or more of the workday (or, 25x or more per hour)

ACTIVITY	N	O	F	C	ACTIVITY	N	O	F	C	ACTIVITY	N	O	F	C
Standing			X		Stooping/Bending		X			Simple Grasping:			X	
Walking		X			Kneeling		X			Left/Right/Both			X	
Sitting		X			Crouching/Squatting		X			Power Grasping:	X			
Twisting (Neck)		X			Crawling	X				Left/Right/Both	X			
Twisting (Waist)		X			Driving	X				Manual Dexterity			X	
Balancing		X			Reaching: Forward			X		Fine Manipulation			X	
Climbing: ft. Stairs/Ladders		X			Overhead		X			Eye-Hand Coordination		X		
					Side			X						

LIFTING	HEIGHT	N	O	F	C
0#–25#			X		
26#–50#		X			
51#–75#		X			
76#–100#					
>100#		X			
CARRYING	**DISTANCE**				
0#–25#			X		
26#–50#		X			
51#–75#		X			
76#–100#		X			
>100#		X			
PUSHING/PULLING	**DISTANCE**				
Pushing Force*: 5 pounds			X		
Pulling Force*: 5 pounds			X		

*Forces determined by ( ) weight of object or ( ) force measurement?

Describe heaviest items lifted and start/end height:
Tools and test equipment lifted 3–5'.

Describe carrying requirements (items, distance):
Tools and materials

Job Requires: ( ) Peak Force (X) Sustained Force

Describe pushing/pulling demands:
Loosen/tighten bolts on flanges, covers on machine guards, adjustment bolts on shafts etc.

ADDITIONAL INFORMATION/COMMENTS:

____________________ Signature of Employer Representative

Project Manager — Title of Employer Representative

__________ Date

FIGURE 17-7. Job requirements and physical demand checklist.

that the employee and the employer disagree on the job's physical requirements. Therefore, if the OT practitioner's description is found to be inaccurate then his or her professional opinion regarding RTW issues might change.

MUSCULOSKELETAL ASSESSMENT

An FCE is not simply an assessment of an injured body part's response to performing the essential job functions; it includes how the individual's whole body responds to performing the essential job functions or the critical components of the job, day in and day out.[5,6] The OT practitioner will assess how the client's aerobic capacity, strength and endurance, and body mechanics over time, respond when working a full day—not just how the injured body part functions. Refer to Box 17-1.

It is important to consider that the client may have other medical or functional issues that are affecting the client's ability to RTW. Individuals may have suffered additional medical issues since the work injury or may have other issues, such as obesity, hypertension, drug dependency, or neurological, cardiac, or orthopedic issues, which can affect the ability to RTW. The OT practitioner must be able to identify these and state whether or not they are interfering with the client's ability to RTW.

When performing the various assessments listed here, the OT practitioner will document careful observations of the client's heart rate changes during the various activities, as well as the client's behavior, noting any observed inconsistent, nonphysiological, or self-limiting behaviors. All of this will be used to determine whether the individual has given a valid and consistent effort during testing.

FUNCTIONAL ACTIVITIES

The OT practitioner will assess the client's ability to perform functional activities that are either specific to this particular job or that the individual may need to be able to perform when looking at any RTW situation. The environment is crucial for assessing the activities a client would normally perform in his or her job. Some industrial rehabilitation centers have an extensive array of simulated environments (Fig. 17-8). Some tasks workers are assessed for may include:

- Ability to climb stairs and/or ladders
- Ability to transition to and from the floor and crawl
- Ability to push and pull dynamically while standing stationary using both the right and left arms (seated and standing) as well as while walking
- Ability to walk distances—walking on a variety of surfaces may be important in certain jobs as well as the type of footwear on the job (steel-toed boots, for instance)
- Ability to safely handle weights—either job specific or, when no job is available, what the client is able to safely dynamically handle. This is not necessarily a new ability of the client to lift weights but, rather, identification of the weights the client is able to effectively handle within his or her pain tolerance day after day.
  - Floor to overhead
  - Floor to shoulder
  - Floor to waist
  - Ability to carry
- Ability to carry weights up and down stairs

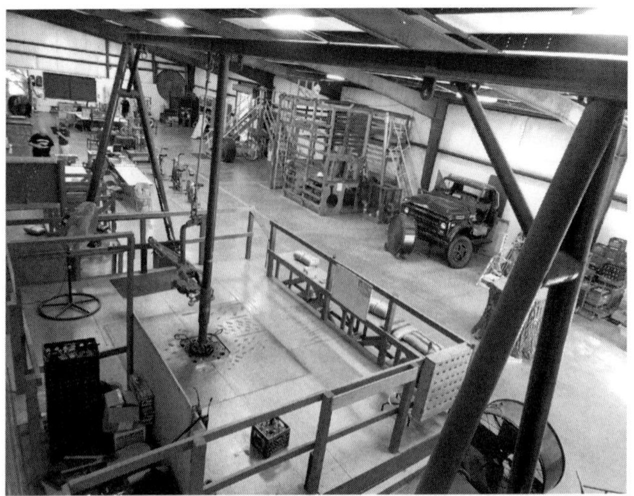

FIGURE 17-8. The Fontana Center, Center for Work Rehabilitation. Note the various simulated environments created in this large space, including a vibrating truck simulator.

STATIC STRENGTH TESTING

A word about the use of static strength testing compared with the use of dynamic lifting assessment is important at this time. In a 1996 court case, Shell Western A&P was sued by the Equal Employment Opportunity Commission (EEOC) for violating the Civil Rights Act of 1964 by having the applicants for employment participate in a physical strength test that was used to discriminate against women for entry-level jobs in the oil fields. The EEOC's contention was that Shell Western:

- Did not have a job analysis or job description to establish the criteria for the physical requirements needed to perform the jobs
- Used static strength tests for arm strength, back strength, and grip strength that were skewed toward men (men have greater static strength than women). There is no correlation between static strength test and a person's ability to dynamically handle weights.
- Did not allow anyone who failed the test to retake the test

Shell Western A&P agreed to settle the case.

In 2005 the EEOC sued the Dial Corporation in the US District Court for the Southern District of Iowa contending that the Dial Corporation violated the Title VII of the Civil Rights Act of 1964 as amended in 2000 by using strength testing to discriminate against women. In the court's decision against the Dial Corporation, the court:

- Upheld that strength testing did discriminate against women. Men have more static strength than women.
- Found no correlation between what a person is able to statically pull and his or her ability to dynamically handle weights

- Upheld that the Dial Corporation had not validated the test protocols to ensure they adequately tested the job requirements
- Upheld that the job simulation component was significantly more stringent than the actual job

Thus, for a defensible test protocol, it is important that the OT practitioner not rely on static strength testing but, rather, develop a reasonable, reliable, and safe way to test dynamic lifting.

Depending on the type of job the client is going to be returning to or the injury he or she has sustained, there are other types of functional activities that will need to be assessed, such as:

- Ability to sustain a variety of postures and positions (lying supine and working overhead or working while sustaining a forward flexed or kneeling position, standing and working overhead, etc.) (Fig. 17-9)
- Ability to swing a sledge hammer against a stable object—hypersensitivity to vibration or jolting
- Ability to repeatedly climb in and out of a motor vehicle of varying heights as well as the ability to sustain vibration over time while seated
- Ability to sustain one's body on a swing rope

The types of functional activities the OT practitioners will have to be able to simulate is limited only by the variety of jobs available within the OT location.

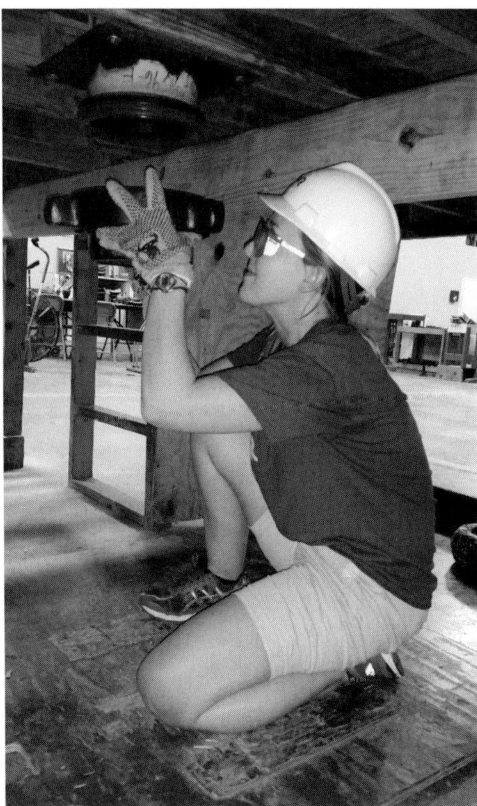

FIGURE 17-9. Worker kneeling and working at eye level.

REPEATABILITY

An FCE is not a record of the maximum a person is able to perform in all these areas of concern but, rather, is documented evidence in the FCR of the client's demonstrated ability to sustain and repeat, day after day, within their pain tolerance. Therefore, it is important that OT practitioners design an activity program that includes reasonable repetitions, reasonable time frames, and reasonable work periods the client is expected to work within. The client must maintain this capacity throughout the 8-hour work day, day after day.

Because even healthy, noninjured individuals will see dramatic decreases in strength, endurance, and aerobic fitness when they become inactive, it is imperative to assess the injured client who has been relatively (or totally) inactive for many months to many years, expecting this same decrease in abilities over time. Clients who have been in the injury management system for long periods routinely state that they can do certain activities on a given day but be in so much pain that they are unable to get out of bed the next several days. It is also reasonable to expect that what a client may able to do on a given day (or morning), he or she may not be able to duplicate on successive days. Thus, it is necessary to see the client for multiple successive days when looking to perform defensible FCEs. Remember, the goal is to identify a level of activity the client is able to sustain in a normal work week—not just on a given day.[5,20]

It is common for ankle or knee joints not to swell after standing and walking, squatting and stair climbing for 1 or even 2 days, only to demonstrate significant swelling on the third day. The same is true for a hand; it may not swell after just 1 or 2 days of work, only to swell significantly on the third day. It is important to test the grip strength of an individual who has suffered an UE injury or a hand injury not only before initiating any activities but also at the conclusion of the 8-hour day's activities so that it can be determined whether the client is experiencing any issues that could adversely affect work performance after a full day's work. His or her ability to hold and swing the sledge hammer, carry a tool box, repeatedly climb ladders, or sustain body weight on a swing rope at the conclusion of the 8 hours of simulated work activity will determine whether or not the client is able to RTW. Identifying how much the joint swells or how much grip strength decreases following the work day will help quantify that the individual is not able to safely RTW at this time and help the physician determine whether additional medical intervention may be needed. By performing the FCE over 3 to 5 consecutive days, the OT practitioner and the client will know how the client will respond to repeated real work activities and therefore feel confident with the results of the evaluation.

There is no way to ensure that an individual, who may continue to have pain and who has been in the injury management system for a significant period, is able to perform over a single 4-hour period or even a single day or that he can reproduce this consecutive 8 hour work day, day after day. Without performing the FCE over successive 8 hour days, all the client has to do to totally discredit the report is state that he was unable to function or even get out of bed the next day.

CROSS CHECKS FOR RELIABILITY

The client is able to control the evaluation to a certain extent because it is based on his or her demonstrated performance or lack of performance of activities, therefore, it is important that every FCE includes cross checks for validity of effort. The occupational therapist and the OTA know more about human anatomy and physiology and function compared with the typical injured worker. The OT practitioner is responsible for documenting an objective observation of a subjective complaint. It is not possible to measure pain objectively. It is the job of the clinician to therefore make careful observations as to how the client performs an activity, what the client's heart rate does, the way the client moves when the individual does not know that he or she is being observed (how the client bends over to drink from the water fountain or walks to or from lunch, what he or she does during break, how he or she gets in or out of their car, etc.). Thus, the OT practitioner should design specific activities where the client is not necessarily aware of being observed. By having the client perform a functional activity that requires him or her to bend, stoop, squat, reach, lift, carry, and so on, similar to what was observed during the musculoskeletal and lifting assessment, the occupational therapist or the OTA is able to determine whether or not the movements or the ROM, coordination, and so on demonstrated when the client thought he was being observed is the same as those when the client had no idea of being observed. See Box 17-2 to learn more about symptom magnification and observation.

DISTRACTION TESTING

One method to objectively identify a client's true abilities is to use distraction testing. For example, if the client did not appear to give maximal effort when being asked to "raise his arms overhead as high as he can" during AROM testing with the goniometer, then a task should be set up later and the client must functionally use that motion in that task. If shoulder flexion is questionable, then client is asked to move an object template from waist to overhead to the floor, working as quickly as possible, with an emphasis on time, not ROM (Fig. 17-10). As the client is distracted by trying to work quickly, not knowing what the OT practitioner is looking for, he may demonstrate significantly more AROM than when initially asked during focused AROM assessment.

During standardized coordination testing a client knows that if he or she drops pegs or works extremely slowly it will demonstrate extremely poor coordination. However, when performing functional activities, if no similar reduced finger dexterity or fine coordination problems are seen, this would be an inconsistency that could indicate that the client is a symptom magnifier. There seems to be a perception in the work injury field that many of the injured workers play games and may not be as injured as they want others to see. Matheson, whom many consider the "father" of this aspect of industrial therapy, found that very few of the individuals

BOX 17-2

Example of the Type II Symptom Magnifier—The Game Player

Client profile:

- 38-year-old driller—light medium type work
- Reported significant back and neck issues
- Negative results of magnetic resonance imaging (MRI) of spine (cervical and lumbar)
- Failed multiple sessions of "conservative" physical therapy
- Entered the clinic with use of a cane and neck brace
- Reported 10/10 pain before any activities

The Center for Work Rehabilitation, Inc., at the Fontana Center in Lafayette, LA, was scheduled to perform a 5-day FCE on a driller for a land drilling company. The individual had reported a neck and back injury. Although MRI results were essentially normal, the client was reporting 10/10 pain with any activity. After the client underwent a musculoskeletal assessment and the morning's functional activities, the OT practitioners documented 27 nonphysiological, inconsistent, or self-limiting behaviors. After the evaluation, the client reported 10/10 pain and did not return to the clinic for the afternoon's activities. The opinion of the occupational therapist was that this individual was a type II symptom magnifier, and as such was consciously magnifying his pain for secondary gain or to control his environment.

A week later, the occupational therapist received a DVD containing videos that were taken by a private investigator. The video was started in the parking lot of the Fontana Center as the individual left the building at lunchtime. It clearly showed the man walking very slowly with a neck brace on and the use of a cane as he carefully climbed into his truck. He was observed to drive 15 minutes north of town where he was observed to exit the vehicle with no neck brace and without the use of a cane. The individual proceeded to get on a horse and ride slowly through his pasture as he inspected his fence line. He remained on the horse for about 30 minutes when he was observed to quickly and smoothly climb off the horse, climb into a backhoe, and then clean out a canal for about an hour. The video clearly showed the jolting and vibration the individual was experiencing while operating the equipment. He was then observed to exit the backhoe machine with the same fluid motion as previously observed. He then backed up his pickup truck and proceeded to use a posthole digger and lift 100 lb sacks of concrete to repair his fence.

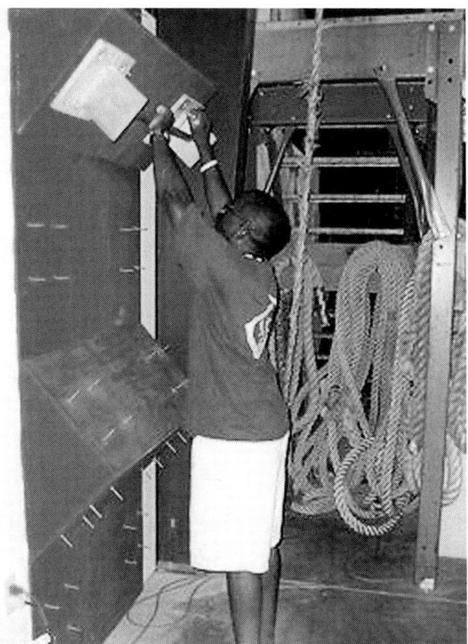

FIGURE 17-10. Distraction testing. Client is unaware during the "timed test" of lifting object from waist to overhead and then to floor, that the OTA is actually looking at AROM shoulder flexion.

in his study (3.8%) who were in the work injury management system were type II symptom magnifiers, "the Game Player", who magnifies his or her pain behaviors in a conscious effort to control the environment or for secondary gain. The Center for Work Rehabilitation, Inc. (CWR) performs approximately 350 FCEs each year. Studies performed there indicate that 1.8% of those evaluated at CWR were found to be type II symptom magnifiers.[17]

It is equally important that the OT practitioner be able to identify when a person is playing games (neither valid nor consistent behaviors) as it is to identify that the individual is giving a valid and consistent effort.

The OTA, once properly trained and has obtained service competency, is able to assist with performing a variety of cross checks with clients. Examples are included in this next section.

Jamar 5-Function Reliability Test: The standard protocol for the Jamar 5-Function Reliability Test is to perform the grip test, starting with the smallest rung and progressing to the largest rung. The client is instructed to give maximal effort on each rung. If the scores are in a bell-shaped curve, the individual passes the 5-Function Reliability test (Fig. 17-11).[21-22]

Distraction Grip Testing: Another means of cross checking the client's grip strength is to use a rapid exchange and varied positioning distraction testing protocol. Studies have shown that an individual is able to consistently give submaximal effort when there is no change of proprioceptive input. By changing how the grip test is performed from the standard assessment protocol (smallest to largest) the OT practitioner will change the proprioceptive feedback. The varied positioning protocol has the OT practitioner starting with the grip handle in the middle position, then in the smallest, then the largest,

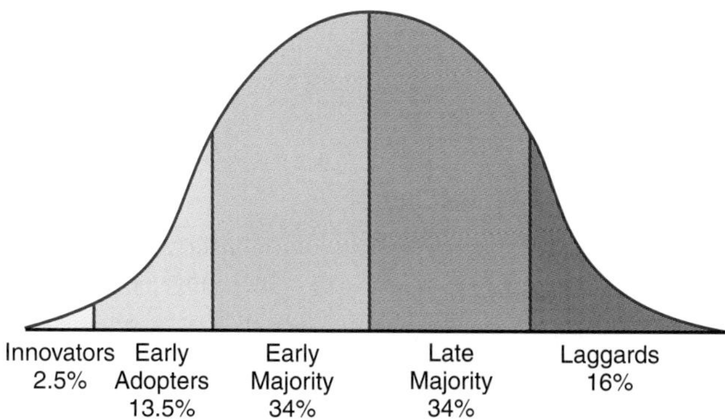

FIGURE 17-11. Jamar 5-Function bell-shaped curve.

then the second smallest, and then the second largest positions. To use the varied position and rapid exchange distraction technique, the OTA will use the same positioning as the varied position stated above but have the client squeeze quick and fast between right and left hands. With all these distractions, the client's grip strength should still not be any greater than the first time the test was performed using the standard protocol. If the results are greater this is a nonphysiological response.[21] See Box 17-3 for the results of the Jamar 5-Function Reliability Test and Distraction Grip Testing as an example of a client with a hand injury not giving maximal effort.

Supine Straight Leg Raise versus seated Straight Leg Raise: Results of a supine SLR and a seated SLR should be essentially the same because both test for neurological issues affecting the sciatic nerve. To perform the test, the client is positioned supine on a mat, and slight AAROM provided while the client brings the hip into flexion (see Fig. 17-12). Next, the client is seated for an SLR. Distract the client with a straight pin, telling her that the OT practitioner is performing a sharp and dull discrimination test. The straight pin is simply a distraction. If there is truly an issue with the sciatic nerve, the client will express the same pain while seated and have

BOX 17-3

Case Study of a Client Who Had a History of a Hand Injury

STANDARD TRIAL

RIGHT HAND	LEFT HAND
20 20 30 30 40	5 25 20 20 20

VARIED GRIP

22 37 42 30 30	15 35 22 25 25

VARIED/RAPID EXCHANGE GRIP

45 66 60 48 54	**45 60 77 45 58**

Failed 5-function reliability test all three times.

Right hand has increases of 110%, 185%, 140%, 150%, 225%, **333%**, 200%, 160%, and 135% compared with standard trials.

Left hand has increases of 300%, 140%, 110%, 125%, 125%, **900%**, 240%, and 385%.

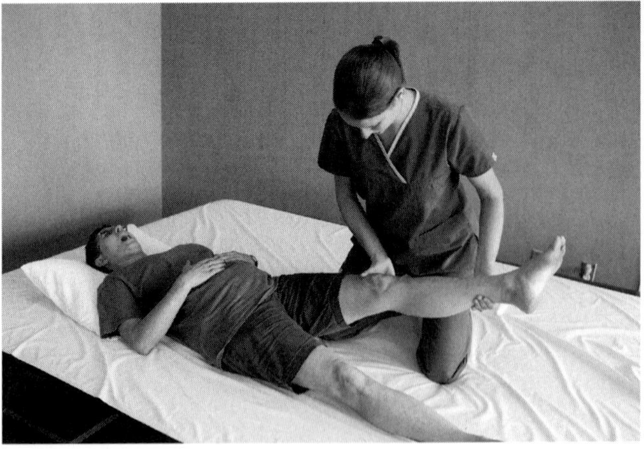

FIGURE 17-12. The client is expressing facial grimacing and has reduced ability to flex her left hip with supine SLR.

reduced hip flexion. If the client does not, then the practitioner has objective evidence that there is no positive response to the sciatic nerve irritation. The OTA is able to further distract the client by having the client dorsiflex her feet while the OTA checks the client's muscle strength. This further stretches the sciatic nerve—if the client truly had a positive supine SLR, then this cross check would also elicit a positive sciatic nerve irritation type response at the same range as the supine SLR demonstrated.[23]

STATEMENT REGARDING ENVIRONMENT

Many individuals do not work in climate-controlled environments but, rather, work outside, where they are exposed to the temperatures and weather associated with the part of the country in which they live and work. However, most therapy clinics are climate controlled. If the assessment is to be performed in a climate-controlled environment, yet the client is going to be working in a non–climate-controlled environment, the FCR should include a statement that indicates the test was not performed in the environment the client will reasonably be expected to work in and therefore may require some additional time to adapt and adjust to the work environment, particularly when the client will be working in an environment where heat and humidity are significant factors. For example, a person may be able to walk on a treadmill at 3 miles per hour for an hour in a climate-controlled environment. However, if he or she attempts this same activity outdoors where the temperature is 98°F and the humidity is 95%, he may not be able to duplicate the same performance. See Box 17-4 for an example of an RTW Protocol.

ONE-DAY EVALUATION VERSUS MULTIPLE-DAY EVALUATION

When dealing with individuals who have been in the injury management system for a significant period and who are still experiencing, in some cases, a significant amount of pain, it is reasonable to expect that these clients will be unable to repeat in the afternoon what they could do in the morning or to repeat the next day what they were able to do the first 8-hour day. Therefore, when performing a partial day or 1-day FCE is it important to state the following:

> *Because the client was seen for only one 4-hour (or 8-hour) day, we are unable to state conclusively whether the client would be able to maintain this work level over a 40-hour work week. Because the client has been in the injury management system for a significant period and relatively inactive, it is reasonable to believe that the client will not be able to maintain the same work level. Therefore, should this information be deemed necessary, a multiday FCE would be recommended.*

BOX 17-4
Return to Work Protocol

One of the largest drilling companies in the United States had a RTW protocol, whether the employee was attempting to RTW following a work related injury or a non-work-related injury or after an illness. The protocol included the following components:

- Obtain a full release to work without restrictions from the treating physician.
- Obtain a full release to work without restrictions from the company's physician.
- Successfully complete a 4 hour FCE and be released to full duty without restrictions (performed at a local physical therapy clinic).

The test protocols did not include simulated activities of real work and was conducted in a climate-controlled environment. The "functional" activities included lifting a box with weights, pushing on a weighted sled, climbing up and down the four-step stairs used to train crutch walkers, climbing an 8-foot ladder (the ceiling was 8 feet high so the employee would climb at most three to four rungs) and performing "nuts and bolts" activities while working from the floor level to the overhead level.

Over a year's time, the drilling company found that 70% of those individuals who completed this entire process and were released to full duty without restrictions were not able to remain at their jobs for even one 12-hour shift on the drilling rig before their symptoms returned or their affected joint started to hurt or swell, and they had to be removed from the job. And these were individuals who were pain-free! Thus, all the non-work-related issues then became work-related issues. In the 20 years that the RTW protocol has been performed at the Center for Work Rehabilitation, Inc. in Lafayette, LA, and Houston, TX, with a revised protocol that includes multiple (3-5 days in succession) 8-hour workdays, using real work activities, conducted in a non-climate-controlled environment, not one person who was released to full duty without restrictions has been unable to remain at work, without modifications or restrictions, for at least the next 4 months of employment.

FUNCTIONAL CAPACITY REPORT

The FCR is the concluding report of the FCE. The report should clearly detail the client's demonstrated abilities in the areas listed below. For each of the areas, the report should identify the job-specific safe limits, or the client's maximal safe and repetitive safe limits. When appropriate, occasional and frequent abilities are to be identified, with some definition as to what this means in each instance. The more specific the written restrictions are, the more useful the report will be.

- Clinic name/address/contact information
- Name of client
- Diagnosis
- Work level to which the client is released
  When the physical requirements are arbitrarily limited by the OT practitioner, on the basis of the client's physical job requirements, a statement regarding this should be included in this section. An example of this is as follows:

  The weights lifted/carried, forces pushed/pulled, stairs and ladders climbed, and positions and postures maintained were all set by the physical job description and not necessarily the client's maximum safe working ability.

- Number of hours of the evaluation
- Bilateral lifting:
  - Floor: Overhead
  - Floor: Shoulder
  - Floor: Waist
  - If the client is unable to squat lift a three-point lift, golfer's lift, or modified golfer's lift may be used to identify the client's ability to lift an object from the floor (see Chapter 21).
  - If the client is unable to lift from the floor, the weights and the work level that the client is able to perform should be identified. For example:
    - Knee: Overhead
    - Knee: Shoulder
    - Knee: Waist
    - Waist: Overhead
    - Waist: Shoulder
  - Unilateral right/left UE lifting, where appropriate
- Carrying:
  - Unilateral, where appropriate
- Standing and walking:
  - Sustained at one time/throughout the day
  - Including footwear and surfaces where important (limestone, level surfaces versus nonlevel surfaces, steel-toed boots, etc.)
- Stair and ladder climbing:
  - Amount of flights in relative succession without stopping
  - Total flights per day
  - Stair climbing while carrying maximum weight and repetitive weight
- Sitting:
  - Vibrational component, where appropriate
- Various postures/positions: Sustained and repetitive for each
  - Stooping
  - Squatting (partial/full)
  - Kneeling
  - Crawling (distances)
  - Bending
- Pushing/pulling while standing and walking
- Push/pull stationary/dynamic
  - Standing right UE: Occasionally and frequently
  - Standing left UE: Occasionally and frequently
- Push/pull stationary/dynamic
  - Seated right UE: Occasionally and frequently
  - Seated left UE: Occasionally and frequently
- Hand function
  - Simple grip: Right/left
  - Firm grip: Right/left
  - Fine manipulation: Right/left
  - Grip strength: Right/left (Compared with average for age/gender)
- Variety of simulated work activities specific to the job:
  - Swinging sledge hammers
  - Swing on a swing rope
  - Work unprotected heights
  - Work while supine with hands overhead
  - Open and close various types of valves: Both lever valves and circular valves
- RTW summary
  - Answer question whether client is able to return to work at former job
  - State the number of hours and then number of consecutive days the assessment was conducted
  - State types of simulated work activities the client participated in
  - Summarize client's description and rating of pain at onset of the evaluation and again at the conclusion of the evaluation
  - Statement of evaluation limitations if any
    - Less than 8 hour/day, multiple days in succession
    - Climate controlled environment versus the climate client will reasonably RTW in
  - Statement regarding reviewing the document with the client during the discharge conference and client's agreement/disagreement
  - Place for client and the occupational therapist to sign
  - Place for the physician to sign if he or she concurs with the FCR

If a clearly written physical job description exists, the FCR will state conclusively whether or not the individual has demonstrated the ability to RTW. If the client is unable to return to his previous job or when no job for the client to return to exists, the FCR will state specifically the client's demonstrated abilities and limitations in all the above listed areas. From this, a vocational counselor is able to identify potential jobs the individual has the physical abilities to perform and then can redirect the individual into another occupation. See Figure 17-13 for a sample FCR.

CENTER FOR WORK REHABILITATION, INC.™
709 KALISTE SALOOM
LAFAYETTE, LA 70508
(337) 234-7018

FUNCTIONAL CAPACITY REPORT

Client: John Smith Date: Jan 15, 2016

Diagnosis: Status post laminectomy and fusion L5 - S1; Chronic pain syndrome

Client can work at the following work level in a safe manner under restrictions as noted in report.

Medium: Lift 50 lbs or less frequently. Lifting 50 lbs frequently equates to heavy level work, however as to not confuse that the client is lifting 100 lbs we will call this medium level work. The weights lifted / carried, forces pushed / pulled, stairs / ladders climbed and postures and positions maintained were all established by the physical requirements of the job and not necessarily the client's physical maximum.

This person is able to:
Never (N); Occasionally (O) 1 - 33%; Frequently (F) 34 - 66%; Continuously (C) 67 - 100%
Safe Height: Overhead (OH); Shoulder (S); Waist (W); Floor (FL); Knee (K).

1. BILATERAL LIFT:
   a. Up to 50 lbs F FL - S b. Up to 40 lbs F FL - OH

NOTE: "Occasionally" is defined in this case as 3 times in relative succession.

2. BILATERAL CARRY:
   a. Up to 50 lbs F W - W

NOTE: "Occasionally" is defined in this case as 3 times in relative succession.

3. CAN THE PERSON PERFORM THE FOLLOWING TASK:

	Task		Comments
a.	Push/Pull Seated & Standing:	Yes	No Restriction per job description - 200 lbs of maximum force right and left; 140 lbs of repetitively sustained force right and left. **200 lbs of force is the maximum capability of the machine.**
	Push / Pull Kneeling:	Yes	No Restriction per job description — 120 lbs of force repetitively using both hands, simulating "cranking" a jack.
b.	Push/Pull Walking:	Yes	No Restriction per job description — 120 lbs of repetitively sustained force.
c.	Bend:	Yes	No Restriction secondary to job description — Recommend performing back extension stretches every 15 minutes.
d.	Squat:	Yes	No Restriction per job description. Client performed both full and ½ partial squatting frequently throughout the day with no problem observed
e	Crawl:	Yes	No Restrictions per job description.
f.	Climb Stairs:	Yes	No Restriction per job description. Client climbed 15 flights of stairs each day.
g.	Carrying While Climbing Stairs:	Yes	No Restriction per job description — 40 lbs maximum and repetitively.
h.	Climb Ladders:	Yes	No Restriction per job description.
i.	Reach above shoulder level:	Yes	No Restriction per job description.
j.	Twisting:	Yes	No Restriction per job description. Recommend avoid spinal tourquing.

4. ASSUMING AN 8 HOUR WORKDAY WITH TWO FIFTEEN (15) MINUTE BREAKS AND 1/2 HOUR MEAL BREAK, I WOULD EXPECT THIS PERSON TO BE ABLE TO: (NOTE: Total does not have to equal 8 hours)
   a. Sit continuously: 2 hours*
   b. Stand continuously: 4 hours
   c. Walk continuously: 2 hours**
   d. Alternately Sit / Stand / Walk: 12 hours***

 Reviewed verbatim with therapist: ________

FIGURE 17-13. Functional capacity report.

Date: Jan 15, 2016
RE: John Smith
Page 2 of 2

*Client was asked to sit continuously for 60 minutes while in our clinic. Client did so with no outward signs or reports of difficulty. Client reported sitting continuously for 2 hours for instance to drive recently, only stopping for a restroom break. We see no reason why he would have difficulty sitting.
**Client was asked to walk continuously for 60 minutes at 3.5 mph while in our clinic. Client did so with no outward signs or reports of difficulty. It may, therefore, be concluded and the client agrees, that client should be able to walk longer, particularly at his own slower pace.
***Although the client was seen for 8 hours maximum while observed clinically, he performed simulated work tasks at a sufficient intensity to approximate the physical work demands expected in a 12 hour work day with no outward signs nor reports of difficulty. It is our belief that the client worked at a level requiring a greater expenditure of energy than he would at his present employment. Therefore, it can be concluded and the client agrees that he should be able to work a 12 hour shift without difficulty.

5. CAN THIS PERSON USE HANDS FOR REPETITIVE ACTIONS SUCH AS:

Simple Grasping:	Firm Grasp:	Fine Manipulating:
Right: Yes	Yes	Yes
Left: Yes	Yes	Yes
Grip Strength:	Right: 130 lbs	Left: 155 lbs
	115 % of Normal	128 % of Normal

6. CAN PERSON NOW RETURN TO FORMER JOB? Yes. Client's job as a Bridge Tender with Reading Railroad is considered a medium level job according to the on-site job visit by Center for Work Rehabilitation, Inc. staff and confirmed by the client. The client has demonstrated the ability to perform all the essential job functions of a Bridge Tender without restrictions.

Mr Smith completed 2 weeks of Work Conditioning and 2 weeks of a Work Hardening Program. He worked 8 hours/day in a non-climate controlled warehouse with concrete floors, temperatures ranged from 60°F to 90°F. Mr Smith has participated in a variety of functional activities including job specific maximum and repetitive lifting, carrying, pushing and pulling, repetitive swinging a 16 lbs sledge hammer, mobility under a load - including walking on unlevel and rocky surfaces, climbing stairs and ladders and work in various positions and postures. **Mr Smith demonstrated the ability to work at a medium work level job of a Bridge Tender with Reading Railroad without restrictions.**

Mr Smith voluntarily decided to see if he could perform the work without any prescription pain medication - taking ½ a pain pill for 2 days then stopping all pain medication and switching to taking only Aleve as needed with no reports of pain increases. At most he states his pain is a dull ache rated 20/100 but often reporting no pain. He has not taken prescription pain medication in the last 5 days.

Our recommendation is to release Mr Smith to full duty at the medium work level as Bridge Tender without restrictions. Because the Reading Railroad return to work process will take several weeks to conclude once he is released by the treating physicians, the plan is to have Mr Smith participate in a structured fitness program at the Center for Work Rehabilitation, working with a certified personal trainer to ensure that he does not lose any of the significant positive gains that he has made. Once Mr Smith is approved to RTW by the medical director for Reading Railroad he will be released to full duty trial work for one week then return to CWR to ensure that all issues are resolved.

I have reviewed the above information with Mr Smith and he agrees this is a fair assessment of his abilities at this time.

John Smith

Paul A Fontana, OTR, FAOTA
Occupational Therapist
Fellow, American Occupational Therapy Association

Katrina R Duhon, MOTR/L
Occupational Therapist

I have reviewed the recommendations contained in this report and concur with the recommendations.

Dr Bob Jones

Date

Reviewed verbatim with therapist: ________

FIGURE 17-13.—continued

SUMMARY

RTW programs are valuable to assist injured workers to continue their rehabilitation in job-specific tasks to either go back to their original employment or to identify those who are unable to do so. This chapter did not intend to provide a step-by-step instruction manual on performing industrial OT programs but, rather, an introduction to the components of these industrial programs and to discuss the role that the OTA plays. The OTA may play a vital role in industrial OT programs; he or she can be responsible for administering assessments for which they are deemed service competent, carrying out interventions, documenting client's performance skills, and informing the occupational therapist when the client is either not progressing as he or she should be, or when the activities are not challenging enough.

REVIEW QUESTIONS

1. A work conditioning evaluation of a client with a right rotator cuff repair 6 months after surgery has revealed these top three problem areas: poor aerobic fitness, decreased ability to lift more than 15 lb secondary to increased pain, and decreased grip strength. Which three of the following types of activities would the OTA reasonably expect to see on the client's daily activity program?
   a. Structured circuit training with emphasis on upper extremity strengthening
   b. BTE Primus™ grip strengthening
   c. Riding a stationary bike for 20 minutes at a time with alternating intervals of 5 minutes at 1.5 and at 2.5
   d. Structured circuit training with emphasis on lower extremity strengthening
   e. Structured circuit training with emphasis on both upper and lower extremity strengthening
   f. Aquatic therapy
2. A client is being seen for a work hardening program after having surgery to repair his left foot fracture. What specific assessments should be done each morning and at the end of the day?
   a. Circumferential measurements of bilateral feet
   b. Volumetric measurements of left leg
   c. Volumetric measurements of left foot only
   d. Objective pain level
3. One important aspect of a successful work conditioning or work hardening program is using an interdisciplinary approach. It is important that in addition to the OT staff working with the client, all those involved in the client's RTW issues be actively engaged in and knowledgeable about the status of the client and his or her situation. Which three of the following are important members of this team?
   a. Referring physician
   b. Company's human resources department
   c. Client's direct supervisor
   d. Attorney
   e. Medical case manager
   f. Client's general physician
4. You are currently working with a client who has spent the past 4 weeks in a work conditioning program at your clinic. At this time, you feel the client should be able to tolerate a work hardening program. Which of the following factors will you assess when transitioning the client from a work conditioning to a work hardening program?
   a. The client has achieved minimal conditioning goals and is able to participate in a few simulated job activities for a limited time during the day.
   b. The client is likely to continue to make sufficient progress toward achieving the highest work level as projected by the OT practitioner.
   c. The client has verbally expressed readiness to advance to a work hardening program.
   d. The client has demonstrated the ability to sustain more than 2 hours of functional activities per day.
5. One occupational therapist is working in an outpatient industrial rehabilitation clinic in charge of supervising three OTAs. Which of the following is NOT a role of the OTA when working in an industrial rehabilitation setting?
   a. Closely monitor and observe the client as he or she completes the designated activity program.
   b. Document client responses to activities.
   c. Implement and modify activities/intervention techniques based on the client's performance.
   d. Independently perform regular reevaluations of the client and make all recommendations for future care based on the client's progress (or lack thereof).
6. Mr. Jones was involved in a motor vehicle accident 1 year ago. Following a series of magnetic resonance imaging, he is referred to a specialist who performs a C4-7 fusion. Today, Mr. Jones presents to your clinic for a full 3-day FCE. During the musculoskeletal assessment, you notice that he is exhibiting some nonphysiological symptoms. Which of the following is an example of a nonphysiological symptom?
   a. Consistent grip strength even during rapid exchange and distraction testing
   b. Intense reports of steady shocking pain (with facial grimacing) when performing AROM exercises, with a rise in heart rate
   c. Reports of neurological symptoms in the shoulder when the wrist is tapped
   d. Ability to climb the ladder one time in 10 minutes
7. You are assisting with preparation for an FCE of a client, and you see that there is no physical job description for this client. Which of the following options *best* depicts what you should do in preparation for the assessment?
   a. Look up the job title in the dictionary.
   b. Call the employer and ask for a job description.
   c. Wait until the client comes and ask him/her about his/her job.
   d. Call the medical case manager or vocational consultant assigned to the case and request his or her assistance in securing a job description in a timely manner.
8. You are asked why it is important to see the client who has had a hand injury for a multiday FCE. Which three of the following six options are correct?
   a. Individuals with hand injuries may not experience an increase in edema/swelling after only 1 day but may see an increase after several full days of activities.
   b. It is important to recheck the individual's grip strength on successive days to see if there is a significant drop in grip strength, which would indicate that there are continued issues with the individual's recovery that could put him or her at risk of another injury.
   c. The doctor wants a multiday assessment.

   d. In addition to needing to recheck the individual's grip strength and edema on successive days, you need to ensure that the individual does not have any other issues that will put him or her at risk of injury, such as poor aerobic fitness, increased fatigue following working 8 hour days, and so on.
   e. We always do a multiple day assessment to ensure defensibility.
   f. Hand injuries impact every aspect of work.
9. The term "symptom magnifier" means:
   a. The client is a malingerer.
   b. The client may be magnifying his pain behaviors for secondary gains.
   c. The client's role has been magnified to that of a patient.
   d. The client's magnification of his pain complaints is a conscious magnification of his attempting to solve what to him or her is an unsolvable problem.
10. When told that in an FCE the client has total control of the outcome, what would your response be?
   a. The client has control of those parts that he or she will participate in.
   b. The practitioner's role is to put the client in a position where the client does not know what is being assessed and is thus able to determine consistency of effort on the part of the client.
   c. All aspects of an FCE are objective by the very nature of the assessment.
   d. OT practitioners have sufficient training to identify when a person is not making a valid effort.

REFERENCES

1. American Occupational Therapy Association. (2014). Occupational therapy practice framework: Domain and process (3rd ed.). *American Journal of Occupational Therapy, 68*(Suppl. 1), S1–S48.
2. Hardison, M. E., & Roll, S. C. (2016). Factors associated with success in an occupational rehabilitation program for work-related musculoskeletal disorders. *American Journal of Occupational Therapy, 71*(1), 7101190040p1–7101190040p8.
3. Brayman, S., Clark, G., DeLany, J., Garza, E., Radomski, M., Ramsey, R., Siebert, C., Voelkerding, K., LaVesser, P., Aird, L., ... & Lieberman, D. (2014). Guidelines for supervision, roles, and responsibilities during the delivery of occupational therapy services. *American Journal of Occupational Therapy, 68* (Supplement 3), S16–S22. Retrieved from http://ajot.aota.org/article.aspx?articleid=1934863http://ajot.aota.org/article.aspx?articleid=1934863
4. Foster, L., & Smith, R. (2010). OT/OTA partnerships: Achieving high ethical standards in a challenging health care environment. *The American Occupational Therapy Association Advisory Opinion for the Ethics Commission*, 1–7.
5. Franklin, B. (Ed.). (2000). *ACSM guidelines for exercise testing & prescription* (6th ed.). Philadelphia, PA: Lippincott Williams & Wilkins.
6. Wilmore, J., & Costell, D. (1994). *Physiology of sports and exercise* (1st ed.). Champaign, IL: Human Kinetics Publishing.
7. Waddell, G., McCulloch, J., Kummel, E., & Venner, R. (1980). Nonorganic physical signs in low back pain. *Spine (Phila Pa 1976)*, 5(2), 117–125.
8. Ogden-Niemeyer, L. & Jacobs, K. (1989). *Workhardening: State of the art.* Thorofare, NJ: Slack.
9. Lechner, D. (1994). Work hardening and work conditioning interventions: Do they affect disability? *Journal of the American Physical Therapy Association, 74*(5), 471–493.
10. Miller-Keane., & O'Toole, M. T. (2003). *Miller-keane encyclopedia & dictionary of medicine, nursing, & allied health* (7th ed.). Philadelphia, PA: Saunders.
11. Dorsey, J., Finch, D., Ehrenfried, H., & Jaegers, L. (2017). *Work Rehabilitation.* American Occupational Therapy Association. Retrieved from http://www.aota.org/About-Occupational-Therapy/Professionals/WI/Work-Rehab.aspx
12. Physician Advisory Committee. (2001). Work hardening/work conditioning treatment guidelines. Retrieved from http://www.owcc.state.ok.us/PDF/Work%20Hardening-Work%20Conditioning%20Guidelines.pdf
13. Hart, D., Berlin, S., Brager, P., Caruso, M., Hejduk, Jr., J., Howar, J., ... & Wah, M. (1994). Development of clinical standards in industrial rehabilitation. *Journal of Orthopaedic & Sports Physical Therapy, 19*(5), 232–241.
14. Mature worker facts. (2016). Retrieved from www.ncoa.org
15. Spitz, B. (2012). Dearie: The remarkable life of Julia Child. New York, NY: *A.A. Knopf Publishing.*
16. Matheson, L., Ogden, L., & Niemeyer. (1986). *Work capacity evaluation—A systemic approach to industrial rehabilitation.* Washington, DC: Education Research Information Center.
17. Matheson, L. (1991). Symptom magnification syndrome structured interview: rationale and procedure. *Journal of Occupational Rehabilitation, 1*(1), 43–56.
18. Matheson, L, personal communication, October, 1984.
19. U.S. Department of Labor. (1991). *The revised handbook for analyzing jobs.* Indianapolis, IN: Author. Retrieved from http://www.vocational.org/Analysis/RHAJ.pdf
20. Resnick, P. (1995). *Guidelines for the evaluation of malingering in post-traumatic stress disorder: Guidelines for forensic assessment.* Washington DC: American Psychiatric Association Publishing.
21. Stokes, H. (1983). The seriously uninjured hand—weakness of grip. *Journal of Occupational Medicine, 25*(9), 683–684.
22. Mathiowetz, V., Kashman, N., Volland, G., Weber, K., Dowe, M., & Rogers, S. (1985). Grip and pinch strength: Normative data for adults. *Physical Medicine and Rehabilitation, 66*(2), 69–74.
23. Main, C. J., & Waddell, G. (1998). Behavioral responses to examination: A reappraisal of the interpretation of "non-organic signs." *Spine (Phila Pa 1976), 23*(21), 2367–2371.

ADDITIONAL REFERENCES

Chapman-Day, K., Matheson, L., Schimanski, D., Leicht J., & DeVries, L. (2011). Preparing difficult clients to return to work. *Work, 40*(4), 359–367.

Faucett, J., & Werner, R. A. (1999). *Non-biomechanical factors potentially affecting musculoskeletal disorders.* Washington DC: National Academy Press.

Fishbain, D. A., Cole, B., Cutler, R. B., Lewis, J., Rosomoff, H. L., & Rosomoff, R. S. (2003). A structured evidence-based review on the meaning of non-organic physical signs: Waddell signs. *Pain Med,* 4(2), 141–181.

Fishbain, D. A., Cutler, R. B., & Rosomoff, H. L. (2004). Is there a relationship between non-organic physical findings (Waddell signs) and secondary gain/malingering? *Clinical Journal of Pain, 20*(6), 399–408.

HIldreth, D., Breidenbach, W., Lister, G., & Hodges, A. (1989). Detection of submaximal effort by use of the rapid exchange grip. *Journal of Hand Surgery, 14*(4), 742–745.

Matheson, L. (n.d.). *The functional capacity evaluation: Disability evaluation* (2nd ed.) Washington DC: Education Resources Information Center.

Matheson, L. (1987). *Presenting and defending Results.* Washington DC: Education Resources Information Center.

Matheson, L. & Hart, D. (1980). Use of maximum voluntary effort testing to identify physical signs in low back pain. *Spine (Phila Pa 1976).*

Neibuhr, B. R., & Marion, R. (1987). Detecting sincerity of effort when measuring grip strength. *American Journal of Physical Medicine, 66*(1), 16–24.

Taanita, H., Suni, J., Pihlajamäki, H., Mattila, V. M., Ohrankämmen, O., Vuorinen, P., & Parkkari, J. (Jan 2012). Predictors of low back pain in physically active conscripts with special emphasis on muscular fitness. *The Spine Journal, 12*(9), 737–748.

The Cooper Institute for Aerobic Fitness. (1972). *Exercise testing and training in apparently healthy individuals: A handbook for physicians.* Dallas, TX: The Cooper Institute for Aerobic Fitness.

Chapter 18

Physical Agent Modalities

Elizabeth A. Fain, EdD, OTR/L

LEARNING OUTCOMES

After studying this chapter, the student or practitioner will be able to:

18.1 Describe the position of the American Occupational Therapy Association on utilization of physical agent modalities

18.2 Describe the regulatory issues guidelines for physical agent modalities as they apply to the role of the occupational therapy assistant

18.3 Identify the occupational therapy ethics that frame the usage of physical agent modalities in occupational therapy practice

18.4 Describe the roles of occupational therapists and occupational therapy assistants in the use of physical agent modalities

18.5 Describe the application, precautions, contraindications, and safety considerations for each physical agent modality and mechanical modality

KEY TERMS

Air speed
Alternating current (AC)
Amplitude
Applicator
Beam nonuniformity ratio (BNR)
Charge
Continuous passive motion machine (CPM)
Contraindication
Diathermy
Direct current (DC)
Duty cycle
Effective radiating area (ERA)
Functional electrical stimulation (FES)
Interferential current (IFC)
Iontophoresis
Megahertz (MHz)
Neuromuscular electrical stimulation (NMES)
Phonophoresis
Physical agent modalities (PAMs)
Pulse duration
Pulse frequency
Pulsed current
Ramp time
Sound head
Transcutaneous electrical nerve stimulation (TENS)
Ultrasound intensity
Ultrasound power
Vasocompression units
Waveform

Physical agent modalities (PAMs) consist of procedures and interventions that are applied to alter specific client factors, such as body functions related to pain and neuromusculoskeletal and movement-related functions, as specified in the *Occupational Therapy Practice Framework, 3rd edition* (OTPF-3).[1] Although PAMs are tools in the occupational therapy (OT) toolkit (or treatment repertoire), it is critical to note that PAMs are intended to be *preparatory methods* to facilitate accomplishing the occupational performance goals. The OT field has a history of passionate discussion about the concerns regarding the use of PAMs. A major argument is that PAMs will cause OT to lose its occupational performance role or focus.[2] The discussion centers around some OT practitioners who use PAMs without a focus on occupation, in the same way that another practitioner might only focus on exercise. However, in 1985, modalities were incorporated into OT practice for those working in hand therapy.[3] The Hand Therapy Certification Commission endorsed the routine use of PAMs as part of therapeutic interventions by occupational and physical therapists with hand therapy certification. As a result of this precedent and the shift in practice, the Representative Assembly of the American Occupational Therapy Association (AOTA) voted to adopt a policy to support the use of PAMs as an adjunctive intervention after a member data survey indicated that 83.4% of its members worked in the treatment of physical disabilities and were most likely to use PAMs.[4]

In 1991, the AOTA wrote a position paper on using PAMs as adjunctive interventions to address occupational performance problems as a means to clarify the appropriate context for application of PAMs in OT; this was updated in 2012.[5] In this paper, the AOTA described the types of PAMs, the roles, ethics, and professional responsibilities that OT practitioners need to understand to be competent, ethical, and to adhere to applicable state laws when utilizing PAMs. The AOTA emphasized that PAMs are to be incorporated as a preparatory method for the clients' occupations or purposeful activities.[5] Although the original term was *adjunctive modality*, the OTPF-3 changed the term to *preparatory method*.[1] Furthermore, OT practitioners must have demonstrated verifiable competence in the application of PAMs in their practices.[5] Components of demonstrating this competence includes obtaining core knowledge for underlying theories and training in biological, neurophysiological, and electrophysiological changes that occur as a result of the application of PAMs. Education in integration of PAMs must also include the application, precautions, contraindications, and safety considerations for the procedural aspect of PAMs. The OT practitioner must also document the synthesis of this preparatory activity into the client's occupational performance activities and goals.

REGULATORY GUIDELINES FOR PHYSICAL AGENT MODALITIES IN OCCUPATIONAL THERAPY PRACTICE

In the United States, the guidelines for PAMs in OT practice vary in each state. It is the OT practitioners' responsibility to be familiar with the practice guidelines in the state in which they practice and to ensure that they have the prerequisite competence in the application of PAMs along with the necessary documentation. "Competence" implies that the OT practitioner has the capacity to safely perform the specific tasks related to PAMs and has met the state's required guidelines to utilize them. Competence requirements vary in each state, region, and country but may include continuing education by preapproved providers, direct observation of a staff member whose training ensures competence, and others.[6] The OT scope of practice for the various states is available for download on the AOTA website as a member benefit. Each state and country has specific guidelines of which the OT practitioner needs to be familiar to ensure compliance with the requirements.

ETHICS FRAMING THE APPLICATION OF PHYSICAL AGENT MODALITIES

The Occupational Therapy Code of Ethics (2015) also addresses principles that guide safe and competent professional practice that must be applied to the use of PAMs.[6] These codes of ethics or principles include numerous standards, but the following standards relate to PAMs that OT practitioners should adhere to.

Beneficence

Principle: OT personnel shall demonstrate a concern for the well-being and safety of the recipients of their services.

- Use, to the extent possible, evaluation, planning, intervention techniques, assessments, and therapeutic equipment that are evidence-based, current, and within the recognized scope of OT practice.
- Ensure that all duties delegated to other OT personnel are congruent with credentials, qualifications, experience, competency, and scope of practice with respect to service delivery, supervision, fieldwork education, and research.
- Provide OT services, including education and training, that are within each practitioner's level of competence and scope of practice.

Veracity

Principle: OT personnel shall provide comprehensive, accurate, and objective information when representing the profession.

- Represent credentials, qualifications, education, experience, training, roles, duties, competence, contributions, and findings accurately in all forms of communication.
- Identify and fully disclose to all appropriate persons, errors or adverse events that compromise the safety of service recipients.

Nonmaleficence

Principle: OT personnel shall refrain from actions that cause harm.

- Avoid inflicting harm or injury to recipients of OT services, students, research participants, or employees.[7]

THE ACCREDITATION COUNCIL FOR OCCUPATIONAL THERAPY EDUCATION STANDARDS RELATED TO PHYSICAL AGENT MODALITIES

In 2016, the Accreditation Council for Occupational Therapy Education (ACOTE) implemented standards that require inclusion of minimum educational standards in the U.S. for PAMs for OT educational programs. A number of ACOTE standards address the use of PAMs for occupational therapy assistants (OTAs), and those documents can be referenced for students and educators. It is also relevant to note that the standard for OT requires demonstration of application, which requires critical thinking about the purpose and application of PAMs.

ROLES OF THE OCCUPATIONAL THERAPY PRACTITIONER FOR USING PHYSICAL AGENT MODALITIES

OT practitioners play a vital role in supporting clients' health, well-being, and participation in life through engagement in occupation.[6] In addressing the application of PAMs, it is important to reflect on the meaning of the core premise of the OT profession. Although there are many perspectives on the meaning of occupation, a general reference point is that occupation consists of the routine activities of everyday life that are meaningful and valuable to individuals and their cultures. Occupation is the core of what people do to occupy themselves for societal and economic contributions in their communities.[9] Since OT practitioners are addressing the person and the interaction within his or her contextual life, it is critical that the OT practitioners do not lose sight of this end goal when including PAMs as a preparatory method. When initiating therapy, OT practitioners must always reflect and ask themselves, "What are the clients' goals?" and "How can OT facilitate the achievement of these goals?" Furthermore, when deciding on the use of any tool to accomplish a client's goals, it is necessary to ask how the use of PAMs will aid the client's ability to engage in his or her occupation. Only when the OT practitioner is able to answer these questions can the decision be made whether to include PAMs as a treatment modality.

THEORETICAL PREMISE FOR USING PHYSICAL AGENT MODALITIES IN OCCUPATIONAL THERAPY PRACTICE

The theoretical framework for application of PAMs aligns with the biomechanical theoretical framework. The biomechanical framework asserts that the focus of OT treatment with PAMs is to improve structural stability, healing, active range of motion (AROM) and passive range of motion (PROM), muscle strength, edema, and endurance. Addressing these areas with the application of PAMs enhances the client's occupational performance by focusing on the core problems that contribute to occupational performance deficits. After the application of PAMs, during the occupational performance and rehabilitation phase, the theoretical frameworks may differ, depending on the setting, the clinician's preference, and the client's goals. However, the integration of several OT theoretical frameworks, such as Person-Environment-Occupation-Performance, Rehabilitation, and Model of Human Occupation, are applicable to providing more client-centered rehabilitation. Ultimately, the application of PAMs is intended to be one of the tools in the toolbox to promote occupational engagement by facilitating pain control, ease of movement, and increased strength.

Another relevant theory to the utilization of PAMs is the pain gate theory, also known as the Melzack and Wall's gate control theory or the opiate system. The pain gate theory explains how modalities aid in pain control; it will be discussed in more detail in the section on transcutaneous electrical nerve stimulation (TENS). Utilization of PAMs potentially facilitates clients engaging more fully in occupational tasks when the pain is controlled.

Wound Healing and Implications for Physical Agent Modalities

Before examining individual PAMs, it is first necessary to review wound healing and the implications for PAMs. Refer to Chapter 8 for a complete discussion of the wound healing process. Roles for OT practitioners in wound care vary by setting, but having a foundational knowledge about wound care is important to the application of physical-agent modalities. Wound healing occurs in response to an injury. The tissue response includes a series of dynamic multisystem responses that include four phases: hemostasis phase, inflammation phase, fibroblastic or proliferative phase, and remodeling or maturation phase.

PAMs commonly used during the inflammation phase include the use of hand held sprayers for gentle debridement and cleaning of the wound (whirlpool therapy, commonly used in the past, has not been proven effective, and may even promote infection) and electrical stimulation with high-voltage pulsed current to increase circulation to the wound area and influence the migration, proliferation, and function of the wound healing cells to promote wound closure. Cold modalities are also effective in reducing the production of inflammatory mediators released by the cell membrane. Shortwave diathermy (SWD) (applying deeper heat to tissues) is also utilized to increase local circulation, reduce swelling, and facilitate tissue healing. Superficial heat is contraindicated (not recommended) during this phase. If ultrasound is used, then it should be utilized in the nonthermal setting.

In the proliferative or fibroblastic phase, use of electrical stimulation, SWD, and light therapy, after careful consideration of the client's condition and risk factors, can facilitate healing. Cold should not be used during the proliferative phase because by causing vasoconstriction (narrowing of blood vessels), it will block the introduction of new cells into the wound area. Heat, however, will increase vasodilation, which helps increase the volume of fibroblastic cells, or cells that produce collagen and aid in wound healing.

During the early remodeling or maturation phase, the OT practitioner must be careful to avoid damaging or disturbing the epithelial tissue. During the later phase of remodeling, continuous or 100% ultrasound may be indicated if scarring is impeding function, ROM, or esthetics.

Although PAMs can be utilized to promote healing, it is important to consider all of the components of wound healing, the goals of the treatment, and which PAMs are effective and which ones are contraindicated. For example, an initial injury may benefit from hydrotherapy or a hand held water sprayer to clean an open wound. Chronic inflammation may benefit from fluidotherapy to decrease joint stiffness, whereas cryotherapy would be contraindicated. Pulsed ultrasound may also be considered to progress wound healing to the proliferation stage.[10] PAMs will be discussed in more detail in the specific section for each of the modalities.

CLASSIFICATION OF MODALITIES

PAMs are classified on the basis of the modality's properties. PAMs are techniques that produce a response in the soft tissue through the application of light or water, the temperature exchange between the modality and the tissue, sound waves, or electricity.[11] Each PAM creates different response and is applicable for different conditions and clients' needs. To most effectively and safely treat the client's condition and occupational performance needs, each modality needs to be considered for its properties and the type of tissue being treated. In addition to considering the properties and application of PAMs, all OT practitioners need to follow the guidelines addressed in Figure 18-1. Before proceeding with a modality, the OT practitioner needs to be able to answer the questions in the guidelines to proceed safely and effectively for the best treatment outcomes. Additionally, the OT practitioner should review the skills required to complete the PAM (see Fig. 18-1), and be competent to perform. These steps precede all of the specific procedural PAM steps that are listed under each modality.

Thermal Modalities

Thermal modalities transfer energy or heat or cold from one object to the tissue that it is in contact with. Heat goes from the warmer modality to the cooler tissue. Cold goes from the cooler modality to the warmer tissue. The heat exchange is based on the temperature difference between the thermal

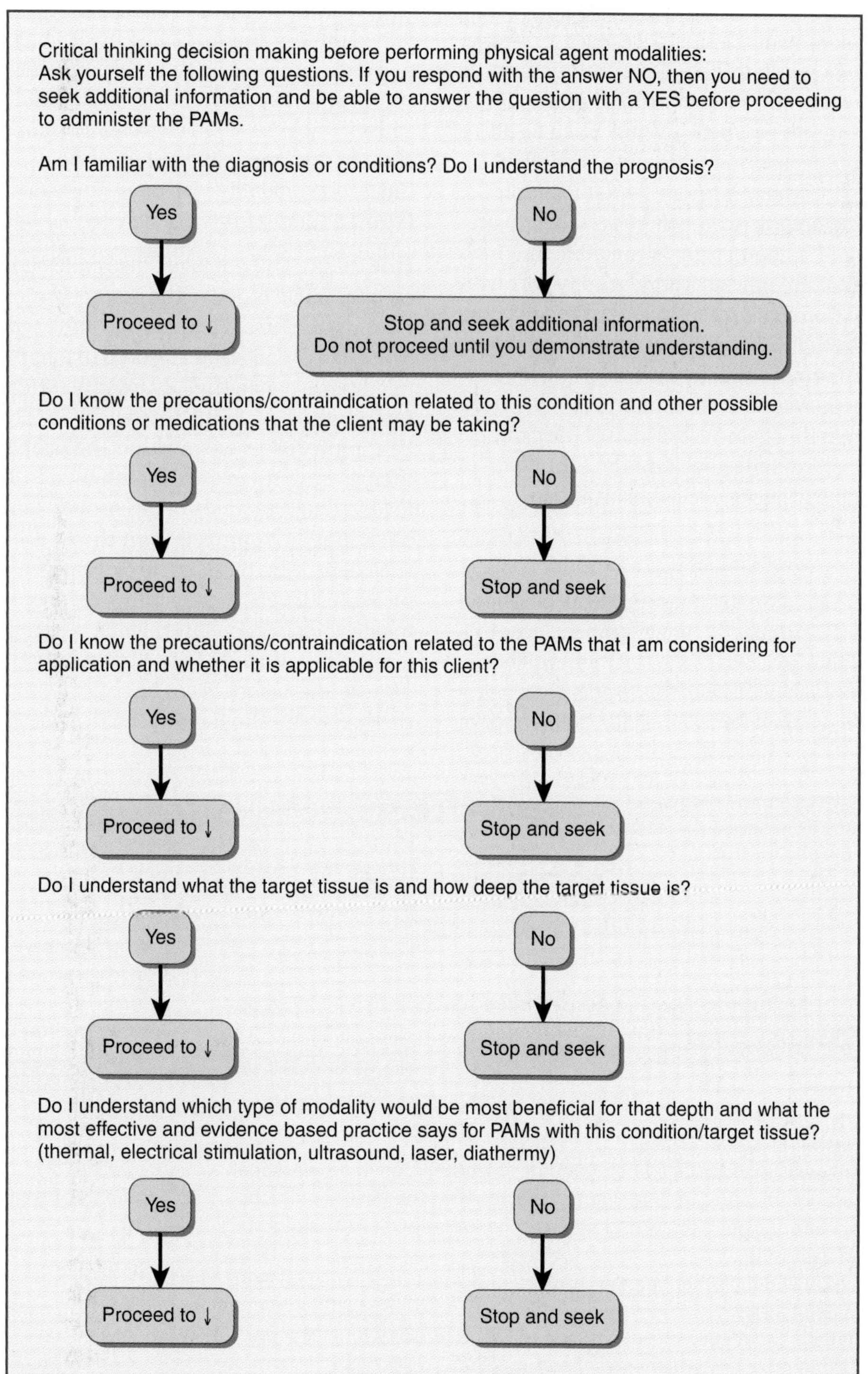

FIGURE 18-1. Critical decision-making tree.

agent and the tissue being treated, time of exposure to the thermal agent, and the conductivity of the tissue along with the intensity of the tissue.[12] The exchange of energy from thermal PAMs and the tissue being treated is impacted by the type of tissue and its level of conductivity. Adipose (fat) tissue, skeletal muscle, bone, and blood, all conduct at different levels and different rates of temperature exchange. Tissue with high water content absorbs and conducts thermal energy most easily.[12]

Conduction is temperature exchange or transfer from direct contact from PAMs to the underlying tissue. The temperature exchange occurs with direct contact between PAMs and tissues with different temperatures. Examples of conduction modalities include moist heat packs and ice massage or ice packs. Transfer of thermal energy through convection is transfer of heat through a moving medium, such as air or water. The delivery of energy occurs through a carrier, which then applies the heat to the treatment tissue. Examples of convection are hydrotherapy (water therapy, where water transfers the heat) and fluidotherapy (a machine in which particles that hold heat are moved around a body part with a constant airflow). Conversion thermal exchange occurs when sound wave energy is changed to a mechanical type of energy to achieve a thermal effect; for example, quickly rubbing the hands together creates friction and results in increased warmth within that tissue. Ultrasound is an example of conversion thermal exchange because the sound waves are transformed to kinetic energy, which warms tissues.[13]

SUPERFICIAL THERMAL MODALITIES

Superficial thermal agents cause a superficial (shallow) change in skin and subcutaneous tissue temperatures to a depth of approximately 1 to 2 cm (0.4 to 0.8 inches). The tissue temperature effect depends on the tissue area being treated, duration of application of the modality, difference in the temperatures of the tissue and the modality, and the conductivity of the treated tissue. The proper temperature elevation of soft tissue is in the range of 104°F to 113° F. If temperature is not elevated to at least 104° F, then the therapeutic range, or altering of cell metabolism, has not been achieved. If the temperature is elevated more than 113° F, then cell death can occur.[14] Superficial heating agents reach their maximal temperature increase to tissue within 8 to 10 minutes if the subcutaneous tissue is well vascularized—that is, if it contains many blood vessels. Skin and subcutaneous tissue temperature increases to a beginning therapeutic temperature of 105.8° F (41° C) after 6 minutes and is maintained up to 30 minutes after application.[12]

When considering thermal modalities for a client, review the properties and changes that the thermal modality causes. Table 18-1 is a reference for properties of heat versus cold thermal modalities when deciding between the two. At times, one modality is strongly indicated; at other times, the OT practitioner must decide which modality to try first.

Hot Pack: The hot pack, also called a heat pack or hydrocollator pack, is one of the most commonly used superficial heating agents. It is a canvas-covered silica gel (or bentonite clay) pack that is stored in a hydrocollator, a device filled with water that is thermostatically controlled at a temperature of 159.8° F to 174° F. Hydrocollators must be monitored to ensure that the proper water levels and temperature ranges are maintained to deliver optimal heat levels. Once heated to the proper temperature, the hot pack may be removed from the hydrocollator for use on the client. The temperature of the hot packs is controlled by water levels, water temperature, and length of time inside the hydrocollator. Once a hot pack has been used, it must be returned to the hydrocollator for at least 20 to 30 minutes before it can be reused. This ensures therapeutic levels of tissue heating.[12]

TABLE 18-1 Indications for Heat Versus Cold

INDICATIONS/BENEFITS OF HEAT	INDICATIONS/BENEFITS OF COLD
↑ Blood flow ↑ Cellular metabolic rate ↑ Inflammatory response ↑ Edema, and prevent adhesion formation ↑ Heat of skin and indirectly ↑ temperature in deeper tissues up to 1 hour following an application Heat is soothing ↑ Extensibility of collagen ↓ Joint stiffness ↑ Relief of muscle spasm Heating modalities are beneficial if applied before other procedures, such as massage, stretching, exercise, and adjusting/manipulating. By stretching the tissue during or immediately after heat treatment, the muscle fibrosis, contracted joint capsule, or scar can increase in extensibility. ↓ Pain, muscle spasm caused by ischemia may be relieved by heat, which increases blood flow to the area of injury. Moist heat causes a greater indirect increase in the deep tissue temperature than dry heat, but dry heat is tolerable up to higher temperatures than moist heat.	↓ Circulation ↓Metabolism ↓ Inflammatory effects ↓ Secondary trauma that can occur following injury ↓ Inflammation because of the effects on blood flow of ice, including vasoconstriction (slowing the hemorrhaging in the area) ↓ Histamine release ↓ Swelling, bleeding ↓ Inflammation ↓ Pain

Hot packs should also be stored in the hydrocollator to prevent them from drying out.

Hot packs come in different sizes and shapes. When choosing a hot pack, consider the body part to which it will be applied to ensure proper contouring and conduction of the thermal heat. After considering all clinical applications of the hot pack, the OT practitioner must properly position and drape the client for the hot pack treatment. A visual inspection of the skin where the hot pack will be applied should be performed and documented. The OT practitioner must also document the sensory status of that area and the client's ability to reliably report concerns or status.[12]

Application: After careful clinical consideration of the client's condition and occupational goals, application of a hot pack as a preparatory activity may be used for conditions such as:

- Decreased ROM or stiffness
- Subcutaneous adhesions
- Contractures
- Chronic arthritis
- Cumulative trauma

Hot packs should be prepared with six to eight layers of towels between the pack and the client's skin. The type of towels and their thickness, and whether hot pack covers are being utilized determine the number of layers needed. Commercial terrycloth covers are generally equivalent to two to four layers of towels. The hot pack is applied with the required towel layers on the client, ensuring comfortable position and that the client is not lying on the hot pack, (the additional pressure against the body while the laying on hot pack could cause overheating of tissue) (Fig. 18-2). The client is instructed on what to expect, what they will experience, and the need to immediately report any sensation of burning or overheating. Skin should be monitored very closely during the first five to ten minutes, because this is when the most rapid change in tissue temperature occurs, then continue to monitor throughout the treatment. Ask the client to provide feedback while ensuring a warm, but not hot, sensation. The towel layers are adjusted on the basis of the verbal feedback from the client and visual inspection of the treatment area. Application time is typically 20 minutes. After removal of the hot pack, the OT practitioner observes and documents the client's skin condition and his or her response.[12] See Box 18-1 for a summary of hot pack application.

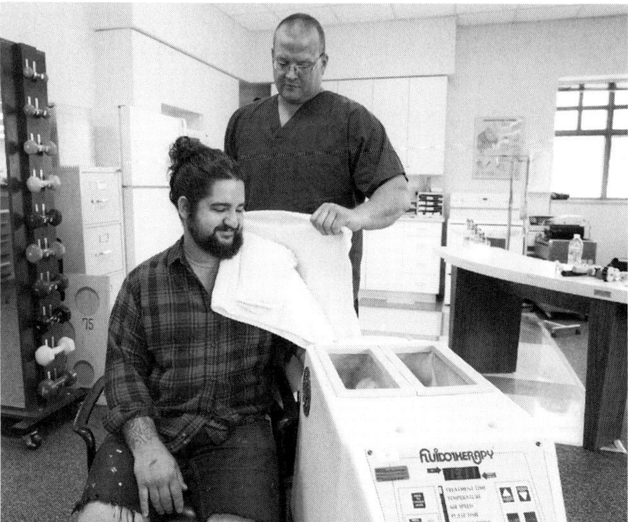

FIGURE 18-2. The OTA places the client's left hand into the fluidotherapy machine and then places the hot pack on the client's shoulder, with appropriate layers of towels and hot pack cover for safety.

Precautions: The terms *precaution* and *contraindication* mean distinctly different things and should not be used interchangeably. Essentially, precautions are comparable to a yellow traffic signal light—proceed with caution after careful critical thinking and in consideration of the client's total clinical condition, comorbidities, and goals. Contraindications are comparable to a red traffic signal light—do not use the modality for clients with specific conditions that are contraindicated. Conditions associated with precautions for hot packs are those that involve diminished sensation or compromised circulation, among others. If a hot pack is used on clients with these types of conditions, then use of that modality requires precaution. This means the OT practitioner must proceed with great care, monitoring the client's status more frequently throughout the treatment session. Monitoring the overt physiological signs,

BOX 18-1

Applying a Heat Pack

1. Evaluate and document the client's occupational performance problems, goals, and status and integrity of the surface that the heat pack is to be administered to.
2. Proceed with application of heat pack after careful chart review for precautions and contraindications along with critical thinking decision making if it is indicated that the heat pack is applicable for this client's condition and is not contraindicated.
3. Explain to the client the procedure and rationale for application of the heat pack. Describe the sensation and time frame to be expected.
4. Obtain heat pack cover applicable for the size and shape heat pack along with six to eight towels.
5. Place the heat pack cover on the heat pack.
6. Place six to eight layers of towels (or two to four layers over the heat pack cover) that will be between the heat pack and the client's skin.
7. Position the client comfortably to ensure he or she is not lying against the heat pack.
8. Monitor the temperature, and inspect the treated area.
9. Upon completion of the 20-minute treatment, reevaluate the client's status and outcomes; proceed with the occupational performance tasks; and document the intervention and the outcomes.

such as respiration, blood pressure, and skin color, is also necessary to ensure that the client is not experiencing adverse reactions to the hot pack.[11]

Contraindications: Contraindications for application of hot packs include clients with significant circulation impairments or edema of undetermined origin; the acute inflammatory phase of healing (the first two days post injury); tumors or cancer; deep venous thrombosis; bleeding conditions; advanced cardiac disease; impaired cognitive status or decreased consciousness; poor thermal regulation; and rheumatoid arthritis (where vigorous levels of heat should be avoided).[11] Hot packs should not be used on clients with any of these contraindications.

Safety Considerations: Basic safety considerations when using hot packs include monitoring the water temperature and the water level in the hydrocollator to ensure adequate heating of the hot packs. Water spillage should be monitored when retrieving hot packs from the hydrocollator to prevent a slip hazard. Tongs should be used when retrieving hot packs out of the hydrocollator to prevent thermal burns.[12]

Fluidotherapy: Fluidotherapy is a therapeutic modality that consists of a closed unit containing finely ground cellulose particles made from corn cob particles. The client places the body part, typically the arm or hand, inside a sleeve that is attached to an opening in the unit. Once the sleeve is fastened on the affected body part, and the body part is inserted into the unit, the machine is turned on and warm air heats and circulates the Cellex™ (cellulose) particles. The heated air and Cellex™ particles massage the affected extremity, providing heat and tactile stimulation to achieve physiological and therapeutic benefits. A thermometer displays the temperature of the unit, which is also easy to control by adjusting the settings. The unit has settings for treatment time. A benefit of fluidotherapy is that the heat is maintained consistently during the treatment session, unlike hot packs and other thermal PAMs that may lose temperature over the treatment time.[10] Fluidotherapy is applicable for conditions with pain, decreased ROM, and arthritis other than rheumatoid arthritis.[13] It may also be used without the heat component to provide sensory input, such as in the case of a peripheral nerve injury or cerebrovascular accident (CVA).

THE OLDER ADULT

Healing is a distinctively different process through a person's lifespan. Healing and wound closure are slower in adults compared with pediatric clients because of the physiological changes that occur with aging. In the geriatric population, collagen has decreased density and cross-linking, which ultimately decreases the tensile strength of the wound closure. The geriatric population may also have decreased circulation, which adversely affects wound healing.[9]

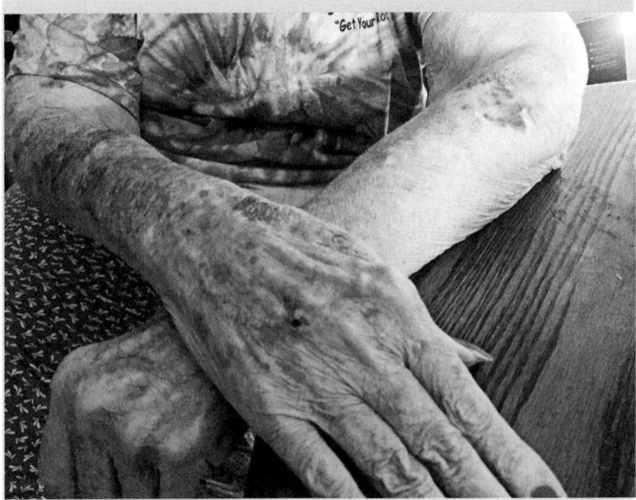

The older adult can have significantly fragile skin.

	HEALTHY OLDER ADULT	OLDER ADULTS WITH COMORBIDITIES
Wound healing	Comparable wound healing with little, if any, delay in wound healing	Older adults often have many comorbidities that impact the wound healing time frame and increase the risk of infection.
Skin integrity	Thin skin but intact integrity	Thin skin tears easily, may bruise easily, and has a greater risk of infection.
Pain	Comparable pain tolerance	These individuals have more complaints of pain but may have difficulty tolerating or expressing pain.

Intrinsic risk factors commonly associated with the older adult population may include the following:

- Immobility
- Poor nutrition
- Poor hydration
- Obesity
- Cachexia or loss of weight
- Muscle atrophy
- Impaired circulation
- Impaired respiratory function
- Chronic diseases, such as:
  - Diabetes
  - Peripheral artery disease
  - Peripheral vascular disease
  - Coronary artery disease
- Renal failure, anemia
- Cancer
- End of life
- Radiation therapy

Extrinsic risk factors commonly associated with the older population may include the following:

- Tobacco use
- Pressure to involved area that compromises circulation
- Desiccation or dry skin that leads to scabs or crusts on the skin
- Presence of eschar or necrotic tissue
- Repetitive trauma, such as high shear forces
- Maceration caused by extreme moisture, such as incontinence or perspiration
- Lack of participation in the wound care

The **air speed,** or rate that the cellulose particles are moving, can be adjusted to the appropriate level for the client to tolerate. Figure 18-2 shows a fluidotherapy machine in use.

Application: Fluidotherapy is easy to use and maintains uniform application of heat to the body area being treated. The timer on the fluidotherapy machine helps set the desirable temperature to preheat the cellulose material before actual treatment time. The unit should be preheated to 100° F to 118° F before the treatment session if heat is desired. The fluidotherapy unit includes a treatment temperature feature that allows the OT practitioner to set the desired temperature, or to just have it at room temperature. If desired, the pulse time feature interrupts the flow of the medium by stopping and starting the medium within a range of 1 second on/off to 6 second on/off ratio of time frame. Alternatively, setting the pulse time to "off" allows for continuous circulation of the medium without stopping.[12] Finally, the treatment time feature sets the time frame for the duration of the fluidotherapy treatment. The display depicts the remaining time left for the treatment and stops when the treatment time is complete. See Box 18-2 for a summary of fluidotherapy.

Precautions: If chronic edema is present, both the dependent position and heat during the treatment may increase the edema. Positioning and active exercises may need to be utilized to counteract the fluid buildup. Additional precautionary considerations are diminished sensation and compromised circulation. The dust from the circulating cellulose can cause sensitivities in clients with respiratory difficulties. Placing a folded sheet over the top of the fluidotherapy machine may prevent some of the emission of the cellulose dust and subsequent breathing difficulties related to the dust.

BOX 18-2
Fluidotherapy Application

1. Ask the client to remove all jewelry and clothing from the body area (typically the arm or hand) being treated.
2. Ask the client to wash and dry the affected body part.
3. If applicable, cover open wounds with a plastic barrier. Insert the body part into the fluidotherapy sleeve, and Velcro® the strap securely to the body part to prevent cellulose particles from falling out of the sleeve.
4. Set the level of cellulose and air circulation as well as heat to the client's therapeutic and comfort level.
5. Instruct client on exercises or positioning during the treatment session. The duration of a treatment session generally is 20 minutes.
6. Upon removal of the extremity from the unit, have a towel ready to wipe cellulose particles back into the unit,[9] and place a small trash can under the unit sleeve to catch any loose particles.
7. Proceed with functional tasks as part of the treatment and established goals.
8. Document the treatment and response.

Contraindications: Fluidotherapy should not be used with clients who have the following conditions: impaired sensation (with heat), poor thermoregulation, open wounds, infections, contagious diseases, tumor/cancer, acute inflammation, and acute edema.[10] For clients who cannot tolerate heat, the OT practitioner can use the fluidotherapy machine without heat for decreasing hypersensitivity of skin as the material circulates around the limb.

Safety Considerations: When setting up clients for treatments, OT practitioners must account for a potentially long preheating period of the unit. Spilled cellulose materials on the floor may create a fall risk. It is important to adhere to the safety standards set by the U.S. Food and Drug Administration (FDA).

Paraffin: Paraffin is melted wax that is mixed with mineral oil in a 6:1 or 7:1 ratio. The paraffin is kept in an electric powered unit that has a heating element to keep the wax melted and in a temperature range of 126° F to 134° F. The temperature needs to be checked and verified that it is in the acceptable treatment range before using the paraffin. The application of paraffin in OT is commonly used with clients' hands because of the size of the heating unit and the ease of use within the clinic and in home programs.

Application: Paraffin is an effective modality because of its ease of use, low cost, and applicability for home use. Paraffin has a variety of applications for several outcomes. It has been noted to be an effective modality for arthritis, systemic sclerosis (systemic connective tissue disease), decreased range of motion, scars, contracture, and pain control.[15]

A paraffin application requires the client to dip his or her hand, or other affected body part, into the melted wax repeatedly to allow the wax to build up. The OT practitioner wraps the body part in plastic or wax paper, followed by a towel or mitt, and the client then waits for a period before the paraffin is removed (Fig. 18-3). Paraffin treatment can be messy, but with proper setup, it can be simple and easy to use. Clients may also use paraffin baths at home by using either a paraffin unit or an electronic cooking pot, such as a Crock-Pot™, dedicated to this use. Although using a double boiler is possible, this is not the preferred method because of the extra setup steps and burn risk from handling hot pots and boiling water. The recipe for making paraffin wax is to melt one, 4-lb block of paraffin, which can be purchased in the canning section of a grocery store, with 1⅓ cups of mineral oil in the paraffin unit. The mixture is heated to reach a temperature between 115° F and 134° F, with 126° F as the optimal temperature for hands. Alternately, pre-mixed paraffin can be purchased, and is available in a variety of scents or scent-free. A candy thermometer can be used to test the temperature before immersing hand(s) into the mixture. Box 18-3 shows the steps for a paraffin dip bath.

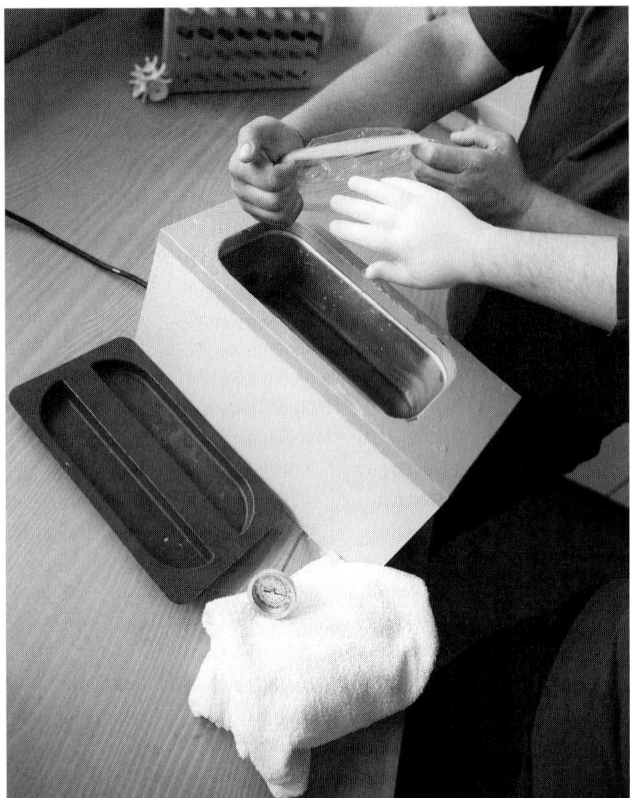

FIGURE 18-3. The OTA directs the client to dip the hand into the paraffin unit, then covers it with plastic before placing in a mitt or wrapping with a towel to maintain therapeutic heat.

Two other paraffin methods are the dip-immersion method and the paint method. The dip immersion method is similar to the steps just described, the difference being that the client dips the hand once and allows a coating to develop (5–15 seconds), before immersing the hand in the unit and keeping it there for up to 20 minutes. This step avoids having to wrap with plastic wrap and towel. This type of paraffin treatment is considered a vigorous heat treatment.[11] The paint paraffin treatment method consists of using a paintbrush to coat an affected body part that cannot be dipped, such as the medial or lateral epicondyle. The OT practitioner paints or coats the client's body part with 10 layers of paraffin, then wraps it with plastic wrap and towel, and positions the client, much like stages 5 to 6 in Box 18-3. Paraffin treatment time is 20 minutes.

Once treatment is complete, the mitt or towel and plastic wrap and then the paraffin coating are removed.[10,11] The client should be instructed to remove the paraffin over a trash can to catch any small pieces that may break off. For home use, the client can place the paraffin back into the paraffin unit for reuse. In a clinical setting with other clients, the paraffin is not reused. When debris is noted in the unit, discarding the paraffin and cleaning out the unit before replacing the paraffin would be advisable.

Precautions: The affected hand is washed and thoroughly dried before treatment. The OT practitioner should ensure that the paraffin removed from a client is discarded to prevent cross-contamination in the paraffin unit. During dipping, it is important to have the client hold his or her hand still to prevent cracking the paraffin coating; this ensures adequate thermal benefits from the treatment.[10] The client should be instructed to avoid touching the bottom or sides of the unit to avoid contact with the heating regulator.

Contraindications: Paraffin use is contraindicated in clients with open wounds, skin infections, sensory loss, and peripheral vascular disease.[13]

Safety Considerations: It is important to understand the manufacturer's directions for use of the paraffin unit; at first,

BOX 18-3
Paraffin Application

1. Ask the client to remove all jewelry from the affected body part.
2. Assess skin integrity, and document any noted areas.
3. Ask the client to wash and dry hands completely. Any water droplets remaining on skin can cause burns.
4. Dip the affected hand into the unit with fingers spread apart. Instruct the client to avoid touching the bottom or the sides of the unit because they may be hotter than the paraffin. Alert the client that the wax will feel very hot and to avoid moving the fingers to ensure that the paraffin can create a solid paraffin coating.
5. Remove the hand from the unit after a few seconds. Wait briefly for the paraffin to cool to a solid coating before immersing the hand back into the paraffin unit.
6. Redip the hand 5 to 10 times for the wrap-and-glove technique.
7. Wrap the client's hand in a plastic bag, plastic wrap, or wax paper. Place a towel or mitt over the wrapped hand. The plastic wrap keeps the wax from adhering to the towel or mitt, and the towel or mitt insulates the heat from escaping quickly.
8. Position the extremity in elevation on an arm trough, and instruct the client to keep the hand still to ensure that the paraffin does not crack and lose heat too soon. The paraffin typically remains in place for about 20 minutes.
9. Upon completion of the paraffin treatment, remove and discard the wax. If the client is performing this at home, he or she can reuse the paraffin.
10. Proceed with functional tasks as part of the treatment and established goals.
11. Document the treatment and response.
12. Cleaning the paraffin unit and replacing the paraffin will depend on the frequency of use and the clinic's policy. At the minimum, paraffin that is used routinely should be replaced monthly, and the unit should be cleaned out to remove possible debris left behind.

the melted paraffin will be hotter than the therapeutic range, and if used during this phase, it could burn the client. Paraffin may take up to 5 hours to melt. The paraffin's temperature should be monitored to ensure that it falls within a range that is between 126° F and 134° F. The temperature should be checked before use with every client. Generally, medical-grade paraffin has antibacterial ingredients that allow use of the remaining paraffin in the unit without cleaning the unit between clients. It is important to adhere to the safety standards set by the FDA.

Cryotherapy: Cryotherapy is the use of cold for therapeutic benefits and consists of ice massage, cold packs, cold baths, or ice bags. Cold is used to control inflammation, pain, and edema, to decrease spasticity, and to facilitate muscle movement in neuromuscular reeducation.[10] Cryotherapy cools the tissue and can be effective for producing analgesia (numbness) and for decreasing edema and muscle spasms by reducing the metabolic activity.[16] Cryotherapy commonly produces four distinct stages, which should be explained to clients so that they understand that these stages are necessary for optimal therapeutic benefits. These four stages are *cold,* which is associated with red skin color (hyperemia), *burning,* deep *aching,* and analgesia or *numbness.* These stages generally occur within 10 to 20 minutes.[11] Cryotherapy impacts nerves through counterirritation and by reducing the metabolic activity of tissue. Blood vessels are constricted if treatment time is generally less than 15 minutes; however, if longer, then blood vessels may vasodilate. When the body switches between vasoconstriction and vasodilation, it is called a "hunting response." The degree of vasoconstriction may impact the edema reduction treatment as a result of the hunting response. Therefore, additional edema reduction techniques, such as active muscle pumping exercises, elevation, light retrograde massage, and manual edema mobilization will be indicated to further reduce the edema.[11]

Application: Cryotherapy is the modality of choice in acute trauma and subacute injury because of its physiological effects on injured tissue. Decreased circulation, decreased metabolism, and decreased inflammatory effects reduce secondary trauma that can occur following injury. Inflammation is also reduced because of the effects of cold on blood flow, including vasoconstriction (slowing the hemorrhaging in the area) and decreased histamine release. Cryotherapy can be therapeutic for inflamed tendons, as in medial or lateral epicondylitis, and painful conditions, such as bicipital tendonitis, or after exercise sessions to minimize soreness and muscle guarding. Other conditions applicable for cryotherapy include acute/subacute inflammation, acute and chronic pain, acute swelling, trigger points, strains, contusions, arthritis flare-ups, and muscle spasticity.[11]

The application of an ice pack, or cold pack, is the most commonly used cryotherapy. If cold is indicated for home use, the best choice is ice cubes in a waterproof bag. Frozen foods in bags, such as peas, are also commonly used as ice bags; however, use on wounds would not be advisable because of the risk of contamination. Box 18-4 includes the steps for cold pack application.

OT Practitioner's Viewpoint

While working with a client who has a nonfunctional and painful hand and had several failed therapy treatments before her admission to the assisted living facility, I had to think carefully about how to approach the treatment session and what to use to increase her ROM and functional usage. Before her fall during an episode of vertigo, she was living alone and was very active. She had enjoyed gardening and performed all of her household chores independently. Her current goal was to go back to her home. I started by conducting a session, where the pros and cons of therapy were discussed, as well as her goals and what we needed to do to accomplish them. Therapy began with tasks that previously were negative experiences with therapy. The current therapy started with a "spa-like session," where she lay on her bed with the call bell within reach; the affected hand was placed in paraffin and a Coban™ wrap was applied, bringing the digits into flexion. We did progressive stretch after the completion of the paraffin treatment, and then followed that with functional tasks that incorporated both hands, such as folding her laundry. During each subsequent session, we ramped up the tasks to more physically demanding tasks. The client was given choices and educated about how the choices were all relevant to her goal of going home. She had concerns about falling again and being on the floor and unable to get assistance. We addressed that by practicing being on the floor after a simulated fall and what she needed to do to be safe and to get help. As she neared to completion of all of her goals, a home visit was performed, and additional instructions were given to ensure safety. This client progressed to having a functional hand and was able to return home to live by herself. ~ Elizabeth A. Fain, EdD, OTR/L

BOX 18-4
Cold Pack Application

1. Wrap the cold pack in a towel, pillowcase, or cheesecloth.
2. Remove clothing from affected area. Assess skin integrity, and document any noted areas.
3. Inform the client of the steps, where the cold pack will be placed, and the four steps of sensory changes (cold, burn, ache, numb).
4. Position the client for comfort, and set the timer for the treatment time of 15 to 20 minutes.
5. At the 2-minute and 5-minute intervals, monitor the client's skin by visual inspection, and ask the client about which sensory stage he or she is experiencing. If there are welts or blanching of skin within the first 4 minutes of treatment, then stop the cryotherapy.
6. After the cryotherapy treatment, remove the cold pack, dry the treatment area with a towel, remove draping and assist the client with clothing, if needed, and proceed with the therapeutic intervention.[11]
7. Document the treatment and response.

An ice massage produces the same benefits and sensory changes as those of a cold pack (Fig. 18-4). The procedure for its application is similar to that for cold pack application, except for the use of a cup of ice, cryocup (a mold to more easily make ice cup) device, or cryostim (metal tube with gel to freeze inside) instead of a cold pack. Ice massage is typically used for small areas. The OT practitioner obtains the cup of ice, cryocup device, or cryostim and use a towel to wipe any melted ice dripping off the treated area. The OT practitioner then places the cup of ice directly on the affected area and uses it to massage the affected area, instead of leaving it in place on the affected area. A roller ice cold and hot trigger point therapy tool may also be used for ice massage; it contains a stainless steel roller ball that retains temperature for application (Fig. 18-5).

Precautions: Cryotherapy should be used with caution in clients with the following conditions: some rheumatoid conditions (increases pain and joint stiffness), paroxysmal cold hemoglobinuria with renal dysfunction and secondary hypertension, very young/very old clients, history of frostbite in the area, and coma.

Contraindications: Cryotherapy is contraindicated in clients with cold-sensitive conditions, such as cold intolerance or allergy to cold (cold urticaria, which may produce hives and joint pain and swelling), Raynaud's phenomenon (causes arterial spasm leading to possible ischemic necrosis), impaired circulation, peripheral vascular disease, open wounds, and local infection.[10,11]

Safety Considerations: When using cryotherapy as a preparatory modality, caution must be used in follow-up activities because analgesia, or numbness, could impact sensation or fine motor skills and require increased efforts for performing the activity. The OT practitioner must monitor the client closely to prevent further trauma.[11] It is important to adhere to the safety standards set by the FDA.

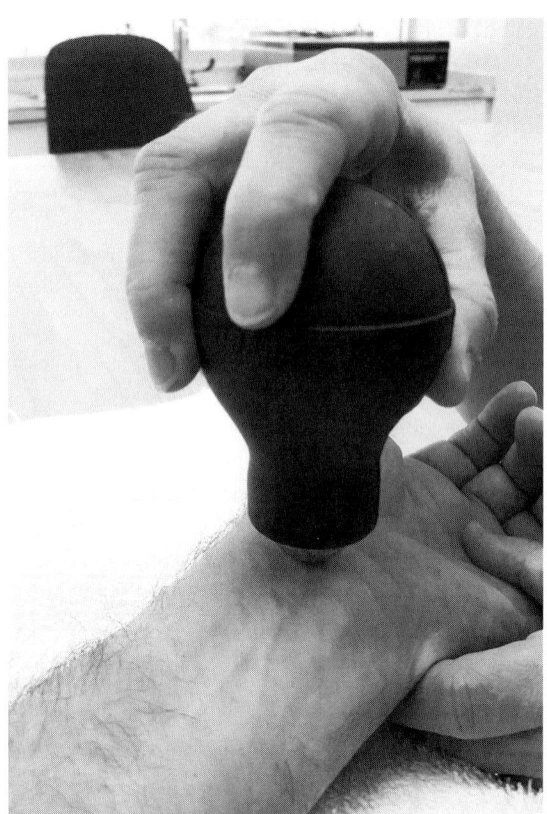

FIGURE 18-5. Roller Ice Cold and Hot Trigger Point Therapy tool that is ergonomically made to hold on to for ease of usage during massage. The roller ball is solid stainless steel that retains the temperature for application.

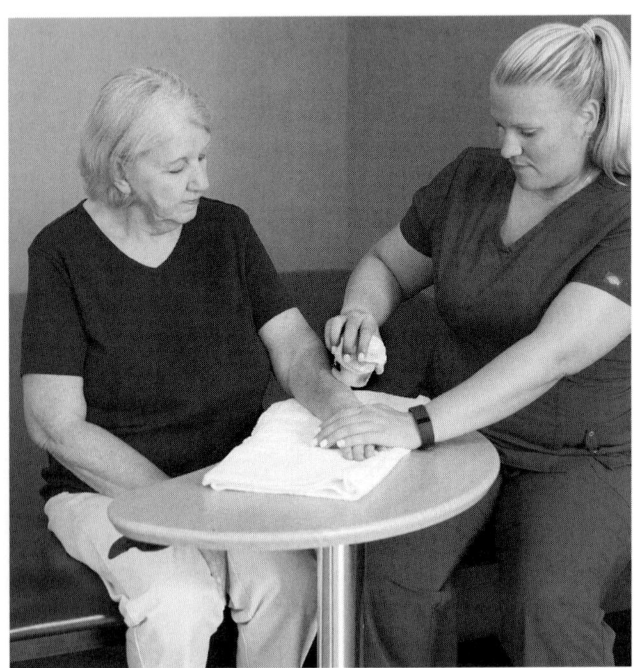

FIGURE 18-4. Ice massage.

Ice Bath: Ice bath or slush consists of a water-and-ice mixture in the temperature range of 50° F to 60° F in a plastic tub, bucket, or sink. It is essential to instruct clients about what to anticipate with regard to sensory changes from cold, aching, pain, and then numbness because this can be very uncomfortable, especially during the first 3 minutes, continuing until 5 minutes of immersion. Total treatment duration is 10 to 15 minutes. This discomfort may impact client compliance; however, this technique is especially helpful for increasing the client's tolerance for potentially painful treatment, such as PROM for loss of ROM or stiffness. If needed, ice baths can start with a higher temperature and progress to cooler temperatures, or the client's fingers can be covered with neoprene finger tips. Generally, the client's tolerance increases with repeated subsequent ice immersion treatments.

Application: Box 18-5 shows the steps for using an ice bath.

COMMUNICATION

Communication in all its forms is important to the OTA, and communication with regard to PAMs is no exception. First, the OTA must communicate with the physician and the occupational therapist for parameters and precautions for the specific client. The OTA must speak up if he or she does not feel comfortable with or competent for independently performing the tasks for PAMs; it is better to take the risk of irritating a coworker or supervisor than to harm a client because of lack of knowledge or training. It is the ethical responsibility of the OTA to not perform tasks that might cause harm to the client. The OTA must also communicate with the client, to educate him or her fully about the chosen PAMs, how the PAMs are preparatory means to the therapeutic task, and why a particular PAM was chosen over another. This can be especially true when cryotherapy, which can be uncomfortable, is chosen over heat therapy, which can be soothing. Other communication needs are met through documentation showing that the modality was administered in a skilled manner, even though it was a preparatory step in therapy.

BOX 18-5
Ice Bath Application

1. After confirming the client's status for possible contraindications, prepare a bucket, tub, or sink with ice-and-water mixture.
2. Assess skin integrity, and document any noted areas.
3. Inform the client of the steps and about the four steps of sensory changes (cold, burn, ache, numb).
4. Position the client for comfort, and place the involved extremity in the ice bath, set the timer for the treatment time of 10 to 15 minutes. Note that lower tolerance may require shorter treatment times or warmer temperatures than 50° F–60° F.
5. Monitor the client's skin by visual inspection, and inquire about the sensory stage during the treatment time at the 2-minute and 5-minute intervals. If there are welts or blanching of skin within the first 4 minutes of treatment, then stop the ice bath.
6. After the ice bath, dry the treatment area with a towel, remove draping and assist the client with clothing, if needed, and proceed with the occupational performance therapeutic intervention.[11] Note that the client's skin will be anesthetized, which may impact fine motor manipulation.
7. Document the treatment and response.

Precautions: Ice immersion is very uncomfortable and may be difficult for the client to tolerate. Skin will be anesthetized after treatment. Immersion should be maintained as withdrawal and repeated immersion prolong the painful stage. The dependent positioning increases the risk of swelling.

Contraindications: Contraindications for ice immersion include the following: cardiac or respiratory system involvement, uncovered open wounds, circulatory insufficiency, and cold allergies or sensitivities, such as Raynaud's phenomenon.

Safety Considerations: It is important to be mindful of the contraindications because the cold temperature and the sensory changes progressing to a painful stage may shock an already compromised system.

Contrast Bath: Contrast baths consist of alternating immersion of a body part into one container with heated water (105° F to 110° F) and then another container with cold water (50° F to 60° F). The primary treatment effect is to alternate between vasoconstriction and vasodilation of cutaneous vessels. The treatment duration is 20 to 30 minutes, and the alternating immersion is repeated, as needed. The duration of hot immersions is typically 3 to 4 minutes, whereas that of cold immersions is 1 to 2 minutes.

Application: Contrast baths are effective for treating subacute or chronic inflammatory conditions (a complex biological response resulting in cells being sent to the site of injury to assist in the healing process, but if they remain longer than necessary, as in chronic inflammation, will eventually cause necrosis), edema (increase of fluid between the skin and other body structures, with various causes), pain reduction, and increasing joint ROM. This treatment can be performed at home by utilizing the kitchen sink. Box 18-6 includes the procedural techniques for the application of a contrast bath.

Precautions: Contrast baths may increase edema because of the gravity-dependent position, but can also decrease

BOX 18-6
Contrast Bath Application

1. After ensuring that the client has no contraindications for contrast baths, proceed with the steps below.
2. Fill two side-by-side tubs or sinks with water. One side should contain warm water (105° F to 110° F) and the other side cold water (50° F to 60° F).
3. Have a timer available to time the immersions.
4. Immerse the client's affected hand in the warm water side first for 3 to 4 minutes.
5. Immerse the same hand in the cold water side for 1 to 2 minutes. Alternate between the two tubs, according to the protocol being utilized, for a total treatment time of 20 to 30 minutes duration.
6. End with the warm immersion if relaxation and vasodilation are desired or with cold immersion if vasoconstriction is desired.
7. Document the treatment and response.

edema via increased circulation as a result of increased blood flow. For edema management, a combination of muscle movement during the baths, and elevation and performance of light retrograde massage after the contrast baths may assist. The OT practitioner should always consider the cause of the inflammation or edema to determine the appropriate use of contrast baths.

Contraindications: Contraindications for contrast baths include acute injuries, hypersensitivity to cold, and those related to cold and heat applications.

Safety Considerations: The OT practitioner should monitor for possible water spillage and ensure that the floor is dry and safe. A towel should be kept at hand for drying, a thermometer to accurately measure the water temperature, and a timer to monitor the duration of immersion treatments.

DEEP THERMAL MODALITIES

Superficial thermal modalities penetrate to the depth of less than 2 cm. However, deep thermal modalities penetrate to a depth of 2 to 5 cm (0.8 to 2 inches). A decision regarding application of superficial or deep thermal modalities is driven by the depth of the target tissue, in addition to other considerations will be discussed.

Ultrasound: Ultrasound has two distinct primary purposes. In medicine, ultrasound is used for diagnosing conditions and imaging structures; in rehabilitation, it is used for producing thermal and nonthermal effects on tissue and deeper structures.[14] Ultrasound that is used in rehabilitation is often termed *therapeutic ultrasound* to clarify its purpose. It has a deeper heat than superficial modalities, such as hot packs, and can be used to heat deeper structures and tissues to promote soft tissue healing.

Although ultrasound can be programmed to provide a superficial effect, it is primarily utilized to give a deeper thermal effect to a depth of up to 5 cm. Ultrasound requires the use of a handheld **sound head** or **applicator,** which is the tool that delivers the ultrasonic energy or sound waves. This tool houses the sound head, transducer, and applicable electronics to aid in the functional delivery of the sound waves. Figure 18-6 shows the use of ultrasound and multiple sound heads.

The piezoelectric effect (the ability to create electric charge in response to mechanical stress) is created when the electrical current passes through the piezoelectric crystal in the sound head of the transducer. The crystal in the sound head oscillates, or moves back and forth, expands, and shortens, thereby creating sound waves that are transmitted through the coupling agent (gel or water) to the tissue. The movement of the sound wave and molecules continues until it is absorbed by the body tissues.

Different tissues and body structures transmit or absorb the ultrasound differently. Body fluid has the lowest resistance and lowest absorption values for the ultrasound waves. Bone has the highest resistance and the highest acoustic absorption for the ultrasound waves.

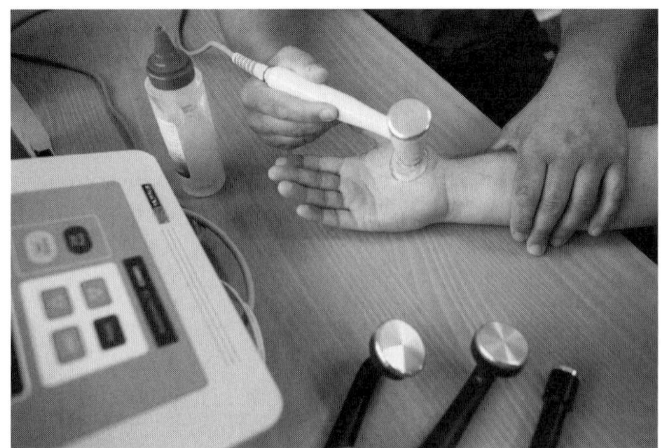

FIGURE 18-6. The OTA is administering ultrasound to the client's thenar eminence. Note the different size ultrasound heads, from small to large, based on the size of the treatment area, pictured at the bottom. The ultrasound sound head or applicator houses crystals and transmits the sound waves for the therapeutic treatment.

Consequently, bone will stop the flow of the ultrasound energy and absorb the energy from the ultrasound wave, resulting in physiological changes. Higher energy levels will heat the tissue and can potentially cause a hot spot, which can be painful and damage the tissue. During ultrasound application, moving the sound head in small, continuous circular motions or back and forth motions will prevent potential damage to tissue. **Beam nonuniformity ratio (BNR)** indicates the variability of the intensity delivered through the ultrasound. BNR is an indicator of the ratio of the highest intensity of the beam to the average intensity of the beam delivery. Optimal BNR should fall between 2 and 5. This indicates that the delivery of intensity is more uniform and less likely to cause hot spots or overheating in one concentrated area. The BNR is expressed as 4:1, which means that the average output intensity is 1 watt per centimeter squared (W/cm^2), and the highest intensity is 4 watts. The lower the BNR, the more uniform the output. The FDA requires that the BNR be indicated on all ultrasound devices.[16] **Ultrasound power** represents the intensity measure by which the ultrasound is delivered to the client. This is represented by watts (W) in clinical documentation. The ultrasound power must be documented in the treatment note to ensure consistency in treatments and to monitor its impact on the client. **Ultrasound intensity** represents the ultrasonic power that is delivered to the client. It is also expressed as watts (W), or for the sound head's effective radiating area (ERA), it is expressed as watts per centimeter squared (W/cm^2).

Application: Application of ultrasound is commonly done via direct contact between skin and a coupling medium, such as ultrasound gel, or through immersion in water. The gel facilitates the transmission to the target tissue. Gel warmers are used to improve the client's comfort level as gel may feel cool at room temperature, but do not impact

EVIDENCE-BASED PRACTICE

A review of the Cochrane Systematic Reviews and Reports found on search engines for application of various PAMs yielded limited evidence-based research and mixed results with regard to the outcomes of different PAMs. Carpal tunnel syndrome is a common entrapment neuropathy that is treated by OT practitioners, and the literature suggests that there has not been much conclusive evidence-based research supporting effective treatments for carpal tunnel syndrome. Ultrasound and paraffin are two PAMs that are frequently used in therapy for carpal tunnel syndrome and were investigated to determine the effectiveness of combining a wrist orthosis with either ultrasound or paraffin treatments. A randomized controlled trial consisting of 47 participants who were randomized into two groups investigated the effectiveness of ultrasound versus paraffin.[18] One group received paraffin therapy weekly, whereas the other group received ultrasound. All participants received a wrist orthosis and completed a questionnaire, physical examination, and received a nerve conduction study of the upper extremities before and after each treatment session. The results yielded statistically significant improvement scores in both groups with regard to their symptom severity. It was also noted that there were statistically significant improvements in the functional status scores and pain scores of the ultrasound therapy group, with a moderate effect noted. This study reported that the combination of ultrasound therapy with a wrist orthosis may be more effective than paraffin therapy with a wrist orthosis. Since this was an exploratory study, further research is suggested to further investigate and explore the efficacy of these two treatments for carpal tunnel syndrome. It is important for the OT practitioner to contribute to the body of research in whatever way possible and to seek out the newest research and use evidence to guide treatment.

Chang, Y.W., Hsieh, S.F., Horng, Y.S., Chen, H.L., Lee, K.C., & Horng, Y.S. (2014). Comparative effectiveness of ultrasound and paraffin therapy in patients with carpal tunnel syndrome: A randomized trial. BMC Musculoskeletal Disorders. *15, 399. doi:10.1186/1471-2474-15-399*

the delivery of the ultrasound. During administration of the ultrasound, it is important to note the essential techniques. Ultrasound gel is applied on skin if the direct method of delivery is used. For the immersion technique, the sound head does not touch the skin, but rather is held about an inch away from the area to be treated, and the water conducts the power. The ultrasound parameters are based on the target tissue. For nonthermal or subthermal levels of ultrasound for tissue healing, a frequency of 3 megahertz (MHz) is used for superficial targets that are less than 2 cm and 1 MHz for deeper targeted tissue.[12]

The **effective radiating area (ERA)** is the circular area on the sound head from which ultrasound energy radiates. This area is smaller in diameter than the actual soundhead. **Pulse frequency** refers to the number of pulses or periods that the ultrasound is delivering; it is expressed in milliseconds. The percentage of time that the ultrasound is on is expressed as **duty cycle**. Duty cycle is the period that ultrasound is being delivered during the treatment time. The duty cycle option consists of continuous or 100% delivery, where as pulsed delivery (20%, 50% or 80%) consists of intermittent or pulsed sound waves for an on-and-off repetitious cycle. Lower percentages indicate lower time of average intensity. The duty cycle is calculated by the following equation:

$$\text{Duty Cycle} = \frac{\text{Pulse duration (on-time)} \times 100}{\text{Pulse period (on-time + off-time)}}$$

This parameter is adjusted to achieve different types of thermal effects. The settings are adjusted to 100% to achieve thermal effects, whereas other pulsed setting produce lower levels of thermal heating effects on tissues.

Intensity is another parameter to consider in the use of ultrasound. An ultrasound setting of 0.5 watts/cm^2 with a 20% duty cycle is a good starting point to promote tissue healing. Using a low duty cycle gives the tissue time to cool down between pulses and still provides an intensity high enough to produce mechanical effects to stimulate cellular activity. If desired results are not achieved, then the setting can be increased to 1.0 watts/cm^2 with a 20% duty cycle if the client with intact sensation does not report feeling heat. During the ultrasound treatment, the sound head needs to be constantly moved to prevent hot spots. The movement of the sound head can be longitudinal or circular. The area to be treated should not be any larger than two to three times the size of the ERA of the sound head. The smallest sound head that covers the target tissue should be used to only treat the targeted tissue.[17] The unit **megahertz (MHz)** expresses one million vibrations per second for the ultrasound wave frequency. One unit of measurement is hertz (Hz) for one cycle per second and is documented in the clinical note for frequency of the ultrasound treatment.[12] Figure 18-7 provides a pictorial view of the depth of sound waves for 3.0 MHz versus 1.0 MHz and will aid in understanding the difference between the two measurements.

Clinical reasoning for decision making with regard to ultrasound application requires reflection on the target tissue, effects of heat on tissues, and the mechanical effects for nonthermal effects.

Heat facilitates the following categories: pain threshold, nerve conduction velocity, blood flow, enzyme activity, and soft tissue extensibility while decreasing muscle spasms. Nonthermal effects of ultrasound facilitate increasing the following categories: cell membrane and vascular permeability,

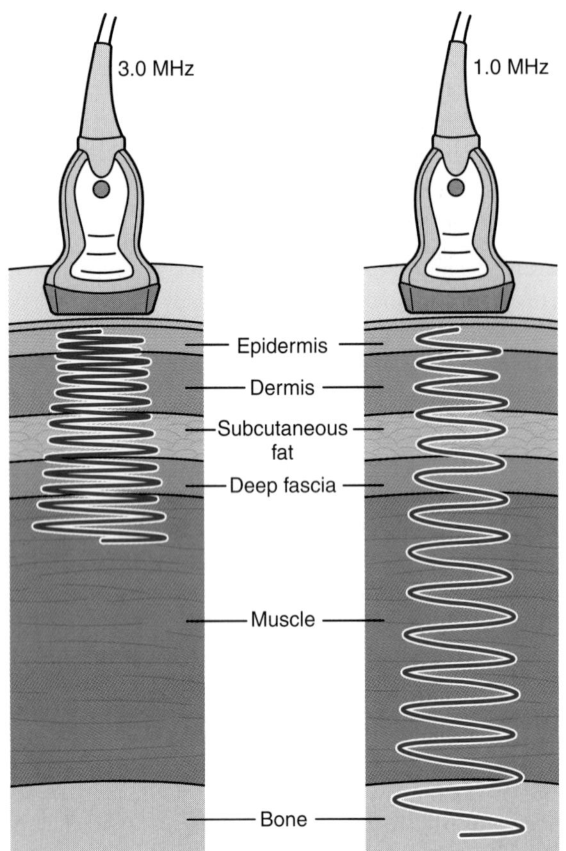

FIGURE 18-7. Depth of ultrasound waves for 3.0 MHz versus 1.0 MHz.

histamine release, inflammatory response, macrophage activity, fibroblast activity or protein synthesis, and wound contraction.[17] The OTA should closely collaborate with the occupational therapist to determine the proper settings for each client, and will demonstrate competence before initial use. Box 18-7 shows the procedure for ultrasound application.

Precautions: The rule of thumb is to limit ultrasound delivery to 14 total treatments because more than 14 treatments can decrease both red and white blood cell counts.[17] Caution should be exercised when treating clients with decreased sensation or decreased circulation.

Contraindications: Ultrasound should not be applied to the eyes or genitals, directly over a bony prominence, near the heart or a pacemaker or its components, and to the epiphyseal growth plate, ischemic tissues, or insensate areas. It is contraindicated for treatments to the abdomen or back during pregnancy, in the presence of thrombus or thrombophlebitis, and in conditions when a tissue temperature rise is contraindicated.[17]

Safety Considerations: OT practitioners should have regular inspections and calibrations of the ultrasound machine and sound heads performed, per the manufacturer's directions. Because the ultrasound treatment produces little, if any, sensation, inspections are essential to ensure that the equipment is working properly. The sound head should be handled with great care because the crystals can be damaged if dropped or hit, and cease to work. Adherence to proper procedural processes is essential to prevent hot spots. The OT practitioner should ensure that safety standards set by the FDA are followed.

Phonophoresis: **Phonophoresis** is the use of ultrasound to enhance the delivery of topically applied drugs. The ultrasound waves deliver drugs through skin for the systemic and/or tissue effects. Medications used in phonophoresis are prepared by the pharmacist per the physician's orders.[12]

Application: In addition to the considerations for the use of ultrasound, the OT practitioner needs to ask the client about possible medication allergies before administering phonophoresis. The acoustical capability of the drug

BOX 18-7
Ultrasound Application

1. After a thorough review of the client's status and indications for ultrasound with the supervising occupational therapist to ensure adherence to precautions and contraindications, proceed with the ultrasound.
2. Position the client for comfort and ease of treating the affected body part.
3. Apply ultrasound gel to the treatment area.
4. Use the sound head with desired ERA half the size of the treatment area.
5. Select the treatment parameters based on the intended treatment outcomes (thermal or nonthermal). Refer to the manufacturer's guidelines and clinical setting protocols for the settings for frequency, intensity, duty cycle, and duration.
6. Clean the sound head with antimicrobial agent that is approved for use at your setting before use.
7. Place the sound head on the treatment area.
8. Turn on the ultrasound machine, and set the treatment settings.
9. Move the sound head continuously over the treatment area. This is to prevent developing "hot spots" in the treatment area. Keep the sound head flat and in full contact with the gel at all times.
10. Upon completion of the treatment, remove the gel from the treatment area.
11. Proceed with functional tasks as part of the treatment and established goals.
12. Reassess the client for changes in status, and document the intervention.
13. Document the treatment and response.

should be checked by applying it with water to the surface of the soundhead transducer, with cellophane taped around the edges of the sound head. If the water moves when the intensity of the sound head is increased, then the medication is acoustically conductive and can be used for the treatment. The most commonly used phonophoresis medications for orthopedic injuries are anti-inflammatories, such as cortisol, salicylates, and dexamethasone. Lidocaine, an analgesic for pain, is also commonly used.[17] As with any prescription medication, a physician's order to use the medication in OT treatment must be received and documented. The procedure for the application of phonophoresis is comparable with that for ultrasound, with the addition of steps and considerations specific to medications. Box 18-8 reviews the steps for the application of phonophoresis.

Precautions: Utilize the same precautions as noted for ultrasound with additional consideration for possible drug allergies because administration of medications is being applied through the ultrasound treatment.

OT practitioners should also speak with the referring physician and/or pharmacist to inquire about a client's allergies, potential medical reactions with clients' medications, and overall condition before administering phonophoresis.

Contraindications: For phonophoresis, the same contraindications as noted for ultrasound are utilized in addition to specifics related to the client's condition, medications, and allergies, which may potentially interact with the medication administered in the phonophoresis.

Safety Considerations: Safety considerations for administering phonophoresis are similar to that of ultrasound application. Refer to the section on ultrasound for safety considerations. The OT practitioner should adhere to the safety standards set by the FDA.

Electrotherapy

Most people have experienced the jolt or shock of electricity whether from touching an electric fence on a farm or from working on a socket. This type of electricity is described as current electricity, in which a stream of loose electrons passes along a conductor. When receiving a shock, the person's hand serves as a conductor when it touches the electricity source. *Current* is the term used to describe how the electrons move along the conductor. The electrical current produces magnetic, chemical, and thermal effects in the tissue.[10] The current flows through the pathway of least resistance and from an area of high concentration to a lower concentration of electrons.[11] **Direct current (DC)** is a continuous flow of unidirectional electrons between the anode (positive) electrode and the cathode (negative) electrode. This type of current accumulates a charge as a result of the unidirectional flow of uninterrupted current. Therapeutically, DC is primarily used for iontophoresis, which delivers medication similar to phonophoresis, using current instead of sound waves. DC is also used to stimulate denervated muscles, and with settings for pause or rest to facilitate muscle movement. This type of electrical stimulation is called electrical muscle stimulation.[11]

Electricity for therapeutic purposes can be set for different settings, flows, pulsed current, waveforms, and amplitudes. The different settings affect both the client's comfort level, as well as the involved tissue or muscle.Table 18-2 presents the properties of electrical stimulation versus ultrasound and will assist the OTA in decision making based on client needs and goals.

NEUROMUSCULAR REEDUCATION

Neuromuscular electrical stimulation (NMES) is the electrical stimulation of muscles. The muscles are innervated with the goal of improving muscle strengthening and

BOX 18-8
Phonophoresis Application

1. Careful, deliberate consultation is required for the medications used with phonophoresis to ensure that there are no allergies or drug interactions and that the medications are mixed appropriately to facilitate drug penetration.
2. After a thorough review of the client's status and indications for ultrasound with the supervising occupational therapist to ensure that precautions and contraindications are adhered to, proceed with the ultrasound.
3. Apply the premixed medication first over the treatment area, and then apply the ultrasound gel liberally over the medication as the second layer.
4. Use the sound head with desired ERA half the size of the treatment area.
5. Select the treatment parameters based on the intended treatment outcomes (thermal or nonthermal). Refer to the manufacturer's guidelines and clinic protocols for the settings for frequency, intensity, duty cycle, and duration.
6. Clean the sound head with antimicrobial agent that is approved for use at your setting before use.
7. Place the sound head on the treatment area.
8. Turn on the ultrasound machine, and set the treatment settings.
9. Move the sound head over the treatment area. This is to prevent developing "hot spots" in the treatment area.
10. Upon completion of the treatment, remove the gel from the treatment area.
11. Proceed with functional tasks as part of the treatment and established goals.
12. Reassess the client for changes in status, and document the intervention.

TABLE 18-2 Benefits of Electrical Stimulation Versus Ultrasound

INDICATIONS/BENEFITS OF ELECTRICAL STIMULATION	INDICATIONS/BENEFITS OF ULTRASOUND
Pain modulation	Thermal effects, particularly in deeper tissues
Muscle contraction	Nonthermal effects
Biofeedback for muscle reeducation	To enhance healing at cellular level
Muscle pumping contractions to decrease edema	
Retardation of atrophy	
Muscle strengthening	
Increasing range of motion	
Facilitation of soft tissue and bone healing	
Creation of ion movement for a chemical effect in the tissues (iontophoresis)	

functional usage of the involved muscle group. NMES is also used with muscle reeducation for muscles with spasticity to enhance ROM and prevent muscle atrophy.[12] The term **charge** is used to describe the volume of electrical energy delivered in each phase. It is charge that influences the strength of the excitatory response.[12] **Pulsed current,** or pulsatile current, consists of current with modulations, meaning the current is turned on and off for brief intervals in short periods. NMES is an example of pulsed **alternating current (AC)** that OT practitioners commonly use.[14] **Pulse duration** is the amount of time that the electrical current stimulus has to be on a body part to generate a motor response; it is measured in microseconds (ms). The most comfortable settings for generating motor responses are between 20 to 200 ms.[12] The **ramp time** consists of the amount of change in pulse intensity or duration from start time to peak intensity. Ramp time is relevant clinically for the purposes of adjusting the electrical stimulation for the client's comfort level and for producing normal muscle contractions instead of tetany (abnormal, involuntary contractions of the muscle).[11] **Waveform** is a visual illustration of the pulse waveform, much like the wave patterns on an electrocardiogram (ECG) for the heart. Waveforms represent the number of phases in a period, the positive or negative charge being delivered, and the duration of the charge being delivered. The waveforms impact the client comfort, muscle fatigue, and the chemical or polarity effects in the tissue.[12]

Application: The application of NMES consists of placing the first electrode on the bulkiest or biggest part of the targeted muscle belly and placing the second electrode distal to the first electrode on the muscle. The OT practitioner may locate the biggest part of the muscle belly through palpation. Palpating the muscle will elicit muscle contraction on the contralateral side with resistance to the desired motion. Correct placement is essential for an effective muscle response. Practice sessions before application on the client would also facilitate success.[12] **Functional electrical stimulation (FES)** is similar to NMES but the distinction is that it is utilized during a functional task (Fig. 18-8). The FES stimulation period is coordinated with performing a functional task, such as stimulating the wrist extensors during an object release, and the off period is when the client is grasping the object. The size of the electrodes impacts the effectiveness and comfort of the electrical stimulation. Smaller electrodes will have higher current density and depth of penetration. In addition, the size of the electrode that best matches the targeted muscle belly should be selected because a larger electrode will stimulate nearby muscles as well, with perhaps an undesired effect. The manufacturer's directions should always be followed.

The types of electrodes vary, but most have gel on the back to help the electrode stay in place on the client's skin. When the electrode is no longer tacky enough to maintain contact with skin, dampen the gel side to increase adherence. Box 18-9 presents the steps for applying electrical stimulation.

Precautions: Precautions for the use of electrical stimulation include hypersensitivity to the electrical stimulation, heart arrhythmias caused by conduction disturbances, congestive heart failure, seizure disorders, sensory loss, vascular diseases, allergies to the gel, tape or electrodes, tissue susceptible to hemorrhage, hematoma, impaired cognition, and immature pediatric nervous systems.[12]

Contraindications: Contraindications for electrical stimulation include placement near demand-type pacemakers, arterial disease, uncontrolled hemorrhage, sites of infection, blood clots, the abdominal or pelvic regions in pregnant

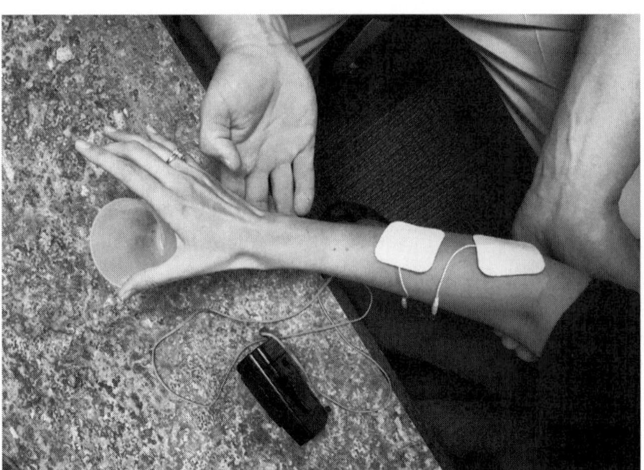

FIGURE 18-8. Functional electrical stimulation.

BOX 18-9
Electrical Stimulation Application

1. Before electrode application, the client's skin needs to be clean and dry. The electrodes will not stick in areas with dense hair; use scissors instead of a razor if possible to carefully trim the hair because shaving with a razor can cause skin irritation, which will prevent optimal use of the modality. Lotion on the skin can also impede the electrodes from adhering to the client's skin and will need to be removed before electrode application.
2. Label the electrodes for specific client application because they can be reused for that client.
3. Place the electrodes at least one width of the size equal to the width of the electrodes apart, and ensure that the electrode is maintaining contact with the client's skin.
4. Hook up the unit to the electrodes. Follow the manufacturer's directions, as units differ.
5. After explaining the modality and what to expect to the client, turn on the electrical stimulation unit. Ask the client to report when he or she first feels the sensation of the electrical stimulation.
6. Instruct the client that you will increase the intensity up to the maximum level of electrical stimulation that they are comfortable with.
7. Give the client the button that enables them to turn off the unit, if needed.
8. Monitor the client frequently to ensure comfort and safety and that the desired effect is occurring.
9. Proceed with functional tasks as part of the treatment and established goals.
10. Document the treatment and response.
11. At the end of the modality use, replace the electrodes on the same original plastic piece and store in an airtight bag with the client's name on it for client-specific application.

women, cancerous lesions, metal implants, a client with history of seizures, the neck and head region, sensory or mental impairment, and unstable fractures.[13]

Safety Considerations: Safety considerations include routine inspection of electrical stimulation units and adherence to protocols for the work setting. Ensure the client has a control or client button available to turn the unit off if problems occur. The OT practitioner should be familiar with the type of unit in use as the setup for the electrode that is the active stimulator may vary for different units. Additionally, some parameters may be preset for different electrotherapy devices, and the only adjustment needed may be the **amplitude,** defined as the maximum amount of current delivered in one pulse. Amplitude determines the intensity of the stimulus and whether the muscle tissue is depolarized. The OT practitioner should refer to the operating manual for his or her electrotherapy unit to be familiar with the specifics related to the operational setup. The practitioner should adhere to the safety standards set by the FDA.

IONTOPHORESIS

Iontophoresis is the delivery of transdermal drugs or chemicals into the tissue via low amplitude DC current. Iontophoresis is similar to phonophoresis, which uses sound waves instead of current to deliver medications.[10] Iontophoresis delivers the medication or chemical based on the principle that similar charges repel each other, resulting in the current pushing the drug into the tissue. This is analogous to putting together two magnets that have the same charge; the magnets will repel each other. In iontophoresis, the transdermal drug delivery occurs by increasing the permeability of skin. A positive attribute for clients regarding iontophoresis is that it is similar to receiving an injection, but without the needle, and is considered a noninvasive method to deliver a medication or chemical.

Application: The iontophoresis unit looks much like an electrical stimulation unit, utilizing an active or medicated electrode into which the medication is inserted. Battery-powered electrodes are also available and are becoming more widely used. They use power from the battery that is attached to the electrode itself instead of from the alternating electrical current that is delivered from electrical stimulation units. The advantage of the battery-powered electrodes is that the client can wear the medicated electrode and receive the benefits while engaged in an activity instead of being restricted by the electrical unit. This enables the client to continue this treatment at home. Iontophoresis is applied with a medicated electrode with continuous DC current. Common medications used for iontophoresis are acetic acid for calcium deposits, dexamethasone phosphate or salicylate for inflammation, and saline for scars.[10] An important consideration is that when a prescription medication is used in iontophoresis, a specific physician's order must be obtained to administer the medication during iontophoresis. Box 18-10 presents the steps used in traditional iontophoresis application, and Box 18-11 presents steps used in integrated electrode iontophoresis patches.

The use of traditional iontophoresis units has been declining following the invention of the battery-powered integrated electrode version. Clients report increased tolerance of the new, slower delivery of the medication or solution. Furthermore, treatment time can vary greatly with the older version, depending on the sensitivity of the client, and only the setup and disconnect time of iontophoresis is billable for OT treatment.

Precautions: Clients should be asked about medication sensitivities or allergies before considering iontophoresis. OT practitioners should also speak with the referring physician and/or pharmacist to inquire about allergies, medical reactions with clients' medications, and condition before

BOX 18-10
Traditional Iontophoresis Application

1. Clean and completely dry the area to which the electrode patches will be applied.
2. Apply the medication/solution to the appropriate patch (refer to the manufacturer's directions).
3. Adhere the medicated patch to the client's skin, taking care to only apply pressure to the outside edge of the patch, and not the center, which contains the medication or chemical. An improper seal can cause blistering of skin or ineffective transmission.
4. Apply the ground patch to the client's skin, at least 4 inches away from the medicated patch, which acts as the return current.
5. Attach the cords of the unit to the appropriate patch. For example, for medications with a negative charge, such as dexamethasone, the OT practitioner must attach the negative (black) connector so that the charges repel and the medication is pushed through the skin barrier. Follow the directions for each medication or solution.
6. Instruct the client on the electric sensation that will be felt and to notify practitioner of any burning or discomfort is felt. Set the machine according to the manufacturer's instructions and for the client's comfort.
7. If the patch crosses or is very close to a joint, such as the volar wrist when treating carpal tunnel syndrome, instruct the client to not bend that joint during the iontophoresis treatment.
8. At the end of the treatment, turn off the machine, and remove both patches. Do not pull on the cords to remove them, as that may damage the cords.
9. Observe and document the client's skin condition (extreme redness or blisters). Continue with OT treatment session.
10. Document the treatment and response.

BOX 18-11
Integrated Electrode Iontophoresis Patch Application

1. Clean and completely dry the skin area to which the electrode patch will be applied.
2. Apply the medication/solution to the appropriate side of the electrode patch (refer to the manufacturer's directions). Some patches require the use of saline in the nonmedication side. Before applying any medicine or solution, carefully view the electrode patch to determine the correct side for medication and the one for saline, if applicable.
3. Adhere the medicated portion of the electrode patch to the client's skin, taking care to only apply pressure to the outside edge of the patch, and not the center, which contains the medication or chemical. An improper seal can cause blistering of skin or ineffective transmission.
4. Depending on the manufacturer, a battery booster may be applied to one side of the patch, left there for the specified amount of time, and then removed. Alternatively, some integrated patches include a self-contained battery. Either type provides enough charge to push the medication slowly through the patch, which is typically worn for 4 hours.
5. The client may continue with other therapeutic activities if iontophoresis is used at the beginning of the session, or it may be used at the end, with the client continuing to wear the electrode patch beyond the therapy session. Be sure to provide instructions to the client about when to remove the patch, how to visually inspect skin, and to contact the OT practitioner if there are any concerns.
6. Document the treatment and response.

administering iontophoresis. DC is used to deliver the medicine and can be more uncomfortable than other types of electrical current; therefore, the client's tolerance for the sensation that DC provides should be assessed. The client should be alerted that the skin underneath the active or medicated electrode may become red. It is also advisable to apply a neutral pH lotion to the treated area afterward. Furthermore, when using dexamethasone, clients with diabetes should monitor their blood sugar before and after treatment and report any adverse effects.[9]

Contraindications: Contraindications for iontophoresis include sensitivities or allergies to the medication or ions being delivered. The medicated electrode should not be applied over skin irritations, bruises, or lacerations. Iontophoresis should not be used with clients who have impaired or absent sensation.[11] The same contraindications for electrical stimulation, which include the placement near demand-type pacemakers, arterial disease, uncontrolled hemorrhage, and sites of infection, blood clots, the abdominal or pelvic regions of pregnant women, cancerous lesions, metal implants, history of seizures for neck and head region, sensory or mental impairment and unstable fractures, should be followed.[13] In clients with poorly controlled diabetes, iontophoresis should not be utilized with dexamethasone or other corticosteroids.

Safety Considerations: Safety considerations include the routine inspection of electrical stimulation units, adherence to protocols for work setting, and making a control or client button available to the client to turn the unit off if problems occur. The OT practitioner should be familiar with the type of unit being used because the setup for the electrode that is the active stimulator may vary for different units. Additionally, some parameters may be preset for different electrotherapy devices, and the only adjustment needed may be the amplitude. The OT practitioner should refer to the operating manual for the electrotherapy unit to be familiar with the specifics related to the operational setup. The same safety considerations as noted for other electrical stimulation should be utilized, if utilizing an electrical AC power unit plugged into the wall outlet. It is important to adhere to the safety standards set by the FDA.[10]

INTERFERENTIAL CURRENT

Interferential current (IFC) consists of two separate channels delivering different frequencies of electrical stimulation simultaneously. The channels are set up so that their paths cross, and they literally interfere with each other. The intersection of these two currents causes amplitude modulation in the tissue,[17] potentially causing deeper effects in the tissue while being more comfortable to clients. The gate control theory of pain also underscores the use of this modality. IFC is primarily used for pain relief because of the functionality of its deeper penetration compared with transcutaneous electrical nerve stimulation (TENS), which is also used for pain treatment and pain relief (described later in the chapter).

Application: IFC utilizes two channels and four electrodes to deliver the current. The four electrodes are applied in a pattern that forms an "X." The center point of the "X" is called a *vector*, and it can be static, fixed, or dynamic. The dynamic vector moves around the treatment field in a sweeping manner. It is also essential that the four electrodes are placed in a crisscrossing manner such that channel 2 forms a direct line opposing each other in a diagonal fashion, and channel 1 does the same thing on the opposite sides. Refer to Figure 18-9 for placement pattern for IFC. IFC is considered to be more applicable for large, deep areas, and TENS is utilized for smaller superficial painful areas.[17] See Box 18-12 for the steps in IFC application.

Precautions: Precautions for the use of electrical stimulation include hypersensitivity to the electrical stimulation, arrhythmias caused by conduction disturbances, congestive heart failure, seizure disorders, sensory loss, vascular diseases, allergies to the gel, tape or electrodes, tissue susceptible to hemorrhage, hematoma, impaired cognition, and immature pediatric nervous systems.

Contraindications: It is important to adhere to the same contraindications for electrical stimulation, which include the placement near demand-type pacemakers, clients with arterial disease, uncontrolled hemorrhage, and sites of infection, blood clots, and abdomen or near pelvic region in pregnant women, cancerous lesions, metal implants, someone with history of seizures for neck and head region, sensory or mental impairment, and unstable fractures.[13]

Safety Considerations: Safety considerations include the routine inspection of electrical stimulation units, adherence to protocols for work setting, and having a control or client button available to the client to turn the unit off if problems occur. The OT practitioner should be familiar with the type of unit being used as the setup for the electrode that is the active stimulator may vary for different units. Some parameters may be preset for different electrotherapy devices, and the only adjustment needed may be the amplitude. The OT practitioner should refer to the operating manual for the electrotherapy unit to be familiar with the specifics related to the operational setup. He or she should adhere to the safety standards set by the FDA.[10]

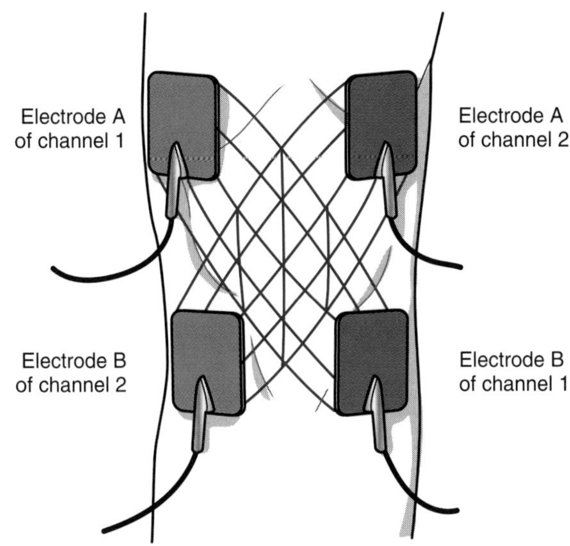

FIGURE 18-9. Note the "X" pattern for interferential current and that the same channels are on the opposite sides of the extremity.

TECHNOLOGY AND TRENDS

Technology has impacted our world in many ways, and PAMs are no exception. Iontophoresis utilizes batteries and is wireless for convenience and portability, as discussed previously. Surgical implants (spinal cord stimulators) are utilized for pain control and functional electrical stimulation for muscle reeducation, especially in clients with spinal cord injuries. Bioness™ also utilizes wireless technology along with an orthotic device to ensure consistent placement of the electrodes for FES. The device is wireless and has a customizable setup for individual clients and can be used during functional activities at home. Bioness™ representatives assist OT practitioners with the prior authorization and setup of Bioness™ devices. The Vectra® NEO unit incorporates electrotherapy, ultrasonography, electromyography, and laser in one unit with a touch screen, protocols, and the capacity for transferrable data. A wireless electrotherapy device that does not have leads and is more client friendly is available. It is anticipated that PAMs will be extended to more applications in the future and have improved convenience for both practitioners and clients.

BOX 18-12
Interferential Current Application

1. Complete the preliminary review for precautions and contraindications along with the indications for IFC for the specific client and his or her condition.
2. Explain to the client the procedural process, the indications, and what to expect during the treatment process.
3. Prepare the client by positioning him or her comfortably and removing clothing and jewelry from the treatment area.
4. Instruct the client regarding maintenance of positioning with minimal to no movement to prevent interference with electrode contact and the focal treatment point.
5. Make sure that the unit settings are on minimal settings.
6. Apply the four self-adhering electrodes (client-specific electrodes) to the leads and the leads to the unit.
7. Locate the center of the client's pain. Visualize this center as the middle of the "X" that you are creating with the four electrodes (see Fig. 18-9 for illustration of the "X" pattern). The two electrodes from channel one are forming one leg of the "X" with opposite sides of the center of the pain point. The other two electrodes from channel two are forming the other leg of the "X."
8. Place the electrodes firmly on the client's skin creating the "X" pattern described in step 6 and depicted in Figure 18-9. Make sure the electrodes have good contact for adequate conductivity.
9. Turn the unit on.
10. Instruct the client that the unit is being turned on and to let the practitioner know when the sensation of pins and needles is beginning to be felt.
11. Instruct the client that the intensity will be increased until it is the most comfortable for the client. No muscular contractions should be elicited with this treatment.
12. Adjust the pulse rate settings for specific treatment problem and goals. Acute pain uses a pulse rate frequency of 80 to 200 pulses per second (PPS). For chronic pain, use a low pulse rate frequency of 1 to 5 PPS.[16]
13. Treatment time is approximately 20 to 30 minutes.
14. Upon completion of treatment, turn off the power, remove the electrodes, and place them in a sealed bag that is labeled for this client.
15. Proceed with functional tasks as part of the treatment and established goals.
16. Assess client's response and status, and document the treatment.

TRANSCUTANEOUS ELECTRICAL NERVE STIMULATION

Transcutaneous electrical nerve stimulation (TENS) utilizes electrodes to deliver pulsed current to stimulate nerves for relieving pain.[17] It is theorized that TENS is effective for pain modulation through the Melzack and Wall's gate control theory, or the opiate system. The gate control theory is based on the premise that the gating mechanism located in the spinal cord allows only one sensation at a time to pass through the brain.[17] When the TENS input is delivered, it overrides the painful stimuli and closes the gate, preventing the painful sensation from traveling to the central nervous system, thereby suppressing the pain.[17]

Application: The electrodes for TENS application are placed such that they surround the area of pain. Settings are set up for the type of pain and comfort level of the client. TENS at the sensory level (no muscle contraction) is applicable for acute or chronic pain during performance of occupational tasks.[11] It is important to follow similar guidelines for preparing the skin site and for the care of electrical stimulation electrodes discussed earlier. Alcohol wipes may help the electrodes to adhere longer or more effectively. Box 18-13 reviews the steps for TENS application.

Precautions: Precautions for the use of electrical stimulation include hypersensitivity to electrical stimulation, arrhythmias caused by conduction disturbances, congestive heart failure, seizure disorders, sensory loss, vascular diseases, allergies to the gel, tape or electrodes, tissue susceptible to hemorrhage, hematoma, impaired cognition, and immature pediatric nervous systems.[10]

Contraindications: TENS, like other electrical stimulation, is contraindicated for use in clients with demand-type pacemakers, placement over carotid sinus, use during the first trimester of pregnancy, and stimulation across the chest for cardiac disease; the head and neck area of clients with epilepsy, treatments for central nervous system disorders, and use in confused or noncompliant clients and children should be avoided.[11]

Safety Considerations: Safety considerations are the same as for electrical stimulation.

DIATHERMY

Diathermy is an application of moderate heat to increase blood flow and heat fibrous tissues. This facilitates the relief of joint stiffness, promotes muscle relaxation, and decreases muscle spasms. Diathermy is has two main classifications based on use: (1) therapeutic medical purposes and (2) surgical cauterization or burning of tissue. Shortwave diathermy (SWD) is one of three types of diathermy and will be the only one described in this text, as it is the most common mode of treatment used by both OT and physical therapy (PT) practitioners. It targets the magnetic fields in tissues,[17] and SWD consists of a generator or box-shaped unit, which houses all of the electrical components that generate the electromagnetic waves. The control panel houses the control buttons for operating the machine. The drum is a hard plastic housing unit containing copper coils that serve the function of applicator for the electrical magnetic field to the tissue. The diathermy drum is similar to the ultrasound transducer sound head because it delivers

BOX 18-13
Transcutaneous Electrical Nerve Stimulation Application

1. Explain the procedure and what to expect to the client if he or she is receiving TENS for the first time. For example, discuss such sensations as "pins and needles," and inform the client that TENS should not cause pain. Explain that TENS does not cause electrocution.
2. Prepare the client with positioning and adjustment of clothing in the treatment area.
3. Before turning the TENS unit on, make sure the settings are at the minimal setting.
4. Label the electrodes for specific client application because they can be reused for that client.
5. Attach the electrodes (client-specific) to the leads, then attach the leads to the TENS unit.
6. Apply the electrodes over the treatment area, with consideration of the pain area, and dermatome.
7. Make sure the electrodes have firm contact with the client's skin.
8. Set the pulse width and rate according to the manufacturer's guidelines and protocols for the condition.
9. Turn the unit on.
10. Tell the client that the intensity will be increased slowly and that he or she needs to inform the practitioner when the sensation of "pins and needles" is felt.
11. Increase the intensity until it is at a comfortable setting for the client. There should not be any muscle contraction with this setting (sensory TENS).
12. Adjust the setting for the pulse width and rate. For acute pain, set a narrow pulse width (75 μsec) with a high pulse rate frequency of 80 to 200 pulses per second (PPS). For chronic pain, set the pulse width 200 μsec with low pulse rate frequency of 1 to 5 PPS.
13. The time frame for application varies according to the level and frequency of pain.
14. If the client uses this at home, then instruct the client in all of the processes for settings and changing the battery, and provide contact information.
15. Document the treatment and response.

the energy to tissues.[17] Refer to Figure 18-10 for a depiction of the diathermy unit.

The diathermy unit is powered by electricity that it converts to a radiofrequency, which is then passed through the coil, generating a fluctuating or alternating magnetic field. This magnetic field, in turn, creates currents in the tissue that is adjacent to the drum. The current in the tissue causes dipoles, or a pair of equal and opposite electric charges separated by small distance. The dipole rotates because of the changing polarity, and the kinetic energy increases in the tissue. This results in an increase in the tissue temperature in tissues that are high in water content, such as muscle; tissues containing less water, such as skin, tendon, and bone, demonstrate a lower rise in tissue temperature.[17]

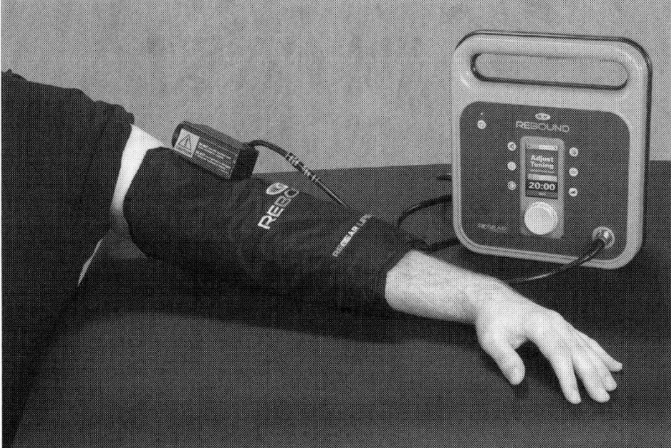

FIGURE 18-10. Shortwave diathermy produces the electromagnetic field, which yields a circular flow of energy for the therapeutic benefits of heat.

Application: Diathermy provides thermal effects with significant temperature increases up to 4 to 5 cm deep in the muscle. Its clinical applications include sensitive soft tissue that cannot withstand the pressure of a hot pack or pressure from a hand held water sprayer. Target tissue is deeper than 1 to 2 cm below skin. Nonthermal effects of diathermy include increased blood flow, vasodilation, relaxation, increased tissue metabolic rate, and pain reduction, if desired, in tissue deeper than 1 to 2 cm beneath skin. Diathermy is most effective for treating a larger area and irregular surfaces, such as the hand, which may be difficult with ultrasound.[17] Box 18-14 reviews the steps for diathermy application.

Precautions: The precautions for diathermy consist of utilizing care with the following: conditions where increased temperature is not desired; over traumatic musculoskeletal injuries with acute bleeding, acute inflammatory conditions, and areas with increased sensitivity to temperature or pain; over fluid filled cavities or organs; and use over wet dressings, over implanted metals, or near other medical electrical devices or equipment. Like other modalities, caution is indicated if the client cannot perceive or report pain or sensory input accurately. Caution is indicated if application of diathermy occurs after application of a thermal modality as the client's sensory perception may be altered. A towel should be used to absorb moisture during the treatment because this could impact the buildup of energy.[17]

Contraindications: Diathermy is contraindicated in ischemic tissue, peripheral vascular disease, metal implants or jewelry; over moist dressings; in clients with cancer, fever, or cardiac pacemakers; in pregnancy; in epiphyseal

BOX 18-14
Diathermy Application

1. Examine the equipment to make sure that the diathermy drum is clean and dry.
2. Prepare the client for the treatment, explaining the treatment session and what to expect with gentle warmth.
3. Remove metal or jewelry from the treatment area.
4. Position the client with a towel under the treatment area and for comfort and modesty.
5. Inspect the treatment area, and document the status before and after treatment.
6. Place the diathermy drum on the treatment area.
7. Turn the device on.
8. Set the pulse duration and pulse frequency low for acute nonthermal effects and high for thermal effects.
9. Set the treatment time (15–30 minutes).
10. Press the start button.
11. Adjust the intensity to the client's comfort level. Monitor at 4 to 5 minutes as the tissue is heating to ensure client's comfort. Continue treatment until treatment goals are achieved.
12. Upon completion of the treatment session, return settings to zero and remove the machine. Inspect the skin for redness or other issues.
13. Proceed with functional tasks as part of the treatment and established goals.
14. Document the treatment and response.

plates in children; over genitals, eyes, and face; in infection sites, and in the abdomen of a client with implanted intrauterine device (IUD).[17] Treatment of the very obese client is contraindicated as excessive heating could occur in the adipose tissue.

Safety Considerations: Diathermy should not be used near any metal in the treatment area. This includes jewelry, watches, and furniture. Metal causes buildup of energy from the treatment. It is important to make sure that the treatment area is dry.[17] The OT practitioner should adhere to the safety standards set by the FDA.

LASER LIGHT

Laser is a commonly used term, which is actually an acronym for *light amplification by stimulated emission of radiation*. Laser is a more coherent (from one small source) and directional flow of light compared with other types of light. The wavelength of the light impacts the depth to which the laser penetrates.[10] Table 18-3 may help in decision making with regard to the use of laser versus diathermy.

TABLE 18-3 Benefits of Laser Therapy Versus Diathermy

INDICATIONS/ BENEFITS OF LASER	INDICATIONS/BENEFITS OF DIATHERMY
Produces no thermal effects Soft tissue and fracture healing Pain management Acute musculoskeletal trauma Myofascial pain Rheumatoid arthritis Carpal tunnel syndrome Low back pain Trigger points Neck pain	If skin or some underlying soft tissue is tender and will not tolerate pressure In areas where subcutaneous fat is thick and deep heating is required Pulsed shortwave diathermy produces the same magnitude and depth of muscle heating as 1-MHz ultrasound When the treatment goal is to increase tissue temperatures in a large area

Application: Laser treatment is utilized for tissue healing in wounds and for management of pain associated with arthritis and neuromusculoskeletal conditions, such as lateral epicondylitis, chronic low back pain, and neck pain.[10] Laser treatment begins with a complete client evaluation and determination of whether laser treatment is applicable, including precautions or contraindications that prohibit administering laser treatment. Following this evaluation, the OT practitioner proceeds with selection of the settings for the laser. The dose for the laser treatment is considered the energy density. The dose is measured in joules per centimeter squared (J/cm^2). The energy density treatment range that is indicated for soft tissue and fracture healing is 5 to 16 J/cm^2.[10] For acute arthritis, the energy density treatment range is 2 to 4 J/cm^2 and for chronic arthritis 4 to 8 J/cm^2.[9] Box 18-15 reviews the steps for laser application.

BOX 18-15
Laser Application

1. Turn the machine on.
2. Adjust the output parameters, as indicated (pulse rate and treatment time)
3. Both the OT practitioner and the client must wear safety goggles if the applicator includes laser diodes. These safety goggles must meet the specifications for the wavelength of the laser.
4. Clean the applicator with antimicrobial agent approved by the facility.
5. Prepare the treatment area by exposing it, and position the client for comfort and modesty.
6. Remove all jewelry and metal from the treatment area.
7. Non-opaque dressing or a thin film over a wound does not need to be removed for the treatment.
8. Apply the applicator to the treatment area with firm pressure.
9. Perform functional tasks as determined by treatment plan and goals.
10. Document the treatment and response.

Precautions: OT practitioners should refer to the recommendations provided with the specific unit being used in their clinic and consider the clinical reasoning related to the specific conditions for which the laser treatment is being applied. The OT practitioner and the client should always wear goggles during the laser treatment.[10] The goggles should be marked with the specific wavelength range that they diminish so that the eyes are protected from that specific band of the laser. Caution should be exercised during low back or abdominal treatments in clients who are pregnant. Extra caution is required in clients with impaired sensation or impaired cognitive status. Laser diodes can also potentially get warm and cause burns if applied for prolonged periods. This is more likely to occur with lower-power light emitting diodes (LEDs) that require longer time to deliver a therapeutic dose of laser light.[10]

Contraindications: General contraindications for application of laser treatments includes direct irradiation to the eyes, malignancy, within 4 to 6 months after radiation treatment, over hemorrhaging regions, or over the thyroid and other endocrine glands.[10]

Safety Considerations: Warning signs should be displayed during laser treatments so that it is clear that laser treatment is being administered. This signage should be visible before entry into the treatment room. Goggles should be worn by both the client and the OT practitioner during the treatment.[10] It is important to adhere to the safety standards set by the FDA.[10]

Mechanical Modalities

Mechanical modalities consist of tools that apply force as part of the treatment. These forces can be applied by the OT practitioner or by a machine. Two of the mechanical modalities discussed here are the vasocompression unit and the continuous passive motion machine (CPM). Both of these mechanical modalities are applied at different stages of the recovery from acute or chronic conditions.

VASOCOMPRESSION UNIT

Vasocompression units, commonly referred to as *intermittent compression units,* are used to reduce swelling, including, but not limited to, the extremities after surgery or for treating chronic conditions, such as lymphedema (Fig. 18-11). The units are designed to apply external forces to the venous and lymphatic systems to move fluid from intracellular tissues to lymphatic capillaries to then be transported out of the body through the lymphatic system.

Application: Compression units are utilized for treating peripheral edema, shaping a residual limb after amputation, increasing lymphatic and venous circulation, and preventing deep venous thrombosis and stasis ulcers. Box 18-16 reviews the steps for vasocompression application.

Precautions: Blood pressure should be monitored before, during, and after the compression treatment. The OT practitioner starts by setting the compression pressure on a lower level to assess the client's tolerance for the compression treatment. The client is positioned with the treated extremity in elevation and the call bell within reach. Any weeping of the lymph fluid and skin condition and changes should be monitored. It is important to note that some lymphedema experts have suggested that compression units should not be utilized with lymphedema because of the risk of damage to lymph nodes. Therefore, careful assessment of all of the contributing factors for the client need to be considered.

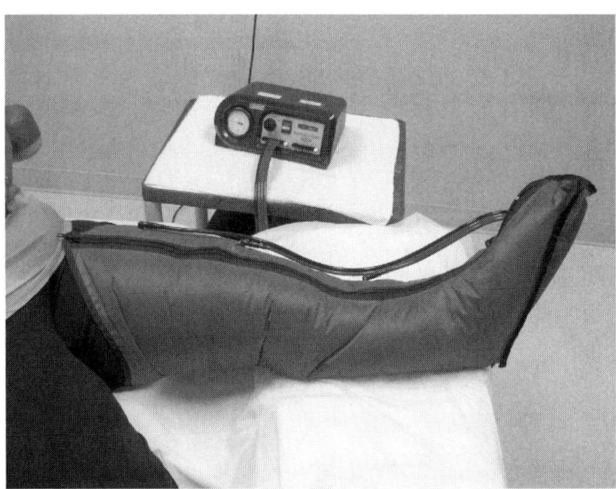

FIGURE 18-11. Compression unit with sleeve on lower extremity in elevated position.

Contraindications: Contraindications for intermittent compression includes malignancy in the treatment area; presence of a deep vein thrombosis; obstructed lymphatic channels, such as sclerotic lymphedema; unstable or acute fracture in the treatment area; heart failure; infection in the treatment area; pulmonary edema; kidney or cardiac insufficiency; and clients who are very young or those who are very old and frail. It is common practice to emphasize that administration of intermittent compression to clients with heart failure, pulmonary edema, and kidney or cardiac insufficiency can be fatal, although there is no evidence in the literature to support this contraindication.

Safety Considerations: The client's blood pressure should be monitored before, during, and after treatment. Normal arterial pressure is 30 millimeters of mercury (mm Hg). Therefore, any pressure that exceeds 30 mm Hg facilitates potential reabsorption of edema and flow of lymph. However, more pressure does not translate to better outcomes. Diastolic blood pressure is the reference point for maximal inflation pressure. Another consideration is the client's tolerance for the pressure on the involved extremity.

CONTINUOUS PASSIVE MOTION MACHINE

The **continuous passive motion machine (CPM)** provides early protected motion to healing soft tissues. The involved extremity is positioned in the machine with straps and careful placement of the moving joint in the hinge or moving component of the CPM. The CPM is used for

BOX 18-16
Vasocompression Application

1. Ask the client to remove all jewelry from the treatment area.
2. Check and record the client's blood pressure.
3. Measure and record the circumferential measurements at specified and documented increments to ensure accuracy of repeated measurements.
4. Drape and position the client in a comfortable position with the affected limb elevated at a 45-degree angle.
5. Place a loose-fitting stockinette over the extremity, smoothing out all of the wrinkles.
6. Place a compression boot or sleeve over the stockinette and affected limb.
7. Connect the rubber hose to the connecting valve on the sleeve.
8. Turn the machine on, and adjust the parameters. One parameter is inflation pressure, which is based on the client's blood pressure, tolerance, and any other special considerations. The on/off sequence or inflation/deflation ratio is usually set to 3:1, which is the ratio of on and off time. A general guideline for reducing edema is 45 seconds on and 15 seconds off or 90 seconds on and 30 seconds off. It is suggested that the first treatment be less invasive so that the client's tolerance for the treatment session can be assessed. The total treatment time varies and is based on the client's condition. Treatment time for traumatic edema is 2 hours, whereas for lymphedema, it is 3 to 4 hours.
9. Once the unit is turned on, then the boot or sleeve is filled with air by a small compressor, thus causing compression forces on the limb. The compression force is maintained for the chosen setting for the inflation/deflation time frame.
10. A call bell is placed within reach of the client, and the client is instructed to call if any discomfort or change in breathing or palpitations is experienced.
11. Monitor blood pressure throughout the treatment.
12. Upon completion of the compression treatment, take repeat measurements at the marked areas.
13. Wrap the involved area with compression wraps after treatment, depending on the client's condition.
14. Utilization of muscle pump action is indicated while in the compression wrap to further aid in the reduction of fluid buildup.
15. Follow up with an occupational performance task with the client in the compression wrap to facilitate functional skills, muscle pump activation for further edema reduction, and application of compensatory techniques, as needed.
16. Document the treatment and response.

treating elbows, shoulders, and knees for contractures or mobilization after surgery to enhance connective tissue strength, facilitate ROM, and evacuate joint hemarthrosis (bloody effusion within the joint space).

Application: The CPM is used after surgery for many conditions that OT practitioners routinely treat, especially trauma, orthopedic conditions, and effects of elective orthopedic surgeries. The CPM is utilized after shoulder and knee replacements. Use of the CPM was shown to result in decreased pain and increased ROM of clients who had undergone arthroscopic rotator cuff repair in a randomized study where an independent examiner took the measurements.[19] The CPM has also been found to be effective in the treatment of various hand injuries that caused decreased ROM and edema; that study yielded statistical significance for better results in edema reduction through application of the CPM compared with limb elevation alone.[20] However other studies have been inconclusive on the outcomes of CPM use. Therefore, utilization of the CPM requires careful consideration.

Application of the CPM varies, depending on the brand of equipment as well as the specific joint to which the CPM is applied. It is suggested that CPM application be tested on an unaffected joint before application to a painful joint to minimize undue fear or stress in the client. CPM units have adjustable Velcro® straps that are marked to aid with the correct application of the unit. See Figure 18-12, for a depiction of CPM placement and how the hinge is centered with the axis of the joint being treated. Box 18-17 reviews the steps for CPM application.

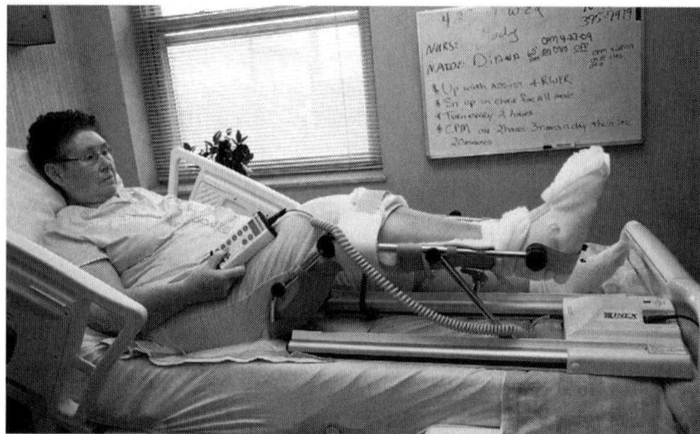

FIGURE 18-12. Continuous passive motion machine may be used on lower extremity or upper extremity.

Precautions: The CPM is applied to a joint that has been cleared for PROM. The CPM must be applied correctly, with the straps securely fastened to provide adequate PROM. The client needs to be positioned comfortably enough to tolerate the required CPM treatment position, especially because that position has to be maintained for the whole treatment period to achieve effective PROM.

Contraindications: Use of the CPM is contraindicated for any joint that has not been medically cleared for PROM, for example, after a rotator cuff repair, where immobilization has been ordered for a set period.

BOX 18-17
Continuous Passive Motion Machine Application

1. Have the CPM strategically placed for application to the applicable joint, and plug it into the outlet for power.
2. The CPM needs to line up with the joint for the axis of the rotation on the CPM unit.
3. Fasten the Velcro® straps for security and comfort to hold the extremity in place during passive range of motion.
4. Adjust the range of motion and speed on the basis of the client's tolerance and the appropriate protocol.
5. Utilize the CPM for the time frame suggested, according to the client's condition, tolerance, and pain level.
6. Document the treatment and response.

Safety Considerations: The hand-held control should be placed within reach of the client because this will enable the client to stop the unit, if needed. The client should be instructed about all aspects of the wearing and care of the CPM unit and what to expect before application.

Competencies

Clinical competence is performing a task correctly and safely. Competence also incorporates theoretical knowledge, cognitive skills, appropriate behavior, maintenance of values, and procedural skills. Although many preparatory components precede the actual administration of PAMs, the focus of this discussion will be on the cognitive and procedural aspects of their application. OT practitioners need to complete this critical thinking decision-making process every time PAMs are being considered for clients. While going through the clinical decision-making process, the OT practitioner must also be aware of the core benefits and special considerations for each modality. Refer to Figure 18-1 for the critical thinking decision-making process before applying PAMs.

Decision Tree for Using Modalities

In addition to reflecting on and responding to the critical thinking decision-making flow chart, the OT practitioner also needs to be able to respond to the following questions to proceed safely and effectively with the treatment and to achieve the best outcomes. Upon completion of these two reflective processes, the OT practitioner will be able to assess his or her skills and knowledge base in the safe and competent application of the PAM.

1. What is the client's condition/functional impairment?
2. What is the target area/tissue/muscle/bone? How deep is this target area?
3. What is the inflammatory state/tissue pathology/limb function that is driving the goal for utilization of a PAM?
4. What are the treatment and functional goals?
5. What are the possible modalities that can be considered?
6. What modalities should be excluded?
7. What is the modality of choice for the type of problem and the type of the surface area being treated?
8. Does the client have any precautions/contraindications that preclude use of the modality of choice?
9. What is the application technique and protocol for this modality with this condition?

Upon completion of response to these questions and to the steps shown in Figure 18-1, the OT practitioner can proceed with administering the modality if his or her licensure or regulation permits it, and if competency has been established.

Documentation and Billing Codes

Documentation has multiple purposes. It is primarily for reimbursement purposes to ensure that the services billed for were rendered, documented, and addressed the treatment goals. Documentation also serves as a legal record of the client's status, progress or lack thereof, and for evidence if needed in any reimbursement claim or litigation. Documentation has various formats, but the essential information that needs to be included in a modality note are the area of the body treated, the client's response, and specifics related to the modality. For example, the following items should be included in documentation specifically for ultrasound treatment:

- Area of the body treated
- Ultrasound frequency
- Ultrasound intensity
- Ultrasound duty cycle
- Treatment variation
- Whether ultrasound was delivered under water
- Client's response to treatment and the follow-up activity

A sample SOAP note is given below. This note is just about the ultrasound portion of the treatment and not about the occupationally based OT to follow. Remember, generally PAMs are a preparatory method, laying the groundwork for another treatment.

S: Reports slowly improving R shoulder ROM and now able to use RUE to brush her hair.
O: *Pretreatment:* R shoulder active abduction ROM 120 degrees, passive abduction ROM 135 degrees. *Intervention:* Ultrasound right inferior anterior shoulder, 2.0 W/cm2, continuous 1 MHz, for 5 min. followed by joint mobility, inferior glide grade IV. *Post-treatment:* R shoulder passive abduction is 150 degrees.
A: Client tolerated treatment well, with increased ROM noted after treatment.
P: Continue ultrasound as above followed by mobilization and ROM to shoulder with ADL retraining.

As another example, the specific parameters for documenting fluidotherapy would include the following:

- Area of the body treated
- Fluidotherapy temperature
- Body part treated

- Time
- Follow-up activity
- Client's response to treatment

Documentation for other PAMs would be the same, except for the specific parameters related to that particular modality. It is advisable to also document skin integrity and significant changes in skin color (e.g., prolonged redness).

Billing codes and reimbursement rules are being updated continually and vary among healthcare systems and third-party payers. The coding system currently consists of International Classification of Diseases (ICD) and Current Procedural Terminology (CPT) codes. ICD codes are used for classifying the client's pathology, whereas CPT codes are utilized to define the treatments rendered by OT practitioners. The CPT code and the ICD code must correlate with each other to qualify for reimbursement. It is also important for the OT practitioner to be familiar with billing and reimbursement patterns and updates. For example, application of cold packs or hot packs is currently not reimbursable unless it is utilized concurrently with another therapeutic procedure to assist with a functional goal.[13]

SUMMARY

PAMs are complex but highly effective tools in the OT practitioner's toolbox. However, it is essential that the OT practitioner be skilled, trained, and aware of their benefits and risks before using PAMs to ensure safe and ethical behavior. It is also critical that the primary focus remains on the client's occupational performance goals, rather than the application of fancy tricks or tools. The roles of the occupational therapist and the OTA must include communication about PAMs to ensure understanding of the application process, skill levels, and adherence to safety, precautions, and contraindications. The OT practitioner completes the assessment, determines the rationale behind the suggestion for a specific modality for a client's condition, and ensures that he or she has a clear understanding of the parameters and application of the modality and of documentation. Both the occupational therapist and the OTA must be in compliance with their practice requirements to administer PAMs.

REVIEW QUESTIONS

1. A client has rheumatoid arthritis in the inflammatory stage in her RUE. During this phase, the OT practitioner established a goal for reducing pain and stiffness. The PAMs for addressing this goal would be:
   a. Ultrasound to right wrist and fingers
   b. Fluidotherapy
   c. Contrast baths
   d. Paraffin
2. The occupational therapist asks you to monitor a client with radial nerve palsy caused by a humeral fracture. The humeral fracture has been treated, but the client continues to have difficulty with wrist and finger extension. The best choice for PAMs to help with the wrist and finger movement is:
   a. Fluidotherapy
   b. Iontophoresis
   c. Neuromuscular electrical stimulation (NMES)
   d. Phonophoresis
3. A client has a diagnosis of glioblastoma in the brain and has flexor synergistic movements in his RUE. The best modality to increase the extensor muscle movement to prepare for functional tasks is:
   a. Iontophoresis
   b. IFC
   c. NEMC
   d. Galvanic current
4. A client has been referred for OT 6 weeks after right carpal tunnel release surgery. Her primary complaints are pain and stiffness, with decreased range of motion at the wrist. Her scar is red and raised 2 to 5 mm with firm pliability. Which physical agent modality would be most beneficial, and which setting would you choose?
   a. Ultrasound pulsed setting
   b. Iontophoresis with acetic acid medication
   c. Ultrasound with continuous setting
   d. Fluidotherapy at 108 degrees
5. You are performing electrical stimulation, and the electrodes are not staying in contact with the client's skin. What can you do to improve the contact between the electrode and the client's skin?
   a. Apply alcohol to the skin.
   b. Apply lotion to the skin.
   c. Moisten the electrodes with water.
   d. Replace the electrodes after each application.
6. Which of the following responses best describes direct current electrical stimulation?
   a. It is used to cool the tissues.
   b. It is used for strong muscles.
   c. It is a continuous unidirectional current flow.
   d. It can only be used to cause muscle contraction.
7. A client is referred for OT after a traumatic fall resulting in a wrist fracture. The client's fracture site is now healed, but she is experiencing continued pain, edema, stiffness, and increased sweating in her hand, as well as decreased hand function. The client carries her hand in a protective mode and has been diagnosed with complex regional pain syndrome. (Complex regional pain syndrome includes such symptoms as significant pain, sensitivity to pressure, edema, and changes in coloration of skin in early stages.) Which modality and treatment activity would you recommend?
   a. Fluidotherapy and massage
   b. Fluidotherapy and functional activities
   c. Ultrasound and resistive activities
   d. DC electrical stimulation and resistive putty
8. Which three of the following are universal precautions applicable to all physical agent modalities?
   a. Decreased cognitive function
   b. Decreased sensory status
   c. Temperature range within range of body temperature
   d. Decreased expressive language skills
   e. Cardiac problems
   f. Pain
9. Which of the following responses indicates the modality and the setting that will reach target tissue that is deeper than 2 cm?
   a. Ultrasound with 1-MHz setting
   b. Phonophoresis with 3-MHz setting
   c. Ultrasound with 3-MHz setting
   d. Cryotherapy with ice massage

10. Which of the following responses best describes the appropriate waveform suited for iontophoresis?
    a. Pulsed wave form
    b. Ultrasound wave form
    c. DC unidirectional wave form
    d. Intermittent wave form

CASE STUDY

Cindy is a 32-year-old administrative assistant referred for OT 8 weeks after a RUE scaphoid fracture. The orthopedist reports that the x-rays indicate that the fracture is healed and recommends that the client can begin therapy. The client has difficulty moving her wrist, and her AROM measurements include: wrist flexion 40 degrees, wrist extension 40 degrees, and difficulty actively making a full fist. The PROM in her fingers consist of the following: metacarpophalangeal (MCP) 0° to 45°; proximal interphalangeal (PIP) 10° to 60°; and distal interphalangeal (DIP) are 5° to 10°. She is unable to use her RUE because of stiffness and pain for activities of daily living (ADLs), instrumental activities of daily living (IADLs), and childcare. She has one child and loves arts and crafts. She wants to be able to resume work and all previous ADLs, and IADLs, including childcare.

1. List the biomechanical problems, occupational performance problems, and assessment tools needed to evaluate and monitor Cindy's progress.
2. List the potential goals for Cindy.
3. Which modalities would best address her functional ROM problems?
4. List the potential theoretical/frame of reference to support usage of PAMs with this client.
5. List some therapeutic activities that the OT practitioner should include in a treatment plan for Cindy.

PUTTING IT ALL TOGETHER — Sample Treatment and Documentation

Setting	Outpatient
Client Profile	Ms. Jones is a 35 y/o female who works in a childcare center as a teacher. She fell and fractured her hand at work when she tripped over toys. She sustained fractures of her metacarpals of her right (dominant) hand (ring, middle, and little fingers). She was casted for 6 weeks after closed reduction of the fractures. The cast blocked her digital flexion of all fingers. Client developed edema and stiffness.
Work History	Works at a childcare center
Insurance	Workers' Compensation
Psychological	Anxious and concerned about recovery and bills
Social	Married and has two children under 6 years of age. Husband works as a consultant from home.
Cognitive	Alert, oriented, has college education
Motor & Manual Muscle Testing (MMT)	WNL for all other extremities except RUE. Cast off and R wrist 10 degrees extension, 15 degrees flexion. MCPs 45 degrees flexion, IPs 20° to 30° flexion and moderate edema with pitting in palm and digits. Pain 5/10 in wrist and hand. Unable to grip dynamometer for testing. Sensory intact in RUE.
ADL	Performs basic ADLs using LUE, unable to assist with RUE for fasteners
IADL	Unable to perform bilateral tasks using bilateral hands. Uses LUE to complete IADLs
Goals	In 4 weeks: 1. Client will fasten fasteners on clothing with adapted techniques 100% of the time. 2. Client will complete laundry tasks independently using both hands 100% of the time. 3. Client will be able to grasp small items needed for ADL and IADL tasks (toothpaste tube, keys, lids and childcare items) 100% of the time. 4. Client will demonstrate decreased pain to 3 or less on a pain scale during functional tasks with compensatory techniques 90% of time.

OT TREATMENT SESSION 1

THERAPEUTIC ACTIVITY	TIME	GOAL(S) ADDRESSED	OTA RATIONALE
Preparatory modality to decrease pain and edema and increase range of motion using contrast baths	10 min	#4	*Preparatory Method; Client Education and Training:* Preparatory/client education and training for contrast baths to do at home and in the clinic. Instruct on UE PROM/AROM to loosen client's joints and muscles for ADLs. Provide exercises client can do in between therapy sessions to increase ROM for ADLs. Monitor pain pre and post modalities and treatments. Instruct in elevation and active muscle pumping to decrease the edema.
ADL session focusing on fasteners with adapted techniques	15–20 min	#1 and #3	*Preparatory Tasks; Client Education and Training:* Discuss adaptations, alternative clothing until fine motor skills improve. Utilize R hand as stabilizer, slowly integrating into more of the fastening task.

Continued

PUTTING IT ALL TOGETHER Sample Treatment and Documentation (continued)

THERAPEUTIC ACTIVITY	TIME	GOAL(S) ADDRESSED	OTA RATIONALE
Retrieving laundry out of dryer putting in clothes basket, folding and putting laundry away	15–20 min	#2	*Occupations; Client Education and Training:* Instruct client in body mechanics, usage of bilateral hands to ensure safety, and increased functional usage of bilateral hands for bilateral tasks.

SOAP note: 4/9/—, 9:00 am -9:40 am

S: Client reported pain 5/10 in R hand at beginning of treatment session.

O: Client participated in 40-minute treatment session for skilled instruction in range of motion, edema management, and fine motor tasks for ADLs and IADLs. Reported pain 4/10 post contrast baths. Client able to complete fasteners with LUE and using RUE as a stabilizer to hold the garment. Client completed laundry tasks using BUE to retrieve items out of dryer and place in the basket. Client instructed to use RUE for the folding tasks. She demonstrated folding tasks with verbal cues from OTA for body mechanics and to prevent proximal motor substitution patterns. Rest break of 5 minutes needed after fine motor tasks.

A: Client able to demonstrate contrast baths & HEP with 100% accuracy. Reported pain decrease 5/10–4/10. Client demonstrated bilateral hand functional skills with some substitution patterns. Client able to correct with verbal cues. Client would benefit from continued OT to address edema, ROM, functional hand usage for ADLs and IADLS.

P: Client to be seen in outpatient clinic for 45 minutes, 1x week for 4 weeks for skilled instructions in HEP, ADLs, and IADLs.

Sue Moore, COTA/L 4/12/—, 12:15 pm

TREATMENT SESSION 2

What could you do next with this client?

TREATMENT SESSION 3

What could you do next with this client?

REFERENCES

1. American Occupational Therapy Association. (2014). *Occupational therapy practice framework: Domain and process* (3rd ed.). American Journal of Occupational Therapy, 68(Suppl. 1), S1–S48.
2. Eliason, M. L., & Gohl-Giesen, A. (1979). A question of professional boundaries: Implications for educational programs. *American Journal of Occupational Therapy, 36,*199–202.
3. Hunter, J. M., Schneider, L. H., Mackin, E. J., & Bell, J. A. (Eds). (1985). *Rehabilitation of the hand.* Philadelphia, PA: Mosby.
4. American Occupational Therapy Association. (1991). *1990 member data survey summary report.* Rockville, MD: American Occupational Therapy Association.
5. Physical agent modalities. (2012). *American Journal of Occupational Therapy, 66,* S78–S80. doi:10.5014/ajot.2012.66S78
6. Burkhart, A., Braveman, B., & Gentile, P. (2002). Evaluating and documenting staff competence for accreditation reviews and staff development. *Administration & Management Special Interest Section Quarterly, 18,* 1–3, 6.
7. Occupational therapy code of ethics. (2015). *American Journal of Occupational Therapy, 69,* 6913410030p1–6913410030p8.
8. American Occupational Therapy Association. (2016). *2011 Accreditation Council For Occupational Therapy Education (ACOTE®) standards and interpretive guidelines (effective July 31, 2013).* Bethesda, MD: American Occupational Therapy Association.
9. Law, M., Polatajko, H., Baptiste, W., & Towsend, E. (1997). Core concepts of occupational therapy. In E. Towsend (Ed.), *Enabling occupation: An occupational therapy perspective* (pp. 29–56). Ottawa, ON: Canadian Association of Occupational Therapists.
10. Cameron, M. (2009). *Physical agents in rehabilitation: From research to practice.*(2nd ed.). Portland, OR: Saunders.
11. Bracciano, A. G. (2008). *Physical agent modalities: Theory and application for the occupational therapist* (2nd ed.). Thorofare, NJ: Slack.
12. Behrens, B., & Beinert, H. (2014). *Physical agents: Theory and practice* (3rd ed.). Philadelphia, PA: F. A. Davis.
13. Starkey, C. (2013). *Therapeutic modalities* (4th ed.). Philadelphia, PA: F. A. Davis.
14. Jacobs, K., MacRae, N., & Sladyk, K., (2014). *Occupational therapy essentials for clinical competence* (2nd ed.). Thorofare, NJ: Slack.
15. Sibtain, F., Khan, A., & Shakil-Ur-Rehman, S. (2013). Efficacy of paraffin wax bath with and without joint mobilization techniques in rehabilitation of posttraumatic stiff hand. *Pakistan Journal of Medical Science, 29*(2), 647–650.
16. Lehmann, J., Masock, A., Warren, C., & Koblanski, J. (1970). Effect of therapeutic temperatures on tendon extensibility. *Archives of Physical Medicine and Rehabilitation, 51,* 481–487.
17. Knight, K. L., & Draper, D. O. (2013). *Therapeutic modalities: the art and science* (2nd ed.). Baltimore, MD: Wolters Kluwer Health/Lippincott Williams & Wilkins.
18. Chang, Y. W., Hsieh, S. F., Horng, Y. S., Chen, H. L., Lee, K. C., Horng, Y. S. (2014). Comparative effectiveness of ultrasound and paraffin therapy in patients with carpal tunnel syndrome: A randomized trial. *BMC Musculoskeletal Disorders, 15,* 399.doi:10.1186/1471-2474-15-399
19. Garofalo, R., Conti, M., Notarnicola, A., Maradei, L., Giardella, A., & Castagna, A. (2010). Effects of one-month continuous passive motion after arthroscopic rotator cuff repair: Results at 1-year follow-up of a prospective randomized study. *Musculoskeletal Surgery, 94*(Suppl 1), S79–S83.
20. Giudice, M. (1990). Effects of continuous passive motion and elevation on hand edema. *American Journal of Occupational Therapy, 44*(10), 914–921.

Chapter 19

Orthotics: Fabrication and Management

Karol Spraggs-Young, OTD, OTR/L, CHT

LEARNING OUTCOMES

After studying this chapter, the student or practitioner will be able to:

19.1 Describe the function of a custom fabricated orthosis

19.2 Compare the different types of orthotic design and materials

19.3 Differentiate between orthotic fabrication and serial casting

19.4 Select the appropriate orthosis in client treatment

19.5 Identify the billing codes for application of an orthosis

19.6 Demonstrate an understanding of the basic principles of orthotic fabrication and fitting

KEY TERMS

Adherence	Prefabricated (P/F)
Casting motion to mobilize stiffness (CMMS)	Resting hand orthosis
Custom fabricated (C/F)	Rigidity
Drape	Serial casting
Dynamic	Static
Memory	Static progressive
Off the shelf (OTS)	Thermoplastic material
Orthosis, orthoses (plural)	Thumb spica orthosis
	Volar wrist orthosis

Orthotic fabrication, previously known as *splinting*, combines the art and science within the occupational therapy (OT) profession. **Orthoses** are a treatment intervention used by OT practitioners to effectively treat a variety of upper extremity diagnoses to improve occupational performance of clients. Orthoses have been used throughout history for immobilization, protection, and assistance with regaining function after an injury or illness.[1] An **orthosis** may be prefabricated or custom fabricated; however, the goals of orthotic intervention are always the same—to assist a client in the return to engagement in occupation. Before fabricating and applying an orthosis, the OT practitioner must have knowledge of the anatomy and physiology of the upper extremity and experience with the principles of orthotic design and construction.

In 2006 and 2007, the Centers for Medicare and Medicaid Services (CMS) collaborated with a group of practitioners from the American Society of Hand Therapists (ASHT) to establish a billing system for orthotic fabrication and fitting.[2] This ASHT task force recommended that the terms *orthosis* and *splint* should no longer be used interchangeably. Instead, the term splint would refer to "a cast or strapping applied to stabilize a fracture or dislocation," and the term orthosis would refer to "a custom molded, custom fitted or prefabricated orthosis."[3] These changes were made to acknowledge and promote the specialized skills and knowledge of OT practitioners who fabricate and fit clients with custom orthoses. Until this change becomes commonplace, some OT practitioners may continue to use the term splint, and not the newer term orthosis.

Orthoses are used for protection, positioning, and improving range of motion (ROM).[4] At any given time, an orthosis may just provide protection, or it may offer all three. Currently, a variety of materials are available for use in orthotic fabrication. The materials range from rigid thermoplastics to softer fabrics with foam padding, elastic and/or Velcro® strapping. With the many options in materials and types of orthosis design, with practice and experience, orthotic fabrication and fitting can be a creative, effective, and rewarding treatment intervention (Box 19-1).

BOX 19-1
Hand Grasp Patterns

The intricate anatomy of the human hand provides both mobility and strength, which allows for a tremendous amount of function. At birth, the human grasp is reflexive, with hands being able to grip an object placed in the palm. As a child grows and progresses through the normal stages of human development, primitive reflexes are replaced by voluntary movement. At around 1 year of age, a child is able to hold a small object with a maturing pincer grasp, using the thumb and the index and middle fingers. Around 2 years of age, the child is able to use the entire hand to manipulate blocks, scribble with a crayon, and hold a utensil. By 5 years of age, the child displays voluntary hand control with writing, manipulating objects, and tying shoelaces.

As adults, the fine motor function in the hand is described in terms of grip and prehension. Normal grasping patterns are classified as cylindrical, hook, or spherical. Prehension, or pinching pattern, is classified as lateral, tip, or palmer. A cylindrical grasp is used for holding such items as canned goods or beverages. A spherical grasp is used for turning a doorknob or to manipulate coins. A hook grip is used for carrying such objects as a grocery bag or a suitcase. Lateral pinch is used when pinching a clothespin or holding a piece of paper. Tip pinch is used to pick up small objects or for holding a sewing needle. Palmar pinch is used for fastening buttons and tying shoelaces. Dysfunction that occurs as a result of an impairment or injury to the wrist and hand will have a profound effect on normal grip and prehension. When treating the client with this type of injury with an orthosis, it is important that the OT practitioner give focused attention to grip and prehension patterns.

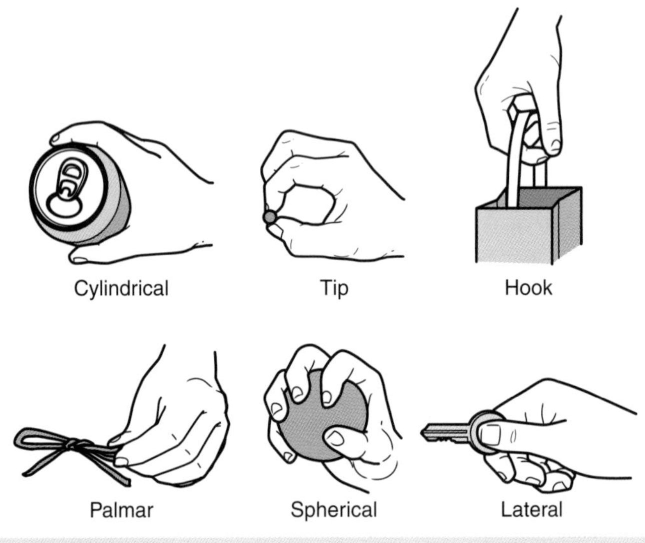

Grasp patterns.

USE OF AN ORTHOSIS FOR PROTECTION

Acute hand injuries, such as fractures, tendon repairs, and trauma, require a period of immobilization and protection during the healing process.

Fractures

For a stable fracture, that is, one that has been reduced or surgically repaired, a protective orthosis offers proper positioning, is lightweight, and may be removed for hygiene. In this application, the protective orthosis can be easily adjusted to accommodate for changes in edema, and the client's wearing schedule can be modified to incorporate hand use in activities of daily living (ADLs) and exercises, when indicated. Common fractures in the wrist and hand that benefit from an immobilization orthosis are distal radius, metacarpal, and phalangeal[5] (Fig. 19-1).

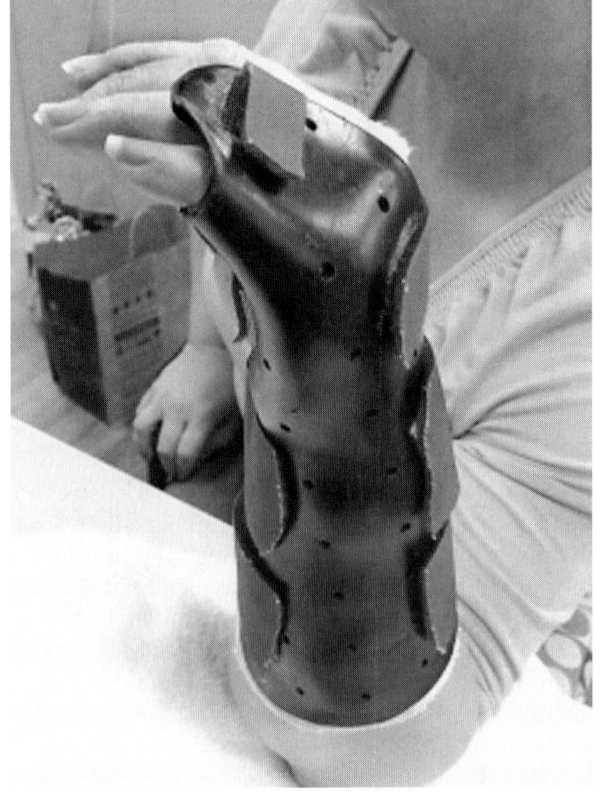

FIGURE 19-1. Ulnar gutter orthosis for Boxer's fracture.

Tendon Repairs

After a tendon laceration and following surgical or nonsurgical intervention, an orthosis is used to protect the injured anatomical structures while allowing the client to progress through restricted ROM exercise protocols. Restricted ROM allows the OT practitioner to move the client's joints and structures that were not injured to avoid joint stiffness. Restricted ROM also allows for gentle motion to the repaired structures to improve tendon glide and to prevent scarring. A protective orthosis is generally used in the treatment of flexor and extensor repairs in the hand and forearm because it can be removed by the OT practitioner during the treatment session and provide protection when the client is not being supervised (such as at home or work)[6,7] (Fig. 19-2).

Trauma

With traumatic hand injuries involving multiple anatomical structures, such as fractures, tendon involvement, amputations, and wounds, an orthosis is used to provide stability to healing structures and is molded to achieve specific positioning goals. For example, with an open metacarpal fracture in the hand, the metacarpophalangeal (MCP) joint will require positioning into MCP joint flexion and interphalangeal (IP) joint extension. The OT practitioner will also need access to the wound for wound care and dressing changes. A cast will not allow for daily removal for dressing changes, but an orthosis provides proper positioning and may be temporarily removed. In the case of trauma, the orthosis allows access for wound care and inspection, edema management, scar management, and ROM to uninvolved structures. When used in cases of trauma, such as amputations, open fractures, and skin grafts, a custom orthosis is lightweight, easy to clean, and adjustable to accommodate for changes in edema and the size of bandages[8] (Fig. 19-3).

USE OF AN ORTHOSIS FOR POSITIONING

Another application for the use of an orthosis is positioning. Several common conditions in the upper extremity benefit from an orthosis to provide positioning to relieve symptoms and promote healing.

TECHNOLOGY AND TRENDS

OT practitioners use orthotic fabrication as a treatment modality to assist individuals in obtaining their occupational performance goals. As advances have been made in the treatment of upper extremity injuries, so have the types of orthotic options for treating these injuries. Now, surgeons and practitioners are finding that early repair and motion to injured bones and soft tissues result in better outcomes. For example, only 10 years ago, a wrist fracture may have been treated with a long arm cast immobilizing past the elbow for 4 weeks, followed by a short arm cast for an additional 4 weeks. This resulted in a stiff elbow, wrist, and hand that would significantly limit function. The OT practitioner and the client would then have to work hard to regain motion in the stiff joints. Now, a wrist fracture can be repaired with an open reduction internal fixation surgery, which uses a plate and screws, thus allowing the client to begin moving in 1 to 2 weeks after surgery. Moving the repaired joint early decreases stiffness and the functional limitations associated with immobilization.

To accommodate these changes in treatment, different types of materials have become available, to make the process of orthotic fabrication and fitting much easier. What used to involve bending metal, sewing leather, and riveting straps can now be accomplished with a variety of low-temperature plastic materials and Velcro®. Low-temperature plastics are offered in a variety of colors, shapes, and thicknesses. Prefabricated orthoses are also now widely available. They can be found in a variety of sizes, designs, and styles to meet the client's needs. Looking through catalogs in the therapy clinic is a great way to see what is available. These catalogs can also be helpful in providing ideas for orthotic design.

As the client makes progress and achieves treatment goals, the practitioner may also determine whether a different type of orthosis may be more beneficial to the client. Therefore, the OT practitioner should keep in mind that to provide the best treatment for the client, it is important to remain current in the procedures, materials, and technology available. Moreover, despite the type of orthosis that is chosen for the treatment, the OT practitioner must always follow the basic principles of orthotic design, fabrication, and fitting when using this treatment modality.

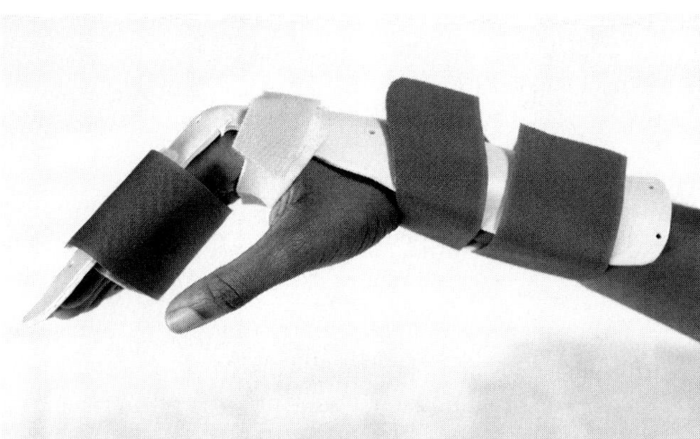

FIGURE 19-2. Dorsal blocking orthosis used when treating a flexion tendon repair.

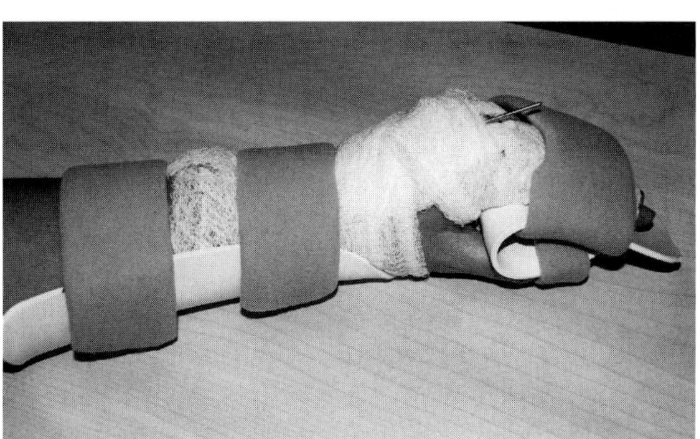

FIGURE 19-3. Custom orthosis molded around bandages and/or pins.

Nerve Compression

Nerve compression injuries, such as carpal tunnel syndrome and cubital tunnel syndrome, require orthotic positioning to relieve pressure on the affected nerve. Studies measuring the amount of pressure in the carpal tunnel show less pressure with the wrist in zero degrees, with pressures increasing as the wrist is flexed or extended.[9] Therefore, a custom orthosis is effective in minimizing the pressure within the carpal tunnel, thus alleviating symptoms of carpal tunnel syndrome[10] (Fig. 19-4). For non-custom orthoses, the wrist angle is often preset at 20° to 35°, and will likely need to be modified to zero degrees for this diagnosis. Likewise, the position of the elbow affects the level of compression on the ulnar nerve. Splinting the elbow in a resting position that limits elbow flexion past 100° to 110° has been shown to decrease stress on the ulnar nerve at the elbow[11] (Fig. 19-5).

Arthritis

In the treatment of arthritic conditions, such as osteoarthritis, rheumatoid arthritis, gout, and scleroderma, orthoses are used to rest inflamed joints and to position against deformity. Gomes-Carrera et al. in a randomized controlled trial found that use of an orthosis, whatever its design, was effective in decreasing thumb pain when used to support thumb carpometacarpal (CMC) joint osteoarthritis[12] (Fig. 19-6). Reports of randomized controlled trials describing the efficacy of orthosis use with rheumatoid arthritis may be difficult to find. However, clinical experience has shown that use of a functional resting orthosis is effective in decreasing inflammation and joint pain and minimizing joint deformities in individuals with rheumatoid arthritis. During an exacerbation of gout or progression of scleroderma, an orthosis will provide a resting position to decrease pain and inflammation (Fig. 19-7).

Awaiting Functional Return

Using an orthosis as a treatment intervention can help improve hand function and thus improve occupational performance.[14] In the case of an individual with radial nerve palsy, a dynamic wrist and MCP extension orthosis will promote grasp/release and normal movement patterns while awaiting nerve return (Fig. 19-8). For an individual with traumatic finger amputation, an orthosis may be fabricated to replace lost length and be used in preparation for prosthetic training (Fig. 19-9). Likewise, a hand-based thumb orthosis may decrease the tone and facilitate grasp in a client with hypertonicity(Fig. 19-10). In the client who has had a cerebrovascular accident (CVA), spinal cord injury (SCI), or traumatic brain injury (TBI), an orthosis is sometimes used to normalize tone and assist with task modification while awaiting return of

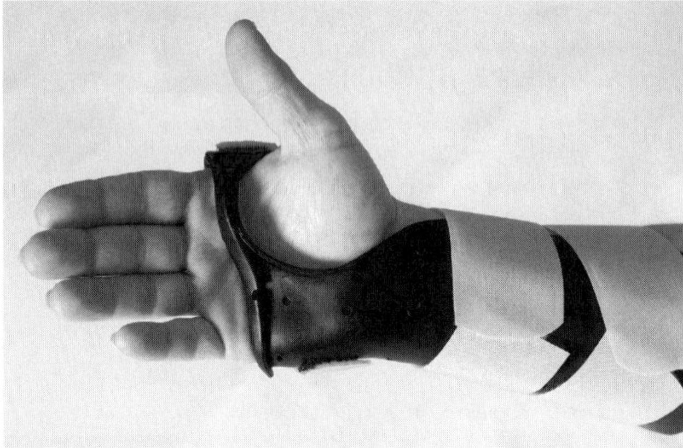

FIGURE 19-4. Volar wrist orthosis used in the treatment of carpal tunnel syndrome.

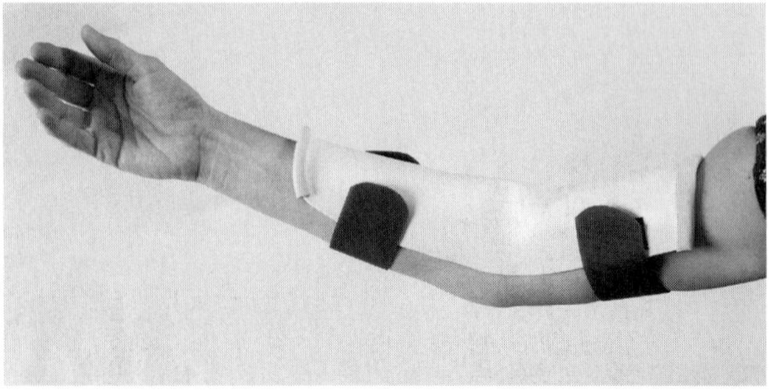

FIGURE 19-5. Elbow positional orthosis used in the treatment of cubital tunnel syndrome.

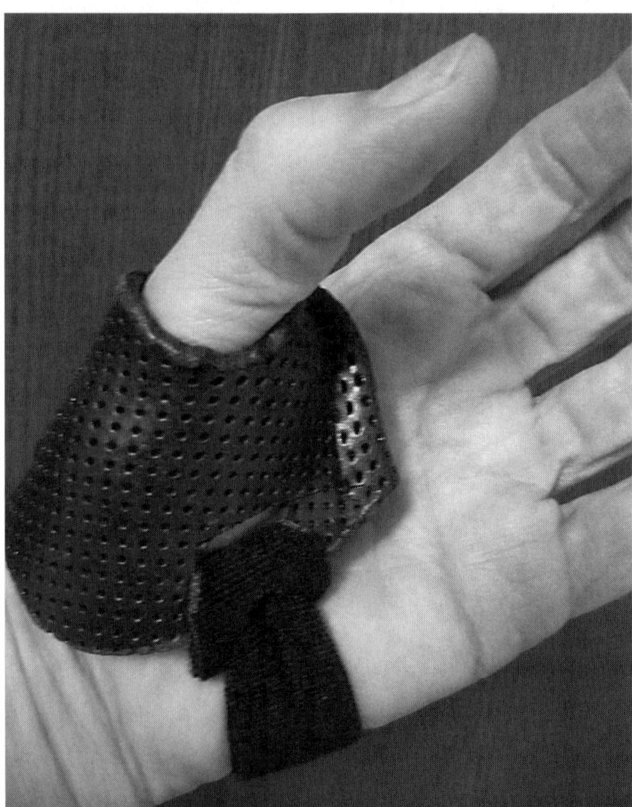

FIGURE 19-6. Custom hand based orthosis used in the treatment of CMC joint osteoarthritis or to support a weakened thumb in the opposition position for pinch.

EVIDENCE-BASED PRACTICE

A research study by Grenier et al.[13] compared three orthoses with differing designs and their effectiveness at improving the functional pinch strength of adults with a diagnosis of thumb CMC joint osteoarthritis. Using a retrospective chart review, the lateral pinch strength of 48 participants was documented, along with the type of orthosis that was issued to the clients. The data was analyzed to determine whether any of the three most common orthotic designs were effective at providing support to the thumb during pinch strength testing. Although a larger sample size is needed, the study concluded that use of an orthosis (of any type) consistently increases the functional pinch strength of individuals with CMC joint osteoarthritis.

Grenier, M-L., Mendonca, R., & Dalley, P. (2016). *The effectiveness of orthoses in the conservative management of thumb CMC joint osteoarthritis: An analysis of functional pinch strength.* Journal of Hand Therapy, 29(3), 307–313.

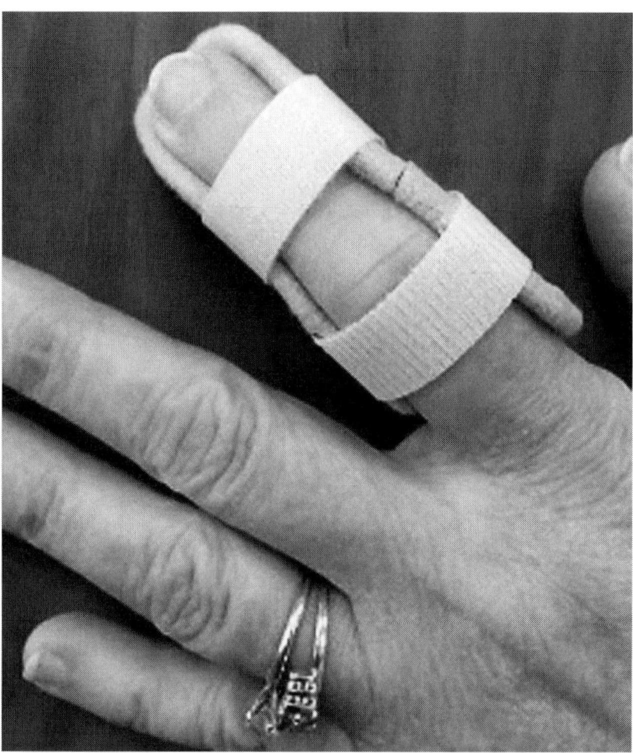

FIGURE 19-7. Finger gutter orthosis.

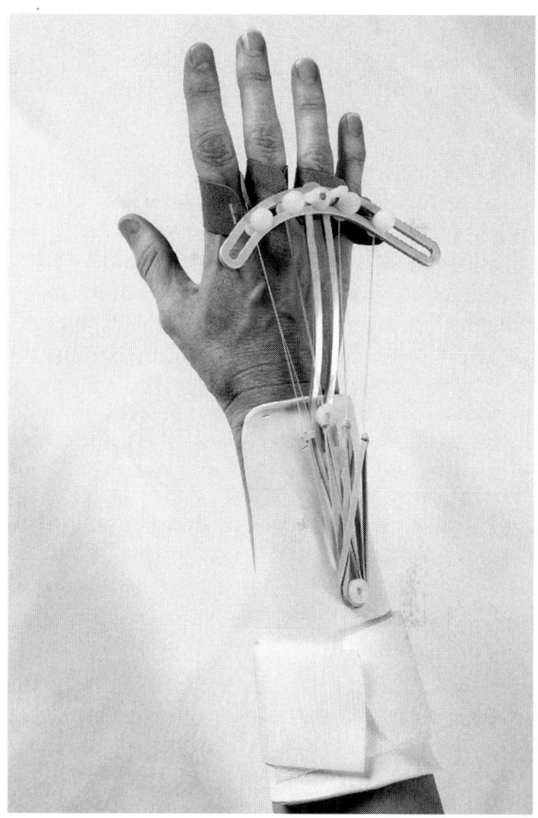

FIGURE 19-8. Dynamic radial nerve palsy orthosis.

upper extremity function. An orthosis is considered assistive technology and is an important part of improving a client's independence with self-care.[15]

USE OF AN ORTHOSIS FOR IMPROVING MOTION

Decreased functional ROM in the upper extremity has the potential to significantly limit a client's occupational performance. A mobilization orthosis may be used to either improve passive motion or compensate for this lack of motion.[16] When considering stiffness that develops in the MCP joints after a metacarpal fracture, an orthosis can be used to help the client gain passive MCP joint flexion to progress with active MCP joint flexion and eventual

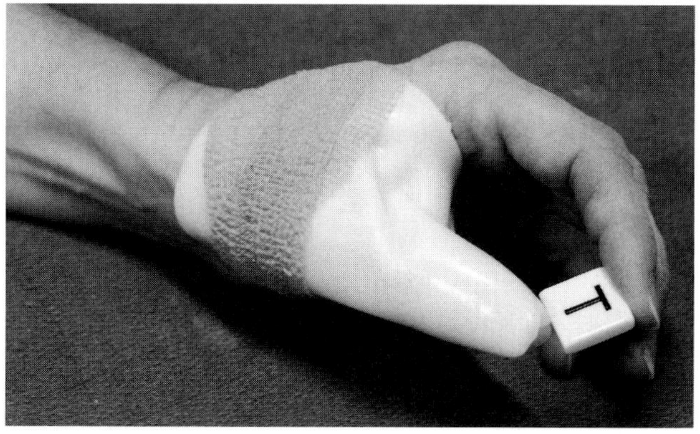

FIGURE 19-9. Thumb post molded to assist with amputation reeducation.

COMMUNICATION

An OT practitioner must obtain a signed order from the physician, or signed plan of care, stating the client's need for a custom-fabricated orthosis. A physician's order is also needed for the insurance to pay for the cost of the orthosis. A client will usually arrive at the first therapy session with a signed order, stating the diagnosis and type of orthosis desired. For example, a client with a radial nerve palsy resulting in wrist drop may have a physician's order that reads: "Occupational therapy for range of motion, strengthening, and to improve functional use of the right wrist and hand, s/p radial nerve palsy from traction injury; dynamic radial nerve palsy orthosis." After the initial evaluation is performed, the plan of care should include orthotic intervention. For the OTA, treatment will then include orthotic fabrication and fitting. However, as the OTA spends time getting to know the client and discusses the treatment plan, the client may become unhappy with the treatment plan. Although the physician's order may clearly state the prescribed orthosis, it is less clear if this is the type of orthosis that the client wants or one that will best suit the client's needs. Consider the following scenario: The client is a 26-year-old male who has just started on a new job. He does not want to have to miss too much work for therapy appointments. He is also self-conscious about his injury and does not want to attract attention to his right wrist and hand. After spending time with the client, the OTA finds that because of its size and bulkiness, the client does not want the dynamic orthosis with the outrigger for extension. The client and the OTA also feel that the client would be more likely to wear an over-the-counter wrist extension brace that is less noticeable. The OTA instructs the client on a home exercise program, and the client agrees to perform active and passive wrist and finger extension exercises at home, with follow-up once weekly. The client is more agreeable to this plan for his treatment.

The OTA must communicate the outcome of this discussion to the occupational therapist and the physician, either through a face-to-face or telephone conversation or via the progress note. The OTA is responsible for this communication and must be able to explain and document why the treatment was changed. This is a typical scenario in OT. As the OTA spends more one-on-one time with the client, the client becomes more relaxed and is able to communicate his or her thoughts and feelings to the OTA. The OTA plays an important role in getting to know the client, and identifying and understanding the client's occupational performance roles and needs. The OTA also plays an important role in advocating for the client and communicating when the treatment goals need to be changed or reevaluated.

gripping (Fig. 19-11). Stiffness that results from scarring after an extensor tendon injury can be addressed with mobilization splinting to improve soft tissue extensibility over the dorsum of the proximal interphalangeal (PIP) joint. With nerve compression injuries and SCI, a mobilization orthosis is helpful in compensating for lost motion (see Fig. 19-9).

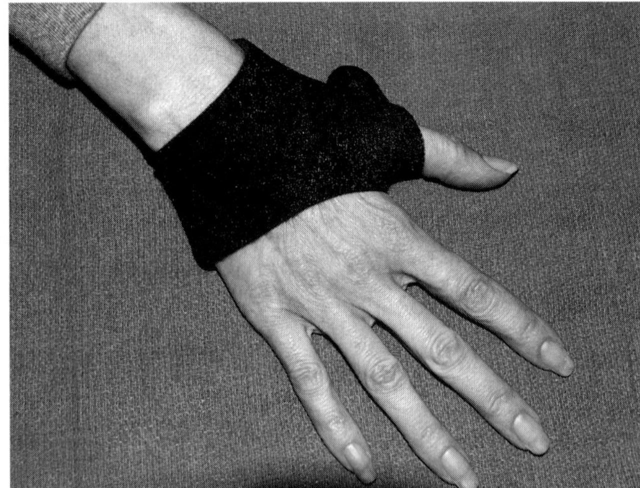

FIGURE 19-10. Neoprene thumb abduction strap.

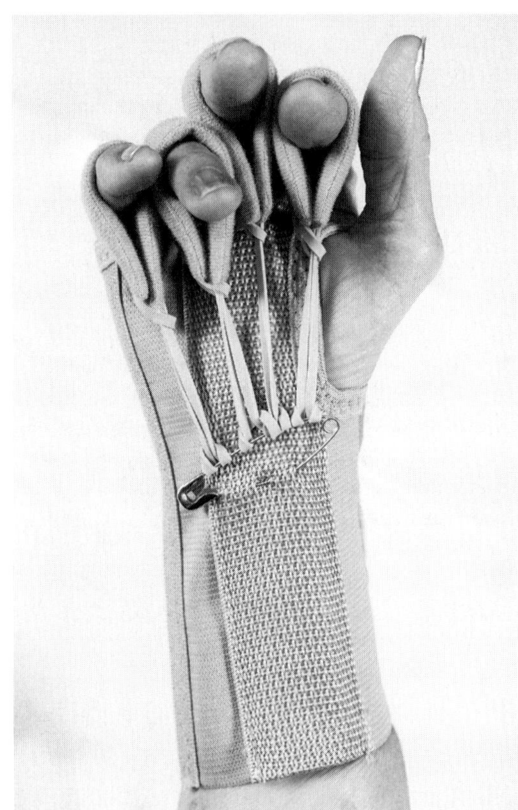

FIGURE 19-11. Dynamic MCP flexion orthosis.

STATIC, STATIC PROGRESSIVE, AND DYNAMIC ORTHOTIC DESIGNS

An orthosis can be classified as **static**, **static progressive**, or **dynamic**. A static orthosis does not have movable parts and is usually designed to protect, restrict motion, and provide proper positioning. A static progressive orthosis is an orthosis that uses inelastic parts to position a joint at the available end ROM with the intent of improving passive range of motion (PROM).[17] A dynamic orthosis has movable or elastic parts and is used to improve motion, provide controlled motion, or compensate for loss of motion.[18] The principles surrounding these different types of orthoses are discussed next.

Static Principles

A static orthosis is used for immobilization, protection, and prevention of deformities. The principles of static orthotic fabrication apply when fabricating and fitting all orthoses because static progressive and dynamic splints use the same orthosis base. The base for a static progressive and dynamic orthosis will be the portion of the orthosis that will be used to support or attach additional components. When fabricating and fitting an orthosis, the OT practitioner must first complete a thorough client assessment, including, but not limited to, ROM, sensation, edema, skin inspection, and hand function. The occupational therapist and occupational therapy assistant (OTA) will also consult each other on the client's potential needs and goals of orthosis application. Several questions must be asked, including the following:

- What is the purpose for the orthosis?
- What anatomical structures are involved?
- How can the orthosis be applied to achieve the best client outcomes?

Even with the application of a static orthosis, such as a resting hand orthosis, an external force is applied to the upper extremity; therefore, the principles of force, pressure, and friction should be considered.[1] As the orthosis is fabricated, it should be kept in mind that a more stable fit is the result of an orthosis base that is three fourths the length of the client's forearm and over one half up the sides of the client's hand or forearm.[16] For fractures, one joint above and one joint below the injury should be stabilized to restrict motion at the injured joint. Areas that may cause too much pressure against the client's skin should be avoided and padding placed at bony prominences to reduce irritation. Padding should be applied before molding the orthosis to ensure proper fit. Adding extra padding to a bony spot after molding will likely only increase pressure to that area. Edges should be smooth and rolled to avoid skin irritation. Strapping should be wide enough to distribute even pressure, slightly angled to avoid a tourniquet effect, and should not restrict motion.

Static Progressive Principles

A static progressive orthosis is used for decreasing joint stiffness and, as reported in the literature, is effective in improving PROM.[17] Based on the physiology of tissue healing, a static progressive orthosis provides a low-load prolonged stretch, which is required for promoting tissue regrowth. Static progressive orthoses use a static base with the addition of inelastic components, which, when applied to the orthosis, assist in holding tissues in a pain-free lengthened position (Fig. 19-12). The tension on the orthosis is increased as the client's tolerance and tissue elasticity improve.[19] Static progressive splinting is now considered more advantageous compared with dynamic splinting for improving ROM.[17]

Dynamic Principles

A dynamic orthosis, also known as mobilization orthosis, is used to improve motion, provide controlled motion, or compensate for loss of motion.[20] A dynamic orthosis uses a

OT Practitioner's Viewpoint

My first client of the morning, Jason, was an 18-year-old male, who had a boxer's fracture to the left small finger. This is a common injury in young males, as it occurs when the small finger metacarpal is fractured because of impact from a closed fist, such as a punch. Jason had a custom orthosis that had been issued for protection. He was wearing the orthosis between exercise sessions and at night to protect his healing fracture. Progress had been made with the AROM in his fingers; however, he still had some stiffness in the MCP joint of his small finger. At his treatment session this morning, we would upgrade his treatment plan to include PROM exercises. After the application of moist heat for 15 minutes, I began applying gentle overpressure to the MCP joint of the small finger into flexion, until Jason reported a stretching sensation. After the stretching, Jason's PROM into flexion improved by five degrees; however, his AROM, the ability to make a fist, was not improving. It appeared that Jason was compensating for his stiffness in the MCP joint of the small finger by increasing the flexion in the PIP and distal interphalangeal (DIP) joints of that finger. At that point, I decided that Jason had to "remember" what bending the MCP joint actually felt like. Therefore, I held the small finger MCP in the flexed position while I instructed Jason to make a fist. This assistance improved Jason's ability to make a fist. I thought, "How can I carry this motor retraining over to his home program?" I decided to use the static protective orthosis as a base to attach gentle dynamic flexion traction to the MCP joint of the small finger. I used a finger loop and a rubber band to make a sling for the small finger that I secured to the splint with Velcro®. Jason was then instructed to apply the finger loop with the traction to the small finger for 15 to 20 minutes four times daily and when performing his fisting exercises. At this point in the treatment, the static, protective orthosis became a dynamic orthosis, used to gain passive motion. Jason returned to therapy several days later and had improved ROM measurements in the flexion of the small finger MCP joint, as well as improved composite finger flexion. As the treatment plan changed, so did the orthosis. The static orthosis could be used as a base for a dynamic component to further improve Jason's ROM. After Jason's ROM and strength improved, he was discharged from therapy with the following instructions: "Next time you become angry, punch a pillow!" ~Karol Spraggs-Young, OTD, OTR/L, CHT

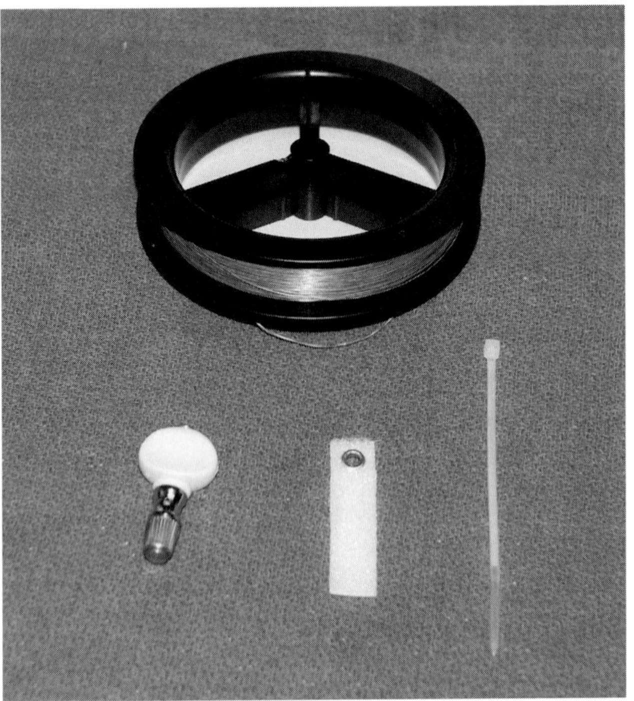

FIGURE 19-12. Static progressive components. *At top*: monofilament, *from bottom left*: guitar tuner, Velcro® loop strip, and zip tie.

static base in which dynamic or elastic components are applied (Fig. 19-13). These components provide continuous tension. When fabricating and fitting a dynamic orthosis, the principles of biomechanics, rotation, torque, and parallel forces should be considered.[18] A dynamic orthosis requires a solid base with an outrigger that provides the structure for the mobilization force. Outriggers can either be high profile or low profile, ensuring that mobilization forces are 90 degrees to the long axis of the joint. High-profile outriggers are attached to the orthosis; however, they are designed to come up and away from the splint to ensure the proper angle of pull during mobilization. Low-profile outriggers also ensure the proper angle of pull; however, they tend to be smaller and are designed to be more streamlined. Outriggers require monitoring and adjusting by the OT practitioner to ensure the proper alignment of pull. The orthosis should be checked at each therapy appointment to find out if gains are made in ROM and if the client has any complaints of discomfort. Although low-profile outriggers are more aesthetically pleasing, they will require more frequent adjustment because they may not be able to maintain the proper angle of pull once changes in ROM are made. The amount of force used in a dynamic orthosis should be sufficient to achieve the goals of mobilization while being comfortable and tolerable to the client.

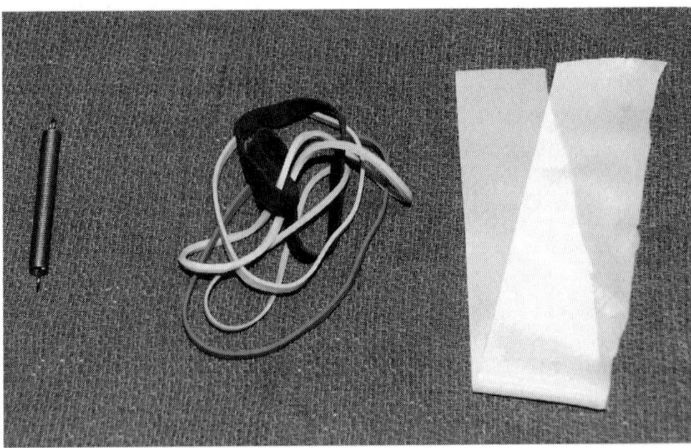

FIGURE 19-13. Dynamic components. *From left*: spring tensioner, rubber bands, and strip of resistive exercise band.

ORTHOTIC DESIGN

In reference to orthotic fitting, the hand surgeon Paul Brand wrote: "We must first realize that a splint, by its very presence on the hand, is doing harm. It is inhibiting the free movement and use of the hand. It is justified only if the specific good that it will do compensates for the general harm and restriction."[21] With this in mind, the OT practitioner must understand the effect that the use of an orthosis has on clients. He or she must consider the principles of construction as well as the needs of the client and the role an orthosis will play in treatment and everyday function.

Form and Function

One way to assess the need for an orthosis is to consider form and function. What form will the orthosis take, and what will be its function? Will the orthosis assist with engagement in functional activities, including the participation in work, leisure, and self-care tasks? The OT practitioner will need to ask the following questions:

1. What is the goal of the orthosis?
2. What does the physician prescription indicate?
3. What is the client's diagnosis?
4. What structures need to be included?
5. What structures do not need to be included?
6. Will the orthosis be static, static progressive, or dynamic?
7. How often will the client wear the orthosis?
8. How long will the client need to use the orthosis?
9. Will the client be able to don the orthosis independently?
10. What is the most cost effective way to achieve the goals?

An orthosis should be comfortable and convenient to use. Although the order for an orthosis comes from a physician and is dependent on the diagnosis, the design should also include input from the client because it is the client who will be using the orthosis. Will the orthosis make the client self-conscious and, therefore, lead to rejection of the orthosis? If an orthosis is not comfortable, not pleasing to the client, or not meeting the client's needs, it will not be used. The conceptual map and table of common orthoses will assist in decision making regarding orthosis design and fabrication (Fig. 19-14).

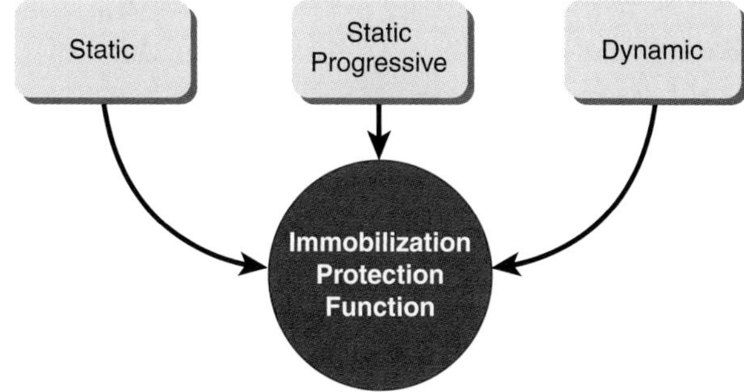

FIGURE 19-14. Concept map.

Precautions and Contraindications

As with all therapeutic interventions, some precautions are involved in orthotic design and application. The client must have sensate skin and be able to perform self-inspection of skin or have a caregiver who can perform skin inspection to identify potential pressure areas, rashes, or numbness caused by the orthosis. The client must be able to attend routine reassessments so that the OT practitioner can ensure progress, monitor or change wearing schedules, and provide adjustments to the orthosis. Edema may be a problem and may require changes in orthosis design and strapping. Contraindications to orthotic use include poor skin integrity, decreased cognitive status, undiagnosed joint instability, pain, and the client's unwillingness to accept responsibility for the use of the orthosis. Age of the client and diagnoses must also be considered. The older client with diabetes and dementia may not be able to remember how to apply the orthosis correctly or may be unable to see well enough to be able to secure the strapping. A younger client with cerebral palsy may not be able to report pain or difficulties with an orthosis and will require a parent or caregiver to assist.[1] If the client is unable to care for himself or herself and requires the assistance of a caregiver, the caregiver should be present during fitting, education, and training. The caregiver must also demonstrate an understanding of the use of the orthosis and be willing to accept responsibility and assist in the application and monitoring of the orthosis. Caregivers in acute and subacute facilities should be educated in the application and monitoring of orthotics. Routine in-services to nursing staff can educate the staff on the purpose of orthosis use and provide helpful hints, such as inhibiting tone before orthosis application. Instructions regarding the use of the orthosis, pictures, and wearing schedules should be placed on the client's chart and potentially in the client's room. The orthosis and straps should be labeled (top, bottom, right, left, and so on), and the rehabilitation department should identify an OT practitioner who can be the contact person should problems arise with orthosis use.

Client Education Regarding Wear and Care

Improper use of an orthosis can result in negative outcomes, including skin breakdown and progressive worsening of joint stiffness. Therefore, it is important that the client understands the rationale behind orthosis use and its significance. The client must agree to the proposed wearing schedule and be able to contact the OT practitioner should problems or questions arise. A client education handout should be provided to the client at their level of health literacy and include instructions on the orthosis wearing schedule, how to care for the orthosis, and how to monitor for skin irritation. A thermoplastic orthosis should not be exposed to a heat source, including the dashboard or seat of a car on a sunny or warm day, because the orthosis will lose its shape. A picture of the client wearing the orthosis can be used as a client education tool. An example of a client education handout is provided in Figure 19-15.

OLDER ADULT

Fabricating and fitting an orthosis for the older adult requires a few additional considerations. The older adult may have arthritic changes, previous injuries, or comorbidities that may require extra care. For example, the older adult who has been referred for a positional night orthosis for rheumatoid arthritis may have an ulnar drift deformity that has been present for years and will be difficult to correct passively. The OT practitioner may only be able to position the hand in comfort and not be able to correct the deformity. This same client may also have peripheral neuropathy with sensory impairment, which will determine the need for a structured wearing schedule with frequent skin checks. Because of age related changes, such as thinning skin, the older adult may often benefit from a softer, prefabricated orthosis, which puts less pressure on the skin, thus avoiding pressure areas or breakdown. When using an orthosis in the skilled nursing setting, the staff and family members must be instructed and demonstrate competency in proper donning or doffing of an orthosis. The OT practitioner is responsible for educating the staff and should assist with developing strategies for caregiver and staff education.

ORTHOTIC CONSTRUCTION

It is best to begin orthotic construction with a pattern. A pattern will assist with a proper fit and ensure that costly material is not wasted. To create the pattern, the involved portion of the extremity is traced, making note of important structures, such as the distal palmar crease, thumb web space, and any anatomical landmarks that will aid in proper fit and design. If the involved extremity cannot be traced, the extremity on the opposite side can be used. Once the extremity has been traced, a quarter to half inch is added around the perimeter of the tracing, for an average-size hand and forearm, and the pattern is cut out. If the client has a larger-than-average hand and forearm, more than a quarter to half inch increase may have to be added to the base pattern. The pattern is then placed on the client and the OT practitioner makes note of any areas that should be

How to Wear and Care for Your Orthotic

The following instructions explain how to wear and care for your orthotic. This orthotic was custom made for you.

When to wear your orthotic (check one)

- ☐ Always wear your orthotic. Removing it may cause damage to the injured area.
- ☐ Wear your orthotic except to exercise and bathe.
- ☐ Wear your orthotic at night and during rest periods only.
- ☐ Wear your orthotic during the daytime only.

Other:

Cleaning your orthotic

- Clean the orthotic with soap and lukewarm water; scrub it with a small brush.
- Rub the inside of the orthotic with alcohol to reduce odor.
- Hand wash the Velcro straps and stockinette with lukewarm, soapy water and then air dry.

Precautions

- Keep away from open flames because it will burn.
- Keep your orthotic away from heat, prolonged sunlight, or water heaters.

If your orthotic causes any of these problems, remove it and call your therapist right away.

- Swelling
- Excessive stiffness, numbness, or pain
- An area of pressure, such as red marks or sores, that remain one hour after removing the orthotic
- Blisters

Talk to your doctor or others on your health care team if you have questions.

FIGURE 19-15. Example of client education handout.

increased or decreased to ensure proper fit. It is important to remember that for proper fit, the orthosis should cover approximately two-thirds the length of the extremity and one half the circumference of the extremity.

The pattern is traced onto the thermoplastic material with either a wax pencil or a scratch awl. A pen may also be used for tracing onto thermoplastic material; however, the tracing will need to be removed with rubbing alcohol before heating the material. The thermoplastic material is slightly warmed by placing it in a splint pan filled with hot water, according to the manufacturer's specifications for the thermoplastic material (temperature and time) that will be used (usually between 155° F and 205° F); then, the material is removed and scissors are used to cut out the shape of the orthosis.

A piece of stockinette is placed on the client's affected side and the client is placed in a position that will allow gravity to assist with draping the orthosis. For example, when making a volar wrist orthosis, the forearm is positioned palm upward. The thermoplastic material is heated, according to the manufacturer's directions, quickly dried off (a pillow case works well and does not leave lint or an indentation like towels and washcloths may), and then applied to the client. A light touch with soft, repetitive strokes is used to mold the thermoplastic material, making sure to avoid leaving fingerprints and unnecessary areas of pressure.

When the orthosis has cooled sufficiently, it is removed from the client, and the finishing touches, which should include rolling and smoothing edges and applying straps, are completed. Rolling edges can be achieved by dipping the edges in the splint pan filled with hot water or by spot-heating with a heat gun. Smoothing the edges is achieved by placing the edges of the orthosis in hot water in the splint pan and then removing the orthosis and using the heel of the hand with a stroking motion to apply even pressure to the edges. To double-check, the OT practitioner should glide his or her finger around all the edges of the orthotic to check for sharp or rough spots, which can cause skin irritation or snag on clothing or other objects. For an orthosis that will require a static progressive or dynamic component, these components should be added, as discussed in the principles above. The orthosis should fit well, be comfortable for the client, and cosmetically appealing. The key to success with orthotic fabrication is practice, practice, practice. For helpful hints see Box 19-2.

Tools for the Clinic

Some essential tools are required for success with orthotic fabrication. Towels, pillowcases, a wax pencil or scratch awl, and a splint pan set at 155° F to 205° F will be needed for heating most thermoplastic materials.[22] If the clinic does not have a splint pan, a large electric nonstick frying pan is an inexpensive and portable substitute; however, caution must be exercised to ensure that the temperature remains constant and does not exceed the manufacturer's guidelines. A utility knife will assist in cutting cold thermoplastic material. A cutting mat should be placed on the countertop so that it does not get damaged by multiple cuts. Flat-edge scissors will provide a smooth edge for cutting warm material, and curved edge scissors will facilitate cutting out contours. A solvent, acetone, or a scratch awl is used to remove coating and allow the thermoplastic material to adhere to itself. A heat gun will help spot-heat the thermoplastic material for finishing and minor adjustments. Great care must be taken with use of the heat gun to avoid melting or burning the

BOX 19-2
Helpful Orthosis Fabrication Hints

*Remember form follows function and that function follows form: What is the goal of an orthosis?

- What is the client's diagnosis?
- Is the orthosis intended to immobilize, protect, facilitate motion, or compensate for lost function?
- What joints should the orthosis cross/immobilize? What joint should be free to move?
- What structures need to be avoided or protected? (pins, wounds, edema)
- What is the safe position and can the client be placed in the safe position?
- Can the client don and doff the orthosis independently?
- What type of material is best for the intended design?

ORTHOTIC MATERIALS

Thermoplastic or soft neoprene materials

- Custom fabricated versus prefabricated
- Thermoplastic properties, such as drape, memory, thickness, and perforation (colors/patterns)
- Drape: Higher drape conforms more easily to contours; less is better for larger joints; more memory means material is more forgiving and easy to reheat
- Thickness: Dependent on needed rigidity and durability
- Strapping materials: Velcro®, padding, neoprene, thickness, elasticity, width, and durability

PATTERNS

- Paper towels make great orthosis patterns.
- X-ray film is also a good template for frequently made orthoses.
- Decide if precut patterns are right for your clinic.

ORTHOTIC DESIGN PEARLS

- Always have a layer of stockinette between the client's skin and hot thermoplastic material.
- Pad bony prominences before molding.
- Issue additional stockinette for daily changes.
- Place the extremity in a gravity-assisted position while molding thermoplastic material.
- For larger joints. such as the elbow, use a compressive wrap to secure the material as it cools.
- Do not press with a heavy hand; rather, gently milk the material to mold to contours.
- Use heel of hand and warm water to smooth edges and flare at the proximal edge to prevent pressure on the forearm.
- Use heat gun and solvent to adhere material together.
- Consider noncoated material if bonding of material is needed.
- Have the client sign a form indicating that he or she received the orthosis and understands that there will be a charge for a replacement.
- Issue an orthosis wear/care information sheet that includes information on cleaning and a wearing schedule.
- When in doubt, contact the physician, or obtain operative/office notes to ensure need for immobilization or protection of structures.

material or burning one's hands on overheated material. The heat gun will also come in handy when heating the sticky back portion of the hook Velcro®, which ensures that the hook will stay put after repeated use. A hole punch, pliers, and a kit with dynamic and static progressive components are also recommended (Fig. 19-16).

Properties of Thermoplastic Materials

A wide variety of thermoplastic materials are available for use with orthotic fabrication. Thicknesses range from 1/16 inch to 1/8 inch, with thinner materials used for finger orthotics or arthritic conditions and thicker materials for larger joints or when more stability is required. Materials can be purchased by the sheet or case and come in various sizes and colors (Fig. 19-17). Perforated materials have become popular because they offer a lighter weight alternative and afford increased comfort to skin. Terms often used to describe the properties of thermoplastic materials are drape, memory, rigidity, and adherence.[18] **Drape** refers to the ability of the material to conform to structures (when heated) without too much handling. A material with the ability to drape is beneficial for smaller joints or when a specific position or contour is required. Materials with high drape may be difficult for the beginning OT practitioner to use because they require a light touch and must be handled gently. **Memory** is the ability of the thermoplastic material to return to its original shape once reheated. Materials with a high degree of memory require continuous coaxing while molding; however, they are frequently used for larger orthoses because they are easier to handle. **Rigidity** refers to the strength of the material when exposed to repeated stress. Materials that offer rigidity are beneficial for an orthosis that will require long-term use or for those that support multiple or larger joints. **Adherence** is the ability of the material to bond to itself. Adherence becomes important when reinforcing an orthosis or adding components to an orthosis.[23] In the case of materials that are self-bonding, the

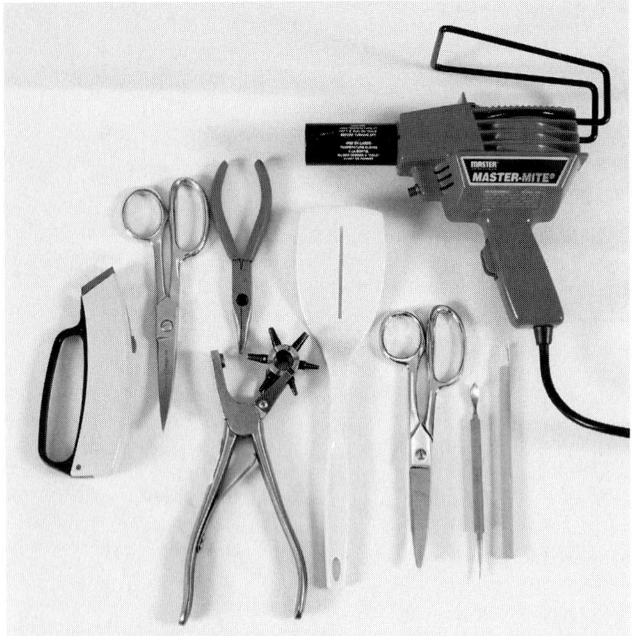

FIGURE 19-16. Tools used in the clinic. *From left*: Box cutter, curved scissors, pliers, hole punch, spatula, straight scissors, scratch awl, wax pencil, and heat gun.

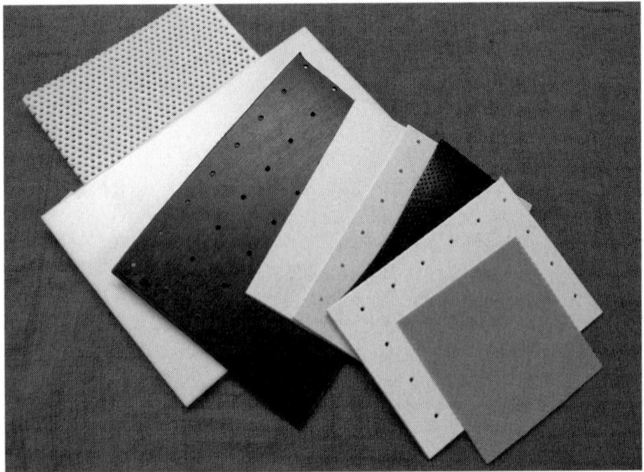

FIGURE 19-17. Thermoplastic materials.

material should be dry, spot-heated with the heat gun (both pieces), and then held or pinched together with pressure. Conversely, materials that are not self-bonding have a coating to prevent the material from sticking to itself by accident during fabrication. For bonding these materials, the coating should be removed with either acetone and/or a scratch awl before spot heating and then the material pressed firmly to achieve bonding.[23] Companies that sell the thermoplastic material provide valuable information regarding the properties of their products through their websites.

Properties of Strapping Materials

Strapping materials come in a wide variety of sizes, widths, textures, and colors. Strapping is an important part of orthotic design because it secures the orthosis in place and provides stability and additional positioning to the digit or extremity (Fig. 19-18). Velcro® strapping comes as hook and loop and is available with adhesive backing, as needed, for easy application. The hook (rough) should be used on the orthosis, and the loop (soft) should be used as strapping. Since the loop is made of softer material, it should be used against the skin or whenever the OT practitioner is concerned about the integrity of the client's skin. It is recommended that the adhesive backing of the hook be cut with slightly rounded edges and be spot-heated with a heat gun before placement on the orthosis so that it stays in place. Wide strapping is used to distribute even pressure over the forearm, and narrow strapping is used on fingers and in the palm of the hand. Strapping that is too narrow may cause areas of pressure and may increase localized edema. Circumferential strapping (wrapping to encompass splint and limb from distal to proximal with an elastic wrap) may aid in edema reduction because it distributes pressure more evenly over the surface of skin. Straps made from elastic and neoprene give added pressure and may be used to secure a small orthosis or to secure an orthosis that is difficult to keep in place. Elastic and neoprene straps also provide overpressure and support, when needed, and are often used in a thumb orthosis for CMC joint osteoarthritis. If losing the straps is a concern, one end of the strap can be riveted to the orthosis. The straps and orthosis may also be labeled to prevent loss and to ensure proper positioning and placement.

CASTING

Casting is commonly used for positioning and protection after fractures; however, casting is beneficial for a variety of other conditions as well. Casting, or the application of a plaster cast to a joint on stretch, promotes tissue growth and elongation and has been shown to inhibit spasticity.[24] Casting has been used by OT practitioners in both the neuro-rehabilitation and orthopedic settings to improve PROM, and is often called **serial casting** due to the common application, removal, and reapplication of a series of

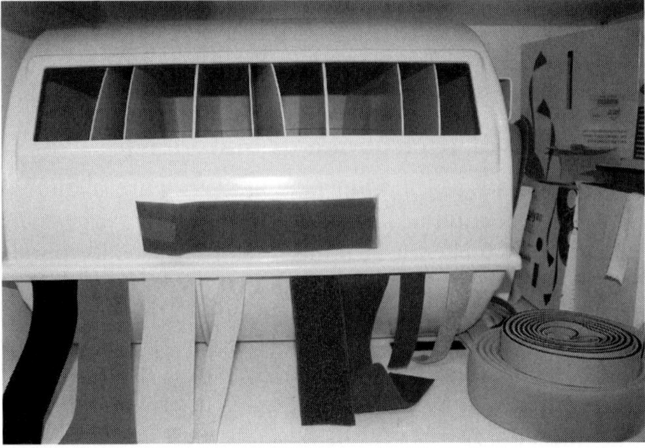

FIGURE 19-18. Strapping materials.

casts. Applying a cast to a stiff joint or tight soft tissue structure assists with stretching these structures over a period of time. The ultimate goal of using casting to gain motion is improvement in the client's function. Although the casting process may appear to be the same in neurological and orthopedic clients, the theory and structures that are targeted are different. The next section discusses casting for the neurological client (tone) and casting for the orthopedic client (joint contracture).

Casting to Decrease Tone: The Client With a Neurological Condition

Individuals with neurological impairments, such as SCI, TBI, CVA, or cerebral palsy may sustain damage to the motor cortex resulting in spasticity or an increase in muscle tone in the upper extremity.[25] In these individuals, casting is used as a treatment intervention to inhibit tone by holding the muscles in a lengthening position. A systematic review of the literature has suggested that serial casting may be an effective treatment approach for clients with neurological impairments;[26] however, additional studies are needed to document the efficacy of this approach used in the upper extremity. At times, the physician will also use botulinum toxin (Botox®) in conjunction with serial casting to gain additional muscle length and reduce tone.[27] The physician administers Botox® injections, and the cast is applied after the Botox® has taken effect to relax the muscles. When casting for tone, an initial assessment should include documentation of active range of motion (AROM), PROM, circulation, and skin integrity.

To fabricate a cast, a stockinette is first applied to the extremity and the bony prominences are padded. The cast padding is applied, followed by plaster or fiberglass cast material, while holding the upper extremity in a stretched position as the cast material dries. The OT practitioner should check skin and circulation regularly because the client with the neurological condition may not be able to alert the OT practitioner about problems. Casts may be applied, removed, and reapplied, as the client's ROM improves. Each successive cast is ideally created with the upper extremity in an increased ROM. It is important to note that serial casting is not effective where bony restrictions are present. Heterotopic ossification (HO), or deposits of extra-articular bone at the elbow, is a common cause of elbow stiffness in the client with neurological dysfunction. Aggressive treatment for HO is not recommended, and therefore, casting may not be effective for the client with HO.[28]

Casting to Decrease Joint Stiffness: The Client With an Orthopedic Condition

Paul Brand first used serial casting to correct the deformities caused by clubfoot in children, and because of the beneficial effects observed, Brand and the occupational therapists at the United States Public Health Service Hospital in New Orleans began using serial casting to improve functional ROM in the hand.[24] Based on the principles of tissue growth and elongation, serial casting is still used today and offers positive results for clients with joint contractures caused by soft tissue or capsular tightness in the upper extremity. It must be kept in mind that serial casting is not effective where bony restrictions are present; therefore, before casting, the physician should rule out structural limitations by using radiography. For serial casting of a stiff joint in the hand, such as the PIP joint, an initial evaluation with ROM measurements is performed. The client's skin integrity, sensation, and circulation should also be assessed. The cast material (plaster or fiberglass) is applied directly to the client's skin to avoid friction or shear forces in the smaller joints. Padding may be placed over bony prominences to avoid areas of pressure. Approximately two layers of 2.5-cm-wide plaster are applied to the finger, and the stiff PIP joint is then held in pain-free end ROM of elongation (Fig. 19-19). The cast is changed every 2 to 3 days to allow for decrease in swelling and changes in ROM.[1] Depending on the diagnosis, exercises may be performed between cast changes. The client is instructed on how to check for circulation and care of the cast. The plaster cast is easy to remove with water soaks and bandage scissors and may be removed at home should problems arise. Cylindrical casting to the PIP is also known for decreasing edema; after the initial application of a finger cast, the client may need to return to the clinic sooner because the cast may slip off as edema decreases. Once the ROM goals have been met through the process of casting, the client may benefit from wearing a cast or orthosis at night to prevent tissue tightness. Recent advances in materials have provided the option of casting tape, which may be lighter weight and easier to change.

In the **casting motion to mobilize stiffness (CMMS)** technique, casting is used to immobilize some joints while encouraging a specific motion to regain motion in the stiff hand. The CMMS technique uses plaster casting to immobilize proximal and distal joints to facilitate transfer of power and to promote motor relearning of specific motions.[29] The client is immobilized in an exact position and encouraged to perform specific active motions within the immobilization cast (Fig. 19-20). Through immobilization of some joints and the performance of isolated active motion, new motor

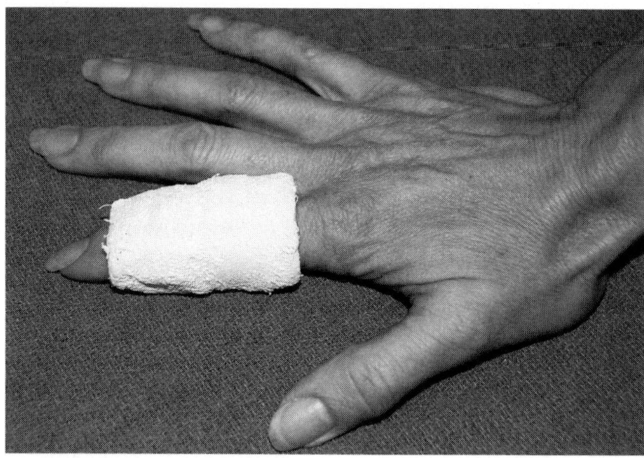

FIGURE 19-19. Casted finger.

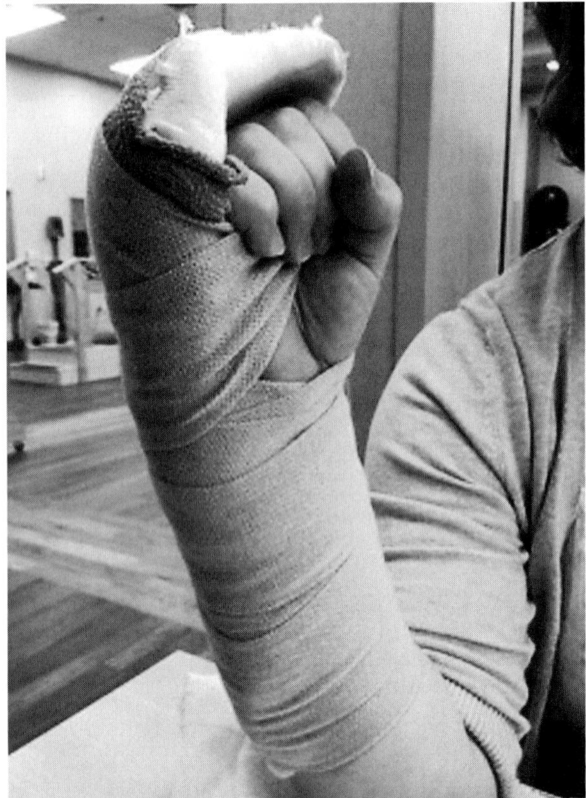

FIGURE 19-20. Hand that has been casted to improve motion.

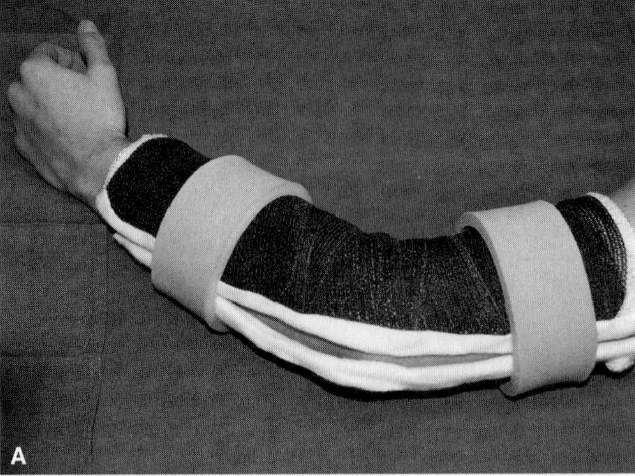

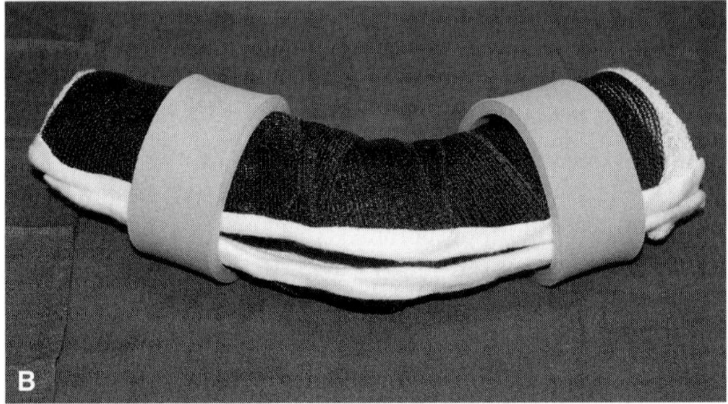

FIGURE 19-21. Bivalved cast. A. Worn by client. B. Cast removed.

patterns are emphasized. The cast is worn from 4 to 8 weeks and changed, as needed, to adjust for fit or ROM gains. The cast is eventually bivalved or cut on both sides for easy removal. The cut sides of the cast are covered in medical tape to avoid sharp edges, the bivalved cast is then wrapped in place on the limb, and the client is slowly weaned from the positional cast. The client is instructed to remove the cast for 1 to 2 hours daily and then increase the time out of the cast until the cast is no longer needed. The weaning process is continued as long as the client is able to maintain the ROM goals that have been achieved with use of the cast (Fig. 19-21).[30] Although the concept of using casting is not new, the idea of using immobilization to produce motion is a relatively new concept. The CMMS technique requires complete understanding of the anatomy and physiology of the upper extremity, and the technique should only be used by a skilled practitioner with experience in application of plaster casts. Clinical evidence supports the efficacy of CMMS in improving motion in the stiff hand, but further research on the benefits of CMMS is needed.[31] However, the author of this chapter has used the CMMS technique with success to treat clients with a stiff wrist and hand.

APPLICATIONS FOR A SOFT ORTHOSIS

A soft orthosis, one made of fabric, neoprene, Velcro®, or strapping, is an excellent alternative for the client who is unable to tolerate a more rigid custom orthosis. A soft orthosis may be purchased through a catalog or a local pharmacy or may be custom made by the OT practitioner. Many have a rigid, yet adjustable center stay (often a metal bar) in the soft orthosis for increased positional choices, especially if the client's ROM is changing. The use of a soft orthosis has been found to be helpful for individuals with arthritis, those with poor skin integrity, and children.[32] Athletes and workers have used soft orthoses beneath work gloves and in sports to achieve protection and stability for the hand as well as increase in functional use. A soft orthosis may be used to treat carpal tunnel syndrome, cubital tunnel syndrome, de Quervain's tendonitis, lateral epicondylitis, rheumatoid arthritis, osteoarthritis, and joint instabilities[33] (Fig. 19-22). Clients with progressive disorders, such as multiple sclerosis or amyotrophic lateral sclerosis, may need the soft orthosis with adjustability to meet their needs for positioning over time. Like a thermoplastic orthosis, application of a soft orthosis will be dependent on the client's diagnosis and will follow the guiding principles of orthotic design; taking into account the client's functional needs and the anatomy and physiology of the upper extremity.

BILLING CODES FOR ORTHOTIC APPLICATION

In the United States, the Healthcare Common Procedure Coding System (HCPCS) codes are assigned to the services a medical practitioner performs and are used to ensure uniformity

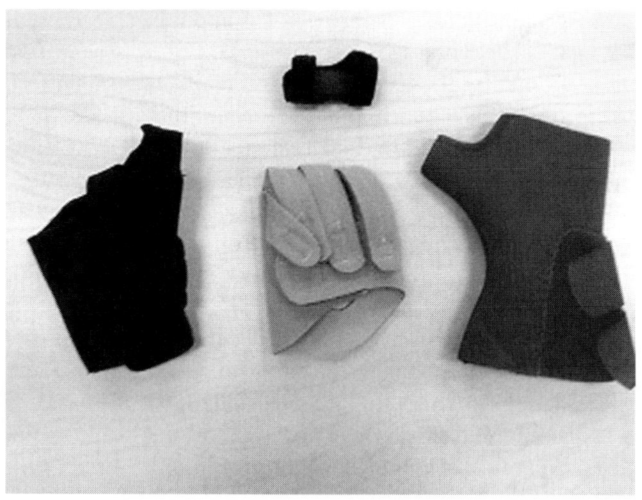

FIGURE 19-22. Variety of soft, over-the-counter orthoses.

in billing. Current Procedural Terminology (CPT) codes are used to bill for "orthotic fabrication and fitting," and "L" codes are used to bill for a custom molded orthosis.[34] The HCPCS "L" codes are inclusive of a practitioner's assessment time, fabrication time, materials, teaching of donning and doffing, and providing instruction in orthosis use. Using a specific "L" code distinguishes between a static orthosis and a dynamic or static progressive orthosis and categorizes an orthosis by the joint it crosses or supports. A static orthosis is considered "not having joints," and a dynamic or static progressive is referred to as having "nontorsion joints, elastic bands, or turnbuckles." The following terms are also used in reference to orthoses: **prefabricated (P/F), off the shelf (OTS),** and **custom fabricated (C/F).** For example, a C/F wrist-hand-finger orthosis (WHFO) is billed as "L3808." For a complete list of "L" codes, see the CMS website or refer to the L-Code section of the ASHT website. Currently, in the United States, Medicare requires a Durable Medical Equipment Prosthetics, Orthotics, and Supplies (DMEPOS) supplier number to bill an "L" code; however, private insurance does not.[35] Before submitting any charges for orthotic fabrication and fitting, the OT practitioner should refer to the policies and procedures for his or her facility and the regulations for the state where he or she practices.

In Canada, an orthosis must be prescribed by a physician and provided through an authorized vendor. For those requiring long-term use of an orthosis, an application and prior approval are required through the governmental agency. For more information regarding reimbursement and billing practices in each Canadian province, see the appropriate website.

INSTRUCTIONS FOR MAKING ORTHOSES

Three orthoses commonly used in OT treatment are the **resting hand orthosis,** the **volar wrist orthosis,** and the **thumb spica orthosis.** The following section describes the fabrication of each type. For a quick reference of orthosis type according to diagnosis, see Table 19-1.

Resting Hand Orthosis

A resting hand orthosis is used to immobilize or position the wrist, fingers, and thumb in a functional position. Clients diagnosed with arthritis, burns, fractures, and trauma can benefit from the use of a resting hand orthosis. The position of the client's wrist and fingers will be dependent on the client's diagnosis and the physician's order. The typical position of the wrist should be between 20 and 40 degrees of wrist extension, with MCP joints at 30° to 70° of flexion and IP joints extended. This position of the fingers is frequently called the *safe position* or the *intrinsic plus position* because it allows the structures in the hand to rest in an elongated position and helps avoid joint contracture or deformity. The thumb is placed in the neutral position, which is 45 degrees of palmar abduction or perpendicular to the tip of the index finger as if holding an object. A resting hand orthosis is applied after an acute injury, trauma, or flare-up

TABLE 19-1 Types of Orthotics Used According to Diagnosis

NAME OF ORTHOSIS	DIAGNOSIS
Resting hand (also called *safe position, resting pan*) can be fixed or movable	Fixed: Arthritis, CVA, burns, traumatic brain injury, trauma Movable: Progressive or changing conditions
Volar wrist (also called *wrist cock up, wrist immobilization*)	Nerve compression wrist fractures, trauma, carpal tunnel syndrome, tendonitis, ligament injuries, wrist sprain, radial nerve palsy, wrist ganglion cysts
Thumb spica (also called *short* or *long opponens, thumb gauntlet, thumb*) *immobilization*)	de Quervain's tenosynovitis, trauma, scaphoid fractures, arthritis, ulnar collateral ligament injuries As opponens, used to support thumb weakness to promote functional opposition
Ulnar gutter	Fractures, wrist ligament injuries
Dorsal blocking	Flexor tendon repairs, nerve repairs, trauma
Metaphalangeal blocking	Extensor tendon repairs, collateral ligament injuries of the fingers, arthritis
Finger gutter	Arthritis, finger fractures, extensor tendon injuries at the finger level, soft tissue injuries, sprains, dislocations

of a condition, such as arthritis, and usually is worn at all times, with removal for dressing changes and hygiene. Clients can reduce wearing time as healing progresses and they are able to begin light use of the wrist and hand for self-care tasks. A client with increased tone or spasticity in the upper extremity as a result of a neurological condition, such as a CVA, TBI, or SCI may also benefit from a resting hand orthosis, which can help position the wrist and hand open for cleaning and hygiene. However, the position of the joint in this client population will be dependent on the amount of tone the client has and how easy it is to position the wrist and fingers within the orthosis. The wearing schedule depends on the diagnosis and the physician's orders. For example, in a client with spasticity or tone, the OT practitioner checks the client's skin for areas of pressure and his or her comfort level and could determine the initial wearing schedule to be for 20 minutes. As the client is able to tolerate the orthosis, the wearing time is increased as the goals regarding orthosis use are achieved. A resting hand orthosis applied for tone may eventually be worn only at night or on a 2-hour-on, 2-hour-off wearing schedule. The orthosis must be frequently checked for fit, and skin must be monitored for pressure injuries or breakdown. The steps below should be followed for fabrication of a resting hand orthosis:

1. Make a pattern of the client's hand by tracing the hand and forearm on a paper towel (long enough to almost reach the elbow). The hand should be positioned with the palm down, the fingers together, and the thumb slightly abducted (Fig. 19-23).
2. Before allowing the client to move the hand, make a dot at the thumb web space, the web space between the index and long fingers, the CMC joint of the thumb, and the ulnar and radial styloid of the wrist. Now, place a line at the level of three fourths of the length of the forearm.
3. Have the client remove the hand, and mark the pattern as follows: point A at the thumb web space, point B at the web space between the index and middle fingers, point C where point A and B intersect, point D at the radial styloid, point E at the ulnar styloid, and point F at the level of the forearm. Make the pattern by adding a quarter inch to the parameter of the hand and a half inch to the forearm. Connect the points as shown in Figure 19-24. The pattern may need to be adjusted according to the size of the client's forearm.
4. Cut the pattern, and place it on the client, making note of any areas that may need to be made larger or smaller.
5. Trace the pattern onto the desired piece of thermoplastic material with either a wax pencil or a scratch awl. Remember that a more rigid material is easier to use with a larger orthosis.
6. Heat the thermoplastic material slightly, and cut out the pattern, making sure not to handle the material too aggressively because this will cause fingerprints and changes in the shape of the material. Be aware of the material sticking to itself while cutting or cut pieces bonding with the pattern. Using the back edge of the scissors in long strokes will also leave a clean smooth line where the cuts have been made.
7. Place a piece of stockinette over the client's forearm, wrist, and hand, and place the client in the desired position, to allow gravity to assist with the drape of the thermoplastic material once applied (Fig. 19-25).
8. Heat the material again until it is pliable and easy to mold onto the client. Mold the material onto the

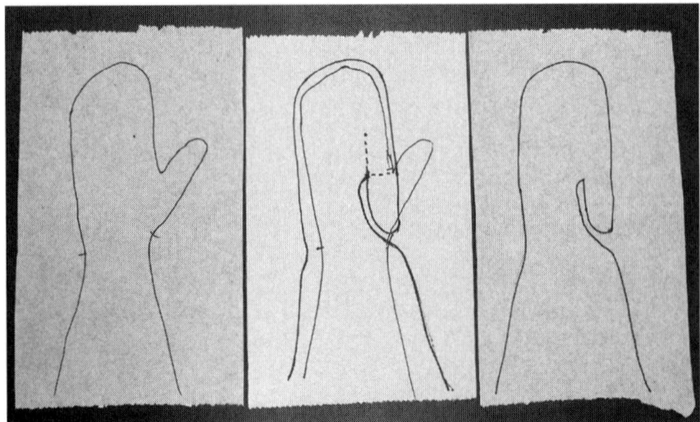

FIGURE 19-23. *From left*: palm-down tracing for pattern of resting hand orthosis, drawing in the orthosis based on the hand plus one quarter to one half inch, just the completed orthosis pattern.

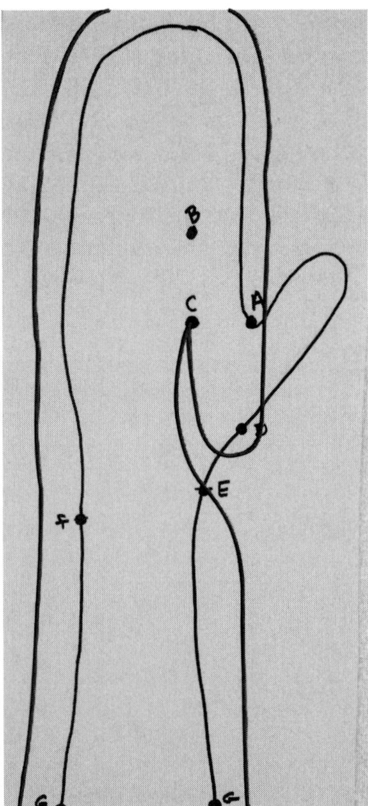

FIGURE 19-24. Pattern for the resting hand orthosis with the points marked.

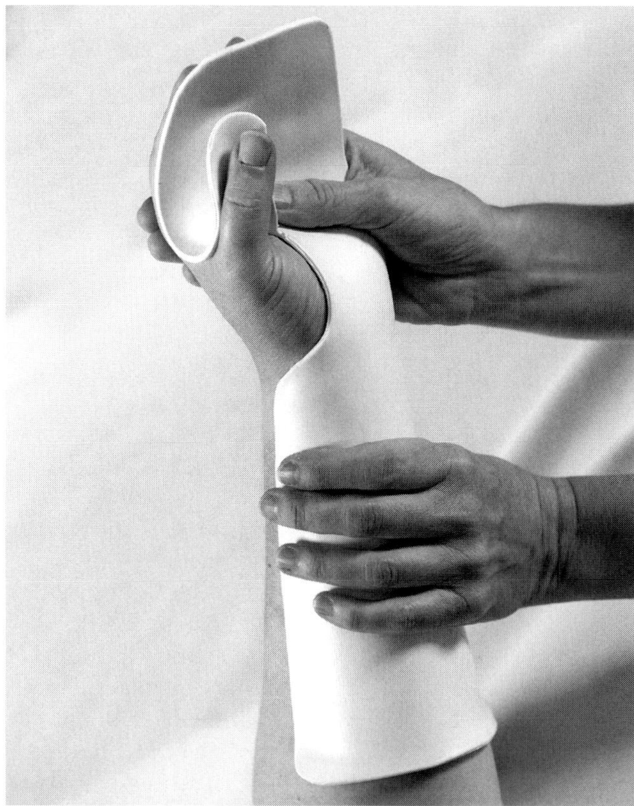

FIGURE 19-25. Position of the hand and wrist while molding a resting hand orthosis.

client by using a light touch and a goniometer, as needed, to ensure the proper angle at the wrist, MP joints, and IP joints

9. When the thermoplastic material has cooled, check the fit of the orthosis, making lines with a pencil or thumbnail to mark the areas that require trimming. Mark the place on the orthosis where Velcro® hook should be applied.
10. Remove the orthosis, and make adjustments. Trim, as needed, and smooth the edges, including flaring at the proximal edge to prevent pressure on the forearm. Apply strapping pieces with rounded corners to the orthosis. The sticky-back hook may be heated with the heat gun before adhering it to the orthosis to ensure secure contact (Fig. 19-26).

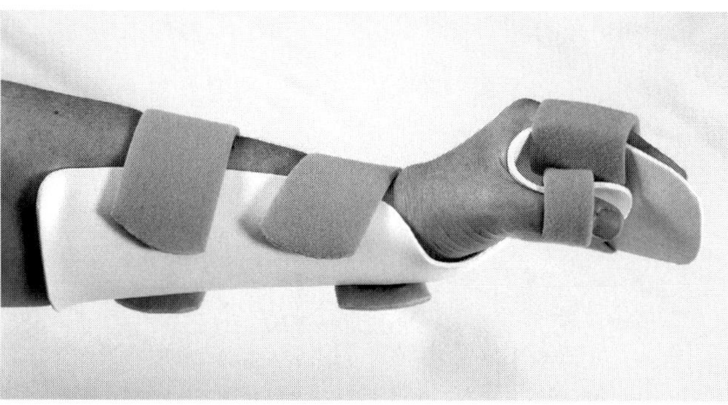

FIGURE 19-26. Completed resting hand orthosis.

11. Provide client education in the form of written, picture, and verbal instructions, including a wearing schedule and precautions.
12. Make a follow-up appointment for the client to have the orthotic checked to monitor for fit and to make any necessary changes.

Volar Wrist Orthosis

A volar wrist orthosis is used to immobilize the wrist in a protected or functional position. Clients who have been diagnosed with arthritis, tendonitis, fractures, and nerve compression injuries, such as carpal tunnel syndrome, can benefit from the use of a volar wrist orthosis. The position of the wrist will depend on the client's diagnosis and the physician's order. The typical position of the wrist should be between 0 and 30 degrees of wrist extension. The wearing schedule also depends on the diagnosis and the physician's orders. A wrist orthosis applied after an acute injury, trauma, or flare-up of a condition, such as arthritis, usually should be worn at all times, with removal only for dressing changes and hygiene. The client decreases the amount of wearing time as healing progresses, and the client is able to begin light use of the wrist for self-care tasks. The orthosis must be frequently checked for fit, and skin must be monitored for pressure injury or skin breakdown. The steps below should be followed for fabrication of a volar wrist orthosis:

1. Make a pattern of the client's hand by tracing the hand and wrist on a paper towel. The hand should be positioned with the palm down, the fingers together, and the thumb slightly abducted.
2. Before allowing the client to move the hand, make a dot at the thumb web space, the radial side of the distal palmar crease, the ulnar side of the distal palmar crease, the CMC joint of the thumb, and the ulnar and radial styloid of the wrist. Now, place a line at the level of three fourths of the length of the forearm.
3. Have the client remove the hand, and mark the pattern as follows: point A at the thumb web space, point B at the radial side of the distal palmar crease, point C at the ulnar side of the distal palmar crease, point D at the radial styloid, point E at the ulnar styloid and, point F at the level of the forearm. Make the pattern by adding a quarter inch to the parameter of the hand and a half inch to the forearm. Connect the points as shown in Figure 19-27. The pattern may need to be made wider, depending on the size of the client's forearm.
4. Cut the pattern, and place it on the client, making note of any areas that may need to be made larger or smaller.
5. Trace the pattern onto the desired piece of thermoplastic material with either a wax pencil or a scratch awl. Remember that a material with more drape will fit to the contours of the hand more easily.

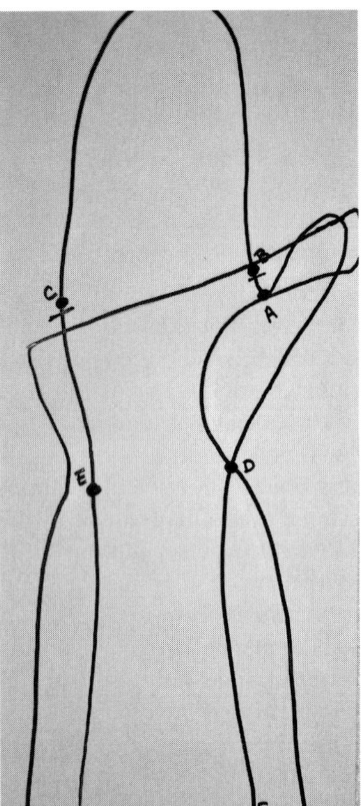

FIGURE 19-27. Pattern for volar wrist orthosis.

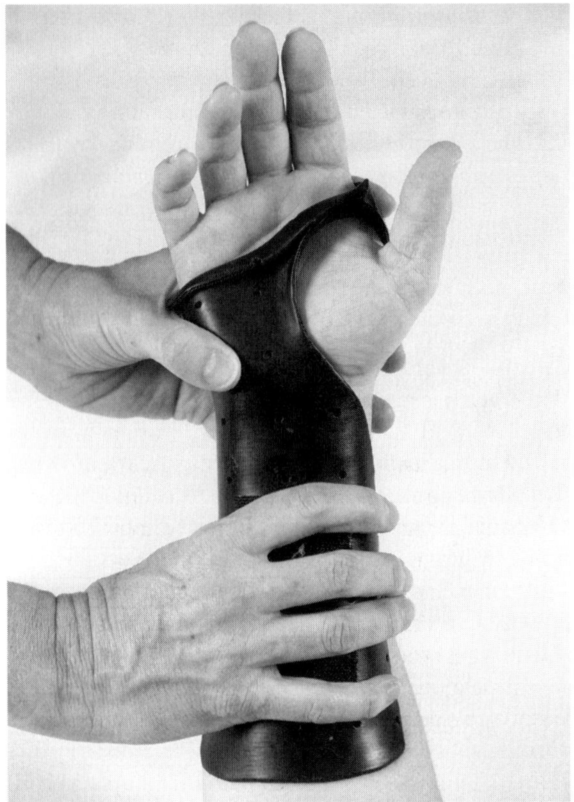

FIGURE 19-28. Position of the wrist while molding a volar wrist orthosis.

6. Heat the thermoplastic material slightly, and cut out the pattern, making sure not to handle the material too aggressively because this will cause fingerprints and changes in the shape of the material. Using the back edge of the scissors will also leave a clean smooth line where the cuts have been made.
7. Place a piece of stockinette over the forearm, wrist, and hand, and place the client in the desired position, allowing gravity to assist with the drape of the splinting material once applied (Fig. 19-28).
8. Heat the material again until it is pliable and easy to mold onto the client. Mold the material onto the client by using a light touch, and fold the material down at the distal palmar crease and at the web space between the thumb and index finger. This is to avoid sharp edges and maintain full finger and thumb function while supporting the wrist. Use a goniometer, as needed, to ensure the desired angle at the wrist.
9. When the thermoplastic material has cooled, check the fit of the orthosis, making lines with a pencil or thumbnail to mark the areas that require trimming. Mark the place on the orthosis where the Velcro® hook should be applied.
10. Remove the orthosis, and make adjustments. Trim, as needed, and smooth the edges, including flaring at the proximal edge to prevent pressure on the forearm. Apply strapping pieces, which have rounded corners to the orthosis. The sticky-back hook may be heated with the heat gun before adhering it to the orthosis to ensure secure contact (Fig. 19-29). Follow the final steps as in the resting hand orthosis.

Thumb Spica Orthosis

A thumb spica orthosis is used to immobilize the thumb in a protected or functional position. Clients who have been diagnosed with arthritis, de Quervain's tenosynovitis, scaphoid fractures, and traumatic injuries, such as an ulnar collateral ligament injury to the thumb, can benefit from the use of a thumb spica orthosis. The position of the thumb and wrist will be dependent on the client's diagnosis and the

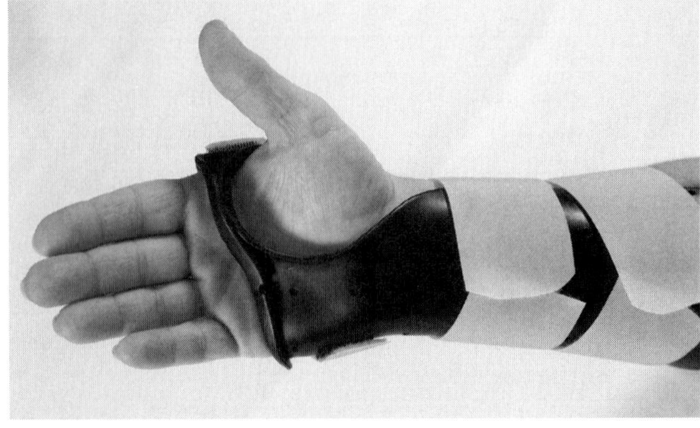

FIGURE 19-29. Completed volar wrist orthosis.

physician's order. A thumb spica orthosis may also be hand-based, which means it will not immobilize or restrict motion at the wrist; this chapter will show the orthosis being made which encompasses the wrist as well as a final version of the hand-based orthosis. The typical position of the thumb CMC should be resting at 30° to 40° of palmar abduction, the thumb MP joint at 0° to 10° flexion, and the IP joint free of the orthosis. The wrist should be positioned in 20° to 30° of extension. At times, this orthosis will be slightly modified when fabricated to hold the thumb in more opposition for supported pinch when the client has thumb weakness to increase functionality. The wearing schedule also depends on the diagnosis and the physician's orders. A thumb spica orthosis applied after an acute injury or trauma, or for tenosynovitis is usually worn at all times, with removal only for dressing changes and hygiene. The client decreases the amount of wearing time as healing progresses and the client is able to begin light use of the wrist for self-care tasks. The thumb opposition position for the orthosis may be worn only for certain functional tasks. The orthosis must be frequently checked for fit, and skin must be monitored for pressure injury or breakdown. Follow the steps below for fabrication of a thumb spica orthosis:

1. Make a pattern of the client's hand by tracing the hand on a paper towel. The hand should be positioned with the palm down, fingers together, and the thumb slight abducted.
2. Before allowing the client to move the hand, make a dot at both sides of the thumb IP joint, the radial side of the distal palmar crease, the ulnar side of the distal palmar crease, the CMC joint of the thumb, and the ulnar and radial styloid of the wrist. Now, place a line at the level of three fourths of the length of the forearm.
3. Have the client remove the hand, and mark the pattern as follows: points A and B at the IP joint of the thumb, point C at the radial side of the distal palmar crease, point D at the ulnar side of the distal palmar crease, point E at the CMC joint of the thumb, point F the ulnar styloid of the wrist, point G at radial styloid, and point H at the level of the forearm. Make the pattern by allowing enough material to wrap around the thumb, adding a quarter inch to the parameter of the hand and a half inch to the forearm. Connect the points as shown in Figure 19-30. The pattern may need to be made wider, depending on the size of the client's forearm.
4. Cut the pattern, and place it on the client, making note of any areas that may need to be made larger or smaller.
5. Trace the pattern onto the desired piece of thermoplastic material with either a wax pencil or a scratch awl. Remember that a material with more drape will be easier to stretch around the contours of the thumb, and, generally, self-bonding material will be easier.
6. Heat the thermoplastic material slightly, and cut out the pattern, making sure not to handle the material too aggressively because this will cause fingerprints and changes in the shape of the material. Using the back edge of the scissors will also leave a clean smooth line where the cuts have been made.
7. Place a piece of stockinette over the forearm, wrist, and hand, and place the client in the desired position, allowing gravity to assist with the drape of the thermoplastic material, once applied.
8. Heat the material again until it is pliable and easy to mold onto the client. Mold the material onto the client by using a light touch, fold the material down at the distal palmar crease, and stretch to fit around the thumb at the web space between the thumb and index finger. Use a goniometer, if needed, to ensure the desired angle at the wrist.
9. When the thermoplastic material has cooled, check the fit of the orthosis, making lines with a pencil to mark the areas that require trimming. Mark the place on the orthosis where the Velcro® hook should be applied.
10. Remove the orthosis, and make adjustments. Trim, as needed, and smooth the edges, including flaring at the proximal edge to prevent pressure on the forearm. Apply strapping pieces with rounded corners to orthosis. The sticky-back hook may be heated with the heat gun before adhering it to the orthosis to ensure secure contact (Fig. 19-31 is the hand-based thumb spica). Perform the final steps as completed with the resting hand orthosis.

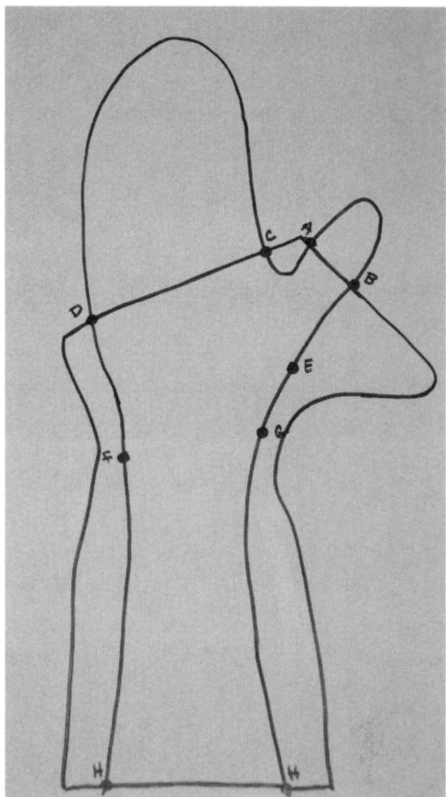

FIGURE 19-30. Pattern for thumb spica orthosis.

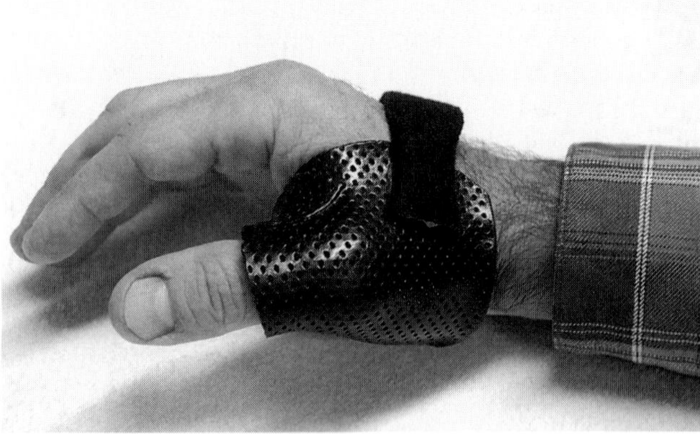

FIGURE 19-31. Completed hand-based thumb spica orthosis.

SUMMARY

As a preparatory measure toward engagement in occupation, the treatment modality of orthotic fabrication and fitting provides a variety of options for the individual with impaired upper extremity function. With the many materials available and designs to consider, this treatment modality is only limited by the creativity of the practitioner and the client as they work together to meet occupational performance goals. Although fitting a client with an orthosis may be intimidating to a student or novice OT practitioner, with time, practice, and adherence to the principles discussed in this chapter, orthotic fabrication and fitting will quickly become a favorite treatment tool for facilitating the client's success in daily occupational performance.

REVIEW QUESTIONS

1. A physician is new to your community and asks if your clinic is able to provide therapy services to his patient population. He specifically asks about fabricating and fitting orthoses. You explain to him that an orthosis is used:
   a. To rest painful joints, to gain motion, and to assist with loss of function
   b. To cause the client discomfort
   c. To decrease function
   d. To replace therapy sessions
2. A client has been referred for a custom orthosis; however, during initial assessment, she is found to have decreased ROM, edema, and impaired sensation in her wrist and hand. Which three of the following are precautions when fitting this orthosis?
   a. Decreased ROM
   b. Edema
   c. Impaired sensation
   d. Poor skin integrity
   e. Application to the dominant hand
   f. The presence of complex regional pain syndrome
3. You are an OT practitioner in an outpatient setting, treating a client who has suffered a CVA. This client presents with a flaccid wrist and hand. He was not fitted for an orthosis while in acute rehabilitation; however, he reports that his hand is getting more swollen and painful and this prevents him from trying to engage in functional activities. Which orthosis would you fabricate for this client?
   a. Finger orthosis for protection
   b. A dynamic shoulder orthosis for stretching the shoulder
   c. WHFO to position the wrist and hand to prevent contractures
   d. A static progressive hand orthosis to gain end range of motion
4. A client with a diagnosis of radial nerve palsy has been referred for a custom orthosis. He presents with inability to extend the wrist and fingers. This loss of motion makes it difficult for him to release objects from his hand after gripping. The goal of the orthosis would be to:
   a. Immobilize the wrist and hand.
   b. Protect skin from exposure to heat and cold.
   c. Gain end ROM in stiff joints.
   d. Assist with function by providing wrist and finger extension while awaiting nerve return.
5. A client has been referred to the clinic for a static orthosis 3 days after he had sustained a fracture to the hand. In this situation, a static orthosis is used for:
   a. Immobilization and protection
   b. To gain motion
   c. To assist with promoting deformities
   d. To dynamically move joints
6. A client was referred to the clinic for a dynamic orthosis 2 weeks after surgically repaired nerves which were damaged when he had sustained a gunshot injury to the arm. In this situation, a dynamic orthosis is used:
   a. For immobilization
   b. To gain stiffness
   c. To compensate for loss of motion and improve function
   d. To statically position joints
7. When fabricating an orthosis, which of the following is a characteristic or property of the thermoplastic materials that you will consider when choosing the material to use?
   a. Drape
   b. Heat
   c. Hardness
   d. Stability
8. Serial casting has been used to treat both orthopedic and neurological conditions. Because of its effect on tissue lengthening, serial casting was *first* used in orthopedic applications to treat which of the following?
   a. Frozen shoulder
   b. Club foot
   c. Wrist sprains
   d. Mobility
9. A client with finger stiffness has been referred for an orthosis to increase the joint ROM in the proximal interphalangeal joint of the index finger. Which of the following statements regarding orthosis fabrication and fitting is true?
   a. Making a pattern is just a waste of time.
   b. Having the proper tools will not assist with orthosis fabrication.
   c. A client education handout should be given to the client for ease in following directions regarding orthosis use.
   d. Orthotic fabrication is not an effective treatment intervention.
10. A client with carpal tunnel syndrome could benefit from a wrist orthosis, but the client's insurance will not pay for a custom-made orthosis. Which three of the following do you recommend?
    a. Tell the client to just pay out of pocket for the custom orthosis.
    b. Inform the referring physician that the client is unable to pay for the custom orthosis.
    c. Make the orthosis, and do not charge the client.
    d. Advise the client where he or she can find a suitable alternative.

e. Explain the purpose of the orthosis, and have the client try a prefabricated version of the orthosis.
f. Recommend that the client borrow an orthosis from a friend who used it for the same condition.

CASE STUDY

Nancy, who is 48 years old, works at a local business performing accounting and data entry work. A mother and homemaker, she is having pain and numbness in her right dominant hand, and it is interfering with her activities at work and at home. Nancy was referred for outpatient OT by her family physician for conservative treatment of carpal tunnel syndrome. On her initial visit, Nancy presented with numbness and tingling in the thumb and the index and middle fingers, stating that the condition worsens at night. Nancy had already undergone positive provocative testing (Phalen's and Tinel's signs). Initially, the practitioner performing the evaluation had provided a home program that included tendon glides, edema management, and postural/ergonomic instruction. The evaluating practitioner thought that a positional orthosis would also help decrease Nancy's symptoms at night. Therefore, an order was obtained for a custom-fabricated orthosis. Nancy is scheduled to see you at her next visit.

1. What will the OT practitioner plan for this treatment session?
2. What type of orthosis should be fabricated and fitted?
3. What joints will the orthosis cross and in what position?
4. What type of "L" code should be used, or how will Nancy's orthosis be charged?
5. Is there an alternative soft orthosis that can be used?

PUTTING IT ALL TOGETHER Sample Treatment and Documentation

Setting	Outpatient OT clinic
Client Profile	Janelle is a 68-year-old female with diabetes who has been referred by the hand surgeon due to arthritic pain in the CMC joint of her right dominant thumb. She was seen last week for her initial evaluation and was fitted with a custom orthosis to position the right thumb while performing tasks that require pinching and manipulation of small objects.
Work History	Retired teacher's assistant who is very active. She enjoys cooking, gardening, and sewing and is a watercolor artist.
Insurance	Medicare primary with BCBS state supplement
Psychological	Recent onset of pain that is limiting engagement in occupation has Janelle concerned, otherwise she is optimistic that the pain will get better with therapy.
Social	Janelle is married to her husband of 42 years. Her husband works part time as a family physician in the community. Janelle has one daughter and three grandchildren who live across the country. She usually sees them in the summer and at the holidays. Janelle teaches art classes and is very active in the local garden club.
Cognitive	No deficits noted. Able to adapt and learn new skills.
Motor & Manual Muscle Testing (MMT)	• AROM is within normal limits in the right thumb with morning stiffness reported • Arthritic changes noted at the base of the thumb with a small nodule present • Right grip strength 55 pounds and the left grip strength 47 pounds • Right lateral pinch 8 pounds and is limited due to report of pain, left lateral pinch 14 pounds • Tip pinch was not tested due to aggravation of symptoms and pain with tip pinching • Pain rating with thumb use is 7/10 and at rest 5/10
ADL	Pain limits thumb use during the performance of self-care tasks and Janelle reports that she has been avoiding use of her thumb for pinching activities, including fasteners and holding utensils. Janelle also has difficulty using her right thumb to administer her insulin injection.
IADL	Pain in the thumb is reported with driving and when holding a paintbrush or sewing needle.
Goals	Within 4 weeks: 1. Client will demonstrate independence with home program which includes orthosis use, paraffin heat, joint protection principles and adaptive equipment to decrease pain with the performance of prehension activities. 2. Client will report a decrease in right thumb pain to 1/10 at rest and with activity with use of orthosis to stabilize thumb CMC joint. 3. Client will demonstrate and apply joint protection principles for self-management of CMC osteoarthritis. 4. Client will have the needed adaptive equipment to decrease thumb pain during the performance of self-care tasks, including administration of insulin injections.

Continued

PUTTING IT ALL TOGETHER Sample Treatment and Documentation (continued)

OT TREATMENT SESSION 1

THERAPEUTIC ACTIVITY	TIME	GOAL(S) ADDRESSED	OTA RATIONALE
Paraffin heat is applied to decrease pain, and client is instructed in use of paraffin heat as part of a home program to decrease stiffness in the a.m. and to alleviate pain.	12 min	#1	*Preparatory Method; Education and Training:* PAM (paraffin heat) can help to decrease arthritic pain. Client is instructed in use of paraffin heat and/or other heat modalities at home to decrease thumb pain and stiffness.
Paraffin is followed by client education, including AROM to thumb and the importance of avoiding resistive activities, which will cause an increase in joint pain. Training in joint protection principles for osteoarthritis.	22 min	#1 and #3	*Preparatory Method; Education and Training:* Emphasis on client education to establish a home program for the acute flare-up of what may become a chronic condition. Patient is trained in joint protection principles and is issued patient education handouts, which include pictures and explanations of how to avoid postures of deformity and to decrease stress on arthritic joints.
Patient education and ADL training to introduce adaptive equipment and to have client use orthosis and adaptive equipment in clinic setting for carry over for home use	18 min	#1 and #4	*Preparatory Task; ADL Training:* Use of adaptive equipment is demonstrated and the client is provided with education regarding use of adaptive equipment to protect arthritic joints. ADL catalog is issued and client is instructed in resources for obtaining adaptive equipment. Focus will be on using orthosis and adaptive equipment to decrease pain and increase independence with insulin injections.
Orthosis checked for fit, and home program for orthosis use reviewed and adjusted as needed	10 min	#1 and #2	*Preparatory Method; Orthotic Fitting; and Training:* Client's orthosis will be checked for fit, adjustments will be made as needed, and use of orthosis at home and with prehension activities will be reviewed. Recommendations for wearing schedule will also be made with client goals and hand use in mind. Pain level with use of orthosis will be assessed while performing activities within the clinic setting.

SOAP note: 10/12/—, 9:00 am–10:02 am

S: Client states, "The black orthotic I am wearing on my thumb has really helped my pain. What else can I do so this does not get worse?"

O: Client was seen this date in outpatient occupational therapy as referred by her MD due to right dominant thumb pain secondary to CMC joint osteoarthritis that is limiting her hand function. Pain reported to be a 3/10 before treatment this date. The client received paraffin heat application for 12 minutes followed by patient education; use of paraffin heat at home, and training in joint protection principles with use of adaptive equipment to decrease thumb pain and improve hand function. Patient completed functional activities in the clinic with orthosis in place and with use of adaptive equipment; built up foam handles, spring assist scissors, adaptive pen, and simulated insulin injections for carry over with adaptations at home. Patient education materials and resources were provided to client who verbalized understanding. Web space of orthosis was heated and rolled to decrease pressure at thumb web space with orthosis use. Remainder of orthosis is fitting well with no signs of irritation or pressure points.

A: Orthosis appears to be assisting with the decrease in thumb pain as evidenced by the client report of a decrease in pain with orthosis use. Client is receptive to information provided and reports that she will begin to incorporate joint protection principles into her daily routine.

P: Will see the client one time next week and continue to address goals established upon the initial evaluation. Next treatment session to review home management of osteoarthritis and monitor/upgrade home program to ensure a continued decrease in thumb pain with use of orthosis, joint protection principles and modifications in ADL performance with use of adaptive equipment. Possible discharge to home program next visit if goals have been achieved.

Jane Brooker, COTA/L, 10/12/—, 11:15 am

TREATMENT SESSION 2

What could you do next with this client?

TREATMENT SESSION 3

What could you do next with this client?

REFERENCES

1. Fess, E., Gettle, K., Philips, C., & Janson, R. (2005). *Hand and upper extremity splinting: Principles and methods* (3rd ed.). St. Louis, MO: Mosby.
2. American Society of Hand Therapists. (2012). American Society of Hand Therapists position statement on the use of orthotics in hand therapy. Retrieved from http://www.asht.org/about/positions.cfm
3. Coverdale, J. (2012). An editorial note on nomenclature: Orthosis versus splint. *Journal of Hand Therapy, 25*, 1–3.
4. McKee, P., & Rivard, A. (2011). Foundations of orthotic intervention. In T. Skirven, L. Osterman, J. Fedorczyk, & P. Amadio (Eds.), *Rehabilitation of the hand and upper extremity* (6th ed.). Retrieved from https://expertconsult.inkling.com/read/skirven-rehabilitation-the-hand-upper-extremity
5. Hardy, M., & Freeland, A. (2011). Hand fracture fixation: Healing skeletal stability and digital mobility. In T. Skirven, L. Osterman, J. Fedorczyk, & P. Amadio (Eds.), *Rehabilitation of the hand and upper extremity* (6th ed.). Retrieved from https://expertconsult.inkling.com/read/skirven-rehabilitation-the-hand-upper-extremity
6. Evans, R. (2012). Managing the injured tendon: Current concepts. *Journal of Hand Therapy, 25*, 173–190.
7. Pettengill, K. (2005). The evolution of early mobilization of the repaired flexor tendon. *Journal of Hand Therapy, 18*, 157–168.
8. Tufaro, P., & Bondoc, S. (2011). Therapist's management of the burned hand. In T. Skirven, L. Osterman, J. Fedorczyk, & P. Amadio (Eds.), *Rehabilitation of the hand and upper extremity* (6th ed.). Retrieved from: https://expertconsult.inkling.com/read/skirven-rehabilitation-the-hand-upper-extremity
9. Weiss N. D., Gordon, L., & Bloom, T. (1995). Position of the wrist associated with the lowest carpal-tunnel pressure: Implications for splint design. *American Journal of Bone and Joint Surgery, 77*, 1695–1699.
10. Evans, R. (2011). Therapist's management of carpal tunnel syndrome. In T. Skirven, L. Osterman, J. Fedorczyk, & P. Amadio (Eds.), *Rehabilitation of the hand and upper extremity* (6th ed.). Retrieved from https://expertconsult.inkling.com/read/skirven-rehabilitation-the-hand-upper-extremity
11. Apfel, E., & Sigafoos, G.T. (2006). Comparison of range-of-motion constraints provided by splints used in the treatment of cubital tunnel syndrome—A pilot study. *Journal of Hand Therapy, 19*, 384–392.
12. Gomes Carreira, A., Jones, A., & Natour, J. (2010). Assessment of the effectiveness of a functional splint for osteoarthritis of the trapeziometacarpal joint of the dominant hand: A randomized controlled study. *Journal of Rehabilitation Medicine, 42*(5), 469–474.
13. Grenier, M. L., Mendonca, R., Dalley, P. (2016). The effectiveness of orthoses in the conservative management of thumb CMC joint osteoarthritis: An analysis of functional pinch strength. *Journal of Hand Therapy, 29*(3), 307–313.
14. McKee, P., & Nguyen, C. (2007). Customized dynamic splinting: Orthoses that promote optimal function and recovery after radial nerve injury: A case report. *Journal of Hand Therapy, 20*, 73–88.
15. Wiclandt, T., McKenna, K., Tooth, L., & Strong, J. (2006). Factors that predict the post-discharge use of recommended assistive technology (AT). *Disability and Rehabilitation, 11*, 29–40.
16. Jacobs, M. A., & Austin, N. M. (2014). *Orthotic intervention for the hand and upper extremity: Principles and process* (2nd ed.). Philadelphia, PA: Lippincott Williams and Wilkins.
17. Schultz-Johnson, K. (2002). Static progressive splinting. *Journal of Hand Therapy, 15*, 163–178.
18. Coppard, B., & Lohman, H. (2014). *Introduction to orthotics: A critical-thinking and problem-solving approach* (4th ed.). St. Louis, MO: Mosby.
19. Flowers, K., & LaStayo, P. (1994). Effects of total end range time on improving passive range of motion. *Journal of Hand Therapy, 7*, 93–102.
20. Fess, E. (2011). Orthoses for mobilization of joints: Principles and methods. In T. Skirven, L. Osterman, J. Fedorczyk, & P. Amadio (Eds.), *Rehabilitation of the hand and upper extremity* (6th ed.). Retrieved from https://expertconsult.inkling.com/read/skirven-rehabilitation-the-hand-upper-extremity
21. Brand, P. (1995). The forces of dynamic splinting: Ten questions before applying a dynamic splint to the hand. In J. Hunter, E. Mackin, & A. Callahan, (Eds.). *Rehabilitation of the hand and upper extremity* (4th ed., p. 1581). Retrieved from https://expertconsult.inkling.com/read/skirven-rehabilitation-the-hand-upper-extremity
22. Patterson Medical. (2015). Patterson Medical hand therapy catalog. Retrieved from https://patersonmedical.com
23. Patterson Medical. (2011). Instructions for use of thermoplastic material. Retrieved from https://content.pattersonmedical.com/PDF/spr/Product/273976.pdf
24. Bell Krotoski, J. (2011). Tissue remodeling and contracture correction using serial plaster casting and orthotic positioning. In T. Skirven, L. Osterman, J. Fedorczyk, & P. Amadio (Eds.), *Rehabilitation of the hand and upper extremity* (6th ed.). Retrieved from: https://expertconsult.inkling.com/read/skirven-rehabilitation-the-hand-upper-extremity
25. Hill, J. (1994). The effects of casting on upper extremity motor disorders after brain injury. *The American Journal of Occupational Therapy, 48*, 219–224.
26. Lannin, N., Novak, I., & Cusick, A. (2007). A systematic review of upper extremity casting for children and adults with central nervous system motor disorders. *Clinical Rehabilitation, 21*, 963–967.
27. Ladwig, J. (2012). Serial casting. *Rainbow Visions Magazines*, p. 1–3. Livonia, MI: Rainbow Rehabilitation Centers.
28. Altman, E. (2011). Therapist's management of the stiff elbow. In T. Skirven, L. Osterman, J. Fedorczyk, & P. Amadio, (Eds.), *Rehabilitation of the hand and upper extremity* (6th ed.). Retrieved from https://expertconsult.inkling.com/read/skirven-rehabilitation-the-hand-upper-extremity
29. Colditz, J. (2002). Plaster of Paris: The forgotten hand splinting material. *Journal of Hand Therapy, 15*, 144–157.
30. Colditz, J. (2011). Therapist's management of the stiff hand. In T. Skirven, L. Osterman, J. Fedorczyk, & P. Amadio, (Eds.), *Rehabilitation of the hand and upper extremity* (6th ed.). Retrieved from https://expertconsult.inkling.com/read/skirven-rehabilitation-the-hand-upper-extremity
31. Glasgow, C., Tooth, L., & Fleming, J. (2010). Mobilizing the stiff hand: Combining theory and evidence to improve clinical outcomes. *Journal of Hand Therapy, 23*, 392–401.
32. Canelon, M. (1995). Silicone rubber splinting for athletic hand and wrist injuries. *Journal of Hand Therapy, 8*, 252–257.
33. Beasley, J. (2011). Soft orthoses: Indications and techniques. In T. Skirven, L. Osterman, J. Fedorczyk, & P. Amadio (Eds.), *Rehabilitation of the hand and upper extremity* (6th ed.). Retrieved from https://expertconsult.inkling.com/read/skirven-rehabilitation-the-hand-upper-extremity
34. American Society of Hand Therapists. (2012). Practice section description of HCPCS codes. Retrieved from http://www.asht.org/practice/durable-medical-equipment-dme/hcpcs-codes
35. Centers for Medicare and Medicaid Services. (2011). *HCPCS level II coding process and criteria*. Retrieved from https://www.cms.gov/MedHCPCSGenInfo/02_HCPCSCODINGPROCESS.asp

unit IV

Health Conditions and Interventions

Chapter 20

Orthopedic Considerations: Spine, Pelvis, Hip, and Knee

Lori Goodnight, MS, OTR/L

LEARNING OUTCOMES

After studying this chapter, the student or practitioner will be able to:

20.1 Identify the general anatomy of the spine, pelvis, hip, and knee

20.2 Discuss common orthopedic conditions and surgical interventions

20.3 Define precautions and safety considerations with orthopedic rehabilitation

20.4 Describe orthopedic occupational therapy intervention techniques to facilitate progress toward performance-based goals

20.5 Discuss the importance of teamwork with orthopedic interventions

KEY TERMS

Aquatic therapy
Artificial disk replacement
Back precautions
Continuous passive motion (CPM) device
Discectomy
External fixator
Foraminotomy
Hemiarthroplasty
Hip movement precautions
Interlaminar implant
Knee resurfacing
Kyphoplasty
Laminectomy
Open reduction internal fixation (ORIF)
Partial knee replacement
Prosthesis
Radiculopathy
Revision surgery
Rigid braces
Spinal fusion
Total hip replacement or arthroplasty (THR)
Total knee arthroplasty (TKA)
Total knee replacement (TKR)
Traction
Weight-bearing

Occupational therapy (OT) has an important role in the recovery and rehabilitation of clients with orthopedic conditions including the spine, pelvis, hip, and knee. The shoulder will be addressed in Chapter 23 due to its complexity. Orthopedics is the area of medicine that focuses on the skeletal system including the related muscles, ligaments, and joints. Clients with orthopedic conditions may be treated in various settings including: acute care hospital, inpatient rehabilitation (an inpatient rehabilitation facility), subacute inpatient rehabilitation (the rehab unit of a long term care facility), long-term care, home health, and outpatient care. The role of OT in orthopedics is to assist clients to manage and overcome functional limitations due to their condition or injury.[1] With pressure to reduce healthcare costs and length of care, OT plays a key role in progressing clients to achieve maximum independence with self-care, safety with functional mobility, and training with adaptive equipment, durable medical equipment, and home/work/leisure modifications to reduce the risk for future injury. OT practitioners work closely with other team members, including staff (orthopedic surgeons, nurses, case managers, social workers, physical therapists, physical therapist assistants, and speech language pathologists), family members, caregivers, and the client to achieve the safest, most appropriate plan of care and discharge placement for each individual. OT practitioners must have good communication with all team members to ensure a successful outcome. This chapter will cover the orthopedic areas of spine, pelvis, hips, and knees by addressing anatomy, injury/diseases, surgeries, and precautions as well as specific and general treatment considerations.

THE SPINE

Because back issues are common, it is important to have knowledge of general anatomy, issues, and common surgeries related to the spine to enhance the OT interventions.

Anatomy of the Spine

The spine is an interconnected complex of bones, nerves, muscles, tendons, and ligaments that all help to provide stability, protect the spinal cord and nerve roots, and also provide flexibility for mobility. This complex mix of strength, structure, and function can become damaged and cause pain, neurological symptoms, or loss of mobility.

The spine has seven cervical vertebrae in the neck, twelve thoracic vertebrae in the upper back, and five lumbar vertebrae in the lower back, sacrum, and coccyx (Fig. 20-1). Each vertebral segment is composed of a cylinder-shaped bone in the front of the spine, called the vertebral body, a soft cartilage disc between each vertebra, and paired facet joints in the back. Each segment is named for its location within the upper, middle, and lower portions of the spine, such as the C6-C7 segment, located in the cervical region, or the L4-L5 segment, located in the lumbar region. The bones in the spinal column surround and protect the spinal cord, which runs behind the vertebral bodies in a canal from the neck down to the top of the lumbar spine. The nerves branch out from the spinal canal and exit the spine through holes in the backs of the vertebrae called foramina.

Back Pain

Low back pain is a significant cause of disability in the United States and worldwide. It is estimated that 70% to 80% of people will experience low back pain at some point in their lives.[2] Any compression of the nerve root in the foramina opening, which can occur due to bone spurs, herniated or degenerated discs, arthritis, fractures or facet joint problems, can cause pain and possible neurological symptoms to radiate along the path of the nerve and into the arm or leg. These symptoms are commonly called **radiculopathy**, and sciatica refers to the pain that radiates along the path of the sciatic nerve from the lower back and down each leg. Ankylosing spondylitis is a type of arthritis of the spine that causes inflammation between the vertebrae and in the joints between the spine and pelvis. Over time, ankylosing spondylitis can fuse the vertebrae together, limiting movement.[3] Spinal stenosis causes narrowing of the spinal vertebrae. The narrowing puts pressure on the nerves and spinal cord and can cause pain, numbness, paresthesia, and loss of motor control.[4] Osteomyelitis is an infection of the bone caused by a bacteria or fungus spread from the bloodstream, open fracture, or surgery. Osteomyelitis of the vertebrae causes severe back pain. People with diabetes, HIV infection, and peripheral vascular disease are more prone to osteomyelitis.[5] Spondylolisthesis is a forward or backward displacement of one of the vertebra, and most often occurs in the lumbosacral area. This may lead to the spinal cord or nerve roots being squeezed causing back pain and numbness or weakness in one or both legs.[6] In between the vertebrae, the intervertebral discs serve as shock absorbers and help facilitate movement of the spine. These discs can degenerate over time and become a source of pain, a condition called degenerative disc disease. The soft inner core of the disc can extrude, called a herniated or ruptured disc, and inflame a nearby nerve root (Fig. 20-2). The entire spine is enveloped in an interwoven network of muscles, ligaments, and tendons. These soft tissues can become strained, which can lead to inflammation, pain, and muscle spasms. Low back pain can be acute (severe), subacute (moderate), or chronic (long-term).

Back Surgery

Usually people only consider surgery for back pain after all other treatments, such as medication, therapy, or injections, have failed to provide relief. Many different surgeries for back pain are available, depending on the condition. **Spinal fusion** is surgery to join, or fuse, two or more vertebrae so there is no movement between them. The two methods of spinal fusion use either bone (from the pelvis or bone bank) or metal implants to hold the vertebrae together until new bone grows between them. **Laminectomy** is a decompression surgery that enlarges the spinal canal to relieve pressure on the spinal cord or nerves. This procedure creates space by removing the lamina (the back part of the vertebra that covers the spinal canal). A **foraminotomy** is a decompression surgery that is performed to enlarge the foramen (passageway where a spinal nerve root exits the spinal canal). **Discectomy** is surgery to remove herniated disc material that is pressing on a nerve root or the spinal cord.[7] **Artificial disk replacement** is a newer surgical procedure for relieving low back pain. Much like hip or knee joint replacements, the intervertebral disk in the spine is replaced with a mechanical device. The device helps to restore motion to the spine by replacing the worn, degenerated disk.[2] An **interlaminar implant** is a U-shaped implant that fits between the spinous processes located in the lumbar

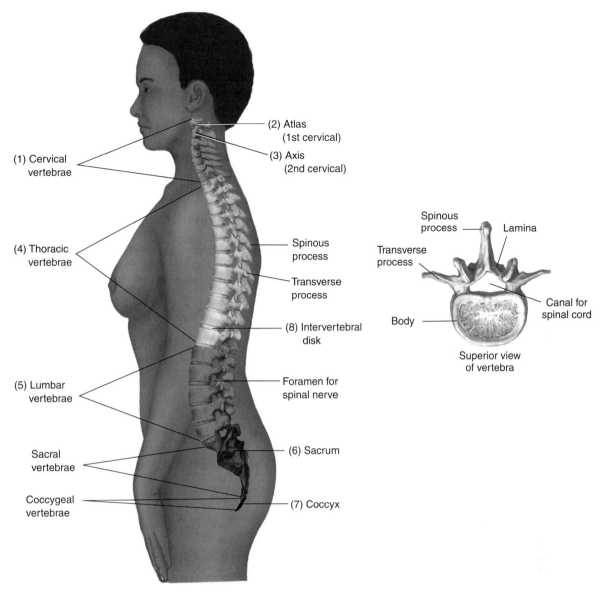

(2) Atlas (1st cervical)
(1) Cervical vertebrae
(3) Axis (2nd cervical)
(4) Thoracic vertebrae
Spinous process
Transverse process
(8) Intervertebral disk
(5) Lumbar vertebrae
Foramen for spinal nerve
Sacral vertebrae
(6) Sacrum
Coccygeal vertebrae
(7) Coccyx
Spinous process
Lamina
Transverse process
Canal for spinal cord
Body
Superior view of vertebra

FIGURE 20-1. Anatomy of the spine, close-up of disc.

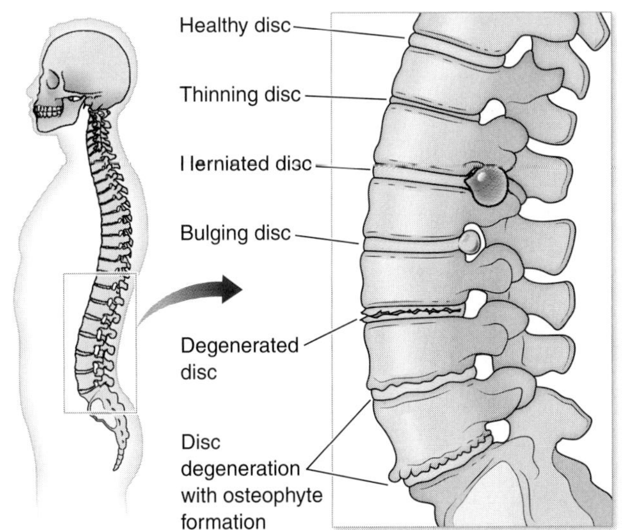

FIGURE 20-2. Degenerative disc disorders: disc thinning and compression, herniated disc and osteophyte (bone spur) formation.

region of the spine. The implant is designed to maintain a fixed distance between the spinous processes to support and stabilize without a reduction in the range of movement and motion.[8] A **kyphoplasty** creates space in a compressed or collapsed vertebrae with a balloon-type device and injection of a special cement to restore the damaged vertebra's height to relieve pain.[9] It is helpful to be familiar with common back surgeries when treating clients.

Some clients will be fitted with a back brace to limit motion in the spine, enhance healing, and decrease pain or discomfort following surgery. Two common types of braces are rigid and corset. **Rigid braces**, such as the thoracolumbar sacral orthosis (TLSO), are form-fitting plastic braces that limit most spinal movement (Fig. 20-3a). They should be worn when the client is up, but may be removed when lying down as long as the client is careful not to twist the spine. Clients should wear only a snug-fitting t-shirt or tank top under the brace to make the brace more comfortable and to keep it off the skin. The TLSO has an

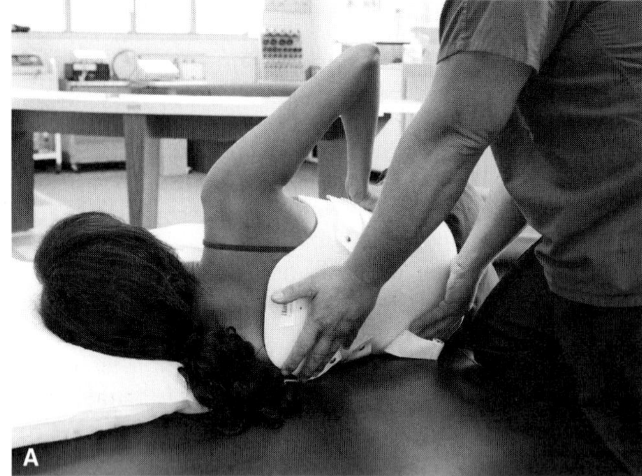

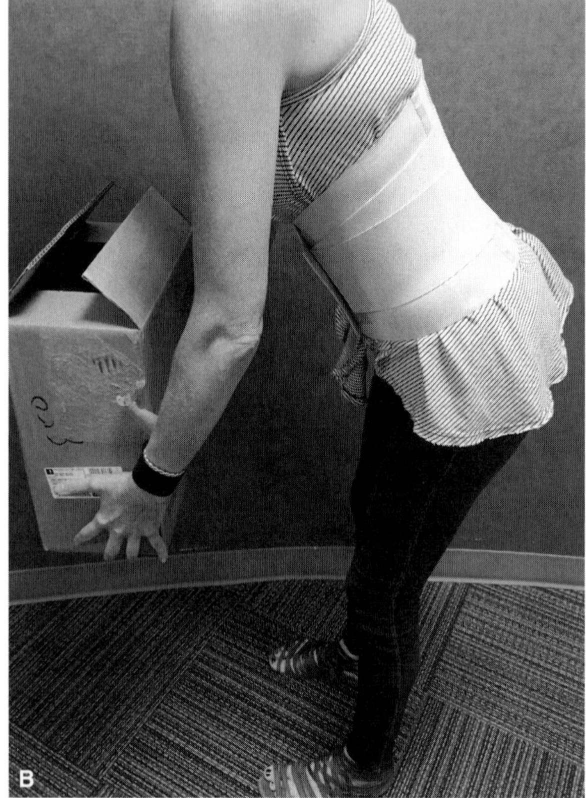

FIGURE 20-3. A. TLSO brace donning. B. Corset brace.

anterior and posterior piece both with identifying marks for the top and bottom. To don/doff the TLSO brace, clients should log-roll to their side in bed and place the posterior piece against their back with the waist indention lined up to the soft space between the waist and hips. Then clients can log-roll onto their back and place the anterior piece on top of their torso. The straps are tightened to prevent gapping between the brace and skin to provide total contact and limit flexion/rotation. The surgeon will specify how long the client must wear the TLSO brace based on individual healing, but it is usually worn 10 to 12 weeks. Another type of brace sometimes recommended is the corset brace because it allows a little motion while still stabilizing the spine (see Fig. 20-3b). The corset brace acts as a reminder to use proper body mechanics during functional activities and lifting. The corset should be donned standing, but can be donned sitting if the client cannot stand.[10]

Intervention

OT intervention for clients with back problems includes both education, training, and functional practice.

EDUCATION AND FUNCTIONAL TRAINING

Multidisciplinary treatment is recommended for back pain.[11] Team treatment emphasizes maximizing pain reduction; improving health-related quality of life, independence, and mobility; enhancing psychological well-being; and preventing secondary dysfunction. OT plays an important role in applying body mechanics education to home, work, and leisure activities. Clients with back conditions must be taught how the back works, how to incorporate proper body mechanics, and how to avoid unnecessary stresses to avoid reinjury. Often after surgery, the client will have to follow certain **back precautions** such as: no bending, no twisting, and specific limits on how much they can lift. General proper body mechanics include (Fig. 20-4):

- Stand smart: Maintain upright posture and a neutral pelvic position. If the client must stand for long periods, place one foot on a low footstool to take some of the load off the lower back. Alternate feet. Good posture can reduce the stress on back muscles.

> **COMMUNICATION**
>
> Good communication is essential with all treatment. Communication involves truly listening, processing information, problem-solving, and responding clearly, effectively, confidently, and professionally. OT practitioners have to communicate well with clients, families, coworkers, supervisors, physicians, and other professionals. Part of good communication also involves clear and effective documentation. Documentation is important for reimbursement, legal purposes, and demonstrating the distinct value of OT. The inclusion of medical necessity and functional outcomes is the key to reimbursement. Electronic documentation offers helpful templates but the practitioner must be sure to describe client responses and functional outcomes tailored to the individual. When using point-of-service documentation, the practitioner must be sure to keep the focus on the client and not the typing. Use good eye contact, and explain how typing during the treatment helps keep the notes accurate so the client understands and still feels connected. Sometimes clients with orthopedic conditions were injured in an accident and are involved in litigation, or there may be a problem in their care and the practitioner's documentation may later be called into question. Documentation is the evidence of the quality of care and intervention the client received.

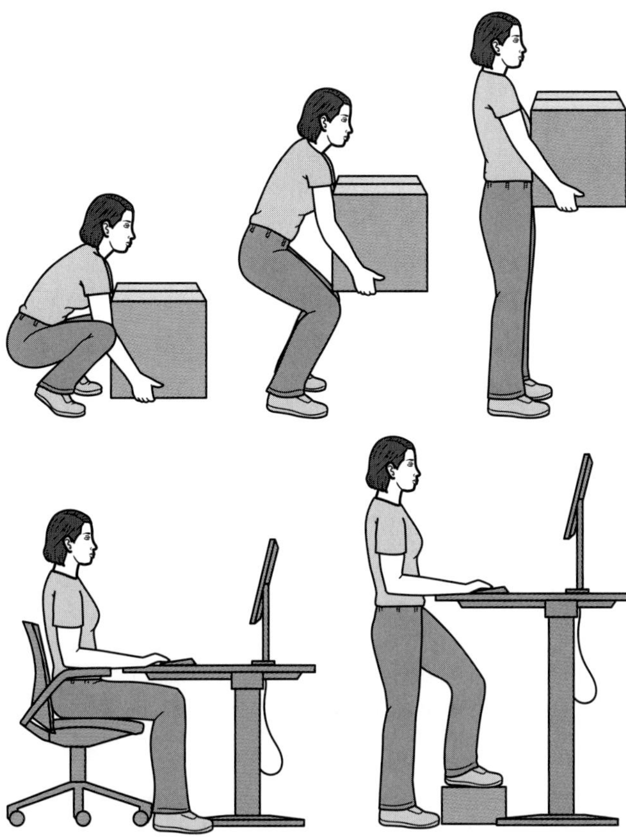

FIGURE 20-4. Body mechanics for lifting, standing, and sitting.

- Sit smart: Choose a seat with good lower back support, armrests and a swivel base. Consider placing a small pillow or rolled towel in the small of the back to maintain its normal lumbar curve. Keep knees and hips level. Change positions frequently, at least every half-hour.
- Lift smart: Avoid heavy lifting, if possible, but if one must lift something heavy, let the legs do the work.
  - Keep the back straight—no twisting—and bend at the knees.
  - Hold the load close to the body.
  - Find a lifting partner, or use lifting equipment if the object is heavy or awkward.
  - Use reachers to avoid bending down or reaching up high (for lightweight items only).
  - Adapt the environment, such as leaving frequently used kitchen items on the counter.
  - After back surgery, lifting is limited to less than 10 pounds, and clients should avoid any strenuous activity until cleared by their surgeon.[12]

TRAINING AND FUNCTIONAL PRACTICE

Another important component of OT treatment for clients with back problems is to teach them to use proper body mechanics with activities of daily living (ADLs) and all other occupations. Most clients, after a back injury or surgery, need to be taught how to compensate or adapt their daily activities. Clients should be taught to use the log-roll technique for bed mobility, similar to the technique used for donning the TLSO. It is best to teach clients with back problems to sit on surfaces that are at a higher level with armrests, such as a raised toilet seat or armchair. They should avoid low couches and toilets that stress the back when bending to get up and down. To avoid back stress while reaching to their feet, teach clients to dress and bathe their lower body while sitting and using adaptive techniques (crossing legs, sitting) or adaptive equipment (long-handled sponge, reacher, sock aid, dressing stick, long shoehorn, and elastic shoelaces). The surgeon must clear clients before they can shower again (due to the surgical incision). To avoid falls in the slippery tub or shower, training to use a raised shower chair or bench is usually recommended. Functional practice of home and workplace lifting, reaching, and carrying techniques is necessary to avoid reinjury. Train clients to use adaptive techniques to avoid back stress for homemaking tasks such as using a reacher to grab a pet's food bowl from the floor or sitting to load/unload the dishwasher or dryer. The practice helps teach clients new routines using the correct way to handle objects safely, and, once cleared by the surgeon, the activity can be graded like exercise so clients gradually increase the amount of weight lifted and learn what they can or cannot handle. Activities can include incorporating body mechanics with lifting and carrying graded weight in boxes, laundry baskets, grocery bags, suitcases, and so on. For any clients injured on the job, the lifting and carrying practice results are important information for their employers and insurance companies (see Chapter 17). Studies show exercise and education reduce the risk for a low back pain episode by 45%, and the risk for time off work due to back pain by 78%.[15]

THE PELVIS

Treating a client with a pelvic fracture requires knowledge of general pelvic anatomy and clinical reasoning during OT interventions to integrate adaptive techniques and safety skills with the physician's recommendations for optimum functioning and recovery.

Anatomy of the Pelvis

The pelvis is a cradle structure of bones at the lower end of the trunk (Fig. 20-5). The two sides of the pelvis are actually three bones (ilium, ischium, and pubis) that eventually grow together (fuse) throughout childhood and adolescence. Strong ligaments join the pelvis to the sacrum at the base of the spine. This creates a bowl-like cavity below the rib cage. Many digestive and reproductive organs are protected within the pelvic region. On each side, a hollow cup (**acetabulum**) serves as the socket for the hip joint. The pelvis is also an attachment point for muscles that reach down the legs and up the trunk to aid mobility. With all these vital structures running through the pelvis, a pelvic fracture can cause substantial bleeding, nerve damage, and internal organ injury. A pelvic fracture is a break in the

EVIDENCE-BASED PRACTICE #1

Evidence-based practice means OT practitioners integrate their own clinical expertise with the best available clinical evidence from research when treating clients. Steps to using evidence-based practice involve: 1) forming a clear clinical question that defines a client's problem, 2) search of the medical literature for the most current and relevant study results on that problem, 3) critical analysis of the study results for validity and clinical usefulness, 4) application of the relevant data to answer the clinical question, and 5) assessing outcome and evaluation of the first four steps to validate your treatment methods and time spent on treatment. All five steps involve an active learning process, well-developed skills of observation, and application to execute these steps.

Evidence-Based Practice Back Example:

1. Problem: Client works as a nurse, diagnosed with lumbar herniated disc from poor body mechanics during work, seen after lumbar laminectomy.
2. Medical literature: Study by Jaromi revealed use of six sessions of training including education on: ergonomics, theory, workstation education, and lifting, resulted in reducing back pain and improving body posture in healthcare professionals.[13]
3. Critical analysis: This study was part of the AOTA Evidence-Based Literature Review Project and qualified as a Critically Appraised Paper (CAP) with statistically significant improvements in body posture and reduced back pain.
4. Application: OTA treatment included education and functional practice incorporating: ergonomics, why back protection techniques are important, workstation adaptations, and appropriate lifting techniques during simulated work tasks.
5. Assessment: Progress was measured by comparing evaluation test results to current testing results for: pain level reported, observed posture during tasks, and level of functional independence incorporating body mechanics with ADLs/IADLs including work-related tasks.

Many professional associations have provided evidence-based practice guidelines for orthopedic conditions, which examine the available literature and make recommendations to guide practitioners. Evidence-based practice guidelines are intended to be used in conjunction with the OTA's clinical reasoning and expertise along with considering the client context and values.

The process of using scientific studies to form clinical guidelines that direct clinical decision making and client care is still evolving, and there are variations in orthopedic clinical practice guidelines. These variations are due to differences in surgical opinions, in service configurations, and the lack of evidence to support clinical practice. This lack of research includes addressing the use of hip precautions and the best ways to deliver postoperative education and care.

Evidence-based practice is only as good as the evidence on which it is based. Much importance rests on well-conducted studies with well-trained professionals using the best study design for evaluating a given outcome. There are many gaps in the evidence, there are key OT questions to be answered, and practitioners must rise to this challenge.[14]

Jaromi, M., Nemeth, A., Kranicz, J., Laczko, T., & Betlehem, J. (2012). Treatment and ergonomics training of work-related lower back pain and body posture problems for nurses. Journal of Clinical Nursing,*21(11–12), 1776–1784.*

What is Evidence-Based Practice? (n.d.). OT Seeker: Evidence-Based Practice Resources. *Retrieved from http://www.otseeker.com/resources/WhatIsEvidenceBasedPractice.aspx*

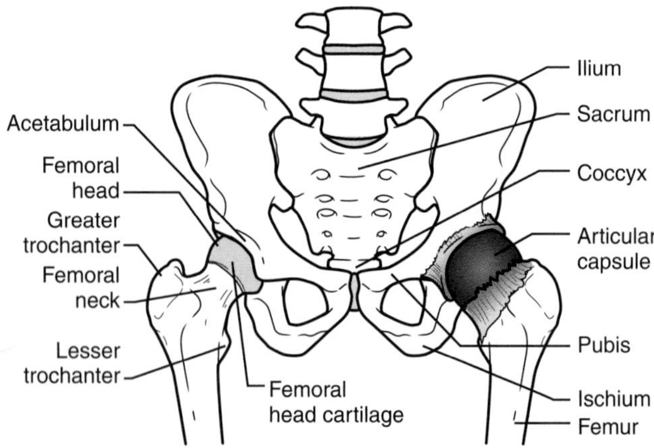

FIGURE 20-5. Note the hip anatomy, as labeled.

bony structure of the pelvis. It is usually caused by falls in older adults, and it may also be the result of strong forces, such as motor vehicle crashes, motorcycle or bicycle accidents, and falls from a significant height. Unstable pelvic fractures may require temporary traction or an external fixator. **Traction** involves using the mechanical force of weight and pulleys set up on a bed frame to put tension on the displaced bone to put it back in position and keep it stable. An **external fixator** has long screws that are inserted into the bones on each side and connected to a frame outside the body to stabilize the pelvis (Fig. 20-6). Surgery is not usually necessary for pelvic fractures, but some may require surgical insertion of plates or screws depending on the type of fracture and the client's condition. Stable fractures

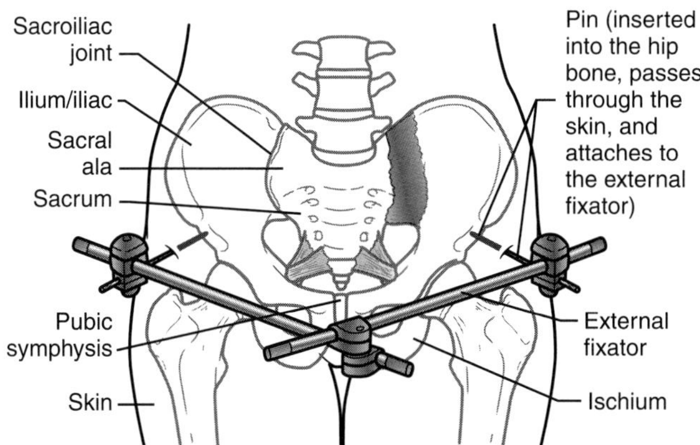

FIGURE 20-6. Pelvic fractures may be treated surgically by placing an external fixator while the bone heals.

will normally heal without surgery, but mobility and daily activities can be painful. Clients will have to use crutches or a walker, and will not be able to put all of their weight on one or both legs until the bones are healed.[16]

Intervention

OT is helpful to teach clients with pelvic fractures how to incorporate proper body mechanics to avoid stress to the pelvis; use adaptive techniques and equipment to aid daily activities; and use safety techniques to avoid reinjury. While movement or **weight-bearing** (how much weight the client can place on the fracture) precautions may be specified by the physician, usually clients can move within their comfort. Mobility starts slowly, and clients may do best with slowly easing each leg to the side of the bed and pushing up to sit until they can tolerate the log-roll technique. It is most comfortable for clients with a pelvic fracture to sit on cushioned chairs that are at a higher level and have armrests to assist with pushing up and down (raised toilet seat or armchair). Teach clients to dress and bathe their lower bodies while sitting and using adaptive equipment (long-handled sponge, reacher, sock aid, dressing stick, long shoehorn, and elastic shoelaces). Much like clients with back issues, clients with a pelvic fracture should avoid bending and twisting, but they also often have pain with crossing and lifting their legs. Pain and abilities will vary with each individual, so clients should be educated to listen to their bodies and avoid painful movements. To avoid falls in the slippery tub or shower, it is usually safest to train clients to sit on a shower chair/bench and lift their legs in/out of tub/shower. A leg lifter can be used if it is painful for clients to lift their legs. Place toiletries within a safe reaching distance in a basket or suction-cupped tray; using a soap-on-a rope or pump soap will avoid the need to bend over to retrieve a fallen soap bar. Functional practice of safe mobility in the home and workplace incorporating safe lifting, reaching, and carrying techniques is helpful to prevent falls and reinjury. Much like treatment of clients with back injuries, clients with pelvic fractures will slowly increase their independence and safety with functional mobility, ADLs, and IADLs during OT training.

THE HIP JOINT

It is important for OT practitioners to have knowledge of general anatomy, problems, and common surgeries related to the hip joint. OT practitioners must be prepared to integrate specific movement and weight-bearing precautions with their interventions to ensure safe and effective treatment.

Anatomy of the Hip Joint

The hip joint is a ball-and-socket type joint formed where the head of the femur meets the pelvis (see Fig. 20-5). The acetabulum of the pelvis is a hollow cup that serves as the socket of the hip joint. A smooth cushion of articular cartilage covers both the femoral head and the acetabulum. The articular cartilage is kept slippery by fluid made in the synovial membrane (joint lining). Since the cartilage is smooth and slippery, the bones move against each other easily and without causing pain. Large ligaments, tendons, and muscles around the hip joint (called the joint capsule) hold the bones (ball and socket) in place and keep it from dislocating.

TECHNOLOGY AND TRENDS

As the mobile device market continues to explode in growth, many OT practitioners are turning to their devices to augment their knowledge and treatments. New applications ("apps") for knowledge resources, client education, and clinical use arrive on the market every day. Apps for knowledge include anatomy apps that contain layered illustrations of bones, muscles, ligaments, and nerves to help both professionals and students review bony prominences, muscle origins, insertions, and nerve and blood supply. Some apps guide practitioners with ICD-10 codes. Ebooks and journal apps give OT practitioners easy access to current knowledge, as well as specific tests, examinations, and outcomes measures to reach objective diagnostic conclusions for musculoskeletal and orthopedic disorders. For clinical use, OT practitioners can also use apps to design individual exercise plans, measure ROM, or obtain assistance with communicating in another language with clients. Some apps also provide client tests or questionnaires to help guide appropriate treatment.

For clients, many new apps provide a cost-effective method for client education on joint anatomy and specific orthopedic conditions to help clients better understand their pathology. Most joint prosthetic companies have apps to illustrate products and surgical techniques. Other apps guide clients through orthopedic rehabilitation, allowing them to sync with their own timelines. Using technology in the clinic can be tremendously beneficial to both the clinician and client.

The hip joint is one of the largest joints in the body and is a major weight-bearing joint. Problems in the hip from disease or injury will significantly affect mobility and ADLs, IADLs, work, and many leisure pursuits.[17]

Common Problems

The many causes of hip pain and disability include arthritis, avascular necrosis, and fractures. Osteoarthritis (OA) is the most common cause of hip pain. It is a chronic, degenerative disorder that occurs with the gradual deterioration of the cartilage in a joint. As the cartilage wears off, the surfaces of the bones become rough, and rubbing together then causes pain, swelling, and loss of motion of the joint. OA mainly affects older adults after years of wear and tear, but younger people may also be affected after trauma, injury, or a genetic defect in the cartilage.[18] Rheumatoid arthritis (RA) is an autoimmune condition in which the body's own immune system attacks its joints, causing destruction of the joint due to severe inflammation. Avascular necrosis is the death of bone tissue due to a lack of blood supply; it can lead to tiny fractures in the hip and eventual joint collapse. Avascular necrosis can be caused by a hip fracture, drugs (excessive long-term steroids), alcoholism, and systemic diseases (systemic lupus erythematosus).[19] Hip fractures in older adults are most commonly caused by falls, but spontaneous fractures may also occur during normal weight-bearing movements if the bones are already weak due to osteoporosis (disease causing decreased bone strength), avascular necrosis, or other conditions.

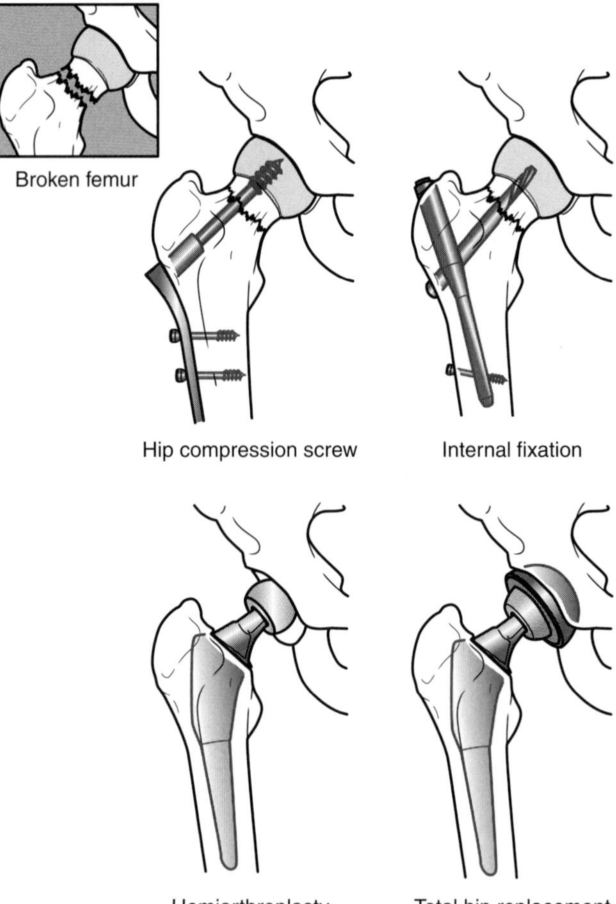

FIGURE 20-7. Types of hip surgery.

Surgery

The main types of hip surgery include open reduction internal fixation (ORIF), total hip replacement (THR) or arthroplasty (THA), hemiarthroplasty, hip resurfacing, and revision (Fig. 20-7). An **open reduction internal fixation (ORIF)** is often used to repair a hip fracture. The fracture is reduced or put back in place, and an internal fixation device is placed on the bone to hold the broken bone together. This involves using screws, plates, rods, or pins depending on the severity of the fracture. Often the surgeon specifies weight-bearing precautions but no **hip movement precautions** (limitations in movement to protect healing joint); clients are just limited by soreness from the surgery but can be encouraged to stretch and move within their comfort for functional tasks. **Total hip replacement** or **arthroplasty (THR, THA)** involves surgically removing the entire hip joint (acetabulum and femoral head and neck) and replacing it with an artificial joint (**prosthesis**) made of different combinations of metal, ceramic, or plastic. During this procedure, the surgeon may use the posterior approach (behind the hip), lateral approach (side of the hip), anterior approach (in front of the hip), or anterolateral approach (midway between the front and side of the hip). The posterior approach allows easier access to the hip joint, but requires cutting through the buttock (gluteus maximus) muscle and detaching some muscle tendons from the femur. This poses an increased risk for postoperative hip dislocation until the muscles heal back together. The lateral approach involves elevating the gluteus medius and vastus lateralis to access the hip joint. Here the risk for dislocation is low, but this approach causes a risk for nerve damage and postoperative muscle weakness. No hip precautions are necessary after the direct lateral approach. The anterior approach is a minimally invasive incision in the groin area that does not require detaching or cutting muscles, and has less chance of dislocation, but it is harder for the surgeon to access the hip, and there is an increased risk for nerve damage. The anterolateral approach involves detachment of about one-third of the gluteus medius from the bone and reattachment. The chance of dislocation is less, but there is an increased risk for muscle weakness and a limp for up to a year. With each approach, the incision may be traditional (single long 10-inch to 12-inch incision with muscles split or detached) or minimally invasive (one or two smaller incisions and fewer muscles around the hip are cut or detached). It is important to know which approach the surgeon used to determine which hip precautions the client must follow.[20]

A **hemiarthroplasty** hip surgery is used to treat a fractured hip. The operation is similar to a total hip replacement, but only involves replacing half of the hip—the ball portion and not the socket portion (*hemi* means half, and *arthroplasty* means joint replacement). A hemiarthroplasty may be unipolar (replacement of the femoral head and neck), bipolar (replacement of the femoral head and neck plus an addition of an acetabular cup that fits in the existing acetabulum), or resurfacing (replacement of the surface of the femoral head). Hip **revision surgery** is performed to repair an artificial hip joint that has been damaged due to an infection, dislocation, or normal wear and tear of the prosthetic hip. Clients who undergo a hemiarthroplasty or hip revision will have to follow hip precautions. The typical life of an artificial hip joint is 10 to 15 years.[21]

Movement Precautions

An important part of OT after a total hip replacement is educating the client on hip precautions specific to his or her type of surgery. Clients typically must follow hip precautions for the first 3 months until the muscles around the hip heal, but sometimes clients have to follow precautions indefinitely if they are prone to dislocating. The surgeon will determine the timeframe and specifics on hip precautions depending on the individual's surgery type, length of incision, muscles cut, and integrity of the surrounding tissue. The two main types of hip precautions are posterior hip precautions and anterior hip precautions.

POSTERIOR HIP PRECAUTIONS

Surgeries that require posterior hip precautions include the posterior approach THR, hemiarthroplasty, and revision (Fig. 20-8).

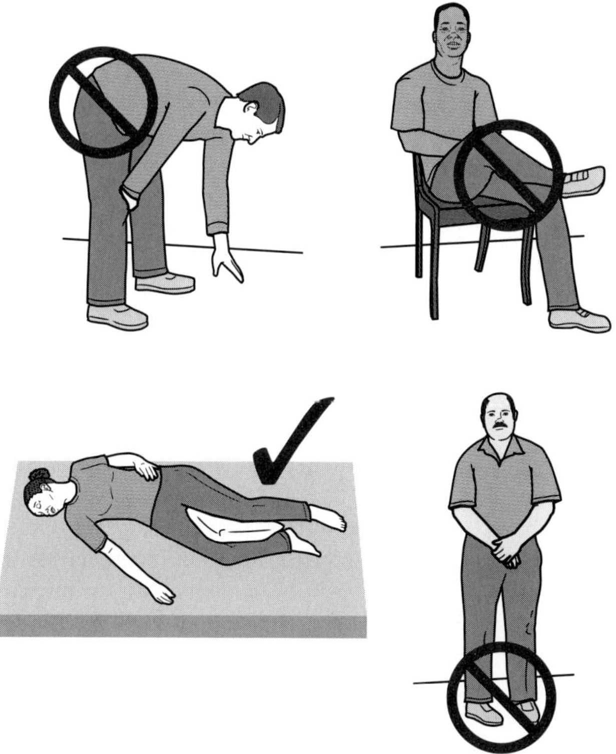

FIGURE 20-8. Posterior hip precautions. Do not bend your hip past a 90-degree angle. Do not cross your legs. Use a pillow between your legs when rolling. Do not twist your hip inward.

1) No Hip Flexion (Bending) Greater Than 90 Degrees: The smaller range of allowable hip flexion (only 90 degrees) limits activities involving bending over or lifting up the affected leg. Clients are only allowed to reach down as far as their knees, so OT practitioners must train them to use adaptive equipment for lower body dressing, bathing, and picking up items from the floor or low cabinets. It takes repetition and training with the use of adaptive equipment (reacher, sock aid, dressing stick, long shoehorn, and elastic shoelaces) while the client is seated. Practicing in a seated position is preferable so clients do not bend over, cross their legs, or lift their leg up in order to reach their feet (as when donning socks or shoes). Instruct clients to pick up and reach items with a reacher instead of bending over, and have them practice with items such as socks, shoes, clothing, or anything they would normally bend over to reach during their occupations. Clients should avoid couches, chairs, and toilets that are low to the ground or even regular height. It is best if the sitting height is above the client's knee level, such as a dining chair or raised toilet seat (around 19 inches). When transitioning from sitting to standing, the client can also slide the operated leg out straight before standing or sitting to increase the hip angle and prevent bending greater than 90 degrees (Fig. 20-9). A few other key areas to train clients occur when transferring to a bed, bathtub, or car. Clients should use a higher bed (bed risers are readily available) and a raised shower chair. After clients sit down, teach them to lean their trunk back and slide back as far as possible, and then swing their operated leg into position without lifting it over 90 degrees flexion. For entering a car, the client should have someone position the seat in a semireclined position, slid back as far as possible from the dashboard before entering the car. Clients should sit down on the seat of the car, leaning their trunk back so as not to break the 90-degree hip flexion precaution, and carefully lift the affected leg into the car, keeping it in line with their torso, while rotating their body into the vehicle.

2) No Hip Internal Rotation (Do Not Turn Leg Inward): Occupational therapy assistants (OTAs) should teach clients not to use the operated leg to kick off shoes or cross legs. The OTA must train clients to lead with their operated leg when making turns to the operated side; do not plant the operated leg and twist the body (because it leaves the operated leg internally rotated). Instruct clients to carefully open a heavy door or refrigerator door because sometimes they forcefully rotate their upper body with the operated leg planted, which leaves the operated leg internally rotated.

3) No Hip Adduction Beyond Neutral (Do Not Cross Legs): Clients should keep their legs spread apart and should not cross them. It is helpful to have clients use a pillow or abduction wedge (triangular foam wedge with straps) between their legs when lying in bed.

ANTERIOR HIP PRECAUTIONS

Surgeries that require anterior hip precautions include anterior and anterolateral approach THR (Fig. 20-10).

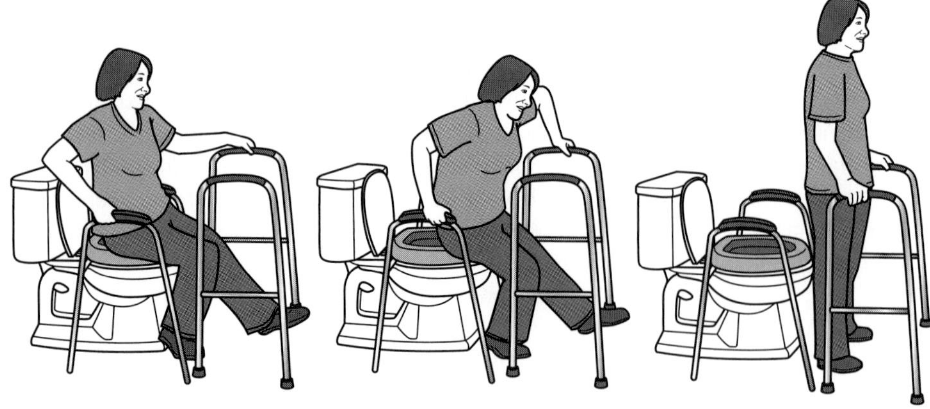

FIGURE 20-9. The client will transfer from a raised height chair with arms by carefully scooting forward, kicking out leg with precautions, and carefully moving to stand, while maintaining hip precautions.

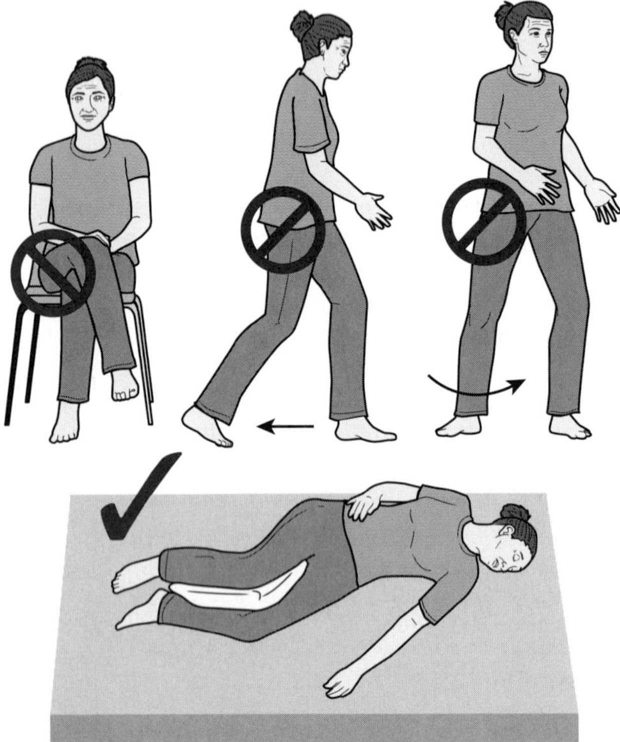

FIGURE 20-10. Anterior hip precautions. Do not cross legs, do not step backward or extend at hip with surgical leg. If backing up, lead with nonsurgical leg. Do not turn surgical leg out (hip external rotation). Use a pillow between legs when rolling.

1) No Hip Extension: Clients should not step or kick backward with their operated leg. Walk with small steps, because large, long steps leave the operated leg in a position of extension. When supine, clients should keep their hip flexed to 30 degrees by placing a pillow under the knee or raise the head of the bed. Clients should not bridge (lift hips while supine) or sleep in the prone position.

2) No Hip External Rotation Beyond Neutral: Train clients to not turn their operated leg out to the side with ambulation, while turning, or during seated activities (toes should be pointed forward). Teach clients to avoid a straddling position when getting out of bed or the bathtub. Instruct client to place a pillow next to the hip/leg to keep the leg from turning/rolling out to the side while in a supine position.

Weight-Bearing Precautions

In orthopedics, weight-bearing is defined as the amount of weight a client can put on the operated limb. Bone healing involves a complex process in which mechanical forces are essential for the regeneration of bone tissue.[22] Weight-bearing can induce osteogenesis (bone formation) to maximize functional outcome and increase achievement of independent living.[23] Before working with an orthopedic client, the OTA must always confirm the client's weight-bearing status. Although weight-bearing helps to heal bone, too much weight-bearing on joints that are not yet stable can cause damage and hinder overall healing. The surgeon will determine the weight-bearing status for each phase of recovery based on stability of the surgical fixation (cemented or uncemented), degree of fracture stabilization, bone integrity, muscle strength, and evidence of bone healing.

The surgeon will choose between using cement (bonding agent) or not with hip or knee replacement surgery. Cemented joints form an immediate strong bond to the bone with less joint pain, but may weaken over time. Uncemented joints have an initially weaker bond but form a strong permanent bond over time as the bone fills in around the prosthesis.[24] When determining the weight-bearing status, the surgeon also has to factor in the degree of fracture stabilization, which is the amount of motion at the fracture site under physiological load. Some fracture patterns are more complex because they result in displacement and spiral lines, which are challenging to fix.

The bone healing process has three overlapping stages: inflammation, bone production, and bone remodeling. Inflammation may last several days and involves bleeding and clotting that provides the initial structural stability. During bone production, fibrous tissue and cartilage develops into hard bone, which is visible on x-rays after several weeks. The final phase of bone healing, bone remodeling, occurs for several months as the bone continues to form, becomes compact, and develops improved blood circulation.[25] As the surgeon sees evidence of bone healing, clients will be allowed to increase their weight-bearing status, so it is important that OT practitioners check the client's chart and stay in good communication with staff for updates on the client's progress. OT practitioners will also consult with physical therapy (PT) practitioners to follow their recommendation of an appropriate assistive device for mobility. Only the PT may progress the client from walker to cane.

LEVELS OF WEIGHT-BEARING

Weight-bearing progresses in the following five levels:

1. Non–weight-bearing (NWB): 0% weight. The leg must not touch the floor and is not permitted to support any weight at all. If clients are unable to hold up their leg by themselves to stand with a walker, a transfer board can be used for transfers. If the practitioner holds up the operated leg, make sure the client doesn't bear weight into the practitioner's hands.
2. Touch-down weight-bearing or toe-touch weight-bearing (TDWB/TTWB): The foot or toes may touch the floor for balance but not support any weight. Practitioners often put their own foot under the client's operated leg while the client is standing to make sure the client is not putting weight through the limb. It may be helpful to instruct clients to think about gently placing their toe on an egg lying on the floor without cracking or breaking the egg, as a means to understand TDWB/TTWB.
3. Partial weight-bearing (PWB): 1% to 50% weight. A small amount of weight may be supported by the operated leg and gradually increased up to 50% of the body weight per surgeon orders. Sometimes a scale is used to determine the amount of weight clients are putting on their operated leg. For example, if the client is 25% PWB and they weigh 200 pounds, the client will be allowed to put up to 50 pounds of weight through their operated leg (weight × % ÷ 100 = WB amount).
4. Weight-bearing as tolerated (WBAT): 50% to 100% of weight. Clients can choose the amount of weight, meaning bear as much as they can tolerate on their affected leg. The amount tolerated may be affected by pain or weakness.
5. Full weight-bearing (FWB): 100% weight. The operated leg can carry 100% of the body weight.

Intervention

OT plays an important role in teaching clients with orthopedic conditions how to incorporate hip precautions, weight-bearing precautions, adaptive techniques and equipment, and safety techniques into their daily activities to enhance independence. Mobility starts slowly, and clients may do best with slowly easing each leg to the side of the bed, with assistance, moving the operated leg and pushing up to sit on the edge of the bed. Clients who do not have posterior hip precautions are allowed to bend over to reach their feet, but may be limited by pain. OTAs can teach clients to dress and bathe their lower bodies with adaptive equipment, but also work on increasing their reach over time. Raised bedside commodes are usually placed over a standard toilet to provide a higher level and armrests to push up/down. To avoid falls in the slippery tub or shower, training clients to use a raised shower chair or bench, non-slip mat, and grab bars is usually recommended. Functional practice of safe mobility in the home and kitchen using a walker with both hands incorporating safe lifting, reaching, and carrying techniques is helpful to prevent falls and reinjury. OT practitioners often encourage the client to use a walker basket, apron, or pockets to carry items so both hands can remain on the walker in the various areas of the home. Clients can also slide items such as a plate or drink along a counter while standing, and then keep both hands on the walker to walk. Clients will slowly increase their independence and safety with functional mobility, ADLs, and IADLs during OT training.

THE KNEE JOINT

OT practitioners should be familiar with general knee anatomy, as well as common knee problems and surgeries they will encounter, along with intervention strategies.

Anatomy of the Knee Joint

The knee is a complex joint with many components (Fig. 20-11). It is a hinge joint formed where the femur, tibia, and patella meet. The ends of the femur, tibia, and the back of the patella are covered with articular cartilage that helps the knee glide smoothly to bend and straighten. Two wedge-shaped pieces of meniscal cartilage act as shock absorbers between the femur and tibia. The bones are connected by ligaments that keep the knee stable. Muscles are connected to bones by tendons.[27] The knee joint is essential to many everyday activities including walking, running, stairs, sitting, and standing.

Common Problems

The bones give strength, stability, and flexibility to the knee. The most common causes of knee disability are OA, RA, and post-traumatic arthritis. OA causes the articular cartilage to wear away, resulting in severe knee pain and stiffness. In RA, the immune system attacks its own tissues and softens the bone. The synovial membrane that covers the knee joint swells and then causes knee pain and stiffness. Post-traumatic arthritis develops after an injury to the knee causing instability and "wear-and-tear" that over time results in arthritis.[28]

Surgery

When pain medication and other treatments (such as corticosteroid injections, braces, electric stimulation, and exercise) are no longer effective, a surgeon may perform a **total knee replacement (TKR)** or **total knee arthroplasty (TKA)** (Fig. 20-12). During the procedure, the surgeon will

EVIDENCE-BASED PRACTICE #2

1. Problem: Client with moderate dementia, fell sustaining a right intertrochanteric hip fracture and is seen after right hip ORIF and has touch-down weight-bearing status.
2. Medical literature: A systematic review found evidence to support the effectiveness of rehabilitation (improved function and ambulation with reduced fall risk) following hip fracture in clients with mild to moderate dementia using a multidisciplinary approach and strategies to manage cognitive and behavioral issues.[26]
3. Critical analysis: Fair- to good-quality ratings for 13 studies that met following inclusion criteria: five randomized clinical trials, seven prospective cohort series, and one retrospective cohort study.
4. Application: OTA treatment included multidisciplinary education and training to enhance carry-over of functional treatment techniques, fall prevention, and safety with touch-down weight-bearing status during transfers. Staff, family, and client included in coordinated training along with PT. Cotreatments with PT and nursing provided to assist with touch-down weight-bearing during functional mobility/transfers. Cognitive treatment strategies included: developing a routine for ADLs; repetition to enhance carry-over of new skills; simple one-step cues; picture labels on bathroom door, closet, and drawers to aid orientation; verbal and visual (handouts) safety reminders to enhance learning. Safety/fall prevention techniques coordinated with nursing staff included: soft mat next to bed at night; pressure bell alarm in bed and chair; toilet program every 2 hours; and, when client left seated, supervised in common area.
5. Assessment: Progress/outcomes was measured by comparing evaluation test results to current testing results for: pain level reported, nursing falls/safety report, functional mobility level, functional ADL level of independence incorporating safety, and return to prior level.

Allen, J., Koziak, A., Buddingh, S., Liang, J., Buckingham, J., & Beaupre, L. A. (2012). Rehabilitation in patients with dementia following hip fracture: A systematic review. Physiotherapy Canada, *64(2), 190–201.*

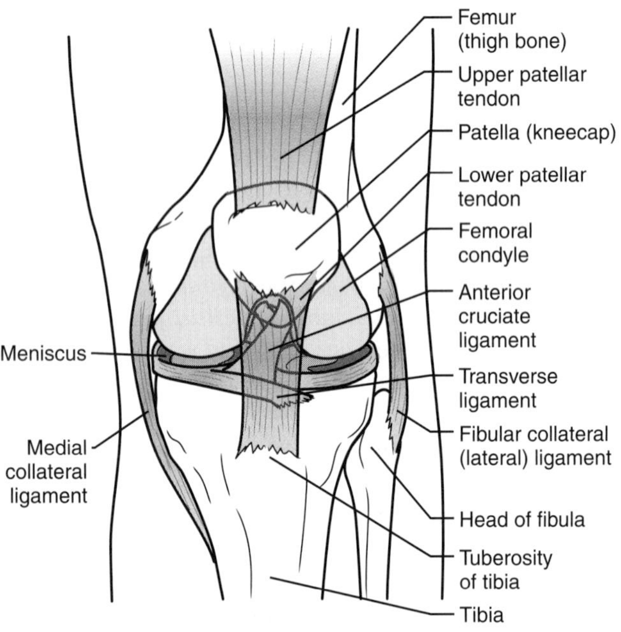

FIGURE 20-11. Anatomy of the knee.

remove the damaged cartilage and bone and reshape the bony surfaces to fit the prosthesis, or artificial joint. The surgeon will cement the prosthetic components into place, including a metal femoral shell, a metal and plastic tibial component, and a plastic patellar component. The prosthetic joint will last usually over 20 years before requiring a revision knee replacement (second knee replacement).[29] Minimally invasive knee surgeries are also performed where only the damaged or arthritic parts of the knee are treated, rather than replacing the entire knee joint. This is called a **partial knee replacement** or **knee resurfacing.** Jagged bone edges or spurs are trimmed and removed. Then only the inner side or outer compartment of the knee joint is replaced with an implant.[30]

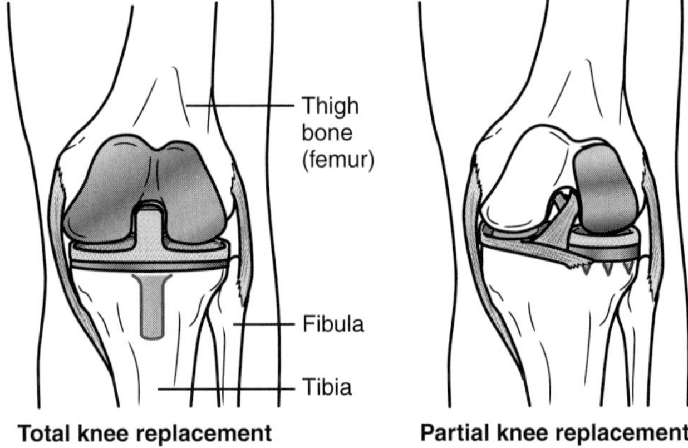

FIGURE 20-12. Total and partial knee replacement.

Intervention

The main goal after knee surgery is to get the knee joint moving. PT focuses on gaining maximum knee range of motion through exercises. The use of a **continuous passive motion (CPM) device** was formerly standard protocol, however, there has been little evidence to indicate use with clients postoperatively, and in fact, use may cause knee swelling to last longer.[32,33] Surgeons may still recommend the device, however, so the OT practitioner should be aware of the machine and its use. While lying in bed, the client's leg is placed in the padded CPM frame. The machine gently

EVIDENCE-BASED PRACTICE #3

1. Problem: Client diagnosed with osteoarthritis is seen after a left TKR and is not wanting to participate with OT.
2. Medical literature: A study by Moffet found an intensive functional rehabilitation (IFR) program was effective in improving functional ability after uncomplicated TKA.
3. Critical analysis: Randomized controlled trial with IFR (n = 38) and control group (n = 39) with significant positive outcomes with: increased ambulation distance in 6 minutes and quality-of-life measures; and less pain, stiffness, and difficulty performing ADLs.
4. Application: OTA treatment included client and family education on the benefits of OT to enhance participation. OTA recommended upgrading client to ultra-high therapy RUG level (at least 720 minutes, PT and OT disciplines, 5 days a week) to enhance rehabilitation outcomes based on research evidence and increased client OT participation.
5. Assessment: Progress/outcomes was measured by comparing evaluation test results to current testing results for: pain level reported, quality-of-life measure, functional mobility level, functional ADL level of independence incorporating safety, and return to prior level.[31]

Moffet, H., Collet, J. P., Shapiro, S. H., Paradis, G., Marquis, F., & Roy, L. (2004). Effectiveness of intensive rehabilitation on functional ability and quality of life after first total knee arthroplasty: A single-blind randomized controlled trial. Archives of Physical Medicine and Rehabilitation. 85*(4), 546–56.*

moves the knee joint to a specified speed and range that is slowly increased over time by the PT. OT practitioners can assist with encouraging clients to flex and extend their knees during ADLs and functional mobility. OT practitioners can progress the client with dressing, bathing, toileting, kitchen mobility, homemaking tasks, tub/shower transfers, and car transfers using the appropriate mobility device that the PT recommends. OT practitioners will determine the client's need for adaptive equipment, such as a shower chair/bench, grab bars, and raised toilet seat/bedside commode. Sometimes OT practitioners may train the client on use of adaptive equipment for lower body dressing and bathing if the client has not achieved full range and needs to be independent. Usually the surgeon wants the client to increase full motion to perform tasks independently without adaptive equipment.

AQUATIC THERAPY

Aquatic therapy is one of the many tools that OTAs use to help clients of all ages, abilities, and diagnoses achieve OT goals. Water can be an excellent environment for clients who have difficulty with muscle strength, muscle tone, weight-bearing, joint pain, joint flexibility, balance, healing, and sensory perception.[34]

1. Muscle strength: Water has high viscosity and provides 12 times the resistance of air, which allows for strengthening of weakened muscles.[35] Clients in water use many more muscles and have stronger muscle contractions than they would by exercising on land. Accessories such as water dumbbells, fins, weighted toys, and other tools help OTAs grade the resistance in the water.
2. Muscle tone: Aquatic therapy is performed in a heated pool normally between 92 and 96 degrees. The heated water helps to normalize muscle tone and reduce stress on the body.
3. Weight-bearing: Water buoyancy decreases the weight-bearing on joints. A 200-lb. person would only weigh 100 lb. in waist-deep water; at shoulder-level depth, that same person would only weigh 20 lbs. (10% of their weight on land).[36] The water can allow increased safety and ease with mobility for clients with weight-bearing restrictions.
4. Joint pain: Water buoyancy reduces joint stress and increases comfort during mobility. In addition, the warm water decreases joint pain.
5. Joint flexibility: The warm water and its massaging effects increase blood supply to sore muscles and promote relaxation. Water buoyancy reduces the effects of gravity allowing for increased joint range of motion. The affected body part will float, making it easier and less painful to move.
6. Balance: The uniform pressure of water along with buoyancy provides support to the body allowing increased time to react without the fear of falling or getting hurt. Water stimulates body awareness, balance, and trunk stability to stay upright. Clients can tolerate increased challenges in the water with reaching, play, walking, kneeling, squatting, and stepping using underwater benches to simulate functional tasks. Accessories such as noodles, floating mats, floatation belts, and vests can allow the OTA to grade the amount of balance required.
7. Healing: Aquatic therapy can facilitate healing to the site of injury. Exercising in water increases vasodilation of blood vessels. Increased blood flow to the injury site results in increased oxygen and nutrient delivery as well as waste product removal—all of which promote the healing process. The hydrostatic pressure in water is helpful in decreasing inflammation and edema. Massager jets can also be used over a healed and closed incision to break down scar tissue formation. In order to avoid cross-contamination with others, no client with an open wound should be in the regular pool without the wound being completely covered from getting wet. Typically, a handheld sprayer is used instead of a whirlpool bath for individual wound care.

8. Sensory-perceptual: Aquatic therapy can also enhance the areas of emotional regulation, cognitive, communication, and social skills. Water activities can be exciting, fun, and a technique to address self-regulating behavior. Incorporating leisure activities, following directions, interactions, and group activities also work on perceptual skills.

All of the skills involved in aquatic therapy are the building blocks of the areas of occupation such as ADLs, IADLs, work, play, education, leisure, and social participation. Aquatic therapy can allow clients to accelerate therapy and participate in rehabilitation activities earlier than they otherwise might on dry land. The healing properties of water offer practitioners a valuable tool to help clients reach their goals.

GENERAL ORTHOPEDIC CONCERNS

Many general concerns are important to consider when working with clients with orthopedic conditions to enhance safety, wellness, and support during OT treatment.

Postsurgical Complications

OT practitioners work closely with clients and are often the ones who become aware of postsurgical complications such as deep vein thrombosis (DVT), infection, and pneumonia. A DVT occurs when the large veins of the body (usually in one of the legs) forms a blood clot. It usually appears as a painful, tender, swollen, redness in the calf muscle. The danger is if the blood clot breaks loose, travels, and becomes lodged in the capillaries of the lung causing a pulmonary embolism. The orthopedic surgeon/internist and all team members should be notified immediately if symptoms appear. The client is usually placed on bedrest and not allowed to move the limb until cleared by the surgeon or internist. Steps to avoid a DVT include a sequential compression device (SCD), which is an inflatable sleeve or boot that provides intermittent air pump pressure around the limb to move venous blood; they are used frequently postsurgery in the hospital. Other ways to avoid a DVT are anticoagulants (blood-thinning medications), compression stockings (tight socks of various compression depending on need), and foot/ankle pump exercises to increase blood flow and venous return in the lower extremity. It is important to keep all incision sites dry, clean, and covered.

To prevent infection, all staff should wash their hands before and after each client treatment. The client will take sponge baths until the surgeon allows him or her to shower. When working on bathing and dressing with clients, OT practitioners can ensure safety and monitor any problems noted at the surgery site such as redness, swelling, and tenderness. If the client has a catheter to drain urine after surgery, always keep the collection bag lower than the client's thigh so the tubing does not back up and cause a urinary infection. After surgery and anesthesia, secretions can pool at the base of the lungs due to immobility, which may lead to lung congestion, infection, or pneumonia. OT practitioners help to minimize this complication by educating clients on deep breathing exercises during activities and mobility. This involves inhaling deeply through the nose and exhaling completely through the mouth. The client may have an incentive spirometer from the hospital, which is a device used to teach clients to take slow, deep breaths. The client breathes in and out through a tube, which moves a ball in the main chamber, and the goal is to keep the ball in the middle of the chamber for a slow, deep breath in. Because OT practitioners works closely and daily with clients with orthopedic conditions, the opportunity exists to help monitor and prevent many surgical complications.

Safety

Clients may have a low hemoglobin (red blood cell) level from blood loss during surgery or have prolonged bedrest that may lead to orthostatic hypotension. This is a quick drop in blood pressure with a change in position from supine to sitting to standing, resulting in lightheadedness, dizziness, and sometimes loss of consciousness. Clients should be progressed slowly out of bed and sit-to-standing tasks, observed closely, and monitored for changes in vital signs (blood pressure, pulse, and oxygen saturation) as needed with change of positioning, especially at the acute stage for safety. Review the normal, age-based ranges for safe levels of hemoglobin, blood pressure, oxygen saturation, blood sugar, and other values to help guide safety for activities (Table 20-1).

Fall Prevention

Regardless of which type of surgery, all clients with an orthopedic condition will have limited mobility and need safety education to prevent falls. It is important to educate the client, family, and staff at each step of recovery. For example, if a client with steel in his or her hip falls, the steel acts like a hammer and often fractures the pelvis. Many falls can be prevented with education on fall-prevention techniques. OT practitioners should follow PT recommendations when using a mobility device, such as a rolling walker, standard walker, or cane, with the client. OT can help determine whether clients need assistance or assistive devices for daily tasks, such as bathing, if mobility has become limited or if medications make the client dizzy. Home environments can be modified to prevent trip and fall hazards by removing loose rugs and clutter, repairing loose flooring or thresholds, and avoiding electrical cords across walkways. Adaptations, such as placing a nonslip mat in the tub and installing shower and toilet grab bars, may help to prevent falls as well. Proper lighting and high-contrast adaptations can aid clients with low vision to see steps and uneven surfaces. Advise clients to avoid slippery wet floors or icy sidewalks. Clients should wear properly fitting, sturdy shoes with nonskid soles. High heels, flip flops, floppy slippers, and slick soles

TABLE 20-1 Activity/Exercise Guidelines

VARIABLE (NORMS)	DO NOT START	STOP
Heart Rate (HR) (68–82 beats/min)	≥120 <50 or angina	≥120 or increase >20 above rest or angina or if HR drops >10
Systolic Blood Pressure (SBP) (<120 mmHg)	>180 <80	≥220
SBP Drop (normally goes up 10–20 mmHg)	Drops >20 Orthostatic hypotension	Drops >10
Diastolic Blood Pressure (DBP) (<80 mmHg)	>100	>100
Respiratory Rate (16–20 breaths/min)	≥30	
Oxygen Saturation (SpO_2) (95–100%)	<90%	Titrate to maintain >90%
Hematocrit (Hct) (male 42%–52%, female 36%–46%)	<25	
Hemoglobin (Hgb) (male 12–18gm/dL, female 12–16gm/dL)	<8	
Platelets (140–440 k/μL)	<20 no exercise 20–30 can do PROM 30–50 can do AROM >50 can do resistive ex	
Glucose (65–110 g/dL fasting) (65–199 random)	<60 >300	

Most conservative values obtained from American College of Sports Medicine, American Association of Cardiovascular and Pulmonary Rehabilitation, and Shore Health System of Maryland.

Contraindications to Activity
Unstable angina
Acute systemic infection
Moderate to severe aortic stenosis
Uncontrolled diabetes
Significant ischemia
Acute pulmonary embolism (PE) (<2 days)
Uncontrolled cardiac dysrhythmias
Deep vein thrombosis (DVT)
Active pericarditis or myocarditis
Recent myocardial infarction (MI) (<2 days)
Always check with the nurse and the medical chart before treatment.

can cause slips, stumbles, and falls. Shoes should cover the back of the heel so the client cannot slide out of them by accident.

Debility

Many clients may have been less mobile for a long time before treatment and as a result display increased weakness and decreased activity tolerance. Whether the issue is their back, hip, pelvis, or knee, they will need to depend on their upper body strength more for functional mobility. If the debility is significant, the client may need a short stay in a rehabilitation unit, especially if they live alone. OT practitioners can address strength and endurance with clients with orthopedic conditions through a progressive resistive upper-extremity exercise program as well as performing everyday tasks to enhance functional mobility and general activity tolerance for ADLs and IADLs. As always, provide the "just-right challenge" for clients as they become stronger and increase functional endurance. For example, the client may start ADLs seated at the edge of the bed, progress to standing with an assistive device (if needed) at counter or sink for ADLs, and then eventually progress to showering with the appropriate adaptive equipment.

Pain

Pain management is crucial to allow maximum client participation with rehabilitation. The OTA must coordinate treatments with the client's pain medication schedule. OT practitioners can also assist with decreasing pain by training the client on proper body mechanics during functional mobility, ADLs, and IADLs. Clients often stiffen up their bodies to guard against pain, but this often causes more pain and reduced movement, blood-flow, and healing. The OTA may also look for signs of fear or hesitation on the client's face. Therapeutic use of self is especially important to use with clients who are experiencing pain. It helps to develop a sense of trust and rapport with the client and educate them on the benefits of movement and activity to reduce pain. Gain the client's confidence by listening and reassuring them that fear and anxiety after surgery is normal. Be honest that it will hurt to move, but reassure clients that all staff will help to make it as comfortable as possible, and the pain will lessen as they move and do more activities. Be sure to support the operated area, discuss each step of the activity, warn the client before moving the operated area, and encourage the client to relax and take deep breaths. Lighthearted joking with clients and distracting them with conversation can also lessen their anxiety and fear of pain. See Chapter 8 for more information on pain.

Cognitive

Many clients experience increased confusion due to multiple factors including stress from trauma, surgical anesthesia, strong pain medications, and change of environment. Clients may have some underlying dementia, which is exacerbated, or may just have temporary confusion. OTAs must be creative with training and safety techniques when clients have cognitive limitations. Return demonstration, illustrations, labels, caregiver training, and repetition are all helpful techniques to develop routines incorporating new learning. Clear, simple handouts with illustrations and simple language can be helpful to reinforce learning as well.

Psychosocial Impact

Management of clients with orthopedic conditions mostly focuses on stabilization of injuries, relieving pain, and restoring physical function. Less attention is focused on client psychosocial status following orthopedic surgery. Poor wound healing, increased postoperative pain, and decreased functional outcomes have been correlated with poor emotional health, such as anxiety, depression, stress, poor coping skills, and poor social support.[38] Acknowledging the influence of psychosocial factors with clients with orthopedic conditions

THE OLDER ADULT[37]

Interventions for older adults with orthopedic conditions are almost always multifactorial to address multiple conditions and impairments. Even healthy older adults with only one clinical disease are likely to have subclinical pathologies. Most older adults experience a gradual decline in physical strength, proprioception, coordination, vision, hearing, and cognitive skills. Comorbidity is the presence of one or more additional diseases or disorders besides the primary focus. Common comorbidities that may contribute to functional disability include cardiopulmonary diseases, neurological conditions, diabetes, cancer, obesity, dementia, affective disorders, ophthalmological disorders, auditory disorders, osteoporosis, and arthritis. Whether the orthopedic client had an acute injury (fall/accident) or subacute functional decline (arthritis/degenerative joint disease) that led to a specific orthopedic surgery, it is important to factor in all underlying medical conditions and impairments during treatment and to prevent recurrent falls.

Two or more comorbidities or health conditions often creates more disability than would be expected, and as the number of impairments increases, so does the functional disability. For example, a client with a hip replacement with weakness on one side from a cerebrovascular accident (CVA) will have an increased work demand to walk or do housework, and if that client also has heart disease, he or she may lack the capacity to compensate for this increased demand. Interventions to increase capacity include oxygen supplementation, breathing exercises, graded exercises, and functional tasks. Interventions to reduce task demands include: using a walker or wheelchair, employing a raised toilet seat, sitting on a shower chair, installing a ramp, obtaining a personal aide, and using energy conservation/work simplification techniques.

In another example, a client with memory problems may have difficulties learning new safety techniques with functional mobility after a hip ORIF and also have poor vision. Compensation techniques may include large-print one-step safety tips, enhanced lighting, removing trip hazards, repetition of new safety routines, placing a soft mat next to the bed or half rails on the bed, creating a toileting program, using a chair/bed alarm, and routine safety checks or supervision.

Another type of potential comorbidity is the possibility of one or more additional diseases or disorders associated with the primary orthopedic focus. Examples of this may be after orthopedic surgery, the client develops pneumonia, infection, increased cognitive impairment, delirium, incontinence, or a DVT. Sometimes OT practitioners pick up on these symptoms because they work closely for long periods every day with the clients. It is important to closely observe and listen to clients and families, and to report any new symptoms to the nurse and physician.

Coexistence of multiple impairments complicates treatment and the natural course of rehabilitation in older adults. It is important for OTAs to treat the whole person, not just the orthopedic diagnosis, and factor in preexisting and potential comorbidities during interventions to obtain the most successful outcome.

promotes successful outcomes. The OT treatment approach should empower clients and encourage positive expectations with respect to recovery and goals, in addition to locating adaptive equipment and methods to overcome any obstacles.

Marked changes in sleep patterns, coping mechanisms, and ability to exercise, perform normal daily tasks, and attend work and social activities are associated with chronic pain and orthopedic problems. Depression, grief, stress, and anxiety are all common emotions clients with orthopedic conditions experience, which can interfere with the rehabilitation process if not addressed.[38] Many clients with orthopedic conditions have been dealing with a chronic disability or the aging process, which can slowly take away their independence, functional mobility, and social and leisure participation for years. Grief over loss of function and displacement from a home environment and family can manifest as depression. Clients can also exhibit stress when dealing with a traumatic fracture, expectations for recovery, anticipated medical bills, and responsibilities. Anxiety is often seen with the client's fear of falling or pain during rehabilitation activities. It is crucial to listen and acknowledge the client's feelings as normal. The process of setting positive goals, maintaining realistic expectations, and celebrating progress with clients are all parts of the OT treatment plan, but are also strategies to keep clients healthy and positive. OT can also encourage healthy habits such as developing a routine for activities and exercise. Providing support, coping skills, and increased independence will help clients gain increased self-efficacy, a person's belief in his or her ability to succeed in a particular situation. A person can develop self-efficacy through mastery of experiences (performing tasks successfully), social modeling (seeing others succeed), and social persuasion (positive encouragement from staff/family/peers to achieve goals).[39] If the client's emotions continue to spiral downward and are getting in the way of their functioning and recovery, the OTA must notify the supervising OT, as well as the physician and nurse for a possible psychiatric consult. The emotional health of the client influences the physical recovery after orthopedic surgery.

Simple questionnaires are available that can determine a client's level of anxiety, stress, depression, and information pertaining to their social support status. Often a simple conversation or question during treatment asking clients about their depression, stress at work or home, methods of coping, fears, and present status of interpersonal support relationships will show them that OT is addressing the whole body, mind, and lifestyle—including any psychological and social issues—and not just the orthopedic issue. This information may also be valuable for the whole multidisciplinary team. OTAs should share information and collaborate with other professionals, such as nurses and physicians for medication management, psychiatrists for counseling, recreational therapists for social/recreational opportunities, and social workers or case managers for support resources. Box 20-1 discusses the importance of assisting clients to return to everyday and leisure activities.

BOX 20-1

Leisure[40]

The goal of orthopedic surgery is to reduce pain and return to everyday and leisure activities. Leisure activities can be a powerful tool to decrease physical or emotional pain and anxiety as well as increase function. Leisure was key in the formation of our profession and is still an integral part of the current *Occupational Therapy Practice Framework: Domain and Process, 3rd edition* (OTPF-3).

Leisure checklists or questionnaires or casual conversation can identify leisure pursuits and hobbies. Incorporating leisure interests while addressing treatment goals can increase participation and motivation, and bridge mental and physical health. Some examples are incorporating playing cards while working on standing balance/tolerance; performing simple cooking tasks while working on kitchen mobility/safety; playing Wii™ bowling to work on balance/reaching skills; and watering plants to work on dynamic standing balance.

OTAs can help identify and resolve challenges that prevent or limit clients from their desired leisure pursuits. Treatment includes education, suggesting assistive devices or alternative approaches, and offering therapeutic activity to restore function. For example, after a posterior approach THR, to avoid internal hip rotation, have the client perform stationary putt-putt instead of a full golf swing or gardening in raised containers to avoid full hip flexion.

There are different risks associated with certain types of leisure and sport activities. Resumption of sports activities should be cleared by the surgeon depending on the type of surgery. In general, the more vigorous the activity, the higher the risk for damaging the orthopedic implant, increasing the wear and tear on the implant, or increasing the risk for loosening or dislocating the implant. High-impact or high-risk sports activities should be avoided such as: high-impact aerobics, high-intensity jogging/running, water skiing, intense hiking, downhill skiing, martial arts, and rough contact sports. Lower-stress activities are much better choices for exercise such as: golf, hiking (on relatively flat surfaces or slight inclines), walking, swimming, table tennis, and bowling.

OTAs have a unique set of skills to: analyze a leisure activity; identify the demands and skills involved; apply medical knowledge of the client's orthopedic condition, strengths, and limitations; use skill-building interventions or adaptations; and grade the activity to meet the just-right challenge. Leisure activities often have elements that build specific skills that directly relate to functional goals and outcomes. Leisure activities are also typically more engaging for the client than rote exercises. OTAs need to incorporate leisure activities in client treatment to stimulate and rehabilitate the mind and body.

As clients experience functional decline, it is common for them to withdraw from more complex activity and social environments and become dependent on others to perform tasks for them. It is important to involve clients in the decision making for rehabilitation and discharge planning to share what is meaningful to them. The act of participation in meaningful activities can help to alleviate depression, anxiety, and stress for many clients. Providing multiple small successes in graded functional activities promotes self-esteem and well-being.

The interpersonal relationship between the OT practitioner and the client is key to helping the client reach his or her full potential. Techniques to build client rapport may vary, such as using humor, giving compliments, sharing common interests, showing respect or admiration of their strengths/talents, listening, or simply repeating the feelings they share. Each client responds differently, and the key is finding ways to intervene that help clients maintain dignity, participation, and a sense of purpose. By understanding the person's behaviors and values, OTAs can more effectively use the client's own belief system to support, develop, and enhance their behavioral change and orthopedic rehabilitation to hopefully restore them to their prior or even better functional level.[39]

Sexual Activity

Sexual activity is an important part of quality of life and should be addressed in orthopedic treatment. It is important for the OTA to normalize sexual activities as one of many ADLs OT addresses with clients. Often OT practitioners are already dealing with personal areas, such as bathing, dressing, and toileting. Using an open-ended question can help open the door to a conversation about sexuality, such as: "People who have had a hip replacement sometimes have concerns or questions about how they'll be affected sexually. Do you have any concerns in this area?" A client who doesn't want to discuss sex is free to refuse, but at least should be given the opportunity to do so. Clients and their partners often have many questions and concerns about sex after surgery, and appreciate the OT practitioner addressing them.

Counsel clients with orthopedic conditions based on their operative stability and what positions are safe for them. With total hip replacements, the safety of sexual positions depends on the approach used by the orthopedic surgeon and the related hip precautions to prevent joint dislocation. It is helpful to give clients a booklet, pamphlet, or information sheet with illustrations of recommended sexual positions to aid education.

Other client recommendations include avoiding excessive pressure directly on any implant, kneeling on a replaced knee, and supporting a partner on his or her replaced joint. Clients may also use pillows for support and comfort of the legs, neck, and back. It is important for clients to check with their surgeons before resuming sexual activity after surgery. Surgeons usually recommend waiting 4 to 6 weeks after surgery to resume sex to allow the wound, muscles, bones, and tissues to heal. Clients are advised to take a mild pain medication about 20 to 30 minutes before sex, which can help relax muscles and prevent minor aches. However, clients should avoid taking medication that is too strong and masks warning pain.

Empathy, sensitivity, and openness are essential aspects of the therapeutic relationship and necessary in addressing sexuality. OTAs should provide a safe environment for clients to express their fears and concerns, and offer assistance with problem-solving sexual issues. Enhancing a client's ability to participate in sexual activity can have a profound effect on their quality of life.[41]

OT Practitioner's Viewpoint

Today's orthopedic client is different from the past. Not only are surgeries more advanced, but the client population is also more advanced. Cutting-edge surgical techniques such as computer-assisted surgery (CAS) and less-invasive procedures allow more precise alignment and sparing of tissue. Clients are often able to progress quickly postoperatively, and OT practitioners must be prepared to assist with advancing clients in a timely manner through each setting. Today's client with an orthopedic condition often has higher expectations from their rehabilitation providers and are more knowledgeable thanks to Internet resources. Many of today's "Baby Boomers" want to stay active through physical exercise, such as skiing, hiking, golfing, and so on. OT practitioners need to be educationally ready to provide current and progressive rehabilitation. ~Lori Goodnight, MS, OTR/L

SUMMARY

OT plays an important role in the rehabilitation of clients with orthopedic conditions at all recovery stages and settings. At each stage or setting, the occupational therapist initiates the client evaluation and with input from the OTA, creates an individual treatment plan with functional, measurable goals. The OTA follows the treatment plan and guides the client through graded functional activities and exercises incorporating not only knowledge of the medical and physical limitations of an orthopedic disability or surgery, but also the cognitive, psychosocial, community, and environmental factors that impact an individual's ability to function independently. The OTA should collaborate closely with the occupational therapist on client progress and adjustments needed to the treatment plan. Although OT is firmly client-centered, it is also important to collaborate with other health professionals, family, caregivers, and sometimes employers to make sure the client's needs are met. OT facilitates clients to manage and overcome functional limitations due to their orthopedic condition or injury. Improving an individual's ability to engage in occupations increases his or her productivity, health, well-being, and life satisfaction.

REVIEW QUESTIONS

1. A client is 2 weeks post–lumbar spine surgery. Which three of the following actions incorporate back precautions that the OTA would recommend?
   a. Reaching in the back seat of a car
   b. Crossing your legs to put on socks/shoes
   c. Log-rolling to the side to push up to sit at the edge of the bed
   d. Lifting a 2-year-old child from a swing
   e. Bending over to tie one's shoes
   f. Sitting in a dining room chair with armrests
2. When adhering to posterior approach hip precautions after a THR, which of the following would be the *most* appropriate OT treatment?
   a. Reaching for cones on the floor
   b. Crossing legs to reach one's shoes
   c. Practicing use of adaptive equipment for lower body dressing
   d. Standing at walker and twisting upper body to reach around to each side
3. An OTA is working with a client who has just had a left anterior approach THR. Which three of the following activities are appropriate treatment activities?
   a. Practice functional mobility while swinging operated leg back to kick a ball.
   b. Practice bridging while lying in bed to pull up pants.
   c. Practice using a raised toilet seat for toilet transfers.
   d. Cross the operated foot over other knee to reach shoe ties.
   e. Practice using a shower chair and grab bar(s) for shower transfers.
   f. Practice reaching in kitchen cabinets while standing at a rolling walker.
4. When preparing for a client to discharge to home who has had THR and has PWB precautions, which of the following would be contraindicated?
   a. Removing throw rugs from floors
   b. Adding nonslip mats to the tub or shower
   c. Practice getting up quickly from supine to sitting to standing
   d. Encouraging the client to use the assistive mobility device recommended by PT
5. Which of the following would be contraindicated for a client who is returning home following back surgery?
   a. Use a long-handled sponge to reach one's feet while seated during bathing.
   b. Place the most used kitchen items in the lower shelves in cabinets under the counters.
   c. Remove all clutter and cords across walkways.
   d. Avoid sitting on low toilets and couches.
6. Clients who are afraid of falling may exhibit which three of the following?
   a. Anxiety
   b. Self-determination
   c. Resistance to therapy
   d. Restriction of physical activities and social participation
   e. Increased self-confidence
   f. Increased functional ambulation
7. The OTA is working with a client after back surgery and the client is complaining of a sudden painful, tender, swollen, redness in the calf muscle. What would be the *best* action to take?
   a. Apply deep-tissue massage to the calf muscle.
   b. Encourage the client to move the leg up and down to work out the pain and tenderness.
   c. Assist the client to get up and walk around on the leg.
   d. Have the client remain in bed and not move the limb, and notify nursing staff and the physician of possible DVT.
8. Regarding OT and total knee replacements, which of the following statements is accurate?
   a. TKR clients should not move their knee joint the first 6 weeks until it has healed.
   b. Only PT works with TKR clients.
   c. OT can assist with encouraging knee mobility during ADLs and IADLs
   d. Clients will have a urinary catheter or diaper to avoid going to the toilet.
9. The OTA is working with a client who had a left hip fracture, resulting in an ORIF, is NWB, but very confused and unable to follow instructions. Which of the following would be the *most* appropriate?
   a. Leave the client in bed until the confusion clears so the client can learn better.
   b. Use a transfer board to transfer the client to a wheelchair.
   c. Perform a stand-pivot transfer with the client.
   d. Buckle the client into wheelchair for safety.
10. An OTA is working with a client who is currently under PWB status after a recent hip fracture. How is this weight-bearing restriction *best* described?
   a. Clients can put as much weight as they can tolerate.
   b. Clients can touch their toe down to help balance.
   c. Clients can only put 50% of their weight on the affected leg.
   d. Clients can only put 75% of their weight on the affected leg.

CASE STUDY

A 54-year-old female childcare worker with 1-year history of lower back pain was diagnosed with degenerative spondylolisthesis and received a L4-L5 spinal fusion with instrumentation (interbody device, screws, rods). She was transferred from the hospital to a skilled nursing facility and evaluated by an occupational therapist. Information from evaluation revealed the client lives alone with a history of depression and anxiety, obesity, and COPD. The client was deconditioned and weak with poor motivation to get out of bed but upset and stressed about her disability. The ultimate goal was for the client to successfully return home alone safely and resume work as soon as possible. Client rapport was built by discussing her love of children and her job at a childcare, as well as by verifying her goals for increased independence, and reviewing the treatment plan, rehabilitation process, and the benefits of activity. OTA goal-directed treatments were coordinated with the client's pain medication schedule and included:

- Education and training on back precautions and body mechanics: Handouts, discussion, demonstration, cues during tasks, repetition/practice incorporating, and family education.
- Bed mobility: Log-roll technique to keep neutral posture (no bending or twisting back); co-treatment with PT until client only requires assist of one; don/doffing TLSO brace while supine; and nursing assistant training to enhance carry-over of techniques.
- Self-care: Training on dressing and sponge bathing while seated at the sink incorporating back precautions and adaptive equipment to reach feet without bending over (long-handled sponge, reacher, dressing stick, long shoehorn, and elastic shoelaces); practicing increasing ability to cross legs to reach feet; once

cleared by surgeon, practicing shower transfers using a shower chair and grab bars simulating her shower at home.

- Functional mobility: Toileting with raised bedside commode over toilet and long-handled toilet aid for hygiene; shower chair transfers with grab bars; kitchen cooking and reaching tasks incorporating back precautions and safety techniques using the rolling walker; homemaking tasks incorporating back precautions, assistive devices, and adaptive techniques (reaching for clothes in the dryer with a reacher, vacuuming using a cane and lightweight vacuum with neutral posture); practicing car transfers with a family member.
- Activity tolerance: Initiated deep breathing exercises; graded upper-extremity range of motion exercises with increasing repetitions; increased standing tolerance for functional tasks, and included standing for leisure interests of playing games and puzzles.

1. What kind of adaptive equipment and environmental adaptations to the home would the OT practitioner recommend for safety?
2. What kind of recommendations on body mechanics and adaptive techniques would the OT practitioner suggest for the client's work environment?

PUTTING IT ALL TOGETHER Sample Treatment and Documentation

Setting	Acute hospital
Client Profile	Client is a pleasant 59-year-old male who is referred for skilled OT services after elective R TKR surgery with self-care and functional mobility deficits. PMH: OA, HTN, COPD, DMII, GERD, back pain, lumbar stenosis, anxiety, depression
Work History	Client works as a mechanic and owns the business.
Insurance	Private insurance covering 5-day hospital stay for OT/PT
Psychological	Anxious about finances and getting back to work
Social	Lives alone in one-level house with three entry steps, tub shower, and daughter in town for 1 week to help, but neighbor can also check in on him
Cognitive	Alert and oriented ×4
Motor & Manual Muscle Testing (MMT)	Good coordination, R hand dominant, BUE MMT 4+/5, SOB and fatigues easily with activity, dynamic standing balance with Min A at RW, tolerates 2 min standing. While sitting, client able to partially cross L leg to reach to midshin, unable to cross R leg, c/o back pain when bending over to reach feet
ADL	Upper-body ADLs with set-up sitting using slow pace; lower body ADLs with Max A to reach feet and Min A standing at walker for peri-care and clothing management over hips
IADL	Standing at sink or closet with RW, WBAT RLE and Min A for balance reaching to simulate kitchen/homemaking tasks ×2 min standing tolerance
STG Goals (2 days)	1. Client to demo LB ADLs with adaptive equipment or adaptive tech with min cues while sitting and standing with Min A for peri-care/clothing management over hips at sink or walker. Client to demo toilet transfers using raised bedside commode over toilet and Min A. 2. Client to demo tub transfer using shower chair and grab bars safely with supervision. 3. Client to demo increased dynamic standing balance and tolerance ×10 min for simple kitchen/closet reaching task with supervision and RW using reacher prn and min cues for incorporating breathing tech/energy conservation/safety tech. 4. Client to demo increased BUE strength to 5/5 and tolerate 15 reps HEP with min cues to incorporate breathing tech to enhance activity tolerance for ADLs and strength for functional transfers.
LTG Goals (4 days)	1. Client to demo Mod I with ADLs/IADLs using adaptive equipment/tech prn to return home alone safely.

OT TREATMENT SESSION 1

THERAPEUTIC ACTIVITY	TIME	GOAL(S) ADDRESSED	OTA RATIONALE
Sponge bath and dressing at sink with training on adaptive equipment	45 min	STG #1	*Occupations; Client Education and Training:* Increasing self-care independence and reducing stress to back with adaptive equipment training
Toilet transfer with b/s commode adjusted to appropriate height	10 min	STG #2	*Occupations; Client Education and Training:* Increasing independence with toileting
Standing at the sink for grooming tasks	5 min	STG #4	*Occupations; Client Education and Training:* Increasing dynamic standing balance and tolerance

SOAP note: 11/15/—, 2:00 pm–3:00 pm

S: "My back hurts when I try to bend over to reach my feet."

O: Client participated in skilled OT in hospital room to address need for adaptive equipment training to enhance LB dressing and bathing. Client performs LB dressing while seated with Min A/cues; performs peri-care and clothing management with Min A for clothing management over hips; using WBAT RLE. Educated client on energy conservation and breathing tech due to SOB

PUTTING IT ALL TOGETHER Sample Treatment and Documentation (continued)

noted with self-care tasks. Adapted bedside commode height over toilet to enhance client independence and safety with toilet transfers requiring Min A for safety. Client tolerated 5 min standing at sink for grooming; educated client on incorporating breathing tech during dynamic standing balance task and client required Min A for balance.

A: Client cooperative with treatment but anxious about returning home soon. Client is making good progress with ADLs, functional transfers, balance, and activity tolerance. He continues to require assistance with functional tasks and would not be safe to return home alone at this point. Client would benefit from family training session with daughter and a social work consult for possible rehab placement upon discharge from hospital.

P: Continue OT daily for 45-60 min to address family training with ADLs/functional mobility, and discuss discharge recommendations/options with OT, client, family, and social worker.

Roberto Gonzalez, COTA/L, 11/15/—, 3:10 pm

TREATMENT SESSION 2

What could you do next with this client?

TREATMENT SESSION 3

What could you do next with this client?

REFERENCES

1. The role of occupational therapy in orthopedics. (2016) Retrieved from http://www.pacificaorthopedics.org/wp10/orthopedics/the-role-of-the-occupational-therapist-in-orthopedics/
2. OrthoInfo. (2010). Retrieved from http://orthoinfo.aaos.org/topic.cfm?topic=A00502.
3. Medifocus guidebook on ankylosing spondylitis. (2015). Retrieved from http://www.medifocus.com/2009/landingp2.php?gid=RH001&?a=a
4. Spinal stenosis. (2014). Journal of Spine. Retrieved from http://research.omicsgroup.org/index.php/Spinal_stenosis
5. Osteomyelitis. (2015). Retrieved from https://www.mayoclinic.org/diseases-conditions/osteomyelitis/basics/definition/con-20025518
6. Spondylolisthesis. (2017). Retrieved from http://orthoinfo.aaos.org/topic.cfm?topic=a00053
7. Ma, C. B. (2015). Spine surgery. Retrieved from https://www.nlm.nih.gov/medlineplus/ency/patientinstructions/000313.htm
8. Types of spine surgery. (2014). Retrieved from http://www.premierortho.com/blog/tag/interlaminar-implant/
9. Marcucci, G., & Brandi, M. L. (2010). Kyphoplasty and vertebroplasty in the management of osteoporosis with subsequent vertebral compression fractures.*Clinical Cases in Mineral and Bone Metabolism, 7*(1), 51–60.
10. Ulrich, P. F. (1999). Back braces. Retrieved from http://www.spine-health.com/conditions/scoliosis/back-braces
11. Hayashi, K., Arai, Y. C. P., Ikemoto, T., Nishihara, M., Suzuki, S., Hirakawa, T., ... & Ushida, T. (2015). Predictive factors for the outcome of multidisciplinary treatments in chronic low back pain at the first multidisciplinary pain center of Japan, *Journal of Physical Therapy Science, 27*(9), 2901–5.
12. Back pain prevention. (2015). Retrieved from http://www.mayoclinic.org/diseases-conditions/back-pain/basics/prevention/CON-20020797
13. Jaromi, M., Nemeth, A., Kranicz, J., Laczko, T., & Betlehem, J. (2012). Treatment and ergonomics training of work-related lower back pain and body posture problems for nurses. *Journal of Clinical Nursing,21*(11–12), 1776–1784.
14. What is evidence-based practice? (n.d.). *OT Seeker: Evidence-Based Practice Resources.* Retrieved from http://www.otseeker.com/resources/WhatIsEvidenceBasedPractice.aspx
15. Steffen, D. (2016). Exercise associated with prevention of low back pain. *JAMA Internal Medicine. 176*(2),199–208.doi:10.1001/jamainternmed.2015.7431
16. Pelvis fractures. (2007). Retrieved from http://orthoinfo.aaos.org/topic.cfm?topic=A00223
17. The hip joint. (2015). Retrieved from http://www.fda.gov/MedicalDevices/ProductsandMedicalProcedures/ImplantsandProsthetics/MetalonMetalHipImplants/ucm241593.htm
18. Cluett, J. (2016). Hip arthritis. Retrieved from http://orthopedics.about.com/cs/hipsurgery/a/hiparthritis.htm
19. Avascular necrosis. (2015). Retrieved from http://www.mayoclinic.org/diseases-conditions/avascular-necrosis/basics/definition/CON-20025517
20. Surgical approaches to total hip replacement. (2015). Retrieved from http://www.hipsforyou.com/typesofsurgicalapproaches.php
21. Hemiarthroplasty of the hip. (n.d.). Retrieved from http://www.eorthopod.com/hemiarthroplasty-of-the-hip/topic/51
22. Ulstrup, A. (2008). Biomechanical concepts of fracture healing in weight-bearing long bones. *Acta Orthopaedica Belgica,74*(3), 291–302.
23. Kreder, H. J. (2009). Improving functional recovery after hip fracture surgery. Retrieved from http://boneandjointcanada.com/wp-content/uploads/2014/05/Surgery-to-improve-function.pdf
24. Cemented or uncemented artificial joints. (2014). Retrieved from http://www.webmd.com/osteoarthritis/tc/cemented-or-uncemented-artificial-joints-topic-overview
25. Bone healing. (2015). Retrieved from: http://www.foothealthfacts.org/footankleinfo/Bone_Healing.htm
26. Allen, J., Koziak, A., Buddingh, S., Liang, J., Buckingham, J., & Beaupre, L. A. (2012). Rehabilitation in patients with dementia following hip fracture: A systematic review. *Physiotherapy Canada, 64*(2), 190–201.
27. Knee joint anatomy. (2010). Retrieved from http://www.joint-pain-expert.net/knee-joint.html
28. Arthritis of the knee. (2014). Retrieved from http://orthoinfo.aaos.org/topic.cfm?topic=A00212
29. Buechel, F. F., Sr.,Buechel, F. F., Jr.,Pappas, M. J., D'Alessio, J. (2001). Twenty-year evaluation of meniscal bearing and rotating platform knee replacements. *Clinical Orthopaedics & Related Research, 388*, 41-50.
30. Knee resurfacing and partial knee replacement. (2016). Retrieved from http://bonesmart.org/knee/knee-resurfacing-and-partial-knee-replacement/
31. Moffet, H., Collet, J. P., Shapiro, S. H., Paradis, G., Marquis, F., & Roy, L. (2004). Effectiveness of intensive rehabilitation on functional ability and quality of life after first total knee arthroplasty: A single-blind randomized controlled trial. *Archives of Physical Medicine and Rehabilitation. 85*(4), 546–56.
32. Maniar, R. N., Baviskar, J., Singhi, T., & Rathi, S. (2012). To use or not to use continuous passive motion post–total knee arthroplasty. *The Journal of Arthroplasty, 27*(2). http://dx.doi.org/10.1016/j.arth.2011.04.009

33. Harvey, L. A., Brosseau, L., & Herbert, R. D. (2014). Continuous passive motion after knee replacement surgery. *Cochrane Database of Systematic Reviews,* (2), CD004260. doi:10.1002/14651858.CD004260.pub3
34. Konlian, C. (1998). Aquatic therapy: Making a wave in the treatment of low back injuries. *Orthopaedic Nursing,18,* 7–85.
35. Pöyhönen, T., Keskinen, K. L., Hautala, A., & Mälkiä, E. (2000). Determination of hydrodynamic drag forces and drag coefficients on human leg/foot model during knee exercise. *Clinical Biomechanics (Bristol, Avon). 15*(4), 256–260.
36. White, K. (2014). Healing through aquatic therapy. Retrieved from www.rehabpub.com/2014/07/healing-aquatic-therapy/
37. Colón-Emeric, C., Whitson, H. E., Pavon, J., & Hoenig, H. (2013). Functional decline in older adults. *American Family Physician, 88*(6), 388–394.
38. Taormina-Weiss, W. (2013). Psychological and social aspects of disability. Retrieved from: http://www.disabled-world.com/disability/social-aspects.php
39. Ayers, D. C., Franklin, P. D., & Ring, D. C. (2013). The role of emotional health in functional outcomes after orthopaedic surgery: Extending the biopsychosocial model to orthopaedics. *Journal of Bone & Joint Surgery, 95*(21), e165.
40. Holst, C. (2011). The power of occupation: The power of leisure pursuits. *Advance for Occupational Therapy Practitioners.*
41. McClure, G. (n.d.). Sex after a joint replacement: The definitive how-to guide. Retrieved from https://www.peerwell.co/blog/2016/05/25/sex-after-joint-replacement-surgery-how-to/

Chapter 21

Arthritic Diseases: Factors, Adaptations, and Treatment

Brenda Kennell, BS, MA, OTR/L, Kelly McCoy Jones, OTR/L, and Amy J. Mahle, MHA, COTA/L

LEARNING OUTCOMES

After studying this chapter, the student or practitioner will be able to:

21.1 Identify the five most prevalent types of arthritis in the adult population

21.2 Describe common areas of physical deficits associated with arthritic conditions

21.3 Describe the functional and psychological impact of arthritis on activities of daily living and instrumental activities of daily living

21.4 Discuss therapeutic interventions used in treating clients with arthritic conditions

21.5 Develop treatment plans for clients with arthritic conditions

KEY TERMS

Arthrodesis
Arthroplasty
Biologics
Bouchard's nodes
Boutonnière deformity
Corticosteroids
Disease-modifying antirheumatic drugs (DMARDs)
Energy conservation
Fusiform swelling
Heberden's nodes
Joint preservation or joint protection
Nonsteroidal anti-inflammatory drugs (NSAIDs)
Osteoarthritis (OA)
Osteotomy
Swan neck deformity
Synovectomy
Ulnar drift
Work simplification

Arthritis is the leading cause of disability among adults in the United States and accounts for 17% of all disability nationwide.[1] Arthritis is not one disease, but a group of approximately 100 different forms and related diseases[2] whose common threads are pain, inflammation, destruction of joints, limited joint motion, and difficulty performing everyday tasks. The umbrella term arthritis includes such varied conditions as:

- Ankylosing spondylitis
- Bursitis
- Carpal tunnel syndrome
- Chronic fatigue syndrome
- Chronic regional pain syndrome
- Infectious arthritis
- Inflammatory bowel disease
- Juvenile arthritis
- Lyme disease
- Myositis
- Osteoporosis
- Paget's disease
- Psoriatic arthritis
- Raynaud's phenomenon
- Reiter's syndrome
- Scleroderma
- Spinal stenosis
- Tendinitis[3]

According to the Centers for Disease Control and Prevention (CDC), the five most common types of arthritis in the United States are osteoarthritis, rheumatoid arthritis, fibromyalgia, gout, and systemic lupus erythematosus (SLE), commonly referred to as lupus.[4] Arthritic conditions may be inflammatory, autoimmune, infectious, or metabolic. In addition to joint pain and disease, there can be erosion and damage to the eyes, skin, and internal organs such as the heart and kidneys.

Arthritic conditions can cause life-changing debility and pain affecting millions of Americans. An estimated one in five adults are diagnosed with an arthritic condition annually in the United States, 60% before 65 years of age.[2] In a May 2010 report issued by the CDC, 37.7% of adults report that arthritis causes limitations, 31.2% say it leads to work limitation, and 25.6% report that it causes severe pain (seven or higher on a zero to 10-point scale).[2] One in five Canadians age 15 or older report having arthritis, and it is the leading cause of disability for women and the third for men.[5] Arthritis not only affects older adults; some forms can begin in infancy or childhood (Box 21-1). Arthritis often begins in middle age, but it may be several years before the

BOX 21-1
Juvenile Idiopathic Arthritis

Arthritis with onset before 16 years of age is called juvenile idiopathic arthritis (JIA), which includes several conditions, including three conditions formerly referred to as variations of juvenile rheumatoid arthritis (JRA).[8-10] According to the American College of Rheumatology, about one in 1000 children in the United States develop some sort of juvenile arthritis, but many will go on to lead active lives.[9] JIA often includes a pattern of exacerbation and remission, but many children will "grow out of it." The most common types of JIA include:

- Systemic onset JIA (formerly called systemic onset JRA)—About 10% of children with JIA have this, with symptoms including a history of repeated fevers of 103° F and an intermittent rash for at least 2 weeks; inflammation of internal organs such as lymph nodes, spleen, liver; and joint swelling. Joint swelling may not appear until weeks after the onset of fever and rash.
- Oligoarticular JIA (formerly called pauciarticular JRA)—Inflammation of one to four joints. This is more common in girls than in boys, and accounts for about 50% of children with JIA. Children with onset before 7 years of age often experience permanent remission, however they are more likely to develop eye inflammation such as iritis or uveitis. Children with later onset may continue to have active arthritis through adulthood.
- Polyarticular JIA (formerly called polyarticular JRA)—Inflammation of five or more joints. This may begin at any age. Some pediatric rheumatologists believe onset in late teens is actually early onset of RA.
- Psoriatic JIA—Presence of both arthritis and psoriasis.
- Enthesitis-related JIA—Inflammation of both joints and enthesis sites (where tendons, ligaments, or joint capsule attach to bone).[9,10]

The primary symptom of JIA may be joint pain and stiffness, but young children often do not report pain. Parents may first notice the fever and rash, followed by the child limping, avoiding use of one or more limbs, or appearing stiff or clumsy; especially in the morning or after a nap. In addition to joint pain and swelling, JIA can include serious eye inflammation that can develop into cataracts or glaucoma if untreated.[8] Bone development can be delayed or accelerated, leading to contralateral limb length discrepancy, a small and misshapen chin, or overall growth delay.[10]

OT can benefit children with JIA. Interventions can include orthotics to protect inflamed joints, education regarding joint protection for the child and family, and recommendations for positioning and activity modifications. For example, the occupational therapy assistant (OTA) may teach children to use a book rest instead of reading with a book in their lap, or help a teacher to position the child's desk in the best spot to avoid excessive neck extension or lateral rotation. The OTA may need to remind the caregivers and teachers that the child needs frequent rest breaks and may struggle with long writing assignments or be able to engage in recess but then be too fatigued to attend in class.

onset of notable symptoms. Incidence of arthritis also varies by gender, and racial and ethnic origin.[6] Many types of arthritis affect more women than men and are unevenly distributed across racial and ethnic origin.[4,7]

The occupational therapy (OT) practitioner is uniquely qualified to make a positive impact on the life of a person with an arthritic condition. The overall goals of OT when working with a client with arthritis are to improve, or prevent further decline in, functional independence; reduce and manage pain; and prevent joint damage and preserve joint integrity; thus improving quality of life. This chapter will primarily focus on the five most common forms of arthritis in the United States: osteoarthritis, rheumatoid arthritis, fibromyalgia, lupus, and gout (Box 21-2).[11,12]

OSTEOARTHRITIS

Osteoarthritis (OA) is also referred to as degenerative joint disease (DJD) or degenerative arthritis.[13] It is the most common chronic condition of the joints and is most prevalent in people 65 years of age and older.[13] With OA, the articular cartilage, the lining that covers the ends of the bones where they meet to form a joint, breaks down or wears away. Cartilage, which is normally a rubbery and smooth-type surface, acts as a natural joint shock absorber. If the cartilage wears away, its ability to provide cushioning is diminished. As the cartilage wears away and the bones are exposed, the bones rub against one another.[13] Often, this is referred to as bone on bone movement (Fig. 21-1). Inflammation can occur secondary to the mechanical irritation of the involved joints.

Deteriorating cartilage affects the shape of the joint. The joint can no longer articulate or function smoothly. Additional problems may occur inside the joint as the cartilage is breaking down, such as spurs (osteophytes), which can develop on the ends of the bones. Spurs can damage surrounding tissues and potentially cause pain.[13] These bony growths can also result in swollen and misshapen joints, such as **Heberden's nodes** and **Bouchard's nodes**, which are seen on the distal interphalangeal (DIP) joints and proximal interphalangeal (PIP) joints of the fingers (Fig. 21-2). In advanced cases of OA, joint changes can result in deformities such as genu varum or genu valgum at the knee (Fig. 21-3).

Osteoarthritis may affect one joint or multiple joints, usually depending on whether it is considered primary or secondary. Primary OA is generalized, commonly occurring in weight-bearing joints such as the spine, hips, and knees, as well as the fingers and thumbs. Primary OA often begins in

BOX 21-2
Types of Arthritis[3]

Adult-onset Still's disease
Ankylosing spondylitis
Back pain
Behçet's disease
Bursitis
Calcium pyrophosphate deposition disease (CPPD)
Carpal tunnel syndrome
Chondromalacia patella
Chronic fatigue syndrome
Complex regional pain syndrome
Cryopyrin-associated periodic syndromes (CAPS)
Degenerative disc disease
Developmental-dysplasia of hip
Ehlers-Danlos
Familial Mediterranean fever
Fibromyalgia
Fifth disease
Giant cell arteritis
gout
Hemochromatosis
Infectious arthritis
Inflammatory arthritis
Inflammatory bowel disease
Juvenile arthritis
Juvenile dermatomyositis (JD)
Juvenile idiopathic arthritis
Juvenile scleroderma
Kawasaki disease
Lyme disease
Mixed connective tissue disease
Myositis (including polymyositis, dermatomyositis)
Osteoarthritis
Osteoporosis
Paget's disease
Palindromic rheumatism
Patellofemoral pain syndrome
Pediatric rheumatic diseases
Polymyalgia rheumatica
Pseudogout
Psoriatic arthritis
Raynaud's phenomenon
Reactive arthritis
Reflex sympathetic dystrophy
Reiter's syndrome
Rheumatic fever
Rheumatism
Rheumatoid arthritis
Scleroderma
Sjögren's disease
Spinal stenosis
Spondyloarthritis
Systemic juvenile idiopathic arthritis
Systemic lupus erythematosus
Systemic lupus erythematosus in children and teens
Systemic sclerosis
Temporal arteritis
Tendinitis
Vasculitis
Wegener's granulomatosis

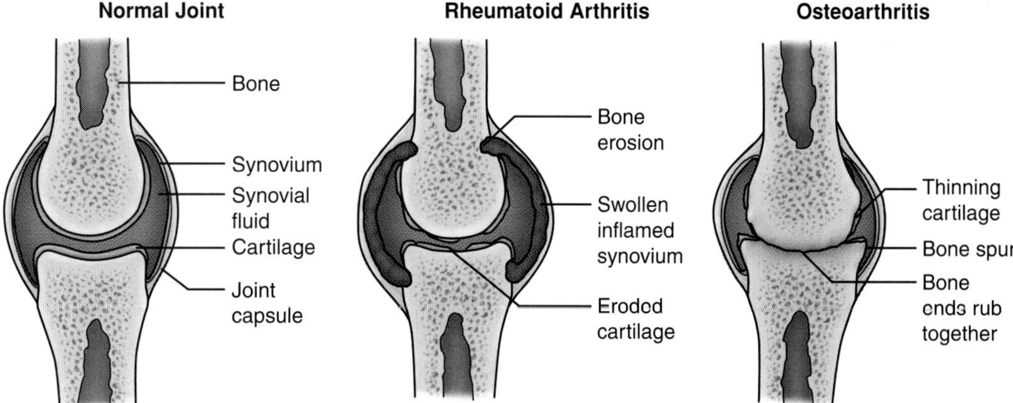

FIGURE 21-1. Compare joint structure and movement in a normal joint versus one with arthritis.

middle age or later, except when the hands are involved. Secondary OA results from an injury, repetitive motion or stress on a joint, or after joint inflammation.[14] This type of arthritis is often seen in younger people whose jobs or leisure activities put stress on their joints. This includes athletes or ballet dancers, people who operate machinery such as jack hammers or pneumatic drills, people who carry heavy loads such as construction workers, and people who work in certain positions such as miners. OA can affect all areas of occupational performance, making it difficult to walk, climb stairs, get in and out of a vehicle, raise up from a seated position, lift objects like a gallon of milk or pot of coffee, dress, bathe, grasp and hold objects, write, and button clothing, just to name a few.

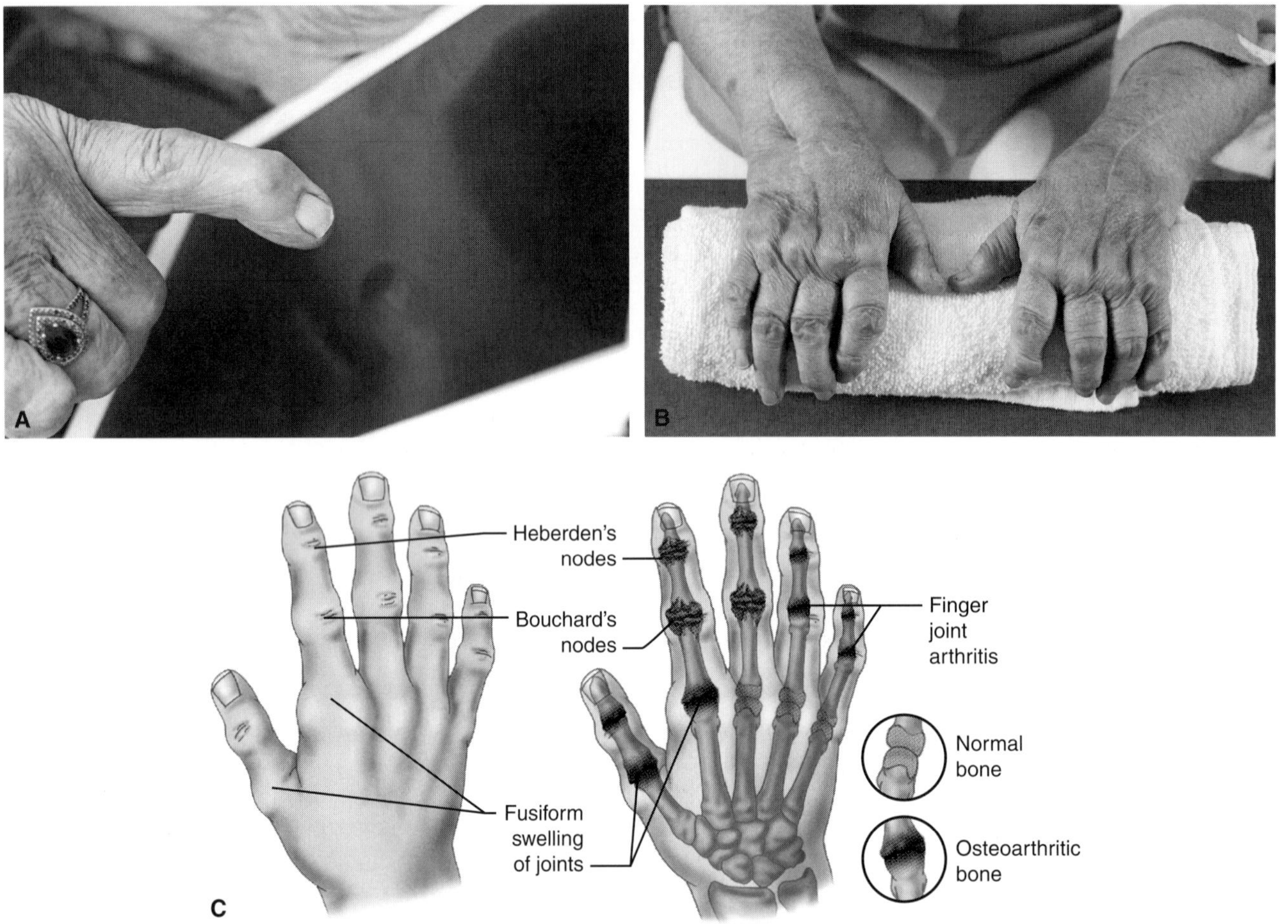

A

B

Heberden's nodes

Bouchard's nodes

Finger joint arthritis

Normal bone

Osteoarthritic bone

Fusiform swelling of joints

C

FIGURE 21-2. Finger nodes. A. Heberden's node (DIP). B. Bouchard's node (PIP). C. Location and structural changes to the joints.

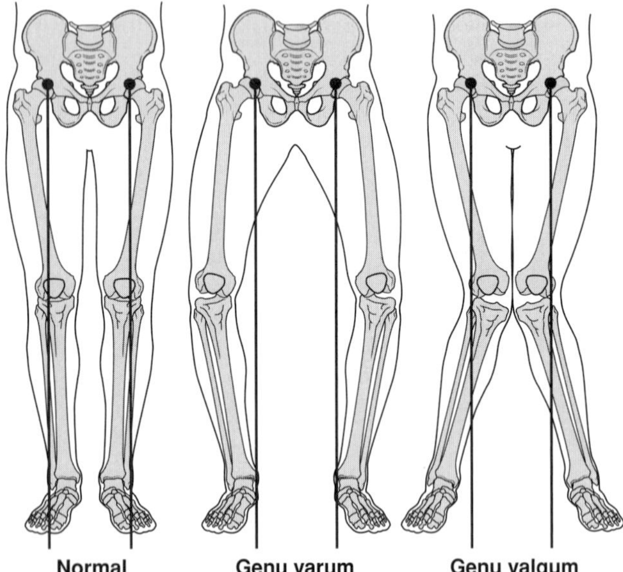

FIGURE 21-3. Normal knee versus knee deformities of genu varum and genu valgum. Note the alignment between the hips and knees, and the areas of increased pressure that cause deformities.

Signs and Symptoms of Osteoarthritis

The signs and symptoms of OA vary depending on the severity of the disease and which joint is affected. Symptoms develop slowly and worsen over time. The most common signs and symptoms are:

- Joint pain, which often increases after activity or as the day goes on
- Joint stiffness, particularly in the morning, or after rest, lasting 20 to 30 minutes
- Decreased range of motion (ROM), which improves after using the joint a bit
- Inflammation, including swelling of fingers, thumb, knees, ankles, toes
- Difficulty performing everyday tasks: activities of daily living (ADLs), instrumental activities of daily living (IADLs), work, and leisure
- Visible joint changes: Heberden's nodes, Bouchard's nodes
- Muscle weakness from decreased activity tolerance[15]

Diagnosing Osteoarthritis

Diagnosing OA should include a detailed health history, history of symptoms, and physical examination of the affected body part. An x-ray can detect bony and joint changes related to OA. Magnetic resonance imaging (MRI) can provide better images and views of cartilage and other structures. Sometimes OA is diagnosed after ruling out other arthritic conditions. For this reason, the physician may order procedures such as blood tests or joint aspiration of synovial fluid (in order to examine joint fluid for evidence of crystals, infection, or synovitis).

Causes and Risk Factors

The specific cause of OA is unknown, but several factors are believed to contribute to its development, including heredity, injury, and lifestyle.[12–14] Some people inherit genes that make them more susceptible to OA, possibly because a gene defect affects the production of cartilage.[14] Since joint alignment may affect the way the joints fit together and cause the cartilage to wear faster, people with genetically inherited joint laxity or hypermobility (often called "double-jointed") are at increased risk for developing OA.[13] Females are more likely to develop OA than males,[2] and risk increases with age. Genetic predisposition does not guarantee that someone will develop arthritis.

Like many other chronic conditions, the cause of OA is complex and may involve multiple factors. Although originally thought that OA was caused simply by mechanical stressors, age, and overuse, it is now clear that lifestyle has a tremendous impact on the potential to develop OA.[13] Risk factors can be classified as modifiable or nonmodifiable. The modifiable risk factors that individuals have some control over include excess body weight, joint injury, knee pain, occupation, and structural misalignment due to muscle weakness.[12] Nonmodifiable factors include gender (women more prone), age (risk increases with age), race (some Asian populations are less likely to develop OA), and predisposition due to genetic factors.[12]

Many lifestyle factors can contribute to this disease, including physiological factors such as obesity, metabolic conditions, and injuries; and the mechanical effects of position, load, and repetitive movement of work and leisure activities. Being overweight puts excess pressure on joints.[14] Each pound of excessive weight adds three pounds of added stress to the knees and six times the pressure to the hips.[13] Excess pressure over time equals greater wear and tear, which leads to breakdown of the cartilage that cushions the joints.[13] Current research is examining a possible link between excess fat tissue and inflammatory effects in joints.[13] Repetitive or prolonged occupational tasks, such as squatting, lifting, pushing, pulling, or gripping can lead to osteoarthritis in affected joints.[12] Sports-related or other wear-and-tear injuries, such as fractures, excessive and repetitive joint compression, as well as OA surgery can contribute to development of osteoarthritis in the future. In addition, metabolic disorders (conditions that affect the body's metabolism) can also contribute to the risk for developing arthritis. Acromegaly is a metabolic disorder in which the pituitary gland produces excessive amounts of growth hormone, and hemochromatosis is another metabolic disorder in which the body absorbs too much iron.[16] Other possible factors are estrogen deficiency or high bone density (leading to increased risk for OA in the knee).[12]

Overview of Treatment

The overall objective in the treatment of OA is similar in many ways to the treatment of the other most common forms of arthritis. In short, the general objective is to reduce pain, improve overall function, reduce the potential for long-term disability, and educate the client on disease management. Medical treatment will depend on the location and severity of the affected joints, as well as the client's vocation and lifestyle. OT intervention includes education and training regarding energy conservation, work simplification, and body mechanics, which will be explained later in the chapter. Lifestyle changes may be discussed with the client, as decreasing weight and increasing exercise may help reduce pain and improve function. Adaptive equipment may be indicated temporarily or long-term for ADLs, IADLs, work, school, or leisure activities. Environmental modifications may be necessary to facilitate transfers or provide appropriate-height work surfaces.

RHEUMATOID ARTHRITIS

Rheumatoid arthritis (RA) is a chronic, polyarthritic disease that may cause premature death or disability, and often leads to an overall decreased quality of life.[18] It is the most common form of inflammatory arthritis, affecting more than 1.5 million people in the United States.[12,18] Rheumatoid arthritis is considered an autoimmune condition and is systemic, meaning that it can affect many joints, the eyes, and internal organs throughout the body. People with RA experience many impairments including, but not limited to, pain, joint deformities, psychosocial

TECHNOLOGY AND TRENDS

The CDC indicates that with the increase in the older population, the incidence of arthritis will increase to 26% of the population by 2040. Furthermore, approximately 11% of all adults in the United States will have arthritis, which *impacts and limits their activities.* The CDC further reports that obesity is one component that impacts the anticipated increase in lifestyles limited by arthritis.[17]

With the anticipated rise in arthritis, OT practitioners have an opportunity to impact this trend through health, wellness, and prevention initiatives. OT practitioners are skilled in the use and education of adaptive equipment and techniques, which if used earlier in the course of the condition, may help to reduce some of the activity limitations of arthritis. OT practitioners are also poised to educate community groups, senior centers, houses of worship, and workers on joint protection and healthy lifestyles, which can help to limit the impact of arthritis.

changes, weakness, motor deficits, muscle atrophy, and cardiovascular impairment. These limitations compromise overall functional status and contribute to increasing healthcare costs.[18] RA may be static or progressive and is often characterized by periods of exacerbation (worsening of symptoms) and remission (lessening of symptoms). Currently, no cure exists for RA, but medical treatment includes prescription **disease-modifying antirheumatic drugs (DMARDs).**[18]

With RA, the immune system's cells do not function correctly and begin to attack healthy tissues. The resulting inflammation produces chemicals that target and cause a thickening of the synovium (tissue that lines the joints) and eventually damages the cartilage and the bone within the joint capsule. Tendons and ligaments that support and align the joints gradually weaken and stretch, thus allowing the joint to lose shape and alignment, which may result in deformities such as subluxation of the base of the proximal phalanges in the metacarpal-phalangeal (MCP) joints (Fig. 21-4c) or **ulnar drift** of the wrist or fingers at the MCP joints (Fig. 21-5). When the intrinsic musculature and protective ligaments in the fingers slip, deformities of the fingers are common. For example, a **boutonnière deformity** occurs with flexion of the PIP joint (see Fig. 21-4a), and a **swan-neck deformity** is caused by hyperextension of the PIP joint (see Fig. 21-4b). Hyperextension deformities are common in the thumb interphalangeal (IP) joint, often combined with flexion deformity at the MCP joint. Stiffness of the thumb carpometacarpal (CMC) joint due to osteoarthritis or rheumatoid arthritis can lead to compensatory hyperextension of the MCP joint.[19,20]

Symptoms of Rheumatoid Arthritis

During an exacerbation of rheumatoid arthritis, the four cardinal signs of inflammation are usually present—heat, swelling, pain, and redness. Since it is a systemic disease,

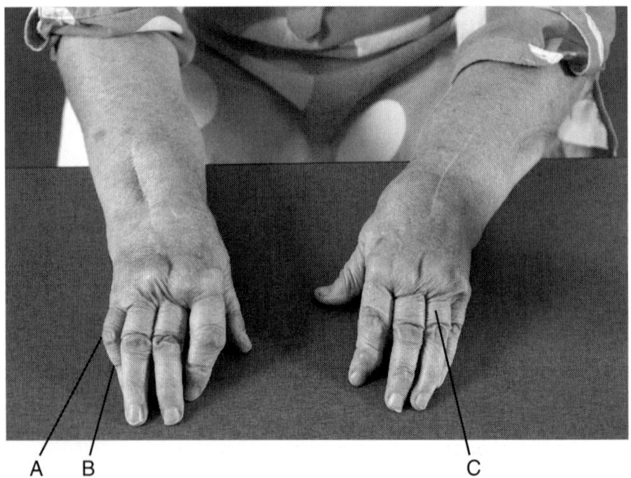

FIGURE 21-4. Common deformities of RA. A. Boutonnière deformity at the PIP. B. Swan neck of DIP in right small finger. C. Subluxation at MCP joints.

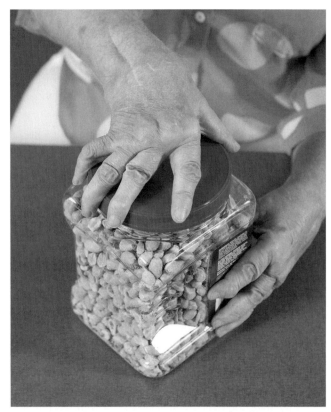
FIGURE 21-5. Ulnar drift at the MCPs, especially noticeable when force is applied to the ulnar direction (for demonstration purposes only; the OT practitioner would not encourage this movement for the client).

additional symptoms may involve other body systems. Signs and symptoms of RA may include:

- Tender, warm, swollen joints
- Morning stiffness lasting several hours
- Rheumatoid nodules (small bumps under the skin)
- Fatigue, fever, and weight loss

The swelling associated with RA is often **fusiform swelling,** where an entire finger or one joint swells and loses the definition of the individual phalanges (Fig. 21-6). Fusiform swelling feels soft and mushy, unlike the firmness seen in the Bouchard's or Heberden's nodes. It is sometimes referred to as "sausage fingers."[21]

Diagnosing Rheumatoid Arthritis

Diagnosis of RA usually involves an extensive history, physical examination, blood tests, and possibly imaging studies. Blood work is looking for an elevated sedimentation rate (ESR) or C-reactive protein (CRP), which may indicate the presence of an inflammatory condition, as well as the presence of rheumatoid factor. Fluid may be aspirated from a joint (arthrocentesis) to differentiate between inflammatory or noninflammatory arthritis. Imaging diagnostics may include x-rays, MRIs, and computerized tomography (CT) scans. History should include questions regarding family history of arthritic conditions, onset of joint symptoms and

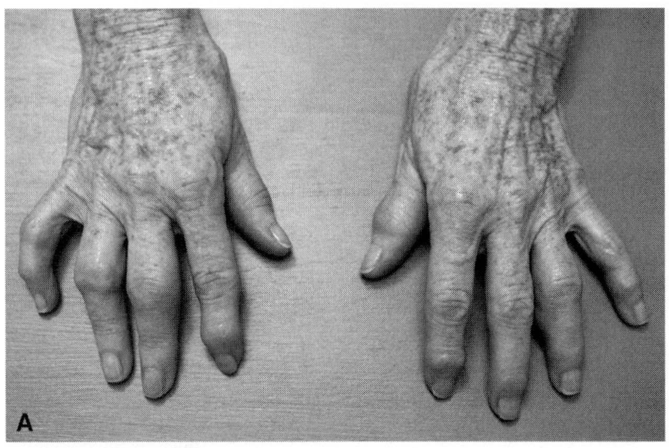

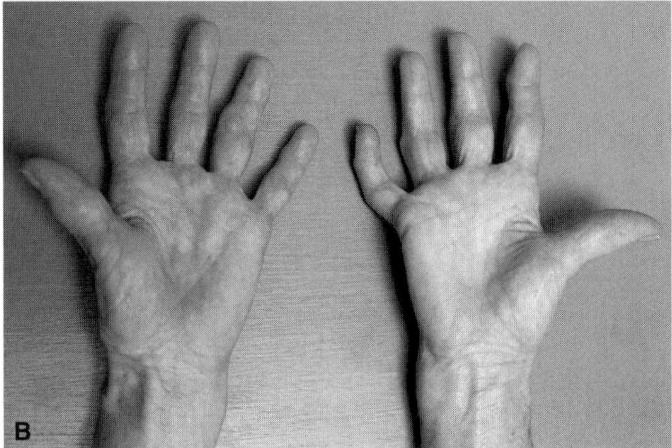

FIGURE 21-6. Fusiform swelling of fingers in (A) dorsal view and (B) volar view.

other systemic complaints, location and duration of pain, and response of pain to different treatments such as over-the-counter (OTC) or prescription medication. Clients may also complain of fatigue, malaise, weakness, muscle tenderness, low-grade fever, and weight loss.[18]

Causes and Risk Factors

While a definitive cause of RA is not yet known, research indicates that genetics definitely play a role. Genes in and of themselves do not cause RA, but instead make one more vulnerable to environmental factors, which may trigger the disease. Other risk factors include gender (women are more likely to develop RA), age (commonly begins between 40 and 60 years of age), and family history.[18]

Overview of Treatment

As with OA the treatment of RA is focused on the reduction of pain, improving overall function, and reducing the potential for long-term disabilities. Medical treatment may include joint replacement or other surgery to repair or remove bone or soft tissue. Pharmaceutical intervention may include **nonsteroidal anti-inflammatory drugs (NSAIDs)**, DMARDs, pain medication, or other medications in severe cases.

OT treatment differs greatly during periods of exacerbation or remission. During an exacerbation of RA, the joints must rest, so therapeutic exercise is limited. Instead, the treatment focuses on client education and reducing pain and inflammation. Fabrication or fitting of orthotics may be necessary to prevent or correct joint deformity, or provide rest to a severely inflamed joint. Education and training in **joint protection** techniques is critical for prevention of joint damage and deformity. The OT practitioner may help the client choose adaptive equipment that will decrease stress on joints and enhance occupational performance. During periods of remission, OT intervention may include gently progressive exercise.[18,21] See Table 21-1 for a helpful guide to compare OA and RA arthritis.

TABLE 21-1 Comparison of Rheumatoid Arthritis and Osteoarthritis[22]

CHARACTERISTIC	RHEUMATOID ARTHRITIS	OSTEOARTHRITIS
Age at which the condition starts	May begin any time in life	Usually begins later in life
Speed of onset	Relatively rapid, over weeks to months	Slow, over years
Joint symptoms	Joints are painful, swollen, and stiff.	Joints ache and may be tender, but have little or no noticeable swelling.
Pattern of joints that are affected	It often (but not always) affects small and large joints on both sides of the body (symmetrical), such as both hands, both wrists or elbows, or the balls of both feet.	Symptoms often begin on one side of the body and may spread to the other side. Symptoms begin gradually and are often limited to one set of joints, usually the finger joints closest to the fingernails or the thumbs, large weight-bearing joints (hips, knees), or the spine.
Duration of morning stiffness	Morning stiffness lasts longer than 1 hour. Can be very difficult to get going in the morning.	Morning stiffness lasts less than 1 hour. Stiffness returns at the end of the day or after periods of activity.
Presence of symptoms affecting the whole body (systemic)	Frequent fatigue and a general feeling of being ill are present.	Whole-body symptoms are not present.

FIBROMYALGIA

Another condition the OT practitioner sees frequently in the clinic is fibromyalgia. Although it is considered an arthritic disease, it is characterized by widespread musculoskeletal pain instead of joint pain or destruction. Sleep deprivation, fatigue, memory impairment, and psychosocial issues accompany this disease. Scientists believe that fibromyalgia amplifies painful sensations by affecting the way the brain processes pain signals.[23]

Symptoms of Fibromyalgia

Symptoms have been reported immediately after trauma or psychological event or develop over time. Most common symptoms are as follows:

- Pain: Noted to be symmetrical and widespread, and is reported as a dull ache lasting at least 3 months.
- Fatigue: Most people affected with this condition awake fatigued, despite sleeping for long periods of time. Among sleep disorders, clients also report restless leg syndrome and sleep apnea.
- Cognitive impairment: Difficulty focusing/attending or concentrating on cognitive tasks, and it is sometimes referred to as "fibro fog."
- Other: People with fibromyalgia also report increased incidence of headaches, depression, and pain/cramping in the lower abdomen.[23]

Diagnosing Fibromyalgia

Fibromyalgia is often misunderstood and misdiagnosed. No definitive laboratory test currently exists to diagnose fibromyalgia, and its symptoms are similar to those of many other conditions, including depression, lupus, and chronic myofascial pain. Because of this, many people are undiagnosed or misdiagnosed for months or even years. Due to the lack of objective evidence, some physicians disregard a client's symptoms altogether. Clients with fibromyalgia also experience psychosocial issues because of the lack of evidence, and others (including some physicians) believe "it is just in the head."A trained physician can diagnose fibromyalgia using the criteria established by the American College of Rheumatology (ACR). This includes a history of widespread pain for at least 3 months, pain on both sides of the body and both above and below the waist, and the presence of other common symptoms such as fatigue. Physicians may also test for tenderness in at least 11 of 18 specific trigger points, but the fluctuating nature of fibromyalgia symptoms can hinder diagnosis (Fig. 21-7).[24]

Causes and Risk Factors

Suspected causes and risk factors are as follows:

- Genetics: Fibromyalgia tends to be hereditary
- Infections: Illness may precede development of fibromyalgia

COMMUNICATION

Clients often need encouragement to be better advocates for themselves when speaking with their physician. Clients will often open up to their OT practitioners about their questions or concerns regarding their condition that need to be addressed by their physician. The OTA can help clients generate a list of questions and concerns to take with them to their follow-up appointments. Although many clients might attend OT sessions by themselves, it is a good idea to invite the caregiver or significant other to some of the sessions for the OT practitioner to provide education.

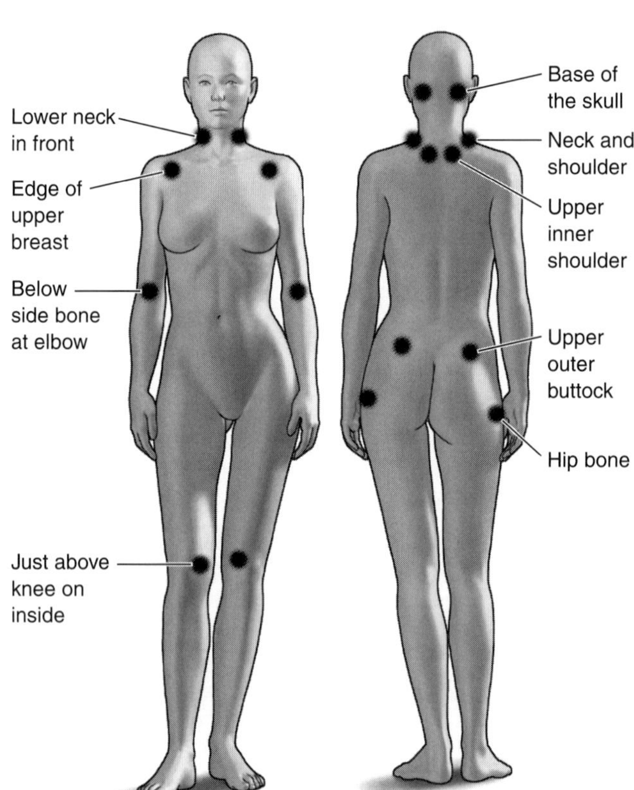

FIGURE 21-7. Fibromyalgia trigger points.

- Physical or emotional trauma: Post-traumatic stress disorder (PTSD) is linked to development of fibromyalgia[23]

Overview of Treatment

The medical treatment of fibromyalgia differs from that of most other arthritic conditions. There is no surgery possible, and treatment is generally directed at relieving pain and addressing other symptoms. Equally important are therapeutic exercises such as swimming, strengthening, and stretching (e.g., yoga, tai chi, Pilates). Alternative approaches to relieve symptoms may include acupuncture, massage therapy, biofeedback, meditation, qi gong, and certain dietary supplements.[25]

LUPUS

While lupus has multiple forms, this chapter addresses SLE because it is considered an arthritic condition. Similar to RA, SLE is both an autoimmune condition and systemic, affecting many body systems and organs as well as the joints. According to the Alliance for Lupus Research,[26] 1.5 million Americans have been diagnosed with lupus, and 90% are women.

Symptoms of Lupus

Symptoms of lupus may be mild or severe, temporary or long-term, and may develop slowly or rapidly. Lupus is sometimes referred to as "the great imitator" since its symptoms mimic those of many other conditions, including RA, fibromyalgia, thyroid dysfunction, diabetes mellitus, and Lyme disease. The most common symptoms include:[26–28]

- Painful, swollen joints
- Extreme fatigue and unexplained fever
- Butterfly-shaped rash over the nose and cheeks (Fig. 21-8)
- Photosensitivity (sensitivity to light and sun)

Other symptoms include:

- Blood-related anemia or abnormal clotting
- Headache, confusion, and/or memory loss
- Raynaud's phenomenon (fingers and toes lose blood supply, become numb, and turn white, blue, or purple when cold)
- Chest pain
- Edema in hands, feet, and around eyes
- Hair loss

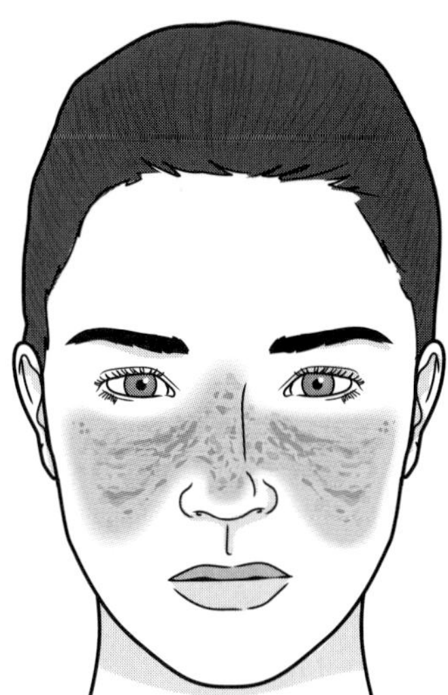

FIGURE 21-8. Characteristic rash of lupus.

Diagnosing Lupus

No single test can diagnose lupus. Instead, the physician will take a detailed history, conduct a physical examination, and may order several tests to also rule out other conditions. Laboratory examinations will include:

- Complete blood count (CBC): May indicate anemia or a low white blood cell count
- Erythrocyte sedimentation rate (ESR): Measures the rate at which red blood cells (RBCs) settle to the bottom of a test tube. An elevated ESR may indicate systemic conditions such as lupus.
- Kidney and liver function tests: May be done to determine how well they are functioning
- Urinalysis (UA): May show increased amount of RBC in the urine, which could indicate that the kidneys are affected by the condition
- Antinuclear antibodies (ANAs): These are produced by the immune system. Although most people with lupus have a positive ANA test, many people with positive ANAs do not have lupus.

Other tests may include chest x-ray, electrocardiogram (ECG), or liver biopsy to assess damage to vital organs that are often affected with this condition.[28]

Causes and Risk Factors

Lupus is most commonly diagnosed in women between 15 and 40 years of age, although it can develop at any age, including infancy. According to the Mayo Clinic,[28] it is believed that lupus occurs as a combination of genetic predisposition and environmental triggers, such as sun exposure, recent infection, and certain medication use. Medication-induced lupus often subsides once the medications are stopped. African American women are three times more likely to develop lupus than Caucasian women. The rate of lupus is also higher for women of Hispanic, Asian, or native American origin.

As a systemic condition, lupus can affect many different organs, body systems, and functions including:

- Musculoskeletal system: Painful, swollen joints
- Integumentary system: The characteristic butterfly rash on the face, as well as skin lesions elsewhere on the body
- Urinary system: Kidney damage is among the leading causes of death for people with lupus
- Cardiovascular system:
  - Blood and blood vessels: Lupus increases the risk for bleeding, blood clotting, anemia, and vasculitis (inflammation of the blood vessels)
  - Heart: Lupus may lead to inflammation of the heart muscle or the lining within or around the heart (myocarditis, endocarditis, and pericarditis). It can also increase the risk for cardiovascular disease and myocardial infarction (MI).
- Respiratory system: Lupus can cause chest pain due to inflammation of the lungs' pleural lining (pleurisy) and increase the risk for pneumonia.

- Brain and central nervous system (CNS): Headaches, dizziness, memory loss, and confusion are common with lupus. It can also cause hallucinations and changes in behavior.
- Reproductive system: Lupus increases the risk for miscarriage, preeclampsia, and preterm birth. Women with lupus are often advised to postpone pregnancy until they have had their symptoms under control for at least 6 months.[26,28]

Overview of Treatment

No longer considered a fatal disease, lupus is generally managed by a combination of medications to control and lessen the symptoms. Due to its chronic nature, some people may also utilize alternative treatments in addition to traditional medicine. This includes vitamins and supplements, yoga, relaxation techniques, and (indoor) aquatic exercise. Lifestyle modifications are very important, especially protection from the sun and avoiding overexertion. If arthritic changes are pronounced, use of orthotics may be necessary.

GOUT

Gout is one of the most painful forms of arthritis, characterized by a sudden and severe onset of pain, swelling, redness, and tenderness in the joints. It is a metabolic condition caused when the bodily waste product uric acid deposits tiny needle-like crystals into the joints and soft tissues.[29,30] For many people, the first episode of gout occurs in the big toe, however, gout can also affect the feet, ankles, knees, elbows, wrists, and fingers.[30] Like some other forms of arthritis, gout is episodic, characterized by periods of exacerbation with painful flareups lasting for days or weeks, followed by remission periods with no symptoms.[29,30] Gout is responsible for approximately 5% of all cases of arthritis.[31] Without proper treatment, gout can lead to severe joint damage and disability.

Symptoms of Gout

Symptoms of gout include:

- Intense pain
- Swelling
- Redness
- Heat/warm joint
- Joint stiffness
- Joint deformity

People with gout develop tophi, which are lumps of uric acid crystals that are deposited in soft tissue. They can be easily seen in the elbow, toe, ankle, knee, ears, and distal joints of the fingers (Fig. 21-9).[30]

Diagnosing Gout

Gout is diagnosed from blood tests for uric acid levels, x-rays for bony changes/abnormalities, and testing of joint fluid to check uric acid crystal levels. Family history is also a contributing factor in the diagnosis of gout.[31]

Causes and Risk Factors

Uric acid occurs as a by-product of the breakdown of purines (a type of protein) in the body. Uric acid may build up either as a result of the body making too much or the kidneys being unable to efficiently filter it. Over time, the uric acid crystals accumulate, settle in the joints, and gout develops. Other factors that contribute to the development of gout are as follows:

- Family history
- Male gender
- Obesity
- Alcohol abuse
- Intake of foods rich in purines (beans, anchovies, liver, salmon, sardines)
- Enzyme defect
- Organ transplants
- Exposure to lead
- Use of diuretics, levodopa, aspirin, or cyclosporine
- Use of the vitamin Niacin[30,31]

Overview of Treatment

Gout is a form of arthritis for which the evidence supports some relief from dietary modifications.[32–34] Recommendations include avoiding or limiting intake of seafood, meat (particularly organ meat), and alcohol, as well as increasing daily dairy intake.[33] The Mayo Clinic publishes a Gout Diet

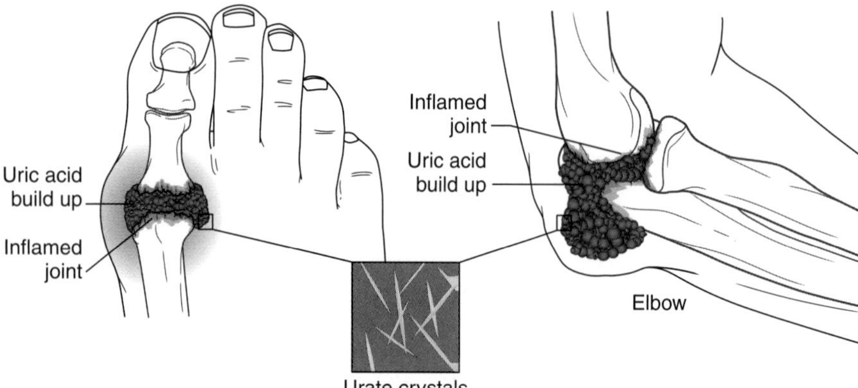

FIGURE 21-9. Acute gout in foot and elbow.

that includes complex carbohydrates (fruits, vegetables, and whole grains), water, low-fat or fat-free dairy products, cherries, and moderate amounts of caffeinated coffee and high-purine vegetables. The diet also limits intake of white flour; sugar; protein from meat, poultry, and fish; and alcohol.[35] Medical treatment of gout involves use of medication, lifestyle changes, and client education.

MEDICAL TREATMENT OF ARTHRITIS AND RELATED CONDITIONS

Treatment approaches vary for the many different types of arthritis. Medication is used for many types of arthritis, to decrease pain and inflammation, and to slow down the disease process and joint damage. Sometimes surgery is necessary to repair or replace joints that have been severely damaged. Dietary recommendations are not necessary for many types of arthritis (except for gout, as mentioned previously), although there are many unsubstantiated claims about relationships between food and arthritis. However, people with all types of arthritis will do better if they keep their weight controlled to avoid excessive load on their joints and body systems. Because of the chronic nature of arthritis and its associated pain, people with arthritis are susceptible to many types of unproven remedies. Examples of treatments that have no evidence-based proof of benefit but also no proven harm, include different diets, vitamins, and mineral supplements. Treatments that can be dangerous include ant venom, bee pollen, and clay enemas.[36] Most people with arthritis will also benefit from lifestyle modifications including decreasing stress and increasing activity levels.

Pharmacological Management

Pharmacological management varies for different arthritic conditions. The most commonly used medications are analgesics and anti-inflammatories. These types of medications are available in different strengths, OTC or by prescription. Analgesic medication is used to decrease pain. It is treating a symptom of arthritis, but not affecting the course of the disease. Anti-inflammatory medications are either **corticosteroids** or NSAIDs. Decreasing inflammation will usually also decrease pain and may slow down destruction and damage to joints and soft tissues. Many medications have both analgesic and anti-inflammatory effects.

OTC analgesics include aspirin, acetaminophen (Tylenol®), and ibuprofen (Motrin®, Advil®). Aspirin and ibuprofen are also anti-inflammatory, but acetaminophen has no effects on inflammation. Opioid (narcotic) analgesics such as hydrocodone and oxycodone are available only by prescription. Previously used just for severe pain, opioids have been found to be effective in the treatment of chronic pain, such as in osteoarthritis.[37] Although they generally do not affect the liver or kidneys like some OTC analgesics, opioids have more potential for dependency and side effects, ranging from dizziness and drowsiness to confusion and constipation. Some opioid medications are also available in a transdermal patch. Individuals need to avoid driving or operating machinery when first starting on an opioid, until they see how they tolerate the medication. Any analgesic medication is more effective when taken at regular intervals, allowing for a steady level of medication in the body. Abruptly stopping an opioid medication can lead to withdrawal symptoms such as anxiety, sweating, insomnia, and nausea.

Corticosteroid medication (cortisone, prednisone, hydrocortisone) mimics the effects of hormones that are naturally produced in the body, but exceeds the body's usual levels. This higher level helps to decrease inflammation and suppress the body's immune system, which is why it is used in inflammatory and autoimmune conditions such as RA and lupus. Corticosteroids for arthritis may be oral, topical, or injected directly into a joint. Although steroids are often seen as a "wonder drug," they can have serious side effects, especially with prolonged use.[38] Oral administration of corticosteroids is most likely to lead to side effects. These can include:

- Fluid retention and swelling in the lower extremities (LEs)
- Elevated blood pressure
- Weight gain, with possible fat deposits in the abdomen, back of the neck, and face
- Effects on mood, memory, and behavior
- Elevated pressure in the eyes (glaucoma)[38]

Long-term use of oral corticosteroids can also lead to infection, cataracts, osteoporosis, bruising, and elevated blood sugar levels. Topical corticosteroids can lead to local irritation, including red or thin skin, or acne. Corticosteroid injections should be limited to 3 to 4 per year due to the possibility of thinning or discoloration of the skin, insomnia, and elevated blood sugar. Clients with arthritis must work together with their healthcare team to evaluate the risks and benefits of corticosteroid treatment. Ways to reduce the risk for side effects include lower or intermittent dosing, making healthy lifestyle choices (e.g., healthy nutrition, sleep), and wearing a medical alert bracelet. People should *never* abruptly stop taking corticosteroids, because the adrenal glands need time to adjust their production of natural hormones. The dosage must be tapered by the physician to avoid withdrawal. Symptoms of withdrawal, including fatigue, lightheadedness, body aches, nausea, and loss of appetite, can range from mild and annoying to serious and potentially life threatening.[39]

Some prescription NSAIDs such as naproxen and ibuprofen are available OTC in lower dosages (Aleve®, Motrin®, and Advil®). Many choices of NSAIDs are available as both generic and brand name, and many people tolerate one type better than others. The most common side effects of NSAIDs are gastrointestinal, such as nausea, vomiting, pain, and in some cases ulcers and bleeding. Severe side effects can include liver and kidney damage and cardiovascular problems. Some types of NSAIDs, however, such as cox-2 inhibitors like Celebrex®, are used with caution in older adults or those with cardiovascular conditions.[40]

Other medication classes are used to treat specific arthritic conditions and are discussed below.

Pharmacological treatment of osteoarthritis is focused on reduction of pain and inflammation. Treatment may begin with OTC analgesics and anti-inflammatory medication, and progress to prescription-strength medication as needed.

Pharmacological treatment of rheumatoid arthritis usually begins with anti-inflammatory medication to decrease inflammation and pain and slow down joint damage. NSAIDs are generally the first approach, though steroids such as prednisone may be used during an acute episode. Aspirin is a powerful NSAID and may be the first choice, but many people have side effects such as tinnitus or gastrointestinal bleeding from the high doses that are needed. Many rheumatologists choose to prescribe DMARDs as soon as the client is diagnosed with RA, because it may take several weeks or even months before they start having a clinical effect. DMARDs help to slow the progression of the disease process itself. Some of these medications have traditionally been used for other conditions, such as Plaquenil for treatment of malaria or Methotrexate as a cancer treatment. Although some clients are able to take DMARDs for several years, they can have serious side effects such as liver damage, bone marrow suppression, and severe lung infections. The newest class of DMARDs are biological response modifiers or **"biologics"** that are often administered through injection or infusion. Biologics such as Humira®, Enbrel®, Orencia®, Remicade®, or Xeljanz® target the parts of the immune system that cause inflammation and damage to joints and tissues. Taking biologics increases a client's risk for infection. They work best when paired with other DMARDs such as methotrexate. Other medications that were commonly used in the past such as cytoxan, penicillamine, and gold salt injections, are now mainly used in aggressive cases that do not respond to other DMARDs.[41,42]

Pharmacological treatment of fibromyalgia is very different, because fibromyalgia does not affect the joints. Since the hallmark symptoms of fibromyalgia are pain, impaired sleep, and depression, pharmacological treatment addresses these factors. Commonly prescribed medications include OTC analgesics or a nonnarcotic pain reliever such as tramadol. Antidepressants such as Elavil® and Cymbalta® are often used both to address depression and promote sleep. Low-dose antiseizure medications, such as Neurontin® and Lyrica®, have also been shown to be effective for treatment of fibromyalgia pain. These drugs limit the release of pain-communicating chemicals from nerve cells in the brain and spinal cord. Dizziness and drowsiness are the most common side effects of these drugs.[43,44]

Since lupus can affect so many different organs and body systems, there are many different types of medication prescribed. Antimalarial drugs such as Plaquenil®, Chloroquine, or Quinacrine may be prescribed as soon as lupus is diagnosed. These medications are not used for treating severe lupus symptoms involving the kidneys or blood vessels. Antimalarials improve muscle and joint pain, skin rashes, fatigue, and fever; and decrease the inflammation of the lining of the heart (pericarditis) and lung (pleuritis). People may take antimalarials for the remainder of their lives, as they have been shown to reduce flares by 50% and prevent lupus from spreading to the kidneys or central nervous system (CNS).[45] Antimalarial drugs may be taken in conjunction with NSAIDs, corticosteroids, and immunosuppressives. Side effects are rare and usually mild and short-term. The most common side effects include rashes, dryness, and discoloration of the skin; and gastrointestinal symptoms such as decreased appetite, bloating, and cramps. NSAIDs may be prescribed for lupus in order to decrease inflammation, fever, and pain; but they increase the risk for gastrointestinal upset, stomach bleeding, and problems with the kidneys or heart. Corticosteroids may be used, but the risk for side effects such as diabetes, hypertension, osteoporosis, weight gain, bruising, and infection, increases with higher doses and long-term use. Immunosuppressive drugs may be prescribed to reduce symptoms, but they increase the risk for infection, cancer, impaired fertility, and liver damage.[45,46]

NSAIDs may be prescribed to reduce inflammation in clients with gout, with higher doses during attacks. Colchicine is a pain reliever often prescribed for gout pain, but side effects can include intense nausea, vomiting, and diarrhea. Corticosteroids may be prescribed to reduce inflammation and pain when a client cannot take NSAIDs or colchicine. Possible side effects of corticosteroids include mood changes, increased blood sugar levels, and hypertension. Xanthine oxidase inhibitors, such as Allopurinol, block the production of uric acid. Side effects for these drugs include rash, low blood count, nausea, and impaired liver function. Other drugs like Probalan® improve the body's removal of uric acid, but they also increase the level of uric acid in the kidneys, which may lead to kidney stones and stomach pain. These medications are often prescribed if the client has several attacks per year or if attacks are extremely painful (Table 21-2).[47]

Surgical Treatment

Many different types of surgical procedures are used for treatment of arthritis and related conditions. When RA causes the synovial tissue in a joint to become severely inflamed, the diseased synovium can be removed through a procedure called a **synovectomy**, which helps to decrease pain and swelling in the joint. Although this may help slow the destruction in the joint, the synovium often grows back after several years, and the procedure may need to be repeated. In an **osteotomy**, the surgeon corrects a bone defect by cutting it and then repositioning the bone. This is often done for clients with osteoarthritis, to correct curvature and improve weight-bearing of lower extremity long bones such as the tibia (Fig. 21-10a). **Resection** or removal of all or part of a bone may be done to help decrease pain and improve function (Fig. 21-10b). Often this

TABLE 21-2 Common Medications for Arthritic Conditions

	OTC ANALGESIC	OPIOID ANALGESIC	NSAID	CORTICOSTEROID	DMARD	BIOLOGIC	ANTIDEPRESSANT	LOW-DOSE ANTISEIZURE	ANTIMALARIAL	IMMUNOSUPPRESSANT	AFFECTS URIC ACID
OA	x	x	x								
RA	x	x	x	x	x	x			x	x (rarely)	
Fibromyalgia	x						x	x			
SLE			x	x					x	x	
Gout			x	x							x

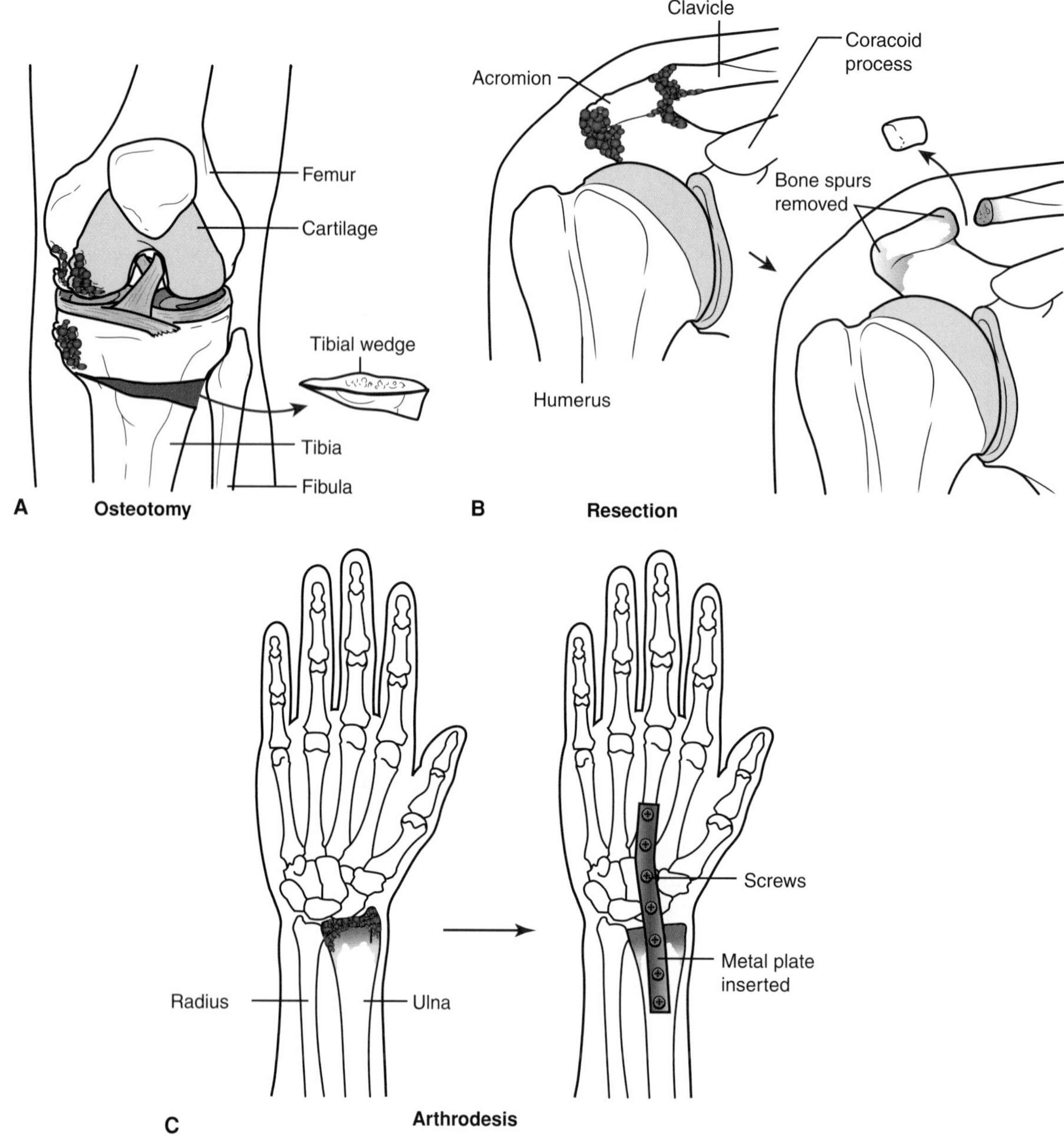

FIGURE 21-10. Common surgeries. A. Osteotomy. B. Resection. C. Arthrodesis.

involves removal of foot bones when walking becomes too painful. It may also involve bones in the wrist, thumb, or fingers. Severe joint pain and instability may be addressed through an **arthrodesis** or joint fusion. Although the person loses movement when a joint is fused, the joint is then less painful and more stable, which may actually increase weight-bearing tolerance. Arthrodesis is most common in the ankle, wrist, thumb, or fingers (Fig. 21-10c).

Arthroplasty means rebuilding of a joint and is commonly referred to as joint replacement. Joint replacements may be partial or total, and are done when the cartilage has eroded and destruction of the articular end of the bone is present. In a total joint replacement, the surgeon removes the ends/surfaces of both bones in the joint, for example, the proximal end of the femur (head, neck, and part of shaft) and the acetabulum of the pelvis and replaces them with metal, ceramic, and/or plastic prosthetic components. A partial joint replacement involves only one of the bones or surfaces, for example, only the femur and not the acetabulum. The most commonly replaced joints are the hip and knee. Successful replacements are also done with the shoulder, ankle, wrist, elbow, and MCP joints. OT intervention is usually included after a joint replacement. Protocols will depend on the surgical approach (e.g., anterior or posterior) and the components used and often include precautions regarding movements and positions. Total hip precautions such as limiting hip flexion, internal rotation, or adduction are addressed in the Chapter 20.[48]

PSYCHOSOCIAL IMPACT

Clients who are diagnosed with an arthritic condition often deal with pain, stiffness, fatigue, and perhaps ultimately, loss of function. Dealing with these issues can affect participation in work, leisure, and ADLs,[49] which can lead to a compromise in psychological well-being.[50] The long-term ramifications of pain and decline in function can also have a negative effect on personal relationships. Research shows that among older adults with arthritis, those with greater pain or disability experienced more psychological distress, higher unemployment, and lower productivity.[51] Studies have shown that divorce rates among couples where one person has a chronic illness are as high as 75%, and the rate may be higher when it is the wife with the chronic condition.[52,53] The OT practitioner must recognize and acknowledge each client's individual challenges, both physical and psychological, and the effect on roles and occupational performance. The occupational therapist and OTA are uniquely qualified to help clients with arthritic conditions who are experiencing these challenges by providing client education in pain management, orthotic devices, adaptive equipment, and modification of work, leisure, and ADL activities. The OT practitioner might also be able to recommend an arthritis support group if there is one close to where the client resides.

OT Practitioner's Viewpoint

When working with clients who have an arthritic condition, it is important to *listen* to the client and not have preconceived ideas of what the client needs. Much of the time, these clients have been dealing with significant pain and loss of function for some time. Therapeutic use of self can be very powerful in working with this population. Creating a space of understanding and caring will go a long way as you develop a relationship with your clients. Find out what is important to them. Ask them, "What are you having trouble doing?" (e.g., when dressing, while cooking, when bathing, during work or leisure activities). They might unload with a great deal of complaints, or they may share solutions with you that they have found work for them. Several times I have been surprised when clients with significant hand deformities tell me that they are able to dress, feed, toilet, bathe, and groom themselves.

With regard to adaptive equipment, joint protection, work simplification, energy conservation, activity modification, and so on, it is most effective to practice techniques and actually use the adaptive equipment versus just "talking" about it or simply giving clients handouts or a catalog. Working with clients to reduce or manage their pain along with coming up with specific solutions to specific problems is the key to successful OT. ~ Kelly McCoy Jones, OTR/L

SAFETY

The most important principle with arthritis is to prevent joint damage. Everyday activities can be dangerous when someone's joints are unstable and/or damaged. Clients need to examine their activities and the tools they use to see if adaptations must be made. It is easier to prevent joint damage than it is to fix it. For this reason, client education and training regarding body mechanics and joint protection is of paramount importance. Clients need to learn to recognize and understand the signals that their bodies send them. Pain is an indication that they are doing too much or that their joints are being stressed. Sometimes people will want to ignore pain, thinking "no pain, no gain," but this is not appropriate for people with active arthritis. Instead they should adopt the "use it or lose it" rule. They need to move their joints to prevent stiffness, but within proper parameters. In addition to overuse, joints may become stressed from repetitive movements or excessive resistance. Skilled training regarding joint protection and body mechanics can help ensure that clients position themselves and their joints in the safest manner when performing any type of task. Clients need to learn to pace and schedule activities according to their stamina and pain levels. Another safety issue relates to medication. Clients and their families need to be knowledgeable about the medications they are taking, such as side effects, risks, contraindications, interactions with other medications or food, and the proper way to wean off or stop a medication. Although the purpose of medication is to slow the disease process and improve quality of life, improper use of medication can lead to life-altering complications.

While OT practitioners should not criticize clients and families about their lifestyle choices, practitioners can help them stay safe by teaching them to recognize the value of evidence-based practice when choosing alternative treatments.

OCCUPATIONAL THERAPY INTERVENTION

After thorough evaluation and development of appropriate treatment goals, the occupational therapist and OTA can formulate a plan to assist clients with arthritis to manage their symptoms and facilitate a return to normal occupational performance patterns. OT intervention varies depending on client status, for example, if the client is in remission or having an exacerbation, or if the client has had surgery, or if conservative treatment is being done to try to prevent surgery. The areas most commonly addressed in intervention include client education and training, adaptive equipment, orthotics, management of pain and edema, work tasks, and exercise.

THE OLDER ADULT

OT practitioners may find that they have a lot of young and middle-aged clients with arthritis, but not as many older adults. This can seem odd, since osteoarthritis is the most common form of arthritis and often begins in the older adult. This issue is of great concern since it is easier to prevent deformity than to correct it, and people who use their joints incorrectly or rely on "splints" that they buy in the drugstore or Walmart are at greater risk for damaging their joints and losing their ability to participate fully in ADLs, IADLs, work, and leisure tasks. A contributing factor may be confusion about what OT practitioners do—people who are older and retired don't think they need OT since they are no longer working. Older adults, caregivers, and physicians may not understand the need for OT when they see the deficits as being temporary, such as after joint replacement surgery.

This disparity in clients served may be because people born between 1925 and 1944, often called "the Greatest Generation," have different attitudes toward health care than Baby Boomers (born between 1945 and 1964), Generation X (born between 1965 and 1984), and Millennials (born between 1985 and 2004). Many older adults view arthritis as just part of aging and not something that they can do anything about. In addition, they tend to view their physicians as "a trusted authority figure to make appropriate healthcare decisions for them."[54] This means that if the physician is not aware of the benefits of OT or does not recommend OT services, the client may not know to ask about it. Although OT practitioners like to think that physicians are all big supporters of therapy, many physicians are more concerned with pharmacological and surgical options and less aware of the value of client education and custom orthotics. In fact, a 2005 study of family physicians in Long Island, New York, found that more than one-half of the respondents were not sure if OT practitioners served clients with serious injuries such as spinal cord injury or traumatic brain injury.[55] In addition, many seniors rely on their children (Baby Boomers) to make their healthcare decisions for them. The children or even grandchildren may search on the Internet, but are more likely to come up with sites for adaptive equipment and prefabricated orthotics.

OT practitioners can reach out to their local physicians to help them understand all that OT has to offer to their clients, including the value of custom-made orthotic devices. Occupational therapists and OTAs can also connect with senior populations through presentations at healthcare facilities and community centers, to educate about joint protection and energy conservation, orthotics, and appropriate adaptive devices. The message to senior citizens can be that they can continue to engage in their chosen ADL, IADL, work, and leisure activities if they get the assistance they need.

Client Education and Training

In treating clients with arthritic conditions, the education is one of the most important and beneficial tools OT practitioners can provide. Education and training can come in many forms, and the OT practitioner may use a combination of many of these.

Verbal instructions and/or discussion—Can help the client better understand the anatomy of a particular joint or body part and what is going on physiologically. It is important that the information is presented on a level that the client and family can understand.

Written information/materials—Handouts or pamphlets, especially with illustrations of equipment or exercises, can help the client and family understand and remember what they are supposed to do or not do. It is also beneficial to provide resources such as helpful websites, magazines, articles, and support groups.

Demonstration—When educating clients on energy conservation, work simplification, and body mechanics, it is not enough just to talk to them or give them handouts. It is important to train by demonstrating techniques and having the client practice and return the demonstration. Clients may be used to doing activities in certain ways, and these may actually be harmful to their joints. It will take practice and determination for them to learn new habits.

JOINT PROTECTION PRINCIPLES

Joint protection is a very important part of managing arthritic conditions. The purpose of joint protection is to reduce joint stress, decrease pain, and preserve joint structure. Joint protection principles include the following:

- **Use the strongest or largest joint possible to accomplish a task.** Show clients how to use the side of the hand, the forearm or the elbow instead of the fingers, the legs instead of the back, and sometimes using the whole body instead of just the arms.
  - Examples: Carrying a purse on the shoulder or at the bend of the elbow instead of holding a handle with the fingers. Closing doors and drawers with the body instead of the arm or hand. Using hips and knees to lift. Pushing a grocery cart rather than carrying a grocery basket. Rolling or sliding objects on a counter or floor rather than lifting and carrying them (Fig. 21-11).
- **Distribute the load over several joints.** This means using both arms to lift, carry, pull, or push objects, and spreading a load across the body instead of just the arms. This can also mean enlarging the handles on objects to spread the grip over all the MCP and IP joints.
  - Examples: Holding a glass or mug with two hands, instead of one hand holding the handle. Carrying flat items (i.e., a computer) on forearms with palms up as opposed to holding the edges. Wearing a backpack or cross-shoulder messenger bag to distribute weight across the upper body instead of on one shoulder (Fig. 21-12). Carrying young children in harness carriers, such as a Baby Bjorn™ instead of one hip.

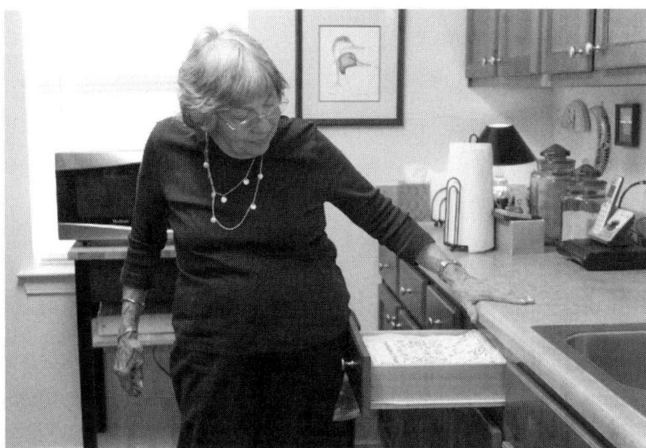

FIGURE 21-11. Use larger movements of the body to accomplish everyday tasks to preserve smaller joints.

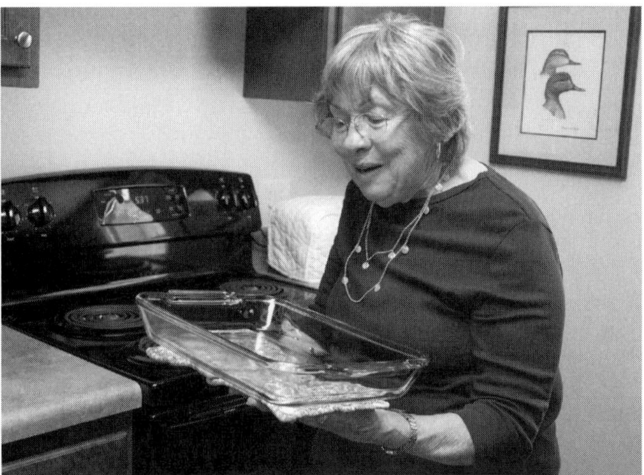

FIGURE 21-12. Distribute the load over several joints. Carry a heavy casserole from underneath, utilizing the stronger muscles and larger joints.

- **Avoid positions of deformity and deforming stress.** This means using each joint in its most stable and functional position and avoiding positions that twist or torque a joint or body part. Internal forces in the hand often pull toward the ulnar side, which can lead to ulnar drift deformities. It is important to limit deviation of the wrist and movement of the fingers in the direction, which occur during activities such as turning knobs, cutting food with a knife, or hammering. It is also important to maintain alignment of all the phalanges and avoid movements into hyperextension, such as pressing tabs or buttons with the distal phalanx of the thumb. It is also important to protect the neck and spine. Simultaneous flexion and rotation at the spine should be avoided, as should craning the head and neck forward, which overstretches the neck extensors and shortens the flexors, leading to "forward head" posture.
  - Examples: *Hands:* Open jars and doorknobs with the left hand and close them with the right hand, and turn hot and cold water taps with opposite hands, to avoid ulnar deviation. Twist open medication bottles or jars using the palm of hand. Hold a spoon in a fisted grasp and stir batter counterclockwise to avoid deviation at the wrist. Carry frying pans with the handle in one hand, and a flat palm underneath. Open boxes of pancake mix with a knife instead of pushing on the tab with the thumb. Get a keyless entry car or using an adapted key holder instead of pressing the button with the thumb. Use a sponge in the kitchen or a nylon mesh scrubber in the shower and squeeze it between two palms or between a flat hand and the side of the sink, instead of wringing out a washcloth. *Spine:* Face doors, cupboards, and drawers when opening them, to prevent pulling or twisting from the side. Avoid leaning the head down or toward a computer screen, especially with laptop computers or tablets held in the lap. Put reading material at eye level instead of looking down at a table or lap. See Figure 21-13 for various tools and techniques to help avoid positions of deformity and stress on joints.
- **Avoid holding joints in one position or repetitive movements for any excessive length of time.** Sustained muscle contraction causes fatigue. Prolonged grip on objects can lead to damage of the small, vulnerable IP joints. Repetitive gripping and pinching tasks can also fatigue muscles, damage joints and soft tissue (i.e., rotator cuff tendons), and lead to painful conditions such as lateral and medial epicondylitis (tennis elbow and golfer's elbow). People with arthritis can learn to use supports to hold objects instead of gripping them. Remember, this applies to not only ADLs and IADLs, but also to work and leisure tasks (Box 21-3).
  - Examples: Use a cookbook stand to hold a book or magazine while reading. Take rest breaks and stretch out the fingers when writing or typing for a long time or engage in leisure activities such

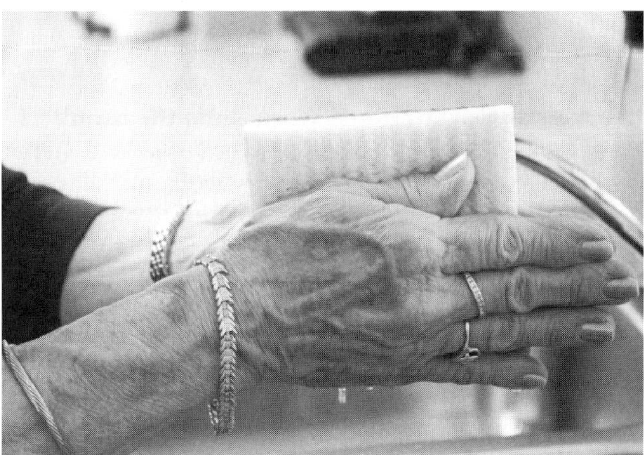

FIGURE 21-13. Avoid positions of deformity. Squeeze a sponge between two palms.

BOX 21-3
Leisure

The ability for people with arthritis to engage in leisure activities may be impacted by pain, stiffness, joint instability or deformity, and depression. This is true for activities that are typically done outdoors and require arm movements, such as golf, gardening, and swimming; or activities that are more fine-motor based and sedentary, such as knitting, reading, and doing crossword puzzles. The OTA can help many clients to adapt their leisure activities by incorporating principles of joint protection, energy conservation, work simplification, and body mechanics. The following are some examples of how the OTA may help clients:

Gardening/Yard Work—To protect back, hips, and knees:

- Using longer handles on gardening tools to avoid bending over
- Sitting on a gardening bench instead of standing and bending
- Raising the garden bed to eliminate bending and crouching

Needlework—To avoid prolonged, tight grasp, and poor positioning of head and shoulders:

- Using a standing frame to hold embroidery or quilting
- Using a table-mounted vise to hold a crochet hook or knitting needles
- Using larger diameter needles and hooks
- Doing rake knitting or arm knitting instead of holding knitting needles
- Putting the stitchery down every few minutes to relax fingers and avoid prolonged grasp

Reading—To avoid prolonged grasp and "forward head" position:

- Using a cookbook stand to support books or magazines
- Listening to books on tape
- Reading books on an e-reader that is properly positioned

Various Game and Craft Activities—To avoid prolonged grasp:

- Enlarged, padded, and/or ergonomic handles on tools such as pens, scissors, paintbrushes, and jewelry-making supplies
- Using a vise to hold woodworking, macramé, or other projects
- Placing playing cards or game tiles on a rack

Outdoor Sports—To avoid injury to weak or unstable joints; excessive fatigue; and twisting, turning, or throwing motions:

- Mounting a fishing pole holder in a boat or on a dock
- Using lighter-weight racquets, golf clubs, bats, balls, and so on, when possible
- Stabilizing a gun on a mounted rack for hunting
- Playing Wii™ versions of sports such as baseball, bowling, or golf until the flareup subsides
- Using flotation devices, noodles, and flippers when swimming

Exercise—To prevent joint damage through excessive impact and fatigue:

- Choosing lower-impact activities such as tai chi, Zumba Gold®, and certain types of yoga
- Pedaling a hand cycle instead of a regular bicycle
- Installing a larger, padded, ergonomic seat on bicycles or exercycles
- Participating in Arthritis Foundation-approved aquatic exercise classes instead of land-based exercise classes

as knitting or crocheting. Change position frequently, moving between sitting and standing. Get out of the car at least once per hour during long-distance drives.

ENERGY CONSERVATION AND WORK SIMPLIFICATION TECHNIQUES

Energy conservation and **work simplification** techniques are based on principles designed to reduce energy demands and eliminate unnecessary work and body motion. In essence, work smarter. The OT practitioner will educate and train the client on easier and more effective ways of performing daily tasks. The following are examples of work simplification and energy conservation:

- **Use automated, lightweight, or ergonomic tools and equipment.** This may mean using electric appliances or larger or padded handles or handles shaped to follow the hand's natural curves and arches.
  - Examples: *For meal preparation activities:* Use an electric can opener, blender, mixer, microwave oven, toaster oven, or water dispenser in refrigerator. *For grooming activities:* Use an electric toothbrush, automated soap and toothpaste dispenser, lightweight blow dryer or curling iron. *For home management activities:* Use a lightweight iron, dustpan with a long handle, or lightweight sweeper. *For leisure activities:* Use an automated card shuffler, ergonomic handle gardening tools, self-threading sewing machines, ergonomic handle tools (e.g., hammers), and electric screwdrivers (Fig. 21-14).
- **Eliminate unnecessary tasks.** If a task cannot be eliminated, it may be able to be done virtually (e.g., shopping) or delegated to a family member, friend, or neighbor. In some cases such as yard work or snow removal, it may be necessary to pay someone else to do it.
  - Examples of ways to eliminate unnecessary tasks: Allow dishes to drip dry. Buy clothes that don't require ironing. Buy prewashed and prechopped fruits or vegetables, or frozen meals.

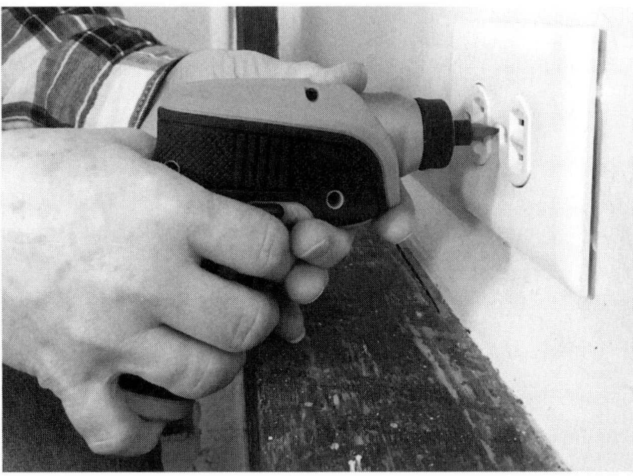

FIGURE 21-14. Using appropriate tools to conserve energy. The lightweight battery powered screwdriver helps to conserve energy. Note that the pistol grip design also helps to protect joints.

- **Eliminate any unnecessary bending, reaching, or walking.** Clients can reduce bending by elevating things and tasks to appropriate height work surfaces.
  - Examples include raised garden beds and raised computer monitors.
- **Sit when possible.** Clients can learn to do certain tasks while seated, including meal preparation, oral hygiene, applying makeup, and getting dressed. They need to be reminded to change position frequently, to take frequent rest and stretch breaks, and use an appropriate height chair or stool.
- **Plan work, and work according to the plan.** Clients can save a lot of energy and wasted movement by planning ahead. Examples including making a list before going to a store (and if possible, organize to match the store layout or in categories), planning meals for the week, researching directions and schedules for planned errands or outings, and assembling all the ingredients for a recipe, or tools for a project, *before* beginning, so it is not necessary to stop midway to get something at the store.
- **Store frequently used items within easy reach.** This may mean putting things that are used daily on kitchen and bathroom counters, and having duplicates of items used in multiple rooms.
  - Examples: Frequently used items should be stored on the lowest shelf above counter height, or the highest shelf below counter height, to minimize bending, stretching, and reaching. It may be necessary to have eyeglasses, tissues, sweaters, or other items located in the bedroom, kitchen, sitting rooms, and so on. In a two-story home, it is advisable to have two vacuum cleaners and also two sets of cleaning supplies to avoid carrying them up and down the stairs.
- **Spread the workload throughout the day/week.** This means alternating heavy and light tasks during the day or throughout the week to prevent exhaustion. It also includes scheduling activities at times when pain is lowest and energy is highest.
  - Example: Housekeeping activities, laundry, and shopping should be split into smaller increments across multiple days.
- **Do not start activities that cannot be stopped.** People with arthritis may need to wait to perform certain activities until help is available, or change the way they are done, if it is not possible to stop the activity when realizing that something is too heavy or hard.
  - Example: A person cannot stop in the middle of carrying a heavy pot full of boiling water from the stove to the sink, or a glass casserole dish from the oven to the dining room.
- **Ask for help when needed.** It is often difficult for people to admit that they need help, especially for routine tasks that they used to be able to do independently. Because of the unpredictable nature of some arthritic conditions like RA, fibromyalgia, and gout, a person may be able to do a task one day and not the next. For this reason, it is important for clients to learn that it is okay to ask for help, and also okay to politely decline offers of help when they do not need it.

BODY MECHANICS PRINCIPLES

Body mechanics principles reflect using the body in the way it was meant to function, with correct postures and movements. Following proper body mechanics principles can help protect the vulnerable joints in the neck and spine, as well as decreasing stress on the joints of the extremities.

- **Maintain proper posture and alignment.** When body parts are properly aligned, it decreases stress on joints in the neck, spine, shoulders, and hips. The client should be taught that the nose, navel, knees, and toes should all be facing the same direction, to avoid twisting injuries. Photos or video of the client may help show proper positioning of the head over the shoulders to avoid "forward head."
- **Have appropriate support.** The spine and limbs need to be properly supported to protect the integrity of the joints. Clients may need to sit in chairs with backs and arms and to use footrests on wheelchairs or on high stools. Footwear should be properly fitted and provide support to the foot and ankle. High-heeled shoes focus all the body's weight on a very small surface and can lead to pain and joint damage in the foot. When standing for long periods, people tend to tilt the pelvis forward or laterally. To prevent this tilt, which can stretch ligaments or compress nerves, teach clients to elevate one leg when standing for a prolonged period. An example of this is resting one foot on the bottom of a grocery cart while waiting in line at the store.
- **Work at the right height.** Working at a surface that is too low causes the client to maintain a position of spinal flexion, and working at a surface that is too high causes the client to maintain a position of spinal

extension. Prolonged time spent in either of these positions can lead to strain on spinal muscles and ligaments. Whether the client is standing or sitting, the ideal height for a work surface is close to waist height. Clients can be taught to sit at a low sink when shaving, brushing teeth, or applying makeup, or to use a bar stool when working at a high counter. Transfers to surfaces that are too low, like toilets, can also put a lot of strain on the spine and LEs. An elevated toilet can raise the height and decrease the strain on the legs. Risers can be put under the legs of surfaces that are not adjustable, such as beds and sofas.

- **Use proper bending and lifting techniques.** Clients may need to be trained how to bend with their legs and not their backs. They can be trained how to squat, center a load to be lifted, and keep it close to their body while rising with their legs. When arthritis affects the hips and/or knees, squatting may not be possible. Clients will need education regarding alternative methods like the golfer's lift or supported bend (Fig. 21-15). When a person cannot bend safely, sometimes it may be necessary to use a reacher to retrieve lightweight objects that are on the floor, or else leave them there.
- **Avoid excessive bending, lifting, or carrying.** Even when using proper body mechanics, excessive bending, lifting, or carrying may put strain on the joints in the spine and limbs. Teach clients that pushing, pulling, rolling, or sliding are preferable to lifting or carrying. Clients should always push a wheeled cart in the store instead of carrying a basket, which puts the entire burden on one side of the body. Objects should be carried at midline and close to the chest if possible. Due to the laws of physics, the farther the load from the axis of movement, the more force required to move or stabilize. This is why clients should hold bags against their torso, instead of carrying bags with handles and arms down at their sides. It is also why picking up heavy items with a reacher can be more stressful to a person's arm than lifting the item itself.

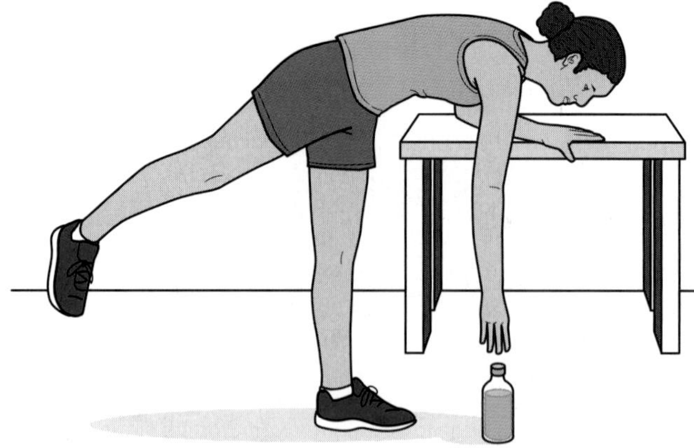

FIGURE 21-15. Golfer's lift.

Adaptive Equipment

Adaptive equipment may be needed due to limited ROM in fingers, arms, spine, and hips. The OT practitioner should never assume that someone needs adaptive equipment just because a client has visible deformities, such as boutonnière or swan neck. Clients are often more capable than their OT practitioners expect. Adaptive equipment and activity modification is supposed to help increase a client's ability to perform activities independently. If the client is not interested in a particular activity or if the equipment makes the activity more difficult or time-consuming, it may not be appropriate. It is also important to remember that clients will have to pay for virtually all adaptive equipment. Many times an OT practitioner, the client, or the family can find something in local big box retail or hardware/home improvement stores that can do the same thing as an expensive piece of adaptive equipment. That is why the OT practitioner needs to make recommendations for commercially available equipment only when it is vital to task performance and there is no way to construct something in a less expensive manner. See Figure 21-16 for samples of inexpensive, simple adaptive equipment. Table 21-3 and Table 21-4 offer common, useful adaptations for individuals affected by arthritis.

EVIDENCE-BASED PRACTICE

The OT treatment of arthritic conditions has not changed significantly over the years, and there is little new research being done on methods to improve function and engagement in occupation. OT practitioners typically first consider the client's ADLs and IADLs when providing treatment, however a recent study is a good reminder to always ask about the occupation of work. The research published in *Arthritis Care and Research* reports how OT has been a useful resource for helping individuals with rheumatoid arthritis or osteoarthritis address work issues. The study was a longitudinal (over 2 years), randomized controlled trial comparing a workplace ergonomic interventions group versus a control group (educational materials only) for individuals with either RA or OA with regard to physical symptoms and work tasks. The group that received the ergonomic intervention in the workplace had less arthritis-related impact on their work, with also fewer symptoms and issues with physical functioning. Overall, there is evidence that supports ergonomic intervention in the workplace as a way to decrease pain and symptoms and improve work productivity.[56]

Baldwin, D., Johnstone, B., Ge, B., Hewett, J., Smith, M., & Sharp, G. (2012). Randomized prospective study of a work place ergonomic intervention for individuals with rheumatoid arthritis and osteoarthritis. Arthritis Care and Research, *64(10), 1527–1535. doi:10.1002/acr.21699*

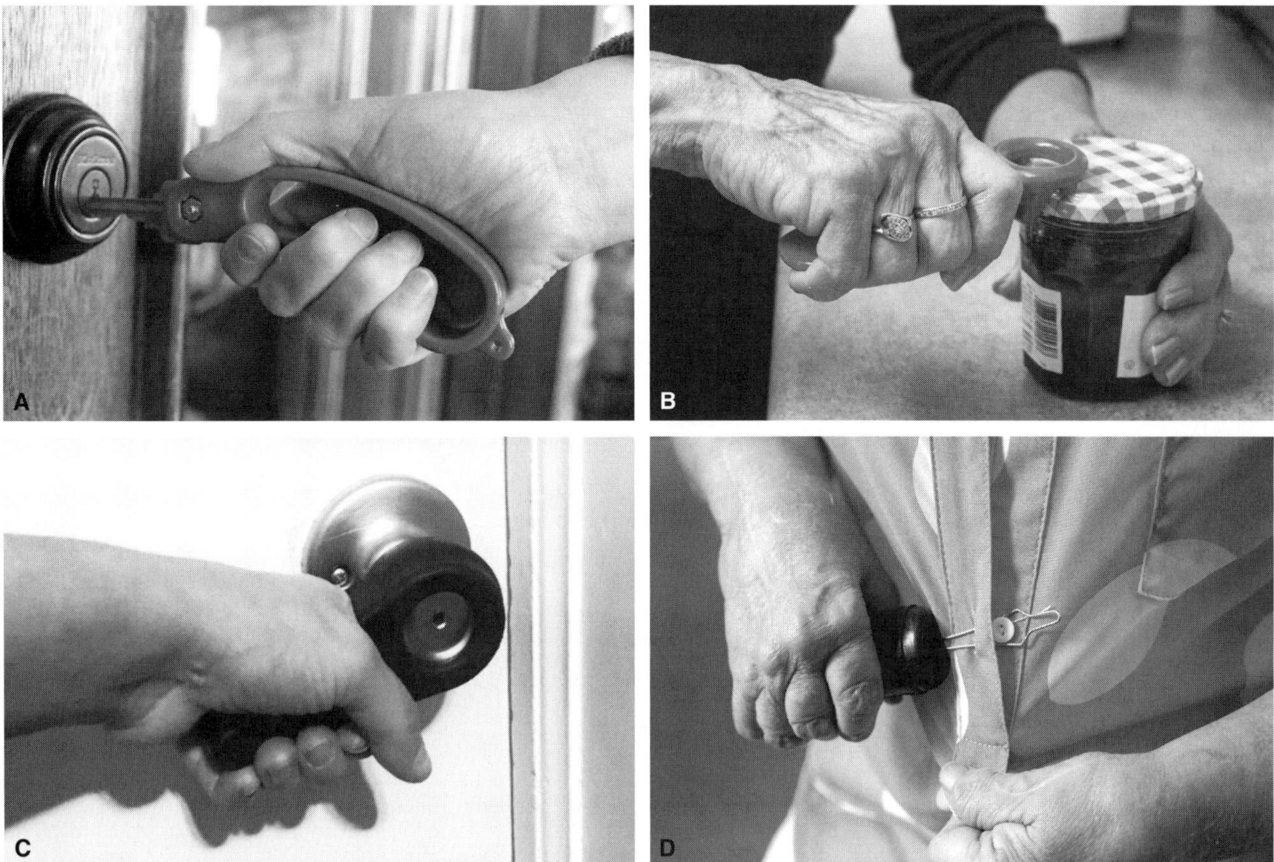

FIGURE 21-16. Adaptive equipment: **A.** Key holder. **B.** Jar key. **C.** Door knob lever handle attachment. **D.** Individual with RA using a button hook.

TABLE 21-3 Common Adaptations for Arthritis Involving the Spine, Hips, Knees, and/or Shoulders

GOAL	PURPOSE OF EQUIPMENT	EXAMPLES
Toileting and toilet transfers	Increased height Stability assistance Compensation for decreased ROM of hips or spine	Raised toilet seat Toilet safety bars Personal hygiene aids (to hold toilet tissue)
Bathing	Compensation for decreased endurance or ROM Compliance with postsurgical precautions (may be temporary)	Shower chair Tub bench Long-handled sponge
Dressing	Compliance with postsurgical precautions (may be temporary) or decreased ROM	Sock aid Long-handled shoehorn Dressing stick Reacher
Grooming	Compensation for decreased ROM of shoulders Compensation for decreased ROM of hips or spine	Long-handled combs or brushes Long-handled razors (for shaving legs), lotion applicators, (toe)nail clippers
Home management	Compensation for decreased ROM Adaptations for lifting	Long-handled items such as sponges, dustpans, or dusters Rolling laundry baskets

Orthotics

Orthotics are an integral part of the OT approach to the treatment and management of arthritic conditions. Orthotics (formerly called splints) are either "soft-goods" made out of neoprene, canvas, or other materials, or thermoplastic material that is prefabricated or custom designed by the occupational therapist or OTA. The goal of using orthotics for arthritic conditions is to put the joint(s) in a position of rest and protection in order to relieve pain, allow the inflammatory process to subside, and manage or prevent further joint deformity/destruction. During an acute flareup, orthotics are

TABLE 21-4 Common Adaptations for Difficulties With Grip or Pinch

GOAL	ADAPTATION	EXAMPLES
Compensate for limited MCP or IP flexion	Built-up handles	Eating utensils Grooming utensils Writing utensils
Compensate for finger or thumb deformities	Adapted handles	Scissors Key holder
Prevent hand fatigue due to prolonged grasp or repetitive motion	Ergonomic handles	Vegetable peelers Hammers, screwdrivers, and other tools Gardening tools
Prevent prolonged grip that can lead to finger deformity	Holders Enlarged tools	Book rests Crochet hook/embroidery frame Lap desk for writing or tablet use
Maintain proper alignment of joints, and avoid positions of deformity	Various methods depending on the tool and joints used	Jar openers Door handle or faucet lever attachments Key holders Right-angle knives (pistol grip) Y-shape vegetable peeler

used to rest the joints and decrease inflammation. Orthotics are typically worn continuously during this period. When the inflammation has subsided and the disease is more subacute, orthotics function to provide support to joints, which are unstable and painful with use. During this stage, orthotics may be worn during certain activities or through the night. Orthotics are also used when joints are grossly deformed and unstable. Although an orthotic cannot *correct* a deformity, it can prevent it from getting worse. During this stage, orthotics are commonly worn during certain activities, but serve little purpose at night. Commonly used orthotics are described in the next section, based on the joints involved.

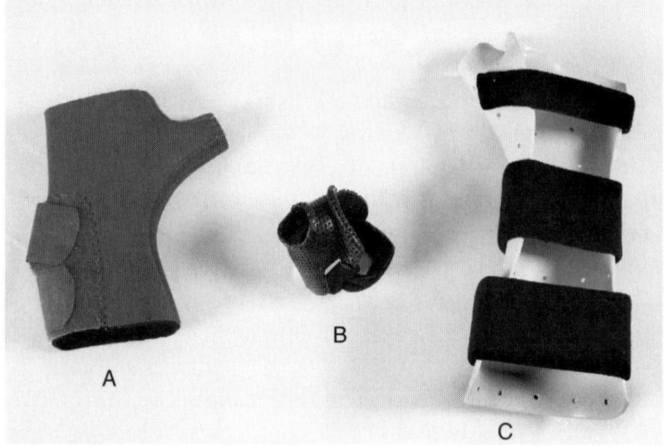

FIGURE 21-17. Orthotics for thumb stabilization. **A.** Benik splint with thumb stabilization bar (custom order). **B.** Hand-based thumb custom-made orthotic. **C.** Long volar, thumb spica custom-made orthotic.

THUMB CARPOMETACARPAL JOINT

The thumb CMC joint may need to be stabilized in a thumb spica orthotic for conditions such as OA and RA. This may be done with a hand-based orthotic or a forearm-based orthotic that also stabilizes the wrist (Fig. 21-17). The MCP and IP joints may or may not also be stabilized. With a flareup of RA, the client may be fitted with a forearm-based orthotic that maintains the wrist in slight extension and the thumb CMC in about 45 degrees of abduction or midway between abduction and extension. With osteoarthritis, which is more chronic, the person may wear a hand-based thumb immobilization orthotic with the CMC joint abducted to a position of comfort.[57]

FINGER AND THUMB INTERPHALANGEAL JOINTS

Orthotics are often worn on one or more IP joints to prevent or correct hyperextension deformities, such as swan-neck deformity and boutonnière deformity. These orthotics often are in a figure-eight pattern, and can be made from thermoplastic material or purchased commercially from manufacturers such as Oval-8 and Silver Ring Splint Company (Fig. 21-18). These orthotics allow flexion at the IP joints but limit hyperextension (extension beyond zero degrees).[57]

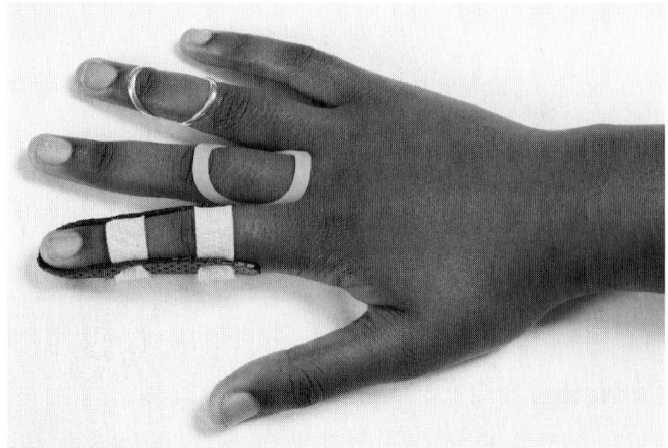

FIGURE 21-18. *From top:* **A.** Ring Finger: SIRIS™ Boutonnière Splint. **B.** Middle finger: Oval-8® Finger Splint. **C.** Index finger: Custom made finger gutter orthosis.

FINGER METACARPOPHALANGEAL JOINTS

Sometimes orthotics are necessary to stabilize the second through fifth MCP joints to rest inflamed joints or to prevent subluxation or ulnar deviation. Orthotics to prevent ulnar deviation are often made from soft material with straps around each finger pulling them in a radial direction (toward the thumb). Ulnar deviation orthotics constructed from thermoplastic material are bulkier and more likely to interfere with hand use during activity, thus potentially affecting compliance. MCP stabilization orthotics can be volar or dorsal, and act by allowing movement in one direction (e.g., flexion) but limiting movement in the other direction (e.g., extension). These orthotics may be hand-based or may incorporate the wrist as well. Examples of a forearm-based orthotic that supports the MCP joints are resting hand and functional position orthotics.[57]

WRIST

Inflammation at the wrist can cause compression on the structures passing through the carpal tunnel at the wrist, including the median nerve. Therefore, wrist orthotics are commonly used for clients with RA and conditions such as carpal tunnel syndrome. The orthotic serves to provide support at the wrist and decrease inflammation. These orthotics are called wrist cock-ups and should hold the wrist in neutral or slight extension. Soft wrist cock-up orthotics are available on the Internet, at pharmacy stores, and in large chain stores. They are often made of canvas or neoprene, fasten with Velcro®, and contain a pliable metal plate (called a spoon) to hold the wrist in extension (Fig. 21-19). Many of these commercially sold orthotics are angled at 20° to 30° of extension, which is not what physicians or OT practitioners typically recommend. The OT practitioner can assist by manually straightening the metal stay to the appropriate angle. Clients may prefer the soft orthotics because they are lighter weight and interfere less with functional activities. The OT practitioner may be responsible for checking the size, adjusting the orthotic to an appropriate level of wrist extension, and for teaching the client when and how to wear and care for the OTC orthotic. OT practitioners often fabricate wrist cock-up orthotics from thermoplastics. Orthotic fabrication is a skill that is covered more in-depth in Chapter 19. Patterns for dorsal or volar-based cock-up orthotics with different degrees of coverage in the palm or the thumbs are available. Styles include radial bar cock-up, thumb-hole cock-up, and long thumb spica. Wrist cock-ups may be worn during activity and/or during the night.

In cases of extreme inflammation through the distal upper extremity, a person may need a resting hand orthosis to protect all the joints of the fingers, thumbs, and wrist. These may be fabricated by the OT practitioner, or a commercially available "soft" orthotic can be purchased (Fig. 21-20). These inhibit any function use of the hand while being worn.

Edema Management

Swelling is one of the cardinal signs of inflammation, and is common in conditions such as RA and fibromyalgia. Swelling, or *edema*, is an excessive amount of fluid in the tissues. In arthritis, edema is the result of the inflammation process, and is different from dependent edema (which is caused by poor circulation), lymphedema (which is an impairment in the lymphatic system), or the initial inflammatory response following an injury. When the edema crowds the structures within the joint, it can result in nerve compression such as in carpal tunnel syndrome. This is often addressed through light compression garments, light massage, and application of modalities such as cryotherapy (to be discussed in the next section). The light compression gloves can be purchased with or without fingertip coverage, and are typically worn at night, and the seam of the gloves should be worn on the outside (Fig. 21-21). Compression gloves should always be checked for proper fit. If they are too tight, they may cut off circulation. Each client is unique, and may or may not benefit from using compression gloves.

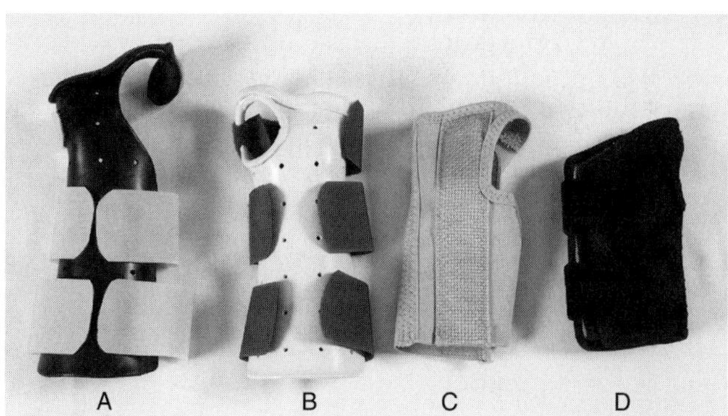

FIGURE 21-19. Wrist orthotics, *left to right:* **A.** Custom fabricated radial bar wrist cock-up orthoses. **B.** Volar thumb hole cock-up orthoses. **C.** and **D.** are commercially available short wrist orthoses.

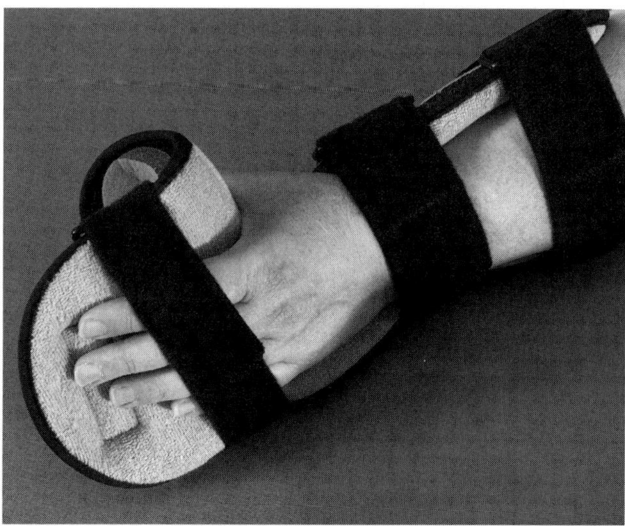

FIGURE 21-20. Soft resting hand orthotic.

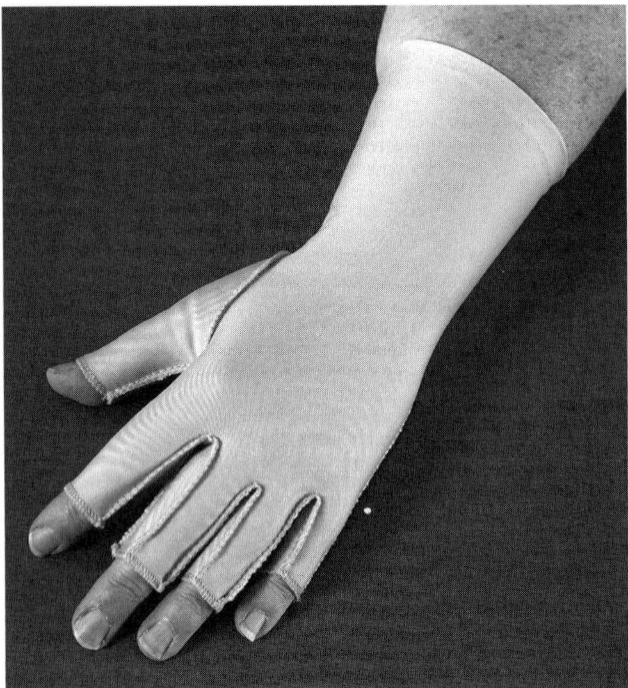

FIGURE 21-21. Edema gloves without fingertips. Note the seams are on the outside.

Therapeutic Exercise and Therapeutic Activity

OT intervention addressing ROM and strengthening differs depending on the client's disease status. When someone is experiencing an exacerbation of RA for example, exercise should focus on gentle active ROM to prevent stiffness but not increase inflammation. When in remission or chronic state, clients can do more stretching exercises to maintain or increase range. Resistive exercises are also contraindicated during periods of active inflammation. In addition, therapeutic activities may include participation in fine motor and in-hand manipulation tasks. OT treatment should always have a focus on function and include purposeful or occupation-based activities.

DURING ACTIVE INFLAMMATION

Slow active movements within the pain free range can be done for the whole body. The focus of these exercises is to prevent stiffness or further loss of motion, not to add repetitions or increase degrees of movement. The client can do these movements from any position. Many clients find it helpful to do this while in bed in the morning, to loosen their joints before getting up and beginning ADLs. It is important that the client perform all movements with their joints in the proper alignment and weak joints being stabilized. If possible, the limbs can be supported and moved in the horizontal plane, to decrease stress on shoulders and spine. Water exercises may be beneficial due to the buoyancy of the water. Tai chi and the ROM dance are great activities that encourage movement. The ROM dance was developed in Wisconsin in 1987 by an occupational therapist and a tai chi instructor, and DVDs and videos are available on the Internet. Participating in ADL and IADL activities as much as possible is also encouraged during this stage (Box 21-4).

DURING CHRONIC STAGE OR REMISSION

At this stage, OT treatment may focus on increasing strength, ROM, joint stability, endurance, and fine motor coordination, in order to improve occupational performance (Box 21-5). Active movements can now stretch just beyond the pain free range, in order to gently increase ROM without damaging joints. Resistive activities involving therapy putty, resistance bands, or light weights can be added. Clients can be taught to do progressive resistive exercises at home with beanbags or water bottles filled to comfort level. If the water bottles are cold, they can also help decrease swelling and discomfort in the hands. Fine motor activities related to the client's occupational roles and routines can also be included. This may include activities like buttoning, assembling nuts and bolts, writing or typing, and meal preparation activities.

At this stage, clients also need to address how to incorporate general endurance and core stability exercises or activities into their lives (Fig. 21-22). They may be introduced to activities in a clinic that they can continue at home or in the community, after learning about pacing and watching for signs of overexertion or joint stress. Activities can include walking, yoga, dance, water exercise, and cycling.

Pain Management

Clients must be taught to respect pain, which is their body's way of communicating that a task is too hard, done too long, or is at risk for causing joint damage. Clients need to learn to distinguish between acute *pain* which is sharp, stabbing, or burning, and is distracting; and *discomfort* which is milder, more achy, and typically does not interfere with thinking, concentrating, or carrying out activities. A certain amount of discomfort may need to be tolerated. Clients can be taught about their "new normal" which may be somewhat uncomfortable, temporarily or even long-term. Clients also need to learn to differentiate between chronic pain or discomfort versus exercise or activity induced pain. The Arthritis Foundation's self-help courses and website teach about the 2-hour pain rule, stating "If you have more joint pain two hours after exercising than before you started, you've overdone it. Ease up at your next workout."[58] OT practitioners advise clients to rethink the level or duration of their activities or exercises so that postactivity pain or discomfort subsides in 30 to 60 minutes.

BOX 20-4
Contraindications of Resistive Exercise

Fast and repetitious movements and resistive exercises with weights, therapy putty, or resistance bands, are contraindicated as they may damage the unstable joints.

BOX 21-5
Sexual Activity

Sexual activity and sexual functioning may be affected by arthritis for multiple reasons, including pain, joint stiffness, fatigue, joint deformity or instability, and depression. People with any type of arthritic condition may be affected. Other arthritic conditions such as scleroderma and psoriatic arthritis can also affect a person's self-image and affect sexuality. A partner may also avoid sexual activity for fear of hurting the person with arthritis. The OTA can help clients and their partners maintain sexual activities by incorporating the principles of joint protection, energy conservation, and proper body mechanics. Below are some suggestions for the OTA to discuss with clients:

POSITIONING

- Using pillows, wedges, or bolsters to support weak or unstable joints in the spine or hips; or to maintain the spine and other joints in proper alignment
- Choosing positions that limit weight-bearing on the upper extremities or the knees
- Considering positions that decrease stress on sore or inflamed joints, such as sidelying or sitting

TIMING

- Scheduling sexual activity to coincide with peak effect of medication
- Balancing rest and activity, so not overdoing it on days when a person wants to engage in sexual activity
- Not engaging in sexual activity when joints are sore from exercise or therapy

STIFFNESS

- Taking a warm bath or shower before sexual activity to loosen joints and relieve discomfort

COMMUNICATION

- For the client: Sharing with a sexual partner which positions, techniques, and movements feel good and which lead to more discomfort
- For the partner: Listening to the partner and showing concern for his or her comfort, but also recognizing the partner as a person with sexual needs and desires

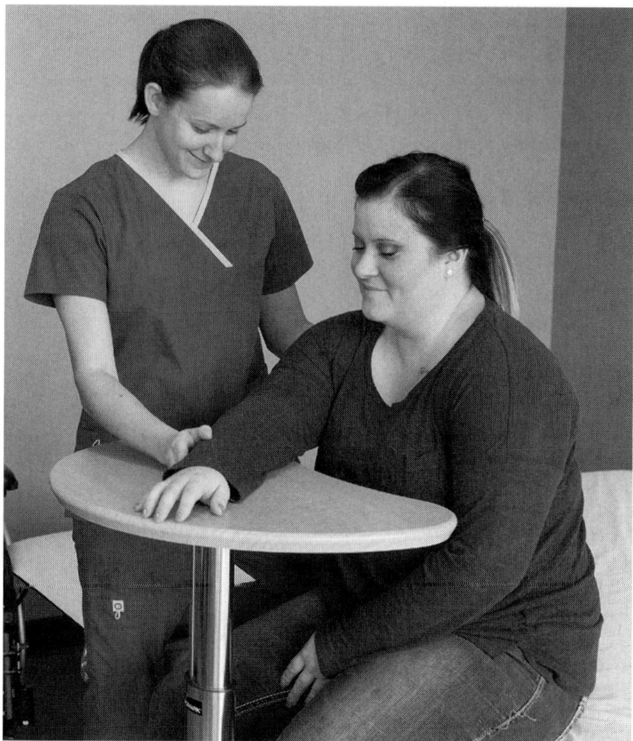

FIGURE 21-22. Gentle ROM exercises: exercising in the horizontal plane.

Physical agent modalities (PAMs) are interventions that are often used by OT practitioners in the treatment of chronic pain that is a hallmark of many arthritic conditions. The American Occupational Therapy Association's position paper on the use of PAMs states that they should be used only "in preparation for or conjunction with purposeful and occupation-based activities and interventions..." and only by practitioners who possess both theoretical background and technical skills in the use of modalities.[58] Use of modalities by OTAs is dependent on demonstration of service competency and adherence to any applicable state regulations (e.g., required courses or training). Thermal modalities (hot and cold) may be used in the clinic and can also be taught to clients for home application. Electromodalities such as electrical stimulation are mainly done in the clinical environment.

THERMAL MODALITIES

These are the most commonly used physical agents. Cold applications (cryotherapy) are used primarily during the acute phases of arthritis, whereas heat applications are used during chronic phases. Cryotherapy is often used at the end of a therapy session to provide pain relief. Ice packs may irritate the skin, so it is best for the client to put a thin wet cloth between the pack and the skin. Cold treatment should be done no more than 15 minutes at a time. Although cold therapy is something that clients can do at home, the OTA must be sure to educate the client and family about precautions and contraindications. An easy way for a client to apply cold at home is to use a bag of frozen peas. It is convenient to keep, and the flexibility of the pack allows it to be molded around an inflamed joint. Another cold alternative is to put a water bottle in the freezer. The person can then take it out and hold it to ease a painful hand.

Heat is also used for pain management, and relief of soft-tissue restrictions and muscle spasms. Heat modalities such as hot packs, paraffin, and fluidotherapy, are often used as preparatory treatments in the clinical setting. While the client is sitting with the heat may be a good time to do client education. Although fluidotherapy and anodyne can only be done in the clinic, clients can apply heat at home through a variety of media and must understand precautions and demonstrate proper technique. When applying a hot pack or heating pad at home, the client must be careful to protect the skin with layers of towels or clothes between the heat and the skin. The heat should not be applied between the client and the bed or table, or the trapped heat can burn the skin. Clients should never go to sleep with a heating pad or a heat patch (e.g., TheraCare®).

Clients who like the paraffin treatment can purchase a unit for home use. These are often available at beauty supply stores or in big box stores.

ELECTROTHERAPEUTIC MODALITIES

The most common modes of electrical stimulation used by the OT practitioner are transcutaneous electrical nerve stimulation (TENS) and interferential current. They are both used for pain relief. Iontophoresis is a transdermal application of a medication or chemicals driven by an electrical current over a painful area. Although TENS and interferential do not require a separate physician's order (apart from the referral to OT), iontophoresis does require a physician's order if it includes a prescription medication. Clients sometimes rent or purchase TENS units for home use and need to be educated in the proper use of these units. The use of physical agent modalities in OT is addressed in depth in Chapter 18.

SUMMARY

As an OTA, it is imperative to understand the functional and psychological impact arthritic conditions can have on clients. Pain, limited mobility, and joint deformity can affect an individual's ability to perform simple ADLs, IADLs, and school, work, and leisure activities. Aside from the biomechanical impairments that affect movement, strength, stability, and endurance, the psychological effects can also be debilitating. Depression and frustration are often seen, and affect the client's roles and satisfaction at home and motivation in treatment. The OT practitioner's role is to recognize and acknowledge this, establish the client's baseline functional level, and adapt the treatment plan accordingly in order to help the client achieve maximal independence and safety in occupational performance.[60]

REVIEW QUESTIONS

1. Which three of the following arthritic conditions often include fever as a presenting symptom?
   a. Rheumatoid arthritis
   b. Gout
   c. Systemic lupus erythematosus
   d. Fibromyalgia
   e. Osteoarthritis
   f. Systemic juvenile idiopathic arthritis
2. Which three of the following are common symptoms of fibromyalgia?
   a. Fusiform swelling of joints
   b. Fatigue
   c. Depression
   d. Memory impairment
   e. Nodules under the skin
   f. Rash
3. A client is referred to the outpatient clinic with a flareup of rheumatoid arthritis affecting her right shoulder, left wrist, and both hands. Which three OT interventions would you *most likely* incorporate into her treatment?
   a. Use of a wrist-hand orthotic
   b. Theraband exercises for shoulder ROM
   c. Moist heat before exercising
   d. Pulling on Velcro® checkers to strengthen her wrist
   e. Doing gentle active range of motion (AROM) exercises in bed before getting up in the morning
   f. Receiving instruction in joint protection techniques
4. Mrs. McCoy, 72 years of age, is a widow and lives alone in a small, one bedroom apartment. She has OA in her hips, knees, and hands. She has difficulty standing for long periods of time. She wants to teach her teenage granddaughter how to make cookies from her favorite family recipe. Which of the following would you recommend for Mrs. McCoy?
   a. Placing a stool in the kitchen to sit while measuring and mixing ingredients
   b. Preparing the dry ingredients the day before her granddaughter arrives
   c. Purchasing a countertop mini convection oven
   d. Purchasing prepared cookie dough
5. Which orthotic would you recommend for a client with osteoarthritis of the thumb CMC joint?
   a. Functional position orthotic
   b. Forearm-based orthotic with wrist in slight extension and thumb in 45-degree abduction
   c. Figure-eight orthotic
   d. Hand-based orthotic with the thumb abducted in a position of comfort
6. The occupational therapist tells you to incorporate cryotherapy and light massage and demonstrate light compression gloves for your client with SLE. What condition are you addressing with this client?
   a. Edema
   b. Spasticity
   c. Joint stiffness
   d. Joint pain
7. Your client with RA complains that in the morning her hands are so stiff that she has difficulty with dressing and grooming activities, thus making her late for work. What do you recommend for her morning routine?
   a. Get up 30 to 60 minutes earlier.
   b. Soak her hands in a sink of warm water for 5 minutes before starting ADLs.
   c. Use a TENS unit for 15 minutes first thing in the morning.
   d. Ask her spouse to assist her with her ADLs in the morning.
8. Your client is having a severe flareup of gout. Which energy conservation tip might be most useful to review with him during your OT session today?
   a. Use long-handled utensils.
   b. Sit when possible.
   c. Avoid prolonged grasp.
   d. Use lightweight tools.

9. In the middle of the OT session, your client with fibromyalgia starts crying and says, "I can't stand this pain anymore. When I get home from work, I am so miserable and tired that sometimes I can't remember what I'm doing when I'm making dinner. I hope I don't burn the house down." What is your *best* response?
   a. "I know just how you feel. It's horrible to be so tired and in pain."
   b. "You think you have it bad? Mrs. Smith over there can't even dress herself."
   c. "It must be frustrating when you feel like this. Let's brainstorm some ideas to lighten your load."
   d. "Why are you still doing all the cooking? What about your husband or kids?"
10. Your client complains that pain and swelling in her hands is preventing her from doing her shoulder exercises. What recommendation would you give her for home?
   a. Take a warm shower before exercising.
   b. Squeeze a stress ball 10 times before exercising.
   c. Do shoulder exercises holding a cold water bottle in each hand.
   d. Do not do any exercises until her hands feel better.

CASE STUDY

Gail is a 54-year-old nurse who works in the neonatal intensive care unit of a hospital. She is married and the mother of three teenagers. She enjoys gardening, cooking, and crocheting in her spare time. For over a year, she has been experiencing pain in her right (dominant) thumb. She notices the pain during many of her everyday activities including using a syringe, writing, and opening various containers (e.g., medications, supplies) at work. She notices pain when lifting pots and casserole dishes as well as when she is gripping wet clothes to pull them out of the washer. Using her gardening tools has become too painful. She has basically had to give up most of the yard work and even the crocheting she enjoys. Gail discussed her concerns with her family physician during her yearly routine physical. Her physician took x-rays and examined her thumb. She tested positive for the "Grind test" (a provocative test used to determine CMC arthritis). Her physician diagnosed her with right thumb basal joint or CMC joint OA.

Gail's primary care physician referred her to an occupational therapist at a nearby outpatient rehabilitation setting. The occupational therapist did a thorough evaluation of Gail's thumb and hand function which included ROM measurements, grip and pinch strength, fine motor coordination test (9-hole peg), and observation of her prehension skills. The occupational therapist fabricated a custom-made hand-based thumb spica splint to be worn during the day to provide proper joint alignment, joint protection, and a position of "rest." Gail was able to do all of her work activities and with a few activity modifications was able do her regular ADL and IADLs. She was even able to put a sterile glove on over her splint for work.

At Gail's second session in OT, she worked with the OTA. The OTA instructed her in a comprehensive home exercise program including ROM exercises and isometric exercises (isometric exercises tense the muscles against resistance without stressing the joints). She was educated and trained via discussion, demonstration, and practice and handouts on joint protection and activity modification. The OTA also discussed and demonstrated, then had Gail try a few pieces of adaptive equipment to decrease joint stress and increase independence with daily tasks such as longer-handled tools for the kitchen, Dycem® for opening containers, and a larger-diameter pen for writing, just to name a few. The OTA had Gail try a paraffin bath as a heat modality to decrease pain and stiffness.

At subsequent treatment sessions, the OTA provided Gail with the paraffin bath before her therapeutic exercises and functional tasks. Once Gail's pain was well under control, additional strengthening exercises were added including resistive therapy putty. Gail was discharged from OT after 6 sessions. Gail felt comfortable with continuing her home exercise program.

1. What do you think Gail should do to continue the progress made in her OT sessions?
2. How can Gail incorporate joint protection in her job?
3. What other household management task might pose a problem for her?
4. If Gail lived in your area, where would she obtain a paraffin bath and paraffin refills?

PUTTING IT ALL TOGETHER — Sample Treatment and Documentation

Setting	Outpatient rehabilitation clinic
Client Profile	Client is a 79 y/o female with bilateral hand OA. Referral is for evaluation and treatment of hands. PMH includes bilateral OA in knees and hips
Work History	Retired for 18 years from the local textile mill, where she worked on a yarn spinning machine for over 35 years
Insurance	Medicare (primary); BCBS (secondary)
Psychological	Dealing with depression re: inability to do as many things as she used to, and pain in hands, hips, and knees. Also dealing with other health issues such as diabetes and glaucoma. Reports lack of energy and less interest in doing the things she used to enjoy.
Social	Widowed. Lives alone and independently at this point. Has a son that comes infrequently to "help" with things. Attends church. Has some support system from church community. Does not have day-to-day help.
Cognitive	Reports becoming forgetful. Likely some age-related cognitive decline.
Motor and Strength	9-hole peg test: R = 32 sec., L = 39 sec. Grip strength: R = 18 lbs., L = 15 lbs. Lateral pinch: R = 6 lbs., L = 5 lbs. 3-point pinch: R = 4 lbs., L = 4 lbs. 2-point pinch: R = 2 lbs., L = 1 lb.

Continued

PUTTING IT ALL TOGETHER Sample Treatment and Documentation (continued)

Physical Characteristics	Bouchard's and Heberden's nodes noted on most PIP and DIP joints bilaterally. Right greater than left. Joint changes noted in CMC and MP joints of bilateral thumbs. Right greater than left.
ROM	Shoulder, elbow, forearm, and wrist ROM WFL. Mildly decreased AROM across all finger and thumb joints bilaterally. Right slightly worse than left. Unable to make a full composite fist bilaterally. Unable to oppose thumb to fifth digits. MMT contraindicated.
Pain	1-2/10 at rest. Pain increases to 6/10 when using hands for most functional tasks, especially those that require grip and pinch. Generally pain is worse in the mornings and on cold days.
ADL	Difficulty with grip and pinch due to pain and decreasing hand strength, affects client's ability to complete ADLs. She chooses clothing based on ease of dressing, and often does a sponge bath instead of showering. Mod A for LB dressing: Due to difficulty donning shoes and socks. Min A for UB dressing: Due to inability to manage clothing fasteners. Min A for grooming: Due to difficulty maintaining grip on utensils such as hairbrush, toothbrush, etc. Min A for toileting: Due to difficulty managing clothing. Mod A for bathing: Due to difficulty with tub transfers and fear of slipping.
IADL	Housework, yard work, and meal preparation are becoming increasingly challenging and frustrating. Client has difficulty using broom and mop and handling the pots and pans while cooking. Client has difficulty with financial management due to difficulty holding a pen while paying bills. She now pays a neighborhood teenager to mow the lawn, but she is still trying to do the housework. Client is really interested in resuming work in her garden to plant vegetables for future canning.
Long-Term Goals	At the end of eight sessions, the client will: 1. Demonstrate at least three joint protection, energy conservation, and work simplification principles independently, while doing preferred ADLs and IADLs. 2. Independently identify three modifications in order to safely continue meal preparation and home management activities. 3. Dress UB and LB with modified independence using AE as needed. 4. Tolerate 15 minutes of gardening without complaint of increased UE pain or stiffness. 5. Demonstrate two pain management techniques to use at home with minimal verbal cues. 6. Complete HEP correctly and independently.

OT TREATMENT SESSION 1

THERAPEUTIC ACTIVITY	TIME	GOAL(S) ADDRESSED	OTA RATIONALE
Fluidotherapy—Both hands	10 min	#3 and #4	*Preparatory Method:* To help improve soft-tissue mobility and decrease pain level, which will lead to increased participation in ADLs and IADLs
Begin education, discussion, and training (demonstration and practice) of joint protection, work simplification, energy conservation, and activity modification	20 min	#1 and #2	*Education and Training:* Develop rapport with client.
Issue and train client in the use of Dycem® for opening containers. Issue cylindrical foam, and train client to use for writing utensil and toothbrush	15 min	#1 and #2	*Education and Training:* To practice with appropriate adaptive equipment

SOAP note: 10/3/—, 3:00 pm-3:45 pm

S: "I really liked that warm blowing treatment for my hands. They felt less stiff and painful afterward."

O: Client participated in 45 minutes of skilled OT to address hand pain, stiffness, and decreased ADLs and IADLs. Client reported less discomfort after fluidotherapy treatment, and hand mobility was slightly increased. After skilled instruction in adaptive equipment use, client was able to write three checks without discomfort and perform grooming activities. Client demonstrated proper joint protection techniques when opening food containers, with occasional verbal cues for technique.

A: Since client benefited from heat modality, further OT sessions will include paraffin treatment that client may be able to continue with at home. Client was engaged and interested in learning techniques to help maintain independence and prevent joint damage. Client's ability to recall and incorporate joint protection techniques indicates excellent potential for independence in chosen ADLs and IADLs.

PUTTING IT ALL TOGETHER Sample Treatment and Documentation (continued)

P: Continue skilled OT to address pain management, joint protection, and energy conservation techniques, as well as explore adaptive equipment possibilities.
Jonas Rimer, COTA/L 10/3/—, 4:55 pm

TREATMENT SESSION 2

What could you do next with this client?

TREATMENT SESSION 3

What could you do next with this client?

REFERENCES

1. Barbour, K. E., Helmick, C. G., Theis, K. A., Murphy, L. B., Hootman, J. M., Brady, T. J., & Cheng, Y. J. (2013). Prevalence of doctor-diagnosed arthritis and arthritis-attributable activity limitation—United States, 2010–2012. *Morbidity and Mortality Weekly Report,62*(14), 869–873. Retrieved from http://www.cdc.gov/mmwr/preview/mmwrhtml/mm6244a1.htm
2. Centers for Disease Control and Prevention. (2016). Arthritis: Addressing the nation's most common cause of disability. Retrieved from http://www.cdc.gov/chronicdisease/resources/publications/aag/arthritis.htm
3. Arthritis Foundation. (2016). Types of arthritis. Retrieved from www.arthritis.org
4. Centers for Disease Control and Prevention. (2016). Arthritis-related statistics. Retrieved from http://www.cdc.gov/arthritis/data_statistics/arthritis-related-stats.htm
5. The Arthritis Society. (2017). Arthritis facts and figures. Retrieved from http://arthritis.ca/understand-arthritis/arthritis-facts-figures
6. S. L. E. Lupus Foundation. (2016). About lupus: Who gets lupus. Retrieved from http://www.lupusny.org/about-lupus/who-gets-lupus.
7. Kvien, T. K., Uhlig, T., Ødegård, S., Heiberg, M. S. (2006). Epidemiological aspects of rheumatoid arthritis: The sex ratio. *Annals of the New York Academy of Sciences, 1069*, 212–222.
8. Mayo Clinic. (2014). Diseases and conditions: Juvenile rheumatoid arthritis. Retrieved from http://www.mayoclinic.org/diseases-conditions/juvenile-rheumatoid-arthritis/basics/treatment/con-20014378
9. Abramson, L. (2015). Juvenile arthritis. American College of Rheumatology. Retrieved from http://www.rheumatology.org/I-Am-A/Patient-Caregiver/Diseases-Conditions/Juvenile-Arthritis
10. National Institute of Arthritis and Musculoskeletal and Skin Diseases. (2015). Questions and answers about juvenile arthritis. Retrieved from http://www.niams.nih.gov/health_info/juv_arthritis/
11. California Department of Public Health. (2016). California arthritis partnership program. Retrieved from http://www.cdph.ca.gov/programs/CAPP/Pages/default.aspx
12. Centers for Disease Control and Prevention. (2016). Arthritis types. Retrieved from http://www.cdc.gov/arthritis/basics/types.html
13. Arthritis Foundation. (2015). What is osteoarthritis? Retrieved from http://arthritistoday.org/about-arthritis/types-of-arthritis/osteoarthritis/what-you-need-to-know.php
14. Cleveland Clinic Foundation. (2016). Diseases and condition: Arthritis.Retrieved from http://my.clevelandclinic.org/health/diseases_conditions/hic_Arthritis.
15. Centers for Disease Control and Prevention. (2016). Arthritis basics: Osteoarthritis. Retrieved from http://www.cdc.gov/arthritis/basics/osteoarthritis.htm
16. Arthritis Foundation. (2016). Arthritis causes. Retrieved from http://www.arthritis.org/about-arthritis/types/osteoarthritis/causes.php
17. Centers for Disease Control and Prevention. (2016). Arthritis data: National statistics. Retrieved from http://www.cdc.gov/arthritis/data_statistics/national-statistics.html.
18. Centers for Disease Control and Prevention. (2015). Arthritis types: Rheumatoid arthritis. Retrieved from http://www.cdc.gov/arthritis/basics/rheumatoid.htm
19. Neumann, D. A., & Bielefeld, T. (2003). The carpometacarpal joint of the thumb: Stability, deformity, and therapeutic intervention. *Journal of Orthopedic & Sports Physical Therapy, 33*(7), 386–399. doi:10.2519/jospt.2003.33.7.386
20. Apfelberg, D. B., Maser, M. R., Lash, H., Kaye, R. L., Britton, M. C., & Bobrove, A. (1978). Rheumatoid hand deformities: Pathophysiology and treatment. *The Western Journal of Medicine, 129*(4), 267–272. Retrieved from https://www.ncbi.nlm.nih.gov/pmc/articles/PMC1238347/
21. Hand Care Center: Shoulder and Elbow Institute. (2016). Rheumatoid arthritis of the hand. Retrieved from http://www.handcarecenter.com/rheumatoid.html
22. WebMD. (2015). Comparing rheumatoid arthritis with osteoarthritis—Topic overview. Retrieved from http://www.webmd.com/rheumatoid-arthritis/tc/comparing-rheumatoid-arthritis-and-osteoarthritis-topic-overview
23. Mayo Clinic. (2015). Diseases and conditions: Fibromyalgia. Retrieved from http://www.mayoclinic.org/diseases-conditions/fibromyalgia/basics/definition/con-20019243
24. Wolfe, R., Clauw, D. J., Fitzcharles, M. A., Goldenberg, D. L., Katz, R. S., Mease, P., ... & Yunus, M. B. (2010). The American college of rheumatology preliminary diagnostic criteria for fibromyalgia and measurement of symptom severity. *Arthritis Care & Research, 62*(5), 600–610. doi:10.1002/acr.20140. Retrieved from http://www.rheumatology.org/Portals/0/Files/2010_Preliminary_Diagnostic_Criteria.pdf
25. WebMD. (2016). Fibromyalgia health center: Fibromyalgia treatments. Retrieved from http://www.webmd.com/fibromyalgia/guide/fibromyalgia-treatments?page=3
26. Alliance for Lupus Research. (2016). What is lupus? Retrieved from http://www.lupusresearch.org/
27. Lupus Foundation of America. (2016). Diagnosing lupus. Retrieved from http://www.lupus.org/answers/entry/common-symptoms-of-lupus
28. Mayo Clinic. (2014). Diseases and conditions: Lupus. Retrieved from http://www.mayoclinic.org/diseases-conditions/lupus/basics/symptoms/con-20019676
29. Centers for Disease Control and Prevention. (2015). Arthritis basics: Gout. Retrieved from http://www.cdc.gov/arthritis/basics/gout.html
30. Cleveland Clinic. (2014). Diseases and conditions: Gout. Retrieved from http://my.clevelandclinic.org/services/orthopaedics-rheumatology/diseases-conditions/hic-gout
31. Illinois Department of Public Health. (n.d.). Healthbeat: Gout. Retrieved from http://www.idph.state.il.us/public/hb/hbgout.htm
32. Shulten, P., Thomas, J., Miller, M., Smith, M., & Ahern. M. (2009). The role of diet in the management of gout: A comparison of knowledge and attitudes to current evidence. *Journal of Human Nutrition and Dietetics, 22*(1), 3–11. doi:10.1111/j.1365-277X.2008.00928.x
33. Choi, H. K., Liu, S., & Curhan, G. (2005). Intake of purine-rich foods, protein, and dairy products and relationship to serum levels of uric acid: The third national health and nutrition examination survey. *Arthritis & Rheumatism, 52*(1), 283–289.
34. Lee, S. J., Terkeltaub, R. A., & Kavanaugh, A. (2006). Recent developments in diet and gout. *Current Opinion in Rheumatology, 18*(2), 193–198.

35. Mayo Clinic. (2015). Gout diet: What's allowed, what's not. Retrieved from http://www.mayoclinic.org/healthy-lifestyle/nutrition-and-healthy-eating/in-depth/gout-diet/art-20048524
36. Shiel, W. C. (2015). Arthritis quackery (unproven remedies and tests). Medicine Net. Retrieved from http://www.medicinenet.com/quackery_arthritis/article.htm
37. Arthritis Foundation. (2016). Arthritis today: Drug guide. Retrieved from http://www.arthritis.org/living-with-arthritis/treatments/medication/drug-guide/drug-class/analgesics.php
38. Mayo Clinic. (2015). Prednisone and other corticosteroids. Retrieved from http://www.mayoclinic.org/steroids/art-20045692
39. Davis, C. P. (2016). Steroid drug withdrawal. Medicine Net. Retrieved from http://www.medicinenet.com/steroid_withdrawal/article.htm
40. Tidy, C. (2014). Anti-inflammatory painkillers. Patient. Retrieved from http://patient.info/health/anti-inflammatory-painkillers
41. Mayo Clinic. (2016). Diseases and conditions: Rheumatoid arthritis. Retrieved from http://www.mayoclinic.org/diseases-conditions/rheumatoid-arthritis/diagnosis-treatment/treatment/txc-20197400
42. Bingham, C., & Ruffing, V. (2016). Rheumatoid arthritis treatment. Retrieved from http://www.hopkinsarthritis.org/arthritis-info/rheumatoid-arthritis/ra-treatment/
43. Mayo Clinic. (2015). Fibromyalgia: Treatment and drugs. Retrieved from http://www.mayoclinic.org/diseases-conditions/fibromyalgia/basics/treatment/con-20019243
44. Fleming, K. C. (2014). Is gabapentin (neurontin, others) an effective fibromyalgia treatment? Retrieved from http://www.mayoclinic.org/diseases-conditions/fibromyalgia/expert-answers/fibromyalgia-treatment/faq-20058273
45. Johns Hopkins Lupus Center. (2016). Anti-malarial drugs. Retrieved from http://www.hopkinslupus.org/lupus-treatment/lupus-medications/antimalarial-drugs/
46. Mayo Clinic. (2014). Lupus: Treatment and drugs. Retrieved from http://www.mayoclinic.org/diseases-conditions/lupus/basics/treatment/con-20019676
47. Mayo Clinic. (2015). Gout: Treatment and drugs. Retrieved from http://www.mayoclinic.org/diseases-conditions/gout/basics/treatment/con-20019400
48. University of Washington Orthopaedics and Sports Medicine. (2016). Basics of surgery for arthritis. Retrieved from http://www.orthop.washington.edu/?q=patient-care/articles/arthritis/basics-of-surgery-for-arthritis.html
49. Katz, P. P., Morris, A., & Yelin, E. (2006). Prevalence and predictors of disability in valued life activities among individuals with rheumatoid arthritis. *Annals of the Rheumatic Diseases: The Eular Journal, 65*, 763–769. doi:10.1136/ard.2005.044677
50. Tsai P., Tak, S., Moore, C., & Palencia, I. (2003). Testing a theory of chronic pain. *Journal of Advanced Nursing, 43*, 158–169. doi:10.1046/j.1365-2648.2003.02690.x
51. James, N. T., Miller, C. W., Brown, K. C., & Weaver, M. (2005). Pain disability among older adults with arthritis. *Journal of Aging Health, 17*, 56–69. doi:10.1177/0898264304272783
52. How a marriage survives when one partner gets sick. (2015). Retrieved from http://www.more.com/relationships/marriage-divorce/how-marriage-survives-when-one-partner-gets-sick
53. Till death do us part—Unless it's the wife who gets sick. (n.d.). Retrieved from http://time.com/83486/divorce-is-more-likely-if-the-wife-not-the-husband-gets-sick/
54. Busari, J. O. (2013). The discourse of generational segmentation and the implications for postgraduate medical education. *Perspectives on Medical Education, 2*(5–6), 340–348. Retrieved from http://doi.org/10.1007/s40037-013-0057-0
55. Weinberg, R. (2005). Family physicians' knowledge and perception of occupational therapy roles: Factors leading to referrals written for occupational therapy services. Touro College.
56. Baldwin, D., Johnstone, B., Ge, B., Hewett, J., Smith, M., & Sharp, G. (2012). Randomized prospective study of a work place ergonomic intervention for individuals with rheumatoid arthritis and osteoarthritis. *Arthritis Care and Research, 64*(10), 1527–1535. doi:10.1002/acr.21699
57. Coppard, B., & Lohman H. (2008). *Introduction to splinting: A clinical reasoning and problem solving approach* (3rd ed.). St. Louis, MO: Mosby.
58. Dunkin, M. A. (2016). How hard should you work out? Arthritis Foundation. Retrieved from http://www.arthritis.org/living-with-arthritis/exercise/how-to/maximize-workouts.php
59. American Occupational Therapy Association. (2008). Physical agent modalities: A position paper. *American Journal of Occupational Therapy, 62*, 691–693. doi:10.5014/ajot.62.6.691
60. Frost, L., & Harmeyer, F. (2011). AOTA fact sheet: Occupational therapy's role in managing arthritis. Retrieved from http://www.aota.org/-/media/corporate/files/aboutot/professionals/whatisot/pa/facts/arthritis%20fact%20sheet.pdf

Chapter 22

Comprehensive Hand Management

Karol Spraggs-Young, OTD, OTR/L, CHT

LEARNING OUTCOMES

After studying this chapter, the student or practitioner will be able to:

22.1 Identify the intricate anatomy of the wrist and hand

22.2 Understand the components of an evaluation of the wrist and hand

22.3 Differentiate between the common diagnoses seen in the wrist and hand

22.4 Discuss the therapeutic interventions used in treating common wrist and hand conditions

22.5 Implement treatment plans for clients with common hand and wrist conditions

KEY TERMS

Axonotmesis
Complex regional pain syndrome (CRPS)
Controlled motion
Desensitization
Dynamometer
Early protected motion
Ergonomics
Graded motor imagery
Isokinetic exercise
Isometric exercise
Isotonic exercise
Lymphedema
Manual edema mobilization (MEM)
Mirror visual feedback (MVF)
Neuropraxia
Neurotmesis
Pinch gauge
Provocative testing
Sensory reeducation
Tenodesis

Occupational therapy (OT) practitioners understand that hand function is important, since individuals in the profession use their hands to care for self and others. Mary Reilly, EdD, OTR, an OT educator and visionary, wrote that, "...man, through the use of his hands, as they are energized by mind and will, can influence the state of his own health."[1] The hand is an amazing structure, with a balance of extrinsic and intrinsic musculature that allows for fine motor coordination while manipulating small objects, and provides the strength and stability to grip and swing a hammer. The shape of the hand, with the longitudinal and transverse arches, also allows for manipulation and gripping of a variety of objects of different sizes. The wrist and hand work synergistically to position and produce motion. Consider the motions produced by **tenodesis;** when the wrist is passively or actively flexed, the fingers extend, and when the wrist is passively or actively extended, the fingers flex (Fig. 22-1). Many OT practitioners spend years learning and specializing in the practice area of hand therapy because hand use is vital to the engagement in occupation. The purpose of this chapter is to provide an overview of the anatomy and common conditions of the wrist and hand.

ANATOMICAL REVIEW

Briefly reviewing the anatomy, the hand has 24 extrinsic muscles that include the flexor and the extensor tendons, and 19 intrinsic muscles that include the lumbricals and interossei. Connective tissue within the wrist and hand keeps these structures secure and enhances their function. The distal radius and distal ulna meet at the wrist along the proximal row of the eight carpal bones and form the distal radioulnar joint (DRUJ).[2] At the DRUJ, the radius rotates around the ulna during the performance of supination and pronation. When a client is gripping, 80% of the force transmits through the radius while 20% transmits through the ulna.[3] During flexion and extension, the proximal and distal row of carpal bones move together, however with radial and ulnar deviation they do not. The required arc of motion

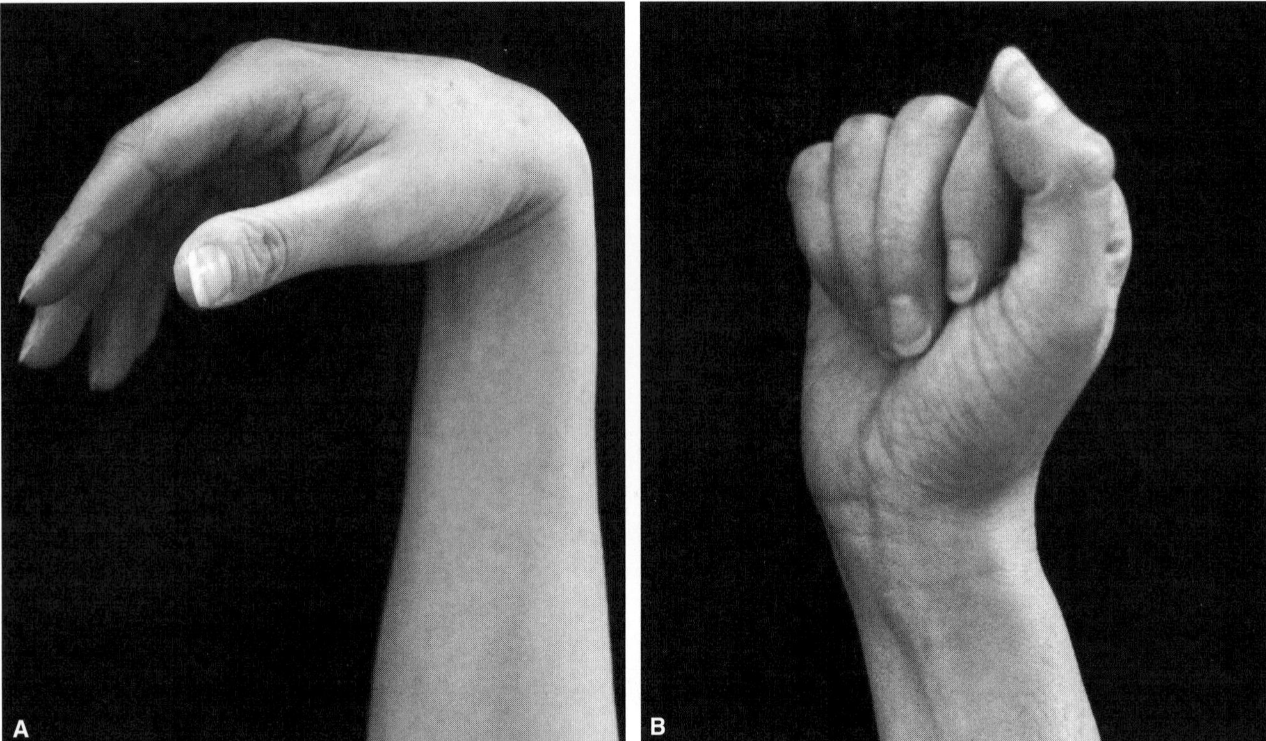

FIGURE 22-1. Tenodesis describes the synergistic movement between the wrist and fingers. **A.** Note that with wrist flexion, the fingers naturally extend thus making it easier to release an object. **B.** Note that with wrist extension, the fingers curl into a flexed position thus making it easier to grasp an object.

for function in the wrist is 40 degrees of flexion and 40 degrees of extension.[4] The carpal bones align with the five metacarpals, which are numbered 1 to 5 starting at the radial side of the hand. The first carpometacarpal (CMC) joint provides the mobility for the saddle joint of the thumb and is the site of commonly seen CMC osteoarthritis. The metacarpal heads meet with the proximal phalanx of each finger to form the hinged metacarpal (MCP) joint or knuckles. The MCP joints have collateral ligaments that provide stability and are stretched while the MCP is flexed, therefore MCP joint flexion is considered a safe position if immobilization is needed (Fig. 22-2).[5] Sagittal bands keep the extensor tendon in position over the MCP joint, while volar plates within the joint provide the stability that protects against too much hyperextension. Moving distally, the proximal phalanx meets with the middle phalanx to create the proximal interphalangeal (PIP) joint. Collateral ligaments and volar plates also provide stability for these joints. Due to the positioning of these soft tissues, the PIP joint should be immobilized in extension to prevent joint contractures. The middle phalanx and distal phalanx form the distal interphalangeal (DIP) joint. Although the arc of motion for this joint is smaller, it also has collateral ligaments for structural support and should be immobilized in extension (Fig. 22-3).

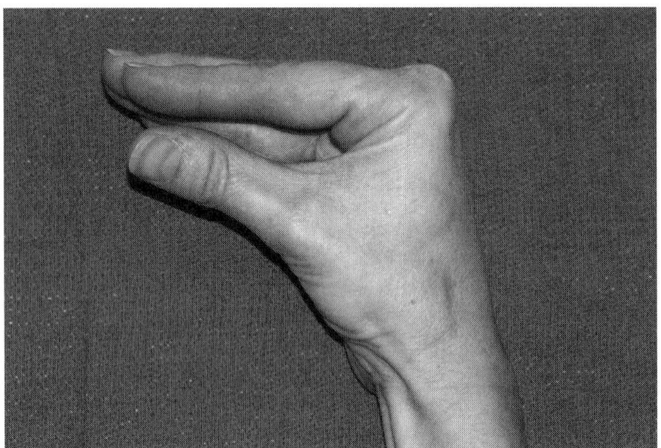

FIGURE 22-2. MCP joint flexion with IP joint extension.

The brachial artery branches into the radial and ulnar arteries at the elbow and supplies vascularization to the wrist and hand. The radial artery at the wrist becomes the superficial and deep branch to the hand, while the ulnar artery also divides into the superficial and deep branch at the wrist, supplying blood to the hand and fingers. Veins in the hand run with the common arteries.

The nerves in the upper extremity (UE) are the median, ulnar, and radial and are considered peripheral nerves because they branch off from the brachial plexus. These nerves provide motor function and sensory function to the wrist and hand. The median nerve provides sensory function to the palm side of the hand, the digital nerves to the thumb, index, middle, and half of the ring finger. The ulnar nerve provides sensory function to the skin over the medial side of the hand and the digital nerves to the small finger and half of the ring finger. The radial nerve provides sensation to the back of the hand (Fig. 22-4).[2] For a complete list of motor innervation see Table 22-1.

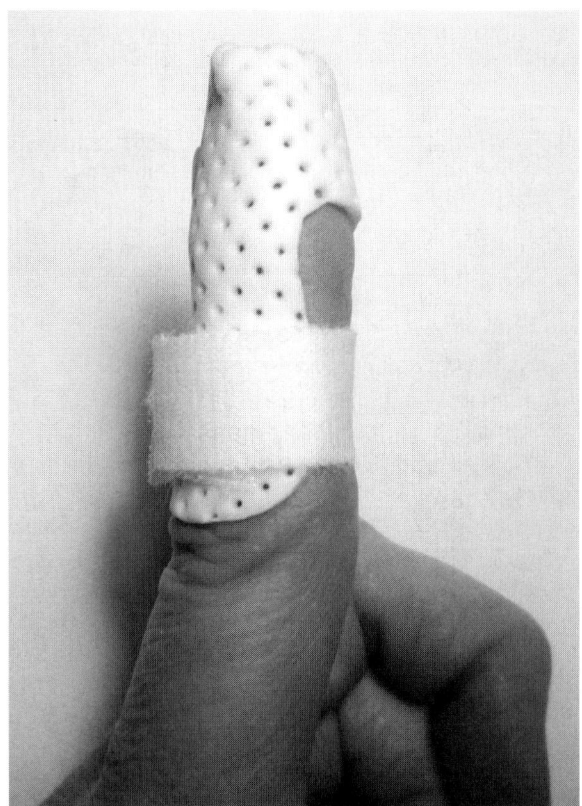

FIGURE 22-3. DIP extension of index finger within a protective orthosis.

ASSESSMENT OF THE WRIST AND HAND

Before developing a treatment plan and providing treatment, it is important to perform a thorough assessment of the client's UE. A thorough assessment will assist in ensuring proper diagnosis and determining the best course of treatment. An assessment of the UE should include a history, noting the mechanism of injury or onset of condition, past medical history, current complaints or symptoms, and a physical examination of the upper extremity making note of any muscle atrophy, skin changes, or abnormal posturing. An assessment of range of motion (ROM), strength, sensation, edema, and vascularity should also be performed.[6] These assessments may be performed by the occupational therapy assistant (OTA) in order to obtain baseline data or to gather information for progress reporting. Once the OTA has completed these assessments, he or she should communicate the results to the occupational therapist. It is important to use all of the information gathered within the context of the client, considering his or her occupational performance roles and personal goals for treatment. The following section describes detailed components of a UE assessment.

Range of Motion

Joint ROM is the amount of motion available at a specific joint, and in the UE it is measured with a goniometer. Active range of motion (AROM) is the amount of motion the client can actively perform without assistance, and passive

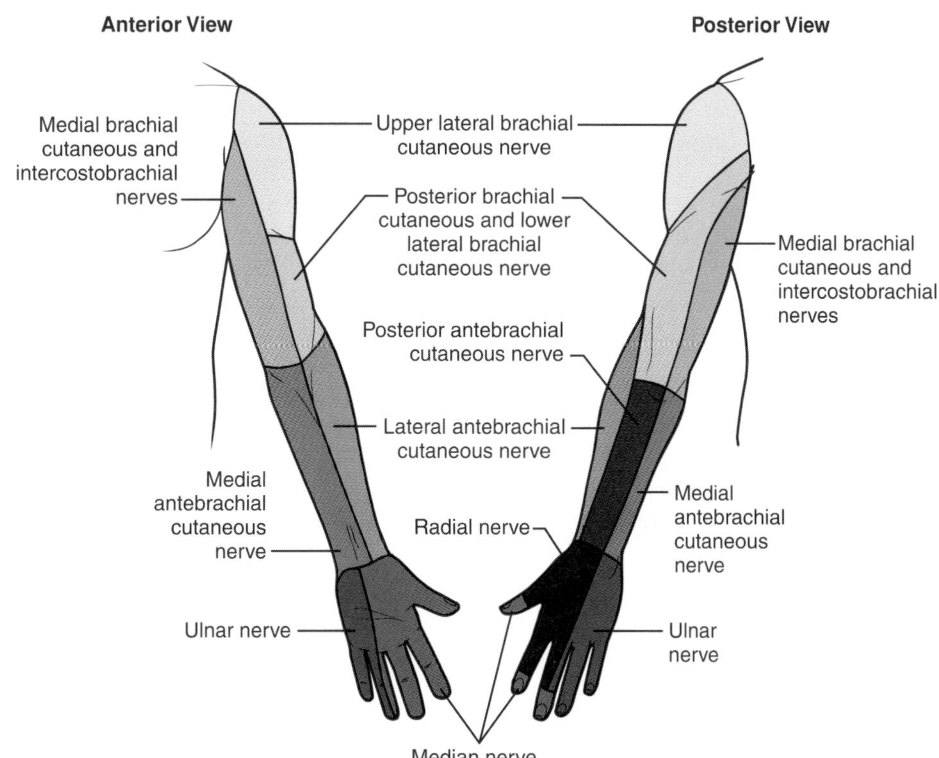

FIGURE 22-4. Cutaneous sensory distribution of the median, ulnar, and radial nerves.

TABLE 22-1 Muscle Action and Nerve Innervation of the Shoulder, Elbow, Wrist, and Hand

MUSCLE	ACTION	INNERVATION
Serratus anterior	Scapular abduction and upward rotation	Long thoracic nerve
Trapezius (upper fibers)	Scapular elevation	Accessory nerve/cranial nerve XI
Levator scapulae	Scapular elevation	C3-C5/dorsal scapular nerve
Trapezius (middle fibers)	Scapular adduction	Accessory nerve/cranial nerve XI
Trapezius (lower fibers)	Scapular depression and adduction	Accessory nerve/cranial nerve XI
Rhomboids	Scapular adduction and downward rotation	Dorsal scapular nerve
Anterior deltoid	Shoulder flexion and scaption	Axillary nerve
Middle deltoid	Shoulder abduction and scaption	Axillary nerve
Posterior deltoid	Shoulder horizontal abduction and extension	Axillary nerve
Coracobrachialis	Shoulder flexion	Musculocutaneous nerve
Supraspinatus	Shoulder flexion, abduction, and scaption	Suprascapular nerve
Latissimus dorsi	Shoulder extension	Thoracodorsal nerve
Teres major	Shoulder extension	Subscapular nerve
Pectoralis major	Shoulder horizontal adduction	Medial and lateral pectoral nerves
Infraspinatus	Shoulder external rotation	Suprascapular nerve
Teres minor	Shoulder external rotation	Axillary nerve
Subscapularis	Shoulder internal rotation	Upper and lower subscapular nerves
Brachialis	Elbow flexion	Musculocutaneous nerve
Brachioradialis	Elbow flexion engages when load is applied, a weak pronator/supinator with resistance	Radial nerve
Biceps brachii	Primary elbow supinator, elbow flexor when forearm supinated	Musculocutaneous nerve
Triceps brachii	Elbow extension	Radial nerve
Aconeus	Assists with elbow extension	Radial nerve
Pronator teres	Primary pronator, elbow flexion when hand is loaded	Median nerve
Pronator quadratus	Unresisted pronation	Anterior interosseous nerve (median)
Supinator	Secondary supinator	Posterior interosseous nerve (radial)
Flexor carpi radialis	Wrist flexion	Median nerve
Palmaris longus	Wrist flexion	Median nerve
Flexor carpi ulnaris	Wrist flexion	Ulnar nerve
Extensor carpi radialis longus	Wrist extension	Radial nerve
Extensor carpi radialis brevis	Wrist extension	Radial nerve
Extensor carpi ulnaris	Wrist extension in supination Wrist UD in pronation	Radial nerve
Flexor pollicis brevis (FPB)	Thumb MP flexion	Two heads/median nerve to the superficial head and ulnar nerve to the deep head
Flexor pollicis longus (FPL)	Thumb IP flexion	Median nerve
Extensor pollicis brevis (EPB)	Thumb MCP extension	Radial nerve
Extensor pollicis longus (EPL)	Thumb IP extension	Radial nerve
Abductor pollicis brevis (APB)	Thumb abduction	Median nerve
Abductor pollicis longus (APL)	Thumb abduction	Radial nerve
Adductor pollicis	Thumb adduction	Ulnar nerve
Opponens pollicis	Thumb opposition	Median nerve

TABLE 22-1 Muscle Action and Nerve Innervation of the Shoulder, Elbow, Wrist, and Hand (continued)

MUSCLE	ACTION	INNERVATION
Opponens digiti minimi	Small finger opposition	Ulnar nerve
Abductor digiti minimi	Small finger abduction	Ulnar nerve
Flexor digiti minimi brevis	Small finger MP joint flexion	Ulnar nerve
Lumbricals	MCP joint flexion/IP extension	First and second median nerve Third and fourth ulnar nerve
Flexor digitorum superficialis (FDS)	PIP joint flexion	Median nerve to index and middle Ulnar nerve to ring and small
Flexor digitorum profundus (FDP)	DIP joint flexion	Median nerve (to index and long fingers) Ulnar nerve (to ring and small fingers)
Extensor digitorum (EDC)	MCP joint extension	Radial nerve
Extensor digiti minimi	Small finger extension	Radial nerve
Extensor indices propreis	Index extension	Radial nerve
Dorsal interossei	Finger abduction	Ulnar nerve
Palmar interossei	Finger adduction	Ulnar nerve

range of motion (PROM) is the amount of motion at the joint when an outside force, such as the OT practitioner, moves the joint. AROM measurements provide information regarding the client's motor control and functional ability, whereas PROM measurements provide the OT practitioner with information about the joint capsule, muscles, and any soft-tissue limitations.[7] When PROM is greater than AROM, weakness, scarring, or a decrease in tendon excursion may be suspected. ROM measurements are expressed numerically. For example, when measuring wrist flexion the neutral starting position would be zero, and the end range would be eighty so the measurement would read: 0° to 80°. Table 22-2 presents a list of normal joint ROM for the UE. In order to ensure validity and reliability, OT practitioners should take goniometric measurements using the same procedures (see Chapter 7).

TABLE 22-2 Normal Joint Range of Motion

Elbow	Flexion	0–150
	Extension	0
	Pronation	0–70/80
	Supination	0–80
Wrist	Flexion	0–75/80
	Extension	0–70
	Radial deviation	0–20
	Ulnar deviation	0–30/35
Thumb	CMC abduction	0–45
	CMC extension	0–20
	CMC flexion	0–15
	CMC opposition	To base of small finger; deficit is measured in centimeters.
	MCP flexion	0–50/55
	IP	0–80
Finger	MCP flexion	0–90
	PIP flexion	0–100
	DIP flexion	0–80

Strength

Manual muscle testing is performed to determine the strength and function of the muscle-tendon units of the wrist and hand. Grades for manual muscle testing are 0 to 5, with 0 being no muscle activity noted, and 5 being normal. The OT practitioner applies manual resistance to the contracted muscle attempting to break the position that the client is holding.[8] The muscle is then graded accordingly. Strength testing is also performed to assess gross grip and pinch strength by using devices called a **dynamometer** and **pinch gauge**, respectively. A 5% to 10% difference in strength usually exists between the client's dominant and nondominant hand for these tests.[9] Strength testing norms have been established, however, to ensure validity and reliability; practitioners within the same clinic should use the same testing procedures. Strength testing requires use of clinical judgment, and at times, may not be performed at the time of the initial evaluation. Strength testing should not be performed on clients with new or unstable fractures or open wounds, and should be performed with caution for painful conditions such as osteoarthritis. For example, testing should be stopped if the client reports pain or if testing causes an increase in pain. If the client has pain with grip or pinch strength testing, this should be documented. Refer to Chapter 9, for more details.

Sensation

Whereas ROM and strength testing can assess joint integrity and nerve-innervated motor function, sensory testing addresses the sensory function of the median, ulnar, and radial nerves and may assist in diagnosing peripheral nerve injuries. Sensory testing also helps to monitor the progression of nerve return. Common sensory tests can be categorized into autonomic response tests, threshold tests, discrimination tests, and functional tests.[10]

SEMMES WEINSTEIN MONOFILAMENT TEST

The Semmes Weinstein monofilament test is for touch-pressure threshold. This test uses monofilaments of varying thickness to determine the client's ability to sense light touch to deep pressure. The monofilaments are applied to the client's fingertip with vision occluded, and the client reports whether or not he or she feels pressure from the monofilament. The monofilaments range from 2.83 being the smallest to 6.65 being the largest in diameter. According to the norms for monofilament testing, 2.83 is the acceptable threshold in the fingertips. Client responses are mapped according to cutaneous nerve innervation.

TWO-POINT TESTS

Dellon described the moving and static two-point tests to assess touch discrimination. These tests use a calibrated tool with 2 mm to 15 mm of distance between two points (Fig. 22-5). The client is tested with vision occluded. Static two-point discrimination is tested starting with 5 mm and stopped at 15 mm if not detected. Normal static two-point discrimination is less than 6 mm. Moving two-point testing starts at 2 mm and ends at 8 mm, as moving sensation is easier to detect than static sensation[11]. Dellon suggests testing for 7 out of 10 correct responses.[11]

MOBERG PICKUP TEST

The Moberg pickup test is a functional test used to incorporate stereognosis or object identification. With the eyes open, the client is asked to pick up 12 common objects while the examiner times the task. The client is then asked to complete the task with vision occluded. Use of the hand is noticed and documented.[12] Although a lack of standardized functional skills assessments to test sensation exists, it is important for OT practitioners to follow standardized procedures within their own clinic. OTAs who perform sensory testing should have obtained training and demonstrate competency in this area.

Inflammation and Edema

Inflammation and edema are sometimes referred to synonymously, and are often confused, because both can cause swelling. Inflammation is the body's natural response to injury and is a common occurrence in the wrist and hand. Edema is excess fluid trapped in the body tissues, typically as the result of a disease or even a medication. The amount of inflammation corresponds with the phases of wound healing. Early on after injury or surgery, inflammation assists with the healing process providing needed nutrients to the tissues. However, persistent inflammation is harmful and may lead to scarring and joint stiffness if unresolved. Assessing a client's inflammation is important to ensure that inflammation is decreasing as an injury heals; assessment is also used to determine the efficacy of the inflammation-reduction techniques used in therapy. Two of the methods for measuring inflammation in the wrist and hand are the volumetric measurement and the circumferential figure-of-eight wrist and hand measurement.

The volumetric measurement is based upon the principle of water displacement and is performed using a volumeter that is specially designed for the UE (Fig. 22-6). The OTA should follow the standardized instructions that come with the volumeter to ensure reliability with testing. Place the volumeter on a level surface, and fill with room-temperature water until it begins to overflow. Ask the client to place his or her forearm of the affected extremity in the pronated position, and then immerse it into the volumeter with the thumb toward the spout and the middle and ring finger web space resting on the bar. Instruct the

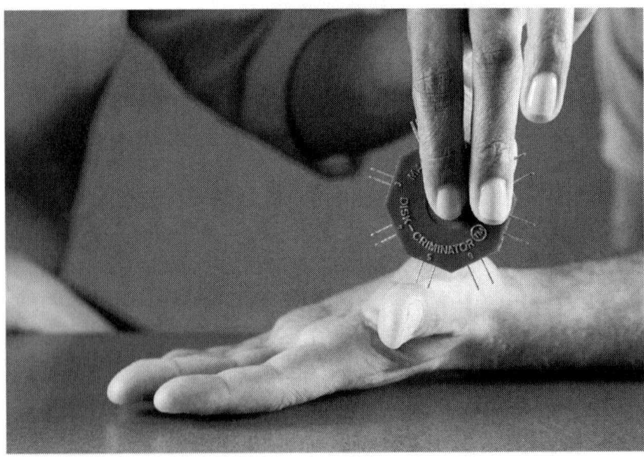

FIGURE 22-5. Two-point discrimination tool used for sensory testing.

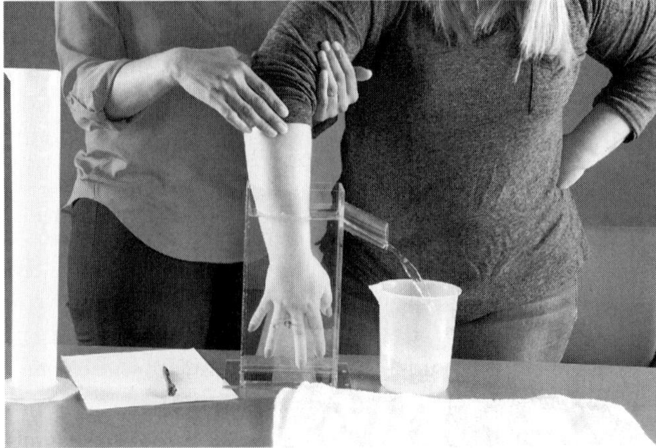

FIGURE 22-6. Volumeter used to measure swelling in the forearm, wrist, and hand.

client not to allow the arm to come in contact with the volumeter. The OTA will then measure in milliliters the water that flows out of the volumeter while the client's hand is immersed using the beaker provided.[9] Measurements should be documented in the client's chart and should be taken at the time of the initial evaluation or when a reassessment of inflammation is indicated. Less water being displaced evidences a reduction in inflammation, while an increase in inflammation is evidenced by more water being displaced.

The circumferential figure-of-eight method involves the use of a tape measure wrapped around the client's wrist and hand, starting at the distal ulnar styloid, placing the tape volarly over the wrist and then diagonally crossing the dorsal wrist toward the fifth MCP joint. The tape is then continued over the distal palmar crease and diagonally over the dorsum of the hand from the index MCP joint to back to the distal ulnar styloid (Fig. 22-7). Circumferential inflammation measurements may also be taken at specific landmarks of the UE such as the distal palmar crease, the distal wrist, mid forearm, and elbow. Documenting the specific location of these measurements and placing the same amount of tension on the tape measure each time will provide accuracy with the circumferential measurements. It is important to remember that inflammation measurements may fluctuate daily and are dependent on position, diet, and exercise, therefore measurements should be taken at the same time of day and consistently compared with the uninvolved extremity.[13]

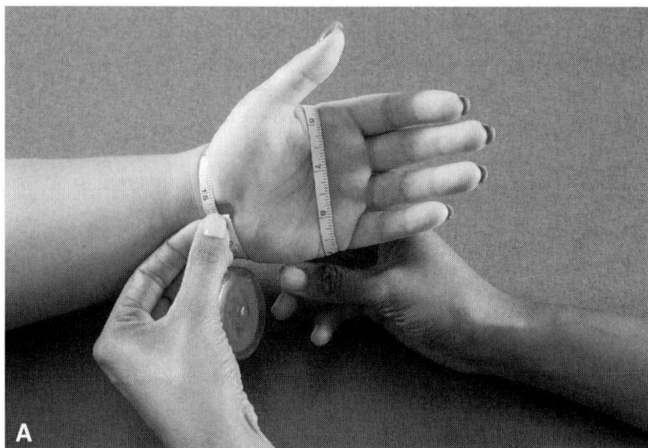

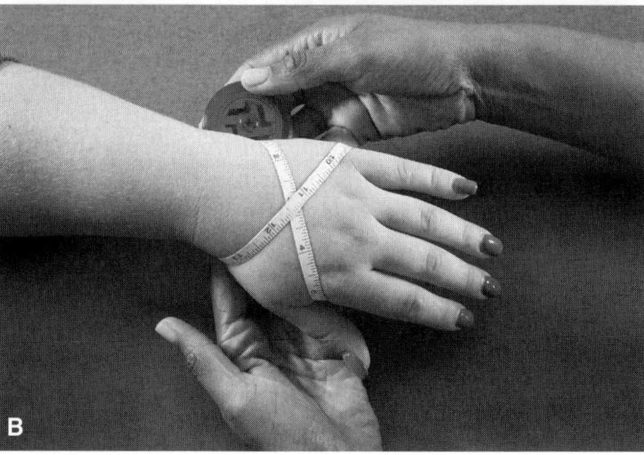

FIGURE 22-7. Figure-of-eight edema measurements using a tape measure. A. Volar aspect B. Dorsal aspect.

Integument

The integumentary system consists of the skin, hair, and nails and is included in an assessment to assist with proper diagnosing and treatment planning. Examination of the client's skin should include palpation of anatomy and bony landmarks and can reveal decreased circulation, infections, wounds, or thick or tight scars, which all will limit hand function. An increase in hair growth or lack of hair growth may indicate sympathetic nerve dysfunction as seen in **complex regional pain syndrome (CRPS).** Abnormal nails, or nails that have changed in structure, may indicate systemic health problems with the kidneys, liver, or the endocrine or respiratory systems. Nail changes can also be a sign of nutritional deficiency (Fig. 22-8). Touch the client's wrist and hand to determine any temperature changes, skin hypersensitivity, muscle atrophy, or the presence of thick scars or nodules.[14] Findings with the integument should be documented and reassessed frequently. Wounds and scars should be described and measured. Commercially available wound measurement guides are available. Photographs of the client's wounds, scars, and skin changes can be used to assist with documentation and to show progress with healing.

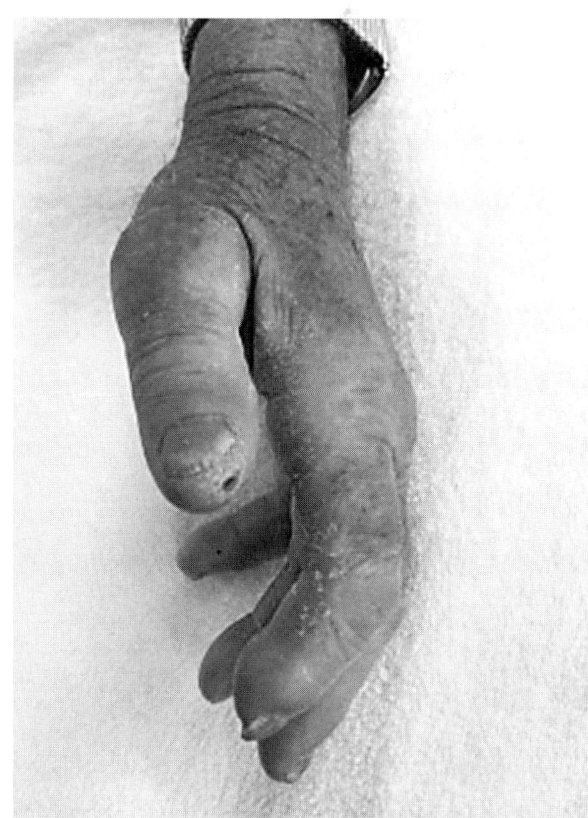

FIGURE 22-8. Client with poor integument.

Observation

From the moment clients enter the clinic, OT practitioners use observation skills to assess their UE functions. OT practitioners examine clients' postures and the positions of their UE. Are clients using the hand to complete paperwork, or are they holding the arm across their body in a protected position? Calloused palms with dirt beneath the nails may indicate repetitive hand use for a laborer, whereas muscle atrophy may indicate lack of hand use or peripheral neuropathy. Blisters at the fingertips may indicate impaired sensation, and needlesticks may indicate the client is a diabetic who uses the fingertips to check blood sugar levels. Arthritic changes and nodules are easily observed and palpated, as are inflammation or edema, tone, and contractures. The resting position of the hand is slight digital flexion, and loss of the natural curve may indicate a flexor tendon injury (Fig. 22-9). The entire UE, including gross motor function, should be inspected and compared with the noninvolved extremity. Observations should be documented within the initial evaluation and as needed in the daily treatment note to monitor and assess change.

Functional Performance

During the initial interview with clients, it is important to determine their ability to engage in their self-care, instrumental activities of daily living (IADL), work, and leisure activities. Traumatic injuries of the UE and pain from tendonitis will both alter the client's ability to dress, bathe, drive, work, and care for others. A change in UE function that interferes with life roles will psychologically affect the client and may influence the healing process. Therefore, it is important to assess and discuss functional abilities at the initial visit, and to begin to address limitations within the first treatment session.[15] Along with an interview, several standardized functional assessments have been designed for use with clients with UE dysfunction. Standardized assessments provide additional information on the client's ability to use the UE while performing a functional task, and also provide an organized way of collecting data, for the purpose of measuring outcomes. In order for a standardized assessment to be acceptable, it should be administered according to the specific instructions and should be reliable and valid.

Reliability and validity are measured in statistical terms. Reliability means the assessment produces consistent results over time and produces consistent results when given by different examiners. Validity means that the assessment consistently measures what it is intended to measure.[16] Standardized assessments for dexterity and coordination include the Jebsen Hand Function Test, the Minnesota Manual Dexterity Test (MRMT), the Purdue Pegboard Test, and the Nine Hole Peg Test (NHPT) (Fig. 22-10). Of these tests, the NHPT has normative data however lacks information on reliability and validity.[17] A variety of standardized assessments have also been designed for use with specific client populations such as those with arthritis, cerebrovascular accident (CVA), carpal tunnel syndrome, and work hardening.

Self-reported outcome measures should also be used at the initial evaluation to document baseline status and change in function over time. Two of the most common self-reported measures are the Disabilities of the Arm, Shoulder and Hand Questionnaire (DASH) and the Patient-Rated Wrist Evaluation (PRWE). The DASH has 30 questions related to UE function with a rating of 1 to 5.[18] The PRWE has 15 questions related to wrist and hand function with a rating scale of 0 to 10.[19] The Quick Disabilities of the Arm, Shoulder and Hand (QDASH) is a shortened version of the DASH with only eleven items assessing the UE. Other self-reported measures include the Patient-Rated Wrist/Hand Evaluation (PRWHE), the Shoulder Pain and Disability Index (SPADI), the Patient-Rated Elbow Evaluation (PREE), and the Michigan Hand Questionnaire. More thorough assessments of function such as the Canadian Occupational

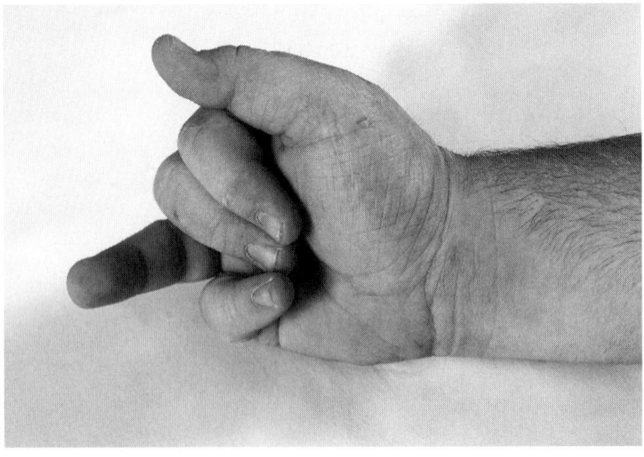

FIGURE 22-9. Hand posturing without flexor tendon intact.

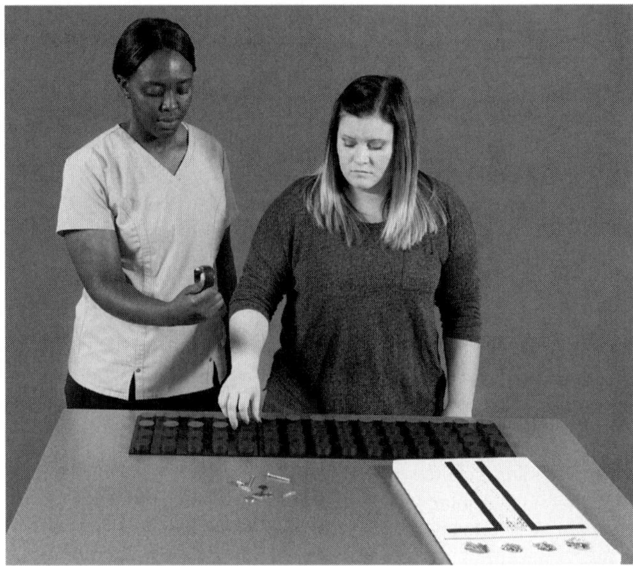

FIGURE 22-10. A variety of hand function tests. *From rear, counterclockwise:* Minnesota Rate of Manipulation Test, Moberg PickUp Test, and Purdue Pegboard Test.

Performance Measure may be used, however they are administered by the OT practitioner and are more detailed, thus requiring more time.[20] Because the use of outcomes measures seem to be specific to each clinic, it is important to discuss outcomes measures with other OT practitioners to ensure that the information gathered for a practice setting is correct.

Provocative Testing and Palpation of Anatomical Structures

When evaluating the wrist and hand, OT practitioners use palpation and **provocative testing** to isolate specific anatomical structures. Perform palpation during the physical examination of the wrist and hand, as it can assist with localizing pain and confirming a clinical diagnosis. Table 22-3 provides a list of suggested areas for palpation. Provocative testing helps "rule out" certain diagnoses, while palpation assists in determining what anatomical structures may be involved. To perform a provocative test, the clinician manipulates the client's anatomical structures in order to reproduce pain or elicit a certain response.[21] Table 22-4 provides an overview of common provocative tests.

Additional provocative tests are described in the literature, however in a systematic review, it was determined that not all provocative tests have the research to validate their use.[24] It is also important to remember that using provocative tests takes practice and should only be used in conjunction with clinical reasoning and the remainder of the information gained during a comprehensive UE evaluation.

TABLE 22-3 Palpation Guide

PAIN WITH PALPATION	POSSIBLE CONDITION	PROVOCATIVE TEST
Radial Side		
Radial styloid	Fracture de Quervain's Arthritis Superficial branch of radial nerve Neuritis	Finkelstein's (see Table 22-5) Tinel's (see Table 22-5) Palpation
Scaphoid in the anatomical snuff box	Fracture Avascular necrosis Scapholunate ligament injury	Watson's test (supinated, pressure over scaphoid tubercle, move hand into ulnar and radial deviation) Palpation
Thumb first metacarpal, phalanges, MP and IP joints	Fracture Sprain/tendon injury UCL/gamekeeper thumb	Ulnar collateral ligament (UCL) stress test to thumb MP with flexion and extension Palpation
First CMC joint	Osteoarthritis	Grind test
Scaphoid-trapezium-trapezoid joint	Synovitis or arthritis	Palpation
First dorsal compartment (APL and EPB tendons)	de Quervain's Tendon rupture	Finkelstein's Observation
Third dorsal compartment (EPL tendon)	EPL tendon rupture or tendonitis	Palpation/Observation for thumb extension
Mid-Dorsal		
Lister tubercle	Fracture EPL tendon rupture or tendonitis	Palpation Resisted thumb extension
Lunate	Kienbock's disease Dislocation, subluxation, instability, or fracture	Palpation
Capitate and capitolunate joint	Fracture Subluxation or instability Dissociation with or without arthritis	Palpation
Index, long and ring: Second, third, and fourth metacarpals, phalanges, CMC, PIP, and DIP joints	Fracture Sprain/ligament injury Volar plate injury Bossing (CMC joints)	Palpation Observation Stress test to MCP joints in flexion
Scapholunate joint	Scapholunate ligament injury or dissociation Dorsal wrist ganglion cyst	Watson's test Observation

Continued

TABLE 22-3 Palpation Guide (continued)

PAIN WITH PALPATION	POSSIBLE CONDITION	PROVOCATIVE TEST
Second and fourth dorsal compartments (ECRB/ECRL and EDC/EIP tendons	Tenosynovitis or impingement between the extensor retinaculum Tendon rupture	Palpation Observation
Ulnar Side		
Ulnar styloid and ulnar head	Fracture Distal radioulnar joint injury	Palpation
Triquetrum	Fracture Lunotriquetral ligament injury TFCC injury	Palpation Lunotriquetral shear test Push off test
Hamate	Fracture	Palpation
Small finger: Fifth metacarpal, phalanges, CMC, MP, PIP, and DIP joints	Fracture Sprain or ligament injury Volar plate injury to PIP joints	Palpation Observation
Distal radioulnar joints	Arthritis Instability TFCC injury	Palpation Push off test
Triangular fibrocartilage complex (TFCC)	TFCC injury Tear of articular disk Ligament disruption Distal radioulnar joint disruption	Push off test
Lunotriquetral joint	Lunotriquetral ligament injury or dissociation	Lunotriquetral shear test
Fifth and sixth dorsal compartments (EDM and ECU tendons)	Tendonitis, tendon rupture, ECU subluxation	Palpation Observation
Volar		
Scaphoid tubercle	Fracture	Palpation
Pisiform	Fracture, arthritis	Palpation
Hook of hamate	Fracture	Palpation
Distal ulnar tunnel	Ulnar tunnel syndrome (Guyon's canal) Nerve or artery injury	Tinel's test (see Table 22-5) Allen's test (see Table 22-5)
Wrist and finger flexor tendons	Tenosynovitis Trigger finger Tendon rupture Dupuytren's Contracture of palmar fascia Volar wrist ganglion	Palpation Resisted flexion Observation

TABLE 22-4 Common Provocative Tests

TEST	HOW TO PERFORM	POSITIVE IF...	
Phalen's test for carpal tunnel syndrome	Practitioner holds the client's wrists in maximal flexion for 1 minute to place pressure on the median nerve through the carpal tunnel	Position reproduces the symptoms of numbness and tingling in the median nerve distribution of the thumb, index, middle, and one-half of the ring fingers	Performing Phalen's test.

TABLE 22-4 Common Provocative Tests (continued)

TEST	HOW TO PERFORM	POSITIVE IF...	
Tinel's test to determine nerve irritation or nerve regeneration or to rule out ulnar nerve compression at the elbow	Practitioner gently taps over the nerve	Client reports tingling in the nerve or the area of nerve distribution	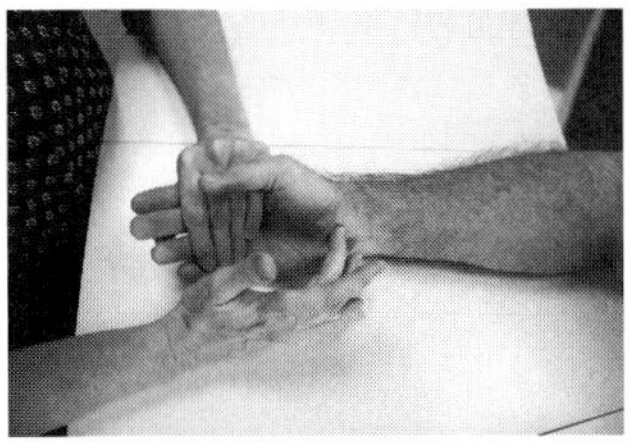 Performing Tinel's test.
Grind test to determine the presence of carpometacarpal (CMC) joint arthritis	Practitioner uses a gentle compression and rotational force to the CMC joint	Compressive force reproduces the client's symptoms or causes complaints of pain	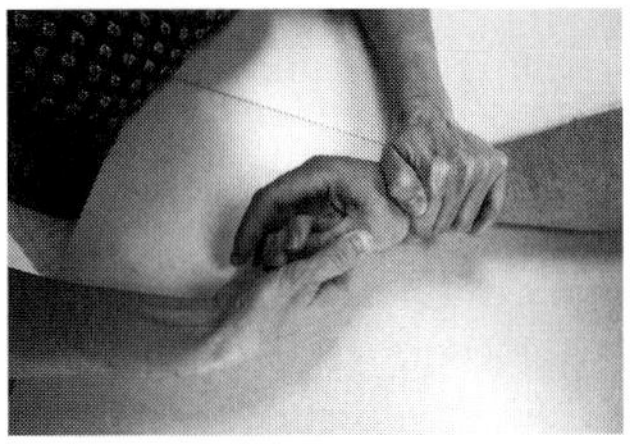 Performing the grind test for CMC joint osteoarthritis.
Finkelstein's test for de Quervain's tenosynovitis	Practitioner has the client flex the thumb into the palm and then combines this motion with ulnar deviation	Test reproduces pain over the first dorsal compartment and the radial side of the wrist[6]	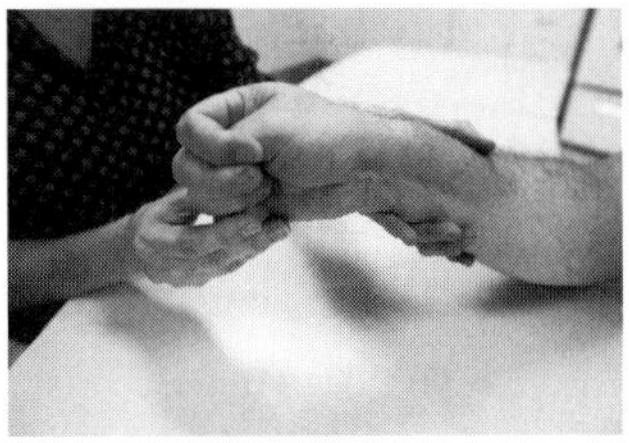 Performing Finklestein's test for DeQuervain's tenosynovitis.
Allen's test to determine the status of arterial flow into the hand	Practitioner has the client make a tight fist while applying pressure over the client's radial and ulnar arteries at the volar wrist. The client next opens and closes the fingers until the skin is white. Practitioner releases pressure on the radial artery, observing hand for return in normal color	Color does not return to the hand once the pressure on the artery has been released[9]	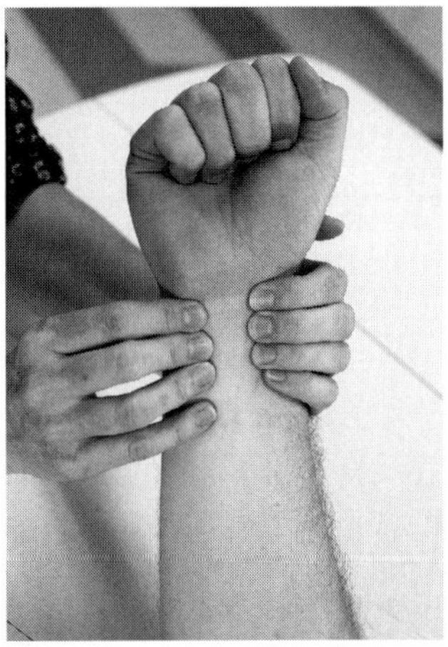 Performing Allen's test for blood flow to the hand.

Continued

TABLE 22-4 Common Provocative Tests (continued)

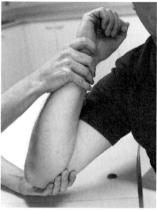

TEST	HOW TO PERFORM	POSITIVE IF...	
Elbow flexion test to rule out ulnar nerve compression at the elbow	Practitioner passively flexes the client's elbow to maximum flexion and holds it there for 1 to 3 minutes	Test causes numbness and tingling in the ring and small fingers[22]	Performing the elbow flexion test.
Push off (or press) test to determine stability at DRUJ and TFCC at the wrist	Practitioner has the client push up from a seated position using the affected wrist	Pushing body weight through the wrist reproduces symptoms or pain[23]	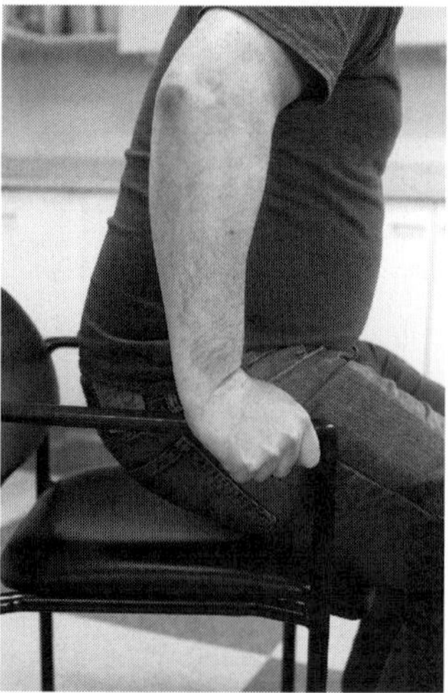 Performing the push off test.

SOFT-TISSUE CONDITIONS

Soft-tissue conditions in the wrist and hand involve the connective tissues including the fascia, muscles, tendons, ligaments, and their associated structures. Soft-tissue injuries, if not treated correctly, can lead to significant stiffness in the hand as the delicate structures in the hand quickly become limited by inflammation, edema, and scarring.

Ganglion Cysts

The most common soft-tissue mass in the UE, ganglion cysts develop on the synovial lining of a joint or tendon sheath. Ganglion cysts can vary in size and are not usually painful. These cysts are usually located on the volar wrist, dorsal wrist, extrinsic extensors, or over the flexor tendon at the level of the proximal phalanx (Fig. 22-11). Ganglion cysts may be associated with osteoarthritis and are surgically removed if they are causing pain and intruding on nearby structures. Clients with ganglion cysts are not usually seen in therapy for conservative treatment, but instead referred to OT after surgery. Treatment after surgical removal of a ganglion includes suture care, scar management, ROM exercises, and progression to strengthening exercises to return the client to functional performance of occupations.[25]

Dupuytren's Contracture

Dupuytren's contracture, also known as Dupuytren's disease, is progressive contraction of the fascia in the palm of the hand. Dupuytren's contracture causes nodules in the palm that may lead to fixed flexion of the MCP and the PIP joints, making it difficult to extend the fingers (Fig. 22-12). Dupuytren's contracture can affect any finger in the hand, however it is usually seen in the ring and small fingers. Risk factors include smoking, diabetes, and having a family history. Dupuytren's contracture is seen most often in males. Treatment for Dupuytren's contracture that is limiting function is either a surgical fasciotomy or closed fasciotomy. In a surgical fasciotomy, the hand surgeon removes the contracted palmar fascia

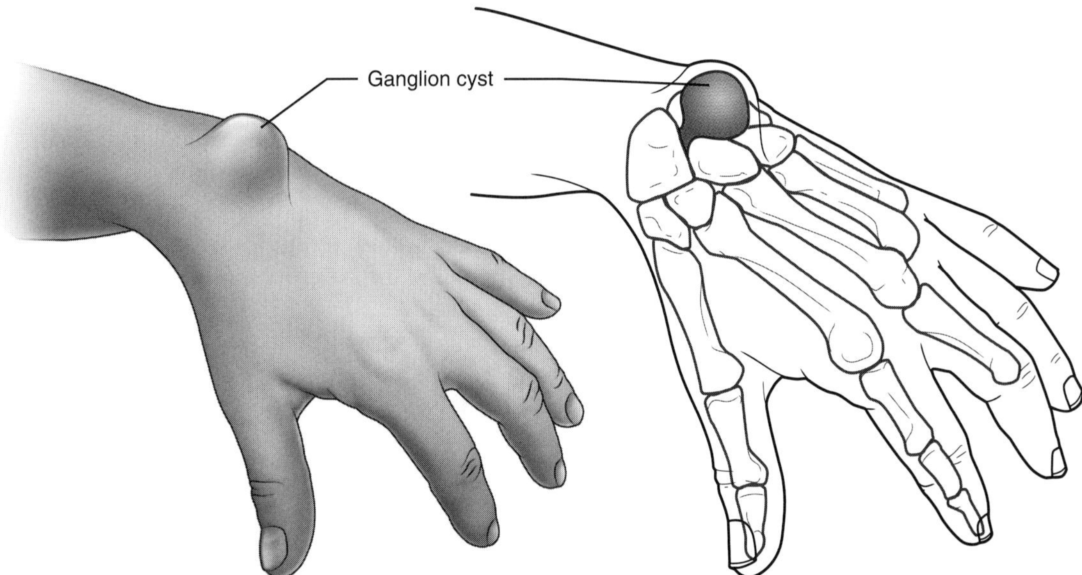

FIGURE 22-11. Ganglion cyst.

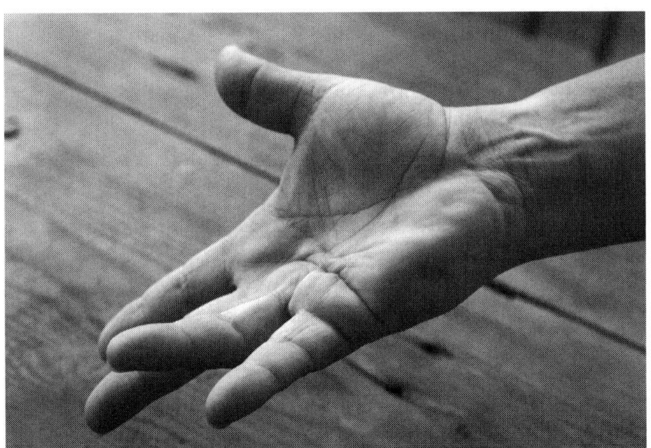

FIGURE 22-12. Dupuytren's contracture.

and associated nodules. With a closed fasciotomy, the client receives a collagenase injection and then returns to the surgeon's office in 24 to 48 hours for a passive manipulation of the contracted fingers.[26] Clients with Dupuytren's contracture are not seen in therapy for conservative treatment, however are referred to OT after an open or closed fasciotomy. Treatment includes a custom extension orthosis, suture care, scar management, ROM exercises, and progression to strengthening exercises to regain functional use of the hand.

de Quervain's Tendinopathy

In 1895, Fritz de Quervain, a Swiss surgeon, described tenosynovitis of the first dorsal compartment. Within the first dorsal compartment over the radial side of the wrist and hand lie the tendons of the abductor pollicis longus (APL) and the extensor pollicis brevis (EPB). Tenosynovitis occurs in this area from thickening and narrowing of the first compartment tunnel or may occur along with inflammation and degeneration of the APL and EPB tendons (Fig. 22-13). de Quervain's tendinopathy is seen most often in women and may be a result of repetitive thumb abduction and wrist ulnar deviation. The provocative test used for de Quervain's tendinopathy is the Finkelstein's test as described earlier. Nonsurgical treatment involves rest of the APL and EPB tendons in an orthosis along with activity modification and client education. Modalities may be used to decrease pain, and AROM exercises are initiated once pain has subsided. Some clients will require a surgical release of the first dorsal compartment in order to alleviate symptoms. After surgery, therapy includes a custom orthosis for postsurgical positioning, AROM with tendon gliding exercises, scar management, and progression to grip and pinch strengthening.[27]

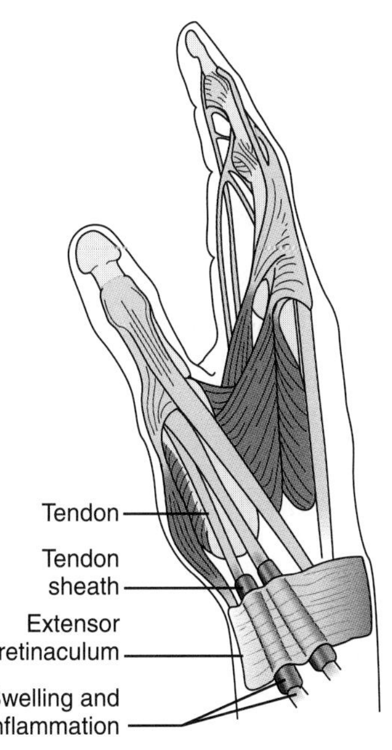

FIGURE 22-13. The site of de Quervain's tenosynovitis.

Trigger Finger

Tenosynovitis of the flexor tendons at the level of the A1 pulley (at the volar plate at the MCP joint) in the palm is called a trigger finger. A trigger finger is characterized as a finger that, once flexed, will lock into position and be difficult to straighten. They can be painful and may be associated with a palpable nodule in the palm. Risk factors include repetitive gripping, diabetes, arthritis, or an associated injury to the palm. Trigger fingers are seen most often in females. If a trigger finger is left untreated, it may lead to significant joint stiffness. Nonsurgical treatment involves a positional orthosis to block full flexion of the affected digit(s) along with client education and activity modification. If the triggering does not improve, the client may benefit from a cortisone injection at the area of pain, or surgical release of the A1 pulley. After surgery, therapy includes AROM with tendon gliding exercises, scar management, and progression to grip and pinch strengthening. A static extension orthosis may be needed if the client has developed finger stiffness.[28]

Tendon Lacerations

Tendon lacerations are usually the result of an injury or accident and will always require surgical repair to improve function. Advances in the understanding of tissue healing have improved the surgical techniques and postsurgical care of repaired flexor and extensor tendons. Postoperative care of the repaired tendon requires good communication among the OT practitioner, client, and surgeon as they work together as a team toward the return to normal hand function.

FLEXOR TENDON INJURIES

According to John Taras, M.D., a hand surgeon known for his expertise with tendon reconstruction, regaining finger motion after flexor tendon injury and repair remains one of the biggest challenges in hand surgery.[29] Flexor tendon injuries are categorized by zone, with zone I at the level of the fingertip and zone V at wrist level, with the thumb having its own zones. Surgical repair is categorized by zone to assist in identifying what other structures may be involved. For example, a repair in zone II usually indicates that both the flexor digitorum profundus (FDP) and flexor digitorum superficialis (FDS) have both been repaired, while a repair of a flexor tendon in zone V, at the level of the wrist, may indicate median nerve involvement. Postsurgical treatment of flexor tendon repairs includes protection in a custom dorsal blocking orthosis, suture care, and the initiation of protected motion as prescribed by the surgeon. The goals of therapy are to protect the healing tendon, prevent adhesions, and promote tendon glide. Although recent research advocates for early mobilization protocols after flexor tendon repairs, flexor tendon injuries still may result in stiffness, scarring, and loss of function.[30] Treating repaired flexor tendons requires the knowledge and skill of an experienced practitioner, and communication with the surgeon, to determine what type of postoperative motion the tendon requires. The OTA will be an important part of the rehabilitation team as he or she works alongside the occupational therapist to assist with orthosis fabrication, suture care, dressing changes, and following postoperative protocols for protected ROM.

EXTENSOR TENDON INJURIES

Extensor tendon injuries are also categorized by zone, with zone I at the fingertip, zone VII at the wrist, and the thumb having its own zones (Fig. 22-14).[27] Surgical repair of extensor tendons may not be as complicated as repair of the flexor tendons, however their intricate anatomy and superficial location over the dorsum of the hand makes them susceptible to scarring and stiffness. Postsurgical treatment includes extension positioning in a custom fabricated orthosis. The goals of therapy are also to provide protection and positioning to the healing tendon. Protocols for extensor tendon repairs usually include a period of immobilization to ensure integrity of the healing tendon.[31] Short arc motion protocols (technique of controlled motion with minimal active tension) may be used, however this will require communication between the practitioner and surgeon, and the client must demonstrate proper understanding. Due to the balance between the flexor and extensor anatomy, the goals of therapy will be to regain extension before flexion.[32] Treating extensor tendon injuries requires a comprehensive knowledge of anatomy and the principles of tissue healing, and progression through protocols should adhere to these principles.

FRACTURES AND DISLOCATIONS

Fractures in the UE are classified by whether the fracture is open or closed, by the location on the bone, by displacement of the fracture, and by the pattern of the break. An

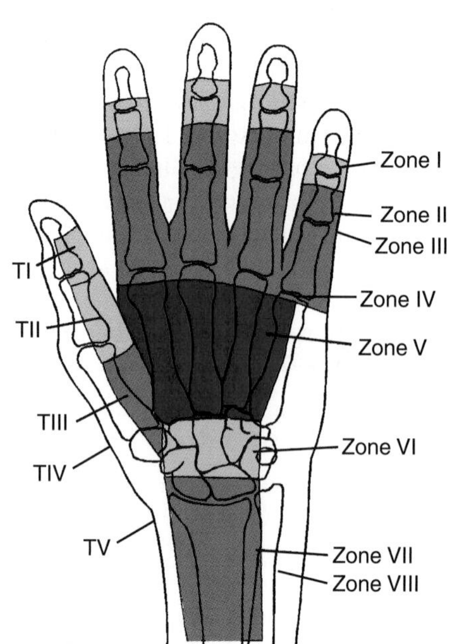

FIGURE 22-14. Zones of the flexor tendons.

open fracture involves a break in the skin, while in a closed fracture the skin is intact. A displaced fracture means that the broken bones have moved out of proper position or alignment. Patterns of fractures include transverse, oblique, spiral, and comminuted.[33] Closed fractures that are not displaced can usually be treated with immobilization. Displaced fractures will require surgery to put the bones back into proper alignment. A fracture treated with surgical fixation of either screws, pins, or plates is considered an open reduction with internal fixation (ORIF). Open fractures require special medical attention as the client with an open fracture will most likely need antibiotics to prevent infection. Fractures heal in three phases. During the first phase, inflammation occurs and bleeding from the fracture site forms a hematoma that will gradually be replaced by granulation tissue at the fracture site. The reparative, bone production, or second phase, occurs within two weeks from the date of injury. The reparative phase occurs when soft callus formation can be seen on x-ray. As the callus formation matures, it will turn into hard callus or bone. The remodeling, or third, phase begins in the middle of the repair phase and continues even after the fracture appears clinically healed (Table 22-5). Clinically healed fractures are no longer painful or swollen. In order to heal in a timely fashion, fractures need a nutrient-rich blood supply to aid in healing. If a client smokes, has diabetes, or has other medical conditions that impair the ability for the body to heal, fracture healing will be delayed. Factors that affect fracture healing are age, diabetes, systemic diseases, infection, osteopenia, and associated injuries.[34] When treating fractures in the UE, the associated soft tissues should always be considered. Associated soft-tissue injuries include injuries to the skin, ligaments, blood vessels, and nerves. These additional injuries may delay or complicate healing as they will also be affected by the inflammatory response of the healing fracture. The OTA should realize the effect the soft-tissue injuries may have on healing as far as time, pain, scarring, and sensitivity, and adjust the client's treatment plan accordingly. Fractures associated with soft-tissue injuries may cause continued swelling and stiffness that does not resolve. Clients who are not making progress as expected should be referred back to their physician for a reevaluation of the healing fracture and the associated injuries.

TABLE 22-5 Stages of Fracture Healing

PHASE	TIMEFRAME
Phase One: Inflammation with hematoma formation	Within 8 hours of injury
Phase Two: Reparative	Soft callus formation 2 to 3 weeks Hard callus formation 3 to 10 weeks
Phase Three: Remodeling	10 weeks to years after injury

Wrist Fractures: The Distal Radius

A fracture to the distal radius is one of the most common fractures in the UE. Distal radius fractures are typically the result of a fall on an outstretched hand (FOOSH); however they also occur in a younger population that engages in contact sports. The physician determines how a distal radius fracture is treated, which may be with a reduction, immobilization in a cast, or with surgery. Regardless of the method for fracture stabilization, the goals for therapy will be the same: to decrease edema, decrease pain, improve ROM, and to assist the client with return to normal hand function. Distal radius fractures that have been treated without surgery will require a period of immobilization; however, clients should be referred to therapy when the fracture is clinically healed. Clients with an ORIF to the distal radius fracture usually begin therapy at two to four weeks after surgery and are fitted with a custom fabricated volar wrist orthosis. Gentle AROM is also initiated at two to four weeks, and activity is progressed as tolerated. Several complications have been documented with treatment of a distal radius fracture including carpal tunnel syndrome, ulnar styloid fractures, and CRPS. It is important to note that because **complex regional pain syndrome (CRPS)** can occur with distal radius fractures, pain-free motion should be emphasized.[35]

OT Practitioner's Viewpoint

When treating a client for the first time, it may be difficult to know where to begin. After an initial evaluation is performed, the treatment plan and goals are established. Goals for the treatment of hand and UE conditions usually include establishing a home exercise program, decreasing pain, improving ROM, and improving function. The OTA will use a variety of treatment modalities to address the goals. Treatment modalities will vary and will depend on the client's diagnosis and the pattern of tissue healing. What treatment modalities should be used when? The following is a scenario of a typical treatment session based upon the goals for a client who is 3 weeks postsurgery to repair a right dominant distal radius fracture.

Deficits: Include decreased wrist flexion, extension, and supination; pain of 4/10 with end-range wrist movements; scar adherence at volar wrist surgical scar with hypersensitivity; mild edema to the wrist; decreased ability to perform light homemaking activities; and unable to return to work until released by physician.

Potential treatment session: The client is greeted as she enters the clinic. She is asked if she is having any problems with the fit of her orthosis, any increase in pain, or any changes in her condition since her last treatment session. The client may also be questioned regarding her current level of pain in order to get a baseline and monitor pain levels throughout treatment. Both the client and OT practitioner wash their hands for infection control. The client is provided

Continued

OT Practitioner's Viewpoint (continued)

with a heat modality such as fluidotherapy or a moist heat pack for 15 minutes. Client education may be provided while the client is "warming up." After the superficial heat treatment, the OT practitioner will perform manual edema mobilization to the fingers, wrist, and forearm followed by soft-tissue mobilization to the volar wrist scar. Gentle passive stretching by the OTA may also be performed. The client will then be asked to demonstrate portions of her home program, to ensure understanding and to answer any questions. Active ROM exercises and functional tasks will be performed in order to improve ROM (i.e. folding towels, turning cards, reaching for lightweight items, manipulating lightweight objects). The OT practitioner will monitor the client during wrist and hand use, to provide cueing to achieve end-range motion, and correct compensation with stronger muscle groups. For example, the stronger finger extensors may be assisting with the performance of wrist extension. At this time in the treatment session, modifications may be made to the orthosis to ensure comfortable fit. The OT practitioner will offer the client encouragement throughout treatment and will emphasize the importance of the home exercise program. When all interventions have been addressed, the client is dismissed and a follow-up appointment is made.

Additional suggestions: If a treatment intervention is not working, do not hesitate to try a different intervention, as long as you are working toward the same goal. And remember, as the client's deficits diminish and the goals are adjusted to accommodate for progress and healing, the therapy interventions will also be adjusted to meet the client's needs. AROM exercises may be replaced with PROM exercises and strengthening. Lightweight object manipulation may increase to lifting objects that simulate work activities. Edema may increase with an increase in activity, therefore compression garments may be required for use to decrease edema. At each therapy session, we reassess the client and his or her progress, keeping in mind the goals established at the time of the initial evaluation. Using a variety of therapeutic interventions will assist in meeting those goals, and will lead to positive client outcomes.
~ Karol Spraggs-Young, OTD, OTR/L, CHT

Carpal Fractures: The Scaphoid

Of all of the carpal bones, the scaphoid is the most common to be fractured. Scaphoid fractures are also a result of a FOOSH and most often seen in young males. The symptoms of a scaphoid fracture are swelling and pain in the anatomical snuff box on the radial side of the wrist (Fig. 22-15). Unfortunately, scaphoid fractures may be difficult to diagnose as the fracture may not be seen initially on x-ray. Fractures to the proximal portion of the scaphoid take a long time to heal because the blood supply to this area is minimal. Scaphoid fractures will often require surgery with an ORIF and bone graft to repair the broken bone. Therapy intervention for a scaphoid fracture involves a custom thermoplastic thumb spica orthosis for protection. As the scaphoid heals, gentle ROM exercises are initiated, with the progression to strengthening and return to normal activities.[36]

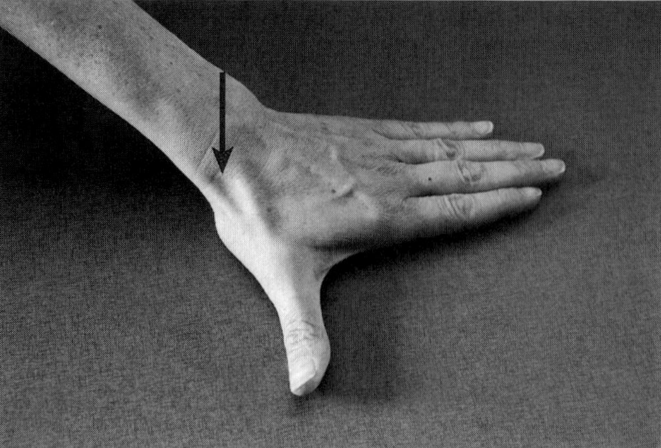

FIGURE 22-15. The anatomical snuffbox, which is the site of pain for a scaphoid fracture.

Metacarpal Fractures: The Boxer's Fracture

The metacarpal bones are essential for providing stability in the palm of the hand. The most commonly fractured metacarpal is the fifth metacarpal or the metacarpal of the small finger. Fifth metacarpal fractures are also known as boxer's fractures as they usually occur with impact to the metacarpal with a closed fist (Fig. 22-16). Metacarpal

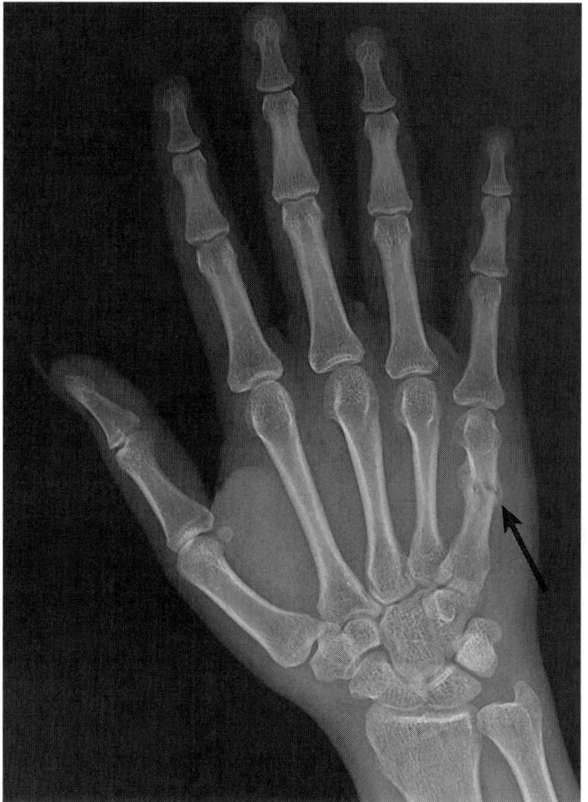

FIGURE 22-16. An x-ray of a 5th metacarpal fracture, also known as a Boxer's fracture.

fractures typically heal quickly, and if they are nondisplaced, require two to three weeks of immobilization before beginning ROM exercises. Rotation of the fractured metacarpal can produce scissoring of the fingers when attempting to make a fist, therefore these types of fractures will require surgery to correct the rotational deformity. After surgery, the client will benefit from a custom orthosis to provide protection. Metacarpal fractures should be positioned in MCP joint flexion after injury or surgery to prevent MCP collateral ligament tightness. As the fracture heals, gentle ROM exercises are initiated, with the progression to strengthening and return to normal activities.[37]

Phalangeal Fractures/Dislocations

The fingers are made up of the proximal phalanx, the middle phalanx, and the distal phalanx. The most common fractures in the finger are at the level of the distal phalanx, which accounts for 50% of all hand fractures.[38] Distal phalanx fractures are often associated with nailbed injuries and are also called tuft fractures. Nondisplaced distal phalanx fractures are positioned in extension in a protective orthosis for three to six weeks. Stable fractures can tolerate gentle AROM at one week. A bony mallet is a distal phalanx fracture that disrupts the extensor tendon along with the fracture, resulting in a fingertip that droops. A bony mallet should be positioned in extension within a custom orthosis for at least six weeks to provide adequate time for the tendon to heal.[35] Distal phalanx fractures that require surgery for proper bone alignment, and to promote healing will benefit from a custom positional orthosis after surgery. When indicated by the physician, a referral to OT will assist in improving motion and regaining functional hand use.

Fractures of the middle phalanx are less common, however, due to the delicate and intricate anatomy at the PIP joint where the middle phalanx and proximal phalanx meet, treatment of these fractures can be challenging. With a stable fracture, the goals of therapy will be to provide a custom positional orthosis for protection, to decrease inflammation, to decrease pain, and to promote tendon glide and joint ROM.[39] With an unstable fracture or one that requires surgery, a positional orthosis will be provided after surgery. If surgical fixation is solid, gentle ROM exercises with blocking and tendon glides (see treatment section later in the chapter) may be initiated within 3 to 5 days of surgery.[34] As with all fractures in the hand, the principles of fracture healing must be considered and progression to normal hand use should follow physician guidelines.

Likewise, proximal phalanx fractures at the level of the PIP joint require special care due to the soft-tissue structures surrounding the PIP joint. Stable and nondisplaced proximal phalanx fractures can be treated with buddy taping or a custom finger orthosis and are encouraged to begin early active motion as tolerated. Displaced proximal phalanx fractures, or those that require surgery will benefit from a custom fabricated positional orthosis and assistance to limit edema and scarring. Unless otherwise instructed by the physician, the position of safety for the PIP joint, within in an orthosis, should be full extension.[37] To avoid joint contractures and stiffness, gentle AROM exercises, including blocking and tendon gliding, should be encouraged as soon as the physician indicates. Complications seen in the treatment of finger fractures include joint contracture, loss of finger extension, infections, stiffness, and CRPS. With this in mind, the OT practitioner should look for any increase in swelling, redness, stiffness, and/or pain. Any change in client status should be communicated to the physician as soon as possible, as early intervention may minimize complications.

Proximal Interphalangeal Joint Dislocations

Many athletes have heard the expression "jammed finger", but what may appear to be a simple jammed finger is often a dislocation at the PIP joint, and when left untreated, results in stiffness, swelling, pain, and the inability to use the hand. Dislocations in the PIP joint of the finger are either classified as volar dislocations, dorsal dislocations, or lateral dislocations and refer to the position of the bone in relationship to the joint. For example, with a dorsal dislocation the middle phalanx will lie dorsal to the proximal phalanx when seen on x-ray.[40] Dislocations are treated similar to fractures, as joint stability is the main goal. With simple sprains to the collateral ligaments, treatment may include buddy taping and ROM. However with unstable dislocations and those requiring surgery, immobilization in specific positions with progression to gentle AROM is the usual course of treatment. Dorsal dislocations may be treated with a dorsal protective finger orthosis with an extension block to allow full flexion. Blocking the joint from going into full extension will decrease the risk for dislocating the joint again, and will allow the tissues to heal. The orthosis is then adjusted weekly until full extension is obtained. Volar dislocations will be positioned in a custom orthosis with PIP joint extension. If the central slip of the extensor tendon is thought to be involved, the client may begin DIP joint flexion within the splint however will be instructed to avoid PIP joint flexion (Fig. 22-17). The severity

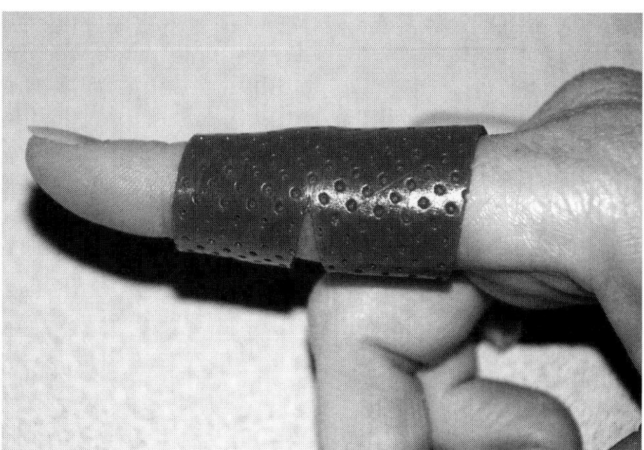

FIGURE 22-17. PIP joint extension orthosis; used in the treatment of PIP joint injuries.

of central slip involvement will dictate the amount of time the orthosis is needed. For those clients having surgery, the goals of therapy will include inflammation management, scar management, decreasing pain, and initiating AROM.[41] Progression through ROM protocols will vary on the type of dislocation and associated injuries to soft-tissue structures. Communication with the physician is important in order to progress the client as healing allows and to have positive functional outcomes.

CONDITIONS OF THE THUMB

The thumb is a unique structure with specialized anatomy that allows for flexibility while manipulating small objects and stability while pinching. The thumb has its own set of thenar muscles that allow for adduction, abduction, opposition, and precise motor control. The collateral ligaments at the MP joint of the thumb contribute to the strength and stability when holding tools or sporting equipment or when opening containers. Injury to the thumb can be limiting, as thumbs are used to participate in everyday activities and for expression (thumbs up).

Ulnar Collateral Ligament Injury to the Thumb

Injury to the ulnar collateral ligament (UCL) of the thumb is also known as gamekeeper's thumb or skier's thumb. This injury occurs with radial deviation and hyperextension of the thumb MP joint, which is often the result of a ski injury when the pole twists and hyperextends the thumb. When a UCL injury is suspected, the laxity at the thumb MP joint is ulnarly stressed in full extension and at 30 degrees of flexion, and then compared with the noninvolved thumb. A stress x-ray is also obtained. A UCL injury is graded from type I to type III. Type I and II injuries are considered incomplete ruptures or sprains, and a type III injury is considered a rupture. Type I and II injuries can be treated with immobilization in a hand-based thumb orthosis for 3 to 6 weeks. Type III injuries will require surgery. A Steiner's lesion is a type III injury that results in the UCL lying on top of the adductor aponeurosis and will require surgery as the UCL will not heal until it is in anatomical position.[42] After surgery for a UCL repair, the thumb is protected in a hand-based thumb orthosis. AROM exercises are initiated at 4 weeks and progression to normal activities between 6 and 10 weeks. Clients may wear a protective orthosis for return to strenuous activities and sports.[35]

Thumb Carpometacarpal Joint Osteoarthritis

One of the most common joints in the hand to develop osteoarthritis is the CMC joint between the trapezium and metacarpal, at the base of the thumb. This is also known as basal joint arthritis. Due to the normal mobility of this joint, it is prone to arthritic changes, which may cause pain, swelling, and the inability to perform a sustained pinch.[43] When the CMC joint develops arthritis, the instability at the joint and the decrease in joint space cause pain when using the thumb for functional activities. CMC joint arthritis is diagnosed by obtaining an x-ray and through clinical examination (Fig. 22-18). This type of arthritis is frequently seen in women older than 50 years of age and may be the result of repetitive use or trauma. Conservative treatment for CMC joint osteoarthritis includes support from a custom fabricated orthosis, which has been shown to be effective at decreasing thumb pain.[44] Use of an orthosis provides support and stability to the thumb CMC joint during the performance of pinching and gripping activities. This support decreases pain by limiting CMC joint motion, and may even provide a tactile reminder to clients to modify the way they perform activities. Home management will include activity modification, joint protection, client education, modalities to decrease pain, and stabilization exercises to prevent deformity.[45] Resistive exercises and activities should be avoided, as they cause more trauma to the arthritic joint. For example, using the painful thumb to open jars, pinch clothespins, or squeeze a tube of toothpaste will put more stress on the CMC joint and eventually cause joint wear and tear and pain. If clients continue to have pain resulting in a decrease in function, they may be candidates for a CMC joint arthroplasty. This procedure reconstructs the arthritic CMC joint. Therapy after surgery includes a custom

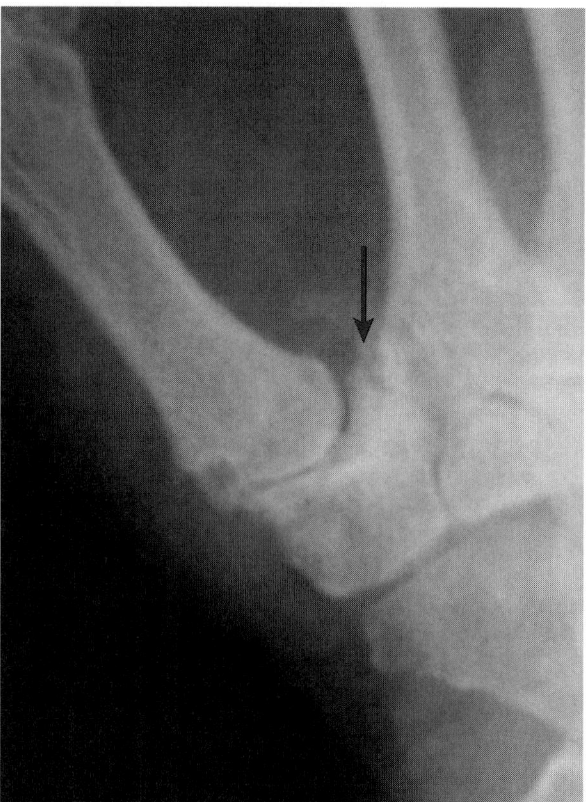

FIGURE 22-18. An x-ray image of thumb CMC joint osteoarthritis. Note the narrowing of the joint space and loss of cartilage resulting in bone on contact against bone.

fabricated orthosis for protection, scar management, edema management, and ROM exercises to assist with return to normal hand use.

NERVE COMPRESSION AND NERVE INJURY

The brachial plexus in the upper arm divides to create the three main nerves that innervate the UE, the median, ulnar, and radial (Fig. 22-19). These peripheral nerves supply motor function to the muscles in the wrist and hand as well as sensation to the forearm, wrist, and hand. Injuries to the nerves in the UE can cause muscle weakness and the loss of sensation resulting in impaired function. Nerve injuries are classified according to severity: **neuropraxia, axonotmesis,** and **neurotmesis.** Neuropraxia, the mildest form, is usually the result of nerve compression or repetitive stress. With neuropraxia, sensory changes may occur, however recovery is expected. Most nerve compression syndromes such as carpal tunnel and cubital tunnel are considered a type of neuropraxia. Axonotmesis is more severe and may be the result of a crush or traction injury. With axonotmesis motor loss is expected, and whereas there is the potential for recovery, it may take a long time. With neurotmesis the nerve has either been lacerated or transected and will require surgery in order to improve. Nerves that have been crushed or compressed will begin to regenerate after the injury/decompression and will regenerate at a rate of 1 mm to 3 mm per day. Nerves that have been lacerated and repaired will take 2 to 3 weeks to begin to regenerate at a rate of 3 mm to 4 mm per day.[46] Although there are many potential compression sites for nerves in the UE, what follows is a discussion of treatment for common nerve compressions and injuries.

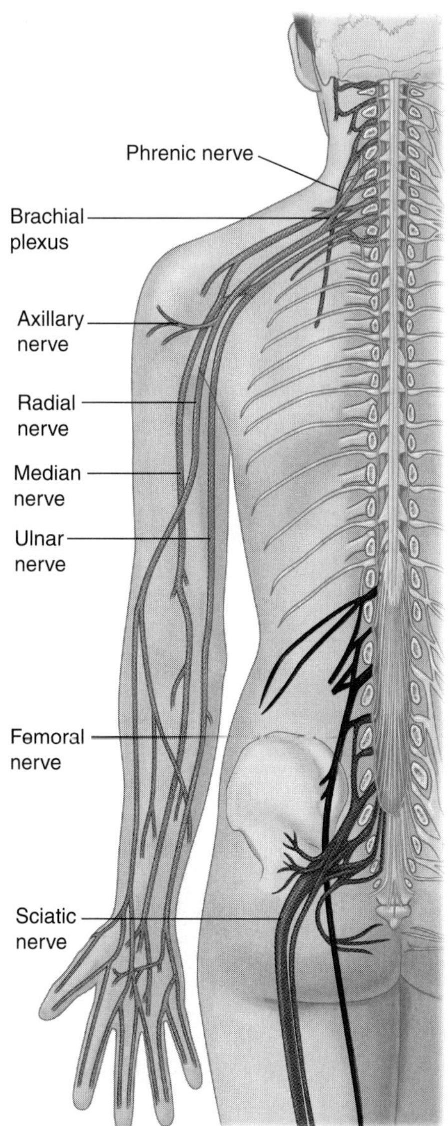

FIGURE 22-19. The brachial plexus and the three main nerves with their muscle innervations: median, ulnar, and radial.

Median Nerve

Compression of the median nerve at the level of the wrist is called carpal tunnel syndrome. Carpal tunnel syndrome is characterized by pain in the wrist and hand primarily at night. It also causes tingling in the thumb, index, middle, and half of the ring finger and weakness in pinch or grip. Sensory changes and weakness are due to the pressure on the nerve that is caused by narrowing in the carpal tunnel. This may be a result of swelling or a thickening of the tendons. When there is pressure on the nerve, it becomes irritated and produces the tingling and numb sensation. The median nerve also innervates the small muscles of the thumb, therefore weakness in these muscles may be evident. Nonsurgical treatment for carpal tunnel syndrome includes use of a wrist orthosis, cortisone injections, activity modification, and client education. Therapy after a carpal tunnel release may not be necessary, however can address scar tenderness, weakness, and return to normal hand function.

A laceration or injury to the median nerve will cause loss of sensory and motor function. Motor loss will be seen in the first and second lumbricals, the superficial head of the flexor pollicis brevis, the abductor pollicis brevis, and the opponens pollicis. Treatment after repair of a median nerve will include positioning in a custom thermoplastic orthosis, scar management, inflammation reduction, and sensory and motor reeducation.[47]

Ulnar Nerve

Compression of the ulnar nerve at the elbow is called cubital tunnel syndrome. Cubital tunnel syndrome is characterized by numbness and tingling in the ring and small fingers that increases with sustained elbow flexion. Nonsurgical treatments for cubital tunnel syndrome includes use of a padded elbow sleeve to decrease pressure on the ulnar nerve, use of an orthosis at night to prevent elbow flexion, activity modification, and client education. Therapy after surgery for cubital tunnel syndrome may include a protective positional orthosis, scar management, ROM exercises, and progressive strengthening for return to normal activities.[48]

The ulnar nerve can also be compressed at Guyon's canal, which is at the level of the wrist. This condition is not as common as carpal tunnel syndrome however is treated in the same manner.[49] After surgical decompression of the ulnar nerve at the wrist, padded work gloves may assist with decreasing scar pain and prepare the client for return to work.

A laceration or injury to the ulnar nerve will cause loss of sensory and motor function. Motor loss will be seen in the third and fourth lumbricals and the interossei, the deep head of the flexor pollicis brevis, and the adductor pollicis. An ulnar nerve injury will result in a claw posture to the hand with a weak prehension pattern or Froment's sign (Fig. 22-20 and Fig. 22-21). Treatment after repair of the ulnar nerve will include positioning in a custom fabricated orthosis, scar management, edema reduction, and sensory and motor reeducation.

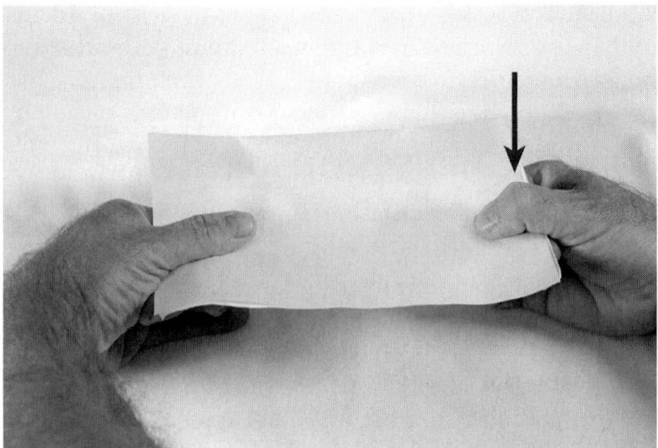

FIGURE 22-21. Froment's sign resulting from an injury to the ulnar nerve characterized by thumb IP joint flexion and MP joint hyperextension.

Radial Nerve

Compression of the radial nerve at the forearm is called radial tunnel syndrome and occurs with repetitive pronation and supination with wrist flexion and extension. Radial tunnel syndrome is characterized by pain medial to the lateral epicondyle over the extensor muscle mass, however is not associated with sensory loss or muscle weakness. Provocative testing for radial tunnel syndrome is resisted middle finger extension with the arm extended and resisted supination (Fig. 22-22). Nonsurgical treatment of radial tunnel syndrome is rest from repetitive activities, activity modification, and if needed a cortisone injection.[50] Surgical release of the radial tunnel may be performed if pain is not relieved with conservative measures. After surgical decompression, therapy will address scar and inflammation management and will progress with ROM with the goal to return to normal activities.[35] A laceration or injury to the radial nerve will result in sensory loss over the dorsum of the hand and loss of motor function to the wrist extensors and the extensors to the fingers and thumb. Treatment after repair of the radial nerve will include positioning in a custom thermoplastic orthosis, scar management, edema reduction, and sensory and motor reeducation. A dynamic functional extension orthosis may be used to assist with function while awaiting nerve return.

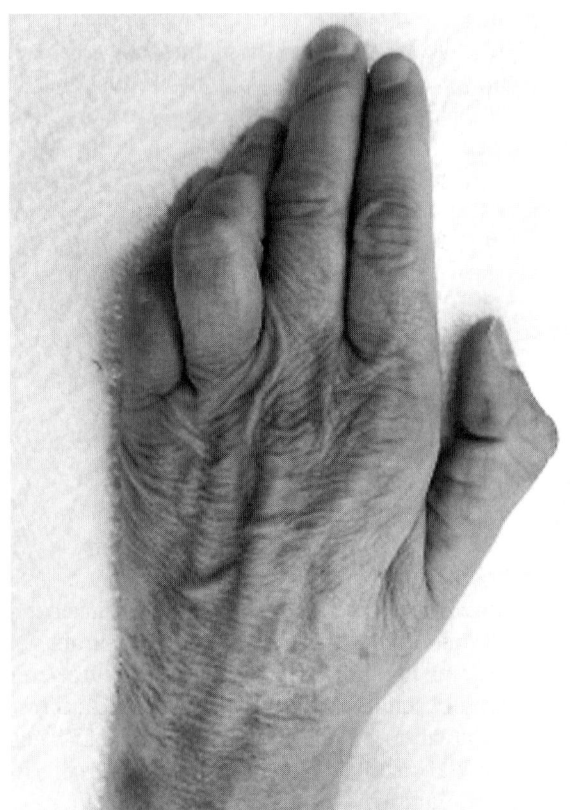

FIGURE 22-20. Claw posture resulting from an ulnar nerve injury.

Digital Nerve Injury

Digital nerve injuries are usually seen in combination with other injuries to the hand, such as tendon lacerations and trauma. On the volar surface, each finger is uniquely

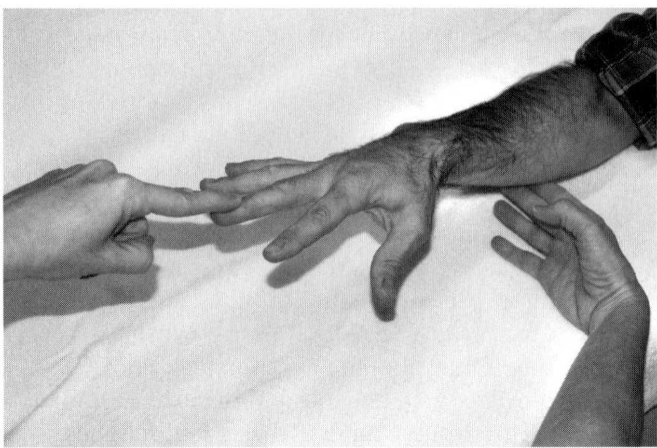

FIGURE 22-22. Performing the provocative test for radial tunnel syndrome.

equipped with a radial digital nerve and an ulnar digital nerve, which contribute to the ability to have discriminatory and localized touch. These nerves, when injured, not only limit function, but also make it unsafe for a person to handle hot, cold, or sharp objects. Digital nerves are usually repaired end-to-end, however they may require a nerve graft if they have lost length or if too much tension will be placed on the repair.[51] Therapy after a digital nerve repair includes a protective orthosis to minimize tension on the repair, scar management, ROM exercises, and **sensory reeducation.** Sensory reeducation is a process of retraining the brain to correctly interpret and to learn to distinguish various sensory inputs from the new nerves, and will be described more in depth later in the chapter. Using the sensory assessments described previously will assist in monitoring nerve return. Expect sensation to return in the following order; pain, deep pressure, moving touch, static light touch, and then discriminative touch.[52]

TRAUMATIC HAND INJURIES

Traumatic hand injuries include crush injuries, amputations, lacerations, fractures, and injuries that include multiple systems; soft tissues, blood vessels, nerves, muscles, tendons, and bones. Traumatic hand injuries are not only a result of work-related accidents, but also occur while participating in everyday activities. They may require multiple staged surgeries to repair damaged structures.[53] It is important for the practitioner treating a client with a traumatic hand injury to have an initial dialogue and frequent communication with the physician to determine what structures have been repaired, how to protect the repaired structures, what structures to mobilize and when, and, what surgeries may be planned for the future. The OT practitioner must also have a thorough understanding of the principles of tissue healing, as the healing of one structure will affect the other. Once referred to therapy, the occupational therapist will complete the initial evaluation and establish the plan of care. Follow-up appointments with the OTA will address the goals of therapy after a traumatic hand injury. These goals typically include wound, inflammation scar and pain management, client education, fabrication of a custom positional orthosis, ADL training, and discussion of the psychological affect of trauma. Progression with ROM will coincide with the phases of tissue healing and will be dependent on the structures that have been repaired. Communication among the team of individuals treating the trauma client—physician, occupational therapist, OTA, nurses, and case manager—is extremely important. Trauma cases are often challenging for the experienced OT practitioner, as they may not follow specific postoperative protocols and rely on a knowledge base of anatomy, physiology, normal tissue healing, and clinical reasoning skills. Likewise, for the OTA involved in the care of a client with a traumatic hand injury, mentoring with the occupational therapist throughout the process will improve confidence and clinical reasoning skills, in the treatment of this type of complex condition.

COMMUNICATION

A debilitating hand injury or condition can physically and psychologically impact the client. Unfortunately, the psychological aspects of hand injuries are often overlooked. Humans use the hands to work, engage in leisure activities, perform self care, and care for others. When the hands are injured, it limits the ability to participate in normal life roles. This change in life roles can psychologically affect the client, which in turn may have a negative effect on treatment outcomes. For example, if clients are overly focused on their pain and impaired status, they may not be able to participate in their home program. Likewise, if clients with a work-related injury feel anger toward their employer, they may unconsciously magnify the symptoms in order to stay away from their stressful work environment. As an OT practitioner, it is important to be aware of the psychology components, in order to facilitate conversations about the psychological aspects of the client's hand injury. When working with the client, consider the following:

- Develop a rapport with the client.
- Allow for honest conversation.
- Include the client in treatment planning and decision-making.
- Encourage the client to take an active role in the healing process.
- Use positive statements and reassurance that pain and the condition will improve.

If working with the client is difficult, share the treatments with another OT practitioner within the clinic, and work together to problem solve on the client's behalf. If the client is not improving or is getting worse, refer the client back to the physician for further workup. Some clients may require referral to a psychologist or collaboration with other healthcare professionals, in order to address their psychological needs.

COMPLEX REGIONAL PAIN SYNDROME

CRPS, previously known as reflex sympathetic dystrophy (RSD), is a chronic pain syndrome that develops either in the upper or lower extremity and is characterized by swelling; stiffness; burning pain; hypersensitivity to cold; changes in skin color; hair and nail growth; and a loss of functional use of the extremity.[54] CRPS symptoms may vary in severity, go away on their own, or last for months. There are two types of CRPS. Type I, the most common, is a result of an illness or injury that did not involve a nerve. Type II, also called causalgia, is the result of an injury to a nerve. CRPS is seen most often in females who smoke, and with clients who have sustained distal radius fractures. Some researchers believe CRPS has a psychological component.[55] After clinical evaluation, the diagnosis of CRPS can be confirmed with an x-ray, bone scan, or diagnostic sympathetic block. Early recognition and treatment of CRPS is important in order to minimize stiffness, muscle atrophy, and disability. For example, one study showed that 80% of clients with CRPS who were treated within the first year showed improvement.[56] The goals of therapy for a client with CRPS will be to minimize the pain and to decrease edema while improving functional ROM. Decreasing the client's pain, and not contributing to an increase in pain, is very important when treating CRPS. The client with CRPS will also require encouragement to use the affected extremity, and therapy should incorporate bilateral hand use, use of the hand for self-care activities, and weight-bearing for motor relearning. Graded motor imagery, sensory reeducation, and orthotic intervention and modalities are all helpful in managing the symptoms of CRPS. The client with CRPS will benefit from the support of a multidisciplinary team in order to address the physical and psychosocial components of this frustrating and painful condition.[57]

CONDITIONS OF THE ELBOW

Clients who present with hand or wrist injuries may also report pain and functional limitations in the elbow as the anatomical structures and biomechanics of the elbow, wrist, and hand are interdependent. A few of the common conditions treated by the OT practitioner include lateral/medial tendonitis, bursitis, and stiffness at the elbow after fractures or dislocations.

Lateral epicondylitis is characterized by pain and tenderness at the lateral epicondyle, which is the point of insertion of the extensor muscles in the forearm. Pain is present with the combined motions of gripping, wrist extension, and elbow extension. Lateral epicondylitis is also known as tennis elbow; however, most clients who present with this condition do not play tennis. Medial epicondylitis affects the medial side of the elbow at the insertion of the flexor and pronator musculature. Medial epicondylitis, also known as golfer's elbow, is characterized by pain in the elbow and wrist on the inside of the forearm with the combined movements of gripping and wrist flexion. Both lateral and medial epicondylitis are considered overuse injuries and are often due to the performance of repetitive resistive motions of the elbow, wrist, and hand. Bursitis at the elbow occurs when the bursa or fluid sac between the olecranon and the skin becomes irritated and fills with additional fluid. The extra fluid, which may have a slow or rapid onset, causes swelling at the back of the elbow. Bursitis usually does not cause pain and is often seen in arthritic conditions or after trauma to the elbow. After a thorough assessment by the OT practitioner, the goals for the treatment of these soft tissue conditions of elbow typically include edema and pain management, ADL training, orthotic fabrication and fitting, and client education with an emphasis on activity modification.

Similar to fractures and dislocations of the wrist and hand, fractures and dislocations of the elbow are usually due to accidents or trauma. Fractures at the elbow may involve the distal humerus, olecranon, or the radial head and are categorized as either stable or unstable. Unstable fractures require surgery to restore stability at the elbow. Dislocations at the elbow occur when the joint surfaces of the elbow become separated and may be simple or complex. Simple dislocations do not involve an injury to the bones; however, complex dislocations involve injuries to the bones and ligaments. A common, simple dislocation seen in children is called "nurse-maid's elbow" and is a result of pulling or swinging a child with an extended elbow. Stable fractures and simple dislocations are treated with a period of immobilization, often in a hinged orthosis that allows for early controlled motion. Fractures and dislocations that are unstable and complex will require surgery. For clients having surgery, the goals of therapy will include edema management, scar management, decreasing pain, and initiating AROM. Progression through ROM protocols will vary on the type of fracture or dislocation and associated injuries to soft tissue structures. Communication with the physician is important in order to progress the client as healing allows.

THERAPEUTIC INTERVENTIONS FOR THE WRIST AND HAND

With an accurate diagnosis and list of treatment goals, the occupational therapist and OTA can begin to work as a team to restore the client with UE dysfunction back to his or her normal occupational performance patterns. *The Occupational Therapy Scope of Practice* includes interventions to promote engagement in ADLs and IADLs as well as social participation. The following are just a few of the interventions that are used by OT practitioners to achieve the goals of improving ROM, strength, and functional use of the UE. These are defined in the scope of practice as preparatory methods and tasks and education and training.[58]

Range of Motion

As discussed earlier in this chapter, joint ROM is the amount of motion available at a specific joint. In reference to treatment, AROM is the amount of motion the client is asked to actively perform without assistance. PROM is performed when the OT practitioner moves the joint through an arc of motion while the client is at rest. When treating a healing fracture, treatment usually begins with AROM as the client can easily control the motion at the injured joint. PROM is then initiated with a stable fracture to gain further joint ROM.[37] When treating a healing tendon, the opposite is true. Healing tendons initially require PROM to promote tendon glide and to prevent joint stiffness. AROM is then initiated when the tendon has healed enough to tolerate tension on the tendon repair.[59] Tension on the tendon repair is created by actively engaging the muscle to contract. The terms **controlled motion** and

early protected motion are also used when providing treatment to address joint ROM. Controlled motion is active motion of an involved joint or previously immobilized structure. For example, initiating gentle AROM exercises in a PIP joint after surgical repair of a proximal phalanx fracture or providing exercises for a client in a hinged elbow brace after an elbow injury would be controlled motion. Another example of controlled motion is the short arc motion protocol that is used when treating tendon repairs. Short arc motion protocols are designed to improve tensile strength of a healing tendon and prevent scarring while the tendon is healing. The short arc motion protocol allows the client to perform gentle active motion within a restricted range or arc of motion. When instructing a client in ROM exercises within a short arc motion protocol, the OTA will discuss the ROM limitations with the occupational therapist and the treating physician. Once the ROM limitations are determined, the OTA will either fabricate an orthosis that allows motion within the predetermined range, or will use a template or goniometer to have the client exercise within the restricted ROM. Controlled motion and short arc motion should only be performed by the OT practitioner who has the knowledge of the anatomy and diagnosis he or she is treating. Likewise, controlled motion and short arc motion should only be performed with a client who is able to demonstrate an understanding of the treatment objectives of this type of exercise. The term early protected motion is used to describe active or PROM that is performed to the uninvolved structures surrounding an injury or immobilized joint. For example, performing AROM exercises to the MCP and PIP joints of a finger with a DIP joint injury would be considered early protected motion.[34]

Other forms of AROM exercises are called tendon gliding and blocking. These exercises promote differential glide between the flexor tendons in the hand and allow for joint ROM to all of the joints in the hand. Tendon gliding exercises are a series of five exercises performed in progression. The client starts with the fingers extended and then moves through the progression of motion as follows:

1. All fingers in an extended position,
2. A "hook" fist (MCPs extended and IPs flexed),
3. To a "rooftop" (MCPs flexed and IPs extended),
4. To a "straight fist" (MCPs flexed, PIP's flexed and DIP joints extended),
5. To a "full fist" (MCP, PIP, and DIP joints flexed),
6. Then returning all fingers to an extended position

To perform tendon gliding exercises with the client, the OTA will have the client rest the forearm and elbow on a supported surface. The OTA will then instruct the client to straighten all of the fingers, keeping the thumb away from the palm. The client will then be asked to perform the exercises just described, making a hook fist, then rooftop, then straight fist, then full fist (composite flexion of the fingers), and returning to the final position with all fingers straight. If the diagnosis allows, tendon gliding may also be performed passively, with the patient or client providing an additional gentle stretch or overpressure with their hands. Observing this series of exercises will also assist the OTA in determining the difference between conditions of the joints and tendons. If the client has limited passive motion, the limitations may be due to a stiff joint; however, if passive motion is greater than active motion, tendon or soft tissue limitations may be present.

Blocking exercises have the client block a joint on the involved hand with the uninvolved hand in order to target motion at a specific joint. For example, holding the MCP joint on the index finger in extension, and instructing the client to perform active flexion at the PIP joint of the index finger, in order to improve ROM at the index finger PIP joint. OT practitioners may use a piece of thermoplastic material, dowel, or small piece of wood to create a "blocking board" to achieve the same outcome. Tendon gliding exercises and blocking exercises are frequently issued as a part of a home exercise program (Fig. 22-23).

It is important to understand tissue healing in order to determine what type of ROM exercises should be performed initially, and as the client progresses. Upon the initial evaluation, the OTA will usually begin with instruction in a home exercise program for ROM. A home exercise program that includes ROM exercises allows clients to be actively involved in their recovery. The OTA will need to review the home exercise program, either verbally or with demonstration at the first follow-up appointment. The OTA will also need to upgrade or modify the home exercise program as the client progresses. Progression through active or passive ROM exercise programs will be dependent on the diagnosis and treatment goals. When treating injuries and conditions in the hand, early ROM decreases inflammation, decreases

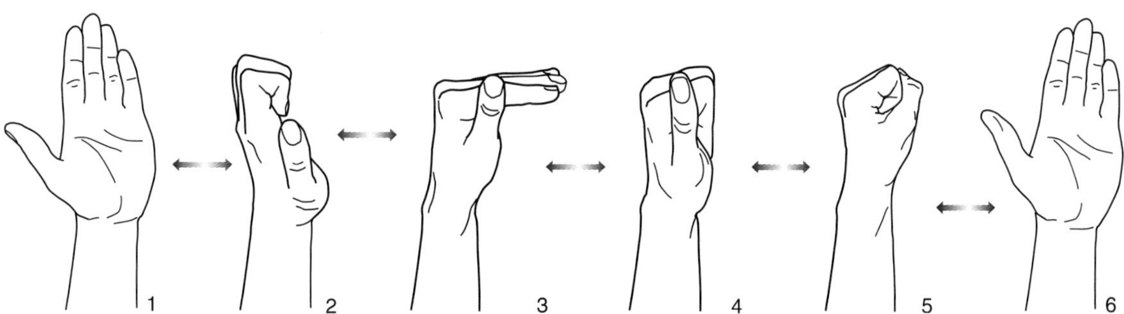

FIGURE 22-23. Series of tendon gliding and blocking exercises.

joint stiffness, and reduces the scarring or adherence of soft-tissue structures.

Wound and Scar Management

Wounds heal either by primary or secondary intention. Wounds that heal by primary intention are clean wounds that have been sutured or stapled for closure. Wounds that heal by secondary intention are usually dirty wounds that are left open to heal on their own. For wounds that are large or for those that will not heal in a timely manner, a skin graft may be indicated.

Wounds are classified by a color system: red, yellow, and black. A red wound is a healthy wound that is showing signs of new tissue growth, with definite edges and the absence of infection. The goals of wound care for a red wound are to promote healthy tissue growth with application of a nonstick dressing, and to avoid friction to the wound bed. A yellow wound has drainage with a creamy exudate or pus. A yellow wound may indicate infection. A black wound indicates necrotic or dead tissue.

The goals of wound care are based on the color system. Goals for a red wound are to promote healthy tissue growth by applying a nonstick dressing and avoiding friction to the wound bed. Goals for a yellow wound are to progress from a yellow to a red wound through cleansing, applying absorbable dressings and preventing maceration, which is caused by excessive moisture. Wounds should be cleansed with soap and water or saline washes. Using hydrogen peroxide on a healing wound can damage the new tissue growth; therefore it should be avoided or mixed with saline before use. A variety of wound care products are available; however, in order to determine the best course of wound care, the OTA should discuss wound care protocols with the physicians and occupational therapists within their clinic.

The goals for treatment of a black wound include debridement with the assistance of hand held water sprayer, topical enzymatic ointments, and wet-to-dry dressing changes.[62]

EVIDENCE-BASED PRACTICE

OT practitioners are aware of the importance of engagement and occupation and the use of purposeful activity as a means to overcome injuries and/or disabilities. When treating UE dysfunction, occupation is an integral part of the assessment and treatment plan as practitioners use the hands to care for self and others. Unfortunately, within the practice setting of the busy outpatient OT clinic, the importance of using purposeful activity can often be overlooked and replaced with exercise programs and passive treatment modalities. The following evidence-based articles examine the issues surrounding the use of occupation-based assessments and treatment, while endorsing the inclusion of occupation based treatment approaches in hand and UE rehabilitation.

This purpose of the study by Che Daud et al. was to determine the efficacy of engagement in occupation as a treatment approach in the rehabilitation of hand conditions. Using a randomized control trial after inclusion criteria was met, 23 individuals with bone, tendon, or peripheral nerve injuries to the hand were treated using a combination of occupation-based intervention (OBI) and therapeutic exercise (TE) and compared to 23 individuals treated with TE alone for the rehabilitation of these hand injuries. When researchers compared the outcomes between the two groups, the combination of OBI and TE produced better recovery than TE alone. Significant differences were found in DASH disability symptoms, total active motion, and neuropathic pain in favor of OBI and TE. The study concludes that the use of OBI in conjunction with TE is a beneficial treatment approach as it is inexpensive, easily accessible, and uses purposeful activity to decrease impairment in the hand and UE. Incorporating daily occupations within a therapeutic exercise program improves abilities and engagement in occupation providing a meaningful and culturally relevant treatment intervention for the treatment of hand and UE conditions.[60]

In the descriptive study by Grice, the author explores the use of occupation-based assessments and interventions used by OT practitioners in the hand therapy setting. This study also examines the perceptions of practitioners pertaining to the use of occupation-based assessments and interventions. A survey was sent to the membership of the American Society of Hand Therapists and consisted of 10 questions. These questions addressed demographic information, the use of occupation-based assessments, impairment-based assessments, and opinions about occupation-based assessment and intervention. A total of 594 surveys were completed and the data was analyzed. The results of the survey concluded that the reasons for not using occupation-based assessments or interventions are time constraints and availability of and familiarity with the assessments. However, the majority of the respondents in this survey reported that occupation-based measures are important and that all hand therapy practice should include them. This study concludes that OT practitioners working in the outpatient hand therapy setting should continue to use and advocate for the inclusion of occupation-based assessments and interventions as they are known to improve patient outcomes.[61]

Che Daud, A. Z., Yau, M. K., Barnett, F., Judd, J., Jones, R. E., & Muhammad Nawawi, R. F.(2016). Integration of occupation based intervention in hand injury rehabilitation: A Randomized Controlled Trial. Journal of Hand Therapy, *29(1), 30–40.*

Grice, K. O. (2015). The use of occupation-based assessments and intervention in the hand therapy setting: A survey. Journal of Hand Therapy: Scientific/Clinical Article *28, 300-306.*

The OT practitioner may perform wound care using a hand held sprayer in the therapy clinic. The gentle agitation loosens dead tissue and cleans the wound. The physician may prescribe topical ointments, which can be used with dressing changes to facilitate softening of a black or necrotic wound. Wet-to-dry dressings are also used, as the wet gauze is applied to the black area of a wound and is allowed to dry. During dressing changes, the dry gauze is then removed, thus debriding nonviable tissue that sticks to the dry gauze. Always follow universal precautions and infection-control principles when performing wound care. Wound care areas must be thoroughly cleansed between each client, and the OT practitioner must wear personal protective equipment, including gloves and eye protection. All wounds should be treated as infectious and contaminated. Therefore, the OT practitioner must be familiar with facility guidelines for infection control and OSHA standards.

The four overlapping stages in the process of wound healing are hemostasis, inflammation, replication and proliferation, and remodeling or maturation. Hemostasis is the body's immediate response to injury and lasts about six hours. The inflammatory phase is characterized by swelling and pain. This is the body's natural response to injury and occurs within six to 48 hours during which neutrophils and macrophages remove bacteria and lay the groundwork for the fibroblasts to produce collagen. The inflammatory phase should last approximately five to seven days. Prolonged inflammation and redness after this time could indicate infection.

Phase three, the proliferative phase, begins around day three to five and lasts anywhere from 14 to 28 days. Inflammation lessens during this phase, and the fibroblasts build collagen fibers, which become scar tissue. This is usually the time when sutures are removed. During the fourth phase, or maturation, collagen fibers mature, or are more organized. This phase begins around day 28 and lasts months to years. Age and medical history will influence the client's progression through the wound-healing process.

Experienced OT practitioners advocate for scar management to begin as soon as treatment to a wound begins.[63] Managing a wound correctly minimizes infection and promotes healthy tissue growth. Proper wound care affords the OT practitioner the opportunity to monitor the wound and to detect thick or hypertrophic scarring as it begins.

SCAR MANAGEMENT

The soft tissues in the hand need to be supple with the right amount of sensitivity to allow for flexibility with gripping and manipulating a variety of objects. Scarring can quickly limit this ability. Although scarring is a natural result of the healing process, excessive scarring will limit ROM, impair sensation, cause pain, and lead to a loss of hand function. For example, a tight scar over the dorsum of the PIP joint will limit full finger flexion and the client's ability to perform a tight grip. A thick scar in the palm of the hand will cause pain when the client uses the palm of the hand to push up from sitting to standing, and a hypersensitive scar at the wrist will cause pain when touched by a watch or a shirt sleeve. It is the OT practitioner's responsibility to monitor and treat scars in order to promote healthy hand function. Initially, a normal scar may be red and raised with minor hypersensitivity to touch and textures that should resolve as the scar matures.

A scar is abnormal if it continues to be hypersensitive or becomes thick, dense, and extends beyond the borders of the original wound bed. Treatment for thick scars includes application of compression to the scar through massage, paper tape, or silicone gel sheeting.[64] Compression garments have been used in the treatment of scarring from burns with success. Compression helps to flatten the scar and assists with reorganization of the collagen fibers during healing. OT practitioners are able to provide anecdotal evidence supporting the use of silicone gel sheeting and paper tape to provide this compression, however the exact mechanism that makes this treatment approach successful is currently unknown.[65]

Instruct the client with a thick, raised scar to perform scar massage at home several times daily. Scar massage may be performed against the scar, to cause friction, or in a circular motion along the scar's length. The amount of pressure applied while massaging will be dependent on the integrity of the scar. (Chapter 28 further explains scar massage. See Figure 28-05.) A thin fragile scar will not be able to tolerate the same amount of pressure as a thick adherent scar. When using compression with silicone gel sheeting or paper tape, the client is instructed to use them for 23 hours a day with removal for bathing and hygiene. If using the gel or tape limits hand function, the client may be instructed to wear them at night, with removal during the day when the hand is in use. The OT practitioner should monitor the scar for any skin irritation or problems, and should instruct the client to decrease the wearing time as the scar matures and becomes supple. Sun exposure may cause scars to become darker; therefore, the client should be instructed to keep scars covered when outdoors and to apply sunscreen for at least one year after injury or surgery. For treatment of hypersensitive scars, see the section on sensory reeducation that follows.

Inflammation Reduction Techniques

Inflammation, or swelling, is the body's natural response to injury. At the initial onset of an injury, inflammation is preparing the tissues for healing and should be soft and easy to move. This type of inflammation can be managed with elevation, ice, gentle compression, and AROM exercises to the uninvolved structures. In the second phase of wound healing, inflammation becomes a problem when it does not resolve. The cellular composition of inflammation in the reparative stage is more protein rich, and if left untreated will cause soft-tissue structures to tighten and contract.[66] Inflammation in this stage of wound healing should be addressed immediately as the long-term effects will be adhesions and a stiff hand. Treatment to address this type of inflammation is manual mobilization, gentle compression, elevation, and AROM exercises. The use of electrical stimulation may be beneficial to increase blood flow and reduce inflammation; however, the OT practitioner should consult with the physician, as it will be dependent on the client and the diagnosis.[62] During the maturation phase of wound healing, inflammation that has not resolved is considered a chronic condition, and would then be considered edema. This type of inflammation/edema will require compression dressings and may benefit from a referral to a lymphedema specialist, depending on the cause.

The lymphatic system helps protect the body from disease and is responsible for moving interstitial fluid back into the bloodstream. **Lymphedema** is the result of mechanical dysfunction within the lymphatic system and is categorized as either primary or secondary. Primary lymphedema is the result of a congenital condition. Secondary lymphedema is a result of surgery, treatment for cancer, tumors, injury to the lymph system, or venous insufficiency.[67] Lymphedema can be minimal to severe and will affect the skin, mobility within joints, and hand function. Its treatment includes manual lymph drainage (MLD), compression bandaging, exercise, and transition to a compressive garment. The client with lymphedema will be instructed in a home program for self-management. Compression pumps and diuretics may be prescribed for the client with severe lymphedema.

Manual edema mobilization (MEM) is a technique used for decreasing edema in the orthopedic population. MEM differs from MLD as it is used in an acute condition to decrease edema in an intact lymph system. The components of MEM include diaphragmatic breathing, light skin massage, exercise, pump point stimulation, and instruction in a home program, which includes light compression wraps. Using a combination of manual circular massage at the shoulder, elbow, and forearm along with AROM exercises that are performed in the direction of proximal (shoulder) to distal (hand), the OT practitioner performs MEM in the clinic, and instructs the client in how to perform the program at home. Contraindications to MEM include infections, active cancer, cardiac conditions, and blood clots, and MEM may alter blood sugar levels and decrease blood pressure.[68] A continuing education course is recommended for OT practitioners desiring to improve their skills in MEM. It is important to remember that clients with primary or secondary lymphedema will not benefit from MEM and should be referred to a specially trained lymphedema practitioner.

Orthotic Fabrication and Fitting

An orthosis is an external support that provides positioning, provides protection, or compensates for loss of function. Orthosis fitting and fabrication is a therapeutic intervention that is used frequently in the treatment of UE dysfunction. During the inflammatory stage of wound healing, an orthosis provides positioning and support to injured structures while maintaining ROM. During the proliferative and maturation stages, an orthosis will assist in decreasing joint stiffness and assist in improving functional ROM. For a complete understanding of orthotic fabrication and fitting, refer to Chapter 19 in this text.

Sensory Reeducation

The cerebral cortex is the part of the brain responsible for higher functions such as motor control and sensation. The goal of sensory reeducation is to ensure that the part of the hand, or impaired portion of the UE, remains active within the cerebral cortex, even if the sensory feedback system is not working.[69] Therefore, sensory reeducation is a learning process and should begin as soon as the client's condition will allow. In order to provide important feedback to the brain, sensory reeducation of a peripheral nerve should be associated with the other senses. For example, when touching a piece of fruit, in the absence of the sense of touch, the client should visualize the fruit and how it tastes, feels, and smells.[70] Researchers found positive outcomes in sensory return with the use of auditory responses to touch using a specially designed glove. They also advocate for **mirror visual feedback (MVF),** which is the use of a mirror to assist the client with visualizing sensory input while watching the uninvolved hand (Fig. 22-24).[71] Sensory reeducation in the absence of sensation should also include instruction in protecting the skin and preventing injuries. For example, clients with impaired sensation in the hand should be instructed to avoid extreme temperatures (hot and cold), avoid sharp objects, and use their vision to compensate for lack of sensation. The client with a nerve injury should also be instructed that sensory return takes time, therefore patience with the process is imperative. (See section on nerve compression and nerve injury for rates of sensory reinnervation.)

In order to modify and upgrade treatment, the OT practitioner should be familiar with the signs of sensory return. To restate, for peripheral nerve regeneration, sensation in the UE returns in the following order: pain and temperature, moving touch, constant touch, touch localization,

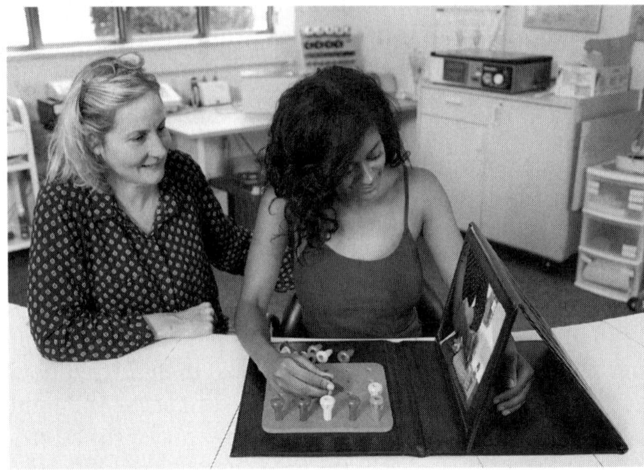

FIGURE 22-24. Mirror box being used with a client during a treatment for sensory reeducation.

two-point discrimination, and stereognosis (object identification). Therefore, when clients begin to complain of an increase in pain or report the ability to feel a cold drink in their hand, sensation may be returning. Once sensation begins to return and the client can detect pressure with the Semmes Weinstein monofilament 6.65, additional sensory reeducation techniques may be used. Dellon described a procedure to assist with sensory reeducation with the goal of localizing moving sensation. Clients are asked to close their eyes and try to detect where they are being touched by the practitioner. If they are unable to specify the area, they are instructed to open their eyes to see where they are being touched. Clients are then instructed to once again close their eyes and to see if they can concentrate on matching the sensory input to the vision of being touched.[72] Once the client is able to identify moving touch, this technique is used with static touch and object discrimination. Additionally, sensory reeducation can be performed with games, incorporated into self-care tasks and using a background medium to discriminate between objects. This author has had success with providing a home program, emphasizing repetition of touch stimulation, a quiet environment, and incorporating bilateral hand use, with and without the assist of visual feedback. An example of this type of program would be instructing the client with impaired sensation to choose a variety of objects (e.g., card, various coins, domino, safety pin). Then, sitting in a quiet room, the client will touch and feel the object with the uninvolved hand and also the hand with sensory impairment. The client is instructed to remember and visualize how the object felt in each hand and how the object should feel. This should be performed for each of the different objects. Clients can also close their eyes and try to identify the objects without using visual cues. Trying to find objects within a bowl of rice and feeling a variety of textures may also be part of a home program for sensory reeducation.

Hypersensitivity in the UE may require sensory reeducation in the form of **desensitization.** Desensitization programs include exposure to stimulation in order to normalize sensory input and to decrease pain. Desensitization programs, such as the program developed by the Downey Hand Center, include the use of textures, immersion particles, and vibration (Fig. 22-25). To initiate a desensitization program, a baseline status is obtained. The client is then introduced to textures, immersion particles, and vibration as tolerated and asked to rate them from most uncomfortable or irritating to the least uncomfortable. This selection then becomes the hierarchy for treatment.[73] Since the goal of desensitization is to decrease pain and improve hand function, the client should be slowly introduced to more uncomfortable textures, immersion particles, and vibration, eventually desensitizing the hypersensitive extremity. Desensitization programs should provide progression toward the more uncomfortable textures as the client improves. A desensitization program for hypersensitivity is frequently used after an amputation at the fingertip level. For a client with this

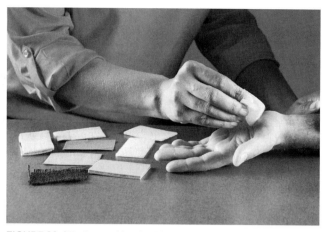

FIGURE 22-25. Desensitization kit used for sensory reeducation.

diagnosis, a desensitization program will begin in the therapy clinic and also be issued as part of a home program. The client is given a variety of textures to run on the tip of the finger. These textures range from soft to rough and may include fleece, moleskin, a piece of terry cloth or velvet, closed cell foam, small grit sandpaper, and Velcro® hook. The textures are rated according to tolerance: comfortable to irritating. The client is then asked to place the hand in the immersion textures, which may include cotton balls, beads, or uncooked split peas, beans, rice, popcorn, or pasta noodles. The immersion particles are also rated according to tolerance; comfortable to irritating. The client is then assigned the textures and particles that are tolerable for five to ten minutes. Instructions for home include rubbing the textures on the fingertip and immersing the hand in the particles for five to ten minutes, three to four times a day. Progression through the program is made as the client tolerates more challenging textures and immersion particles. Home exercise programs for desensitization may also include exposure to vibration, however from clinical experience, vibrators with multiple settings that are tolerable to the client are difficult to obtain and issue for home use.

Physical Agent Modalities

A physical agent modality (PAM) is any intervention that produces a change in soft tissue through the use of temperature, sound, or electricity. Modalities are used in OT to prepare the client for engagement in purposeful activity. Cold packs, paraffin heat, hot packs, fluidotherapy, whirlpool, ultrasound, neuromuscular electrical stimulation (NMES), and transcutaneous electrical nerve stimulation (TENS) are all modalities that are used in UE rehabilitation. For complete coverage of physical agent modalities, please refer to Chapter 18. There are contraindications to using modalities, and the OT practitioner must have knowledge of the client's medical history and consider how the modality may impact their condition. Furthermore, PAMs should always be used as an adjunct to occupation-based treatment. Regulatory boards in several states dictate competency requirements in order to use PAMs, therefore they should always be performed within the guidelines and regulations of the OT practitioner's state, province, and/or and facility.[62]

Ergonomic Design

Treating the client who is an injured worker can be a challenge, as the wrist and hand are often used for repetitive tasks with the performance of work activities. **Ergonomics** is the study of the musculoskeletal system and how to modify tools and work environments to ensure the body works efficiently and safely. Having knowledge in the area of ergonomics will assist in treating the client who will be returning to work. To begin an ergonomic assessment, obtain a job description and review it with the client, as he or she knows the requirements that are needed to perform their job. If possible, complete a job analysis by videotaping or watching the actual job being performed, making note of risk factors including work environment temperatures, repetition, time cycles for completion of tasks, postures, vibration, and required lifting.[74] Suggestions for modifications in tool use, posture, grip, and workstation design can then be made, to ease with the transition of returning to work. As the occupational therapist and OTA spend time in treatment with the client, they may identify further needs in the area of ergonomics. Clients may discuss portions of their job that may be difficult to perform or may cause exacerbation of their symptoms. The OT practitioner will assist in problem-solving and make recommendations as needed. Recommendations often include the use of padded gloves to decrease exposure to vibration, ergonomic handles on tools to place the wrist in neutral when gripping, and modifications in seat and table height to promote proper posture. For the OT professional unfamiliar with ergonomics, there are a variety of resources available in print and online. Many OT practitioners choose to specialize in this field. The specialized practice of ergonomics provides consultation to industries collaborating with design engineers to adapt work environments and establish prevention programs in order to decrease stress on the worker.

Joint Protection

Joint protection principles are often used in chronic conditions that affect the hands and upper extremities. They are typically included in the treatment of rheumatoid arthritis and osteoarthritis, but may also be used with the client who has sustained an injury. The goals of joint protection principles are to provide education to the client in order to reduce joint stress and pain and to ensure integrity of joint structures. Joint protection principles should include an explanation and examples of the following: respecting and minimizing pain, avoiding positions of deformity/joint stress, using the larger more stable joints, avoiding sustained postures, and pacing activities.[76] Joint protection principles also encourage the use of adaptive equipment to decrease joint pain, to prevent further deformity or injury, and to increase independence with the performance of self-care tasks. See chapter 21 for more information on arthritis.

TECHNOLOGY AND TRENDS

The brightly-colored tape is seen on the skin of athletes in every sport and venue. This elastic tape, known as Kinesio Tape®, has become a popular treatment intervention for OT practitioners when treating conditions of the upper extremity. For many years, athletic trainers have used taping to stabilize joints during sports. In 1973, chiropractor Kenzo Kase developed Kinesio Tape®, as an alternative tape; it is less rigid than other tape and mimics the elastic properties of skin and muscle. Dr. Kase developed this tape to decrease pain, improve lymphatic flow, facilitate and inhibit muscle function, and to provide joint support.[75] Like most treatment interventions, the application of Kinesio Tape® will be dependent on the client, the treatment goals, and the diagnosis. When applied to the skin, the elastic tape can stay in place for 3 days. The tape can also withstand exposure to water, so it does not have to be removed for bathing. Copious research is beginning to emerge about the efficacy of this treatment intervention, and it is often used in UE rehabilitation. For more information regarding use of Kinesio Tape®, visit www.kinesiotaping.com.

Instruction in Use of Adaptive Equipment and Activity Modification

It is important to remember that the use of adaptive equipment along with activity modification will facilitate the use of the client's UE during the performance of functional activities. Incorporating the injured extremity into functional activities is beneficial for physical and psychological healing, therefore the use of adaptive equipment to improve occupational performance should be addressed within the first few treatment sessions.[15] Currently, adaptive equipment is readily available including tools, pens, and self-care aids with built-up handles. Padded work gloves, ergonomic tools, and modifications in workstation design will also assist with the client's return to work. If a tool is not available, OT practitioners are uniquely equipped to use creativity to fabricate a piece of adaptive equipment or to suggest alternative ways of performing tasks. Suggestions for activity modification for a client with lateral epicondylitis may include carrying groceries in a single paper bag close to the chest to avoid combined elbow and wrist extension, which occurs when carrying several plastic bags at one time. For the musician, activity modification may include decreasing the time in practice sessions or using adaptive equipment that evenly distributes the load of an instrument when practicing for long periods. Performing postural exercises during frequent rest breaks and placing a computer monitor directly in front of the client are also ways to modify activities for a data entry operator. Activity modification should be discussed during the therapy session, along with exploration of the client's adaptive equipment needs, in order to accomplish self-care, IADL, leisure, and return-to-work goals that have been established as part of the treatment plan.

Strengthening Exercises

After injury or immobilization, muscles in the UE become weak and may even have to work harder due to scarring and joint stiffness. Resistive exercises are used in therapy, and as part of a home exercise program to improve strength. Strengthening exercises can be classified as isometric, isotonic, or isokinetic.[77] **Isometric** exercises are performed when the muscle contracts, however the joint does not move. Isometric exercises are beneficial for arthritic conditions and when the joints surrounding the muscle should not be stressed.[45] An example would include pushing the hand into the table without moving the hand or wrist or tightening up on a ball that does not squeeze (e.g., basketball) for finger flexion. Isometric exercises are also used with arthritic conditions to keep the muscles active without placing stress on the arthritic joints. **Isotonic** exercises are performed with weights or elastic bands and provide a constant amount of resistance throughout the full ROM. Isotonic exercises are used after a fracture is healed to strengthen the muscles surrounding the involved joints. Isotonic exercises are performed after a wrist fracture, using a light resistive band to strengthen the muscles in the forearm. As the client is able to tolerate an increase in resistive activities, a stronger elastic band or weight is used. **Isokinetic** exercises provide a changing resistance with a constant velocity, which allows for maximal force throughout the full ROM. Isokinetic exercises require specialized equipment to produce the varying resistance and constant velocity. This type of strengthening program is not as common in the treatment of UE injuries as the specialized equipment may not be available to the OT practitioner. Before initiating a strengthening program, it is important to review the diagnosis and client condition, as the type of strengthening program will depend on the diagnosis and the stage of tissue healing. Strengthening exercises should also involve muscle groups that work synergistically to perform functional activities. For example, squeezing therapy putty is preferred over squeezing a ball, as it allows greater ROM, has finger flexors working synergistically with wrist extension stabilizers, and the amount of resistance is easy to monitor and adjust (Fig. 22-26). Using weights while reaching in diagonal patterns also facilitates the use of the UE, within normal movement patterns, thus strengthening muscles for carryover during the performance of functional activities.

Graded Motor Imagery

Graded motor imagery is a technique to treat chronic pain in the UE.[78] Graded motor imagery uses three steps to influence the sensorimotor cortex in the brain; laterality training, imagined hand movements, and MVF. The first step, laterality training, asks the client to identify pictures of hands as either right or left. The client is assessed for time and accuracy. The client continues with laterality training until he or she is able to identify the images correctly and without pain. The goal of laterality training is to reestablish the concept of "right" and "left" within the brain. In the second phase, imagined hand movements, clients imagine that they are moving their own hand to match the images on the cards. In order to decrease the association between pain and movement, clients try to imagine the movement is done without pain. Once clients are able to imagine the images without pain, they progress toward use of a mirror box for mirror visual feedback (see Fig. 22-24). When using the mirror box, clients are instructed to place the painful hand inside the box and the uninvolved hand outside of the box. They are then instructed to move the uninvolved hand and watch the mirrored hand motions. If clients do not experience pain, they are then instructed to move both hands while watching the mirror.[78] Graded motor imagery has been used with clients diagnosed with CRPS; however, more research is needed to support the efficacy of this treatment technique with other diagnoses.

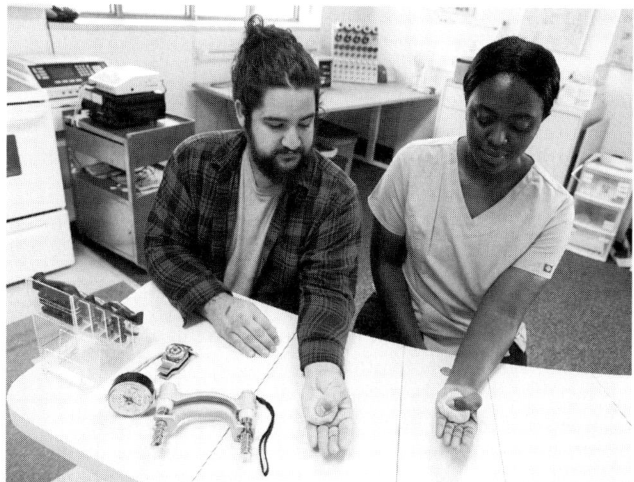

FIGURE 22-26. Client using therapyputty for range of motion and grip strengthening.

SUMMARY

This chapter reviewed the anatomy of the wrist and hand, discussed the principles of tissue healing, explored common diagnoses seen, and discovered the variety of treatment modalities available to the OT practitioner when treating conditions of the hand and UE. OTAs are well equipped to collaborate with the occupational therapist to provide a comprehensive evaluation, determine the functional deficits of the client, and to collaborate to address these deficits through treatment planning and implementation. This knowledge is the basis for OT treatment interventions and will assist in returning the client with a UE condition to his or her occupational performance roles.

REVIEW QUESTIONS

1. The occupational therapist completed a careful evaluation on the hand of an injured worker as he uses his wrist and hand to perform gripping and the manipulation of small

objects. An OTA will see the client on the first return appointment. Which three of the following should this treatment session include?
a. A sensory evaluation
b. Review of the home exercise program
c. A discussion regarding activities that exacerbate symptoms
d. A client-reported outcome measure
e. Modalities that the client is requesting and that are part of the plan of care
f. A workplace evaluation

2. The client is a 52-year-old female who lacerated her extensor tendon in the left middle finger and is three days after a tendon repair. What is her treatment likely to include?
a. A dynamic orthosis for flexion
b. ROM and strength testing
c. A protective orthosis, suture care, and dressing changes
d. Ergonomics and return-to-work training

3. You have a new client who is being seen after a tendon laceration and repair in your outpatient clinic. For this client, which of the following statements regarding strength testing is true?
a. Strength should always be assessed on the first therapy visit.
b. Strength testing should only be performed when the client's condition is stable.
c. Only the treating occupational therapist may perform strength testing.
d. Strength is tested on a scale from 1 to 10.

4. After reviewing the initial evaluation, you find that your client has muscle strength of zero in the right dominant wrist extensors. Which three of the following *best* describe your client?
a. Has normal strength at this time
b. Is able to take resistance when pulled into extension
c. Is unable to lift the wrist up against gravity
d. Is unable to flex the wrist
e. Has difficulty using a hairbrush or screwdriver
f. Is able to actively grasp and release a foam ball

5. A self-reported outcome measure is usually performed at the time of evaluation and at the time of reassessment. The OTA can help to gather this data, which:
a. Measures progress over time
b. Provides information from the caregiver's perspective
c. Provides an objective measure comparable to ROM measurements
d. Wastes the therapist's and client's time

6. You received an order from the physician to fabricate an orthosis for a client with a fracture. Which of the following terms are used to describe fractures in the upper extremity and may be written on the order:
a. Closed, open, displaced
b. Painful, swollen, red
c. Hot, itchy, uncomfortable
d. Cold, mild, severe

7. Your client had a flexor tendon repair to the right dominant hand one week ago. Which of the following is the *most likely* current course of treatment for the client?
a. Active exercises and no protective orthosis
b. Sutures in place with a dorsal blocking protective orthosis
c. A protective extension orthosis just to the finger
d. A cast over the ulnar two digits with the MP joints flexed

8. Mr. Stein has difficulty placing his hand into his jeans pocket due to the inability to extend his ring finger. Which of the following conditions is Mr. Stein *most likely* experiencing?
a. Dupuytren's contracture
b. Carpal tunnel syndrome
c. de Quervain's
d. Rotator cuff impingement

9. Mrs. Mullis is recovering from hand surgery, and comes to her outpatient OT appointment noting increased pain in her incision. The OTA uncovers the incision and is immediately concerned about infection. Which of the following are the visual signs of infection in a wound?
a. Tight, red, purple
b. Open, blue, painful
c. Black and dry
d. Yellow and exuding pus

10. An OTA has been working with a client with painful CMC joint osteoarthritis. Which of the following does the treatment plan *most likely* include?
a. A supportive brace, modalities for pain relief, and instruction in joint protection principles
b. A strengthening program, wound care, and graded motor imagery
c. Graded motor imagery, electrical stimulation, and edema management
d. Edema management, wound care, and ice

CASE STUDY

Lindsay is a 28-year-old female with recent onset of pain at the radial side of her wrist and thumb. Lindsay is married and has an eight-month-old baby. She also works as a hairdresser part time. Lindsay's pain is worse at rest after she has been performing activities that require combined wrist and hand movements. Lindsay was seen by her family practice physician and referred to outpatient OT for treatment to her right dominant wrist and thumb pain. The evaluating therapist indicated that Lindsay had a positive Finkelstein's test.

1. What do you think Lindsay's diagnosis is?
2. What would be the goals of Lindsay's treatment?
3. What type of therapeutic interventions should be used?
4. Create a treatment session for Lindsay, and carefully consider the types of treatment interventions you will use. In what order will you provide these treatment interventions? Are there any precautions or contraindications?

PUTTING IT ALL TOGETHER — Sample Treatment and Documentation

Setting

Outpatient occupational therapy clinic

Client Profile

Suzanne is a 59-year-old female s/p left distal radius fracture from a fall while teaching an exercise class. She is now 2½ weeks s/p ORIF for the distal radius fracture. She was seen by her physician earlier in the week, and her sutures were removed. She was issued a prefabricated removable wrist brace and was instructed to begin AROM to the left wrist and fingers.

Work History

Teaches an exercise class with emphasis in dancing. Assists her husband on the weekends as they own a parking lot near the local stadium and sell parking spaces during events.

Insurance

Private insurance with preauthorization required after 20 visits. Preauthorization is also required for any custom orthosis.

Psychological

Has a positive attitude, but is anxious to return to her exercise program

Social

Lives at home with her husband who works full time. He has two older children that live in the area and three grandchildren under the age of 8. She has a cat and is very active in her church community. Volunteers delivering meals on wheels two days per month.

Cognitive

No deficits noted, however does not like to have too much "down" time

Motor, Integument, Sensation, Pain, and Manual Muscle Testing (MMT)

- AROM left wrist: Flexion 20 degrees, extension 30 degrees, ulnar deviation 5 degrees, radial deviation 10 degrees, pronation 80 degrees, supination 40 degrees
- AROM left digits: Limited into composite flexion due to mild inflammation with 0.5 cm from fingertips of all digits to distal palmar crease
- Thumb MP joint: Flexion 0–45 degrees, and IP 0–30
- Remainder of left UE AROM is within normal limits
- Volumetric measurement of the left wrist and hand is 25 mL greater than the right
- Scar at volar wrist from surgical repair is tight and hypersensitive to touch
- Pain at rest is a 2/10 and with activity is a 4/10.
- Strength has not been assessed due to the acuteness of the condition

ADL

- Dressing difficulty: Buttons, zippers, socks, shoe tying, fastening bra
- Bathing difficulty: Having a difficult time reaching under the right arm
- Sleeping difficulty: Unable to find a comfortable sleeping position, pain with pushing up from sit to stand
- Unable to tolerate her shirtsleeve rubbing on her wrist scar

IADL

- Currently requires assist with homemaking activities, driving, meal preparation, and unable to perform regular work activities

Goals

Within 4 weeks:

1. Client will have an increase in thumb and finger active ROM to within normal limits for independence with fastening buttons and zippers.
2. Client will have an increase in left wrist flexion and extension by 20 degrees for using the left hand when bathing the right side of the body.
3. Client will have an increase in left wrist supination by 30 degrees for opening doors and containers.
4. Client will have a decrease in volumetric edema measurement to within normal limits to facilitate an increase in composite flexion for gripping objects.
5. Client will have a decrease in scar hypersensitivity in order to tolerate her clothing against her scar/skin at the wrist.
6. Client will have a decrease in reported pain to 0/10 with rest and activity for return to pushing up from sit to stand.
7. Client will demonstrate independence in her home exercise program addressing ROM, scar, and edema management to increase participation in ADL's.
8. Client will tolerate strength testing at 4 weeks s/p ORIF and her home exercise program will be upgraded to include strengthening as indicated.

OT TREATMENT SESSION 1

THERAPEUTIC ACTIVITY	TIME	GOAL(S) ADDRESSED	OTA RATIONALE
Fluidotherapy preparatory heat to allow active ROM to the fingers and wrist. Fluidotherapy also acts to desensitize the scar. Heat set to 110 degrees in attempt to keep swelling to a minimum.	15 min	#1, #2, #3, #5, and #6	*Preparatory Method:* PAM (fluidotherapy) can improve soft-tissue extensibility to allow for greater AROM. Fluidotherapy can also be used to desensitize scars.

Continued

PUTTING IT ALL TOGETHER Sample Treatment and Documentation (continued)

THERAPEUTIC ACTIVITY	TIME	GOAL(S) ADDRESSED	OTA RATIONALE
Manual Edema Mobilization in conjunction with scar/soft-tissue mobilization to decrease edema and desensitize volar wrist scar	18 min	#4, #5, and #6	*Preparatory Method; Education and Training:* Manual Edema Mobilization will assist in decreasing edema in wrist and fingers while soft-tissue work also assists in softening and desensitizing scars. A decrease in edema and scarring will improve ROM and functional use of the extremity.
Therapeutic exercise and activities to facilitate return to normal hand use and to use tissues that have been heated and stretched to maintain motion gained	26 min	#1-#7	*Preparatory Task and Training:* Performed after the heat and soft-tissue mobilization. PROM to thumb and digits with gentle overpressure followed by AROM to the thumb, digits, and wrist in all planes of motion. Also completed functional tasks with gentle gripping, reaching, turning, and manipulating objects to use ROM gained in treatment. Trained in HEP for carryover at home. HEP is checked with each visit to ensure adherence to program and to make any necessary changes/upgrades.

SOAP note: 9/3/—, 10:00 am–10:59 am

S: Client states, "I hope I will be able to turn my palm up so I can help my husband collect parking money."

O: Client participated on this date in outpatient OT to address limitations in ROM, pain, edema, and scarring related to ORIF distal radius fracture. Client received fluidotherapy prep heat at 110 degrees for 15 minutes followed by manual edema mobilization to decrease edema localized to digits and wrist. Scar and soft-tissue mobilization were performed to decrease scar hypersensitivity and to improve ROM at the wrist. Client educated in AROM exercises with blocking and tendon glides to thumb and fingers followed by gentle PROM and overpressure to digits by OTA. AROM was then completed at the wrist in all planes of motion with the client gently gripping a small cylinder to isolate wrist motion and to prevent compensatory motions from the long finger flexors and extensors. HEP was reviewed and encouraged throughout treatment.

A: Client presented with gains in wrist AROM all planes of motion and finger ROM was WNL after therapy this date. Pain has now decreased with 1/10 at rest and 0/10 with activity. Client appeared fearful to use the left digits however was more confident after performing functional activities within the clinic setting.

P: Will continue 2 times weekly per initial plan of care to improve AROM in the left wrist and hand for carryover into increased independence with the performance of self-care tasks.

Jane Brooker, COTA/L, 9/3/—, 3:15 pm

TREATMENT SESSION 2

What could you do next with this client?

TREATMENT SESSION 3

What could you do next with this client?

REFERENCES

1. Reilly, M. (1961). Slagle lecture. Retrieved from https://www.asht.org/
2. Hansen, J. (2014) *Netter's clinical anatomy* (3rd ed.). Philadelphia, PA: Saunders.
3. Kijima, Y., & Viegas, S. (2009). Wrist anatomy and biomechanics. *The Journal of Hand Surgery, 34,* 1555–1563.
4. Ryu, J., Cooney, W., Askew, L., An, K., & Chao, E. (1991). Functional ranges of motion of the wrist joint. *The Journal of Hand Surgery, 16,* 409–419.
5. Fess, E., Gettle, K., Philips, C., & Janson, R. (2005). *Hand and upper extremity splinting: Principles and methods* (3rd ed.). St. Louis, MO: Mosby.
6. Kenney, R., & Hammert, W. (2014). Physical examination of the hand. *The Journal of Hand Surgery, 39,* 2324–2334.
7. Norkin, C., & White, J. (1985). *Measurement of joint motion: A guide to goniometry.* Philadelphia, PA: F. A. Davis.
8. Hisop, H., & Montegomery, J. (1995). *Daniels and Worthingham's muscle testing: Techniques of manual examination* (6th ed.). Philadelphia, PA: W. B. Saunders.
9. American Society of Hand Therapists. (1982). *Clinical assessment recommendations.* Mount Laurel, NJ: ASHT.
10. Krotoski, J. B. (2011). Sensibility testing: History, instrumentation, and clinical procedures. In T. Skirven, L. Osterman, J. Fedorczyk, & P. Amadio (Eds.), *Rehabilitation of the hand and upper extremity* (6th ed.). St. Louis, MO: Mosby.
11. Dellon, E. S., Mourey, R., & Dellon, A. L. (1992). Human pressure perception values for constant and moving one- and two-point discrimination. *Journal of Plastic and Reconstructive Surgery, 90,* 112-117.
12. Moberg, E. (1958). Objective methods of determining the functional value of sensibility of the hand. *Journal of Bone and Joint Surgery, 40,* 454–476.
13. Pellicchia, G. (2003). Figure of eight method of measuring hand size: Reliability and concurrent validity. *Journal of Hand Therapy, 16,* 300–304.
14. Seftchick, J., Detullio, L., Fedorczyk, J., & Aulicino, P. (2011). Clinical examination of the hand. In T. Skirven, L. Osterman, J. Fedorczyk, & P. Amadio (Eds.), *Rehabilitation of the hand and upper extremity* (6th ed.). St. Louis, MO: Mosby.
15. Powell, R., & von der Heyde, R. (2014). The inclusion of activities of daily living in flexor tendon rehabilitation: A survey. *Journal of Hand Therapy, 27,* 23–29.

16. Portney, L., & Watkins, M. (2009). *Foundations of clinical research.* Upper Saddle River, NJ: Prentice Hall.
17. Yancosek, K., & Howell, D. (2009). A narrative review of dexterity assessments. *Journal of Hand Therapy, 22,* 258–270.
18. Kennedy, C. A., Beaton, D. E., Solway, S., McConnell, S., & Bombardier, C. (2011). *Disabilities of the arm, shoulder and hand (DASH). The DASH and quick DASH outcome measure user's manual* (3rd ed.). Toronto, Ontario: Institute for Work & Health.
19. MacDermid J. C., Tottenham, V. (2004). Responsiveness of the disability of the arm, shoulder, and hand (DASH) and patient-rated wrist/hand evaluation (PRWHE) in evaluating change after hand therapy. *Journal of Hand Therapy, 17,* 18–23.
20. Law, M., Baptiste, S., Carswell, A., McColl, M., Polatajko, H., & Pollock, N. (1998). *Canadian occupational performance measure* (3rd ed.). Ottawa, Ontario: CAOT Publications.
21. LaStayo, P., & Howell, J. (1995). Clinical provocative tests used in evaluating wrist pain: A descriptive study. *Journal of Hand Therapy, 8,* 10–17.
22. Rekant, M. (2011). Diagnosis and management of cubital tunnel syndrome. In T. Skirven, L. Osterman, J. Fedorczyk, & P. Amadio (Eds.), *Rehabilitation of the hand and upper extremity* (6th ed.). St. Louis, MO: Mosby.
23. Vincent, J., MacDermid, J., Michlovitz, S., Rafuse, R., Wells-Rowsell, C., Wong, O., & Bisbee, L. (2014). The push-off test: Development of a simple, reliable test of upper extremity weight-bearing capability. *Journal of Hand Therapy, 27,* 185–191.
24. Valdes, K., & LaStayo, P. (2013). The value of provocative tests for the wrist and elbow: A literature review. *Journal of Hand Therapy, 26,* 32–43.
25. Budoff, J. E. (2010). Mucous cysts. *Journal of Hand Surgery, 35,* 828–830.
26. Hurst, L. (2011). Dupytren's disease. In T. Skirven, L. Osterman, J. Fedorczyk, & P. Amadio (Eds.), *Rehabilitation of the hand and upper extremity* (6th ed.). St. Louis, MO: Mosby.
27. Jebson, P. J. L., & Kasdan, M. L. (1998). *Hand secrets.* Philadelphia, PA: Hanley and Belfus.
28. American Society of Hand Therapists. (2014). What is a trigger finger? Retrieved from https://www.asht.org/sites/default/files/downloads/2014/trigger_finger_2014.pdf?
29. Taras, J., Martyak, G., & Steelman, P. (2011). Primary care of flexor tendon injuries. In T. Skirven, L. Osterman, J. Fedorczyk, & P. Amadio (Eds.), *Rehabilitation of the hand and upper extremity* (6th ed.). St. Louis, MO: Mosby
30. Evans, R. (2012). Managing the injured tendon: Current concepts. *Journal of Hand Therapy, 25,* 173–190.
31. Howell, J., Merritt, W., & Robinson, S. (2005). Immediate controlled active motion following zone 4–7 extensor tendon repair. *Journal of Hand Therapy, 18,* 182–190.
32. Sameem, M., Ignacy, T., Thoma, A., & Strumas, N. (2011). A systematic review of rehabilitation protocols after surgical repair of the extensor tendons in zones 5-8 of the hand. *Journal of Hand Therapy, 24,* 365–373.
33. Hardy, M. A. (2004). Principles of metacarpal and phalangeal fracture management: A review of rehabilitation concepts. *Journal of Orthopedic Sports Physical Therapy, 34,* 781–799.
34. LaStayo, P., Winters, K., Hardy, M. (2003). Fracture healing: bone healing, fracture management, and current concepts related to the hand. *Journal of Hand Therapy, 16,* 81–93.
35. Cannon, N. (Ed.). (2001). *Diagnosis and treatment manual for physicians and therapists: Upper extremity rehabilitation* (4th ed.). Indianapolis, IN: The Hand Center of Indiana.
36. Ibrahim, T., Qureshi, A., Sutton, A., & Dias, J. (2011). Surgical versus nonsurgical treatment of acute minimally displaced and undisplaced scaphoid waist fractures: Pairwise and network meta-analyses of randomized controlled trials. *The Journal of Hand Surgery, 36,* 1759–1768.
37. Meals, C., & Meals, R. (2013). Hand fractures: A review of current treatment strategies. *The Journal of Hand Surgery, 38,* 1021–1031.
38. Wadsworth, M. C., Barch, E., & Erickson, M. (2011). *The wrist and hand: Physical therapy patient management using current evidence.* Current Concepts of Orthopaedic Physical Therapy (3rd ed.). LaCrosse, WI: APTA.
39. Feehan, L. (2011). Extra-articular hand fractures, part II: Therapist's management. In T. Skirven, L. Osterman, J. Fedorczyk, & P. Amadio (Eds.), *Rehabilitation of the hand and upper extremity* (6th ed.). St. Louis, MO: Mosby.
40. Shah, C. M., & Sommerkamp, T. G. (2014). Fracture dislocation of the finger joints. *The Journal of Hand Surgery, 39,* 792–802.
41. Chinchalkar, S., & Gan, B. S. (2003). Management of proximal interphalangeal joint fractures and dislocations. *Journal of Hand Therapy, 16,* 117–128.
42. Kevin J., Little, K. J., & Jacoby, S. M. (2011). Intra-articular hand fractures and joint injuries. In T. Skirven, L. Osterman, J. Fedorczyk, & P. Amadio (Eds.), *Rehabilitation of the hand and upper extremity* (6th ed.). St. Louis, MO: Mosby.
43. Poole, J. U., Pellegrini, V. D. (2000). Arthritis of the thumb basal joint complex. *Journal of Hand Therapy, 13,* 91–107.
44. Gomes Carreira, A., Jones, A., & Natour, J. (2010). Assessment of the effectiveness of a functional splint for osteoarthritis of the trapeziometacarpal joint of the dominant hand: A randomized controlled study. *Journal of Rehabilitation Medicine, 42*(5), 469–474.
45. Valdes, K., & von der Heyde, R. (2012). An exercise program for carpometacarpal osteoarthritis based on biomechanical principles. *Journal of Hand Therapy, 25,* 251–263.
46. Mary Bathen, M., & Gupta, R. (2011). Basic science of peripheral nerve injury and repair. In T. Skirven, L. Osterman, J. Fedorczyk, & P. Amadio (Eds.), *Rehabilitation of the hand and upper extremity* (6th ed.). St. Louis, MO: Mosby.
47. Koo, J., & Szabo, R. M. (2004). Compression neuropathies of the median nerve. *Journal of the American Society for Surgery of the Hand, 4,* 156–175.
48. Woo, A., Bakri, K., & Moran, S. (2015). Management of ulnar nerve injuries. *Journal of Hand Surgery, 40,* 173–181.
49. Aitken, J. (2008). Entrapment neuropathy of the ulnar nerve. *Journal of Hand Therapy, 21,* 300–301.
50. Markiewitz, A., & Merryman, J. (2005). Radial nerve compression in the upper extremity. *Journal of Hand Surgery, 5,* 87–99.
51. Slutsky, D. (2011). New advances in nerve repair. In T. Skirven, L. Osterman, J. Fedorczyk, & P. Amadio (Eds.), *Rehabilitation of the hand and upper extremity* (6th ed.). St. Louis, MO: Mosby.
52. Bell-Krotoski, J., Weinstein, S., & Weinstein, C. (1993). Testing sensibility, including touch-pressure, two-point discrimination, point localization, and vibration. *Journal of Hand Therapy, 6,* 114–123.
53. Rizzo, M. (2011). Complex injuries of the hand. In T. Skirven, L. Osterman, J. Fedorczyk, & P. Amadio (Eds.), *Rehabilitation of the hand and upper extremity* (6th ed.). St. Louis, MO: Mosby.
54. Mayo Clinic. (2015). What is CRPS? Retrieved from http://www.mayoclinic.org/diseases-conditions/complex-regional-pain-syndrome/basics/definition/con-20022844
55. Ciccone, D., Bandilla, E., & Wu, W. (1997). Psychological dysfunction in patients with reflex sympathetic dystrophy. *Pain, 71,* 322–333.
56. Koman, A., Li, Z., Patterson-Smith, B., & Smith, T. (2011). Complex regional pain syndrome type I and type II. In T. Skirven, L. Osterman, J. Fedorczyk, & P. Amadio (Eds.), *Rehabilitation of the hand and upper extremity* (6th ed.). St. Louis, MO: Mosby
57. Galer, B., Henderson, J., Perande, J., & Jensen, M. P. (2000). Course of symptoms and quality of life measurement in complex regional pain syndrome: A pilot study. *Journal of Pain and Symptom Management, 20,* 286–292.
58. American Occupational Therapy Association. (2013). *Occupational therapy scope of practice.* Retrieved from http://www.aota.org/-/media/Corporate/Files/AboutAOTA/OfficialDocs/Position/Scope-of-Practice-edited-2014.PDF
59. Chesney, A., Chauhan, A., Kattan, A., Farrokhyar, F., & Thomas, A. (2011). Systematic review of flexor tendon rehabilitation protocols in zone II of the hand. *Journal of Plastic and Reconstructive Surgery, 127,* 1583–1592.
60. Che Daud, A. Z., Yau, M. K., Barnett, F., Judd, J., Jones, R. E., & Muhammad Nawawi, R. F. (2016). Integration of occupation based

intervention in hand injury rehabilitation: A randomized controlled trial. *Journal of Hand Therapy, 29*(1), 30–40.

61. Grice, K. O. (2015). The use of occupation-based assessments and intervention in the hand therapy setting: A survey. *Journal of Hand Therapy: Scientific/Clinical Article*, 28, 300-306.
62. Bracciano, A. G. (2008). *Physical agent modalities: Theory and application for the occupational therapist* (2nd ed.). Thorofare, NJ: Slack.
63. Davidson, J. (1998). Wound repair. *Journal of Hand Therapy*, 11, 80–94.
64. Reiffel, R. S. (1995). Prevention of hypertrophic scars by long term paper tape application. *Journal of Plastic and Reconstructive Surgery, 96*, 1715–1718.
65. Von Der Hyde, R., & Evans, R. (2011). Wound classification and management. In T. Skirven, L. Osterman, J. Fedorczyk, & P. Amadio (Eds.), *Rehabilitation of the hand and upper extremity* (6th ed.). St. Louis, MO: Mosby.
66. Vilecco, J. (2011). Edema. In T. Skirven, L. Osterman, J. Fedorczyk, & P. Amadio (Eds.), *Rehabilitation of the hand and upper extremity* (6th ed.). St. Louis, MO: Mosby.
67. Artzberger, S. (2006). Edema reduction techniques: a biologic rationale for selection. In C. Cooper (Ed.), *Fundamentals of hand therapy: Clinical reasoning and treatment guidelines for common diagnoses of the upper extremity*. St. Louis, MO: Elsevier.
68. Artzberger, S., & Priganc, V. (2011). Manual edema mobilization: An edema reduction technique for the orthopedic patient. In T. Skirven, L. Osterman, J. Fedorczyk, & P. Amadio (Eds.), *Rehabilitation of the hand and upper extremity* (6th ed.). St. Louis, MO: Mosby.
69. Elbert, T., & Rockstroh, B. (2004). Reorganization of human cerebral cortex: The range of changes following use and injury. *Neuroscientist, 10*, 129–141.
70. Merzenich, M. M., & Jenkins, W. M. (1993). Reorganization of cortical representations of the hand following alterations of skin inputs induced by nerve injury, skin island transfers, and experience. *Journal of Hand Therapy, 6*, 89–104.
71. Rosen, B., & Lundborg, G. (2011). Sensory re-education. In T. Skirven, L. Osterman, J. Fedorczyk, & P. Amadio (Eds.), *Rehabilitation of the hand and upper extremity* (6th ed.). St. Louis, MO: Mosby
72. Dellon, A. L. (1978). The moving two-point discrimination test: Clinical evaluation of the quickly adapting fiber/receptor system. *Journal of Hand Surgery. 3*, 474–481.
73. Barber, L. (2011). Desensitization of the traumatized hand. In T. Skirven, L. Osterman, J. Fedorczyk, & P. Amadio (Eds.), *Rehabilitation of the hand and upper extremity* (6th ed.). St. Louis, MO: Mosby.
74. Ulin, S., & Armstrong, T. (2011). Analysis and design of jobs for control of work-related upper limb musculoskeletal disorders. In T. Skirven, L. Osterman, J. Fedorczyk, & P. Amadio (Eds.), *Rehabilitation of the hand and upper extremity* (6th ed.). St. Louis, MO: Mosby.
75. Copee, R. (2011). Elastic taping (kinesiotaping method). In T. Skirven, L. Osterman, J. Fedorczyk, & P. Amadio (Eds.), *Rehabilitation of the hand and upper extremity* (6th ed.). St. Louis, MO: Mosby.
76. Pedretti, L. W. (1996). *Occupational therapy: Practice skills for physical dysfunction* (4th ed.). St. Louis, MO: Mosby.
77. Purkayastha, S., Cramer, J., Trowbridge, C., Fincher, A., & Marek, S. (2006). Surface EMG amplitude-to-work ratios during isokinetic and isotonic muscle actions. *Journal of Athletic Training, 41*, 314–320.
78. Priganc, V., & Stralka, S. (2011). Graded motor imagery. *Journal of Hand Therapy, 24*, 164–169.

Chapter 23

Orthopedic Considerations: The Shoulder

Salvador Bondoc, OTD, OTR/L, BCPR, CHT, FAOTA, and
Luis de Leon Arabit, OTD, MS, OTR/L, BCPR, C/NDT, PAM

LEARNING OUTCOMES

After studying this chapter, the student or practitioner will be able to:

23.1 Describe the anatomical and biomechanical considerations in shoulder treatment

23.2 Describe common shoulder orthopedic conditions in terms of their pathomechanics and general treatment considerations

23.3 Explain the assessment process for shoulder conditions

23.4 Discuss the unique role of occupational therapy in the management of shoulder orthopedic conditions

23.5 Relate the intervention approaches/methods and precautions to managing postsurgical shoulder orthopedic conditions

KEY TERMS

Arthroscopy
Bursa
Bursitis
Capsuloligamentous complex
Cryotherapy
Immobilization
Impingement syndrome
Joint laxity
Kinematics
Modalities
Repair and remodeling phase
Reverse total shoulder arthroplasty
Rotator cuff
Rotator cuff disease
Rotator cuff muscles
Shoulder instability
Synovial joints
Tendinitis
Tendinopathy
Tendinosis

Occupational therapy (OT) practitioners understand that the profession focuses on holistic care within every occupation, body function, and structure. Why, then, is a chapter that isolates one specific area of the upper body needed? The occupational therapy assistant (OTA) is mindful of treating the whole person; however, the shoulder, although an incredibly important joint for function and independence, is so easily mishandled. The shoulder is elegant in its design in that it provides wide arcing mobility while having the stability to maintain function. Shoulder pain and dysfunction can inhibit all the areas of occupation, including activities of daily living (ADLs), instrumental activities of daily living (IADLs), rest and sleep, education, work, play, leisure, and social participation. This chapter focuses primarily on shoulder anatomy and function, as well as orthopedic conditions and treatment, but further information on neurological shoulder conditions and management can be found in Chapter 33.

THE SHOULDER

The shoulder performs a multitude of functions in a wide range of occupations. These functions may be categorized in the following manner:

1. Reaching to bring the hand to an object (e.g., reaching for a cup)
2. Supporting the distal upper limb and the hand while manipulating, stabilizing, or transporting an object (e.g., opening a jar)
3. Funneling of body forces to accelerate and project the upper limb, such as during a throwing or striking motion (e.g., shooting a basketball or hitting a volleyball)
4. Supporting the body weight with the upper limb (e.g., leaning for support when rising from the bed)

The shoulder may compensate for a weakness or loss of mobility in the distal joints of the upper limb from the elbow to the fingers as well as the decreased or loss of lower limb function. Such compensatory action may lead to pain syndromes or dysfunctions of the shoulder, if not corrected. For reference, Table 22-1 from Chapter 22 notes every muscle of the shoulder with actions and nerve innervation as well as those of the elbow, wrist, and hand.

ANATOMY AND BIOMECHANICS

The shoulder complex consists of three bones: clavicle, scapula, and humerus. These bones articulate into three **synovial joints** (e.g., joints separated by synovial fluid and cartilage and encapsulated by a synovial membrane) which are the glenohumeral, acromioclavicular, and sternoclavicular joints (Fig. 23-1). Table 23-1 outlines each shoulder joint, its structural type, and its bony articulations. These joints work in synergy when producing functional movement. Therefore, a restriction or pathology in one can impact the function of the other and the overall function of the shoulder complex.

The shoulder complex also consists of two articulations or quasi-joints—the scapulothoracic and the acromiohumeral (subacromial) articulations. The scapula, which glides over the thorax, is essential in the dynamic stability of, and is intimately linked to, the function of the glenohumeral joint (GHJ). Movements of the humerus at the GHJ require the coupling of movements at the scapulothoracic articulation. For instance, as the humerus moves into shoulder flexion, the motion at the scapula (upward rotation) increases.[1] Thus, alterations in the stability and positioning of the scapula can cause functional disruptions in glenohumeral movement.[2] Table 23-2 demonstrates the synergy, known as scapulohumeral rhythm, between certain humeral movements at the GHJ, scapular movements and their prime movers.

An understanding of biomechanical relationships of the bones and joints of the shoulder complex and the muscles that support their functions is key to the successful management of conditions in the shoulder complex that impact occupational performance.

Muscles

The muscles that aid in shoulder movement include:

- *Serratus anterior:* Fixes the scapula into the thoracic wall and aids in rotation and abduction
- *Deltoid:* Different fibers of the muscle responsible for different actions, including humeral flexion and abduction and assisting the pectoralis muscle
- *Levator scapulae:* Rotates the scapula downward and elevates the scapula
- *Pectoralis major:* Humeral flexion, internal rotation, adduction
- *Pectoralis minor:* Medially rotates the scapula, protracts the scapula and moves the scapula inferiorly
- *Trapezius:* Scapular depression, upward rotation, elevation, and adduction
- *Rhomboid major and minor:* Downward rotation and retraction of the scapula
- *Teres major:* Humeral adduction, internal rotation, extension
- *Latissimus dorsi:* Humeral adduction, internal rotation, extension

Four muscles—supraspinatus, infraspinatus, teres minor, and subscapularis—make up the **rotator cuff** (Fig. 23-2). It stabilizes the shoulder and holds the head of the humerus into the glenoid cavity to maintain the principle shoulder joint.

- *Supraspinatus:* Humeral abduction—most active in first 15 degrees of movement
- *Infraspinatus:* External rotation, shoulder stability

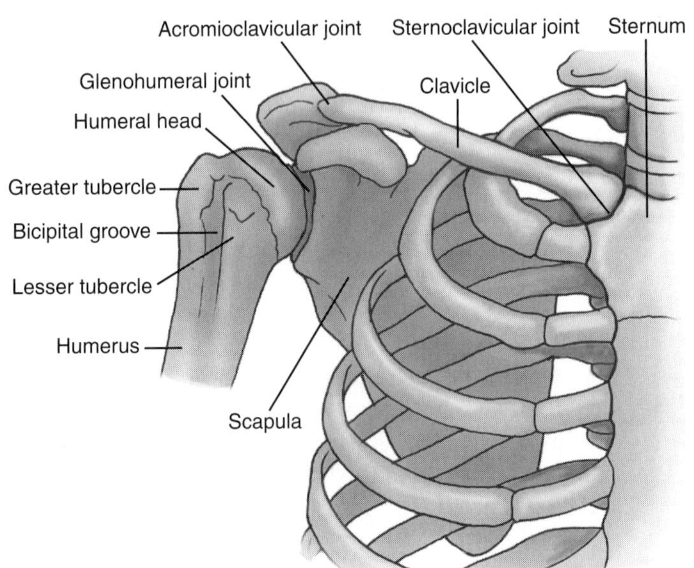

FIGURE 23-1. The anatomy and anatomical relationships among joints.

TABLE 23-1 Shoulder Joint, Structures, and Articulations

JOINT	JOINT TYPE	PROXIMAL BONE	DISTAL BONE
Sternoclavicular	Saddle shaped	Sternum (cartilage of the first rib)	Sternal (proximal) end of the clavicle
Acromioclavicular	Plane	Acromial (distal) end of the clavicle	Acromion of the scapula
Glenohumeral	Modified ball-and-socket	Glenoid fossa of the scapula	Head of the humerus

TABLE 23-2 Shoulder Scapulohumeral Rhythm

HUMERAL MOTION	SCAPULAR MOTION	SCAPULAR PRIME MOVERS
Flexion (with scaption* at the latter ranges)	Protraction (with upward rotation)	Serratus anterior Pectoralis major Pectoralis minor
Abduction or scaption	Upward rotation	Serratus anterior Upper trapezius Lower trapezius
Extension (with adduction)	Retraction (with downward rotation)	Trapezius Rhomboids

Scaption

*"Scaption" refers to the humeral motion 30° to 45° off the frontal plane.

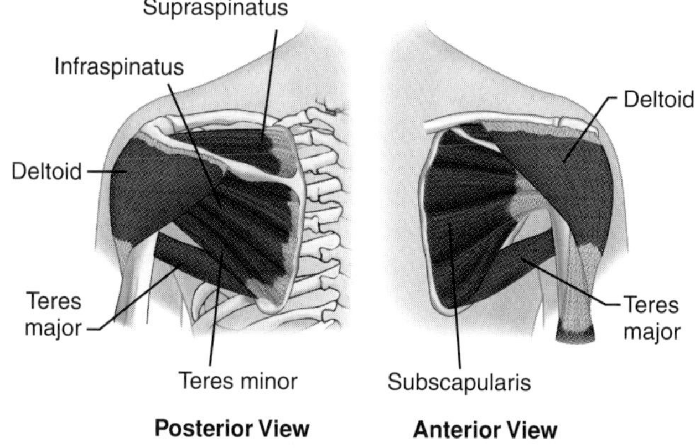

FIGURE 23-2. The four rotator cuff muscles.

- *Teres minor:* External rotation
- *Subscapularis:* Internal rotation

Kinematic Link

The complex functions identified at the beginning of the chapter are not isolated to the shoulder but inherently require the coordination of the entire body segment. This coordination involves the principle of kinematics. **Kinematics** is the study of motion, and a kinematic link is the relative motion which one part of a system (arm) has in relation to another part (trunk). Several studies point to the relationship between the upper extremity segments with the trunk postural segments, with the shoulder complex providing the kinematic link between these segments.[3,4] One simple illustration of this kinematic link is the shoulder complex mobility when the trunk is flexed versus when the trunk is appropriately extended. Flexion of the trunk restricts the ability of the scapula to glide over the rib cage during upward and downward rotations. The OTA may see this functionally with a client with rounded shoulders who cannot get his or her arms above 90 degrees at the shoulder, such as when a client has difficulty donning a shirt or combing the hair.

COMMON SHOULDER CONDITIONS

Shoulder pain is considered the third most common musculoskeletal condition after back and neck pain.[5] According to the Centers for Disease Control and Prevention, nearly 1.2 million people visited emergency departments in the United States in 2014 because of a shoulder condition.[6] The causes of musculoskeletal conditions of the shoulder vary but may be interrelated. Pathologies to the shoulder may occur as a result of sudden trauma, repetitive trauma from overuse, a gradual deterioration caused by age-related wear-and-tear, or disease-related degeneration (e.g., rheumatoid arthritis). Some conditions of the neck or cervical spine may also manifest with shoulder pain and dysfunction. It is important to rule out cervical pathology through an extensive evaluation, which may require referral to or consultation with specialists before addressing the shoulder pain.

Rotator Cuff Disease

The dynamic stability of the GHJ relies heavily on the health and function of the **rotator cuff muscles**—supraspinatus, infraspinatus, teres minor, and subscapularis, as a coordinated group (see Fig. 23-2). During shoulder movement, the rotator cuff muscles work together to maintain the stability of the humeral head and keep it appropriately centered on its axis of rotation about the glenoid fossa. The rotator cuff muscles work to counterbalance the deltoid, which produces a superior translation (upward movement) of the humeral head during such movements as flexion or abduction. Without the balancing counterforce exerted by the rotator cuff (acting as humeral depressors), the humeral head would impinge against and pivot about the coraco-acromial arch during humeral elevation (flexion, abduction). The lack of stability of the GHJ as a result of muscle imbalance has been identified to contribute in a variety of rotator cuff pathologies.[7] In addition to the collective function of the rotator cuff muscles, each muscle performs specific functions as noted above—that is, the supraspinatus abducts/elevates, the infraspinatus and teres minor rotate externally, and the subscapularis rotates the humerus internally. **Rotator cuff disease** can present in many different ways as described in the following sections.

Shoulder Instability

The vertical orientation and the shallowness of the articulating surfaces and the relatively loose surrounding capsuloligamentous structures are the reasons for the inherently unstable GHJ. As stated previously, the balance of muscles acting on the GHJ is crucial to a stable shoulder during functional performance. **Shoulder instability** is common in clients with hyperlax joints, but it may also occur in clients with normal **joint laxity** (loose ligaments). The most common mechanism for shoulder instability is trauma resulting from falls, athletics, or work-related injuries.[7] The degree of shoulder instability may range from unidirectional to multidirectional and from subluxation (mild slipping out of the fossa) to complete dislocation. Recurrent instability is common especially in the adolescent population[7] and may lead to persistent pain and disability into adulthood. In severe cases, and depending on the client's expectations, occupational choices, and lifestyle, surgery is indicated to avert pain and recurrent dislocations.

The objective of shoulder surgeries—be it open or arthroscopic—to treat shoulder instability is to tighten the glenohumeral capsule (Fig. 23-3). In the earlier stages of postsurgical rehabilitation, the OT practitioner must take precautions to avoid applying excessive stress while preventing scar adhesions and promoting restoration of normal glenohumeral kinematics. Further treatment will be described below.

Shoulder Impingement

Damage to the rotator cuff happens when the mechanical stress on the tissue exceeds its tensile strength (resistance to breaking under stress) and may range from degenerative inflammation to partial or complete tears. Repetitive strain or overuse leads to microtears and is often marked by an acute inflammatory reaction or **tendinitis.** Over time, when the rate of damage exceeds the rate of healing, the tendon degenerates, weakens, and becomes prone to further rupture. This tendon degeneration, which is also known as **tendinosis,** typically occurs at the supraspinatus and infraspinatus as a result of poor blood supply.[8] **Tendinopathy** refers to disease of the tendon. The clinical presentation includes tenderness on palpation and pain, often when exercising or with movement.

An inflammation of the **bursa,** which are fluid-filled sacs that surround and protect the shoulder, may also accompany the tendinitis or tendinosis. Often, **bursitis** (inflammation or irritation of the bursa) or shoulder tendinitis, is referred to as **impingement syndrome,** in the absence of an apparent rotator cuff tear (Fig. 23-4). Impingement specifically refers to the tendons and bursa becoming irritated, trapped, or compressed by movements at the shoulder. Weakness and damage to the components of the rotator cuff cause muscle imbalance and instability to the GHJ, especially during overhead motions. Structures between the humeral head and the coraco-acromial arch, such as the supraspinatus tendon, the subacromial bursa, and the long head of the biceps, become prone to impingement when the superiorly directed forces of the deltoid muscle are no longer counteracted effectively by the rotator cuff. Thus, bursitis, continuous damage to the rotator cuff, and tendinopathy of the long head of the biceps are secondary effects of glenohumeral instability.[9]

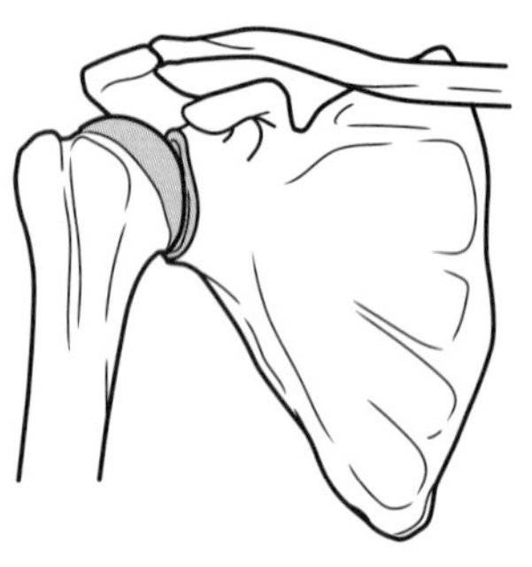

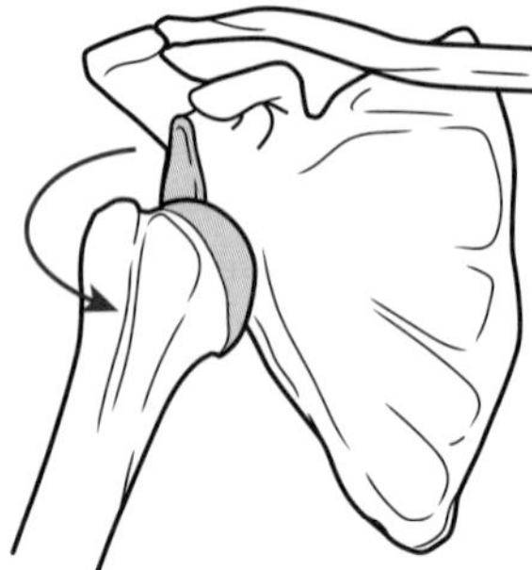

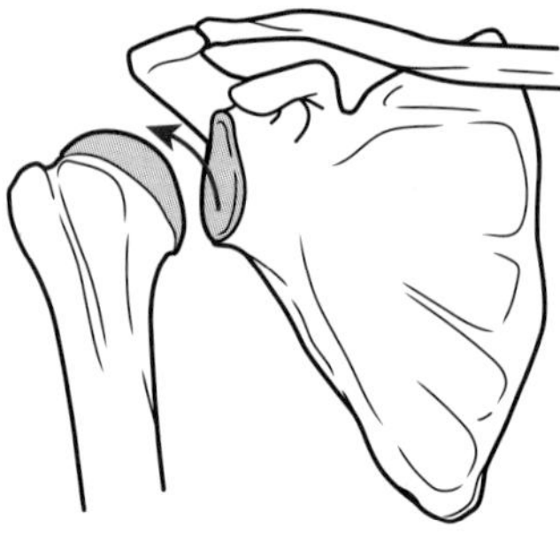

FIGURE 23-3. Glenohumeral configuration in normal and dislocated positions.

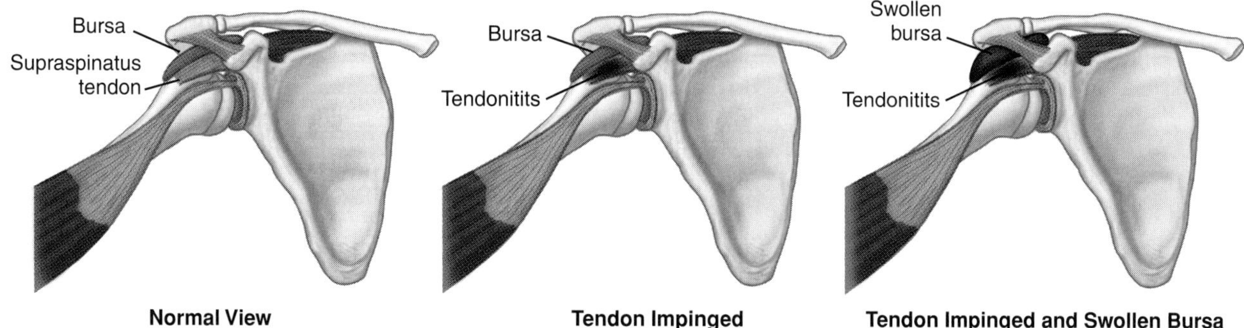

FIGURE 23-4. Impingement syndrome.

When the OT practitioner assesses the client with impingement syndrome, it is important to determine whether the condition is bursitis or a tendinopathy to appropriately apply the correct intervention modalities. This will be further elaborated in the "Shoulder Assessment" section.

Rotator Cuff Tear

Tears to the rotator cuff may be acute or chronic in nature and may be full or partial. Chronic tears of the rotator cuff are typically an extension of the shoulder impingement where microtears (tendinosis) leads to larger tears. Acute tears, in contrast, are associated with a singular, accelerating traumatic event, such as a fall on an outstretched hand (FOOSH) in the case of an older adult or a forceful overhand throw in the case of a younger adult. In acute situations, the rotator cuff tear may accompany other injuries, such as fractures and dislocations. Therefore, the approach to rehabilitation for acute tears would be different from chronic tears. Furthermore, the choice of medical–surgical management may vary, depending on a multitude of factors, including the location and cause of the tear, a host of client-specific variables (e.g., age, prior and expected level of function), and the physician's treatment philosophy.[10]

Frozen Shoulder (Adhesive Capsulitis)

Given the limited articulation between the humeral head and the shallow glenoid fossa, a series of connective tissue, known as the **capsuloligamentous complex (CLC)**, surrounds and supports the GHJ to provide stability by limiting the amount of translation (movement) and rotation of the humeral head away from the glenoid fossa.[14] This complex is both resilient and elastic and contains the synovial fluid that lubricates the GHJ surfaces. In adhesive capsulitis or frozen shoulder, the synovium of the GHJ becomes inflamed (synovitis), and the soft tissue becomes thick with fibrous adhesions (fibrosis).[15] These, in turn, cause pain and significant loss in shoulder range of motion and can grossly impact a client's performance in all areas of occupation.

Frozen shoulder may be idiopathic (primary) or secondary to past shoulder injuries or health conditions that may be systemic or indirectly related to the shoulder, such as diabetes, thyroid disease, cerebrovascular accident,

THE OLDER ADULT

Shoulder problems occur frequently in older adults.[11] According to the U.S. Centers for Disease Control and Prevention, as adults age their bodies become less resilient and more susceptible to injuries, such as those caused by falls.[12] Although hip, knee, and head injuries account for the majority of the results of these falls in the older adult, the shoulders have an increased risk for damage as well.

Shoulder dislocation more often results in more rotator cuff issues among older adults compared with younger adults, according to a study in the *Journal of the American Academy of Orthopedic Surgeons*.[13] Injury to the rotator cuff musculature is more likely experienced by older adults because the cuff becomes weaker, more brittle, and tears more easily as a result of aging.

When older adults fall, it results in shoulder fractures, dislocations, and rotator cuff injuries, and more likely than not, surgical intervention will be required. It is important to note that healing of underlying injured structures usually takes a prolonged period. Older adults who suffer shoulder damage are more likely to experience limited mobility and ROM, which impairs their ability to participate in meaningful daily occupations.

To prevent falls and injuries to body parts, especially shoulders, it is recommended that older adults be aware of the importance of home safety and ensure a fall-free environment. They should consult with their healthcare provider to make sure that they have the correct and proper medications and, if possible, to obtain a fall risk assessment. Older adults should participate in exercises that strengthen their upper extremities and lower extremities to improve their balance and reflexes. They should get a vision checkup, eat a healthy diet, and have a balanced lifestyle of work, play, and leisure. However, despite these prevention measures, in the event older adults suffer a fall, it is of utmost importance that they seek immediate medical attention. This is especially true if they notice changes such as diminished shoulder ROM, pain, weakness, or numbness in the arm. In the older adult, this might be indicative of an undiagnosed condition, such as a fracture, rotator cuff tear, dislocation, or a frozen shoulder. It is highly recommended that older adults develop and engage in daily routines, habits, and occupations that keep them active, healthy, and pain-free.

and cardiopulmonary conditions.[16] Frozen shoulder undergoes four distinct stages; stage 1 may mimic other rotator cuff diseases and is marked by pain at end-range of shoulder motion; stage 2 is the "freezing" stage, where a client complains of significant pain and discomfort and at least 25% loss of range of motion (ROM) in two planes; stage 3 is the "frozen" stage, where the shoulder is significantly stiff, but with lesser discomfort; and stage 4 is the "thawing" stage, where the stiffness remains, but the joint may be stretched with the least amount of discomfort.[15] A client with frozen shoulder may be referred for OT at any given stage of the condition. Comprehensive history and examination are helpful to discern the stage and determine the appropriate approach to rehabilitation. Generally, stages 1 and 2 are primarily pain management with ROM, when possible, and then increased ROM as tolerated in stages 3 and 4.

Shoulder Fractures

Fractures commonly occur in any of the three bones of the shoulder complex, but the most common type of fracture is the proximal humerus fracture. Most of these fractures occur in older adults as a result of a fall on an outstretched hand (FOOSH).[17] Depending on the client's bone integrity, impact of the fall, and speed of body acceleration, the extent of fracture may range from nondisplacement to significant displacement with two or more parts. The most common classification system is Neer's four-segment system, which simply defines the fracture by the number of displaced parts. Developed by Dr. Charles Neer in 1970, the system continues to be used to guide evaluation and treatment.[18]

Rehabilitation of shoulder fractures largely depends on the stability of the fracture (following fixation, as needed) and the phase of fracture healing. Complex fractures are often immobilized with a sling for 4 to 6 weeks, whereas nondisplaced and minimally displaced fractures may only require 1 to 3 weeks of **immobilization** (no movement allowed). The direction, pace, and intensity of therapeutic intervention may also depend on the decision to treat conservatively or through surgery options to reduce and stabilize the fracture. Conservative non-operative management is often reserved for stable and nondisplaced or minimally displaced fractures. Non-operative management may also be the only option available to clients with certain health (comorbid) conditions that could put them at risk of further debility or death if they were to undergo surgery.

Surgical or operative options include percutaneous pinning (pins and screws to repair fractures), K wire fixation (sharpened, smooth stainless-steel pins used to hold bone fragments together), open reduction with locked plate fixation (plate with screws), intramedullary nailing (shaft through length of humerus with nail fixation), and hemiarthroplasty (broken humeral head is replaced with an artificial joint and the fractured bone is reconstructed around the artificial joint).[19] It is important for the OT practitioner to seek information from the referring physician before commencing the treatment process. At a minimum, the OT practitioner should know the answers to the following questions:

- What was the approach to surgery?
- What structures were repaired?
- How were they repaired?
- How stable is the fracture fixation?
- How long should the shoulder be immobilized in a sling?
- When can active motion begin?
- What is the weight-bearing status?

As a general rule, the OT practitioner must set an early goal of establishing active motion with normal joint kinematics while protecting the healing structures and facilitating the healing process.

Brachial Plexus Injuries

A potential consequence of shoulder orthopedic trauma is injury to the brachial plexus. The brachial plexus is a network of peripheral nerves originating from the spinal roots C5 through T1 and innervating the upper extremity (refer to Fig. 22-19). Clients who sustain a brachial plexus injury manifest paralysis of various muscles of the arm and hand, pain, and/or sensory impairments. The prognosis for recovery depends on the severity of the injury from a neuropraxia (mild traction or pull) to complete severance. Severe injuries resulting from total attenuation (excessive stretching), avulsion (nerve torn from attachment at spinal cord), or rupture require surgical repair of the nerves to facilitate resumption of motor and sensory functions. The rehabilitation of the orthopedic trauma will have taken into primary consideration the nerve injury and/or repair.[20]

Disruptions of the brachial plexus may also occur as a result of nontraumatic events, such as tumors and radiation, but they are less common in the adult population.

Cervical Radiculopathy

Compression of the spinal nerve roots originating from the neck, such as those that form the brachial plexus, may cause a variety of signs and symptoms that are often mistaken for a shoulder orthopedic condition. More particularly, clients may report pain radiating from their neck down to the upper back or to the arm. They also exhibit weakness, especially in the shoulder and arm muscles. Clients may experience specific tender spots or trigger points in the upper back muscles, such as the trapezius, levator scapulae, and rhomboids, as well as in muscles that support the neck, such as the sternocleidomastoid, scalenes, and the cervical components of the erector spinae. Additionally, clients with cervical radiculopathy may report persistent tension headaches along with stiffness of the neck. Consequently, in addition to limited shoulder and arm ROM, the client will also exhibit restricted head/neck movements and postural difficulties that significantly impact occupational performance.

The OTA must collaborate with the occupational therapist to evaluate the need for additional referral to another provider who can best address the cervical condition. Depending on the cause and severity of the cervical radiculopathy, clients may respond well to manual therapy and postural training. These types of interventions are often within the purview of physical therapists and chiropractors. However, depending on their respective state practice acts, OT practitioners with advanced training or demonstrated competency in manual therapy may also provide manual interventions that directly address the cervical pathology. OT practitioners should remain true to the practice of occupation and use interprofessional collaboration to address the health and functioning needs of clients with cervical radiculopathy.

MEDICAL AND SURGICAL MANAGEMENT

The diagnosis of shoulder conditions typically begins with a history and physical examination by a physician. In the case of acute conditions, predisposing events, such as trauma, infection, or systemic condition, may readily rule out the pathology. In the case of chronic conditions, history of pain and weakness are hallmarks of clinical manifestation. Clients may describe some predisposing event, such as a fall or a seemingly minor trauma in the remote past; however, it is also common to note that clients would experience pain with activity with increasing frequency and decreasing time intervals between remissions. It is often in this scenario that OT practitioners can contribute to the diagnosis and evaluation of the shoulder condition. Orthopedic screening tests (later discussed) that are sensitive and specific to the shoulder may be utilized to determine the need for further referral and diagnostic imaging. For either acute or chronic cases, diagnostic imaging procedures, such as radiographs (x-rays), magnetic resonance imaging (MRI), and/or diagnostic ultrasonography are often recommended and may be utilized to determine structural integrity of the shoulder anatomy.[21] Blood work to identify the levels of antibodies, erythrocyte sedimentation rate (which increases with inflammation), and other inflammatory markers are used to determine the presence of an infection or an inflammatory disorder, such as rheumatoid arthritis.[22]

Upon diagnosis, the decision to manage the client surgically, and/or nonsurgically (non-operatively) could depend on a variety of factors, including, but not limited to, the status of the injury and the extent of involvement with key neurovascular structures, potential for anatomical and functional recovery, the client's health status (e.g., presence of comorbidities), the client's age and lifestyle, and the impact on the client's overall health, well-being, and quality of life. In addition, in the era of evidence-based practice/evidence-based medicine, interventions that are proven effective and efficient and the preferences of the client must be considered. These decisions are further guided by the physician, in collaboration with a healthcare team and the client.

Conservative Management

Conservative management has two general indications: (1) when it is the more effective, efficient, and less complicated option; and (2) when the benefits of surgery outweigh the risks to the client's health (which include death). In many instances, clients who directly benefit from conservative management also respond well to education and self-management. In particular, a home exercise program and strategies for balancing rest with modifications to one's activities are sufficiently effective, along with prescription or over-the-counter pain medications. However, in the case of clients with more significant injuries or impairments but who are not good surgical candidates and whose only option is through conservative management, prevention of further injury and secondary complications is key. In this particular case, clients and/or their caregivers must be sufficiently educated on proper immobilization of the healing structures (sling, rest), mobilization of the noninvolved structures (e.g., wrist and finger joints) through ROM because they tend to become stiff when the shoulder is immobilized, and managing the pain and edema with appropriate modalities. **Modalities** are preparatory methods and interventions such as ice and heat, as used to manage pain, stiffness, and edema and are thoroughly addressed in Chapter 18.

Surgical Management

Surgical management is often indicated for clients who have sufficient physical health and cognitive status to fully benefit from postsurgical care. Many surgical options, from simple to complex, are available, and the final decision is based on the type of injury and the structures involved. The choice of the surgical approach is also dependent on the client's preference, the surgeon's skill and/or preference, and the client's postsurgical expectations. Certain surgeries require a longer healing time, a longer rehabilitation period, or both. Best practice dictates that a surgeon must have a discussion with the client about the choices, evidence-based outcomes, and potential complications, including failure of the surgery. Common surgeries in the shoulder complex are discussed below.

ARTHROSCOPY

Arthroscopy is a procedure that involves small incisions through which a scope (miniature camera) and miniature surgical instruments are inserted into the joint. The advantage of this procedure is immediate visualization of both intact and damaged tissues and faster recovery time. Arthroscopic surgeries are typical in rotator cuff repairs and capsular surgeries for instability.

ARTHROPLASTY

Arthroplasties or joint replacements are indicated when one or both joint surfaces are so irreparably damaged that the joint is significantly limited, painful, and debilitating. In the shoulder, arthroplasties may be total (conventional or reversed) or partial (hemiarthroplasty). The outcomes for each type of surgery varies, depending on the nature of the

OT Practitioner's Viewpoint

As an occupational therapist, I see a variety of shoulder surgeries on a typical day in the acute orthopedic floor. What has been interesting is the variety of shoulder revision surgeries that are also referred to OT. Shoulder revision is not a typical straightforward diagnosis. Shoulder revisions are conditions in the acute setting, where the client had to undergo a second surgery or may have had multiple shoulder surgeries in the past secondary to complications related to persistent dislocations, infections, or perhaps a replacement of old or worn out shoulder hardware. Treating shoulder surgery revisions requires careful rehabilitation considerations and must be based on the orthopedic surgeon's preferences. I make sure that I follow the orthopedic surgeon's prescribed orders. Depending on the extent of the shoulder revision performed, I speak to and clarify with the orthopedic surgeon what exactly he or she wants us to do from a rehabilitation standpoint at this acute stage. More often than not, orthopedic surgeons order strict adherence to no active shoulder movement or ROM. What does the OT practitioner do in this instance besides educating the client on the necessary shoulder precautions and modifications in his or her ADLs? Most orthopedic surgeons would order what they call "six-pack hand exercises." These exercises are essentially designed to decrease swelling and edema that may be present in the distal extremities after surgery. These exercises also help prevent further secondary complications or any muscle atrophy that may possibly occur after surgery. ~ Luis de Leon Arabit, OTD, MS, OTR/L, BCPR, C/NDT, PAM

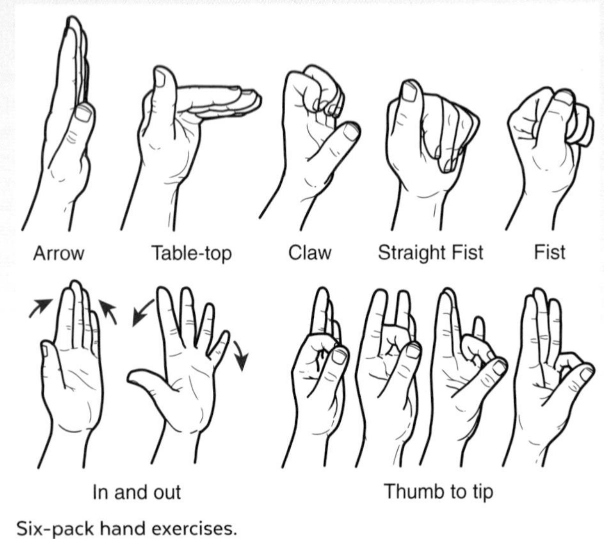

Six-pack hand exercises.

repair itself, the client's condition and expectations, and postsurgical care.

OPEN REPAIR

With the advent of arthroscopic procedures, open surgeries are often reserved for larger and more complex injuries, such as trauma on the shoulder caused by a fall or a motor vehicular accident, resulting in comminuted fractures with extensive soft tissue injuries (tendons, ligaments) and nerves. Examples of indications for open approaches include reduction of fractures with internal fixator devices (e.g., plates and screws) as well as shoulder replacements (partial or full).

THERMAL CAPSULORRHAPHY

Thermal capsulorrhaphy is a procedure specifically developed for shrinking the glenohumeral capsule through the use of a heat probe and is often indicated for nontraumatic shoulder instability or frequent dislocations.

OCCUPATIONAL THERAPY ASSESSMENT

The OT evaluation for shoulder conditions consists of multiple components and begins with obtaining a history of the existing condition and related medical status, as well as establishing the client's occupational profile. Then, the evaluation proceeds with clinical observations, physical examination, and an analysis of occupational performance. The evaluation is primarily completed by an occupational therapist, but components may be delegated to the OTA, depending on state regulations, insurance parameters, facility guidelines, and the documented skill of the practitioner. It is most prudent for both the occupational therapist and the OTA to collaborate throughout the OT process to deliver the best care possible to the client.

History and Intake Information

The OT practitioner's clinical and professional reasoning processes commence immediately at the initial encounter. The OT practitioner starts by obtaining information about the client's age and medical diagnosis and then may determine the association between age and the condition. Certain diagnoses tend to have age determinants. For instance, nontraumatic shoulder instability is more common in adolescents, whereas fall-related shoulder fractures tend to be associated with older adults. In addition to learning about what the injury (condition) is, the OT practitioner should seek to understand the mechanism of injury. Helpful questions include the following:

1. *When did your symptoms (e.g., pain) begin? Were there any predisposing events (e.g., fall, car accident, etc.) that could possibly explain your condition? Has your condition gotten worse, better, or stayed the same?*
   These questions help the practitioner understand the acuteness or chronicity of the condition and/or whether the condition is progressive in nature. Many soft tissue conditions, such as tendinitis, may come and go, depending on the nature of clients' life routines as well as presence of chronic conditions that predispose them to musculoskeletal conditions. For instance, clients who have diabetes have been identified as being at risk for recurring tendinopathies[23] with slower healing rates.
2. *What activities or movements tend to aggravate or worsen your symptoms? What activities or movements*

have you avoided since you started noticing your symptoms?
Answers to these questions provide a more specific indication of the potential source of pathology, and the OT practitioner can then analyze the movements involved in a given activity and understand the mechanics of the movements. For example, if the effort to reach overhead, combined with adduction–internal rotation, is painful, there is a possibility of impingement syndrome.

3. *What was your typical routine like before your symptoms began? How has your routine been since your symptoms began?*
It is also worthwhile to determine what the client's occupational routines throughout the day are to understand whether the condition is caused by overuse or repetitive strain resulting from assuming/maintaining awkward postures. A person who waits tables during the day and bartends at night is predisposed to having shoulder pain as a result of microtrauma and overuse.
4. *What interventions have been working until now or have worked in the past?*
Similar to question 1, this question gives the OT practitioner an idea of the nature of the condition. If over-the-counter pain control medications provide some relief to the client, the OT practitioner should determine whether those agents have anti-inflammatory properties. If so, the OT practitioner should consider the presence of an inflammatory event (e.g., bursitis, tendinitis, etc.). The same reasoning may be applied when the client reports rest in response to question 2.
5. *What has resolved, and what continues to linger?*
It is not uncommon for clients to report weakness and/or distally radiating pain. It will be important during the physical examination/clinical observation phase of the assessment to perform tests that may point to an additional or alternative source of pathology, such as a nerve entrapment.

Clinical Observation and Physical Examination

Physical examination and associated clinical observations provide the most crucial information for determining the direction of intervention planning and implementation. To be effective, the OT practitioner must have a thorough understanding of the biomechanics of the shoulder and be able to discern deviations from normal patterns of movement. The OTA in collaboration with the occupational therapist must appreciate the biomechanical issues to better execute the intervention plan.

OBSERVATIONS

The OT practitioner may begin the assessment with a clinical observation of the client's posture. *Is the client overprotective of the injured/impaired arm by limiting its movements and keeping the limb tucked close to the body? Are there asymmetries in the resting posture between the impaired and healthy upper limbs?* The practitioner should observe the posture at both the sagittal plane (divides the body into left and right halves) and the frontal plane (front and back halves). The sagittal plane provides direct visualization of the humeral head and the acromioclavicular joint. From the frontal plane, the practitioner should observe and palpate for the bony prominences and alignment of the scapula in relation to the spine, the neck and upper back muscles, and the position of the clavicle. Any abnormal rotation of the spine in the transverse plane should be noted. The planes, axes, and descriptions of movements can be found in Table 23-3 and Figure 23-5.

ORTHOPEDIC EXAMINATION

A variety of orthopedic screening tests are indicative of specific shoulder pathologies. In a comprehensive review of orthopedic screening tests (OSTs) for the shoulder,[24] the following are recommended:

1. For suspected impingement syndrome, perform the Hawkins-Kennedy test, followed by assessment of the integrity of the supraspinatus and the infraspinatus.
2. For suspected rotator cuff tear, perform the supine impingement test, followed by assessment for the external rotation lag sign for infraspinatus tear or the bear hug test and belly press test for subscapularis tear. The OT practitioner is advised to seek further training on how to perform OSTs to determine signs of labral tears and glenohumeral shoulder instability. See Table 23-4 for a summary of procedures in the aforementioned tests.

Although these tests have been studied for their diagnostic properties, the practitioner should only report the presence of positive or negative findings and collaborate with the

TABLE 23-3 Planes and Axes

PLANE	AXIS	DESCRIPTION
Sagittal/Anteroposterior	Coronal or frontal, lateral	Bisects the body from front to back, dividing it into left and right halves Flexion and extension movements usually occur in this plane.
Coronal/Frontal/Lateral	Sagittal or anteroposterior	Bisects the body laterally from side to side, dividing it into front and back halves Abduction and adduction movements occur in this plane.
Transverse/Horizontal	Vertical	Divides the body horizontally into superior and inferior halves Rotational movements usually occur in this plane.

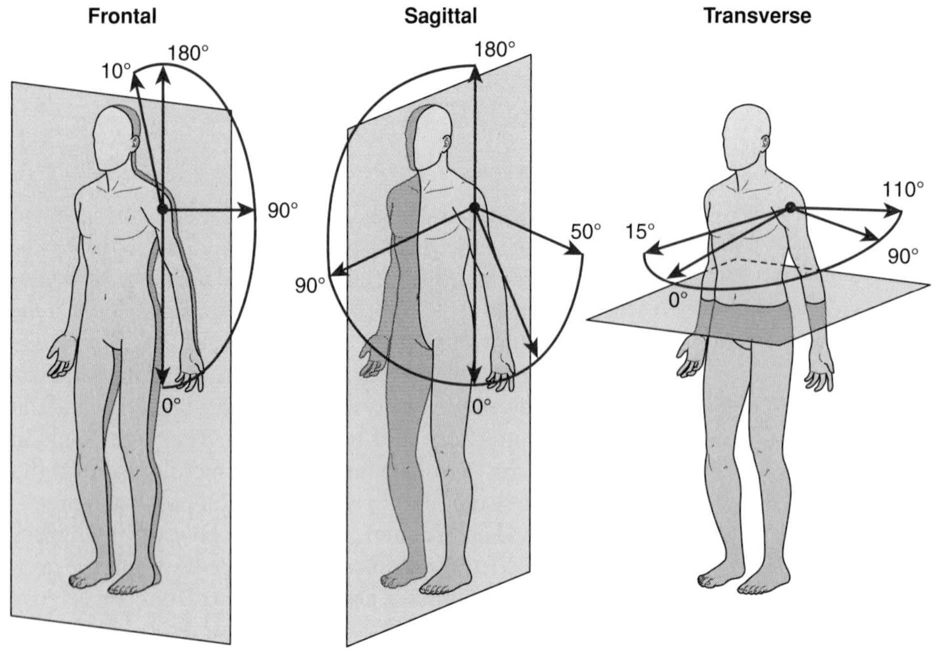

FIGURE 23-5. Body planes, with focus on shoulder movement.

TABLE 23-4 Common Tests

TEST	PROCEDURE	
Hawkins-Kennedy Test	Flex the shoulder to 90 degrees, passively internally rotate the shoulder. This procedure may be repeated with increasing horizontal adduction. A positive sign is reproduction or magnification of pain symptoms.	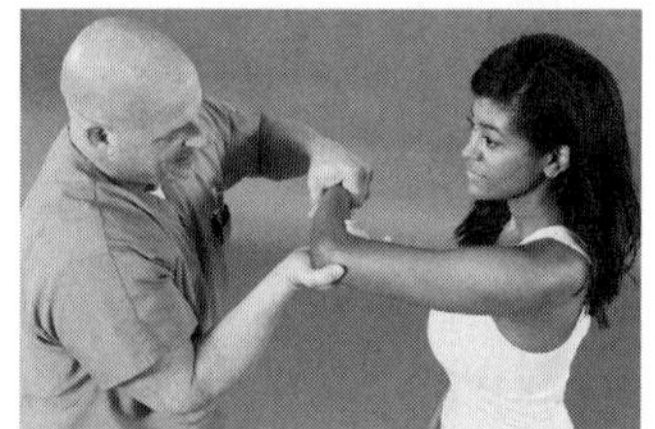 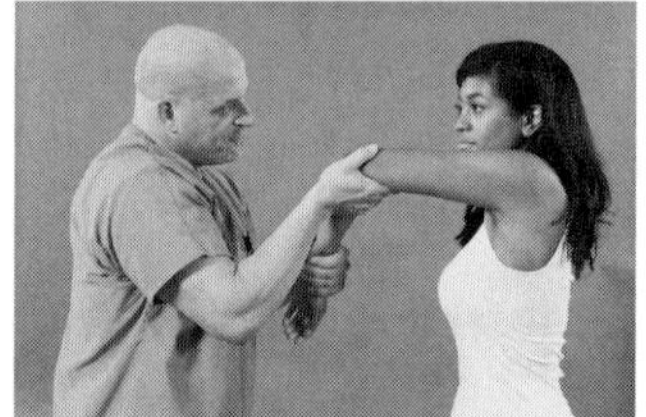
Infraspinatus Test	Instruct the client to hold the shoulder adducted and in neutral to 30 degrees of external rotation, with elbow flexed to 90 degrees, and apply resistance toward internal rotation to test for infraspinatus integrity. A positive sign is reproduction or magnification of pain symptoms and/or the inability to hold the position, especially when resisted.	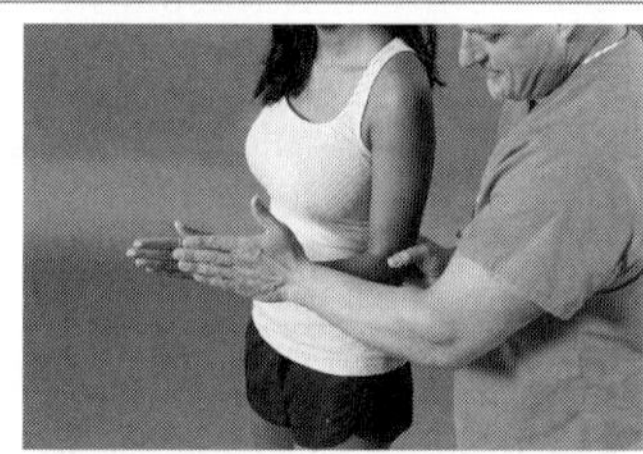
Supraspinatus Test (Empty Can Test)	Position and instruct the client to hold the shoulder in 30 degrees of abduction/scaption with the humerus internally rotated (thumb pointing down), and apply downward resistance to test for supraspinatus integrity. A positive sign is reproduction or magnification of pain symptoms and/or the inability to hold the position, especially when resisted.	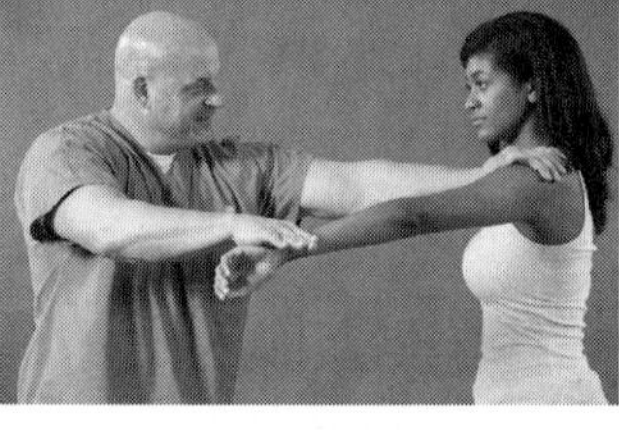

TABLE 23-4 Common Tests (continued)

TEST	PROCEDURE	
Supine Impingement Test	With the client in the supine position, stabilize the scapula while passively flexing the shoulder to its maximum range. A positive sign is reproduction or magnification of pain symptoms, especially as the end range is reached.	
Bear Hug Test	Position the client's hand to the opposite shoulder and slightly elevate the shoulder so that the elbow is pointed forward ("bear hug" position) and instruct the client to hold this position in place. Apply upward resistance to the forearm so as to lift the hand of the opposite shoulder. A positive sign is reproduction or magnification of pain symptoms and/or the inability to hold the position, especially when resisted.	
Belly Press Test	Instruct the client to place (or the practitioner positions) both hands on the client's belly with the elbows pointing outward. Upon cue, instruct the client to press the belly. Observe for asymmetrical positioning of the shoulder, signs of apprehension, or reports of pain magnification as indicators of a positive sign.	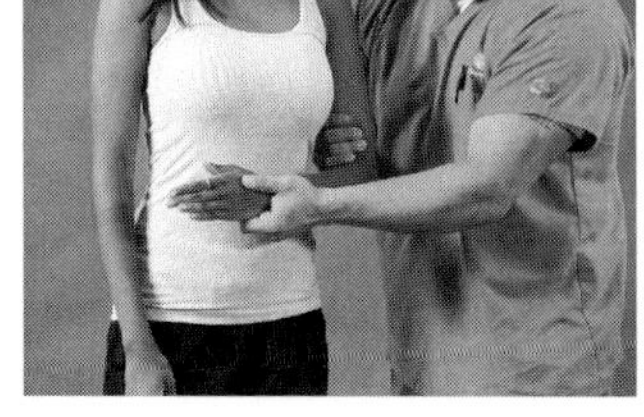

referring physician for any changes in the plan of care. The OT practitioner must be cautious not to interpret the findings because it is beyond the scope of practice of the OT practitioner to render a medical diagnosis.

Outcome Measures

Self-reported outcome measures are valid and reliable tools to document functional changes over time. For shoulder conditions, a variety of outcome measures have been developed, each with well-established clinimetric properties (ability to accurately measure client care items). Two common measures widely seen in evidence-based literature are the Disabilities of Arm, Shoulder and Hand (DASH) questionnaire and its shorter version, the Quick-DASH questionnaire[25], and the Shoulder Pain and Disability Index (SPADI).[26] The DASH is a 30-item, self-report questionnaire designed to measure physical function and symptoms and to monitor changes in symptoms and function over time.[25] The SPADI asks about pain and disability on a scale of 0 to 10 for various functional tasks, such as reaching and putting on pants. Both measures are available through open access sources online.

Analysis of Occupational Profile

Integral to the OT process is a process of synthesizing multiple sources of data and analyzing the accomplishment of desired/preferred occupations.[27] Part of this analysis is an observation of task performance in context to further understand which movements are efficient and which ones are problematic (Fig. 23-6). The following is an illustration of such an analysis.

In the client's occupational profile, if performing laundry is part of the client's role expectation, the OT practitioner would begin by understanding the tasks inherent in this occupation. For example, the task of folding clothes involves reaching and grasping for clothing and encompasses shoulder flexion or abduction and lifting and sustaining both shoulders in varying degrees of elevation. The OT practitioner must then be able to observe the client in this activity and determine the inherent movements in the folding activity that are therapeutic, effective, and restoring to the client versus those that limit the client's movement or cause pain. Depending on the specified shoulder condition and the client's context or setting, the OT practitioner must take into consideration the preferences of the referring physician (e.g., orthopedic surgeon, if applicable), the stages of healing, and the necessary precautions, as well as client factors.

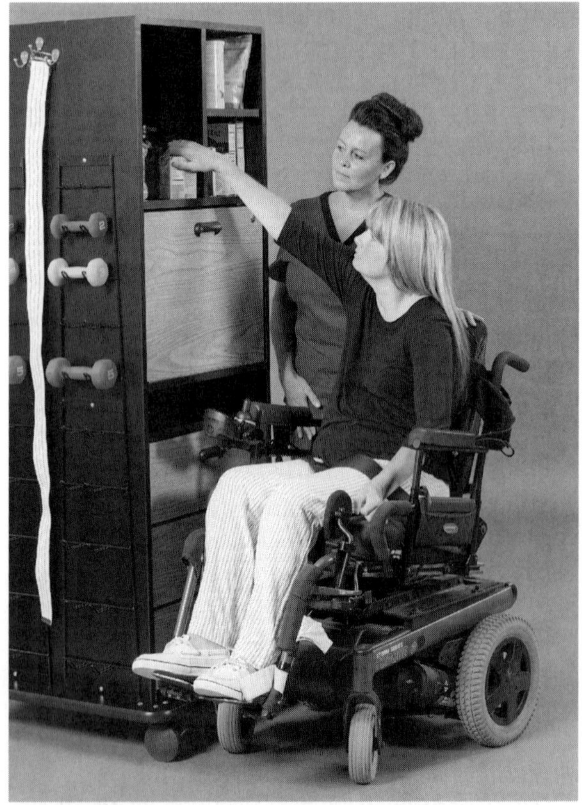

FIGURE 23-6. Client reaching to shelf, with OTA observing the height the client must reach to, in order to elicit pain.

OCCUPATIONAL THERAPY INTERVENTIONS

The OT practitioner establishes the plan of care in collaboration with the client. Before the implementation of the intervention plan, the occupational therapist and the OTA discuss the plan of care, including a plan for ongoing collaboration until the conclusion of the OT services. The ongoing intraprofessional collaboration is crucial to monitor how the client is progressing and to determine the need for a change or discontinuation of services and for additional consultation with and/or referral to other services. Throughout the process of intervention implementation, the OT practitioner must use the evaluation findings as primary consideration along with the client's stage of healing and the onset of the condition. For an acute condition or exacerbation of a chronic condition with shoulder implications (e.g., diabetes, congestive heart failure, chronic obstructive pulmonary disorder), the OT practitioner's goal is to initially protect the healing structures and to gradually transition the client to resuming usual routines, with or without task and environmental modifications. For chronic onsets, the OT practitioner's goal is more oriented toward secondary prevention—that is, teaching the client how to prevent recurrence of the condition and how to self-manage the current symptoms. Furthermore, based on the evaluation findings, the OT practitioner should consider the client's age, routines and lifestyle, values and interests, and past medical/surgical history and comorbidities because these factors may impact the process and the duration of functional recovery.

Specific to postsurgical conditions, the OT practitioner must also consider the healing of tissues that were involved in the repair. Surgeons base their protocols on normal physiological healing of tissues and, as such, set specific timelines for the various stages of rehabilitation—from immobilization to return to usual activities. As the client progresses through physiological healing, the rehabilitative intervention progresses in terms of the level of intensity and the repertoire of activities that the client is capable of performing pain-free. Often, postsurgical protocols simply outline two elements—period of immobilization and progression of active/passive exercises. The OT practitioner must understand the surgical procedures, integrate knowledge of healing, and interpret the exercise guidelines within the protocols to determine the appropriate task and environmental modifications when performing desired occupations. For instance, if the protocol calls for pendulum exercises, the OT practitioner may translate the pendulum position (leaning forward at the trunk with the shoulder hanging straight down)as an opportunity to teach the client various self-care task modifications performed in the pendulum position, such as donning/doffing a button-up shirt, applying deodorant, and/or cleaning the underside of the arm during hygiene tasks.

In the next segments, three phases of postsurgical or post-acute rehabilitation, acute/immobilization, repair and remodeling/mobilization, and return/reintegration will be discussed, as well as the contexts that may be addressed in each phase.

Acute/Immobilization Phase

The acute phase of rehabilitation usually starts from day 1 and lasts for up to a period of 4 to 6 weeks. It is characterized by immobilization to allow soft tissues to heal and, in postsurgical cases, maintain the integrity of repaired tissues. The goals of this phase are to help the client manage pain, to reduce inflammation and edema, to reduce muscular inhibition, and to promote resumption of select occupations. Furthermore, the OT practitioner must promote health literacy.

The client's clinical picture at the acute phase is usually one of pain and apprehension. In postsurgical cases, inflammation and edema/swelling and some bruising or hematoma are common. If seen in an acute care environment, clients may experience lethargy, nausea, and vomiting, as well as a temporary state of altered mental status brought about by the effects of anesthesia or analgesia from the surgery. Some may also experience a temporary loss of sensation and distal motor impairment on the operated extremity caused by the interscalene nerve block applied before surgery. It is imperative that the OT practitioner be aware of the postsurgical precautions and the status of the client before commencing any intervention at this phase. The practitioner must monitor vital signs and laboratory values to assess the readiness of the client for skilled OT intervention. Communication with the nursing staff and the rest of the team is crucial.

COMMUNICATION

"When can I shower?"
"When can I take the brace off?"

These are just two typical questions among others raised by clients referred to OT after shoulder surgery in the acute postsurgical setting. The answer to these questions is usually dependent on the orthopedic surgeon's preferences. However, as an OT practitioner, it is important to understand and inform the client that it is not advisable to shower at this very early stage and to thus expose and wet the operated shoulder because this may increase the risk of infection and other complications. Refer to the section on Sling/Shoulder Immobilizer and Bathing for more details under the section Acute/Immobilization Phase.

In the acute postsurgical setting, clients who have undergone shoulder surgeries are usually kept in a shoulder immobilizer right after surgery. This shoulder immobilizer is essential and keeps the operated shoulder in the most optimal position after surgery. It is important to instruct and remind the nurse and all other healthcare providers who come in contact with the client to ensure that a pillow is placed behind the elbow of the operated shoulder in the supine and sitting positions to prevent the scapula from going into retraction and causing damage to the repaired structures.

EDUCATION AND TRAINING

Treatment interventions at the acute phase would include education and training about the importance of tissue healing through immobilization/activity restriction, as well as task modifications. Ideally, family training should be started on day 1 because clients typically remain in the hospital overnight and are discharged the following day unless there are unforeseeable complications. It is customary for postsurgical clients to be immobilized with a sling for a period of 3 to 4 weeks. The sling or immobilization device may be removed by trained personnel for short periods for purposes of therapy and hygiene.

SLING/SHOULDER IMMOBILIZER

Slings or shoulder immobilizers become a temporary necessity but should be treated as part of the client's daily routine. When the client is deemed safe to independently perform exercises unsupervised, knowing how to safely don and doff the sling/shoulder immobilizer is a crucial step (Fig. 23-7). During doffing, the Velcro® strap on the shoulder immobilizer must be loosened. The client should be instructed to use the nonsurgical arm to pull the shoulder strap over the head or to take the strap out of the connector loop. The client is taught how to unfasten the waist strap of the immobilizer as well as the lower arm strap by using the nonsurgical arm. It is important to gently and carefully pull the sling/abductor pillow from underneath and out to the front to prevent any movement on the surgical arm. The elbow should be straightened and the arm kept supported on the lap or a pillow. The shoulder is maintained in neutral rotation. The sling and the abductor pillow may be separated to readjust the pillow to sling, as needed. The client is taught to use the nonsurgical arm to place the waist strap going from surgical side toward the nonsurgical side. The client must be careful to slide the abductor pillow with the attached pocket/pouch underneath between the waistline

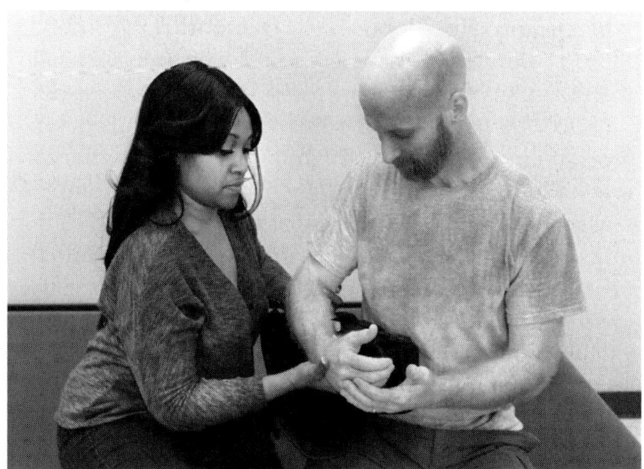

FIGURE 23-7. Donning immobilizer.

and the surgical arm without undue movement on the operated shoulder. It is important to ensure that the curved side of the abductor pillow rests under the breast/chest line. The client's elbow is gently placed back as far as possible in the pouch/pocket, ensuring no unnecessary movements that cause stress and tension on the operated shoulder. The lower arm strap is fastened, the shoulder strap pulled over the head, and the strap adjusted, as needed. The padding on the shoulder strap should be positioned where the strap comes across the side of the neck for comfort and to prevent any skin irritation. Last, the waist strap is fastened.

CRYOTHERAPY

Pain and inflammation may be controlled through the combined use of pharmacological and nonpharmacological strategies such as **cryotherapy** or ice packs, as well as through meditation and relaxation techniques. Cryotherapy is applied as often as possible (as often as 20 minutes on, 20 minutes off) and should be continued as long as inflammation exists.

EXERCISES

Depending on the surgeon's preferences, clients may be taught pendulum exercises early on (Fig. 23-8). These exercises involve the client bending forward, with the arm hanging down, and then performing very gentle swinging and rotational movements of the whole arm with a straight elbow. The arm should stay relaxed. Clients who are not able to tolerate the dependent/hanging position early in the recovery process may be instructed to perform a closed-chain "modified pendulum" by propping the hand on a beach ball that positions the shoulder at approximately 30 degrees or doing finger walks in a small circle on a table surface (Fig. 23-9).

In addition to pendulum exercises, clients may also be instructed to exercise by lifting their injured arm with the noninjured arm with passive forward flexion up to 90 degrees while in the supine position and perform external rotation from the belly to 0° to 20°. Scapular exercises, such as shrugs, pinches (scapular retraction), and gentle circumductive (rotational or circular) movements, can ease muscle guarding/spasms and promote increased blood flow. Distal joint exercises, such as active assisted elbow ROM and active forearm, wrist, and finger exercises, should also be incorporated because they can help with edema management. It is important to emphasize the precautions and contraindications at this stage, such as those for shoulder active range of motion (AROM) exercises. As the client improves toward the late stages of the acute phase, the practitioner will continue to progress the ROM with assisted flexion beyond 90 degrees, external rotation up to and beyond 20° to 30°, and gradual increments of shoulder extension to reach behind the back. The client may also be progressed from active distal extremity exercise to light strengthening, as appropriate. As treatment progresses, the OT practitioner must be mindful of where in the capsule the surgery took place and consider the type of movements that could put significant tension on the healing capsule. For example, when the anterior capsule is repaired, external rotation with abduction rotates and displaces the humeral head more anteriorly. Such movement, while

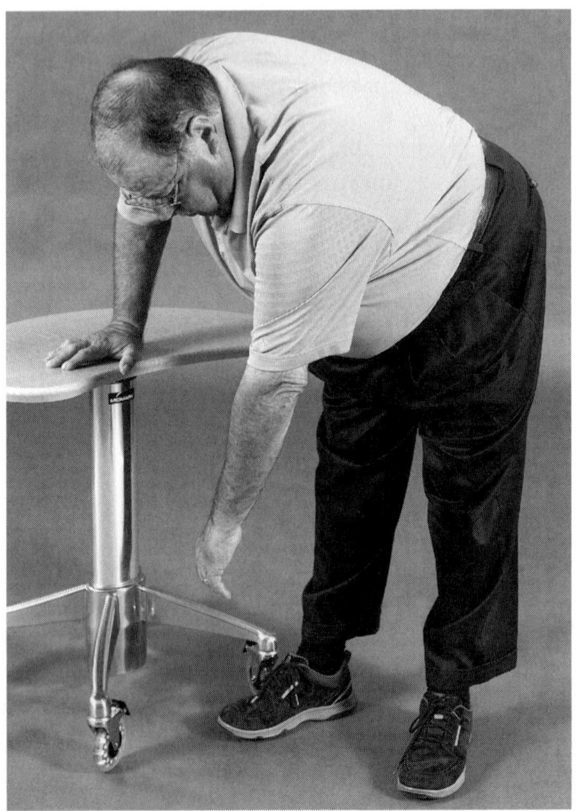

FIGURE 23-8. Pendulum exercises.

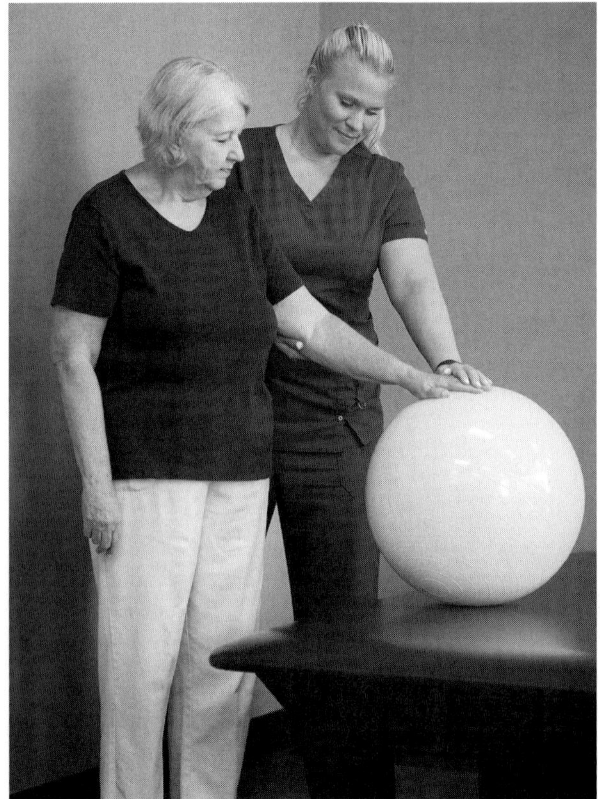

FIGURE 23-9. Modified pendulum exercises.

EVIDENCE-BASED PRACTICE

WHEN EARLY MOBILIZATION IS TOO EARLY FOR ROTATOR CUFF REPAIRS

The two general approaches to postoperative rotator cuff rehabilitation are early mobilization and delayed mobilization. Postsurgical stiffness is common and with surgeries becoming more sophisticated, OT practitioners are bound to see more early mobilization protocols as a way to improve outcomes. However, the practitioner is also advised to be aware of the current state of evidence. When is early mobilization too early? Two systematic reviews offer guidance. Chang et al. pooled the results of six randomized controlled trials (n = 482) and concluded that early passive ROM (e.g., pendulum exercise, passive forward flexion) prevented postsurgical stiffness but cautioned about the likelihood of improper healing for large tears.[28] Kluczynski et al. however, found that early active mobilization was associated with risks of improper healing and structural defect with small or large repairs.[29]

Often surgeons and OT practitioners alike are concerned that when performing pendulum exercises, clients may perform them incorrectly and that it would lead to premature stress on the healing rotator cuff. A study by Long et al. found that performing large pendulums of approximately 51cm in diameter or greater elicited 15 percent of maximum voluntary contraction on the supraspinatus and infraspinatus.[30]

The clinical bottom line is that it is safe to provide PROM exercises early in recovery, especially for those with smaller tears. However, the OT practitioner should be cautious about applying large-amplitude passive exercises too soon because it could trigger voluntary muscle contractions. Furthermore, early AROM should be avoided in the early stage of recovery.

Chang, K., Hung, C., Han, D., Chen, W., Wang, T., & Chiang, K. (2015). Early versus delayed passive range of motion exercise for arthroscopic rotator cuff repair: A meta-analysis of randomized controlled trials. American Journal of Sports Medicine, *43, 1265-73. doi:10.1177/0363546514544698*

Kluczynski, M., Isenberg, M., Marzo, J., & Bisson, L. (2015). Does early versus delayed active range of motion affect rotator cuff healing after surgical repair? American Journal of Sports Medicine, *44(3), 785-791. doi:10.1177/0363546515582032;*

Long, J. L., Ruberte Thiele, R. A., Skendzel, J. G., Jeon, J., Hughes, R. E., Miller, B. S., & Carpenter, J. E. (2010). Activation of the rotator musculature during pendulum exercises and light activities. Journal of Orthopedic Sports Physical Therapy, *40(4), 230-237.*

necessary for a variety of tasks such as fixing hair, should be introduced gradually.

Ultimately, the aim of rehabilitation is to restore scapulohumeral balance where the muscle forces acting on the GHJ produce a net reaction that maintains the alignment of the humeral head to the center of the glenoid fossa. To achieve this, the OT practitioner must be accurate and careful with examining the shoulder movement in context and identifying which movement direction tends to produce pain, discomfort, and/or dysfunction. Because of the kinematic linkages between the shoulder complex and the trunk, it is crucial to give consideration to the client's core strength during the rehabilitative phase. At the minimum, the OT practitioner must address the client's posture and how it impacts the functioning of the shoulder.

OCCUPATIONS

The OT practitioner should also foster engagement in select occupations by teaching modifications in self-care with minimal to nonuse of the postsurgical shoulder. Changes in environmental setup and adapting tasks with assistive devices may also be recommended to increase the ease of performing these tasks. Full bathing may need to be substituted with safer sink-baths, especially until incisions and open areas have fully healed. Many IADLs, including driving, are not recommended at this phase. Precautions include no lifting, carrying, pushing, or pulling of objects, as well as strict adherence to non–weight-bearing precautions. The basic self-care areas and corresponding treatment recommendations are discussed below.

Rest and Sleep: Sleep is one of the areas of occupation that easily gets disrupted as a result of pain and postsurgical discomfort. Clients are often instructed to sleep on a recliner or an adjustable bed for comfort, ease of rising up, and safety. Clients are also instructed to sleep with the sling or shoulder immobilizer for a period of 4 to 6 weeks or until discharged by the surgeon. Because of potential disruptions of sleep, clients may have a diminished sense of wellness and may experience decreased concentration, increased irritability, and lowered appetite. Therefore, a primary goal for the practitioner should be promotion of restful sleep. The following strategies for sleep preparation and participation are recommended:

- One hour before scheduled sleep, engage in quiet and pleasant activities, such as light reading or listening to soothing music.
- Prepare the environment by diminishing potentially alerting stimuli—for example, dimming the lights in the sleep area and turning off the television, adjusting the room temperature, and discontinuing use of electronic devices.
- When lying down, use a pillow under and behind the arm and shoulder for support.
- Try to use relaxation and meditation techniques as part of sleep preparation.

Bathing: During this phase, the practitioner may instruct the client to gently clean the underarm area daily with soap and water using a damp wash cloth. The underarm must be dried well with a towel and must always be kept clean and dry. Instruct the client to use the unaffected arm for washing. A long-handled sponge with a bendable handle can be used to wash the back and legs to prevent twisting out to the surgical side. Depending on the needs of the client, a tub transfer bench or shower chair may be recommended for use. It is also recommended that the client use a shampoo and liquid soap in a pump bottle. If assistance is needed, the client must have a designated caregiver or family member who can be instructed by the OT practitioner in assisting the client.

Toileting: Depending on the needs of the client, a raised toilet seat, toilet safety frame, or a bedside commode may be recommended. A grab bar positioned on the nonsurgical side inside the bathroom may help during sit-to-stand activities and for ease during toileting tasks and for clothing management. If needed, a toilet aid or bidet may be recommended to ease the performance of toilet hygiene. A long-handled toilet aid will assist with reaching for hygiene tasks, especially if the dominant shoulder has had the surgery/injury.

Upper Body Dressing: When donning upper body clothing, it is recommended that the client don the sleeve on the surgical arm first with the assistance of the nonsurgical arm. The client must make sure to pull the sleeve up as far as possible on the surgical arm followed by threading the nonsurgical arm into its sleeve and adjusting the garment, as needed. During doffing, the garment should be removed from the nonsurgical arm first and then the nonsurgical arm used to remove the clothing from the surgical arm. Front opening garments and oversized shirts/clothing are recommended for ease of use. Clients and their families may also be taught to modify personal clothing by cutting the seams or removing buttons/zippers and applying Velcro®.

When donning a bra, it is recommended that the client hook the bra in the front first, then slide hooks to the back. The arm strap is donned first on the surgical arm with the use of the nonsurgical arm, pulling the strap as far as possible. The nonsurgical arm is put into its strap and adjusted, as needed. During doffing of the bra, the client should unhook the bra band with the nonsurgical arm, remove the strap from the nonsurgical arm first, and then use the nonsurgical arm to remove the strap from the surgical arm. Other modifications for this activity include using Velcro® instead of hooks, a dressing stick, a sports bra, or a bra with front-opening Velcro®.

Lower Body Dressing: It is highly recommended that the client sit during donning and doffing of underwear, pants, and socks. The client is instructed to cross the leg on the surgical arm side on top of the other leg. Using the nonsurgical arm, the leg is placed inside the underwear/pant leg, followed by the other leg on the nonsurgical side. For pulling up pants, some clients may use suspenders, a dressing stick, or a pant clip to assist on the surgical side. For doffing the lower body garment, the client is instructed to remove the pant leg from the nonsurgical side first, followed by the pant leg from the surgical side. Other recommendations for lower body dressing include the use of loose sweat pants with elastic waistband and other stretchy but loose garments. Adaptive equipment, such as a reacher, sock aid, long-handled shoehorn, or dressing stick, may be recommended as appropriate.

TECHNOLOGY AND TRENDS

Reverse total shoulder arthroplasty (rTSA) is a surgical procedure in which the ball-and-socket prosthesis construction is reversed, wherein the ball is fitted on the glenoid side, and the cup is situated on the humeral side. This type of surgery is indicated for clients with glenohumeral joint arthritis, complex fractures associated with severe rotator cuff tears, and failed total shoulder arthroplasty or hemiarthroplasty. This surgical procedure is excellent to gain both function and pain control.[31] The precautions observed with this type of surgery differ from the straightforward total shoulder arthroplasty or hemiarthroplasty, where abduction and external rotation is contraindicated. In rTSA, adduction and internal rotation are contraindicated; therefore,some activities, such as tucking in a shirt and reaching behind to don a belt, are not encouraged, especially in the immediate postoperative phase and through at least the first 12 weeks, depending on the orthopedic surgeon's orders.

Feeding: For feeding activity for which the surgical side is used, the OT practitioner may recommend stabilizing containers and jars by placing them between the thighs and opening the lids using the nonsurgical arm. Commercially available jar and bottle openers, both powered and manual, are good options. Bags and packets can be stabilized using the surgical arm and then using the nonsurgical arm to tear them open. The OT practitioner may recommend the use of adaptive feeding equipment, such as nonskid or nonslip mats, plate guards, rocker knife, sporks, nonspillable cups, scoop bowls, and partitioned plates, although these items can be expensive for a temporary condition. The client may also be advised to have a caregiver precut foods and to use ready-made finger foods.

Personal Hygiene and Grooming: The practitioner may recommend to the client to purchase flip-top tubes of toothpaste instead of the customary ones with a screw-on cap. The client is instructed to place the toothbrush on the counter to apply the toothpaste using the nonsurgical arm. For women, the OT practitioner may recommend the use of headbands and men may be advised to keep their hair short. Roll on antiperspirant deodorants are recommended over spray deodorants for reaching with the nonsurgical arm. Nails can be trimmed using a nail file, by getting a manicure, or asking a family member to assist.

Leisure: Many adults with shoulder pain have active leisure interests, such as softball, golf, woodworking, and volleyball. Before resumption of such activities, care should be taken to ensure that the injury is well into the later stages of healing. The OTA can assist the client to identify more sedentary leisure interests for a time, such as computer games, reading, or knitting.

Sexual Activity: Sexual activity is a topic which is often not brought up during the evaluation or treatment process, although it can be extremely important to many adults, no matter their age. Shoulder pain and immobility, especially when chronic, can lead to difficulties with sexual activity. The OTA can assist with research, education, and communication about alternative positioning for the client and his or her partner, use of pillows, use of external tools, or a focus on intimacy.

Summary of the Acute Phase: All of the above strategies may be used as needed through the phases of recovery. The goal of OT in the acute phase is to transition the client toward prior and preferred occupational routines and gradual resumption of usual occupations. Therefore, it is crucial for the OT practitioner to give utmost consideration to not just occupational performance itself but to the development of occupational routines. Such routines should also incorporate other forms of occupations and not just self-care, including light recreation/leisure activities and social participation (e.g., scheduling visits or communication with family, friends, etc.). Portable computing devices (e.g., tablets, smartphones) are helpful pieces of technology to serve both the recreational and the social participation needs of clients. In addition, with social platforms such as Skype and FaceTime, healthcare providers, including OT practitioners, may engage in telehealth/telerehabilitation (according to state or province practice guidelines). However, IADLs and community mobility should be kept at a minimum at this time.

Mobilization/Repair and Remodeling Phase

The intermediate phase of rehabilitation typically corresponds to a period when repaired soft tissues have sufficient tensile strength, when the fixated bone has sufficient rigidity, and/or when strained soft tissues are no longer inflamed. Depending on the extent of the injury and/or surgery, this phase may commence weeks 4 to 6 post-acute onset or postsurgically. The goal of this stage is to gradually transition the client to being more active, and resuming light activities with the impaired arm.

EXERCISES

A number of exercises are suggested at this stage of recovery, as noted in Table 23-5. Beyond this table, another popular exercise for the shoulder is with the overhead pulley (Fig. 23-10). Significant care must be taken with the pulley to have the thumb pointing upward and the shoulder in some external rotation. The OTA should also educate the client on careful use of this tool because it can easily overstretch and cause additional pain and inflammation.

As clients progress through their exercises and activities, they may continue to experience pain and brief inflammation as a reaction to tissue stress. Although this is a typical reaction, the practitioner must monitor whether the signs and symptoms persist for more than 48 hours. If so, the client's rest and activity/exercise cycle must be adjusted by decreasing the intensity, adjusting the interval between activities and exercises, and/or distributing the frequency. For example, if initially, the practitioner recommends that the above exercises be done three times daily at three sets of 10 repetitions each (total of 90 repetitions), this may be adjusted to five times daily every 3 hours at two sets of 8 to 10 repetitions (total of 80–100 repetitions).

MODALITIES

As a proactive measure, clients may continue to use cryotherapy after every exercise session to reduce pain and inflammation brought on by tissue stress reaction. It is also appropriate at this stage to introduce superficial heat to warm surface tissue before the initial exercise.

TABLE 23-5 Exercises Allowed in Immobilization and Mobilization

IMMOBILIZATION (WEEKS 1–4)	MOBILIZATION (WEEKS 4–10)
Pendulum exercises	Active low intensity, low resistance tasks (e.g., wiping table, self-feeding, etc.)
Passive forward flexion progressing to 90 degrees up to 120 degrees by weeks 4–6	Passive forward flexion progressing to full range An overhead pulley or finger ladder or wall climbs may be used as an adjunct
Active assisted/passive and pain free external rotation from belly to neutral, progressing to 20° to 30° by weeks 4–6	Active external rotation with pain free passive stretch at the end of active range progressing to 45° to 60° by weeks 8–10
Shoulder slight extension to neutral position, progressing to comfortable extension during arm swing when walking without sling	Gradual extension to reach behind the back, progressing from buttocks to sacrum to the lumbar curve by weeks 8–10
Scapular shrugs (elevation) and pinches (retraction)	Scapular exercises with light resistive bands, including protraction (forward press) and retraction and downward rotation (rows) as well as "salutes" to encourage upward rotation

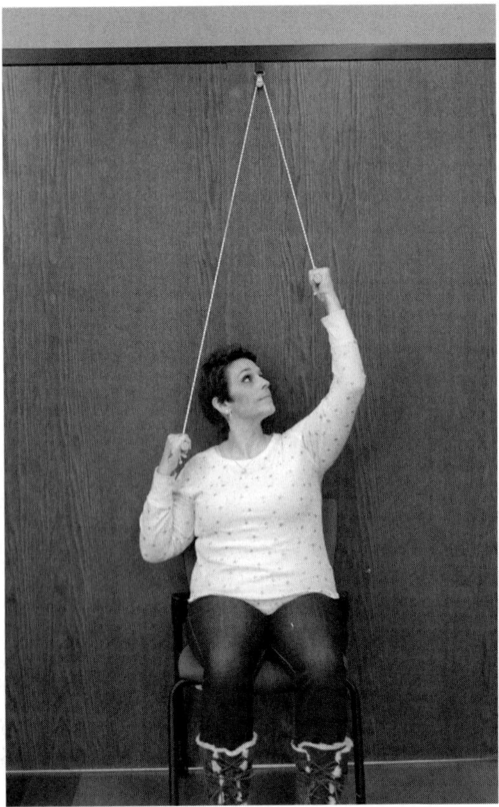

FIGURE 23-10. Overhead pulley exercises.

AEROBIC EXERCISE

One strategy that is widely reported in the literature to facilitate increased rate of healing is aerobic exercise.[32] Aerobic exercise benefits clients who have been deconditioned from decreased activity during the immobilization phase. The practitioner should use judgment in terms of intensity of aerobic exercise in relation to the client's cardiorespiratory conditions. As a baseline, 20 to 30 minutes of low intensity aerobic exercise is recommended with clients rating their perceived exertion as "moderate." For clients at this stage, stationary cycling or brisk walking is appropriate. Upper extremity ergometer (also known as the "arm cycle") should be used with caution because it can irritate the subacromial structures, especially if the shoulder is positioned at 90 degrees of elevation with internal rotation.

OCCUPATION, REST, AND ACTIVITY

During this phase, the client will be weaned off the sling. In some cases, surgeons may instruct clients to discontinue the sling without a gradual weaning off period. In such cases, the practitioner must monitor whether the client is overusing the arm through reports of pain and inflammation. Then, resumption of sling use at certain times of the day is recommended when there is high likelihood of overusing the arm and gradually wean the client off over a period of 1 to 2 weeks.

Conversely, the client may be apprehensive about not wearing the sling and reinjuring the arm and may feel more secure with the sling in place. In such cases, the OT practitioner may provide the client with a tapering schedule and suggestions for the types of activities that can be attempted without the sling. One strategy is to walk around the house without the sling on and allow the arm to swing. The client should be educated on typical patterns of healing and informed that residual pain and inflammation is not an unusual response to tissue stress and that gradual stress is necessary to rehabilitate the healing tissues.

The client should be encouraged to continue performing basic self-care activities, to transition into light home management tasks, and to continue with light recreational activities. However, the client should avoid heavy lifting, pushing-pulling, and jerking/abrupt motions. When driving is a concern for the client, the OT practitioner must perform a basic predriving assessment, which may include trunk mobility, balance and postural control, transferring in/out of the car, and reaching and manipulating car controls with the engine off. When necessary, the OT practitioner should collaborate with a certified driving rehabilitation specialist to determine behind-the-wheel driving readiness (see Chapter 16 for details). It is important to note that medical clearance for driving activity is determined by a qualified healthcare provider, such as a physician, and ultimately driving licenses are issued and administered by the state Department of Motor Vehicles.

Return/Reintegration Phase

This phase of rehabilitation may begin as early as weeks 8 to 10 and is marked by the gradual transition into resistive activities and resumption of or return to usual activities. Part of the goals for this phase is to improve muscular strength, power, and endurance, with a gradual return to more advanced functional activities and progression to optimal weight-bearing, as appropriate. At this time, clients may continue to experience some residual pain/discomfort; the practitioner would be wise to determine whether this is a result of faulty kinematics resulting from muscle imbalance and/or lack of joint ROM. Therefore, before the client progresses to more physically demanding activities, such as those that increase demand for ROM and strength, the OT practitioner must evaluate the balance of muscle forces at any given task. Deep heat modalities and manual therapy (ROM, joint mobilization) may be of particular use when coupled with targeted exercises. The following should be considered first with regard to exercise prescription:

- Perform rotator cuff strengthening, especially the external rotators using resistive bands progressing to diagonal patterns. Tie together the ends of a 3-foot-long resistive band, making a loop. Attach this to a door knob or a stabilizing object. Have the client stand perpendicular to the door with the shoulder being exercised away from the door knob. The client should stand holding the resistive band and keeping the elbow bent and close to the side (Fig. 23-11). Then he or she slowly rotates the arm outward in external

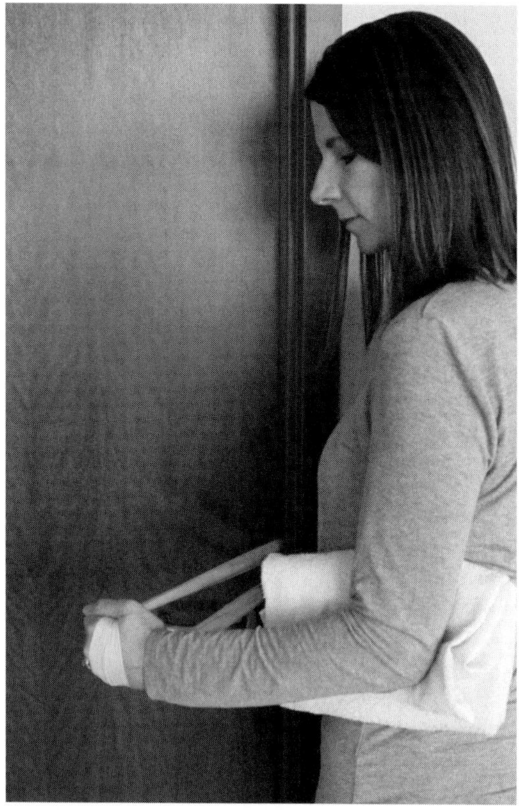

FIGURE 23-11. External rotation exercise with resistive band.

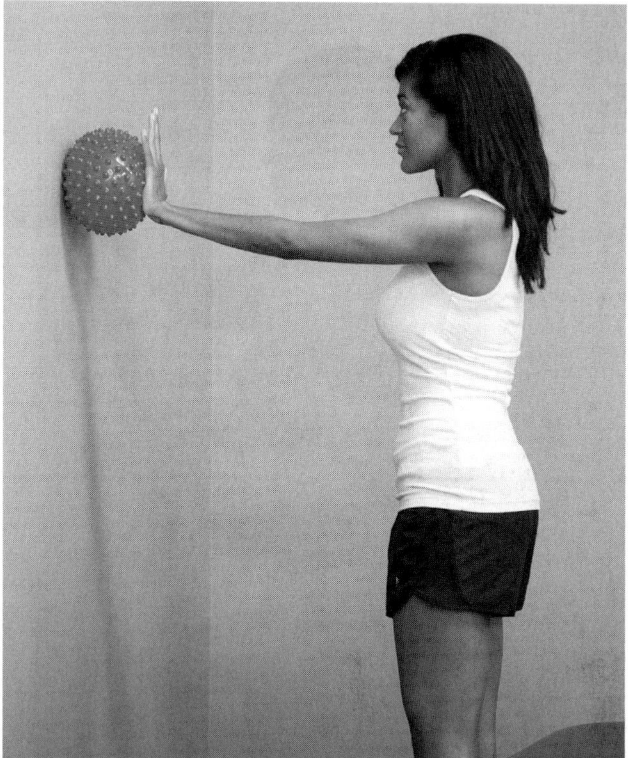

FIGURE 23-12. Scapular stabilization exercises.

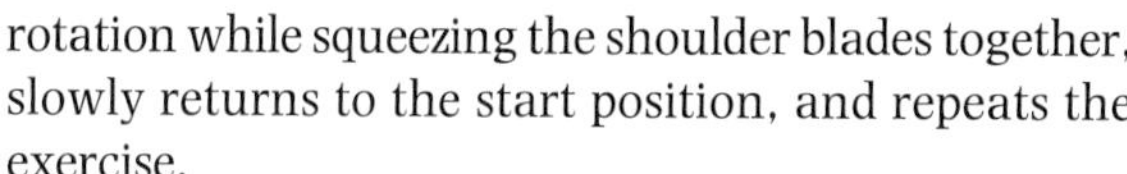

rotation while squeezing the shoulder blades together, slowly returns to the start position, and repeats the exercise.

- Scapular stabilization exercises in prone and upright positions to increase lower trapezius and serratus anterior activity during upward rotation and rhomboids during downward rotation (Fig. 23-12). Have the client keep his or her hand on a ball up against a wall while keeping the back and neck straight. In this position, shoulder blades should be completely squeezed and the elbow straight, with the client leaning slightly toward the wall. Instruct the client to gradually change position by protracting the shoulder blades (by lengthening the arm). Have the client hold this position for 2 seconds and again go back to the initial position. The exercise is repeated 10 times, but the OT practitioner should make sure that it is pain-free.
- Core strengthening and postural education. Have the client sit against the backrest of a chair, with the buttocks and the thoracic curvature of the spine touching the backrest evenly. Encourage the client to align the head at the center and just above the shoulders. Have the client look slightly up and arch the back to straighten the spine. The client then pulls the shoulder blades together and slightly lowers the chin. Finally, instruct the client to pull the belly button inward and hold this for a few seconds. From here, the client may be instructed not to use a back support and focus on maintaining an upright alignment. Additional exercises, such as rotation of the upper trunk and hiking the hip side to side, may be incorporated. Throughout this process, make sure that the client is not holding his or her breath. The same procedures may be done in the standing position, this time starting with the buttocks and the upper back resting against the wall. Gradually, the occiput and the calves may glide backward against the wall to create a "plumb line" posture. (A plumb line is a string suspended overhead with a small weight, attached at the end near the floor, often used as a reference of alignment for the body when examining posture.)

Generally, when providing therapeutic exercises, practitioners must consider a number of variables and not just the exertion–rest cycle. Gschwind et al. recommended that the exercise should begin with "moderate" intensity, according to the client's rate of perceived exertion (RPE)—rated on a scale of 1 to 10, with 1 being "very easy" and 10 being "extremely difficult." The OT practitioner must ensure that the client completes the ROM and that he or she is technically correct. To maximize muscle strength, the OT practitioner should provide both concentric and eccentric modes and allow for 2-minute rest breaks in-between. See Table 23-6, which is a summary table of the exercise recommendations.[33]

Another important goal of this phase is achieving the ability to carry out prior occupations, which includes gradual transition to the worker role. The OT practitioner must continually monitor and assess the client's performance in

TABLE 23-6 Therapeutic Exercise Guidelines[33]

EXERCISE VARIABLE	RECOMMENDATIONS
Intensity	Beginner (moderate: 5-6/10 RPE)
Quality	Technically correct movement
Quantity	Maximal range of motion 10–15 repetitions with moderate resistance (beginner) 8–12 repetitions hard resistance until muscle fatigues (advanced) 2–3 sets of concentric contraction 2–3 sets of eccentric contraction
Rest	2 minutes between sets

various tasks and be ready to problem-solve with the client through an analysis of activity demands and the environment. Clients must experience a sense of self-efficacy through small successes in resuming prior tasks and roles.

In the case of many postsurgical clients, once the surgeon deems that the client has healed, he or she may opt to set the follow-up appointment at 3 to 6 months later. It is conceivable that client may still require ongoing rehabilitation, but the OT practitioner should emphasize self-management and surveillance.

For clients who have high physical work demands or those who engage in competitive sports, strengthening and high intensity mobilization may be introduced no sooner than week 12 to allow for optimal soft tissue healing and to avoid reinjury. Referral for functional capacity evaluation and work hardening programs may be appropriate before return to work and athletic training before return to sporting activities. Driving and community-based activities can be performed without restriction.

PSYCHOSOCIAL IMPACT OF SHOULDER ISSUES

Temporary or chronic pain of the shoulder, whatever the degree of severity, can lead to a feeling of hopelessness, depression, and decreased quality of life. The shoulder is vital for so many occupations that it is nearly impossible to keep from attempting to use it functionally during the day. One role for the OTA is giving clients the tools and education to remain independent despite shoulder pain and immobility. Problem-solving with the client on particular tasks that are difficult and require assistance will almost immediately increase clients' hopefulness and encouragement. Use of helpful tools, such as a long-handled shoehorn for reaching the shoes with elastic shoelaces or a dressing stick to pull up bra straps and assist with pulling up pants, can be vital. If the OT practitioner notes that depression seems to be worsening, then talking to the client, caregivers, and perhaps the referring physician may be appropriate.

COMPENSATORY STRATEGIES

At times, the shoulder weakness, instability, or pain cannot be managed through standard rehabilitation. This may be seen in clients with progressive diseases, such as amyotrophic lateral sclerosis or multiple sclerosis, those with severe post-cerebrovascular accident conditions, those with rheumatoid arthritis, and those with nonsurgically appropriate rotator cuff tears. Management of these types of shoulder issues tend to be focused on maintaining comfort through positioning and gentle ROM, maintaining function through use of adaptive equipment and techniques, and management of pain through modalities and pain medications. Caregiver and client education may be needed on active assistive ROM within comfort limits and on ways to avoid increasing pain during occupations. Positioning assistance in the bed, in the wheelchair, and when ambulating can be recommended, such as use of supportive armrests on the wheelchair or extra pillows in the bed. Adaptive equipment and techniques will be determined by the functional tasks the client wishes to perform but may include all areas of occupation. Equipment demonstration and education in use will increase functional performance.

OCCUPATIONAL THERAPY VERSUS PHYSICAL THERAPY

OT practitioners working in the field should note that while they may be able to treat shoulder impairments, it is equally important to acknowledge that interventions for shoulder conditions are not solely or entirely under their domain of practice. Physical therapists and physical therapist assistants (PTAs) are equally equipped to treat a variety of shoulder conditions. It is vital to delineate what physical therapists and PTAs do as part of their intervention versus what OT practitioners do. OT practitioners bring a distinct occupational perspective into the rehabilitation of shoulder conditions. A physical therapist or PTA working on a client with shoulder impairment would focus on exercises to improve ROM and strength; an OT practitioner would focus on interventions to improve the ability and the quality of the shoulder to move into various ROM positions with enough strength to participate in client-identified meaningful occupations. In the past, some departments would divide the rehabilitation of a client with the OT practitioner managing the upper body and the physical therapist managing the lower body. This is certainly not best practice because occupations do not get performed in isolation, and one of the basic tenets of OT is a focus on holistic care.

SUMMARY

OT practitioners understand that the profession focuses on every occupation, body function, and body structure, as well as client roles, routines, and quality of life. The shoulder is a very important joint for function and independence, and shoulder pain and dysfunction can inhibit all life occupations. Whatever the age, disability, or condition of the individuals that the OTA chooses to work with, shoulder management will be a consideration and a part of treatment.

REVIEW QUESTIONS

1. A client has difficulty initiating humeral abduction. In addition to the deltoid muscles, what rotator cuff muscle should be evaluated to determine potential source of dysfunction?
   a. Supraspinatus
   b. Infraspinatus
   c. Teres minor
   d. Subscapularis
2. A client has been referred for shoulder stiffness. This client has been wearing a sling much longer than what was prescribed by her physician provider. The client is able to shrug her shoulders and protract and retract her scapula with little to no problem. However, shoulder abduction, flexion, and internal and external rotation are diminished. The *most likely* explanation is stiffness of the connective tissues surrounding the:
   a. Sternoclavicular joint
   b. Acromioclavicular joint
   c. Glenohumeral joint
   d. Scapulothoracic articulation
3. A client is referred to OT with the diagnosis of shoulder pain resulting from impingement syndrome. If the client wants to know what is wrong with her shoulder, the *most* appropriate response should be:
   a. "You should ask your doctor."
   b. "I'm sorry I am just an occupational therapy assistant and can't answer that question."
   c. "Your doctor diagnosed you with shoulder impingement, which means that there are inflamed soft tissues that are getting pinched when you move in certain way."
   d. "Your doctor diagnosed you with shoulder pain as a result of impingement syndrome."
4. A client who was to undergo a rotator cuff repair was referred for preoperative intervention. Following an OT evaluation, preoperative education was identified as a need. Which three of the following is the *minimum* information that the OTA must provide to the client?
   a. Cryotherapy
   b. Activity precautions
   c. Surgical procedures; edema management
   d. Exercise postsurgery
   e. Wound care
   f. Immobilization precautions
5. You are an OTA working in outpatient rehabilitation. After the occupational therapist completes the initial evaluation on a client 3 weeks after a rotator cuff repair, he states that the client's occupational performance of specific ADLs needs further assessment. Which of the following is an appropriate OTA role during the ongoing assessment process?
   a. Perform orthopedic screening tests.
   b. Observe the client's performance in self-care tasks and perform a task analysis to identify which tasks are most challenging for the client.
   c. Interview the client on what activities are meaningful to him or her.
   d. Assess the client by using the Barthel Index.
6. You are seeing a client in subacute/short-term rehabilitation setting 10 days after ORIF of a proximal humerus fracture. She identified increased independence in self-care routines as her goal. Which would be the *most* appropriate short-term goal for the next 1 to 2 weeks?
   a. Client will be able to dress independently.
   b. Client will be able to complete meal preparation.
   c. Client will be able to drive independently.
   d. Client will be able to have a full bath with the aid of adaptive equipment.
7. After going through 6 weeks of short-term rehabilitation, a client who underwent shoulder arthroplasty was discharged home with home health services. The client's therapy protocol transitions to the "mobilization phase." Which three of the following intervention methods are appropriate at this stage?
   a. Restorative range of motion exercises
   b. Zumba classes for aerobic activity
   c. Light self-care and home management activities
   d. Cryotherapy and moist heat, as needed
   e. Return to work
   f. Return to driving
8. In addition to pendulum exercises, which of the following exercises are typically indicated for a client 10 days after ORIF of a proximal humerus fracture?
   a. Active shoulder flexion
   b. Elbow flexion and extension with 2-lb weights
   c. Scapular shrugs and pinches
   d. Passive stretching in all planes of motion
9. You are an OTA working in a skilled nursing facility. After completing the initial evaluation on a client 1 week after a total shoulder arthroplasty secondary to rheumatoid arthritis, the occupational therapist discussed with you the goal of instructing the client on how to properly doff and don the shoulder immobilizer. What would be the *best* method to remove the abductor pillow of the shoulder immobilizer?
   a. Gently pull the abductor pillow of the shoulder immobilizer from underneath and out to the front of the client.
   b. Gently pull the abductor pillow of the shoulder immobilizer laterally outward from the client.
   c. Gently pull the abductor pillow of the shoulder immobilizer directly in the front of the client.
   d. Gently pull the abductor pillow of the shoulder immobilizer medially and inward from the client.
10. Clients who undergo shoulder surgery often have rest and sleep disruptions. Rest and sleep is one of the occupations that needs to be addressed by OT practitioners to promote a sense of wellness and quality of life. All of the following are important recommendations that the OT practitioner should make to the client to promote better rest and sleep *except*:
    a. When prone, use a pillow under and behind the arm and shoulder for support.
    b. Engage in quiet and pleasant activities, such as listening to soothing music and light reading, at least 1 hour before scheduled sleep.
    c. Diminish potentially exciting stimuli by dimming lights, turning off television, and adjusting the room temperature.
    d. Try relaxation and meditation techniques.

CASE STUDY

Lucille is a 77-year-old retired grade school teacher living in a two-bedroom senior housing unit. She became a widow in her 50s and never remarried. Lucille has two cats and occupies her time going to casinos, taking bus trips on weekends, and volunteering at the local library twice a week. One of her three children (her son), who remained single, lives nearby and routinely accompanies her to appointments and assists her with grocery shopping. Lucille had rotator cuff tears in both shoulders and received multiple cortisone injections. Her right (dominant) shoulder progressively worsened with pain and decreased range of motion because of advancing osteoarthritis. She was losing sleep because of pain and anxiety and was increasingly worried about her independence. Although her son was generous with his time, Lucille did not want to place any more burden on him. She and her orthopedic surgeon agreed on a trial of physical rehabilitation before resorting to surgery.

Lucille was referred to outpatient rehabilitation services, where she was evaluated by an occupational therapist. Lucille's main motivation for undergoing therapy was to manage her pain. The occupational therapist attempted to establish Lucille's occupational routines and interests to determine appropriate time frames and schedules for performing simple ROM exercises as part of her home program. More importantly, the occupational therapist collaborated with Lucille on prioritizing her occupations and determined the activities that Lucille could continue to do, which ones could be outsourced, and which ones could be delayed. In addition, Lucille's son was becoming increasingly concerned about her ability to drive, given her limited range of motion and pain. Furthermore, Lucille's sense of well-being was diminished because she had to give up some of her commitments to the library and her socializing with friends.

Lucille was being seen by the OTA twice weekly initially to review her exercises and attempt some task modification strategies in day-to-day activities. On her fifth visit, her OTA discussed Lucille's progress with the surgeon. Although her pain had diminished to an extent and a few strategies in self-care were being carried out, it became apparent that surgery was inevitable. The OTA and occupational therapist, in consultation with the surgeon, shifted the therapy plan of care to preoperative education.

Lucille underwent a total shoulder arthroplasty for her right shoulder. Before the surgery, Lucille received basic instructions on safety precautions, including immobilization and management of pain and inflammation, as well as education on postoperative functional expectations.

Lucille was admitted for 2 days and was discharged to short-term rehabilitation (STR) for 7 to 10 days. Before transitioning to STR, her occupational therapist reviewed the same preoperative instructions and ensured that there was adequate documentation in her discharge paperwork for the rehabilitation staff to follow up. While Lucille was in STR, the OTA trained Lucille on simple pendulum exercises and passive ROM exercises according to the protocol outlined by her surgeon. The OTA also worked with Lucille on simple strategies for dressing, basic hygiene, and positioning while at rest and sleeping. Collaboration with the physical therapist and her son on safety was critical, especially when he had to take her to appointments.

It was important for Lucille's psychosocial well-being to remain in contact with her friends; thus, at the suggestion of the practitioners, her son got her a tablet to be used as a way to keep in touch with friends, to consult with the OT practitioners on the progression of her exercises, and to engage in quiet recreation by using game apps and the e-reader function on the tablet.

Lucille continued her therapy at home for 6 weeks. The home care practitioner initially consulted with the STR practitioners and continued to consult with the surgeon regarding exercise and activity progression. By the time the home health services were about to conclude, Lucille was being weaned off from her immobilization device. The home care practitioner discussed with Lucille and her son a referral for outpatient services.

At postoperative week 8, Lucille continued to make steady progress. Her initial evaluation at the outpatient clinic showed that Lucille has regained nearly 50% of her AROM against gravity. But more importantly, Lucille resumed all of her self-care at a modified independent level, continued to engage in alternative recreational tasks at home using her tablet, and took up knitting as well. As a precautionary measure, her OTA discussed strategies to protect her left shoulder through activity and environmental (ergonomic) adaptations.

Lucille was getting anxious about resuming her volunteer work, so her OTA suggested that she go for social visits to reacquaint herself with the environment. Driving could not be resumed until it was cleared by the surgeon; however, Lucille's OTA instructed her on safely transferring in and out of the driver's side of her car.

Lucille's son who had taken days off from his work also began the process of resuming his normal routine. This was an important part of assisting Lucille's transition to past roles, notwithstanding her new/modified routines.

Lucille continued her outpatient therapy for approximately 8 weeks. She was discharged at postoperative week 16 with a home program to ensure her range of motion was maintained and her strength returned. Lucille also began reporting back to her volunteer work but reduced her hours there because she had joined a knitting club. Lucille was very satisfied with the outcome of her surgery and that she no longer had pain.

1. What should the focus of rehabilitation be for Lucille? What are the goals?
2. What outcomes should an OT practitioner anticipate regarding Lucille's conservative management?
3. What are the psychosocial considerations for managing Lucille's expectations?
4. What is the role of OT in preoperative education?
5. What clinical criteria should the practitioner consider to help Lucille wean off from the immobilization device?
6. What strategies should be taught to Lucille to help her transition to increased independence in her home management, leisure, sexual expression, and social participation?
7. What are the clinical criteria for discharging a client?
8. What information must be emphasized with the client before discharge?

PUTTING IT ALL TOGETHER — Sample Treatment and Documentation

Setting	Acute setting, referral from hospital orthopedic surgeon, where client underwent a right total shoulder arthroplasty 12 hours ago
Client Profile	Joan is a 77-year-old right-handed female who underwent a right total shoulder arthroplasty secondary to osteoarthritis
Work History	Retired elementary school teacher
Insurance	Medicare/HMO
Psychological	Pleasant and cooperative
Social	Became a widow in her 50s and never remarried; currently lives in a 2-bedroom senior housing apartment
Cognitive	Intact
Motor & Manual Muscle Test (MMT)	Client presents with pain, numbness on her operated R shoulder • WFL AROM on LUE; loss of motion in the R shoulder • MMT R shoulder: grossly 0–1/5; elbow, forearm, wrist and fingers: 3/5 • MMT LUE: 5/5 • Ambulates with Min A due to unsteady balance
ADL	• Self-feeding: Mod I using one hand • Bathing: Max A for sink baths; full bath unable due to precautions • UB Dressing: Max A • LB Dressing: Min A • Grooming: Mod I using one hand • Toileting: Min A • Functional Mobility: Min A with bed mobility; ambulated with Min A holding onto the LUE; transfers to tub and toilet, Min A
IADL	Min A using one hand techniques since client is right handed; would need retraining and practice to use the LUE
Goals	Due to shorter acute hospital stay, goals are set for completion within 2–3 days in the orthopedic floor with or without complications. 1. Client and her son will verbalize independent and accurate knowledge of shoulder precautions, proper positioning, and modifications in ADLs using references provided by practitioner. 2. Client will be able to perform her home program with supervision and use of handout. 3. Client will don/doff UB garment and shoulder immobilizer with Min A; don/doff LB garment without fasteners with Min A. 4. Client will complete toileting with supervision, using nonsurgical LUE. 5. Client will complete bed mobility and transfers in the bathroom with supervision.

OT TREATMENT SESSION 1

THERAPEUTIC ACTIVITY	TIME	GOAL(S) ADDRESSED	OTA RATIONALE
Perform education and training on shoulder precautions, positioning, modifications in ADLs, safety at home	10 min	#1	*Education and Training:* Of client and family in preparation for safe discharge; safety awareness
Perform shoulder pendulum exercises as prescribed and ordered by orthopedic surgeon 3X with 10 repetitions each	15 min	#2	*Preparatory Tasks:* For strengthening and exercise to increase active control over RUE
Upper body dressing and lower body dressing	15 min	#3	*Occupations:* Functional task performance; ADL performance; Increase independence before discharge
Toileting and toilet transfer	15 min	#4	*Occupations:* Functional task performance, safety awareness, increase independence before discharge.

Continued

PUTTING IT ALL TOGETHER Sample Treatment and Documentation (continued)

SOAP note: 12/2/—, 9:00 am–9:57 am

S: Client states, "When do you think I can use this arm?" Son was present during the treatment session.

O: Client participated in skilled therapy session to address ADLs specifically UB and LB dressing, toileting activities, functional mobility, education on shoulder precautions, positioning, safety ADL modifications, and instructions on pendulum exercises on the right surgical shoulder. Client had 0/10 pain level due to medications provided earlier in the morning by the nurse. Client was trained to properly perform bed mobility techniques rolling toward the nonsurgical left side to sit at the edge of the bed with Min A. Vital signs were monitored with BP at 135/87 and HR at 80 with oxygen saturation levels at 95. Client received instruction to safely ambulate toward the bathroom with Min A on the nonsurgical left side, and on how to safely transfer toward the toilet with correct hand and foot placement and ensuring that the shoulder is kept in place with the shoulder immobilizer.

Client was able to doff and don LB garment with Min A provided during toileting. Able to perform toilet hygiene with SBA for thoroughness using the LUE. Client returned to the room and instructed on how to don/doff shoulder immobilizer properly as well as instructions on UB garment modifications. Son present and was educated on how to assist client on UB dressing as well as possible modifications and adaptations. While shoulder was out of the immobilizer, pendulum exercises were commenced in forward, sideways and circular motions with noted guarding and rest breaks provided as needed. A handout on shoulder pendulum exercises was provided to the client and her son and discussed with them to assess understanding.

A: Client was very pleasant and cooperative, requiring assistance for her ADLs, functional mobility, and shoulder pendulum exercises. Client appeared to be motivated to follow through with recommendations and exercises and wishes to return home soon. Client would benefit from one more session of skilled OT intervention for reinforcement and follow through with pendulum exercises, modified ADLs, and functional mobility training.

P: Continue to work on client and family education and instructions on shoulder precautions, pendulum exercises, UB and LB dressing, toileting, and functional mobility; provide handouts on precautions as a reference before discharge.

Jonah Bonassera, COTA/L, 12/2/—, 4:30pm

TREATMENT SESSION 2

What could you do next with this client?

TREATMENT SESSION 3

What could you do next with this client?

REFERENCES

1. Scibek, J., & Carcia, C. (2012). Assessment of scapulohumeral rhythm for scapular plane shoulder elevation using a modified digital inclinometer. *World Journal of Orthopaedics, 3*(6), 87–94.
2. Kibler, W. (1998). The role of the scapula. *American Journal of Sports Medicine, 26*(2), 325–337.
3. Tanaka, H., Hayashi, H., Inui, H., Ninomiya, H., Muto, T., & Nobuhara, K. (2016). Influence of combinations of shoulder, elbow and trunk orientation on elbow joint loads in youth baseball pitchers. *Orthopaedic Journal of Sports Medicine, 4*(7 Suppl4). http://doi.org/10.1177%2F2325967116S00204
4. Park, W., Kim, Y. H., Lee, T. R., & Sung, P. S. (2012). Factors affecting shoulder–pelvic integration during axial trunk rotation in subjects with recurrent low back pain. *European Spine Journal, 21*(7), 1316–1323. doi:10.1007/s00586-012-2280-5
5. Butler, M. (2007). Common shoulder diagnoses. In C. Cooper (Ed.), *Fundamentals of Hand Therapy*. St. Louis, MO: Mosby.
6. Centers for Disease Control and Prevention. (2014). *National hospital ambulatory medical care survey: 2010 emergency department summary tables*. Retrieved from http://www.cdc.gov/nchs/data/ahcd/nhamcs_emergency/2010_ed_web_tables.pdf
7. D'Addesi, L., & Dantuluri, P. K. (2011). Shoulder instability. In A. O. T. M. Skirven (Ed.), *Rehabilitation of the hand and upper extremity* (Vol. 2, pp. 1189–1196). Philadelphia, PA: Mosby.
8. Budoff, J. (2006). Tendinopathy of the rotator cuff and proximal biceps. In T. Trumble, J. Budoff, & R. Cornwall (Eds.), *Hand, elbow, shoulder: Core knowledge in orthopaedics* (pp. 573–592). St. Louis, MO: Mosby.
9. Post, B., & Benca, P. (1989). Primary tendinitis of long head of the biceps. *Clinical Orthopaedics and Related Research, 246*, 117–125.
10. Wilk, K., Crockett, H., & Andrews, J. (2000). Rehabilitation after rotator cuff surgery. *Techniques in Shoulder and Elbow Surgery, 1*(2), 128–144.
11. Millett, P. J., & Weiss, B. D. (2015). Pain when reaching overhead: Four common shoulder problems in older adults. Retrieved from http://www.nursingandhealth.asu.edu
12. Stevens J. A., & Olson, S. (2000). Reducing falls and resulting hip fractures among older women. *MMWR Recommendations and Reports, 49*(RR-2), 3–12.
13. Murthi, A. M., & Ramirez, M. A. (2012). Shoulder dislocation in the older patient. *Journal of the American Academy of Orthopaedic Surgeons, 20*(10), 615–622.
14. Cohen, B., Romeo, A., & Bach, B. (2003). Shoulder injuries. In S. Brotzman, & K. Wilk (Eds.), *Clinical orthopaedic rehabilitation* (2nd ed.) (pp. 125-250). St. Louis, MO: Mosby.
15. Kelley, M. (2011). Therapist's management of the frozen shoulder. In T. Skirven, A. Osterman, J. Fedorczyk, & P. Amadio (Eds.), *Rehabilitation of the hand and upper extremity* (6th ed) (Vol. 2, pp. 1181–1188). Philadelphia, PA: Elsevier.
16. Questions and answers about shoulder problems. (2014). National Institute of Arthritis and Musculoskeletal and Skin Disorders. Retrieved from http://www.niams.nih.gov/Health_Info/Shoulder_Problems/default.asp
17. Palvanen, M., Kannus, P., Parkkari, J., Pitkäjärvi, T., Pasanen, M., Vuori, I., & Järvinen, M. (2000). The injury mechanisms of osteoporotic upper extremity fractures among older adults: A controlled study of 287 consecutive clients and their 108 controls. *Osteoporosis International, 11*(10), 822–831.
18. Carofino, B., & Leopold, S. (2013). Classifications in brief: The Neer classification for proximal humerus fractures. *Clinical Orthopaedics and Related Research, 471*(1), 29–43.
19. Wheeless, C. (2015). *Proximal humeral fracture*. Retrieved from http://www.wheelessonline.com/ortho/proximal_humeral_fracture
20. Shin, A.Y., Spinner, R.J., Steinmann, S.P., & Bishop, A.T. (2005). Adult traumatic brachial plexus injuries. *Journal of the American Academy of Orthopaedic Surgeons, 13*(6),382–396.

21. O'Brien, M., Leggin, B., & Williams, G. (2011). Rotator cuff tendinopathies and tears: Surgery and therapy. In T. Skirven, A. Osterman, J. Fedorczyk, & P. Amadio (Eds.), *Rehabilitation of the hand and upper extremity* (6th ed) (Vol. 2, pp. 1157–1173). Philadelphia, PA: Elsevier Mosby.
22. Hegman, K. (2011). *Occupational medicine practice guidelines: Evaluation and management of common health problems and functional recovery in workers* (3rd ed). Elk Grove, IL: American College of Occupational and Environmental Medicine.
23. Abate, M., Schiavone, C., Salini, V., & Andia, I. (2013). Occurrence of tendon pathologies in metabolic disorders. *Rheumatology, 52*(4), 599–608.
24. Hegedus, E., Goode, A., Campbell, S., Morin, A., Tamaddoni, M., & Moorman, C. T. III, & Cook, C. (2008). Physical examination tests of the shoulder: A systematic review with meta-analysis of individual tests. *British Journal of Sports Medicine, 42*, 80–92.
25. Franchignoni, F., Vercelli, S., Giordano, A., Santoro, F., Bravini, E., & Ferreiro, G. (2014). Minimal clinically important difference of the disabilities of the arm, shoulder and hand outcome measure (DASH) and its shortened version (QuickDASH). *Journal of Orthopedic Sports Physical Therapy, 44*(1), 30–39.
26. MacDermid, J. C., Solomon, P., & Prkachin, K. (2006). The Shoulder Pain and Disability Index demonstrates factor, construct and longitudinal validity. *BMC Musculoskeletal Disorders, 7*, 12.
27. American Occupational Therapy Association. (2014). Occupational therapy practice framework: Domain and process (3rd ed.). *American Journal of Occupational Therapy, 68*(Suppl. 1), S1–S48.
28. Chang, K., Hung, C., Han, D., Chen, W., Wang, T., & Chiang, K. (2015). Early versus delayed passive range of motion exercise for arthroscopic rotator cuff repair: A meta-analysis of randomized controlled trials. *American Journal of Sports Medicine, 43*, 1265–1273.
29. Kluczynski, M., Isenberg, M., Marzo, J., & Bisson, L. (2015). Does early versus delayed active range of motion affect rotator cuff healing after surgical repair? *American Journal of Sports Medicine, 44*(3), 785–791.
30. Long, J. L., Ruberte Thiele, R. A., Skendzel, J. G., Jeon, J., Hughes, R. E., Miller, B. S., & Carpenter, J. E. (2010). Activation of the rotator musculature during pendulum exercises and light activities. *Journal of Orthopedic Sports Physical Therapy, 40* (4), 230-237.
31. Bondoc, S. & Arabit, L. L. (2016). Occupational therapy in the acute rehabilitation of post-surgical shoulder arthroplasty. *AOTA CEA, OT Practice, 21*(07).
32. Emery, C.F., Kiecolt-Glaser, J. K., Glaser, R., Malarkey, W.B., & Frid, D. J. (2005). Exercise accelerates wound healing among healthy older adults: A preliminary investigation. *Journal of Gerontology, 60*(11), 1432–1436.
33. Gschwind, Y., Kressig, R., Lacroix, A., Muehlbauer, T., Pfenninger, B., & Granacher, U. (2013). A best practice fall prevention exercise program to improve balance, strength/power, and psychosocial health in older adults: Study protocol for a randomized controlled trial. *BMC Geriatrics, 13*, 105.

Chapter 24

Amputations and Prosthetics: Components, Training, and Treatment

Claribell Bayona, OTD, OTR/L and Jordan Tucker, PT, DPT

LEARNING OUTCOMES

After studying this chapter, the student or practitioner will be able to:

24.1 Describe the causes and types of upper and lower extremity amputations

24.2 Explain the various phases of rehabilitation of the client with amputation and the important focus areas of each phase

24.3 Explain the role of the occupational therapy assistant regarding functional considerations and activities of daily living in relationship to rehabilitation following amputation

24.4 Identify the types of prosthetics and their indication for use

24.5 List various new technologies and treatments that assist in postamputation rehabilitation

KEY TERMS

Amputation	Shrinker
Disarticulation	Socket
Mirror therapy (MT)	Suspension
Phantom limb pain (PLP)	Targeted muscle reinnervation (TMR)
Phantom limb sensation	Terminal device (TD)
Physiatrist	Transfemoral amputation
Proportional control	Transhumeral amputation
Prosthesis/Prosthetic device	Transradial amputation
Prosthetic socks	Transtibial amputation
Prosthetist	

The loss of parts of a limb, a whole limb, or multiple limbs causes a change in a person's engagement in occupations. Limb loss or loss of part of a limb is also referred to as **amputation.** The occupational therapy assistant (OTA) has the important role of helping to restore a client's ability to participate in their occupations after limb loss. Along with limb loss comes the need for extensive education of both the client and the client's family. The OTA provides education and training regarding activities of daily living (ADLs) and instrumental activities of daily living (IADLs) adaptations, functional mobility, adaptive equipment, skin care, use of a **prosthesis** (an artificial device that replaces a body part), and changes in energy expenditure. Limb loss is an event that spans all age groups and can affect each client differently. This chapter provides basic information on amputation and intervention. The OTA may seek further training for specialization in myoelectric prosthetics and advanced technology.

In the United States, it is estimated that 1.2 to 2 million people have some type of amputation or limb loss. This number is projected to be 3.6 million by the year 2050.[1] For the upper extremity (UE), the most common cause of limb loss is trauma, and for the lower extremity (LE), the most common cause is vascular disease.[2,3] Limb loss may also be caused by other factors, such as cancer, infection, or a congenital defect. With each of these causes of limb loss come some specific considerations.

For those clients who have experienced limb loss as a result of a vascular disease, the OTA has an important role in assisting the team in the client's education regarding the management and complications of the disease. Many clients with vascular disease have diabetes as a comorbidity, so it is important to take both these diagnoses into consideration when working with this population. In fact, research shows that clients with diabetes are at a 10 times higher risk of limb loss than those without diabetes.[3] Individuals with vascular disease and/or diabetes may have complicating medical issues, such as decreased or absent protective sensation, nail pathologies, bony deformities,[4] or decreased ability for wound healing. All of these issues may lead to additional medical concerns that may lead to the client's inability to wear a prosthesis or require further amputation. Unfortunately, over half of persons whose first amputation resulted from factors related to diabetes are likely to have a second amputation of the contralateral limb within two to three years.[5,6] To help prevent further amputation or functional decline, skin care is an important area of focus for the OTA when working with someone whose limb loss had vascular causes. The OTA should teach the client about general skin care as well as skin care and skin inspection specifically related to prosthetic wear.[7] Additionally, it is also important to remember that clients with compromised circulation may have decreased cardiovascular endurance and functional activity tolerance and that this may affect the intervention plan and implementation.[8]

CAUSES OF AMPUTATIONS

When an amputation is a result of a traumatic cause, such as an accident during work or recreation, a motor vehicle accident, or injury from military or other similar activities, there are some things to keep in mind. First, the manner in which the amputation occurred may have an effect on the client's emotional coping ability.[9] It is also important to consider if other medical conditions that may have occurred during the trauma would complicate the rehabilitation process. These may include, but are not limited to, other injured limbs, brain injury, fractures, soft tissue injury, or spinal cord injury.[9] Additional medical diagnoses will alter intervention plans and the client's goals.

Another cause of amputation is congenital limb loss, which is more likely to occur in the UE and may be caused by genetic or environmental factors.[3] Because clients with a congenital limb loss have it from birth, they may have coping issues that need to be addressed differently as they grow and self-image becomes important. Parents may also need increased support as important caregivers.[7] By the time clients reach adulthood, most are well used to the amputation and generally quite functional. They may require the services of the OTA when the amputation is a secondary diagnosis to a new cerebrovascular accident (CVA) or accident or for training on a new type of prosthetic.

Among cancers being the cause for amputation, the most common are osteosarcoma and Ewing's sarcoma. These cancers occur mostly in later childhood through early adulthood.[3] Because of this, the OTA needs to take into consideration the age of the client and any specific psychosocial needs they may have. Additionally, clients may be receiving other medical treatments, such as chemotherapy and radiation, affecting their rehabilitation course while coping with the side effects of these treatments.

Types of Upper and Lower Extremity Amputations

The different types of UE and LE amputations are referred to by the level at which the amputation occurs. Figures 24-1 and 24-2 depict UE amputation levels and LE amputation levels. These figures include other, often older, versions of terms, in parentheses, that may still be heard in the clinic. For **transradial, transhumeral, transtibial,** and **transfemoral amputations,** various lengths of residual limbs may be present. These amputations may be referred to as "short" or "long" amputations. For example, the medical record may say that the client has a "short transradial" amputation—that is, a large section of the limb was removed, leaving the client with a shorter residual limb.[10,11] The length of the residual limb may have an effect on the client's function, so surgeons attempt to conserve as much of the limb as possible.[12] The term **disarticulation** refers to amputation at a joint line (between bones). Note that with both UE and LE amputations, the more proximally the amputation is performed, the greater the loss of function the client will experience.[8]

Multiple Amputations and Military Considerations

Several additional scenarios need to be considered when working with clients with amputations, such as more than one amputation or the client being in the military. Clients with multiple amputations require special consideration because they require greater energy demands for ADLs,

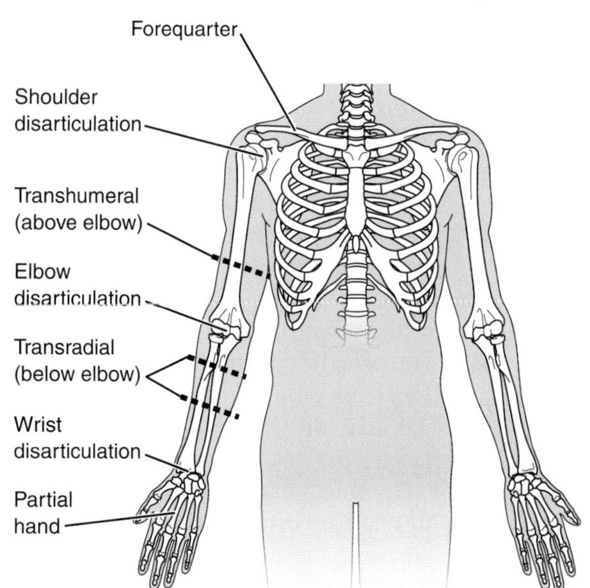

FIGURE 24-1. Levels of upper extremity amputation.

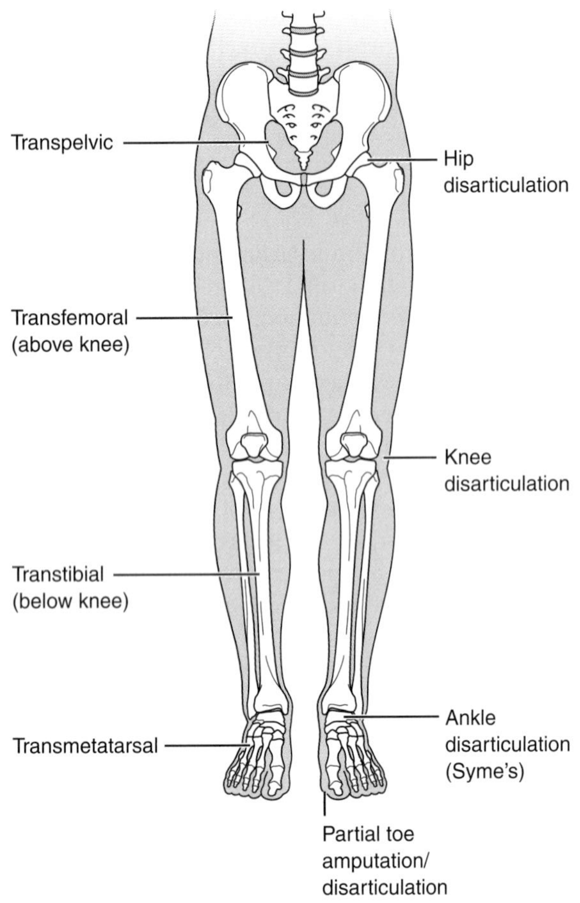

FIGURE 24-2. Levels of lower extremity amputation.

donning/doffing prosthetics, and functional mobility.[13] Clients with bilateral UE amputation work closely with occupational therapy (OT) practitioners and their **prosthetist** (the medical professional who is trained to fabricate and fit a prosthetic) to find the best prosthetic setup to allow for maximum independence and function.[13] Clients with bilateral LE amputation may rely more on a wheelchair for mobility and require their upper extremities for more assistance with ambulation and transfers. Because of this increased use of the UEs, these clients are at an increased risk of overuse injuries of the shoulder, elbow, wrist, and hand.[13] Finally, clients with both UE and LE amputations work with OT practitioners to overcome challenges with prosthetic management.[13]

One cause of traumatic and multiple amputations is warfare injury, and in recent years, many of those traumatic amputations have been caused by landmines and improvised explosive devices. Because of the nature of these blast injuries, soldiers are experiencing multiple limb amputations, internal organ damage, and traumatic brain injuries,[14] as well as additional skin issues caused by shrapnel and skin grafts, which may complicate the prosthetic fitting and its use.[15] Other considerations for these clients include posttraumatic stress disorder, sleep disorders, depression, and pain.[13] Also of interest, after Operation Desert Storm, the U.S. military realized that an amputation does not necessarily result in discharge from the military, and because of advanced technology and the proactive supportive team approach, soldiers may have the option to return to their military career.[16] Military clients are typically younger and more physically fit compared with clients in the general population and likely require a different rehabilitation approach.[13] For instance, military clients may have more active interests and certainly a more active job before their amputation compared with other clients, and the OTA can tap into the military clients' physicality to assist with goal setting and for a focus on occupations. Military clients are generally very self-reliant and want to be given strategies and tools that can help them be fully independent. Finally, these clients may experience psychological barriers to rehabilitation following amputation.

Clients with amputations are at the center of a team of rehabilitation professionals from the disciplines of medicine, nursing, OT, physical therapy (PT), social work, counseling, and prosthetics. Each team member has an important role in helping the client.

PSYCHOSOCIAL IMPACT

Following traumatic or surgical limb loss, clients may experience many changes that affect them psychosocially, including alterations in self-awareness, performance skills, social interaction skills, and performance patterns, such as their habits, routines, rituals, and roles. Individuals may also experience a grieving process after the loss of a limb and go through the typical emotional stages of grief, as well as depression and anxiety.[9] The stages identified for clients with limb loss are shock and disbelief, denial, anger, guilt, bargaining, yearning, and finally acceptance of the loss.[9] The client may or may not experience all of these stages in that order or may skip some because each client deals with loss differently. Clients may even seem as though they are progressing toward acceptance and then experience an event that may bring them back to the beginning stage of the process. Some may move through this process toward acceptance of their amputation quickly, whereas some others may take much more time. It is important that an OTA provides support to clients regardless of their grief stage. The OTA should not expect one typical course of emotional reaction and coping from any of the clients.[9] Many factors may influence a client's emotional reaction to amputation. Gender may be a contributing factor because it can influence a client's role in the family and can also influence a client's self-awareness; women are more likely to want to cover up a prosthesis compared with men.[9] For all clients, values, beliefs, and spirituality, as well as age, education, and life experiences, are going to play an important role in coping.[9] It is important for an OTA to work closely with the client and take into account these emotional reactions and help the client in the most appropriate way. The OTA may be able to help identify positive outlets for clients' emotions, help them with coping skills, assist in developing acceptance of new body image with and without the prosthesis, educate and involve their support system, and refer clients to outside help, if appropriate.[8,9]

Peer visitors and support groups are other great resources for clients to increase social participation, develop a network of support, and improve their functional outcomes. Many great local or Internet resources are available to the OTA and their clients. One example is Amputee Coalition, a national organization that has education, publications, and support networks to assist clients, families, and medical professionals.[16] Finally, the OTA can work with clients to ensure that they can make adaptations to their functional tasks and leisure activities so that they can continue to participate in all of their occupations.[8] Leisure will be addressed in more detail later in the chapter.

POSTSURGICAL CONSIDERATIONS

As with any medical procedure, some effects and complications that may occur following amputation surgery need to be taken into account when considering the client's rehabilitation process.

Pain

Pain is a common effect of amputation surgery. Clients require management of postoperative pain to be able to fully participate in their rehabilitation process and understand all the new information that is presented to them. Working with the medical team is important in ensuring that the client's pain can remain at a manageable level so that he or she may get to fully participate in the treatment sessions and not be limited by pain.[17]

PHANTOM PAIN OR SENSATIONS

One complication following amputation surgery may be the development of **phantom limb sensation** or **phantom limb pain (PLP)**. This phenomenon presents as the client perceives a sensation in a specific part of, or throughout, the whole limb that was amputated.[17] The sensations may present as pulling, tingling, numbness, or other sensations. For example, following a below-elbow amputation, a client may report experiencing a tingling sensation in the pinky finger. PLP is similar to phantom sensations, but the sensation the client feels is specifically pain.[17] These sensations or pain may occur immediately after surgery or years later.[18] Some factors that have been found to increase the likelihood of developing phantom sensations include female gender, UE amputation, pain before amputation, and pain in the residual limb (not PLP).[18] Currently, there is no definitive evidence that can identify a specific cause of phantom sensations. Recent research has pointed to possible causes at the level of the peripheral nerve, the level of the spinal cord, or the level of the brain.[18] Although it was once thought that PLP was a psychological condition, recent research does not support this theory.[18] Currently available treatments for phantom sensations and pain are varied and include medication, transcutaneous electrical nerve stimulation (TENS), mirror therapy (MT), biofeedback/behavioral treatment, and surgical intervention.[18] MT will be more fully explained later in this chapter.

It is important for OTAs to educate clients regarding development of phantom sensations and PLP. The OTA

COMMUNICATION

The care and rehabilitation of the client with an amputation or multiple amputations requires a large team of healthcare professionals to ensure that all of the client's needs are met. To successfully return the client to maximal independence, it is important that all members of the team communicate effectively and efficiently.

The members of the rehabilitation team caring for a client with limb loss may include some or all of the following, depending on the needs of the client: occupational therapist, OTA, physical therapist, physical therapist assistant (PTA), prosthetist, recreation therapist, physician, nurse, social worker, and counselor. First, think about all the ways in which an OTA can communicate with the members of this team. What methods of communication are available, and what information would be most important to communicate? What is the OTA's preferred method of communication with other members of the rehabilitation team? What are the possible consequences of inefficient communication among members of the rehabilitation team?

Imagine working with a client who sustained upper and lower extremity amputations, as well as a brain injury, and requires care provided by all members of the rehabilitation team. Because of the busy nature of this particular hospital, opportunities to sit down and discuss this client's care with the rehabilitation team are rare. What can the OTA do in this situation to ensure that quality communication takes place and the care of the client remains consistent across all disciplines?

Think about the other team members with whom OTAs will need to communicate to provide optimal care for their clients. What is the best way to communicate with individuals, such as the prosthetist or the physiatrist (physician with specialty in rehabilitation), who may not always be in the hospital and may not be easy to reach? While considering this scenario, think about the rules and regulations regarding electronic communications; in today's world, this is often an easy way to communicate.

Finally, remember that the most important members of the team are the client and the client's support system. The OTA should consider how he or she might change the teaching methods with regard to skin care, skin inspection, and use of the prosthesis if the client has a brain injury and thus memory deficits and difficulty following directions. What things could the OTA do to change his or her communication with this client and the support system to ensure that there is carryover of this new information?

should directly ask the client if he or she is experiencing these phantom sensations or pain. The OTA should be direct with clients who may not tell their healthcare team about the phantom sensations because they may believe they are abnormal or have a psychological basis.[17] The team will try to treat the phantom sensations as they are occurring. Intervention strategies will be discussed later in the chapter. An awareness of the client's PLP or sensation is important for many reasons. First, the PLP may interfere with the client's rehabilitation process. Additionally, the pain and sensations may lead the client to think that a limb is still present when it is not. This creates a fall or injury hazard if the client goes to bear weight on or reach for a supporting surface with a limb that is no longer present. This is an important education area to help clients understand the potential dangers of their phantom sensations.[17] Finally, knowing if the client is experiencing phantom sensations is important because this issue can be addressed in the treatment sessions.

Changes in Sensation

Finally, it must be kept in mind that both the hand and the foot are very important for obtaining sensory information from the environment. The hand is necessary for functional tasks such as ADLs and IADLs, and the foot is needed for gait and balance. Lack of these limbs changes the way clients function and interact with their world, and this change in sensory input should be considered when completing the rehabilitation process.[17]

TYPES OF PROSTHETICS

First, the OT practitioner must be knowledgeable about some general terms when speaking about prosthetics. The **socket** is the piece of the prosthesis that fits around the residual limb to attach the prosthesis to the residual limb.[19] **Suspension** refers to the way the socket is held onto the residual limb.[19] UE prostheses have various shoulder, elbow, and hand components, and LE prostheses have different hip, knee, and ankle/foot components.

The term **terminal device (TD)** refers to the most distal component of the prosthesis that acts as the hand. It can be disconnected at the wrist, and the client can change the TD depending on which activity is being performed. The two general types of TDs are passive and prehensile. The passive TD is a static hand that often serves a cosmetic purpose for the client, and the prehensile TD provides an active grasp.[20] Depending on how the prehensile TD is operated, it may have a voluntary opening (VO) device, where the TD is held closed by a rubber band or a spring and the pull on a cable opens it, or a voluntary closing (VC) device, which works in the reverse manner: the pull on the cable closes the device.[20] TDs are either body powered or myoelectric. Body-powered prosthetics have VO or VC TDs, which include hooks, split hooks, and hands. In the myoelectric prosthetic, the TD is the externally powered hand. UE and LE prostheses can have different distal components. The distal portion of the LE prosthetic is referred to as the *foot*.

Cost of Prosthetics

The prices of prosthetics vary greatly, depending on the level and type of amputation. The higher the technology, the greater is the cost. The out-of-pocket cost for a simple, nonfunctional cosmetic UE prosthetic is approximately $5000; and a simple body-powered functional prosthetic costs approximately $10,000. A moderately priced myoelectric UE prosthetic costs around $20,000 or higher, depending on the amount of limb loss, and a very advanced myoelectric prosthesis costs about $100,000.[21] A basic LE prosthetic costs $7000 to $10,000, and an advanced technology LE prosthetic can cost $50,000 to $70,000.[22] It should also be kept in mind that the client will likely need to replace the prosthetic several times throughout his or her lifetime because the devices do wear out over time.

Clients with health insurance may copay 10% to 50% of the cost of a prosthetic.[21] Clients should thoroughly discuss all prosthetic options with their individual insurance companies to find out what is covered. The client should ask for the pricing to be bundled, if possible, so that visits to the prosthetist for the needed adjustments are covered and not billed separately.[16] The Amputee Coalition has resources available via its website to assist with understanding the insurance and funding options.

Types of Upper Extremity Prosthetics

The client's level of UE amputation determines the type of prosthesis and components for which the client can be fitted (Fig. 24-3). Another factor that impacts the type of prosthesis and TDs is the clients' vocational and leisure interests.[23,24] Each of the components of the prosthetic and TD has its pros

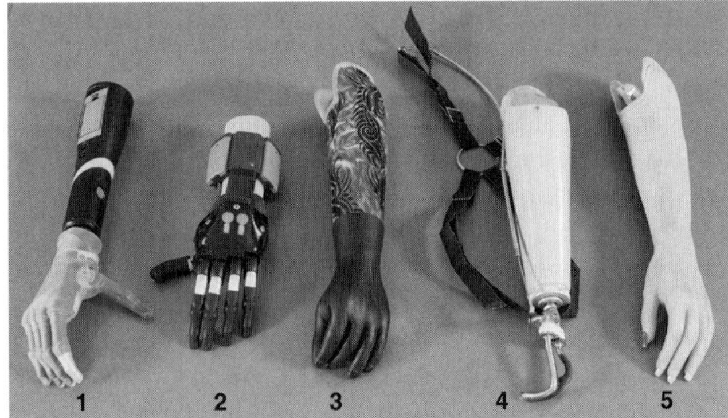

FIGURE 24-3. Types of upper extremity prostheses. *From left to right:* The prosthetics shown here are (1) i-limb™ myoelectric hand with multiarticulating digits (Touch Bionics); (2) i-limb™ digits hand (Touch Bionics); (3) a myoelectric prosthesis with the sensor hand speed (Ottobock®). The thumb, index and middle finger are the controlled digits; (4) body-powered prosthesis for a client with a transradial amputation. The terminal device is a voluntary opening (VO) split hook; and (5) passive functional prosthesis for a client with a transradial amputation.

and cons, which may change as the client uses the prosthesis functionally over time. Insurance restrictions, coverage, and finances may restrict choices, but the OTA and the other members of the healthcare team should work with the client to ensure that he or she chooses the best option.

PASSIVE FUNCTIONAL PROSTHESIS

The passive functional prosthesis is similar in appearance to the nonaffected limb and is passive (no movement) in nature. Although it does not provide the client with grasping ability, it can be used to stabilize as a gross assist and to carry items. They can be made of latex, PVC (polyvinyl chloride) material, or silicone and are light in weight.

BODY-POWERED PROSTHESIS

The body-powered prosthesis consists of a harnessing system and uses the client's gross body movements to control an excursion on a cable attached to the harness, which then moves the TD and elbow locking mechanism (for the client with transhumeral amputation). This device is very durable and resistant to many environments and materials (e.g., water and dust), and its maintenance cost is low. Cable tension felt through the harness provides some proprioceptive feedback to the user when using the TD. One drawback to the body-powered prosthesis is that it becomes nearly impossible for clients to perform proficiently when shoulders are in the end ranges of flexion (e.g., task that require reaching overhead) because of the way the TD is opened and closed by the shoulder muscles.

MYOELECTRIC PROSTHESIS

The myoelectric prosthesis uses electrical motors to move the TD (hand or hook), wrist, and elbow. These motors are powered by a battery system that must be charged and replaced, as needed. The client controls this prosthesis through the use of myoelectric signals, which are picked up by electrodes in the prosthetic socket fitted over the residual limb. For example, if a client has a long transradial amputation, the myoelectric prosthesis fits over the residual limb, and has electrodes placed inside which align with the muscles in the forearm. The client is trained to contract a specific muscle (causing a myoelectric signal), which is in contact with an electrode that is wired to open the device. A different muscle is used to rotate the wrist, and so on. Because of the amount of electronics (e.g., battery and motors), the prosthesis tends to be heavier and the repair process is more complicated and time consuming. The grip force of the hook or hand is significantly improved, unlike in the body-powered prosthesis, and it can be used in more positions, such as overhead reaching. This prosthesis is susceptible to damage if exposed to moisture.

HYBRID PROSTHESIS

The hybrid prosthesis typically combines the use of body-powered components to operate the elbow and then uses myoelectric signals to operate a TD (wrist rotator, hand, or hook). It provides the user with the ability to control the elbow and the wrist and/or hand simultaneously. It is lighter in weight, and good grip force is maintained through the use of myoelectric TD. The clients that are fitted with this prosthesis are usually those with a transhumeral or humeral neck amputation.

ACTIVITY SPECIFIC PROSTHESIS AND TERMINAL DEVICE

Used to perform a specific task or activity, activity-specific prostheses are available in a wide number of options. Leisure TDs can include attachments for riding a bike, paddling a kayak, swinging a bat or a golf club, playing basketball, and gardening. If the client is returning to work, some TDs serve as tools or handles for tools, such as hammers, screwdrivers, or nail holders. It is important to communicate with the prosthetist and relate the client's work and leisure goals to ensure that the client is aware of his or her options and can choose the best TD and then be trained on how to use it (Table 24-1).

Types of Lower Extremity Prosthetics

Depending on the level of amputation and the functional goals for a client, many varieties of LE prostheses are available (Fig. 24-4). Each of the components has its advantages and disadvantages, which may change as the client uses the prosthesis for a longer period. There are sometimes limitations on selecting components based on insurance regulations and functional potential, but that is a topic the OTA would be able to discuss with the client, the physical therapist or PTA, and the prosthetist. The healthcare team

TABLE 24-1 Types of Upper Extremity Prosthetic Components

COMPONENT PART	TYPES AVAILABLE
Suspension	Harness-based systems Self-suspending sockets Suction sockets
Elbow	Motion Control Utah arm LTI Boston arm Ottobock Dynamic arm Ottobock Axon Arm Ergo Ottobock Axon Arm Hybrid
Wrist	Wrist rotators Multiflex wrist options
Hand	Hooks Split hooks Ottobock Sensor Hand i-limb™ Quantum i-limb™ Revolution i-limb™ Ultra i-digits™ Quantum Livingskin™ Bebionic hand Michelangelo hand M-fingers

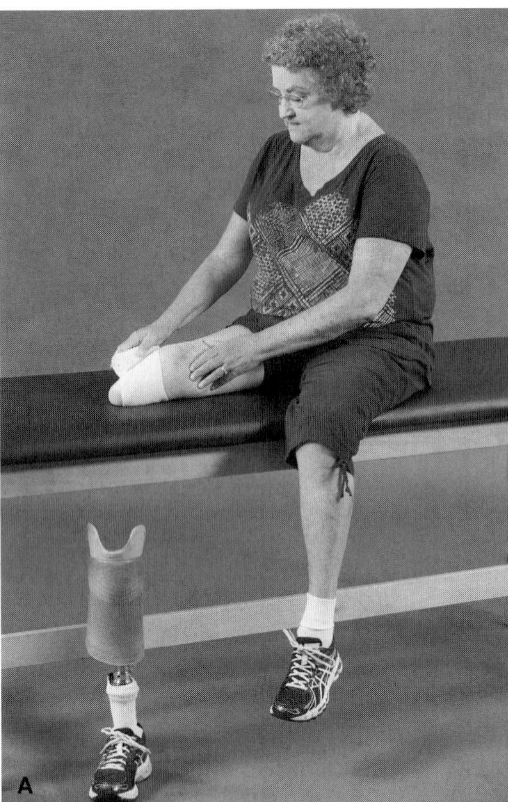
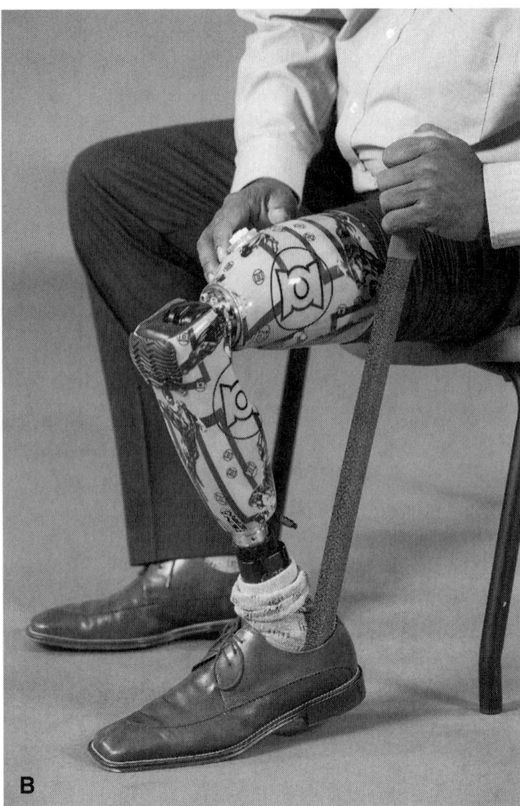

FIGURE 24-4. Clients with lower extremity amputation with their prosthetic limbs. **A.** The client on the left has a transtibial amputation and her prosthesis is placed on the floor beside her while she wraps her limb for edema management and shaping. **B.** The client on the right has a transfemoral amputation and is wearing his prosthesis (note the knee component). The client is also using a long-handled shoe horn to assist with donning his shoes.

works with the client to ensure that he or she chooses the best prosthesis. As mentioned earlier, not all clients are suitable candidates for a LE prosthesis. Some clients may only use a prosthesis for transfers or very minimal ambulation; this obviously affects the type of components that are chosen[19,25]

As an active client progresses to more advanced functional goals (e.g., running), he or she may require other options available to meet these functional needs. Specialty prosthetics are available for various sports and athletic endeavors, generally through self-pay or fundraising.

Additional **prosthetic devices** are available for a client with a partial toe or partial foot amputation. Such prosthetics are contained in the shoe to assist with gait, replace the missing parts of the foot, and prevent abnormal changes in the foot.[26] Another important consideration when working with clients with partial foot amputation is to be aware that the toes play a key role in balance and that without toes, a client's standing and dynamic balance may be affected. This is important to keep in mind when completing ADL tasks with clients because these tasks may need to be adapted to prevent a fall.

General Prosthetic Issues

Some general concepts are important to keep in mind when working with clients with amputations, especially with regard to the donning, doffing, and functional use of the prosthesis. If a client has been wearing a particular prosthesis for a long time, the client or the caregivers are the best people to tell the OTA how to don/doff it and how the practitioner can best help. However, if the client is new to using a prosthetic, the OTA may need to guide him or her in the donning and doffing, and this will become part of the treatment sessions and eventually part of the client's ADLs.

First, it is good to understand the basic types of UE/LE suspensions, which refers to the method of attaching the prosthetic to the residual limb. Most importantly, it must be ensured that the client does not begin ambulating or performing functional tasks when wearing the prosthesis until the suspension is fully engaged or secured on the residual limb because the client may fall or develop pain or skin issues.[25] The types of suspension system vary, depending on how the prosthesis is secured.

With any suspension system using a liner, the liner is turned inside out, placed distally on the limb, and then rolled up so that it is right-side out. If the client is using a pin suspension, the pin helps the prosthetic attach more securely to the residual limb. With the pin, there are often a certain number of "clicks" that need to be heard before having the client weight bear or use the limb functionally. Too few clicks means that the pin is not fully engaged in the locking system, and too many clicks may mean the client may be putting too much weight or stress on the distal residual limb during use, leading to possibility of skin breakdown. The OTA should speak with the client's healthcare team to find out exactly how many "clicks" should be heard.[27]

A client may need to wear **prosthetic socks** (also called stump socks) to fill the space between a socket and the residual limb. Unlike typical socks, prosthetic socks are shaped similarly to the residual limb and are sometimes cut to best accommodate the limb and the socket. Socks are never worn touching skin but are, instead, placed over the type of suspension the client is using. Socks are rated according to the "ply," which refers to the sock's thickness. When a limb is larger in size (because of edema), one sock may be used on the limb, but when a limb is smaller in size (because of changes in limb volume or shape), more socks may need to be added to ensure a proper fit. Prosthetic socks may need to be adjusted several times when initially donning a prosthesis. This is especially true when a client is new to a prosthesis and the limb has not stabilized in shape and size.[26] The OTA may need to work with the client to help him or her figure out how many socks to use at various points during the day.[27] Additionally, a client may need to change the ply of the sock throughout the day as the size of the limb changes with natural fluctuations. If a client is wearing too many socks, it is time to speak with the prosthetist regarding an adjustment to the socket itself because the limb has achieved a more consistent, smaller size, and a new prosthetic/socket is warranted.[26] Too many socks may bunch up, cause sweating and moisture on skin, or cause shearing irritation.

A transtibial prosthesis can often be donned in the sitting position, followed by standing to ensure the residual limb is fully in the socket.[27] As transfemoral sockets need to be worn higher on the limb, the client may need to don the prosthesis before dressing. Clients may need to wear loose-fitting shorts or cut-off pants to properly don the prosthesis.[27] Donning a transfemoral prosthesis may be performed in many positions, such as sitting, standing, or even lying down. If performed standing, the client must have adequate balance and strength to safely do so to avoid a fall.[26,27]

Generally, a UE prosthetic is donned sitting or standing, but the client may need to use the bed or a table as support. Some clients with bilateral UE amputations may roll around on the bed or floor to more easily don the devices and attach the straps properly.

When working with a client with a transfemoral (or higher) amputation, the OTA helps the client learn how to properly use the prosthetic knee. One of the important skills that the client needs to develop is safely locking and unlocking the knee. The OTA should ensure that the client knows how to lock and control the knee unit when in weight-bearing positions. The knee unit is designed to support weight only when fully engaged, so the knee not being fully locked may lead to it buckling and then to a fall.[28] Some clients may need verbal cues to properly activate the locking mechanism on the knee. Knowing how to unlock a knee is important because the client can then safely and effectively work on functional tasks that involve the standing-to-sitting transition. The OTA needs to work with the rehabilitation team members to ensure that he or she knows how to instruct the client in locking and unlocking the knee component.

Finally, it must be kept in mind that when assisting a client in removing the prosthesis, the limb is placed within the client's reach so that he or she may don it again later, if needed for ADLs. It is important to create the habit of removing the sock and suspension (liner), and then performing a skin check for areas of redness, blisters, or a rash.

PHASES OF REHABILITATION OF THE CLIENT WITH AMPUTATION

After an evaluation by the occupational therapist, the OTA is responsible for implementing the treatment plan and guiding the client through the rehabilitation process, which occurs in several phases, as described in this section. The goal during the four phases of rehabilitation is to educate and train the client to return to being independent with his or her occupations. The phases may overlap at times and might take place in one setting or in multiple settings. It is important for the OTA to know the phase of rehabilitation the client is in to implement the proper care and training to achieve the best outcomes.

Phase One: Early Management and Wound Healing

During this phase, the focus is on promoting wound healing, controlling incisional and PLP, and maintaining the range of motion (ROM) of the involved and noninvolved limbs (as indicated). This phase is also the time when the client and the caregivers are educated on the prosthetic rehabilitation process, the different kinds of prosthetic devices available, and the stages of grieving the loss of a limb and changes in body image.[23] Clients can quickly and easily develop contractures in either the UE or LE if they are not encouraged to frequently move the affected limb and to position the limb in such a way as to not encourage the development of contractures. For the UE, it is important to make sure that the client is avoiding positions of shoulder adduction, shoulder internal rotation, forearm supination, and elbow flexion.[29] For the LE, the client should avoid knee flexion, hip flexion, or excessive hip abduction or adduction for prolonged periods.[7] Extended positioning for clients with either UE or LE amputation can deter functional progression and prevent the use of a prosthesis until the ROM deficit can be corrected. Finally, although the ROM concern is likely related to the involved side, as indicated above, careful monitoring of the uninvolved limb is also important to maintain function, especially as the client may have to remain in positions, such as sitting, for an extended period unlike in the past.

LIMB CARE

Education on proper limb care, including wound management, skin care, limb wrapping, and the use of **shrinkers** (elastic sock used to shape the limb and control edema), help prevent infection as the wound begins to heal. It also maintains good skin integrity, which is necessary for future tolerance and use of a prosthesis. This education and training can be performed by any OT practitioner and ideally also includes family members or caregivers.

Wound Management: During the initial stages of wound healing after an upper limb loss, the OTA can be involved in performing wound care and dressing changes following the physician's guidelines. (See Chapter 8 for full details regarding the stages of wound healing.) When the wound has stopped draining, the client may be able to initiate application of antibacterial ointment with gentle massage and wound debridement, if necessary.[23] An elastic bandage is used for compression and limb shaping, followed by the use of a shrinker once the sutures are removed. As the wound closes and the scar matures, the client learns how to don and doff a silicone liner that provides constant pressure on the site to prevent the formation of hypertrophic scar tissue. Delayed wound healing prevents a client from initiating use of a prosthesis, so the OTA should encourage changes to a healthy lifestyle, such as smoking cessation, which can assist in the wound healing process.[8] Sometimes, a wound may take over six months to heal, especially when there are vascular issues or slow healing, as with diabetes. Other healthy habits, such as proper nutrition, increased activity levels, and care of secondary medical conditions, should also be encouraged by the OTA.

Postoperative Prostheses: Some clients receive an immediate postoperative prosthetic (IPOP), which is a plaster/fiberglass prosthetic applied in the surgical suite, or an early postoperative prosthetic (EPOP) applied 5 to 7 days after the surgery. The benefits of these prosthetics are early weight-bearing and mobility; in the case of upper extremity, IPOPs/EPOPs are vital to keeping the client able to perform tasks two handed. If the prosthetic fitting occurs too long after surgery, some clients simply learn to perform tasks one handed. If the surgeon decides not to use an early prosthetic on the LE, the healing period can be greater than 12 weeks, and there is greater risk of clients experiencing limb weakness, body deconditioning, joint stiffness, or injury to the residual limb as a result of falling while trying to move about on one leg.[30]. Some clients get physical and psychological benefits from having a limb fitted early on in their recovery and thus build tolerance of the prosthetic more quickly.

Another option is a removable rigid dressing, also made of plaster, fiberglass, or a combination, which may be put on right after surgery.[31] Removable and nonremovable rigid dressings have the advantages of controlling edema, shaping and protecting the limb, reducing pain, and protecting the wound from injury and contamination.[31]

Skin Care: Skin hygiene is necessary to maintain good skin integrity and to promote wound healing. It is important to keep the skin of the residual limb clean and dry and to apply fragrance-free lotion to moisturize it and prevent dryness, which can lead to skin breakdown. Lotion should never be applied directly before donning the prosthesis. The OTA should teach the client how to use, on a daily basis, a long-handled mirror to inspect the skin of the residual limb, which is not easily visible, following bathing. By performing a mirror inspection, the client can ensure prevention of skin breakdown by quickly identifying any nonhealing or pressure injuries on the residual limb, which can then be addressed by the physician and/or the nursing staff. The daily skin care routine is important not only early on in the rehabilitation process but also throughout the time the client uses a prosthesis. Once a prosthetic device is introduced, the client must be instructed on skin inspection for areas of too much pressure from the prosthesis (redness, tenderness, excess moisture), which may lead to skin breakdown.[8] The importance of proper nutrition and healthy habits should also reinforced because they are crucial for skin healing and rebuilding.

Limb Wrapping: Limb wrapping is essential for protecting the wound/incision site, managing edema, and shaping the residual limb in preparation to wearing a prosthetic device. An elastic bandage is used for wrapping the residual limb using the figure-of-8 technique. This technique provides compression and shaping distally to proximally, and as the wound heals, a shrinker is introduced to provide compression and to shape the limb. Both the client and his or her caregivers require education on proper donning/doffing of the elastic bandage and shrinker.

Instructions for Figure-of-8 Wrapping: The wrapping process begins by placing the end of the bandage diagonally at the distal end of the residual limb. The wrap should encircle the limb from behind and wrap diagonally upward to cross over the end of the bandage. This figure-of-8 wrapping process should continue with each pattern overlapping the previous one by approximately two thirds the width of the bandage. The wrap should be brought above the next most proximal joint above the level of the amputation for more appropriate suspension of this bandage.[32] Secure the end of the bandage with tape instead of metal clips to avoid causing any issues with skin integrity.

When using the figure-of-8 wrapping technique, oblique turns should be maintained as opposed to circular turns. Circular turns can cause a tourniquet effect, and this could affect the vascular status of the residual limb (think about what happens when wrapping a rubber band too tightly on the fingertip). Proper wrapping is important to prevent formation of an undesirable limb shape, which would complicate prosthetic fitting and wear. The wrap should be worn daily and rewrapping done every 4 hours, or more frequently if it bunches up or begins to slip.[32] Various versions of wrapping exist; see Figures 24-5 to 24-6 for examples of wrapping procedures.

Shrinkers: The client begins to use a shrinker once the residual limb has healed almost completely; by then, the incision line will have healed and the sutures have been

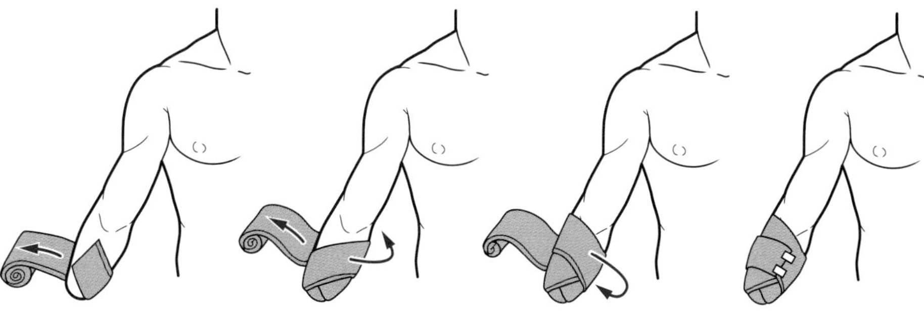

FIGURE 24-5. Limb wrapping for client with transradial amputation.

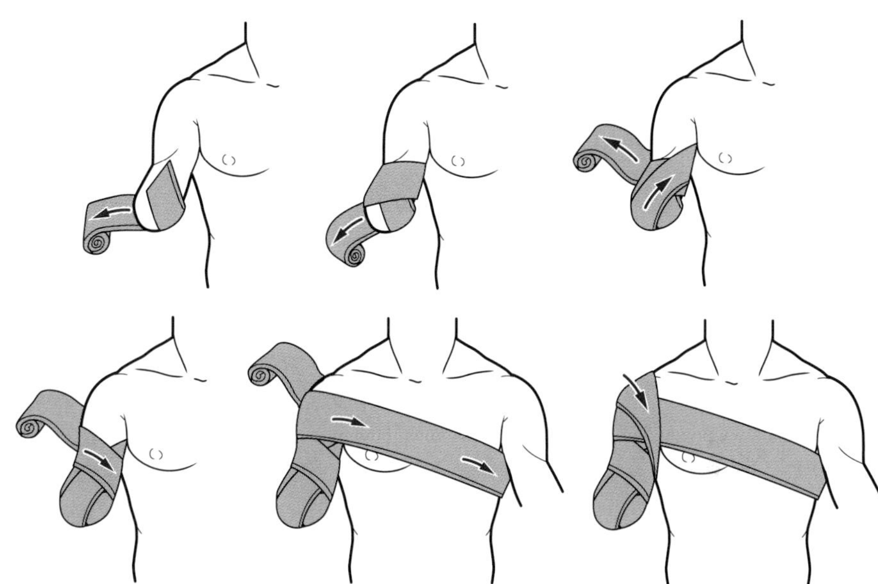

FIGURE 24-6. Limb wrapping for client with transhumeral amputation.

removed. The shrinker is a piece of tight elastic fabric shaped similarly to the residual limb, and is worn at night to control edema and to shape the residual limb, both of which are important for fitting the limb into the prosthesis. Ensure that the client is cleared by his or her physician before applying a shrinker. Depending on the client, someone with a LE amputation may require the use of a shrinker the rest of his or her life because of various factors, such as activity levels, food and drink intake, and temperature, which may all affect the size of their limb on a daily basis. Clients with UE and LE amputations may not need the shrinker for an extended period once the size and shape of the residual limb stabilizes, to consistently fit into the prosthetic device.[33] It is important to note that donning a shrinker requires tension, which could stress the incision site if it has not completely healed. The shrinker should fit snugly, and the client may need to have different sizes of shrinkers as the limb decreases in size and changes shape. In the initial stages after an amputation, the limb is larger because of edema, which decreases over time. Also, as time progresses, the muscles in the limb atrophy, causing the limb to further reduce in size. The limb also goes through changes in size daily, being larger each morning and becoming smaller throughout the day as the pressure from the prosthetic helps disperse fluid in the limb. If the client's shrinker is not fitting tightly enough, the OTA should work with the rehabilitation team to determine the best size to use.

Once a client has been cleared to wear a shrinker, the OTA must reinforce the importance of using the shrinker, if needed. Clients may become frustrated if they cannot fit the limb into the prosthetic socket and may have their rehabilitation time extended if they are unable to wear the prosthetic. Additionally, if the shape of the limb is not optimal, the client may be unable to wear the prosthesis because of discomfort or skin breakdown caused by pressure of the socket on excess areas of skin or prominent bone.

Finally, the OTA should make sure that the client knows how to properly don and doff the shrinker and understand the appropriate care of the shrinker, as part of the client's ADL skills, including when to wear and when not to wear it. The prosthetist assists in devising a plan to use the shrinker (e.g., hours, correct use) to achieve the optimal limb size. The shrinker can be pulled on, much like a sock. If the client is unable to don it independently, he or she should be able to direct the caregiver about donning and doffing of the shrinker (Fig. 24-9).

DESENSITIZATION

Desensitization is a process that decreases the sensitivity of an area to various stimuli; it is a therapeutic technique that is used to decrease and normalize the body's response to

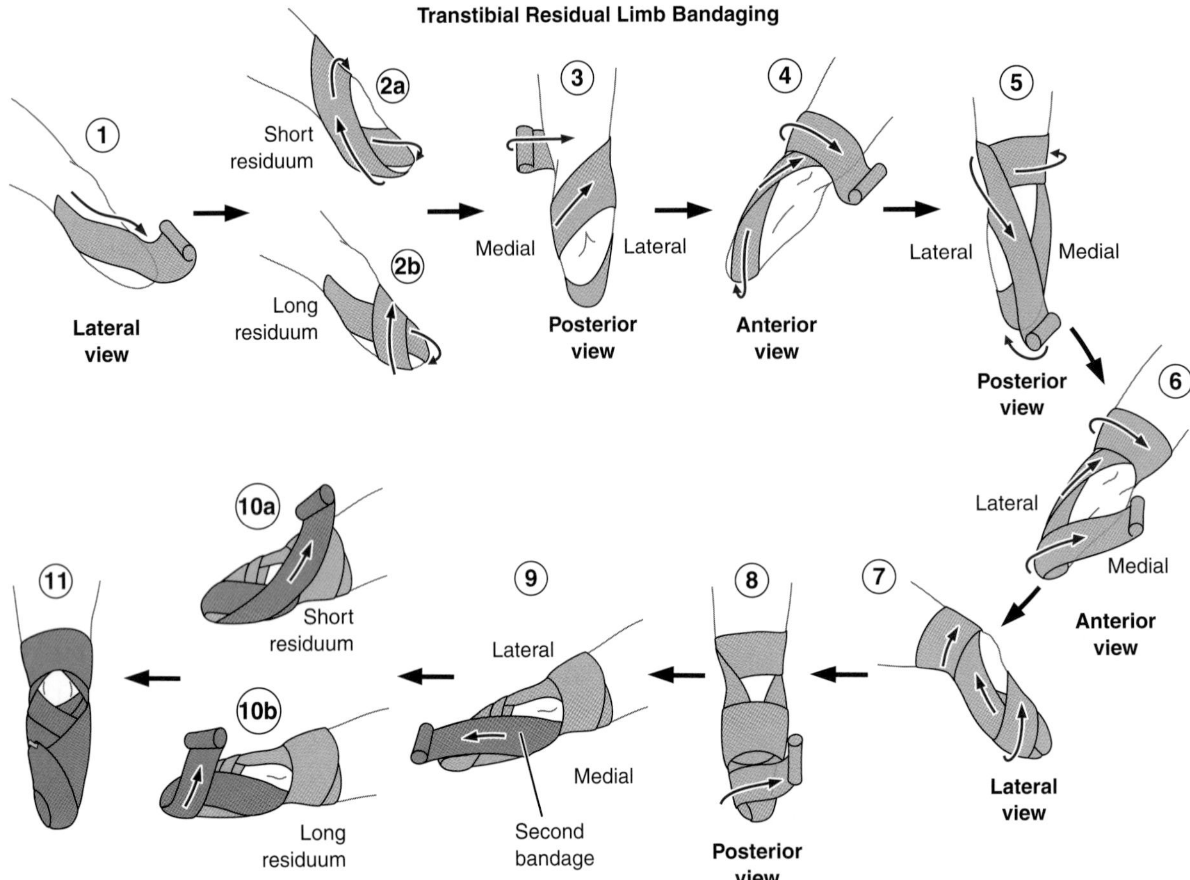

FIGURE 24-7. Limb wrapping for client with transtibial amputation.

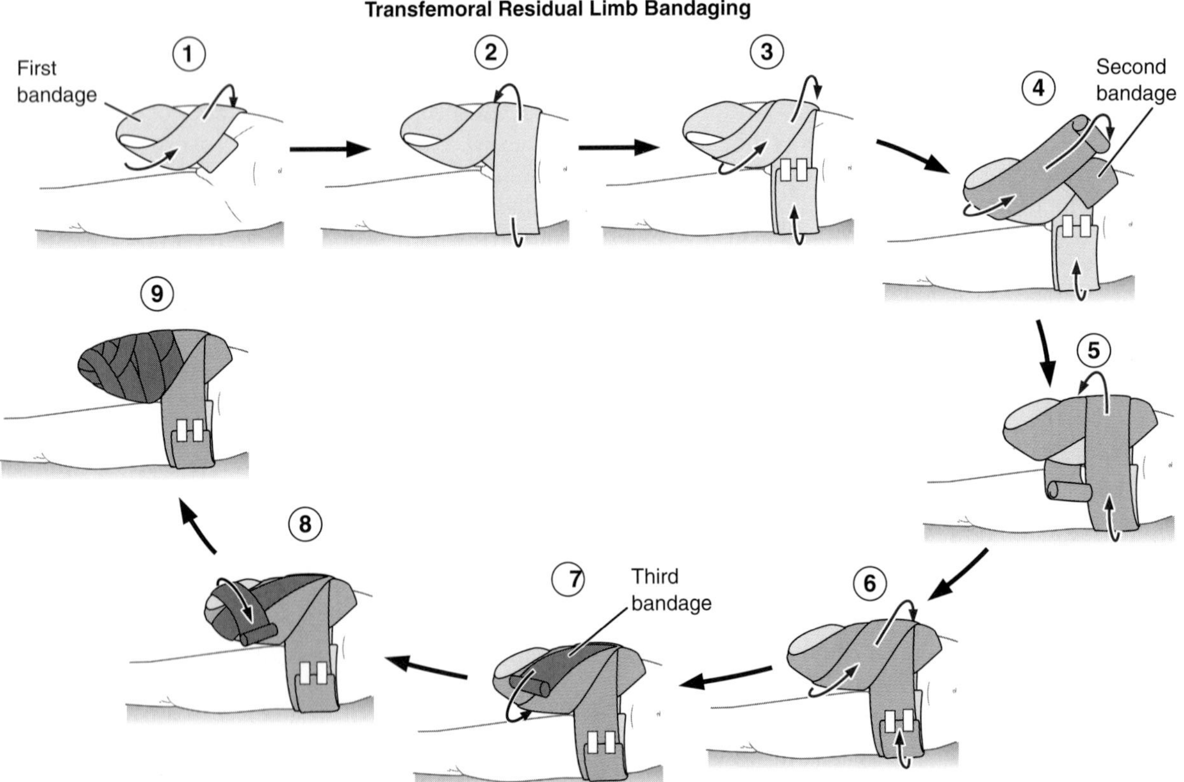

FIGURE 24-8. Limb wrapping for client with transfemoral amputation.

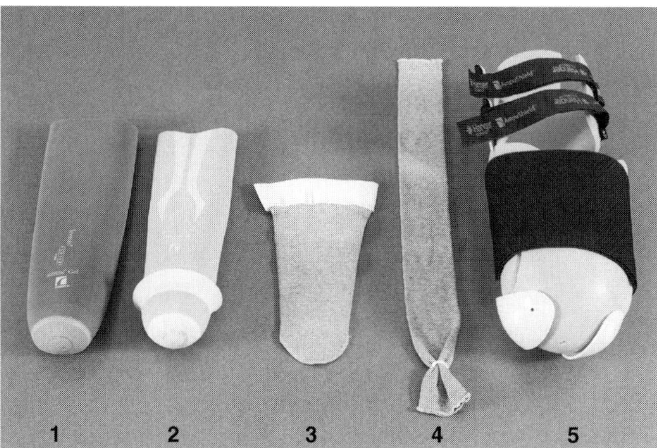

FIGURE 24-9. Various items used by clients with lower extremity amputation. *From left to right:* Pictured are (1) a silicone gel liner worn over the limb; (2) a silicone suction liner which allows the client to keep their limb in the prosthesis with suction; (3 and 4) two types of lower extremity shrinkers; and (5) rigid removable dressing worn postoperatively to assist with edema management and limb shaping, protection of the limb, and contracture prevention.

particular sensations. The use of desensitization techniques on the residual limb is critical for increasing tolerance to wearing a prosthetic socket. After surgery, skin or the scar may be hypersensitive, and desensitization techniques help the client tolerate the increased sensory input resulting from placing one's body weight onto the residual limb. Education and training on these techniques should be provided to both the client and the caregivers. Desensitization should be performed three times a day for 20 to 30 minutes as tolerated.[27] The use of graded sensory stimuli help regulate the sensory input. Clients are advised to begin with different textures, gradually progressing from soft to rough materials. The client can combine the stimuli of textures with additional stimuli of tapping, massage, and vibration. Massage to the limb may be performed with a massage cream or lotion. Medical supply companies sell several types of vibrators, such as a vibrating mitt, a vibrating tube that can be wrapped around the end of the limb, or a small handheld mini-vibrator. Tapping can be accomplished by using a fingertip or other solid, blunt object to repeatedly tap the surface of the residual limb. At first, the client may report that the resulting sensations feel strange, but over time, the body accommodates to the new sensations. The timeframe required for sensory stimulation varies between individuals. The client can also submerge the residual limb in a container of items with different textures, such as dry beans or rice, and graded to tolerance. This process is very helpful in reducing pain and hypersensitivity in the residual limb, and it should be implemented first in the therapy clinic and then continued at home.

Phase Two: Preprosthetic Program—Preparation and Training

The second phase of rehabilitation includes increasing the client's endurance, strength, and functional abilities so that he or she may begin to perform ADLs without using the prosthesis. This serves as the foundation for the tolerance and successful training of the client with a prosthesis in the next phase of rehabilitation.

ENDURANCE

It is necessary to educate the client with limb loss to perform exercises that promote cardiovascular and aerobic fitness, such as walking, jogging, low impact aerobics, upper body ergometer (an upper extremity exercise machine), wheelchair propulsion, and aquatic exercise. Selection of the aerobic exercise may depend on the specific limb loss. Adapted exercises are also available, such as wheelchair basketball, wheelchair tennis, adapted water and snow-skiing, use of weight machines with cuffs and loops, and bicycles propelled with the UEs, to name a few. Aerobic exercise improves the body's ability to take oxygen in and perform daily tasks with more comfort and less fatigue in preparation for prosthetic training and the rehabilitation process. The client may be severely lacking endurance from extended hospitalization because of the injury or because of comorbidities that may have led to the amputation.[33]

STRENGTHENING AND RANGE OF MOTION

OTAs should educate clients and caregivers on ways to incorporate passive range of motion (PROM), active assistive range of motion (AAROM), and active range of motion (AROM) exercise programs for the involved and uninvolved limbs to maintain joint integrity and prevent stiffness or joint contractures. A strengthening program for the upper body, lower body, and core should be implemented at this time. This should include the use of elastic bands and cuff weights to build proximal strength of the affected and nonaffected upper limbs to prepare for wearing a prosthesis for prolonged periods. Increasing postural awareness is a key component of minimizing overuse injuries of the neck, upper extremities, and back because of the client potentially using abnormal patterns of movement to compensate following the amputation.[27] Having the client perform isometric (no joint movement with muscle contraction) and isotonic (joint movement and muscle contraction) strengthening exercises in front of a mirror provides the needed visual feedback to minimize compensatory body movements.[27] For a client with a LE amputation, it is important to work on the upper body and UE strength and endurance because he or she needs to rely on the UEs more while moving through the rehabilitation process.

FUNCTIONAL TRAINING: ACTIVITIES OF DAILY LIVING

The OTA educates and trains the client with upper limb loss in the use of assistive/adaptive equipment to perform feeding, bathing, grooming, dressing, and toileting. Initial education focuses on one-handed techniques to perform self-care tasks while maintaining good body mechanics. If a client has lost the dominant hand, training for change of hand dominance begins during this phase, and if the client has had bilateral UE hand amputation, then he or she will require a universal cuff. The universal cuff is an adaptive device that is used by the client when hand grasp is absent.

It is introduced to facilitate self-feeding and use of grooming tools with the dominant residual limb at the wrist. The client is educated on the use of a bath mitt with a Velcro® fastener to be placed on the residual limb to assist in washing the body and to increase incorporation of the affected limb during bathing. Education on the use of Dycem® (a nonslip material) is important to facilitate holding items in place while opening and/or grasping them. The OT practitioner is able to use creativity to develop and adapt devices for a specific client's needs, depending on the client's level of amputation and desires. Ultimately, clients select which equipment is best suited for their needs and what they are willing to use. Most clients prefer to limit the amount of adaptive equipment they use because of the inflexibility of specific equipment being used in different environments.[27] For example, a client may prefer to use an adapted technique for self-feeding rather than adaptive equipment that would have to be transported to every meal outside of the home.

For clients with a LE amputation, training in use of durable medical equipment, such as a shower chair, tub bench, raised toilet seat, and 3-in-1 commode, is crucial for performance of toileting and bathing with increased independence and safety in the bathroom. Teaching this client to use a long-handled reacher is important for the prevention of falls because the client does not have to bend down from a standing position or lean too far forward while seated in a wheelchair to reach the desired object.

MYOSITE TESTING

If the client has been identified as a potential user of upper limb myoelectric prosthesis, it is during this phase two that testing for electromyographic (EMG) signals on muscles sites should be performed. Typically, the flexor muscles are used to close the TD and the extensor muscles to open the TD. The goal is to identify two specific muscles on the residual limb that can generate two clear signals. The client is then trained by the OTA and the prosthetist in using the specific musculature to activate and perform basic myoelectric prosthetic functions (with a demonstration/practice unit), such as grasp and release of objects.

Phase Three: Prosthetic Training

The goal during the prosthetic training phase is to train the client how to operate the prosthesis and ultimately incorporate it in the performance of their daily tasks. The OTA focuses on training the client on how to don/doff the prosthesis, care for the prosthesis, control the prosthesis, and achieve independence by using the prosthesis for all daily activities (Fig. 24-10).

- The client must first learn how to don/doff the prosthesis and identify the components of the prosthesis and their uses.
  - If the client is wearing a body-powered prosthesis, he or she should learn how to don/doff the harness and prosthetic and adjust it.

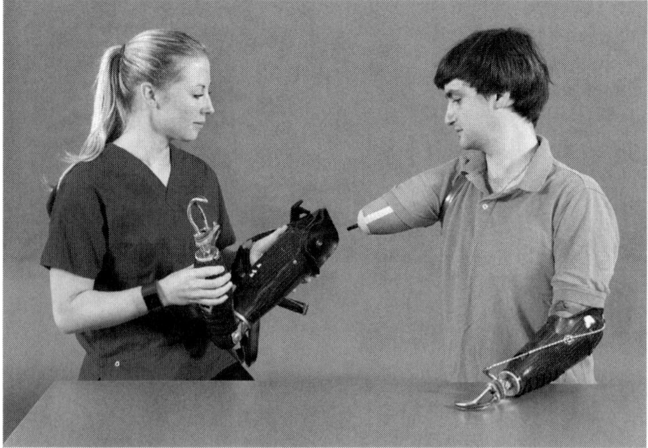

FIGURE 24-10. Upper extremity prosthetic donning. This client has both transradial and transhumeral amputations. The pin on the liner on the right upper extremity holds his residual limb in the prosthetic socket.

  - For the client with transradial amputation using a body-powered prosthesis, education should focus on using bilateral shoulder movements to open and close the TD and prepositioning of the TD by adjusting the TD attachment at the wrist level.
  - For the client with a transhumeral amputation using a body-powered prosthesis, education should focus on how to don and doff the harness and adjust it.
  - In addition, the client is trained on using shoulder joint movements to lock and unlock the elbow and how to operate the TD by using shoulder movements.
- For the client using a myoelectric prosthesis, education should include how to remove and insert the battery, charge it, and care for the prosthesis. Education begins on how to turn the TD on and off and how to control the TD for basic movements and then move on to proportional control during prosthetic training.
- The OTA also works with the client on training and adapting functional activities while now using the prosthesis, such as dressing, meal preparation, or laundry.

CONTROLS TRAINING

The client who is using a body-powered prosthesis must learn to control the following body motions before training with the prosthesis.

- Scapular abduction—In combination with humeral flexion, provides the tension needed to open the TD.
- Chest expansion—Obtained by inhaling deeply, expanding chest and then relaxing. This is used by clients with transhumeral, forequarter, and shoulder disarticulation amputations.
- Scapular depression, humeral extension and abduction—These movements are used by the client with transhumeral amputation to operate the internal locking elbow.
- Humeral flexion—This movement in combination with scapular abduction allows the TD to open.

- Elbow flexion/extension—These movements are important for the client with transradial amputation to maintain ROM at the elbow and allow the affected limb to reach in various planes.

Prosthetic controls training is initiated after learning the above movements, and it should be a gradual process. The client should be progressed accordingly with rest breaks, as needed, to minimize fatigue and frustration.

TRAINING FOR BODY-POWERED PROSTHESIS CONTROL

After education and training on how to use biscapular movements to operate the elbow locking mechanism and opening/closing of the TD, the next step is prepositioning of the wrist TD. This is achieved by using the nonaffected limb to passively rotate the TD. If the client has bilateral UE limb loss, he or she can place the TD against a surface to assist in turning it or place it against the side of the leg or knee, if seated. For the client with transhumeral amputation, learning to lock the elbow is an important component of training to achieve control when positioning prosthesis to perform any task. After the training in prepositioning of the wrist and elbow, the OTA trains the client on using the prosthesis to reach, grasp, place, and release different-sized objects, ideally progressing from hard to softer objects. For example, it is easier to control the hold on a hard plastic cup than a thin, disposable plastic cup. Such objects as wooden blocks and balls, foam, or plastic cups can be used during control training, and the OTA should progress the client to pick up and release these objects at different heights. Verbal and tactile cues should be used to train the client to develop awareness in the use of proper body mechanics, maintenance of upright posture, and avoiding the use of compensatory movements. Repetitive drills should be performed first with the body-powered prosthesis to work on improving control of opening and closing the TD as well as positioning the elbow, if applicable. Once the client becomes proficient in these, then he or she should be progressed to drills that require the use of bilateral hand integration, and training in the use of the prosthesis during ADL tasks should be initiated during this phase.

TRAINING FOR MYOELECTRIC PROSTHESIS CONTROLS

During training in the use of a myoelectric prosthesis, it is important to identify which muscle sites are used for the opening and closing of the hand. For the client with transradial amputation, typically, the wrist extensors are used for opening the TD and the wrist flexors are used for closing the TD (myoelectric hand).

For the movement, the client with transhumeral amputation using a hybrid prosthesis—that is, elbow locking mechanism operated by biscapular movements and a myoelectric TD (hand)—the biceps muscle is used to close the TD and the triceps muscle to open the TD once the elbow has been locked. When using a prosthesis with an electrical elbow, wrist, and hand, the client with transhumeral amputation can use the biceps muscle for elbow flexion and the triceps muscle for elbow extension. Then, the client can switch to the wrist mode and use the biceps muscle for turning the wrist into pronation and the triceps muscle for supination, followed by the use of the biceps muscle for closing of the TD and the triceps muscle for opening of the TD. For a client with shoulder disarticulation and forequarter amputation, the deltoid, trapezius, and pectoralis muscles may be used for operating the prosthesis. Which muscles are used to operate the prosthesis is determined during myosite testing and in collaboration with the prosthetist because it is the prosthetist who is responsible for placement of electrodes inside the prosthetic socket to pick up the client's EMG signals. The first goal of training with the myoelectric prosthesis is the client learning to isolate muscle signals to operate the TD. Some companies offer computer-based hardware and software in combination with electrodes from the socket, which can be used, if available, for training in separation and operation of myosite signals to operate a TD.[34] Once the client has achieved the ability to separate the muscle signals, training in mastering proportional control begins.

Proportional control is a term used to describe the proportional relationship of the elicited strength of the selected muscle contraction to the speed and grip force of the TD.[34] Because there is no sensory input coming from the prosthetic, learning proportional control helps the client avoid "crushing" objects or dropping them unexpectedly when they learn to grade their muscle contractions while operating the TD to grasp and release different-sized objects of different materials (e.g., plastic, metal, soft foods).

The use of repetitive drills in training the client to use the TD to pick up different-sized objects with different textures can be very effective. Muscle fatigue during training should be taken into consideration, and implementation of rest breaks is important. During the use of repetitive drills, the client learns to master how to control the muscle contractions used to control the gripping force of the TD.[32] The client is also trained to use various grips that can be programmed in the myoelectric hand (e.g., lateral pinch, gross grasp, tip to tip pinch, and how to switch between grasps). Once the client has achieved good control of the myoelectric TD for prepositioning, grasping, and releasing different-sized objects and switching between grasps through the use of repetitive drills, bilateral hand integration drills should be initiated. By using bilateral hand drills, the OTA educates the client to incorporate both UEs when picking up objects. Using ADL tasks to train the client on incorporating the affected extremity is the goal during this training phase. It is important to note that establishing a good relationship with the prosthetist is essential to ensure the best outcomes for the client. The prosthetist can assist in myosite testing and educate the OTA on the settings of the electrode sensitivity and settings of the myoelectric hand (e.g., what muscle contractions are necessary to change grips and which grips have been programmed in the hand to be used). It is recommended that the OTA read the clinician's manual for each TD that the client will be using to become familiar with the different settings, hand grips, and options that the TD provides to the client. The knowledge is beneficial when training the client to become proficient in the use of the myoelectric prosthesis to perform ADLs and IADLs.

CONSIDERATIONS FOR THE CLIENT WITH PARTIAL HAND AMPUTATION

Technology in prosthetics for the client with partial hand amputation has advanced in recent years. Prostheses to increase the functional use of the affected hand beyond the esthetic/passive realm are now available.[34] Collaboration with the prosthetist is important in determining which prosthesis is appropriate for a specific client, given his or her goals. The OTA can train the client to use the remaining hand musculature to operate the prosthesis, whether through a biomechanical approach or a myoelectric approach.

ACTIVITIES OF DAILY LIVING TRAINING WITH A PROSTHETIC

Training a client with unilateral upper limb loss in performing ADLs with a body-powered prosthesis or a myoelectric prosthesis includes training the client to use the prosthesis as a gross assist to hold and stabilize objects. The nonaffected UE will always be the dominant extremity for all activities performed.[32] Education on prepositioning of the prosthesis and the TD is crucial to achieve the best outcomes during ADL task performance. The client should be trained to position the prosthesis in a way that resembles how a regular limb would be used in the task. Activities that should be practiced are as follows:

- Dressing: Donning lower body clothing (keeping TD closed while pulling up pants and also managing fasteners), donning shoes, buttoning shirts, and tying shoelaces
- Feeding: Managing utensils to cut foods and feed self
- Opening different types of containers: Jars and bottles
- Meal preparation: Cutting different kinds of food (fruits/meats), setting the table, item retrieval in the kitchen, and managing pots and pans
- Folding clothing: Short- and long-sleeved shirts, pants, socks, undergarments, towels, and linens

Training of the client with bilateral upper extremity limb loss is more involved and takes more time because the client may be totally dependent on the prostheses to perform daily tasks. Because of this dependence, it is important for the OTA to train the client to use the prostheses efficiently early on.[32] The OTA also needs to teach the client to make adaptations for some tasks, such as bathing, when a prosthetic cannot be worn.

PROSTHETIC TRAINING FOR THE CLIENT WITH LOWER EXTREMITY AMPUTATION

Once a client is cleared to begin using his or her LE prosthesis, the OT and the PT teams work together to increase the client's independence while using the prosthesis. The OTA should ensure that the client is independent with donning and doffing the prosthesis as part of ADLs and reinforce the importance of ongoing skin inspection. Skin inspection becomes even more important when the client is starting to wear the prosthesis because the prosthesis may produce increased pressure on skin. The OTA then works with the client on the performance of ADLs and IADLs while adapting to the use of the LE prosthetic. It is also important to educate the client on changes to balance and proprioception. With the loss of a LE, the client now has a changed center of gravity, which can increase the risk of falls, if balance is not properly managed. The ability to manage balance will impact how the client retrieves items from high and low surfaces during dressing, meal preparation, doing laundry, grocery shopping, and house cleaning. The physical therapist/PTA and the occupational therapist or the OTA address balance, although the OTA focuses on occupational performance of desired tasks that require balance to perform. Additionally, with the removal of sensory input from the LEs, the client initially has altered balance, which has to be accommodated for in the rehabilitation process. This decrease in balance is typically initially addressed by use of an assistive device (AD) as the client begins to function again in the standing position.

During treatment sessions, clients may be using a variety of ADs when ambulating with a prosthesis. These may include a standard walker, a rolling walker, forearm crutches, axillary crutches, quad cane, or single point cane. There are variations on all of these items as well. It is important to help the client learn how to properly use the AD not only with ambulation, but also when performing functional tasks. Common errors when ambulating with a prosthesis along with an assistive device include relying on the AD too much or leaning forward onto the AD, resulting in increased trunk flexion. When working on ADL and IADL training, ADs may seem to get in the way. For example, while performing tasks in the kitchen, clients may take unnecessary risks by potentially not using their ADs or not using them in the correct and safest manner. This may mean leaving the crutch by the sink and hopping to the refrigerator to save time. The OTA can assist the client in adapting that ADL or IADL to make it both safe and functional while continuing to use the most appropriate AD to complete the task. Clear communication with the healthcare team is also important to make sure that everyone knows the ultimate goal for an ambulation device for the client because this may change the treatment activities.

Phase Four: Advanced Prosthetic Training

As the client approaches the advanced prosthetic training phase, he or she should be able to don/doff the prosthesis independently, tolerate wearing the prosthesis during the course of a whole day, and operate the basic controls of the prosthesis well. The goal during this phase is for the OTA to train the client in incorporating the prosthesis efficiently during ADLs and IADLs.[34]

THE OLDER ADULT

Many factors go into the decision made by the medical team with regard to the type of prosthesis a client will receive.[35] Consider a 78-year-old client who has recently undergone a surgical below-knee amputation secondary to diabetes. The team would need to assess many things before deciding that this client was an appropriate candidate for a prosthesis. First, it would be important to look at the client's current medical status. Some diagnoses, such as vascular or cardiac disease, could place the client at an increased risk of injury while using a prosthesis. As noted in this chapter, walking with a prosthesis takes substantially more effort compared with baseline ambulation, so the client's cardiovascular system has to be assessed to determine if it can tolerate the increased stress. Clients with diabetes and vascular compromise also often have trouble with healing of wounds and have more fragile skin. Using a prosthesis places increased pressure on the tissues of the residual limb, so the team would need to make sure that the client's skin could tolerate this increased pressure and that the client has the cognitive skills to complete regular skin inspections to limit the risk of severe wounds developing from use of the prosthesis. Circulatory compromise may lead to increased pain and decreased tolerance of the increased pressure on the residual limb from the socket. The team would need to look at the client's premorbid status to determine whether a prosthesis would be appropriate and which type. If the client was nonambulatory before the amputation, the team would need to assess if ambulation would be an appropriate goal.[35,36]

Walking with a prosthesis can be hard to learn; the need for the use of socks and liners, skin inspection, and the extra safety awareness has to be taken into account. The team needs to determine whether a client has enough cognitive capacity to use the prosthesis safely. However, the team should also assess the client's support system and caregivers to decide if they may be able to provide support to the client in the use of the prosthesis. Finally, the goals and motivation of the client need to be taken into consideration. If the client has no desire to use a prosthesis, that is a decision that the team and the OTA need to accept and then continue with teaching functional adaptations to help the client perform ADLs and IADLs independently and safely.[35-37] Although there may be many reasons to not recommend a prosthesis for an older adult, the OTA must also keep in mind that every client is unique and that many older adults would benefit from and can safely use a prosthesis. The client may benefit from a prosthesis for limited function, such as for transfers to access the community or transfers at home from different surfaces, such as the toilet seat or the car seat.[37] Always make sure to speak with older adult clients about their therapy goals to ensure that they have all the tools they need to reach their functional goals. It will be important for them to maintain safety and independence as much as possible in their environments.

Advanced Prosthetic Training for the Client With Upper Extremity Amputation

The following are examples of ADL and IADL activities that the client is trained in performing while using the UE prosthesis:

- Meal preparation: Setting the table, item retrieval in the kitchen, and managing pots and pans
- Folding clothing: Short- and long-sleeved shirts, pants, socks, and undergarments
- Laundry: Placing clothing in washer/dryer, retrieving it, and carrying it to and from different places
- Home management: Cleaning of table, use of broom incorporating prosthesis, and using tools to fix items in the house
- Grocery shopping: Retrieving items from shelves, carrying grocery bags, and retrieving money from the wallet to pay for food items

The client is also trained in the use of proper body mechanics and energy conservation techniques to decrease biomechanical stress to the intact limb and to incorporate the prosthesis without using compensatory movements. Ambulating with a LE prosthetic and using an UE prosthetic may be tiring and cause increased energy expenditure. Some clients may lean forward while walking or laterally at the trunk with UE prosthetic use to compensate. Without learning the correct techniques for prosthetic use and working on strengthening both the intact and amputated residual limb, the client may experience unnecessary discomfort that impacts function. This phase also focuses on educating the client to use the prosthetic in meaningful tasks in all occupations, not just ADLs. The client learns to use the prosthesis efficiently by performing tasks that require bimanual use and multiple steps to complete.

Advanced Prosthetic Training for the Client With Lower Extremity Amputation

For the client with lower limb loss, this phase of prosthetic training includes the use of the LE prosthesis during such tasks as grocery shopping, meal preparation, laundry, household cleaning, bed making, and working tasks that require standing and dynamic movements. The OTA educates the client on the use of modified techniques, such as the attachment of a bag to a rollator and/or rolling walker or use of a backpack to carry items in the community if the client is using an AD to ambulate. The focus during this phase is increasing the client's independence in home and community management tasks while using the LE prosthesis with or without ADs to ambulate.

Once a client has become more comfortable and independent with basic ambulation, PT practitioners will start to work on more advanced skills, such as negotiating stairs, curbs, ramps, and uneven surfaces. The client also works on balance skills and, if appropriate, begins working on progressing to a lower-level AD or no AD. This is

OT Practitioner's Viewpoint

As an OT practitioner, I often work closely with physical therapists in my outpatient clinic. One day, while I was working, one of the physical therapists approached me regarding a client. The client, a female in her 30s, had undergone bilateral transfemoral amputations. Although the client was progressing well with her PT, the physical therapist was concerned that she would not be able to properly instruct her client on how to use her forearm crutches to do all of her IADLs and ADLs and would benefit from OT. I explained to the physical therapist what the focus of the OT treatment would be for this particular client, given her level of amputations and how the client would benefit from OT services to increase her independence with ADLs and IADLs. At the end of the conversation, I encouraged the physical therapist to speak to the client's physiatrist (a doctor specializing in rehabilitation medicine) to obtain a referral for the client to be seen by an OT practitioner. I was then able to work with the client on how to prepare meals, perform grocery shopping, and carry objects while using the forearm crutches. This was also a great opportunity to teach energy conservation principles and proper body mechanics techniques during ADL and IADL performance. I only had to see the client for a few treatment sessions, and the client was able to gain more independence by working with OT. Always make sure to advocate for your clients and your profession, and do not hesitate to ask your colleagues to refer their clients for OT treatment if you believe a client would benefit from OT services to help them achieve their goals. ~Claribell Bayona, OTD, OTR/L

also a time when clients may start to work on safely falling and on floor transfers. The OTA consults with the physical therapist or the PTA to be sure that all team members are on the same page. Clients may also work on returning to leisure activities with the use of the prosthesis.[20] The OTA helps pull all of these skills together, works to adapt various tasks, as needed, to make them possible for the client to perform, and works on more difficult ADLs. The OTA should always ensure that he or she is working with the client's rehabilitation team so that all advanced skills that the client requires for ADLs are addressed.

FUNCTIONAL CONSIDERATIONS IN ALL PHASES

A key part of the OT rehabilitation process in every phase is the retraining for and adaptations of ADLs and IADLs, both with and without the prosthetic. The following section will describe the use of techniques and adaptive equipment during functional activities while also considering energy expenditures to complete these daily tasks.

Activities of Daily Living

It is the role of the OTA to help clients with amputations learn how to perform ADLs. Some ADLs allow the use of the prosthetic, but others can be performed with the residual limb only.

BATHING

The UE prosthesis is not used during bathing because components of a body-powered and myoelectric prosthesis could be easily damaged by water. The OTA educates clients with transhumeral amputation to use a wash mitt with a Velcro® fastener on the residual limb to incorporate the affected UE when washing the nonaffected side. For these clients, the length of the residual limb determines whether they can use the bath mitt effectively during bathing. The installation of shampoo and soap containers on the wall is beneficial because they can be accessed by pushing buttons with the residual limb or other parts of the body (if the client has a short transhumeral amputation or shoulder disarticulation). When washing the body, if the residual limbs do not have enough length for placement of a bath mitt that can be fastened by Velcro®, bath sponges placed on higher and lower portions of the wall and are attached to a suction cup are useful to the clients with bilateral UE amputations.

For increased safety during bathing, the client with lower limb loss should be educated on the use of a shower chair. The client with bilateral lower limb loss is taught to use a tub bench because it provides a larger surface to sit on and facilitates transfers from a wheelchair or toilet without the use of the prosthesis. Installation of grab bars is recommended to maintain safety during tub or stall shower transfers.

DRESSING

The OTA trains clients with unilateral UE limb loss in the use of the prosthesis to fasten clothing by using the TD. The TD holds the waistband of the pants, while the intact extremity places the belt through the loop, tucks in the shirt, and fastens the pants. The TD can be used to hold the material at the end of the zipper, and then the sound hand pulls up the zipper. A button hook device can be used to button the cuff buttons on the unaffected side, or the buttons can be fastened before donning the shirt. The button hook device is very helpful to clients with transhumeral or higher amputation, and to clients with bilateral UE loss.[32] Elastic shoe laces can be used when donning/doffing shoes but if the client prefers to use non-elastic shoelaces, the OTA can educate the client on the use of the one-handed technique or using the prosthesis to tie the shoelaces.[34]

SELF-FEEDING

For a client with an UE amputation, training includes a mix of one-handed techniques, adaptive equipment, and/or modified techniques. Clients may benefit from a rocker knife, a roller knife, bendable or curved utensils, or specialty terminal devices, such as a utensil. A great deal of practice is needed to manage utensils with a traditional hook TD.

Depending on the level of amputation, the client may be able to manage only using the residual limbs. For example, one client with double UE congenital amputation was taught from a young age to balance a fork between his two residual limbs and swivel it to bring food to his mouth.

GROOMING

A client with an UE amputation may have difficulty with grooming tasks, such as reaching the back of the head for brushing or combing hair or holding a toothbrush or razor. As with other ADLs, a client with one UE amputation may benefit from retraining the remaining limb and hand to complete tasks. Adaptive equipment, such as a long-handled comb, comb with a curved handle, or large-handled toothbrush may be useful. There are specialty TDs available, as well as TDs that replace the traditional TD, usually with a quick disconnect device.

TOILETING

A client with an UE amputation of the dominant hand may not want to or be able to use the prosthetic for toilet hygiene and may work on retraining the other hand to perform such hygiene tasks. A client with double amputations may have a specific TD that works best for hygiene tasks or use tools, such as a toilet aid or a bidet. A higher toilet seat or bars/handles may assist a client with a LE amputation to get off the toilet easily, either with or without the prosthetic on. A client with double LE amputations may transfer forward from the wheelchair to the toilet, facing the toilet tank (see Fig. 13-31 in Chapter 13).

SEXUAL ACTIVITY

OTAs are experts in addressing ADLs, and it is important not to exclude addressing sexuality as one of the ADLs to be discussed during the rehabilitation process. Most important, and the first step, is that a trusting relationship must be formed between the client and the OTA.[38] Sexuality and intimacy are often seen as private matters, so clients and partners may be reluctant to discuss them. Therefore, an OTA who develops a trusting and supportive relationship with the client may assist him or her in addressing these issues. Research has repeatedly established that healthcare providers acknowledge that it is important to discuss sexual activity after amputation, but few actually do discuss it with their clients.[39] This is related to many factors, including the provider's lack of comfort and knowledge of subject, the provider not seeing it as his or her job (and sometimes referring the client to another practitioner for such matters), the client not asking about sexuality, which leads the provider to assume that the client has no questions or concerns, and lack of private space to discuss the issue. As mentioned previously, the client may not feel comfortable discussing sexuality with practitioners, leading to the topic never being addressed during the healing process.[39,40]

Once the OTA has developed a trusting relationship with the client, several areas related to sexuality may need to be addressed. As a result of the amputation, the client may be experiencing an alteration in body image.[41] Therefore, the OTA needs to work with the client to develop acceptance of his or her body changes. This may impact the client's partner as well, so it is important to involve the partner in education regarding body image and general sexuality. It is important to discuss with the client his or her values and beliefs about sexuality and to consider the relationship status. A client who is married may have different concerns from those of a client who is still dating and anxious about when to reveal their amputation and prosthesis to potential partners. The OTA may also need to take into account comorbidities that accompany the cause of amputation, such as vascular disease or cancer. However, unlike some other medical diagnoses, sexual functioning itself may not be affected, so the physical adaptations need to be addressed.[40]

The amputation of a limb may cause changes to the mechanics of sensuality and sexuality. An UE amputation may affect the acts of stroking, caressing, and masturbation, and a concurrent UE and LE amputations may affect certain sexual positions being possible.[42,43] Pain in the residual limb must also be considered when discussing sexual positions. The OTA may need to work with the client and the partner to adapt the performance of sexual acts and to find a way that suits the needs of the relationship. The OTA may need to have a discussion with the prosthetist about adaption to the prosthetic or an additional prosthetic to facilitate resumption of sexual activity.[28,42,43]

Instrumental Activities of Daily Living

Completion of IADLs can be challenging for clients using UE or LE prostheses. The OTA can offer options to support IADL performance in the home and in the community.

MEAL PREPARATION

During training in meal preparation, the OTA should educate the client on use of energy conservation techniques and principles of body mechanics to minimize biomechanical stress during retrieval of items. The client begins training to cook without the use of a UE prosthesis, using one-handed techniques and one-handed equipment (e.g., one-handed cutting board and can openers). Once the client begins using the prosthesis, he or she should be educated on incorporating the prosthesis to retrieve items from higher- and lower-level shelves, manipulate pots and pans, and cut foods while using the prosthesis. The client with a LE prosthesis may require a rolling cart for transporting items in the kitchen or a stool to sit on for energy conservation.

OPENING CONTAINERS

The OTA will train the client to hold the container with the TD and open the container with the sound hand. For the client with bilateral UE limb loss, the use of Dycem® on the table surface can be helpful to stabilize the bottle or container when using a TD to twist the top off.

HOME MANAGEMENT, PET CARE, AND CHILD CARE

The OTA can assist the client to adapt items for a UE prosthetic for cleaning and vacuuming with a TD and potentially to add straps or buildups for easier grasp. The client may require adaptations for laundry tasks, such as putting items to be folded on the table and carrying the laundry basket. During pet care, the client may want to attach the leash to a belt instead of trying to hold it and to use automatic feeding/watering devices and self-cleaning litter boxes to avoid daily chores associated with pets. Children's clothing can be altered with Velcro® to avoid small snaps and buttons, and clients may want to carry an infant in a baby carrier attached to them if use of the UE prosthetic is unreliable at first. The OTA should address each specific concern, as needed, during the therapeutic process.

The client with a LE amputation requires consideration of balance, safety, and potential use of walker/crutches/wheelchair when performing cleaning and laundry tasks. A reacher or dressing stick will avoid bending and help get items off the floor and out of the washer/dryer. Some clients prefer to get assistance for heavy cleaning and do the day-to-day tidying themselves. Clients may prefer to use a wheelchair for the daily dog walking to save energy or may consider using a dog walking service. It may be difficult to carry infants and maintain balance while using a walker or crutches, so for such clients, a baby sling may be necessary. Keeping up with toddlers who can be very active may be challenging, and the parent may want to employ a child harness for temporary safety and control.

SHOPPING AND DRIVING

Community reintegration is part of the advanced prosthetic training phase, and the OTA educates and trains the client on how to use the prosthesis during all components of shopping, including item retrieval, placing groceries in bags, and retrieving money or the credit card from the wallet. The client is evaluated for return to driving and is trained in using adaptive equipment to drive, including to manage steering the vehicle safely and to operate the pedals, as needed. Driving rehabilitation and retraining can be performed by an OT practitioner who is a driving rehabilitation specialist or a certified driving rehabilitation specialist (see Chapter 16).

Work

The OTA provides education to the client on the use of activity-specific TDs for many different activities, including work performance. The activity-specific TD that the client is fitted with and trained on depends on the client's specific work demands. It is important for the OTA to have knowledge of the various activity-specific TDs that are available for the client and how the client plans to use it to return to being independent with performing a specific task. The client with an amputation may be planning to return to work at the same job with no adaptations, require adaptations for the same job, move to a different job within the same company, be retrained to a new type of work, or need to retire or pursue disability. Certainly, a construction worker who lays brick and stone may find it more difficult to return to his job after any amputation compared with a worker in a call center. The OTA may address aspects of work tasks, such as balance, strength, coordination, and use of adaptations and adaptive equipment. At times, return to work may depend on the reason for the amputation; for example, a client with an amputation as a result of diabetes may also have numerous other health concerns in addition to diabetes. The client may require a referral to a work hardening program tailored to his or her specific job duties, vocational rehabilitation for job training, and/or further education to pursue a new career.

Leisure

Finally, the *Occupational Therapy Practice Framework, 3rd edition* (OTPF-3) includes leisure as part of the occupation domain along with ADLs, IADLs, rest and sleep, education, work, play, and social interaction.[38] The loss of a limb can present challenges in returning to leisure/recreational activities. The OTA plays an important role in helping the client with amputation return to engaging in leisure activities. As the client progresses through the rehabilitation process, he or she begins to be more proficient in performing basic ADLs, and it is important for the OTA to include the return to recreational activities as a goal during treatment sessions because these activities not only impact the physical well-being of the client but psychological well-being as well.[32] As the client prepares for reintegration into the community, the leisure activities that the individual returns to vary for each person. Some clients with upper limb loss may prefer performing the activity using only one hand. Other clients may be interested in using a prosthetic adaptation or equipment modification to participate in the leisure activity. The OTA should become familiar with the different prosthetic devices available for leisure/recreational activities, such as swimming, baseball, cycling, fishing, golf, kayaking, gardening, and playing musical instruments. Therapeutic Recreation Systems is a company that manufactures adaptive TDs for a multitude of leisure/recreational and competitive activities. Communication with the client and the prosthetist is essential to determining which adaptive prosthesis will be effective to return the client with limb loss to achieving independence in his or her chosen leisure task. Once the client has acquired the activity-specific prosthesis, the OTA begins to train the individual in the use of the prosthesis in the leisure task. It is also crucial for the OTA to provide education and resource information on opportunities to engage in leisure/recreational activities. The Amputee Coalition website is a great resource to encourage clients with limb loss because it provides information on sports programs that are geared to such individuals. The Orthotic and Prosthetics Assistance Fund is a not-for-profit organization that promotes physical fitness through recreation. This group provides an opportunity for users of orthotics and prostheses to participate in their First Clinics, which are held throughout the year at no cost all over the United States. The OTA's role in educating the client with limb loss in these recreational programs will further empower the individual

EVIDENCE-BASED PRACTICE

The articles included here represent information gathered on individuals with limb loss and the use of prosthetics to participate in leisure and recreational activities. Leisure and recreational activities are an important component in a client's ability to return to health, well-being, and participation in physical activities. The literature shows a gap in research between the use of sports and adaptive prostheses and increasing physical activity and maintaining an active lifestyle. OT practitioners are important advocates in bridging this gap by learning about the sports and adaptive prostheses that are available and by facilitating clients to become more active and motivated to use them to return to participation in leisure and recreational activities. The role of the OTA includes the use of evidence-based practice, gathering of outcomes, and increased collaboration with manufacturers to identify the best prostheses for clients who are interested in returning to leisure, sports, and recreational activities.

- The number of young clients with traumatic amputations is expected to rise in the coming years as a result of armed military conflicts and dangerous hobbies, and this has increased the need for specialized sport prostheses. Lower limb prostheses and prosthetic adaptations for cycling, golfing, running/jogging, skiing/snowboarding, and swimming; prosthetic adaptations for sports; and prostheses for clients with upper limb amputations for baseball, cycling, fishing, golfing, kayaking, and skiing are discussed in the article.[44]
- Overall, clients with LE amputation as a result of vascular issues participated less in leisure activities after the amputation than before the amputation; however, their leisure satisfaction was actually higher than that of similar-aged individuals without amputation. Some of the barriers to participation in leisure activities included lack of time because of ongoing medical appointments, lack of accessibility, other ongoing medical issues (e.g., declining eyesight), lack of resources to allow participation, fear of exclusion following amputation, lack of knowledge about available leisure activities and how to adapt them.[45]
- A systematic review of 12 articles indicated that 68% of individuals with amputations are generally inactive compared with 40% of the general population. A decrease also occurs in the level of leisure activities after lower limb amputation, although people's satisfaction with their new physical status remains high. Barriers to becoming more active after an amputation were physical limitations, lack of confidence, older age, and overweight; these factors affected participation if the individuals found it physically demanding and embarrassing. More barriers than motivations exist to adopting or maintaining a physically active lifestyle. The crucial takeaway for rehabilitation professionals is playing a role in helping people with amputations overcome their fears and anxieties about participation in physical activities.[46]

Bragaru, M., Dekker, R., & Geertzen, J. H. (2012). Sport prostheses and prosthetic adaptations for the upper and lower limb amputees: An overview of peer reviewed literature. Prosthetics and Orthotics International, 36(3), 290-296.

Couture, M., Caron, C. D., & Desrosiers, J. (2010). Leisure activities following a lower limb amputation. Disability & Rehabilitation, 32(1), 57-64.

Deans, S., Burns, D., McGarry, A., Murray, K., & Mutrie, N. (2012). Motivations and barriers to prosthesis users participation in physical activity, exercise and sport: A review of the literature. Prosthetics and Orthotics International, 36(3), 260-269.

to engage with peers in a social and active environment. This will improve their socialization skills and emotional well-being in addition to improving their physical fitness as they return to participating in leisure activities.

Gait and Energy Expenditure

Although OT may not have a role in specific gait training with clients with amputations, the OTA will be completing functional activities with them that will involve standing and ambulation. It is important to find out from the PT team and the prosthetist about any gait corrections they are working on with the client and that OT practitioners could help carry over into their treatment sessions. For example, a client might find it hard to bend the knee on the prosthesis when walking but is able to when cued. The OTA may be asked to help make sure that while performing functional tasks, that client is focusing on bending the prosthetic knee.

Another important consideration relating to gait and ADLs is energy expenditure. Although research findings vary, walking with a prosthesis increases energy demand and oxygen consumption.[13,26] For example, walking with a transfemoral prosthesis may increase a client's energy demands up to 50% or more.[13,26] This increased energy expenditure is an important factor to be considered in both treatment planning and client education. The OTA needs to explain to clients that ADLs may take longer and that they may be more tired than they were before their amputation when completing functional tasks. This is also an excellent time to instruct them in energy conservation methods, such as taking breaks, breaking down larger tasks into smaller parts, or sitting down to perform tasks typically performed while standing.

REASONS FOR LIMITED PROSTHETIC USE

It is important to keep in mind that not all clients may be candidates for a limb prosthesis and that some may only use a prosthesis for basic functional tasks and limited weight-bearing. Additionally, even clients with a prosthesis will not always be able to wear it during occupational tasks, either because of the task itself (e.g., bathing and showering) or other reasons, such as skin issues, prosthetic fit, or pain. Some clients with UE amputations choose not to wear the prosthesis because they feel they can manage fine without it. For example, one client stated that she only used her UE prosthesis when cutting roses in her garden (because she could not feel the thorns) and transitioned very well into using one-handed and adapted techniques for all other occupational tasks. Another client with a LE amputation may experience too much pain because of arthritis in the shoulders and hands to tolerate crutches or a walker during functional use of the prosthesis for ambulation and may find that pain decreases dramatically with the use of the power wheelchair for ADL and IADL tasks.

It is important to train the client in performing functional tasks with and without the LE prosthesis to promote as much independence as possible for various conditions. With 54% of LE amputations resulting from vascular conditions, the remaining intact limb is at a greater risk for future amputation, with 55% experiencing an amputation of the second leg within 2 to 3 years.[47] Therefore, some clients with LE amputations are encouraged to use a wheelchair for part of the day. Concerns regarding clients who may need long-term wheelchair use include the following:[47]

- Age
- Comorbidities/medical history
- Cardiovascular tolerance
- Skin integrity and circulation (Is the client at risk for wound development with the prosthesis?)
- Upper-body strength
- Condition or strength of the intact leg
- Fitness level
- Body weight and body type

Additionally, the level of a LE amputation greatly impacts the amount of energy expenditure required for occupations. A client with a transfemoral will need to use significantly more energy to ambulate compared with a client with a transtibial amputation.[47] Some clients may use a wheelchair during the training phase as they make progress with strength, endurance, stability, and balance.[47]

NEW TREATMENTS AND TECHNOLOGIES

In rehabilitative treatments, new methods are constantly being researched and developed for improved treatments and outcomes for clients. When working with any specific population, it is important to stay on top of any advances in the field. The following are some of the newer advances in the care of clients with amputations.

Mirror Therapy

The prevalence rate of chronic PLP after amputation has been shown to be 80%, and this often limits the individual's ability to participate in rehabilitation, ADLs, and IADLs.[33] The presence of PLP has also been found to be greater in clients with UE amputation compared with those with LE amputations. According to some research studies, clients with upper limb loss have reported that their quality of life, social functioning, and mental health status are much more affected compared with those of clients with LE loss.[48] Furthermore, if the PLP is not managed, the client is more likely to develop depression, which could greatly affect their participation in therapy sessions and ADLs.[49] Although current management of PLP relies on the use of medications, the use of **mirror therapy (MT)** has been shown to be effective in reducing PLP and does not require the use of medications. In MT, the client sits parallel to a mirror or a mirror box, and the view of the affected limb(s) is blocked. The client then performs movements with the nonaffected limb in front of the mirror and looks at the image. This image forms an illusion and tricks the brain into thinking that there are two intact limbs (see Fig. 33-6). This facilitates cortical reorganization in the brain and reduces PLP.[50] Movements can include basic motor movements at each joint, use of objects (grasp and release), and sensory stimulation with different textures. Descriptions of protocols for MT vary in the literature; however, MT has been shown to be effective for clients with limb loss when performed several times a day for a minimum of 15 minutes during each session. MT is also easily performed both in the clinic and at home with inexpensive supplies.

Target Muscle Reinnervation for the Client with Upper Extremity Amputation

A new development in surgical procedures is enhancement of the use of myoelectric signals to allow more intuitive control of an advanced prosthesis. The current prostheses available for clients with UE limb loss provide the user with little sensory feedback and no sense of touch. A new procedure, **targeted muscle reinnervation (TMR),** uses the residual nerves from the amputated limb and transfers them to remaining muscles that have not been biomechanically functional since the amputation.[51] TMR has been performed on clients with shoulder disarticulation amputations, using the pectoralis muscle as the target area for the nerves.

The reinnervated muscles then serve as amplifiers to the amputated nerve motor commands; when the client thinks about closing or opening his or her hand, the reinnervated muscle contracts, and the myoelectric signal is then used to operate the myoelectric hand.[51] Nerve reinnervation requires approximately 3 months of recovery after surgery, and then training can begin in use of a prosthesis. Benefits of this procedure include increased myoelectric muscle sites to operate a prosthesis, reduced PLP, prevention of symptomatic neuromas, intuitive use of prosthesis when operating multiple joints (elbow, wrist, and hand), and more proficient and faster use of the prosthesis when performing ADLs and IADLs.[51,52] The OTA works with the prosthetist and trains the client to use the prosthesis as efficiently as possible to return to independence in performing everyday tasks.

Components of a Computerized Lower Extremity Prosthesis

The foot and the knee are two components of LE prostheses, where computer-assisted technology is most commonly utilized. Foot components that assist in providing dorsiflexion for the client to help with clearing the foot with walking and functional mobility are now available. Additionally, some clients may use a microprocessor knee component that allows them to make quick adjustments to the knee to allow for smoother ambulation and mobility. The microprocessors also allow for reciprocal stair negotiation because of the increased control they can provide to the client.[26] Technology is improving constantly; so the OT practitioner should keep watching for continued advancements in LE prostheses.

TECHNOLOGY AND TRENDS

The loss of an upper extremity can have a devastating effect on an individual's ability to perform daily activities. Myoelectric multiarticulating hands (bionic hands) have been created to duplicate the functions of the hand. Matching the complexity of the hand is a very difficult challenge to conquer, but manufacturers of the bionic hands have been gradually improving their products with regard to the weight of the hands, the speed of the motors used, and battery life.[53] Use of myoelectric signals from the remaining muscles of the limb is the most widely used technique for operating a bionic limb. The procedure of targeted muscle reinnervation amplifies muscles signals and provides enhanced control of the myoelectric limb. The use of pattern recognition control of multifunctional myoelectric prosthesis has been researched on clients with transradial amputations. This approach uses the pattern recognition of electromyography (EMG) signals in the remaining musculature of the residual limb. Once a pattern of EMG signals has been identified, a command signal is sent to a prosthesis controller, which then matches the intended movement with the prosthetic function.[54] This provides a more intuitive control of the prosthesis and reduces training time because the client does not have to switch between muscle signals to operate different components of the prosthesis (e.g., wrist rotators and different hand grasps), as is the case in a conventional myoelectric-powered prosthesis without the use of pattern recognition.

Other procedures that will involve the implantation of bipolar differential EMG electrodes within the muscle are being researched and will increase the number of controls sites available to operate a prosthesis.[25] The most promising technology presently being researched is the use of intraneuronal electrodes, which will integrate the bionic limb into the biological system. These electrodes would interface directly with the nerves of the residual limb and carry a bidirectional flow of information between the bionic limb and the user.[25]

SUMMARY

The number of people with limb loss in the United States is expected to be 3 million by the year 2050,[1] and many of those clients will need rehabilitation to assist them in achieving independent function. The OTA plays an integral part in the rehabilitation team when treating clients with UE and LE amputations. The OTA's role in treating this client population begins right after the amputation and continues until the client becomes independent in ADLs and IADLs while using the prosthetic device or devices. Early on, the OTA will be instrumental in assisting with limb care, ADL adaptation, emotional coping, and preparation for use of the prosthesis. Once a client starts to use the prosthesis, OT practitioners assist in the training of donning and doffing the device and training in performing ADLs with the use of the prosthesis. Finally, as the client becomes more and more independent, the OTA works with the client on higher-level activities, including home management and return to work and community tasks. Reinforcing proper limb care and monitoring a client's emotional coping are crucial throughout the phase of rehabilitation.

As with any specific diagnosis in rehabilitation, there is a lot to learn when it comes to the terminology and the specific equipment used with clients with amputations. Over time and with experience, the OTA can become more familiar with the terminology and the evolving technology. Many prosthetic options are available, ranging from those that are best for performing basic ADLs to those made for high-level task performance. Constant communication with the client's rehabilitation and healthcare team will ensure that a client is fitted with and trained in the use of the most appropriate prosthetic device for him or her. It is also important to maintain consistent communication with the client and his or her support system as the team works to increase the client's independence. The OTA may find that some clients are not interested in using a prosthesis at all, so it is important to work with the team to meet the goals of such clients.

Limb loss affects clients of any age and health status; working with these clients provides a great variety of learning experiences and opportunities to be creative to ultimately help clients achieve their goals.

REVIEW QUESTIONS

1. A client recovering from bilateral transfemoral amputation wants to try meal preparation. The client tells the OTA that he will not use the walker that the physical therapist would like him to use. The physical therapist is working with another client and not available to speak with. Which of the following is the *best* initial action for the OTA to take when responding to this situation?
   a. Postpone working on meal preparation activity with the client until the physical therapist can be reached.
   b. Tell the client that he must use the walker until the physical therapist can be reached for consultation.
   c. Have the client sit at a table when working on meal preparation.
   d. Have the client work on meal preparation while standing without the walker.

2. A client with traumatic transradial amputation of the dominant arm is participating in OT after receiving the prosthesis. The occupational therapist has incorporated a goal into the treatment plan to facilitate independence with feeding and meal preparation. Which of the following is the *best* procedure for the OTA to recommend the client to use when cutting meat?
   a. Hold a regular knife with a builtup handle in the terminal device, and hold the plate with the nondominant hand.
   b. Hold a regular knife with the terminal device to cut the meat and a regular fork with the nondominant hand.
   c. Use a rocker knife with the nondominant hand, and hold the plate with the terminal device.
   d. Hold a regular knife with the nondominant hand, and hold a regular fork in the terminal device.
3. A client with unilateral transhumeral amputation is ready to begin prosthetic training with a body-powered prosthesis. During the first session, after the initial evaluation, the client mentions to the OTA that she would like to work on folding clothing during the session. What should the OTA explain to the client is the recommended sequence of training with the prosthesis?
   a. Use of bimanual drills before repetitive drills
   b. Use of repetitive drills before practicing folding clothing
   c. Folding clothing multiple times before doing repetitive drills
   d. Performing meal preparation before doing bimanual drills
4. The OTA walks into the client's inpatient rehabilitation room on the third day following his upper extremity amputation, and the client states, "I am having pain in my fingers even though I know they aren't there. Is there anything we can do about it?" Which three of the following would be the *best* treatment strategy to try for this client complaint?
   a. Use of weight-bearing techniques
   b. Use of transcutaneous neuromuscular stimulation (TENS)
   c. Speaking with the physician regarding this complaint so that she can consider medication management
   d. Recommend wearing a prosthesis to reduce the phantom limb pain
   e. Use of repetitive residual limb movements
   f. Use of mirror therapy
5. The OTA is treating a 65-year-old client with a lower extremity amputation. Without looking at the chart, the OTA knows that the *most likely* cause of this amputation is:
   a. Cancer
   b. Vascular disease
   c. Trauma
   d. Congenital
6. An OTA is working with a client in donning the lower extremity prosthesis. The OTA feels that the client's prosthesis is not fitting properly and the client has a little too much room between the limb and the socket. What would be the next best short-term choice for the OTA?
   a. Continue with the treatment hoping the limb will swell to fill the space.
   b. Have the client not wear the prosthesis for today's session.
   c. Suggest removing the prosthesis and adding socks to fill the space.
   d. Call the prosthetist to schedule an appointment for an adjustment.
7. Which of the following reasons is the *most* important for the OTA to review energy conservation with clients with lower limb amputation?
   a. Walking with a prosthesis places more demand for energy and oxygen on the system.
   b. All of these clients are older and therefore get more tired.
   c. Clients get tired from all the medications they take.
   d. Clients get 3 hours of therapy every day and are likely to be tired.
8. While in the inpatient rehabilitation setting, which three of the following should be the focus of the early OT treatment plan for the client with upper limb loss?
   a. Having the client do repetitive drills with the prosthesis
   b. Educating the client on the use of assistive/adaptive equipment during self-care tasks
   c. Increasing the client's ROM and strength
   d. Training the client on how to fold clothing with the prosthesis
   e. Teaching the client to don/doff the prosthesis
   f. Educating the client on one-handed techniques
9. When is it important to address shaping of a residual limb with a client?
   a. Before the client gets the prosthesis
   b. When the client is having phantom pain
   c. Only in the first week of prosthesis wearing
   d. Only when the client cannot fit into the prosthesis
10. During initial training of a client with transradial amputation on how to use a myoelectric prosthesis, the client asks the OTA, "I want to learn all the grips that this hand has." What concepts should the client be educated on at this point in the training?
    a. How to change to different grasp patterns available for the myoelectric hand
    b. Prepositioning of the terminal device (TD)
    c. Proportional control of TD
    d. Desensitization of the residual limb

CASE STUDY

Today, the OTA has two clients with amputations on his caseload. The clients were both involved in the same car accident in which a drunk driver hit their car while they were going through an intersection. The driver, Joe, is a 35-year-old who sustained a right upper extremity transhumeral amputation as well as a mild brain injury. Joe works full time as an information technology consultant and enjoys lifting weights and running to stay in shape. He also has 2-year-old twins and shares household duties evenly with his wife. Joe has no other past medical history. The passenger, Pamela, is 70 years old and sustained a left below-knee amputation. Pamela's past medical history includes diabetes mellitus and a right hip replacement 5 years ago. Her diabetes is moderately controlled, and she has been working with her endocrinologist to improve the control of her blood sugar levels. She recovered well from her hip replacement and lives alone in a one-level condo that has one step without railing at the entrance. She has been driving local distances and active in her church and her local senior center.

Considering these two clients, think through what the focus should be by the OTA for each of the stages of rehabilitation of a client with an amputation.

1. What part of the treatment plan will be the same for each of these clients, and what will be different?
2. What would be the predicted final functional status of each client? Why?
3. What ADLs and IADLs will the OTA need to the focus on for each client?
4. What areas of leisure may need to be adapted for each client?
5. What emotional areas may need to be addressed with each client?

PUTTING IT ALL TOGETHER — Sample Treatment and Documentation

PREPROSTHETIC TRAINING

Setting	Outpatient clinic
Client Profile	29 y/o male who suffered multiple rib and leg fractures, and internal injuries following a motor vehicle accident. Presents with R transhumeral amputation, LLE injury and skin graft, RLE femur fx, ambulates with one Lofstrand crutch for balance
Work History	Worked full-time for a moving company before the accident. Currently on disability
Insurance	Worker's Comp. Approved for 30 visits for OT. Submit for more visits after 30th visit
Psychological	Motivated to become independent again
Social	Not married. He has two children, ages 6 and 9 y/o and is the primary caregiver of his children.
Cognitive	Intact
Motor & Manual Muscle Testing (MMT)	LUE PROM and AROM and MMT is WNL. RUE (dominant) transhumeral amputation. PROM/AROM is limited at shoulder in all planes. MMT is 2+/5.
ADL	Feeding: Dependent for cutting foods, awkward when feeding himself with nondominant hand Dressing: Difficulty donning/doffing lower body clothing, tying shoelaces, difficulty managing upper body fasteners (e.g., zippers, buttons) Bathing: Using shower chair, requires assistance to wash back and left side of the body
IADL	Presents with difficulties with food shopping and meal prep, including cooking. Difficulties with home management (e.g., cleaning, performing laundry).
Goals	1. Pt will demonstrate carry over of exercise program for R shoulder PROM/AROM and strengthening in preparation for prosthetic fitting by 4 weeks. 2. Pt will use assistive equipment to increase independence with upper and lower body dressing with Min A by 4 weeks. 3. Pt will increase ability to cut foods from dependent to modified (I) by using modified techniques and a rocker knife to cut foods by 4 weeks.

OT TREATMENT SESSION 1

THERAPEUTIC ACTIVITY	TIME	GOAL(S) ADDRESSED	OTA RATIONALE
Educate client and family members on PROM/AROM exercise program to be performed at home.	15 min	#1	*Education and Training:* Training and education on PROM and AROM Ther Ex to increase ROM in shoulder and facilitate use of RUE with and without prosthesis
Educate client on use of rocker knife with the L hand to cut foods. Educate client to pick up different-sized objects using a fork with the L hand.	15 min	#3	*Education and Training:* Training and education on use of adaptive equipment for increased (I) with feeding task
Educate client on hemi-dressing techniques to use when donning/doffing upper and lower body clothing. Educate client on modified techniques to manage clothing fasteners (e.g., belts, buttons, shoelaces).	15 min	#2	*Education and Training:* Training and education to facilitate independence with dressing task

SOAP note: 9/18—, 1:00 pm–1:45 pm

S: Client arrived on time and stated, "I have to learn how to use my L arm for a lot of things now."

O: Client participated in skilled OT outpatient session for education and training with ADLs and HEP for preprosthetic training due to RUE amputation. Client and caregiver were provided with handout for HEP for RUE PROM/AROM exercises, and handout was reviewed. Client and caregiver demonstrated good carryover of given HEP during treatment session. Rocker knife provided and educated client on how to use it with the L hand to cut a piece of fruit. Client worked on using a fork to pick up different sized pieces of foods using the L hand. Client also instructed on use of hemi-dressing techniques to don/doff upper and lower body clothing. Client demonstrated good ability to don shirt and pants using hemi-dressing techniques. Client instructed on how to place belt in pants before donning for increased (I) when fastening belt and pants and how to use one handed technique for tying shoelaces. Instruction on use of button/zipper pull was provided, and client demonstrated use of buttonhook with min assist for buttoning smaller buttons on a shirt.

Continued

PUTTING IT ALL TOGETHER Sample Treatment and Documentation (continued)

A: Client noted to have significant limitations in PROM/AROM in R shoulder flexion and abduction and encouraged to incorporate given HEP daily at home. Client demonstrated fair ability to cut foods with rocker knife and use L hand to feed himself with a fork. Discussed with client importance of using L hand to perform ADL tasks during preprosthetic training phase to increase efficiency in use of L hand.

P: Skilled OT treatment to continue 2X a week for 45-minute sessions. OTA to provide continuous education on use of AE as needed to increase independence with ADL and IADLs and prepare client for prosthetic training.

Mariana Kiernan, COTA/L, 9/18/–, 4:00 pm

TREATMENT SESSION 2

What could you do next with this client?

TREATMENT SESSION 3

What could you do next with this client?

REFERENCES

1. Ziegler-Graham, K., MacKenzie, E. J., Ephraim, P. L., Travison, T. G., & Brookmeyer, R. (2008). Estimating the prevalence of limb loss in the United States: 2005 to 2050. *Archives of Physical Medicine and Rehabilitation, 89*(3), 422–429.
2. Shurr, D., & Cook, T. (2002). Upper limb prosthetics. In D. Shur & J. W. Michael (Eds.), *Prosthetics and orthotics* (2nd ed, pp. 143–168). Upper Saddle River, NJ: Prentice Hall.
3. Varma, P., Stineman, M. G., & Dillingham, T. R. (2014). Epidemiology of limb loss. *Physical Medicine and Rehabilitation Clinics of North America, 25*(1), 1–8.
4. Mayfield, J. A., Reiber, G. E., Sanders, L. J., Janisse, D., & Pogach, L. M. (2004). Preventive foot care in diabetes. *Diabetes Care, 27,* S63–S64.
5. Limb Loss Statistics. (n.d.). Retrieved from http://www.amputee-coalition.org/limb-loss-resource-center/resources-by-topic/limb-loss-statistics/limb-loss-statistics/#6.
6. Nielsen, C. (2007). Etiology of amputation. In M. M. Lusardi & C. C. Nelson (Eds.), *Orthotics and Prosthetics in Rehabilitation* (2nd ed, pp. 519–531). St. Louis, MO: Saunders Elsevier.
7. May, B. (2002). *Amputations and prosthetics: A case study approach* (2nd ed). Philadelphia, PA: F. A. Davis.
8. Keenan, D., & Glover, J. (2006). Amputations and prosthetics. In H. M. Pendleton & W. Schultz-Krohn (Eds.), *Pedretti's occupational therapy: practice skills for physical dysfunction* (7th ed, pp. 1149–1193). St. Louis, MO: Mosby Elsevier.
9. Belon, H. P., & Vigoda, D. F. (2014). Emotional adaptation to limb loss. *Physical Medicine and Rehabilitation Clinics of North America, 25*(1), 53–74.
10. Schuch, C., & Pritham, C. (n.d.). International Standards Organization terminology: Application to prosthetics and orthotics. *JPO Journal of Prosthetics and Orthotics, 6*(1), 29–33.
11. Pepe, J., & Lusardi, M. (2007). Amputation surgeries for the lower limb. In M. M. Lusardi & C. C. Nelson (Eds.), *Orthotics and Prosthetics in Rehabilitation* (2nd ed, pp. 563–592). St. Louis, MO: Saunders Elsevier.
12. May, J. (2014). Amputation. In S. B. O'Sullivan, T. J. Schmitz, & G. D. Fulk (Eds.), *Physical rehabilitation* (6th ed, pp. 1001–1029). Philadelphia, PA: F. A. Davis.
13. Wong, C. K., Benoy, S., Blackwell, W., Jones, S., & Rahal, R. (2012). A comparison of energy expenditure in people with transfemoral amputation using microprocessor and nonmicroprocessor knee prostheses: A systematic review. *JPO: Journal of Prosthetics and Orthotics, 24*(4), 202–208.
14. Wallace, D. (2012). Trends in traumatic limb amputation in Allied Forces in Iraq and Afghanistan. *Journal of Military and Veterans Health, 20*(2), 31.
15. Kapp, S., & Miller, J. (2009). Lower limb prosthetics. In P. F. Pasquina & R. A. Cooper (Eds.), *Care of the combat amputee* (pp. 553–580). Retrieved from http://www.cs.amedd.army.mil/Portlet.aspx?ID=3e4c64b4-3b35-483f-900b-a394a0ae45eb
16. Amputee Coalition. (2015). A team-based approach to amputee rehabilitation. Retrieved from http://www.amputee-coalition.org/military-instep/amputee-rehab.html
17. Lusardi, M. (2007). Postoperative and preoperative care. In M. M. Lusardi & C. C. Nelson (Eds.), *Orthotics and prosthetics in rehabilitation* (2nd ed, pp. 593–641). St. Louis, MO: Saunders Elsevier.
18. Subedi, B., & Grossberg, G. T. (2011). Phantom limb pain: Mechanisms and treatment approaches. *Pain Research and Treatment, 2011,* http://doi.org/10.1155/2011/864605
19. Seymour, R. (2002). *Prosthetics and orthotics: Lower limb and spinal.* Philadelphia, PA: Lippincott Williams & Wilkins.
20. Gailey, Jr., S. R., & Clark, C. (1992). Physical therapy management of adult lower-limb amputees. In H. K. Bowker & J. W. Michael (Eds.), *Atlas of limb prosthetics: Surgical, prosthetic, and rehabilitation principles* (2nd ed). Retrieved from: http://www.oandplibrary.org/alp/
21. Cost Helper. (2017). Prosthetic arm cost. Retrieved from http://health.costhelper.com/prosthetic-arms.html
22. Cost Helper. (2017). Prosthetic leg cost. Retrieved from http://health.costhelper.com/prosthetic-legs.html
23. Miguelez, J., Conyers, D., Lang, M., & Gulick, K. (2009). Upper extremity prosthetics. In P. F. Pasquina & R. A. Cooper (Eds.), *Care of the Combat Amputee* (pp. 607–640). Retrieved from http://www.cs.amedd.army.mil/Portlet.aspx?ID=3e4c64b4-3b35-483f-900b-a394a0ae45eb
24. The Management of Upper Extremity Amputation Rehabilitation Working Group. (2014). *VA/DoD clinical practice guideline for the management of upper extremity amputation rehabilitation.* Retrieved from http://www.healthquality.va.gov/guidelines/Rehab/UEAR/
25. Fergason, J. (2007). Prosthetic feet. In M. M. Lusardi & C. C. Nelson (Eds.), *Orthotics and prosthetics in rehabilitation* (2nd ed., pp. 643–657). St. Louis, MO: Saunders Elsevier.
26. Edelstein, J., & Wong, C. (2014). Prosthetics. In S. B. O'Sullivan, T. J. Schmitz, & G. D. Fulk (Eds.), *Physical rehabilitation* (6th ed.) (pp. 1364–1402). Philadelphia, PA: F. A. Davis.
27. Smurr, L., Gulick, K., Yancosek, K., & Ganz, O. (2008). Managing the upper extremity amputee: A protocol for success. *Journal of Hand Therapy, 21,* 160–176.
28. Verschuren, J. E., Zhdanova, M. A., Geertzen, J. H., Enzlin, P., Dijkstra, P. U., & Dekker, R. (2013). Let's talk about sex: Lower limb amputation, sexual functioning and sexual well-being: A qualitative study of the partner's perspective. *Journal of Clinical Nursing, 22*(23-24), 3557–3567.
29. Wise, M. (2007). Rehabilitation for persons with upper extremity amputation. In M. M. Lusardi & C. C. Nelson (Eds.), *Orthotics and prosthetics in rehabilitation* (2nd ed, pp. 859–874). St. Louis, MO: Saunders Elsevier.
30. Rheinstein, J. (2017). Post-op prostheses offer benefits after amputation surgery. Retrieved from http://www.amputee-coalition.org/resources/post-op-prostheses-benefits/

31. Fairley, M. (2005). Focus on IPOPs, EPOPs: Does early mobility benefit amputees? The O & P edge. Retrieved from www.oandp.com
32. Meir, R. H., & Atkins, D. J. (2004). *Functional restoration of adults and children with upper extremity amputation.* New York, NY: Demos Medical.
33. Ries, J., & Vaughan, V. (2007). Rehabilitation of persons with recent transtibial amputation. In M. M. Lusardi & C. C. Nelson (Eds.), *Orthotics and prosthetics in rehabilitation* (2nd ed) (pp. 711–744). St. Louis, MO: Saunders Elsevier.
34. Smurr, L. M, Yancosek, K., Gulick, K., Ganz, O., Kulla, S., Jones, M., ... & Esquenazi, A. (2009). Occupational therapy for the poly-trauma casualty with limb loss. In P. F. Pasquina & R. A. Cooper (Eds.), *Care of the combat amputee* (pp. 493–533). Retrieved from http://www.cs.amedd.army.mil/Portlet.aspx?ID=3e4c64b4-3b35-483f-900b-a394a0ae45eb
35. Kurichi, J. E., Kwong, P. L., Reker, D. M., Bates, B. E., Marshall, C. R., & Stineman, M. G. (2007). Clinical factors associated with prescription of a prosthetic limb in elderly veterans. *Journal of the American Geriatric Society, 55,* 900–906.
36. Sheehan, T. P. (2005). When are prostheses the right choice for older amputees? *inMotion, 15*(6), 14–16.
37. Wells, G. (2012). To fit or not to fit. *The O&P Edge, 14*(12). Retrieved from http://www.oandp.com/articles/2012-12_01.asp
38. American Occupational Therapy Association. (2014). Occupational therapy practice framework: Domain and process (3rd ed.). *American Journal of Occupational Therapy, 68*(Supplement 1), S1–S48.
39. Geertzen, J. H., Van Es, C. G., & Dijkstra, P. U. (2009). Sexuality and amputation: A systematic literature review. *Disability and rehabilitation, 31*(7), 522–527.
40. Ide, M. (2004). Sexuality in persons with limb amputation: A meaningful discussion of re-integration. *Disability and rehabilitation, 26*(14-15), 939–943.
41. Mathias, Z., & Harcourt, D. (2014). Dating and intimate relationships of women with below-knee amputation: An exploratory study. *Disability and rehabilitation, 36*(5), 395–402.
42. Verschuren, J. E., Enzlin, P., Geertzen, J. H., Dijkstra, P. U., & Dekker, R. (2013). Sexuality in people with a lower limb amputation: A topic too hot to handle? *Disability and rehabilitation, 35*(20), 1698–1704.
43. Verschuren, J. E., Geertzen, J. H., Enzlin, P., Dijkstra, P. U., Dekker, R., & van der Sluis, C. K. (2013). Addressing sexuality as standard care in people with an upper limb deficiency: Taboo or necessary topic? *Sexuality and Disability, 31*(2), 167–177.
44. Bragaru, M, Dekker, R., & Geertzen, J. H. (2012). Sport prostheses and prosthetic adaptations for the upper and lower limb amputees: An overview of peer reviewed literature. *Prosthetics and Orthotics International, 36*(3), 290–296.
45. Couture, M., Caron, C. D., & Desrosiers, J. (2010). Leisure activities following a lower limb amputation. *Disability & Rehabilitation, 32*(1), 57–64.
46. Deans, S., Burns, D., McGarry, A., Murray, K., & Mutrie, N. (2012). Motivations and barriers to prosthesis users' participation in physical activity, exercise and sport: A review of the literature. *Prosthetics and Orthotics International, 36*(3), 260–269.
47. Bury, E. (2012). Balancing loss and gain: A deeper understanding of amputations, prosthetics and the clinical considerations of wheelchair fittings. *Mobility Management.* Retrieved from https://mobilitymgmt.com/Articles/2012/11/01/Amputations-Prosthetics.aspx?Page=2
48. Davidson, J. H., Khor, K. E., & Jones, L. E. (2010). A cross-sectional study of post-amputation pain in upper and lower limb amputees, experience of a tertiary referral amputee clinic. *Disability and Rehabilitation, 32*(22), 1855–1862.
49. Ephraim, P. L., Wegener, S. T., MacKenzie, E. J., Dillingham, T. R., & Pezzin, L. E. (2005). Phantom pain, residual limb pain, and back pain in amputees: Results of a national survey. *Archives of Physical Medicine and Rehabilitation, 86*(10), 1910–1919.
50. Rothgangel, A., Braun, S., Witte, L., Beurskens, A., & Smeets, R. (2015). Development of a clinical framework for mirror therapy in patients with phantom limb pain: An evidence-based practice approach. *Pain Practice, 16*(4), 422–434.
51. Kuiken, T. A., Miller, L. A., Lipschutz, R. D., Lock, B. A., Stubblefield, K., Marasco, P. D., & Dumanian, G. A. (2007). Targeted reinnervation for enhanced prosthetic arm function in a woman with a proximal amputation: A case study. *The Lancet, 369*(9559), 371–380.
52. Cheesborough, J. E., Souza, J. M., Dumanian, G. A., & Bueno, R. A. (2014). Targeted muscle reinnervation in the initial management of traumatic upper extremity amputation injury. *Hand, 9*(2), 253–257.
53. Clement, R. G. E., Bugler, K. E., & Oliver, C. W. (2011). Bionic prosthetic hands: A review of present technology and future aspirations. *The Surgeon, 9*(6), 336–340.
54. Li, G., Schultz, A. E., & Kuiken, T. A. (2010). Quantifying pattern recognition–based myoelectric control of multifunctional transradial prostheses. *IEEE Transactions on Neural Systems and Rehabilitation Engineering, 18*(2), 185.

Chapter 25

Chronic Disease Management: Utilizing a Self-Management Approach

David H. Benthall, MS, OTR/L and Cathrine Balentine Hatch, MS, OTR/L

LEARNING OUTCOMES

After studying this chapter, the student or practitioner will be able to:

25.1. Recognize population trends related to chronic disease and their implications on health care in the United States

25.2. Understand the chronic diseases discussed in the chapter, including physiological mechanisms, risk factors, and their impact on occupational performance

25.3. Discuss self-management and the benefits of using a self-management approach in occupational therapy practice

25.4. Identify lifestyle modifications and self-management strategies for improved health outcomes and quality of life in clients with chronic disease

25.5. Apply intervention approaches with clients to compensate for symptoms and facilitate necessary modification of roles and routines

25.6. Develop treatment intervention plans for clients with various chronic diseases

KEY TERMS

Canadian Occupational Performance Measure (COPM)
Chronic disease
Chronic fatigue syndrome (CFS)
Chronic obstructive pulmonary disease (COPD)
Congestive heart failure (CHF)
Diabetes
Fibromyalgia
Health literacy
Health management and maintenance
Lifestyle modification
Obesity
Self-management
Self-management support
Self-monitoring
Transtheoretical Model of Behavior Change (TTM)

"Patients with chronic conditions self-manage their illness. This fact is inescapable ... The question is not whether patients with chronic conditions manage their illness, but *how* they manage."[1] With the increasing prevalence of chronic diseases in society, healthcare systems must be prepared for how to best collaborate and support individuals as they self-manage chronic disease on a day-to-day basis. This chapter will focus on the importance of self-management of chronic disease within the home and community and the pivotal role of occupational therapy assistants (OTAs) in helping clients maintain participation in everyday occupations while adapting to daily life with chronic disease.

Chronic disease is defined as a persistent or life-long condition that can be controlled and self-managed over time, but is not curable.[2] According to the Centers for Disease Control and Prevention (CDC) *half* of all adults (117 million) living in the community in the United States have one or more chronic health conditions, including heart disease, chronic obstructive pulmonary disease (COPD), diabetes, cerebrovascular accident (CVA), cancer, arthritis, kidney disease, human immunodeficiency virus (HIV) infection, and/or chronic fatigue syndrome (CFS); and half of these adults are actually living with two or more chronic health conditions.[2] This percentage continues to increase as people age.[3] See the box "The Older Adult" for more details on the prevalence of chronic diseases in aging individuals. The CDC states that 86% of health care costs in the United States are related to the treatment of chronic diseases, which are the nation's leading cause of death and disability.[2] Faced with this reality, the staggering percentage of healthcare costs will only continue to grow given the population trends of older Americans. With healthcare reform's shift toward health promotion, improving quality care, and reducing healthcare costs, occupational therapy (OT) practitioners must gain a deeper understanding of how chronic disease impacts participation in daily life and how to best empower clients using a self-management approach to improve quality health outcomes.[4]

SELF-MANAGEMENT

Living with a chronic disease is physically, socially, and psychologically challenging. Although treatment of acute illnesses is typically geared toward returning clients to their prior level of function, treating chronic disease is a complex, dynamic, and continuous process that requires self-management of the condition on a day-to-day basis and over the duration of clients' lives. **Self-management** is defined as the "individual's ability to manage the symptoms, treatment, physical and psychosocial consequences and lifestyle changes inherent in living with a chronic condition."[7] The California Healthcare Foundation estimates that 90% of the management of a chronic disease must come directly from the person who has the disease, emphasizing the need for clients to be engaged partners in managing their personal health goals.[8,9] Components of effective chronic disease self-management are based on empowering individuals with knowledge of their chronic condition, developing problem-solving skills to recognize and navigate lifestyle changes, and emphasizing the collaborative partnership developed between clients and healthcare providers. A growing body of evidence demonstrates that adoption of self-management strategies improves clients' ability to cope with chronic disease, facilitates behavior change, increases quality of life, and ultimately reduces healthcare costs.[7,9]

Management of chronic diseases does not easily fit into most traditional healthcare models, in which the client takes on a more passive role as a recipient of care from the healthcare provider. In contrast to the traditional medical model, which primarily focuses on reaction-based care and the view of the physician as expert, effective models for self-management of chronic disease rely on collaboration between practitioner and client to provide individuals with the knowledge and strategies to manage their condition over time. Essentially, the individual living with a chronic disease becomes his or her own manager and expert of the condition, and the healthcare professional becomes a consultant supporting clients in this role.[1] Healthcare providers focusing on self-management support must recognize that the client is in control of decision making when responding to his or her condition and that empowerment is fundamental in promoting behavior change. **Self-management support** by healthcare professionals aims to increase a clients' skills and confidence in their care, providing ongoing assessment of progress, goal setting, and problem-solving[10] (Fig. 25-1). Self-management support is most effective when healthcare professions tailor interventions to the needs of the individual client.[1]

In addition to clients being supported as active and informed participants in their plan of care, successful

THE OLDER ADULT

The prevalence of chronic disease increases as people age, further impacting the older adult population. More than half of older adults (65+ years of age) have at least one chronic condition, and many are managing multiple chronic diseases simultaneously. Statistics show that as of 2012, 30% of older adults were living with some type of heart disease, 20% had diagnosed diabetes and 72% had hypertension (or were taking preventative medications for hypertension).[3] The older adult population is projected to more than double from 43 million in 2012, to 92 million by 2060.[3] This rapid population growth coupled with the steady increase of life expectancy in Americans poses a significant challenge for how healthcare systems will manage the vast needs associated with caring for an aging population.

One option is the use of smart technology to monitor chronic conditions. A recent review article noted that, "Baby boomers have begun to widely adopt smart devices and have expressed their desire to incorporate technologies into their chronic care."[5] In fact, older adults also have expanded the way they use smartphones and tablets in the past few years, with health information seeking being the second most frequently executed task besides making phone calls.[6] The authors reviewed 40 articles identified eight strategies to support technology use for self-management, including:[5]

1. Self-monitoring: Self-monitoring of the various biometrics, symptoms, medication, or healthy behaviors
2. Client education: Education of clients related to disease outcomes, self-monitoring, interpretation of measurements, benefits and risks of healthy behaviors, and medication and side effects
3. Reminders: Reminders for medication, self-monitoring, or behavior change
4. Automated feedback: Feedback content including motivational messages, educational messages, or how clients' values compare with a clinical guideline
5. Coaching: Active coaching involving structured and predefined sessions with healthcare providers through in-person, over-the-telephone, and virtual interactions for the purposes of education, motivation, and discussion about self-management strategies
6. Goal setting: Individualized goal setting for the treatment or behavior change
7. Treatment plan: Treatment plan outlining a protocol to follow when clients experience exacerbations of symptoms
8. Social support: Sharing of the self-management progress to engage family members and friends

This review highlights the incorrect assumption many practitioners may make about their older clients. Smart phones and other technology can be a viable option to manage chronic diseases and should be implemented when appropriate.

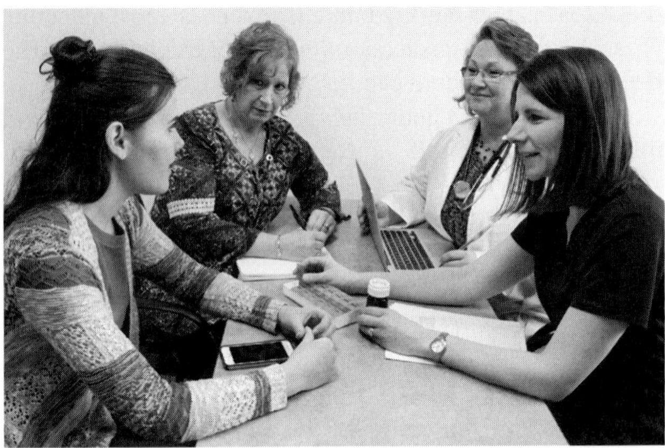

FIGURE 25-1. Self-management support. Collaborative approach to self-management between client, caregiver, primary care provider, and OT practitioner.

approaches to chronic disease self-management put an emphasis on clients:

1. Learning key behavioral skills including goal setting, self-monitoring, and decision making
2. Utilizing community resources
3. Developing strong partnerships with healthcare providers
4. Taking action to promote behavior change[9]

Effective self-managers are encouraged to embrace management of their condition(s) in collaboration and partnership with their healthcare team. The overarching goal of establishing and maintaining this transactional relationship among client, disease, healthcare providers, and community is to achieve improved health outcomes while optimizing the client's quality of life. Thus, healthcare practitioners working with clients with chronic conditions must embrace a supportive partnership and strive to help them integrate self-management into their daily choices, habits, roles, and routines.

ROLE OF OCCUPATIONAL THERAPY IN SELF-MANAGEMENT

The OT profession is ideally positioned to address chronic disease self-management based on its holistic understanding of the client, environmental context, and specific demands of chronic diseases on daily activities. Chronic diseases impact every aspect of daily life, including how a person engages in basic and instrumental activities of daily living (IADLs), social participation, functional mobility in the home and community, leisure performance, sexual activity, sleep and rest, employment, and overall life participation. Living with a chronic condition not only affects a person's physical abilities but also has a wider-reaching social impact associated with depression and other psychological effects on health.[11] Consider the challenges of a gardener who must adapt to life with rheumatoid arthritis, an avid church-goer who no longer has the endurance to attend services because of COPD, a local book club member who is having difficulty reading because of the effects of diabetes, or a grandmother who must relearn lifelong cooking habits after her diagnosis of congestive heart failure (CHF). To say that managing day-to-day life with a chronic disease is challenging is an understatement. Chronic disease disrupts the flow of everyday life and often results in the loss of ability to perform meaningful occupations and fulfill valued roles. OT supports the client not only in managing the disease but also in managing the challenges of day-to-day life. OT recognizes that "self-management is about being in charge of one's life and managing one's condition instead of being managed by that condition."[12]

OT practitioners are particularly well equipped to work with individuals toward effective chronic disease management, given their approach to understanding how habits and routines structure daily life. The foundation of chronic disease self-management is grounded in how individuals successfully create, integrate, and maintain health management behaviors within daily life and in the context of their environment. The notion of how individuals learn and embed new health management behaviors requires OT practitioners to understand performance patterns. As identified in the *Occupational Therapy Practice Framework, Domain and Process, 3rd edition* (OTPF-3), "performance patterns are the habits, routines, roles, and rituals used in the process of engaging in occupations or activities that can support or hinder occupational performance ... Practitioners who consider clients' performance patterns are better able to understand the frequency and manner in which performance skills and occupations are integrated into clients' lives. Although clients may have the ability to engage in skilled performance, if they do not embed essential skills in a productive set of engagement patterns, their health, well-being, and participation may be negatively affected."[13] When considering chronic disease self-management, OT practitioners are working with clients and their caregivers to implement new health management behaviors not simply one time, but repeatedly, routinely, and habitually often over the course of the person's life.

Consider the example of Susan, a 53-year-old single mother of two teenage boys, who has recently been diagnosed with type 2 diabetes. After meeting with her physician, receiving formal education about diabetes, and even taking a 6-week diabetes management program at the local hospital, Susan continues to experience difficulty modifying unhealthy behaviors and incorporating diabetes self-management into the new habits and routines within her daily life. Although Susan understands the basic components of healthy food choices, medication management, and exercise to control diabetes, modifying lifelong behaviors and establishing new habits and routines is extraordinarily difficult. Now consider the approach of an OT practitioner in supporting Susan with her health management goals. What aspects of Susan's daily life might an occupational therapist or OTA consider? The questions may include: What is the family culture surrounding mealtime routines? Does Susan enjoy cooking? What is Susan's method for developing a grocery shopping list? Does income impact her food choices? How are medications organized in the home? Are there natural times during the day to incorporate physical activity? What daily activities and occupations does Susan enjoy performing? These are just a few considerations for OT practitioners to have a better contextual understanding of Susan's day-to-day life, ability to self-manage her chronic disease, and identify areas for intervention to support better health management and maintenance (Fig. 25-2).

The OTPF-3 identifies **health management and maintenance** as an IADL that comprises "developing, managing and maintaining routines for health and wellness promotion, such as physical fitness, nutrition, decreased health risk behaviors and medication routines."[13] OTAs are involved in the treatment of clients with chronic diseases across the continuum of care, including hospital-based settings, rehabilitation centers, outpatient clinics, long-term care facilities, and the client's home and community. Approaches to chronic disease self-management, including assessment, interventions, and outcomes, can be applied in all practice settings; however, in collaboration with the supervising occupational therapist, OTAs must adjust the scope of treatment based on the clinical setting and functional capacities of the client. Treatments are most effective when clients are in their natural environments, such as the home, community, or workplace, where OTAs can assist clients to generalize knowledge and to incorporate self-management strategies into their daily habits, roles, and routines.[14] By the time of discharge, the goal of OT services is to transition the management of the chronic condition to the client or the caregiver as he or she assumes responsibility of day-to-day management.

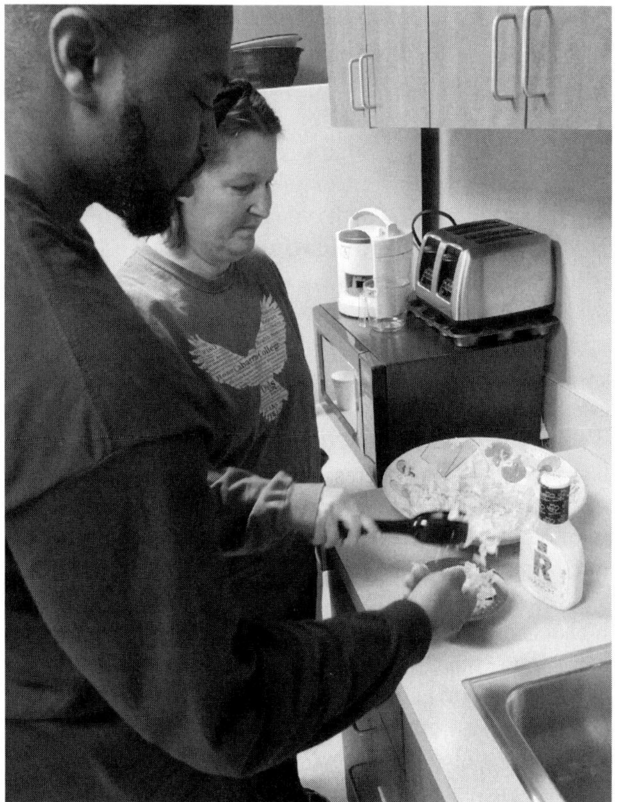

FIGURE 25-2. Health management and nutrition. Susan is performing a meal preparation activity guided by an OTA.

As the number of people living with chronic diseases increases, OTAs will directly impact how clients participate in valued occupations while self-managing and adapting to daily life with a chronic condition. This chapter will further explore the OTA's role in chronic disease management and demonstrate how OT's approach to practice allows clients with chronic diseases to participate in life and meaningful occupations as fully as possible. See "Evidence-Based Practice" to learn more about the evidence that supports OT's role in chronic disease management.

CHRONIC DISEASE CONDITIONS

Practitioners must have an understanding of the chronic diseases their clients are managing on a daily basis. The following section provides an overview of common chronic conditions affecting adults and older adults, including diabetes, CHF, COPD, fibromyalgia and CFS, and obesity. This overview of conditions is not exhaustive but represents a sample of the most pervasive chronic diseases. Although other chronic conditions, such as arthritis, CVA, and cancer, are not described in detail in the following section, self-management principles and the OT practitioner's role in treatment, presented later in the chapter (see Chapters 21, 33, and 29 respectively), still may apply to these conditions as well. While considering these conditions, it is important to realize that many chronic diseases not only have similarities with regard to risk factors, medical treatment, and impacts on occupational performance but also that it is very common for an individual to be living with more than one of these conditions.

Diabetes

Diabetes is a group of diseases characterized by the presence of elevated blood sugar, or hyperglycemia. Risk factors associated with diabetes include age, family history, obesity, hypertension, history of gestational diabetes in women, decreased physical activity or sedentary lifestyle, and ethnicity.[19,20] Depending on the type, diabetes is the result of having issues either with how insulin is produced and/or used in the body. Over time, high blood glucose often results in complications related to impaired function and failure of body organs. If diabetes is poorly controlled, clients are at higher risk for developing other serious conditions, such as heart and cerebrovascular disease, kidney failure, vision loss, and even premature death.[19,20]

EVIDENCE-BASED PRACTICE

Research studies of OT self-management and lifestyle modification interventions have shown introductory evidence for improving functional outcomes in individuals with chronic disease, including ADLs, functional self-efficacy, social or work function, psychological health, stress management, fatigue management, and quality of life.[15-17] In a systematic scoping review of the effectiveness of OT in treating clients with chronic disease, Richardson, et al. found that OT practitioners made moderate contributions in self-management strategies and that interventions directed toward behavior change in individuals with chronic disease were the most consistent strategies used among OT practitioners. The most frequently used self-management interventions included "goal setting, barrier identification, problem-solving, goal modification, peer support, action planning and self-regulation."[15]

Qualitative research studies have also explored the experiences of individuals living with chronic diseases. A 2004 qualitative study was conducted to understand the occupational experiences of individuals with COPD and the benefits of an OT intervention in improving occupational engagement.[18] Researchers found that despite participants' feelings of uncertainty related to the course of COPD and the activity limitations of daily life, utilizing an OT intervention based in self-management principles improved their knowledge of COPD, increased their perceived ability to take control of their diseases, decreased anxiety and mental burden, and facilitated reengagement in meaningful occupations.[18] As noted above, OT demonstrates effectiveness in not only helping client's self-manage chronic disease, but enabling participation in the meaningful occupations of daily life.

Richardson, J., Loyola-Sanchez, A., Sinclair, S., Harris, J., Letts, L., MacIntyre, N., ... & Martin Ginis, K. (2014). Self-management interventions for chronic disease: A systematic scoping review. Clinical Rehabilitation, 28, 1067–1077.

Hand, C., Law, M., & McColl, M. A. (2011). Occupational therapy interventions for chronic diseases: A scoping review. American Journal of Occupational Therapy, 65, 428–436.

Clark, F., Azen, S. P., Zemke, R, Jackson, J., Carlson, M., Mandel, D., ... & Lipson L. (1997). Occupational therapy for independent-living older adults. A randomized controlled trial. JAMA, 278(16), 1321–1326.

Chan, S. C. C. (2004).Chronic obstructive pulmonary disease and engagement in occupation. American Journal of Occupational Therapy, 58, 408–415.

An individual living with diabetes must incorporate routines for the monitoring and maintenance of appropriate blood glucose into everyday life. This monitoring and maintenance can be very different for each individual, depending on the type of diabetes and the severity of the condition. A person can develop type 1 diabetes, formerly known as *insulin-dependent diabetes mellitus* or *juvenile-onset diabetes*, at any age. Type 1 diabetes results from the destruction of beta cells in the pancreas that produce the body's insulin, the hormone needed to lower blood sugar. The cells are initially compromised by the immune system, and their ability to produce or secrete insulin is diminished or completely eliminated. For blood glucose to be managed, individuals with type 1 diabetes get their insulin via injection or pump.[19,20] At least 90% of individuals with diabetes have type 2 diabetes, once called *non–insulin-dependent diabetes mellitus* or *adult-onset diabetes*. The person with type 2 diabetes has developed insulin resistance, which causes muscle, liver, and fat cells to use insulin inappropriately. Over time, the beta cells that produce insulin are not able to keep up with the demand. At this point, intervention is needed to maintain therapeutic levels of blood glucose. As determined by a medical provider, the individual may have to check blood glucose levels multiple times per day. Medication management is vital to maintaining appropriate blood glucose levels. This can involve wearing and utilizing an insulin pump or may require taking pills or administering insulin injections, again possibly having to do so several times per day. Individuals may also have to understand how to adjust insulin dosages on the basis of glucose levels, time of day, and/or mealtime routines. Because of the chronic nature of the disease, individuals may be required to track and log glucose levels and adapt to changes in pharmacologic management as their disease changes.

The mechanism through which the body receives insulin can vary, but regardless of whether an individual takes insulin orally or via pump or injection, maintaining balanced glucose levels and avoiding hypoglycemic and hyperglycemic episodes lower the risk of developing other complications. Individuals with type 2 diabetes are encouraged to make **lifestyle modifications,** such as establishing healthy dietary and physical activity habits, as a means for glucose control.[19] Thus, it is important that people with diabetes and their caregivers learn how one's body responds to abnormal glucose levels and become aware of associated changes in behavior or appearance. Regardless of where they are or what they are doing, individuals with diabetes must be prepared with necessary medications and/or foods when experiencing hyperglycemic or hypoglycemic episodes. Having an emergency preparedness plan and responding to these situations in a timely manner reduces the development of a more severe and emergent medical concern.

Someone who has poorly controlled diabetes over a long period is likely to experience complications associated with the disease. Thus, not only must persons with diabetes work to control and maintain glucose levels, they must also address and manage other complications and related symptoms, as discussed below. For those individuals who develop multiple disease-related complications, disease management and life participation in daily occupations become more complex. Identifying symptoms related to diabetes and treating complications early is critical in slowing or preventing the progression of the disease. Progression of these complications can result in more serious problems that demand more intense medical interventions.

Depending on the nature of the complication, the individual's activities, roles, and routines must be altered. For example, in *diabetic retinopathy*, a common vision impairment associated with uncontrolled diabetes, the blood vessels in the retina are damaged and may result in vision loss[19] (Fig. 25-3). Individuals who develop diabetic retinopathy must adapt to their vision impairment by modifying tasks, using assistive devices, and/or receiving assistance, as necessary. Significant vision loss may result in a person being unable to participate in valued occupations as desired or at all; changes, coupled with the decreased ability to visually engage in one's environment, can also result in negative emotional and psychosocial responses.

Individuals with uncontrolled diabetes may also experience sensory changes (i.e., numbness, tingling) and nerve pain in the upper and lower extremities called *diabetic neuropathy*. Developing adaptive responses to sensory loss and environmental challenges will reduce the risk of injury and maintain safety. Individuals with more significant sensory loss may also be asked to perform regular foot checks to reduce the risk of wound development or other skin issues. Individuals with diabetic neuropathy are recommended to wear supportive footwear at all times when ambulating, even in their home environment. Because of poor sensation, individuals with diabetes can step on something as small as a rock or splinter and not experience a typical pain response. If they are unable to feel their feet, they are less likely to determine whether they are hurt or if a wound has developed. Poor lower extremity circulation, which is common in individuals with diabetes, also means that wounds heal at a slower pace. Foot wounds can quickly lead to *infection*, *sepsis* (severe blood infection), or even *gangrene* (death of body tissue as a result of poor blood supply), if unmanaged. Amputation of a limb is a severe consequence of an infection in individuals with diabetes. Thus, performing daily foot care (e.g., inspecting, washing, drying thoroughly, and applying lotion), maintaining trimmed toe nails, and wearing proper footwear are essential to minimize risk of wounds and infections in individuals with diabetes.

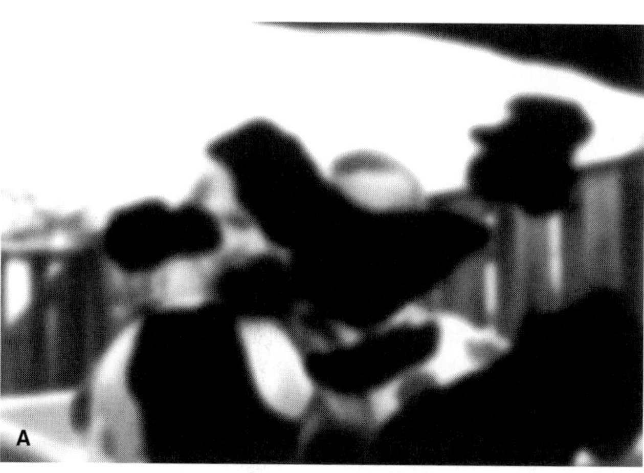

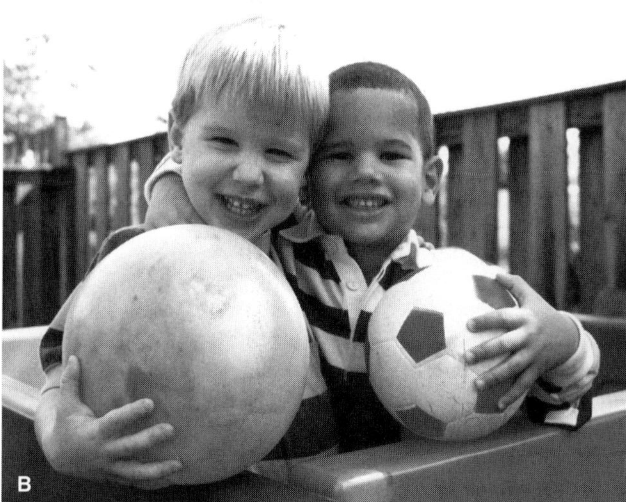

FIGURE 25-3. A scene as it might be viewed by a person with (A) diabetic retinopathy and (B) with normal vision. *(National Eye Institute, National Institutes of Health, Bethesda, MD.)*

Last, individuals with uncontrolled diabetes have an increased likelihood of developing kidney disease. They will benefit from making dietary modifications to minimize the progression of kidney damage. Making these changes to diet may significantly affect one's engagement in individual and group food-related occupations. People who experience severe kidney disease may require dialysis to maintain optimal kidney function. Dialysis can cause fatigue and weakness following the procedure and further limit one's ability to participate in desired or necessary occupations.

Congestive Heart Failure

Congestive heart failure (**CHF**) is a condition in which the heart progressively loses its ability to effectively pump the blood and oxygen that the body needs. This disease can be caused by a variety of conditions, such as hypertension, coronary artery disease, and myocardial infarction, all of which weaken the heart and diminish its ability to act as an efficient pump.[21] Risk factors for CHF include smoking, obesity, hypertension, high cholesterol level, physical inactivity, and long term stress levels, as well as genetic factors, such as heredity, gender, and age, with more men having the disease compared with women. Because CHF is incurable, treatment is focused on minimizing symptoms and optimizing quality of life. Management of the disease with medication must be a priority, but a strong emphasis should also be placed on how individuals make positive lifestyle modifications and self-monitor symptoms of the disease on a daily basis to prevent CHF exacerbations and reduce the risk for hospitalizations.

Managing daily life with CHF can be complex and challenging. Symptoms that must be managed and monitored include hypertension, edema, dyspnea (shortness of breath), and fatigue. Heart failure in one or multiple chambers of the heart often results in fluid accumulation in the lungs and other parts of the body if not treated and managed properly. Although the body often does attempt to compensate for the weakened functioning of the heart via physiological changes, such as the enlargement of heart chambers, increased cardiac muscle mass, and increased heart rate, over time, the heart still is not able to pump effectively enough to meet the demands of the body.[22] The eventual result is fluid accumulation in the lungs, abdomen, and lower extremities that can be visibly apparent and/or noted with weight gain. Sudden weight gain or loss can be a sign of heart failure and must be treated immediately. In the case of fluid overload, medical intervention is needed to remove the excess fluid from the body to slow the progression of the disease. Interventions can include a procedure being done to physically remove excess fluid and/or adjustments being made to medications (e.g., diuretics) to facilitate increased fluid output. In the case of the latter, people will experience increased urination and must be prepared to accommodate for this in their daily routines. In fact, as the disease progresses, individuals may be maintained on medications that cause frequent urination.

For individuals to most successfully manage their condition, they must not only incorporate effective medication management routines and self-monitoring habits but also consider lifestyle modifications, including physical activity and healthy food choices. It must be noted that modifying already established and existing behaviors is harder than introducing new lifestyle choices. Some of these choices include maintaining healthy eating habits, limiting caffeine and alcohol intake, increasing physical activity, controlling weight, quitting smoking, managing blood pressure, reducing stress, and incorporating healthy sleep habits.[22] One of the most challenging areas of daily life that CHF impacts are mealtime routines. Modifying unhealthy eating habits and adopting meal preparation strategies that improve nutrition is a challenge for most individuals despite diagnosis of a chronic condition. Individuals with CHF must monitor sodium and fluid intake and incorporate a balanced diet into their daily life, which requires ongoing support and education. It is also known that building physical activity into a one's lifestyle can improve cardiopulmonary functioning and assist with weight management.

In addition to fluid retention, other signs of CHF exacerbation include sudden weight gain, fatigue, wheezing or coughing, dyspnea, decreased appetite, and sleep pattern changes.[22] It is often recommended at some stage of disease progression that individuals weigh daily and inform their physician if they have gained or lost more than 3 lbs in 1 day or more than 5 lbs in a week. People with CHF may benefit from keeping a daily diary of their symptoms to track changes in their chronic condition over time. Diaries support the individual in self-monitoring his or her condition and increase the ability to identify problematic symptoms as early as possible.

As CHF progresses, participation in all areas of occupational performance can be impacted. Whether someone is engaged in basic ADLs or IADLs, functional mobility, leisure performance, and sleep or rest, symptoms, such as fatigue, weight gain, and dyspnea, can all significantly impact how someone participates in a given occupation. Over the course of living with such a condition, the individual may have to consider how to modify his or her approach to tasks, making decisions about which tasks will be done at what times to fulfill the roles and activities he or she considers top priority at any given time, all the while incorporating specific self-management responsibilities associated with CHF. Not only will the person with CHF have to make these types of decisions throughout life, but those decisions will have to evolve and shift as the condition progresses, functioning declines, and desires and priorities change.

Chronic Obstructive Pulmonary Disease

Chronic obstructive pulmonary disease (COPD) is an irreversible lung disease in which individuals experience progressively difficult breathing when air flow in the lungs is disrupted by damage to the alveolar walls and thickening of the airways. The obstruction in air flow challenges normal breathing and is made worse by physical exertion.[23] Several risk factors are associated with the development of COPD, including cigarette smoking, which accounts for 80% to 90% of diagnoses; genetics; and exposure to air pollution, second-hand smoke, and other airborne irritants.[24] In many cases, COPD can be prevented by avoiding these risk factors.

Given the progressive nature of COPD, living with the disease means that one will experience challenges in completing daily tasks and valued routines.[24] Many symptoms associated with COPD, including wheezing, chronic cough, dyspnea, and increased presence of mucus, can impact functioning. Early in the course of the disease, individuals may only experience some of these symptoms when engaged in activities that are physically demanding. With progression of the disease comes higher risk for more frequent respiratory infections, which result in worsening of symptoms that are triggered with less physical strain. In its severe stages, people with COPD experience shortness of breath even at rest, causing significant disruption to all areas of occupational performance.[18] Although the disease is incurable, many available medications may be used to address COPD-related problems.

Management of medications is an integral part of daily life for individuals with COPD, including use of supplemental oxygen and a variety of breathing treatments to minimize shortness of breath. When someone is at risk for or experiencing *hypoxia*, resulting from the inability to provide adequate oxygen to the body without assistance, oxygen may be used continuously or on an as-needed basis. Supplemental oxygen will likely be prescribed to most people living with COPD some time in their lives. The logistics of having to use and manage oxygen can greatly affect someone's ability to participate in activities and roles in the desired manner. Whether use of oxygen is prescribed for a short period or for long-term use, individuals and/or their caregivers must be armed with the skills and knowledge required to manage the prescribed regimen. They must (1) be prepared with all necessary equipment and supplies for the designated time it will be needed, especially if they will be away from home; (2) recognize symptoms that indicate need for administration, if used as needed; (3) safely manipulate and handle tanks, concentrators, liter flow devices, and tubing and know when/how these items need to be replaced; (4) know how to store reserves safely; and (5) have an emergency preparedness plan if there is a power shortage. Individuals must also be prepared to self-administer other prescribed medications, such as inhalers or nebulizers, which may be needed to relieve symptoms and support functioning. Individuals should be able to recognize when prescribed breathing treatments are needed and know how they are to be administered.

Dyspnea and fatigue associated with COPD can affect every aspect of the individual's life. Participation in ADLs, functional mobility in the home and community, sexual functioning, and leisure performance are all impacted by disease progression, altering how clients maintain engagement in valued occupations of daily life. To a person with COPD, daily routines, such as making a cup of coffee, brushing one's teeth, or even maintaining a conversation for longer than 5 minutes, may feel like climbing a mountain. Additionally, required use of supplemental oxygen and management of oxygen tubing may increase the challenges with performance of tasks such as sexual activity and home management.[25] Severe stages of COPD ultimately result in shortness of breath even when the person is at rest. Decline in physical functioning can be accompanied by changes in psychosocial health because individuals may feel less control over routine ADLs that once may have been basic or automatic.[18] The resulting feelings of depression and anxiety around the loss of ability to fulfill roles can further impact one's participation and quality of life. See Chapter 26 for further information on COPD and COPD interventions.

Fatigue and Pain Syndromes

Fibromyalgia and **chronic fatigue syndrome (CFS)** are chronic conditions that both do not have a clear or specific etiology. Once they develop, either can significantly impact a person's participation in all aspects of life. The approaches to their medical management are similar. Risk factors identified as potential contributors to the development of fibromyalgia and CFS are multifactorial; they can be psychological, physical, biological, nutritional, or environmental in nature.[26] Age, gender, poor diet and nutritional choices, sleep problems, physical inactivity, overexertion, long-term levels of stress, infection, and exposure to environmental toxins are just a few risk factors that may contribute to the symptoms. Understanding and addressing these risk factors may not only reduce the chance of developing a chronic condition but also slow the progression or reduce the frequency and/or severity of flare-ups.

Fibromyalgia is a chronic condition characterized by widespread pain. Individuals often experience a regular and constant presence of pain generalized throughout the body.[26] Diagnosing fibromyalgia involves eliminating other possible diagnoses while meeting a specific set of criteria developed in 2010, including specific scores on widespread pain and symptom severity scales, symptoms at similar level for over 3 months, and no other disorder that could explain the symptoms.

In addition to pain, common symptoms of fibromyalgia include muscle spasms, headaches, morning stiffness, fatigue, sleep disturbances, irritability, anxiety, depression, and cognitive problems associated with being consumed and/or distracted by other symptoms.[26,27] Fibromyalgia causes pain and tenderness in the joints, tendons, and ligaments throughout the body, including in one's limbs, neck, and back. Pain sensations may include, but are not limited to, aching, burning, stabbing, and feelings of pins and needles.[28] Individuals with fibromyalgia have to deal with ongoing pain as well as accompanying fatigue. In fact, some consider the secondary symptom of fatigue to be more difficult to live with than the pain directly related to fibromyalgia.[27]

Individuals with CFS experience extreme fatigue that does not improve with rest and may actually worsen with activity. Like fibromyalgia, CFS is also challenging to detect because there are no tests that can directly diagnose the disease, and the symptoms of CFS can mirror those of other conditions. Beyond fatigue, symptoms include headache, cognitive issues related to memory and concentration, complaints of joint and muscle pain, feeling ill after exertion, tender lymph nodes, and sore throat, as well as disrupted and nonrestorative sleep.[29-31]

Living with pain and/or fatigue greatly influences one's participation in daily activities and ability to fulfill life roles. It may be necessary for people with fibromyalgia or CFS to modify their routines for completing ADLs in such a way that is tolerable and achievable. They may consider completing tasks at certain times of day when the energy level is optimal, incorporating rest breaks, using specialized equipment, or having assistance, when appropriate. Making these adjustments to meet self-care needs affects one's ability to engage in other valued occupations that are related to leisure, work, caregiving, and so on. Furthermore, one's psychosocial state affects one's ability to participate in valued activities and should be considered in the treatment plan.

Given the chronic and debilitating nature of fatigue and pain syndromes, it is vital that individuals living with these conditions understand the risk factors and lifestyle choices that support optimal functioning and quality of life. Addressing these risk factors may not only reduce the chance of developing a chronic condition but also slow the progression or reduce the frequency and/or severity of flare-ups. A variety of medications can be used for symptom management, such as pain relievers and antidepressants.[27,30] Supplements are sometimes explored as a means of symptom relief. Medical interventions are often focused on fostering positive lifestyle changes to overcome and minimize the presence of contributing factors that can cause flare-ups and/or influence progression of the conditions. Positive changes might include working to optimize diet and nutrition, improving both the quantity and the quality of sleep, increasing activity level over time, taking measures to reduce depression, and enhancing stress management.[27]

Obesity

Obesity is a condition characterized by an atypical measure of fat content that has the potential to negatively impact one's health.[32] According to the World Health Organization (WHO), individuals with a body mass index (BMI) greater than 25 are considered "overweight," and those who exceed 30 are considered "obese." Obesity is a significant risk factor for many other chronic conditions, including diabetes, heart disease, some cancers, and musculoskeletal problems; this risk continues to increase with further elevation of BMI.[33] Childhood obesity continues to be a serious and growing concern, as children who are obese are not only at more risk for chronic health problems in adulthood but also at higher risk for premature death.

Participation challenges may extend across several domains and include a wide variety of occupations. Participation in daily tasks is made harder by associated complications, decreased endurance and activity tolerance, and size restraints. Medical care for obesity involves responding to complications associated with the condition (e.g., osteoarthritis, breathing disorders, and sexual dysfunction). Daily roles and routines often must be altered to account for functional limitations and to fulfill necessary life roles. Engagement in social, leisure, or other activities may also be made more complicated or impossible because of the social stigma surrounding individuals who are overweight.

In the majority of cases, obesity is a preventable and reversible condition. The modern world has seen changes, such as increased consumption of high-fat foods and a rise in work behaviors, lifestyle activities, and living environments that foster more sedentary behavior. It is important to recognize that obesity is a disease that results from the interplay of personal (biological, genetic, psychological) and environmental (physical, social, cultural) factors. Nutritional choices and participation in food-centered occupations, whether shopping, preparing, or consuming foods are influenced by someone's disease and his or her response to it. OT practitioners should consider both the physical and social aspects of mealtime participation, family occupations surrounding mealtime routines, and the sociocultural importance of food. While facing some or all of these challenges, individuals may also be working to manage other chronic conditions because of the high rates of comorbidities with obesity. See Chapter 27 for further details.

THERAPEUTIC PROCESS TO CHRONIC DISEASE MANAGEMENT

The experiences and daily challenges of individuals living with chronic disease have been described in this chapter. Having a thorough understanding of how chronic disease impacts occupational participation both enhances therapeutic relationships with clients and supports best practice. Helping individuals work toward effective chronic disease management requires OT practitioners to take a self-management approach to practice. This approach is grounded in a perspective that focuses on empowering clients with the problem-solving skills that will allow them to manage their disease over the course of their life. As experts in habits, routines, rituals, and roles, OT practitioners play a pivotal role in addressing chronic disease self-management with the goal of integrating wellness, maintenance, and prevention strategies into daily life. This section discusses the therapeutic process OTAs should use when working with clients with chronic conditions.

Collaboration of Occupational Therapist and Occupational Therapy Assistant

Effective delivery of healthcare services occurs when the occupational therapist, the OTA, the client, and the caregivers are working in partnership to achieve shared goals. The integration of practitioners and clients as partners leads to a plan of care that is not only client centered but is client driven as well.[13] Given the complex, dynamic, and ongoing nature of chronic disease management, this type of collaborative partnership between the client and the OT team is especially important when working within the continuous and ever-changing process that is self-management.

Occupational Therapy Assessment

OT practitioners bring their own individual perspectives, experiences, and skill sets to practice. Thus, maintaining the collaboration between the occupational therapist and the OTA through the entire therapeutic process is ideal to optimize client outcomes. This collaboration should start in the assessment stage. Evaluation of a new client in any healthcare setting starts with reviewing the medical record to understand the individual's diagnosis, secondary health conditions, precautions, relevant test results, and social history. The clinical assessment of the client incorporates the development of both an occupational profile and an analysis of occupational performance (see Chapter 6 for further details). The purpose of the OT assessment is to fully understand the client's level of functioning, as well as his or her barriers or limitations to health, well-being, and participation in daily occupations.[13] OTAs can and should contribute to the assessment of individuals with chronic conditions in collaboration with the supervising occupational therapist. Although this may formally occur in the first session with the client, OTAs can utilize their assessment skills through the entire treatment process.

Developing a client's occupational profile is especially critical when working with individuals with chronic diseases. Whether a client has recently been diagnosed or has been living with a chronic disease for quite some time, having a more complete picture of the client's past and current contexts, roles, routines, abilities, interests, perspectives, and priorities will allow OT practitioners to better identify problems and work toward outcomes that are most important to the client.[13] Embracing the interrelatedness of all elements of the profile positions OT practitioners to support clients in their efforts to achieve positive health outcomes and participate in life as they desire.[13] Having a thorough understanding of the valued occupations and roles of the client, along with any functional or structural body changes that may impact performance, allow OT practitioners to better partner with and support their clients in working toward the achievement of goals. Discussion should not be limited to the most common ADLs; areas as personal device care, caregiving tasks, and sexual activity, which might be more meaningful or important to the client, should also be included. OTAs have a critical role in developing the occupational profile because they may be the clinician who interacts with and provides treatment to the client most frequently over time. OTAs are well positioned to develop lasting partnerships with clients with chronic diseases and to contribute to an occupational profile that enhances and informs the therapeutic process.

Analysis of occupational performance for individuals with chronic conditions involves observing daily occupations and health management tasks that are challenging to the client, administering standardized assessments to measure occupational performance, selecting appropriate outcome measures, and collaborating with the client to determine realistic and achievable self-management goals that can be successfully integrated into daily habits and routines. Examples of self-management tasks include managing medications (e.g., insulin, inhaler, nebulizer, pill box), self-monitoring activities (e.g., monitoring blood pressure, weight, blood sugar, foot inspection, energy conservation), nutrition (e.g., preparing grocery lists, making healthier food choices, meal preparation tasks), physical activity (e.g., participation in valued occupations, home exercise), and problem-solving in the context of varying capabilities.[34] The OT practitioner assesses the client's baseline performance of new self-management tasks and supports the development of an intervention plan that addresses learning of new tasks in context of existing habits and routines.[35] Understanding the client as an occupational being within the context of the client's environment is especially important for individuals with chronic diseases because they will be seen over time in different stages of life and in different stages of their diseases. Results of the assessment should be shared with the client and used to determine goals and expected functional outcomes.

Common questions or considerations in the assessment of a client with a chronic condition include the following: Does this individual have a diagnosis of one or more chronic conditions? What is the client's level of understanding of the condition in relationship to health and wellness? What techniques are the individual currently employing to self-manage the condition? How do the client's chronic condition impact daily functioning? How does existing habits and routines support or hinder self-management performance? What is the client's readiness for change in the management of the condition?[34] Incorporation of these questions in the assessment process yields a greater understanding of how the client views his or her health and related conditions, as well as how chronic disease is impacting participation in daily life occupations.

Making a lifestyle change is a complex process that occurs over time, not in a single moment. Thus understanding a client's preparedness to make change is important to ensure that the plan of care and intervention design optimizes likelihood for success. It also helps the practitioner avoid interventions that the client may not be ready to accept.[36] To assess readiness for change or the client's intrinsic belief they can succeed in making a lifestyle change, consider asking the client the following questions:

1. On a scale of 0 to 10 (10 being the highest), rate how important it is to make an identified behavior change (e.g., physical activity, weight loss, improved medication management, etc.)
2. What are the health benefits to making this change?
3. When do you want to take action to make the behavior change?
4. What barriers have limited your success in the past to make the identified change?
5. On a scale of 0 to 10, rate how confident you are to carry out the identified behavior change.[36]

The **Transtheoretical Model of Behavior Change (TTM)** can be used by OT practitioners to understand a client's readiness for change (Fig. 25-4). The TTM is an evidenced-based model that describe the five intentional stages a person often goes through when making a behavior change.[37] This model can help OT practitioners best

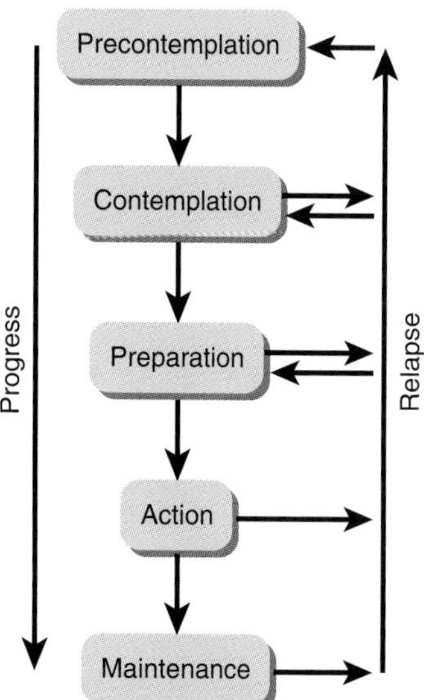

FIGURE 25-4. Transtheoretical Model of Behavior Change. Looking at the five stages of behavior change.

determine what stage of change a client is in, develop goals, and tailor interventions to areas of occupation that are relevant to the client. The five stages include the following:

1. *Precontemplation:* The client is not considering making a change.
2. *Contemplation:* The client may see some benefits of changing but is experiencing ambivalence.
3. *Preparation:* The client has decided to try and make a change and has taken some behavioral steps in this direction.
4. *Action:* The client initiates the behavior change plan.
5. *Maintenance:* The client works to maintain the changed behavior and has changed the behavior for more than 6 months.

Relapse can occur within any stage of the behavior change model and could prompt the cycle to start again.[37] OT practitioners must recognize that not all clients are in the same stage of life or in the management of their chronic condition. For example, the OT practitioner who assumes that the newly diagnosed client with type II diabetes is ready to initiate change (action stage) may receive resistance if the client has not gone through the process of problem-solving (contemplation stage) and making the decision for the desired behavior change (preparation stage). Thus, understanding where the client is along the continuum of behavior change better informs the practitioner regarding which intervention approach would be most successful. Refer to Table 25-1 for further discussion of appropriate strategies OT practitioners can use based on the TTM stages of behavior change.

TABLE 25-1 Transtheoretical Model of Behavior Change—Intervention Strategies[38]

STAGE	APPROPRIATE STRATEGIES
Precontemplation: Client is not considering trying to make a change.	Provide appropriate information as to why change may be helpful, presented in a nonauthoritarian manner by way of simple information.
Contemplation: Client sees some benefits in changing but is also experiencing or aware of benefits of not changing.	Encourage client to: Analyze the arguments for and against change (e.g., complete a pros/cons list). Reflect on different options for change and the likely effect of each. Consider whether there are any very small ways he or she could begin to take steps in the direction of change, which seem achievable and reasonable to him or her.
Preparation: Client has decided to try to achieve change.	Encourage client to: Plan change carefully rather than make a rushed decision. Break plan down into achievable goals. Write down commitment to change. Think about where the client can get support for following his or her plans.
Action: Client is taking action to achieve change.	Encourage client to: Follow his or her plan, monitor, and review progress. Reward and congratulate self on successes (even small ones). Remind self of the benefits that will ensue if goals are achieved and identify those benefits as they happen (even if only partially achieved). Pace self at a level where he or she will be able to sustain motivation and recognize there is a life outside of the plan. Learn from things that do not turn out as expected. Make use of appropriate support. In case of a relapse, recognize the progress made.
Maintenance: Client is consistently enacting the desired behavior change.	Encourage client to: Recognize that development is an ongoing process. Maintain and review plans until absolutely sure they are no longer required. Think about whether there is a way he or she can help others make positive changes in light of the experience.
Termination: Client has made the behavior change permanent.	Encourage client to: Celebrate his or her success. Think about whether there is a way he or she can help others make positive changes in light of the experience.
Relapse: Client reverts back to an undesired behavior.	Use the model to show the client that the situation is not hopeless or beyond their control. If there is a lapse, he or she should try not to return to the starting place, but instead, recognize their progress and implement a new plan, learning from the relapse. Encourage a mentality of learning from relapses rather than judging. Remind client of the work through normal stages on the path to change. The process should be understood as a cycle—a person may go through the stages several times before a permanent change is made and the goal is achieved.

Formal assessments can be used in the evaluation to further understand the client's perceptions of his or her abilities. The ***Canadian Occupational Performance Measure, 4th edition*** (COPM) is an evidence-based assessment to measure a client's self-perception of barriers that impact occupational performance in everyday living.[39] The COPM is a client-centered tool that has individuals prioritize the everyday activities that they need, want, or are expected to do but are having challenges with performing.

The tool measures three areas of occupational performance problems utilizing self-report from the client including the following: (1) rating the importance of the problem; (2) rating the client's perceived performance of the activity; and (3) rating the client's satisfaction with performance. Use of the COPM influences goal writing by the OT practitioner and helps tailor interventions to clients' self-identified performance concerns. The COPM is used as an outcome measure intended to be performed at the initial assessment, appropriate times throughout the intervention process, and at the conclusion of services.

Self-Management Approach to Intervention

People with chronic disease must learn to manage a long-term condition over the course of their entire lives. OT practitioners must recognize that self-management is a process and that this process is one of active participation that has to evolve as the person and the disease changes. The strategies in Box 25-1 describe actions that, if adopted, support individuals to be more successful self-managers. Individuals employing these strategies demonstrate problem-solving skills and are better able to negotiate the changing demands of life with chronic disease.

BOX 25-1
Effective Strategies for Self-Management[40]

Clients should:

1. Review and revise common assumptions about their health and wellness
2. Successfully mourn the multiple losses that the long-term condition has forced upon them and contemplate potential future losses
3. Actively learn about what being ill means for them in a practical sense
4. Actively learn about their condition and what healthcare professionals recommend for its management
5. Keep daily life as "normal" as possible
6. Develop new routines to support healthy daily living and actively engage in day-to-day problem-solving
7. Deal constructively with the reaction of others to changing health
8. Make new plans for life in light of changing circumstances
9. Confidently express points of view and negotiate self-management goals with healthcare clinicians, give reports of progress and successfully inform the team when challenges may develop

To support clients in becoming successful self-managers of chronic disease, OT interventions must be focused on embedding health-supporting behaviors into clients' habits and routines. Chronic disease self-management is not achieved through verbalizing understanding of education provided by a healthcare provider. It is also not displayed through a one-time demonstration of skills during therapy sessions. Self-management requires clients to generalize new learning to everyday living tasks and the challenges they will encounter living with chronic disease.[41] Generalization suggests that clients can spontaneously, habitually, and automatically integrate self-management performance into their daily lives and existing routines. Thus, observing a client's performance or return-demonstration in a clinical environment does not indicate that performance will be incorporated into the client's natural environment. Implementing new tasks, behaviors, and techniques require conscious attention and mental effort to build them into daily life and daily habits.[42]

To generalize knowledge, strategies, and techniques across tasks and environments, OT practitioners should focus interventions on establishing and/or modifying existing performance patterns to support self-management goals. The OTPF-3 states: "Practitioners who consider clients' performance patterns are better able to understand the frequency and manner in which performance skills and occupations are integrated into clients' lives. Although clients may have the ability to engage in skilled performance, if they do not embed essential skills in a productive set of engagement patterns, their health, well-being and participation may be negatively affected."[13]

COMMUNICATING EFFECTIVELY WITH CLIENTS

Education should not be limited to traditional models where information and technical skills are passed down from the practitioner to the client. Instead, self-management interventions center on empowering clients with healthcare knowledge and how they can most successfully self-identify problems, make their own healthcare decisions, take appropriate actions, and modify behaviors as they encounter changes in their disease.

Health literacy, or the client's ability to obtain, process, and understand health information, is critical to consider when working with clients with chronic conditions. Individuals older than 65 years not only bear the greatest burden of developing a chronic condition(s), but 30% of this population has inadequate health literacy skills to understand their condition and implement strategies to manage that condition in daily life.[43] Low health literacy is directly linked to higher hospitalization rates and increased healthcare costs.[44] Everyone at some point in time has difficulty understanding healthcare information. Navigating healthcare systems and information is an incredibly complex task; thus, simplifying education is an important communication strategy to support clients with self-management goals. OT practitioners are encouraged to utilize common or plain language that is easily understandable to the client.

Breaking down complex information, avoiding technical terms, writing clearly, and asking the client to repeat back information using their own words are simple strategies to support good communication and support clients in their understanding of healthcare information. As an OT practitioner, building positive healthcare relationships with clients and using effective communication improves clients' coping, confidence, and the ability to balance the responsibilities of self-management in daily life.[45] See Chapters 4 and 5 for more detailed information.

One evidence-based strategy to better engage clients in self-reflective problem-solving is through motivational interviewing. Motivational interviewing is a client-centered communication style targeted at facilitating behavior change in individuals who may be ambivalent, hesitant, or resistant to change.[46] Motivational interviewing, which is widely used in psychology, can be applied in different contexts and used by other professionals, including OT practitioners. In contrast to the view of the clinician as the expert, motivational interviewing relies on self-reflective practices that support the client assuming responsibility for what, when, and how change will be implemented. The clinician facilitates clients moving toward behavior change by evoking motivation in a collaborative, nonjudgmental, and client-centered manner. The four guiding principles of motivational interviewing include resisting the righting reflex (e.g., the urge to correct clients), understanding the client's motivations, listening with empathy, and empowering the client utilizing hope and encouragement.[47] Additionally, common strategies used in motivational interviewing include utilizing open-ended questions to retrieve useful information from the client, reflective listening, affirming clients' beliefs, summarizing information, asking permission to give advice, evoking change talk, and restating what the client says using his or her own words to create shared understanding.[46]

When considering a self-management approach to OT practice, utilizing motivational interviewing can effectively support clients toward behavior change. Instead of the practitioner imparting knowledge to the client, this communication style empowers clients to participate in problem-solving daily challenges and barriers. Lastly, this technique can be used to help clients develop action plans by breaking down goals into achievable and attainable steps. Use of action plans support clients in taking ownership toward the behavior changes they wish to see in their daily lives and optimizes success with the overall self-management of chronic disease. Refer to Table 25-2 for further discussion of strategies to minimize resistance.

UNDERSTANDING PSYCHOSOCIAL IMPLICATIONS OF CHRONIC DISEASE

The challenging work of self-managing chronic disease falls primarily on the individual with the condition and his or her family. As previously explored in this chapter, living with a chronic disease is a job, and the day-to-day challenges of this work will persist through the duration of the client's life. Thus, OTAs must be aware of not only the physical challenges the individual faces but also the emotional and mental strain endured while living with chronic disease. Psychosocial implications of living with chronic disease can increase an individual's level of emotional distress, anxiety, and depression and may require attention to enhancing coping skills for continued self-management and satisfaction with life engagement. In addition, individuals living with chronic disease may commonly experience feelings of guilt, fear, and anger/resentment for loss of occupational roles.[21,48] Consider the emotional well-being of a mother who feels she can no longer attend her son's baseball games because of pain and fatigue caused by fibromyalgia. Consider the feelings of burden an older adult with advanced COPD may experience when needing basic assistance because even making a sandwich causes shortness of breath. It is well understood that being unable to engage in basic daily occupations can negatively impact health and can affect social relationships and social identity.[49] Thus, OT practitioners should not only appreciate the physical challenges of daily life but also the psychosocial implications of living daily life with a chronic disease. It is important that OTAs are sensitive to clients' varying states of readiness and motivation and understand that changing lifelong habits and routines are hard.[40] In recognizing the complexities of behavior change, OTAs should eliminate labeling clients as "noncompliant" and advocate

TABLE 25-2 Motivational Interviewing—Eliciting Change Talk[47]

Clients tend to move toward behavior change when offered a guiding communication style instead of being directed to do so. Change talk elicits the client's motivations and encourages problem-solving rather than resistance from your clients. Compare the difference in questions posed by the healthcare professional, and consider which type of communication is more likely to elicit change talk:

DEFENSIVE QUESTIONS	GUIDING QUESTIONS
"Why don't you want to ...?"	"Why might you want to make this change?"
"Why can't you ...?"	"If you did decide to make this change, how would you do it?"
"Why haven't you ...?"	"What are the three most important benefits that you see in making this change?"
"Why do you need to ...?"	"What are you already doing to make this change?"
"Why don't you ...?"	"On a scale of 1 to 10, how ready do you feel to make this change?"

for more client-centered language, such as "adherence" or "concordance," which promotes a partnership between the client and the practitioner.

Establishing health-supporting behaviors and integrating them into clients' daily habits and routines requires time, consistency, encouragement, and reinforcement. Making this level of commitment to clients with respect to appreciating the psychosocial implications of living with chronic disease promotes best practice.

RECOGNIZING CAREGIVER NEEDS

This chapter largely focuses on the individual client as the person responsible for adopting self-management and lifestyle modification principles into daily life. However, caregiver participation and support in the treatment process is fundamental to improving efficacy of OT interventions and supporting clients to generalize education into their everyday lives. OT practitioners understand that the clients are not only the individual with the chronic disease, but also the family caregivers and the social structure surrounding that individual. OTAs should actively incorporate caregivers into treatment sessions as lifestyle modification and health management requires consistent and ongoing daily monitoring over the duration of clients' lives. Caregivers should be incorporated into interventions as their direct involvement may be required to support implementation of self-management strategies. Maximizing the involvement of caregivers in the therapeutic process best supports the client with chronic disease and creates a community of support that can surround the client at home and in the community.

TABLE 25-3 Dealing with Resistance[47]

Recognizing Resistance Behaviors
Arguing (e.g., challenging, hostility)
Interrupting
Negativity/Denial (e.g., blaming, minimizing, disagreeing)
Withdrawal/Ignoring
Ways to Generate Resistance
Using the righting reflex (e.g., correcting/directing the client what to do)
Using a judgmental or confrontational approach
Insisting on change
Discounting the client's feelings/motivations
Ways to Prevent or Minimize Resistance
Understanding the client's motivations and desires
Emphasizing personal choice and autonomy
Offering clients options/choices for change with their permission
Incorporating clients in problem-solving barriers/challenges
Using reflective listening

Intervention Planning and Implementation

As identified in the OTPF-3, OT practitioners utilize all types of intervention approaches to assist clients with chronic disease to self-manage their condition, including health promotion, remediation/restoration, maintenance, modification, and prevention. Tailoring intervention approaches to the specific goals of the client is a hallmark of OT and ideally situates the profession to address chronic disease and foster self-management. Interventions can involve a variety of methods, including, but not limited to, (1) teaching health management strategies and self-monitoring skills, (2) incorporating energy conservation and activity modification techniques, (3) developing coping strategies, and (4) adapting behaviors to support lifestyle modifications related to health, wellness and prevention.[12,16] Given the ever changing and dynamic nature of chronic disease, OT practitioners should utilize multiple intervention approaches during treatment sessions to better prepare the client with chronic disease to self-manage his or her condition over time. Table 25-3 provides specific examples of interventions to implement when working with clients with chronic disease.

SELF-MONITORING OF SYMPTOMS

Self-monitoring of symptoms is an important component of effective chronic disease management. Self-monitoring is a method of self-observation that requires actively analyzing one's actions, thoughts, and feelings with the goal of achieving desired health outcomes. Developing self-monitoring strategies increases self-awareness of the disease's impact on daily life and empowers individuals to make informed choices. Symptoms that need to be monitored are disease dependent and can vary, depending on the state of disease the client is experiencing. Refer to Table 25-4 for disease-specific symptoms that require self-monitoring for effective self-management.

Self-monitoring can require individuals to assess symptoms at predetermined intervals as recommended by a physician. This may include task-oriented self-monitoring, such as assessment of vital signs (e.g., blood sugar, blood pressure, oxygen saturation, heart rate). Refer to the Chapter 26 to review skills in measuring vital signs. Clients may require training in *personal device care,* an ADL, which includes proper use, maintenance, and cleaning of personal care items. Personal care items can include equipment, such as blood glucose meter, electronic blood pressure cuff, and pulse oximeter, needed for self-monitoring of chronic conditions. In addition to teaching clients strategies to measure vital signs and to properly use medical devices, OTAs can also assist clients to create a daily vital signs diary. The diary serves to track progress over time and can assist clients to take increased ownership of self-monitoring his or her disease on a daily and habitual basis. Clients can use this tracking method to monitor changes in health and better communicate with healthcare professionals when changes occur.

Self-monitoring of chronic disease also requires individuals and caregivers to become more self-aware of physiological and behavioral changes associated with their chronic diseases. For example, a client with diabetes experiencing symptoms of hypoglycemia, such as sweating, dizziness, blurred vision, hunger, and shakiness, can avoid a potential life-threatening situation by recognizing symptoms earlier,

TABLE 25-4 Intervention Approaches for Chronic Disease Self-Management[13]

OTPF-3 APPROACHES	DEFINITION (OTPF-3)	INTERVENTION APPROACHES
Health Promotion	"An intervention approach that does not assume a disability is present or that any aspect would interfere with performance. This approach is designed to provide enriched contextual and activity experiences that will enhance performance for all people in the natural contexts of life"	Consult with dietitian about providing after-school cooking classes for parents and their children to foster healthy family eating habits. Provide exercise and nutrition classes at local senior center to facilitate healthy lifestyle modifications for older adults. Address a diabetes caregiver support group on stress management techniques and coping skills.
Remediation/ Restoration	"An intervention approach designed to change client variables to establish a skill or ability that has not yet developed or to restore a skill or ability that has been impaired"	Address deconditioning in the client with CHF posthospitalization. Incorporate energy conservation and activity modification into existing routines to reduce shortness of breath for the client with fibromyalgia. Develop written diary for clients with diabetes to monitor daily vital sign assessments. Teach meal planning skills to the client with diabetes by creating a weekly grocery list according to dietary guidelines/restrictions. Teach diaphragmatic breathing techniques to improve/ restore breathing capacity for clients with COPD.
Maintenance	"An intervention approach designed to provide the supports that will allow clients to preserve the performance capabilities they have regained, that continue to meet their occupational needs, or both. The assumption is that without continued maintenance intervention, performance would decrease, occupational needs would not be met, or both, thereby affecting health, well-being and quality of life"	Support weight management principles through ongoing incorporation of nutrition and home exercise program into daily routine. Maintain daily schedule to administer oral, injectable, or inhaled medications, as prescribed by physician. Connect clients with community resources and social supports to facilitate ongoing self-management efforts (e.g., smoking cessation programs, exercises classes, senior citizen centers). Coordinate telehealth services for ongoing monitoring of chronic disease symptom management.
Modification	"An intervention approach directed at 'finding ways to revise the current context or activity demands to support performance in the natural setting, [including] compensatory techniques ... [such as] enhancing some features to provide cues or reducing other features to reduce distractibility'"	Adapt occupations or environments to support activity participation. Trial a talking glucometer adaptive device for successful monitoring of blood sugar for clients with diabetic retinopathy. Teach task simplification techniques to help a person continue to cook for his or her family. Introduce durable medical equipment/adaptive equipment for bathroom safety. Initiate pill box alarm application on smartphone for organization of medication administration. Ensure large-print medication labels for individuals with visual impairment.
Prevention	"An intervention approach designed to address the needs of clients with or without a disability who are at risk for occupational performance problems. This approach is designed to prevent the occurrence or evolution of barriers to performance in context. Interventions may be directed at client, context, or activity variables"	Incorporate daily self-monitoring techniques to include vitals and symptom management of: • Weight • Blood pressure • Heart rate • Oxygen saturation • Shortness of breath • Edema • Fatigue • Pain • Skin integrity Teach fall prevention techniques to clients with diabetic neuropathy and sensory impairment. Perform preventative home safety screening and consultation for clients at risk for chronic disease. Promote occupational engagement in caregivers to prevent burnout.

measuring blood sugar level with glucometer, and quickly ingesting simple carbohydrates, such as raisins, juice, hard candy, or glucose tablets (Fig. 25-5). Supporting clients in developing the knowledge and skills around activity engagement that might exacerbate disease-related symptoms and how to best respond in those situations is also important. Even when energy conservation and work simplification strategies have been put in place, there will be times when individuals experience symptoms during performance, for example, shortness of breath with dressing, fatigue with grocery shopping, pain with bathing a baby, or hypertension with sexual activity. In the previously given examples, good self-monitoring facilitates problem-solving on how to respond based on the symptoms they are experiencing, whether this means stopping the activity, further modifying or adjusting their participation, or contacting the appropriate persons for assistance. Improving self-awareness of symptomatic changes associated with daily life with a chronic disease increase clients' ability to accurately self-monitor their condition over time.

To support clients to develop and generalize problem-solving skills, OTAs might include role-play scenarios in their interventions with clients. An example of a role-play scenario is to ask the client: "In what context or situation would you contact your local healthcare provider when experiencing a health-related change?" The OTA might also ask the client to explain and demonstrate how to contact his or her physician. Both these scenarios support the client in being not only better at self-monitoring, but also better at self-advocating. Clients who are better able to recognize changes in their personal health and contact their physicians when new symptoms develop may be less likely to require hospitalization if treatments can occur on a timely basis.

Self-monitoring of symptoms must become a routine aspect of daily life for people living with chronic disease. Interventions should be targeted at helping clients develop the necessary self-monitoring skills and embed them into already established routines. Strategies for incorporating self-monitoring into daily life may consider times of day during which habits and routines are well established, for example, around sleep/wake or meal times, as well as times at which potential for disruptions in routine are minimal.[50] OTAs may also consider compensatory strategies to support effective self-monitoring practices, including use of (1) assistive devices, such as talking glucometers to assess blood glucose for someone with diabetic retinopathy or long-handled mirrors to perform more thorough skin checks; and (2) visual or auditory cues, such as picture reminders or alarm clocks for maintenance of self-monitoring schedules for someone who may have memory deficits (Table 25-5).

OTAs can assist clients with organizational strategies to maintain healthcare appointments in the community with their primary care providers and healthcare specialists. Ultimately, equipping clients with self-monitoring skills has the potential to minimize exacerbations, slow disease progression, and reduce the risk for hospitalization.[1] OTAs who work with individuals toward becoming successful self-monitors support their clients in actively assuming responsibility for their health, contributing to positive health outcomes for both clients and the healthcare system in general.[51]

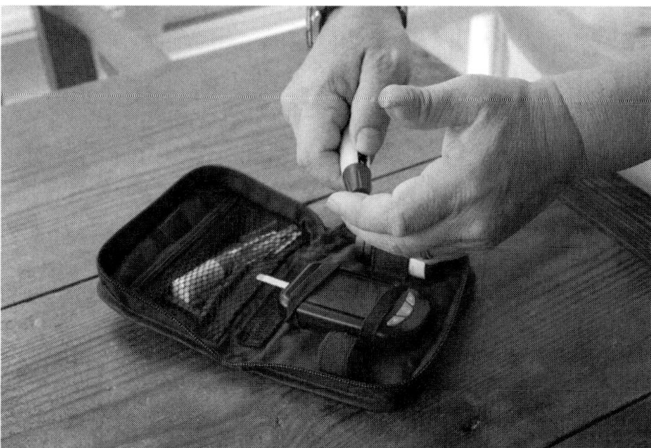

FIGURE 25-5. Self-monitoring. Measuring blood glucose using a glucometer is an important aspect of self-management for a person with diabetes.

TABLE 25-5 Disease-Specific Self-Monitoring Tasks

CHRONIC CONDITION	SELF-MONITORING
Congestive heart failure	Daily weight Edema Shortness of breath Fatigue Blood pressure Sodium Intake
Chronic obstructive pulmonary disease	Oxygen saturation (pulse oximeter) Shortness of breath Fatigue Self-pacing/energy conservation Use of supplemental oxygen
Diabetes	Blood sugar (glucometer) Sliding-scale insulin dose (recording) Behavioral responses to hyperglycemia/hypoglycemia Nutrition: Sugar/carbohydrate intake Foot/skin integrity Sensory impairment
Fibromyalgia/Chronic fatigue syndrome	Pain response to daily activity Fatigue Shortness of breath
Obesity	Nutrition tracking Physical activity tracking Pain, fatigue, shortness of breath

MEDICATION MANAGEMENT

Medication management is identified as an IADL that supports the health management and maintenance of clients with chronic diseases.[50] Understanding medications and developing strategies for safe medication administration is critical to managing chronic diseases and preventing adverse health events or hospitalizations. Given the significant role that medications play in the management of chronic diseases, OT practitioners should routinely incorporate medication management into the plan of care and work with clients to develop habits and routines that support safe self-administration of medications. It is also essential that OT practitioners work with clients to establish medication routines that are individualized and consider the larger context of day-to-day life. OT interventions must be targeted at helping people develop successful routines and prepare clients with the problem-solving skills to maintain medication adherence when routines are disrupted.

OT practitioners are skilled in analyzing and addressing the performance components of medication management. While being knowledgeable about common medications to treat chronic diseases as well as side effects and potential impact on other areas of occupation, OT practitioners should refrain from specific teaching on medications because it does not fall within their scope of practice. Performance areas that OT practitioners may address include obtaining medications, opening and closing containers, following or reading prescribed schedules, organizing medications, administering correct quantities, reporting adverse medication effects, and integrating medication management into the habits and routines of daily life. OT practitioners address these performance areas by assessing performance skills and functional abilities, such as vision, hearing, memory, problem-solving, executive function, dexterity, motivation, mobility, and communication. Practitioners may incorporate assistive aids or compensatory strategies for medication management, such as pill box organizers, medication alarms, or medication diaries (Fig. 25-6). OT practitioners may work with pharmacists to arrange for bubble-pack medication options to simplify medication administration, increasing the text size on prescriptions for individuals with visual impairment, removing child-proof caps for clients with impaired dexterity, and facilitating home-delivery options for the client with community mobility challenges. The OT practitioner should also consider aspects of the physical environment that support or hinder medication administration and recommend environmental cues that can facilitate greater independence in medication management. Common examples might include assessing for optimal lighting in the home, situating pill boxes in common and easily accessible areas in the home, or utilizing visual/auditory/tactile cueing techniques (e.g., placing a written reminder by the morning alarm clock or using a low-tech alarm system). As individuals are using smartphone technology more frequently, OT practitioners can explore "apps" or alarm clock settings with clients to support medication management. The most important factor for the OT practitioner to address is how clients are integrating medication management into their daily habits and routines. OT practitioners should be familiar with the time of day and location in the home where their clients manage their medications and incorporate strategies that are tailored to the client. Understanding the bigger picture of a client's day-to-day life offers context into how medication management can be optimized and supported through the development of routines.

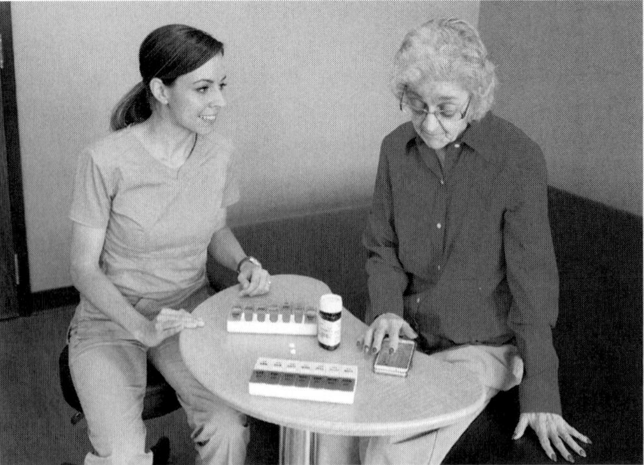

FIGURE 25-6. Medication management. Use of pill box organizers and smart phone to facilitate safe administration of medications.

ENERGY CONSERVATION AND ACTIVITY MODIFICATION

In response to functional changes caused by disease progression and/or associated symptoms, individuals living with chronic conditions must learn to modify their approach to participation to continue to fulfill life roles and complete self-care and other valued activities.[14] Energy conservation and work simplification strategies are common interventions that OT practitioners teach clients to support continued engagement in desired and necessary occupations despite functional changes. Through the use of energy conservation and work simplification strategies, individuals learn to modify their approach to support successful activity completion. Practitioners should collaborate with clients to determine which occupations are most important to meet one's needs and fulfill valued roles. Questions can be asked to determine which of these strategies to incorporate to allow for easier and safer participation in valued occupations:

1. Can the activity be done in a different way to make it easier or safer?
2. Can the activity be done in a different position or with use of supports for positioning to reduce symptoms during participation?
3. Can the activity be done at a different time or on a different day when the individual may have more energy or is not in as much pain?

4. Can equipment be used to assist with activity completion?
5. Can rest breaks and breathing techniques be incorporated into habits and routines to address fatigue?
6. Can the activity or task be prepared for or organized in a different way or done in a different space or place to minimize or eliminate barriers to participation?
7. Can assistance be given by another person to optimize safety and/or minimize strain?
8. Can medication or modalities, such as moist heat or cold pack, be used before, during, or after activity engagement to reduce symptoms?

Even if the OT practitioner is focused on supporting participation in one or a few specific occupations, he or she should facilitate the desired engagement within the context of all of the client's daily habits, routines, and responsibilities. This approach is particularly relevant when working with clients with chronic diseases, as the symptoms they experience can compound and cause greater functional limitations over the course of the day, week, and so on. Thus, it is important that OT practitioners work with clients to prioritize their most valued activities and roles to best support them to participate in all desired occupations. This sometimes means having conversations that may initially be uncomfortable for the client and/or the practitioner, for example, talking about sexual activity. OT practitioners should be sensitive to the fact that despite the physical and functional changes experienced by individuals with chronic conditions, many still want and plan to remain sexually active. Since for many adults, sexual activity occurs in the evening, the client may be too fatigued to desire to participate. OT practitioners may take different approaches to discuss sexual concerns, for example, by making general comments about how other clients have indicated that having a chronic disease has impacted their sexual health or by asking open-ended questions, such as "What worries do you have about your sexual activity?" Communicating with clients to identify the importance of fulfillment related to sexual health and then working with clients to support their desired engagement should be incorporated into OT practice.[25]

Individuals with one or multiple chronic conditions experience a variety of symptoms that impact daily participation, such as fatigue, pain, shortness of breath, and anxiety. The presence and severity of these and other symptoms can vary from moment to moment or day to day and will become more prominent over time with regard to causing functional limitations. The goal of utilizing energy conservation and work simplification interventions is to help the client integrate these strategies into established habits and routines, making modifications as necessary to support meaningful participation. While implementing a self-management approach to intervention, OT practitioners should not only be working with clients to address their immediate challenges but should also be working to teach clients the problem-solving skills that will allow them to generalize knowledge to apply energy conservation and work simplification strategies to other occupations. Fostering this type of self-management will allow clients to optimize engagement in valued activities and roles over the course of their lives, even in the face of changing demands, shifts in priorities, and progression of their diseases.

LIFESTYLE MODIFICATION

There is a paradigm shift in health care in the United States away from treatment of disease and toward prevention-based interventions and the promotion of healthy lifestyles.[52] Engaging clients in the adoption of healthy lifestyles can have a positive impact on slowing chronic disease progression and assist in avoiding long-term complications or comorbidities.[51] Health-promoting behaviors, including physical activity, healthy diet, coping/stress management, social and leisure participation, self-care, and spiritual and psychological well-being are documented lifestyle factors that can improve health-related quality of life and assist with the daily self-management of chronic disease.[53]

The OT profession has historically recognized that health promotion, wellness, and prevention are important approaches that enable clients to achieve greater health, independence, and autonomy. One of the most widely regarded OT research studies, the Well Elderly Study, was performed to evaluate the effectiveness of preventive OT services in 361 independent-living older adults.[17] This randomized controlled study compared three groups over a 9-month treatment period, including an OT treatment group, a social activity control group, and a nontreatment control group. The OT treatment group received individualized prevention-based OT treatment that focused on "health through occupation" (e.g., performing meaningful daily activities to promote a healthy and satisfying lifestyle). Examples of treatment sessions included home and community safety, transportation utilization, joint protection principles, adaptive equipment, energy conservation, and exercise and nutrition. The social activity group participated in activities designed to facilitate social interactions. Participants in the social activity group engaged in community outings, craft projects, film-watching, and games. The nontreatment control group received no intervention. The results showed clearly that the treatment group that received individualized OT services improved in areas of function and quality of life, whereas the nontreatment groups declined in function over the 9-month intervention period. The Well Elderly Study demonstrated that receiving individualized and preventive OT treatment could mitigate against the health risks in older adulthood and allow individuals to construct routines that would be health promoting and meaningful.[17] Additionally, approximately 90% of the therapeutic gain from OT treatment observed in a 6-month follow-up study was retained in study participants demonstrating that integrating health-promoting habits and routines into client interventions can offer long-lasting benefits for health and independence.[54]

As evidence indicates, OT practitioners are well poised to address health promotion, wellness, and prevention-based interventions in clients with chronic diseases. Addressing health-related lifestyle requires OT practitioners to not only look at personal choices and individual responsibility but also consider an individual's predetermined personal, cultural, environmental, and health factors that contribute to everyday behaviors.[53] Otherwise known as *lifestyle modification*, new and health-supporting routines can be developed in clients when OT practitioners demonstrate the ability to address potential risk factors for chronic diseases. Common examples of lifestyle modifications that OT practitioners might address in clients with chronic diseases include increasing physical activity and maintaining a healthy diet.

Maintaining a healthy diet is critical to promoting health and wellness in all people. For those living with chronic disease, it is vital that modifications are made in a person's diet to reduce health complications and the risk of exacerbation and to slow disease progression. Depending on the diagnosis, the client may have specific dietary requirements and restrictions that should be followed. For example, a client living with CHF is required to make modifications such as reduction of salt and fluid intake to minimize fluid retention and weight gain that could trigger an exacerbation. An OTA might work with clients to modify meal time habits and routines by engaging the client in meal preparation with healthy food choices, helping to create grocery lists that support a healthy diet, and teaching the client to read nutrition labels. Food and associated mealtime routines are embedded within a larger social and cultural context that extends beyond meeting an individual's nutritional needs. Making modifications toward a healthier diet can be a complex and complicated process. It is important that OT practitioners work with clients to get a holistic understanding of what their habits, roles, and routines are around food-related occupations. Some contextual factors that should be considered are sociocultural meaning tied to meals, how family and/or friends may be impacted by dietary changes, financial and time constraints, and other limiting factors that might affect access to healthier foods and ingredients.

Just as it is challenging to make changes toward maintaining a healthier diet, modifying one's life to incorporate more consistent and regular physical activity and exercise can be equally challenging. OT practitioners should consider how to include exercise and physical activity in interventions with clients to promote health and to manage chronic diseases. Building physical activity into a person's lifestyle not only supports optimal functioning but can minimize impairment and slow disease progression (e.g., improving cardiopulmonary functioning and assisting with weight loss). Individuals who have been sedentary for a long period will need support to incorporate physical activity in daily life, grade and progress the amount of activity, and then support the maintenance of participation in those activities and exercise over time. Ideally, physical activity interventions incorporate activities/occupations that are meaningful to the client and that can be easily embedded in clients' daily routines. Initially, it may be helpful to focus on opportunities to increase physical activity during the natural flow of the individual's day before focusing on introducing exercise specific activities. For example, a client may have decreased receptiveness to daily performance of an upper body home exercise program but may be interested in walking 200 feet to check the mail box or standing for 15 minutes to wash dishes (Fig. 25-7). OTAs may also consider introducing clients to community exercise programs to increase community mobility opportunities and build social connections with group participants. If clients may benefit from more exercise-based activity, practitioners should consider all contextual factors that could either support or hinder their regular and consistent participation and develop a plan that is best designed for success. It is important to be aware of any activity restrictions or precautions that should be followed during physical activity and ensure that training related to following these recommendations is incorporated into interventions. Examples of restrictions or precautions may include limitations on frequency, duration of physical activity, maximum levels of exertion, and

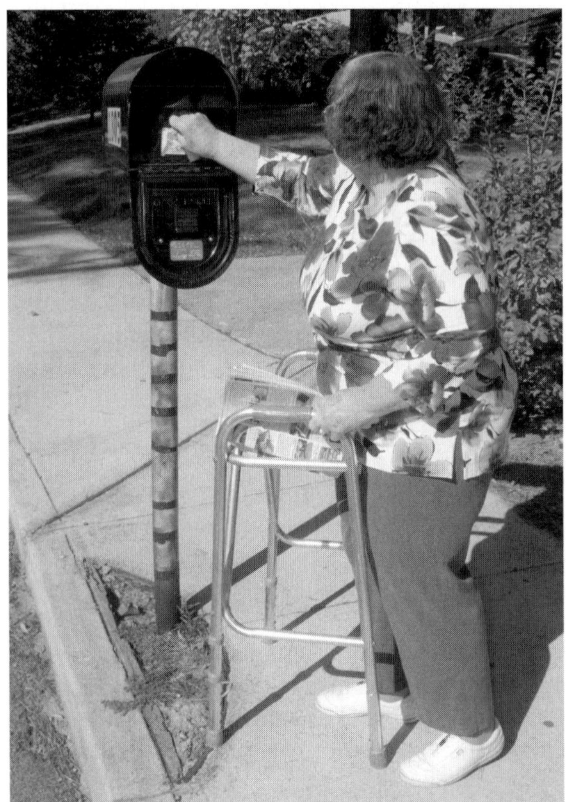

FIGURE 25-7. Lifestyle modification. Incorporating physical activity into daily habits and routines is an important aspect of chronic disease self-management. *(Courtesy CDC/Amanda Mills.)*

oxygen or other medication administration before, during, or after activity.

Individualizing the plan of care to incorporate the client's personal history, interests, and lifestyle goals is critical to supporting self-management of chronic disease. Equipping clients with the tools to generalize knowledge and problem-solving skills related to lifestyle modification is essential to promoting behavior change and integrating self-management into daily life.

TECHNOLOGY AND TRENDS

OT has historically treated clients with chronic disease in traditional practice settings, including hospital-based settings, rehabilitation centers, and the client's home and community. However, as healthcare continues to evolve, OT practitioners have newfound opportunities to address prevention and health promotion through new technology as well as in emerging practice areas. Telehealth technology and emerging practice areas, such as primary care, are two newer areas where the OT profession is already making an impact.

Telehealth is a service delivery model where healthcare professionals use virtual communication technologies to deliver healthcare services and education to clients at a location that is physically distant.[55,56] Telehealth is often used for clients who may live in rural areas or have decreased access to healthcare providers, thereby allowing healthcare services to occur in the client's natural setting. OT practitioners are increasingly utilizing telehealth technology to optimize the client's healthcare experience. OT practitioners are demonstrating the ability to evaluate, treat, consult, and monitor health behaviors in clients using telehealth technology and this helps clients develop new skills, modify physical environments, incorporate assistive technology and adaptive equipment, and create/maintain health-promoting habits and routines. Self-management of chronic diseases ideally fits within the telehealth service delivery model as clients with chronic conditions require ongoing education and support to integrate self-management behaviors into the habits and routines of daily life. Telehealth has been shown to increase client access to healthcare services, improve health outcomes, promote health and wellness initiatives, and facilitate coordination of clients' health care.[57] OTAs demonstrate the knowledge to utilize telehealth technology in their practice but must maintain compliance with supervision guidelines relevant to state/province and national practice guidelines and ethical standards to practice.[58]

With regard to primary care, healthcare reform, has refocused efforts in health care to improve the integration and coordination of healthcare services for clients. The common goals of healthcare reform are to improve the healthcare experience of the client, improve population health, and reduce overall healthcare costs.[56] Primary care has been highlighted as one emerging practice area where OT practitioners can contribute to the holistic care of clients with chronic diseases.[59] Primary care is defined as the "provision of integrated, accessible health care services by clinicians who are accountable for addressing a large majority of personal health care needs, developing a sustained partnership with patients and practicing in the context of family and community."[60-62] Traditional primary care models have historically focused on symptom reduction, disease management, and basic preventive medicine. However, primary care models are evolving to offer a more integrated and coordinated experience for clients. Emerging standards for comprehensive primary care promote collaborative practice among interdisciplinary team professionals, shared decision making between the client and the healthcare team, and sustained partnerships with clients and their families.[60] Thus, primary care is evolving from a singular physician-patient model to a more dynamic and team-based approach to improve the healthcare experiences of clients. Utilizing interdisciplinary partnerships in emerging primary care models opens doors for the OT profession to reach a wider population and initiate care with clients before hospitalizations may occur. OT practitioners are well prepared and ideally situated to contribute to primary care teams whether in the physician office or preferably in the client's home environment and community. In addition, OT practitioners can make a significant impact in primary care by understanding how habits and routines contribute to the management of chronic conditions and the development of healthy lifestyles.[60] OTAs demonstrate the complex clinical skills to practice in primary care but must maintain compliance with supervision guidelines and ethical standards to practice. Advocacy is also needed to further OT's role in this emerging practice area.[63]

SELF-MANAGEMENT EDUCATION

Even if chronic disease is not identified as the primary diagnosis on the OT plan of care, there is a responsibility to include self-management education into the treatment plan regardless of the clinical setting. Many clients who are treated by OT practitioners have diagnoses of chronic diseases as secondary conditions but may be referred for OT services for different reasons. For example, an OTA may treat a client with COPD in a skilled nursing facility after a fall that resulted in hip replacement surgery. Primary interventions for this client in a rehabilitation setting would most likely focus on restoring independence in various areas of occupation and assisting the client's return to his or her former level of functioning. However the OTA, in collaboration with the supervising occupational therapist, must account for the impact that COPD as a chronic disease may have on a client's functioning. The client's diagnosis of COPD must be taken into consideration and addressed by the treating OTA, with self-management being a component of the treatment plan of care. OTAs are in an ideal position to advocate for incorporation of self-management interventions into the plan of care because OTAs generally spend more direct treatment time with the client. Additionally, OTAs may observe challenges in occupational performance related to chronic diseases not specifically identified in the initial evaluation. In these situations, OTAs should be comfortable collaborating with their supervising occupational therapist and advocating for goals and treatment plans that address self-management based on OTA supervision guidelines.[64]

COMMUNICATION

OTAs are encouraged to utilize their interdisciplinary team in addressing self-management of chronic diseases with clients. In addition to OT, common chronic disease interdisciplinary teams may include physicians, nursing staff, dietitians, pharmacists, psychologists, social workers, physical therapists, physical therapist assistants, recreational therapists, and speech language pathologists. Interdisciplinary teams offer collaborative care, in which each individual discipline uses its professional knowledge to contribute to common and shared goals for the client.

Effective coordination of client care cannot exist without the foundation of communication within the interdisciplinary team. For example, improving independence in medication management may be a common team goal for a client with CHF, and it can be addressed in different ways by multiple disciplines on the healthcare team. A registered nurse offers expertise in monitoring drug interactions and polypharmacy; education on medication administration, including proper dosage, frequency, and side effects; and evaluation of the therapeutic responses to medications. A social worker may contribute to the shared goal of improving medication management by assessing the client for adequate social and community support, determining financial needs for accessing medications, and evaluating the health beliefs of the client with regard to medication adherence. An OT practitioner is critical to supporting medication management by analyzing the performance skills required for the activity, identifying environmental barriers and support, and developing organizational and compensatory strategies to integrate the medication regimen into the client's daily routine. The combination of these interventions shared by the interdisciplinary team serve to reinforce the common goal of medication management to the client and demonstrate how multiple professions can work together with their own skill sets to teach self-management principles. Teaching chronic disease self-management is most effective through an interdisciplinary team-based approach. Collaborating with the interdisciplinary team, as described above, requires OTAs to have knowledge of the other disciplines, respect for their professional knowledge, and a commitment to communication with team members. It has been specifically noted that OTAs should partner with and incorporate certified nursing assistants into the plan of care, when possible, to offer opportunities for clients to practice skills related to self-management (e.g., personal care, home exercise program, medication management) initiated by the occupational therapist and the OTA.

OT Practitioner's Viewpoint

In my first year of practice, I had an excellent opportunity to develop my practice skills and understanding of chronic diseases while working with my client Mr. P, in hospice care. When I met Mr. P in his home, he was mostly bedridden in the advanced stages of chronic diseases, including COPD and a CVA. He lived with his wife, who was his primary caregiver, in a rural community in North Carolina. In building a partnership with Mr. P, I learned that as a young adult, he had served in the military before becoming an aeronautical engineer. He graduated top of his class and worked several years as a professor at his local college. Mr. P had two children and enjoyed spending time with his family, meeting with his local men's group, volunteering at a local homeless shelter every week, and creating model airplanes. Mr. P was an active person and shared his passion for cooking with his wife.

When I met him, Mr. P was 75 years old and had begun receiving hospice services after a devastating CVA and long-term complications of COPD. Once an active and vital individual, Mr. P now exhibited right-sided weakness, significant limitations in mobility, and new-onset hearing loss. The functional limitations of his CVA were only further complicated by his COPD, which had progressed to a stage that made breathing difficult during all tasks and mobility.

At the time of the hospice referral, Mr. P had been bedbound for 6 months, was unable to transfer out of his hospital bed, and was confined in one area of the kitchen that had sufficient space for his hospital bed and oxygen equipment. He was on continuous flow of 6L to 8L of oxygen. Mr. P was an excellent self-advocate and requested OT and physical therapy to assist him in his goal to be able to transfer out of his bed and have better access to his home and activities that he had enjoyed so much. These activities included sharing a meal with his wife, sitting in his favorite recliner, working on his model airplanes, and possibly going outside again. Mr. P shared with me that he felt like his hospital bed was a physical barrier in his life, limiting his ability to engage in the activities that were meaningful to him. Although I knew this was a big challenge, given the advanced stage of his chronic disease, I was prepared to assist Mr. P with reaching his goals.

During my initial assessment of Mr. P, I learned that his oxygen saturation levels would plummet to unsafe levels (<80% peripheral capillary oxygen saturation [SpO_2]) with even minimal physical exertion, such as basic bed mobility. For several sessions, I worked with Mr. P on improving activity tolerance with energy conservation techniques, self-monitoring his levels of dyspnea with physical exertion, and utilizing deep breathing strategies. I worked with Mr. P to safely tolerate a transfer with a battery operated patient lift. I also evaluated him for use of a reclining wheelchair and explored functional positioning techniques that would support Mr. P's activity participation goals. Mr. P became more successful over multiple OT sessions learning how to incorporate self-monitoring and self-awareness strategies when engaging in physically exerting tasks. He embraced energy conservation as part of living with advanced COPD

OT Practitioner's Viewpoint (continued)

and took control over his disease. After determining that Mr. P could tolerate the power lift transfer and sit in a semireclined position for a period while maintaining safe oxygen saturation levels, my interventions began to evolve in two ways. I was able to proceed to family caregiver training and education on safe performance of transfers in the home and safe monitoring of oxygen levels so that the caregivers could support Mr. P in achieving his goals. I also worked with Mr. P to modify and set up the physical environment to facilitate his participation in meaningful occupations. Mr. P and I worked collaboratively toward setting up tables at appropriate heights so that he could work on his model airplanes. We worked on energy conservation techniques so that Mr. P could participate in making meals with his wife and tolerate sitting at the dining table for an evening meal. We worked together to adapt the living room space to perform power lift transfers to Mr. P's favorite recliner. We practiced on safely using a ramp to get his wheelchair outside of his home. We focused on the occupations that were meaningful to Mr. P and that enhanced his quality of life and sense of satisfaction. Understanding chronic disease and how OT practitioners can work with clients to embrace self-monitoring and self-management strategies allowed me to support Mr. P in reaching his goals.

On his last Christmas, Mr. P was able to dine with his family, watch his grandchildren open presents, and have a meaningful time with his family. He was not confined to his hospital bed or to his kitchen. I learned many lessons from working with Mr. P but mainly that OT can offer a unique perspective for individuals with chronic diseases. Through my understanding of habits, roles, and routines, I was able to identify Mr. P's goals and incorporate self-management strategies to support participation in his most meaningful occupations. I learned that the focus of OT was not only ADLs but a person's participation in the meaningful occupations of daily life as well. ~ David H. Benthall, MS, OTR/L

SUMMARY

The fundamental approach of OT toward occupation-centered practice and client-centeredness puts the profession in an ideal position to advocate for the role of OT practitioners in the management of chronic diseases. This chapter discussed the importance of self-management and how OT practitioners should help clients with chronic diseases integrate self-management strategies into everyday practice. It must be understood that "patients with chronic conditions self-manage their illness. This fact is inescapable. Each day, patients decide what they are going to eat, whether they will exercise, and to what extent they will consume prescribed medication."[1] Regardless of setting or primary diagnosis, when working with individuals with chronic disease, OT practitioners should take full advantage of their unique perspective, knowledge, and skill set to support clients in becoming the best self-managers they can be. Through the skilled nature of understanding clients as occupational beings, OT practitioners are well positioned to facilitate a greater quality of life that allows individuals living with chronic diseases to continue life participation and engagement in meaningful occupations as fully as possible.

REVIEW QUESTIONS

1. A client was recently diagnosed with diabetic neuropathy. When working with the client on goals targeted at fall prevention and safe meal preparation, the OTA should educate the client on associated symptoms that should be expected. Symptoms of neuropathy include:
   a. Numbness, tingling, or stabbing pain throughout the upper and/or lower extremities
   b. More difficulty seeing the print clearly in the daily newspaper
   c. Dizziness upon getting out of bed in the morning
   d. Edema/swelling throughout the lower extremities
2. Mr. Jones lives with CHF. To minimize the risk of exacerbation that could result in hospitalization, Mr. Jones must monitor which three of the following conditions?
   a. Joint tenderness and fatigue
   b. Shortness of breath
   c. Weight gain
   d. Signs of hyperglycemia or hypoglycemia
   e. Hypertension
   f. Dizziness
3. Ms. Smith was recently discharged home from the hospital with the addition of four new cardiac medications. Historically, she had been able to manage her medication regimen without difficulty but is now expressing concerns about her ability to organize and remember the different times of day to self-administer the newly prescribed medications. The OTA should consider which of the following factors when working with Ms. Smith to improve medication management?
   a. How to integrate the new medication into established routines during leisure tasks
   b. What equipment is needed to safely prepare meals to be eaten with certain medications
   c. Which assistive devices would best support the ability to organize and access the kitchen for meal prep
   d. What compensatory strategies might be necessary to adhere to the prescribed schedule
4. Michael, a 35-year-old truck driver, recently had a fall when trying to get into the driver's seat and fractured his femur. The fracture required surgical repair. Michael is receiving home health OT. In reading the assessment, the OTA notes that Michael is obese and that the occupational therapist has written a goal of increasing physical activity as part of his daily routine. The OTA determines that the best approach in working toward this goal with Michael would be to use motivational interviewing to support behavior change because Michael has expressed some ambivalence toward exercise. Michael states, "I've been large my entire life. I don't think I can change it now." Knowing this about Michael, why is motivational interviewing a good strategy to utilize?
   a. Motivational interviewing allows the OTA to take the lead in informing Michael why exercise is important for weight loss.
   b. Motivational interviewing is designed to force someone like Michael to make a change as soon as possible.

c. Motivational interviewing supports clients in identifying their own strategies toward behavior change with support and guidance from the therapist.
d. With motivational interviewing, OT practitioners can create a written action plan based on the client's problems.

5. Jan is a mother of two and works as a teller in a bank. Last month, she was diagnosed with fibromyalgia and was referred for OT services because she was having more and more trouble completing caregiving and work tasks on a daily basis. The OTA focused on teaching Jan strategies for adapting and modifying how she participates in daily activities by considering such elements as self-pacing, activity modification, fatigue avoidance, organizational skills, adaptive equipment, and environmental supports or barriers. What are these strategies called?
   a. Energy conservation techniques
   b. Pursed lip breathing
   c. Coping strategies
   d. Sensory integration strategies
6. Working with clients to foster lifestyle modifications is especially important when working with people with chronic diseases. Which three of the following are considered lifestyle modifications that OTAs should encourage clients with chronic disease to incorporate into their daily lives?
   a. Stress management and coping strategies
   b. Work simplification strategies
   c. Self-monitoring techniques
   d. Physical activity and exercise
   e. Adaptive equipment use for ADLs
   f. Healthy diet choices
7. Given that individuals with chronic conditions are at risk for more frequent hospitalizations, it is even more critical that OT practitioners use communication strategies with clients, regardless of health literacy level, to better support them in becoming effective self-managers. Which of the following strategies should be used to minimize concerns related to communicating with a client with low health literacy?
   a. Providing lengthy written handouts with as much detail as possible
   b. Using common language, avoiding technical terms and having the client and/or caregiver repeat back information
   c. Explaining ideas in multiple ways during the same session so that clients will understand at least one portion of the discussion
   d. Speaking at a higher volume to ensure the client can hear you
8. Individuals who have chronic disease must learn to live with that disease over the course of their entire lives. It is for this reason that the OT practitioner should use a self-management approach to intervention when working with people with chronic diseases. Which of the following characteristics of a self-management approach is *most* important when considering the long-term nature of chronic disease?
   a. Teaching generalization and problem-solving skills
   b. Addressing deconditioning after hospitalization for an exacerbation
   c. Embedding medication management into preexisting habits and routines
   d. Demonstrating energy conservation skills during ADLs
9. Assessment of vital signs is an important clinical skill that OTAs must possess to be able to safely monitor clients during sessions and modify interventions, as needed. It is equally important when working with someone with chronic disease to be prepared to use this knowledge to teach standardized self-assessment of vital signs when developing chronic disease self-management strategies. Of the intervention strategies below, what should be the *initial* focus of teaching self-assessment of vital signs for a person with a recent diagnosis of COPD?
   a. Teaching clients self-advocacy skills for effective communication with healthcare providers
   b. Creating a daily vital signs diary
   c. Developing self-awareness strategies for clients to understand their body's responses to activity
   d. Teaching compensatory strategies that should be used in response to atypical vital signs experienced during activity
10. Ben has diabetic retinopathy, which is making self-monitoring of his diabetes challenging in the home environment. What is the *best* compensatory strategy that the OTA should recommend to increase Ben's independence in the daily self-monitoring of his diabetes?
   a. Hanging pictures to provide visual cues for monitoring of physiological/behavioral signs of hypoglycemia or hyperglycemia
   b. Monitoring weight change and edema with the use of a large-print digital scale
   c. Performing skin checks with a long-handled mirror
   d. Checking blood glucose levels, as scheduled, with a talking glucometer

CASE STUDY

Mr. Banks is a 67-year-old retired factory worker who lives in the small town where he was born and raised on a tobacco farm. Mr. Banks is one of eight siblings who shared responsibilities working on the farm to support the family when Mr. Banks was younger. After completing his sixth grade, Mr. Banks was required to drop out of school and completely devote his time to working and supporting his family. He has been a smoker since age 9 years and now currently smokes two packs per day. Mr. Banks was diagnosed with diabetes 20 years ago.

Shortly after his wife's death 3 years ago, he joined an interdisciplinary medical program that provides community-based care. The program allows Mr. Banks to attend a day center 2 days per week, and there he can see the physician, nurse, and pharmacist, as well as rehabilitation staff, social worker, and a dietitian on a regular basis. He now lives alone with his dog, Sparkles, in his mobile home. A homecare aide comes twice a week to assist with bathing and light housekeeping. Mr. Banks still drives around in his immediate community and receives occasional assistance from a neighbor with IADL tasks.

In the last 2 years, Mr. Banks has been diagnosed with COPD and CHF and now requires oxygen on an as-needed basis. His blood sugar continues to be poorly controlled because of lack of medication adherence and failure to follow dietary recommendations. The development of peripheral neuropathy has contributed to decreased sensation and numbness in Mr. Bank's hands and feet. One day, when Mr. Banks was ambulating in the home without proper footwear, he received a small splinter in his left foot that remained undetected for several weeks. An infection developed in his left foot, eventually resulting in amputation of his left great toe.

Over the last year, Mr. Banks has been hospitalized on three occasions for CHF exacerbations and has had a short-term stay at a skilled nursing facility as a result of excessive weight gain (25 lbs in less than 2 weeks), difficulty breathing, and deconditioning that further limited his independence and ability to continue to live safely in his home. Once rehabilitation concluded, Mr. Banks was discharged back home, where he was assessed by OT practitioners.

In the evaluation, it was learned that Mr. Banks had limited understanding of his chronic diseases and struggled with self-monitoring tasks related to diabetes, COPD, and CHF. The OT practitioners observed that Mr. Banks was overwhelmed by organizing and administering his 17 different daily prescription medications since discharge from the hospital. He presented with high risk for falls in the home because of the cluttered environment and his neuropathy, as well as decreased activity tolerance associated with shortness of breath and fatigue. Self-management goals were developed with the client around these occupational performance problems. The occupational therapist and the OTA collaborated to determine the best plan of care to support Mr. Banks' personal goal of improved self-management of his chronic diseases. The treatment goals included increasing client knowledge of chronic disease diagnoses and potential consequences of uncontrolled diseases, creating a vital signs self-monitoring diary to be integrated into the client's daily routine, developing compensatory strategies and safe use of adaptive equipment to improve medication management, incorporation of energy conservation techniques during daily self-care activities, adoption of home safety principles to reduce risk for falls, and self-initiation of home exercise program to improve cardiovascular health.

Mr. Banks worked with his OTA for a period of 2 months, with regular supervisory visits by the occupational therapist. Chronic disease education, which was consistently integrated into each session, provided self-management strategies for diabetes, CHF, and COPD. The focus of the OTA's interventions was to help Mr. Banks establish habits and routines that would support his desired goal of living independently at home while equipping him with the problem-solving skills to actively manage his chronic disease. The interventions included (1) introduction of pill box organizer with alarm system to facilitate medication management, (2) teaching Mr. Banks how to self-monitor daily vital signs by using electronic monitors (e.g., electronic blood pressure cuff, pulse oximeter, glucometer, digital weight scale) and recording results in a written diary, (3) developing grocery lists and teaching meal preparation skills based on dietary guidelines, (4) incorporating adaptive equipment during lower body bathing and dressing to decrease fatigue, (5) performing deep breathing exercises to alleviate shortness of breath, (6) teaching diabetic foot care inspection, and (7) developing a home exercise program to increase physical activity and reduce the risk of falls within the home and in the community. Despite recommendations to quit smoking and education provided through community smoking cessation programs, Mr. Banks was not ready to give up smoking at this time. The OTA reviewed oxygen safety and recommended precautions, such as making sure the oxygen valve was turned off when smoking and that the client maintained a safe distance away from the tank—ideally outside. Although Mr. Banks returned demonstration of self-management techniques with relative success during intervention sessions, it was evident that he required ongoing sessions and reinforcement to generalize education to everyday habits, roles, and routines. Building self-advocacy skills were also integral to the OT intervention. As a result, Mr. Banks became more comfortable with notifying healthcare providers when problems arose or when daily vital signs were abnormal.

With the consistency of the OT intervention, Mr. Banks was able to develop a greater level of control of his chronic diseases and to self-manage those diseases on a daily basis. Mr. Banks developed adaptive strategies for medication management without missing daily dosages, incorporated energy conservation and deep breathing techniques into daily self-care routines, participated in the home exercise program on a daily basis, and maintained a written diary for self-monitoring of vital signs. At the time of discharge, the occupational therapist, in collaboration with the OTA, was able to assess Mr. Banks had met the self-management goals set in the original plan of care. Mr. Banks was not only able to resume living alone at home with his dog but was also able to integrate new health-promoting behaviors into his ongoing self-management of chronic disease.

1. As the OTA working with Mr. Banks in the community-based program, how might you have worked with Mr. Banks and the interdisciplinary team to assist him in better controlling his blood sugar and reducing the risk of associated complications?
2. What could the hospital-based OT practitioners working with Mr. Banks have done differently to better incorporate self-management of chronic disease into his care plan and interventions to reduce future exacerbations and rehospitalizations?
3. Refer to the "Putting it all Together" feature for an additional example of a treatment session, including sample documentation. Consider writing treatment plans for sessions 2 and 3 as an individual learning activity.

PUTTING IT ALL TOGETHER Sample Treatment and Documentation

Setting	Client's home
Client Profile	Mr. A is an 82 y/o gentleman with diagnosis of type II diabetes, CHF, and osteoarthritis. He was referred to home health OT services following a hospitalization due to symptoms related to uncontrolled diabetes.
Work History	Mr. A worked at a family owned bakery for 55 years in New York before retiring.
Insurance	Medicare Part A & Part B
Psychological	Undiagnosed intellectual disability
Social	Following retirement in New York, Mr. A moved to North Carolina to live with his sister where he has remained for the past 10 years. Mr. A does not drive, but he lives within walking distance to a local shopping center. On a typical day, Mr. A can be found at one of the many shops visiting friends and/or the business owners where he is very well known. Hobbies include going to the local movie theater, shopping on his own at the grocery store, and grabbing a slice of pizza at his favorite Italian restaurant. Mr. A values the ability to access the local shopping center where he receives regular social interaction and can participate in meaningful occupations.
Cognitive	Mild deficits noted in short-term memory, problem-solving, and sequencing requiring education/instruction to be broken down into simple step-by-step directions for optimal comprehension.

Continued

PUTTING IT ALL TOGETHER Sample Treatment and Documentation (continued)

Motor & Manual Muscle Testing (MMT)	UE Testing: 140 degrees AROM bilateral shoulder flexion-WFL-No functional deficits noted 4+/5 shoulder strength/elbow/wrist/grip LE Testing: 110 degrees AROM bilateral knee flexion-limited by pain associated with OA 5/5-bilateral hip/knee/ankle strength-No functional deficits noted
Sensory	Vision: Diabetic retinopathy resulting in blurred/dark vision Hearing: Wears bilateral hearing aids Touch: Mr. A reports mild numbness and tingling throughout feet Absent sensation to light touch in feet Diminished dull and sharp sensation in feet with poor localization
ADL	Mr. A reports Mod I or better in performance of all ADLs in the home; however, assessment results revealed that performance of lower body ADL tasks is noted to either be completed inconsistently or without good quality due to increased time needed and pain experienced during task completion. Due to osteoarthritis in his bilateral knees, Mr. A exhibits difficulty with routine performance of diabetic foot care, including daily washing and drying/nail care/skin checks. Foot care inspection revealed excessive dry skin with callous on plantar surface of L foot. There was an obvious odor indicating poor hygiene and self-management of diabetic foot care placing Mr. A at risk for wound development. Deficits in functional reach, as well as chronic bilateral knee pain, limit Mr. A's self-monitoring and management of diabetic foot care.
IADL	Health Management & Maintenance: Mr. A is noted to excel in incorporation of exercise into daily habits/routines. OT assessment reveals difficulty with self-monitoring of daily blood glucose levels, performance of medication management, and adherence to a diabetic diet. Mr. A's sister provides support for household and financial management in the home. He does not drive, but exhibits good community mobility to shop at local grocery store.
Functional Mobility	Mr. A ambulates within the home and community with 4-wheeled walker. He is at increased risk for falls associated with diabetic neuropathy in bilateral feet.
Goals	Within 6 weeks: 1. Mr. A will perform lower body bathing with Mod I utilizing adaptive equipment and with decreased self-report of pain to <3/10. 2. Mr. A will demonstrate three safety measures and falls precautions for functional mobility activities within the home and community to compensate for sensory deficits. 3. Mr. A will verbalize and demonstrate three self-management strategies for diabetic foot care to minimize risk of skin breakdown. 4. Mr. A will incorporate medication dosing into his morning self-care routine, self-administering morning medications correctly at least 6/7 days during a 1 week period. 5. Mr. A will create and maintain a written diary log to self-monitor daily blood glucose levels at least 6 days during a 1 week period.

OT TREATMENT SESSION 1

THERAPEUTIC ACTIVITY	TIME	GOAL(s) ADDRESSED	OTA RATIONALE
Client education on diabetic foot care principles and principles for self-management of chronic disease	20 min	#3	*Education and Training:* Performance of skin inspection; Reviewed self-monitoring strategies for diabetic foot care with verbal and written instruction
Falls prevention training in context of shower transfers and DME setup	10 min	#2	*Education and Training:* Shower transfer training to reduce falls risk; Training and setup in bathroom DME/AE
Completion of diabetic foot care hygiene including training in use of adaptive equipment/ compensatory techniques	25 min	#1 and #3	*Occupations; Education and Training:* Trained and educated on AE options/ compensatory strategies for ADL tasks to minimize bilateral knee pain.

SOAP note: 12/2/—, 1:05 pm-1:55 pm

S: At OTA arrival, Mr. A presented seated in recliner of his home reporting that "I've already bathed this morning, but had a hard time washing my feet. My doctor says I need to take care of them better."

PUTTING IT ALL TOGETHER **Sample Treatment and Documentation (continued)**

O: OTA performed foot inspection for Mr. A who has difficulty with reaching/viewing bottom of feet given bilateral knee pain. Mr. A had notable dry skin throughout bilateral feet, untrimmed toe nails, as well as a callous on the plantar surface of the L foot. Education was provided today on strategies to monitor/maintain daily foot care for diabetes self-management including need to: inspect & wash feet on daily basis, dry feet completely after washing, apply lotion daily, and maintain trimmed toenails on a weekly basis per instructions from primary care provider. Mr. A was provided a long handled mirror to facilitate daily foot inspection with training provided. Mr. A returned demonstration of foot care inspection using AE with cueing needed to compensate for visual deficits. He was able to recall and verbalize 3/5 diabetic foot care instructions discussed today, and was receptive to new learning. OTA provided a written list of foot care instructions and posted in Mr. A's bathroom where he typically performs lower body bathing routine. Mr. A demonstrated ability to transfer in/out of the shower utilizing grab bars safely with distant supervision. Mr. A owns a shower chair, but has historically preferred to not utilize device during shower routine. OTA demonstrated safe techniques for utilizing shower chair during shower routine to facilitate improved functional reach of bilateral feet as well as reduce risk for falls. Even when seated, Mr. A continued to report 5/10 pain when attempting to reach bilateral feet for performance of lower body bathing. Mr. A was issued a long handled sponge as well as a long handled toe washer today and was provided instruction in use of both devices to perform diabetic foot care regimen. Mr. A was receptive to use of lower body bathing adaptive equipment and was able to demonstrate use of both devices while seated on shower chair requiring Min A and consistent verbal cueing. He reported slightly improved pain (3/10) with use of device and minimized need for excessive bending. OTA educated Mr. A on adaptive equipment and compensatory strategies to support performance of lower body bathing and diabetic foot care including with Mr. A demonstrating receptiveness to strategies.

A: Mr. A was receptive to training in use of lower body bathing adaptive equipment today, but required consistent cueing and reinforcement for proper use of devices for thorough hygiene. Mr. A is limited by learning disability as well as limited social support, making carry over of self-management skills challenging. Slow progress noted today with mild improvement in self-report of pain level with use of adaptive equipment for lower body bathing. Mr. A would benefit from continued skilled OT services to maximize understanding of diabetic foot care principles and reinforce teaching of adaptive equipment/compensatory strategies for lower body bathing.

P: OTA will continue plan of care with progression of diabetic self-management instruction; exploration of strategies for independent performance of foot hygiene; reinforcement of instruction in adaptive equipment needs to facilitate lower body bathing, given poor generalization of learned skills. Mr. A continues to be homebound due to weakness and pain. Plan includes training on use of long handled mirror for daily foot care inspection, strategies for applying lotion to bilateral feet, and need for "soapy soles" suction cup device for washing plantar surface of feet.

Meredith Webb, COTA/L, 5/2/—, 3:35 pm

TREATMENT SESSION 2

What could you do next with this client?

TREATMENT SESSION 3

What could you do next with this client?

REFERENCES

1. Bodenheimer, T., Lorig, K., Holman, H., & Grumbach, K. (2002). Patient self-management of chronic disease in primary care. *JAMA, 288*, 2469–2475.
2. Centers for Disease Control and Prevention. (2014). *Chronic disease prevention and health promotion: Chronic disease overview.* Retrieved from http://www.cdc.gov/chronicdisease/overview/index.htm
3. Administration on Aging, Administration for Community Living, & U.S. Department of Health and Human Services. (n.d.). *Profile of older Americans: 2013.* Retrieved from http://www.aoa.gov/Aging_Statistics/Profile/2013/docs/2013_Profile.pdf
4. Metzler, C. A., Hartmann, K. D., & Lowenthal, L. A. (2012). Health policy perspectives—Defining primary care: Envisioning the roles of occupational therapy. *American Journal of Occupational Therapy, 66*, 266–270.
5. Kim, B. Y., & Lee, J. (2017). Smart devices for older adults managing chronic disease: A scoping review. *JMIR mHealth and uHealth*, 5(5), e69. http://doi.org/10.2196/mhealth.7141
6. Smith, A. (2015). U.S. smartphone use in 2015. Chapter one: A portrait of smartphone ownership. Washington, DC: Pew Research Center. Retrieved from http://www.pewinternet.org/2015/04/01/chapter-one-a-portrait-of-smartphone-ownership/
7. Barlow, J., Wright, C., Sheasby, J., Turner, A., & Hainsworth, J. (2002). Self-management approaches for people with chronic conditions: A review. *Patient Education and Counseling, 48*, 177–187.
8. California Healthcare Foundation. (2015). *Patient self-management.* Retrieved from http://www.chcf.org/topics/patient-self-management.
9. Trappenburg, J., Jaarsma, T., Os-Medendorp, H., Kort, H., Hoes, A., & Schuurmans, M. (2013). Self-management: One size does not fit all. *Patient Education and Counseling, 92*, 134–137.
10. Institute of Medicine. (2003). *Priority areas for national action: Transforming health care equality.* Washington, DC: National Academies Press.
11. Carrier, J. (2009). *Managing long-term conditions and chronic illness in primary care: A guide to good practice.* New York, NY: Routledge.
12. American Occupational Therapy Association. (n.d.). The role of occupational therapy in chronic disease management. Retrieved from https://www.aota.org/~/media/Corporate/Files/AboutOT/Professionals/WhatIsOT/HW/Facts/FactSheet_ChronicDiseaseManagement.pdf
13. American Occupational Therapy Association. (2014). Occupational therapy practice framework: Domain and process, 3rd Edition. *American Journal of Occupational Therapy, 68*(Supplement 1), S1–S48.

14. Coppola, S., & Wood, W. (2009). Occupational therapy to promote function and health-related quality of life. In J. Hodgkin, B.R. Celli, & G.L. Connors (Eds.), *Pulmonary rehabilitation: Guidelines to success.* St. Louis, MO: Mosby Elsevier.
15. Richardson, J., Loyola-Sanchez, A., Sinclair, S., Harris, J., Letts, L., MacIntyre, N., ... & Martin Ginis, K. (2014). Self-management interventions for chronic disease: A systematic scoping review. *Clinical Rehabilitation, 28,* 1067–1077.
16. Hand, C., Law, M., & McColl, M. A. (2011). Occupational therapy interventions for chronic diseases: A scoping review. *American Journal of Occupational Therapy, 65,* 428–436.
17. Clark, F., Azen, S. P., Zemke, R, Jackson, J., Carlson, M., Mandel, D., ... & Lipson L. (1997). Occupational therapy for independent-living older adults. A randomized controlled trial. *JAMA, 278*(16), 1321–1326.
18. Chan, S. C. C. (2004). Chronic obstructive pulmonary disease and engagement in occupation. *American Journal of Occupational Therapy, 58,* 408–415.
19. Centers for Disease Control and Prevention. (2014). National diabetes statistics report: Estimates of diabetes and its burden in the United States, 2014. Atlanta, GA: U.S. Department of Health and Human Services.
20. Escott-Stump, E. (2008). *Nutrition and diagnosis-related care* (6th ed). Philadelphia, PA: Lippincott Williams & Wilkins.
21. Foster, E. R., Cunnane, K. B., Edwards, D. F., Morrison, M. T., Ewald, G. A., Geltman, E. M., & Zazulia, A. R. (2011). Executive dysfunction and depressive symptoms associated with reduced participation of people with severe congestive heart failure. *American Journal of Occupational Therapy, 65,* 306–313.
22. American Heart Association. (2015). About heart failure. Retrieved from http://www.heart.org/HEARTORG/Conditions/HeartFailure/AboutHeartFailure/About-Heart-Failure_UCM_002044_Article.jsp
23. Celli, B. R. (2009). Pathophysiology of chronic obstructive pulmonary disease. In J. Hodgkin, B. R. Celli, & G. L. Connors (Eds.), *Pulmonary rehabilitation: Guidelines to success.* St. Louis, MO: Mosby Elsevier.
24. American Lung Association. (2015). Understanding COPD. Retrieved from http://www.lung.org/lung-disease/copd/about-copd/understanding-copd.html
25. Miracle, A. W., & Miracle, T.S. (2009). Sexuality in late adulthood. In B. R. Bonder & V. D. Bello-Haas (Eds.). *Functional performance in older adults* (pp. 409–426). Philadelphia, PA: F.A. Davis Company.
26. Green, W. (2012). *50 things you can do today to manage fibromyalgia.* Chichester, UK: Summersdale. Retrieved from http://www.ebrary.com
27. Wentz, K. (2013). *Health, medicine and human development: symptom fluctuation in fibromyalgia: Environmental, psychological and psychobiological influences.* Hawthorne, NY: Walter de Gruyter.
28. Wolfe, F., Clauw, D. J., Fitzcharles, M. A., Goldenberg, D. L., Häuser, W., Katz, R. S. ... & Winfield, J. B. (2011). Fibromyalgia criteria and severity scales for clinical and epidemiological studies: A modification of the ACR preliminary diagnostic criteria for fibromyalgia. *The Journal of Rheumatology, 38*(6), 1113–1122.
29. Svoboda, E., & Zelenjcik, K. (2010). *Immune system disorders: Chronic fatigue syndrome: Symptoms, causes and prevention.* New York, NY: Nova Science Publishers, Inc.
30. Campling, F., & Sharpe, M. (2008). *Facts: Chronic fatigue syndrome* (2nd ed.). Oxford, UK: Oxford University Press.
31. Jason, L. A., Lapp, C., Kenney, K. K., & Lupton, T. (2010). An innovative approach in training healthcare workers to diagnose and manage patients with CFS. In E. Svoboda & K. Zelenjcik (Eds.), *Immune system disorders: Chronic fatigue syndrome: Symptoms, causes and prevention* (pp. 175–184). New York, NY: Nova Science Publishers, Inc.
32. Ogden, C. L., Carroll, M. D., Kit, B. K., & Flegal, K. M. (2012). Prevalence of obesity in the United States, 2009–2010. NCHS data brief, no 82. Hyattsville, MD: National Center for Health Statistics.
33. World Health Organization. (2015). Obesity and overweight fact sheet. Geneva, Switzerland: WHO. Retrieved from http://www.who.int/mediacentre/factsheets/fs311/en/
34. Siebert, C., Hart, E., & Moore, S. (2015). Delivering distinct value: Supporting self-management of chronic conditions. Short course presented at NCOTA Annual Conference, Raleigh, N.C.
35. Siebert, C. (2016). The occupational therapy evaluation process in home health. In. K. Vance (Ed.), *Home health care: A guide for occupational therapy practice.* Bethesda, MD: AOTA Press.
36. Miller, P. A., & Cook, A. (2008). Interventions along the care continuum. In S. Coppola, S. J. Elliott, & P. E. Toto (Eds.), *Strategies to advance gerontology excellence: Promoting best practice in occupational therapy.* Bethesda, MD: AOTA Press.
37. Prochaska, J., Redding, C., & Evers, K. (2008). The transtheoretical model and stages of change. In K. Glanz, B. Rimer, & K Viswanath (Eds.), *Health behavior and health education* (pp. 98–121). San Francisco, CA: John Wiley & Sons.
38. Lowry-Lehnen, T. (2014). Prochaska and DiClemente's transtheoretical model of change (PowerPoint presentation). Retrieved from http://www.slideshare.net/lehnent/prochaska-and-di-clementes-transtheoretical-model-of-change
39. Law, M., Baptiste, S., Carswell, A., McColl, M., Polatajko, H., & Pollock, N. (2005). *Canadian Occupational Performance Measure* (4th ed). Ottawa, Ontario: CAOT Publications.
40. Deacon, M. (2008). Mental health promotion: The key to the effective management of long term conditions. In M. Presho (Ed.), *Managing long term conditions: A social model for community practice.* Chichester, UK: Wiley-Blackwell.
41. Seibert, C., & Vance, K. (2013). Occupational therapy plans of care affecting chronic condition outcomes. Short course presented at NAHC Annual Conference, Washington D.C.
42. Siebert, C. (2016). Sustainable outcomes in home health. In K. Vance (Ed.), *Home health care: A guide for occupational therapy practice.* Bethesda, MD: AOTA Press.
43. Gazmararian, J. A., Williams, M. V., Peel, J., & Baker, D. W. (2003). Health literacy and knowledge of chronic disease. *Patient Education and Counseling, 51,* 267–275.
44. Baker, D. W., Gazmararian, J. A., Williams, M. V., Scott, T., Parker, R. M., Green, D., ... & Peel, J. (2002). Functional health literacy and the risk of hospital admission among Medicare managed care enrollees. *American Journal of Public Health, 92,* 1127–1183.
45. Disler, R. T., Gallagher, R. D., & Davidson, P. M. (2012). Factors influencing self-management in chronic obstructive pulmonary disease: An integrative review. *International Journal of Nursing Studies, 49,* 230–242.
46. Miller, W. R, & Rollnick, S. (2002). *Motivational interviewing: Preparing people for change* (2nd ed). New York, NY: Guilford.
47. Rollnick, S., Miller, W. R., & Butler, C. C. (2008). *Motivational interviewing in health care: Helping patients change behavior.* New York, NY: Guilford.
48. Loggenburg, D. (2008). Psychosocial consequences of living with a long term condition. In M. Presho (Ed.), *Managing long term conditions: A social model for community practice.* Chichester, UK: Wiley-Blackwell.
49. Christiansen, C. H. (1999). Defining lives: Occupation as identity: An essay on competence, coherence, and the creation of meaning—The 1999 Eleanor Clarke Slagle lecture. *American Journal of Occupational Therapy, 53,* 547–558.
50. Sanders, M. J., & Van Oss, T. (2013). Using daily routines to promote medication adherence in older adults. *American Journal of Occupational Therapy, 67,* 91–99.
51. Guillen, A. (2010). Shift from physician-driven care to patient-managed self-monitoring and care for chronic diseases related to metabolic disorders. Conference proceeding: Annual International Conference of the IEEE Engineering in Medicine and Biology Society. IEEE Engineering in Medicine and Biology Society. Annual Conference, 2010, 854–6857.
52. Hwang, J. E. (2010). Promoting healthy lifestyles with aging: Development and validation of the Health Enhancement Lifestyle Profile (HELP) using the Rasch measurement model. *American Journal of Occupational Therapy, 64,* 786–795.

53. Peralta-Catipon, T., & Hwang, J. E. (2011). Personal factors predictive of health-related lifestyles of community-dwelling older adults. *American Journal of Occupational Therapy, 65*, 329–337.
54. Clark, F., Azen, S.P., Carlson, M., Mandel, D., LaBree, L., Hay, J., ... & Lipson, L. (2001). Embedding health-promoting changes into the daily lives of independent-living older adults: Long-term follow-up of occupational therapy intervention. *Journal of Gerontology: Psychological Sciences, 56B*, 60–63.
55. American Occupational Therapy Association. (2013). Telehealth [Position paper]. *American Journal of Occupational Therapy, 67*, S69–S70.
56. Cason, J. (2015). Health policy perspectives—Telehealth and occupational therapy: Integral to the triple aim of health care reform. *American Journal of Occupational Therapy, 69*, 1–8.
57. Cason, J. (2012). Health policy perspectives—Telehealth opportunities in occupational therapy through the Affordable Care Act. *American Journal of Occupational Therapy, 66*, 131–136.
58. American Occupational Therapy Association. (2015). Code of ethics. Retrieved from http://www.aota.org/-/media/Corporate/Files/Practice/Ethics/Code-of-Ethics.pdf
59. Muir, S. (2012). Health policy perspectives—Occupational therapy in primary health care: We should be there. *American Journal of Occupational Therapy, 66*, 506–510.
60. American Occupational Therapy Association. (2014). The role of occupational therapy in primary care. [Position Paper]. *American Journal of Occupational Therapy, 68*(Supplement 1), 1–10.
61. National Institute of Medicine. (1994). Defining primary care: An interim report. Washington, DC: National Academies Press.
62. Patient Protection and Affordable Care Act of 2010, 42 U.S.C. § 256A-1(f) (2010).
63. Lamb, A. J., & Metzler, C. A. (2014). Defining the value of occupational therapy: A health policy lens on research and practice. *American Journal of Occupational Therapy, 68*(1), 9–14.
64. American Occupational Therapy Association. (2014). Guidelines for supervision, roles and responsibilities during the delivery of occupational therapy services. *American Journal of Occupational Therapy, 68*, S16–S22.

Chapter 26

Cardiopulmonary Conditions and Treatment

Renee Causey-Upton, OTD, MS, OTR/L, Cathrine Balentine Hatch, MS, OTR/L, and David H. Benthall, MS, OTR/L

LEARNING OUTCOMES

After studying this chapter, the student or practitioner will be able to:

26.1 Describe common cardiopulmonary conditions and how to provide effective occupational therapy services for these populations

26.2 Identify intervention precautions for common cardiac and pulmonary conditions

26.3 Educate clients on energy conservation techniques to decrease fatigue and support occupational engagement

26.4 Discuss how to correctly monitor and assess vital signs during occupational therapy intervention

26.5 Recognize signs and symptoms of exercise and activity intolerance

KEY TERMS

Active expiration
Angina pectoris
Cardiomyopathy
Chronic obstructive pulmonary disease (COPD)
Congestive heart failure (CHF)
Coronary artery bypass graft (CABG)
Cystic fibrosis (CF)
Diaphragmatic breathing
Energy conservation
Hypertension
Idiopathic pulmonary fibrosis
Myocardial infarction (MI)
Pursed-lip breathing (PLB)
Work simplification

According to a 2016 report, cardiovascular disease is the leading cause of death, globally resulting in greater than 17.3 million deaths each year; this number is predicted to increase to more than 23.6 million by 2030.[1] Heart disease is the number-one cause of mortality in the United States and worldwide. Over 370,000 people die each year in the United States due to cardiac disease, or approximately 1 out of every 7 deaths are attributed to these diagnoses.[1] The overall annual costs of heart disease are substantial. Combined direct costs of heart conditions, such as inpatient hospital stays and medications, equal $108.7 billion in healthcare expenditures each year in the United States. Indirect costs such as lost productivity and mortality add another $98.6 billion in annual expenses.[2] Nationally, there are approximately 26.6 million (11.3%) adults who are diagnosed with heart disease.[3]

Pulmonary conditions are another leading cause of decreased function, healthcare expenditures, and mortality for Americans as well as the larger global community. As of statistics available in 2015, chronic lower respiratory diseases including **chronic obstructive pulmonary disease (COPD)** were the third leading cause of death in the United States.[4] Deaths from COPD are expected to increase significantly in coming years if preventive measures are not taken. COPD is projected to become the third leading cause of death globally by 2030.[5] In 2013, the national economic costs of respiratory diseases were $161 billion, including both direct costs as well as indirect costs of mortality.[6] The World Health Organization[5] estimates that 65 million people worldwide have moderate to severe COPD.

Cardiopulmonary conditions have a significant impact on functional ability and quality of life. These conditions can lead to a variety of limitations such as decreased activity tolerance, declines in strength, dyspnea or shortness of breath (SOB), poor psychosocial health, and reduced participation in valued occupations. This chapter will focus on the most common cardiac conditions including myocardial infarction, diagnoses that require open heart surgery, and congestive heart failure, while COPD will be the main pulmonary condition discussed. Cardiac and pulmonary conditions will be reviewed in detail, with a discussion of intervention approaches for the occupational therapy (OT) practitioner to follow in the associated rehabilitation sections. Knowledge of cardiac and pulmonary conditions are vital for occupational therapy assistants (OTAs) due to the high prevalence of these conditions as both primary and secondary diagnoses among adult clients who receive OT services. OTAs providing care to these populations must follow appropriate medical precautions associated with each condition and monitor clients' vital signs for safety throughout intervention sessions.

CARDIAC CONDITIONS AND SURGICAL PROCEDURES

The heart is a muscle that pumps blood throughout the entire body and the main organ of the circulatory system. The heart consists of four hollow areas: two upper chambers (atria), and two larger and lower chambers (ventricles). Refer to Figure 26-1 for a depiction of the heart chambers and other general cardiac anatomy. The heart also has four valves (pulmonary, tricuspid, mitral, and aortic) that are designed to open and close in a specific sequence to control blood flow in a single direction. The left ventricle is the largest compartment of the heart, and the area where most heart attacks occur. During circulation, the venous system returns deoxygenated blood to the right atrium, where it is pumped to the right ventricle and then on to the lungs to become oxygenated again. This oxygen-rich blood is returned from the lungs to the left atrium, where it is then sent to the left ventricle and pumped throughout the body to all the organs. Oxygenated blood provides the oxygen and nutrients needed for normal and successful functioning of the organs throughout the body. Coronary arteries supply the various areas of the heart itself with blood needed for nourishment to support its proper functioning. Heart disease results from blockages within coronary arteries, abnormalities of cardiac structures and/or function, or from diseases of the actual heart muscle. Cardiac conditions can lead to many limitations that affect occupational performance, as will be discussed next in the sections that follow.

Myocardial Infarction

Acute coronary syndrome (ACS) is a condition in which blood flow to the heart has been reduced. ACS includes **myocardial infarction (MI)** and other conditions, such

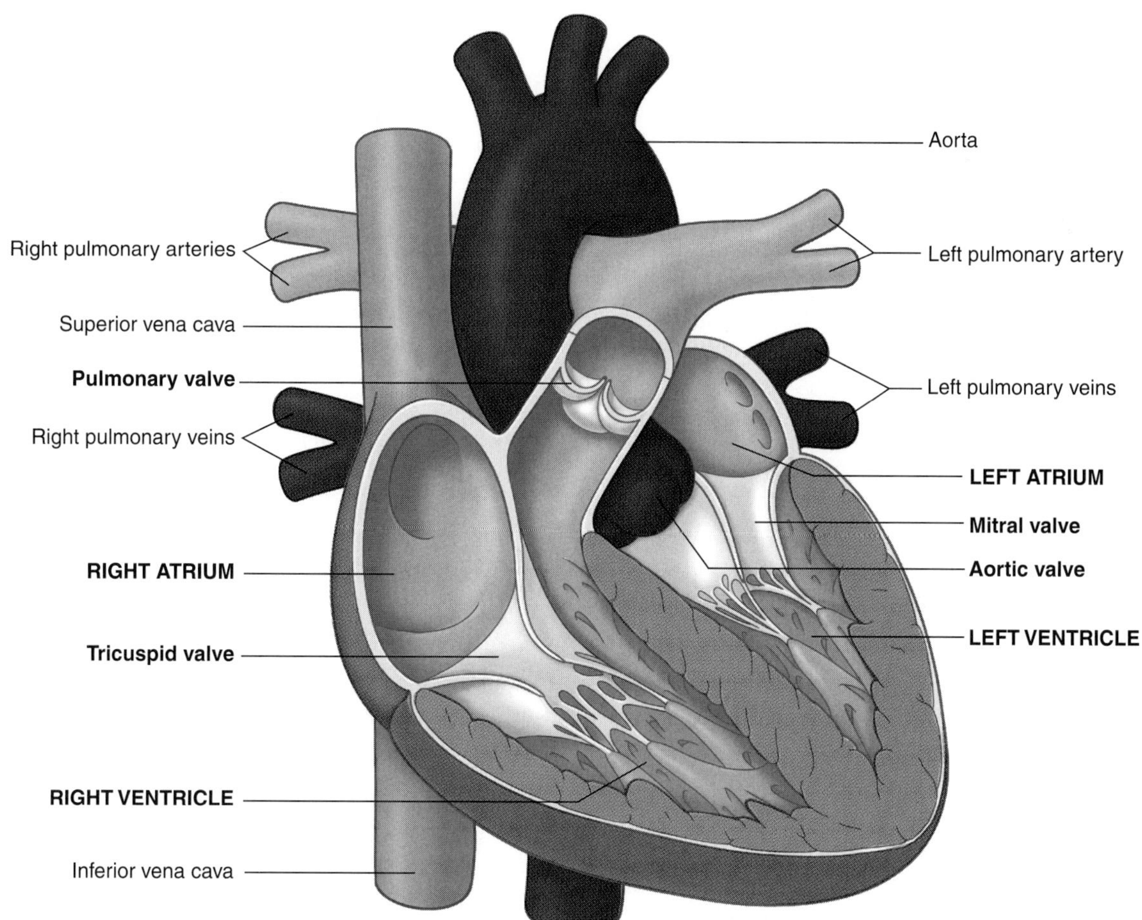

FIGURE 26-1. The heart has four chambers: right atrium, right ventricle, left atrium, and left ventricle.

as angina (chest pain), that result from reduced blood flow. MI, also known as a heart attack, occurs when a portion of the heart muscle has reduced blood flow that is sustained for an extended period. This reduction in blood flow limits oxygen that is necessary for heart functioning and leads to damage and necrosis, or death, of cardiac tissues. Coronary artery disease (CAD) is a related condition that results from narrowing and hardening of the coronary arteries. CAD most often occurs due to atherosclerosis as fatty deposits and plaque line the walls of the arteries that supply blood to the heart. If CAD is left untreated, a plaque can rupture and create a blood clot at the site of the rupture with resulting MI due to blockage of a coronary artery.[7] Spasm of a coronary artery can also result in temporary reduction in blood flow that can lead to an infarction if the spasm does not resolve quickly. According to the American Heart Association, approximately 550,000 new incidences of MI occur each year in the United States as well as an additional 200,000 recurrent heart attacks.[2] It is estimated that approximately 15% of all persons who experience an MI each year will die of the event.[2]

Symptoms of MI can include pain or pressure in the chest that may radiate to other areas such as the teeth, jaw, ear, arm, or even the middle of the back.[7] Other common symptoms are nausea, vomiting, SOB, diaphoresis (excessive sweating), and fatigue. While chest pain or discomfort is the most common heart attack symptom for both women and men, women may experience a heart attack without chest pain and are more likely than men to have other symptoms such as SOB, nausea and vomiting, fatigue, and/or back or jaw pain.[8] Women also often associate their symptoms to other conditions, such as reflux or the flu, rather than a heart attack, which can cause them to delay seeking treatment.[8] The severity or duration of symptoms may differ across clients. These symptoms do not always indicate MI, but should be taken seriously. When MI is suspected, it is imperative that treatment is sought immediately to reduce the risk for death and to achieve better cardiac outcomes through salvaging as much heart muscle as possible. MI is evaluated with an electrocardiogram, referred to as either an EKG (in the United States) or ECG (in the rest of the world), to help determine whether or not a heart attack is in progress or has occurred in the past. Blood tests are also commonly used to assess for various proteins and enzymes that can increase during a heart attack. See Table 26-1 for a description of common cardiac diagnostic tests.

The two types of MI are non–ST-segment elevation MI (NSTEMI) and ST-segment elevation MI (STEMI). ST elevation refers to elevation of the ST segment on an EKG. See Figure 26.2 to view a normal EKG reading. When the heart beats, an electrical signal causes the atria to contract followed by activation of the ventricles. Activation of the atria is reflected on an EKG in the P wave where atrial depolarization is observed, while activation of the ventricles is observed in the QRS wave complex with depolarization of the ventricles. Repolarization of the atria occur here as well, but this is often not observed on an EKG due to low amplitude

TABLE 26-1 Common Cardiac Diagnostic Tests

CARDIAC TEST	EXPLANATION OF CARDIAC TEST
Blood tests	Blood is drawn to assess for cardiac enzymes (such as Troponin) when MI is suspected. Blood tests can also measure electrolyte levels, blood counts, blood clotting time, and other factors that relate to heart attack and heart disease risk.
Coronary angiography	This test is used to diagnose CAD. A catheter is inserted through the groin and is threaded up to the heart itself. A radioactive dye is pushed through this catheter and into the coronary blood vessels to permit visualization of these vessels.
Echocardiogram	Ultrasound imaging of the heart is used to record the structure, size, as well as movement of the heart musculature and valves. A stress echocardiogram examines the heart at rest, followed by an examination of the heart during exercise. Medication can be provided to mimic exercise effects on the heart if exercise is not safe for a client.
Electrocardiogram (ECG or EKG depending on country)	Electrodes are positioned on the body to detect heart rate and heart rhythm.
Holter monitoring	A small, portable EKG machine records heart rate and rhythm over time, typically 24 to 48 hours during regular daily activities.
Nuclear stress test	Clients exercise to their maximum tolerance on a treadmill. A radioactive substance is injected in the bloodstream when clients feel they will only be able to tolerate 1 more minute of exercise in order to provide diagnostic information about the heart.
Transesophageal echocardiogram	A small probe is inserted in the mouth and through the esophagus, finally resting behind the heart. This test can detect several disorders and conditions, such as clots, masses in the heart itself, valvular disorders, and cardiac arrhythmias.

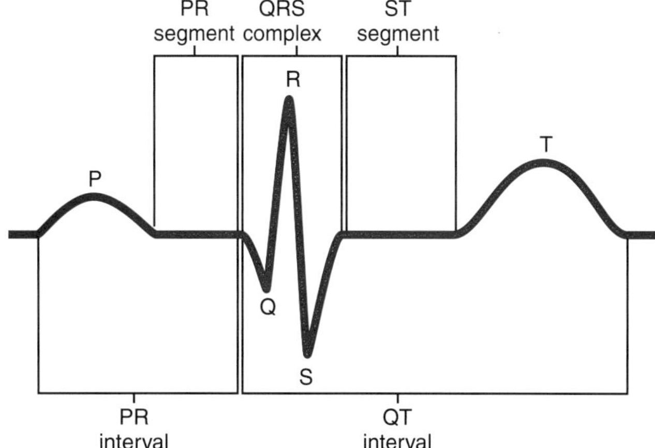

FIGURE 26-2. A basic EKG reading with labeled waves and segments: P wave, Q wave, R wave, S wave, QRS wave complex, ST segment, and T wave.

of this process that is overshadowed by the power of the QRS wave complex.[9] Repolarization of the ventricles occurs in the T wave or recovery wave as the ventricles refill with blood. Typically, the ST segment is observed to be flat on a normal EKG. When the segment is elevated, this can indicate that a STEMI has occurred.

The severity of an MI varies depending on the type, location, and the size of the infarct. See Figure 26-3 to view the general anatomy of the heart and areas that may be affected during MI. The coronary artery is blocked completely during a STEMI, resulting in a greater amount of tissue necrosis, but the coronary artery is only partially blocked during a NSTEMI which leads to less cardiac tissue death.[10] This type of infarction is harder to distinguish from unstable angina because markers are often not present on an ECG; typically cardiac enzymes measured by drawing blood are needed to diagnose a NSTEMI. An MI occurring in the anterior wall of the heart has a poor prognosis, as this results in greater tissue damage than those that occur in the inferior wall or other areas.[10] The larger the size of the infarct, the greater the loss of healthy cardiac tissue, which also results in a poorer prognosis.

RISK FACTORS

Many risk factors for MI are modifiable, while others are not. Modifiable risk factors include smoking, hypertension, high cholesterol, obesity, low activity levels, stress, and high blood glucose.[11] In addition, cocaine use has also been associated with increased risk for heart attack. Nonmodifiable factors include family history of heart disease, previous heart attack, and increased age. Clients should be educated on risks for MI and encouraged to make lifestyle changes to alter modifiable factors for a first or recurrent heart attack. The Framingham Heart Study is a national, longitudinal project that identified major cardiovascular disease risk factors at a time when little was known about what caused heart disease. More information about this pivotal study and continuing research can be found at: https://www.framinghamheartstudy.org/.

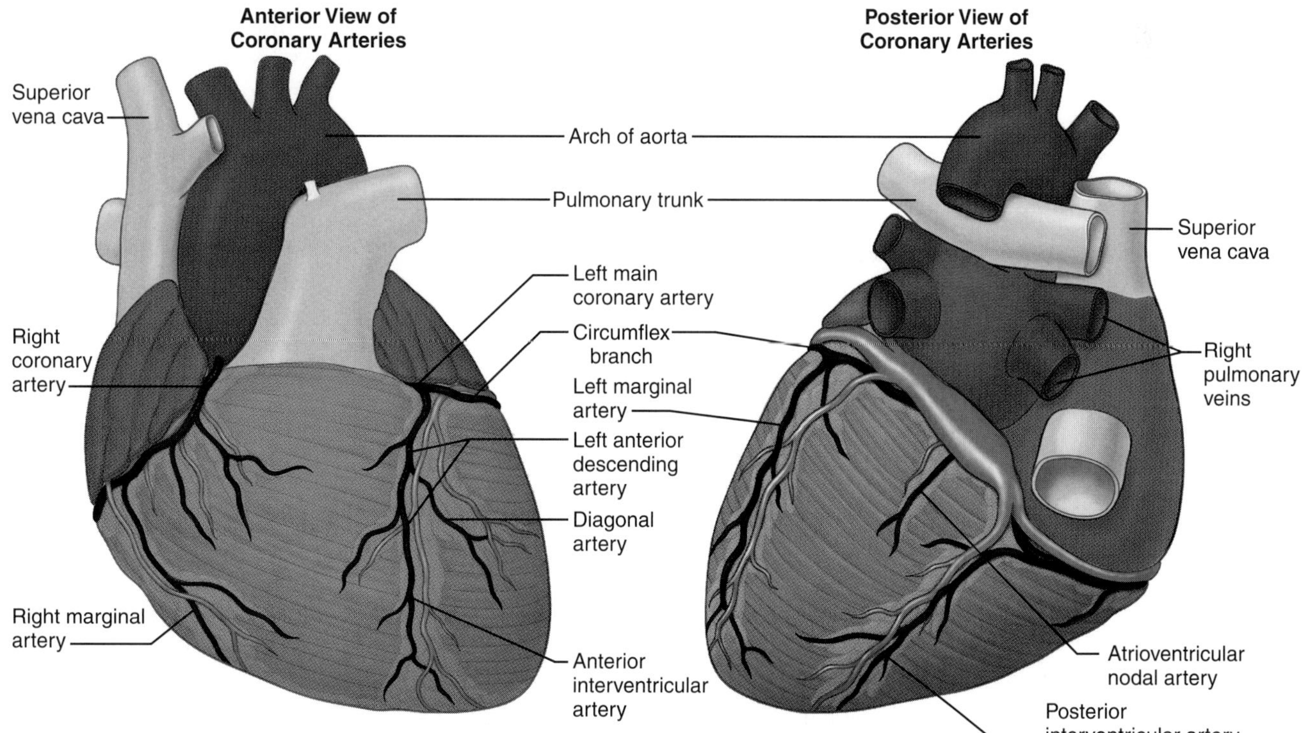

FIGURE 26-3. The general anatomy of the anterior and posterior heart. Coronary arteries that are occluded will determine where damage to the heart occurs.

MEDICAL MANAGEMENT

Common medical interventions for acute MI can include medication as well as procedures to improve blood flow in an occluded artery. Anticoagulants or anticlotting medicines, such as aspirin, can be taken during MI to slow blood clotting and limit the size of a thrombus (or blood clot) that is restricting blood flow. Other common medications include angiotensin-converting enzyme (ACE) inhibitors, beta blockers, and calcium channel blockers. ACE inhibitors have a vasodilating effect that increases blood flow and decreases the amount of work that the heart must perform. Beta blockers reduce heart rate and blood pressure, as well as decrease oxygen demands of the heart muscle.[12] Calcium channel blockers can work as vasodilators and also decrease the force of contraction of the heart muscle, which lowers the effort required by the heart to pump blood.[12]

Percutaneous coronary intervention (PCI), also known as balloon angioplasty, is a common procedure used to open blood vessels that have been occluded in order to restore proper blood flow. Sometimes PCI is performed in isolation, but other times a stent is also inserted inside the artery to maintain a fuller opening for unobstructed blood flow. Stents without medication are called bare-metal stents, while those that include medication are called drug-eluting stents. Drug-eluting stents release medication in a controlled manner that typically occurs over the first 30 to 45 days after they are implanted and interferes with the proliferative phase of vascular healing in order to limit thrombus formation.[13] PCI involves inserting a balloon catheter into the coronary artery directed to the area that has been occluded. The end of the catheter that includes the balloon is positioned at the site of the occlusion and is inflated outward to push the plaque material toward the sides of the arterial walls, creating a larger opening for blood flow. When a stent is used, the device is placed over the balloon catheter before insertion and the balloon is deflated once the stent is in place so that it remains in the artery after the catheter is removed. Decreased incidence of restenosis (closure of the artery) with resulting reduced need for repeat PCI has been found for using a stent compared with angioplasty alone as a single intervention.[14] Drug-eluting stents have been found to have lower risk for restenosis than bare-metal stents as well as reduced rates of thrombus formation at the stent site.[15] The size of the occluded vessel, client risks, cost, and other factors help to determine which approach is best to treat individual clients.

Some clients are not candidates for PCI due to heavy calcification of plaques within coronary arteries. For these clients, an atherectomy may be needed to physically remove plaques from the vessel for dilation to support better blood flow. This approach may also be used before an angioplasty or stenting to provide access for these procedures when complex lesions or severe calcification are present.[16] Atherectomy involves similar procedures as PCI with the addition of a laser or rotating blade that cuts apart calcifications and then removes them from the vessel with a suction device. This procedure can provide more optimal expansion of a stent within an artery due to this removal of plaque.[14] Access for any form of PCI, including angioplasty, stenting, or atherectomy, is most often obtained through the femoral artery at the groin; the radial artery in the upper extremity (UE) is another option for access during PCI.[17] Following these approaches, the client is required to maintain the affected extremity in extension for approximately 4 to 8 hours after the procedure while on bedrest. At the next OT session, clients should be able to resume activities of daily living (ADLs) and functional mobility as well as gentle exercise without resistance.

Open Heart Surgery

Management of many cardiac conditions can require open heart surgery. Advanced CAD, congenital disorders, and diagnoses that necessitate cardiac valve replacement such as endocarditis (an infection of the inner lining, or endocardium, of the heart), rheumatic disease (a variety of conditions affecting the joints and muscles including the heart), cardiomyopathy, or MI, can all require this procedure to access the structures of the heart. See the Risk Factors (for open heart surgery) section for further discussion about conditions that can lead to open heart surgery. Invasive surgical approaches involve a midline sternotomy, a procedure that opens the chest through the sternum to allow the surgeon to reach the heart effectively, in addition to the use of a heart-lung bypass machine. Minimally invasive techniques can utilize smaller incisions and/or approaches that do not require the heart to be stopped during surgery.

A **coronary artery bypass graft (CABG)** involves replacing occluded coronary arteries with grafts of arteries or veins from other parts of the body. See Figure 26-4 for a depiction of common graft sites for this procedure. This is often referred to by healthcare professionals as a "cabbage" surgery. During the procedure, clients are placed on a cardiopulmonary bypass machine to maintain oxygenation while the heart is stopped. The surgeon takes the artery or vein graft and attaches it to the aorta and the portion of the coronary artery that is not clogged in order to bypass the obstructed portion and restore blood flow to the heart. When the graft is successfully attached, the heart is restarted and the surgeon closes the sternum and the incision. Grafts often come from either the saphenous vein or an internal thoracic artery (ITA), which has also been previously called the internal mammary artery. The ITA has been found to remain patent, or open and unobstructed, longer than the saphenous vein and also has been linked to greater survival rates.[18] The radial artery is another graft site that is sometimes used for CABG. The site where the graft is removed will need to be monitored for healing. For example, clients with a saphenous vein graft will have two or more incisions on the medial portion of the lower extremity (LE). For an ITA, incisions are in the chest area and the artery can be accessed with small openings for a minimally invasive approach. When the radial artery is used for grafting, clients will have incisions on the anterior surface of the forearm between the elbow and the wrist.

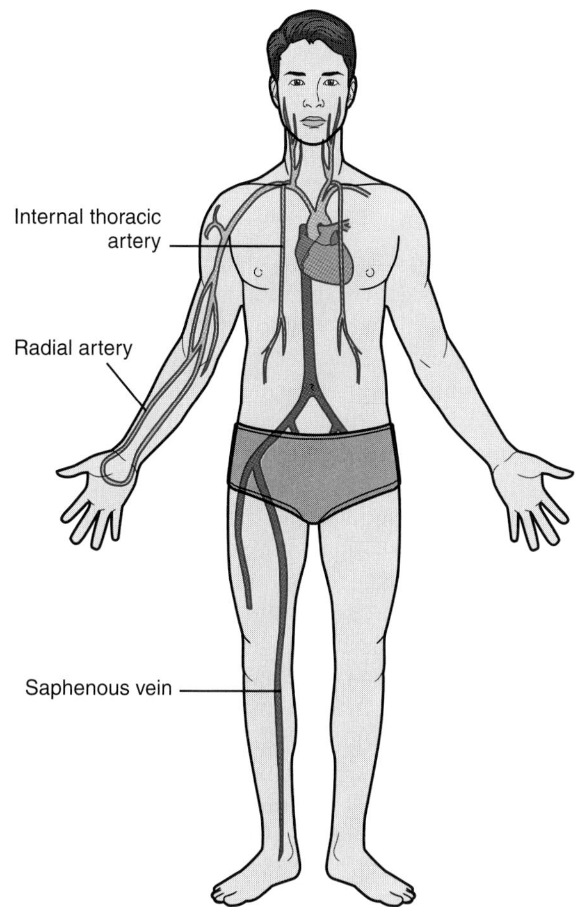

FIGURE 26-4. Graft sites for the saphenous vein, internal thoracic artery, and radial artery.

Following a sternotomy, clients will have sternal precautions for approximately 4 to 6 weeks, however some clients may have precautions for up to 12 weeks. Standard sternal precautions and recommendations may vary by setting and by surgeon, so OTAs should refer to their facility policy and surgeons for specific guidelines. Examples of these include:

- **Clients should avoid completing asynchronous movements with the UEs.** Asynchronous movements involve moving one arm without the other, such as by reaching to put a plate in a cabinet with one arm only. This should be avoided due to the risk for sternal shifting or clicking while the sternum is still healing. Move the arms together instead to complete daily tasks when possible.
- **Clients should avoid any activities that cause feelings of sternal clicking or shifting to protect the sternum as it heals.** Sternal shifting and/or clicking is a sensation that the sternum is moving apart and can sometimes even be heard as a "clicking" or popping sound.
- **Clients should avoid shoulder flexion beyond 90 degrees and other excessive shoulder movements while sternal precautions are in place.**
- **Clients should not lift anything heavier than 5 to 10 pounds and should be cautious of their UE weight-bearing as well as pushing/pulling with the arms during mobility.**
- **Clients may be provided with a small pillow after surgery to hold against the sternum when they cough and during transitions for mobility.** Some surgeons may want clients to hold this pillow against their chest while moving into sitting from supine, as well as during sit to stand. Clients should be advised to hold the pillow lightly, and should avoid squeezing the pillow tightly against the sternum while it is still healing.

Another form of CABG that does not require stopping the heart for the surgical procedure is called off-pump coronary artery bypass (OPCAB). A midline sternotomy is still required, but one advantage of the OPCAB is that the client is able to avoid postperfusion syndrome (neurocognitive impairment) that can sometimes accompany CABG.[19] This syndrome can include deficits such as decreased attention, difficulty concentrating, short-term memory loss, and slowed mental processing. Postperfusion syndrome is typically short-term, although the greater the length of time the client spends on cardiopulmonary bypass, the longer and more severe neurocognitive impairments can be. Endoscopic atraumatic coronary artery bypass (endo-ACAB) is a less-invasive approach to open heart surgery.[19] In this procedure, the heart is accessed through an incision that is made between the ribs. Because a sternotomy is avoided, clients are able to resume their regular activities sooner with less recovery time for the endo-ACAB approach compared with a typical CABG. See Table 26-2 for an overview of common surgical approaches for CABG.

Another indication for open heart surgery is valve repair or replacement. When damage occurs to one of the valves, the heart must work harder to pump effectively. If the valve damage is minor, the heart may be able to compensate for this deficit; if the damage to the valve is significant, this can lead to more severe outcomes and may require surgical intervention.[19] Valve replacements can be performed either

TABLE 26-2 Approaches for Coronary Artery Bypass Surgery

SURGICAL APPROACH	EXPLANATION OF APPROACH
Coronary artery bypass graft (CABG)	A midline sternotomy is performed. The heart is stopped, and the client is placed on a cardiopulmonary bypass machine to sustain oxygenation.
Off-pump coronary artery bypass (OPCAB)	The surgery is performed on a beating heart following a midline sternotomy, and a cardiopulmonary bypass machine is not used.
Endoscopic atraumatic coronary artery bypass (endo-ACAB)	The surgical incision is made between the ribs. A cardiopulmonary bypass machine is not used.

through a sternotomy or through minimally invasive approaches that involve the use of smaller incisions. Similar to CABG surgery, clients may require the use of a pulmonary bypass machine or less commonly, the surgeon may perform the procedure on a beating heart. Clients who receive a sternotomy would be required to follow the sternal precautions discussed previously. Replacement heart valves are made with manufactured materials (for mechanical valves) or with tissue from pigs, cows, or cadavers (for bioprosthetic valves). Mechanical valves last longer than those made from tissue, but they place clients at higher risk for clotting at the replacement site.[19] An annuloplasty is an approach for valve repair that attempts to tighten the annulus (base of the heart valve) to restore proper functioning without replacing the valve itself. When a valve becomes too small due to stenosis, surgeons can use techniques to open the valve either by dilating or enlarging the valve using similar techniques with a cardiac catheter, discussed previously in this chapter for balloon angioplasty.

RISK FACTORS

Many risk factors for conditions requiring open heart surgery are similar to other cardiac conditions such as CAD and MI. Advanced stages of CAD can also require open heart surgery when less-invasive approaches, such as PCI, are no longer sufficient to correct the condition. Smoking, high blood pressure, obesity, reduced activity levels, stress, diabetes, and high cholesterol can lead to conditions that will require CABG in order to restore blood flow to areas of the heart. Increasing age, family history of cardiac conditions, as well as male gender also increase risk. Heart valves can become damaged due to endocarditis, rheumatic disease, cardiomyopathy, atherosclerotic heart disease (a condition that causes hardening and narrowing of cardiac arteries), or MI.[20] Valves can also be damaged as a result of congenital diseases or malformations. Some risk factors that can lead to open heart surgery are modifiable, such as high cholesterol or reduced activity levels, while others cannot be altered.

MEDICAL MANAGEMENT

Following open heart surgery, surgical sites will need to be monitored for potential infection. Sternal incisions as well as any artery or vein graft sites should be assessed for proper healing. Access sites for other procedures, such as PCI, will also need to be checked to ensure that there are no skin concerns. After cardiac surgery, clients may be required to take certain medications to prevent future complications. For example, clients will require long-term adherence to anticoagulants to prevent clotting after heart valve replacement with a mechanical valve. After MI, clients may be prescribed ACE inhibitors, beta blockers, or calcium channel blockers indefinitely. Clients with hypertension or increased cholesterol may be prescribed medication to lower blood pressure and lipids to prevent future cardiac events. Other risk factors that can be controlled pharmacologically, such as diabetes, may also require long-term adherence to prescribed medicines. Some clients may need additional intervention in the future that will require surgical approaches. For example, bioprosthetic valves do not last as long as mechanical valve replacements, so clients may require more than one replacement in their lifetime.

Congestive Heart Failure

Congestive heart failure (CHF) is characterized as a chronic and progressive condition in which the heart loses its ability to pump effectively to meet the body's need for blood and oxygen. CHF can result from many different cardiovascular abnormalities including CAD, hypertension, and MI, which weaken the heart so that it cannot pump blood efficiently throughout the body.[21] Any of the heart's four chambers can be affected by heart failure, which often results in fluid accumulation in the lungs as well as edema in the LEs and abdomen, if not treated appropriately. With CHF, the heart is unable to maintain its standard workload, prompting several physiological changes in compensation for the weakened heart, including enlargement of the heart chambers, increased muscle mass in the heart, and increased heart rate.[22] In combination, these changes may mask the symptoms of heart failure, but eventually the heart is no longer able to sustain the heightened workload. As a result, fluid begins to accumulate throughout the LEs, abdomen, and lungs. Medical intervention is then required to remove excess fluid from the body and slow the progression of the disease. In addition to observed edema created by excess fluid, common signs of heart failure include sudden weight gain, SOB, wheezing/coughing, fatigue, decreased appetite, and changes in sleep patterns.

RISK FACTORS

Risk factors for CHF are associated with smoking, obesity, hypertension, cholesterol levels, physical inactivity, and long-term stress levels. Genetic factors, including heredity, gender, and age also affect an individual's risk for CHF, and men have higher incidence rates of CHF than women. Prevention of heart failure has been linked to lifestyle changes such as smoking cessation, weight management, consuming a heart-healthy diet, physical fitness, stress management, limiting caffeine and alcohol intake, and promoting healthy sleep habits.

MEDICAL MANAGEMENT OF CONGESTIVE HEART FAILURE

CHF slowly damages the heart structure, limiting its ability to efficiently provide blood throughout the body. Heart failure can be treated to improve symptoms and quality of life, but it is not curable. The primary treatments of heart disease include both medication management and lifestyle interventions to reduce the frequency of CHF exacerbations. Medications commonly used include: anticoagulants, antiplatelet agents, ACE inhibitors, angiotensin II receptor blockers, beta blockers, calcium channel blockers, cholesterol-lowering medications, vasodilators, and diuretics. Refer to Table 26-3 for further description of common cardiac medications and

TABLE 26-3 Common Cardiac Medications and Purposes

CARDIAC MEDICATIONS	COMMONLY PRESCRIBED	PURPOSE FOR MEDICATION
Anticoagulants	Coumadin® Heparin Lovenox® Innohep® Aspirin	Prevent formation of blood clots
Angiotensin-converting enzyme (ACE) inhibitors	Perindopril Benazepril Lisinopril Captopril	Treat hypertension and CHF
Beta blockers	Timolol Propranolol Metoprolol Atenolol	Treat hypertension, cardiac arrhythmias, and chest pain (angina)
Calcium channel blockers	Amlodipine Diltiazem Felopdipine Nisoldipine Verapamil	Treat hypertension, prevent coronary artery spasms, and control heart rate
Antiarrhythmatics	Procainamide Cordarone® Lidocaine Amiodarone	Treat abnormal heart rhythm
Vasodilators	Hydrazaline Nitrates Isordil® Minoxidil	Treat angina, lower BP, control CHF
Diuretics	Lasix® Hydrochlorothiazide	Reduce edema, lower blood pressure

their purposes. The goal of medication management is to maintain optimal cardiac function and reduce exacerbations; however, surgical procedures may be necessary if medication management or lifestyle interventions are no longer working. Physicians may use implantable devices for treatment of cardiac dysfunction, including valve replacement, defibrillator implantation, and left ventricular assistive device (LVAD). More extensive heart surgeries may also include angioplasty, coronary artery bypass, or even heart transplant. None of the medical interventions listed earlier in the chapter can be completely successful without adoption of lifestyle changes and making healthier choices. Lifestyle changes may include smoking cessation, changing eating habits, managing blood pressure, increasing physical activity, and weight management.[22]

Impact of Cardiac Conditions on Occupational Performance

Cardiac conditions can influence all areas of occupational performance with reduced independence in ADLs, higher-level occupations, and functional mobility. Many conditions will share some similar effects, while others can create unique limitations. Most people with cardiac conditions will experience fatigue and reduced activity tolerance. This is due to multiple factors, such as decreased functioning of heart tissue and reduced physical activity during hospitalization or exacerbations. Strength in both the UEs and LEs can also be affected for clients with cardiac conditions due to reduced activity levels, fatigue, and even SOB. SOB is common for clients with CHF due to fluid that collects around the lungs. People with other cardiac conditions, especially in the acute phases, can also experience difficulty breathing.

Some clients with heart conditions will experience edema in the extremities, specifically those who have CHF. Edema can limit ADLs and other occupations by reducing available range of motion (ROM), making the extremities heavier to actively lift during daily occupations, as well as altering the size and shape of the extremities. It may be difficult to don and doff clothing that fits more tightly than normal due to swelling. Dietary changes are almost always indicated for clients with cardiac conditions. In particular, clients with CHF must closely monitor their sodium intake to reduce swelling and decrease high blood pressure. Other conditions, such as MI and CAD, require healthier food choices to decrease cholesterol, treat obesity, and lower blood pressure as appropriate to prevent future cardiac events.

Psychosocial Impact of Cardiac Conditions

Psychosocial symptoms can occur in response to both acute and more chronic cardiac conditions. Anxiety and depression are common for these populations, and some clients may even develop posttraumatic stress disorder in response to a dramatic event such as a near-death experience from a cardiac episode. Clients with cardiac conditions may become depressed due to the inability to fully participate in previously valued occupations and as they cope with adjusting to a new lifestyle. Anxiety can occur due to fear of future cardiac events during activities such as sexual activity, shoveling snow or climbing stairs, or in response to SOB. Anger is a personality trait that can be present before heart disease as a contributing cause of the condition, or after in response to the disease; similarly, anxiety and depression can both contribute to and/or develop after the onset of heart disease.[22] The presence of anxiety, depression, as well as anger and hostility can affect the course of the disease with less favorable outcomes.

Other Cardiac Conditions

Hypertension occurs when there is an excessive amount of force being exerted against the walls of arteries as blood is pumped throughout the body by the heart. Over time, the blood vessels can become weak and overly stretched. In new standards published in late 2017, blood pressure is now considered to be:

- Normal at less than 120 mmHg (millimeters of mercury) systolic over less than 80 mmHg diastolic
- Elevated at 120-129 mmHg systolic over less than 80 mmHg diastolic
- Hypertensive stage 1 at 130-139 mmHg systolic over 80-89 mmHg diastolic
- Hypertensive stage 2 at greater than or equal to 140 mmHg systolic over greater than or equal to 90 mmHg diastolic.[23]

About 70 million adults in the United States, or approximately 1 out of 3 adults, have a diagnosis of hypertension.[24] The annual cost associated with high blood pressure as of 2014 is $48.6 billion, including direct costs of health care as well as indirect costs, such as financial losses due to missed days of work.[2] Hypertension is a serious diagnosis as it is a contributing risk factor for many other cardiovascular conditions such as heart attack and cerebrovascular accident (CVA). Blood pressure should be monitored for safety during exercise and also for long-term management of hypertension. Individuals can improve blood pressure by eating healthier, participating in regular exercise, using stress-management techniques, decreasing alcohol intake, avoiding tobacco use, and complying with prescribed medications.[25] Clients can also experience hypotension when blood pressure is too low. Blood pressure is considered hypotensive when the systolic, or top number, is less than 90 mmHg and/or the diastolic, or bottom number, is less than 60 mmHg. Low blood pressure can lead to dizziness, fatigue, nausea, and even fainting. OTAs should educate clients with high and low blood pressures on the importance of blood pressure monitoring and creating healthy lifestyle changes to manage their condition. They should also monitor blood pressure before, during, and after intervention sessions to ensure that the client is tolerating activities within safe blood pressure levels.

Cardiomyopathy (CM), when the heart muscle becomes enlarged, thick, or rigid, includes several conditions. The three more common types of CM are dilated, hypertrophic, and restrictive; the most common form is dilated CM.[26] CM can be hereditary or develop over time as a result of a variety of factors and conditions, such as family history of CM, coronary artery disease, hypertension, or even aging. In dilated CM, the left ventricle of the heart enlarges, becomes weak, and does not pump blood effectively. This leads to decreased cardiac output as well as increased risk for blood clots.[19] For hypertrophic cardiomyopathy (HCM), the left ventricle and intraventricular septum enlarge and thicken. This can lead to blood flow blockages as well as impacting the ventricles' ability to relax and fill with blood.[27] HCM is the most common genetic heart condition, often linked to sudden death in athletes, and is estimated to affect more than 1 million persons in the United States and 36 million or more persons worldwide.[28] Clients with HCM should avoid vigorous exercise and instead engage in low to occasional moderately intense activities. When restrictive CM is present, the heart muscle becomes stiff and rigid, losing the ability to pump blood effectively throughout the body. This form of CM is less common than dilated or hypertrophic CM. The various types of CM can lead to a variety of negative outcomes, such as reduced activity tolerance, SOB, cardiac dysrhythmias, edema from resulting heart failure, and even death. Treatment for CM varies by type but may include medications, devices implanted surgically, or even heart transplant in severe cases.[29] Some recommended lifestyle changes include limiting alcohol consumption, losing weight, smoking cessation, and decreasing dietary sodium.[30] OTAs can educate clients with cardiomyopathy on these healthy lifestyle choices. They should also monitor vital signs closely for this population under supervision of an occupational therapist, and adjust activity levels for safety, especially for clients with a diagnosis of HCM.

Angina pectoris is characterized by chest pain or tightness that results from reduced blood flow in coronary arteries, most commonly as a result of CAD. Other symptoms can include pain in the jaw, neck, or left UE. Between 2009 and 2012, approximately 3.4 million persons 40 years of age or older in the United States had angina.[31] The two main types of angina are stable and unstable. Stable angina occurs during physical activity and resolves with rest or medication. Common pharmacological interventions for this condition include nitrates, such as nitroglycerin, as vasodilators to open arteries, restore appropriate blood flow, and reduce chest pain.[32] Unstable angina does not have a predictable pattern and occurs even outside of exertional activities. This form of angina typically results from plaque fissure or rupture within an artery that leads to thrombus formation; the resulting thrombus creates an arterial occlusion that limits blood flow.[33] Unstable angina is also more dangerous because it may indicate that a heart attack is imminent.[19] Lifestyle modification is recommended to manage cardiovascular risk factors for clients with angina, such as decreasing high blood pressure, lowering cholesterol, smoking cessation, managing diabetes, participating in regular exercise, and losing weight for those who are obese.[34]

Another cardiac condition that may be present is an abnormal heart rhythm or arrhythmia. The heart can have irregular beats, beat too fast (tachycardia), or beat too slow (bradycardia). Atrial fibrillation is when the heart flutters, producing ineffective pumping. This can last seconds or, if lasting continuously, can be life-threatening. Pacemakers are implantable devices which monitor and help control arrhythmias, and an implantable defibrillator shocks the heart when atrial fibrillation is detected.

OT practitioners have a role in educating clients about appropriate lifestyle modifications for this condition as well as monitoring angina. Rest and/or nitrates are indicated for clients with stable angina, but unstable angina can indicate an emergency. OTAs should treat any chest pain seriously by stopping treatment and notifying nursing staff immediately in inpatient settings. For other settings, such as home health or outpatient facilities, the OTA should assist the client to take nitroglycerin if this has been prescribed by the physician. If chest pain does not go away quickly after resting or within 3 to 5 minutes of taking nitroglycerin, another nitroglycerin pill should be taken and the OTA should call 911 because a medical emergency could be imminent.[7] Some physician instructions allow clients to wait to see if chest pain goes away after the second pill and then call 911 if the client requires a third pill for chest pain. OTAs should check with their facility policies and physician instructions for further guidelines; however, 911 should be contacted immediately if a heart attack is suspected. If the client is in an inpatient setting and heart attack is suspected, the in-facility emergency number should be called for immediate medical assistance.

Cardiac Rehabilitation

Cardiac rehabilitation is an interprofessional approach to treating cardiac diagnoses across the continuum of care from acute illness to long-term maintenance. The interprofessional team may consist of physicians, nurses, OT practitioners, physical therapy practitioners, dietitians, case managers, pharmacists, and other healthcare staff as appropriate. Secondary prevention is a key part of cardiac rehabilitation to reduce the risk for recurrent cardiac episodes and to improve quality of life. The American Association of Cardiovascular and Pulmonary Rehabilitation (AACVPR) has published best practice guidelines for cardiac rehabilitation. The most current version of these guidelines at the time this chapter was written are published in the fifth edition of *Guidelines for Cardiac Rehabilitation and Secondary Prevention Programs.* The general goals of cardiac rehabilitation are to:

- Restore independence with ADLs and other valued occupations.
- Increase strength and endurance within safe cardiac parameters.
- Modify risk factors through healthy lifestyle changes to prevent future cardiac events.
- Increase quality of life and overall occupational performance and engagement.
- Support psychosocial adjustment to living with cardiac disease.[35]

PHASES OF CARDIAC REHABILITATION

Cardiac rehabilitation spans the entire continuum of care, beginning with acute hospital inpatient therapy and then progressing to outpatient care followed by community-based

EVIDENCE-BASED PRACTICE

Both cardiac and pulmonary rehabilitation are well supported by high-quality research evidence. An overview of Cochrane systematic reviews found that exercise-based cardiac rehabilitation for low-risk cardiac clients reduced readmissions to the hospital as well as improved health-related quality of life.[36] Exercise-based cardiac rehabilitation was defined as exercise training for an independent intervention, or combined with psychosocial and/or educational interventions. The research included 148 randomized controlled trials (RCTs) with 98,093 participants. A systematic review examining the effectiveness of exercise-based cardiac rehabilitation for clients with coronary heart disease found reduced mortality due to cardiovascular disease and decreased incidence of rehospitalization.[37] This review included 63 RCTs with 14,486 total participants. The AACVPR (2013) provides the following evidence-based guidelines based on quality research evidence: clients with a diagnosis of ACS, following CABG, or after PCI should be referred to a cardiac rehabilitation program; home-based cardiac rehabilitation can be an appropriate substitute for supervised cardiac rehabilitation in an outpatient setting for low-risk clients; and cardiac rehabilitation can be appropriate for medically stable outpatient clients with a

Continued

EVIDENCE-BASED PRACTICE (continued)

history of heart failure.[19] Similar to cardiac rehabilitation, pulmonary rehabilitation programs are also supported by high-level research evidence in the literature.

A recent meta-analysis of pulmonary rehabilitation for persons with COPD found statistically significant improvements in quality of life, dyspnea, fatigue, emotional function, and exercise tolerance. This research was strong with inclusion of 65 RCTs and a total of 3,822 participants for the meta-analysis.[38] Moderate evidence is also available to suggest that pulmonary rehabilitation can reduce hospital readmission and decrease mortality rates following a COPD exacerbation.[39] Recommendations provided by the AACVPR (2011) from quality evidence are that pulmonary rehabilitation programs should include the following interventions: exercise training, endurance training of the upper extremities, education on self-management and prevention of exacerbations, and psychosocial intervention.[40] The AACVPR also reports that current evidence demonstrates decreases in SOB, improvements in quality of life, and psychosocial benefits for clients who complete pulmonary rehabilitation programs.

While strong evidence exists to support cardiac and pulmonary rehabilitation in general, high-quality evidence that specifically examines OT for clients with cardiac and pulmonary disease is very limited in the literature. A scoping review of RCTs examined the impact of community-based OT interventions on chronic diseases, and only one study included in the review focused specifically on cardiac disease. This review found that a multidisciplinary cardiac rehabilitation program that included OT resulted in improvements of 18 points on a 105-point scale that measured health-related quality of life compared with an improvement of only 4 points on the same scale for the control group.[41,42] A study utilizing observational methods found reduced resting heart rate and improved quality of life following a 9-week OT program for older adult clients after MI.[43] There is greater evidence available regarding OT and COPD than for cardiac diagnoses, although this evidence is limited as well.

A recent study examined the impact of OT on clients with COPD using an RCT design.[44] The results found that clients did not improve in occupational performance or satisfaction with performance as measured by the Canadian Occupational Performance Measure (COPM) compared with a control group. The COPM assesses clients' perceptions of their performance and satisfaction, rather than objectively measuring actual performance, which could have affected the study's results. Clients in the intervention group did report lower levels of perceived exertion than the control group during an individually chosen occupation. A previous RCT from 2005 found that receiving activity training by an occupational therapist combined with exercise resulted in higher functional status than exercise alone or combined with education for clients with COPD.[45] Another lower-level study found some reductions in activity limitations for clients with COPD who received OT compared with pulmonary rehabilitation that did not include OT.[46]

Cardiac and pulmonary rehabilitation are evidence-based interventions for clients with cardiac and pulmonary disease. OTAs have the knowledge and skills to address the multifaceted needs of these clients through training in adaptive occupational techniques, addressing client factors that can improve performance, educating clients about lifestyle changes and self-monitoring of symptoms, training clients in breathing and relaxation techniques, among many other beneficial interventions. More research is needed to determine and demonstrate the effectiveness of OT intervention for clients with cardiopulmonary conditions to support evidence-based practice.

Anderson, L., Thompson, D. R., Oldridge, N., Zwisler, A. D., Rees, K., Martin, N., & Taylor, R. S. (2016). Exercise-based cardiac rehabilitation for coronary heart disease. Cochrane Database of Systematic Reviews, *1. doi:10.1002/14651858.CD001800.pub3*

McCarthy, B., Casey, D., Devane, D., Murphy, K., Murphy, E., & Lacasse, Y. (2015). Pulmonary rehabilitation for chronic obstructive pulmonary disease. Cochrane Database of Systematic Reviews, *2. doi:10.1002/14651858.CD003793.pub3*

Puhan, M. A., Gimeno-Santos, E., Scharplatz, M., Troosters, T., Walters, E. H., & Steurer, J. (2011). Pulmonary rehabilitation following exacerbations of chronic obstructive pulmonary disease. Cochrane Database of Systematic Reviews, *10. doi:10.1002/14651858.CD005305.pub3*

American Association of Cardiovascular and Pulmonary Rehabilitation. (2013). Guidelines for cardiac rehabilitation and secondary prevention programs *(5th ed.). Champaign, IL: Human Kinetics.*

Puhan, M. A., Gimeno-Santos, E., Scharplatz, M., Troosters, T., Walters, E. H., & Steurer, J. (2011). Pulmonary rehabilitation following exacerbations of chronic obstructive pulmonary disease. Cochrane Database of Systematic Reviews, *10. doi:10.1002/14651858.CD005305.pub3*

American Association of Cardiovascular and Pulmonary Rehabilitation. (2011). Guidelines for pulmonary rehabilitation programs *(4th ed.). Champaign, IL: Human Kinetics.*

Hand, C., Law, M., & McColl, M. A. (2011). Occupational therapy interventions for chronic disease: A scoping review. American Journal of Occupational Therapy, *65(4), 428–436. doi:10.5014/ajot.2011.002071*

Austin, J., Williams, R., Ross, L., Moseley, L., & Hutchison, S. (2005). Randomised controlled trial of cardiac rehabilitation in elderly patients with heart failure. European Journal of Heart Failure, *7(3), 411–417.*

Jianu, A., & Macovei, S. (2011). The occupational therapy impact on the recovery of convalescent elderly people after an acute myocardial infarction. Palestrica of the Third Millennium, Civilization and Sport, *13(10), 23–26.*

Martinsen, U., Bentzen, H., Holter, M. K., Nilsen, T., Skullerud, H., Mowinckel, P., & Kjeken, I. (2016). The effect of occupational therapy in patients with chronic obstructive pulmonary disease: A randomized controlled trial. Scandinavian Journal of Occupational Therapy. *Advance online publication. doi:10.3109/11038128.2016.1158316Jhjlh*

Norweg, A. M., Whiteson, J., Malgady, R., Mola, A., & Rey, M. (2005). The effectiveness of different combinations of pulmonary rehabilitation components: A randomized controlled trial. Chest, *128(2), 663–672. doi:10.1378/chest.128.2.663*

Lorenzi, C. M., Cilione, C., Rizzardi, R., Furino, V., Bellantone, T., Lugil, D., & Clini, E. (2004). Occupational therapy and pulmonary rehabilitation of disabled COPD patients. Respiration, *71(3), 246–251. doi:10.1159/00007742244*

Ainsworth, B. E., Haskell, W. L., Hermann, S. D., Meckes, N., Bassett, D. R., Tudor-Locke, C., ... & Leon, A. S. (2011). Compendium of physical activities: A second update of codes and MET values. Medicine and Science in Sports and Exercise, *43(80), 1575–1581.*

cardiac rehabilitation. Some clients who have significant functional limitations may need an additional step in the rehabilitation process, with a transitional placement in a skilled nursing facility or inpatient rehabilitation unit immediately following an acute hospital stay to increase independence with daily tasks and support return to home. During phase I cardiac rehabilitation (inpatient), clients must receive a significant amount of information in a short amount of time. The typical length of an acute stay after uncomplicated cardiac events, such as an MI or CABG, has been reduced to only 3 to 5 days.[20] Therapy in this phase focuses on mobilizing the client, completing ADL retraining, and providing extensive education on risk factors and ways to modify these to decrease incidence of future cardiac episodes. Clients should also be provided home programs as appropriate for their medical condition. Topics of these home programs may include: energy conservation, risk factors and ways to reduce these, cardiac and sternal precautions, lifestyle modification, sexual activity, safe activity and exercise guidelines, signs and symptoms of exercise intolerance, and stress-reduction techniques. Refer to the sections that follow for detailed information about interventions OTAs facilitate to address the needs of clients with cardiac conditions.

Phase II cardiac rehabilitation (outpatient) is a formal outpatient program that lasts approximately 6 to 12 weeks. This phase focuses on continued risk monitoring and reduction to decrease risks for future cardiac events. Supervised exercise is a major component of outpatient cardiac rehabilitation to continue increasing strength and endurance for daily life tasks. Phase III cardiac rehabilitation (community-based) focuses on maintenance of health-promoting activities and exercise to support gains made from cardiac rehabilitation and to maintain healthy lifestyle choices. Formal maintenance programs typically provide lower levels of supervision and often offer services in a group format. Many clients forgo Phase III cardiac rehabilitation due to limited insurance coverage of these programs, or may transition out of these formal programs over time.[19] These clients can complete a maintenance program on their own at home or through a local gym, where they continue to build on their outpatient exercise program.

GENERAL FUNCTIONAL MOBILITY

Clients with cardiac conditions may experience declines in functional mobility due to the strength and endurance impairments that are common for these populations, as well as other factors such as reduced mobility from initial bedrest after a cardiac event. OTAs should ensure that clients are medically stable and cleared by the physician before initiating intervention. In the acute hospital setting, the occupational therapist will have determined this during the initial evaluation, but the medical status of cardiac clients can change quickly. It is important to have open and frequent communication with nursing staff and the physician to ensure that clients are medically able to participate in therapy. In the acute phase of cardiac rehabilitation, a client's vital signs will be tracked in several ways such as through telemetry for heart rate and rhythm and pulse oximetry for oxygen saturation. In addition, clients may have other lines such as an intravenous line (IV) that will need to be managed during bed mobility and transfers. OTAs will need to monitor clients' vital signs during activity to ensure that these are within safe ranges. Before discharge, clients should be taught how to monitor their own vital signs and response to activity so that they will be able to engage in mobility and other tasks within safe and appropriate ranges when they leave the hospital. Refer to the Assessment of Vital Signs and Activity Tolerance section of this chapter for further information regarding how to assess vital signs and exertion with activities.

Activity levels for functional mobility should be gradually increased in relation to the client's response to these levels and within appropriate metabolic equivalents (METs). METs are a measure of the body's oxygen consumption during activities. MET levels have been tested and established for many activities and are used as a guideline for promoting safe activity, specifically for clients who have experienced a cardiac event. Refer to the first Addressing Activities of Daily Living and Other Occupations section of this chapter for further discussion of MET levels. Established MET levels are not exactly the same for all individuals because they do not take into account environmental factors, skill level of individuals, or their physical conditions. OTAs need to consider these factors when progressing a client in both functional and exercise programs. A progression of activities for a client after a cardiac episode may include bedrest initially with gentle bed mobility, and progress to sitting up in a chair after completing a short functional transfer that minimizes exertion. A client who tolerates light activities in bed or sitting can progress to regularly transferring to a bedside commode or using a urinal in standing for toileting. As clients continue to improve, they can be more mobile around their room and progress to completing longer transfers such as going into the bathroom for toileting tasks. Clients continue to increase the length and frequency of functional transfers within and outside of the room as their condition improves.

MOBILITY FOR STERNAL PRECAUTIONS

Clients who have had a sternotomy must adhere to sternal precautions during functional mobility. Clients with sternal precautions must avoid pushing or pulling with the UEs during mobilization, and should use gravity and momentum to assist during transfers. When clients need to roll in bed, they should bend their knees and hips and log-roll these to the side at the same time as their trunk, allowing the weight of the LEs to assist with turning over. When transferring from supine to sitting, clients should roll onto their side and allow momentum to assist with sitting up by utilizing a pendulum-like motion as they lower their legs off the side of the bed, bringing their trunk up into sitting at the same time. The client should avoid pushing or pulling on the rail during all bed mobility tasks. For sitting to standing, clients should scoot forward on the surface they are sitting on and lean forward to increase ease with standing, but should not push with the arms to assist. Some clients may need to avoid using an assistive device such as a walker or cane for functional mobility during this time because they may inadvertently bear too much weight through their UEs. Providing handheld assistance as well as assistance with a gait belt allows therapy staff to better assess and control UE weight-bearing during mobility. Because clients are unable to use their arms to assist with mobility during the early phase after a sternotomy, they may need more help with transfers. Staff should never pull on the UEs when assisting with mobility as this can apply pressure on the healing sternum. In the hospital, the head of the bed or the entire bed can be raised to increase ease with transfers. Low chairs should be avoided, and chair height can be raised by adding folded blankets or pillows to the seat of the chair. Before discharge home, clients should be trained in how to transfer from surfaces that will be similar to what they will encounter at home. Clients should be educated on ways to adapt their home to increase ease with mobility as needed, such as adding pillows and blankets to chairs or using risers to increase the height of a low bed or chair.

ADDRESSING ACTIVITIES OF DAILY LIVING AND OTHER OCCUPATIONS

OTAs must be mindful of MET levels as they engage clients in ADLs and other occupations across the continuum of cardiac care. In phase I, clients must begin with lower MET-level activities due to the acuteness of their medical condition and slowly progress to more difficult occupations. See Table 26-4 for examples of MET levels for various occupations, such as ADLs, leisure, IADLs, and sexual activity. In the acute phase after MI, clients are often advised to perform activities in the 2 to 4 MET-level range,[7] and may begin with tasks as low as 1 MET level in the earliest days of hospitalization, especially in the Intensive Care Unit

TABLE 26-4 Examples of Metabolic Equivalent Levels[47]

MINIMAL: <1.5	LIGHT: 1.5 - <3.0	MODERATE: 3.0 - <6.0	VIGOROUS: ≥6.0
<u>Self-Care</u> • Having hair or nails done by another person seated (1.3) • Passive sexual activity, light effort, kissing, hugging (1.3) <u>Home Activity</u> • Knitting, sewing, wrapping presents with light effort in sitting (1.3) <u>Leisure</u> • Sitting and laughing (1.0) • Sitting playing a traditional video or computer game (1.0) • Sitting, writing, reading a book or newspaper (1.3)	<u>Self-Care</u> • Bathing seated (1.5) • Eating seated (1.5) • Sitting on toilet, eliminating in sitting or standing (1.8) • Grooming such as washing hands, brushing teeth, or shaving in sitting or standing (2.0) • Showering and toweling off in standing (2.0) • Dressing and undressing in standing or sitting (2.5) • Hairstyling in standing (2.5) • Active sexual activity, vigorous effort (2.8) <u>Home Activity</u> • Ironing (1.8) • Washing dishes in standing (1.8) • Laundry: folding or hanging clothes, loading and unloading the washer and dryer (2.0) • Putting away groceries (2.5) • Mowing lawn, riding mower (2.5) <u>Walking</u> • Walking very slowly at less than 2.0 mph on a level surface (2.0) • Walking slowly at 2.5 mph on a level surface (2.8) <u>Exercise</u> • Activity promoting video game such as Wii Fit with light effort (2.3)	<u>Home Activity</u> • Cleaning, sweeping carpet or floors (3.3) • Making bed, changing linens (3.3) • Cooking or food preparation, moderate effort (3.5) • Sweeping garage, sidewalk, or other outside areas (4.0) • Yard work, moderate effort (4.0) <u>Walking</u> • Walking at 2.5 mph on a level surface (3.0) • Walking at a moderate pace of 2.8 to 3.2 mph on a level surface (3.5) • Stair climbing, slow pace (4.0) <u>Exercise</u> • Resistance training, multiple exercises, 8–15 repetitions (3.5) • Calisthenics, moderate effort (3.5) • Activity-promoting video game such as Wii Fit with moderate effort (3.8) • Circuit training, moderate effort (4.3) • Upper body exercise, stationary bicycle with arms only, moderate effort (4.3) • Bicycling, stationary, light to moderate effort (4.8) • Water aerobics and water exercise (5.3)	<u>Home Activity</u> • Yard work, vigorous (6.0) • Scrubbing bathroom, vigorous effort (6.5) • Carrying groceries upstairs (7.5) • Moving household items upstairs, carrying boxes or furniture (9.0) <u>Walking</u> • Stair climbing, fast pace (8.8) <u>Exercise</u> • Resistance training, vigorous effort (6.0) • Video exercise workouts, vigorous effort (6.0) • Bicycling, stationary (7.0) • Calisthenics, vigorous effort (8.0)

TABLE 26-4 Examples of Metabolic Equivalent Levels[47] (continued)

MINIMAL: <1.5	LIGHT: 1.5 - <3.0	MODERATE: 3.0 - <6.0	VIGOROUS: ≥6.0
	• Stretching, mild (2.3) • Calisthenics, light effort (2.8) • Upper body exercise, arm ergometer (2.8) Leisure • Card playing in sitting (1.5) • Chess game in sitting (1.5) • Sitting and talking in person or on the phone, light effort (1.5) • Reading in standing (1.8) • Drawing, writing, or painting in standing (1.8) • Seated arts and crafts, light effort (1.8) • Standing arts and crafts, light effort (2.5)	Leisure • Seated arts and crafts, moderate effort (3.0) • Standing arts and crafts, moderate effort (3.3)	

(ICU). Most clients with coronary heart disease are restricted to a maximum 4 MET levels or less during the inpatient phase of cardiac rehabilitation.[35] A typical progression of functional activities moves from light tasks, such as light grooming in bed or sitting up in a chair, to more difficult ADLs. Clients may transition next to completing UE ADLs followed by participating in a seated shower or total body sponge bathing and dressing as their condition improves. At discharge, it is hoped that the client will have achieved independence with most ADL tasks if medical status and functional progression allow.

Clients should be trained in adaptive techniques for completing occupations that will limit exertion and increase independence with valued activities. Adaptive equipment should be introduced as needed to increase function and reduce straining with activities. For example, a reacher would be useful for LE dressing for those after an MI or CABG to avoid bending over and the associated risk for holding their breath during exertion if a client is unable to bring the LEs up for dressing. Clients who have sternal precautions must follow these precautions during all ADL tasks, such as complying with lifting restrictions, limiting shoulder flexion or abduction to 90 degrees or less, and avoiding asynchronous movements (one side lifting, pushing, or pulling) of the UEs. See Figure 26-5 for a depiction of a client incorporating sternal precautions into daily occupations. For example, clients may need to pick up items in the kitchen with two hands to avoid reaching only with one arm such as by picking up a pitcher of lemonade with one hand on the handle and the other supporting underneath the bottom of the pitcher.

Clients may also need to have a family member place clothing items on a lower shelf to avoid overhead lifting when gathering items for dressing in the mornings. In the weeks following a sternotomy, clients should limit excessive overhead flexion of the UEs as well as excessive chest expansion.[19] For example, clients should only reach as high as needed to comb hair and pull on a shirt, being careful not to flex the shoulders greater than 90 degrees. Women who wear intricate hair designs that require raising the arms excessively for styling hair will need assistance with this

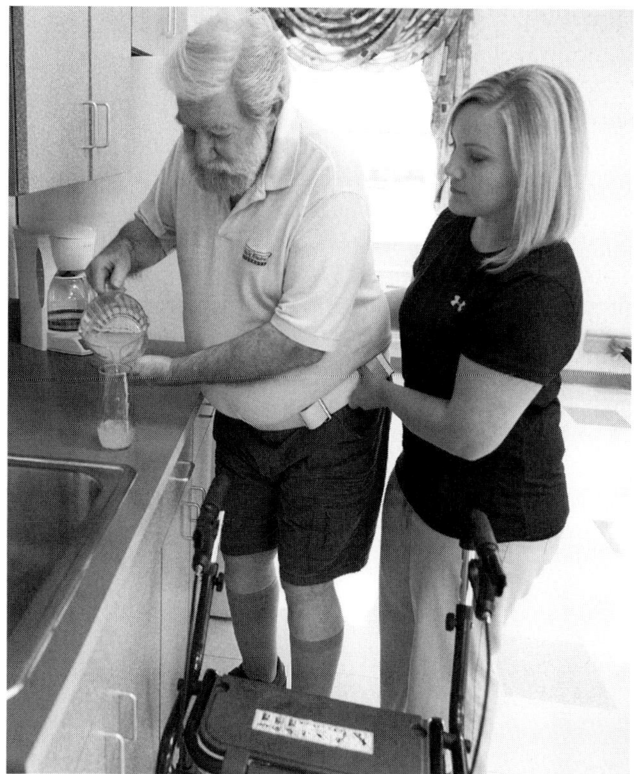

FIGURE 26-5. Clients must use adaptive techniques to complete daily occupations while sternal precautions are in place.

task. Clients who have difficulty donning a shirt without exceeding shoulder flexion of 90 degrees or those who have difficulty pulling shirts down in the back without great chest expansion may benefit from a dressing stick or reacher to assist with these components of dressing. Chest expansion is also a risk during other tasks, such as fastening a bra or even during toilet hygiene. One technique to decrease the risk for pulling on the sternum is to encourage clients to tuck the chest in, keep the arms close to the body and to internally rotate the shoulders slightly during tasks that would normally encourage the following movements: pushing the chest out, extending the arms behind the body, and shoulder external rotation (such as fastening a necklace). OTAs should discuss occupations that clients will need to complete at home and problem solve to develop techniques as needed to support clients to maintain compliance with their sternal precautions.

Other occupations, such as leisure tasks, will need to follow the same activity progression discussed previously for self-care occupations. Clients would need to start with activities that have lower MET requirements before engaging in more physical leisure tasks. Some examples of lower-level MET activities include reading, watching television, playing computer or card games while seated, and completing light crafts while sitting down. Clients could then progress to craft activities that require more effort, or completing some of the tasks mentioned previously in a standing position or at a more vigorous pace. As clients improve, they can continue proceeding to more difficult tasks, such as playing Wii Fit® or other video games that require movement. If cleared by their physician, clients may later return to vigorous leisure tasks such as gardening and sports. OTAs can make recommendations regarding safe activities for clients to engage in while recovering, as well as adaptive strategies to support engagement in occupation. For example, leisure supplies can be stored in areas that will allow clients to access these without raising their arms above their head. The OTA may suggest that clients care for smaller Tumbler tomato plants or a few small pots of flowers during the wait to return to caring for an entire flower or vegetable garden. OTAs are skilled at identifying adaptive ways to complete valued occupations, and suggesting alternate activities when it is not possible or safe for a client to engage in an activity in the early cardiac phase. Clients should also be trained to monitor their vital signs and feelings of exertion during all occupations, including leisure. For a full discussion of vital signs and activity monitoring, refer to the Assessment of Vital Signs and Activity Tolerance section of this chapter.

Due to fatigue that is common for clients with cardiac conditions, this population may need to take frequent rest breaks during both occupations and exercise and may initially also need to complete tasks seated. Energy conservation techniques can be useful to compensate for declines in activity tolerance, and clients should be educated on these approaches. For example, clients can use a shower stool for bathing at home and can complete this task at night to decrease energy expenditure for getting ready the next morning. Paper plates and cups can decrease difficulty with cleaning up after meals by reducing the amount of dishes to wash. Adaptive, yet easy to find tools can be purchased for higher-level occupations, such as a lightweight vacuum or a broom with a long-handled dustpan for cleaning. See the Energy Conservation Techniques section of this chapter for more details about these general approaches.

Most clients with heart conditions will need to make healthy dietary changes to reduce the risk for cardiac disease. Changes to diet will necessitate alterations in previous routines for making shopping lists as well as completing grocery shopping, meal preparation, and eating. OTAs should educate clients on healthier meal options and ways to incorporate these lifestyle changes. Clients can be asked to create a healthy shopping list with guidance from the OTA while they are in the hospital to prepare for life after discharge. Clients should also be advised to check nutritional guidelines at restaurants and on food labels at the grocery store to make better food choices. OTAs can also educate clients on useful resources, such as websites that provide heart-healthy recipes. If the facility has a kitchen area, clients can be engaged in meal preparation tasks in the inpatient setting or after discharge in their home environment. Referral to a dietitian would be appropriate for detailed review of sample meal plans and appropriate portion sizes for eating.

Clients may also have questions regarding sexual activity after a cardiac event or surgery, but may be embarrassed to discuss these with healthcare providers. Members of the healthcare team should be sensitive and assure clients that questions about sexual activity are common concerns for those with cardiovascular conditions. Some of the most common problems encountered by this population include avoiding sexual activity due to anxiety or fear, having decreased libido, and experiencing impotence.[35] Clients who are medically appropriate to resume sexual activity should be encouraged to return to this occupation. Those who have not been cleared to engage in intercourse can still be encouraged to be intimate with their partner in other ways, such as holding hands, hugging, and kissing. Clients should be supported to discuss their concerns openly with both their healthcare team as well as their partner. A scientific statement on sexual activity from the American Heart Association recommends that sexual activity be discontinued after open heart surgery until 6 to 8 weeks after surgery, and clients after MI are advised to wait until they can tolerate activities with MET levels of 3 to 5 without symptoms before resuming this occupation.[48] If clients are experiencing difficulty with sexual activity after medical clearance, OTAs can offer suggestions for activity modifications and also make referrals to appropriate members of the healthcare team. For example, an OTA can suggest less strenuous positions for the client with the cardiac condition and recommend resting before sex or engaging in this occupation at a time of day when the client typically has more energy.

STRENGTH AND ENDURANCE TRAINING

Clients across all phases of cardiac rehabilitation can benefit from strength and endurance training within safe parameters. In the acute phase of cardiac rehabilitation, clients should exercise within lower MET levels of 2 to 4 to allow for proper healing and safe progression of exercise tolerance. Clients who have undergone a sternotomy will be required to follow sternal precautions during exercise and will be limited to gentle active ROM exercises within these precautions, stopping if the client feels any sternal clicking. In the outpatient phase of cardiac rehabilitation, clients will further increase to higher MET levels during activities. Strength training may also begin in the outpatient phase depending on the client's condition. For example, a client with a NSTEMI could begin with light weights such as 5 pounds in the outpatient setting.[7] However, clients who have undergone a sternotomy should not engage in resistive UE exercises until at least 5 weeks after surgery.[20] After a PCI, clients are safe to begin resistance training 2 to 3 weeks after the procedure if they have already completed 2 weeks of supervised endurance training.[49] The American College of Sports Medicine provides specific exercise guidelines for various cardiac conditions in the ninth edition of *ACMS's Guidelines for Exercise Testing and Prescription,* and this textbook is a useful resource for OTAs who treat clients with cardiac issues.

Gentle aerobic exercise can be initiated during phase I for cardiac clients, such as functional mobility to and from the bathroom with assistance or mild chair aerobics for short time frames. For example, beginning with 2 minutes of gentle exercise followed by 1 minute of rest and completing 2 to 3 intervals of this training would be appropriate in the early acute phase with progression to 8 to 10 minutes of total exercise.[7] This program could include hand and wrist ROM exercises, biceps curls, shoulder flexion to 90 degrees, or combinations of other gentle activities without resistance. Initially, these exercises may be completed in bed or sitting supported in a chair. As the client's cardiac condition improves and activity tolerance increases, they can complete exercises sitting on the edge of a bed and may eventually be able to do so while standing with appropriate assistance for balance and safety.

Clients' vital signs should be monitored before, during, and after exercise to maintain safety with activity. Any abnormal responses to exercise should be relayed to nursing staff as well as the physician and may indicate a need to end the session. Clients who exhibit signs and symptoms of exercise intolerance such as chest pain, nausea/vomiting, SOB, and diaphoresis (excessive sweating) should stop activity, and nursing staff should be notified. See the Signs and Symptoms of Exercise and Activity Intolerance section of this chapter for a complete discussion. Poor responses to exercise can also include abnormal changes in blood pressure or significant alterations in heart rate. Systolic blood pressure should not increase by more than 40 mmHg with exercise, and a drop in systolic blood pressure of more than 10 mmHg is also considered to be an abnormal response to exercise.[20] Heart rate should not increase by more than 30 beats per minute with exercise to support safe progression of activity levels.

STRESS MANAGEMENT AND COPING TECHNIQUES

Clients may experience stress as a result of their condition or as a contributing factor for heart disease. Clients should be educated on stress management techniques to decrease anxiety/depression and reduce the risk for future cardiac events. Multiple techniques can be utilized, such as visual imagery, exercise within safe parameters, deep breathing, utilizing social support, and gentle progressive muscle relaxation (PMR). Listening to relaxing music may provide relaxation by itself, or can be a useful support for other relaxation techniques. During visualization, clients imagine being in a peaceful, relaxing environment while they have their eyes closed to remove themselves cognitively from a stressful situation. This visualization can initially be guided verbally by the OTA by describing a peaceful setting to the client. Once clients become independent with this technique, they would be able to imagine the relaxing environment without assistance from the OTA. PMR for clients with cardiac conditions involves gently tightening and releasing the muscles throughout the body to achieve a state of relaxation. Clients begin with tightening the muscles of the forehead, and slowly work their way through their muscle groups all the way down to their feet. Clients with cardiac conditions must be cautious to avoid severe tightening of the muscles and holding their breath during PMR as this can increase abdominal pressure and pressure within the chest cavity. Another relaxation technique that can be used for stress reduction is mindfulness meditation. This approach involves sitting quietly and focusing on one's thoughts, breathing, emotions, and sensory experiences without passing judgment. For example, someone using mindfulness meditation would acknowledge thoughts and emotions as they pass, but would not allow these to pull their focus away from a relaxed state. A physical or imaginary focal point, such as an object or an imagined peaceful environment, can be used to promote relaxation. In addition, clients with anxiety and/or depression should be referred to their physician for pharmacological intervention and other services outside the scope of OT that may be needed to address these needs.

LIFESTYLE MODIFICATION EDUCATION

Education is an important part of OT intervention for clients with heart conditions. For those who have undergone CABG, PCI, and other surgical approaches, it is important to provide education on continued cardiac risk factors and ways to reduce these so that clients do not view their procedure as a permanent "cure" for their cardiac condition.[20] If lifestyle changes are not implemented, clients can require further medical intervention in the future as symptoms return. Topics for lifestyle modification education include: weight reduction, healthy eating, lowering high blood pressure, adhering to appropriate physical activity levels, adhering to prescribed medication, managing comorbidities such as diabetes, smoking cessation, addressing psychosocial health, and managing stress. Postsurgical precautions that were discussed earlier in this chapter, such as sternal limitations following CABG, will also require education and training from OT to implement these precautions into daily occupations. All of these educational areas will necessitate that clients adapt their current occupational routines to incorporate needed changes to maintain a healthier lifestyle. See Chapter 25 for further information.

ADDRESSING EDEMA

Clients with CHF can experience significant swelling and edema, especially in the LEs and abdomen. Swelling should be monitored to avoid affecting circulation with clothing that is too tight; clients may need larger clothing items or may need to have openings on articles of clothing widened to protect the skin and increase comfort (such as widening elastic bands on socks). Loose clothing that can be pulled on rather than fastened with zippers and buttons can make it easier for clients to dress themselves and may decrease the risk for creating areas of pressure on the skin when edema is present. Clients who have abdominal swelling may need to use alternative techniques for LB dressing, such as propping the LEs on a stool to don socks or using a reacher to put on pants, in order to increase independence and comfort with ADLs.

ADDRESSING SHORTNESS OF BREATH

Feelings of breathlessness are common for clients with CHF due to additional fluid around the lungs. Other cardiac conditions can result in SOB and additional oxygen needs. For example, some clients may need oxygen therapy after MI during hospitalization. Oxygen therapy has been a standard of care for most clients after heart attack, but newer evidence is showing that this may be harmful for those who do not have low oxygen saturation and is best indicated only for those clients with hypoxemia.[50] OT practitioners should follow physician orders for use of oxygen both at rest and during activity for cardiac clients. Clients with cardiac conditions, especially CHF, may need to sit and sleep with the head of the bed elevated to reduce feelings of breathlessness. Some clients may have a habit of sleeping on multiple pillows to increase ease with breathing, and a foam wedge may also be effective. In particular, clients with CHF should be encouraged to complete ADLs sitting up rather than lying down and should not be returned to supine immediately after exercise or other strenuous activity. Lying down after exertion can increase preload (ventricular blood volume), and clients should be positioned sitting up to decrease pulmonary congestion, which negatively affects ventilation.[19]

PULMONARY CONDITIONS

The respiratory system includes the lungs and other organs that bring in oxygen for the body and also remove carbon dioxide. Air is inhaled through the nose or mouth and then transported from the throat (pharynx) through the trachea to the two bronchial (bronchus) tubes, which are connected to each lung. The bronchial tubes divide to enter each lobe of the lungs and then subdivide further into smaller bronchi. The right lung consists of three lobes (superior, middle, and inferior), while the left lung only has two lobes (superior and inferior) to accommodate the position of the heart in the chest cavity. The bronchioles are the smallest parts of the bronchial tubes and connect to alveoli, or air sacs. The alveoli contain capillaries that allow blood to pass through. Red blood cells take oxygen from the lungs and transport it throughout the body wherever it is needed for the body to function properly. These same red blood cells also transport carbon dioxide back to the lungs so that it can be removed from the body during expiration. The diaphragm is the most important muscle for breathing and is located near the bottom of the chest cavity. When we breathe, the diaphragm moves downward to create suction within the chest, pulling in air to expand the lungs. See Figure 26-6 for a depiction of the respiratory system.

Chronic Obstructive Pulmonary Disease

COPD is a lung disease that involves thickening of the airways and damage to the alveolar wall in the lungs, making it challenging for individuals to breathe.[51] COPD is a permanent

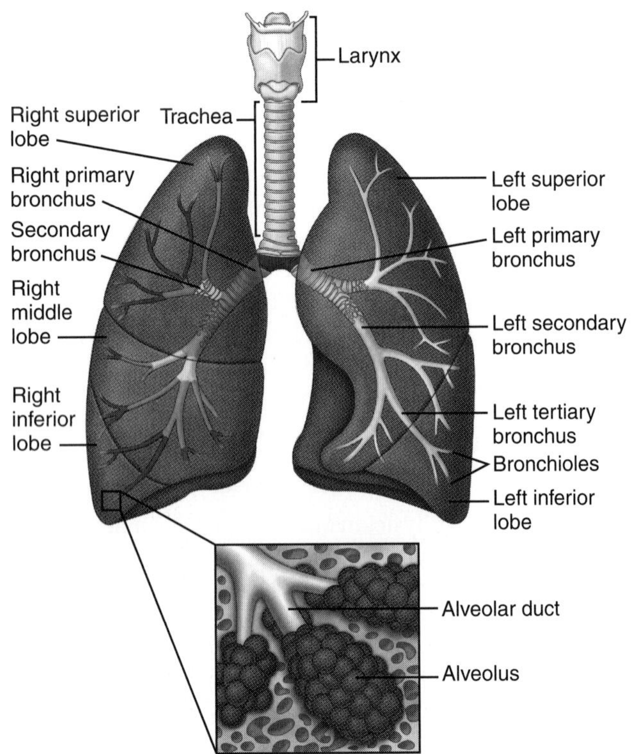

FIGURE 26-6. The general anatomy of the respiratory system.

and progressive condition that includes chronic bronchitis, peripheral airway disease, and emphysema. Clients who have chronic bronchitis have inflammation in the bronchi that results in increased mucus secretion. Increased mucus makes breathing more difficult, and the client is not able to inhale enough oxygen to meet the body's needs. Clients who have chronic bronchitis as their main underlying cause of COPD are sometimes referred to as "blue bloaters" because their low oxygen levels and high CO_2 levels cause the skin to turn blue, or cyanotic, and they experience bloating as a result of increasing lung obstruction. Emphysema differs from bronchitis in that the alveoli are affected rather than the bronchial tubes. The alveoli are destroyed, which interferes with the body's ability to exchange oxygen and carbon dioxide, resulting in extreme SOB. Clients with emphysema are sometimes referred to as "pink puffers" because they hyperventilate (breathe quickly) in an attempt to compensate for poor oxygenation of the blood, and they usually have a pink or even flushed complexion as they typically do not experience cyanosis.

Because COPD is a chronic rather than acute condition, the diagnosis is typically found in the medical history portion of a client's medical record and may or may not be listed as the primary diagnosis. COPD is the third leading cause of death in the United States and results in disability and long-term challenges to daily living.[52] General common symptoms of COPD include chronic cough, dyspnea (shortness of breath), fatigue, wheezing, cyanosis (blueness of the lips or fingernail beds), frequent respiratory infections, and/or increased mucus production. Initially, symptoms of mild COPD may be difficult to recognize in individuals as airflow limitation is minimal and SOB only occurs with physical exertion. As the disease progresses, recurrent respiratory infections may occur, resulting in increased coughing and mucus production that causes SOB with moderate activity levels. Severe COPD is characterized by SOB at rest with ongoing and potentially severe respiratory-related complications.[53]

RISK FACTORS

Risk factors associated with COPD include smoking; air pollution; inhalation of irritating fumes, chemicals, and dust; passive exposure to cigarette smoking; and genetics. It is estimated that 80% to 90% of COPD diagnoses are caused by cigarette smoking.[52] In nonsmokers, occupational exposures are the leading predictive factor in COPD diagnosis. Workplace environments including coal mines and the cotton textile industry are examples of occupations with high-risk exposure to irritants, chemicals, and/or dust. COPD is preventable through smoking cessation, avoidance of secondhand smoke, protection from irritating fumes or chemicals, and promoting clean air initiatives. COPD has historically been more prevalent among men than women in the past, but now both genders are almost equally affected by the condition due to increased exposure to chemicals and dust as well as higher rates of smoking among women.

THE OLDER ADULT

Older adults are disproportionately affected by both cardiac and lung conditions. Advanced age is a risk factor for numerous cardiac-related diagnoses such as myocardial infarction, congestive heart failure, and hypertension. Older adults are also more likely to develop lung conditions associated with smoking, such as COPD, due to higher rates of smoking among this age group in their younger years. Whereas current smoking rates among those 65 years of age and older is low at 8.5%,[54] this generation of males had the highest rates of smoking in U.S. history during the 1960s at 54%, with an additional 21% of males also being prior smokers during this same time frame.[55] Not surprisingly, adults older than 65 years of age have the highest incidence of COPD. In earlier years, less was known about the harmful effects of smoking. More recently, smoking has been linked to lung disorders, heart conditions, cancer, and other diagnoses. Increased awareness of these harmful effects combined with other factors has led to lower rates of smoking currently among middle-age and young adult populations compared with older generations during these same stages in life.

Often older adults feel that the benefits of quitting smoking are limited. However, this population can achieve some of the same great outcomes experienced by younger populations through smoking cessation, even if they have been smoking for many years. Smoking cessation for older adults has been linked to increased life expectancy, improved quality of life, and increased ease of breathing.[55] Risks for various health conditions, such as CVA, heart disease, lung disease, and cancer, have been found to decrease significantly when older adults quit smoking.[55] OTAs should educate older adults on the cardiac and pulmonary risks of continued smoking, as well as the great benefits of quitting to dispel the myth that older clients cannot benefit from smoking cessation.

MEDICAL MANAGEMENT OF CHRONIC OBSTRUCTIVE PULMONARY DISEASE

COPD is a chronic and progressive disease. Medical management of COPD does not cure the disease, but it can reduce or alleviate symptoms to allow for greater quality of life. Common medications involved in treatment of COPD include:

1. *Bronchodilators* (e.g., anticholinergics, beta agonists) are medications that help to relax the bronchi and bronchioles around the airways making it easier to breathe. Most bronchodilators are taken using an inhaler or nebulizer that delivers medications directly to the lungs offering quick relief of symptoms to individuals experiencing difficulty breathing.
2. *Anti-inflammatories* (e.g., steroids, corticosteroids) are mostly inhaled medications that help clear mucus away from the lungs and open airways.

3. *Antibiotics* are used to treat bacterial and viral lung infections, which can be common in individuals with COPD.

Supplemental oxygen may be prescribed for individuals at risk for hypoxia (inadequate oxygen supply to the body) to allow for continued participation in ADLs, functional mobility, and therapeutic exercise. If handled properly, oxygen tanks, cylinders, and concentrators are safe. However, improper management of oxygen can present a severe safety hazard. See Box 26-1 for tips for safe handling of oxygen.

IMPACT ON OCCUPATIONAL PERFORMANCE

COPD has a significant influence on all areas of function. SOB is one of the most common, and possibly the most distressing, symptoms that clients with COPD experience. Over time, clients may develop postural abnormalities due to hyperinflation of the lungs, which alters the position of the ribs and scapulae, or from chronic use of a forward-leaning position to decrease feelings of SOB. Clients diagnosed with COPD also have declines in strength and activity tolerance. Muscle atrophy (wasting) occurs from disuse as clients begin limiting their activity levels due to fatigue and SOB. Avoiding activity leads to further declines in endurance over time. Postural control (the ability to maintain balance during activity) has been found to be worse for clients with COPD than for those without this condition, unrelated to strength or endurance deficits found among this population.[56]

Clients with COPD are commonly underweight due to reduced appetite from fatigue and SOB. A client with COPD may also burn more calories during breathing than a client without this condition, as this process requires increased effort for those with a COPD diagnosis. Cognitive changes can occur with COPD as a result of resting hypoxemia in later stages of the disease.[57] This can result in decreased safety during occupations, memory deficits, poor reasoning skills, and other cognitive declines. Clients can experience reduced independence and participation in all occupations such as ADLs, IADLs, rest and sleep, work, leisure, and social participation as a result of the functional deficits mentioned previously.

BOX 26-1
Tips for Safe Oxygen Handling

Oxygen Safety Tips (American Lung Association)

Avoid open flames in the presence of oxygen use (e.g., matches, cigarette lighters, candles, and burning tobacco). Oxygen is nonflammable, but it does support combustion.
Maintain 5-foot distance between oxygen and heat sources (electric or gas heaters).
Store cylinders safely. Cylinders should be upright and secure, in an approved cart or device for storage.
Turn off oxygen supply valves when oxygen is not in use.
When using oxygen, avoid using lotions or creams containing petroleum. The combustion of flammable products containing petroleum can also be supported by the presence of oxygen. Use water-based products instead.
Always follow the instructions of the oxygen supply company regarding safe usage.
Be aware of oxygen tubing as it presents a fall hazard.

PSYCHOSOCIAL IMPACT OF PULMONARY DISEASE

Psychosocial symptoms, such as anxiety and depression, are common among clients with COPD. This may be due to the debilitating symptoms caused by the disease as well as the inability to fully participate in valued occupations. Clients can become very anxious due to feelings of SOB that often accompany exertion, although breathlessness and anxiety can also occur at rest. Depression can result in decreased motivation and engagement in life activities. Clients may have fears about death related to their condition, and they may also be angry about their diagnosis and declining health status. For some clients, body image can be altered due to the need to wear a nasal cannula for delivery of supplemental oxygen.

Other Pulmonary Conditions

Idiopathic pulmonary fibrosis (IPF) is a progressive lung condition of unknown cause where the lungs become fibrotic, scarred, and stiff over time. This hardening of the lungs prevents them from contracting and expanding effectively for breathing. IPF is a restrictive lung disease that is characterized by fatigue, chronic dry cough, worsening dyspnea, and decreased activity tolerance. Incidence of IPF is estimated to be 6.8 to 8.8 cases per 100,000 people in the United States.[58] While IPF is less common than other cardiopulmonary diagnoses, such as MI or COPD, it is a severely debilitating and fatal condition. IPF has a poor prognosis with a short life expectancy of only 3 to 5 years after the condition is diagnosed.[19] Clients with IPF, especially in later stages of the disease, can have significant declines in oxygen saturation levels, even when they are provided with high-flow oxygen due to decreased flexibility of the lung tissues for proper breathing.[40] Clients with this condition will need guidance in energy conservation techniques and appropriate breathing to combat significant fatigue and dyspnea. OTAs should monitor clients with IPF closely for oxygen desaturation and fatigue; these clients may need frequent rest breaks during intervention sessions. Clients may also need access to water or throat lozenges, if safe and appropriate, to decrease coughing that often accompanies exertion for this population.

Cystic fibrosis (CF) is a genetic condition characterized by increased production of very thick mucus that blocks airways needed for breathing. This buildup of thick, sticky mucus creates an environment that supports the growth of bacteria; clients with this condition suffer from frequent lung infections and resulting hospitalizations. Clients with CF are living longer, although the average life expectancy for this condition is still only 40 years of age.[59] CF affects areas outside of the lungs as well, such as pancreatic functioning and appropriate digestion of food and absorption of nutrients. As a result, clients can become malnourished. Other symptoms include coughing, wheezing, SOB, fatigue, and decreased activity tolerance. Some practitioners see CF as a pediatric illness because the condition is diagnosed in childhood, however, more than one-half of all persons with CF are older than 18 years of age according to the Cystic Fibrosis Foundation.[60] According to a 2013 report, this condition affects approximately 30,000 children and adults in the United States and 70,000 persons worldwide.[60] Due to frequent hospitalizations clients with CF may experience as a result of recurring infection, OTAs are likely to encounter adults with this condition in the acute care setting. Clients with CF will need training in energy conservation, breathing techniques, and adaptive approaches to continue involvement in valued life activities. Good nutrition should be encouraged as a part of daily routines as well as adhering to appropriate hand-hygiene practices. Recent guidelines for infection prevention and control for those with CF recommend that healthcare providers enact contact precautions (wearing a gown and gloves) when caring for clients with CF to protect clients from potential infection.[61] These guidelines also advise that clients with CF should not be within 6 feet of other clients with the condition because of the risk for cross-infection. Due to health concerns, providing group therapy sessions for clients with CF would be contraindicated.

A variety of neuromuscular and chest wall disorders can also lead to impairments with breathing. These conditions can cause rapid and shallow breathing as well as weakness of the respiratory muscles; the position of the respiratory muscles in these conditions can even create a mechanical disadvantage for breathing.[40] Weakness of muscles used for breathing can also decrease the ability to cough to clear secretions from the lungs, negatively affecting respiration. Examples of neuromuscular disorders include conditions such as muscular dystrophy, multiple sclerosis, amyotrophic lateral sclerosis, and myasthenia gravis. All of these conditions can result in severe weakness of the respiratory muscles as well as other muscles throughout the body. These clients may have difficulty lying flat, usually have dyspnea, and may require mechanical ventilation. Kyphoscoliosis is an example of a chest wall disorder that causes both an exaggerated outward curvature of the thoracic spine (kyphosis) as well as lateral spinal curvatures (scoliosis). This condition alters the position of the chest wall and rib cage, restricting the ability of the lungs to fully expand for breathing.[62] Clients with neuromuscular and chest wall conditions will need training in energy conservation techniques as well as appropriate coughing strategies to assist with clearing secretions. Clients with these disorders will not be able to tolerate longer episodes of activity and will require frequent rest breaks; excess muscle fatigue should be avoided with these populations. Clients often need respiratory support through devices such as continuous positive airway pressure (CPAP) or bilevel positive airway pressure (BiPAP) to maintain oxygenation. CPAP delivers a single constant pressure that clients both inhale and exhale out against, while BiPAP delivers pressure for both inhaling and exhaling. Both devices help to keep airways open for breathing. Some clients will need these devices during waking hours, and others may only need them at night. OTAs should check orders in the medical record to determine when these devices are needed. Clients with these conditions also may not be able to tolerate lying flat and may need to have the head of the bed elevated during activities and/or at rest to support breathing and reduce SOB.

Pulmonary Rehabilitation

According to the American Thoracic Society and the European Respiratory Society, "pulmonary rehabilitation is a comprehensive intervention based on a thorough client assessment followed by client tailored therapies that include, but are not limited to, exercise training, education, and behavior change, designed to improve the physical and psychological condition of people with chronic respiratory disease and to promote the long-term adherence to health-enhancing behaviors".[63] AACVPR has established guidelines for best practice in pulmonary rehabilitation that can be used to support effective rehabilitation programs for clients with multiple pulmonary conditions. The current guidelines from AACVPR at the time this chapter was written are published in the fourth edition of the *Guidelines for Pulmonary Rehabilitation Programs.* The pulmonary rehabilitation team is interprofessional and should include physicians, respiratory therapists, occupational and physical therapists, dietitians, psychologists, and other healthcare providers as needed. The general goals of pulmonary rehabilitation are to:

- Increase independence with ADLs, functional mobility, and other valued occupations.
- Reduce anxiety and improve coping skills to manage SOB.
- Improve strength, activity tolerance, balance, and use of appropriate breathing patterns to support maximal function.
- Enhance overall quality of life and occupational engagement.
- Decrease the symptoms of pulmonary disease through interprofessional collaboration.
- Educate clients and their caregivers to support carry-over of therapy recommendations to maintain functional gains made through pulmonary rehabilitation over time.[64]

PHASES OF PULMONARY REHABILITATION

Pulmonary rehabilitation follows the continuum of care from the acute hospital and/or inpatient rehabilitation to outpatient settings, followed by community-based care. During the acute and inpatient phase, intervention is focused on increasing independence with ADLs and functional mobility, training in appropriate breathing techniques, addressing psychosocial needs, and preparing for discharge. Outpatient pulmonary rehabilitation involves supervised exercise, education, and increasing independence with ADLs as well as higher-level occupations through training in energy conservation, appropriate breathing patterns, and adaptive techniques. The outpatient stage typically lasts between 8 and 12 weeks. Pulmonary function tests are often used to assess lung functioning and are sometimes used to determine whether or not a client qualifies for outpatient pulmonary rehabilitation. See Table 26-5 for a description of common pulmonary function tests. The community-based portion of pulmonary rehabilitation is a maintenance phase of rehabilitation. Similar to cardiac rehabilitation, clients may complete a formal maintenance program of lower-level supervision with exercise, or they may continue maintenance activities on their own either at home or through a local gym or YMCA. Singing has been found to be an enjoyable and useful treatment, as it requires breath control and can strengthen diaphragm muscles. Refer to the sections that follow for a detailed discussion of intervention techniques for clients with pulmonary conditions.

ADDRESSING ACTIVITIES OF DAILY LIVING AND OTHER OCCUPATIONS

Clients with pulmonary disease can experience extreme fatigue and dyspnea during occupational tasks that limit their performance. Other outcomes of lung disease, such as decreased strength and balance, also reduce independence with valued activities. In addition, cognitive deficits from hypoxemia can interfere with ADL performance as well. Clients may need training to use compensatory strategies, such as checklists, to compensate for memory deficits. Clients should be educated on the importance of using their prescribed oxygen during ADLs and other occupations to maintain oxygen saturation greater than or equal to 90%. Some clients are afraid to wear their oxygen tubing during bathing tasks, however, this is safe to do and will limit oxygen desaturation with exertion. For those clients who do not currently wear oxygen, saturation levels below 90% both at rest or during activity should be reported to the physician as oxygen prescription may be indicated. During exertion, some clients have a habit of holding their breath. This requires training to develop appropriate and safe breathing patterns with activity.

TABLE 26-5 Common Pulmonary Function Tests

PULMONARY FUNCTION TEST	WHAT IT MEASURES
Forced vital capacity (FVC)	Amount of air forcefully exhaled after a maximum inhalation
Forced expiratory volume in the first second (FEV_1)	Amount of air forcefully expelled in the first second of exhalation after a maximal inhalation
Diffusing capacity for carbon monoxide (DLco)	Ability of the lungs to diffuse carbon monoxide, calculated by the difference in the amount of carbon monoxide that was inhaled compared with what was exhaled

Clients should be encouraged to sit when possible during occupations to limit fatigue and conserve energy for other activities. While leaning forward slightly can decrease SOB, extreme forward leaning to complete tasks such as putting on shoes actually decreases the ability of the diaphragm to work effectively for breathing. Clients should be encouraged to sit for LE dressing and cross one foot over the opposite knee or to prop their foot on a stool to prevent extreme forward flexion during bathing and dressing tasks. Adaptive equipment such as a sock aid, long–handled sponge, or long shoehorn should be introduced as appropriate to increase occupational independence and to reduce fatigue. For example, a reacher can be used to assist with putting on pants but can also be used to pick items up off the floor. Encourage clients to wear comfortable, loose clothing because tight clothes can increase difficulty with breathing. Because shower steam can cause coughing and/or SOB, lowering the temperature of the water and using a ventilation fan before, during, and after showering is a good approach to limit the amount of steam that develops in the bathroom. A terry cloth robe can be used to passively soak up water from bathing and requires less energy than using a towel to dry off. An electric razor can be used for both men and women to make shaving easier, and allowing hair to air dry rather than using a hair dryer also reduces fatigue with grooming. See Figure 26-7 for a depiction of a client using energy conservation techniques to complete grooming tasks.

Energy conservation techniques and adaptive methods can also be used to increase engagement in valued leisure occupations. Clients should be advised to wear their oxygen as prescribed when engaging in leisure tasks to reduce SOB and prevent desaturation. Activities may need to be planned for times of the day when clients feel their best, with more active leisure tasks scheduled after taking any prescribed inhalers or nebulizer treatments. Because the weather can impact breathing, clients will need to attend to the temperature outside and adjust their schedules to avoid extreme heat or very cool temperatures. Adaptive methods can also be used to alter the activity demands of a leisure task to increase performance. Tasks can be completed seated or with fewer activity demands. For example, a client who loves to play golf and is still able to partake in this activity could use a golf cart to maneuver from one hole to the next, as well as remain seated except for when it is his or her turn to golf. As a client's illness progresses or on days when the client is not feeling as strong, he or she could play on a 9-hole golf course, switch to putt-putt golf, or even transition to Wii® golf if needed. A client who enjoys bowling can switch to a lighter bowling ball, utilize pursed-lip breathing techniques while bowling, and rest by sitting down between turns. Leisure occupations help to support quality of life, and should be addressed by OTAs

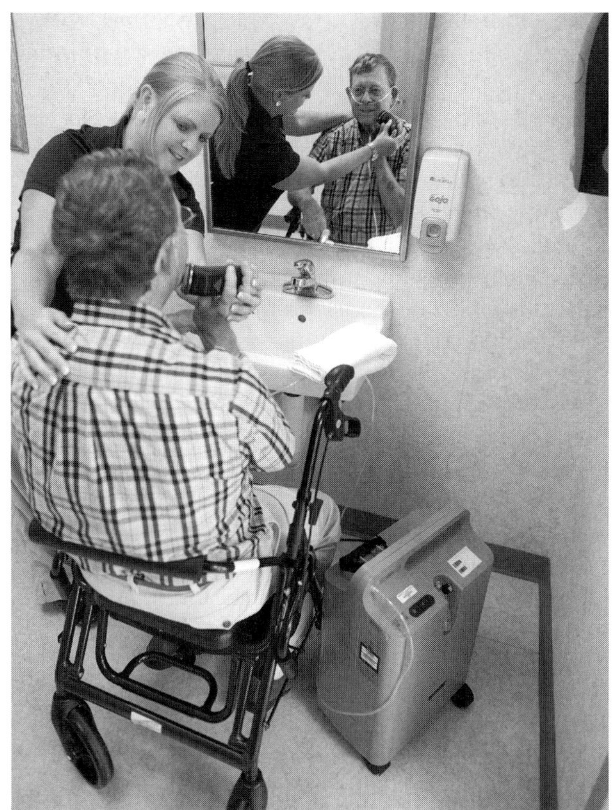

FIGURE 26-7. Implementing energy conservation strategies can reduce fatigue and increase independence for clients with both pulmonary and cardiac disease.

using the same techniques available for self-care and other valued occupations.

Clients may need to eat smaller meals more frequently throughout the day to avoid fatigue with eating and to support proper nutrition. Chewing slowly with the mouth closed helps prevent swallowing air during eating. Clients with COPD should also be trained to use appropriate breathing and swallowing patterns to reduce the risk for aspiration. Clients should be instructed to breathe in, exhale partially, swallow food, and finish exhaling before breathing in again to avoid pulling food particles into the lungs. While some clients prefer to eat without their oxygen, clients should be advised to wear their prescribed oxygen during all meals to maintain oxygenation and to reduce SOB. Some clients with advanced COPD may become so fatigued with meals that they may need to have an altered diet, such as softer foods that require less energy to chew and swallow or eating several smaller meals throughout the day rather than three larger ones. The need for dietary adjustment should be assessed by an occupational therapist and/or speech language pathologist to make appropriate recommendations.

Adaptive techniques and approaches to conserve energy are available for higher-level occupations as well. Adaptive equipment, such as a lightweight vacuum or long-handled duster, can be used to reduce fatigue with cleaning tasks. Presorting laundry and using a reacher to load/unload a washing machine and dryer can increase independence for washing clothing. Difficult cleaning or yard work activities may need to be delegated to other family members, and clients may also consider hiring someone to assist with these more strenuous tasks. Ergonomic and lightweight tools can also make outdoor tasks easier. Clients who do plan to complete yard work tasks should do so in the early morning or evening to avoid hot temperatures in warmer months and should also plan to avoid outdoor work when pollen, mold, or pollution counts are high (these can be monitored by watching local news channels).

Sexual activity can be affected significantly by chronic lung disease, and this is an area that should be addressed by OTAs. Clients and their partners may have fears about the lung condition, or the client may have difficulty engaging in this occupation due to fatigue, SOB, and other symptoms. OTAs can make recommendations to reduce the energy required for sexual activities and decrease SOB, as well as suggesting preparatory methods for preparing to engage in this occupation. Clients who have prescribed inhalers or nebulizers would benefit by using these before sex to increase ease with breathing as well as wearing prescribed oxygen during sexual activity. Using controlled coughing techniques to clear sputum for those who have increased secretions would also help support better breathing. Positions that may support breathing and reduce fatigue for clients with lung disease could include lying supine with the upper body elevated on pillows, side lying, or seated positions.[65] Clients should be advised to avoid positions that would increase difficulty with breathing, such as lying completely flat or being positioned in a way that requires significant energy to maintain.[65] Engaging in sexual activity at a time of day when the client feels best would also support participation in this occupation. Clients and their partners should be encouraged to communicate openly about their concerns, and referrals should be made to appropriate members of the healthcare team as needed to address areas that are beyond the scope of OT.

STRENGTH AND ENDURANCE TRAINING

Strength and endurance should be addressed because weakness is common for clients with pulmonary conditions. The causes of weakness for this population are multifactorial and can result from hypoxemia, decreased activity levels, chronic steroid use to reduce respiratory inflammation, and overall systemic inflammation.[40] Inflammatory markers from systemic inflammation are thought to be factors that lead to muscle dysfunction and reduced exercise tolerance.[66] Clients with pulmonary conditions often use accessory muscles from the upper shoulder to assist with breathing, which can make it difficult for them to complete activities with the UEs if they are not supported for sitting. Accessory breathing muscles include muscles in the neck and shoulders for inhaling and the muscles of the abdomen and chest when one is forcefully exhaling. If these muscles are activated during breathing, clients will fatigue easier and may have trouble maintaining balance without support.

During acute pulmonary exacerbations, OTAs should engage clients in light UE strengthening exercises and mild aerobic activities to improve endurance. As always, safety is a priority and clients may need to complete both activities in sitting to prevent falls. When clients improve, the frequency, duration, and intensity of exercise can slowly be increased over time. Clients should engage in progressive resistive strengthening exercises with the use of free weights or exercise bands. Other equipment can be utilized as well, such as a UE ergometer commonly known as an arm bike. In addition, clients with pulmonary disease often have LE weakness. Engaging clients in LE strengthening can improve standing tolerance and safety during functional mobility. If clients are not receiving physical therapy services or if deficits relate to functional tasks, it would be appropriate for OT practitioners to include LE strengthening exercises in addition to addressing UE strength. UE and LE exercise for strength training could progress from using light resistance bands for 1 to 2 sets of 10 to 12 repetitions of each exercise, to completing multiple sets of increased repetitions with greater resistance as the client improves. Aerobic exercise could include an UE ergometer and functional mobility for increasing lengths of time with fewer rest breaks. Other tasks, such as Wii® games or various seated therapeutic activities, could be used for aerobic exercise with progression to standing, longer duration of participation in the activity, and fewer rest breaks. Try to incorporate exercise into the client's desired occupations, instead of simply performing straight exercise routines, if possible.

BREATHING TECHNIQUES

In coordination with use of energy conservation, breathing retraining can be used as a strategy for clients with lung disease to reduce SOB, facilitate relaxation, decrease anxiety, promote controlled breathing, and assist with performance of everyday functional tasks. OT practitioners teach clients individualized breathing techniques to support ongoing participation in valued occupations. Performance of breathing techniques requires a sense of self-awareness by clients of their body's response to activity. When clients are able to observe and recognize changes in breathing function, they can develop control over how and when to initiate breathing techniques during functional activity to reduce the impact of dyspnea.

Before strenuous activity, clients may benefit from using their prescription inhaler or receiving a nebulizer (breathing) treatment. This can be especially beneficial in the hospital setting before OT sessions to increase ease with breathing. Clients should also be advised to continue this approach at home to maximize breathing during difficult tasks, such as using their inhaler before showering or exercising. Timing breathing treatments and inhalers before difficult tasks can help reduce SOB and associated anxiety with exertion. Healthcare staff members who treat clients with pulmonary conditions should avoid wearing scented lotions and perfumes as these can cause coughing and difficulty breathing for pulmonary clients. Clients themselves and their visitors should also be asked to avoid these strongly scented products to reduce lung irritation. Keeping areas cooler with fans or air conditions can also increase ease with breathing. Some clients also find that a slight forward-leaning position, such as the position clients use when completing functional mobility with a walker, can reduce SOB through improved use of the diaphragm. This position could be mimicked at the edge of the bed or up in a chair using a bedside table to rest the UEs to achieve slight forward flexion. As discussed previously in this chapter in relation to participation in outdoor occupations, clients should avoid completing tasks outside during high temperatures and must also be mindful of pollen, mold, and pollution counts (monitored by watching local news channels) to increase ease with breathing.

Pursed-lip breathing (PLB) and **active expiration** are two different breathing strategies often recommended by OT practitioners for individuals with pulmonary conditions. PLB is used to control and maintain a client's breathing pattern when experiencing SOB. PLB encourages individuals to slow their breathing, improves respiratory muscle recruitment, reduces respiratory rate, and increases oxygenation.[67] Active expiration is a breathing technique that is advocated by the AACVPR as another approach to relieve SOB and improve the effectiveness of the lungs for breathing.[40] To use active expiration, clients contract the abdominal muscles while they exhale. Diaphragmatic breathing is a strategy used to promote increased use of the diaphragm muscle and reduce overuse of the accessory muscles for breathing. According to the AACVPR, strong evidence support is lacking for diaphragmatic breathing, and they recommend the use of active expiration in lieu of diaphragmatic breathing.[40] However, some sources do continue to support diaphragmatic breathing as an approach to reduce dyspnea and increase self-awareness of one's own breathing patterns.[19,5] See Box 26-2 for a step-by-step description of all three breathing techniques. OT practitioners often cue clients for performance of breathing-retraining techniques during individual intervention sessions. However, mastery of breathing retraining occurs when clients recognize their own symptoms of dyspnea, initiate breathing techniques to manage SOB, and generalize those same techniques to new and novel situations. Education and demonstration of breathing-training techniques requires consistent reinforcement by OT practitioners for clients to incorporate strategies into habits and routines of daily life. Self-utilization of breathing techniques during participation in meaningful occupations can also signify a sense of control and autonomy over the impact of chronic disease.

COUGHING TECHNIQUES

Clients with a variety of pulmonary conditions can benefit from training in coughing techniques to clear secretions from the lungs. Conditions such as COPD and CF result in excess secretion, while clients with neuromuscular disorders may not be able to clear normal amounts of mucus

BOX 26-2
Breathing Techniques

Pursed-Lip Breathing (PLB)

- Use during activities that make one short of breath. If already experiencing dyspnea, use to regain control of breathing.
- Relax neck and shoulder muscles in supine or seated position.
- Breathe in slowly through the nose as if smelling a flower.
- Purse the lips as if to whistle and slowly exhale through the pursed lips.
- It should take twice as long to exhale as it does to inhale.
- Practice exhaling during the most strenuous part of an activity (e.g., bending/lifting).
- Continue until control of breathing has returned.

Diaphragmatic Breathing

- Lie comfortably in a semireclined or supine position.
- Lean head forward to promote use of the diaphragm and decrease use of upper respiratory muscles.
- Place a hand on the abdomen just below the rib cage.
- Inhale deeply while forcing the hand to rise with the expanding diaphragm.
- Exhale slowly and gently push in with the hand that is on the abdomen.
- Stronger pressure or a weight can be placed on the abdomen to increase strength.
- Stop the exercise if dizzy or lightheaded.

Active Expiration

- Sit, stand or lie comfortably.
- Place a hand on the abdomen just below the rib cage.
- Inhale deeply while the hand rises with the expanding diaphragm.
- Exhale slowly while keeping the abdominal muscles tightly contracted.
- Repeat the steps.
- Stop the exercise if dizzy or lightheaded.

from their lungs due to weakness. A deep cough will remove mucus that is further down into the lungs while a huff cough helps to clear secretions in the upper respiratory tract. For deep coughing, the client should inhale deeply and hold for 1 to 3 seconds, and then use the abdominal muscles to cough hard once or twice to move mucus up the respiratory tract. Coughing more than one to two times can irritate the lungs, so this should be avoided for deep coughing. For a huff cough, clients should take a deep breath and then use the abdominal muscles to cough as they open their mouth to say "huff" several times while coughing.[68] This can be repeated two to three times to clear airways for breathing. The huff cough can be used following a deep cough to remove mucus that has been moved further up the respiratory tract. Coughing techniques are preparatory tasks that should be used in preparation for, but not in lieu of, engaging clients in occupational tasks.

Clients with significant amounts of secretion or difficulty clearing their lungs due to severe weakness may need intervention beyond OT services, such as the use of a pulmonary vest (high-frequency chest wall oscillation) with respiratory therapy to vibrate the chest area and loosen secretions for easier removal with controlled coughing. Percussion and postural drainage are other techniques to clear the lungs. Clients are positioned to promote drainage of mucus from a part of the lungs, and then percussion is performed over this part of the lung to help the mucus move into larger airways to be coughed up and expelled. Following the pulmonary vest or percussion, a cough assist device may be implemented to simulate a natural cough for clients with significant weakness. This can be completed by using a machine that causes rapid inflation of the airway followed by quick deflation. When clients cough up secretions, a suction device may help remove secretions from the mouth, and any changes to the sputum (mucus or phlegm that has been coughed up from the lungs) should be reported to nursing staff. For example, increased sputum production or changes in the color, odor, or thickness of sputum can indicate potential lung infection.

ENERGY CONSERVATION TECHNIQUES

For most individuals with a chronic disease, fatigue, SOB, and anxiety are common elements of everyday life that impact participation in meaningful activities. Engagement in occupations such as showering, preparing a family meal, sexual activity, or attending a social function with friends may appear simple to the client without significant impairment. However, the most basic tasks of daily life can become challenging to those with pulmonary and other diseases. When living with a chronic condition, a task like preparing a family meal could require double the amount of time and result in exhaustion due to the physical demands of the task. The progressive nature of many pulmonary conditions unfortunately forces individuals to reevaluate their priorities of daily life and reconsider participation in habits, roles, and routines that were once deemed important.

To help clients navigate functional changes associated with cardiopulmonary diseases, OT practitioners teach individuals skills in **energy conservation** and **work simplification.** Energy conservation and work simplification are methods for adapting and modifying how one participates in valued occupations by considering elements such as self-pacing, activity modification, fatigue avoidance, organizational skills, adaptive equipment, and environmental supports/barriers. Box 26-3 contains a list of general energy conservation and work simplification principles that can be utilized with clients. Using energy conservation strategies allows clients to simplify their work, while at the same time being able to accomplish the activity that is meaningful to the client. For the homemaker, making simple suggestions, such as sitting to prepare cooking ingredients, distributing cooking tasks throughout the day, or placing common cooking items in accessible locations in the kitchen can minimize dyspnea and fatigue, while also supporting the client's ability to complete a valued daily occupation with autonomy and control. The goal of energy conservation and work simplification education for OT practitioners is for clients not only to incorporate strategies into existing routines, but to generalize their knowledge into new activities or problem areas they experience. Utilizing energy conservation and work simplification techniques can support engagement in meaningful occupation, thus leading to a greater quality of life for people living with a chronic disease.

STRESS MANAGEMENT AND COPING TECHNIQUES

Psychosocial symptoms such as anxiety and depression are common for clients living with pulmonary disease. When clients feel that they are unable to catch their breath, this is very distressing and can lead to fear and panic if they do not have the training to mitigate this anxiety before an episode occurs. Depression and feelings of being overwhelmed by their condition also have negative effects on psychosocial functioning for clients with pulmonary conditions. Relaxation techniques, such as visualization and PMR, can be effective for decreasing anxiety and promote coping as well. For visualization, clients close their eyes and imagine being in a peaceful and relaxing environment to distract them from a stressful situation. PMR and mindfulness meditation are two techniques clients can use to promote relaxation. Some clients may need pharmacological intervention to improve psychosocial functioning when anxiety is frequent and severe. OTAs should discuss concerns regarding anxiety and depression with the supervising occupational therapist as well as the nurse and physician.

BOX 26-3
Energy Conservation and Work Simplification

- Sit, when possible, during activity.
- Take consistent rest breaks.
- Spread heavy and light tasks throughout the day.
- Plan ahead and gather all items needed for starting a task.
- Keep items within easy reach.
- Work at one's own pace.
- Eliminate unnecessary tasks.
- Use adaptive equipment as needed.
- Limit excessive bending, lifting, or twisting.
- Minimize arm movements above the shoulder.
- Support elbows on table when working in one place.
- Use proper body mechanics and posture.
- Push, pull, or slide objects on counter space rather than lifting.
- Prioritize tasks that are most important.
- Share workload with friends and family.
- Allow enough time to complete a task without rushing.
- Stop and rest before becoming tired/short of breath.

OT Practitioner's Viewpoint

I learned a great deal about the importance of multifactorial approaches for intervention early in my career as an occupational therapist when I worked with a client who had advanced COPD. Mrs. A was a widow with two children, and she also had a sister who lived near the skilled nursing facility where she resided. Mrs. A had been a homemaker all of her life and was married for 52 years. Her sister, children, and grandchildren visited her often in the skilled nursing facility.

When I first met Mrs. A, she was very anxious and did not leave her room often to participate in facility activities. She spent a large part of the day in bed, and when certified nursing assistants (CNAs) did assist her to the wheelchair, they often left her sitting up for longer periods of time than she could tolerate. Mrs. A had lost weight because her appetite had decreased and she became SOB when eating. Mrs. A did not tolerate showers well due to anxiety and SOB, which increased the time needed for CNAs to assist her in daily self-care activities. She also often screamed for help to get to the bathroom for toileting, even when she had just pressed her call bell moments before. The CNAs found her to be a difficult client, and they came to dread working with her in their daily shifts. While Mrs. A's oxygen saturation levels would decrease at times to as low as 86%, this was rare and she would often feel short of breath and state "I can't breathe" even when her levels were 90% or higher. Feelings of breathlessness was another trigger for severe anxiety for Mrs. A.

When I began working with Mrs. A for OT services, I knew that I would need to incorporate a multifactorial approach to address her needs. The initial evaluation revealed that she had decreased independence with bathing, dressing, toileting tasks, and functional mobility as well as reduced participation in feeding and activities within the facility. She demonstrated reduced functional activity tolerance, decreased standing balance, and severe SOB. Mrs. A also had significant anxiety as well as depression, which were both observed by myself and documented previously in her medical record. In addition to client factors, I knew that environmental barriers within the facility as well as knowledge and behavior of staff members would also need to be addressed. For example, showering schedules did not align with the time of day when Mrs. A had the most energy, and staff members leaving her sitting up in

OT Practitioner's Viewpoint (continued)

her wheelchair for several hours at a time were factors that needed to be altered. Staff beliefs that Mrs. A was a difficult client also did not encourage empathy for the client's experiences.

One of the first limitations in occupational performance that was addressed for Mrs. A was toileting because she identified this as her highest concern. CNA staff also identified this as a concern due to Mrs. A yelling for help as soon as she called for assistance with her call bell. This did not allow staff enough time to get to her room before she started screaming, and this created a stressful work environment as well as severe anxiety for the client. One solution for decreased independence with toileting was to complete training for bed mobility and functional transfers so that Mrs. A would be able to get to the bathroom more quickly with assistance when she did need to use the restroom. She was also placed on a toileting schedule that was followed by CNA staff so that they would check on Mrs. A during time frames in which she would normally ask for help and assist her with toileting before this became an emergency. I also trained Mrs. A to use various relaxation techniques, such as deep breathing and visual imagery, so that she could employ these techniques when she became anxious to decrease the frequency of panic attacks. In addition, she was also trained to use pursed-lip breathing to decrease SOB with activities or when she started becoming anxious. Staff members were educated on the experience of having COPD, including the significant anxiety and SOB that results even when a client may have a normal oxygen saturation level. CNA staff members were more understanding and no longer viewed Mrs. A as a "difficult client."

Other areas of need for Mrs. A such as showering and self feeding, were addressed through a combination of approaches. CNAs were educated on the importance of timing Mrs. A's morning ADLs after she had received a breathing treatment and during a time of day when she typically had more energy. The exhaust fan was turned on before and during the shower to reduce steam that caused difficulty with breathing. The client was scheduled to receive five small meals a day rather than three larger meals to encourage greater caloric intake with less fatigue. Mrs. A was also assisted with lying down to take a nap before dinner so that she would be well rested and better able to tolerate sitting up in her wheelchair for meals in the dining room. Mrs. A also completed interventions to address reduced activity tolerance and standing balance that included occupation-based, purposeful, and preparatory methods to improve these client factors. As a result of increased endurance and balance, better breathing techniques, less anxiety, and better understanding from staff members about appropriate time frames for sitting up in the wheelchair, Mrs. A was able to participate more in activities in the facility and spend increased time out of her room engaging with others.

Through working with Mrs. A, I learned about the importance of using a multitude of approaches to address client needs. Some factors within the individual, such as functional activity tolerance, can be altered to improve performance. At other times, compensatory approaches may be needed such as changing the time of day in which a client completes an occupation. Barriers in the environment may need to be removed, and this includes both physical limitations as well as addressing social issues such as viewing someone as a "difficult client." Healthcare providers should always consider their own attitudes and behavior to seek ways to change these to meet client needs. ~ Renee Causey-Upton, OTD, MS, OTR/L

REFERRAL TO OTHER HEALTHCARE DISCIPLINES

Due to the significant and varied deficits often experienced by clients with COPD, clients may need other services beyond OT. OTAs should discuss with their supervising occupational therapist any needed referrals to other disciplines. For example, clients with postural control deficits may need a referral to physical therapy to address balance or to introduce a mobility device for safety. Clients may have swallowing deficits that could be addressed by speech language pathology. Respiratory therapy (in addition to nursing staff) may need to be contacted if clients are having desaturation during therapy; the respiratory therapist in conjunction with the physician may determine that oxygen delivery should be raised to a higher level during therapy sessions. Caution must be taken in adjusting oxygen settings for all clients, but especially those with COPD due to the restrictive nature of the condition and the inability of the lungs to expand fully to tolerate higher levels of oxygen delivery. A specific order from the physician with exact parameters is needed for any oxygen level adjustments during activity; oxygen levels need to be returned back down to the normal level as soon as the client's oxygen saturation and respiratory rate allow.

ASSESSMENT OF VITAL SIGNS AND ACTIVITY TOLERANCE

Assessment of vital signs is an important clinical skill for OTAs. Not only is it necessary for safe monitoring of clients in response to therapeutic activity, but OTAs must also use this knowledge to teach clients standardized vital assessments when developing self-management strategies. As already discussed, chronic disease affects all aspects of a client's daily life, including a client's physical, mental, and emotional functioning, and vital assessments are considered the baseline indicators of a client's health status.[69] Incorporating vital assessments into interventions promotes safety during therapy sessions, teaches clients the importance of self-monitoring the impact of cardiac and pulmonary disease on daily life, and allows clients to take achievable steps toward self-management of their own

COMMUNICATION

Clear and frequent communication among members of the healthcare team is vital for achieving the best outcomes for clients with cardiac and pulmonary conditions. Typical members of the healthcare team include: nurses, CNAs, physicians, occupational therapists, OTAs, physical therapists, physical therapist assistants, dietitians, respiratory therapists, speech language pathologists, and other providers, as needed. Both verbal and written communication must be clear, accurate, and complete. Communicating important information to the interprofessional team not only leads to changes in care to better support the client, but could have health implications as well. For example, when a client presents with chest pain, nursing staff should be notified because this could indicate signs of exercise intolerance or even an MI. Any new symptoms observed during an OTA session should be relayed to nursing staff and the physician, as well as included in written OTA documentation. A client with a pulmonary condition who has decreased oxygen saturation may need to begin wearing oxygen if this has not yet been prescribed, or may need to have a higher dosage of oxygen delivered during therapy sessions. This information should be shared with the physician and respiratory therapy staff who can make needed adjustments to oxygen delivery when appropriate. Clients who express interest in smoking cessation should be referred to their physician for any needed pharmacological intervention to assist with this process. Smoking is a risk factor for both cardiac and pulmonary conditions, so it is very important for the OTA to share any interest in quitting smoking with the client's physician. The OTA should also communicate any relevant observations from therapy sessions to the supervising occupational therapist and other rehabilitation team members. For example, notifying the speech language pathologist that the client was less SOB after receiving a breathing treatment 30 minutes before a feeding intervention would be pertinent information to share. This information should also be documented in the client's daily note so that other members of the interprofessional team will be aware of progress from the intervention session. Any techniques that allow the client to be more independent with ADLs should be relayed to certified nursing assistants so the client can carry over skills that were learned from the OTA and also perform daily tasks more independently with less SOB. OTAs must also have open communication with the client and appropriate family members. Clients should be educated on appropriate expectations about their condition, any precautions they must follow, and when to resume their regular activities. Education should be provided in multiple formats and reinforced over time to ensure understanding and carryover of recommendations. For example, a client who is being educated on sternal precautions needs this information verbally, in writing, via demonstration, and through implementing these precautions in daily life activities. To ensure that client needs are being fully met, it is imperative that OTAs have good communication with all members of the interprofessional team as well as with clients and their families.

disease. Skilled intervention OTAs can use with clients related to vital assessments include:

1. Create a daily vital signs diary to be implemented by the client.
2. Develop self-awareness strategies for clients to understand their body's physical response to occupational performance.
3. Teach compensatory strategies in response to atypical vital signs, teaching self-monitoring skills for vital signs using electronic monitors (e.g., digital blood pressure monitor, pulse oximeter for measurement of blood oxygen saturation and heart rate, or glucometer for measurement of blood glucose levels)
4. Teach clients self-advocacy skills for effective communication of vital assessments with healthcare providers.

Primary vital signs include assessment of heart rate, respiratory rate, oxygen saturation, and blood pressure, and will be addressed in further detail. Table 26-6 offers general guidelines for monitoring of vital signs and key measures. However, the physician may determine and set individual vital sign guidelines based on internal and external factors related to the client. OTAs should understand common vital sign ranges and communicate with their supervising occupational therapist and the physician when assessment results of vital signs are abnormal. Other measures of exercise and activity tolerance can be included as well, such as maximum-age adjusted heart rate and rate of perceived exertion/dyspnea. These measures will be discussed in the following sections along with common vital signs.

Heart Rate

The pulse is determined by the speed of a person's heartbeat (beats per minute) and results when the heart contracts and pushes blood throughout the arterial system. Heart rate is most accurately measured when palpating an artery close to the body's surface such as the carotid, brachial, or radial arteries. The radial artery is used most commonly; it is located on the volar surface of the wrist, lateral to the radial head. When manually measuring a client's heart rate, OTAs should palpate the radial artery using the pads of their second and third fingers and then determine whether the pulse is regular (beating in a consistent pattern) or irregular (not beating in a consistent pattern). If the pulse is steady or regular, count the number of beats for 20 seconds and multiply that number by 3. The more common practice of counting for 10 seconds can have a high rate of error. If the pulse is irregular, count the number of beats for a full 60 seconds. The average resting pulse rate in adults is 70 beats per minute and ranges between 60 and 100 beats per minute. In adults, *tachycardia* is a pulse rate that exceeds 100 beats per minute, and *bradycardia* is a pulse rate less than 60 beats per minute.[69] The OTA should assess clients' heart rate before, during, and after engagement in activity to gain a full understanding of their physiological response to physical activity.

TABLE 26-6 Monitoring of Vital Signs[19]

VITAL SIGN	NORMAL VALUE	ABNORMAL VALUE
Blood pressure (BP)	Less than 120/80 mmHg Systolic: 90-120 mmHg Diastolic: 60-80 mmHg	Hypotension: Less than 90 mmHg systolic and/or 60 mmHg diastolic Prehypertension: 120-129 mmHg systolic, less than 80 mmHg diastolic Hypertension stage 1: 130-139 mmHg systolic, 80-89 mmHg diastolic Hypertension stage 2: Greater than 140/90 mmHg
Pulse heart rate (HR)	60-100 bpm	Bradycardia: Less than 60 bpm Tachycardia: Greater than 100 bpm
Oxygen saturation (SpO_2)	95%-100% SpO_2	Hypoxemia: Less than 90% SpO_2
Respiratory rate (RR)	12-20 breaths/min	Tachypnea: Greater than 20 breaths/min Bradypnea: Less than 12 breaths/min

Pulse oximeters are commonly used devices that assess heart rate and oxygen saturation. Whereas the device is convenient for quick assessment of vital signs, it should be noted that certain factors such as tremors or excessive movement, cold hands, or use of nail polish could cause inaccurate readings. When using the pulse oximeter, the client's hand should rest on his or her chest at heart level, on a tabletop, or on his or her lap to minimize excessive motion. Clients can be taught by the OTA how to assess their own pulse before, during, and after activity to better understand their body's response to activity.

CALCULATING MAXIMUM AGE-ADJUSTED HEART RATE

Maximum age-adjusted heart rate (MAHR) can be used to determine safe parameters for heart rate during exercise and other activities. MAHR becomes more appropriate in the outpatient setting after clients have been progressing in tolerance to MET levels. To calculate the MAHR, subtract the client's age from 220; the resulting difference is the client's MAHR. For example, a 65-year-old male would have an MAHR of 155, derived from 220 minus 65 ($220 - 65 = 155$). To calculate an appropriate heart rate range for exercise, multiply the MAHR by 50% and 85%. In the previous example, the exercise range for heart rate would be 78 to 132 beats per minute. This was derived from multiplying 155, the MAHR, by 0.50 and 0.85, respectively. When a client is taking a beta blocker, such as Toprol or Metoprolol, the heart response can be altered, so MAHR may not be an accurate way to determine an appropriate level of activity for these clients.[7] In these cases, the rate of perceived exertion may be a better indicator of exercise and activity responses. Refer to the Rate of Perceived Exertion and Dyspnea section of this chapter for more information.

Respiratory Rate

Respiratory rate is the number of breaths per minute and is inspected by measuring the rise and fall of the client's chest. The primary muscles of respiration are the diaphragm and

TECHNOLOGY AND TRENDS

Hospital lengths of stay have decreased in recent years for the acute care setting. Shorter hospital stays have resulted in clients being discharged while they may still be in an acute phase of recovery. OTAs must be prepared to provide care across a continuum to meet the needs of clients with cardiac and pulmonary disease. Earlier discharge from acute care settings is providing opportunities for OTAs to treat clients in other settings outside the hospital. This same trend is also affecting clients by requiring them to take responsibility for their health at an earlier stage, a process that is supported by recent technology.

TRENDS

Clients are requiring more care in nonhospital settings and are needing access to outpatient cardiac and pulmonary rehabilitation sooner. In addition to earlier utilization of outpatient rehabilitation, other new models of care are being explored and implemented to meet clients' needs and to reduce costs. Contemporary models of care share several features such as providing individualized care, utilizing telehealth, providing clients with supplemental educational materials, and community or home-based delivery of services.[70] Telehealth is an approach to client care that allows providers to deliver services through virtual technology, reaching clients who may be in geographic areas that are remote or a great distance from healthcare professionals. Refer to the Technology and Trends section in Chapter 25 for more information about telehealth. Contemporary models of care can support clients to be more compliant with exercise programs and lifestyle changes, as well as permit access to healthcare providers who would otherwise be unavailable for clients in more rural locations. OTAs can meet client needs via telehealth with the appropriate supervision from an occupational therapist. Providing supplemental materials, such as handouts, videos, or other educational formats are beneficial for carryover of recommendations provided by the OTA and occupational therapist. These materials serve as reminders for clients to correctly implement recommendations to support their

Continued

TECHNOLOGY AND TRENDS (continued)

best health. When care is delivered in the home, OTAs can provide care in the client's natural environment and make recommendations that fully translate into the home setting.

TECHNOLOGY

Because clients are leaving the inpatient setting more quickly, they must become involved with self-management of their own condition at an earlier phase. Self-management education is a collaborative process between healthcare providers and clients that involves active learning and development of problem-solving skills.[40] This supports clients to become active participants in managing their condition even after inpatient or other formal rehabilitation programs are completed. Several devices are currently available to assist clients with the self-management process. Wristband tracking devices are able to track exercise activities, and some also monitor heart rate. Clients can use these devices to track their heart rate for safe activity levels as well as to record fitness progress for a healthy heart and lungs. Other electronic features can be used for health as well, such as phone "apps" that track physical activity or that provide healthy recipes to control weight or reduce cholesterol. Other "apps" are available to track nutritional intake as well as healthy eating habits. Clients can also use electronic calendars to schedule exercise sessions throughout the week to make this a priority for their time use. OTAs can educate clients about available "apps" and devices that may be useful for clients to support healthy lifestyle changes for self-management of cardiac and pulmonary disease.

intercostal muscles. To assess a client's respiratory rate, count the number of breaths, both inspiration and exhalation, that occurs in 1 minute. A typical adult's respiratory rate ranges from 12 to 20 breaths per minute and is influenced by factors such as age, activity level of the client, and/or diagnosis of lung condition (e.g., COPD, asthma, lung cancer, emphysema). *Bradypnea* is defined as a persistent respiratory rate slower than 12 breaths per minute, and *tachypnea* is defined as a persistent respiratory rate faster than 20 breaths per minute.[69] It is important for clients to understand how to self-monitor and control their respiratory rate in order to maintain safe participation in occupational performance areas. OTAs help clients better understand how physical exertion during daily activities affects respiration and ways to incorporate energy conservation techniques and breathing techniques (PLB/active expiration) to facilitate participation in valued occupations in safe ways. Boxes 26-2 and 26-3 offer examples of breathing techniques and energy conservation strategies.

Oxygen Saturation

Oxygen saturation refers to the concentration of oxygen in the blood or the percentage of hemoglobin-binding sites in the bloodstream occupied by oxygen.[71] Normal oxygen saturation levels range from 95% to 100% SpO_2 and can be easily measured through noninvasive pulse oximeter devices. Pulse oximeters are portable, battery-powered devices that can quickly provide oxygen readings and allow clients to track oxygen saturation over time. OTAs utilize pulse oximeters when working with clients to determine baseline oxygen level readings as well as oxygen saturation levels with exercise/functional activity. OTAs utilize pulse oximeters to measure clients' response to activity and teach clients self-monitoring strategies as related to their breathing condition. Clients should be returned to a resting position and led through PLB exercises when oxygen saturation drops below 90% SpO_2 during intervention sessions. The supervising occupational therapist and physician should also be notified if a client's oxygen saturation drops below 80% as organ function (e.g., brain/heart) could be compromised.

Blood Pressure

Assessing a client's blood pressure measures the pressure that blood is pushing against artery walls in the heart. Blood pressure is composed of two numbers: *systolic pressure* and *diastolic pressure.* Systolic pressure is the top number on a blood pressure reading and measures the pressure inside the arteries when the heart contracts. Diastolic pressure is subsequently the bottom number on a blood pressure reading and measures the pressure inside the arteries when the heart is at rest between heartbeats and refilling with blood. A normal adult blood pressure reading is less than 120/80 mmHg according to the American Heart Association.

Measuring a client's blood pressure is a typical skill performed by OTAs during their academic training and later as practitioners. For routine measurements, the client may sit or lie in a supine position. However, assessment of the client in standing position may be necessary to understand the effect of postural changes on blood pressure. Measurement of blood pressure requires use of a sphygmomanometer (blood pressure cuff) and stethoscope. First, place the blood pressure cuff comfortably around the client's UE approximately 3 cm above the antecubital fossa. The client's arm should be resting at heart height and legs should not be crossed. Palpate for the brachial artery, which is typically medial to the biceps brachii tendon. Inflate the cuff to a pressure approximately 30 mmHg above the point where the palpable pulse disappears. Press the bell of the stethoscope lightly over the brachial artery, deflate the cuff slowly, and record the reading at which the client's pulse first becomes audible. This reading is taken as the *systolic pressure.* Continue to listen for the pulse as deflation of the cuff proceeds. The *diastolic pressure* reading will be the last audible pulse. See Figure 26-8 for a depiction of UE landmarks for blood pressure monitoring. If a blood pressure reading cannot be obtained from a client's upper arm, the OTA can assess blood pressure from the forearm. The blood pressure cuff is wrapped around the distal forearm, and the stethoscope bell is placed over the radial artery.[72] Contraindications do exist for assessing blood pressure. OT practitioners should take necessary precautions and avoid obtaining blood pressure in the same arm of a client who has lymphedema, mastectomy, IV line,

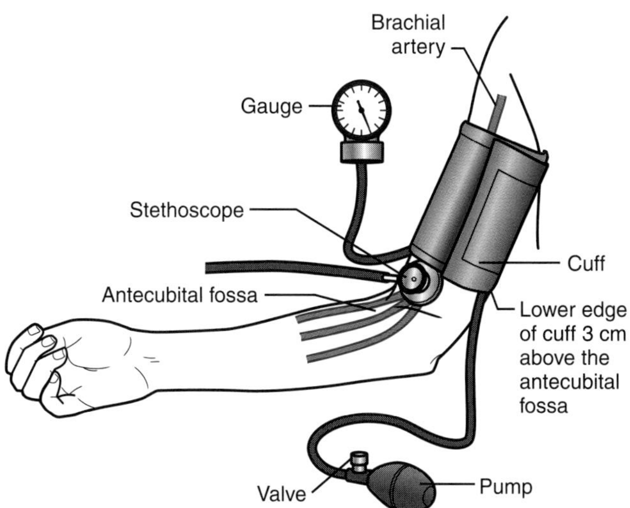

FIGURE 26-8. Upper-extremity landmarks for blood pressure monitoring.

or arteriovenous fistula needed for dialysis treatment. Utilize the other arm if a client presents with any of these conditions. Taking blood pressure on the same arm repeatedly in a short amount of time can falsely raise the blood pressure reading, and this should be avoided. The OTA should also ensure that the blood pressure cuff fits the client appropriately to obtain an accurate reading. For example, a larger cuff will be needed for clients who are obese, and a smaller cuff will be needed for clients who are more petite. For clients who are obese, the blood pressure can be taken in the forearm and wrist. Also, be aware that blood pressure may be elevated if the client just engaged in activities or if they are feeling anxious.

Rate of Perceived Exertion and Dyspnea

In addition to monitoring vital signs such as oxygen saturation as well as respiratory rate and heart rate, it is important to also determine the client's rate of perceived exertion (RPE) and rate of perceived dyspnea (RPD) during exercise and functional tasks. A common measure of both exertion and dyspnea is the Borg scale. The scale established by Borg ranges from 6 to 20 and measures increased feelings of exertion experienced by the client.[73] A modified version of this scale published by the AACVPR measures exertion along with dyspnea from a minimum 0, which indicates no feelings of exertion or dyspnea, to a maximum level of 10 to reflect extreme dyspnea and fatigue.[74] The range of this scale may be easier for clients to understand and use due to client experiences with other common scales that rate factors, such as pain, from 0 to 10. Client ratings of 3 to 5 would be considered an appropriate range for activity, whereas ratings greater than or equal to 6 would demonstrate high feelings of dyspnea or fatigue that indicate the need for taking a rest break. Clients should not continue tasks when they have an RPE or RPD of greater than 6. Other measures of feelings of SOB and fatigue exist, such as using a simple visual analog scale (VAS) to ask clients to rate these factors on a line that ranges from 0 to another maximum level, such as 10. Clients who have severe cognitive impairments will be unable to utilize these self-report measures to report RPE and RPD. When cognitive impairments limit the ability to provide RPE and RPD, clinicians should rely on vital signs, client report of being tired or having difficulty breathing, as well as physical appearance to determine feelings of SOB and fatigue.

Signs and Symptoms of Exercise and Activity Intolerance

Acute signs and symptoms of exercise intolerance can include chest pain as well as pain that refers to other areas of the body, such as the teeth, jaw, ear, or UEs. Clients may also exhibit SOB, extreme fatigue, and diaphoresis. Nausea and vomiting may occur during exercise or other strenuous activity, and this can indicate client intolerance to their current level of exertion. Weight gain of 3 to 5 pounds in a short period of time, such as 1 to 3 days, can also indicate intolerance to the current activity program.[7] When clients demonstrate potential signs and symptoms of exercise intolerance, intervention should be stopped and nursing staff should be notified to assess the client's medical status. Future intervention sessions may need to be altered to include lower-level activities and slowly increase to tasks with higher MET levels. See Box 26-4 for a quick reference guide for signs of intolerance to activity.

BOX 26-4
Signs of Intolerance to Activity

Signs and symptoms of intolerance to exercise and activity:

- Chest pain
- Pain that radiates to the teeth, jaw, ear, or upper extremities
- Severe shortness of breath
- Extreme fatigue
- Diaphoresis
- Nausea and vomiting
- Weight gain of 3 to 5 pounds in a short time

SUMMARY

Cardiopulmonary conditions are common diagnoses that OTAs will encounter across the care continuum, especially in the acute care setting. OTAs must have the knowledge and skills to provide safe and effective interventions for these populations. An understanding of appropriate precautions and vital signs are necessary for providing care to clients with cardiac and pulmonary conditions. A combination of preparatory, purposeful, and occupation-based techniques provides a strong approach to meeting the needs of cardiopulmonary clients to promote optimal occupational functioning.

REVIEW QUESTIONS

1. Brad has recently undergone open heart surgery for coronary artery bypass grafting due to severe obstruction of a coronary artery. Which of the following approaches would be the safest way for the OTA to teach Brad to complete bed mobility while the sternum is still healing?
   a. Brad should be instructed to bend his knees and hips and log-roll these to the side at the same time as his trunk, allowing the weight of the LEs to assist with turning over.
   b. Brad should be advised to pull on the bed rail to assist with rolling over onto his side.
   c. Brad should be trained to pull on the OTA's arm to assist with rolling over onto his side so that the assistant can monitor how much force he is using for pulling.
   d. Brad should be taught to use an overhead trapeze to allow his upper extremities to assist with rolling and scooting in bed.
2. Based on current research, which three of the following statements regarding the evidence to support cardiac and pulmonary rehabilitation including OT is *most* accurate?
   a. Pulmonary rehabilitation including OT is supported in the literature by research, but cardiac rehabilitation is not.
   b. Pulmonary rehabilitation and cardiac rehabilitation including OT are both well supported in the literature.
   c. Pulmonary rehabilitation including OT is supported by strong research evidence, but cardiac rehabilitation is not.
   d. Cardiac and pulmonary rehabilitation overall are supported by strong research evidence in the current literature.
   e. Cardiac and pulmonary rehabilitation are evidence-based interventions supported by strong research, but evidence for OT with cardiac and pulmonary populations is currently lacking.
   f. Occupational therapy for clients with cardiac and pulmonary conditions is well supported by research evidence, but cardiac and pulmonary rehabilitation programs are not supported overall by current research.
3. Mary has been recently hospitalized due to an exacerbation of COPD. She has been having severe anxiety due to extreme shortness of breath during functional tasks. What is an appropriate way that the OTA can teach her to breathe to reduce shortness of breath during daily occupations?
   a. Mary should be taught to inhale deeply and then hold her breath while completing the most difficult portion of an ADL task.
   b. Mary should be advised to breathe out during the easier portion of ADL tasks, and then inhale with exertion.
   c. Mary should be instructed to inhale for 2 counts through her nose, and then slowly exhale for 4 counts through pursed lips.
   d. Mary should take quick, shallow breaths during exertion.
4. Clients with pulmonary diseases, such as COPD and IPF, can experience coughing during activities or even without exertion. Episodes of coughing can lead to extreme fatigue and shortness of breath. Which three of the following would be the *best* approach for reducing coughing related to exertion?
   a. Sitting to complete morning ADL tasks
   b. Drinking fluids after exercising
   c. Using a reacher to pick up items off the floor to avoid bending over
   d. Using PLB and active expiration breathing techniques
   e. Using throat lozenges while completing functional mobility
   f. Avoiding strongly scented ADL products
5. Mark experienced a recent MI, but was cleared medically by his physician for OT services. During an OT session, he began having nausea, shortness of breath, extreme fatigue, and chest pain. What action should the OTA complete in response to these symptoms?
   a. The OTA should continue intervention but reduce the amount of exertion required by the client to grade the activity down and reduce fatigue.
   b. The OTA should continue intervention at the same level but should monitor the client's vital signs more closely for safety.
   c. The OTA should stop intervention immediately and notify nursing staff because these are signs and symptoms of exercise intolerance, as well as possible signs of a heart attack.
   d. The OTA should continue intervention because this is a normal response to physical activity after MI.
6. Susan was recently diagnosed with a new condition and has been working closely with her OTA to implement strategies to mitigate limitations caused by her diagnosis. She has been experiencing fatigue, swelling in her LEs, weight gain, and coughing. Susan has been having trouble sleeping at night and has had to raise the head of her bed due to shortness of breath when she lies down flat. Which of the following conditions align with the symptoms Susan has been experiencing?
   a. COPD
   b. CHF
   c. MI
   d. CABG
7. Vital signs are important to monitor during OT intervention sessions to ensure that clients are participating within safe medical parameters. Which of the following readings would be considered abnormal when measured during low MET level activities?
   a. Respiratory rate: 28 breaths/min
   b. Blood pressure: 118/78 mmHg
   c. Oxygen saturation: 93% SpO_2
   d. Pulse heart rate: 75 bpm
8. Percutaneous coronary intervention (PCI) can be used to open up blood vessels that have been occluded within the heart. Following this procedure, clients have activity precautions related to the access site for the PCI. Which of the following restrictions are required after PCI?
   a. Avoid any asynchronous movements of the upper extremities for 4 to 6 weeks.
   b. Avoid lying down after exertion to prevent increasing preload, or ventricular blood volume.
   c. Avoid lifting, pushing, or pulling with either upper extremity for 4 to 6 weeks.
   d. Remain on bedrest, and maintain the affected extremity in extension for approximately 4 to 8 hours.
9. An OTA is reviewing a client chart before beginning an intervention session. In the orders section of the chart, the OTA notes that blood tests have been ordered to assess Troponin levels. The OTA checks with nursing staff and does not see the client for intervention because:
   a. The client is being assessed for a potential MI and may not be safe to see for intervention until cleared by the physician.
   b. The client is having a COPD exacerbation and will not be able to tolerate intervention.
   c. Troponin may indicate that the client has dangerously high blood pressure.
   d. Troponin may indicate that the client has dangerously high blood glucose levels.

10. After a recent COPD exacerbation, Mr. James has transitioned from needing oxygen on an as-needed basis to requiring it at all times. In addition to seeing Mr. James in the hospital to address deconditioning, the OTA needs to reeducate Mr. James and his wife on important safety measures to take when using oxygen. Which of the following safety tips is *true* regarding safe oxygen use?
    a. Be around open flames with oxygen use.
    b. Store cylinders in an approved rack.
    c. Oxygen tubing has no impact on fall risk.
    d. Leave oxygen valves on when not in use.

CASE STUDY

Mr. Coffman is a 63-year-old male with a history of hypertension, osteoarthritis, and COPD. He recently had a COPD exacerbation and a moderately sized STEMI. Mr. Coffman has been a smoker for the last 40 years, but has recently considered quitting due to his worsening health condition. He is currently being treated in an acute care hospital setting for his recent MI and COPD exacerbation. At home, he wears 2 liters of oxygen at night, but he has been prescribed continuous oxygen at 4 liters since his hospitalization. Mr. Coffman spent 1 day in the intensive care unit and was then moved to the telemetry unit because his condition was improving. His physician has ordered OT evaluation and intervention to address the client's decreased independence with ADLs and other occupations, shortness of breath, reduced functional activity tolerance, anxiety due to poor breathing patterns, and fatigue with daily activities.

Mr. Coffman has been married for 35 years to his wife Betsy, and they reside in a two-level house with three steps to enter the home. The main bedroom and bathroom are on the first floor, so he does not have to go upstairs when he first discharges home after his hospitalization. He has three children and seven grandchildren. His children live nearby and are willing and able to help him if needed. Mr. Coffman's parents passed away several years ago, but all four of his siblings are still living and he visits with them often. He enjoys socializing with friends and customers at a local farmer's market. Mr. Coffman has a high school education and has not completed any college courses.

Mr. Coffman was independent with all self-care activities, functional mobility, and driving until his most recent hospitalization. He was also able to help with light home-management tasks, although his wife does most of the cooking, cleaning, and laundry in their home. Mr. Coffman enjoys yard work, such as mowing and tending to his large garden, but he has found this to be increasingly difficult over the last few years. He enjoys spending time with his grandchildren, and he often attends their baseball games and other activities. Mr. Coffman had to retire early from his factory position due to his health conditions, but he still works for several hours 2 days a week at a local farmer's market during produce seasons.

The occupational therapist completed the initial evaluation with contributions from the OTA to gather objective data, and a plan of care was established for the OTA to follow with skilled interventions. Self-care occupations that were identified as priorities to address in intervention included total body bathing and dressing, as these were areas that the client needed assistance with in the hospital. Mr. Coffman was also very concerned with managing his large garden and completing other yard work at home. He also wanted to be able to continue his work at the farmer's market because this was a highly valued occupation that held value even beyond working. Gathering the occupational profile at the initial evaluation, the occupational therapist discovered that the farmer's market was a place for socializing with other friends who both worked at and attended the market. The initial evaluation revealed that the client had normal strength, ROM, postural control, and fine motor skills. However, Mr. Coffman had decreased functional activity tolerance and was also noted to use ineffective breathing patterns. He became anxious with activity, although he maintained oxygen saturation above 90% during the evaluation with 4 liters of oxygen via nasal cannula. His other vital signs were within normal parameters.

The OTA monitored Mr. Coffman's vital signs closely throughout intervention sessions to ensure that his heart rate, oxygen levels, and respiratory rate were within safe parameters. Rate of perceived exertion and dyspnea were also included along with attention to MET levels due to his recent MI. Mr. Coffman was able to tolerate increasingly difficult occupational and exercise activities throughout his hospital stay. Mr. Coffman was trained in energy conservation techniques to reduce his fatigue with daily activities. Education also included adaptive techniques, such as crossing one foot over the opposite leg for LB dressing and sitting for bathing tasks. Adaptive equipment was introduced to decrease exertion and limit forward leaning to support better breathing. For example, Mr. Coffman was advised to use a reacher to pick up items off the floor. He was trained in PLB and active exhalation to reduce shortness of breath and to prevent anxiety during daily occupations. He was also trained in stress-management techniques for further anxiety reduction and to address stress as a cardiac risk factor. Mr. Coffman was educated on other cardiac risk factors and the importance of smoking cessation related to both COPD and his recent heart attack.

The OTA discussed concerns regarding yard work, gardening, and work activities at the farmer's market with the client. It was determined that other arrangements would need to be made to care for the yard and large garden due to Mr. Coffman's various medical conditions. Family members were contacted and were willing to assist with these tasks, with plans to hire someone for yard and garden management if these became too time-consuming for the client's family. Mr. Coffman was educated on some modified gardening techniques so that he could still participate in this valued occupation at home. Throughout his hospital stay, he was slowly weaned off oxygen and had returned to only using 2 liters at night, or as needed throughout the day if he became very SOB.

Through skilled OT intervention, Mr. Coffman gained back his independence with ADL tasks using adaptive techniques and appropriate breathing patterns. He was able to return to completing light home-management tasks using energy conservation and adaptive techniques as needed. Mr. Coffman's oldest grandson has begun mowing the yard for him each week, and his children and grandchildren are taking turns assisting with managing the large garden. Mr. Coffman has a few small tumbler tomato plants in hanging baskets growing on his back porch so that he is still able to participate in gardening within the limitations of his conditions. He has been able to return to selling produce at the farmer's market and takes rest breaks as needed to avoid becoming overly fatigued. Mr. Coffman pays a neighbor to set up and take down his produce stand for the market to prevent becoming overly exhausted. He has learned to use stress-management techniques to reduce anxiety related to shortness of breath, as well as to lower his stress levels to decrease the risk for a future cardiac event. He has successfully quit smoking, and his family has been cooking and eating healthier meals, further decreasing the risk for another MI. Mr. Coffman is continuing to progress in his exercise program and functional activity tolerance through outpatient pulmonary rehabilitation services.

1. What vital signs and other client factors would need to be monitored while providing OT intervention for Mr. Coffman?
2. What signs and/or symptoms would cause one to stop intervention or contact the physician with one's concerns?
3. How does OTA intervention for cardiopulmonary clients vary across the continuum of care from acute to outpatient rehabilitation?

PUTTING IT ALL TOGETHER Sample Treatment and Documentation

Setting	Acute care hospital, day 3 of admission
Client Profile	Mr. F, 67-year-old male, experienced a mild STEMI and COPD exacerbation, history of hypertension and diabetes mellitus type II
Work History	Retired teacher, 1 year of college education, volunteers 1 to 2 days a week at a local food pantry
Insurance	Medicare
Psychological	Anxiety due to SOB, no other psychological conditions
Social	Married, lives in a two-level home with four steps to enter
Cognitive	No limitations present.
Motor & Manual Motor Testing (MMT)	Client presents with normal strength and ROM BUE as well as good postural control, but has reduced functional activity tolerance. • WFL AROM in BUE • MMT RUE: 5/5 throughout • MMT LUE: 5/5 throughout • Close supervision for functional mobility due to fatigue • Client needs frequent rest breaks and can only stand for short periods of time. Also experiences reduced O_2 saturation at times.
ADL	Supervision for toileting including transfer, Min A bathing, Min A LB dressing, Supervision UB dressing, Mod I grooming, independent feeding
IADL	Max A with all due to fatigue and SOB as well as MET limits in the acute cardiac phase. IADLs to be addressed after acute phase.
Goals	Within 1 week: 1. Client will be Mod I for bathing and total body dressing with AE as needed and O_2 sats greater than or equal to 90%. 2. Client will be Mod I with toilet hygiene and clothing management with adaptive techniques as needed. 3. Client will be Mod I with functional mobility including toilet transfer with O_2 sats greater than or equal to 90% to increase independence with self-care activities. 4. Client will be independent with PLB and EC/WS techniques during daily self-care activities.

OT TREATMENT SESSION 1

THERAPEUTIC ACTIVITY	TIME	GOAL(s) ADDRESSED	OTA RATIONALE
PLB education and training through verbal instruction, written handout, demonstration, and return demonstration from client	10 min	#1, #3, and #4	*Education and Training:* Preparatory task and training to use appropriate breathing techniques during functional tasks to reduce SOB and maintain normal O_2 saturation
Bathing on shower seat in shower area in room, handheld shower, education on EC/WS for bathing verbally, through demonstration, and return demonstration during showering	15 min	#1 and #4	*Occupations; Education and Training:* Functional task performance to increase I with bathing tasks Preparatory task and training to use EC/WS techniques during bathing to reduce fatigue

PUTTING IT ALL TOGETHER Sample Treatment and Documentation (continued)

THERAPEUTIC ACTIVITY	TIME	GOAL(s) ADDRESSED	OTA RATIONALE
Upper and lower body dressing education on EC/WS for bathing verbally, through demonstration, and return demonstration during dressing	15 min	#1 and #4	*Occupations; Education and Training:* Functional task performance to increase I with dressing tasks Preparatory task and training to use EC/WS techniques during dressing to reduce fatigue
Toilet transfer, clothing management and hygiene, toilet in room with raised toilet seat and grab bars	10 min	#2 and #3	*Occupations:* Functional task performance to increase I with toileting tasks and toilet transfer
Education on general EC/WS techniques for all ADLs and review of techniques for bathing and dressing, verbal instruction and handout	15 min	#1 and #4	*Occupations; Education and Training:* Preparatory task and training to use EC/WS techniques to decrease fatigue during daily occupations

SOAP note: 7/12/—, 8:00 am–9:00 am

S: Client states, "I feel a little tired" after completing transfer to bathroom for showering.

O: Client participated in skilled OT in the acute care setting to address ADL performance, ineffective breathing patterns with SOB, and reduced functional activity tolerance. No c/o pain. Client educated on PLB techniques verbally, with handout and thorough demonstration. Client returned demonstration of PLB with Min verbal cues for proper technique. Client was able to ambulate to bathroom with supervision, however was fatigued when he reached the shower seat and his oxygen saturation had dropped to 88%. O_2 saturation returned to 91% with PLB and rest in approximately 45 seconds. Client was educated on EC/WS techniques for bathing while completing showering task. He required Min A for bathing and drying after shower due to fatigue. He was able to complete UB dressing with supervision and LB dressing with Min A. O_2 saturation was greater than or equal to 90% during these ADL tasks using PLB and rest breaks as needed. Client completed toilet transfer with supervision using raised toilet seat with grab bars, and clothing management and hygiene with supervision. Client educated on general EC/WS techniques along with review of bathing and dressing via handout and verbal instruction.

A: Client demonstrated increased independence with bathing, dressing, and toileting this date compared with initial evaluation. He maintained O_2 saturation greater than or equal to 90% except for dropping to 88% one time and needing a short recovery period to return to 90%. Client demonstrated understanding of PLB and EC/WS techniques but requires further training to become independent with these approaches for carryover at home after discharge. He is progressing steadily toward all goals and is making good functional progress. Client will benefit from continued skilled OT services for ADL retraining, transfer training, and training for PLB and EC/WS techniques to decrease fatigue and SOB with ADL tasks and return client to prior level of function.

P: Complete LB AE training at next session to increase independence with total body bathing and dressing. Continue retraining for ADL tasks with incorporation of EC/WS and PLB techniques. Recommend referral to outpatient cardiac or pulmonary rehabilitation program upon discharge to further address client's functional limitations and decreased independence with IADL tasks.

Mary Stivers, COTA/L, 7/12/—, 1:02 pm

TREATMENT SESSION 2

What could you do next with this client?

TREATMENT SESSION 3

What could you do next with this client?

REFERENCES

1. American Heart Association. (2016). Heart disease, stroke and research statistics at-a-glance. Retrieved from https://www.heart.org/idc/groups/ahamah-public/@wcm/@sop/@smd/documents/downloadable/ucm_480086.pdf
2. Blackwell, D. L., Lucas, J. W., & Clarke, T. C. (2014). Summary health statistics for U.S. adults: National Health Interview Survey, 2012. National Center for Health Statistics. *Vital Health Statistics, 10*(260). Retrieved from http://www.cdc.gov/nchs/data/series/sr_10/sr10_260.pdf
3. U.S. Department of Health and Human Services. (2016). *Health, United States, 2015* (Report No. 2016-1232). Atlanta, GA: Author. Retrieved from http://www.cdc.gov/nchs/data/hus/hus15.pdf#019
4. World Health Organization. (2016). Burden of COPD. Retrieved from http://www.who.int/respiratory/copd/burden/en/
5. National Heart, Lung, and Blood Institute. (2013). Disease statistics. In U.S. Department of Health and Human Services, *NHLBI fact book, fiscal year 2012*, (pp. 33–52). Retrieved from http://www.nhlbi.nih.gov/about/documents/factbook/2012
6. Cox, C. (2017). How much does the U.S. spend to treat different diseases? Retrieved from https://www.healthsystemtracker.org/chart-collection/much-u-s-spend-treat-different-diseases/?_sf_s=disease#item-start
7. American Heart Association. (2016). Heart attack symptoms in women. Retrieved from http://www.heart.org/HEARTORG/Conditions/HeartAttack/WarningSignsofaHeartAttack/Warning-Signs-of-a-Heart-Attack_UCM_002039_Article.jsp#.Vztv4PkrJhF
8. Garcia, T. B. (2015). *12-Lead ECG: The art of interpretation.* Burlington, MD: Jones & Bartlett Learning, LLC.
9. Thomason, T. R., Siroky, K., & Ryan, L. (2015). 12 lead ECGs: Ischemia, injury, infarction [Continuing education course]. Retrieved from http://lms.rn.com/getpdf.php/2151.pdf
10. Huma, S., Tariq, R., Amin, F., & Mahmood, K. T. (2012). Modifiable and non-modifiable predisposing risk factors of myocardial infarction—A review. *Journal of Pharmaceutical Sciences and Research, 4*(1), 1649–1653. Retrieved from www.jpsr.pharmainfo.in
11. de Lemos, J. A., O'Rourke, R. A., & Harrington, R. A. (2011). Unstable angina and non-ST-segment elevation myocardial infarction. In V. Fuster, R. A. Walsh, & R. A. Harrington (Eds.), *Hurst's the heart* (13th ed., Vol. 2, pp. 1328–1353). New York: McGraw Hill.
12. Dehmer, G. J., & Smith, K. J. (2009). Drug-eluding coronary artery stents. *American Family Physician, 80*(11), 1245–1253. Retrieved from www.aafp.org/afp
13. Douglas, J. S., & King, S. B. (2011). Percutaneous coronary intervention. In V. Fuster, R. A. Walsh, & R. A. Harrington (Eds.), *Hurst's the heart* (13th ed., Vol. 2, pp. 1430–1457). New York: McGraw Hill.
14. Tsigkas, G. G., Karantalis, V., Hahalis, G., & Alexopoulos, D. (2011). Stent restenosis, pathophysiology and treatment options: A 2010 update. *Hellenic Journal of Cardiology, 52*, 149–157.
15. Toomey, M. I., Kini, A. S., & Sharma, S. K. (2014). Current status of rotational atherectomy. *Journal of the American College of Cardiology, 7*, 345–353. doi:10.1016/j.jcin.2013.12.196
16. Rao, S. V., Turi, Z. G., Wong, S. C., Brener, S. J., & Stone, G. W. (2013). Radial versus femoral access. *Journal of the American College of Cardiology, 62*(17, Suppl), S11–S20. doi:10.1016/j.jacc.2013.08.700
17. Sabik, J. F., Bansilal, S., & Lytle, B. W. (2011). Coronary artery bypass. In V. Fuster, R. A. Walsh, & R. A. Harrington (Eds.), *Hurst's the heart* (13th ed., Vol. 2, pp. 1490–1503). New York: McGraw Hill.
18. Smith-Gabai, H. (2011). The cardiac system. In H. Smith-Gabai (Ed.), *Occupational therapy in acute care* (pp. 75–119). Bethesda, MD: AOTA Press.
19. American Association of Cardiovascular and Pulmonary Rehabilitation. (2013). *Guidelines for cardiac rehabilitation and secondary prevention programs* (5th ed.). Champaign, IL: Human Kinetics.
20. Foster, E. R., Cunnane, K. B., Edwards, D. F., Morrison, M. T., Ewald, G. A., Geltman, E. M., & Zazulia, A. R. (2011). Executive dysfunction and depressive symptoms associated with reduced participation of people with severe congestive heart failure. *American Journal of Occupational Therapy, 65*, 306–313. doi:10.5014/ajot.2011.000588
21. American Heart Association. (2015). About heart failure. Retrieved from http://www.heart.org/HEARTORG/Conditions/HeartFailure/AboutHeartFailure/About-Heart-Failure_UCM_002044_Article.jsp
22. Centers for Disease Control and Prevention. (2011). Vital signs: Prevalence, treatment, and control of hypertension. United States, 1999–2002 and 2005–2008. *Morbidity and Mortality Weekly Report, 60*(4), 103–108. Retrieved from http://www.cdc.gov/mmwr/index.html
23. Whelton, P. K., Carey, R. M., Aronow, W. S., Casey, Jr., D. E., Collins, K. J., Dennison Himmelfarb, C., ... & Wright, Jr., J. T. (2017). ACC/AHA/AAPA/ABC/ACPM/AGS/APhA/ASH/ASPC/NMA/PCNA guideline for the prevention, detection, evaluation, and management of high blood pressure in adults [manuscript ahead of print]. *Journal of the American College of Cardiology*. doi:10.1016/j.jacc.2017.11.006
24. American Heart Association. (2014). Prevention & treatment of high blood pressure. Retrieved from http://www.heart.org/HEARTORG/Conditions/HighBloodPressure/High-Blood-Pressure-or-Hypertension_UCM_002020_SubHomePage.jsp
25. American Heart Association. (2016). Dilated cardiomyopathy (DCM). Retrieved from http://www.heart.org/HEARTORG/Conditions/Conditions_UCM_001087_SubHomePage.jsp
26. National Heart, Lung, and Blood Institute. (2015). Types of cardiomyopathy. Retrieved from https://www.nhlbi.nih.gov/health/health-topics/topics/cm/types
27. Hypertrophic Cardiomyopathy Association. (2015). How common is hypertrophic cardiomyopathy? Retrieved from http://www.4hcm.org/content.asp?contentid=149
28. Mayo Clinic. (2015). Disease and conditions: Cardiomyopathy. Retrieved from http://www.mayoclinic.org/diseases-conditions/
29. Wexler, R., Elton, T., Pleister, A., & Feldman, D. (2009). Cardiomyopathy: An overview. *American Family Physician, 79*(9), 778–784. Retrieved from www.aafp.org/afp
30. Will, J. C., Yuan, K., & Ford, E. (2014). National trends in the prevalence and medical history of angina: 1988 to 2012. *Circulation Cardiovascular Quality and Outcomes, 7*, 407–413. doi:10.1161/CIRCOUTCOMES.113.000779
31. Nossaman, V. E., Nossaman, B. D., & Katowitz, P. J. (2010). Nitrates and nitrites in the treatment of ischemic heart disease. *Cardiology in Review, 18*(4), 190–197. doi:10.1097/CRD.0b013e3181c8e14a
32. Sami, S., & Willerson, J. T. (2010). Contemporary treatment of unstable angina and non-ST-elevation myocardial infarction (part 1). *Texas Heart Institute Journal, 37*(2), 141–148. Retrieved from http://www.ncbi.nlm.nih.gov/pmc/articles/PMC2851417/
33. Wee, Y., Burns, K., & Bett, N. (2015). Medical management of chronic stable angina. *Australian Prescriber, 38*(4), 131–136. http://dx.doi.org/10.18773/austprescr.2015.042
34. Graham, I. M., Fallon, N., Ingram, S., Leong, J. G., O'Doherty, V., Maher, V., & Benson, S. E. (2011). Rehabilitation of the patient with coronary heart disease. In V. Fuster, R. A. Walsh, & R. A. Harrington (Eds.), *Hurst's the heart* (13th ed., Vol. 2, pp. 1513–1530). New York: McGraw Hill.
35. Anderson, L., & Taylor, R. S. (2014). Cardiac rehabilitation for people with heart disease: An overview of Cochrane systematic reviews. *Cochrane Database of Systematic Reviews*, 12. doi:10.1002/14651858.CD011273.pub2
36. Anderson, L., Thompson, D. R., Oldridge, N., Zwisler, A. D., Rees, K., Martin, N., & Taylor, R. S. (2016). Exercise-based cardiac rehabilitation for coronary heart disease. *Cochrane Database of Systematic Reviews*, 1. doi:10.1002/14651858.CD001800.pub3
37. McCarthy, B., Casey, D., Devane, D., Murphy, K., Murphy, E., & Lacasse, Y. (2015). Pulmonary rehabilitation for chronic obstructive pulmonary disease. *Cochrane Database of Systematic Reviews*, 2. doi:10.1002/14651858.CD003793.pub3
38. Puhan, M. A., Gimeno-Santos, E., Scharplatz, M., Troosters, T., Walters, E. H., & Steurer, J. (2011). Pulmonary rehabilitation

following exacerbations of chronic obstructive pulmonary disease. *Cochrane Database of Systematic Reviews*, 10. doi:10.1002/14651858.CD005305.pub3

39. American Association of Cardiovascular and Pulmonary Rehabilitation. (2011). *Guidelines for pulmonary rehabilitation programs* (4th ed.). Champaign, IL: Human Kinetics.
40. Hand, C., Law, M., & McColl, M. A. (2011). Occupational therapy interventions for chronic disease: A scoping review. *American Journal of Occupational Therapy*, 65(4), 428–436. doi:10.5014/ajot.2011.002071
41. Austin, J., Williams, R., Ross, L., Moseley, L., & Hutchison, S. (2005). Randomised controlled trial of cardiac rehabilitation in elderly patients with heart failure. *European Journal of Heart Failure, 7*(3), 411–417.
42. Jianu, A., & Macovei, S. (2011). The occupational therapy impact on the recovery of convalescent elderly people after an acute myocardial infarction. *Palestrica of the Third Millennium, Civilization and Sport, 13*(10), 23–26.
43. Martinsen, U., Bentzen, H., Holter, M. K., Nilsen, T., Skullerud, H., Mowinckel, P., & Kjeken, I. (2016). The effect of occupational therapy in patients with chronic obstructive pulmonary disease: A randomized controlled trial. *Scandinavian Journal of Occupational Therapy*. Advance online publication. doi:10.3109/11038128.2016.1158316Jhjlh
44. Norweg, A. M., Whiteson, J., Malgady, R., Mola, A., & Rey, M. (2005). The effectiveness of different combinations of pulmonary rehabilitation components: A randomized controlled trial. *Chest, 128*(2), 663–672. doi:10.1378/chest.128.2.663
45. Lorenzi, C. M., Cilione, C., Rizzardi, R., Furino, V., Bellantone, T., Lugil, D., & Clini, E. (2004). Occupational therapy and pulmonary rehabilitation of disabled COPD patients. *Respiration, 71*(3), 246–251. doi:10.1159/00007742244
46. Ainsworth, B. E., Haskell, W. L., Hermann, S. D., Meckes, N., Bassett, D. R., Tudor-Locke, C., ... & Leon, A. S. (2011). Compendium of physical activities: A second update of codes and MET values. *Medicine and Science in Sports and Exercise, 43*(80), 1575–1581.
47. Levine, G. N., Steinke, E. E., Bakaeen, F. G., Bozkurt, B., Cheitlin, M. D., Contin, J. B. ... & Stewart, W. J. (2012). Sexual activity and cardiovascular disease: A scientific statement from the American Heart Association. *Circulation, 125*, 1058–1172. doi:10.1161/CIR.0b013e3182447787
48. American College of Sports Medicine. (2014). *ACMS's guidelines for exercise testing and prescription* (9th ed.). Philadelphia: Lippincott Williams & Wilkins.
49. Cabello, J. B., Burls, A., Emparanza, J. I., Bayliss, S., & Quinn, T. (2013). Oxygen therapy for acute myocardial infarction. *Cochrane Database of Systematic Reviews, 8*(CD0071670). doi:10.1002/14651858.CD007160.pub3
50. Celli, B. R. (2009). Pathophysiology of chronic obstructive pulmonary disease. In J. Hodgkin, B. R. Celli, & G. L. Connors (Eds.), *Pulmonary rehabilitation: Guidelines to success*. St. Louis: Mosby Elsevier.
51. American Lung Association. (2015). Understanding COPD. Retrieved from http://www.lung.org/lung-disease/copd/about-copd/understanding-copd.html
52. Chan, S. C. C. (2004). Chronic obstructive pulmonary disease and engagement in occupation. *American Journal of Occupational Therapy, 58*, 408–415.
53. Centers for Disease Control and Prevention. (2016). Burden of tobacco use in the U.S. Retrieved from http://www.cdc.gov/tobacco/campaign/tips/resources/data/cigarette-smoking-in-united-states.html
54. American Lung Association. (2010). Smoking and older adults. Retrieved from http://ala1-old.pub30.convio.net/stop-smoking/about-smoking/facts-figures/smoking-and-older-adults.html?referrer=https://www.google.com/
55. Roig, M., Eng, J. J., MacIntyre, D. L., Road, J. D., & Reid, W. D. (2011). Postural control is impaired in people with COPD: An observational study. *Physiotherapy Canada, 63*(4), 423–431. doi:10.3138/ptc.2010-32
56. Thakur, N., Blanc, P. D., Julian, L. J., Yelin, E. H., Katz, P. P., Sidney, S., ... & Eisner, M. D. (2010). COPD and cognitive impairment: The role of hypoxemia and oxygen therapy. *International Journal of Chronic Obstructive Pulmonary Disease*, 5, 263–269. http://dx.doi.org/10.2147/COPD.S10684
57. Nalysnyk, L., Cid-Ruzafa, J., Rotella, P., & Esser, D. (2012). Incidence and prevalence of idiopathic pulmonary fibrosis: Review of the literature. *European Respiratory Review, 21*(126), 355–361. doi:10.1183/09059180.00002512
58. Campbell, P. W., & Marshall, B. C. (2013). *Patient registry annual data report: 2013* [Booklet]. Retrieved from https://www.cff.org/2013_CFF_Patient_Registry_Annual_Data_Report.pdf
59. Cystic Fibrosis Foundation. (2015). About cystic fibrosis. Retrieved from https://www.cff.org/What-is-CF/About-Cystic-Fibrosis/
60. Saiman, L., Siegal, J. D., LiPuma, T. J., Brown, R. F., Bryson, E. A., Chambers, M. J., ... & Tullis, E. (2014). Infection prevention and control guideline for cystic fibrosis: 2013 update. *Infection Control and Hospital Epidemiology, 35*(S1), S1–S67.
61. Donath, J., & Miller, A. (2009). Restrictive chest wall disorders. *Seminars in Respiratory Critical Care Medicine, 30*(3), 275–292.
62. Spruit, M. A., Singh, S. J., Garvey, C., ZuWallack, R., Nici L., Rochester, C., ... & Wouters, E. F. M. (2013). An official American Thoracic Society/European Respiratory Society statement: Key concepts and advances in pulmonary rehabilitation. *American Journal of Respiratory Critical Care Medicine, 188*(8), e13–e64. doi:10.1164/rccm.201309-1634ST
63. Causey, R. (2013). Pulmonary rehabilitation in skilled nursing facilities. *OT Practice, 18*(21), 13–17.
64. Levack, M. M. (2014). Sexual wellbeing for people with chronic obstructive pulmonary disease: Relevance and roles for physiotherapy. *New Zealand Journal of Physiotherapy, 42*(2), 170–176.
65. Yende, S., G., Waterer, W., Tolley, E. A., Newman, A. B., Bauer, D. C., Taaffe, D. R., ... & Kritchevsky, S. B. (2006). Inflammatory markers are associated with ventilator limitation and muscle dysfunction in obstructive lung disease in well functioning elderly subjects. *Thorax, 61*(1), 10–16. doi:10.1136/thx.2004.034181
66. Coppola, S. & Wood, W. (2009). Occupational therapy to promote function and health-related quality of life. In J. Hodgkin, B. R. Celli, & G. L. Connors (Eds.), *Pulmonary rehabilitation: Guidelines to success*. St. Louis: Mosby Elsevier.
67. Fink, J. B. (2007). Forced expiratory technique, directed cough, and autogenic drainage. *Respiratory Care, 52*, 1210–1221. Retrieved from http://www.rcjournal.com/
68. Ball, J. W., Flynn, J. A., Solomon, B. S., & Stewart, R. W. (2015) Vital signs and pain assessment. *Seidel's guide to physical examination*. St. Louis: Elsevier/Mosby. Retrieved from http://www.ebrary.com
69. Redfern, J., & Briffa, T. (2011). Cardiac rehabilitation—Moving forward with new models of care. *Physical Therapy Reviews, 16*(1), 31–38.
70. Tiep, B. L., & Carter, R. (2009). Therapeutic oxygen. In J. Hodgkin, B. R. Celli, & G. L. Connors (Eds.), *Pulmonary rehabilitation: Guidelines to success*. St. Louis: Mosby Elsevier.
71. LeBlond, R. F., Brown, D. D, Suneja, M., & Szot, J. F. (Eds.). (2015). *DeGowin's diagnostic examination* (10th ed.). New York: McGraw-Hill Education/Medical.
72. Borg, G. (1982). Psychophysical bases of perceived exertion. *Medicine and Science in Sports Exercise, 14*, 377–381.
73. American Association of Cardiovascular and Pulmonary Rehabilitation. (2004). *Guidelines for pulmonary rehabilitation programs* (3rd ed.). Champaign, IL: Human Kinetics.

Chapter 27

Bariatric Factors and Management

Lisa Pierce, COTA/L, LLCC, CEAS

LEARNING OUTCOMES

After studying this chapter, the student or practitioner will be able to:

27.1 Identify the factors that contribute to the body mass index scale and its interpretation
27.2 Identify the risk factors that contribute to obesity
27.3 Describe the medical and surgical procedures used to assist clients who are obese to lose weight
27.4 Explain the roles of the interdisciplinary healthcare team with the client who is obese or morbidly obese
27.5 Describe the role of the occupational therapy assistant in facilitating the client who is obese to establish new habits and routines
27.6 Select multiple occupational therapy interventions appropriate for use with this client population

KEY TERMS

Bariatric	Obese
Body mass index (BMI)	Panniculus
Lipedema	Pitting edema
Lymphedema	Stemmer's sign
Maceration	Super obese
Morbidly obese	

The number of obese and overweight people in the United States is on the rise, and obesity-related conditions are some of the leading causes of preventable deaths in the United States. According to the World Health Organization (WHO), the prevalence of obesity worldwide tripled from 1975 to 2016, with 39 percent of adults 18 or older considered overweight as of 2016.[1] Occupational therapy assistants (OTAs) will encounter clients who are not only **obese** (over 20% higher than expected weight) but who are **morbidly obese** (100 pounds or more overweight). These clients have most likely been ridiculed and discriminated against by family, peers, and society, and may have also experienced negative comments from healthcare providers. OTAs must be sensitive to the needs of the clients who are obese as well as the needs of healthcare professionals and caregivers who work with this population. It is important to realize that obesity is a chronic disease and that OTAs cannot cure the situation, but can assist in restructuring and adapting the client's lifestyle to be more productive.

The term **bariatric** refers to a branch of medicine that deals with all stages of obesity—from its cause to its treatment. Obesity occurs when the caloric intake is consistently greater than the activity level performed on a daily basis. One of the measuring tools used to determine whether a person is overweight versus obese is the **body mass index (BMI)** (Table 27-1).[2]

BMI can be used as an assessment and screening tool and to monitor for overweight and obesity, however the results can differ depending on the client's overall status. For example, BMI can underestimate or overestimate the amount of body fat a client has depending on the musculature or the amount of edema. A weight lifter could have an excessive amount of muscle mass, whereas an older adult would most likely have less due to muscle wasting. Clients with edema have less amounts of fat compared with clients without edema. Therefore, clinical judgment must be used when interpreting BMI because of situations that may affect its accuracy.

How to calculate BMI:

1. Weight × 703 (imperial conversion factor)
2. Height × height

TABLE 27-1 BMI Standard Weight Categories[3]

BMI	WEIGHT STATUS
Below 18.5	Underweight
18.5–24.9	Normal/healthy weight
25.0–29.9	Overweight
30.0–39.9	Obese
40.0–49.9	Morbidly obese
50.0 or 59.9	Super obese
60.0 and above	Super-super obese

3. Divide the weight answer by the height answer to get the BMI.
   Example: A female who is 5 ft. 7 in. tall and weighs 263 lbs.
   1. $263 \times 703 = 184{,}889$
   2. $67 \times 67 = 4{,}489$
   3. $184{,}889 \div 4{,}489 = 41.18$

After referring to Table 27-1, the client in the previous example who has a BMI of 41.18 would be categorized as morbidly obese. The National Institutes of Health furthermore designates any person 100 pounds or more overweight as morbidly obese.[4] The connection between BMI and risk for disease varies from person to person. A client that presents as overweight can have multiple risk factors, whereas a client who is obese may present with fewer, depending on other risk factors.

RISK FACTORS

Despite the stigma of obesity, overeating is not its only cause. Several contributing factors may lead to obesity, including genetics, lifestyle, emotions/depression, lack of sleep, medications, age, and some medical conditions (Table 27-2).[4–8] Certain hormone problems that can cause obesity and are not necessarily linked to overeating include hypothyroidism (underactive thyroid), Cushing's syndrome, and polycystic ovary (ovarian in some cases) syndrome (PCOS).[9] With hypothyroidism, the client may have an underactive thyroid gland with decreased metabolism, weakness, and feeling tired, which may cause weight gain. Cushing's syndrome is a condition in which the body's adrenal glands make too much of the hormone cortisol, or it may also develop if the client takes high doses of certain medicines, such as prednisone, for long periods. People who have Cushing's syndrome gain weight around the neck, face, and trunk/stomach primarily. PCOS is a condition that affects about 5% to 10% of women of childbearing age, and between 40%–80% of women with this condition are classified as overweight or obese.[10]

MEDICAL TREATMENT

Multiple treatment strategies are available that should be considered when working with a client who is obese, including physical activity, dietary, behavioral, pharmacological, and surgical procedures.[11] There are many "fad" diets and supposed "treatments" for weight loss that can

TABLE 27-2 Contributing Factors That May Lead to Obesity[9]

Genetics	Genes may affect where and how much of the fat is distributed as well as partially affect the client's resting metabolic rate.
Lifestyle	A person develops and changes habits from childhood to adulthood, whether good or bad. These may include eating style, activity levels, and overall lifestyle.
Environment	Work schedules, lack of access to healthy foods, lack of access to safe outdoor spaces or gym facilities, food advertising, oversized food portions.
Emotional	Some people tend to eat more when they are experiencing anger, sadness, boredom, and stress. Over a period of time, this can cause weight gain.
Lack of sleep	A body requires a certain amount of sleep to maintain proper balance. If a client does not get enough sleep, they can develop hormonal changes that could increase appetite and cravings for carbohydrates.
Medications	Some of the medication one might take could contribute to weight gain. These medications include but are not limited to corticosteroids, antidepressants, and seizure medications. The medications can change the rate at which the body burns calories, increase appetite, and cause fluid retention, all which can lead to weight gain.
Age	Obesity can occur at any age. As people age, they are more susceptible to weight gain due to reduction in muscle mass, becoming less active, having decreased metabolism, and hormone changes.
Medical conditions	Some medical conditions can contribute to obesity. Musculoskeletal (e.g., arthritis), cardiac (e.g., atrial fibrillation), and respiratory (e.g., COPD) conditions can limit the amount of activity that is tolerable. If the amount of intake is not controlled to compensate for the decreased amount of activity, weight gain will likely ensue.

have harmful effects on the body through poor nutrition and severe calorie restriction, slower metabolism, and rapid weight loss. The OTA can encourage clients to work with qualified healthcare professionals to assist with weight management and lifestyle changes.

Physical Activity

Physical activity should always be a part of a treatment program with the client who is obese. Clients must maintain strength and mobility to prevent further weight gain. When initially starting an activity, the client might require initial clearance by a physician, supervision for adequate performance, injury prevention, and encouragement for follow-through with the task. Some clients may start with moving in the water or walking to begin to increase their endurance in a gentle way. For most clients who are obese, the initiation of activities would begin at a slow pace and increase in time and intensity as the client presents with increased endurance, strength, motivation, as well as weight reduction.

Dietary Treatment

Dietary treatment consists of education on the types and the amount of food that would benefit the client's nutritional balance and weight-loss goals. It is beneficial for the client to meet with a dietitian for education and counseling on the amount of caloric intake and types of foods that would be appropriate for the client's needs. The OTA can assist the client in organizing kitchen cabinets, preparing and packaging proper-portion meals (set by a dietary team) ahead of time, and educating and assisting with organizing shopping lists and maintaining food diary logs.

TECHNOLOGY AND TRENDS

As technology has made life easier, it has also led people to become increasingly sedentary. From early childhood onward, many are drawn to television, movies, phones, tablets, computers, games, and so on, which are typically used in a sitting or lying position. Rarely does one walk to the store, harvest food, or perform many more active routines as were completed in the past. Most communities are set up for driving versus walking or biking between locations. It may not be as much about total calorie consumption but about how the body uses those calories. The OTA can assist the client who is overweight or obese to use technology to help with management. Behavioral strategies through technology might be a tracker of steps taken, an online food/exercise journal, or even recommending a height-adjustable desk for standing. Phones can be set with reminders to get up and move every hour or more. Some individuals have set personal rules that the television is only on for a certain period a day or only when accompanied by movement or exercise. The OTA can assist with leisure exploration for pursuits that are more active yet enjoyable, or gaming that involves movement such as the Wii® system. The OTA is in a position to recommend increased activity, exercise, and movement with technological options to assist all clients.

Behavioral Strategies

Behavioral strategies provide techniques to help the client comply with the new diet and physical activity. This is a very important part of the treatment not only for the client but also for the family and friends. Family members and friends can inadvertently become food "enablers" to the obese client by providing nonhealthy foods, encouraging unhealthy eating (e.g., "Don't you want some more cake?"), and offering comfort verbal responses (e.g., "You look fine the way you are!"). If clients who are obese do not identify with the life event or behaviors that have contributed to the development of poor habits, they will experience a vicious cycle of weight loss and gain. The more psychologically and emotionally damaged the client feels, the greater chance of poor eating habits, social isolation, decreased motivation, and negative self-worth. It is beneficial to the client to seek professional counseling and assistance, such as from a psychologist, clergy member, or fitness trainer, to address and recognize the causes and contributing factors. The OTA can educate and assist the client in keeping a daily journal for a set period of time. Generally, have clients record when they get the urge to eat, specifically, what is happening at that particular time, their mood, what they consumed, and how they felt after consumption. Keeping a journal can increase awareness and possibly assist with recognizing the triggers to overeating. It would be beneficial for the OTA to provide education to the family members and friends about the importance of positive, appropriate support and techniques on how they can assist the client with this lifestyle change.

Pharmacological

Several weight-loss medications are currently available by prescription or over-the-counter. Most of the medications have side effects (e.g., headache, dry mouth, constipation, insomnia, diarrhea, oily stools, gas, flatulence) and should only be used by clients who present with an increased medical risk from the obesity and are under the care of a physician. The assumption is that the medical benefit would outweigh the side effects of the medication.

Surgery

Surgery is usually reserved for clients who are morbidly obese who have tried other methods of weight loss, have failed, and present with comorbid conditions. Bariatric surgeries alter the digestive process; the different types include:[15]

1. Restrictive operations that limit food intake by reducing the amount of food the stomach can hold (separating the stomach into two pouches—one smaller than the other) and slowing the passage of

EVIDENCE-BASED PRACTICE

Nearly every time a client is diagnosed with type 2 diabetes, the drug of choice is Metformin, and he or she is also typically prescribed lifestyle modifications that may include diet and exercise. A number of studies have been performed on the effects of Metformin and physical activity. Several studies have suggested that, compared with either intervention alone, the combination of Metformin and exercise often is no better, and sometimes even worse, at improving glycemic control.[12] Metformin has been shown to increase heart rate and lactic acid concentrations, which is considered the opposite of what would be expected with an exercise routine.[13] Some studies have found better blood sugar control if the exercise was after the breakfast meal than before it in a fasting mode. Certainly, factors such as insulin sensitivity and other cardiovascular disease risk factors, and other outcomes such as fitness and exercise metabolism all need to be considered as well.[12] It would seem that beyond the blood sugar effects, exercise has other positive benefits to a client with diabetes such as improved body image and well-being, improved quality of life, weight loss, cardiovascular fitness, and decreased impact on joints. There have also been studies noting that for overweight and obese individuals with type 2 diabetes an intensive behavioral intervention that focused on weight loss and increased physical activity resulted in fewer hospitalizations, fewer days in the hospital, and less use of prescription medications.[14] It is a complicated issue that is still being researched and affects millions of clients on a daily basis.

Boulé, N. G. (2016). Exercise plus Metformin in the fight against diabetes. Exercise and Sports Sciences Reviews, *44(1),2.*

Boulé, N. G. (2011). Metformin and exercise in type 2 diabetes. Diabetes Care, *34(7), 1469–1474. doi:10.2337/dc 10-2207.*

Espeland, M. A., Glick, H. A., Bertoni, A., Brancati F. L., Bray, G. A., Clark J. M. ... & Zhang, P. (2014). Impact of an intensive lifestyle intervention on use and cost of medical services among overweight and obese adults with type 2 diabetes: The action for health in diabetes. Diabetes Care, *37(9), 2548–2556. http://dx.doi.org/10.2337/dc14-0093*

food to the stomach. Types of restrictive operations include:

- Adjustable gastric banding (ABG) or lap band surgery: Attaching an inflatable band around the top portion of the stomach and tightening it like a belt. This can be altered by the surgeon after the procedure by increasing/decreasing the amount of saline in the band through a port under the skin. Problems that can occur after band placement include nausea, vomiting, acid reflux, heartburn, stomach ulcer, gastritis, gas bloat, trouble swallowing, dehydration, diarrhea, constipation, and weight regain. The band may deflate if a leak occurs in the tubing, the port, or the band itself.
- Vertical banded gastroplasty (VBG): Utilizes a combination of band and staples to separate the stomach to create the small pouch. Ongoing nausea and vomiting is common if too much food is consumed.
- Vertical sleeve gastrectomy (VSG): Removes a large portion of the stomach (gastric sleeve). Common side effects of VSG are diarrhea, vomiting, and dumping syndrome (sweating, flushing, lightheadedness, rapid heart rate, palpitations, upper abdominal fullness, nausea, diarrhea, cramping, and active audible bowels sounds).

2. A malabsorptive operation does not limit food intake, but bypasses the intestines. By avoiding the intestines, the surgery allows for less caloric absorption and increased weight loss. However, one must be mindful that this also limits absorption of nutrients as well. There is only one type of malabsorptive operation:
   - Biliopancreatic diversion (BPD or duodenal switch): This is the most complicated operation. It involves removal of the lower portion of the stomach, then connects to the small intestines and bypasses the duodenum and jejunum. Side effects can be diarrhea, nausea, vomiting, flatulence, nutritional deficiencies, and dumping syndrome.
3. Combined restrictive/malabsorptive operations (RGB): This is the most common type of bariatric surgery; it combines restrictive and malabsorptive procedures.
   - Gastric bypass (Roux-en-Y or RNY): This is the most common bariatric procedure performed. The procedure takes the top portion of the stomach, creates a small pouch, then attaches it directly to the small intestine. Common problems following gastric bypass include gallstones, kidney stones, hypoglycemia (low blood sugar), diarrhea, anemia (low iron), dumping syndrome, and nutritional deficiencies.
4. Gastric balloon: Either one or two inflated balloons are inserted into the stomach to cause the client to feel full sooner and eat less food. The balloons are generally left in about 6 months, and are meant to jump-start a weight-loss program.
5. Vagal nerve block (VBloc): A rechargeable neuroregulator device is implanted under the skin. Flexible leads are placed around the vagus nerve that intermittently block signals, reducing hunger and increasing feelings of fullness. Complaints are rare, but do include tingling of the throat, pain, heartburn, nausea, difficulty swallowing, belching and/or abdominal cramping.

Financial Costs of Obesity

The financial cost for a person who is obese from medical services, durable medical equipment (DME), to everyday clothing is often far more expensive than that of an average-weight person. Clients who are obese may face limitations for medical services secondary to those not covered by insurance, as some procedures could be viewed as "cosmetic" services, and the client would have to pay for them out of pocket. An example might be excess skin removal after weight loss. DME is usually more expensive due to the amount of and higher quality of materials utilized in making of the equipment. Clothing could cost more due the amount of fabric utilized and, depending on the size, could be difficult to find and may have to be custom made. Barriers may also exist within the home that might prevent the client from remaining at that location. The client may not have the finances to have reinforced flooring placed, to purchase heavy-duty furniture to accommodate their weight, or widen doorways that the client might not be able to pass through. A wheelchair lift on a vehicle is generally rated to 500 pounds, but a heavy-duty power wheelchair can be over 525 pounds by itself. Transportation is another large expense that the client may face. Depending on a client's overall size, he or she might not be able to drive their car secondary to girth and be forced to rely on other means of transportation. The cost of traveling could be more expensive if traveling by bus or plane, as some facilities require the person to purchase an extra ticket to accommodate girth.

IMPAIRMENTS AND CLIENT FACTORS

The client who is obese certainly faces numerous impairments and client factors that could impede occupation and performance of activities of daily living (ADLs) and instrumental activities of daily living (IADLs). Impairments and complications that can occur with obesity are addressed in the following sections.

Physical/Motor

Impairments in body structures and body functions can be some of the most debilitating and challenging factors for the client who is obese. One example of a physical challenge is joint stability. An average person's body and joints endure significant stress on any given day; this is especially true of a client who is obese. The excessive amount of weight, weight distribution, and activity on the joint can cause problems not only with the cartilage between the joints but with the muscles and ligaments. Osteoarthritis (OA) is one potential risk to the joints of a client who is obese. As the cartilage between the joints deteriorates from excessive force (weight) and repetitive movements, the joint space becomes smaller and ligaments become lax. Clients who are obese tend to compensate for the joint issues when performing functional mobility. Over a period of time, the OTA will likely notice the client walking with "stiff legs" (quadriceps avoidance) with very little, if any, bend at the knee. Quadriceps avoidance limits the amount of quadriceps control of the knee flexion and creates an increased amount of impact shock through the joint.[16] This increased shock leads to damage in the joint.

> **THE OLDER ADULT**
>
> Obesity presents with several medical complications and can affect one's quality of life. However, the older adult that is obese may have an escalated decline in physical function due to decreased muscle mass, decreased strength, and arthritis. A complicating factor is primarily related to sarcopenia, the progressive loss of muscle and gain in fat that come with aging.[17] What exactly constitutes obesity in older adults, who naturally undergo changes in body composition as they age? BMI may be misleading with the elderly because of the higher percentage of fat and the lower percentage of lean muscle mass. Weight-loss treatment for the older adult can be complicated, as obesity provides some benefits as well as harm. Some of the benefits of obesity in older adults include an increase in bone density; increase in hormonal factors—which can be beneficial by stimulating bone growth and remodeling; and extra cushioning around the trochanter to provide hip fracture protection during a fall. Some of the negative aspects include an increase in arthritis (especially OA) from years of heavy weight-bearing on joints; urinary incontinence that is related to BMI; cancer (especially breast cancer in women); and metabolic disorders. When treating an older adult, the treatment approach would be different than that for a younger person, primarily because of the importance of preventing loss of muscle with intentional weight loss.[17] People of all ages who lose weight intentionally lose fat and, to a lesser extent, skeletal muscle, but older clients have already lost some muscle mass and the overall effect can be exaggerated.[17] Further changes in body composition can be limited by consuming a diet with high-quality protein and by performing resistance and weight training.

Another physical challenge the client who is obese faces is management of the panniculus (sometimes mistakenly called pannus), which is the excessive adipose (fat) tissue in the lower abdominal region that hangs down, creating an increased pull against the client's lower back. This can create pain by adding increased pressure on the lower extremities (LEs), hinder daily activities, interfere with ambulation, and cause lymphedema. Urinary stress incontinence can also result from pressure on the pelvic and abdominal organs from the weight of the panniculus. Depending on the severity of the panniculus, hygiene and skin integrity may also present problems. When working with the client who is obese with a panniculus, it is important to educate him or her and demonstrate compensatory techniques to assist with hygiene and **maceration** (excessive moisture in contact with the skin) management (Box 27-1). The panniculus severity is graded on the appearance of the panniculus as seen in the following table and figure (Table 27-3 and Fig. 27-1).

HYGIENE MANAGEMENT

Most clients who are obese have to learn compensatory techniques to assist them when performing ADLs. Hygiene under the panniculus is a very important area to address

BOX 27-1
Moisture Management Tip

Some hospital settings carry products in their wound care supplies that wick away moisture, however they are often expensive. If unable to utilize a product, the client can use a soft, clean white bath towel. Instruct and/or assist the client in folding the towel lengthwise and placing it under the panniculus to provide a barrier. It is important to remind the client to monitor and change the towels frequently when excessive moisture is present.

TABLE 27-3 Panniculus Severity Grades

GRADE	PANNICULUS APPEARANCE
Grade 1	The panniculus covers the hairline of the pubic symphysis region.
Grade 2	The panniculus covers the entire genital region.
Grade 3	The panniculus covers down to the upper thigh area.
Grade 4	The panniculus covers down to the mid-thigh area.
Grade 5	The panniculus covers down to the knees and below.

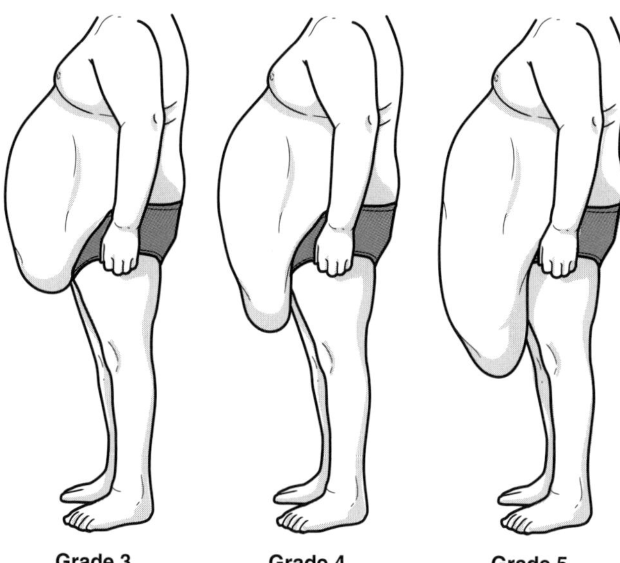

FIGURE 27-1. Three of the stages of panniculus: Grades 3, 4, and 5.

due to the moisture and the constant pressure to the area. Depending on the severity of the panniculus and the client's respiratory status, have the client lie in supine position or a slight Trendelenburg position (supine with feet higher than the head), if available, to assist with positioning the panniculus in reverse position. Doing this not only allows for thorough cleaning of the area beneath the panniculus, but also provides pressure relief. Some clients utilize a bath towel versus a washcloth to bathe the area due to its size and location. Utilizing a bath towel enables the client to hold both ends of the towel to control cleaning movements and reach the area more thoroughly.

Sensory

Most clients who are obese present with pain and sensitivity as well as proprioception issues. For example, a client with a grade 3 or greater panniculus could develop back pain due to the forward pull of the tissue as well as skin sensitivity with maceration and possible nerve compromise. Excessive pain and sensitivity can also contribute to an increase in sedentary lifestyle. The OTA must address pain by providing positioning and pressure-relieving devices, such as foam, gel, and low air-loss or alternating pressure specialty cushions and mattresses; encouraging low-impact exercise and functional mobility; and engaging in discussion with the interdisciplinary team in reference to pain medication. Clients who are wheelchair users or bedbound can present with decreased sensation and may become unaware of lines and tubes under their bodies and in their skin folds. Therefore, the OTA must be aware of catheter tubing placement, take precautions with the use of bedpans, and monitor for ill-fitting seating devices as prolonged pressure can initiate skin breakdown. The OTA must also educate the client to be aware of these risks and consistently monitor for excessive redness and skin breakdown.

Emotional

Obesity, whether primary cause or secondary, can trigger emotional responses, which include depression, eating disorders, poor body image, low self-esteem, hopelessness, guilt, social isolation, sexual dysfunction, anger, boredom, and feelings of worthlessness.[18] Many clients who are obese use food as a defense mechanism to deflect unwanted feelings, and food can become a coping strategy over time. It is important to assist the client in recognizing the root problem that has brought on the emotion and assist in the method for dealing with this problem. The OTA can assist the client with coping mechanisms, such as problem-solving, relaxation techniques, physical activities or hobbies, and seeking support groups. However, many clients can benefit from behavioral and psychological counseling as part of the interdisciplinary approach. The role of the psychologist is important not only for the behavioral treatment but also for presurgical and postsurgical support, should the client have bariatric surgery.

Complications

Obesity can increase one's risk for developing any number of serious health complications. Some of the complications associated with obesity include, but are not limited to, heart disease, diabetes, respiratory issues, deep vein thrombosis, pulmonary embolism, lymphedema/lipedema, and skin breakdown. The following sections will discuss implications of the disease and OTA's role when treating the client.

HEART DISEASE/CARDIOVASCULAR DISEASE

Cardiovascular disease (CVD) is the narrowing or blocking of blood vessels that affect the heart muscle, valves, or rhythm. A group of disorders that are classified as CVD include:[9,19]

- Cerebrovascular disease: A disease of the blood vessels that supply the brain
- Coronary artery disease: A disease of the blood vessels that supply the heart muscle
- Peripheral arterial disease: A disease of the blood vessels that supply the arms and legs
- Rheumatic heart disease: Damage to the heart muscle and valves from rheumatic fever
- Congenital heart disease: Malformation of the heart structure at birth
- Deep vein thrombosis/pulmonary embolism: Blood clots

The client who is overweight or obese with hypertension (high blood pressure), elevated glucose levels (high blood sugar), and elevated lipids (fats, oils, and cholesterol) has a higher risk for developing CVD. Studies have shown that clients with a BMI greater than 30 have an increased risk for developing CVD as well. This development is caused by an increase in the cardiac workload due to fluid retention and weight gain. The increased cardiac workload is thought to be due to the physiological changes that occur in the heart because of increased blood volume and flow. Weight loss and increased activity can reduce progression and promote regression of CVD.[20]

DIABETES

Diabetes has two classifications, type 1 and type 2. Type 1 is a genetic condition that is generally diagnosed at a younger age, in which the body does not produce the insulin hormone. Type 2 generally occurs in adults due to obesity and other lifestyle factors, in which the body does not produce enough insulin to offset blood glucose levels. Clients who are obese are most commonly diagnosed with type 2 diabetes, which is usually associated with poor diet and lack of exercise. Excessive weight gain adds extra stress to the body's ability to maintain proper blood glucose levels and can cause the body to become resistant to insulin.[21,22] Type 2 diabetes can be managed through diet and exercise in the early stages of prediabetes, but generally requires the client to take oral medication and/or inject insulin in the later stages. In some clients, weight reduction, a change in diet, and increased exercise routine can reduce the amount of insulin and prevent diabetes if they are prediabetic.

RESPIRATORY ISSUES

An increase in the amount of fat tissue in the abdominal wall and around the organs limits movement of the diaphragm, decreasing lung expansion and capacity. The diminished lung expansion with inspiration may cause abnormal ventilation perfusion (amount of air and blood that reaches the alveoli) and arterial hypoxemia (low oxygen in the blood).[23]

Some types of respiratory disease and symptoms associated with obesity are:

- Aspiration pneumonia: An inflammation of the lung and bronchial tubes after inhalation of a foreign matter, potentially due to gastroesophageal reflux disease (GERD)
- Asthma: Chronic lung disease that inflames and narrows the airways
- Chronic obstructive pulmonary disease (COPD): An inflammation and thickening of the airways preventing adequate air exchange
- Pulmonary embolism (PE): Blood clot in the lung
- Obstructive sleep apnea syndrome (OSAS): Cessation or decrease in breathing during sleep caused by a partially blocked or narrowed airway
- Obesity hypoventilation syndrome (OHS): Lower oxygen and higher carbon dioxide levels in the blood due to poor breathing

When treating clients with compromised respiratory systems, the OTA should monitor vital signs before beginning, during, and upon completion of treatment, especially if exercise is a part of the treatment program. The most common vital signs monitored are:

- Pulse rate (heart rate, HR)[24] measures the number of times the heart beats per minute, heart rhythm, and strength of pulse. Normal pulse rate for a healthy adult is 60 to 100 beats per minute (with an average of 70).
- Respiratory rate (RR) measures the number of breaths per minute. Normal range for an adult is 12 to 20 breaths per minute.
- Blood Pressure (BP)[25,26] measures the force of the blood pushing against the artery walls. Chapter 26 has detailed instructions for taking blood pressure. The American Heart Association recommendations/ guidelines are as follows:
  - Normal: Systolic less than 120, diastolic less than 80
  - Prehypertension: Systolic 120 to 129, diastolic less than 80
  - Stage 1 hypertension: Systolic 130 to 139, diastolic 80 to 89
  - Stage 2 hypertension: Systolic 140+, diastolic 90+
  - Hypertensive crisis: Systolic 180+, diastolic 120+[26]
- Oxygen saturation (SpO_2) measures the client's oxygen levels in the blood. This can be measured by utilizing a pulse oximeter (pulse ox) on the finger or earlobe. Values less than 90% SpO_2 can be considered low (normal is 95 to 100% SpO_2). A client wearing dark nail polish may not have an accurate reading; in this case, remove the nail polish or take the oxygen saturation levels via the earlobe.

All vital sign ranges are only guidelines. OT practitioners should check the medical record and observe each client to determine the "normal" for that particular client, as medical conditions can cause a variance. One example of a variance could be a client with COPD. Normal target

SpO_2 would be lower for this client than the average client due to hypercapnia (CO_2 retention—elevated levels of carbon dioxide).

DEPRESSION

Depression has two components: psychological (cognitive), which affects mood, and physical (somatic), which affects appetite and sleep.[18,27] Studies have shown that depression can be 25% more likely to be present in the obese than in the general public, and it may be associated with poor self-image, lower self-esteem, and social isolation.[27] Having a poor body image or distorted body image (unrealistic view of one's body) is often associated with depression and eating behaviors. Some studies have suggested that gender and race also play a role, indicating that non-Hispanic white women who have depression have a higher rate of obesity than the same group without depression, and that the correlation does not exist in "non-Hispanic black and Mexican-American women".[27] Therefore, an uncertainty exists whether depression causes obesity or obesity causes depression. The OTA does not actively treat the depression itself, but can offer many ways to increase activity levels and improve quality of life. The OTA can assist by encouraging the client in active leisure pursuits and the ability to independently perform all areas of occupation.

DEEP VEIN THROMBOSIS AND PULMONARY EMBOLISM

Obesity is one of the risk factors for development of deep vein thrombosis (DVT), which is a clot that develops in the vein and prevents normal circulation.[28,29] A BMI that is greater than 39 places increased pressure on the veins in the legs and pelvic region. This, along with potentially decreased mobility and activity, increases the chance for development of a DVT. A major concern with DVT is a risk for dislodgement of the clot from its original site. If it dislodges, it may travel through the circulatory system to blood vessels in the lungs and cause blockage, otherwise known as a PE. PEs can be very serious and are potentially fatal. Clients with DVTs are usually started on anticoagulant therapy and/or receive inferior vena cava (IVC) filter placement. An IVC filter is an umbrella-shaped vascular filter that is implanted in the inferior vena cava via surgery to prevent venous emboli from entering the cardiopulmonary circulation.

Symptoms of a possible DVT include swelling, warmth, redness, and tenderness or pain in the leg at a specific site, often in the calf. If suspicious of a DVT, the OTA should have the client lie down and should notify the occupational therapist, nurse, or other medical professional (depending on the setting) regarding the concerns. The client is usually then placed on bedrest until cleared by the physician. Once the physician determines that the client has reached therapeutic levels of the blood thinner, the physician will recommend that OT treatment resume. Until cleared by the physician, the OTA should limit mobility, prevent rubbing of the affected limb, omit application of compression garments or obtaining blood pressure in the affected extremity, and avoid heat modalities to the area. The OTA is often the first professional to notice a potential DVT as he or she often sees the client for bathing and dressing, and may notice the associated abnormalities (Table 27-4).

LYMPHEDEMA AND LIPEDEMA

The lymphatic system transports bacteria, fluid from the tissues, and waste products to the lymph nodes, where filtration occurs. The protein-rich fluid (lymph) is then transported to the heart and back into circulation. **Lymphedema** usually presents as swelling in the lower part of the arms and legs with the client who is obese, but can encompass the entire extremity. Research has shown that obesity can be a risk factor for Type II lymphedema (Type II is classified as secondary acquired).[30,31] Lymphedema can initially appear as **pitting edema** (soft swollen area that leaves an indentation after gentle pressure applied and released). **Stemmer's sign** is a test for lymphedema, however it can present with false negative. The Stemmer sign is a thick fold of skin at the base of the second toe or finger. If the skin cannot be pinched and lifted, it could be a positive indication of lymphedema. If left untreated, lymphedema can result in decreased function of the limb, weeping, chronic infection (cellulitis), and skin breakdown.

The OTA can treat clients with lymphedema under the guidance of an occupational therapist, however, extra training and, in some cases, certification must first be obtained. Depending on the severity of lymphedema, management can be extremely complicated, and further education will be required. There are several institutes and companies that offer education in the management of lymphedema. Treatment of lymphedema could include: manual lymph drainage (a massage technique), application of compression wraps to the affected extremity, skin care, and range of motion (ROM) exercises to increase lymph flow.

Lipedema is characterized by a bilateral symmetrical increase in the stored fat, generally of the LE.[32] Lipedema may appear similar to lymphedema due to the increased size of body mass, however, it is a hormone-driven condition that progresses rapidly with weight gain, especially in females, and usually around puberty. Lipedema usually affects the hips, buttocks, and thighs, but seldom involves the feet. The accumulation of fat tends to be worse in people who are obese, but also affects people who are a normal weight. It

TABLE 27-4 DVT and PE Comparison

DVT SYMPTOMS	PE SYMPTOMS
Redness	Sudden onset of shortness of breath
Painful	Coughing up blood
Affected area swollen	Irregular/rapid heartbeat
Warm to touch	Discomfort with deep breath
	Chest pain

OT Practitioner's Viewpoint

I was honored to treat a client in the home health setting who was obese, had challenging medical issues with lymphedema, and was only 28 years of age. The client's lymphedema had gone untreated for several years, cellulitis developed, wounds occurred, and the client became basically bed bound due to the girth of his bilateral LEs. This client was also experiencing depression. Having extensive lymphedema training, I began to treat the client's bilateral LEs. The client's body began to respond well to the treatment as noted by a reduction in size and increased active movement of LEs. The client began to actively participate in ADLs and strengthening sessions, and was able to perform transfers. Upon discharge, the client was referred to an outpatient clinic for continued care of lymphedema, and returned home with his family. He was able to perform self-care tasks, ambulate with a walker, and, most importantly, he felt good about himself again, as he could function in society. ~ Lisa Pierce, COTA/L, LLCC, CEAS

should not be mistaken for obesity, as dieting does not make any difference to the condition.

Women often describe a feeling of heaviness in the LEs, which become painful in the advanced stages, and the LEs bruise easily. However, unlike lymphedema, clients with lipedema are not usually at risk for infections. An OTA can treat clients with lipedema after receiving specialized training. Treatment of lipedema could consist of ROM exercises, skin care, and lymph drainage. Due to the painfulness of the condition, drainage would need to be light and compression wraps mostly omitted. Some clients may seek a liposuction procedure for removal of fatty deposits (Table 27-5).

SKIN INTEGRITY AND PRESSURE INJURIES

Clients who are obese are at high risk for skin breakdown and pressure injuries.[31–33] Wound healing is noted to be slower due to poor nutrition, tension on wound edges, reduced perfusion (delivery of blood/fluid to the tissue), and emotional stress. Clients who are obese may experience maceration within the skin folds that can develop a fissure (narrow opening or slit in the skin), intertrigo (yeast infection within the skin folds), or dermatitis (inflammation of the skin). It is very important to assist and educate clients who are obese in hygiene and moisture management.

Pressure injuries are another common occurrence with the client who is obese due to weight and decreased mobility. This usually occurs with prolonged positioning over bony prominences with poor blood supply to fatty tissues, however it can also occur within the skin folds or from improper fit of the wheelchair. The OTA can assist the client with:

- Obtaining a proper wheelchair and pressure-relieving cushion (through a DME company and seating specialist or seating clinic)
- Educating and training the client on skin inspections to include adaptive equipment such as skin inspection mirror, if needed
- Education and training on weight shifting for pressure relief
- Education and training on the importance of turning and repositioning of the client with limited mobility as well as avoidance of certain positions when wounds are involved

TABLE 27-5 Lymphedema and Lipedema Comparison Table

LYMPHEDEMA	LIPEDEMA
Positive Stemmer sign	Negative Stemmer sign
Not symmetrical	Symmetrical
Foot involved	Foot noninvolved
Not painful to touch (normally)	Painful to touch
No bruise	Easy to bruise
No hormonal disturbances	Hormonal disturbances
Pitting edema	Nonpitting edema
Skin feels firmer	Skin feels rubbery

TREATMENT AND INTERVENTIONS

Treatment and interventions for obesity can be complicated for the client as well as the caregivers. In the following sections, the OTA will explore techniques to assist with caregiver fatigue and injury prevention as well as treatment approaches for the client who is obese.

Safe Handling for Caregivers

In most settings, the common complaint from caregivers is the inability to roll, position, and transfer the client who is obese due to lack of physical assist, lack of appropriate equipment, and lack of knowledge on techniques. As OT practitioners, it is important to educate caregivers and employees on safe handling techniques and make equipment recommendations to accommodate the client. If possible, it is better to make accommodations before arrival of the client at the facility or home from the hospital to allow time to obtain the proper equipment, training, and setup. There are several devices to assist with turning, repositioning, and transferring of the obese client who has limited mobility.

TURNING AND REPOSITIONING

Turning and repositioning of the client who is obese and who has limited mobility can put an increased strain on the healthcare practitioner or caregiver's body. Some facilities utilize sheets or draw sheets to turn and reposition the client. If this method is used, it is important to obtain enough physical assistance to properly roll and/or turn the client's body as a unit to maintain proper body alignment. Utilizing this technique evenly distributes the client's weight and decreases the amount of strain on both the client and caregiver. It is important to educate the caregivers on safe and proper body mechanics when performing tasks.

Suggestions for repositioning:

- Obtain enough physical assistance to safely turn the client, while being sensitive to the client's feelings regarding the need for extra staff and to avoid embarrassment for the client.
- Use the draw sheet lengthwise under the client to evenly distribute the body weight; this lessens the amount of strain for the caregiver and client.
- Use dense foam wedges instead of pillows for positioning. Dense foam will support more weight and maintain better alignment than pillows. Pillows are normally made with cotton or soft foam filling, therefore they are unable to provide enough support for positioning.
- Educate the caregivers and client on the importance of turning and repositioning. If a client is in one position for a prolonged period, this could initiate development of skin breakdown. Because of limited mobility, clients who are obese must be monitored closely for skin breakdown.

TRANSFERRING THE CLIENT WHO IS OBESE

When first meeting a client who is morbidly obese, it is easy to assume that the client is unable to independently transfer or ambulate. However, some clients have developed compensatory techniques to allow them to remain at a functional level. It is always best to allow clients to demonstrate or attempt to demonstrate their method of functional mobility if possible. When utilizing any transfer device, the OTA must make sure that the device can accommodate the client's weight. Assistive devices, transfer equipment, and mat tables have weight limits. Specialized equipment for the bariatric client is often labeled "EC," expanded capacity and includes the specific weight limit.

When performing any transfer with the client who is obese, it is important to first assess the client, available DME, and surroundings for safety. See Chapter 13 for more specific details about performing transfers. Ask these questions before initiating the transfer: Is the client stable for the type of transfer being performed? Can the client assist in the transfer? How many people are required to safely perform the transfer? Is there enough room to safely perform the transfer? Is there appropriate DME to accommodate the client's weight? The OTA should not judge the amount of assist required by reviewing a previous transfer; the client could have had a change in medical status or may not be feeling as strong that day.

Safe Transfer Guidelines:

- Have enough physical help to assist with transfer.
- Utilize transferring devices when possible (e.g., properly rated transfer board, patient lifts).
- Review step-by-step the intentions of the transfer with the client beforehand.
- Make sure to lock all wheels on the bed or wheelchair before transfer.
- Rolling a client in bed: Assist clients in turning their head in the direction of the roll. Once the head is turned, follow with the shoulders, hips, and LEs.
- Utilize a gait belt, when feasible, with any standing transfers.
- Instruct caregivers to be aware of body positioning at all times. Educate them to keep their knees and hips slightly bent, their back in alignment, and their stomach muscles contracted when transferring the client.
- Avoid twisting and jerking movements. Instead, perform small, smooth, steady steps toward the chair or bedside commode.

Devices Used for Transfers: When utilizing a transfer board for transfers to a wheelchair or bedside commode, it is important to prevent shearing (force or pressure against skin to cause skin compromise) during the transfer. Some methods to assist with reduction of shearing include: place the transfer board in a pillowcase to prevent skin-to-board contact, use a draw sheet or pad as a barrier between the skin and the transfer board, or have the client wear lower body clothing. Clients with increased upper-extremity (UE) strength can perform modified push-up scoots across the transfer board. Bariatric transfer boards have weight limits up to 600 pounds, while standard transfer boards can hold 250 to 300 pounds, depending on the brand.

A bariatric stand assist lift allows the caregiver to safely lift and transfer the client from one seated surface to another (bed, chair, and toilet) with minimal physical effort. The client must be able to sit at the edge of the bed and tolerate weight through the legs to utilize this lift. Bariatric stand assist lifts have weight limits up to 600 pounds, however the OTA must also be aware of girth limits.

An extra-wide walker can be utilized for standing transfers, and generally have weight limits up to 400 pounds, however be aware of girth limits (Fig. 27-2).

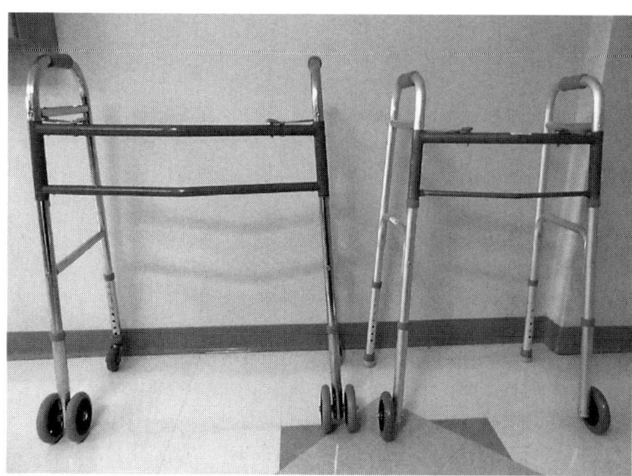

FIGURE 27-2. Bariatric and regular-size rolling walkers.

Glide lateral air transfer devices can also be used for safer transfers. Once the client is in a supine position, assist in rolling side to side for placement of the pad. Then, once the deflated pad is under the client, secure all straps across the client, attach air hoses, and inflate. The client can be transferred, in supine position only, from one flat surface to another with ease and with no skin shearing. The devices must be deflated once the transfer is complete and before changing of position. The glide lateral air device has weight limits up to 1,000 pounds (Fig. 27-3).

Z-Sliders® are comprised of plastic sheeting material folded over into a tube used to perform lateral transfers and reposition clients. The Z-Slider® is to be placed between the draw sheet and the bedsheet with the arrows pointing in the direction of the move. Once in place, the client can be pulled by a draw sheet laterally or pushed in the direction of the desired move as the Z-Slider® rolls upon itself. Upon completion of the transfer, remove the Z-Slider®; it can also be used to slide the client up in the bed.

Lifts and slings for the client who is obese can be used to lift the client dependently from one surface to another. The client is placed in the sling by rolling in bed, then the straps are attached, and the hoist lifts the client. The lifter can roll on the floor, be attached to a freestanding frame, or be mounted in the ceiling. Be aware of weight limits of each lift and the sling as they vary. Some lifts and slings can accommodate up to 1,000 pounds, but many have a 600 pound limit. Lifters can be found in hospitals, nursing homes, client homes, and some community facilities (to include pools). However, lifters for bariatric clients are limited in most facilities or unavailable, especially in community locations. Most lifters are not transportable due to the size and weight of the lift or availability of transport vehicle and physical assist. However, there are some portable lifters that are collapsible that have a weight limit up to 450 pounds.

The turn and position system (TAPS) is a system that assists with turning and repositioning the client who is immobile and obese. The system is made with low-friction material to reduce the amount of stress and strain on caregivers and reduce the shear and friction with turns and boosting of the client's body. The TAPS comes with a low-friction glide sheet to cover the bed and has Velcro® anchors to assist with positioning, dense foam wedges to help stay in the side-lying position, a top glide sheet that has boost straps, and microclimate disposable body pads. The TAPS sizes XL/XXL have a weight limit of 800 pounds.

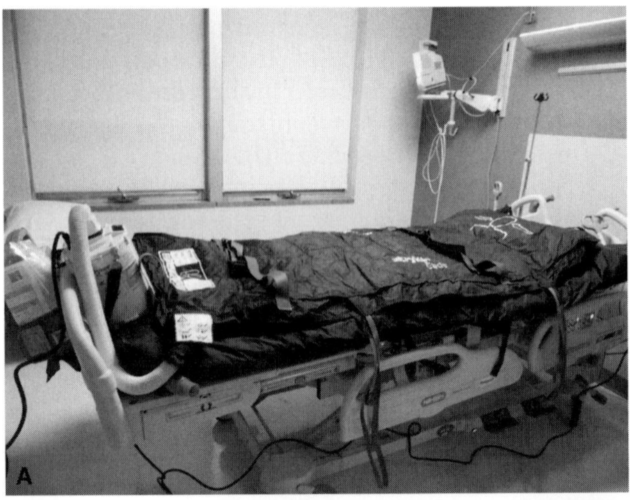

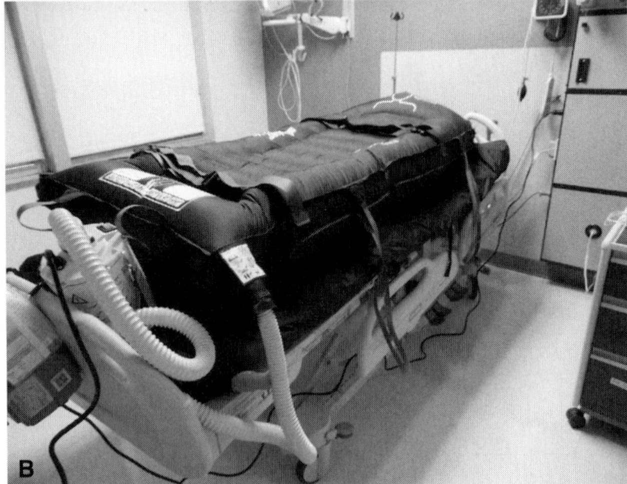

FIGURE 27-3. Glide lateral air transfer device. **(A)** Deflated and **(B)** inflated.

Treatment Approaches

OT treatment approaches for clients with obesity will focus on ADL and IADL performance, joint mobility and stability, safe handling education, social isolation and depression, decreased skin integrity, behavioral management skills, and trunk and limb strengthening. OTAs will use their skills to plan client-specific treatment interventions based on the OT evaluation and goals that are set.

EDUCATION AND TRAINING

The OTA can provide caregiver education and training on transfers, bed mobility, and daily care of the client with obesity to prevent injury and caregiver fatigue. The OTA may also present inservices with demonstration to support groups, staff teams, and out-of-town family. It is beneficial to have hands-on demonstration of the transfers, bed mobility, and certain aspects of daily care. Education and training on prevention of injury and/or caregiver fatigue should include extra physical help and/or use of equipment and creating a support system, whether it involves friends, family, neighbors, or community programs. The OTA also can create documentation logs for daily food consumption and exercise routines to encourage a healthy lifestyle (Table 27-6).

RESPIRATORY FUNCTION WITH ENERGY CONSERVATION

Because many clients who are obese present with shortness of breath (SOB) upon minimal exertion, it is necessary to educate the clients in proper breathing techniques and also techniques to conserve energy when performing a task. See Chapter 26 for a number of techniques. The OTA may have a client who presents with difficulty with self-pacing while performing tasks. Some clients hold their breath when

TABLE 27-6 Daily Food/Fluid Intake and Weight Log (Example)

DAY	SUN	MON	TUES	WED	THURS	FRI	SAT
Breakfast							
Lunch							
Dinner							
Snacks							
Amount of fluid							
Weight							
Feelings							

performing difficult tasks, leading to increased SOB. The OTA should encourage the client to quietly count out loud when performing tasks, which ensures proper air exchange. This technique can also work with positive results for clients who become SOB when ambulating or performing transfers.

ENERGY CONSERVATION DURING ACTIVITIES OF DAILY LIVING

The OTA can assist the client in establishing a new routine to conserve energy for daily tasks. Performing the daily routine can be taxing and requires extra energy for the client who is obese. Encourage clients to pace themselves, break the task down to perform in smaller steps instead of all at once, spread harder tasks over a longer period, focus on breathing, and plan ahead. A few examples of energy conservation techniques with occupations are:

- Bathing: Plan the bathing task around the client's energy level, and gather all items needed before beginning the task. The best time of day for bathing may be different each day. Encourage the client to perform the task in a seated position, and watch the temperature as too hot can cause fatigue.
- Grooming: Obtain all toiletries needed before beginning the task; perform in a seated position with UEs supported (on counter), if possible. The client should utilize an electric razor and electric toothbrush, unless he or she uses oxygen. These devices, along with hair dryers, can present the risk of a spark or fire.
- Dressing: Obtain all items needed before beginning the task; avoid tight clothing; perform lower body dressing before standing to pull underwear and pants up at the same time; and utilize adaptive equipment as necessary.
- Meals: When preparing meals, have all necessary items within reach before beginning the task; perform in a seated position, if possible; prepare small/quick meals instead of long taxing meals; and utilize adaptive equipment (electric can opener, long-handled reacher, rolling cart for transport of items).
- Mobility: Utilize a mobility device to get from one side of the home to another, outside to the mailbox, down to the neighbor's home, or through the store as needed. A power wheelchair requires less energy than a walker or a manual wheelchair.

Cardiovascular Function with Activity Tolerance: During exercises or any strenuous activity, closely monitor vital signs such as blood pressure, heart rate, and respiratory rate of the client. Also, keenly observe the client, noting changes in skin color, profuse sweating with clammy skin, or dizziness. When initiating an exercise program, the client may perform it from bed level at first, progressing to supported sitting, then unsupported sitting, to eventually standing to perform the exercise. The amount of repetitions and intensity may be low initially and progress as the client tolerates them. An OTA could assist the client in establishing a daily log to document and monitor status and improvements (Table 27-7).

TABLE 27-7 Daily Exercise Log (Example)

DAY	TYPE OF ACTIVITY/EXERCISE	MINUTES PERFORMED	FEELINGS AFTER ACTIVITY/EXERCISE
Sunday			
Monday			
Tuesday			
Wednesday			
Thursday			
Friday			
Saturday			

Skin Function With Activities of Daily Living: Skin integrity is extremely important for any client, and certainly the client with obesity is at high risk for skin maceration and wounds. The following are considerations with ADL tasks:

- Educate the client in skin monitoring and moisture management, especially between skin folds and the sacral region.
- Encourage the client to obtain and use mirrors with extended curved arms to perform daily skin inspection to include between the toes.
- Educate the client on techniques to manage excessive moisture and hygiene between skin folds, under the panniculus and under the LEs to include toes.
- Utilize a clean, dry towel or sock between skin folds. Monitor and change the towel or sock frequently.
- When bathing large skin fold areas, encourage the client to utilize a hand towel or bath towel to bathe the areas. The towels are long and soft enough for the client to bathe thoroughly and can "hook" under the panniculus for hygiene.
- Utilize a long-handled bath sponge for cleaning between toes. Dry feet thoroughly before donning socks and shoes.
- Encourage the client to utilize a terry cloth robe to assist with drying and to conserve energy with the task. Educate clients that utilizing fabric softener when washing clothes can decrease the ability of a towel and robe to absorb moisture.
- Encourage the client to wear nonrestrictive moisture-wicking clothing and looser-fitting socks and shoes.

Durable Medical Equipment: The bariatric client will require specialized equipment for care and to avoid safety risk. Some types of DME used are bariatric bedside commodes either with or without drop arms (Fig. 27-4), bariatric walkers (Fig. 27-2), bariatric manual wheelchairs (Fig. 27-5), heavy-duty scooters and power wheelchairs, bariatric scales, bariatric beds with specialty mattresses and an over–the–bed trapeze, and a bariatric rolling shower commode chair (Fig. 27-6). It is important to realize that most bariatric equipment is heavy and difficult to maneuver even without the client; therefore, obtaining enough help is as important as using proper body mechanics. The client's home must be assessed to ensure that equipment will be functional within the space provided and that the condition of the home can withstand the weight of the equipment. For example, a 500-pound client in a 500-pound heavy-duty power wheelchair is 1,000 pounds of force on the floor of a home. Not all floors can withstand that amount of weight in one spot. The width of doors must be assessed to ensure that the equipment will fit inside the house or the intended room. For instance, a manual wheelchair with a seat size of 28 inches wide can be 37 inches wide push rim to push rim, which is much too large for a standard door (36 inches). The true opening once the door width is accounted for is only about 34 to 34.5 inches. Standard door widths of 36 inches does not mean all homes have this size door, and some doors can be 32 inches or less; bathroom doors on older homes can be as small as 19 inches. Since power wheelchairs have the wheels tucked under

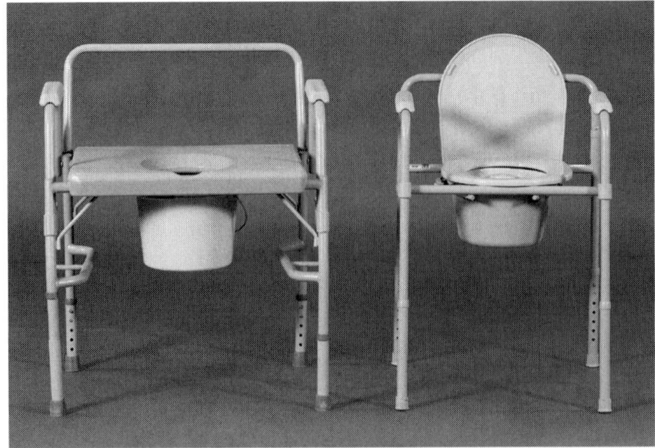

FIGURE 27-4. Bariatric and standard bedside commodes.

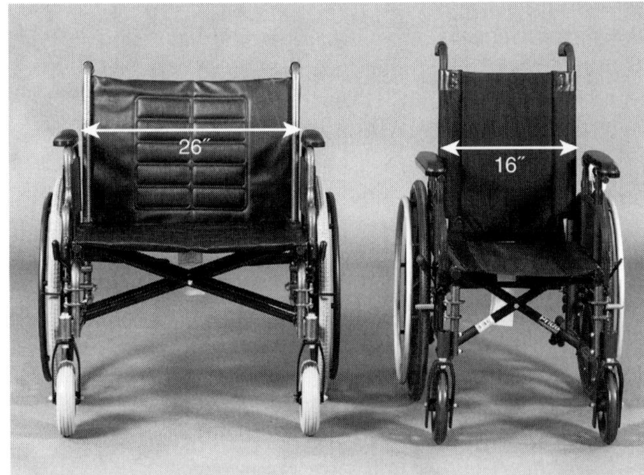

FIGURE 27-5. Bariatric and standard manual wheelchairs.

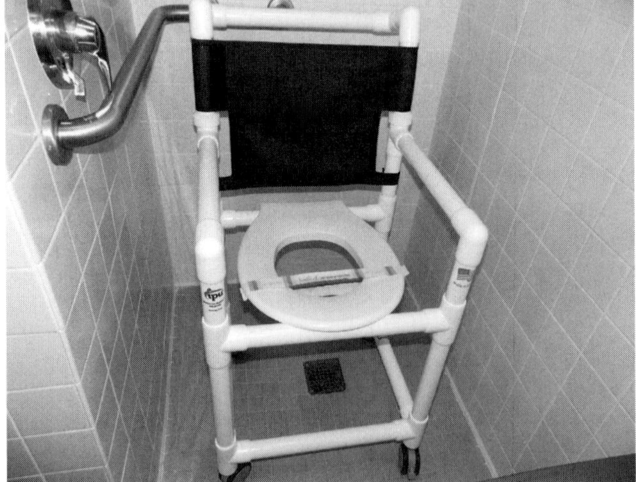

FIGURE 27-6. Bariatric rolling shower chair in the shower.

the seat instead of out to the side like manual wheelchairs, they tend to be narrower, with the armrests as the widest point. Some clients have to remove one or both armrests (even to the point of holding the joystick in their lap) to get through standard doors. A specialty seating clinic can assist with matching the client to effective and functional seating and mobility equipment, and OTAs should familiarize themselves with vendors online and in the area for other types of equipment.

MODIFICATION OF TASKS

Many clients who are obese will require some type of modifications to improve function for occupational performance. Modifications can include, but are not limited to, adaptive equipment, structural/environmental modifications for access, social/sexuality issues, and habit/routine options.

Activities of Daily Living: The client will most likely require some level of assistance when performing ADLs due to decreased activity tolerance, decreased endurance, limited functional mobility, extremity limitations, and structural barriers secondary to obesity.

Bathing: Some clients who are obese perform sponge baths due to the inability to safely transfer in and out of the shower. Other problems that could be encountered are the shower or bathroom may be too small, doorways may not be large enough to maneuver through with an assistive device, or the client has decreased overall endurance. It is important with these clients to stress hygiene, especially between skin folds. Clients who can take a shower would benefit from a bariatric shower chair or bariatric transfer tub bench. The equipment would decrease pressure on the joints and conserve energy when performing bathing and increase the ability to reach lower areas and between skin folds safely with or without adaptive equipment. Some types of adaptive equipment that would be beneficial are a long-handled bath sponge; a handheld shower hose with a wand that also has an on/off control; a bath mitt (depending on grasp); large, soft towels, and a long-handled mirror for skin inspections. The client can also utilize a hair dryer on the cool setting to dry between skin folds, use a drying machine for the shower on a cool setting, and limit use of powders in folds as this can cause "caking" that can lead to a breeding ground for bacteria. If available, moisture-wicking material can be used between skin folds.

Dressing: This task causes fatigue in most clients who are morbidly obese, due to their limited mobility, decreased endurance, inability to fully raise UEs, and limited elbow flexion due to girth of UEs. Recommendations to assist the client in the dressing task would include having the client: don large, nonconstricting clothing that slips on or opens in the back; avoid multilayer dressing as this causes increased fatigue; and use slip-on shoes with Velcro®, magnetic closures, or elastic laces. Take caution with the use of socks with clients who are obese, especially if the LEs are edematous or if the client has lymphedema. Most socks have elastic openings, and they may not be large enough for the client, which can cause pressure areas and constrict lymph flow. Recommendations for adaptive equipment and dressing tips can include a long-handled reacher, long-handled shoehorn, dressing stick, and a bariatric sock or stocking aid (Fig. 27-7).

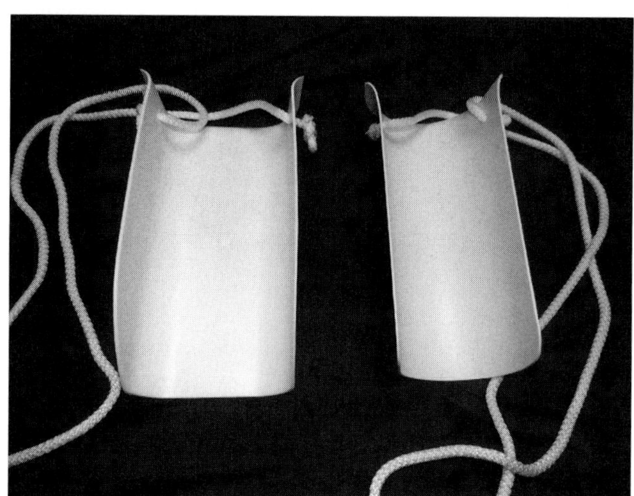

FIGURE 27-7. Bariatric and standard sock-aid.

COMMUNICATION

Society tends to "look down" on a person who is obese, and often views obesity as a result of laziness and personal failure. Therefore, people who are obese not only suffer from medical conditions but also receive harsh criticism by the media and society in general, as well as their healthcare team. Some clients who are obese avoid the doctor to avoid this criticism, which has the potential to exacerbate medical conditions. Through the years, medical science has explored causes and determined that obesity is not only caused by high caloric intake and sedentary lifestyle but can also be hereditary. Scientists have identified several genes that contribute to weight gain and can lead to obesity.[34] According to Herrera and colleagues, there are "different effects on different individuals in the same environment, highlighting an underlying, inherited susceptibility to obesity and fat-distribution."[34] Certainly for many clients who are obese, the battle with weight and health does not come down to simply willpower. It can be difficult for any practitioner to treat all clients fairly, justly, and respectfully when society, the workplace, and potentially their own beliefs are pushing toward ridicule and prejudice. A careful examination of values and the OT Code of Ethics can assist to guide the OTA through these murky waters. The OTA should strive to communicate compassion for all clients, treat all clients with dignity and respect, and maintain a focus on the holistic roots of OT.

Toileting: Most standard commodes are too low or cannot accommodate the weight of the client who is obese. The OTA can recommend use of a bariatric bedside commode (BSC) or a bariatric drop arm commode with an extra wide seat, and place the commode frame over the standard toilet at an elevated height. The client can utilize arms of the BSC or the elevated extra-wide toilet seat to assist with ascending and descending from the commode. Take caution with the use of a regular bedpan with the client, as it can cause discomfort and increased chances of pressure areas.

Toilet Hygiene: This task is difficult for the client because of UE limitations and limited trunk mobility due to girth. In some settings, the client with immobility simply uses cloth or disposable underpads due to lack of bariatric bedpan or staffing issues. If the client is mobile, there are several different toilet aids that can be recommended to assist with the task. The purpose of a toilet aid is to assist the client in reaching and cleaning areas too difficult to independently reach. Toilet aids have extended curved handles and can be equipped with spring clips, push-button grasp/release, or slotted hooks to hold any tissue or premoistened wipes. (See Chapter 14 for a variety of toilet aids.) Another type of adaptive equipment that can assist with toilet hygiene is a bidet. Bidets attach to the toilet, have either a heated pulse wash or water spray to assist with cleansing the area, and typically will blow dry the area as well.

Sexual Activity: Sexual activity with all clients, including the obese, appears to be a difficult subject for the client and most medical professionals. Clients who are obese have sexual needs and desires and may wish to act on them; however, at times, physical and psychological components present a problem. Women more than men may experience poor body image and low self-esteem. Many women are worried about their physical appearance (e.g., size of their buttocks or stomach), fear of being ridiculed, and rejection, and, therefore, tend to avoid sexual encounters. Men may present with a challenge of erectile dysfunction or adipose (fat) tissue causing penile retraction, which, in turn, can cause depression from lack of performance. At times, the client who is super obese may have other underlying medical problems that would prevent orgasm, erection, or ejaculation.

The OTA may be able to educate on various adapted positions and techniques to trial, such as lifting/moving the panniculus or using assistive devices such as a penile pump or vibrator. Dense foam wedges may provide support and positioning as well. The client's view/interpretation of sexuality should be explored and needs/preferences established, as meaning could vary. Some clients might be longing for the personal touch of affection and intimacy, and some could be looking for sexual encounters. The OTA can assist clients with coping mechanisms, offering handouts and education, keeping a journal, documenting their feelings with any changes in weight, and seeking support groups. As with many occupations, sexuality and intimacy issues are best addressed with a team approach to include behavioral and psychological counseling, if available.

Functional Mobility: Clients who are obese could present with functional mobility challenges, depending on their level of obesity and overall health condition. Some treatments an OTA could assist with include: strengthening exercises; balance and endurance activities; transfer training to/from the bed, chair, shower, and toilet; wheelchair mobility for environment accessibility; and manipulation of mobility device while performing a self-care task (e.g., toilet transfer). Some clients may not realize that fatigue could be more easily managed with a mobility device, and that it may also increase safety while decreasing risk of falls. Some clients may have pain or SOB with ambulation, which forces them to be more sedentary than desired. A power mobility device may assist to keep the client active and engaged in their desired occupations instead of limited by decreased mobility.

Instrumental Activities of Daily Living: IADLs are higher-level skills that some clients who are morbidly or super obese need assistance with due to decreased functional mobility, endurance, activity tolerance, and structural as well as environmental barriers.

Meal Preparation: Most clients who are obese are unable to stand for long periods, which hinders shopping and meal preparation. Therefore, clients tend to go for "quick fix" snacks, which often end up being unhealthy food choices. The OTA can recommend healthy frozen dinners, healthy "one-pot" crockpot meals, or Meals on Wheels as alternatives. The OTA can encourage the client to look online, in magazines, or in cookbooks for a variety of healthy recipes, as well as to educate the client in compensatory techniques to perform simple meals and conserve energy. Other options are to purchase precut fruits and vegetables, and to perform meal prep from a seated position, if possible.

Driving and Community Mobility: Driving can be a challenge for some clients who are obese, especially for the morbidly or super obese. Some clients are unable to reach the steering wheel due to girth, get into/out of the car, reach the foot pedal, or utilize a standard seat belt. Hand controls may replace the brake/gas pedals, and larger seat belts or extensions may be available. A certified driving instructor referral may be required (details found in Chapter 16). If clients cannot transport themselves, the OTA can assist with researching other avenues for transport. Some of the other transportation options are ride sharing companies, taxis, or public transportation. However, depending on the mobility and size of the client, not all transport options are possible. One must consider the doors, seats, aisles (if public transport), cost, and if there is accommodation for assistive mobility devices and physical assist if needed. Some public transportation lifts and ramps will only lift 600 pounds; when the client weighs 450 pounds and the power wheelchair weighs 500 pounds, transportation can be a problem.

Home Management: Home management is another area in which OTAs can assist the client. OTAs can assist with energy conservation, encourage use of disposable items versus items that require washing (e.g., dishes), assist in making a cleaning schedule through the day/week/month, and adapting cleaning tools (longer handle, lighter weight, less scrubbing) to better assist the client. OTAs can also encourage and assist the client in making a call list of contacts for help with housekeeping, lawn and garden work, and car and household repairs.

Rest and Sleep: The client with obesity issues may have difficulty getting adequate or quality sleep, either because of disordered breathing, difficulty with rolling and repositioning, or due to an unsupportive mattresses for his or her weight. It may be difficult to find a bed mattress and frame that is sturdy enough for the weight, and a regular hospital bed may be too narrow. Many clients sleep with breathing devices for sleep apnea and other issues, and must manage the hoses and reaching, putting on, and taking off the accompanying masks.

Education and Work: A study from 2015 looked at the hiring and employment practices in relation to the obese and found significant discrimination of this population. Workers who were obese were considered to be less suitable for employment.[35] Obesity stigmatization and discrimination may be found in the workplace, schools, and many other public places. Desk chairs may be too small or ill-fitting, restroom stalls may be too small, and clients may potentially have difficulty performing certain job tasks when the tasks require long periods of standing or high levels of activity. Colleges often have long distances to walk between classes, stairs in dorms and buildings, and they may be less accessible for mobility devices. The client could utilize Vocational Rehabilitation services for assistance with job training and placement and options for job and school support.

Leisure: While clients who are obese may be sedentary, many are also very active. Excess weight may not mean that the client is not also very strong, and there are athletes of all sizes participating in sports and active leisure. A client who is more sedentary due to fatigue or pain may perform activities that require less energy such as reading or time on the computer. The OTA may also encourage the client to use leisure tasks to be more active, such as going for walks, biking, or swimming. Time with grandchildren, chair yoga at the senior center, or a goal of walking the full length of a greenway trail may be options both to be active and to increase social participation.

Environmental Modifications: The client who is obese will be presented with many environmental challenges, some of which may be modifiable in his or her own environment with significant renovations and cost; however, some public areas are simply not accessible. Some challenges might include the following:

- Door openings that are not wide enough for safe passage with or without an assistive device
- Furniture that is too small or unable to support the client's weight (especially in waiting areas)
- Transportation limitations due to inability to transfer in and out of a vehicle safely
- Driving limitations due to steering wheel position (panniculus obstructing safe distance from steering wheel)
- Building access limitations due to inability to climb stairs
- Hallways that are too narrow to pass or turn with or without a device
- Beds that are too small (unable to turn self)
- Bathrooms that are too small in the home or community
- Restaurant booths or chairs that do not accommodate weight or girth
- Movie or concert seats that do not accommodate weight or girth
- Weight limit as well as girth size limits with medical imaging equipment (CT scanner, MRI, Doppler, and standard x-rays)

Some of these challenges can be modified but may have an expense to the client. Examples of modifications may include:

- Remodeling the home to widen doorways
- Replacing the bathtub with a large walk-in shower
- Purchasing furniture that can accommodate the client's weight and girth
- Obtaining a bariatric bed that would allow independent repositioning
- Building a ramp to accommodate the client's weight and size of both the client and the wheelchair or other device
- Obtaining mobility devices (bariatric electric scooter or heavy-duty power wheelchair) to assist with mobility within the home and community
- Rearranging cabinets to allow ease for obtaining items and conserving energy
- Contacting transportation facilities that have transportation vans to assist with wheelchair use. However, depending on the weight of the client, the Emergency Medical Services (EMS) might have to be contacted for medical transport, as a wheelchair lift on a transportation van may have a weight limit.

Lifestyle: Clients who are obese must encounter and be willing to commit to a lifestyle change if they are serious about losing weight and becoming more independent. The OTA can assist the client in techniques to help with this change by encouraging the client to:

- Keep self-monitoring logs or utilize fitness apps (e.g., My Fitness Pal) to pay attention to what is consumed and to recognize what triggers cravings.

- Keep exercise logs or utilize fitness apps (e.g., FitBit, S Health) to note progress with activity levels.
- Place junk food out of reach, or simply do not purchase it.
- Identify and control stimuli that cause the overeating or inactivity.
- Join an exercise group, or start walking with a friend. Accountability is a key factor in making and maintaining changes.
- Work on improving self-image and maintaining positive lifestyle changes.
- Enjoy nonfood rewards when a positive transformation takes place, such as purchasing a new piece of clothing, going to the movies with family, or going on an adventure that has a weight limit which has been reached (e.g., snorkeling).
- Participate in stress-reduction activities; this can be as simple as relaxation, breathing techniques, or massage. (Caution: If clients have a distorted body image, they may not feel comfortable with massage.)
- Search for positive alternative for cravings (e.g., substitute music for food).
- Participate in outside hobbies, like simple gardening, bird watching, or going to ball games.
- Join a support group or a community treatment program.

SUMMARY

Obesity-related conditions are some of the leading causes of preventable deaths in the United States.[2] There are several contributing risk factors, both modifiable and nonmodifiable, that could lead to obesity. Recognizing the modifiable risk factors and seeking help are two of the best ways to prevent or control obesity. Treatment can consist of increased physical activity, dietary changes, recognizing and modifying behaviors that trigger negative habits, medication, and surgical procedures. Obesity can present with several medical complications, and clients who are obese must be aware of their own body and recognize signs or changes as they occur and seek treatment. The OTA will be able to address the needs of the client who is obese and their caregivers by utilizing various treatment approaches discussed in this chapter.

REVIEW QUESTIONS

1. A client who is 350 pounds now requires a manual wheelchair for mobility and ADL/IADL tasks due to a medical change in condition. The client lives in a single-wide trailer with a ramp. Which of the following considerations must be addressed *before* supplying the wheelchair?
   a. Width of outside and inside doors
   b. Covering over the porch at the top of ramp
   c. Potential weight gain
   d. Material of wheelchair seat
2. A client who is active, has completed sprint triathlons, and has no particular health concerns can still have a very high BMI and be considered morbidly obese. What is the *most likely* reason for this?
   a. They simply eat too much.
   b. The BMI can be less reliable with muscular clients.
   c. They are getting older, and their metabolism is changing.
   d. The BMI is not accurate.
3. Which three of the following are contributing risk factors that may lead to obesity?
   a. Only walking one mile a day
   b. Lack of sleep
   c. Too many natural vitamins
   d. Emotions/depression
   e. Certain medications
   f. Lifting weights
4. You have a client who is receiving OT after her second bariatric surgery. She really wants help to succeed. Which of the following is an OT treatment intervention that should be considered when assisting the client with prevention recurrence?
   a. Diet and lifestyle modification
   b. Daily workouts
   c. Referral to a psychologist
   d. Medication management
5. A 45-year-old client with morbid obesity is in the acute care hospital. He lives in a single wide trailer with four steps to enter, has few financial resources because of his inability to work, lives with his older parents, and is regaining strength after a bout with pneumonia. He can stand with Min A, but can only ambulate 5 feet at a time. Which three of the following would be required for the client to safely go home next week?
   a. A bariatric power wheelchair
   b. A bariatric rental manual wheelchair
   c. A bariatric bedside commode
   d. Widening all interior doorways
   e. Continued OT and physical therapy to assess and adapt the home and daily tasks
   f. A cane
6. When treating a client with obesity and a compromised respiratory system, the OTA should closely monitor which three of the following?
   a. Respiratory rate
   b. Stride rate
   c. Oxygen saturation
   d. Daily weight
   e. Hemoglobin levels
   f. Heart rate
7. While working with a home health client who is super obese, the OTA begins to suspect the client has a DVT due to localized redness and pain. What should the OTA immediately do?
   a. Continue treating as per the plan of care (POC) set by the occupational therapist.
   b. Continue treating as long as the OTA does not rub the area in question.
   c. Have the client lie down until the next physician visit.
   d. Have the client lie down, and notify the occupational therapist, RN, or MD of the suspicions.
8. A client with grade 3 panniculus presents with maceration of the genital region. What would the OTA *most likely* address first?
   a. Provide DME contacts
   b. Provide education on moisture management, skin care, and hygiene
   c. Provide diet tips to lose weight
   d. Provide exercise logs

9. Clients who are morbidly obese and immobile are at greater risk for skin breakdown. While working on ADLs with a wheelchair-bound client, the OTA notices pink-red areas on the buttocks and sacral region. What should the OTA do to assist the client with maintaining skin integrity and preventing skin breakdown?
   a. Educate the client to keep areas moist with lotion.
   b. Educate the client on the importance of being seated at 90 degrees.
   c. Educate the client on the importance of daily skin hygiene and inspection.
   d. Educate the client to stay on his sides in bed and out of the wheelchair for the greater part of the day.
10. Caregiver fatigue and injuries are common when caring for the client who is obese and also immobile. As an OTA, what should be the *first* focus to assist the caregiver with fatigue reduction and injury prevention?
   a. Educate caregivers on the proper use of patient lifts when performing transfers.
   b. Provide caregivers with the adaptive equipment and techniques to safely assist with the ADL task.
   c. Provide and encourage the use of back braces when working with the obese client.
   d. Assist caregivers in self-awareness of their limitations and capabilities.

CASE STUDY

Grace is a 49-year-old female client who is super obese. She was admitted to the hospital from a skilled nursing facility (SNF) where she had resided for the past 5 months. The client presented to the hospital with multiple medical problems that included acute respiratory failure requiring ventilation, obesity hypoventilation syndrome, obstructive sleep apnea, super obese with BMI of 82, sepsis, panniculitis, bipolar disorder, hypertension, chronic pain, and depression with an anxiety component.

Upon medical stabilization, a referral was made for OT to evaluate and treat. Prior level of functioning: Client was able to assist with approximately 50% of ADLs and transfer to wheelchair with Min A. Current level of functioning: Client noted to be dependent for all ADLs, transfers, and functional mobility, fatigue upon minimal exertion, BUE strength 2+/5. The OT course of treatment initially was to address safe handling for staff and client, begin UE ROM and increase to strengthening exercises as tolerated, tolerate EOB sitting for 5-minute intervals, and instruct in energy conservation techniques and adaptive equipment as indicated.

1. What would be the safest transfer, initially, for the hospital staff and caregivers to perform?
2. What would be the initial treatment course for Grace and why?

PUTTING IT ALL TOGETHER — Sample Treatment Session and Documentation

Setting	Inpatient rehabilitation facility
Client profile	Client is a 38-year-old morbidly obese female, requires IV antibiotics for acute cellulitis in both lower extremities with lymphedema
Work history	Cashier at local diner, 28 hours per week, for the past 8 years
Insurance	None
Psychological	Depression due to medical status
Social	Single, lives with mother in a single-story house, leaves home only for work and shopping for groceries.
Cognitive	No issues
Motor and Manual Muscle Testing (MMT)	BUE ROM WFL and strength 5/5
ADL	Bathing: UB—Min A, LB—Max A Dressing: UB—Indep, LB—Max A (client prefers sandals vs. shoes) Toilet hygiene: Unable to perform adequately due to girth
IADL	Client reports problems with cooking due to decreased endurance and limited standing ability.
Goals	Client to be seen for 2 weeks to address the following goals: 1. Client will increase ADL performance of lower body ADLs to a Min A with or without use of AE and compensatory strategies × 2 weeks. 2. Client will perform adequate toilet hygiene and peri-care to a Mod I level with or without use of AE × 2 weeks. 3. Client will independently incorporate energy conservation techniques to assist with ADL and IADL performance × 2 weeks. 4. Client will perform simulated cooking task utilizing energy conservation techniques and modifications at Mod I level × 2 weeks.

Continued

PUTTING IT ALL TOGETHER Sample Treatment Session and Documentation (continued)

OT TREATMENT SESSION 1

THERAPEUTIC ACTIVITY	TIME	GOAL(S) ADDRESSED	OTA RATIONALE
Educate and train client in energy conservation techniques for ADL performance. Provide handouts, practice, and review with client.	10 min	#3 and indirectly #1, #2, #4	*Education and Training:* Increased ADL performance and activity tolerance.
Educate and train client on adaptive equipment and compensatory techniques to assist with LB bathing to include panniculus area. Client to return demonstration. AE and techniques to include long-handled bath sponge, wet wipes, and use of large, soft towel for bathing/drying under panniculus. Demonstrate usage of AE, compensatory strategies, and educate on moisture management to maintain skin integrity.	30 min	#1 and indirectly #2	*Occupations; Education and Training:* AE, compensatory strategies and moisture management to increase independence with ADL performance, promote good hygiene, and maintain skin integrity

SOAP note: 06/22/—, 1:40 pm–2:20 pm

S: Client presents slightly withdrawn upon arrival for tx, but willing to participate.

O: Client participated in skilled OT in room at edge of bed for education and training in energy conservation, skin care, and adaptive equipment. Handouts provided. Client acknowledged understanding by verbalization and return demonstration. Setup provided for bathing. Client performed lower body bathing utilizing a long-handled bath sponge, from chair level with Min A for techniques for using AE. Client performed skin care under panniculus and placed towel for moisture management from semiseated position with Mod A.

A: Client demonstrated ability to incorporate energy conservation techniques 75% of treatment, requiring occasional verbal cuing for redirection of task. She was able to utilize AE to assist with bathing, but would benefit from further repetition.

P: Continue treatment as per plan of care set by occupational therapist. Next visit, continue to address energy conservation techniques, review lower body bathing and use of AE, and educate and address lower body dressing and toileting hygiene with use of AE.

Susie Jackson, COTA/L, 06/22/—, 2:25 pm

TREATMENT SESSION 2

What could you do next with this client?

TREATMENT SESSION 3

What could you do next with this client?

REFERENCES

1. World Health Organization. (2017). Obesity and overweight fact sheet. Retrieved from http://www.who.int/mediacentre/factsheets/fs311/en/
2. Centers for Disease Control and Prevention. (2015). About adult BMI. Retrieved from http://cdc.gov/healthyweight/assessing/bmi/adult_bmi/index.html
3. Why use BMI? (2017). Retrieved from https://www.hsph.harvard.edu/obesity-prevention-source/obesity-definition/obesity-definition-full-story/
4. National Institutes of Health, A.D.A.M. Medical Encyclopedia. (n.d.). Overweight. Retrieved from https://www.nlm.nih.gov/medlineplus/ency/article/003101.htm
5. About obesity. (n.d.). Retrieved from http://obesity.ygoy.com/about-obesity/causes/
6. Centers for Disease Control and Prevention. (2015). Insufficient sleep is a public health problem/features/CDC. Retrieved from http://www.cdc.gov/Features/dsSleep/index.html
7. National Health, Lung, and Blood Institute. (2012). What causes overweight and obesity? Retrieved from http://www.nhlbi.nih.gov/health/health-topics/topics/obe/prevention
8. National Health, Lung, and Blood Institute. (2012). What are the health risks of overweight and obesity? Retrieved from http://nhlbi.nih.gov/health/health-topics/topics/obe/prevention
9. What causes overweight and obesity? (2012). Retrieved from https://www.nhlbi.nih.gov/health/health-topics/topics/obe/causes
10. Sam, S. (2007). Obesity and polycystic ovary syndrome. *Obesity Management*, 3(2), 69–73. http://doi.org/10.1089/obe.2007.0019
11. National Health, Lung, and Blood Institute. (2012). How are overweight and obesity treated? Retrieved from http://nhibi.nih.gov/health/health-topics/topics/obe/prevention
12. Boulé, N. G. (2016). Exercise plus Metformin in the fight against diabetes. *Exercise and Sports Sciences Reviews, 44*(1), 2.
13. Boulé, N. G. (2011). Metformin and exercise in type 2 diabetes. *Diabetes Care, 34*(7), 1469–1474. doi:10.2337/dc 10-2207

14. Espeland, M. A., Glick, H. A., Bertoni, A., Brancati, F. L., Bray, G. A., Clark, J. M. ... & Zhang, P. (2014). Impact of an intensive lifestyle intervention on use and cost of medical services among overweight and obese adults with type 2 diabetes: The Action for Health in Diabetes. *Diabetes Care, 37*(9), 2548–2556. http://dx.doi.org/10.2337/dc14-0093
15. National Institute of Diabetes and Digestive and Kidney Disease. (2011). Bariatric surgery for severe obesity. (NIH Publication No. 08-4006 ed.). Bethesda, MD: National Institute of Health. Retrieved from http://www.niddk.nih.gov/health-information/health-topics/weight-control/bariatric-surgery-severe-obesity/Pages/bariatric-surgery-for-severe-obesity.aspx?utm
16. Torry, M. R., Decker, M. J., Viola, R. W., O'Connor, D. D., & Steadman, J. R. (2000). Inter-articular knee joint effusion induces quadriceps avoidance gait patterns. *Clinical Biomechanics (Bristol, Avon), 15*(3), 147–159. doi:S0268003399000832
17. Cetin, D. C., & Nasr, G. (2014). Obesity in the elderly: More complicated than you think. *Cleveland Clinic Journal of Medicine, 81*(1), 51–61.
18. Engstrom, D. (n.d.). Obesity and depression. Retrieved from http://www.obesityaction.org/educational-resources/resource-articles-2/obesity-related-disease/obesity-and-depression
19. Wright, J. G., Chaudhari, A., Doria, J., Kennedy, J. D., Kink, F., Leonard, T. N., & Simmons, P. (2002). Obesity: Facts, figures, guidelines section three. West Virginia Health Statistic Center. Retrieved from https://www.wvdhhr.org/bph/oehp/obesity/credits.htm
20. Batsis, J. A. (n.d.). Cardiovascular disease—Obesity and the heart. Retrieved from http://www.obesityaction.org/educational-resources/resource-articles-2/obesity-related-diseases/cardiovascular-disease-obesity-and-the-heart
21. Diabetes and obesity. (2017). Diabetes.uk.com: The global diabetes community. Retrieved from http://www.diabetes.co.uk/diabetes-and-obesity.html
22. Rogers, J. Z., & Still, C. D. (n.d.). Obesity and type 2 diabetes. Retrieved from http://www.obesityaction.org/educational-resources/resource-articles-2/obesity-related-diseases/obesity-and-type-2-diabetes
23. Mandal, A. (2013). Obesity and respiratory disorders. Retrieved from http://www.news-medical.net/health/obesity-and-respiratory-disorder.aspx
24. Brown, A. (2013). How to manually check your heart rate. Retrieved from http://www.livestrong.com/article/268875-how-to-manually-check-your-heart-rate/
25. Description of high blood pressure. (2015). Retrieved from http://www.nhilbi.nih.gov/health/health-topics/topics/hbp
26. Hypertension clinical guidelines. (2017). Retrieved from http://professional.heart.org/professional/ScienceNews/UCM_496965_2017-Hypertension-Clinical-Guidelines.jsp
27. Pratt, L. A., & Brody, D. J. (2014). Depression and obesity in the U.S. adult household population, 2005–2010. *NCHS Data Brief, 167*, 1–8.
28. Mayo Clinic. (2014). Deep vein thrombosis (DVT). Retrieved from http://www.mayoclinic.org/diseases-conditions/deep-vein-thrombosis/basics/definition/con-20031922
29. Centers for Disease Control and Prevention. (2015). Venous thromboembolism (blood clots): Facts. Retrieved from http://www.cdc.gov/ncbddd/dvt/facts.html
30. Hardy, D. (2015). What is lymphoedema? Retrieved from http://www.lymphoedema.org/menu3/Index.asp
31. Fife, C., Benavides, S., & Otto, G. (2007). Morbid obesity and lymphedema management. *Lymph Link Newsletter, 19*(3), 1–3. Retrieved from http://klosetraining.com/wp-content/uploads/2013/10/Morbid-Obesity-And-Lymphedema-Management-CE-Fife-MD-July-2007.pdf
32. The Lymphoedema Support Network. (2015). Lipoedema. Retrieved from http://www.lymphoedema.org/Menu7/Index.asp
33. Hahler, B. (2006). An overview of dermatological conditions commonly associated with the obese patient. *Ostomy/Wound Management, 52*(6), 34–36, 38, 40.
34. Herrera, B. M., Keildson, S., & Lindgren, C. M. (2011). Genetics and epigenetics of obesity. *Maturitas, 69*(1), 41–49. http://doi.org/10.1016/j.maturitas.2011.02.018
35. Flint, S. W., Čadek, M., Codreanu, S. C., Ivić, V., Zomer, C., & Gomoiu, A. (2016). Obesity discrimination in the recruitment process: "You're not hired!" *Frontiers in Psychology, 7*, 647. http://doi.org/10.3389/fpsyg.2016.00647

ACKNOWLEDGMENTS

Special thank you to Amy Mahle and Amber Ward for the guidance provided with the development of this chapter.

Chapter 28

Burns Across the Continuum of Care

Heather S. Dodd, MS, OTR/L, Susan Hardesty, MS, OTR/L, and Amy J. Mahle, MHA, COTA/L

LEARNING OUTCOMES

After studying this chapter the student or practitioner will be able to:

28.1 Explain the functions of the skin
28.2 Identify the depth of burns and the impact on function with regard to activities of daily living and recovery
28.3 Describe types of skin grafts, the rationale for using a specific skin graft, and the precautions related to their use
28.4 Discuss the goals of orthoses and positioning to prevent scar contractures and loss of range of motion
28.5 Identify key concepts for success with burn rehabilitation
28.6 Explain the various types of range of motion as a primary treatment intervention
28.7 Provide education to client/and or family about the importance of participation and compliance in range of motion to gain independence in activities of daily living and instrumental activities of daily living
28.8 Describe trending outpatient treatment modalities
28.9 Explain how a burn can alter a person's self-image as well as life occupations

KEY TERMS

Allograft (homograft)	Keloid scar
Autograft	Partial-thickness burn
Burn	Scar contracture
Deep partial-thickness burns	Scar maturation
Eschar	Skin substitutes
Escharotomy	Superficial burn
Fasciotomy	Superficial partial-thickness burns
Full-thickness burn	Total body surface area (TBSA)
Heterotopic ossification (HO)	Xenograft
Hypertrophic scar	

A burn injury is typically an unexpected "event" and can range from a finger blister sustained while cooking to the more severe, traumatic burn sustained in a car accident or house fire. By definition, a **burn** is a type of injury to the skin caused by heat, chemicals, electricity, friction, or radiation resulting in a wound. All burns, regardless of type, are painful at some point, whether in the initial moments following the injury and/or in the rehabilitation phase. People who survive burns experience a variety of physical impairments that can include loss of range of motion (ROM); loss of self-care skills because of pain, immobility, and edema; loss of endurance because of time in the hospital; and the increased effort required to move the body because of weakness, pain, stiffness and fatigue. In addition to pain, some of the emotional components that follow a burn injury include anxiety, regret, sadness, fear, hope, and resolve.[1] Individuals with burn injuries experience significant psychosocial factors, such as depression, anxiety, poor self-esteem, and posttraumatic stress disorder. Above all, postburn scarring can permanently change a person's appearance and skin function.

According to the American Burn Association Burn Incidence Fact Sheet, there were 40,000 burn-related hospital admissions and 486,000 burn injuries receiving medical treatment in 2015. Burn injury is a significant cause of disability, morbidity, and mortality in the United States, with 3,275 deaths per year.[2]

Burns are multifaceted injuries that require time, effort, and multiple interventions to enable the client to overcome challenges and return to desired occupations. The client with a burn injury is forever changed by the experience.[1] Occupational therapy (OT) starts as early as day 1 of the burn injury and will continue with the client through the entire recovery and rehabilitation periods, through to functional independence, scar maturation, and, when indicated, scar reconstructive surgery. The length of time from a person sustaining a burn injury to gaining functional independence and **scar maturation** (complete healing of the scar through all phases) can be up to 2 years or more depending on the burn's size, location, and severity.[3] This fact is important because regardless of practice area—from acute care to acute rehabilitation, to a skilled nursing facility to an outpatient clinic or home health—occupational therapy assistants (OTAs) will most likely have opportunities to work with clients with burn injuries being a primary or secondary issue. Of interest to note, current terminology also refers to clients with a burn injury as "burn survivors," per the Model Systems Knowledge Translation Center[4] and the terminology will be used interchangeably throughout this chapter.

IMPAIRMENTS AND CLIENT FACTORS

Most people think of the heart, liver, or brain when they think of vital organs. When one of these vital organs is damaged in an accident the effects are obvious and immediate. However, to many it is a surprise that skin is the body's largest organ. When this vital organ is injured, as in sustaining a burn injury during a traumatic event, a person initially may be able to perform functionally. Many stories from burn survivors describe the minutes after a burn as being fully functional. People who have sustained burns are often the ones who call 911, work to put the flames out, and walk into the hospital. However, as time passes and the mind and body realize that one is "safe" from immediate danger, the fully functional picture starts to change because skin is an organ that performs important work to maintain a person's health, and that work is significantly compromised following a burn injury. "The complex nature of burn injury, both acute and chronic, and the physical and psychological ramifications for the burn patient make it mandatory that a multidisciplinary team of providers work in concert to provide the optimal care for this truly complex patient."[5] The team may include the burn surgeon, nurse, anesthesiologist, respiratory therapist, occupational therapist, OTA, physical therapist, physical therapist assistant, dietitian, psychologist/psychiatrist, pharmacist, recreational therapist, and social worker.

Skin Anatomy and Function

To understand the effect of burns, it is essential to understand the functions of skin, which include providing protection from infection-causing pathogens, conserving body fluids, regulating body temperature, producing vitamin D, providing a cosmetic covering, allowing for sensation, and resisting contact with stresses that would otherwise harm soft tissue under the skin.[6]

Skin is made up of three layers: the epidermis (thin top layer), the dermis (thick second layer), and the hypodermis, which is underneath the dermis. The average skin depth is 1 to 2 mm. See Figure 8-6 for an illustration of the skin. The **epidermis** contains the cells that produce pigment, fight infection, and make new skin cells about once every month. The **dermis** is a thick layer that in addition to being the origin of the hair follicles, sweat glands, oil glands, and nerve endings (which provide information about touch, pressure, vibration, and skin tension) it also houses blood capillaries and is comprised of collagen—a fibrous connective tissue that allows stretchability while providing strength to withstand tearing.[7] The **hypodermis** is mostly composed of fat, which provides cushioning, helps regulate body temperature, and connects skin to muscles and bones. In reflecting on the anatomy and physiology of skin, one can see that when skin is damaged by a burn, many of these functions are compromised or cease to exist. For example, if the burn affects the epidermis, skin loses the ability to produce new skin cells or proper pigmentation. If the burn is deeper and affects the dermis, the natural collagen that allows skin to stretch is replaced by scarring, which can cause contractures resulting in significant difficulties with ROM and function.

Types of Burns

Burn damage to skin may be limited to the epidermis or include the dermis, subcutaneous fat, muscle, bone, or internal organs, depending on the extent of the injury. The mechanisms of burns vary, and burn severity can be heightened, depending on the mechanism, duration of exposure, and intensity of the source. The different mechanisms of injury for burns include thermal, electrical, chemical, and radiation. Burns are generally classified by the depth of the burn wound, as either superficial, partial-thickness, or full-thickness. Contact with fire or flame is the most frequent cause of severe burns, accounting for 44% of cases, with estimated annual cost of US $7.5 billion in 2014.[8] Fire or flame-related types of burns typically are more of deep partial and full-thickness burns in nature. Electrical and chemical burns can be quite complex. They may result in amputation as well as neuropathic, long-term symptoms that may remain for years.[6]

SUPERFICIAL BURNS

Superficial burns, also known as *first-degree burns,* involve only the epidermis and appear like simple sunburn. Characteristics of a superficial burn include pain upon touch, redness, and possibly edema. Healing takes place in 3 to 5 days without scarring.[9] First-degree burns rarely need medical attention (Table 28-1). Old unfounded remedies, which include applying butter to a burn, are not advised; instead, proper first aid for a minor burn includes running cool (not cold) water over the burned area for at least 10 to 15 minutes (ice should never be applied because it can cause more injury), drying the area with a clean cloth or sterile gauze, applying aloe vera cream or an

TABLE 28-1 Burn Depth and Characteristics

	SUPERFICIAL BURN	SUPERFICIAL PARTIAL-THICKNESS BURN	DEEP PARTIAL-THICKNESS BURN	FULL-THICKNESS BURN
	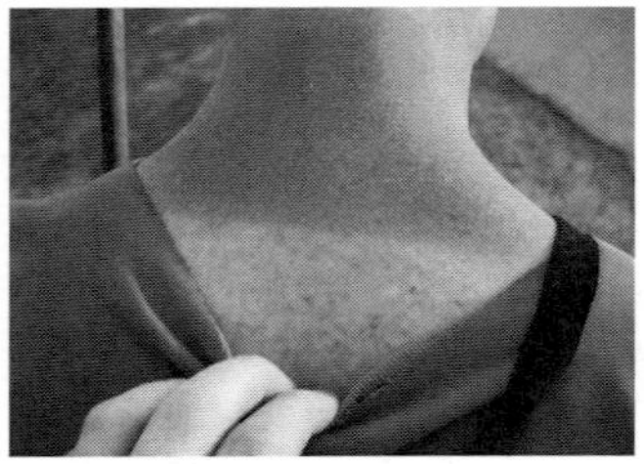 Superficial burn.	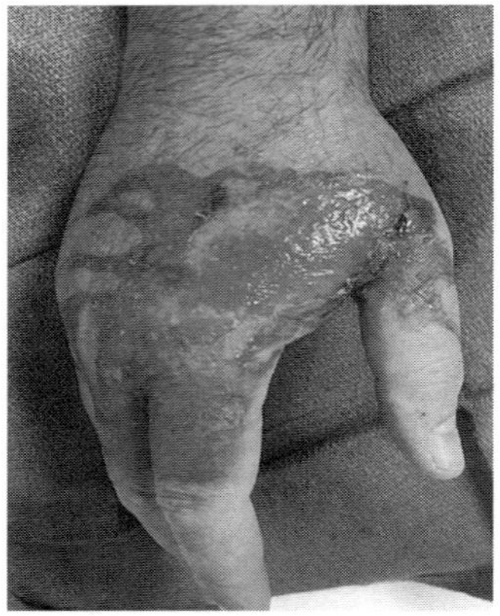 Superficial partial-thickness burn.	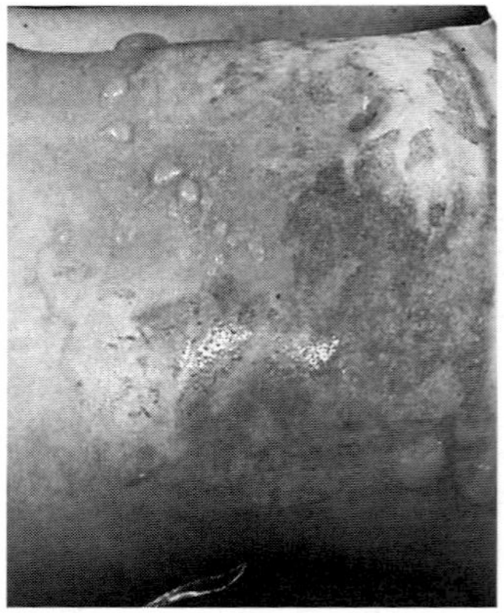 Deep partial-thickness burn.	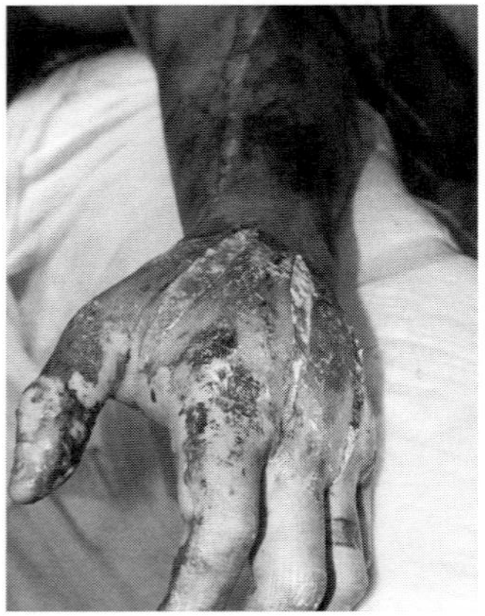 Full-thickness burn after escharotomies.
Skin layers affected	Epidermis only	Epidermis and top of dermis	Epidermis and deeper into dermis	Epidermis and entire dermis
Symptoms	Painful, no blisters, red, blanches to touch	Painful, blisters, moist, red, blanches to touch with brisk capillary refill	Less painful, sloughed skin, dryer, pale red, may blanch with slow to no capillary refill	No pain, pale, brown, white, red, leather-like, dry, no blanching, thrombosed vessels
Healing	Heals in 3 to 5 days	Heals before 21 days	Heals in greater than 21 days. Usually needs surgery via skin grafting to heal.	Will not heal (unless small), requires surgical skin grafting to heal
Scarring	No scar	Risk of pigment change (color difference)	Scarring, risk for hypertrophic scarring and contractures	High risk for hypertrophic scarring and contracture

antibiotic ointment, and loosely covering with nonstick gauze bandage.[10]

PARTIAL-THICKNESS BURNS

Partial-thickness burns, also called *second-degree burns,* extend through the epidermis and into the dermis. These burns are further subdivided into superficial or deep, depending on how far into the dermis the burn extends. Severe sunburns and contact burns from exposure to hot liquids or touching a hot surface tend to result in superficial or deep partial thickness burns (see Table 28-1).

Superficial partial-thickness burns involve the entire epidermis and the top part of the dermis. Characteristics of a superficial partial thickness burn include bright red appearance of skin, blisters, moist surface, pain, and blanching to touch with brisk capillary refill (the speed at which color and blood return to the area). Healing usually takes place by 21 days.

Deep partial-thickness burns involve the entire epidermis and go deeper into the dermis. Characteristics of a deep partial-thickness burn include a surface that may be slightly moist or dry; they usually do not have blisters because skin has already sloughed; and they may blanch to touch, but capillary refill will be slow or absent. Swelling begins, and the area usually appears dry, pale, and red or waxy-white in color. Pain associated with a deep partial-thickness burn tends to be less than that from a superficial partial-thickness burn because the nerve endings and other skin appendages are damaged. Healing will likely take longer than 21 days. Wounds that take longer than 21 days to heal tend to show long-term fragility (frequent breakdown) and hypertrophic scarring (thick scarring) and cause loss of motion when near a joint. Surgery soon after the injury to remove the burned tissue (excision) and apply a skin graft is recommended for optimal cosmetic and functional outcome.

FULL-THICKNESS BURNS

Full-thickness burns involve both layers of skin (epidermis and dermis) and extend to the hypodermis, or subcutaneous fat. Characteristics of a full-thickness burn include a surface that is firm, dry, and leathery and a variety of possible colors, depending on the cause of the burn, that may range from charred (black), pale white, yellow, or nonblanching red (see Table 28-1). Edema appears within hours of the injury as a result of a fluid shift from the capillaries to the interstitial space. The risk of infection increases because the infection-fighting power of skin has been destroyed. Pain is absent because the nerve endings in the skin are destroyed; yet motor function is usually intact. Many burn survivors with full-thickness burns delay seeking medical attention because they have little to no pain and full movement. It is not until they develop a fever (signaling infection) or another person recognizes the seriousness of the burn that they realize they require medical help. Full-thickness burns also cause an increase in metabolic rate. A high metabolic rate means the body is burning nutrients at a very rapid rate, and this is a problem for this client population because of the seriousness of the injuries; clients may also experience difficulty with oral intake of food to meet the significant increase in nutritional requirement and need supplemental nutrition. The physiological changes (edema, infection risk, and metabolic demands) caused by full-thickness burns necessitate skilled medical care with a focus on early fluid resuscitation, infection control, and nutrition.

Depending on their size and depth, full-thickness burns can affect every organ and body system. Healing without surgery is not possible unless the burn area is very small. Early excision of the burn, or cutting the damaged skin away, is recommended. The burn may require multiple surgeries depending on the size.

Subdermal burns, often called *fourth-degree burns,* involve all layers of skin and subcutaneous tissue—fat and muscle or bone. Characteristics of subdermal burns can present as mummified or firm, charred, dry, and leathery tissue. No pain is present. Amputation or advanced surgical flaps are often required, depending on the location.[9] Amputations can occur because of necrotic tissue or sepsis and are most common in high-voltage electrical injuries.[11]

MEDICAL MANAGEMENT OF THE BURN

"The burn did not overcome you; therefore, you can overcome the burn"—a burn survivor.

The trauma of a burn begins with its unexpected nature. Survival, both physical and psychological, begins with proper medical management. The severity of the burn injury depends on the burn's cause, the duration of contact with the cause, and the amount of body surface area involved. Initial care of clients with more severe burn injuries begins in the emergency department or burn center. The medical team works to establish the facts surrounding the burn injury and medically stabilize the client. Their evaluation of the client starts with the airway, breathing, and circulation. Lung injury (smoke inhalation) is the leading cause of death in the burn population. Inhalation injury adds additional complexity to the medical management of the burn, and the functional long-term impact can be deconditioning and loss of lung function leading to acute or chronic reduced activity tolerance. The most common complications of burns involve infections and scarring. Scar formation is a normal phase of wound healing, yet the way in which a person forms scars can be influenced depending on the treatment.[12] Scarring and infection will be discussed later in the chapter.

Severity of Burn

The physical presentation and severity of a burn wound varies, depending on its size and depth. Client evaluation continues with estimating the "size" of the burn, which is often based on its total body surface area (TBSA) percentage. The "rule of nines" is the common way to estimate

TBSA of burn wounds in adults. The body surface is divided into areas that equal approximately 9% (Fig. 28-1). For example, a person's hand is equal to approximately 1% of his or her body surface area, and an adult arm approximately consists of 9% of a person's TBSA.

This percentage, coupled with the age and premorbid health of the client, guides the degree of fluid resuscitation that is necessary. Individuals who experience greater than 10% of TBSA are at risk of shock resulting from fluid loss.[13] The greater the percentage of TBSA and the presence of inhalation injury (which includes toxins), the greater are the mortality rates and length of hospital stays.[8] A typical length of stay in the hospital can be estimated as 1 day for each percent of body area burned.[14] As the TBSA increases, the chance for greater loss of function and mortality rates increases. Overall, the survival rate for admissions to burn centers in the United States was 96.8% over 9 years of data.[2]

Related Burn Complications

Clients with more than 20% TBSA of burns experience capillary leak (excessive plasma) that occurs as a result of vasoactive substances that are released by the burn wound. Maximum capillary leak and burn edema occur within 24 hours after the burn. Multiple physiological processes are also occurring during this period. The client is closely monitored for symptoms of burn shock, which would ultimately lead to death. Shock occurs when the organs of the body are not receiving enough blood flow (as with low blood pressure, blood going to heart and brain over organs, capillary leak and edema), depriving them of oxygen, and causing the accumulation of waste products.[15] Damage to skin places the client's body temperature regulation at risk (because skin helps regulate body temperature), and the burn team works to prevent hypothermia, which is a dangerously low body temperature. Hypothermia also increases the metabolic response, and therefore medical personnel work to maintain the client's normal body temperature.[7] An increased metabolic rate results in constriction of blood vessels, slowing of heart rate, and increase in glucose release to help the body to get warm through the shiver response.[16] Simply put, the body works harder to maintain proper temperature, which requires more stored energy to be used. Temperature regulation can continue to be at risk for clients during recovery, and an OT practitioner caring for clients with burns must continually be aware of hyperthermia or hypothermia throughout the rehabilitation process.

Full-thickness burns that enclose all sides of an arm or leg and the trunk may cause vascular or respiratory compromise. This is caused by the firm, leathery qualities that are characteristic of a full-thickness burn coupled with the edema that occurs within the first 24 to 48 hours. When

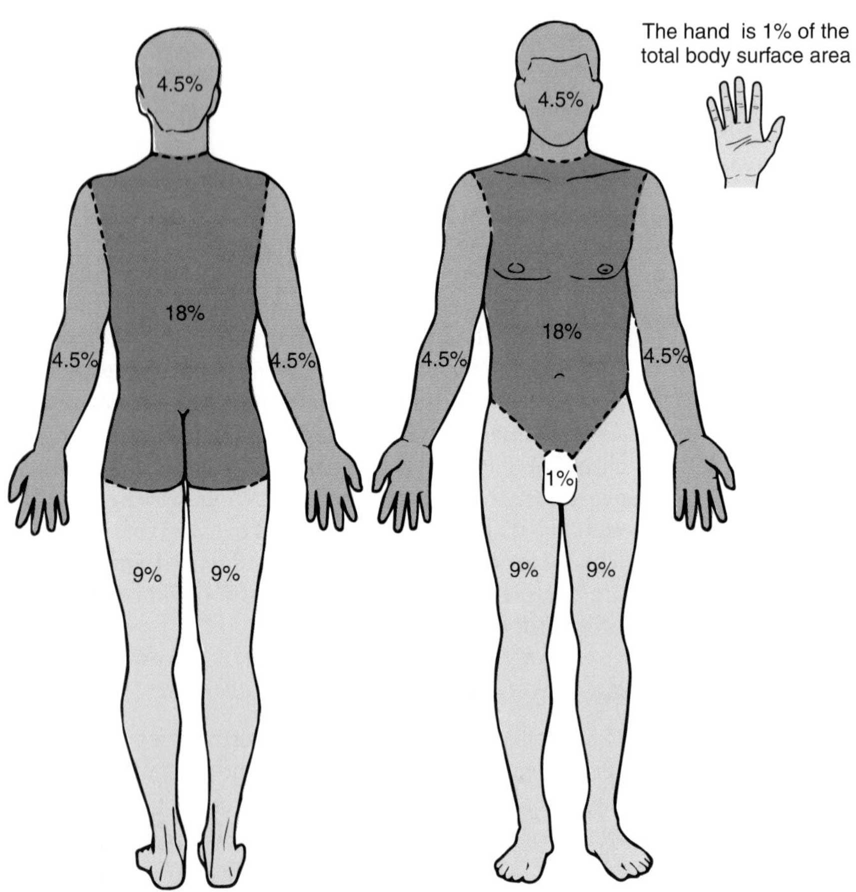

FIGURE 28-1. The rule of nines.

the client's venous pressure inside the fixed-volume area exceeds 30 mmHg, compartment syndrome (caused by high pressure in an enclosed space) and cell death inside the affected body part begin to occur. Compartment syndrome can be seen in the forearm, hand, leg, abdomen, or other areas. The nursing staff monitors the pulse of the client's affected extremity on an hourly basis by using a Doppler stethoscope and alerts the physician if consistent Doppler monitoring demonstrates weak or absent pulse. The treatment to prevent permanent damage (should a weak or absent pulse occur) is an **escharotomy,** which is a surgical incision made through the **eschar** (dead tissue) within the burn wound to release the pressure of the swollen tissues and restore blood flow[17] (Fig. 28-2). Another treatment may be a **fasciotomy,** which is a similar procedure in which the fascia is cut through to relieve the tension/pressure.

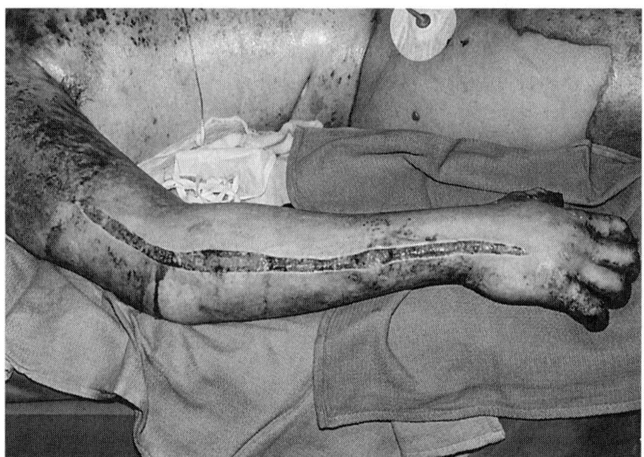

FIGURE 28-2. Escharotomy is an incision into the skin to release edema and avoid potential compartment syndrome.

Wound Care and Infection Control

Wound care and infection control are fundamental components of the medical management of burns and are essential in optimizing wound closure, which leads to client rehabilitation and increased occupational performance.

INFECTIONS AND SEPSIS

Infection in a burn wound is a serious issue because it delays healing and can cause formation of additional scar tissue. Ideally, prevention of infection is the primary goal.[18] Newer practices, such as wound excision and the use of handheld shower spray units for debridement, rather than immersion hydrotherapy, have helped decrease the development of infection in burn wounds.[19] Wound excision involves cutting away necrotic (dead) or scar tissue, either for increased healing or in preparation for a skin graft. Possible causes of infection may include the client's own flora on intact skin or gastrointestinal sources, or they may be outside sources, such as the hands of healthcare providers, family, or equipment and surfaces surrounding the client. Infections may be found in the burn wound itself or may be systemic (throughout the body). Effective treatment of burn infections requires the medical team to identify the source of infection and apply the appropriate topical antibiotics to the wound or other antibiotics for sepsis (systemic infections). Signs of sepsis include tachypnea (abnormal, rapid breathing), hypotension (low blood pressure), oliguria (low urine output), hyperglycemia (high blood sugar), and/or mental confusion.[19] Strict hand washing before and after client care is standard practice. When a client has exposed wounds, wearing a gown, mask, cap, and gloves is required for infection control.

STAGES OF WOUND HEALING

Burns heal through a series of overlapping and variable processes that begin in response to tissue injury. The four general phases of wound healing are hemostasis, inflammation, replication/proliferation, and synthesis/remodeling. The general stages of wound healing are explained in detail in Chapter 8. With burn wounds, the scarring process (fourth stage) is the most difficult because of the trauma to tissues and the propensity to develop hypertrophic scarring. A contracture can develop as scar tissue is formed during the healing process, which prevents functional movement in a joint, impacting performance of activities of daily living (ADLs) and instrumental activities of daily living (IADLs).[20] Contractures can develop quickly after burns because of the body's attempts to heal and form scars. The OT practitioner's role in scar and contracture management will be discussed later.

BURN WOUND HEALING FACTORS

The factors that can affect burn healing can be slightly different from those related to other injuries. The specific burn-related factors include the following:[21]

1. *Older age:* Older adults can have more fragile skin with less efficient physiological functioning because of decreased blood supply in some areas of skin.
2. *Nutrition:* After a burn, the body uses a tremendous amount of energy to heal. Clients who are unable to self-feed because of serious medical issues or severe pain often require a nasogastric feeding tube (from the nose to stomach).[22] Additional protein and other nutrients may be required.
3. *Infection:* An infected wound may have delayed healing or be nonhealing, and the infection must be cleared before healing can occur.
4. *Other illnesses:* Diabetes can cause changes in blood vessels, circulation, and peripheral nerves and a higher risk of infection.
5. *Medications:* Steroids and other medications can cause wounds to heal more slowly.

TYPES OF WOUND COVERAGE

Burns can be severe enough that there is no skin to heal, necessitating alternative solutions to manage. The type of coverage used on the burn wound depends on the depth and appearance of the wound. One option is temporary coverage, which initially "tricks" the wound into thinking that the coverage is skin. A variety of temporary **skin substitutes** are used to obtain wound closure and reduce pain in partial-thickness burns. The temporary skin adheres to the clean partial-thickness burn, thereby reducing pain and facilitating healing. As the wound heals, the temporary skin lifts off and can be trimmed away.

Two types of common temporary skin substitutes are used when a burn will likely heal on its own. One is a **xenograft,** a tissue graft from another species, usually porcine (pig) and/or biosynthetic wound dressings. These are applied on a clean wound and aid in reducing fluid loss and pain. The second type is cadaver skin, referred to as **homograft** or **allograft.** Cadaver skin is used as a temporary wound coverage until the client is ready for an **autograft,** a graft of the client's own skin. The homograft is used to cover a wound that is too large for an autograft until some healing has occurred to shrink the wound to the size required. The client's body will eventually reject the homograft, so it cannot be permanent; the duration of use can vary, depending on rate of healing. The homograft adheres to the healthy wound bed, reduces fluid loss, and allows for assessment of wound bed readiness. This assessment of the wound bed is important because if the homograft does not adhere, the client's own skin will not "take" or adhere either. However, if the homograft adheres properly, there is a good chance that the client's own skin will "take" when the autograft is applied.

Permanent wound coverage consists of a skin graft, or autograft. This graft is taken from a site on the client's body and transferred to a completely different site.[17] Three common types of autograft are as follows:

1. *Split-thickness sheet skin graft (STSG) and meshed graft:* This skin graft is the most commonly used permanent wound covering. It is taken from an unburned area of the body, usually the thigh, abdomen, buttocks, or back, using a small machine called a *dermatome,* a tool with a sharp razor blade. The machine harvests a strip of skin for transfer to the burn wound. This donor skin consists of the entire epidermis and the top part of dermis, hence the name of the graft. The donor site, which is now a superficial partial-thickness injury, is usually painful, will heal on its own within 7 to 10 days, and may leave a scar.[17] The STSG can be in the form of a sheet graft or a meshed graft. A sheet graft (strip of smooth-looking skin) is commonly preferred for use on hands, neck, and face because it appears similar to normal skin and has less of a chance of contracture (Fig. 28-3). Meshed autografts are the most widely used for coverage of full-thickness injuries. Meshed skin is put through a machine that creates small slits in skin, allowing it to be stretched to cover a larger area. Although meshing at 1.5:1 or 2:1 allows for the donor skin to expand and cover a bigger area, these grafts are more prone to contracture—they have less dermis per square inch because of the holes.[1]
2. *Full-thickness sheet graft (FTSG):* This type of autograft is ideal and is used for reconstruction in small areas, such as eyelids and in the web spaces of the fingers. The donor skin includes the entire epidermis and the dermis; therefore, the donor site is "primarily closed" and stitched back together.
3. *Cultured epithelial autograft (CEAs):* Clients with large burn TBSA have limited donor sites to complete wound closure. CEAs are grafts that are made from epithelial cells after a full-thickness skin biopsy specimen is obtained and sent to a laboratory, where the epithelial cells are grown into sheets of cells that are then prepared for transplantation. Cell growth takes about 3 weeks before the sheets can be placed on the client. These grafts are fragile and have an unpredictable pigmentation long after healing.[17]

INTERVENTIONS FOR BURNS

An interdisciplinary burn team has long been recognized as vital to successful outcomes with burn survivors.[23] The focus of burn rehabilitation is to complete therapeutic interventions that prevent or minimize scarring and contractures and prepare the person for future occupations, including social activities, which can be particularly challenging following a burn injury. Education, training, modalities, therapeutic techniques, and orthoses are tools used to progress the client through the burn healing process and manage scarring. Occupational therapists and OTAs facilitate learning and retrain clients in the performance components needed to prevent deformity and maximize independence with ADLs. Anticipation of potential scarring and contracture and delivery of effective treatment interventions are key to maximizing a client's functional outcomes and are optimized with a supportive team.[12] In many

TECHNOLOGY AND TRENDS

ARTISS [Solutions for Sealant] is a fibrin "glue" used in place of staples to secure an autograft to a wound bed. ARTISS [Solutions for Sealant] is made from two substances found in human plasma. Several years ago, a person could have 200 staples in the arm to hold the autografts in place for the first 48 to 72 hours, but now with the use of ARTISS [Solutions for Sealant], staples are minimally used, and depending on how the grafts look, the client may be able to move sooner after surgery.

Other technology, such as carbon dioxide and pulsed-dye lasers, are options for hypertrophic, hyperpigmented, and/or hypersensitive scars. They can also help with pliability of scar tissue for increased ROM. This is typically done in an outpatient setting, beginning 3 months after the burn injury, by a plastic surgeon. Compression garment therapy and scar management education (silicone) is continued to be utilized by OT services concurrently.

cases, part of the "team" can be a specialized burn practitioner whom OT practitioners contact at regular intervals for advice.

Scar Management Overview

The location and depth of a burn provides a predictable pattern of possible deformity from wound and burn **scar contracture** (tightening of the skin) starting on the first day.[24] Therefore, the burn team must develop, implement, and follow an aggressive, yet thoughtful, rehabilitation plan through until scar maturation. The longer a burn wound takes to heal, especially longer than 3 weeks, the more likely hypertrophic scar and burn scar contractures will form.[6] This is important for OT practitioners to understand so that anticipation of burn scar formation and subsequent action to reduce the contracture risk is followed. **Hypertrophic scarring** is characterized by its dark red–purple "angry" color; it is thick, firm to the touch, and itchy; it results from the complex processes that are required to heal a large burn wound. Instead of forming neatly, the scar tissue forms randomly and creates the rough texture. Over time, within 1 to 2 years, all scars mature and become lighter, softer, and flatter to a certain extent.[6] However, therapeutic interventions that optimize ROM, functional ability, and appearance of the scar are essential to implement *before* the scar matures.

Multiple factors influence tissue repair and wound/scar remodeling or contracture.[25] In the early phases of wound healing (the first 3 weeks), OT practitioners can encourage, educate, and facilitate a client's healing and wound care by focusing therapeutic interventions around creation and fitting of orthoses, ADLs, family/caregiver involvement, functional mobility, the practice of standard precautions, and reinforcement of proper wound (skin) care practices. These areas will be addressed further in the chapter.

As the client and the burn team work toward the ultimate goal of wound closure and a functional outcome, educating the client about what a burn scar can look like is useful in helping the client understand the rationale behind certain treatments, such as the importance of moving through pain and sleeping in stretched positions. The longer a burn wound takes to heal, the more likely the area will scar. The severity with which a person will scar is unpredictable and highly variable (Fig. 28-3). A guiding practice thought for OT practitioners is: *Scar contracture is easier to minimize or prevent than to fix.*

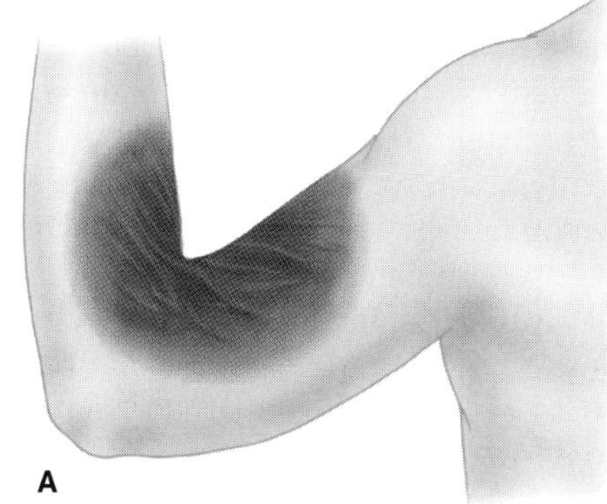

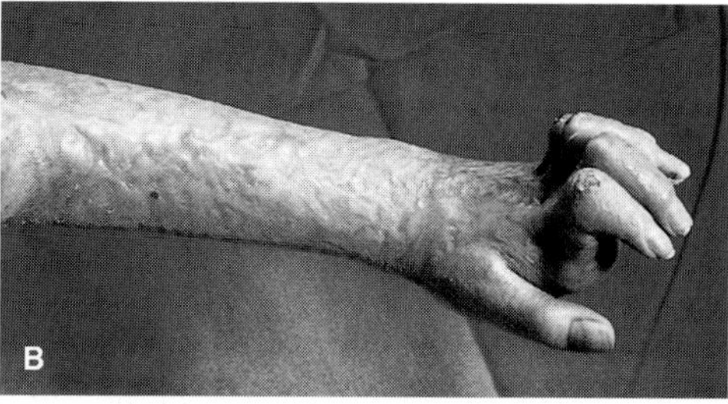

FIGURE 28-3. Scarring can be unpredictable and variable, often impacting function. **A.** Elbow flexion contracture. **B.** Scarring on volar side of forearm, hand, and fingers.

Phases of Recovery

Although burn recovery certainly follows some different stages, experts suggest that it is best to view burn rehabilitation as a continuum and realize that significant crossover occurs regarding what the burn team does to support the client throughout.[26] The initial stage of burn care is sometimes called "critical care" or "acute care" stage. The acute care stage is when the client is first admitted to the hospital or burn unit and typically includes the first 72 hours. The next phase is the surgical and postoperative stage, which can extend for weeks, depending on the severity of the burns and the need for surgery. This means the client may still be in the acute care setting, or may have transitioned to another setting, such as inpatient rehabilitation or home. The medical focus at this stage is on prevention of infection and wound healing. The third phase is where the focus shifts to rehabilitation, and can be divided between inpatient and outpatient (or early and late).[26] At this phase, the wounds have typically healed, and it can also be the most challenging phase for all involved.[27] Some challenges might include contracture management, pain, and psychosocial factors (as the reality sets in with the change of environment). When the client is discharged from the inpatient unit it is crucial for him or her to continue with therapy and to be monitored for depression, anxiety, and anger because as circumstances change (change going from hospital environment to home environment), these issues may emerge, if they have not already.[26]

Acute Phase Intervention Techniques

During the acute phase of a burn, the rehabilitation approach depends on the severity of the burn; determining the severity includes an assessment of burn depth, TBSA, and other medical factors, such as smoke inhalation injury. Yet the primary therapy goal in this phase, regardless of the severity, is the prevention of deformity. OT interventions include, but are not limited to, manual therapy techniques, therapeutic activity and exercise, neuromuscular reeducation, and orthosis fabrication and management. Specific manual techniques include scar management, active assistive range of motion (AAROM), edema reduction, positioning, scar massage, composite stretching, joint mobilization, and client/family education/support. Specific therapeutic activities can include ADL retraining, functional mobility retraining, ROM completion before and during functional tasks, and endurance activities. Neuromuscular reeducation can take form in facilitating postural control and center of balance to desensitization of a newly healed burn.

USE OF ORTHOSES

Immediately after a burn, the three primary reasons why a person may develop limitations in ROM and mobility are (1) edema, (2) tight eschar, and (3) pain.[28] In many cases, orthoses may be utilized in preventative, protective, or corrective phases during the wound healing process to assist clients with burn injuries.

Preventive Orthoses: In the preventive phase, orthoses are often applied to minimize further damage or provide protection. Clients are often intubated and sedated within an intensive care unit (ICU) setting of a burn center, delaying the start of active ROM; however, the OTA may be able to start passive range of motion (PROM) with the client and educate the family on PROM and positioning. Depending on the severity and mechanism of the burn, clients may have exposed bones and tendons when presenting to the burn center, which will be protected by the orthosis. When the client is awake and not sedated, and as edema and pain set in, an orthosis for the hand is often recommended to prevent contracture. This is because clients in intense pain may not actively move their hands as recommended and often prefer a flexed position of comfort. All of these are reasons to acutely splint a hand, elbow, or shoulder that shows an area of potential contracture. Orthoses have been present in burn rehabilitation for centuries and are an integral part of a comprehensive rehabilitation program.[28] Several types of orthoses are used within a burn center, depending on the burn location as well as the location of the line of "pull" or tension near a joint. Orthoses are used most commonly as positioning devices to counteract the active and ongoing contracture of wounded tissue through to healing and scar tissue through its maturation.[28] Acutely, hand orthoses are fabricated bedside by the OT practitioner and applied to assist in proper positioning for prevention of scar contracture and edema control. These orthoses are typically antideformity hand splints that put the hand in an intrinsic-plus position (metacarpophalangeal [MCP] joints at 70 degrees flexion, interphalangeal [IP] joints at neutral and wrist at 20 degrees extension) (see Chapters 19 and 22 for photos and illustrations of orthoses). Orthoses may be static, that is, they are designed to preserve a position of choice, such as an end ROM, by immobilizing the joint.[28] They also may be dynamic, which can provide low-load long stretch to the affected joint and assist to provide effective tissue mobilization; this orthotic must be checked frequently for proper alignment.[29] Maintaining the client's hand in an antideformity position when an OTA or other team member is not present to complete the daily exercises lowers the risk for continued loss of ROM. These preventive orthoses are worn all day and all night and only removed for wound care and daily ROM exercises if the client is intubated and/or unable to participate in a home exercise program (HEP). Soft or padded firm neck collars are also options to prevent neck contractures when a client is immobilized in the bed. As the client becomes more involved in his or her HEP for daily ROM, orthotic wearing time will decrease so that the client can be more independent in performing ADLs.

Protective Orthoses: Protective orthoses may be applied as the client's healing process progresses. As described previously, clients with burn injuries undergo several stages of healing and may require surgical intervention to close poorly healing wounds. OT practitioners will also create orthotics for clients within the operating room after the surgeon has applied the skin grafts. Postoperative orthoses provide joint immobilization, protection of the graft site from shearing, and positions the client in an antideformity position. These are also considered protective orthoses.

Orthoses can be fabricated to be used on any or all extremities or areas that may develop a scar contracture, including the hand, wrist, elbow, axilla, neck, ankle, and knees. Wearing and time frames of use vary from one burn center to another, but often orthoses can be worn several days postoperatively to allow the skin graft to heal properly before any ROM is resumed. This is one area of OT that is unique to burn practitioners because they have the experience of working in an operating room as part of the surgical team.

Orthoses prevent deformity and optimize ease of movement by keeping the affected body part "on stretch" during times of rest and OT practitioners establish a wearing schedule based on how the client is performing. The OT practitioner encourages and educates the client to move and utilize the affected (burned) extremity. Yet pain often limits all movement, and the OT practitioner is left to determine which is better—(1) no orthosis, which would allow movement that the client will likely not do because of pain, which can result in the client holding his or her body part in a position that favors deformity; or (2) applying the orthosis, thereby guaranteeing no active movement but facilitating the client's rest in the best position for healing. For the burn population, the position of comfort (flexed or fetal position) can be the position of deformity.[30]

The OT practitioner should also be aware of some precautions regarding orthotic use during active range of motion (AROM). Elbow extension orthosis straps should be wide (to disperse pressure) and loose enough to easily place a finger under the strap. Pressure from the most proximal strap—near the triceps—can compress the radial nerve leading to radial nerve palsy, which is the inability to actively perform wrist and finger extension. All orthoses can migrate out of their intended position because of client movement, smoothness of the orthosis material, and variability of dressings; therefore, frequent readjustment/repositioning is common and necessary.

Orthosis Contraindications and Precautions: OT practitioners should consider orthosis contraindications and precautions to prevent the development of joint and skin problems. Acutely, because of increased edema from fluid resuscitation and the initial burn, the orthosis should be fabricated to be adjustable to the changing body size and level of swelling. If an orthosis or an underlying joint is not properly padded with gauze or foam, a pressure injury (decubitus ulcer or skin breakdown) could occur (typically to the posterior elbow or heel). To avoid this, a client who is wearing a dorsiflexion or foot-drop orthosis should never have his or her heel placed on top of a pillow but have the calf supported and the heel clear. Orthoses should be assessed daily to ensure skin integrity and proper positioning. OTAs should educate and train the client, the family, and nurses or caregivers about the proper application of the orthoses and about signs of poor fit. Another precaution to possible joint discomfort is to avoid the overuse of an orthosis. The use of an orthosis for a client's extremity should be monitored on a daily schedule. For example, if a client is maintained in constant elbow extension orthosis for an extended period without ROM or proper positioning, he or she may develop **heterotopic ossification (HO).** This is an abnormal calcification process occurring in and around damaged joints, most often in the elbow or shoulder, severely limiting joint movement and interfering with the ability to perform everyday tasks.[6] There can be three types of heterotopic ossification: traumatic, neurogenic, and genetic. Burns fall under the traumatic subtype, and therefore the term is *HO*. In other conditions, such as spinal cord injury and traumatic brain injury with neurogenic central nervous system insults, the term used is *neurogenic heterotopic ossification (NHO)*.[31] This calcification process can be quite painful and could potentially relate to a permanent loss of ROM to a joint involved with HO (or requiring surgical intervention). Orthosis schedules are necessary for gaining functional ROM without further skin and joint damage, and education is essential for the client and caregivers to be aware of potential problems related to orthosis use. Schedules should be written with detailed directions and pictures and be visible to the client and caregivers so that orthoses can be applied correctly (Table 28-2).

RANGE OF MOTION, POSITIONING, EDEMA REDUCTION, AND PRESERVATION OF FUNCTION

AROM is optimal to preserving function after a burn. To facilitate AROM in a client with a burn, OTAs must be aware of normal movement patterns and motor functions. Immediately after a burn, clients will exhibit full motor functioning in the affected area, unless he or she has had a previous injury to that site or sustained an additional injury when the burn occurred. Document motor function, or lack thereof, during the assessment. Depending on the severity of the burn, edema, pain, fear, or medication side effects can cause the client's full motor functioning to quickly change, thereby increasing the risk of contracture. Because of the preexisting factors, as well as systemic changes, scarring can occur within the first few months after the initial injury or surgical procedure. If medically advised, stretching should be performed five to six times per day.[32]

Although burn scar formation is a normal part of the wound healing process, it is still possible to minimize or prevent contractures and deformity by minimizing healing time and maximizing scar management interventions. The following is a guide to acute intervention techniques identified by body part; positioning, edema reduction, preservation of function and AROM, AAROM, PROM, and scar massage are the guiding interventions.[12] If the burn crosses multiple joints, it is important to stretch across all joints simultaneously for maximal benefit.

Hand: If a client exhibits a deep burn on the hand and requires surgery, an intrinsic plus or safe position orthosis for a burn injury (0° to 20° wrist extension, 70° to 90° MCP

TABLE 28-2 Recommended Orthosis Positions

Neck burn (anterior and lateral)	No pillow behind head, a towel roll behind neck can be used for comfort. Neck extended 10° to 20°. Focus on neck extension. Remind "teeth together, lips together" to avoid mouth opening to lessen neck stretch.
Dorsal hand burn	Safe position orthosis (wrist 0° to 20° extension, metacarpals 70° to 90° flexion, full IP extension)
Volar hand burn (palmar)	Palmar extension orthosis (0° to 20° wrist extension, MCP/IP full extension)
Dorsal AND volar hand burn	Alternate between safe position orthosis and palmar extension orthosis, as indicated
Shoulder (axilla-anterior/posterior)	80° to 120° abduction and 30° to 60° of horizontal adduction (into scaption to protect the brachial plexus)
Elbow/Knee	Full extension of elbow and knee. Neutral position ("hand shake" position or supination of forearm) If range of motion is lacking because of heterotopic ossification, then the elbow can be splinted at 90 degrees of flexion for functional use
Ankle	Neutral dorsiflexion using multipurpose orthosis (MPO) (foot/ankle orthosis). Nothing should touch the heel if in an MPO.

flexion, full extension for the IP joints, and thumb in neutral) is fabricated for use immediately after autografting. The orthosis is also used at night to position a client's hand "on stretch" when not in use. Elevation and movement of the hand to decrease edema is strongly encouraged. The OT practitioner instructs the client and his or her family on functional task completion (using the affected hand, when possible), which is reinforced by the burn team. When pain limits functional use and therapy is repeatedly not tolerated, the OT practitioner can consider the use of a hand continuous passive motion (CPM) machine which provides regular movement in a controlled fashion. The CPM can never replace the practitioner stretching, but can allow the client to begin to tolerate therapy. A dynamic flexion hand orthosis is often considered as well.

Wrist: Clients tend to hold a burned wrist in a flexed position. Education on the risk of the loss of wrist extension along with proper positioning (0° to 20°) and AAROM/AROM is stressed. An orthosis is used when education and functional tasks are not effective and loss of wrist extension is progressive.

Forearm: Early in burn recovery, individuals tend to rest with their palms down in pronation, a typical sleeping position. Therefore, one of the most common forearm burn limitations is supination. Client education is key, along with teaching the client and his or her family stretch patterns into supination frequently completed in therapy. A static progressive supination orthosis can also be utilized.

Elbow: The goal for the elbow is full extension, followed by flexion. Elbow flexion is usually easy to preserve because people want to eat, scratch the head, and sleep in the fetal position. However, full elbow extension is easily limited because of the less frequent need to fully extend the elbow compared with flexion, but it is very important for functional reach, self-care, and mobility. An elbow extension orthosis is an effective tool to use after stretching, at night, or anytime the person needs sustained stretch.

Shoulder: Preserving shoulder flexion and abduction is one of the hardest burn scar contractures to prevent. People reach and raise the arms multiple times a day, yet rarely does one keep the shoulders stretched overhead for hours at a time. Positioning and orthosis use that hold the healing skin on stretch are interventions to preserve shoulder motion (Fig. 28-4). Manual and therapeutic interventions such as AROM, through encouragement from family, a posted exercise program, and the use of pulleys, are effective in preserving function and preventing contractures. It is necessary to protect the client's brachial plexus when a client is positioned with shoulders in abduction. Typically, this position is used when a client has burn injuries to the upper torso, axilla, or shoulder. A client should not be placed and secured into an extreme stretch position that can strain the brachial plexus of the arm and cause neuropathy. The best way to prevent brachial plexus injuries is by providing education to the nursing staff and client's family that helps with positioning and orthosis wear. It is also important to instruct clients that if numbness, tingling, or weakness is felt in the positioned arm, the client must tell someone. The nurse or a family member is instructed on how to assess the client's positioning and change the position or remove the orthosis if the symptoms (numbness, tingling or weakness) do not improve. Keeping the client's arm "forward," or slightly horizontally adducted into scaption to avoid extreme shoulder abduction is one of the best preventions for preventing brachial plexus injuries.

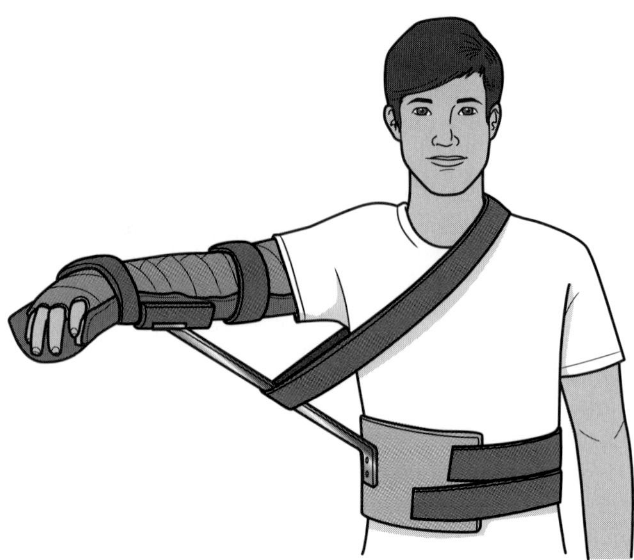

FIGURE 28-4. Airplane or axilla splint for burns to stretch axilla and under shoulder.

Neck: The skin of the neck is mobile to allow multidirectional movement. Almost everything a person performs tends to occur in the front of the body, from eating, to texting, to reading, or to driving. Prevention of a neck flexion contracture is critical because of the functional limitations caused by the inability to look up or side to side. Additionally, burn scar formation on the front of the neck can lead to pulling of facial skin and ultimately deformity of the burn scar. Most clients with a burn on the neck use a cervical collar or custom neck orthosis and no pillow on the bed mattress.

STRENGTHENING

To facilitate strengthening in the client with an acute burn, preserving endurance and prior movement is the focus. AROM, AAROM, self-care independence, and mobility out of bed for all meals, when possible, is facilitated by the OT practitioner and supported by the burn team. Clients are encouraged to be out of bed as soon as they are medically fit to do so, and this can assist with "a feeling of well-being, and a sense of confidence and achievement."[26] Use of weights may not be indicated for this population during the acute phase because ADL and functional mobility tasks may be significantly fatiguing. See Table 28-3 for carryover options of positioning, orthoses, and home programs.

TABLE 28-3 Carryover

CONCEPTS FOR CARRYOVER OF PROPER POSITIONING, ORTHOSIS MANAGEMENT, AND HOME EXERCISE PROGRAM	
Positioning	Use photographs or descriptive drawings when able. It is quick and easy to take a digital photograph of the client in the proper position for edema control and then post it for nursing staff and family to use as a reference.
Orthosis Application and Proper Fit	Photographs work well. If the client is an outpatient or going to a rehabilitation facility and he or she or a family member has a phone with camera, suggest taking a picture of each step of application for later reference. A video and audio instructions can be recorded as well.
Written Communication	Dry erase boards or personalized handouts with pictures are effective in communicating about the wearing schedule for the orthosis, activity out of bed (e.g., "All meals should be eaten in chair out of bed"), and HEP to client, family, and nursing staff.
Inpatient Treatment	Nurses are key for communication of needs. Having a "nurse huddle" or plan of care discussion with the nursing team is important to relay orthotic schedules, positioning, and client's OT goals. They also are good for follow-through and continuance of care when the OT practitioners or family are not available bedside.
Outpatient Treatment	Client and family understanding of continued need for involvement in the HEP is essential for success. HEP programs should be written and provided with drawn diagrams of "end goals" for ROM and graded therapeutic activities if previous and/or baseline ROM is not reachable.

Rehabilitation Phase Intervention Techniques

The rehabilitation phase is divided into inpatient and outpatient phases and takes place typically after the burn wounds have healed. Depending on the severity of the burn, the client may have been in acute care throughout the first phase or may be coming back to acute care after initial discharge for more surgery and inpatient rehabilitation.

SCAR MANAGEMENT

In the later stages of wound healing, the synthesis and remodeling phase, the wound is closed and scar remodeling is progressing. This process of scar remodeling toward scar maturation continues for 12 to 18 months during which time the texture, height, and color of the scar is changing and can be influenced by therapeutic interventions to achieve the best movement and appearance possible. Scar maturation characteristics include a softer texture and a less red (less vascular), more flesh-like color. When scar maturation occurs, the scar is in a more static, unchanging state, similar to that of normal skin. OT practitioners will educate their clients on the fact that once the scar matures, surgery is really the only option to make any change in that scar; therefore, it is important to get as much movement out of that scar *before* it matures.

Scar management techniques vary and include use of massage, silicone products, scar management education and training, and compression use. Daily scar massage with use of manual deep tissue pressure and prolonged pressure and stretching can soften the scar tissue, which, in return, will aid in skin pliability and also help with pain control. The client's spouse or family members should be educated and trained about how much pressure and amount of time to massage the client if he or she is not able to do this independently, although active participation by the client is preferable. The mechanical action of massage helps to soften the scar by promoting collagen remodeling and reducing hypersensitivity[6] (Fig. 28-5 A/B). Products that may decrease hypertrophic or keloid scarring, such as silicone gel sheets, hydrogel, and silicone gel, are also available. Current practice guidelines in burn clinics includes:[33]

- Gels or gel sheets should be applied to burn scars that have a high probability of forming hypertrophic scars.
- Only immature scars should be treated with gels or gel sheets, as mature burn scars have not been shown to respond.
- No clear benefits to using gel versus gel sheets or non-silicone versus silicone products exist with respect to the treatment effect, but the use of silicone gels appear to cause fewer adverse reactions compared with gel sheets.

When introducing a silicone product to a client, education and precautions should be provided because rash and skin infections may occur.

CORRECTIVE ORTHOSES

Corrective orthoses may be required, depending on how the client is healing from a burn injury. As noted previously, everyone heals differently from a burn injury. Clients may experience a hypertrophic or keloid scar because of genetics; scar contracture with loss of functional ROM; traumatic injuries, such as amputations or tendon damage. In a **keloid scar**, there is overgrowth of tissue beyond the original wound; such scars can be firm or rubbery and can vary in color. When deep burns occur to the dorsum of the proximal interphalangeal (PIP) joints, the fingers are at risk of extensor hood disruption, and subsequent boutonnière deformities can occur.[6] This could lead to permanent loss of function and disfigurement of the digit if not managed

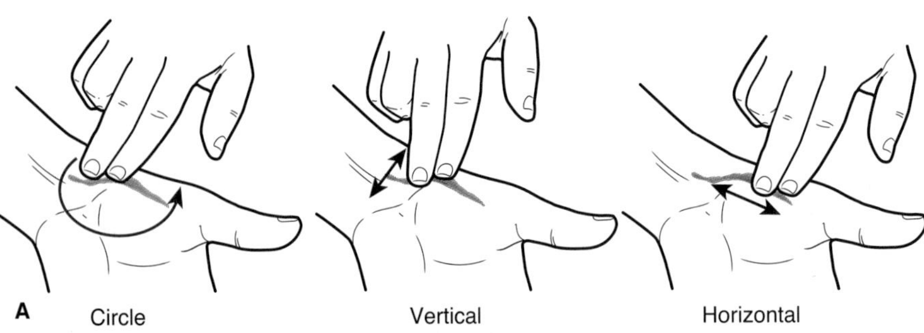

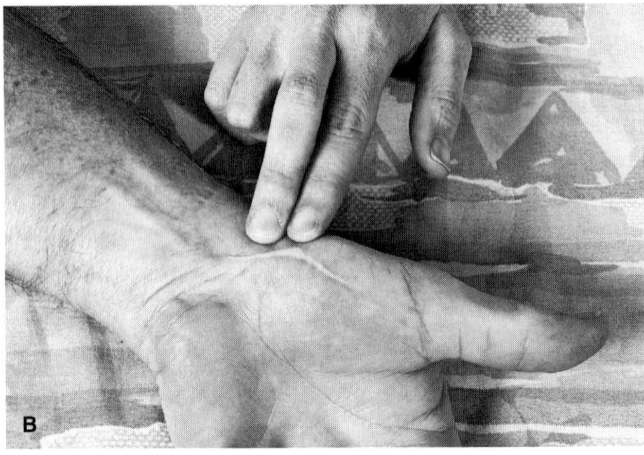

FIGURE 28-5. A. Scar massage, causing friction, can be performed in a circular motion along the length of the scar, vertically across the scar, or horizontally along the scar. **B.** The amount of pressure will vary with the integrity of the scar, sensitivity and skin irritation, and pain. The fingers remain in constant contact with the skin and do not slide; the intent is to move the layers of skin to disrupt the scar formation.

appropriately. OTAs will become familiar with the fabrication of simple orthoses, such as a gutter shape to prevent boutonnière deformities, and other more complicated orthoses with training and experience. Often, a client may require referral to a plastic surgeon for reconstructive surgery to address both physical limitations and aesthetic concerns. OTAs may often be involved in this reconstructive process because corrective orthoses may be needed. Corrective orthoses, such as dynamic MCP flexion splints, elbow extension splints applied after contracture release, or laser therapy, can also be considered progressive orthoses.

The fabrication of dynamic splints requires more complex splinting skills because they are used to mobilize a joint or allow a client to exercise a joint against the supported resistance of the orthosis.[28] The OT practitioner may also use commercially made dynamic orthoses to mobilize or provide resistance at the affected joint. Orthotic fabrication in either the preventative, protective, or corrective phases of wound healing can be an art form in that OTAs use their creativity to achieve the client's fullest potential with their ROM.

RANGE OF MOTION

PROM and AAROM are the second most effective and widely used therapeutic interventions for burn rehabilitation. These techniques can be done with the client in the supine, sitting, or standing position and are often used in conjunction with AROM and functional tasks. PROM can help the client achieve more motion than AROM alone. Slow sustained stretch, which involves pushing the extremity into further motion and holding the stretch at "end range," and scar massage with PROM all improve ease of motion and aim to prevent scar contractures. Counting during the stretch (distraction) and allowing breaks gives the client control and improves tolerance because stretching can be painful.

STRENGTHENING

As the client heals and ROM is improving, strengthening via resistive bands, free weights, functional tasks, which are strenuous, and work simulation tasks can be completed. The client works daily, often multiple times a day with and without therapy, on a strengthening program. Strengthening and stretching are coupled together to preserve or improve full ROM. Strengthening optimizes a client's power to move his or her joints "through" the scar, preventing the scar from adhering and deforming the burn survivor.

The key to a successful HEP is the client. OT practitioners serve as coaches, teachers, and cheerleaders to promote functional independence, strengthening, and scar management. The client must be an active participant in the creation and follow-through of any HEP. Traditional barriers to participation in therapy may include the complexity of the regimen (the number and timing of medicines, frequency of ROM, following guidelines for exercise, and wearing compression garments) and failure on the client's part to understand the importance of adherence, which may arise from poor communication by the burn team. Adherence to therapy may also be affected by the client's perception of barriers to adherence and the need to make lifestyle changes to accommodate a recommended regimen of treatment.[34] A client's former habits and routines need to change for the healing process to continue. For example, if the client was particularly sedentary, a workaholic, averse to exercising or lacked proper self-care, adherence may be affected.

NERVE REEDUCATION/DESENSITIZATION

Another important part of the rehabilitation phase is desensitization. Sensory reeducation is achieved by performing desensitization techniques. In addition to touching and massaging the scars, applying different textures and varying pressures to the scar will assist to alleviate neuropathic pain and allow the client to normalize the scarred skin. These techniques also help with decreasing hypersensitivity of the burned skin.

Once a client's wounds are well closed and the scar tissue has matured, OT practitioners often introduce heat modalities in the outpatient treatments. Some clients complain of arthritic pain, joint tightness from contractures, and hypersensitivity of the scar and surrounding skin. The use of heat modalities may assist in diminishing these ailments. Fluidotherapy is a device that will heat the skin and joints but will also aid in desensitization and pliability through dry heat. Other heat modalities such as paraffin and hot packs are better for the client than ice or cold therapeutic modalities, which can be contraindicated because of the decreased circulation to the burned area. Of course, precautions of regulation of the temperature of the modalities should be considered by the OTA so that the client does not get burned again. Paraffin has mineral oils can help during scar massage and aid in improving the pliability of skin.

TRENDING TREATMENT MODALITIES AND OUTPATIENT SERVICES

Clients with burn injuries often require outpatient services following hospital discharge because of the late effects of the burn and the constant changes in skin. Once home, clients begin to experience both the functional as well as the social consequences of a serious burn injury. Changes in self-image, work roles, and social relationships all have a direct effect on motivation and compliance with therapy recommendations.[6] OTAs will continue to assist with orthotic progression, scar management modalities, client and family education and training, and the application of vascular compression garments in an outpatient setting. Orthoses will be modified not only for comfort and fit but also to progress a client's ROM as scar maturation occurs. Many other options to help with breaking down active scar tissue are available, such as scar management techniques, use of compression garments, and laser therapy. OTAs should be familiar with each so they may provide them to clients, educate about their use, and complete training.

Compression Therapy

Vascular compression garments may be fabricated for clients to reduce their symptoms of itching, neuropathic nerve pain, to edema, and also, protect skin grafts. Poor venous return to burned extremities is evident by the presence of edema in the limb and vascular pooling (as evidenced by erythemic skin color), and clients may report throbbing, itching, stinging, and pain.[6] Clients are generally instructed to wear compression garments 23 hours each day, and better results are observed if compression garments are initiated as early as 2 weeks following wound closure.[35] OTAs may measure and sew these garments to provide a custom fit for clients of varying sizes, or they may obtain them from a medical supplier. Early compression can be achieved with the application of Isotoner™ gloves or elastic bandage wrapping. As the skin graft sites are well healed, compression intensity and tightness are increased. Typically, a client with skin grafts will wear compression garments with 20 mmHg to 30 mmHg pressure. Compression garments should interfere with clients' abilities to move and perform ADLs. Because of the tightness of the compression garments and the necessity to wear them, it is important that the OTA assist with teaching the client how to don and doff the garments. Compression garments may be more easily put on by using a compression stocking donner device. Some garments are made with zippers to help with donning, or the client may need the assistance of a caregiver. Clients with burn injuries may need to wear the compression garments 6 months to 2 years, depending on the severity of their symptoms. Wearing pressure garments can be uncomfortable and challenging; problems with full movement, appearance, fit, comfort, social acceptance, swelling of extremities, rashes, and blistering are common.[36]

Some dispute exists over the effectiveness of pressure garment therapy because recent research has shown that challenges include accurate assessment of pressure applied by the garments in varying areas of the body, potential lack of client adherence to wearing schedules, expense of the garments, and lack of evidence for timing (prophylactically or as an established treatment for hypertrophic scarring)[35] (Fig. 28-6).

Sun Protection and Skin Care

Following continued skincare and sun protective measures is a battle clients with burn injuries will have to fight throughout their lifetimes. Acutely, the healed skin will be fragile and at risk for tearing easily. Once well healed, the skin will continuously feel dry and itchy, and it will require constant moisturizing to prevent skin breakdown. A physician can recommend the best type of lotion for clients to relieve dry skin, and care should also be taken to not use scented lotions. Clients are at high risk for reburning of the skin upon sun exposure, and the client should avoid long periods of direct sun exposure. OTAs will assist in the education of sun protection needs, such as the daily use of a sunscreen cream of at least SPF 50 (sun protection factor 50), at least during the first year, regardless of weather conditions. The OTA may also provide education about sun protective clothing options.

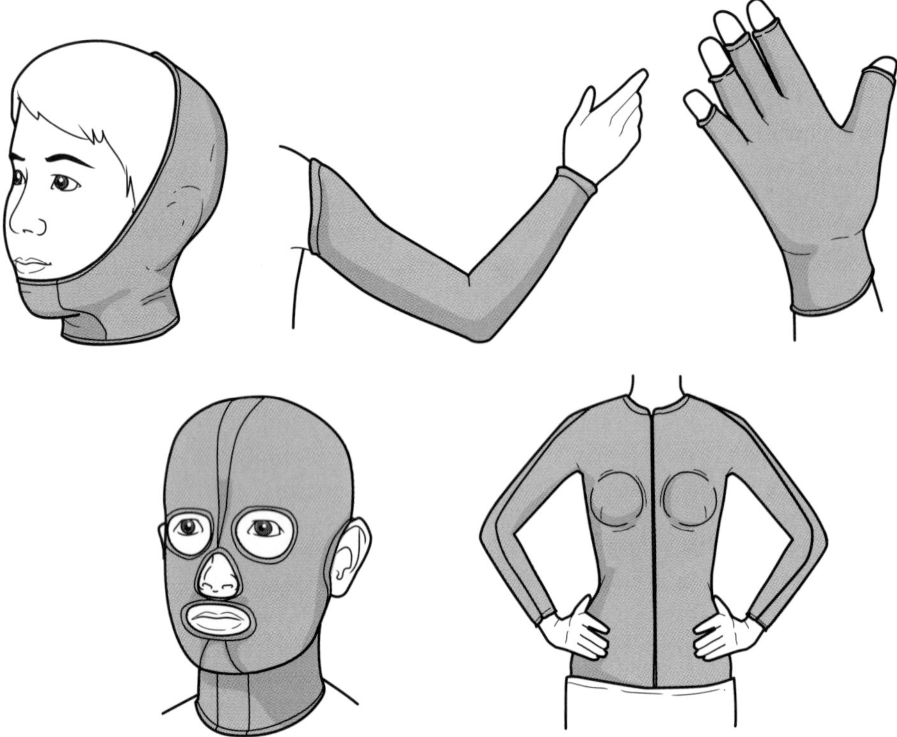

FIGURE 28-6 Burn pressure garments.

> **OT Practitioner's Viewpoint**
>
> Although it is recommended that clients with burns wear compression garments for a certain amount of recommended time (3 months for partial-thickness burns or 1 to 2 years for deep partial-thickness and full-thickness burns), it is important to understand that every client heals differently. I had a client come for an outpatient burn clinic visit not wearing his compression garments. He stated he was having minimal vascular symptoms and did not need them anymore. Rather than insisting that the client wear the garments, I assessed the need for continued vascular support and found that he had healed well enough to no longer require the garments. Compression garments are quite expensive and sometimes not covered by insurance. The garments are also potentially hot, itchy and uncomfortable, and many clients do not want to wear them. Necessity for the use of garments should be questioned on a regular basis. ~ Heather S. Dodd, MS, OTR/L

PSYCHOSOCIAL FACTORS FOR BURN REHABILITATION

How a burn injury occurs involves multiple reasons and mechanisms. Sometimes, underlying psychosocial or cognitive impairments can increase the probability of being burned. Self-inflicted burns (self-mutilation or suicide attempt) are a small portion of burn injuries overall, and those individuals may have a history of psychiatric illness and difficulty with family.[37] Individuals with self-inflicted burns experience a higher total burned surface area, longer hospitalizations, more infection complications, and a higher mortality rate.[37] Burns can also be caused by abuse (e.g., cigarette burns, scalding) and attempted arson or homicide. When a client has a burn injury, with either minimal or significant result in relation to the TBSA and depth, the burn may leave lifelong psychological effects. The most commonly identified psychiatric sequela to burn injury is posttraumatic stress disorder (PTSD). Rates of PTSD among clients with burn injuries have been cited as ranging from 7% to 45%.[38] OTAs are instrumental in developing rapport and motivating clients to participate in therapy in order to be independent in their ADLs/IADLs, as clients who are more engaged in their occupations experience higher life satisfaction. Understanding a client's previous psychological state and current emotional needs is important in order to promote the client's success in his or her phase of rehabilitation. Burn injuries often result in disfigurement and scarring and at times even amputation, leading to social stigmatization. The term "social death" (when an individual feels as though he or she is not accepted by society as being fully human) also describes the public response to clients with burn injuries, alluding to the significant impact on social functioning.[38] Many resources are available to clients with burn injuries to help overcome the social stigma and psychological impacts of burns.

THE OLDER ADULT

In 2015, Jones, Buchanan, and Harcourt[39] conducted a qualitative study on older adult clients with burn injuries (ages 51 to 71 years), via semistructured interviews to better understand the lived experience as adults age. The study identified four themes as follows:

1. "Time and adjusting to an altered appearance"—Participants who were burned as children were more well-adjusted to the change in appearance compared with those who sustained burns as an adult.
2. "Living with a visible difference in the eyes of others"—Older adults stated they still felt stigmatized by society as not being "normal." For some, this limited their social interaction to avoid negative and unwanted attention; however, most had gained coping skills to deal with negative reactions.
3. "Me, myself, and I"—Several study participants expressed a lack of peer or emotional support, which they desperately needed, especially in the years following the burn injuries, that has continued into their older years.
4. "The importance of maintaining appearance"—One participant stated that during hot flashes that occur in menopause, the scarring on her face turned red. Several reported that despite directives from their physicians, they purposefully exposed their scars to the sun so the skin pigmentation would darken and not be as noticeable. Some noted that the regular changes that occur with aging were even more noticeable with burn scars.

The OTA should remain supportive of the client with an old or new burn, because psychosocial adjustment is difficult, even into the older years. OTAs can help guide the clients they are working with in the initial phases of burn recovery to counseling and peer support resources and teach the client to positively interact in social situations (e.g., to smile at an individual who is staring). These resources may help alleviate some of the social isolation and loneliness that can occur at any age.

Cognition

A client who understands the burn rehabilitation process in terms of scar contracture and maturation and continued need for ROM and participation in ADLs/IADLs will increase his or her probability of returning to daily life at a quicker rate. Medical advances have resulted in the decline of burn-related mortality, leading to an overall rise in surgeries, disfigurement, and physical impairment. The subsequent emotional and physical toll may be great, as evidence suggests that clients with burn injuries are at risk not only for PTSD but also for depression, chronic pain, and multiple interpersonal problems, especially those who experience visible disfigurement as well.[38] If a client has baseline cognitive impairments, continued education and demonstration of ROM will need to be expressed to family and caregivers. Written information, pictures and/or modified instruction may be necessary. OTAs will often provide graded activities throughout the client's treatment to ensure the client is able to understand the importance of meeting his or her goals.

Pain

Burn pain is complex and the necessary medical treatments are painful as well; the OTA must respect the client's pain. Pain management includes understanding pain (e.g., type, timing, description), treating pain with medications or behavioral approaches, and the client learning to cope with pain.[40] The medical team will try to alleviate as much associated pain as possible with medications, being careful not to overmedicate the client, so he or she may participate in ADLs and the HEP. Clients' discomfort during medical procedures impedes wound care, increases the risk of wound infection, decreases the ability to perform the usual ROM exercises, increases psychological stress, and is associated with longer hospitalizations.[41]

Pain throughout the course of the burn and recovery process can also interfere with sleep, mood, and the ability to work.[42] The OT practitioner may work in conjunction with nursing staff to develop a schedule for daily therapy to ensure that pain medication is often provided before therapy so the client can address ROM goals through prolonged stretching and exercise while receiving the benefits of some pain relief.

Uncontrolled acute pain has been shown to increase the incidence of mental health disorders in clients, such as depression and PTSD. This can also decrease the client's compliance with rehabilitation therapy and negatively affect the client's confidence in the burn team.[43] OTAs will often relay the concern about the client's increased pain and decreased ability to participate in therapy to the multiple team members who are engaged in the client's care. OT practitioners can work together with the other members of the burn team to develop strategies for pain relief beyond medications, such as relaxation techniques, distracting a client with videos, or playing favorite music, depending on the client's age and needs. Relaxation techniques can be cognitive, such as cognitive restructuring (changing one's thinking to reassure self the pain is temporary) including meditation, or physical, including deep breathing techniques, yoga, and progressive muscle relaxation.[42] Clients may benefit from hypnosis (via a psychologist) and pacing of activities to avoid overdoing it.[42] Being patient with the client and respecting his or her level of pain is necessary and critical to proceed with treatment goals. When working with burn survivors who have had a history with drug and/or alcohol abuse, it often is difficult to determine "real" pain from drug-seeking behaviors. See further discussion in Chapter 8 about pain.

Anxiety

Anxiety is also a factor following a burn injury and affects every client differently. Often, the recurring sensations of feeling the initial burn will deter a client from willingly being involved in the wound care and therapy his or her injury requires. It is important for the OT practitioner to be able to identify the difference between pain and anxiety in order to effectively motivate a client as well as to communicate this information to the medical team. The client may have anxiety about the future, role fulfillment, finances, and many other current and future aspects of burn management. Sometimes anti-anxiety medication will help a client regain control of his or her daily tasks and independence. Another way an OTA may help alleviate or reduce a client's anxiety is having the client choose his or her OT schedule, or integrating such techniques as adding music during therapy sessions.

Self Image

Whatever the severity or location of a client's burn injury, his or her initial thought is, "What will I look like?" Burns can heal in different ways due to multiple factors, such as genetics, scarring, skin grafting, and pigmentation changes. Clients who have been disfigured by a burn injury have additional challenges and increased anxiety. They must deal with the aesthetic changes to their appearance, which often result in unwanted stares, unsolicited questions, and comments from people they already know as well as from strangers they encounter in their daily lives.[6] OTAs will often be involved, along with other burn team members, in explaining to clients what may happen acutely as well as what their skin may look like in 2 years. Once a scar has matured, a plastic surgeon can address surgical and aesthetic options. Self-image is important to both men and women alike. OTAs are often involved with community reintegration programs that educate the client's family and friends about how to adapt to the changes in the client's life. Peer support and resources for support groups for the survivor and/or the family are available to help the client adjust to the changes in their appearance and emotional needs.

COMMUNICATION

Peer support has been well established as a positive coping strategy that can affect recovery of individuals with traumatic conditions, such as spinal cord injury, cerebrovascular accident, and burns. Phoenix SOAR® (Survivors Offering Assistance in Recovery®) is a peer-support program designed to ensure that clients with a burn injury and their families do not go through the experience alone. Phoenix SOAR® connects compassionate and caring volunteers with the newly injured and their family to talk openly, share experiences, and offer encouragement. The one-on-one program is available in over 60 hospitals and burn centers in the United States. More information about the program can be found at the website www.phoenix-society.org.

Sexual Activity

Another occupational performance area that OTAs should be mindful of, and may address by answering questions or providing education, is the client's concern of returning to sexual activity and intimacy. Burn injury survival means coping with more than just the physical changes and disabilities often encountered after burn injury. The client may feel unattractive, unlovable, or ugly after sustaining a burn. The burn may cause pain, stress, depression, and anxiety, which may need to be managed before the client can feel free to be intimate. Certainly issues, such as sexuality and intimacy, are significant facets of quality of life for many clients, especially those who have sustained a potentially disfiguring burn.[44] OTAs may discuss sexual positioning needs, self-image concerns, or also suggest referral to counseling resources.

ROLE OF THE OCCUPATIONAL THERAPY ASSISTANT IN BURN CARE

Clients with burn injuries who have good rapport with their therapy staff tend to experience the most successful recoveries. OTAs are integral members of the rehabilitation team and their responsibilities vary from day to day, which is both rewarding and exciting as each day brings new challenges. OTAs are often the primary motivators for clients to gain independence in their occupations and to regain confidence in their life roles.

Common Occupational Therapy Goals for Inpatient and Outpatient Treatments

Beyond the medical management of a client's wound, the burn therapy team plays a significant role in the daily life of a client with a burn injury. During the initial assessment and evaluation of the client, the occupational therapist will discuss the client's primary treatment goals and needs with the OTA. Initially, biomechanical needs, such as ROM and positioning, are the focus to prevent loss of ROM from a burn scar contracture. These are typical goals that an OTA may address within the first weeks of a burn injury:

- Client/family will verbalize understanding of burn rehabilitation process.
- Client will be independent in HEP for ROM.
- Client will increase AROM/PROM of upper extremities in order to be independent with ADLs and reduce potential for burn scar contracture.
- Client will maintain proper positioning for edema control to optimize wound healing.

These goals would vary dependent on the status and stability of the client. Daily ROM, positioning, orthosis use, HEP education, and client involvement will be the focus of the OTA's treatments primarily until the client has met functional ROM and focus on maintaining ADLs/IADLs can be addressed.

ACTIVITIES OF DAILY LIVING

Every day, people get out of bed, bathe, dress, and feed themselves, and go about their normal daily routines. When a client sustains a burn, especially to the hand, these tasks become much more challenging. The task of buttoning a shirt following a burn injury can be a lengthy process. The OT practitioner may suggest clothing with Velcro® closures, pull-over upper body or pull-on lower body clothing, and selecting comfortable, soft fabrics that do not irritate healing skin. Uncontrolled scarring or noncompliance with exercise programs often result in contractures, which impair motion and skin flexibility. When this occurs, previous performance patterns cannot be completed without compensatory techniques or adapted equipment.[6] OTAs are highly involved in teaching clients ways to adapt if they have significant contractures, experience weakness, fatigue, or pain, or if they are missing digits or limbs; OTAs will also work with the client to determine the best way for the client to become independent in these tasks. With the use of sock aids, dressing sticks, and modified devices, such as builtup handles on utensils, clients with burn injuries can begin to regain their independence (see Chapter 14 for examples of adaptive equipment). Strengthening in the rehabilitation phase will be important for gaining as much functional use of the upper extremity as possible in preparation for tackling ADLs, IADLs, and returning to work responsibilities. The therapy team should grade and modify each task related to the client's engagement in ADL tasks and strengthening programs as a way to continually motivate the client toward meeting his or her goals and prevent discouragement that might occur, such as if the client is unable to complete simple grooming tasks as they had previously. OTAs will observe the client's involvement in ADL tasks, including toileting, bathing, self-feeding, and functional mobility to determine the client's ability to return to his or her previous residence. In addition, the OT practitioner will work with the client in performing all desired occupations to help the client be aware of precautions. For example, when bathing, the client should be aware of the proper temperature of water. In addition, clients may have itchy skin, and the OTA may suggest bathing in lukewarm water because it does not dry out skin and using colloidal oatmeal, which may provide temporary relief. The OTA may also suggest applying fragrance free moisturizers several times throughout the day.[37] Often, further adaptive equipment and home medical equipment will need to be recommended by the therapy team before discharging a client home safely.

INSTRUMENTAL ACTIVITIES OF DAILY LIVING

IADLs can also be an important area for the OTA to address when the client is returning home or ready to begin returning to previous role participation. If the initial burn was caused by a cooking incident, the client may be fearful to be in the kitchen or feel unsafe around the stove. The OTA will need to address alternative ways to prepare meals with fearful clients, potentially beginning with preparation of cold snacks and increasing tolerance to being near heat sources in the kitchen. The client with safety issues may not be able to perform meal preparation independently. The presence of contractures, pain, and weakness may limit a client's ability to clean the home and perform laundry tasks. Alternatives might be using a dressing stick to more easily reach into the washer, a long-handled dust pan, pacing chores that are fatiguing, and performing chores after taking pain medications. Pet care can be a challenge; food bowls may need to be placed higher for easier reach, self-cleaning litter boxes can be utilized, and caregivers and friends may assist with walking a dog. Clients who were taking care of children or others as a role before the burn may require additional assistance from others to manage these tasks or adaptations from the OTA for task management. Some adaptations might include a baby carrier to hold an infant when a hand/arm has been burned, specific sun protection products to be used when on the child's soccer field, or hiring someone to temporarily assist with caregiving tasks.

REST AND SLEEP

More than 50% of people who have had severe burn injuries report difficulty sleeping, and insomnia is the most common issue.[45,46] Insomnia includes difficulty falling asleep and maintaining sleep, poor sleep quality, waking up too early, or having nightmares. Sleep may also be difficult because of pain, depression, anxiety, itching, or side effects of medications. Lack of sleep has further consequences, such as difficulty handling stress, poor concentration, delayed wound healing, or intensifying pain. Standard OT interventions for sleep include creating a good sleep routine—avoiding daytime napping, creating and maintaining a schedule for sleep, avoiding caffeine or exercise before bedtime, removing televisions from the bedroom, reducing the use of electronic devices before sleep, and performing progressive muscle relaxation. If difficulty with sleep persists, the medical team should be notified because medications can be prescribed to address this issue.[45,46]

LEISURE

Some previously loved leisure tasks may be physically difficult after a burn, for example, playing softball with decreased shoulder ROM or crocheting with the effects of a hand burn. The OTA can research options for adapted leisure activities in the community based on the nature of the restrictions of the particular client. Adapted sports clubs exist all throughout the country and may have adaptive sports equipment to trial as well as a social network. Some clients may be uncomfortable in social leisure situations, such as going to a bar, participating in a religious social activity, or a joining a bowling team. The OTA may role play social situations where others may stare at the burn or make comments and discuss options to handle difficult scenarios. Because of fatigue and decreased endurance, less intense leisure options, such as playing card or board games, reading, or a doing a craft, may be explored with the client while he or she is healing.

EVIDENCE-BASED PRACTICE[46]

Sleep is an ADL that has been studied very little in the burn population, as the primary focus tends to be on more medically urgent aspects of burn medical care and rehabilitation. However, sleep is well known to be an important aspect for both physical and mental health and healing. Associated mental health conditions for burn clients are posttraumatic stress disorder, anxiety, and depression; poor sleep routines negatively affect these conditions. A 2013 study addressed the concerns of the burn client's sleep in postburn rehabilitation phase "to determine the quality and nature of sleep patterns in postburn clients along with the various relevant social, clinical, and demographic parameters associated with such altered patterns."[46] Clients from a burn hospital (n=818) in India were given a questionnaire (the Pittsburgh Sleep Quality Index [PSQI], a subjective assessment of sleep) at 12 months after a burn injury, in which they reported current sleep patterns versus their preburn sleep patterns. One significant finding was that the highest portion of individuals reporting sleep disturbances were those with postburn neck contractures. The study found the following significant differences in the patterns of sleep:

1. Increased duration of time spent awake in bed before falling asleep
2. Abnormal postures because of contractures/pain, making falling asleep more difficult
3. Nightmares
4. Short bouts of sleep punctuated by frequent awakening
5. Difficulty breathing
6. Arising late in the morning and not feeling well rested

Implications for OT include a continued focus on contracture management and client compliance, discussing sleep routines with clients in all phases of burn care, and providing appropriate interventions for creating sleep habits and routines, including identifying aspects to promote stress reduction, and referring for counseling, as appropriate.

Masoodi, Z., Ahmad, I., Khurram, F., & Haq, A. (2013). Changes in sleep architecture after burn injury: "Waking up" to this unaddressed aspect of postburn rehabilitation in the developing world. The Canadian Journal of Plastic Surgery, *21(4), 234–238.*

RETURN TO WORK

Beyond aesthetic issues, some burns result in functional impairment, which may further intensify a client's social isolation, result in financial hardship, and limit the individual's ability to fulfill the roles they occupied before the injury.[38] Returning to work is often a primary concern for adults with burn injuries because they carry large financial burdens after they sustain the injury, not only because of the medical bills but also because of being out of work for a long time while their wounds heal. An important consideration is that the cost of burn injuries is not limited to in-hospital charges. Disability and productivity loss from burn injuries are associated with significant financial burden as well.[8] OTAs and the interdisciplinary team determine the client's previous role in the workplace and its associated responsibilities, including lifting requirements, environmental considerations, and length of the work day. Dynamometer measurements along with other objective measures are assessed to determine lifting restrictions. Environmental considerations, such as sensitivity to hot or cold environments or work that involves being outdoors all day, are all limiting and impactful factors when determining when a client is physically ready to return to work. Often, the client's endurance has decreased after a long hospital stay, and the individual is unable to tolerate long work hours; this may necessitate a trial return to work. In 2012, it was reported that 72% of previously employed individuals had returned to a form of work at 3.3 years after a burn injury.[47] This delay may have resulted from physiological or psychosocial limitations. There are multiple factors to consider when addressing the client's desire to return to work to avoid further injury. (See Chapter 17 for more information on work rehabilitation.)

The client who cannot return to work may be interested in volunteer opportunities, which the OTA can research and potentially facilitate. A client who is socially anxious could make calls from home for a charity fundraiser, and could then slowly progress to volunteer work outside of the home. Additionally, the client may be able to volunteer as a peer mentor (see Communication box).

SUMMARY

Burn rehabilitation requires an understanding of physiology, wound-healing processes, scar management, the vascular system, and orthosis needs.[6] OTAs in burn centers are integral members of an interdisciplinary team that is committed to the care of clients with burn injuries and their rehabilitation. This setting enables OTAs to use their creativity through the fabrication of orthoses and possibly compression garments to meet the specialized needs of their clients; it is also an opportunity to develop rapport with clients, motivating them to maximize their potentials. Burn survivors can demonstrate impairment in their performance skills, specifically, motor, process, and social interaction skills, because of the psychological and physical toll of the burn injury. The unique skills and training of an OTA are especially effective when working with the burn population because OTAs facilitate engagement in daily life through skilled interventions that promote health and occupational performance.[3]

REVIEW QUESTIONS

1. While cooking at the stovetop, Ms. Thornton had a seizure, which resulted in her hand coming into contact with the hot burner, thus sustaining a full-thickness burn. She does not recall the event and appears lethargic. What is the *first* thing the OT practitioner should do when Ms.Thornton is seen at the burn center for treatment?
   a. Let her pain subside before beginning ROM.
   b. Fabricate and apply a hand orthotic.
   c. Wait for family to come to assess her previous level of functioning.
   d. Position her hand so that it is comfortable and by her side.
2. A client sustained a flame burn to the anterior neck in a gas grill explosion. Which is the *best* position in bed for the client?
   a. On her side
   b. On her stomach
   c. On her back, with two pillows behind her head
   d. On her back, flat, with no pillows behind her head
3. Mr. Lowe sustained a significant burn—70% total body surface area (TBSA) flame burns as well as an inhalational injury—from a house fire. He is in the intensive care unit and remains intubated and sedated. He has circumferential burns to his hands and arms. As the OTA is stretching his upper extremities, she notices that his heart rate increases and blood pressure rises during PROM to his right elbow. What is the OTA's *most* important concern?
   a. That there may be a fracture to his arm
   b. That he may have developed heterotopic ossification
   c. That he has a pressure injury
   d. That he needs more sedation
4. An OTA is treating a client in the outpatient burn clinic.The client has autografts to her right hand from a grease burn sustained a month ago, and today she is complaining of increased tightness. Which three of the following options should the OTA suggest that she should do to increase ROM?
   a. Continue HEP for ROM and stretching.
   b. Massage the hand.
   c. Apply ice packs to the hand.
   d. Rub moisturizer cream on the hand.
   e. Use a contrast bath.
   f. Use overhead pulleys.
5. A young adult male expresses to the OTA that he would have rather not to have survived his injury that caused him to lose his arm. What should the OT practitioner do to help him?
   a. Tell him that you understand his frustrations.
   b. Ignore the comment as this would be a Health Insurance Portability and Accountability Act (HIPAA) violation.
   c. Tell the interdisciplinary team involved in his care.
   d. Have the resident physician prescribe an antidepressant.
6. Mrs. Ha sustained a steam burn while cooking at home. She presents to the burn clinic with raised blisters and is in moderate pain. What kind of wound care should be suggested to the client?
   a. Autografting for the hand
   b. Letting the blisters dry up
   c. Applying cultured epithelial autograft
   d. Applying a topical cream to keep the wound moist
7. A client is returning to work as a construction worker after he had an autograft to his legs 6 weeks ago. What is the *most* important thing he should do to prevent edema when returning to work?
   a. Wear sun protection lotion or clothing.
   b. Wear compression garments to his legs and donor sites.
   c. Take hourly breaks to elevate his legs.
   d. Drink a lot of fluids to stay hydrated.
8. At initial evaluation and assessment of a client with a significant burn, what is the primary focus the OTA should have to develop an appropriate treatment plan?
   a. A full understanding of the client's prior and current functioning with ADLs
   b. Understanding current AROM
   c. Knowing the client's pain tolerance
   d. Determining where the client will be discharged to
9. When a client sustains a full-thickness burn circumferentially to an extremity, what is the biggest concern?
   a. Loss of sensation
   b. Loss of joint ROM
   c. Compartment syndrome
   d. Body temperature loss
10. Once a client's burned skin is ready for scar management, which three of the following are suggested to decrease a scar contracture?
   a. Transcutaneous electrical nerve stimulation
   b. Silicone
   c. Massage
   d. Traction
   e. Neuromuscular electrical stimulation
   f. Paraffin

CASE STUDY

John is a 17-year-old male with a 30% TBSA burns (both deep partial and full-thickness) to chest, abdomen, right side of face, neck, back, and upper arms to wrist bilaterally (hands were spared). He was given fluid resuscitation and a nasogastric feeding tube immediately. The injury occurred at work during a fall on the ice while carrying hot grease to the oil dumpster. John, a high school senior, lives 2 hours from the Level I trauma and burn center and was transported from the local hospital.

The occupational therapists at the burn center completed an evaluation of John's burn wounds and medical status within the first 24 hours of his arrival. The ultimate goal was for John to successfully return to being an independent high school senior. John's parents were present at his bedside on the burn unit. They were divorced but had a good relationship in caring for their son. The OT evaluation determined his immediate need for proper positioning, client/family education regarding the burn rehabilitation process, and developing therapeutic goals. John was positioned with his shoulders in flexion to 90 degrees and his elbows fully extended. Neck extension was facilitated by putting no pillows behind his head. These positioning goals were written on a communication board in his room for the nurses and family to follow. A treatment plan was developed and included daily ROM/stretching of BUE's, positioning to optimize healing and decrease edema, and education of John and his parents on the rehabilitation process. John was a social individual, and he was disappointed about missing school events as a senior. The burn team provided emotional support, and John was encouraged to focus on bigger school events, such as the prom and graduation in the future.

John endured several operative grafting procedures. Within 4 days of his admission, surgeons debrided the burn and applied homograft/allograft to all burned areas. He then returned to the operating room on his 18th birthday for his second grafting procedure: split-thickness autografts applied to arms, neck, chest, abdomen, and right side of back. The OT staff was active during the surgeries, stretching him before surgery in the operating room when he was asleep and fabricating and applying orthoses for his arms and neck to promote optimal autograft adherence and healing.

From the beginning of his hospital stay, therapy was complicated by poor pain tolerance. It was important for the OT and physical therapy practitioners, nurses, and his family to encourage him to engage in his recovery. Anxiety and frustration from John and the family was apparent due to his need for increased time and support to tolerate the daily process of recovery that included ROM, mobility, positioning/orthoses, and dressing changes, all of which signaled "pain!" to John. He became withdrawn, and his therapy participation was minimal unless he was in an individual session with a practitioner. The burn team utilized his past interests and social demeanor to improve his participation. He initially required multiple practitioners to help him walk because of pain and deconditioning. His situation of dependence and altered physical appearance was the opposite of how he viewed himself before his injury. As his hospitalization continued, he reported that he felt none of his friends cared anymore. He slowly regained his strength for walking, yet he continued to avoid feeding himself or independently completing his self-stretching program. Three weeks after his burn injury, he was discharged to acute rehabilitation. He was then discharged home with his mother a little more than 1.5 months after his burn.

It was important for John to continue his rehabilitation, but the burn center was 2 hours away from his home, and he wanted desperately to be near his friends and family. He was set up with OT near his home, with weekly follow-up at the burn center. The burn center OT practitioners spoke to his hometown OT practitioners frequently and aided in establishing appropriate treatment goals and modalities.

John began to develop significant hypertrophic scarring to his arms and neck. This limited his ability to fully extend his elbows, move his shoulders, or turn his head functionally. Within 2 weeks of returning home, he and his family agreed to five-times-a-week intensive outpatient therapy at the burn center, which required weekly stays at a nearby hotel. As aggressive daily therapy continued, multiple therapeutic techniques were used to increase the ROM. John had serial casting applied to his elbows and an airplane orthosis to his shoulders was fabricated; John was fitted with custom compression garments with silicone inserts. Ultrasound, scar massage, Kinesio® taping, and moist heat, combined with intense manual stretching by OT practitioners and PT practitioners was also completed. Three months after the burn, physicians recommended surgical scar release to his shoulders, elbows, and neck.

Even after intense rehabilitation, John had developed contractures—his right shoulder movement was 90 degrees abduction and 75 degrees of flexion, and his neck rotation was 30 degrees towards the left. He underwent surgical scar revisions to the right arm and neck (left side to follow). He then returned to acute rehabilitation for a short stay while he adjusted to his new surgical wounds and the orthoses to his neck and arms.

He was discharged to his hotel during the week with his mother and continued this path of surgical releases and outpatient therapy five times per week until 6 months after his injury, when he returned home for continued therapy twice a week at the burn center and twice a week closer to home. He continued to undergo multiple scar revision surgeries and subsequent OT for several years.

1. What life roles changed for John?
2. What types of interventions would an OTA perform with John?
3. What impact do you think John's injury had on his family?
4. Why do you think John said that none of his friends cared anymore?
5. What do you think his eventual outcome might have been?

PUTTING IT ALL TOGETHER — Sample Treatment Session and Documentation

Setting	Inpatient rehabilitation burn unit
Client Profile	Ms. H, 42 y/o, experienced partial and full thickness burn injuries to torso, neck, face, RUE (volar forearm spared), R hand and RLE due to flames in a house fire (38% TBSA). Significant inhalation injuries. Found unconscious in kitchen during fire. R hand dominant.
Work History	Self-employed as a hairdresser; owns a salon
Insurance	Private
Psychological	Depression, anxiety, high risk for PTSD
Social	Single. Many close friends in her community. One adult son lives 2 hours away. Owns two cats (one perished in the fire).
Cognitive	Normal
Integument & ROM	Client presents with postsurgical wounds that have been recently autografted and are nearly completely healed. Decreased neck ROM with beginning of flexion contracture. 95 degrees R AROM shoulder flexion & abduction (PROM 110 degrees) -15 degrees R AROM elbow extension (165 degrees with flexion contracture), PROM - 10 degrees (170 degrees) 100 degrees R AROM elbow flexion 15 degrees R AROM wrist extension (PROM 25 degrees) 15 degrees R AROM finger extension (20 degrees PROM) LUE: AROM WNL & MMT 4+ throughout Slow, cautious movements with RUE
ADL	Mod A bathing, Mod I self-feeding, Min A grooming, Mod A dressing
IADL	Dependent for all

PUTTING IT ALL TOGETHER Sample Treatment Session and Documentation (continued)

Goals Within 4 weeks:

1. Client will perform UB dressing with Mod I.
2. Client will increase AROM shoulder flexion and abduction by 10 degrees to improve functional ADL & IADL tasks and reduce burn scar contracture.
3. Client will increase AROM wrist extension by 10 degrees to improve functional ADL & IADL tasks and reduce burn scar contracture.
4. Client will be independent in HEP to increase strength and endurance for ADL tasks.

OT TREATMENT SESSION 1

THERAPEUTIC ACTIVITY	TIME	GOAL(s) ADDRESSED	OTA RATIONALE
PROM with stretch	10 min	#2, and indirectly #1, #3, and #4	*Preparatory Method:* OTA applies gentle stretch to right shoulder in direction of flexion and abduction with hold for 1 minute × 5. R wrist extension PROM held for 1 min × 5.
Education for client in HEP, with demonstration, handout and return demonstration.	20 min	#2, #3, and #4	*Education and Training:* To help facilitate AROM movement of RUE and alleviate burn scar contracture so client can perform ADLs.
Functional activity – Grooming and bathing while standing at sink	25 min	#2, #3, and #4	*Occupations:* Grooming/bathing increases ROM, balance, strength, well-being, and increases independence.

SOAP note: 3/11/—, 8:00 am–8:58 am

S: Client states, "I feel gross."

O: Client participated in skilled OT to improve ROM, exercise to increase strength and endurance, and functional ADL activities in room. Client noted she received pain medication 30 minutes before session and pain is 2/10. After receiving PROM to right shoulder into flexion and abduction with prolonged stretch of 1 min x 5 for each movement, an increase in 5 degrees each was noted. Client was also given PROM to wrist extension on the right, for 1 min x 5, with ROM increase of 3 degrees. After demonstration, client was able to complete the UE HEP with Min A to adapt for RUE and to recall exercises with use of a handout. Client performed bathing task in standing at the sink for 5 min x 3 with rest breaks of 2–3 min and with Min A with use of a wash mitt and long handled sponge to bathe UB and back thoroughly. Client required Min A for management of grooming supplies and bringing right wrist into effective position for tooth brushing.

A: Client was engaged and an active participant in therapy session with increased AROM noted at both right shoulder and wrist after stretch. An electric toothbrush may assist with difficulty in wrist positioning during tooth brushing. Client continues to have excellent rehab potential due to improvements in endurance and strength as well as cooperation despite some pain. Client would benefit from further therapy to address goals and work toward modified independence.

P: Continue to work with client on increasing ROM through stretching, ADL performance and HEP to increase endurance and strength for ADL performance. OTA to also educate client's nursing staff on ways to have client stand more often when not in therapy.

Justin Cannon, COTA/L, 3/11/—, 4:50 pm

TREATMENT SESSION 2

What could you do next with this client?

TREATMENT SESSION 3

What could you do next with this client?

REFERENCES

1. Coleman, III., J. J. (2006). Principles of burn reconstruction. In B. M. Achauer & R. Sood (Eds.), *Achauer and Sood's burn surgery reconstruction and rehabilitation* (pp. 1–8). Philadelphia, PA: Elsevier.
2. American Burn Association. (2016). Burn incidence and treatment in the United States: 2016. Retrieved from http://www.ameriburn.org/resources_factsheet.php
3. Weber-Robertson, K. (2006). Physical therapy principles for the burn patient. In B. M. Achauer & R. Sood (Eds.), *Achauer and Sood's burn surgery reconstruction and rehabilitation* (p. 357). Philadelphia, PA: Elsevier.
4. Model Systems Knowledge Translation Center. (2016). Burn. Retrieved from http://www.msktc.org/burn
5. Cinat, M. E., & Smith, M. M. (2006). Acute burn management. In B. M. Achauer & R. Sood (Eds.), *Achauer and Sood's burn surgery reconstruction and rehabilitation* (p. 59). Philadelphia, PA: Elsevier.
6. Monafo, W. W., & Bessey, P. Q. (2000). Wound care. In D. N. Herndon & J. H. Jones (Eds.), *Total burn care* (pp. 88–89). Edinburgh, UK: Harcourt Publishers Limited.
7. William, W. G., & Phillips, L. G. (2000). Pathophysiology of the burn wound. In D. N. Herndon & J. H. Jones (Eds.), *Total burn care* (pp. 63–67). Edinburgh, UK: Harcourt Publishers Limited.

8. Prochazka, M., Thornton, S., & Dodd, H. (2011). Enabling life roles after severe burns. In C. H. Christiansen & K. M. Matuska's *Ways of living: Intervention strategies to enable participation* (pp. 359–378). Bethesda, MD: AOTA Press; 2011.
9. Veeravagu, A., Yoon, B., Jiang, B., Carvalho, C., Rincon, F., Maltenfort, M., ... & Ratliff, J. (2014). National trends in burn and inhalation injury in burn patients: Results of analysis of the nationwide inpatient sample database. *Journal of Burn Care & Research, 36*(2), 258-265.
10. Mayo Clinic. (2016). Burns: First aid. Retrieved from www.mayoclinic.org/first-aid/first-aid-burns/basics/art-20056649
11. Tarim, A., & Ezer, A. (2012). Electrical burn is still a major risk factor for amputations. *Burns, 39*(2), 354–357.
12. Sood, R. (2006). Preface. In B. M. Achauer & R. Sood (Eds.), *Achauer and Sood's burn surgery reconstruction and rehabilitation.* Philadelphia, PA: Elsevier.
13. Summit Medical Group. (2017). Burn: Partial thickness (second degree). Retrieved from http://www.summitmedicalgroup.com/library/adult_health/aha_first_aid_for_second-degree_burns/
14. Calota, D. R., Nitescu, C., Florescu, I. P., & Lascar, I. (2012). Surgical management of extensive burns treatment using allografts. *Journal of Medicine and Life, 5*(4), 486–490.
15. Medical Dictionary. (2016). Shock. Retrieved from http://medical-dictionary.thefreedictionary.com/burn+shock
16. Ruffalo, D. (2002). Hypothermia in trauma—The cold, hard facts. Modern Medicine Network. Retrieved from http://www.modernmedicine.com/modern-medicine/content/hypothermia-trauma-cold-hard-facts
17. Knipe, C., Gabehart, K., Zieger, M., & Sood, R. (2006). Acute nursing management. In B.M. Achauer & R. Sood (Eds.), *Achauer and Sood's burn surgery reconstruction and rehabilitation* (pp. 89, 93–96, 98, 100–108). Philadelphia, PA: Elsevier.
18. Rafla, K., & Tredgett, E. E. (2011). Infection control in the burn unit [Abstract]. *Burns, 37*(1), 5–15.
19. Church, D., Elsayed, S., Reid, O., Winston, B., & Lindsay, R. (2006). Burn wound infections. *Clinical Microbiology Review, 19*(2), 403–434.
20. Model Systems Knowledge Translation Center. (2016). Scar management. Retrieved from http://www.msktc.org/burn/factsheets/Wound-Care-And-Scar-Management
21. Kramer, L. (2012). Factors affecting the healing of burns. Retrieved from www.burn-injury-resource-center.com
22. Hildreth, M., & Gottschilich, M. (2000). Nutritional support of the burn patient. In D. N. Herndon & J. H. Jones (Eds.), *Total burn care* (p. 237). Edinburgh, UK: Harcourt Publishers Limited.
23. Nakamura, D. (2006). Occupational therapy principles for the burn patient. In B. M. Achauer & R. Sood (Eds.), *Achauer and Sood's burn surgery reconstruction and rehabilitation* (p. 371). Philadelphia, PA: Elsevier.
24. Evans, E. B., Alvarado, I. M., Ott, S., & McElroy, K. (2000). Prevention and treatment of deformity in burned patients. In D. N. Herndon & J. H. Jones (Eds.), *Total burn care* (p. 443). Edinburgh, UK: Harcourt Publishers Limited.
25. Garner, W., & Nabavian, R. (2006). Normal wound healing. In B. M. Achauer & R. Sood (Eds.), *Achauer and Sood's burn surgery reconstruction and rehabilitation* (p. 18). Philadelphia, PA: Elsevier.
26. Procter, F. (2010). Rehabilitation of the burn patient. *Indian Journal of Plastic Surgery, 43*(Suppl), S101–S113.
27. Reeves, S. U., & Deshaies, L. (2013). Burns and burn rehabilitation. In Pendleton, H. M. & Schultz-Kron, W. (Eds.), *Pedretti's occupational therapy: Practice skills for physical dysfunction* (pp. 1110–1148). St. Louis, MO: Elsevier.
28. Richard, R., & Ward, S. (2005). Splinting strategies and controversies. *Journal of Burn Care and Rehabilitation, 26*(5), 392–396.
29. Serghiou, M., Ott, S., Whitehead, C., Cowan, A., McEntire, S., & Suman, O.E. (2016). Comprehensive rehabilitation of the burn patient. Retrieved from http://plasticsurgerykey.com/comprehensive-rehabilitation-of-the-burn-patient/
30. Judson, A. B. (1891). Prevention of short leg of hip disease. *JAMA, 16,* 511. Retrieved from https://books.google.com/books?id=TNg5AQAAMAAJ&printsec=frontcover#v=onepage&q&f=false
31. Nauth, A., Giles, E., Potter, B. K., Nesti, L. J., O'Brien, F. P., Bosse, M. J., ... & Schemitsch, E. H. (2012). Heterotopic ossification in orthopaedic trauma. *Journal of Orthopaedic Trauma, 26*(12), 684–688. http://doi.org/10.1097/BOT.0b013e3182724624
32. Hall, S., Kowalske, K., & Holavanahalli, R. (2016). Scar management after burn injury. Model Systems Knowledge Translation Center. Retrieved from msktc.org/burn/factsheets/wound-care
33. Nedelec, B., Carter, A., Forbes, L., Shu-Chuan, H., McMahon, M., Parry, I., ... & Boruff, J. (2014). Practice guidelines for the application of nonsilicone or silicone gels and gel sheets after burn injury. *Journal of Burn Care & Research, 36*(3), 345–374.
34. Aronson, J. K. (2007). Editors' view: Compliance, concordance, adherence. *British Journal of Clinical Pharmacology, 63*(4), 383–384.
35. Atiyeh, B. S., El Khatib, A. M., & Dibo, S. A. (2013). Pressure garment therapy (PGT) of burn scars: Evidence-based efficacy. *Annals of Burns and Fire Disasters, 26*(4), 205–212.
36. Ripper, S., Renneberg, B., Landmann, C., Weigel, G., & Germann, G. (2009). Adherence to pressure garment therapy in adult burn patients. *Burns, 35,* 657–664.
37. Macedo, J., Rosa, S. C., & Silva, M. G. (2011). Self-inflicted burns: Attempted suicide. *Revista do Colégio Brasileiro de Cirurgiões, 38*(6), 387–391. https://dx.doi.org/10.1590/S0100-69912011000600004
38. Cukor, J., Wyka, K., Leahy, N., Yurt, R., & Difede, J. (2014). The treatment of posttraumatic stress disorder and related psychosocial consequences of burn injury: A pilot study. *Journal of Burn Care & Research, 36*(1), 184–190.
39. Jones, B.A., Buchanan, H., & Harcourt, D. (2015). The experiences of older adults living with an appearance altering burn injury: An exploratory qualitative study. *Journal of Health Psychology, 22*(3), 364–374.
40. Wiechman, S., & Mason, S. (2011). Managing pain after burn injury. Model Systems Knowledge Translation Center. Retrieved from http://www.msktc.org/burn/factsheets/Managing-Pain-After-Burn-Injury
41. Thompson, E. M., Andrews, D. D., Christ-Libertin, C. (2012). Efficacy and safety of procedural sedation and analgesia for burn wound care. *Journal of Burn Care & Research, 33*(4), 504–509.
42. Model Systems Knowledge Translation Center. (2014). Managing pain after burn injury. Retrieved from https://www.phoenix-society.org/resoruces/entry/managing pain
43. Retrouvey, H., & Shahrokhi, S. (2015). Pain and the thermally injured patient—A review of current therapies. *Journal of Burn Care & Research, 36*(2), 315–323.
44. Rimmer, R., Rutter, C., Lessard, C., Pressman, M. S., Jost, J. C., Bosch, J., ... & Caruso, D. (2010). Burn care professional's attitudes and practices regarding discussions of sexuality and intimacy with adult burn survivors. *Journal of Burn Care & Research, 31*(4), 579–589.
45. Model Systems Knowledge Translation Center. (2013). Resources offered by the MSKTC to support individuals living with burn injury. Retrieved from http://www.msktc.org/lib/docs/Booklet/Burn_Booklet.pdf
46. Masoodi, Z., Ahmad, I., Khurram, F., & Haq, A. (2013). Changes in sleep architecture after burn injury: "Waking up" to this unaddressed aspect of postburn rehabilitation in the developing world. *The Canadian Journal of Plastic Surgery, 21*(4), 234–238.
47. Mason, S.T., Esselman, P., Fraser, R., Schomer, K., Truitt, A., & Johnson K. (2012). Return to work after burn injury: A systematic review. *Journal of Burn Care & Research, 33*(1), 101–109.

Chapter 29

Oncological Care and Treatment

Joanna Edeker, PT, DPT and Brittany Lorden, MHS, OTR/L, CLT

LEARNING OUTCOMES

After studying this chapter the student or practitioner will be able to:

29.1 Describe the pathophysiology of cancer

29.2 Describe the role of an occupational therapy practitioner in the management of clients with cancer

29.3 Explain why cancer rehabilitation is beneficial

29.4 List primary precautions to be aware of with a client with cancer

29.5 Develop treatment intervention plans and exercise recommendations for a client with cancer

KEY TERMS

Benign tumor	Hospice care
Cancer	Metastasis
Cancer rehabilitation	Oncology
Cancer-related fatigue (CRF)	Palliative care
Chemotherapy-related cognitive dysfunction	Survivorship
Chemotherapy-induced peripheral neuropathy (CIPN)	Tumor
	Quality of life (QoL)

Cancer is defined by the American Cancer Society as "a group of diseases characterized by the uncontrolled growth and spread of abnormal cells."[1] These abnormal cells form a tumor in most cases. **Oncology** is the branch of medicine concerned with the diagnosis and treatment of cancer.[1] Cancer is a disease with a broad spectrum; presentations are very different, depending on the type of cancer and its location in the body.[1] This chapter will familiarize occupational therapy assistants (OTAs) with cancer rehabilitation, but it will not be all inclusive because of the broad spectrum of the disease. **Cancer rehabilitation** involves an interdisciplinary team and may be on an inpatient or outpatient basis. The OTA will work with the cancer survivor and the supervising occupational therapist to set and meet goals and, most importantly, increase **quality of life (QoL).** With the growing number of cancer survivors, occupational therapy (OT) practitioners will most likely treat a client with a cancer diagnosis or a history of cancer at some point in their careers, regardless of the setting in which they are practicing. In this chapter, the term "cancer survivor" will be used interchangeably with "client," because it is a term frequently used by national cancer organizations, and is not meant to disregard person first language.

CANCER STATISTICS

According to the National Comprehensive Cancer Network (NCCN), cancer is the second leading cause of death in the United States, with 1.1 million new cases of cancer diagnosed each year.[2] The 5-year cancer survival rates are improving and are now greater than 55%. Increasing survival rates are attributed to earlier diagnosis of cancer and advances in treatment options for cancer.[3]

It is estimated that the number of cancer survivors in the United States will increase by 37% by the year 2022[4] (Fig. 29-1). The number of cancer survivors by 2025 is predicted to be over 18 million. Whether the client presents with impairments from the cancer itself, from cancer treatments, or from late effects of cancer and cancer treatments, OTAs will need to know how to treat this client population.[3]

TYPES OF CANCER

Most types of cancer cells form a mass called a **tumor,** however, not all tumors are cancerous. A cancerous tumor is a malignant tumor, whereas a noncancerous tumor is a

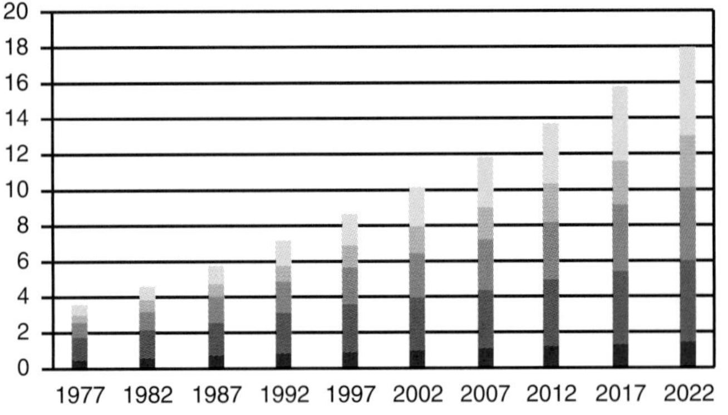

FIGURE 29-1. Individuals who survive cancer (>5 years) represent a growing population and future trend.

THE OLDER ADULT

With an increase in the aging population in the United States and individuals with cancer living longer, a phenomenon called the "silver tsunami" of cancer is developing. The number of older clients with cancer is increasing significantly as a result of improving cancer treatments that extend life, better screening tools that detect cancer earlier, and increasing numbers of those of the aging baby boomer generation. According to research by Bluethmann, Mariotto, and Rowland, as of January 2016, it was estimated that 62% of the cancer population was older than 65 years and it has been predicted to increase to 73% by 2040.

Health problems increase with age, even in those without a cancer diagnosis. When cancer is accompanied by age-related comorbidities, it makes cancer treatment planning more complex, and weighing the risks and benefits of cancer treatments for the geriatric population requires the involvement of everyone (client, physician, family, OT practitioners, physical therapy (PT) practitioners, etc.).

Ongoing research involving older clients with cancer will assist physicians to gain better understanding of appropriate cancer treatments for this population and possibly of the long-term effects of cancer treatments.[5]

benign tumor. Cancers are described by the type of tissue in which they originate (Table 29-1).

Metastases

Cancerous cells from the tumor can break away and travel to other parts of the body, where they may continue to grow and form more tumors called **metastases** (Fig. 29-2). Even when cancer spreads to another part in the body, it is still named after the part of the body where it started. For example, breast cancer can metastasize to the brain. Even though it has now spread to the brain, it is still referred to as *breast cancer with metastases to the brain*. Benign tumors do not metastasize.[6]

MOST COMMON TYPES OF CANCERS

The most common types of cancer are breast, prostate, lung, and colon cancers (Fig. 29-3).

Breast

Breast cancer is the number one cancer diagnosed in women. Although less common, breast cancer can also occur in men. Mammography is the best modality for early detection for breast cancer. When diagnosed early, the 5-year survival rate for those with breast cancer is 99%.[1]

Lung

Currently, lung cancer has the highest mortality rates for both men and women in the world, although the incidence of lung cancer diagnoses is declining (Fig. 29-4). The decreasing rates of lung cancer most likely have resulted from increasing rates of smoking cessation, reduction in secondhand smoke as a result of bans on smoking in public places, and asbestos, which is a known cancer-causing agent, no longer used in construction and being removed from most old buildings, if present.[1]

Prostate and Colon

Prostate cancer is common in men, but not necessarily fatal if it is diagnosed and treated early. Although about 1 in 7 men will be diagnosed with prostate cancer in his lifetime, only 1 in 38 will die of this disease.[1]

Risk factors for developing colorectal cancers include poor diet, obesity, smoking, and lack of exercise. Colorectal cancer is the third most common cancer diagnosed in both men and women in the United States and the third highest mortality rate, but the incidence of new cases is decreasing. Screening for colorectal cancer is an important part of cancer prevention and should begin at age 50 years for both men and women. Early detection of colorectal cancer through screening makes the treatment less extensive (as far as surgery and recovery time are concerned), than if detected after symptoms are present, and provides more successful survival rates. This decline can be attributed to

TABLE 29-1 Types of Cancer

TYPE OF CANCER	SITE OF ORIGIN	EXAMPLES
Carcinoma	Within an organ	Skin, mouth, lungs, breast, prostate, colon and rectum, pancreas, ovaries, liver, kidneys
Sarcoma	Within connective tissues Rare form of cancer	Bones, muscles, tendons, cartilage, nerves, fat, blood vessels
Lymphoma	Within lymphatic tissue	Lymph nodes, spleen, thymus gland, bone marrow
Leukemia	Within blood-forming tissue Does not form a tumor	Granulocytes, monocytes, lymphocytes

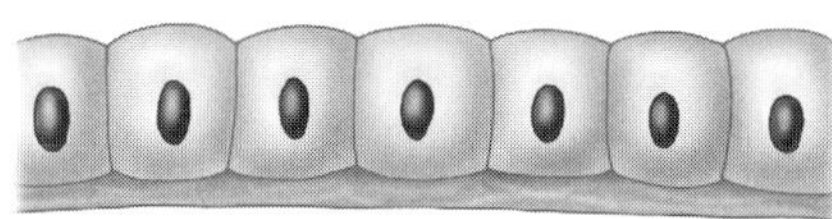

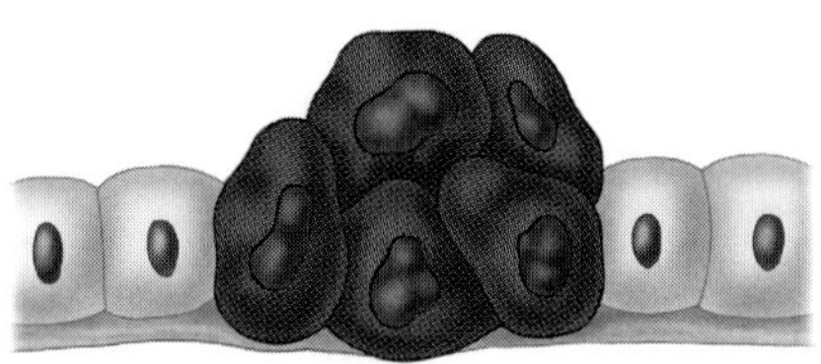

FIGURE 29-2. Metastases or cancer cell versus normal cell.

prevention of colorectal cancer made possible by screening. Several recommended methods are used for screening of colorectal cancer, including fecal occult blood test (FOBT), stool DNA test, sigmoidoscopy, colonoscopy, computerized tomography (CT) colonography, and double-contrast barium enema (Table 29-2).[1]

Although cancers of the central nervous system (CNS) are not among the most common types, they are included here because of the extensive impairments that they cause. Clients with brain tumors and spinal cord tumors have concurrent neuro-oncological conditions affecting the nervous system. Successful outcomes for clients with neuro-oncological conditions depend on immediate referral for rehabilitation to improve the client's independence with functional mobility.[6,7]

Brain

Brain tumors can be primary tumors or metastatic tumors. The brain is a common site for metastases. Similar to a cerebrovascular accident (CVA) or traumatic brain injury (TBI), brain tumors can affect any part of the brain, and the area of the brain affected will determine the impairments caused to the individual. For instance, a brain tumor located in the occipital lobe may affect that individual's vision. There are different types of primary brain tumors, including, but not limited to, glioblastomas and meningiomas. Glioblastoma multiforme (GBM) tumors tend to be highly malignant, and a 2009 study reported that only 10% of clients with GBMs may live 5 years or longer. Meningiomas are typically benign tumors and grow slowly. They account for nearly one third of primary brain tumors.[8]

Spinal Cord

Spinal cord tumors may be primary spinal cord tumors or the result of metastases from another type of cancer. Similar to a traumatic spinal cord injury or disease (SCI/D), a spinal cord tumor can affect any level of the spinal cord and can be complete or incomplete. Spinal cord tumors present with symptoms similar to a SCI/D, but will be a nontraumatic injury instead of a traumatic injury to the spinal cord.[6,7]

CANCER STAGING AND GRADING

Cancers are classified into grades and stages. This helps predict the client's prognosis, or chances of recovery, and guides the appropriate intervention to treat the cancer. The grade and stage of the tumors are determined by oncologists and pathologists.

Once the tumor is staged, a grade of I, II, III, or IV is assigned (Table 29-3). The tumor grade is a system used to classify cancer cells in terms of how abnormal they look under a microscope and how quickly the tumor is likely to spread and grow.

Grade I and II tumors resemble normal cells. They tend to grow and multiply slowly, and they are generally considered the least aggressive type of tumor. Grade III and IV tumors have cells that do not look like normal cells of the same type. They tend to grow rapidly and spread faster than in tumors with a lower grade (I or II).[9,10]

TNM Staging System

The TNM staging system, the most common staging method for cancer reporting, assesses tumors in three ways: the extent of the primary tumor (T), the absence or presence of regional lymph node involvement (N), and the absence or presence of distant metastases (M) (Table 29-4).[9,10]

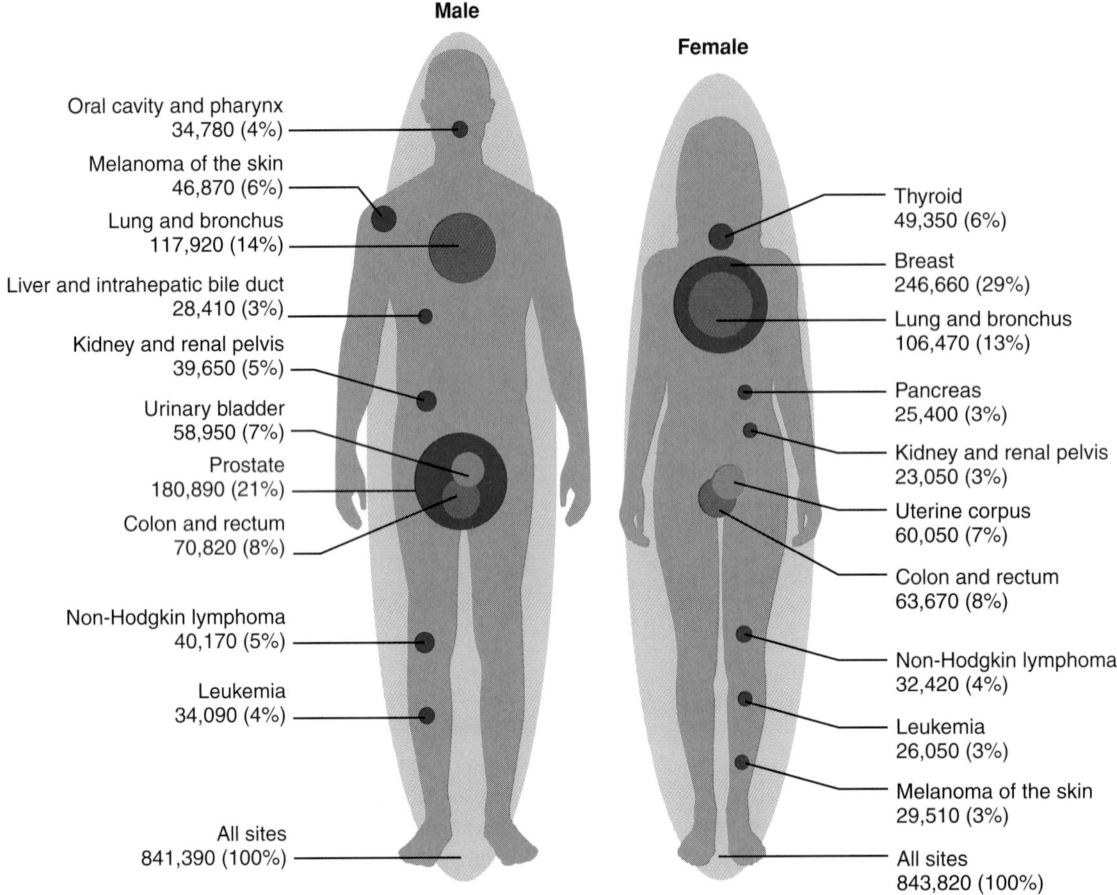

FIGURE 29-3. The most common new cancer cases by gender. *(American Cancer Society, Inc., Surveillance Research, 2016.)*

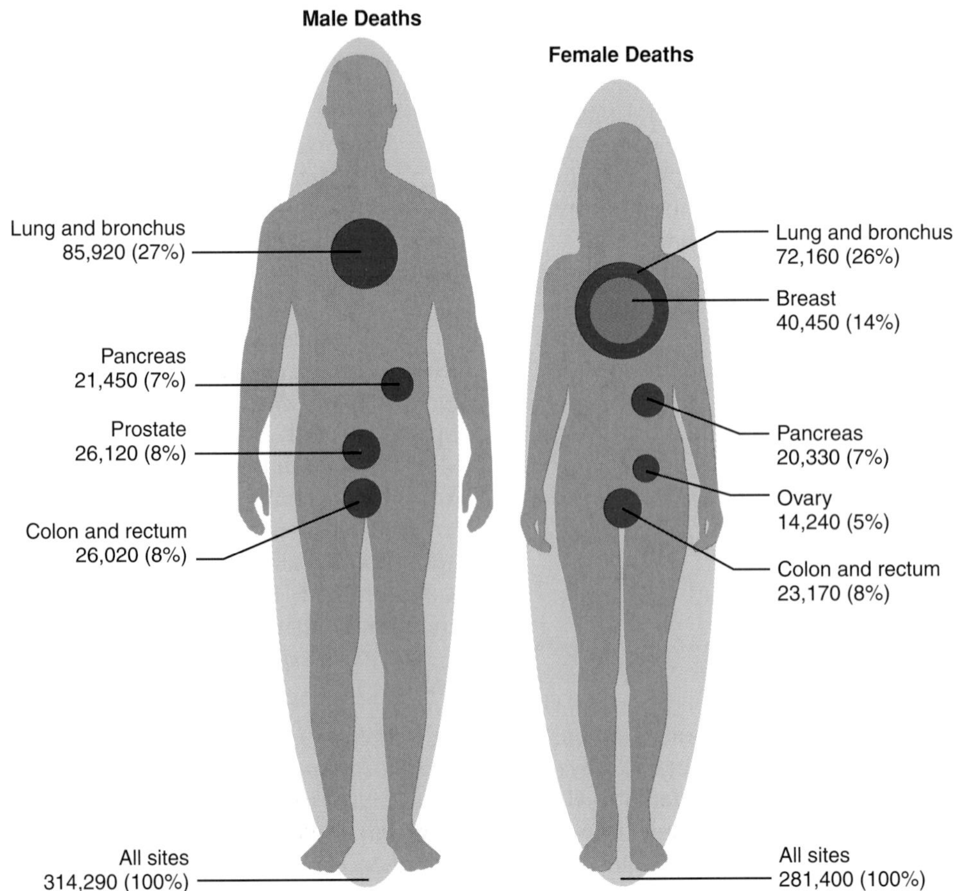

FIGURE 29-4. Cancers with the highest mortality rates. *(American Cancer Society, Inc., Surveillance Research, 2016.)*

TABLE 29-2 Screening Methods for Colon Cancer

SCREENING TOOL	METHOD	FREQUENCY
Fecal occult blood test (FOBT)	Can be performed at home or in laboratory Looks for blood in feces	Every year
Stool DNA test	Performed at home and mailed to laboratory Looks for DNA abnormalities	Every 3 years
Sigmoidoscopy	Scope with a camera is inserted through anus into colon Only views lower part of colon	Every 5 years
Colonoscopy	Scope with a camera is inserted through anus into colon Views upper and lower part of colon	Every 10 years
Computerized tomography (CT) colonography (virtual colonoscopy)	CT images of colon and rectum taken internally	Every 5 years
Double-contrast barium enema	Radiography of colon and rectum	Every 5 years

TABLE 29-3 Cancer Grading

I	Well differentiated (low grade)
II	Moderately differentiated (intermediate grade)
III	Poorly differentiated (high grade)
IV	Undifferentiated (high grade)

TABLE 29-4 TNM Cancer Staging[11]

T	Refers to the size and the extent of primary tumor
N	The number of nearby lymph nodes that have cancer; indicates the absence or presence of lymph node involvement.
M	Absence or presence of metastases
Number system	Either an X or number is assigned to each T, M, or N. A client's stage might be T3N1M0, and this system gives the client more information about the cancer. The numbers are based on the following descriptions: ▪ X: Cannot be measured ▪ 0: Not present ▪ 1, 2, 3, or 4: Higher numbers indicate more significant effects (larger tumor, more lymph nodes involved, or more metastases, respectively)

CANCER TREATMENTS

Following diagnosis of cancer, the most common treatments involve surgery, radiation, and chemotherapy. An individual with cancer may undergo any of these treatments, all of these treatments, or a combination of any two of the treatments. The client's oncologist determines the most appropriate cancer treatment(s) on the basis of the type, stage, and grade of the cancer and the individual's current state of health and comorbidities. For instance, the oncologist may deem a client "not a surgical candidate" if the oncologist feels that the risks of the surgery outweigh the benefits of the surgery. This may also be the case with initiating chemotherapy. The client, as well as his or her family, will be a part of the final decision-making process with regard to what treatment route will be taken.

Surgery

Surgery is often the first treatment option if the tumor can be removed from the body. However, in cases where only a portion of the tumor can be removed surgically, radiation and/or chemotherapy may be used before or after surgery.

Radiation

Radiation is the use of radioactive materials aimed directly at tumors or the surrounding tissue to kill cancer cells. Radiation can be used to shrink the tumor, or it can be used to alleviate a client's symptoms. When the goal of radiation is to shrink the tumor, the associated symptoms are expected to be alleviated as well.[12] For example, a client with a spinal cord tumor is also having low back pain and lower extremity weakness because of the tumor compressing on the spinal cord. As a result of radiation treatment for the cancer, the client will possibly experience a decrease in low back pain and increase in lower extremity strength. This occurs as a result of the decrease in pressure against the spinal cord as the tumor shrinks. OT can also contribute to the alleviation of impairments through strengthening of weak muscles and addressing pain management while the client is concurrently receiving radiation therapy.

Chemotherapy

Chemotherapy is the use of drugs to destroy or slow the growth of cancer cells. Once administered, these drugs travel throughout the body in the bloodstream to reach the cancer cells. Because chemotherapy is a systemic treatment, and not specifically directed toward cancer cells, it kills healthy cells as well. Chemotherapy drugs can be given orally or intravenously (Fig. 29-5). A client with cancer must be strong enough, even before chemotherapy is administered, to be able to tolerate the side effects of drugs.

Each type of cancer treatment has a variety of side effects, and each individual responds differently. These cancer treatments can be lifesaving but can also create impairments in the client. It is difficult to anticipate which side effects an individual will experience; however, there are some side effects that are common to radiation and chemotherapy (Table 29-5).[13]

TABLE 29-5 Common Side Effects of Cancer Treatment

RADIATION (RADIOTHERAPY) SIDE EFFECTS	CHEMOTHERAPY SIDE EFFECTS
Immunosuppression	Nausea
Fatigue	Vomiting
Skin irritation/burns	Hair loss
Soft tissue fibrosis	Neuropathies
Delayed wound healing	Mouth sores
Edema	Low blood cell counts
Hair loss	Loss of appetite

REHABILITATION

Cancer, as well as cancer treatments, can cause a variety of medical and functional impairments in the client with cancer (Table 29-6). The benefits of rehabilitation for clients with cancer include improved mobility, improved performance of activities of daily living (ADLs), decreased pain, decreased fatigue, improved QoL, improved safety for discharge, preserved dignity, and establishment of resources and supportive services.[14]

The rehabilitation approach to the treatment of cancer originated with the National Cancer Act of 1971.[15] This legislation declared cancer rehabilitation as an objective, and it directed funds to the development of training programs and research projects. In 1972, the National Cancer Institute sponsored the National Cancer Rehabilitation Planning Conference, which identified four objectives for the rehabilitation of clients with cancer: psychosocial support, optimization of physical functioning, vocational counseling, and optimization of social functioning.[15]

TABLE 29-6 Potential Impairments in Cancer Survivors

MUSCULOSKELETAL	NEUROMUSCULAR	FUNCTIONAL
Tendonitis	Neuropathy	Fatigue
Adhesive capsulitis	Myopathy	Psychiatric
Spondylosis	Myelopathy	Cognitive
Fracture	Pain	Autonomic
Impending fracture	Radiculopathy	Cardiac
Arthritis	Plexopathy	Endocrine
Osteoporosis	Cerebropathy	Gastrointestinal
Bony metastases	Neuropathy	Urinary
Pain		Debility/frailty
		Lymphedema
		Balance

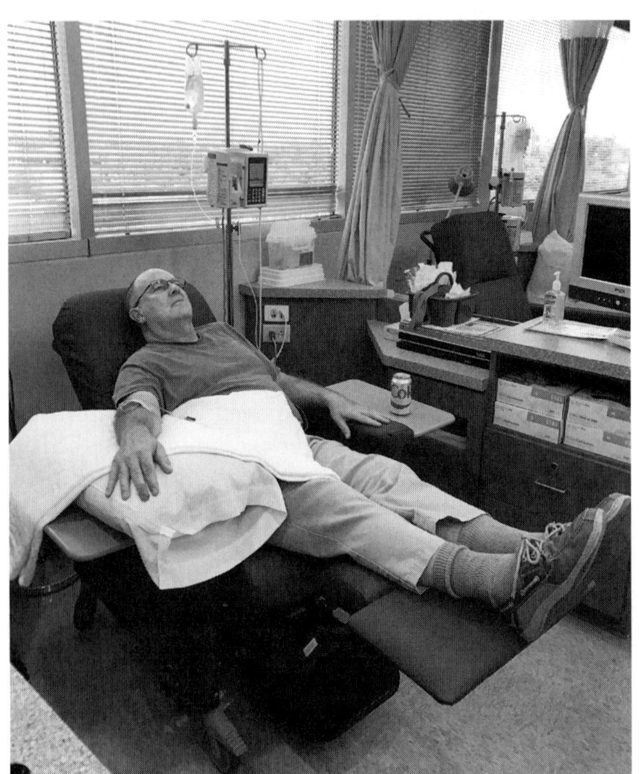

FIGURE 29-5. Client receiving chemotherapy via infusion.

Cancer rehabilitation can be defined as a process that assists the client with cancer to obtain maximal physical, social, psychological, and vocational functioning within the limits created by the disease and its resulting treatment.[16] Rehabilitation requires an interdisciplinary team approach because of the variety of potential problems clients may face during the course of illness. The healthcare team must develop rehabilitation goals within the limitations of the client's illness, environment, and social support, in which goals are objective, realistic, attainable; involve the client and family in goal setting; be collaborative with professional members of the team and with the client and the client's support network; provide services to clients throughout the course of illness and during all stages; and create treatment plans that are individualized to meet each client's unique and specific needs.[16]

Dietz identified four categories of cancer rehabilitation that address the scope and course of the illness (Table 29-7).[17]

- *Preventive interventions:* To lessen the effect of expected disabilities, emphasize client education, improve the client's physical functioning and general health status, and assist with the early identification of adjustment issues
- *Restorative interventions:* To return clients to previous levels of physical, psychological, social, and vocational functioning
- *Supportive interventions:* To teach clients to make accommodations for their disabilities and to minimize debilitating changes caused by ongoing disease
- *Palliative interventions:* To focus on minimizing or eliminating complications, providing comfort and support, pain control, prevention of contractures and pressure sores, prevention of unnecessary deterioration from inactivity, and psychological support for the client and family members.[17]

The purpose of rehabilitation of cancer survivors is similar to that of clients with other diseases. However, the pathology of the tumor, the anticipated progression of disease, and any associated cancer treatments must be considered carefully when setting goals. When tumor progression and treatment cause a functional decline or when the disease causes a fluctuation in abilities, rehabilitation assumes a supportive role, and the goals are adjusted to accommodate the client's limitations.[18]

When working with this population, it is imperative to remember that clients who participate in rehabilitation programs have been shown to make functional gains, even though they have significant medical comorbidities,[18] and can still be expected to make improvements with regard to their functional mobility and QoL. This can be seen in both inpatient and outpatient settings.

TABLE 29-7 Cancer Rehabilitation Objectives[17]

REHABILITATION APPROACH	EXAMPLES
Preventive	Smoking cessation Education on adaptive equipment following pathological fracture of hip before surgery
Restorative	Strengthening Independence with ADLs Rehabilitation of hemiplegic upper extremity
Supportive	Adaptive strategies, such as one-handed dressing techniques
Palliative	Pain management Family education and training Range of motion Pressure injury prevention

COMMUNICATION

Oncology rehabilitation is a growing field that provides services to a growing population. Nonetheless, some practitioners still ask, "What can be done for this population, and how?" The amount of new research related to this population has demonstrated the need and the importance of rehabilitation in the oncology population. Despite supporting evidence, it may be difficult to clearly portray to insurance companies the need for OT for clients with cancer because this population may not show progress with OT as quickly (or at all) compared with clients with other diagnoses. To address this challenge, it is first necessary for the OTA to appreciate the needs of these clients for skilled OT. Next, the OTA must clearly communicate and document this need. It is fairly common for a medical doctor to conduct a peer-to-peer meeting with an insurance company representative to demonstrate a client's need for continued therapy. The OT practitioner may need to be a client advocate and verbally communicate a client's need when written documentation is not enough.

PREHABILITATION

Cancer prehabilitation is rehabilitation that starts at the time of initial diagnosis, before any cancer treatment begins. Prehabilitation starts early with the goals of decreasing the morbidity of cancer-related impairments and cancer treatment–related impairments. It includes physical and psychological assessments and is an important aspect in the continuum of care because it has been shown to decrease impairments and improve outcomes of clients with cancer. For example, urinary incontinence is a common impairment after prostatectomy for prostate cancer.[19] Research shows that strengthening of pelvic floor muscle through prehabilitation delays the occurrence of postsurgical urinary incontinence.[20] Research on the psychological aspect of prehabilitation has demonstrated that depression may be decreased and immunity may be improved if psychological support starts immediately after diagnosis and before surgery.[21]

SURVIVORSHIP

According to the National Coalition for Cancer Survivorship, **survivorship** begins at the time of cancer diagnosis and continues throughout the client's lifespan. Survivorship is no longer defined as beginning when a client reaches remission. The survivorship experience encompasses care for clients through the entire journey, including care for those living with, through, and beyond a cancer diagnosis.[22] The goal of survivorship is to decrease the risk of recurrence and prevention of new cancers, optimize health by reducing the consequences of cancer and cancer treatments, facilitate recovery, and nurture resiliency and well-being.[23]

TECHNOLOGY AND TRENDS

As an increasing number of individuals are diagnosed with cancer, it creates a greater demand for products that are more aesthetically pleasing to help clients adapt to treatment side effects, such as lymphedema, hair loss, or need for an ostomy bag. Lymphedema sleeves now come in a variety of colors and patterns. Fashionable robes have been created for individuals with breast cancer who are being treated with radiation. An online company, Cancer Be Glammed, connects cancer survivors with designers and manufacturers specializing in unique items for clients with cancer, such as mastectomy bras, headscarves, and clothing with easy port access for chemotherapy. For those individuals with an ostomy, modified clothing, such as stretchy pants or maternity pants and shirt styles with patterns or ruching, may be necessary to conceal the ostomy bag.

Integrative oncology is a holistic approach to assist clients in promoting wellness, reducing cancer's impact, and maximizing both quantity and quality of life. This approach consists of dietary and lifestyle changes that are evidence based. It addresses the physical, emotional, and spiritual needs of both clients and their families. Healing touch, yoga, qigong massage, massage therapy, deep relaxation classes, mindfulness classes, and tai chi are some approaches that might be involved in an integrative oncology program. There are physicians and other healthcare professionals with specialization in integrative oncology. The aims of utilizing this approach are to reduce side effects of cancer treatment, introduce use of vitamins and supplements, develop a plan to reduce cancer risk factors, answer questions regarding alternative or complementary care, and, most importantly, to improve health and wellness.

Art classes, writing classes, music therapy, support groups (including long-term survivors, newly diagnosed clients, and family members), financial counseling, smoking cessation classes, nutrition classes, and breast reconstruction support groups are more therapeutic opportunities that benefit this population.

Especially important for cancer survivors of childbearing age is the development of a fertility preservation plan. Cancer treatments may affect fertility, and reproductive endocrinologists can work with clients on a plan.

Health care for cancer survivors is continuing to improve and become more standardized. The Survivorship Training and Rehabilitation (STAR) program connects clients with cancer with rehabilitation services by identifying the impairments experienced before, during, and/or following cancer treatment. This is an interdisciplinary, outpatient program that provides certification training and is available to hospitals, rehabilitation centers, and individual practitioners.

IMPLICATIONS FOR OCCUPATIONAL THERAPY—INTERVENTIONS FOR CLIENTS WITH CANCER

The OT practitioner may treat the client with cancer at any point through the cancer treatment process and for a multitude of reasons. An OT referral may be made for a client with cancer for a reason unrelated to the cancer diagnosis, or for a cancer survivor 20 years after remission for an impairment resulting from the cancer diagnosis, or for an impairment completely unrelated to the cancer diagnosis. The client with cancer may receive OT services for prehabilitation before cancer treatment begins (to increase strength, activity tolerance, improve performance of ADLs and instrumental activities of daily living [IADL]) or acutely after surgery and/or during radiation treatments.

Activities of Daily Living Training and Adaptive Techniques

Thorough assessment of a client's impairments and disabilities is paramount before the team proceeds with rehabilitation. Emphasis is initially placed on restoring or maximizing the client's independence with ADLs, mobility, cognition, and communication. Issues of survivorship and community reintegration, including returning to work, are considered next. Knowing and continuing to address the goals of the client with cancer are key throughout the continuum of care. These may change along the course of treatment, so updating information and maintaining communication about goals is important.[24]

The occupational therapist should assess the individual's performance skills with regard to basic ADLs and IADLs, and the OT practitioner should then promote increased independence through use of adaptive equipment or compensatory strategies, such as in hemi-dressing (one-handed dressing techniques), or address the underlying deficits causing dysfunction in ADL performance. For example, the OT practitioner can educate and train the client on the use of a reacher to thread lower body garments onto the feet or can address the strength and flexibility components required to perform lower body dressing.

SEXUAL ACTIVITY

The side effects from cancer treatment can have a significant impact on both client's and caregiver's feelings about sexuality and intimacy. The loss of hair, removal of one or both breasts, significant fatigue, low energy, nausea/vomiting/diarrhea, and other symptoms can cause challenges in relationships, a lowered desire for sexual activity and changes in the client's own sense of self. Self-esteem may be lower due to the aforementioned issues as well. Sexual activity may be painful due to scar tissue, early menopause symptoms or radiation in the pelvic area, and the partner may decrease intimacy in a desire not to cause pain.[25] The breasts may feel different or numb after surgery as well. A few of the chemotherapy drugs can be found when tested in vaginal fluids, and to be safe, partners should wear condoms for 2 weeks after each round of chemotherapy.[25] Clients should ask their physician if there are any specific precautions for sexual activity during the treatment process, and may be more prone to infections such as a urinary tract infection when sexually active. The OT practitioner can offer practical options for weakness, pain, or mobility concerns such as alternate positions or adapted toys, as well as suggest a focus on intimacy while not feeling well, such as holding hands, talking, hugs, massage and kissing.

Energy Conservation and Work Simplification

Some techniques, such as energy conservation and work simplification, may help enhance the client's performance of ADLs. Energy conservation is the practice of using a strategy to reduce the amount of energy expended with an activity. The OT practitioner can educate the client with cancer on energy conservation strategies that can be used in the performance of ADLs, such as the following:

- Try to eat smaller, more frequent meals and snacks throughout the day, rather than eating three large meals. This can increase the overall intake, needed by the body, limit fatigue caused by eating a large meal, and maintain energy levels throughout the day.
- Allow frequent, short rest periods within or between activities to avoid fatigue. Activities lasting longer than 10 minutes should be performed in the seated position.
- Avoid sitting on low chairs because more energy is required to get out of them.
- Consider the best time of the day for each activity.
- Use slow, smooth movements instead of fast, jerky movements.
- Use proper breathing techniques.
- Avoid extreme temperatures.
- Consider use of a bath bench or shower chair.
- When climbing stairs, make sure that the entire foot is on the step, and put both feet on each step.
- Consider a high stool with back support to sit on while working in the kitchen.
- Use light-weight pots and pans.
- Select foods that eliminate preparation.[26]

Cardiovascular Exercise

Along with energy conservation, exercise plays a vital role in the rehabilitation process. Exercise provides a number of health benefits for the general population but is especially beneficial for cancer survivors. Avoiding inactivity is the primary goal relating to exercise because "some physical activity is better than none," according to the 2008 U. S. Department of Health and Human Services Physical Activity Guidelines for Americans.[27] Specifically related to the cancer population and exercising, the American College of Sports Medicine's guidelines indicate that exercise improves QoL, decreases fatigue level, increases psychological well-being and physical functioning, and provides the typical cardiovascular and strength improvements. According to the "American College of Sports Medicine Roundtable on Exercise Guidelines for Cancer Survivors," the exercise prescription goal does not change for this population and should be made as exercise recommendations would be made for a population with any other diagnosis. The recommendation is 150 minutes of moderate to intense exercise or 75 minutes of vigorous exercise a week. Standard exercise precautions and goals are appropriate for this population but may need to be adapted on an individual basis, as is appropriate for all populations. Adjustments may be based on prior aerobic status and comorbidities.[28]

The OT practitioner can use the modified Borg rate of perceived exertion scale (Fig. 29-6) to ensure that the

OT Practitioner's Viewpoint

Treating clients with cancer can be emotionally challenging at times, but also extremely rewarding, for OT practitioners. It is tough to see a client decline as he or she approaches the end of life, yet it is overwhelmingly rewarding to help a client be well enough to go home to be with family until death occurs. We do not do what we do for acknowledgment, but when an individual OT practitioner is mentioned by name in a client's obituary, we know we have impacted a life!

A particular client came to us just after being diagnosed with stage IV glioblastoma (brain tumor). She could not use her right side at all and had lost all independence. Before admission, she had been working full time as a hospital administrator. She worked diligently during her OT to regain strength and balance, independence with functional mobility, and dignity. She was discharged home, where she had support of her husband, and with mobility equipment and durable medical equipment (DME) including a wheelchair, rolling walker, right ankle foot orthosis to assist with dorsiflexion, bedside commode, and shower chair. She kept all her outpatient appointments after discharge and continued to make progress. She was able to ambulate using a quad cane and worked on higher-level home management tasks, including preparation of lunch for her "favorite therapists." She was discharged from outpatient OT when she reached her goal of being able to vacuum her home. She also reached the point where her husband was able to return to work and she was able to manage at home by herself.

Unfortunately, a few months later, she experienced some complications that she was not able to overcome. She did return to inpatient rehabilitation again for a short stay upon the request of her family. She went home with hospice care, where we visited her, and she was able to thank us for our assistance and support throughout her journey. As both friends and therapists, we later attended her funeral. The family was extremely grateful for our "excellent and authentic care, support, and friendship," as stated in her obituary. ~ Brittany Lorden, MHS, OTR/L, CLT and Joanna Edeker, PT, DPT

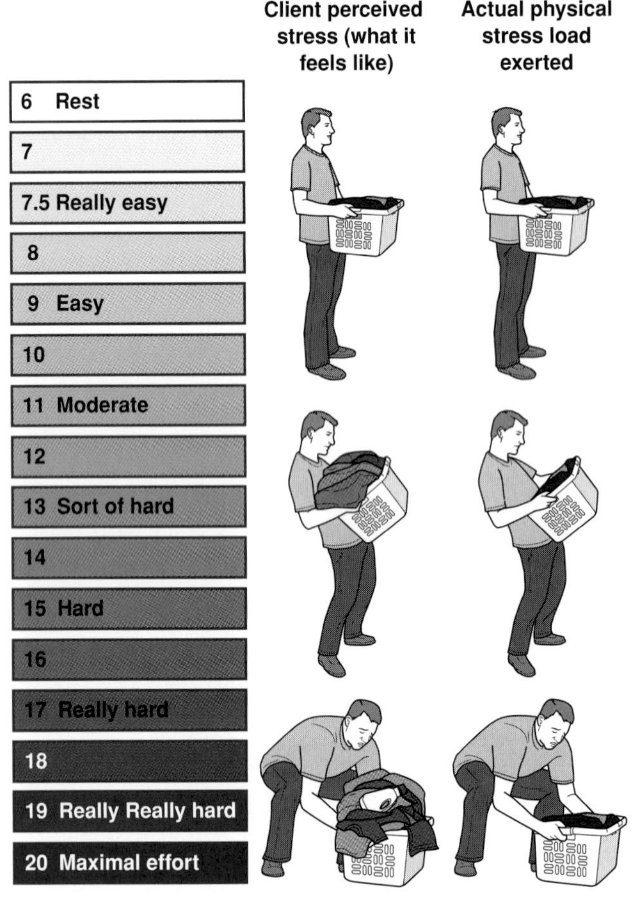

FIGURE 29-6. Modified Borg scale rating of perceived exertion. Notice the differences between actual workload and perceived exertion.

cancer survivor is exercising within the appropriate cardiovascular pulmonary parameters.

Strength Training

The OT practitioner will initiate a strength training program based on the client's needs and goals and can advance or adjust it, as needed. Strength training for cancer survivors should include two to three sessions a week for major muscle groups and also should include stretching.[29] These recommendations are generally appropriate for the cancer survivor but the intensity or duration may need to be adapted for each individual, depending on the acuity and location of the cancer. The most common problems associated with cancer treatments that OT practitioners need to be mindful of during exercise include increased risk for fractures, cardiotoxicity (heart damage due to chemotherapy), and musculoskeletal impairments related to treatments. Although risks do exist for cancer survivors when exercising, it is safe to exercise through the entire cancer treatment process.[29]

Pain Management

Pain is a major impairment in clients with cancer and may negatively affect QoL. Bone, musculoskeletal, neuropathic, inflammatory, and complex cancer pain are different types of pain present in this population. Pain management incorporates various approaches to prevent, reduce, or stop the sensation of pain. Depending on the type and degree of pain, pharmacological and nonpharmacological options are

EVIDENCE-BASED PRACTICE

The importance of exercise for clients diagnosed with cancer cannot be overemphasized. Research has demonstrated the inverse relationship between exercise and certain cancers. Increasing levels of physical activity has been proven to reduce the risk of colon cancer, breast cancer, endometrial cancer, and lung cancer. Exercise may also decrease the risk of cancer recurrence.[30-34]

Colon cancer: Researchers are finding that adults who increase exercising (by increasing intensity, duration, or frequency) decrease their risk of developing colon cancer, especially compared with those who are inactive. Research has also shown that exercising after a colon cancer diagnosis decreases recurrence risks and increases the survival rate.[30,33]

Breast cancer: Inactive women are at a greater risk of developing breast cancer compared with premenopausal and postmenopausal women who exercise regularly. Studies have shown that adolescent females who engage in moderate to vigorous physical activity decrease their risk of developing breast cancer. Exercise lowers hormone levels, which, in turn, lowers the risk of tumor development. There is ongoing research on the benefits of moderate exercise after breast cancer diagnosis in improving survival rates.[32]

Endometrial cancer: The risk of developing endometrial cancer decreases with physical activity. Increased level of hormones are also related to endometrial cancer.[34]

Lung cancer: There is evidence that increased physical activity decreases the risk of lung cancer; the more intense the activity, the better are the benefits.[31]

Slattery, M. (2004). Physical activity and colorectal cancer. Sports Medicine, 34*(4), 239–252.*

Tardon, A., Lee, W., Delgado-Rodriguez, M, Dosemeci, M., Albanes, D., ... & Blair, A. (2005). Leisure-time physical activity and lung cancer: A meta-analysis. Cancer Causes and Control,16*(4), 389–397.*

Holmes, M., Chen, W., Feskanich, D., Kroenke, C., & Colditz, G. (2005). Physical activity and survival after breast cancer diagnosis. Journal of the American Medical Association, 293*(20), 2479–2486.*

Meyerhardt, J., Giovannucci, E., Holmes, M., Chan, A. T., Chan, J. A., Colditz, G. A., & Fuchs, C. S. (2006). Physical activity and survival after colorectal cancer diagnosis. Journal of Clinical Oncology, 24*(22), 3527–353.*

International Agency for Research on Cancer. (2002). IARC handbooks of cancer prevention. weight control and physical activity *(Vol. 6). Lyon, France: IARC Press.*

available, and a combination of the two may provide the best results. Timing and dosage of pain medications will depend on each client and his or her varying activity levels during the day, and pain medication dosages are determined by the client's physician. It is often helpful to have a client time the intake of pain medication around OT sessions to prevent pain from being a barrier during treatment.

Nonpharmacological pain management options may include the use of modalities, such as the following:

- Manual therapy (e.g., trigger point release, manual traction, joint/soft tissue mobilizations, desensitization exercises, therapeutic massage, etc.)
- Exercise (e.g., active range of motion (AROM), stretching, etc.)
- Relaxation techniques (e.g., guided imagery deep breathing)
- Integrative techniques (e.g., massage, acupuncture, essential oils, etc.)
- Repositioning for comfort (e.g., if a client has low back pain while sleeping, the OT practitioner can teach the client how to sleep in a different position and/or use pillows to relieve back pain)
- Desensitization techniques to address neuropathic pain
- Fluidotherapy[35]

Refer to "Contraindications for Use of Modalities" in this chapter and to the discussion on physical agent modalities (PAMs) in Chapter 18. A pain scale can be used to obtain a subjective pain measurement from the client with cancer for documentation (see Chapter 8 for examples of various pain scales).

Functional Mobility

OT practitioners educate and assist clients to transfer and move safely, whether it is by using an assistive device, a wheelchair, or ambulating. The OT practitioner along with the PT practitioner will assess the safest technique to transfer for ADLs and progress the client accordingly to use the least restrictive device. Unlike other populations in rehabilitation, a client with cancer may experience fluctuating fatigue levels or a progressively worsening disease process, making it necessary for the OT practitioner to accommodate the client's needs at different levels. The goal may even be for the family to be able to independently assist the client in transfers.

Education and Training

The OT practitioner will continually provide education and training to the cancer survivor and his or her caregiver(s). Home exercise programs, appropriate exercise techniques, precautions/contraindications, pressure relief strategies, skin management, transfer training, ADL techniques, recommended supervision level, and DME are all areas to consider when providing education. Proper positioning with pillows in the supine or side-lying positions may be needed for pressure relief and/or pain management. The OT practitioner treating a client who is currently undergoing radiation treatment may find the client fluctuating between a stand pivot transfer and a squat pivot transfer as a result of fatigue. The OT practitioner would educate and train the caregiver in both techniques and recommend a drop-arm bedside commode as opposed to a standard bedside commode to take into account the varying levels of independence.

If the client is being discharged home from an acute care hospital, an inpatient rehabilitation center, or a skilled nursing facility, the OT practitioner will be an important part of the team to provide education and training for a safe discharge home. For instance, if the client will need assistance to go to the bathroom after he or she returns home, the OT practitioner will train the caregiver(s) how to provide the appropriate assistance, through verbal instructions, demonstration, and teach-back, in preparation for a safe discharge home. The OT practitioner may want to consider the client's shifting levels of fatigue as well as independence, depending on the cancer treatment and the cancer disease process, in providing education and recommending DME.

HOW DO CANCER AND CANCER TREATMENTS AFFECT FUNCTION?

Cancer and cancer treatment can both cause a number of deficits that result in an individual's decreased independence in ADLs and IADLs.

Cancer-Related Fatigue

Cancer-related fatigue (CRF) is defined as "a persistent, subjective sense of physical, emotional, or cognitive tiredness or exhaustion related to cancer and cancer treatment that is not proportionate to activity and interferes with normal functioning."[2] CRF is an effect of the cancer itself as well as that of the cancer treatments and is the most common complaint of clients with cancer. It can be a debilitating impairment. CRF is not the feeling of needing a nap or even a few naps a day but, rather, a feeling of exhaustion from which one cannot recover. Surprisingly, research has shown that exercise is the most effective way to treat CRF.[36] Educating clients and caregivers is key to helping clients understand that exercise, as opposed to the former mentality of rest, is the solution to battle CRF.

Chemotherapy-Related Cognitive Dysfunction

Chemotherapy-related cognitive dysfunction, more commonly known as "chemo brain" or "chemo fog" is a possible side effect of certain chemotherapy drugs that impairs cognitive function and may present during or after treatment. Symptoms of "chemo brain" may include the following:

- Forgetfulness
- Difficulty concentrating
- Difficulty multitasking
- Feeling disorganized
- Difficulty with learning new skills[37]

"Chemo brain" is an impairment that has become more acknowledged by the medical community in recent years.[37] It is not a new phenomenon to clients; however, in more recent years, research has focused more attention on examining this deficit. When it starts, how long it lasts, and how much trouble it causes can all vary from one individual to another. OT practitioners need to be aware of this impairment and assist clients with adjusting to these changes.[37] For example, if a client's memory has been affected by "chemo brain," the OT practitioner can recommend that the client use the microwave or make sandwiches, instead of cooking in the oven or on the stovetop. This may prevent a house fire because there is a risk of the client forgetting to turn off the oven or stove after cooking. Education and training on use of a memory notebook, smartphone, or tablet as an external aid may also be beneficial. The client can use any of these options as a medication log or to remember physicians' names and appointment times. A pill box can also be a method of keeping medications organized when an external aid is needed.

Chemotherapy-Induced Peripheral Neuropathy

The American Cancer Society identifies **chemotherapy-induced peripheral neuropathy (CIPN)** as a disabling side effect of cancer treatment, in which the chemotherapy agents used to treat cancer also damage the peripheral nerves. Because chemotherapy involves systemic treatment of cancer, it can destroy both cancer cells and healthy cells, including different nerve cells; it usually affects the nerves farthest from the trunk initially. Table 29-8 shows the most common symptoms of CIPN. CIPN can cause pain and impair an individual's performance of ADLs and IADLs. For example, peripheral neuropathy of the feet affects balance, which impairs standing and walking. Peripheral neuropathy affecting the hands impairs fine motor skills. This can make fastening clothing more difficult, make it impossible to don/doff clothing for toileting, or become a safety hazard during meal preparation. The OT practitioner may be the first clinician to note that the client with cancer has new-onset tingling of fingers and sharp pains down the arms or is having difficulty grasping an object. If so, the OT practitioner should immediately notify the client's oncologist.[38]

Currently, there is no definitive method for the prevention of CIPN, however, research is ongoing to explore prevention. Typically, with presentation of symptoms of CIPN, chemotherapy is discontinued or the dosage modified. The oncologist, along with the client, determines the plan of treatment following manifestation of side effects.

TABLE 29-8 The Most Common Chemotherapy-Induced Peripheral Neuropathy (CIPN) Symptoms

Constant or intermittent pain	Muscle atrophy/weakness
Burning	Trouble swallowing
Tingling ("pins and needles") or electric/shock-like pain	Constipation
Loss of sensation or numbness	Trouble urinating
Fine motor coordination deficits or dropping objects	Blood pressure changes
Balance problems	Decreased or no reflexes
Sensitivity to cold or heat and/or touch or pressure	

SPECIAL CONSIDERATIONS

As with most diagnoses, cancer requires special considerations that the OT practitioner should keep in mind. These include knowledge and monitoring of lymphedema, vital signs, laboratory values, weight-bearing restrictions, seizures, swallowing precautions, and infection control.

Lymphedema

Lymphedema is an accumulation of lymph fluid, superficial to the skin, resulting from impaired lymphatic circulation. Impaired circulation can be caused by a number of factors, but in the cancer population, it is usually caused by lymph node dissection, radiation of the lymphatics, or a tumor that has spread into a lymphatic structure.[39] Lymphedema may occur immediately after treatment or sometimes will not appear until months or even years after treatment. Lymphedema is a chronic disease that is treated in two phases—the decongestion phase (phase I) and the maintenance phase (phase II). The goal of the decongestion phase is to decrease the size of the area affected to a normal volume by using continuous skin care, manual lymph drainage (MLD) at least once a day, daily exercises, and 24-hour specialized compression bandaging (Fig. 29-7). Specialized therapy practitioners are trained to perform complete decongestive therapy (CDT), which consists of skin care, MLD, compression therapy, and decongestive exercises, to treat lymphedema. CDT is used to treat lymphedema to lessen its effects as opposed to curing it. In phase II, the goal is to maintain the normal volume of the area using continuous skin care, MLD as needed, daily exercises, and elastic compression garments worn during the day.[39] At the end of phase II treatment, clients with lymphedema as a result of cancer treatment will most likely need to use some type of compression ongoing and will be trained by the practitioner to determine individual needs (compression at night and/or compression during the day to maintain normal volume).

Vital Signs

Pulmonary complications of cancer and cancer treatment may include bronchial obstruction (airway obstruction), pleural effusion (fluid accumulation in the tissues that line

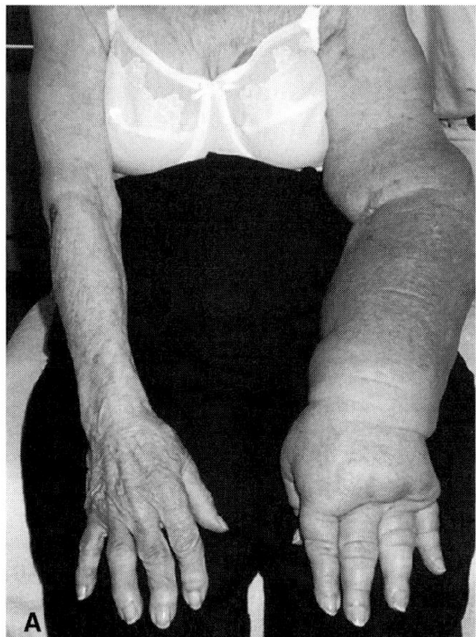

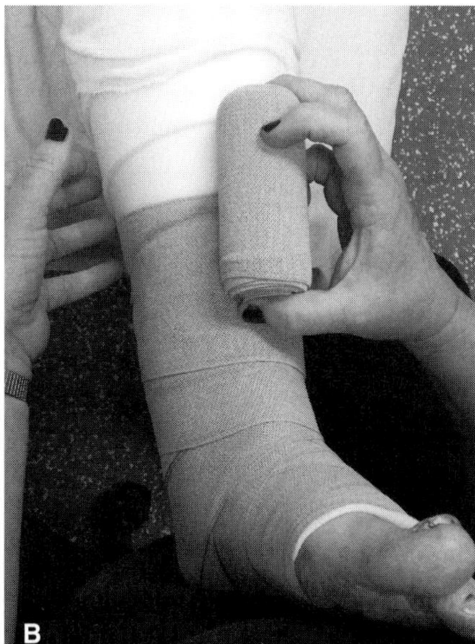

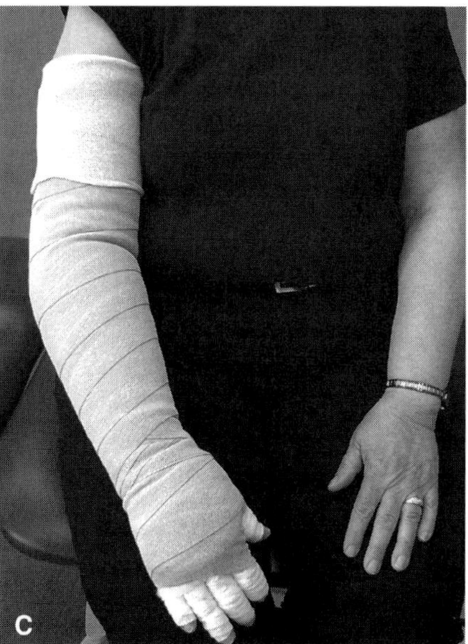

FIGURE 29-7. (**A.**) Lymphedema of the left upper extremity, (**B.**) compression bandaging of the left lower extremity, and (**C.**) right upper extremity has been completely wrapped in the layered compression bandages.

the lungs and chest), pneumothorax (collapsed lung), phrenic nerve paralysis (paralysis/palsy of the nerve innervating the diaphragm), pulmonary embolisms (PEs; blockage of the lung's artery by a clot that traveled from elsewhere in the body via the bloodstream), and pneumonia (Fig. 29-8). The significance of these complications to the OT practitioner is the client's decreased exercise capacity, shortness of breath, and pain. Oxygen saturation (SpO_2) should be monitored and maintained to a level greater than 90 percent. If there is a physician order for oxygen, supplemental oxygen should be administered as ordered. Symptoms, such as dizziness and shortness of breath, should also be monitored. The OT practitioner should monitor the client's vital signs intermittently, especially if the client becomes symptomatic. Energy conservation education and implementation during treatment can assist the client who has pulmonary complications. Education of deep breathing techniques, such as pursed-lip breathing, active exhalation, and diaphragmatic breathing, are also beneficial in addressing pulmonary symptoms.[40,41] (See Chapter 26.)

Brochial obstruction	Cancer of the bronchus will cause an obstruction
Pleural effusion	Cancer or cancer treatment can cause fluid accumulation
Pulmonary embolism	Cancer can cause the blood to clot or a tumor can present as a blocked artery
Phrenic nerve paralysis	Muscle that controls breathing (diaphragm muscle) has been paralyzed

FIGURE 29-8. Pulmonary complications of cancer and cancer treatments.

OTHER COMPLICATIONS

Cardiac complications may be a side effect of radiation or chemotherapy. Injury to the heart muscles and the coronary arteries may cause the client to present with angina on exertion during treatment sessions. The OT practitioner should monitor for symptoms of chest pain, rate of perceived exertion (e.g., in the modified Borg RPE assessment), and dizziness. In clients identified as high-risk, a cardiology workup and clearance from a physician is recommended before starting an exercise program.[42]

Gastrointestinal complications may present as nausea, vomiting, diarrhea, poor nutritional intake, and poor appetite. The OT practitioner may need to contact the oncologist if a client mentions that he or she no longer has an appetite. The OT practitioner may also educate the client on consuming five smaller meals daily or modifying his or her diet to allow for increased nutritional intake.[43] See Box 29-1, Nutritional Strategies.

Renal complications may cause fluid and electrolyte disorders, which are a significant cause of morbidity in clients with cancer. Renal complications, in the client with cancer, may be caused by the underlying cancer or its treatments. Electrolyte or fluid imbalances resulting from renal complications may cause edema (which is different than lymphedema) in any or all limbs, hands/feet, abdomen, and so on.[43]

Laboratory Values

Chemotherapy may cause low blood cell counts by damaging the blood-producing cells in bone marrow. The OT practitioner should review the client's hemoglobin level, red blood cell count, white blood cell count, and platelet count

BOX 29-1
Nutritional Strategies

The National Cancer Institute recommends the following:

- Avoid carbonated drinks, such as sodas, and foods that cause gas, such as beans, peas, broccoli, cabbage, brussels sprouts, green peppers, radishes, and cucumbers.
- Increase calories by frying foods and using gravies, mayonnaise, and salad dressings.
- Take supplements high in calories and protein.
- Choose high-protein and high-calorie foods to increase energy and help wounds heal. Good choices include eggs, cheese, whole milk, ice cream, nuts, peanut butter, meat, poultry, and fish.
- If constipation is a problem, increase fiber by small amounts and drink lots of water. Good sources of fiber include whole-grain cereals (e.g., oatmeal and bran), beans, vegetables, fruit, and whole-grain breads.

Other helpful strategies are as follows:

- Use nutritional supplement drinks between meals.
- Make changes in diet, such as eating small meals throughout the day.
- Use Teriyaki sauce or barbeque sauce to help cover up the metallic taste that is often caused by chemotherapy.
- Use plastic ware instead of metal utensils to get rid of the metallic taste caused by chemotherapy.

before initiation of and during the rehabilitation program. Anemia (low red blood cell count) can cause decreased exercise tolerance and/or fatigue, angina symptoms, dizziness, pale skin, and tachycardia (rapid heart rate). If a client has anemia, the OT practitioner should be aware that the client may not perform as well as he or she did in a prior treatment session, whether it was on the previous day or during the previous week. If the above symptoms are observed without a diagnosis of anemia, the OT practitioner may need to notify the client's physician. If the symptoms are due to anemia, a blood transfusion may be warranted. Neutropenia, also called leukopenia (low white blood cell count), places a client at a higher risk of infection because of the decrease in cells that fight infections. If the client has an extremely low white blood cell count, the oncologist may consider the client immunocompromised, at which point the client is more susceptible to infections. Common examples of infections clients with cancer are at an increased risk for are pneumonia, urinary tract infections, gastrointestinal infections, and cellulitis.[43] OT practitioners can educate clients to be diligent in hand washing, avoid coming into contact with individuals with symptoms of contagious illnesses, and possibly avoid public places, especially during flu and cold season, or wear a mask while in public. OT practitioners may need to wear a mask while in the client's private environment, for instance, if providing home health care to a client who is immunocompromised, to avoid passing on any infection to the client.

Thrombocytopenia (low platelet count) increases the client's risk of bleeding and bruising. In this instance, the OT practitioner should be cautious not to bump into or nick the client. The bruising or bleeding will be excessive compared with a client with a normal platelet count (Table 29-9).[42,43]

Weight-Bearing

Myeloma and lymphoma are cancers that directly affect bones. However, metastasis is the most common process affecting bones in clients with cancer. Breast, lung, prostate, renal, and thyroid cancers are the most common cancers that metastasize to bone.[43]

If metastases to bone are present, they can cause orthopedic complications. Weakened bones place clients at a higher risk of developing osteoporosis.[43] Both metastases and primary bone cancers predispose bone to an impending, pathological fracture (a fracture from bone weakened by a disease state). A pathological fracture can happen easily, without warning, and may also cause a client to fall. A fracture resulting from weakened bone will only further complicate a client's medical course, including, but not limited to, reduced mobility and increased risk for falls, as well as being a source of unwarranted hospitalizations. A fracture also causes extreme pain, may necessitate surgery, and may

TABLE 29-9 Symptoms of Abnormal Laboratory Values

BLOOD CONDITION	DESCRIPTION OF LAB RESULTS	SYMPTOMS/EFFECTS
Anemia	Low red blood cell count	Dizziness Pale skin Tachycardia Angina symptoms Decreased exercise tolerance Fatigue
Neutropenia/leukopenia	Low white blood cell count	Decrease in cells that fight infections Higher risk of getting infections
Thrombocytopenia	Low platelet count	Decrease in cells that stop bleeding Increased risk of bleeding and bruising

limit weight-bearing through the affected bone. For example, a client with multiple myeloma with bones that are in a weakened state falls and lands on her right side with resulting right arm and right leg fractures. She is now non–weight-bearing on her right leg and right arm, going from being completely independent to requiring assistance with ADLs and IADLs and being confined to a wheelchair for mobility. For an individual with strong, healthy bones, this same fall would likely be inconsequential, permitting the individual to return to his or her previous level of functioning (Table 29-10). Figure 29-9 shows the most common causes of bone metastases.

Seizures

The presence of primary brain tumors or metastases to the brain increases the chance of a client with cancer having a seizure, although this risk is based on the location and size of the tumor. About 50% of clients with brain tumors or metastases are affected by seizures. A client with cancer is at a greater risk for seizures when the brain tumor has a central location, is slow growing, and has multiple lesions.[44]

Swallowing

Clients with head and neck cancer and those with brain tumors will most likely have significant impairments in swallowing function, which may increase the risk of aspiration secondary to the underlying cancer or its treatments. Some clients may have had a removal of part of the tongue, jaw, or other structures vital for swallowing. Radiation to the head and neck will lead to fibrosis (deposits of connective tissue or "scarring") of key muscles and structures used in the swallowing mechanism, possibly making it unsafe to swallow thin liquids. If so, swallowing exercises, compensatory strategies, and/or thickened liquids are required.[45]

TABLE 29-10 Systemic Complications and the Role of the OTA

BODY SYSTEM	COMPLICATION	EFFECT ON CLIENT	OTA ROLE
Pulmonary complications	Bronchial obstruction Pleural effusion Pneumothorax Phrenic nerve paralysis Pulmonary embolisms (PEs) Pneumonia	Decreased exercise capacity Shortness of breath Pain	Monitor oxygen saturation. Maintain oxygen saturation greater than 90%.
Cardiac complications	Clients with a history of radiation or chemotherapy may also have sustained injury to the heart muscle and the coronary arteries.	Angina on exertion	Monitor for symptoms of chest pain. Assess rate of perceived exertion. Monitor dizziness. In high-risk clients, cardiology workup and clearance from a physician is recommended before starting an exercise program.
Renal complications	Fluid and electrolyte disorders are a significant source of morbidity in clients with cancer. These disorders may be due to the underlying cancer or its treatments.	Anemia (low red blood cell count) Cognitive changes Fatigue Fluid and electrolyte balances	Monitor for cognitive changes. Monitor for extreme changes in fatigue level.
Hematological precautions	Chemotherapy can cause low blood cell counts by damaging the blood-producing cells in the bone marrow.	Anemia (low red blood cell count) Neutropenia/leukopenia (low white blood cell count) Thrombocytopenia (low platelet count)	Review hemoglobin, white blood cell count, and platelet count before initiation and during the rehabilitation program.
Orthopedic complications	Fracture	Pain	Possible weight-bearing restrictions
Infectious disease complications	Pneumonia Urinary tract infection Gastrointestinal infections Cellulitis Immunocompromise		Use appropriate protective precautions.

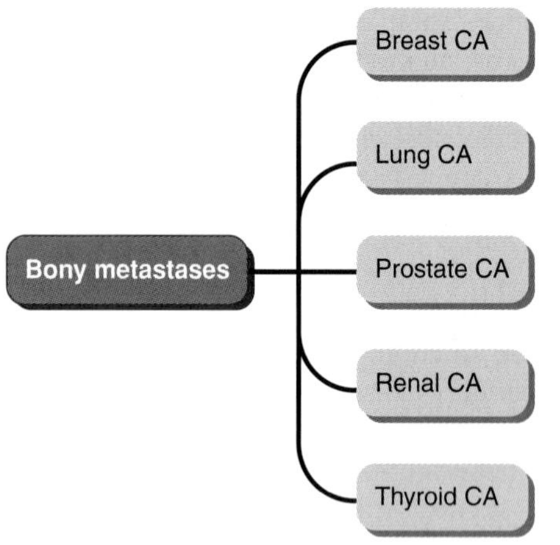

FIGURE 29-9. Common cancer (CA) causes of bone metastases.

MODALITIES

PAMs are utilized for various outcomes in the rehabilitation process, including pain management and circulation. Specific PAMs used may include heat therapy, cryotherapy (ice/cold), ultrasound (deep heat via sound waves), and transcutaneous electrical nerve stimulation (TENS).[46]

Indications for Clients With Cancer

Heat therapy has the physiological effects of decreasing pain and causing vasodilation (increased blood flow), and it is indicated for inflammation, pain, and muscle spasms. Cryotherapy has the physiological effects of vasoconstriction (decreased blood flow), decreasing inflammation, decreasing pain, and it is indicated for an acute or chronic pain from muscle spasms, limitation of motion secondary to pain, and edema. Ultrasound is indicated for pain, inflammation, and tissue healing. TENS is indicated for pain and, as indicated in some evidence, for increased circulation. Neuromuscular electrical stimulation (NMES) is indicated to facilitate muscle contractions, decrease spasticity and spasms, increase strength, and enhance local circulation. These modalities can benefit a client with cancer for pain management, increased functional use of extremities, increased soft tissue and joint mobility, and enhance the rehabilitation process.[46] See Chapter 18 for further details on PAMs.

Contraindications

For most PAMs, malignancies are listed as a contraindication because of the unknown effects of changes in blood flow and movement of cells and their impact on the cancer.[46] However, some physicians no longer consider the use of modalities on a client with cancer a contraindication but, rather, a precaution. Because no research currently supports the contraindication reversal, it is crucial to discuss modality options with the physician and the occupational therapist before initiating intervention. The emerging trend is to weigh the benefit against the risk. If a client with stage IV cancer will have decreased pain with the use of ultrasound to a shoulder, for instance, the benefit outweighs the risk. NMES applied over metastases would not be ideal, but heat applied over metastases may be approved by a physician, especially if the benefits of heat outweigh the so-called risks.

DURABLE MEDICAL EQUIPMENT

DME is sometimes covered by insurance; however, each individual's insurance benefits vary and may or may not cover the expenses of DME. DME typically includes bedside commodes, shower chairs, tub transfer benches, canes, walkers, wheelchairs, hospital beds, transfer boards, and mechanical lifts. In the client with cancer, especially for clients with poorer prognoses, it can be difficult to justify the need for specialized DME, such as custom wheelchairs, to a third-party payer. A client with cancer may be an appropriate candidate for a custom wheelchair. For instance, if a client with cancer who has a high-level spinal cord tumor with tetraplegia and who is able to independently perform functional mobility when provided with a power wheelchair may be deemed an appropriate candidate for a custom wheelchair. Sometime an appropriate DME item for the condition or need is not always a "funded" item, and the OT practitioner will have to advocate for his or her client. When requesting specific DME for a client with cancer, it is important to be aware of the client's prognosis to plan for the most appropriate DME based on the client's needs now and in the future.

PALLIATIVE AND HOSPICE CARE

The primary goal of **palliative care** or palliative medicine is to alleviate suffering and improve the QoL for clients with advanced illnesses; it is similar to, but not the same as, hospice care. Palliative care offers support and coping strategies to clients and their families. Palliative medicine can be offered simultaneously with all other appropriate medical treatments. For example, a client can undergo radiation treatment and receive palliative care services at the same time. Palliative medicine focuses on pain control, management of physical symptoms, management of psychological issues, and addressing spiritual concerns. Palliative medicine strives to achieve the best QoL for clients and their families. It is appropriate for clients with life-limiting illnesses and uncontrolled physical symptoms. Clients and/or their family members who wish to discuss advance care planning, goals of therapy, comfort-directed therapy, and withdrawal of mechanical ventilation/artificial nutrition and/or other forms of artificial life support will also benefit from palliative care. Although palliative medicine is covered by Medicare, Medicaid, and private insurance companies, eligibility for these services is not based on a client's ability to pay.[47]

The goal of all hospice agencies in the United States is to provide comfort to the client. **Hospice care** focuses primarily on end-of life care. Hospice services typically do not provide treatments that are meant to diagnose or cure an illness. Hospice does not hasten a client toward death, nor does it work to extend life, if it means that the individual will continue to suffer. Instead, it strives to ease the difficulties during the last stages of terminal illnesses. To qualify for hospice care, "a patient must have certification from two physicians that he or she has less than 6 months to live if his or her disease runs its natural course."[47] The client's physician and the hospice medical director can provide this certification. If a client stays on hospice care for more than 6 months, the hospice team will reassess that there is still evidence indicating that the client's condition is terminal. Benefits of participating in hospice care include exposure to a variety of disciplines that may help address the challenges that the client and his or her family are experiencing. Hospice services offered locally vary, but may include skilled nursing facilities, DME, 24-hour on-call staff for emergencies, bathing and personal care assistance, spiritual care services, management of pain and other symptoms, social work visits, trained volunteer support, core medical services with the client's physician and the hospice physician, assistance with appropriate community resources, assistance with transitioning to a hospital if it becomes necessary, assistance with advance care planning, and bereavement support for families and loved ones.

Client and Family Goals

An OT practitioner may be involved in providing family education in an inpatient setting before the client's transition to hospice and communicate with hospice services regarding recommendations for care and/or DME. Family education would include the necessities for a safe transition home. Hospice staff may include an occupational therapist, who would participate in a one-time home assessment and family education session or offer recommendations for DME. OT services are not commonly provided through hospice and would usually be a one-time session.[47]

Hospice services, which comprise different levels of care, may include the following:

- *Routine home care*: Accounts for the majority of hospice days of care. The hospice staff visits on an intermittent basis at a frequency designed to meet the care, teaching, and support needs of the client and family.
- *Continuous care:* Provided only in a time of crisis and is to be used only as necessary to maintain the client at home.
- *Short-term general inpatient care:* Available for the client requiring pain control or acute and chronic symptom management. It may be provided in a hospital, nursing facility, or hospice inpatient unit.
- *Inpatient respite care:* Designed to provide relief to the caregivers of clients being cared for at home. It may be provided occasionally for up to 5 days at a time. Care may be provided in a nursing home, acute care facility, or hospice inpatient unit.

Some hospice services in the U.S. are covered by reimbursement from Medicare, Medicaid, and private insurance. Those on Medicare or Medicaid may be eligible for a special hospice benefit. Payment for services not covered by insurance is based on the client's ability to pay, such as a sliding scale. Those eligible for care are not denied hospice services because of inability to pay. Hospice providers may be for-profit or not-for-profit; the latter also operates on contributions from individuals, foundations, corporations, communities of faith, and civic organizations to help pay for services not covered by third-party payers. However, each community's hospice services vary, so it may be beneficial for OTAs to research their local hospice and its services (Table 29-11).[47] In Canada, the term hospice palliative care is used; the goal is to "relieve suffering and improve the quality of living and dying."[48] The qualifying features for receiving care in Canada are slightly different than the U.S., with care provided additionally to those at risk of developing a life limiting illness and/or regardless of prognosis.[48]

PSYCHOSOCIAL FACTORS AND QUALITY OF LIFE

One of the goals of rehabilitation in the oncology population is to restore QoL. By always maintaining client-centered goals, the OT practitioner helps enhance the client's QoL by facilitating his or her return to preferred occupations, such as cooking for the family or engaging in a game of golf. Assessment tools validated for clients with cancer, include the Cancer Rehabilitation Evaluation System (CARES) and Functional Assessment of Cancer Therapy (FACT), are available to assess an individual's QoL.[48-50]

TABLE 29-11 Hospice Care and Palliative Care in the U.S.

HOSPICE CARE	PALLIATIVE CARE
Terminal illness (less than 6 months to live)	Does not have to be terminal
Does not provide treatments that are meant to diagnose or cure an illness	May include medical treatments with intention to cure illness
Emphasizes family	Relieves suffering
Provides comfort	Improves quality of life (QoL)

SUMMARY

Currently an estimated 12 million cancer survivors worldwide are functioning less than optimally, either because of the cancer itself or because of the toxic and debilitating side effects of treatments received to combat the cancer. A great need exists to improve knowledge of these deficits and to address them to optimize cancer survivors' independence and QoL. The OTA and the occupational therapist have important roles in this area of care for clients with cancer.

REVIEW QUESTIONS

1. The OTA is treating a client for a short time who had a heart attack and then was newly diagnosed with cancer. The client states that he wants to cancel all of the appointments he has scheduled because he does not think he needs to exercise anymore following the new cancer diagnosis. What should the OTA advise the individual with newly diagnosed cancer?
   a. To eat whatever he wants
   b. To sleep until he feels fully rested
   c. To maintain exercise regimen and increase activity, as recommended by the OTA
   d. Immediately stop taking all prescription medicines
2. The OTA is treating a client who is about to begin chemotherapy. Which three of the following would the OTA use to explain to the client how chemotherapy is administered and its side effects?
   a. Administered intravenously or through an x-ray machine
   b. Causing nausea but no vomiting
   c. Administered via a patch, which would cause an increase in white blood cell count
   d. Causing hair loss and short-term memory problems
   e. Administered as a topical cream, which would cause mouth sores
   f. Administered orally, which would cause impaired balance while standing
3. A client has a history of breast cancer with bilateral mastectomies and chemotherapy. She has recently noticed that it is getting difficult to button her shirt and to perform her favorite leisure activity of knitting. Which three of the following are appropriate treatments that the OTA can provide?
   a. Fluidotherapy for the hands while performing fine motor manipulation of objects
   b. Static stretching of finger and wrist muscles to increase fine motor grip
   c. Task practice of knitting
   d. Issue builtup eating utensils
   e. Alternate moist heat and cold packs to bilateral hands
   f. Strengthen shoulder girdle muscles
4. What would be an appropriate goal to set for a cancer survivor?
   a. Educating the family on providing all care
   b. Eliminating use of all DME
   c. Promoting dependence on caregiver and allowing the client to rest
   d. Increasing independence in mobility with or without an assistive device
5. The OTA has a client who is curious about hospice and palliative care services that are available. When the OTA encouraged her to ask her physician, he told the client that to qualify for hospice services in the U.S., an individual must be in the terminal phase of an illness with a life expectancy of:
   a. 2 weeks or less
   b. 6 months or less
   c. 12 months or less
   d. 2 years or less
6. The OTA has a client who was recently diagnosed with breast cancer. She will be starting radiation therapy next week. What is a common side effect of radiation that can be expected as she continues OT while undergoing radiation?
   a. Increased energy
   b. Increased fatigue
   c. Weight gain
   d. Immediate upper extremity weakness
7. The client has just finished chemotherapy and is complaining of extreme fatigue. What should the OTA teach the client about combating cancer-related fatigue?
   a. Exercising paired with energy conservation
   b. Sleeping until no longer fatigued
   c. Drinking lots of caffeine
   d. Taking frequent naps throughout the day
8. The client reports that he wants help planning out his day to be more efficient. The OTA would educate him that energy conservation techniques include:
   a. Exercising just before bedtime
   b. Having frequent, short rest periods to avoid fatigue
   c. Eating three large meals a day
   d. Exercising in really hot temperatures
9. The OT practitioner writes an exercise program for the client who is a cancer survivor. What type of exercises will the OTA be educating the client to perform?
   a. Physical activity limited to aerobic exercises on a treadmill
   b. Aerobic exercises, strength training, and stretching
   c. Sitting exercises only
   d. Heavy weight lifting
10. A 34-year-old client with a 5-year history of brain tumor presented to the emergency department with sudden-onset significant left-sided weakness and neglect impacting his ability to safely move in the home or care for himself. He was referred to home care at the time of disease progression. Which three of the following are the appropriate treatments for the OTA to perform?
    a. Left upper extremity strengthening
    b. Obtaining a physician's order for NMES for neuromuscular reeducation of the left upper extremity
    c. Fabricating an orthotic for the left upper extremity and educating the family to ensure that the arm is kept in the sling 10 to 12 hours per day
    d. Educating family to perform all ADLs for the client to promote energy conservation
    e. Visual exercises to attend to midline
    f. Keeping the client in a wheelchair for all ADLs and IADLs, even though the home health physical therapist has cleared the family to help the client ambulate in his home

CASE STUDY

Pam is a 76-year-old female, diagnosed with stage III colorectal cancer with metastases to the nearby lymph nodes in her pelvis and groin. She is a retired waitress with a history of cigarette smoking (quit at age 50) and a family history of cancer. Pam lives alone in a rural town (except for her beloved pets). She has a two story house with a full bath on the first level, two bedrooms, and one bathroom upstairs. She has a daughter and grandchildren nearby and two daughters who live out of state. She has to travel over an hour to the closest hospital for healthcare visits (oncology, radiotherapy, chemotherapy). Due to the location of her cancer, she is not a candidate for surgery and opted for intensive radiation and chemotherapy. Part way through her 6 weeks of almost daily radiation, and after her first week-long chemotherapy infusion, she is extremely fatigued, dehydrated, and has a very low blood pressure. She barely has energy to walk to the bathroom, talk on the phone, and can no longer walk up the stairs to her bedroom. She has no appetite, and is also experiencing very painful blisters in her mouth and throat from the chemotherapy. The home health nurse referred her for home health OT.

1. What are Pam's immediate needs?
2. What referrals might be helpful?
3. Are there any safety concerns for Pam?
4. What transportation options might be available for her to travel to and from her 5 day per week radiotherapy appointments?
5. What can be changed in her home environment to assist her in basic ADLs?
6. What do you recommend to help Pam meet her nutritional needs?

PUTTING IT ALL TOGETHER Sample Treatment and Documentation

Setting	Inpatient rehabilitation
Client Profile	55 y/o female s/p 1 week glioblastoma multiforme resection
Work History	2nd grade teacher
Insurance	Private insurance
Psychological	Appropriately tearful at times
Social	Married with two children. Lives with spouse that works full time. Pt will have 24-hour assist and supervision at discharge
Cognitive	Slightly impulsive; impaired problem-solving and memory
Motor & Manual Motor Testing (MMT)	R shoulder: 2+/5 R elbow: 3−/5 R wrist: 3/5 R hip: 2+/5 R knee: 3−/5 R ankle: 1/5 LUE and LLE strength is within normal limits at grossly: 4+/5 Poor midline orientation Impaired trunk control Mild right-sided inattention Static sitting balance Min A Assistance × 2 to stand in the parallel bars
ADL	Toilet transfers and toileting with Max A Dressing with Max A
IADL	Dependent
Goals	1. Client will increase RUE strength to ≥ 3/5 to perform self-feeding and upper body dressing with Min A within 2 weeks. 2. Client will perform toilet transfer and toileting with Min A within 2 weeks.

OT TREATMENT SESSION 1

THERAPEUTIC ACTIVITY	TIME	GOAL(s) ADDRESSED	OTA RATIONALE
Perform RUE movement with Saebo mobile arm support	18 min	#1	*Preparatory Task:* For increased functional use of RUE and increased I with ADLs
Client to cross midline to grasp items placed to right with verbal cues for attention to R using RUE.	12 min	#1	*Therapeutic Activity:* For increased functional use of RUE and increased I with ADLs

SOAP note: 8/13/—, 1:15 pm–1:45 pm

S: "I want to work on my right arm so I can do more things for myself."

O: Client seated in w/c at start of session in room with head rotated toward L side. No complaints of pain. Client transported to gym by OTA, and client's RUE positioned in Saebo mobile arm support with resistance set to 6. Client was able to move through horizontal abduction, horizontal adduction, and shoulder protraction and retraction x10 each with short rest periods. Using arm support, client crossed midline to grasp family pictures to place onto scrapbook pages placed to R of client with Min verbal cues required for attention to R using RUE. Client demonstrated increased RUE strength, coordination, and attention for increased functional use of RUE and increased independence with ADLs.

Continued

PUTTING IT ALL TOGETHER Sample Treatment and Documentation (continued)

A: Client invested in therapeutic activities and demonstrated increased strength with use of Saebo mobile arm support from previous session. Client demonstrated increased attention to R with fewer verbal cues required to attend. Client progressing in independence with ADLs.

P: Continue to address RUE strength and coordination and R side attention for client's continued I for safe d/c home.

Grace Ezra, COTA/L, 8/13/—, 1:54 pm

TREATMENT SESSION 2

What could you do next with this client?

TREATMENT SESSION 3

What could you do next with this client?

REFERENCES

1. American Cancer Society. (2015). Cancer facts and figures 2015. Retrieved from http://www.cancer.org/research/cancerfactsstatistics/index
2. National Comprehensive Cancer Network. (n.d.). NCCN clinical practice guidelines in oncology: Cancer-related fatigue. Retrieved from http://www.nccn.org/professionals/physician_gls/pdf/fatigue.pdf
3. DeSantis, C. E., Lin, C. C., Mariotto, A. B., Siegel, R. L., Stein, K. D., Kramer, J. L., ... & Jemal, A. (2014). Cancer treatment and survivorship statistics. *CA: A Cancer Journal for Clinicians, 64*(4), 252–271.
4. de Moor, J. S., Mariotto, A. B., Parry, C., Alfano, C. M, Padgett, L., Kent, E. E., ... & Rowland, J. H. (2013). Cancer survivors in the United States: Prevalence across the survivorship trajectory and implications for care. *Cancer Epidemiology, Biomarkers, and Prevention, 22*(4), 561–570.
5. Bluethmann, M., Mariotto, B., & Rowland, J. (2016). Anticipating the "silver tsunami": Prevalence trajectories and comorbidity burden among older cancer survivors in the United States. *Cancer Epidemiology, Biomarkers, and Prevention, 25*(7), 1029–1036.
6. Ragnarsson, M. D., Kristjan, Thomas, M. D., & David, C. (2003). Cancer rehabilitation medicine. In *Holland-Frei cancer medicine* (6th ed). Hamilton, Ontario, Canada: BC Decker.
7. Loblaw, D. A., Perry, J., Chambers, A., & Laperriere, N. J. (2005). Systematic review of the diagnosis and management of malignant extradural spinal cord compression: The Cancer Care Ontario practice guidelines initiative's neuro-oncology disease site group. *Journal of Clinical Oncology, 23*(9), 2028–2037.
8. American Brain Tumor Association. (n.d.). Retrieved from http://www.abta.org/brain-tumor-information/
9. Sobin, L. H., & Fleming, I. D. (1997). TNM classification of malignant tumors, fifth edition, Union Internationale Contre le Cancer and the American Joint Committee on Cancer. *Cancer, 80*(9), 1803–1804.
10. American Cancer Society. (n.d.). Retrieved from http://www.cancer.gov/about-cancer/diagnosis-staging/prognosis/tumor-grade
11. National Cancer Institute. (2017). Staging. Retrieved from https://www.cancer.gov/about-cancer/diagnosis-staging/staging
12. Mustian, K. M., Griggs, J. J., Morrow, G. R., McTiernan, A., Roscoe, J. A., Bole, C. W., ... & Issell, B. F., (2006). Exercise and side effects among 749 patients during and after treatment for cancer: A University of Rochester Cancer Center Community Clinical Oncology Program study. *Supportive Care in Cancer, 14*(7), 732–741.
13. Macquart-Moulin, G., Viens, P., Bouscary, M. L., Genre, D., Resbeut, M., Gravis, G., ... & Moatti, J. P. (1997). Discordance between physicians' estimations and breast cancer patients' self-assessment of side-effects of chemotherapy: An issue for quality of care. *British Journal of Cancer, 76*(12), 1640.
14. Cromes, G. F. (1978). Implementation of interdisciplinary cancer rehabilitation. *Rehabilitation Counseling Bulletin, 21*, 230–237.
15. National Institutes of Health. (2015). Cancer rehabilitation symposium. Rehabilitation clinical models for cancer care. [Slides 6 and 16]. Bethesda, MD: NIH.
16. Silver, J. K., Baima, J., & Mayer, R. S. (2013). Impairment-driven cancer rehabilitation: An essential component of quality care and survivorship. *CA: A Cancer Journal for Clinicians. 63*(5), 295–317.
17. Diets, J. H. (1980). Adaptive rehabilitation of the cancer patient. *Current Problems in Cancer, 5*(5), 1–56.
18. Yoshioka, H. (1994). Rehabilitation for the terminal cancer patients. *American Journal of Physical Medicine and Rehabilitation, 73*, 199–206.
19. Silver, J. K., & Baima, J. (2013). Cancer prehabilitation: An opportunity to decrease treatment-related morbidity, increase cancer treatment options and improve physical and psychological health outcomes. *American Journal of Physical Medicine and Rehabilitation, 92*, 715–727.
20. MacDonald, R., Fink, H. A., & Huckabay, C. (2007). Pelvic floor muscle training to improve urinary incontinence after radical prostatectomy: A systematic review of effectiveness. *BJU International, 100*, 76–81.
21. Cohen, L., Parker, P. A., & Venice, L. (2011). Presurgical stress management improves postoperative immune function in men with prostate cancer undergoing radical prostatectomy. *Psychosomatic Medicine, 73*, 218–225.
22. National Coalition for Cancer Survivorship. (n.d.). Our mission. Retrieved from http://www.canceradvocacy.org/about-us/our-mission/
23. Hewitt, M., Greenfield, S., & Stovall, E. (Eds). (2006). *From cancer patient to cancer survivor: Lost in transition.* Washington, DC: National Academies Press.
24. National Comprehensive Cancer Network. (n.d.). NCCN clinical practice guidelines in oncology: Survivorship. Retrieved from http://www.nccn.org/professionals/physician_gls/pdf/survivorship.pdf
25. Lee, M. T. (2016). Sexual healing after cancer. Retrieved from https://www.slideshare.net/drmarthalee1/sexual-healing-after-cancer
26. Lyons, M., Orozovic, N., Davis, J., & Newman, J. (2002). Doing-being-becoming: Occupational experiences of persons with life-threatening illnesses. *American Journal of Occupational Therapy, 56*(3), 285–295.
27. Physical Activity Guidelines Advisory Committee. (2008). *Physical activity guidelines advisory committee report, 2008*. Washington, DC: U.S. Department of Health and Human Services.
28. Doyle, C., Kushi, L., Byers, T., Courneya, K. S., Demark-Wahnefried, W., Grant, B., ... Andrews, K. S. (2006). Nutrition and physical activity during and after cancer treatment: An American Cancer Society guide for informed choices. *CA: A Cancer Journal for Clinicians, 56*, 323–353.
29. Schmitz, K. H., Courneya, K. S., & Matthews, C., (2010). American College of Sports Medicine roundtable on exercise guidelines for cancer survivors. *Medical Science Sports Exercise, 42*(7), 1409–1426.
30. Slattery, M. (2004). Physical activity and colorectal cancer. *Sports Medicine, 34*(4), 239–252.
31. Tardon, A., Lee, W., Delgado-Rodriguez, M., Dosemeci, M., Albanes, D., ... & Blair, A. (2005). Leisure-time physical activity and lung cancer: A meta-analysis. *Cancer Causes and Control, 16*(4), 389–397.
32. Holmes, M., Chen, W., Feskanich, D., Kroenke, C., & Colditz, G. (2005). Physical activity and survival after breast cancer diagnosis. *Journal of the American Medical Association, 293*(20), 2479–2486.

33. Meyerhardt, J., Giovannucci, E., Holmes, M., Chan, A. T., Chan, J. A. Colditz, G. A., & Fuchs, C. S. (2006). Physical activity and survival after colorectal cancer diagnosis. *Journal of Clinical Oncology, 24*(22), 3527–353.
34. International Agency for Research on Cancer. (2002). *IARC handbooks of cancer prevention. Weight control and physical activity* (Vol. 6). Lyon, France: IARC Press.
35. Goodwin, P. J. (2014). Pain in patients with cancer. *Journal of Clinical Oncology, 32*(16), 1637–1639.
36. Blaney, J. M., Lowe-Strong, A., Rankin, J., Campbell, A., Allen, J., & Gracey, J. H. (2010). The cancer rehabilitation journey: Barriers to and facilitators of exercise among patients with cancer-related fatigue. *Physical Therapy, 90,* 1136–1147.
37. Boykoff, N., Moieni, M., & Subramanian, S. (2009). Confronting chemo brain: An in-depth look at survivors' reports of impact on work, social networks, and health care response. *Journal of Cancer Survivorship, 3*(4), 223–232.
38. American Cancer Society. (n.d.). CIPN. Retrieved from http://www.cancer.org/treatment/treatmentsandsideeffects/physicalsideeffects/chemotherapyeffects/peripheralneuropathy/peripheral-neuropathy-caused-by-chemotherapy-treating-cipn
39. Foldi, M., & Foldi, E. (2006). *Foldi's textbook of lymphology* (2nd ed). Munich, Germany: Elsevier Gmb H.
40. Stevens, R., & Hudson, W. (1934). Bronchial obstructions: Its diagnosis and treatment. *Radiology, 22*(3).
41. American Lung Association. (n.d.). Retrieved from http://www.lung.org/lung-disease/pneumonia.
42. Fialka-Moser, V., Crevenna, R., Korpan, M., & Quittan, M. (2003). Cancer rehabilitation particularly with aspects on physical impairments. *Journal Rehabilitation Medicine, 36,* 153–162.
43. Cristian, A., Tran, A., & Patel, K. (2012). Patient safety in cancer rehabilitation. *Physical Medicine and Rehabilitation Clinics of North America, 23,* 441–456.
44. Schaller, B., & Stephan, R. (2003). Brain tumor and seizures: Pathophysiology and its implications for treatment revisited. *Epilepsia, 44*(9), 1223–1232.
45. Crozier, E., & Baran, S. (2010). Head and neck cancer. *Otolaryngology for the Internist, 94*(5), 1031–1046.
46. Pope, G., Mockett, S., & Wright, J. (1995). A survey of electrotherapeutic modalities. *Physiotherapy, 81,* 82–91.
47. National Comprehensive Cancer Network. (n.d.). NCCN clinical practice guidelines in oncology: Palliative care. Retrieved from http://www.nccn.org/professionals/physician_gls/pdf/palliative.pdf
48. Canadian Hospice Palliative Care Association. (2017). About us: The Canadian hospice palliative care association. Retrieved from http://www.chpca.net/
49. Black, J. F., & Kishner, S. (2015). Retrieved from http://emedicine.medscape.com/article/320261-overview.
50. Courneya, K. S., & Friedenreich, C. M. (2001). Framework PEACE: An organizational model for examining physical exercise across the cancer experience. *Annals of Behavioral Medicine, 23,* 263–272.

Chapter 30

Human Immunodeficiency Virus: Factors and Considerations

Sharon D. Novalis, PhD, OTR/L

LEARNING OUTCOMES

After studying this chapter, the student or practitioner will be able to:

30.1 Explain the mechanism of autoimmune diseases, human immunodeficiency virus (HIV), and acquired immunodeficiency syndrome (AIDS)

30.2 Identify common medical issues related to autoimmune diseases, HIV, and AIDS

30.3 Discuss the clinical and social climate involving the history of HIV/AIDS

30.4 Describe various HIV/AIDS-related conditions relevant to the *Occupational Therapy Practice Framework: Domain and Process, 3rd edition*

30.5 Identify applicable occupational therapy treatment interventions associated with HIV/AIDS-related conditions

30.6 Review current evidence-based research

KEY TERMS

Acquired immunodeficiency syndrome (AIDS)
Antiretroviral therapy (ART)
Autoimmune disease
Human immunodeficiency virus (HIV)
Opportunistic infections

More than 36.7 million people worldwide are infected with the **human immunodeficiency virus (HIV)** currently, and in 2015, 2.1 million new infections were reported worldwide.[1] HIV attacks the immune system but HIV infection is not an autoimmune disorder (where the body attacks its own immune system). Without treatment, HIV infection advances in stages, overwhelming the immune system and progressing over time. The immune system functions to protect the body against abnormalities, infections, and diseases through a series of complex responses at the cellular level. A description of the standard process within the immune system might include the body's identification of abnormal cells (e.g., a virus), production and release of antibodies/antigens, isolation and/or elimination of abnormal cells, and the regulation of each of the individual components of this complex immune system.[2-4] When a breakdown occurs within the immune system, the result may involve misidentification of healthy cells as abnormal or diseased, which triggers the release of antibodies that attack and/or eliminate the healthy cells. As the system continues to become increasingly imbalanced through a continued series of faulty responses, healthy cells that comprise other components (e.g., cellular components), structures (e.g., skin, tissue, organs), and systems (e.g., the central nervous system) become affected. In specific cases, such as with HIV infection, unhealthy cells are replicated, weakening the immune system, resulting in an immune disease (disorder).[3] In the presence of an immune system disorder, the immune system triggers a response that actively destroys healthy cells.

In some cases, the trigger is not an external source, such as a virus, but an abnormal response as the body begins to attack itself. This is called **autoimmune disease,** and more than 23.5 million Americans are affected. Researchers have identified more than 80 different types of autoimmune diseases or autoimmune disorders.[2,3] Diagnosis of a specific type of autoimmune disease is largely dependent on the affected body process and the impact of the disease in terms of its symptomatology and/or the body component (body part) affected. Several examples of diseases that have autoimmune disorder components and are covered in other chapters:

1. Multiple sclerosis—Chapter 32
2. Systemic lupus erythematosus—Chapter 21
3. Rheumatoid arthritis—Chapter 21

4. Type 1 diabetes—Chapter 25
5. Myasthenia gravis—Chapter 31

This chapter will focus primarily on the role of the occupational therapy assistant (OTA) in treating clients and caregivers impacted by HIV infection and acquired immunodeficiency syndrome (AIDS).

HUMAN IMMUNODEFICIENCY VIRUS

HIV targets the CD4 T lymphocytes, also known as *CD4 cells* or *T cells*. CD4 cells have a key role within the immune system in that they trigger the immune response to fight infection and disease (Fig. 30-1). When HIV is introduced into the body, it attacks CD4 cells, and in the process, the virus continues to replicate itself. The three stages of HIV infection are (1) acute HIV infection, (2) clinical latency, and (3) AIDS.[1] Each stage will be described in more detail in various sections in the chapter.

Because of the advances in medical treatment options, not all individuals infected with HIV will develop AIDS. It can take 10 to 15 years for an HIV-infected person to develop AIDS; antiretroviral drugs can slow down the process even further.[5]. However, if left untreated, an individual infected with HIV becomes vulnerable to other infections, called **opportunistic infections,** and diseases, including, but not limited to, candidiasis (thrush), herpes simplex, herpes zoster, cytomegalovirus, tuberculosis, HIV dementia, HIV wasting syndrome, pneumonia, Kaposi's sarcoma, cervical cancer, and lymphoma. At the final stages of the HIV infection, wherein symptoms, infections, and/or diseases become clinically apparent (with additional indicators, such as an extremely low CD4 cell count) and as the complexity of symptoms increases to include the presence of opportunistic infections and disease(s), the medical diagnosis becomes known as **acquired immunodeficiency syndrome (AIDS)**. Regardless, occupational therapy (OT) practitioners have an important role in helping those who are identified as belonging to at-risk groups, which include individuals (client and caregiver) living with the impact of the chronic components of HIV, those dealing with the side effects of treatment associated with HIV/AIDS, and those individuals who have an HIV infection that has advanced to AIDS.

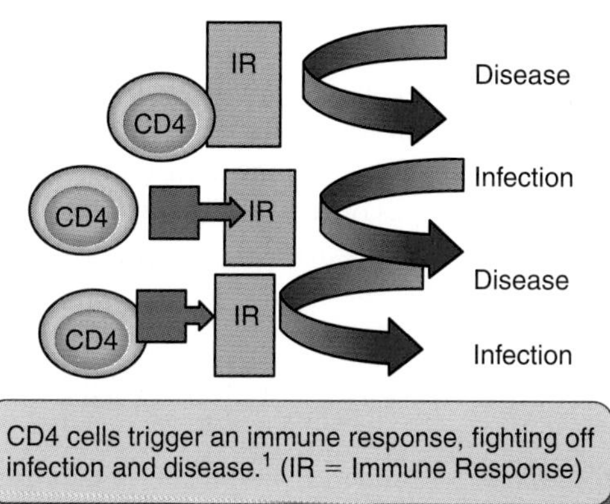

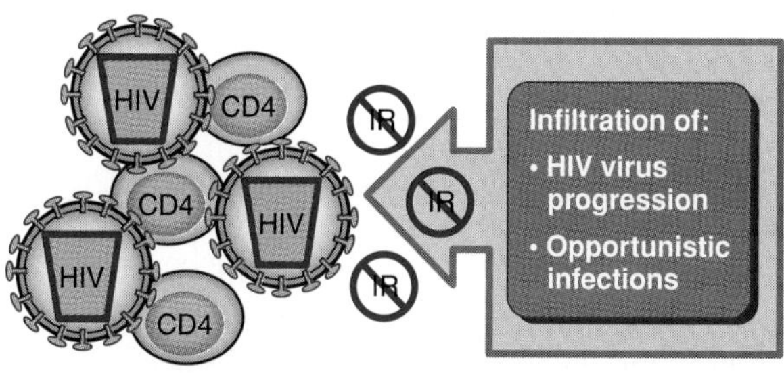

FIGURE 30-1. T-cells and infection response.

CAUSES AND RISK FACTORS

HIV is primarily contracted through exposure to specific body fluids from another individual who is infected with HIV. Those body fluids include blood, semen, preseminal fluids, rectal fluids, and vaginal fluids. Additionally, HIV can be transmitted to a fetus as well as to an infant during childbirth or through the breast milk of an individual who is infected.[6,7]

Worldwide, the primary method of HIV transmission is through sexual contact with an infected individual. Increased risk of exposure to HIV occurs when an individual:

- Has unprotected sex (anal, vaginal, or oral) with a person who is infected
- Shares needles or syringes with a person who is infected
- Has a sexually transmitted disease/infection
- Has multiple sex partners
- Has a diagnosis of hepatitis, tuberculosis, or malaria
- Exchanges sex for drugs or money
- Is exposed as a fetus or infant (at childbirth or is receiving breast milk from an infected person)
- Received a blood transfusion or clotting factor in the United States anytime from 1978 to 1985[8]

SIGNS AND SYMPTOMS

The symptoms related to the initial HIV infection (stage 1) include fever, fatigue, swollen lymph nodes, diarrhea, weight loss, cough, and/or shortness of breath. This typically lasts from 1 to 3 weeks. In the second stage, clinical latency, an individual may be asymptomatic for up to 10 years (or longer) after contracting HIV infection. During this latent period, transmission of the virus to other individuals is still possible. This becomes an increasingly important consideration in view of the Centers for Disease Control and Prevention (CDC) report indicating that 14% of individuals in the United States with HIV infection are unaware that they are infected.[9]

Diagnostics

Diagnosis of HIV is obtained via a blood test that detects the presence of the virus, and subsequently, in combination with clinical presentation of symptoms, the CD4 cell count is obtained to gather indicators of the progression and severity of the HIV infection. Individuals with a healthy immune system typically have CD4 cell count values between 500 and 1600 cells/mm^3. A lowered (below 200 cells/mm^3) CD4 cell count gives an indication of the severity of the infection. The presentation of clinical symptoms that include one or more opportunistic infections and/or cancers is indicative of HIV that has advanced to AIDS regardless of the CD4 cell count values[10] (Box 30-1).

MEDICAL TREATMENT

An individual can limit risk of exposure to HIV infection by having an increased awareness of the risk factors discussed previously. Protected sex, such as with appropriate use of condoms, awareness of a sex partner's HIV status, and use of sterile needles or syringes (e.g., not shared with anyone) are all methods of reducing the risk of exposure. Additionally, because healthcare workers, such as OTAs, are frequently exposed to clients' body fluids, taking measures, such as standard precautions,[11] are important to prevent transmission of HIV secondary to an occupational exposure. Standard precautions (previously called universal precautions) include hand hygiene procedures and use of personal protective equipment. Where there is any question as to the potential for exposure to any client's body fluids, regardless of known diagnoses, these precautions are to be employed by the OTA to prevent exposure to and transmission of infectious diseases, including, but not limited to, HIV. Additionally, caution should be utilized in an environment where needles, syringes, and potentially contaminated sharps are present, whether within a healthcare facility or within a community environment, such as a client's home.

An additional step in reducing exposure to and transmission of HIV is through periodically getting tested for the virus. The CDC recommends that every individual between the ages of 13 to 64 years be tested at least once and ideally as part of the routine healthcare examination. For individuals at greater risk (based on list presented earlier), the frequency of recommended testing increases to every 3 to 6 months. Additional guidance related to testing before pregnancy and during the first and third trimesters, is provided to women who are pregnant or plan to become pregnant, particularly for at-risk individuals.[6,10]

Testing for HIV is an important measure to reduce exposure to and transmission of the virus. An individual's knowledge of his or her HIV status allows the individual to make informed choices that might include limiting further behaviors that increase personal risk and/or put others at risk for exposure to the disease. Additionally, obtaining an HIV-positive result may potentially impact the type of medical treatment that would be considered beneficial for an individual as well as others in intimate contact with the individual (e.g., a sexual partner).

BOX 30-1
Physical Manifestations and Opportunistic Infections/Diseases Associated With HIV/AIDS

Pneumonia
Coughing
Shortness of breath
Toxoplasmosis
Brain infection
Encephalopathy/encephalitis
Neurological disorders
Memory loss
Depression
Cognitive impairments
Mycobacterium avium complex infection (with fever, diarrhea, weight loss)
Yeast infection/pain with swallowing/pharyngitis
Fungi-related diseases (causing symptoms, such as fever, cough, anemia)
Peripheral neuropathy
Primary central nervous system lymphoma
Kaposi's sarcoma (metastatic)
Systemic lymphoma (metastatic)
Neoplasms
Cytomegalovirus retinitis (blurred/distorted vision)
Decreased strength
Decreased range of motion
Extreme fatigue

Antiretroviral Therapy

Antiretroviral therapy (ART) is designed by the physician in collaboration with the client and considers applicable clinical factors of the individual, such as comorbidities; viral load; side effects of drugs; financial burden, which can impact adherence to regimen; drug interactions; and drug resistance, which is related to mutating strains of HIV. Upon assessment of the individual client and individual client factors, a complete regimen of treatment is prescribed. The medication regimen, which typically comprises several different medications selected from over 25 potential medications, is then devised, in accordance with the US Department of Health and Human Services (DHHS) guidelines, to reduce the amount of HIV within a person's body. Conceptually, controlling or reducing the amount of HIV will limit the amount of damage to the healthy components of an individual's immune system, thereby reducing associated symptoms and disease progression. ART can contribute to the reduction of HIV transmission in that a lower amount of HIV that could be transmitted is present within a person's system. ART is the primary method that enables individuals with HIV to live longer with the illness and subsequently avoid the progression of the disease into the complex disease processes of AIDS. The DHHS recommends ART for anyone who is infected with HIV. The urgency of those recommendations increases as an individual's CD4 counts decrease because the reduction in CD4s is indicative of advancing illness and disease.[3,12]

ART has proven to be very effective in the treatment of HIV, but it does not "cure" infection with the virus. Conversely, although ART does not cure HIV infection, it can be effective in preventing HIV from advancing to the disease process of AIDS. The actual success of ART is indicated by the individual's HIV viral load becoming undetectable through blood tests. This reduction in viral load typically indicates that the treatment has been effective. ART treatment requires a daily, lifelong commitment.

Individuals who are known sexual partners of those infected with HIV or other individuals who may be at high risk of HIV infection may be candidates for a drug regimen known as pre-exposure prophylaxis (PrEP). Some communities may not have access to PrEP. This is a daily medication treatment/regimen that requires adherence by the partner. Additionally, other methods of reducing the risk of exposure to HIV, such as appropriate use of condoms, are critical to the success of the PrEP methodology.

Side Effects of Medical Treatment

ART and/or PrEP treatment options for those affected or potentially affected by HIV and/or AIDS have many obvious benefits. However, individuals considering these options must take into account the potential side effects of the medications, particularly in considering the exponential, clinical combinations of some of the 25 different medications included in the prescribed ART or PrEP. Common side effects of ART drugs include, but are not limited to, the following:

- Anemia
- Diarrhea
- Dry mouth
- Fatigue
- Headache
- Nausea/vomiting
- Pain
- Peripheral neuropathy
- Rash
- Weight loss

Additional complications can occur when premorbid or comorbid conditions are present, resulting in an exacerbation or initiation of a disease, such as diabetes or cancer. These negative results have very serious consequences. Whether these conditions are known prior or subsequent to ART or PrEP, such results require clinical attention because they may result in serious disability and/or death.

STATISTICAL INFORMATION

In addition to understanding the nature and treatment of HIV/AIDS, it is important for the OT practitioner to be aware of the current status of HIV/AIDS globally and within the United States.

Global Occurrences

The latest estimates from 2015 indicate that approximately 36.7 million individuals worldwide are living with HIV/AIDS[5] (Table 30-1). Of these individuals, it is estimated that approximately 19 million worldwide are unaware that they are infected with the virus. It is further estimated that 3.2 million of this group are children under the age of 15 years, many of whom contracted HIV in utero from an infected mother or during childbirth or breastfeeding.[12] However, some individuals ages 15 years and younger may be sexually active and may be injectable drug users, or they may already be married in accordance with culturally accepted practices.[12] Additionally, it is estimated that approximately 17 million people are receiving ART globally,[11,13] with approximately 740,000 of these being children 15 years of age or younger. The World Health Organization (WHO) estimates that three out of five individuals with HIV are not receiving ART (approximately 22 million).[5,12] Worldwide, it is estimated that there have been 39 million deaths as a result of HIV/AIDS since 1981, which is the year of the first reported case.

These statistics, as well as the most current information related to global occurrences, indicates that the worldwide HIV epidemic continues to grow with the tens of thousands affected annually. Although many worldwide initiatives have addressed educational needs related to transmission of this disease, focus in provision of treatment has been increased substantially, in part as a result of the continued increase in numbers of individuals still contracting this infection.[12]

TABLE 30-1 2016 Worldwide Estimates of Individuals Living With HIV/AIDS[12]

AREA	LIVING WITH HIV
Sub-Saharan Africa	25.8 million
Asia/Pacific	5 million
North America & Central/ Western Europe	2.4 million
Latin America	1.7 million
Eastern Europe & Central Asia	1.5 million
Caribbean	280,000
Middle East & North Africa	240,000

AT-RISK GROUPS

Through an examination of the estimated number of new HIV infections worldwide,[12,13] groups most at risk were also identified as follows:

- Men who have sex with men
- Sex workers
- Injectable drug users (sharing needles, improper use of needles)
- Prisoners
- Transgender people
- Women
- Children

In considering the individuals belonging to at-risk groups, it is important to note that the risk for HIV infection is sometimes associated with behaviors that put these individuals at risk, such as unprotected sex, not the identity of the individuals, such as a person's sexual orientation or ethnicity. Additionally, environmental, cultural, and socioeconomic factors can influence the risk among the groups previously indicated.[12,13] Although the social implications associated with HIV/AIDS will also be mentioned in subsequent sections of this chapter, it is important to note that a variety of studies on subgroups of individuals with HIV and associated at-risk behaviors have been published. Those subgroups would include women with a history of childhood sexual abuse,[14] HIV-positive adults with a history of childhood sexual abuse,[15] homosexual and bisexual men with at-risk behaviors and a history of childhood sexual abuse,[16] adolescents and young adults with HIV with posttraumatic stress and trauma,[17] to name only a few. It is important to stress the significance of the behaviors that put an individual at risk, such as unprotected anal, vaginal, and/or oral sex or sharing needles/syringes with a person who is infected with HIV, as opposed to the person's identity, for example, sexual orientation, gender, or ethnicity. Second, as will be examined more closely within this chapter, the facets of OT intervention may include more than the effects of the infection itself but may potentially include the management and/or healing associated with the individual's personal history, such as the historical presence of trauma or abuse.

At this point, in consideration of the clinical manifestations, complexities of the infection and its treatment, and the statistical indications of prevalence globally, it likely that OT practitioners may be involved in the individual's treatment at any stage/phase of the disease. The OT practitioner may be called upon to address a variety of symptoms/manifestations across the lifespan. However, to provide an even greater perspective, a discussion of the clinical and social climate associated with the initial "discovery" of HIV/AIDS is important in that the perceptions of some individuals (including those in healthcare roles) remains influenced by the historical aspects of this disease.

HISTORY OF HIV/AIDS

To fully appreciate the various aspects of the role of OT practitioners in providing interventions for those with HIV/AIDS and/or their caregivers, it is equally important to be aware of the history of the disease in terms of the clinical timeline and social climate.

Several theories exist concerning the origin of HIV. One well-known and established theory is that of transfer of the virus from chimpanzees (simians), infected with a similar virus called simian immunodeficiency virus (SIV)[18,19] to humans through hunting, butchering, and/or eating the meat of an infected monkey. Again, the primary issue would be exposure to the blood of the infected animal. In this case, the theory suggests that SIV then adapted to the human host, morphing into HIV.

Other theories on the transfer of SIV to humans include transmission via the oral polio vaccine because the development and growing of the vaccine included the use of primate tissue.[19] Various other theories, including conspiracy theories, suggest the use of contaminated needles or syringes during administration of such vaccines.

There is still much debate about whether it is necessary to continue to study the origins of HIV. General agreement exists, however, regarding location and timing of the first reported cases related to HIV/AIDS within the United States.

Clinical Timeline

In June 1981, the CDC reported five different cases of young gay men in Los Angeles presenting with numerous unusual infections, indicative of their failing immune systems.[8] These cases were quickly followed by similar cases reported from other areas of the country, leading to 270 reported cases of what turned out to be HIV-related infections with symptoms indicative of what is now known to be AIDS. Of the 270 reported cases in 1981, primarily among gay men, 121 of these individuals subsequently died within that same year. By the end of 1982, infants were now among those found with this virus. In these cases, transmission was thought to be either through blood transfusions or through a still unknown mechanism. By 1983, it was apparent that HIV/AIDS was a disease affecting more than just gay men and that it affected people of all sexual orientations/preferences, gender, and ages; infection involved more than specific forms of sexual contact and involved contact with other body fluids, such as blood. In 1983, discussion ensued regarding policies and procedures related to collecting and utilizing blood and blood products, as it was now known that HIV/AIDS could be transmitted through exposure to or transfusion of blood.[20]

Social Climate

Because the initial reports of HIV in the United States involved young gay men, the disease was quickly surrounded by stigma, discrimination, and fear and was referred to as "gay-related immunodeficiency disease." [21] In 1982, the infection was more appropriately described as being caused by "human immunodeficiency virus" because it clearly affected men, women, and children, regardless of sexual orientation. Despite its renaming, HIV infection continued to engender stigma, discrimination, and fear. Social attitudes and personal beliefs also impacted the social and clinical "climate." A subgroup of individuals who were at risk, namely illegal drug users, were also marginalized.

Even today, an underlying stigma persists in relation to those with HIV/AIDS and the "type" of individual or lifestyle of an individual who would contract HIV. There are some who, through personal and/or religious constructs, would subscribe to the belief that HIV/AIDS is a divine punishment. Even among those with less extreme beliefs, there are some who stigmatize and discriminate against individuals identified as being at risk for contracting the disease, namely, those who are homosexual, or bisexual, and/or are intravenous drug users. Additionally, considering the global presence of HIV infection, cultural influences can impact how individuals might avoid transmission, how individuals who are infected with HIV are viewed, and whether or not they will be able to access appropriate treatment. One example of this would be from Swaziland in South Africa, where the perpetuation of cultural influences, has placed women and children (viewed as subordinate beings) at risk because they are forced into intergenerational sex, polygamy, and child marriage. Such cultural influences also perpetuate social and financial challenges, with many infants being born to mothers who are infected with HIV, which results in higher transmission rates. Avert.org[12] provides further details of the complexities associated with the transmission and the treatment of HIV in Swaziland. This country has received global attention because of the ongoing epidemic and the cultural factors that must be addressed to facilitate a decrease in the transmission of this infection.

SOCIAL IMPLICATIONS AND ADVOCACY

Because of the stigma and discrimination against individuals who are homosexual, bisexual, or transgender and/or are intravenous drug users, in part because of the perception that they are more likely to have HIV infection, these populations may be reluctant to get tested for HIV, disclose their HIV status, and take antiretroviral drugs. An unwillingness to be tested for HIV means that more people are diagnosed later, when HIV infection may have already progressed to AIDS. This makes treatment less effective, increasing the likelihood of transmission of HIV to others and early death.[22] Stigma may present in many forms, including the following:[22]

- Self-stigmatization: Fear of discrimination, shame about the condition
- Governmental stigmatization: Discriminatory laws, rules and policies, such as outlawing homosexuality
- Healthcare stigmatization: Potential breaches of confidentiality, fear of disclosing personal or sexual information, fear being treated differently
- Employment stigmatization: By coworkers and employers, resulting in social isolation, ridicule, discriminatory practices, termination, or refusal of employment
- Restrictions on travel, entry, and stay: Some countries still deport those with HIV or have mandatory testing or reporting
- Community stigmatization: Fear of losing family and friends after disclosure

As well as being made aware of their rights, clients living with HIV can be empowered to take action if these rights are violated. Adopting a human rights approach to HIV/AIDS is important as stigmatization blocks access to HIV testing and treatment services, making spread and transmission more likely.[22] OTAs can find support groups and advocacy options to empower their clients with HIV/AIDS. They should also speak out against ill-treatment, discrimination, and prejudice. Some clients find new purpose through peer mentoring and advocacy efforts (Fig. 30-2).

OCCUPATIONAL THERAPY AND HIV/AIDS

The degree to which an understanding of the history of HIV/AIDS is relevant to the OTA is substantiated by the response of the American Occupational Therapy Association (AOTA) to the social and clinical climate of the 1980s to 1990s. In March of 1990, the AOTA released a special issue of the *American Journal of Occupational Therapy* (AJOT) that was specifically dedicated to the topic of HIV infection and AIDS. The articles in this issue encouraged open dialogue about the role of OT as well as the impact of individual OT practitioners' views, fears, attitudes, and beliefs on the types and ways in which OT services were delivered.[21,23-25]

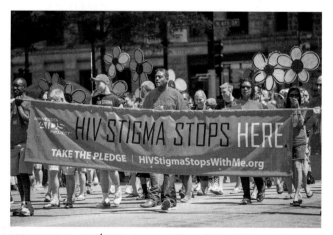

FIGURE 30-2. HIV/AIDS advocacy efforts. *(© Tony Webster, Portland, OR, United States [CC BY 2.0 (http://creativecommons.org/licenses/by/2.0)], via Wikimedia Commons.)*

Pizzi suggested that "personal (and) professional transformations" needed to occur for OT practitioners to become true role models for healthcare and in once again establishing the value of OT services specifically for those with HIV infection and AIDS.[25] Pizzi provided an avenue to look deeper into the role of the OT practitioner; he broadened that scope to encourage personal examination of relationship and responsibility as human beings. (As an aside, it is also interesting to note that in 1990, there was already reference to HIV infection as a "chronic disease" or "chronic illness").[25]

The special issue of the AJOT further considered the ethical issues and responsibilities associated with provision of treatment to those with HIV/AIDS,[24,26] as well as potential legal concerns regarding the same.[27]

Having laid the groundwork regarding OT practitioners' approach and concerns, both personally and professionally, the special issue of the AJOT further provided practice articles related to models of OT as applied to the clinical approach to those with HIV/AIDS;[23] behavioral impact of the disease;[27] relationship of at-risk groups, such as those with hemophilia, intravenous drug users, and children with perinatal HIV infection;[28-31] treatment programs (day treatment programs);[32] education regarding safe sex practices;[33] and, last, OT practitioner stress and burnout related to loss and grief in working with those with HIV/AIDS.[34]

OT Practitioner's Viewpoint

This chapter provided a number of details related to the social and clinical climate experienced by those living with HIV/AIDS. As is evidenced by the release of position papers by the AOTA, OT practitioners have been challenged personally and professionally to respond to the individuals affected by these diseases.

As OT practitioners continue to broaden their scope and knowledge related to HIV and the conditions associated with transmission, including social and cultural conditions, they can be better prepared socially and clinically to address their clients' occupational needs. Given that therapeutic use of self includes approaching the client with empathy and taking on a role of collaborator, OTAs will need to identify and acknowledge any potential barrier (socially and clinically) to utilizing this approach with clients.

An OTA might benefit from exploring his or her clinical knowledge regarding the transmission and development of the manifestations of HIV/AIDS as a way to understand the potential areas of OT that would be of benefit to the client.

Equally, an OTA might benefit from expanding his or her cultural awareness as it applies to beliefs, sexual orientation, gender issues, socioeconomic issues, and so on and the potential impact it has on the prevalence of HIV. This broadening of perspective will promote a more complete, client-centered approach within the OT process to ensure meaningful delivery of treatment. - Sharon D. Novalis, PhD, OTR/L

Position Paper 1996

That the AOTA recognized the need to release such a special issue of the AJOT is clearly indicative of the social as well as clinical climate of the time related to HIV/AIDS, clients with HIV/AIDS, and the many and varied concerns, beliefs, attitudes, and fears of practitioners, as well as the continued identification of at risk groups and the expanding role of OT in provision of care. Although practice-related articles were published after the 1990 special issue,[35] a social and clinical climate of stigmatization, discrimination, and fear remained so much so that in 1996, the AOTA published a document entitled "Position Paper: Providing Services for Persons with HIV/AIDS and Their Caregivers."[36] While acknowledging the presence of fear regarding the transmission of the disease, as well as the stigmatization and discrimination among some and potential for personal beliefs surrounding individuals with HIV/AIDS, the AOTA succinctly and directly reminded OT practitioners of their professional and ethical responsibility to provide OT services in an equitable manner to all individuals in need of such services "regardless of age, gender, ethnicity, religion, disability, condition, income, place of residence, sexual orientation and current life circumstances."[36]

In this position paper,[36] the AOTA pointed out that the needs of those with HIV/AIDS were varied in terms of the severity, duration, episodes of infection and that those needs could be related to any and all "performance areas" (e.g., domains including client factors, performance skills, performance patterns, and context/environment),[36] as well as location (acute care facilities, inpatient/outpatient settings, day treatment/community facilities, extended/skilled service settings, long-term care, hospice, and/or the client's/caregiver's home). Additionally, the AOTA specifically identified the inclusion of caregivers/family (including "nontraditional" family members) as an "important part of the health care team."[36]

The AOTA[36,37] clearly acknowledged the "current climate of stigma, fear, prejudice, misinformation, and discrimination surrounding HIV/AIDS ...." To the degree that the release of such a position paper was deemed necessary by the AOTA should give an indication as to the need for such guidance to be provided to OT practitioners. This position paper also provided a conceptual framework of sorts in terms of maintaining a holistic view and approach in providing OT services to those in need.

Today, exploration of a variety of topics related to OT services for those with HIV/AIDS, including practitioner anxiety,[38] attitudes,[39] practice related to community wellness,[40] assessment measures of daily life performance,[40,41] intervention strategies and implications,[20,42-45] settings,[46] and specific groups affected by HIV/AIDS,[20,44,47-49] continues. These citations are only a representation of vast growing body of research related to providing services to those with HIV/AIDS. Although several of these references will be explored further in this chapter, it is important to note that the topics and the nature of research related to OT services for those with HIV/AIDS and caregivers has grown increasingly similar to the topic and nature of research associated with other diseases that do not have the historical social stigma. Additionally, because of the advances in knowledge related to prevention of transmission of the virus as well as the treatment options that are now available for those with HIV/AIDS, the body of knowledge related to the needs of older adults with HIV/AIDS continues to expand.[46,50] Such growth in the evidence that includes identification, assessment, intervention, demographics, and the range of physical, psychological, and spiritual needs of individuals with HIV/AIDS and caregivers is further indication of the need to approach the client holistically. Experts recognize the impact of what can now potentially, with appropriate medical care, be a chronic illness spanning decades. The need for OT services is varied and wide.

OCCUPATIONAL THERAPY SERVICES

The remainder of this chapter will explore the role of OT practitioners in providing services to individuals with HIV/AIDS and their caregivers with a specific focus on the involvement of the OTA.

Treatment Settings

OTAs should be aware of the potential for providing services to clients with HIV/AIDS within acute care hospitals, trauma units, intensive care units (ICUs), transitional units, rehabilitation hospitals, skilled nursing facilities, outpatient settings, day treatment facilities, behavioral health units/facilities, day camps, schools (pre-, elementary, secondary, and high schools), and the client's home. Additionally, OTAs should be aware that the reasons for referral to OT may or may not be directly related to the client's HIV/AIDS status. The setting may or may not be indicative of the status of the HIV or AIDS progression. In some instances, the setting may be required because of other types of disease- or trauma-related injuries that are of primary concern, such as cerebrovascular accident (CVA) or injury from an industrial accident, and the diagnosis of HIV or AIDS may be a secondary diagnosis. In other cases, the HIV or AIDS diagnosis may be part of the eligibility requirements for a day treatment program for those with the disease.

Assessments

OT research continues to explore the use of various known assessment tools for their applicability to clients with HIV/AIDS.[42,43] HIV/AIDS–specific assessment tools are also available for use by OT practitioners, most notably, the Pizzi Assessment of Productive Living for Adults with HIV Infection and AIDS (PAPL).[51] Use of an instrument, such as the PAPL, is a holistic, comprehensive evaluative assessment that incorporates all aspects potentially relevant to the individual's occupational performance. Although it includes the physical, cognitive, and day-to-day functions of the person, it also includes exploration of the things that have meaning and value for the client, psychosocial aspects of the impact of HIV/AIDS in the client's life, and the client's hopes and aspirations. There are other applicable assessments that address occupational role (e.g., as worker

EVIDENCE-BASED PRACTICE

Although this chapter includes many references to the available literature from a variety of sources, including peer-reviewed scientific and clinical studies, the following presents an example of the potential influence of evidence on actual clinical practice.

An OTA is quite likely to work with a female client living with HIV/AIDS. The OTA could be involved in searching for information that could facilitate a more meaningful treatment session with the client, particularly as the OTA continues to build on clinical experience in working with these clients. Beauregard & Solomon[21] provided a summary of a qualitative study that examined four themes that emerged related to the experiences of women living with HIV/AIDS. The authors further provided discussion about the potential impact in OT practice.

In this case, the OTA might particularly be drawn toward addressing the physical challenges identified within this article. In conjunction with the OT assessment, it is possible that based on the evidence, exploration of sleep hygiene, activity tolerance, and even meal preparation/consumption will be addressed. Additionally, on the basis of the results of this study, it would be reasonable to consider planning of the daily routine with the client to maximize efficiency and energy levels to better meet the demands of ADLs/IADLs and employment.

Another reasonable consideration might be alternatives for social engagement. For example, the use of FaceTime or Skype might offer a client some alternatives for communication that still has a face-to-face component, and therefore, a relevant source of socialization that would accommodate a physical challenge that limits activity.

This is only one example of utilizing the information presented in a peer-reviewed journal to help guide the clinical considerations and/or treatment provided. The exploration of the available evidence can assist the OTA in gaining clinical competence and can broaden the OTA's clinical treatment options.

Beauregard, C., & Solomon, P. (2005). Understanding the experience of HIV/AIDS for women: Implications for occupational therapists. Canadian Journal of Occupational Therapy, *72(2), 113–120.*

or student), are occupation based (e.g., the Canadian Occupational Performance Measure), and/or client factor–specific characteristics (e.g., strength, pain, range of motion).

Addressing Occupations

By reviewing the information obtained through the evaluation and the occupational profile, the OTA identifies the client's required and/or preferred occupations. Additionally, as the OTA initiates treatment, the client's other secondary occupations of importance may emerge. Utilization of the *Occupational Therapy Practice Framework, 3rd edition* (OTPF-3) to conceptually organize the discussion of occupation identifies eight key categories of occupation: activities of daily living (ADLs), instrumental activities of daily living (IADLs), rest and sleep, education, work, play, leisure, and social participation.[37] Dependent on the priorities established within the treatment plan, the OTA may be involved in provision of OT services that are relevant to any of these categories. Additionally, the type and methods of interventions delivered will also be impacted by the client's status within the continuum of the disease process. For example, treatment related to the completion of ADLs might include pacing of task performance for an individual with early manifestations of HIV, work simplification and compensatory strategies for an individual dealing with the side effects of ART, or routinization of tasks and caregiver education and training with an individual with progressive AIDS-related dementia. This example further emphasizes the need for utilization of the OTA's skills in activity analysis, clinical reasoning, therapeutic use of self, and applied selection of activity/occupation to address client goals.

To reinforce these points, consider the task of completing laundry. The OTA needs to understand what aspects of HIV are manifesting in the client to provide treatment appropriately. Equally important, the OTA must be able to analyze the activity of laundry completion to determine which aspects of this task would potentially be problematic given the client's condition. Of course, completing laundry has many cognitive aspects (sorting by appropriate material and color group, selecting the appropriate settings on the washer/dryer, following any special care instructions on the clothing label, measuring appropriate amounts of detergent and softener, etc.). If the client had a cognitive impairment associated with HIV, the OTA would need to determine which components of the task could be adapted, modified, and/or routinized for the client's successful engagement.

As with any activity, beyond the cognitive aspects, there are many other components related to task completion, such as the physical components related to sensory and movement functions. For example, if the client has muscle weakness or incoordination, the OTA, through appropriate activity analysis, would be able to select certain aspects of the laundry task so that it can be utilized as a rehabilitation task (therapeutic activity) or adapt or modify the methods for the client to be able to successfully complete the task. A simple example of an adaptation or modification might be to utilize a table or a cart to place the laundry detergent and softener on while measuring the amounts. A second example might be to transport smaller portions of laundry to avoid overutilizing muscles that are weak.

In either of these examples, the OTA would need to apply clinical reasoning to reasonably and meaningfully ascertain the client's manifestations/clinical presentation of symptoms with the known components of the activity being applied.

Utilizing the skills associated with activity analysis and clinical reasoning can be further enhanced by the OTA's employment of therapeutic use of self. OTPF-3 describes therapeutic use of self as an approach that also engages aspects of clinical reasoning to provide client-centered treatment.[37] The OTA must be aware of what is of importance to the client, the factors that might affect the client's engagement, and what approach will facilitate the greatest, most effective clinical outcome of meaning for the client.

Continuing the example of the laundry task, the client might have an underlying motivation and belief related to the performance of laundry for the family. In not being able to successfully complete that task, perhaps the client will feel diminished in his or her role as family caregiver or provider. The OTA's awareness of the meaning attributed to the task for each individual client will facilitate an appropriate, therapeutic approach to support the client in the required rehabilitation, adaptation, or modification. As will be discussed further, even though many of the ADLs/IADLs are considered basic, the actual components of the tasks can be quite complex and even overwhelming to a client who is impaired in some way and unable to completely, independently complete the task. Therapeutic use of self will facilitate a collaborative and empathic relationship with the client as he or she moves forward through the therapy process.

Although ADLs, such as dressing, toileting, and bathing, are generally thought of as basic, everyday necessary tasks, not all of these tasks need to be performed completely by the client. Client circumstances, preferences, and/or values may dictate that OT treatment time be spent in other areas, even though the client may be experiencing difficulty completing basic ADLs. Where possible, the OTA should also consider the types of treatments that result in transferable skills across various occupations. Many preparatory and compensatory treatment strategies can be applied to various occupations. For example, energy conservation/work simplification strategies could be applied to dressing and bathing as well as to performing pet care.

Strategies related to functional mobility are also important. Although physical therapy (PT) may be involved in areas related to ambulation and mobility, OT may also be utilizing various strategies that relate to performance of occupations. For example, in the case of a client who may be experiencing sensory loss associated with peripheral neuropathy, a physical therapist might instruct the client to utilize a specific technique to negotiate uneven terrain safely while using a cane for balance and safety. The OTA would want to have this client utilize the same strategy while negotiating various floor surfaces (e.g., carpeting, tile, shower mat, etc.) or while engaging in outdoor activities (e.g., gardening, home maintenance, walking to the mailbox to retrieve mail, and so on). However, the OTA may also utilize additional strategies for specific tasks as addendums to the techniques provided by the PT practitioner. The OTA might provide compensatory methods or adapted techniques to transporting items (mail, gardening tools, etc.) while using the assistive device that add to the functionality of the ability to ambulate safely.

The client's need for compensation strategies or adapted performance techniques may be caused, in part, by fatigue, effects of peripheral neuropathy, muscle weakness, muscle atrophy, incoordination, or impaired function of the cardiovascular and/or respiratory systems (refer to Table 30-1 for potential clinical manifestations). Where such impairments are present, the OTA needs to determine whether a compensation strategy or adapted performance technique would benefit the client. Examples related to functional mobility might include installation of grab bars in the toilet and shower areas, use of a raised toilet seat, tub bench/shower chair, hand held shower, risers for chairs, couches and bed, use of a hospital bed, and provision of rest areas in the house and/or yard that are easily and safely accessible.

The client may also have a cognitive impairment that affects his or her safety awareness and/or judgment, orientation, sequencing, and so on. Utilization of memory aids that promote safety, orientation, and appropriate sequencing can be very helpful. Cue cards used as reminders for hand placement, brake negotiation, sequence of transfer techniques all can add to the efficiency and safety for functional mobility.

In considering the subcategories of ADLs, it is possible that the OTA could be involved in treatment related to swallowing/eating. Again, because one of the manifestations associated with HIV/AIDS is pharyngitis, which can make swallowing painful, it may result in the client's reluctance to take in nourishment. Due to other issues related to cognition and motor planning/sequencing, it is also possible that the OTA will work on self-feeding tasks with the client and/or caregiver. Treatment approaches might include exploration of cooking activities that utilize recipes that would be appropriately tolerated by the client. Cognitive strategies might include routinization of the mealtime preparation/activity, provision of appropriate background environment that does not detract from the awareness required to self-feed (e.g., limits the distractions so that the client can focus on the task at hand). The use of adapted utensils, plates, and drinkware facilitate successful cognitive negotiation of these occupations (e.g., straws, cups with lids, and disposable dinnerware/flatware), and prepackaged mealtime necessities, including meals). All of these strategies promote some self-sufficiency and independence, while understanding that additional support/caregiver support may also be a required option.

Varying levels of engagement are possible for different IADLs. Ideally, the OTA will select interventions that help the client maintain independence in performing the tasks.

TECHNOLOGY AND TRENDS

Though there are many advancements related to identification and treatment of HIV/AIDS, OTAs should explore the various available technologies that can assist a client in successful functional performance of occupations. OTAs should consider the following suggestions:

- Many devices (e.g., smartphones and tablets) have a plethora of applications ("apps") that could be useful to a client. For example, calendars, notes and alarms could be used for successful medication management, scheduling of appointments, and follow-through with tasks in ADLs.
- Health and wellness apps allow users to track steps, distance, heart rate, and other indicators. These values can be tracked over time to encourage successful engagement in wellness programs.
- FaceTime and Skype allow for "face to face" interaction, promoting social engagement and support. Internet capabilities, in general, might afford a client a variety of employment opportunities that might not otherwise be available, particularly if the client is challenged by manifestations of HIV/AIDS.

Devices can be preset/preprogrammed for use with furnace, air conditioner, coffee maker, lighting, etc., to promote safety and efficiency. Although many of these technologies are utilized by the general public, these applications can be extremely useful (not just convenient) to an individual with impairments of cognitive or physical function.

For IADLs, the levels of complexity are visible in the individual components of each of the items represented, and each component has multiple steps. There is also the potential for a great deal of meaning to maintaining independence in these items for the client. One example of evidence related to the meaning of such occupations is that of pet care (Fig. 30-3). A qualitative study by Allen et al.[44] examined the experiences associated with pet ownership among seven men with HIV/AIDS. The results indicated that there were effects from the disease on the participant's daily/life routines, affect, and physical health related to pet care. Although the authors pointed out the various effects that are presumably typical of all pet owners, the factors that were reported as being influenced by the presence of HIV/AIDS and associated complications were related to a motivation to persist despite challenges. In particular, participants commented on the unconditional nature of the relationship with a pet that was not impacted by the presence of the illness. Additionally, participants indicated that pets counteracted the effects of stigma or isolation. The presence of a pet, for some, did cause a contemplation of long term planning and care for the pet, which is also indicative of the meaningfulness of the occupation of pet ownership.

Naturally, the implications associated with successful management of occupations identified within OTPF-3 vary. These implications are also an important reason for the increasing importance of including a client-identified support

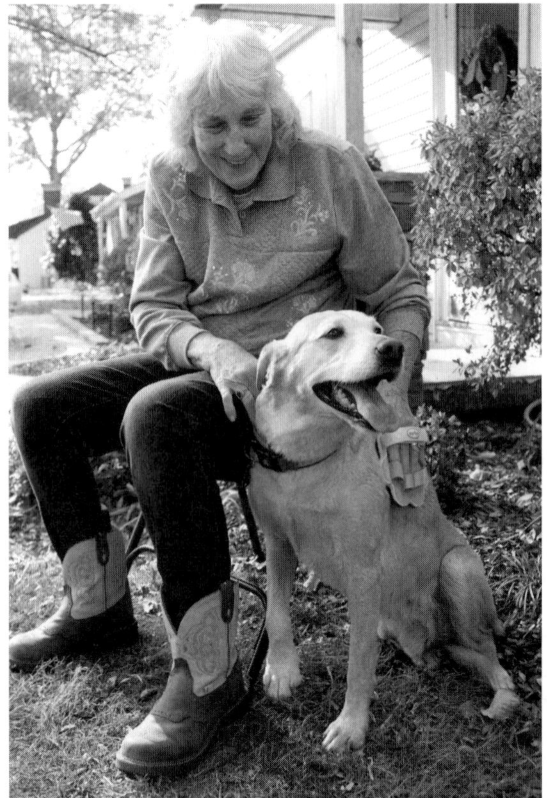

FIGURE 30-3. Pet care as a meaningful occupation.

and/or caregiver, much as is the case for all individuals whether or not an illness is present. Tasks related to a client's responsibility for self and others, such as financial management, are multifaceted and may require the client to consider compensatory strategies to maintain or improve management skills. Such skills may include budgeting, use of online banking reminders, direct deposit, automated bill paying, and so on. The client may also need to consider long-term planning related to delegation of portions of (or total) task completion to others. Failure to do so could negatively impact the client and others for whom the client may have responsibility, such as a spouse, partner, or dependent children.

As the OTPF-3 points out, IADLs may require "more complex interactions than those used in ADLs."[37] These interactions can include all areas of client factors and functions because of the complexities involved. For example, the IADL of health management in reference to self might include setting appointments or maintaining healthy routines, both of which could easily include cognitive and physical functional components. The OTA might engage a client in development of a reminder calendar of appointments or easily accessible contact information for medication management and health provider access. Treatment might include budgeting of time or funding, or arranging access for participation in activities that would promote the client's health and wellness (e.g., access to a support group). Even the psychosocial aspects of navigating public transportation would be within the possible realm of treatment options for those clients who are challenged by such social situations.

All of the occupations identified in the OTPF-3 may be pertinent and relevant to a client, and the level and degree of engagement in these occupations will be, in part, dependent on where the client is in relation to status of his or her HIV/AIDS and the effects of any associated medical treatment. The interaction and balance of these occupations and addressing the abilities of the client to engage successfully in these occupations are likely to be components of the treatment plan. The importance of sleep, ability to perform job duties, participation in leisure activities, and engagement in social activities or sexual activity are all client driven either out of necessity or preference, or both. Helping the client achieve a healthy and fulfilling balance in these occupations may be in the content of the OT treatment provided by the OTA.

Addressing Client Factors

Although an OTA will spend a great deal of time addressing issues related to body function and structure, it is important not to lose sight of the impact that values, beliefs, and spirituality may have on the client or the caregiver. For example, personal values may directly impact what priorities are determined for treatment, which occupational roles will be addressed, and in what manner. These examples may all be positive motivators for the client to actively participate in treatment.

In some instances, values, beliefs, and spirituality may have such an impact that the client is not motivated to actively participate in treatment and may actually refuse treatment instead. For example, a client may have religious beliefs that view illness and/or disease as punishment for a certain lifestyle or "sin." In this instance, the client may be encased in guilt or shame and will be more difficult to actively engage in any treatment, seeing his or her life circumstances and diagnosis as a judgment.

In either event, being aware of what the client values, being sensitive to personal beliefs, and being open and supportive to expressions of spirituality that are of a healthy benefit to the client and do no harm to others are important. This importance is not only to promote all aspects of the client's health balance but also as a means of acknowledging the client's individual choices.

A blending of values, beliefs, and spirituality may create benefits related to body functions and structures. For example, some individuals practice mindfulness as a part of spirituality. Mindfulness focuses on what is occurring in the moment, using meditation and breathing exercises, and connecting the way one thinks to the way one feels in order to interrupt negative thought patterns. Mindfulness-based cognitive therapy has been shown to be effective in improving the quality of life and emotional status of individuals with HIV infection.[46] Gonzalez-Garcia et al. further suggested that the results of their randomized controlled trial indicated positive effects of mindfulness-based cognitive therapy on psychological stress, symptoms of anxiety, and depression and potentially promoted increased CD4 cell count, thereby facilitating reaching old age in spite of HIV infection.[46] It is understood that to achieve optimal health, wellness, and engagement, ideally, all body functions and body structures would be functioning normally and in synergy and balance with each other.

In addition to the examples that are provided in the OTPF-3, Table 30-2 provides different examples of these various types of interventions and their application to the categories of body functions and body structures embedded in the performance of occupations.

Mental functions, which are closely tied to the client's ability to regulate and navigate various psychosocial factors associated with disease and impairment, are also important client factors to consider in treatment. Depression and anxiety are known to be experienced by many individuals who have HIV infection.[52] Psychological factors might also impact the client's consideration of treatment options, particularly when the prognosis is poor.[21] It is possible that the OTA will be involved in providing treatment that is focused on coping strategies, development of support systems, and/or development of self-esteem in order to support the client in reducing depression, anxiety, or related manifestations. Those strategies might include identification of supportive services and relationships, identification of client strengths and areas of functionality/accomplishment, provision of feedback related to the client's progress, and providing appropriately paced interventions that facilitate the client's success.

Addressing Performance Skills

Being able to differentiate one skill from another and adequately describe the action as well as the impact on performance of specific occupations or activities is important. This helps establish overall status of the client, provide rationale for the OT intervention, determine necessary modifications to the treatment plan, and establish the methods employed by the client in performing the specific occupation or activity.[37] Performance skills involved in participation in occupation and activities may be compromised in clients with HIV/AIDS.

Outcomes of Occupational Therapy

Ideally, the outcomes of the OT process are measurable by OT practitioners as well as the client or the caregiver and are meaningful to both. Those outcomes that are targeted at the beginning of the OT process through the evaluation of the client by the occupational therapist may have measurability at various levels, actual performance of specific occupation or activity, body functions/structures that support this performance, and/or improvement in the performance skills of the applied body function.

OT outcomes for those with HIV/AIDS will depend on the status of the client's disease stage. These outcomes could be related to mental/cognitive functions, physical functions, and/or functional task needs (e.g., employment strategies versus home management strategies). Furthermore, the presence of AIDS-related disease(s), relevant comorbidities, and the impact and response to medical treatments also can be factored into the outcomes being measured. Unfortunately, it is quite possible that a client already had other health-related issues before becoming infected with HIV. For example, if a client had diabetes before being diagnosed with HIV, the potential complications associated with neuropathy would be of serious consideration. Outcomes, therefore, might be related to successful management of tasks, for example, utilizing compensatory strategies to protect skin, such as skin inspection, utilizing a thermometer to measure temperature of water, using protective coverings (e.g., gloves, and so on). Obviously, there will also be instances where OT is closely linked to whether or not the medical treatments are successful for clients. If a client is receiving ART, the outcomes may still be rooted in the components of physical function, cognitive function, psychosocial well-being, and/or functional performance in the client's specific and required environment (at home, at place of employment, successful completion of child care, and so on). Ultimately, the OT interventions prescribed and delivered will address the determined needs of the client, with client and/or caregiver involvement, to sustain occupational performance through participation in daily life roles as well as to improve the client's quality of life.

TABLE 30-2 Examples of Interventions and Their Application to the Performance of Occupations

BODY STRUCTURE/FUNCTION	INTERVENTION TYPE	EXAMPLES
Structures related to movement/ joint range of motion	Preparatory tasks	Active range of motion exercises (e.g., yoga-based motion)
	Occupation-based	Basic IADLs (e.g., placing clean laundry onto hangers in closet)
	Client education	Joint protection strategies/modifications (e.g., using adapted kitchen utensils)
Structures related to movement/ control of voluntary movement	Preparatory tasks	Sequential fine motor active range of motion (e.g., tip to tip prehension/opposition of all digits)
	Occupation-based	Basic ADL prep or IADL tasks: (e.g., organizing make up drawer; counting change)
	Client education	Compensatory strategies (e.g., using adapted wide grip handles secondary to fine motor control deficits)

THE OLDER ADULT

Because of the advancements in the treatment of HIV infection through ART, HIV is now considered more of a chronic health condition.[50] This also means that clients are now living into late life within the home setting, community settings, and health care facilities, similar to those without HIV infection. Considerations in OT treatment would include, as with all clients, consideration of comorbidities that could have an impact on the current health status, prognosis, and functional performance.

An example, provided within the chapter, discusses the potential impact of a preexisting comorbidity—diabetes with peripheral neuropathy. Treatment considerations for a client with HIV would still be focused on compensatory strategies and protection related to skin integrity, balance, and safety.

Another example might be of a client who has a cardiac or pulmonary disease as a comorbidity. Because of the nature of HIV and the potential for opportunistic infections, the OTA would want to be aware of the risk for exacerbations related to, for example, chronic obstructive pulmonary disease and the impact on functional performance. This client may benefit from energy conservation/work simplification, including the application of these principles to the home environment; the client is able to maintain engagement in daily life tasks while taking into consideration the actual complexities of living with HIV and comorbidities.

Rosenfeld et al.[50] reported a worrisome finding regarding the community of aging individuals living with HIV.[50] Before the availability of ART, the prognosis for those with HIV was poor in that HIV would eventually lead to AIDS resulting in death. Rosenfeld et al.[50] conducted a qualitative study, in which the aging participants with HIV indicated that they were in "uncharted territory" and were "uncertain" about aging with HIV, as no substantial group had done this before. This finding brings up serious considerations for the OT practitioner because of the complexities related to aging as well as living with HIV (both in all aspects of the OTPF-3). The OTA may well be a collaborator with these clients to navigate both internal and external environments for successful and meaningful life engagement as the clients continue to go through the aging process.

COMMUNICATION

The OTPF-3 defines advocacy as "efforts directed toward promoting occupational justice and empowering clients to seek and obtain resources to fully participate in daily life occupations. The outcomes of advocacy and self-advocacy support health, well-being, and occupational participation at the individual or systems level."[36]

The OTA certainly has the opportunity to advocate by collaborating with clients to obtain appropriate accommodations and coverage of services. Additionally, OTAs can advocate for improved care services, improved awareness, and elimination of the stigmatization associated with HIV/AIDS. Political action committees (through national and state OT associations) that lobby for reform, funding, and programming are all relevant forums for OTA involvement in becoming mechanisms of change and support for individual clients as well as communities affected by HIV/AIDS.

Client and Caregiver Education and Training

The educational needs of the client and the caregiver are broad and vital to the successful carryover of OT interventions. The client and caregiver have a variety of needs, and since interventions are provided in settings across the continuum based on the status of the disease (acute versus more chronic in presentation), the OTA must use numerous educational and training methods.

For example, a client who initially presents with fatigue, muscle weakness, and associated depression would likely benefit from education in principles of energy conservation and work simplification. As the OTA incorporates this education into the treatment session, including active application of the principles within that session (training), the OTA is able to observe the client's performance, establish the client's understanding of these principles, and provide feedback and adjustments, where necessary. As the client utilizes these principles in all contexts (healthcare facilities, in leisure pursuits, employment environments, and home), theoretically, the client will be able to sustain a longer duration and more efficient and enjoyable period of engagement in activity/occupation. Client education and training empowers that client with strategies, resources, and tools that allow him or her to choose when and if the educational concepts will be applied. Although many components of topics that can be a part of client education may help address acute issues, these components may also be applied throughout the client's management of episodic and/or chronic manifestations of HIV/AIDS as well.

Wherever possible and appropriate, the involvement of the caregiver in client education and training sessions should be considered. When a caregiver must learn specific handling techniques, range of motion, or transfer strategies, for example, the session should also include the active involvement of the caregiver in the performance of those techniques and/or strategies. Additionally, where the client and the caregiver share environments (e.g., sharing a home), providing the caregiver with the rationale for certain types of strategies or adjustments that the client might employ may facilitate provision of support by the caregiver. Even the most basic adjustments may impact the typical routine of a caregiver and may be a source of added frustration. For example, energy conservation/work simplification strategies that would include rearranging where kitchen items are placed and stored may impact how the caregiver also uses the kitchen. Explaining the rationale of techniques and strategies may allow the caregiver to weigh the benefits of the modifications in comparison with maintenance of previous routines and be supportive of such modifications.

SEXUAL ACTIVITY

One additional area related to client education involves sexual activity, which remains a topic that OT practitioners frequently bypass.[53,54] Numerous aspects related to sexual activity may enter the realm of treatment for a client with HIV/AIDS, including education on safe sex practices, application of protection for safe sexual intimacy, positioning considerations that facilitate a pleasurable experience for the client and the partner, considerations of pacing/energy conservation, physical functions and impairments, compensatory strategies, and adapted techniques. OT practitioners will need to consider specific client factors, including sexual orientation, to select appropriate strategies and educational sessions for the client. Sexuality would also include the client's self-expression, potential for other forms of intimacy, impact on social engagements, and many aspects of ADLs (e.g., selection of clothing). Considering the therapeutic use of self, the OTA will benefit from collaborating with the client on determining specifically what client-centered needs are present as he or she relates to the presence of HIV, thereby avoiding assumptions and potentially ineffective treatments.

OTHER CONSIDERATIONS FOR THE OCCUPATIONAL THERAPY ASSISTANT

The life expectancy of a person who was diagnosed at an early stage of HIV, receives and responds to ART, and maintains a healthy lifestyle is actually similar to that of the general population.[55] However, HIV will remain a chronic illness for that individual, who will likely experience side effects associated with ART that also pose challenges that may be addressed in part by receiving OT services. In either event, OTAs may be involved in the treatment of those who are dealing with the effects of a chronic illness, with exacerbations of symptoms, and at-risk for changes in condition. An OTA may also work with other clients who may not have been diagnosed with HIV early enough or may not respond favorably or effectively to ART. In these cases, the individual will likely progress from HIV infection to AIDS and may subsequently die as a result of AIDS-related diseases and complications. Because there are continued at-risk groups and social anxieties associated with individuals and individual behaviors, the psychological/psychosocial environment may also present challenges for both the client and the OTA.

OTAs are at risk of the effects of the stressors associated with working with clients with chronic illness and in environments that may present social challenges. An OTA may be in a circumstance that causes him or her to question personal beliefs or address social stigmas. Even the act of carrying out what the OTA views as a personal and professional obligation to provide care may be questioned by others who do not hold similar personal or professional views. The OTA must find healthy ways to manage personal stress while still assisting clients.

There will be instances, regardless of the population, setting, or circumstances, in which the OTA will experience some version of loss in working with clients. OTAs will work with grieving clients who are terminally ill because of AIDS-related disease and complications. OTAs will work with caregivers who are also grieving this anticipated loss of their spouse/partner, parent, sibling, friend, and so on. The OTA may also experience similar feelings of loss or associated grief in working so closely with those clients and clients' supportive others.

When there are stressors associated with client care and environment or when feelings of loss or grief cannot be expressed or addressed, OTAs as well as other healthcare workers and caregivers may experience burnout.[56] Symptoms can include physical and/or emotional exhaustion and reduction or loss of positive approaches to interventions and even to clients themselves. Inaccuracies may also emerge in the treatment process, leading to ineffective and careless intervention. The OTA may become anxious and depressed as well.

Just as it is important for the OTA to approach clients and their caregivers with awareness, empathy, and compassion, it is equally important that OTA directs the same awareness, empathy, and compassion to himself or herself. With such awareness, the OTA may seek out support, seek healthy means of addressing personal and professional needs, and facilitate wellness that can lead to a productive and rewarding life, both personally and professionally.

SUMMARY

Because of the advances in medical diagnostics and available treatments, some immune diseases/disorders must now be approached in terms of a long-term chronic illness. As the course of what has been discovered regarding HIV infection over the last 35 years has continued to develop, it is recognized that through early diagnosis and client compliance to appropriate treatment regimens, a client with HIV infection can live a full and productive life. Unfortunately, despite the many medical advancements, there are still many health concerns related to HIV infection, including side effects of treatment.

Individuals who have been diagnosed with HIV infection, those with AIDS, and those caring for these individuals can all benefit from OT. The role of the OTA is to competently deliver the services within the scope of practice based on the treatment plan developed by the supervising occupational therapist. Additionally, the OTA should bring to the attention of the occupational therapist any changes in the client's condition and/or reports of additional areas of concern mentioned by the client/caregiver.

The OTA can have a meaningful impact on the quality of life of the client with HIV/AIDS and his or her caregivers.

Many opportunities exist for provision of services because of the potential variation in age range and age-appropriate needs at various points in the manifestation/progression of the disease (from infancy to end of life), in varied treatment settings, and across a wide array of potential symptomatology. In each case, OT has value as it offers interventions that are occupation based, client centered, and ultimately designed to facilitate the client's ability to live as independently and completely as possible with meaning and satisfaction.

REVIEW QUESTIONS

1. An OTA is scheduled to see a client in the behavioral health unit of an acute care hospital. The client was mandated to undergo a psychiatric inpatient assessment following a suicide attempt. The client is a 42-year-old male recently diagnosed with AIDS-related lymphoma with a very poor prognosis. The OTA coleads groups with the occupational therapist. Which of the following is a group that this client will likely be offered?
   a. Community reentry group to build social and leisure resources
   b. Cooking group and financial management group to build IADL skills
   c. Self-esteem group, stress management, community resource identification to address issues related to self-esteem, to facilitate healthy relationships and coping strategies, and to build supports for utilization in the community
   d. This client is not included in groups but instead is provided one-on-one treatment only.
2. Donna, a 35-year-old recovering from heroin addiction (clean for the last 2 years), had been diagnosed with HIV at age 27 years. Because of her drug habit, she was initially inconsistent with compliance to her antiretroviral therapy (ART) regimen. She has severe residual peripheral neuropathy in her hands and legs. The interventions would include:
   a. Desensitization of the extremities to reduce the client's complaints of "pins and needles" feeling
   b. Electrical stimulation to fatigue the muscles associated with the altered sensation
   c. Compensatory strategies in client-relevant occupations secondary to the presence of peripheral neuropathy
   d. Education regarding heroin addiction and its social implications
3. Millie, a 62-year-old female, was sent to the rehabilitation center for further rehabilitation following a right total hip replacement. Millie is HIV positive secondary to receiving a blood transfusion in 1979 following a traumatic multivehicle accident, which had claimed the life of her husband. The course of treatment will likely involve which three of the following?
   a. ADL techniques that include hip precautions
   b. A review of anticipated manifestations of HIV-related illnesses
   c. Preparation for continued stay at the center secondary to her age and comorbidities
   d. Care staff education for all of Millie's toileting and personal hygiene needs so that your risk of exposure to HIV is reduced
   e. Functional mobility for home negotiation, including the use of adaptive equipment (tub bench, raised toilet seat, etc.)
   f. Home management tasks that incorporate compensatory strategies for coping with limitations in functional mobility
4. The OTA is currently providing OT services to David, a client in the outpatient setting, seen following a long rehabilitation course from multiple injuries sustained in a motorcycle accident. David is HIV positive. During the treatment session, where focus is on passive range of motion and stretching to the bilateral upper extremities, the OTA is acting strangely, and uses gloves even though not warranted. Which of the following would be the appropriate behavior of the OTA?
   a. Use double gloves instead.
   b. Perform completely hands-off treatment, avoiding all physical contact.
   c. Treat David as any other client, with standard precautions.
   d. Avoid this situation completely by refusing to treat the HIV-positive client.
5. Steven, a coworker and an OTA, has been employed at the same rehabilitation center for the last 8 years. Steven is very dependable, very organized, and very professional in his presentation. Sometimes, others joke with him that he is a "neat freak." He has a good sense of humor and jokes right back. Recently, Steven has been under the weather, presenting with a dry cough that has lasted over the past 2 weeks. He is also looking a little run down and fatigued and has actually verbalized that he is a bit tired. His eyes have been "bothering" him as well and by just observing him, the OTA can tell he is straining to see the computer screen to complete his documentation. Others in the department have noticed the same. This morning, upon entering the therapy office, the OTA overhears two coworkers talking about Steven, pondering whether or not he is gay and then whether he might be HIV positive. The *best* course of action would be to:
   a. Join the conversation, agreeing with the coworkers because the OTA actually feels the same way.
   b. Join the conversation and defend Steven because he is a friend.
   c. Talk with Steven and let him know that people are talking about him behind his back so that he can defend himself if he so chooses.
   d. Speak with the department manager about the situation, providing a complete overview and details, including discomfort with the conversation that was overheard.
6. A new client complaining of fatigue, painful joints, and muscle weakness (preliminary diagnosis is fibromyalgia) is assigned to the caseload of the OTA in the outpatient setting. The OTA has never met the client before, and although the occupational therapist completed the evaluation and the client has actually received three treatment sessions already, it is today during the treatment session that the client states that she is HIV positive. The client begins to cry, indicating that she feels shameful and guilty, and states that she had "brought this on herself." Which of the following would be the *best* response?
   a. To let the client know that sharing this information with the occupational therapist is important in the event that there are any modifications that need to be made to the treatment plan in light of this diagnosis because the previous three treatments may have had an incorrect focus.
   b. Ask the client to explain why she feels she "brought this on herself" and agree with her conclusion.
   c. Go back to the therapy office and let everyone know of this new information so that they can protect themselves.

   d. Respond with empathy (therapeutic use of self), giving the client time to express herself in a space that gives her privacy and facilitates a confidential conversation, and when client is able, indicate that a discussion with the occupational therapist needs to occur in order to make sure that the appropriate treatments are being provided.
7. In the above scenario, numerous other clients witnessed a portion of the client's tearfulness. Everyone begins to ask why she was crying. Which of the following would be the *best* response?
   a. "It is confidential, sorry."
   b. "Unfortunately, she just found out that she is HIV positive, and she blames herself."
   c. "She just got some bad news. She'll be okay."
   d. "One of things I appreciate about you is what a caring person you are. I know you realize that I need to maintain the confidentiality of all of those that I treat, including you. Thank you, though, for being such a caring and understanding person." Then, direct focus back to the treatment session.
8. The OTA is working in a subacute rehabilitation hospital setting. This is Paul's fifth admission into the hospital. He has a progressive AIDS-related dementia and is now presenting with severe memory impairment and difficulty carrying out basic ADLs; he is also combative at times. Paul's life partner of 28 years, Robert, visits every day, spending most of the day with Paul. Robert is very attentive to Paul and has a very calm demeanor. However, whenever Paul "lashes out," Robert becomes tearful and will typically go out into the hallway to regain his composure. Which of the following would be the *best* response?
   a. Continue to provide treatment to Paul, as he is the client.
   b. Continue Paul's treatment, including Robert in those sessions, when possible, but also approach Robert to offer education, strategies, resources, support, and/or referral to other service providers in order to address Robert's needs and concerns.
   c. Leave the room to go speak with Robert and then come back and complete the treatment session with Paul.
   d. Continue the treatment with Paul but document Robert's response to Paul's behavior and bring it up at the next week's clinical team meeting.
9. The occupational therapist has provided comprehensive evaluation and a complete treatment plan, which should be initiated with a new client today. Portions of the evaluation include an ADL/IADL assessment, which resulted in setting goals related to the client's presentation of decreased activity tolerance. In this case, the client is a 51-year-old female who is HIV-positive being treated with an ART regimen. Which three of the following would be the *most* appropriate treatments to be initiated?
   a. Begin UE strengthening exercises to increase activity tolerance.
   b. Provide active education session in energy conservation/work simplification for ADL/IADL tasks.
   c. Utilize functional mobility tasks as an aerobic exercise.
   d. Provide education in the manifestations of HIV/AIDS progression.
   e. Begin ADL retraining to address activity tolerance.
   f. Utilize electrical stimulation to facilitate muscle strength passively.
10. David, a 52-year-old man, has been on an ART therapy treatment regimen for approximately 6 years. David has done well with the treatment but recently was diagnosed with non–HIV-related pneumonia. David was hospitalized with dehydration, generalized weakness, and initially with delirium associated with the dehydration. David was evaluated by the occupational therapist and the discharge plan is to return home. Which three of the following would David's OT treatment likely focus on?
   a. ADL retraining to address functional performance
   b. ADL retraining to provide education on energy conservation
   c. Home management tasks that incorporate work simplification and compensation strategies
   d. Functional mobility secondary to delirium
   e. Exploration of support services secondary to delirium
   f. Referral for placement secondary to manifestations of AIDS-related symptoms.

CASE STUDY

Joshua is a 57-year-old social worker who lives alone in a small apartment just outside of the cultural district of Philadelphia. Joshua has worked for the Philadelphia AIDS Task Force for the last 30 years. This chosen place of employment was largely the result of the number of friends he lost to AIDS in the 1980s and most notably, his first partner, Daniel, in 1983. Joshua, then only in his mid-20s, had been overwhelmed by grief and loss but also anger and fear. He had witnessed and experienced numerous acts of discrimination, some of which were violently directed toward the gay and lesbian community, all the while dealing with the devastating losses caused by AIDS.

Joshua was determined to make a difference and became an advocate for gay rights, and, as a means to address his fears regarding HIV infection and a way to honor the lives of those he had lost, he took a position with the Task Force.

When you read through the occupational profile, you will find that Joshua finds his work rewarding, and he does believe he has made a difference in the lives of many of the people that he has served. He is also seen many changes in the medical treatment and consequently the prognosis of those with HIV infection. He laments that these advances came too late for so many.

Joshua maintains an active social life, as he has for most of his life. He certainly is aware of precautions associated with the transmission of HIV infection and has taken those precautions the majority of times during any sexual activity.

Joshua has many friends but prefers to reside alone with his terrier mix Chloe. He finds her to be a faithful companion, and he makes every effort to be the same through the loving care he provides.

Joshua is responsible for all of his ADLs and IADLs. He prides himself on his attention to detail and level of organization in his personal life as well as his professional role. He does enjoy a variety of outdoor activities and enjoys taking any visiting friends on sight-seeing tours to all of the historic places in the Philadelphia area.

Joshua has been referred to OT because of manifestations associated with his recent diagnosis of HIV infection. Joshua presents with extreme fatigue, mental exhaustion, and muscle weakness and is emotionally distressed. Joshua is fully aware of the medical treatment options that will likely allow him to live a relatively healthy life into his 70s. Still Joshua expresses his anger, fear, and depression, speaking of his embarrassment about being diagnosed with HIV and his anxiety regarding the potential for needing assistance to take care of his responsibilities in the future.

Joshua has difficulty performing his ADL routine or any activity for that matter for a period longer than 20 consecutive minutes. He reports that activity beyond that span of time leaves him with a debilitating weakness and fatigue that completely "interferes and interrupts" any activity. He is most concerned about his ability to work to support himself and equally concerned about his general ability to care for himself.

1. What do you think Joshua and the OT practitioner would identify as the priority in Joshua's treatment plan?
2. What goals do you think would be associated with those priorities?
3. What treatment interventions would you introduce to Joshua?
4. What compensatory strategies would you introduce to Joshua?
5. Would you engage anyone else in Joshua's session (with Joshua's permission), or given Joshua's desire to independently maintain his life, would you forgo the inclusion of anyone else?

PUTTING IT ALL TOGETHER — Sample Treatment Session and Documentation

Setting	Home health, referred from acute care hospital where client received care for 4 days
Client Profile	Mrs. S, 45 y/o, diagnosed with HIV in 2001; did not receive follow up treatment and was diagnosed with AIDS in early 2013.
Work History	Was employed as a grocery clerk until mid/late 2013; has been on disability/SSI since early 2014
Insurance	Medicaid; Federal insurance program participant
Psychological	Depression; anxiety disorder
Social	Married; Mrs. S. and her husband both attend Narcotics Anonymous (NA) meetings and have been in recovery for the last 3 years. They have two adult children, both of whom live out of state. Mrs. S. has a number of close friends, primarily from her NA group.
Cognitive	Short-term memory is impaired; Mrs. S. has difficulty processing multistep and sequential tasks; higher-level cognitive tasks are now avoided by Mrs. S.
Motor & Manual Muscle Testing (MMT)	Mrs. S. presents with full AROM; MMT is 3+/5 for movements at the shoulder (flexion/extension) and elbow (flexion/extension). Mrs. S. is right hand dominant. Gross grasp/grip strength WNL bilaterally. Additionally, throughout testing of ROM, MMT, and hand strength measures, client reports overall fatigue and weakness. Client does not use any assistive devices, but does ambulate between the rooms of her home with deliberate and slow movement while holding onto furniture or doorways for support. Decreased discriminatory sensation in bilateral UEs noted.
ADL	Mod A for UB bathing; Mod A for UB dressing and grooming particularly with tasks that require sustained reach overhead (e.g., using the blow dryer; putting on a sweatshirt/long sleeve pullover blouse). Min A for LB bathing and dressing. (Client wears slacks with elastic waist band.)
IADL	Mod A for cooking due to cognitive and motor impairments; requires Mod A and verbal cues for medication management; requires Mod A for bill paying/banking tasks; requires Min A with homemaking (dusting/laundry/vacuuming) but takes frequent breaks and does receive assistance from her husband.
Goals	Within 3 weeks: 1. Client will require Min A for UB dressing utilizing compensatory strategies. 2. Client will require Min A for UB bathing utilizing AE and compensatory strategies. 3. Client will demonstrate independence in use of compensatory strategies for medication management. 4. Client will verbalize accurate understanding of energy conservation techniques applicable to homemaking tasks. 5. Client will demonstrate follow through with energy conservation techniques in home management with minimal verbal cues.

PUTTING IT ALL TOGETHER Sample Treatment Session and Documentation (continued)

OT TREATMENT SESSION 1

THERAPEUTIC ACTIVITY	TIME	GOAL(s) ADDRESSED	OTA RATIONALE
Provide client education and training (verbal, written, and demonstration) on energy conservation techniques for homemaking tasks.	30 min	#1, #2, #4, and indirectly #5	*Preparatory Method; Education and Training:* Education on energy conservation techniques provided in the three forms of verbal, written, and demonstration facilitates retaining of information and appropriate application. The techniques associated with energy conservation can apply to all areas of client's function (not just limited to homemaking tasks). Beginning with this type of education may lead to improved quality of life as client is able to attend to a greater variety of tasks with less fatigue.
AROM and AAROM for UE function including compensatory strategies to facilitate movement, strength, and stability	15 min	All	*Preparatory Task; Education and Training:* Movements through full range of motion, applied during functional tasks, utilized compensatory strategies to facility strength, stability, and coordination of movement during functional tasks.
UB ADL retraining, employing energy conservation techniques and compensatory strategies	15 min	#1, #2, #4, and indirectly #5	*Education and Training; Task Performance Training:* Provide training, apply energy conservation/compensatory strategies to ADL to facilitate independence and decrease fatigue. Provide client with knowledge/tools for future application during changes in health status.

SOAP note: 9/15/—, 12:00 pm–1:00 pm

S: Client states, "I am so tired of not being able to take care of such simple things," and "I guess this will only get worse." "He helps me a lot" (referring to her husband).

O: Client participated in skilled OT session in her home. Husband was present and encouraged participation in session. Client participated in the discussion of energy conservation techniques and verbalized appreciation for the printed material as well secondary to short term memory deficits. OTA and client practiced the compensatory strategies for UE function in medication management and upper body ADLs. Client required Mod A to obtain pill bottles from overhead cupboard. Client also required Mod A to manipulate the pill bottles to obtain the medications. Client was able to utilize the compensatory strategies of utilizing the table surface for stability during the table top activities (sorting the make-up and/or sorting medications).

A: Client fully engaged in education regarding energy conservation. Client was able to demonstrate appropriate application of the principles during UB ADL and medication management tasks with Min A and min verbal cues. Client also was able to verbally generalize the information to other tasks (such as pet care) and methods of applying these techniques in order to successfully complete tasks. The printed patient education material was beneficial as client referred to them often in her conversation and as a means to double check her work in applying the principles to tasks. Client would benefit from further graded strategies to employ depending on her level of fatigue/weakness. Client would also continue to benefit from the support of her husband due to her short-term memory impairments.

P: Next visit, continue to address the energy conservation and compensatory strategies to be utilized to facilitate increased independence in ADLs and IADLs. Explore possible adaptive equipment (e.g., shower chair, pill sorter) to facilitate ease of tasks and to decrease fatigue/need for current levels of assistance.
Josh Gabour, COTA 9/15/—, 1:15 pm

TREATMENT SESSION 2

What could you do next with this client?

TREATMENT SESSION 3

What could you do next with this client?

REFERENCES

1. UNAIDS. (2016). Fact sheet–Latest statistics on the status of the AIDS epidemic. Retrieved from http://www.unaids.org/en/resources/fact-sheet
2. American Autoimmune Related Diseases Association, Incorporated. (2015). Autoimmune information. Retrieved from www.aarda.org/autoimmune-information/
3. National Institutes of Health. (2015). Autoimmune diseases. Retrieved from https://www.nlm.nih.gov/medlineplus/autoimmunediseases.html
4. American Autoimmune Related Diseases Association, Incorporated. (2015). Autoimmune information: Autoimmune statistics. Retrieved from www.aarda.org/autoimmune-information/autoimmute-statistics/
5. World Health Organization. (2016). HIV/AIDS. Retrieved from www.who.int/mediacentre/factsheets/fs360/en
6. Department of Health and Human Services. (2015). National Institute of Arthritis and Musculoskeletal and Skin Diseases: Understanding autoimmune diseases. Retrieved from niams.nih.gov/Health_Info/Autoimmune?default.asp
7. Centers for Disease Control and Prevention. (2015). HIV transmission. Retrieved from http://www.cdc.gov/hiv/basics/transmission.html
8. National Institute of Health: National Institute of Allergy and Infectious Diseases. (2015). HIV/AIDS. Retrieved from www.niaid.nih.gov/topics/hivaids/Pages/Default.aspx
9. Centers for Disease Control and Prevention. (2015). HIV/AIDS fact sheets. Retrieved from www.cdc.gov/hiv/library/factsheets/index.html
10. Department of Health and Human Services (2015). AIDS.gov. Retrieved from https://www.aids.gov/
11. Occupational Safety and Health Administration. (2011). OSHA fact sheet: OSHA's bloodborne pathogens standard. Washington, DC: Occupational Safety and Health Administration. Retrieved from www.osha.gov/OshDoc/data_BloodborneFacts/bbfact01.pdf
12. AVERTing HIV and AIDS: AVERT.org. (2016). Global information and advice on HIV and AIDS. Retrieved from http://www.avert.org/about-hiv-aids
13. United Nations Programme on HIV/AIDS. (2015). Fact sheet 2014. Retrieved from www.unaids.org/sites/default/files/en/media/unaids/contentassets/documents/factsheet/2014/20140716_FactSheet-en.pdf.
14. Aaron, E., Criniti, S., Bonacquisti, A., & Geller, P. A. (2013). Providing sensitive care for adult HIV-infected women with a history of childhood sexual abuse. *Journal of the Association of Nurses in AIDS Care, 24*(4), 355–367.
15. Persons, E., Kershaw, T., Sikkema, K. J., & Hansen, N. B. (2010). The impact of shame on health-related quality of life among HIV-positive adults with a history of childhood sexual abuse. *AIDS Patient Care and STDs, 24*(9), 571–580.
16. Brennan, D. J., Jellerstedt, W. L., Ross, M. W., & Welles, S. L. (2007). History of childhood sexual abuse and HIV risk behaviors in homosexual and bisexual men. *American Journal of Public Health, 97*, 1107–1112.
17. Radcliffe, J., Fleisher, C. L., Hawkins, L. A., Tanney, M., Kassam-Adams, N., Ambrose, C., & Rudy, B. J. (2007). Posttraumatic stress and trauma history in adolescents and young adults with HIV. *AIDS Patient Care and STDs, 21*(7), 501–508.
18. AIDS Institute. (2015). Where did HIV come from? Retrieved from www.theaidsinstitute.org/education/aids-101/where-did-hiv-come-0
19. AVERTing HIV and AIDS: AVERT.org. (2015). Origins of HIV and AIDS. Retrieved from http://www.avert.org/origin-hiv-aids.htm
20. United States Department of Health and Human Services. (2015). A timeline of AIDS. Retrieved from https://www.aids.gov/hiv-aids-basics/hiv-aids-101/aids-timeline/
21. Beauregard, C., & Solomon, P. (2005). Understanding the experience of HIV/AIDS for women: Implications for occupational therapists. *Canadian Journal of Occupational Therapy, 72*(2), 113–120.
22. AVERTing HIV and AIDS: AVERT.org. (2016). Stigma, discrimination, and HIV. Retrieved from www.avert.org
23. Atchison, B. J., Beard, B. J., & Lester, L. B. (1990). Occupational therapy personnel and AIDS: Attitudes, knowledge, and fears. *American Journal of Occupational Therapy, 44*, 212–217.
24. Hansen, R. A. (1990). The ethics of caring for patients with HIV or AIDS. *American Journal of Occupational Therapy, 44*, 239–242.
25. Pizzi, M. (1990). The transformation of HIV infection and AIDS in occupational therapy: Beginning the conversation. *American Journal of Occupational Therapy, 44*(3), 199–203.
26. Peloquin, S. M. (1990). AIDS: Toward a compassionate response. *American Journal of Occupational Therapy, 44*, 271–278.
27. Cornblatt, M. S., Ayres, M. J., & Kolodner, E. L. (1990). A legal perspective on AIDS. *American Journal of Occupational Therapy, 44*(3), 244–246.
28. Weinstein, B. D. (1990). Assessing the impact of HIV disease. *American Journal of Occupational Therapy, 44*(3), 220–226.
29. Weinstein, B. D., & de Neffe, L. S. (1990). Hemophilia, AIDS, and occupational therapy. *American Journal of Occupational Therapy, 44*(3), 228–232.
30. O'Rourke, G. C. (1990). The HIV-positive intravenous drug abuser. *American Journal of Occupational Therapy, 44*, 280–283.
31. Anderson, J., Hinojosa, J., Bedell, G., & Kaplan, M. T. (1990). Occupational therapy for children with perinatal HIV infection. *American Journal of Occupational Therapy, 44*, 249–255.
32. Gutterman, L. (1990). A day treatment program for persons with AIDS. *American Journal of Occupational Therapy, 44*, 234–237.
33. Sladyk, K. (1990). Teaching safe sex practices to psychiatric patients. *American Journal of Occupational Therapy, 44*, 284–286.
34. Piemme, J. A., & Bolle, J. L. (1990). Coping with grief in response to caring for persons with AIDS. *American Journal of Occupational Therapy, 44*, 266–269.
35. Atchison, B. J. (1992). Clinical assessment and treatment of HIV: Rehabilitation of a chronic illness. *American Journal of Occupational Therapy, 46*, 1047–1047.
36. American Occupational Therapy Association. (1996). Position paper: Providing services for Persons with HIV/AIDS and their caregivers. *American Journal of Occupational Therapy, 50*(10), 853–854.
37. American Occupational Therapy Association. (2014). Occupational therapy practice framework: Domain & process (3rd ed.). *American Journal of Occupational Therapy, 68*(Suppl. 1), S1–S48.
38. All, A. C., & Fried, J. H. (1996). HIV/AIDS: Factors influencing anxiety concerning HIV/AIDS in rehabilitation workers. *Journal of Rehabilitation, 62*(4), 17–21.
39. Johnson, C., & Sim, J. (1998). AIDS and HIV: A comparative study of therapy students' knowledge and attitudes. *Physiotherapy, 84*(1), 37–46.
40. Phillips, I. (2002). Occupational therapy students explore an area for future practice in HIV/AIDS community wellness. *AIDS Patient Care and STDs, 16*(4), 147–149.
41. Merritt, B., Gahagan, J., & Kottorp, A. (2013). Research paper: HIV and disability: A pilot study exploring the use of the Assessment of Motor and Process Skills to measure daily life performance. *Journal of International AIDS Society, 16*(17339), 1–8.
42. Ranka, J. L. & Chapparo, C. J. (2010). Assessment of productivity performance in men with HIV associated neurocognitive disorder (HAND). *Work, 36*, 193–206.
43. Lal, S., Jarus, T., & Suto, M. J. (2012). A scoping review of the Photovoice method: Implication for occupational therapy research. *Canadian Journal of Occupational Therapy, 79*(3), 181–190.
44. Allen, J. M., Dellegrew, D. H., & Jaffe, D. (2000). The experience of pet ownership as a meaningful occupation. *Canadian Journal of Occupational Therapy, 67*(4), 271–278.
45. Robinson, R., Okpo, E., & Mngoma, N. (2015). Interventions for improving employment outcomes for workers with HIV (Review). *Cochrane Database of Systematic Reviews, 2015*(5), CD010090.
46. Gonzalez-Garcia, M., Ferrer, M. J., Borras, X., Muoz-Moreno, J. A., Miranda, C., Puig, J., ... & Fumaz, C. R. (2014). Effectiveness of mindfulness-based cognitive therapy on the quality of life, emotional status, and CD4 cell count of patients aging with HIV infection. *AIDS Behavior, 18*, 676–685.
47. Lapointe, J., James, D., & Craik, J. (2013). Occupational therapy services for people living with HIV: A case of service delivery in a primary health care setting. *Occupational Therapy Now, 15.5.*, 22–24.

48. Beagan, B. L., Chiasson, A., Fiske, C. A., Forseth, S. D., Hosein, A. C., Myers, M. R., & Stang, J. E. (2013). Working with transgender clients: Learning from physicians and nurses to improve occupational therapy practice. *Canadian Journal of Occupational Therapy, 80*(2), 82–91.
49. King, E., De Silva, M., Stein, A., & Patel, V. (2009). Interventions for improving the psycho-social well-being of children affected by HIV and AIDS. *Cochrane Database of Systematic Reviews, 2009,* (2), CD006733.
50. Rosenfeld, D., Ridge, D., & Von Lob, G. (2014). Vital scientific puzzle or lived uncertainty? Professional and lived approaches to the uncertainties of ageing with HIV. *Health Sociology Review, 23*(1), 20–32.
51. Pizzi, M., & Teaford, G. (2013). HIV infection and AIDS. In H. M. Pendleton & W. Schultz-Krohn (Eds.), *Pedretti's occupational therapy practice skills for physical dysfunction* (7th ed.) (pp. 1246-1266). St. Louis, MO: Elsevier Mosby.
52. American Occupational Therapy Association. (2014). Guidelines for supervision, roles, and responsibilities during the delivery of occupational therapy service. *American Journal of Occupational Therapy, 68*(Suppl. 3), S16–S22.
53. Bellani, M., Furlani, F., Gnecchi, M., Pezzotta, P., Trotti, E., & Bellotti, G. (1996). Burnout and related factors among HIV/AIDS healthcare workers. *AIDS Care, 8*(2), 207–221.
54. Morrison, M. F., Petitto, J. M., Have, T. T., Gettes, D. R., Ciappini, M. S., Weber, A. L., ... & Evans, D. L. (2002). Depressive and anxiety disorders in women with HIV infection. *American Journal of Psychiatry, 159,* 789–796.
55. McGrath, M., & Lynch, E. (2014). Occupational therapists' perspectives on addressing sexual concerns of older adults in the context of rehabilitation. *Disability and Rehabilitation, 36*(8), 651–657.
56. McGrath, M., & Sakellariou, D. (2016). Why has there been so little progress made in the practice of occupational therapy in relation to sexuality? *American Journal of Occupational Therapy, 70,* 7001360010.

Motor Unit and Myopathic Diseases: Considerations and Treatment

Amber L. Ward, MS, OTR/L, BCPR, ATP/SMS

LEARNING OUTCOMES

After studying this chapter, the student or practitioner will be able to:

31.1 Describe the differences between various diseases described in the chapter

31.2 Explain Guillain-Barré syndrome and how it differs from the other diseases in the chapter

31.3 Discuss occupational therapy treatments for motor unit and myopathic diseases

31.4 Describe how exercise plays a role with each disease

KEY TERMS

Chronic inflammatory demyelinating polyneuropathy (CIDP)
Electromyography (EMG)
Guillain-Barré syndrome (GBS)
Motor neuron
Muscular dystrophy
Myasthenia gravis (MG)
Myelin
Myotonia
Neuromuscular junction
Plasmapheresis
Post-polio syndrome

All of the diseases of the motor unit that will be covered in this chapter are or can be progressive in nature, with the vast majority having no medical treatment besides symptomatic and therapeutic care. Because of this, the occupational therapy (OT) practitioner is extremely important in the care and maintenance of function for these clients. This chapter will focus on diseases including Guillain-Barré syndrome, post-polio syndrome, myasthenia gravis, and poliomyelitis, various muscular dystrophies, including limb girdle, facioscapulohumeral, Duchenne, Becker, and myotonic, and diseases such as Charcot-Marie-Tooth and spinal muscular atrophy. The commonality of all these diseases is a disruption in the motor unit. The motor unit consists of a **motor neuron** (a cell body located in the spinal cord) and all the muscle fibers it innervates (Fig. 31-1). Each disease disrupts the motor unit in a different way, which will be described as well as how the occupational therapy assistant (OTA) might manage and assist a client with the disorder. Due to similarities in management, the OT treatments will be combined into one section after the all diseases are described. The only exception is Guillain-Barré syndrome, which is treated by the OT practitioner in a somewhat different way and will have its own section.

GUILLAIN-BARRÉ SYNDROME

Guillain-Barré syndrome (GBS) is different from other diseases of the motor unit because it presents as significantly and quickly progressive, leaving the client in a dependent state over the course of a few days to weeks, followed by a slow, steady, and long recovery. Guillain-Barré syndrome is not a slowly progressive disorder over a lifetime, but rather an acute and life-threatening event that causes severe muscle weakness, including the muscles of speech, swallowing, and respiration. GBS can affect anyone at any age, although it usually occurs after a viral infection of the respiratory or gastrointestinal (GI) systems. Occasionally it can be seen after an immunization or surgery. The syndrome is rare,

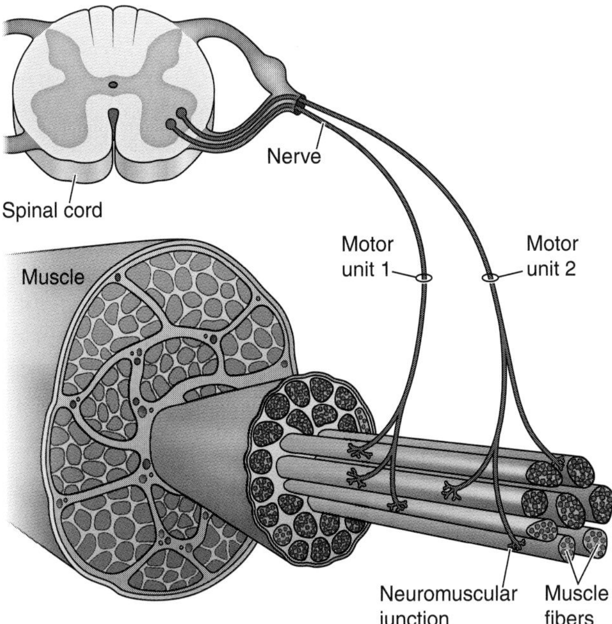

FIGURE 31-1. Motor unit and muscle fibers.

however, afflicting only about 1 person in 100,000.[1] Most clients will reach the stage of greatest weakness within the first 2 weeks after symptoms appear, and by the third week of the illness 90% of all clients are at their weakest.[1]

GBS has six known subtypes, which the OTA may see in a client chart, specifically:[2]

1. Acute inflammatory demyelinating polyneuropathy (AIDP): The most common form of GBS, and the term that is often used synonymously with GBS.
2. Miller Fisher syndrome (MFS): A rare variant of GBS that usually affects the eye muscles first.
3. Acute motor axonal neuropathy (AMAN): Prevalent in China and Mexico. The disease may be seasonal, and recovery can be rapid.
4. Acute motor sensory axonal neuropathy (AMSAN): Similar to AMAN, but also affects sensory nerves with severe damage to the axons. Recovery is slow and often incomplete.
5. Acute panautonomic neuropathy: The rarest variant of GBS, sometimes accompanied by encephalopathy (brain disease/damage causing changes in brain functioning). It is associated with a high mortality rate, owing to cardiovascular involvement.
6. Bickerstaff's brainstem encephalitis (BBE): Characterized by acute onset of ophthalmoplegia (paralysis of eye muscles), ataxia, disturbance of consciousness, and hyperreflexia. The course of the disease can be seen only one time or be remitting-relapsing. BBE, despite its severe initial presentation, usually has a good prognosis.

With GBS, the body's immune system begins to attack itself, specifically at the myelin sheath surrounding the axons (nerve fibers which conduct the impulses) of peripheral nerves. **Myelin** acts as an insulator, and allows the nerve information to pass effectively over long distances via the axon. Without myelin, the axons do not pass information effectively from the nerve cell to the muscles. In diseases in which the peripheral nerves' myelin sheaths are injured or degraded, the nerves cannot transmit signals efficiently.[1] That is why the muscles begin to lose their ability to respond to the brain's commands. Because the signals to and from the arms and legs must travel the longest distances, they are most vulnerable to interruption with GBS. Therefore, numbness, muscle weakness, and tingling sensations usually first appear in the hands and feet and progress proximally.[1] Clients with GBS quickly become weak in all muscle groups, many to the point of complete immobility, may become completely unable to swallow and require supplemental nutrition via an intravenous (IV) line or nasogastric tube, and may require full respiratory support up to and including tracheostomy with a ventilator. Many clients with GBS have pain, either from the inflammation of the nerves or immobility and stiffness from not moving. A full symptom list includes:[3]

- Prickling, "pins and needles" sensations in fingers, toes, ankles, or wrists
- Weakness in the legs that spreads to the upper body, and may result in total paralysis
- Unsteady walking or inability to walk or climb stairs
- Difficulty with eye or facial movements, including speaking, chewing, or swallowing
- Severe pain that may feel achy or cramplike and may be worse at night
- Difficulty with bladder control or bowel function
- Rapid heart rate
- Low or high blood pressure
- Difficulty breathing

To confirm a diagnosis of GBS, two tests may be performed: a lumbar puncture to determine elevated fluid protein levels, and/or an **electromyography (EMG),** which is an electrical test of nerve and muscle function (Fig. 31-2).[1] These tests, along with symptoms, will lead to a definitive diagnosis.

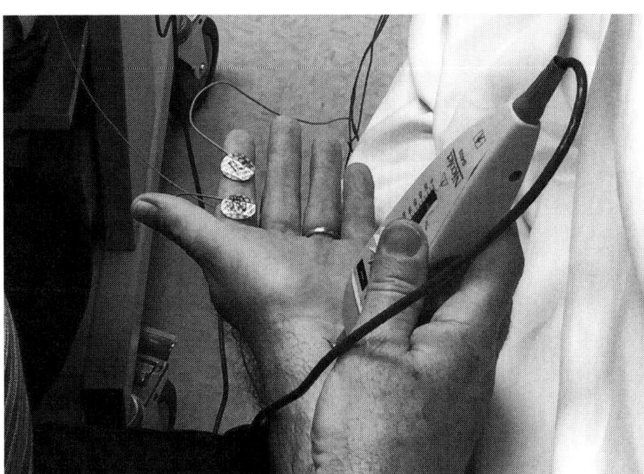

FIGURE 31-2. EMG test being performed.

Presentation, Progression, and Life Expectancy

Some clients with GBS will become only slightly weak (difficulty standing, bilateral foot drop, or bilateral hand weakness), yet others will lose all voluntary muscle function, including that of the respiratory system, and require mechanical ventilation. About one-third of those affected can maintain the ability to ambulate, and are considered mild.[4] Generally, both sides of the body are equally weak, and normal reflexes are diminished. If clients seek medical attention when they first have symptoms of severe and rapid muscle weakness, they generally do not die of Guillain-Barré syndrome. Fatalities are generally from complications of respiratory symptoms such as pneumonia. The rehabilitation process can be a long one as clients regain muscle strength and control. Depending on how weak a client became during the acute stage of illness will determine the length of his or her recovery process; the average is 3 to 6 months.[5] Two-thirds of those who have GBS will recover completely, but some will have lingering weakness or pain.[5] Secondary complications from being in the hospital bed for weeks can also be an issue for clients with GBS, and may include contractures, atrophy, pressure injuries, and pain. The pain can include backache, paresthesias (abnormal sensations such as "pins and needles"), and muscular pain, and for some clients, the pain actually comes before the other symptoms. Sensory disturbances and fatigue can last for years.[4] About 5% to 10% of clients have one or more relapses during the recovery period, in which case they are then classified as having **chronic inflammatory demyelinating polyneuropathy (CIDP).**[2] CIDP is closely related to GBS in symptoms, and is often considered the chronic counterpart of acute GBS. Some clients with CIDP have relapses followed by spontaneous recovery, yet others may have many "attacks" with partial recovery in between relapses.[6]

Research, Medical Treatment, and Exercise

GBS has no known cure, however, medical therapies that lessen the severity of the illness and accelerate the recovery in most clients exist. Currently, plasma exchange, also called **plasmapheresis,** and high-dose immunoglobulin therapy are used. Both are equally effective, but immunoglobulin is easier to administer. Plasmapheresis is a method by which whole blood is removed from the body and processed so that the red and white blood cells are separated from the plasma, or liquid portion of the blood. The blood cells are then returned to the client via an IV line without the plasma, which the body quickly replaces. Although scientists are still studying why this plasma exchange is effective in some clients, the technique seems to reduce the severity and duration of the Guillain-Barré episode. The success may be because plasmapheresis can remove antibodies and other immune factors that could contribute to nerve damage. In high-dose immunoglobulin therapy, doctors administer intravenous injections of the proteins that, in small quantities, the immune system uses naturally to attack invading organisms. Researchers have found that giving high doses of these immunoglobulins to clients with GBS can lessen the immune attack on the nervous system.[4] Researchers do not know why or how this works, although hypotheses have been proposed such as activation of immune cells. The use of steroid hormones has also been tried as a way to reduce the severity of GBS, but controlled clinical trials have demonstrated that this treatment not only is ineffective but may even have a negative effect on the disease.[1]

Exercise is very important for recovery as the client may be significantly weak after the disease process, and at times cannot move a muscle after the initial wave of the illness. Strengthening will be an important part of the client's routine for 6 months to 1 year and beyond, as the client regains muscle control and endurance. Clients can have periods of extreme fatigue if they push too hard, so all exercise should be under the direction of a physician and OT practitioner, be submaximal, and carefully monitored to start. Submaximal exercise is less than maximal exertion, in the case of progressive diseases; the level of effort may need to change at each session to avoid pain and over-exertion. For some, even completing basic ADLs is an extreme workout in the beginning.

MYASTHENIA GRAVIS

Myasthenia gravis (MG) is an autoimmune disease that occurs when the immune system attacks the body's own tissues. In MG, that attack interrupts the connection between nerve and muscle, which is called the **neuromuscular junction.**[7] During normal muscle function, when impulses travel down the nerve, the nerve endings release the neurotransmitter acetylcholine. Acetylcholine travels from the neuromuscular junction and binds to acetylcholine receptors that are activated and generate a muscle contraction. In myasthenia gravis, antibodies block, alter, or destroy the receptors for acetylcholine at the neuromuscular junction, which prevents the muscle contraction from occurring. These antibodies are produced by the body's own immune system.[8]

Myasthenia gravis is a progressive disorder, which if caught early and treated, can reverse or remain stable, and if not treated, will continue to progress. The cause of MG is unclear. Researchers suspect viruses or bacteria might trigger the autoimmune response; the thymus gland also sometimes seems to play a role in the disease. Although MG is not hereditary, genetic susceptibility appears to play a role.[7]

A diagnosis of MG can be confirmed in several ways, including:

- Blood test for specific antibodies
- Office test: Edrophonium test or Tensilon test (a drug that when given to persons with MG can make them stronger) is an examination performed by specialists to evaluate an improvement in strength that may be consistent with MG.
- EMG studies can provide support for the diagnosis of MG when certain characteristic patterns are present.[9]

Presentation, Progression, and Life Expectancy

Although MG may affect any voluntary muscle, muscles that control eye and eyelid movement, facial expression, and swallowing are most frequently affected. The arms, legs, trunk, neck, vocal cords, and diaphragm can be affected as well. The onset of the disorder may be sudden or slow, and symptoms often are not immediately recognized as MG. The degree of muscle weakness involved in MG varies greatly, ranging from a type limited to eye muscles (ocular myasthenia), to a severe or generalized form in which many muscles, at times including those that control breathing, are affected.[8]

The hallmark symptom of MG is muscle weakness that gets worse with exertion or sustained activity and improves with rest.[7] This may mean that symptoms are worse later in the day; that is, if speaking is affected, it will be worse with prolonged talking, or if arms are affected, the weakness will be worse after reaching and holding tasks. MG affects women more often than men and tends to begin at younger ages. The average age of onset in women is 28; the average age of onset in men is 42.[8] Most people with MG have a normal life expectancy and with consistent symptom management can live a relatively disability-free life.[8] It is important for the treatment team to educate the client on factors that can increase exacerbations (and are potentially under client control), and for the OTA to assist with management of these factors during occupational performance; they include:[10]

- Fatigue, insufficient sleep
- Stress, anxiety
- Illness
- Overexertion, repetitive motion
- Pain
- Sudden fear or extreme anger
- Depression
- Extreme temperatures (hot or cold weather, hot showers or baths, sunbathing, saunas, hot tubs)
- Humidity
- Sunlight or bright lights (affects eyes)
- Hot foods or beverages (affects mouth and throat)
- Some medications, including beta blockers, calcium channel blockers, and some antibiotics
- Alcoholic beverages
- Quinine or tonic water
- Low potassium levels or low thyroid hormone levels
- Some chemicals, including some household cleaners, insecticides, and pet flea sprays
- Exposure to chemical lawn treatments

Research, Medical Treatment, and Exercise

MG is treatable with drugs that suppress the immune system or boost the signals between nerve and muscle.[7] Generally, clients will be given an anticholinesterase medication (to increase the amount of acetylcholine in the blood, which can increase strength) or an immunosuppressant medication to avoid the production of harmful antibodies.[10] Certainly, any immunosuppression can lead to a higher risk for infections. A thymectomy to remove the thymus gland may be helpful in many cases. The relationship between the thymus gland and myasthenia gravis is not yet fully understood. The prevailing theory is that "the thymus gland may give incorrect instructions to developing immune cells, ultimately resulting in autoimmunity and the production of the acetylcholine receptor antibodies, thereby setting the stage for the attack on neuromuscular transmission."[8] Another medical therapy used to treat myasthenia gravis is plasmapheresis (removing blood plasma). This therapy may be used to help individuals during especially difficult periods of weakness.[8] Most people with MG are able to manage their symptoms and lead active lives, whereas a few experience remission lasting many years.[7]

Clients with MG can exercise when symptoms are well-controlled as long as they do not overexert themselves and avoid extremes in temperature. When having an exacerbation or weakness, the normal daily routine with energy conserving strategies will generally be enough exercise.

POST-POLIO SYNDROME/ POLIOMYELITIS

Polio, or poliomyelitis, is a potentially deadly infectious disease caused by the poliovirus that generally attacks children younger than 5 years of age. The virus spreads from person to person and can invade an infected person's brain and spinal cord, causing paralysis. In 1988, a global polio eradication initiative (GPEI) was developed and launched by numerous worldwide organizations and has decreased the number of polio cases by 99%.[11] Endemic (stable/prevalent over long periods) transmission is continuing in Afghanistan, Nigeria, and Pakistan. Failure to stop polio in these last remaining areas could result in as many as 200,000 new cases every year, within 10 years, all over the world.[11] In the United States, polio was rampant in the 1940s and 1950s, with over 35,000 people affected each year.[12] In 1955 the polio vaccine was offered, and by 1979 it was eradicated in the United States. Currently 10 to 20 million people worldwide are living with the aftereffects of polio.

People who seemed to fully recover from the initial onset of polio can develop new muscle pain, weakness, or paralysis 15 to 40 years later, which is called **post-polio syndrome** or **PPS**.[13] Most often, polio survivors start to experience gradual new weakening in muscles that were previously affected by the polio infection. Some individuals experience only minor symptoms, yet others develop visible muscle weakness and atrophy. The symptoms of PPS are:

- New onset of weakness in previously involved muscles and at times, originally uninvolved muscles
- Muscle pain
- Becoming easily exhausted or fatigued
- Muscle wasting and muscle atrophy
- Trouble breathing and/or swallowing
- Sleep-related breathing problems
- Susceptibility to cold temperatures[14]

PPS is rarely life-threatening, but the symptoms can significantly interfere with an individual's ability to function independently. Respiratory muscle weakness, for instance, can result in trouble with proper breathing, affecting daytime functions and sleep. Weakness in swallowing muscles can result in aspiration of food and liquids into the lungs and lead to pneumonia.[15] Many people with polio who recovered once from the disease and have been used to a certain level of functioning with the residual deficits from when they were children, now must deal with the disease all over again. For these clients, the new changes can be difficult to accept, and the OTA will have a valuable role in maintaining levels of independence with occupations.

The cause of PPS is unknown, but current theories range from the fatigue of overworked nerve cells, to possible brain damage from a viral infection, to a combination of mechanisms. The new onset of muscle weakness from PPS appears to be related to the "degeneration of individual nerve terminals in the motor units" which occurred during the original polio episode.[15] In an effort to compensate for the loss of these motor neurons, surviving cells sprouted new nerve-end terminals and connected with other muscle fibers. Years of high use of these recovered but overly extended motor units adds stress to the motor neurons, which over time lose the ability to maintain the increased work demands. This results in the slow deterioration of the neurons, which leads to loss of muscle strength. This hypothesis explains why PPS occurs after a delay following the initial polio episode and has a slow and progressive course.[15]

Presentation, Progression, and Life Expectancy

The weakness caused by PPS is slowly progressive, but continuous. A small change in muscle control may lead to a large functional change (e.g., a small amount of hip extensors affected may cause the client to be unable to move from sitting to standing), and clients with PPS will require OT to address those changes. Life expectancy is rarely affected by PPS, although weakness in respiratory or swallowing muscles will lead to increased risk for aspiration pneumonia or breathing difficulties.

Research, Medical Treatment, and Exercise

Currently no effective pharmaceutical treatments exist that can stop deterioration or reverse the deficits caused by the syndrome itself. However, a number of controlled studies have demonstrated that nonfatiguing exercises may improve muscle strength and reduce overall feelings of fatigue.[15] Most of the clinical trials in PPS have focused on finding safe therapies that could reduce symptoms and improve quality of life.[15]

Exercise is safe and effective when carefully prescribed and monitored by the OTA or other therapy staff. Exercise is more likely to benefit those muscle groups that were least affected by polio. Cardiopulmonary endurance training such as swimming or biking is usually more effective than strengthening exercises, especially when activities are paced to allow for frequent breaks and strategies are used to conserve energy. Heavy or intense resistive exercise and weight-lifting using polio-affected muscles is contraindicated, as this can further weaken rather than strengthen these muscles.[15] Exercise should be reduced or discontinued if it causes additional weakness, excessive fatigue, or unduly prolonged recovery time. As a general rule, no muscle should be exercised to the point of causing ache, fatigue, or weakness.[15]

BECKER AND DUCHENNE MUSCULAR DYSTROPHIES

Becker and Duchenne muscular dystrophies are basically different mutations of the same gene with a significant difference in severity of presentation. **Muscular dystrophies** in general are a group of genetic disorders causing muscle weakness via degeneration of voluntary muscles. Becker and Duchenne both affect boys only, although women can be carriers of the abnormal gene, and some of these women are affected and may show symptoms. The gene which is defective in these two particular muscular dystrophies provides instructions for making a protein called dystrophin.[16] This protein is located primarily in skeletal muscles and in cardiac muscle, where it is part of a group of proteins that work together to strengthen muscle fibers and protect them from injury as muscles contract and relax.[16] Becker muscular dystrophy (BMD) is caused by mutations that lead to an abnormal version of dystrophin that retains some function. Mutations that cause the more severe Duchenne muscular dystrophy (DMD) typically prevent any functional dystrophin from being produced.[16] Skeletal and cardiac muscle cells without enough functional dystrophin become damaged as the muscles repeatedly contract and relax with use. The damaged cells weaken and die over time, causing the characteristic muscle weakness and heart problems seen in DMD and BMD.[16]

Both disorders cause difficulties with voluntary motor control at the muscle level, although men with BMD often walk into their 30s, and boys with DMD stop walking at around 8 to 10 years of age. The first signs of BMD may be trouble walking fast, running, or climbing stairs. Boys with DMD may be late walkers, and as toddlers have more difficulty getting off the floor, running, and climbing stairs. Diagnosis is made with genetic testing, EMG, symptoms, and biopsy.[16]

Presentation, Progression, and Life Expectancy

Table 31-1 shows the differences in presentation of DMD and BMD.

For both diseases, the effect is on bilateral voluntary muscles, with more proximal weakness than distal, which is progressive. By adulthood, clients with DMD are totally dependent on caregivers for most activities of daily living (ADLs), although the majority can retain control over their power wheelchair, phone, and computer with adaptations.

TABLE 31-1 Presentation of Duchenne and Becker Muscular Dystrophies

AVERAGE	DUCHENNE	BECKER
Age of diagnosis/onset	2-5	Teens
Age of stopping ambulation	9-12	20s to 30s
Age of life expectancy	20s to 40s	40s to 60s
Progression	Faster	Slower, more varied

Generally, in adulthood, many men with DMD can still control their power wheelchair with a smaller joystick or control a mouse for a computer, but are severely limited in most other functionality. In contrast, in adulthood, many men with BMD are still ambulating, working, and performing all daily care tasks without assistance. Many men with DMD and BMD can have cardiac issues, which can be a cause of death along with respiratory weakness. By early adulthood to the mid-20s, most clients with DMD are using BiPAP or volume ventilation with a mask or have a tracheostomy with a ventilator.

Many men with DMD battle spinal scoliosis from proximal weakness, and generally spinal rod surgery in their teenage years is recommended to manage their positioning and medical needs. Once in a wheelchair full time, the risk for scoliosis increases to ultimately affecting 77% of young men.[17] The surgical procedure to manage scoliosis generally involves the insertion of rods and screws along the spine for support, along with a bone graft at times to stabilize the spine as well. Those clients who decline rod surgery often face positioning challenges in adulthood as the scoliosis becomes significant, with increased respiratory and gastrointestinal issues from abnormal sitting postures (Fig. 31-3).

Adults with DMD often have symptoms of pain, anxiety, fatigue, and depression, which can significantly influence health-related quality of life[18] The OTA can certainly address pain management with wheelchair seating, positioning and pressure relief in the bed, chair and bathing systems, passive range of motion (PROM), and contracture management. Anxiety can be caused by shortness of breath that the respiratory therapist and pulmonologist will manage, or medications may help decrease anxiety. The OTA can work with clients on options to increase function with adaptive equipment and techniques, technology use and integration, and to increase involvement in family and community events, which may decrease depression and increase quality of life.

Adults with DMD typically want to be more independent, but may feel frustrated because they require more care and assistance from others, such as their parents. As muscle weakness progresses, clients with DMD are at risk for becoming more isolated or socially withdrawn.[19] Some clients with DMD may have learning disabilities and present with behavioral challenges that can make attending college or sustaining employment difficult. College used to be just a dream for young men with DMD as the life expectancy was generally in the late teens and 20s. Now, unless there are cardiac issues, many young men with DMD are living into their 30s and 40s with ventilators, going to college, having careers, and getting married. They still require total support, however, and must have family or caregiver support 24/7.

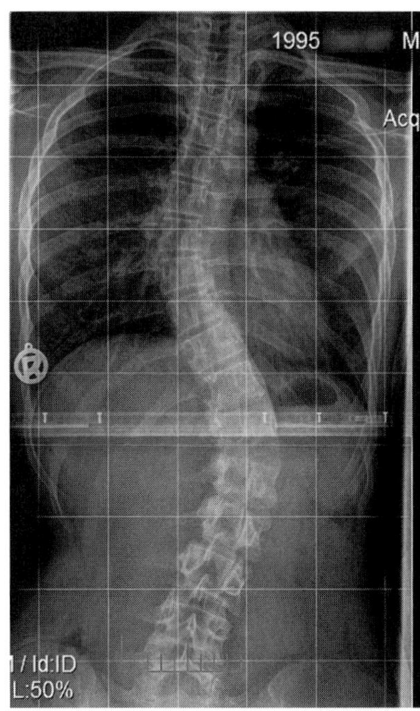

FIGURE 31-3. Client with DMD with scoliosis and without rods.

Adults with DMD typically are nearly dependent for all ADL and instrumental activities of daily living (IADL) tasks, and rely on technology and caregivers for assistance. Through the use of technology, the client may control many aspects of their environment through their computer and smartphone. With BMD, clients generally have difficulty with safe bathing, toileting, dressing, and other self-care tasks by their 20s and 30s as it gets harder to move from sit to stand or to ambulate. Equipment management and adaptation for self-care challenges are paramount for these men to maintain independence.

Research, Medical Treatment, and Exercise

Medical treatment for BMD and DMD used to be more symptom management than treating the disease, but there are many new research studies underway that hold some promise for disease modification. Corticosteroids have been found to slow the course of the disease in DMD, but not in BMD. A new corticosteroid called Emflaza™ (deflazacort) was released in 2017 for treatment of those with DMD ages five and up. It contains a glucocorticoid with anti-inflammatory and immunosuppressant properties. The drug reduces the rate and overall loss of muscular strength and function, and ensures longer term cardiac and respiratory function. It also has been shown to reduce the incidence of scoliosis and/or age of onset.[20] Some preliminary evidence indicates that treatment with angiotensin-converting enzyme (ACE) inhibitors and beta blockers can slow the course of cardiac muscle deterioration in DMD and BMD if the medications are started as soon as abnormalities on an echocardiogram (ultrasound imaging of the heart) appear, but before symptoms occur.[21] In late 2016, the Food and Drug Administration (FDA) granted accelerated approval of a drug called Exondys 51™ (eteplirsen) given via IV line, that can slow progression of DMD in one genetic variant that affects about 13% of cases.[21] Overall health management goals for men with DMD may include:

- Preservation of strength
- Minimization of obesity and osteoporosis (side effects of steroids)
- Treatment of cardiomyopathy
- Prevention of contractures
- Adaptation for functional deficits
- Preservation of respiratory function
- Avoidance and treatment of scoliosis[17]

Exercise is a debated treatment for DMD and BMD, but the most up-to-date literature shows that exercise can be helpful within certain parameters.[21–25] Flexibility and stretching must be a part of the daily routine for anyone with DMD/BMD to maintain range of motion (ROM), decrease pain, and maintain as much functional movement as possible. Cycling, walking on flat ground, and swimming are all good activities for exercise with BMD. High-resistance strength training is not recommended, however submaximal aerobic exercise can be appropriate.[22] For clients with BMD, exercise can help build skeletal muscle, keep the cardiovascular system healthy, and contribute to feeling better.[23] Two recent studies show that a combination of strength and aerobic training has the potential to safely improve functional ability in clients with BMD.[24,25] Boys and men with DMD tend to become obese both from being sedentary as well as from steroid use, so staying active as possible and carefully monitoring nutrition is important throughout the progression.

CHARCOT-MARIE-TOOTH DISEASE

Charcot-Marie-Tooth disease (CMT) is caused by defects in the genes for proteins that affect axons or in the genes for proteins that affect myelin.[26] In both cases, the damaged nerve fibers result in peripheral neuropathy. The nerve fibers in the legs and arms, which are the longest, are affected first, and motor and sensory fibers are both affected. CMT causes weakness, numbness in the extremities, and often pain, usually starting in the feet. More than 30 genes have been implicated in CMT, each one linked to a specific type (and in many cases, more than one type) of the disease.[26]

OT Practitioner's Viewpoint

Sexual activity, sexuality, and intimacy are often uncomfortable topics to discuss, but important, and all do come up in the career of the average OTA. Recently, I found out about a young man with Duchenne muscular dystrophy in his 20s who had asked a young woman with significant disabilities to marry him. This gentleman is completely dependent for all care, drives a power wheelchair, uses a BiPAP for breathing, and relies on his mother for all care. His bride-to-be is completely dependent as well, also uses a power wheelchair, and relies on her father for all care. After the wedding, they will all move in together and the couple will begin their married life. All intimacy between groom and bride will be initiated by the couple, but will have to be facilitated by their caregivers, including holding hands, kissing, and lying together in bed. What a strong and amazing set of people to make love work, and allow these two people to be together in all aspects of their married life. How easy it would have been for the caregivers to create barriers that would have prevented this marriage from working out for the couple. - Amber L. Ward, MS, OTR/L, BCPR, ATP/SMS

Presentation, Progression, and Life Expectancy

In the most common kinds of CMT, symptoms usually begin before 20 years of age. These symptoms may include:

- Foot contractures/deformities with very high arched feet, hand contractures/deformities with metacarpophalangeal (MCP) hyperextension, distal interphalangeal (DIP)/proximal interphalangeal (PIP) flexion (claw position) (Fig. 31-4).
- Loss of muscle in the legs and arms (distal first)
- Foot drop with the need for orthoses
- Numbness in the feet/hands
- Pain from overuse and from the disease process
- Difficulty with balance[27]

A diagnosis of CMT is established through a thorough neurological evaluation by an expert in neuropathy, including a complete family history, physical examination, nerve conduction tests, and appropriate genetic testing. Genetic testing can provide the exact cause for most people who have CMT.[27] CMT affects about 2.8 million people of all races and ethnic groups worldwide.[28] Some individuals have a more severe form with faster progression and are in a wheelchair by 20 years of age, yet others continue with more distal weakness for many years with a slower progression. CMT is generally not life threatening, although it can cause significant disability.

Research, Medical Treatment, and Exercise

Research through the Muscular Dystrophy Association (MDA) and other organizations is ongoing in the areas of genes, proteins, and molecular markers that may play a

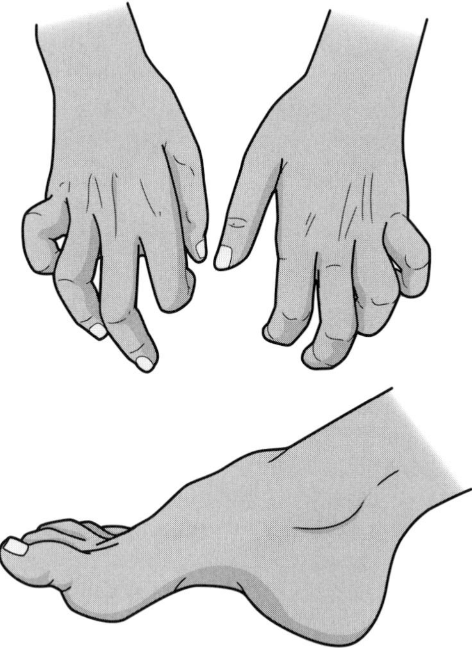

FIGURE 31-4. High arches and claw hands in CMT disease.

role in CMT. Although no drugs are currently available to help slow the progression of CMT, symptom management can be helpful for pain and cramping. Generally, muscles affected by the disease cannot strengthen, however, aerobic exercise and gentle core strengthening are possible. Clients may have weakness from deconditioning as well as the disease process. Exercise for CMT revolves around four modalities: balance, stretching, endurance, and strength.[29] Endurance activities can be aerobic activity in the pool, recumbent bike riding, or a mini-cycle to use with the arms or legs while sitting in a wheelchair. Strengthening should be gentle, and submaximal exercise is required to avoid further pain and to prevent overuse.

MYOTONIC DYSTROPHIES

Myotonic muscular dystrophy (MMD) is a disorder that affects muscle strength as well as some organ function and causes **myotonia** (the inability to relax a muscle at will). The two major types of myotonic muscular dystrophy, MMD1 and MMD2, are both caused by genetic defects, and can be passed on to male and female children equally. MMD1 may either begin at birth or in childhood (early onset) or in adolescence/early adulthood (adult-onset). It is characterized by slow progressive weakness, cardiac abnormalities, and, sometimes, mild to moderate cognitive difficulties. MMD1 tends to affect the distal muscles (hands/feet) first. MMD2 has an onset from 8 to 60 years of age, and tends to involve the proximal muscles (shoulders and hips), rather than the distal muscles. In general, MMD2 is not as severe as MMD1. However, it may affect walking ability earlier than MMD1, because it causes early weakening of the hip muscles.[30] See Table 31-2 for differences between the two types.

MMD1 diagnosis can often be tentatively made from the symptoms, and characteristic facial features (facial weakness, drooping eyelids) and male pattern balding (seen as significant hair thinning in women). MMD2 is more difficult to diagnose and usually requires an EMG, along with a DNA blood test, which will be definitive.[33]

TABLE 31-2 Comparison of MMD1 and MMD2[31,32]

FEATURE	MMD1	MMD2
Age of onset	Birth to adulthood	8–60 years
Facial weakness	Prominent	Mild
Drooping eyelids	Prominent	Mild
Neck muscle weakness	Common, early	Common, early
Hip and thigh weakness	Late	Early
Distal muscle weakness	Prominent	Mostly hands
Weakness anywhere	Can occur	Can occur
Muscle pain	Can occur	Often occurs
Myotonia	Occurs	Occurs
Enlargement of calf muscles	Does not occur	Occurs
Early cataracts (of the eyes)	Occurs	Occurs
Early balding in males	Common	Common
Cardiac rhythm abnormalities	Common	Variable
Cardiac muscle degeneration	Can occur, especially late in disease course	Not common
Excessive daytime sleepiness	Common	Variable
Cognitive impairment	Occurs often; can be mild to severe	Can occur; generally mild
Respiratory abnormalities	Common, particularly sleep-disordered breathing and inadequate breathing	Not common
Gastrointestinal disturbances	Difficulty swallowing, constipation, diarrhea, gallstones can occur	Not common
High blood sugar because of insulin resistance	Can occur	Can occur

Presentation, Progression, and Life Expectancy

Symptoms of both types of MMD beyond weakness can include overall apathy, diabetes, daytime sleepiness, and executive function problems; a spectrum that involves drive, motivation, focusing, planning, and the ability to suppress short-term gains for long-term goals.[32] Cognitive impairment can occur at the severe end of the MMD1 spectrum. In MMD1, there may be difficulties with vision/cataracts, weakness of the mouth and tongue muscles, which make speech hard to understand, and weakness of the facial muscles, which limits facial expression.

MMD2 tends to be less severe than MMD1 and has less impact on life expectancy. MMD1 is much more variable, and the prognosis for an affected individual is difficult to predict. Some clients may experience only mild stiffness or cataracts in later life. In the most severe cases of MMD1, respiratory and cardiac complications can be life threatening even at an early age. In general, the younger an individual is when symptoms first appear, the more severe symptoms are likely to be. However, prognosis for both types is as variable as the symptoms of the disease.[32]

Research, Medical Treatment, and Exercise

The major focus in MMD research has been done using animal and cellular models with MMD1. However, many experts believe the findings from the MMD1 experiments will have implications for MMD2 as well. In both conditions, the underlying defect is an expansion of DNA (an increase in repeats of a DNA sequence from one generation to the next). In MMD1, the expansion occurs in the chemical sequence in a gene on chromosome 19. In MMD2, the expansion occurs in the chemical sequence in a gene on chromosome 3.[34]

Treatment is aimed at managing symptoms and minimizing disability. Drugs are available to manage most of the symptoms, such as daytime sleepiness, myotonia, and insulin resistance. Cataract surgery may be required in middle age.

Exercise, including ROM, strengthening, and aerobic, is important for the management of MMD. This helps to maintain strength in the muscles and also keep the cardiovascular system healthy. ROM exercises are important in maintaining joint function and may play a role in reducing pain that is caused by muscular imbalance or tightness. Because clients with myotonic dystrophy often have heart problems, any exercise program should be undertaken under the guidance of a cardiologist.[33] Studies have shown neither positive benefit nor negative effects from exercise with this population as far as disease modification, however, deconditioning can play a role with dysfunction.[35,36]

LIMB-GIRDLE MUSCULAR DYSTROPHY

Limb-girdle muscular dystrophy (LGMD) is a term for a group of over 20 subtypes that are caused by mutations of the genes for various proteins, which have specific functions in relation to the muscle. The voluntary muscles most affected are those most proximal, specifically the muscles of the shoulders/shoulder girdles, upper arms, pelvis/hip girdle, and thighs.[37] The severity, age of onset, and features of LGMD vary among the many subtypes of this condition and may be inconsistent even within the same family.[37] Signs and symptoms may first appear at any age and generally worsen slowly with time. In the early stages of LGMD, affected individuals may have an unusual walking gait, such as waddling or walking on the balls of their feet, and may also have difficulty running. As the condition progresses, people with LGMD may require further mobility assistance from a walker or wheelchair.

Muscle wasting may cause changes in posture or in the appearance of the shoulder, back, and arm. Weak shoulder muscles tend to make the scapulae protrude from the back, a sign known as scapular winging (Fig. 31-5). Affected individuals may also have lordosis (excessive lumbar curve) or scoliosis (Fig. 31-6). Some develop joint contractures that can restrict movement in their hips, knees, ankles, or elbows. These deformities can result in pain and functional impairment, interfering with ambulation, ADLs, and quality of life.[38]

Cardiomyopathy, a weakening of the heart muscle, occurs in some forms of LGMD. Some affected individuals experience mild to severe breathing problems related to the weakness of the diaphragm.[39] Diagnosis is made with blood tests, EMG, DNA testing, and at times muscle biopsy.

Presentation, Progression, and Life Expectancy

Some forms of the disorder progress to loss of walking ability within a few years and cause serious disability, yet others progress very slowly over many years and cause minimal disability. LGMD can begin in childhood, adolescence, young adulthood, or even later. Both genders are affected equally. When LGMD begins in childhood, some physicians say the progression is usually faster and the disease more disabling. When the disorder begins in adolescence or

COMMUNICATION

Because many of the diagnoses covered in this chapter are also covered by the MDA, it is important for the OTA to have good communication with this resource. The MDA provides a newsletter, webinars, ongoing research, and a website (www.MDA.org), as well as many clinics that offer loaner equipment options. Because many MDA clinics have a loaner closet, this may be tapped by savvy OTAs for their clients, as long as the client is registered with the MDA. Some loaner closets even have power wheelchairs, recliner lift chairs, or rolling shower commode chairs for those with limited financial resources. The MDA staff can provide advocacy support for college, work, or community needs as well as education and in-services for practitioners, teachers, and groups.

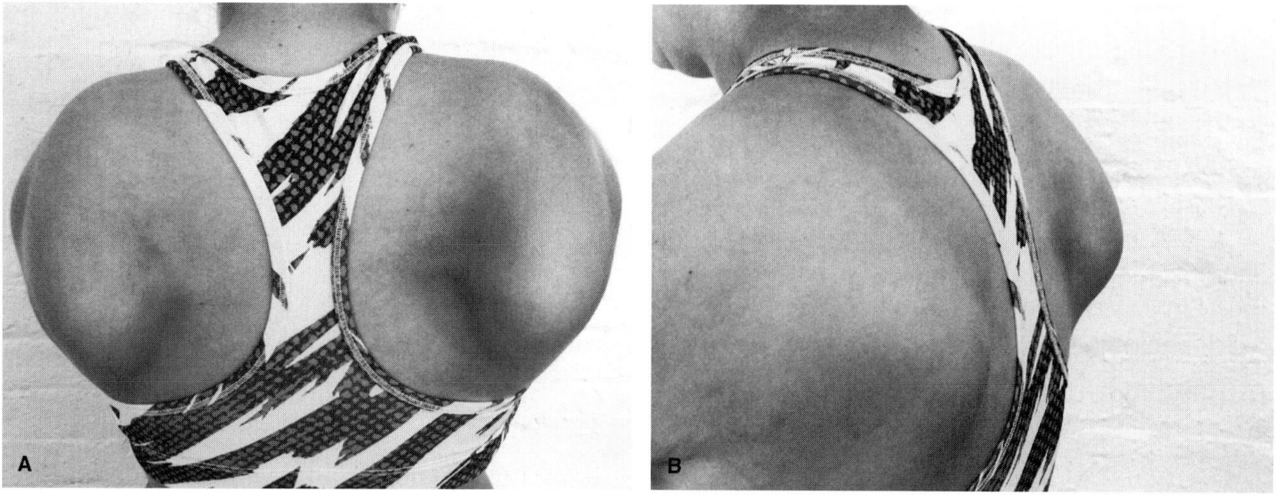

FIGURE 31-5. Client with scapular winging. **A.** From the back. **B.** From the side.

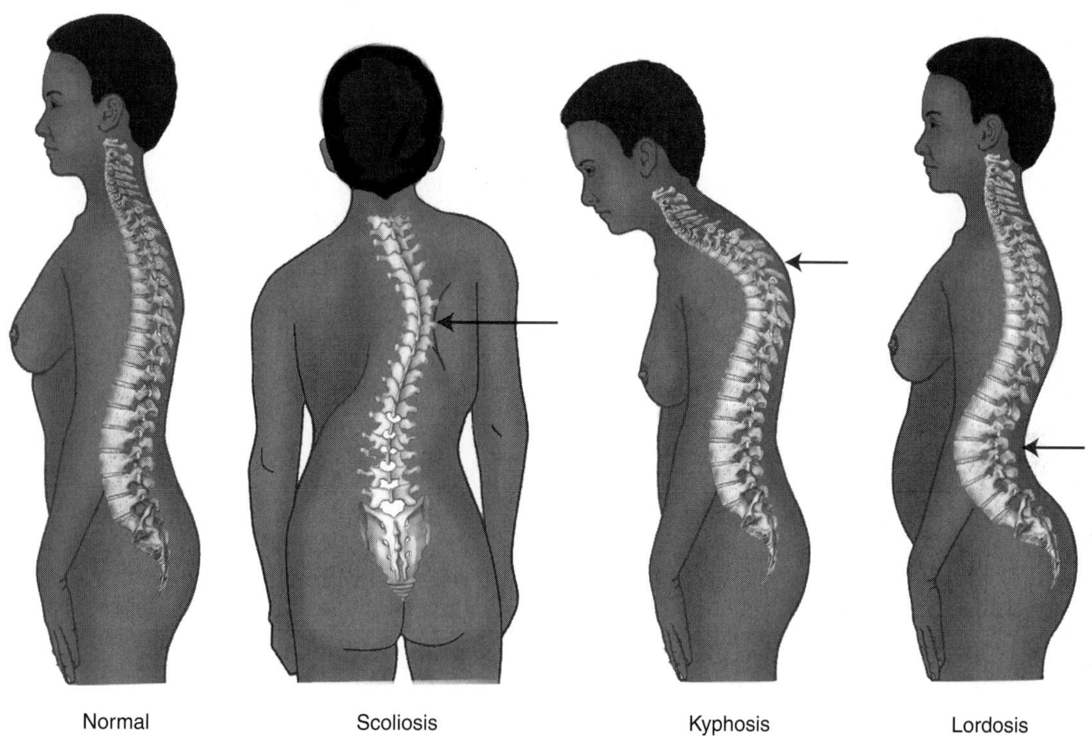

FIGURE 31-6. Normal, scoliosis, kyphosis, and lordosis spinal postures.

adulthood, it is generally not as severe and progresses more slowly.[37] Unless it is a cardiac issue, LGMD is generally not life threatening.

Research, Medical Treatment, and Exercise

Ongoing research is extensive and includes gene and drug therapy. One type of gene therapy, antisense therapy, may block faulty gene expression; another is premature stop codons, which help with the full expression of genes that make certain proteins and which are skipped in the disease process; the last is stem cell therapy.[39] A drug called ATYR1940 is currently being tested both in LGMD and facioscapulohumeral muscular dystrophy; it is a protein which seeks to decrease inflammation to alter the body's immune response (that damages muscle). Because no specific disease-modifying drugs for the treatment of LGMD currently exists on the market, medical management involves symptom management for pain and cardiac issues. OT is important for all occupations with these clients, including ADLs, IADLs, work and leisure management, as well as ROM and energy conservation.

Researchers have somewhat different opinions on the relative value or danger of various exercise regimens in people with LGMD. In LGMD, certain kinds of stress-causing exercises may actually hasten muscle damage.[38] These may include high-intensity exercise and significant muscle strain with weights. The available evidence, however, suggests that clients with LGMD would benefit from gentle strengthening and aerobic fitness training programs.[38] Some experts recommend swimming and water exercises as a good way to keep muscles as toned as possible without causing them undue stress. The buoyancy of the water helps protect against certain kinds of muscle strain and injury.[37]

FACIOSCAPULOHUMERAL MUSCULAR DYSTROPHY

Facioscapulohumeral muscular dystrophy (FSHD) is a genetic muscle disorder that begins before 20 years of age, and atrophy begins with the muscles of the face, shoulder girdle, and upper arms.[40] Many of those affected by FSHD are unable to lift their arms for more than a few seconds, lose the ability to show any facial expressions, and experience serious speech impediments.[40] Later, weakness can spread to abdominal muscles and hip/leg muscles. Symptoms can include:

- Shoulder girdle weakness
- Facial weakness
- Abdominal muscle weakness with lordosis
- Hip and lower-leg weakness
- Pain and inflammation
- Mild hearing loss/visual changes
- Cardiac problems (rare), respiratory function problems.[41]

Diagnosis is made by blood tests, EMG, nerve conduction tests, DNA testing, and, at times, muscle biopsy. FSHD can be confused with other disorders that may have similar symptoms such as polymyositis.[40]

Presentation, Progression, and Life Expectancy

FSHD may be inherited through either the father or the mother, or it may occur without a family history. It is almost always associated with a genetic mutation that leads to a shorter than usual segment of DNA on chromosome 4. The segment is not part of any particular gene, but it nevertheless seems to interfere with the correct processing of genetic material.[41] FSHD can take 30 years to become seriously disabling, however, some people do not even notice symptoms until very late in life. Estimates are that about 20% of people with FSHD eventually use a wheelchair at least some of the time.[41] In a 2009 study looking at pain and quality of life with FSHD, more than one-half of the clients complained of at least moderate pain. Frequent pain locations were upper back and shoulders, lower back, and hips.[42] The progression is generally very slow. FSHD is not life limiting, unless there are cardiac or respiratory function problems in the very late stages.

Research, Medical Treatment, and Exercise

Medical treatment is often symptom-based management, although researchers are beginning some drug studies that target strength and disease modification as well as exercise and strength. Normal participation in sports and work appears not to harm their muscles, but insufficient evidence fails to establish that it offers benefit.[43]

Exercise standard of care includes regular submaximal exercise such as swimming, and gentle aerobic activity with the addition of low-resistance strength training. No high-resistance strength training should be prescribed, and eccentric contractions (such as going down stairs slowly) are to be avoided.[44] Persistent pain and cramping (>24 hours) after an activity or exercise indicates the client has overdone it and is at risk for contraction-induced injury or "overwork weakness." Maintenance of good ROM and flexibility is important to prevent pain, maintain ambulation, and prevent contractures and deformities.[44]

SPINAL MUSCULAR ATROPHY

Spinal muscular atrophy (SMA) is characterized by the loss of motor neurons and classified as a motor neuron disease. The most common forms of SMA are caused by a mutation in the survival motor neuron 1 (SMN1) gene on chromosome 5, and a mutation in this gene leads to a deficiency of the survival motor neuron protein (SMN).[45] In SMA types 1 to 4, symptoms vary on a continuum from severe to mild, based on how much SMN protein the motor neurons contain. The more SMN protein there is, the later in life symptoms begin, and the milder the course of the disease is likely to be.[45] The weakness associated with SMA is usually symmetrical and more proximal than distal, with sensation preserved. Tendon reflexes are absent or diminished overall. Weakness in the legs is greater than in the arms, and the severity of weakness generally correlates with age of onset. Diagnosis is rendered through a blood test for an enzyme called creatine kinase, and genetic testing is also performed along with a nerve conduction test.[45]

Presentation, Progression, and Life Expectancy

In SMA type 1, children have a short life expectancy and generally die in early childhood. In SMA type 2, symptoms begin in babies at approximately 7 to 18 months of age, as they learn to sit unassisted (most), but not to stand or walk independently. At the strongest end of this category are those who can stand with a standing frame or long leg braces, but are not able to walk independently. Bulbar weakness with swallowing difficulties may lead to poor weight gain in some children and adults; they have difficulty coughing and clearing tracheal secretions. They will have nocturnal hypoventilation (difficulty with respiration due to diaphragm weakness) problems, which will require BiPAP or volume ventilation with a mask as support. Scoliosis eventually develops, and bracing or spinal surgery is generally needed. Joint contractures commonly evolve over years, and these clients are generally very small in stature from limited weight-bearing and movement. The lifespan of clients with SMA 2 varies widely; individuals might die at an early age or live well into adulthood. As with all forms of SMA, weakness increases over time.

In SMA type 3, muscle weakness begins in older children and teens, who learn to stand and walk normally as children, but lose the ability to stand and walk as the disease presents itself later in life. Although some with type 3 stop walking in adolescence, others walk well into their adult years. Scoliosis can develop in these clients. Swallowing difficulties, cough, and nocturnal hypoventilation are less common problems than in SMA 2, but may occur. Muscle aching and joint overuse symptoms are common. Life expectancy is generally normal.

SMA type 4, or adult-onset SMA, begins in the late teens or adulthood, and the life span is generally normal. Symptom onset can be as young as 18 years of age, but generally after 35 years of age. Clients will have mild muscle weakness, tremors, twitching, muscle aches, and fatigue. They generally maintain walking, although they may have a waddling gait. Life expectancy is not affected.[45]

Research, Medical Treatment, and Exercise

Some of the research currently occurring is in the realm of gene modification therapies to try to make clients with SMN stronger and more productive. Researchers are also working to create a synthetic SMN1. Drug and exercise studies are also under way, including some with stem cells injected into mice and animal model studies.[30] The U.S. Food and Drug Administration on Dec. 23, 2016, approved the antisense therapy nusinersen (brand name Spinraza™) for the treatment of all forms of SMA. Spinraza™ is designed to treat the underlying defect in SMA, which means it potentially may be effective at slowing, stopping, or even reversing the symptoms of SMA. Spinraza™ targets the intermediate step between DNA and the protein manufacturing stage within cells, causing increased production of SMN protein.[46] Some clients have reported improvements in strength and a regaining of lost muscle strength and control. Traditionally, the role of exercise in SMA is to assist in improving a client's flexibility, function, independence, and quality of life. No evidence supports traditional strength training, although new research is underway to develop exercise guidelines to match the muscular improvements documented with Spinraza™. It may be best for clients with SMA to exercise by practicing the movements and tasks they want to perform throughout the day; this is called functional exercise. It can consist of any movement or position one would like to strengthen in order to improve functionality, for example, reaching, dressing, and bathing. These activities are dependent on age, amount of neuromuscular involvement, and stage. Although exercise is important, excessive exercising may cause overfatigue and damage.[47] Clients with SMA 3 and 4 with later onset will generally be used to exercising and sports, although they may have to focus more on submaximal exercise with less overexertion depending on symptoms and fatigue. They are able to perform as much physical activity as is comfortable; swimming and adaptive sports may be options and can be a great way to stretch, exercise, and move functionally.

OCCUPATIONAL THERAPY TREATMENT

The traditional OT program for a client with a disability is often a biomechanical model that works toward improving strength. While in certain cases this approach may be possible with some of the diseases noted in this chapter, many are progressive and require a different focus. This may be adaptive or compensatory and addresses functional changes that have occurred due to disease progression in all areas of occupation. The treatments for Guillain-Barré syndrome are noted first, and then the treatments are noted by occupation and other categories for the other diseases.

Occupational Therapy Treatment for Guillain-Barré Syndrome

The OT practitioner is often involved very early in the acute stage of GBS for treatments including ROM, orthotic fabrication, proper positioning in the bed and wheelchair for avoidance of pressure injuries, and client/caregiver education and training. Even as the weakness from GBS is still progressing, the OT practitioner may begin to assist. Orthoses fabricated may be a resting hand orthosis for positioning and contracture management or a wrist cock-up orthosis for wrist stability and support (see Chapter 19 for information on fabrication of both). It will be important to involve the caregivers in performing ROM early and often to keep the client from developing significant contractures as he or she weakens. Although Guillain-Barré syndrome does not cause contractures specifically, the client may quickly develop them from immobility in the hospital, and the OTA plays a vital role in prevention. Pain may be a significant factor, and the OTA may trial a TENS unit, massage, or moist heat to manage it (see Chapter 18 for details on modalities). Clients may have significant anxiety as they lose functional abilities and will require reassurance that the team will work to recover their ability to participate in desired occupations and roles.

As the client begins to recover, the OTA may begin hand-over-hand grooming, face washing, or applying lotion to the hands while grading the amount of assistance given. In severe cases, the client must relearn all movements and regain all motor control for every voluntary muscle group, so the movements may be dependent at first. Because of this dependence, a cotreatment with the physical therapy practitioner or assistance from a rehabilitation aide may be needed, with the client sitting supported on the edge of the bed, to address grooming and self-feeding. Educating and training caregivers and clients on bed positioning and pressure injury avoidance will be important, as they can be taught safe rolling, use of pillows for positioning, and turning every 2 hours. The potential for a decrease in function due to "overdoing it" is very real with GBS, and the OTA should carefully monitor the client's fatigue and stop at the first signs. Heart rate, respiratory rate, and blood pressure may also need to be monitored. As the client begins to recover sensation and motor control, activities may be progressed from PROM to active-assisted range of motion (AAROM) to active range of motion (AROM). Initially, active movement should be performed at low repetitions and resistance with frequent rest breaks.[48] Generally, after acute hospital discharge, the client will transition to an inpatient rehabilitation facility for further therapy. With milder cases, the client may be able to go home with home health or outpatient therapies. In either case, the therapy will generally address functional mobility, endurance and balance, bed mobility and transfers, ROM and gradual strengthening, and occupational performance. The OTA will work to expand activities gradually, with a focus on increasing time and repetitions instead of resistance. Exercising to exhaustion will delay recovery without benefit to the client. For example, if the client requires moderate assistance to sit at the edge of the bed and has upper body weakness, then a light grooming and dressing program with some hand-over-hand assistance while positioned in the bed or wheelchair may be appropriate. If the client can stand with minimal assist, then perhaps a functional activity at the counter in the kitchen with periods of sitting and standing, as tolerated, would work well. The OTA should expand all activities gradually, and of paramount importance is to adapt all tasks. At times, adaptive equipment, such as a universal cuff to hold a utensil, a mobile arm support or counter-balance arm sling (deltoid aid) to assist to lift the arm, or a long-handled shoehorn with adapted shoes will assist with functionality and ADL performance (Fig. 31-7). Some clients respond well to OT in the pool for weightlessness and gentle exercise, yet others are negatively affected by the heat. Certainly, it is important to teach the client to build in rest periods, home safety and safe transfers, and practice with the client fine and gross motor tasks that can be performed when not in therapy.

Each person with Guillain-Barré syndrome recovers differently and has a different level of severity, so the OTA role will vary with this population. Some clients may be in acute rehabilitation or a skilled nursing rehabilitation unit for months, and others may walk out of the hospital. Home health and/or outpatient therapy are generally required to continue progress toward function and to regain full independence after the more intense rehabilitation. A client's home may need to be quickly modified with a ramp or grab bars for the shower and toilet to allow the client to return home while still using a wheelchair or walker.

Recovery may occur over 6 months to 2 years or longer. Certainly the psychosocial, economic, and personal impact of potential years of recovery can be significant. Particularly frustrating consequences of GBS are long-term recurrences of fatigue and/or exhaustion as well as abnormal sensations, including pain, paresthesias, and muscle aches. These can be aggravated by "normal" activity and can be alleviated by pacing activity and rest.[49] Energy conservation and work simplification will be extremely important to these clients and may include using a shower seat for bathing, stool for grooming, sitting to dress and cook, taking fewer trips through the home for laundry and cleaning, spacing out chores, taking naps, and monitoring activity levels for fatigue.

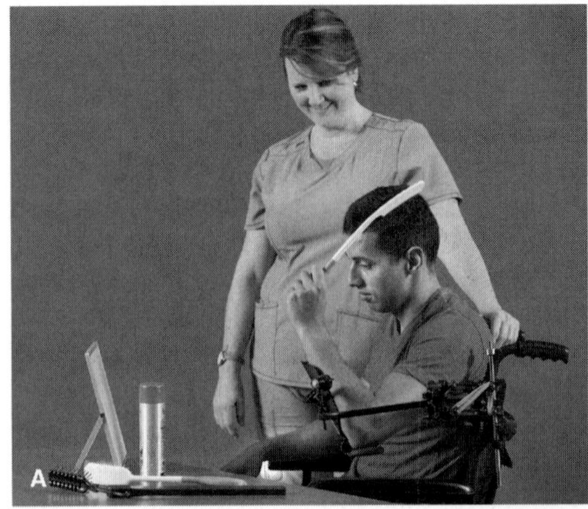

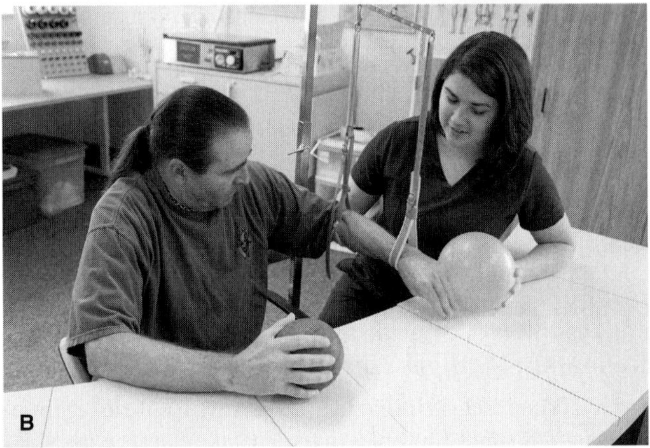

FIGURE 31-7. **A.** Mobile arm support in use for grooming. **B.** Deltoid aide supports the weight of the arm, so even small amounts of strength can be seen during attempts to move the arm.

Occupational Therapy Treatment for Other Progressive Motor Unit Diseases

The OT practitioner may help individuals in all phases of the fluctuating or progressive disease process by providing adaptations, strategies, and techniques for occupations as required. Treatment may vary depending on new symptoms over time and how the client is affected functionally. An OTA may see a client as part of an MDA clinic, the acute hospital, inpatient rehabilitation, long-term acute care (LTAC), skilled nursing facility (SNF), outpatient clinic, or home health. Many times treatment for these diseases is short-term adaptive and accommodating versus rehabilitative due to disease progression, although pain and contracture management or an acute event may require increased

EVIDENCE-BASED PRACTICE

A study by Matsuda and colleagues in 2015 examined both the prevalence of and risk factors for falls as a function of medical diagnosis and age among adults aging with physically disabling conditions, specifically multiple sclerosis, muscular dystrophies, PPS, and spinal cord injury.[50] Factors that distinguished participants who reported falling from those who did not varied across diagnostic groups: mobility level and imbalance were the important factors for participants with MDs; age and self-reported vision problems were important factors for those with PPS.[50] Findings from this study also suggest that the prevalence of falling peaks in middle-age groups (55 to 64 years of age) in individuals with PPS and at a slightly younger age (45 to 54 years of age) in those with MD.[50] Although older adults are often the target for fall-prevention programs, the results of this study suggest that OT practitioners should begin asking about falls and providing fall-prevention information to middle-aged clients with disabilities, even though these clients may not consider themselves at risk for falls. Because many of the disorders discussed in this chapter are slowly progressive, the client may be loath to change habits, and using a device, however small, may be seen as "giving in" to the disease. The OTA has a large job at times in "selling" the adaptation or equipment that could make the client's life dramatically easier, save energy, prevent falls, and decrease frustration.

Matsuda, P. N., Verrall, A. M., Finlayson, M. L., Molton, I. R., & Jensen, M. P. (2015). Falls among adults aging with disability. Archives of Physical Medicine and Rehabilitation, 96*(3), 464–471.*

length of treatment. Fatigue control and energy conservation can be issues as clients are forced to change the ways they have "always" performed a task. Adaptive equipment may be needed to accommodate for changes in weakness over time, and also depends on client needs to perform certain tasks. Many adaptive equipment solutions for specific client needs can be found in Chapter 14.

ACTIVITIES OF DAILY LIVING: BATHING AND TOILETING

Many clients will experience fatigue and weakness that will make standing during bathing less safe. The additions of a shower seat or tub bench, handheld shower hose, and grab bars will make bathing safer and help the client conserve energy. Long-handled sponges with bendable handles will assist with reaching all body parts, and pump bottles for shampoo and soap can prevent the need for lifting, flipping, opening, or squeezing containers for those with hand weakness. More dependent clients, such as those with DMD or SMA 2, may require a more supportive solution, such as a rolling shower commode chair in a roll-in shower or a tub slider system for dependent bathing and toileting. External catheters to collect urine are useful for overnight and dependent urine management for males. Many clients have hip and leg weakness and will require higher toilets or commodes plus handles or bars. Hand weakness will make toilet hygiene difficult for some, and a toilet aid or bidet could assist.

ACTIVITIES OF DAILY LIVING: DRESSING AND GROOMING

Adaptive equipment, such as a reacher to retrieve items overhead in the closet or a dressing stick to put on a shirt, will often be needed due to weakness and decreased AROM for dressing and grooming tasks. Long-handled and/or lightweight items, such as a comb or shoehorn, a dressing stick, reacher, or other adaptive equipment may be needed to accommodate for weakness in the shoulders. For hand weakness, Velcro® can be used in place of small bra hooks, buttons, and zippers, and will allow easier fastening; elastic or magnetic shoelaces will avoid tying; and foam can be placed around makeup brushes. Power seat elevation in the power wheelchair or raised height seat surfaces, such as a stool, will assist with dressing tasks for those with weak leg muscles. Sitting on a walker seat or stool in the bathroom will save energy and avoid balance issues with grooming; some clients make a grooming station at the kitchen table where they can prop their elbows for easier reaching, and have easy access to a mirror on a stand, water, a spit-cup, and all other grooming items.

ACTIVITIES OF DAILY LIVING: FEEDING, EATING, SWALLOWING, AND BREATHING

Swallowing can potentially be an issue for clients with MG, FSHD, and MMD due to weakness of neck, face, and swallowing muscles. Swallowing is not generally a problem for clients with most of the other diseases until mechanical ventilation is required, but some clients with DMD or SMA 2 will require physical assistance due to weakness much earlier. Some clients with hand weakness require larger-handled or bent utensils and adapted knives. Using long straws and cup holders may eliminate the need to lift the cup. Many clients will use BiPAP or volume ventilation support for weakened respiratory muscles throughout the course of their disease, especially later in life. As men with DMD reach their early 20s, and their respiratory function continues to decline, most will use full-time BiPAP or choose a ventilator with a tracheostomy and feeding tube. Clients with SMA 2 will often require ventilator support as adults.

ACTIVITIES OF DAILY LIVING: FUNCTIONAL MOBILITY, TECHNOLOGY, AND DEVICES

Many clients will use a walker in the home and a manual wheelchair pushed by family for longer distances in the early stages of their disease process. They may also require a power wheelchair for functional mobility in and out of the home. A power wheelchair or scooter will become necessary for safe mobility when weakness in the hip muscles and legs cause falls. Safety will be a goal as weakness increases and mobility changes from walking to wheelchair use. Home modification options and a home safety check may be required, including a ramp and ways to gain full home access.

As young men and women with DMD and SMA 2 become adults, supportive and functional power wheelchair options and adaptations and mounts for computers, phones, and games are required. Equipment and support will also be needed in the home for the nearly total care they require for desired occupations. As adults, all clients with these disorders will require power wheelchairs with significant adaptations to maintain control for positional changes and driving; these evaluations will be performed at a specialty seating clinic. Many wheelchair manufacturers are including Bluetooth and/or infrared control on higher-end power wheelchairs via the upgraded electronics. This allows whichever way the client operates the chair (hand, head, switches, etc.) to control the mouse for a computer (Bluetooth) or the television controls (infrared). Bluetooth in the joystick can also control a smartphone or tablet, which then can control many other home automation items. The OTA may be involved with setting up computer and phone access systems, or can refer clients for a consultation with an assistive technology specialist to integrate their phone, TV, wheelchair, and computer as well as offer control over the home such as lights, thermostat, doors, locks, and alarm systems.

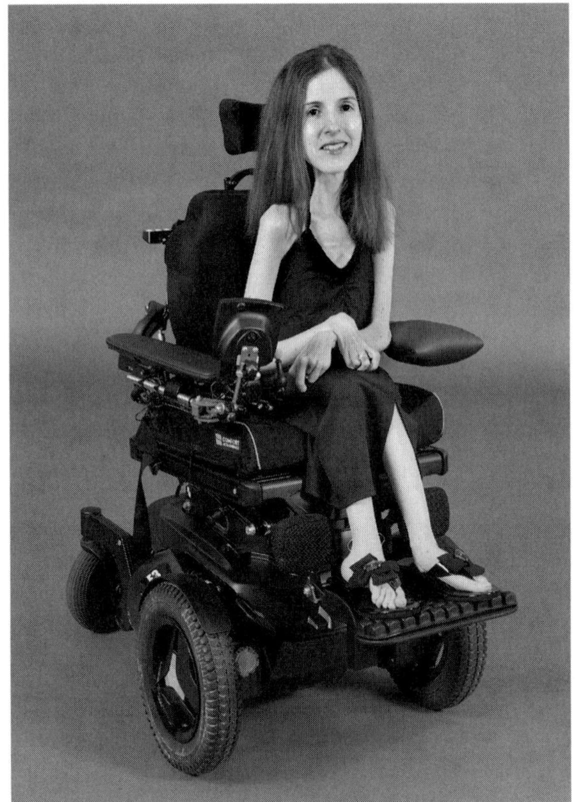

FIGURE 31-8. Client with SMA 2 as an adult.

ACTIVITIES OF DAILY LIVING: SEXUAL ACTIVITY

The OT practitioner should discuss sexuality issues with all clients, including adaptations for disability and energy conservation. Many clients with motor unit disorders may already have spouses and children when they are diagnosed; the disease process can change their feelings about themselves and their physical abilities during intimacy and sexual activity. The OTA can offer options for adaptation of sexual activity such as alternate positions, fatigue management, adaptive equipment such as wedges, and a focus on intimacy when sexual activity is too difficult due to pain.

Clients who are diagnosed at a younger age may have significant difficulties with sexuality when parents are the caregivers (Fig. 31-8). Imagine being in a position to have a parent have to assist with hygiene from a sexual encounter or after a date. Independence, dating, social, and sexuality topics can certainly be important client issues for the OTA to manage as needed. Expectations are changing as life expectancy is increasing for young adults with DMD and SMA, and many live alone with paid caregivers, get married, and/or have children. Some clients with disabilities can be socially isolated and have more contact in the online realm than in person. The OTA can offer education and training on ways to remain safe with online chats, dating, and other encounters.

INSTRUMENTAL ACTIVITIES OF DAILY LIVING

Fatigue management may require work simplification and energy conservation techniques, such as spreading out cleaning tasks or yard work over the week instead of performing them all in 1 day, or sitting to cook in the kitchen instead of standing. Pain from joint instability and overuse especially in the shoulder can mean that adaptive equipment to work in a less painful ROM could be helpful. Because of hand weakness and/or pain, many clients have fine and gross motor challenges that require adaptation for tasks such as managing packaging and containers, opening pill packs/bottles, and feeding pets. Other helpful items may be a lightweight pliers for opening sugar packets and Ziploc bags, larger pens for writing, jar and bottle openers, a dressing stick to get wet laundry out of the washer, a reacher to grab items off the floor, a key-turning assist, and a device for turning a round-knob door. The OTA will provide education and training on adapted techniques and adaptive equipment to manage those functional tasks and many others. Safety issues with cooking may require the client to slide heavy pots of food on the counter on top of a towel from stove to sink instead of lifting, or to use a rolling cart to carry a laundry basket. Long-handled items will assist with reach, and reorganization of the closets and kitchen will assist to increase ability to reach all necessary items. Clients who are more dependent will direct home management and other tasks if needed or use home automation options.

REST AND SLEEP

A hospital bed that is adjustable at the head, feet, and total height may assist clients with breathing and positioning as well as transfers and pressure relief. Some clients prefer an adjustable-style bed or a bed of a certain mattress type for comfort. A consideration is that a plush mattress chosen for comfort may make rolling more difficult for clients due to weakness. Once clients can no longer roll themselves or if they have any pressure injuries, a bed with a special air mattress on top or other pressure-relieving surface will be helpful. Many will require assistance for rolling in bed, including every 2 to 3 hours through the night. Lateral rotation beds are available to assist with rolling the client, which work well for repositioning and pressure relief, but can be very expensive. The burden on the rest and sleep of both the client and caregivers can be substantial.

EDUCATION, WORK, VOLUNTEER, AND DRIVING

During college, clients with hand/arm weakness and pain may require a computer for writing and taking notes, voice-to-text for papers, and increased time for testing. Using the phone may require hands-free and automated options. Clients with DMD or SMA 2 may require mouse options with a modified option at the hand, a head mouse or eye gaze, onscreen keyboards, and/or voice-to-text programs for their computers. Many clients will require adaptations from the OT practitioner for assistance with college, work, and volunteer opportunities, with a potential referral to vocational rehabilitation as well. Some adults who are unable to work or have a disability status through the Social Security Administration still have the ability to volunteer, and the OTA may be able to assist with finding the right community match for a particular client. Many adults with later-onset diseases are already working, and will require adaptations for work tasks such as typing, mouse and phone use, desk ergonomics, standing for long hours, and walking from the parking lot to the work space. Decisions about when to stop working, family finances, and the disability process may also be important to discuss or refer to a social worker. Community mobility and driving will be a concern as the weakness continues to progress; many clients will require options for increased safety for both (see Chapter 16).

LEISURE AND SOCIAL PARTICIPATION

Many adults with a long-term disability are very isolated socially and require encouragement to do more than stay in the home and play video or computer games. A study by Bendixen and colleagues found that participation in recreational and social activities was significantly lower in older children and adults with DMD than with younger individuals, with a significant decline over time.[51] They found that as individuals age, social isolation occurs with decreasing time spent with friends and in the community.[51] The OTA can work with these clients on other opportunities such as volunteerism, support groups, and supported employment.

Some clients with later-onset diseases may have long histories with active sports and recreation and will have a difficult time managing to continue in the same way when they have increasing weakness. One strategy is to focus on what the client really enjoys most about the activity. One example is playing golf, which requires strength, balance, endurance, and motor control. Does the client love hitting the ball, or is the experience as much about being outside with buddies on a beautiful day? Could the client ride in the cart, keep score, and tease friends? Could the client take a grandchild or neighbor to a driving range and educate them on proper technique? Could the client watch golf on television with friends? The OTA is often able to find leisure opportunities through exploration of strengths and interests for many clients. Some clients will require assistance to develop and explore other leisure interests or adaptations to perform new tasks.

POSITIONING, TRANSFERS, AND SAFETY

Bed mobility can be a challenge, and a hospital bed or adjustable bed, leg lifter, and trapeze or side rail may be helpful. Getting comfortable with positioning in the bed, recliner, or wheelchair can be difficult when the client is relying on a caregiver to move them, and the OTA can assist

THE OLDER ADULT

Until more recent times, many people with DMD, SMA 2, and polio would never have lived to experience any of the normal aging issues that an older adult without significant disabilities is expected to have. These issues are arthritis, changes in vision and hearing, osteoporosis, heart disease/hypertension, and memory loss. Older adults with long-term physical conditions, such as post-polio syndrome or muscular dystrophy, can face more of these health problems than their peers without such conditions.[52] Smith and colleagues surveyed 1,594 people with disabilities such as multiple sclerosis, post-polio syndrome, muscular dystrophies, and spinal cord injury twice, 3½ years apart. Overall, participants with long-term physical disabilities reported slightly greater rates of chronic health problems than adults without physical disabilities, and people who already had one health problem at the beginning of the study were much more likely to get other health problems over the next 3 years.[52] Arthritis was the most common reported problem. In another study of self-reported fatigue in people with the same types of disabilities as the study by Smith and colleagues, it was noted that people with disabilities reported greater fatigue than those without disabilities and a higher risk for fatigue as they age compared with normal cohorts.[53] Other considerations as clients with disabilities get older is the age of their caregivers and their ability to provide long-term care. The OTA will certainly have a role with the older adult with and without a long-term disability in assisting to maintain quality of life and functional performance of desired occupations.

with positioning options using pillows, wedges, and bolsters. Transfers from sitting to standing can be easier by placing risers under chair legs to make the chairs taller. Once clients are using a power wheelchair for mobility, press-over or stand-pivot transfers may be accomplished with the power seat elevation feature, if available. A pivot disc will assist when clients have difficulty moving their feet for the transfer; over time, clients may transition to a transfer board or a patient lifter with sling. Some families manage by lifting the client themselves, especially if the client is small in stature. See Chapter 13 for more information on transfers.

Safety can be an important issue as clients and caregivers have strategies for mobility, transfers, and daily tasks that have worked for years, and suddenly do not due to changes in strength or condition. Clients may have frequent falls, fatigue, and injuries before being willing to seek an adaptation or adaptive equipment. The OTA can assist clients to be proactive with the future in mind for all aspects of their occupations.

ENDURANCE, STRENGTH, FATIGUE, AND ENERGY CONSERVATION

To compensate for decreased endurance and fatigue, adaptations may include using a reacher for obtaining objects overhead, a stool in the kitchen, or a shower seat (Fig. 31-9). Strategies such as performing activities for shorter periods may be required to avoid tiring out the eyes during reading or the voice during speaking for clients with those issues. Throughout the client's lifetime, energy conservation and work simplification will be required to manage fatigue and for pacing of tasks.

Treatment for overstretched and overused muscles such as those around the shoulder girdle may include pain management as well as education and training on adaptive equipment, which could assist with decreasing the pain and increasing function.

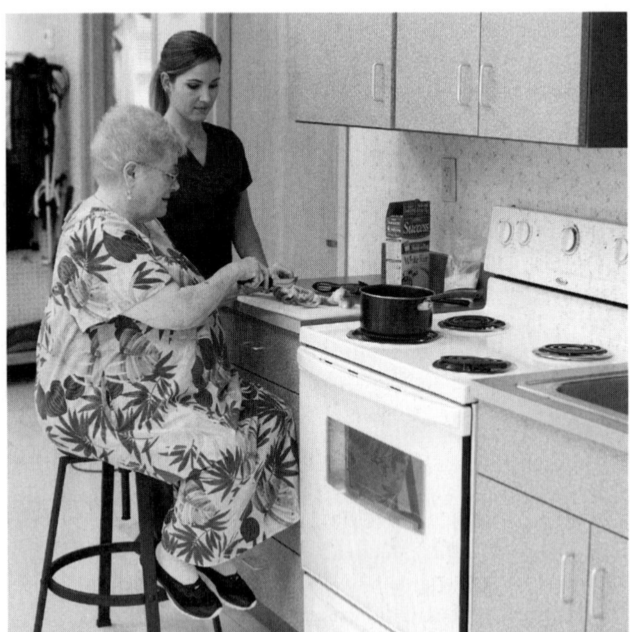

FIGURE 31-9. A client with CMT sitting on a tall stool to cook and to save energy.

Teaching the client to perform safe exercise will be important, with a focus on cardiovascular fitness, such as swimming or riding a recumbent bike. In 2010, Larsson and Lexell studied the effects of an individualized, interdisciplinary rehabilitation program for clients with post-polio syndrome. They found that most participants felt it was a turning point in their sense of control and development of new skills to manage their changed function and decreased strength.[54] Contractures can be a significant issue both with pain and positioning for many clients, and the client must perform daily ROM exercises as well as utilize orthotics fabricated by the OT practitioner, as required. One goal is to prevent contractures, especially at the shoulder and in the hands through a daily ROM program. The role of the OTA with many of the diseases in this chapter is to instruct in supportive and safe exercise, AROM education and training for flexibility, and assisting to remain active with safe and supportive mobility.

ORTHOTIC MANAGEMENT AND FABRICATION

Wrist supports that hold the hand in a supported position for using a keyboard, writing, or drawing can help compensate for weak wrist muscles. Resting hand orthoses may be needed overnight to maintain arches and avoid hand and finger contractures. An adult with SMA 2 may use a thoracic-lumbar-sacral-orthotic (TLSO) for trunk support that would be fabricated by an orthotist. Creation of custom hand orthoses by the OT practitioner may also be helpful. One example is for individual finger extension for computer or iPad®/tablet use. Another is to manage excessive claw-hand position with an orthotic for a client with CMT to hold the MCP joints in a slightly flexed position (Fig. 31-10). A padded wire frame cervical collar may be required for cervical weakness to assist with head control in some clients (Fig. 31-11).

TECHNOLOGY AND TRENDS

Power wheelchairs are becoming more and more sophisticated, and getting better at meeting the needs of clients with significant and progressive disorders. For those clients on ventilators, an inverter can be added that taps the wheelchair batteries to run the ventilator, giving increased time to be out of the house and away from a plug. The inverter also comes with a second cigarette plug adaptor port for charging other items such as a phone. Some wheelchairs allow control over the smart phone functions via the joystick or chair control. Others will allow Bluetooth control over the computer or laptop mouse with the joystick or chair control. Another item allows a cord to attach in the charging port of the power wheelchair which has a USB plug for charging devices on the other end. Technology in the standard market is significantly farther ahead, but wheelchair technology is starting to catch up for what is at least possible, if not paid for, by insurance.

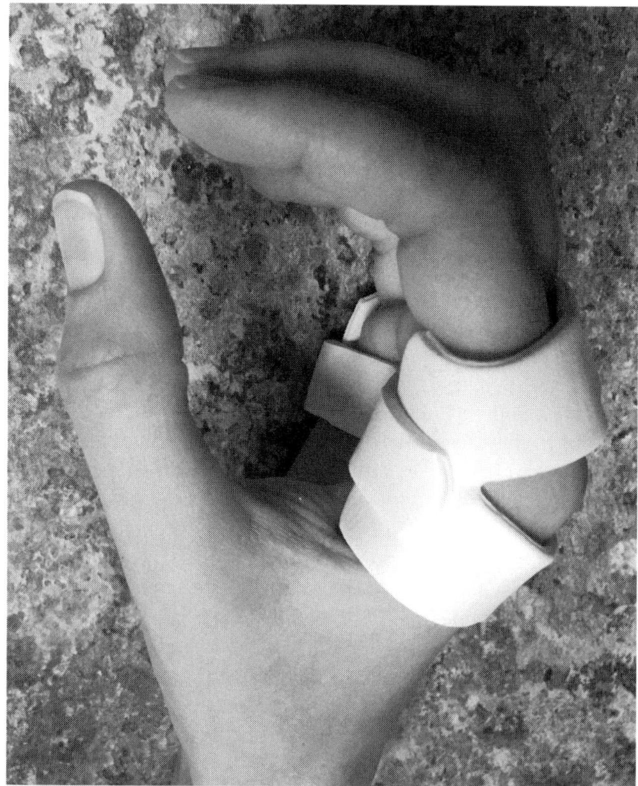

FIGURE 31-10. MCP blocking splint on client with CMT prevents excessive hyperextension at the MCP, thus increasing hand grip and functionality.

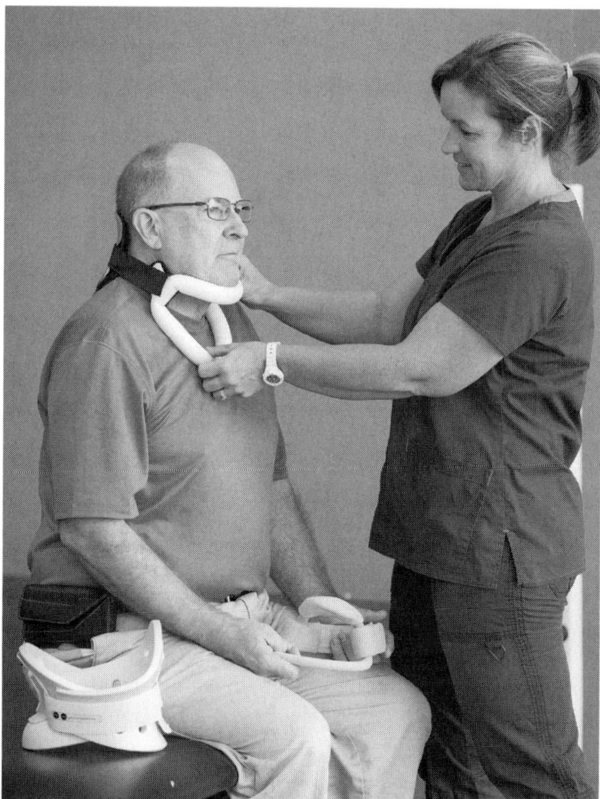

FIGURE 31-11. Padded wire frame cervical collars on a client and in his lap, which are adjustable in height and width, and a nonadjustable cervical collar on the mat.

SUMMARY

Although the needs of the population with motor unit diseases can vary widely, the management of changes due to disease progression is constant. Many times, ongoing OT intervention will not be required, but simply different techniques or problem-solving for new changes in strength may be needed. Because many of these diseases are rare, the OTA may need to use this chapter as a reference once in the field and when a client with a certain diagnosis is on the caseload. Most of these diseases are a covered diagnosis under the MDA (except for post-polio and Guillain-Barré syndromes), and the MDA can offer resources, information, loaner equipment, and research for the client as well.

REVIEW QUESTIONS

1. A client has recently been diagnosed with myasthenia gravis, and is having difficulty with IADL tasks, specifically with putting away groceries and retrieving items from higher shelves and in the closet. Which items and techniques might the OTA offer?
   a. Using a stool for energy conservation in the kitchen
   b. Using a reacher and dressing stick in the kitchen and bedroom
   c. Using grocery bag holders in the kitchen
   d. Using a power wheelchair for mobility
2. A young adult with Duchenne muscular dystrophy might use which item on his power wheelchair for controlling the mouse on his computer?
   a. Mobile arm support
   b. Bluetooth mouse control through the joystick
   c. Eye gaze computer system
   d. Gel armrest pads
3. An older woman with SMA type 4 adult-onset has always exercised as part of her daily routine, and she is nervous about continuing and doing damage to her muscles. What should the OTA tell her about exercise?
   a. Any exercise is fine for SMA type 4.
   b. Perform stretching and ROM exercises only.
   c. Do as much physical activity as is comfortable without overdoing it.
   d. No exercise is recommended.
4. For most muscular dystrophies, the diagnostic process is lengthy and will include which of the following?
   a. Symptoms and problem list only
   b. Genetic testing only
   c. Biopsy and blood work only
   d. EMG or nerve conduction tests, blood work, and genetic testing
5. The OTA is treating an older male client with LGMD who is having significant difficulty with self-care at home. What types of problems might he be having?
   a. Reaching to pull up pants, getting off toilet, donning and doffing shirt, getting in and out of bed
   b. Using buttons and zippers, picking up pills, opening a bottle
   c. Opening packages for cooking, opening sugar packets, and turning a screwdriver
   d. Performing self-feeding and grooming tasks

6. All progressive disorders have something in common with respect to equipment and adaptive techniques given by the OTA. The OTA must have which of the following?
   a. Patience, due to behavioral challenges
   b. Strength, to transfer the obese client
   c. Creativity, to manage the condition over time
   d. Rigidity, to not be dismayed by clients not improving
7. A new client with Guillain-Barré syndrome just got to the inpatient rehabilitation hospital, and she looks like a client with quadriplegia because she has very little active control. How might the OTA begin treatment with her in the first session?
   a. Utilize hand-over-hand grooming while sitting up in the hospital bed.
   b. Utilize pain management strategies including ice and ultrasound.
   c. Use the assisted cough procedure.
   d. Sit to stand at the edge of the bed for dressing.
8. Scoliosis and other back deformities are seen *most* often in which three of the following client diagnoses?
   a. MMD
   b. Guillain Barré syndrome
   c. SMA 2
   d. Post-polio syndrome
   e. DMD
   f. LGMD
9. Post-polio syndrome can be a challenging disorder because clients have been functioning for many years at a certain level, and now they are getting worse again. Which three of the following changes might they have to face with post-polio syndrome?
   a. Decreased ability to ambulate with a need for a power wheelchair
   b. Decreased transfer ability for sit to stand
   c. Decreased need for caregiver support
   d. Increased need for caregiver support
   e. Continued ability to manage all job tasks
   f. Laxity of joints
10. You are covering for another OTA at the MDA clinic and are about to see a client with MMD. You remember some about the disorder, but are not sure what to expect. The client walks in with complaints of difficulty opening bottles, pulling up zippers, and fastening buttons. Based on these complaints, you know the client will also *most likely* have difficulties with:
   a. Sit-to-stand
   b. Shoe tying
   c. Rolling in bed
   d. Controlling a power wheelchair

CASE STUDY

Megan is a 35-year-old woman with CMT who is married, has two children 2 and 4 years of age, and works full time as a cashier at Walmart. She frequently has pain in her hands and feet, some numbness in her fingers and toes, and stands all day at her job. She wears bilateral ankle-foot orthoses, and is beginning to have a slight claw deviation in her hands with hyperextension at the metacarpals, and flexion at the proximal and distal finger joints. She is having difficulty with fastening her own clothing as well as her children's, and struggles to perform the evening cooking and other chores after a long day at work. She has messy writing, and her hand cramps when texting or using the computer. She has difficulty opening jars and bottles, and some difficulty bagging heavier items at work such as gallons of milk and juice.

1. What pieces of adaptive equipment and adaptive techniques could the OT practitioner offer Megan at her OT appointment?
2. What are some IADL and work adaptations the OT practitioner could offer?
3. What child care options could the OT practitioner offer?
4. What energy conservation techniques could the OT practitioner suggest?

PUTTING IT ALL TOGETHER Sample Treatment and Documentation

Setting	Outpatient hospital setting, OT clinic
Client profile	Joey is a 28-year-old young man with Guillain-Barré syndrome who has been recently discharged from the inpatient rehab hospital to home. He was 4 weeks in acute care, 3 of those on a ventilator in the ICU. He spent 3 weeks in inpatient rehab. He can ambulate with Min A with a walker. He has significant contractures in his shoulders from prolonged hospitalization, which are often painful and make him less functional.
Work history	Finished high school; never attended college; worked at a big-box store before the illness; lives with parents
Insurance	Private insurance through work
Psychological	Occasional depression and anxiety; not on medication
Social	Lives with his parents who are still working; has one younger sibling in college
Cognitive	Within normal limits
Motor and Manual Muscle Testing (MMT)	UEs have 90 degrees AROM in shoulder flexion on the right and 70 degrees on the left with pain and 3-/5 strength at shoulders. He has 3/5 strength throughout the rest of his UEs. Client is right-hand dominant. Static sitting balance good, static standing balance fair, dynamic standing balance poor.
ADL	Supervision for self-feeding with built-up handles for utensil, Min A rest of ADLs primarily due to shoulder weakness, pain, and contractures. Min A sit to stand and for transfers.
IADL	Mod-Max A for all IADLs

PUTTING IT ALL TOGETHER Sample Treatment and Documentation (continued)

Goals Within 3 weeks:

1. Increase active shoulder flexion bilaterally to 120 degrees to increase ADL performance.
2. Improve dynamic standing balance to fair for ADL/IADL tasks in standing.
3. Increase standing tolerance to 5 min at a time for increased ADL/IADL performance.
4. Demonstrate independence to perform/direct AAROM/AROM to BUE to increase ADL performance.

OT TREATMENT SESSION 1

THERAPEUTIC ACTIVITY	TIME	GOAL(s) ADDRESSED	OTA RATIONALE
Perform PROM with sustained stretch to bilateral shoulders with pain management strategies including ultrasound	20 min	#1	*Preparatory Methods:* PROM performed to B shoulders with prolonged stretch and ultrasound to increase ROM and decrease pain.
Standing during task involving snack prep in the kitchen, with 2-min rest breaks in between	20 min	#3	*Occupations and Activities:* Client will increase strength and endurance as well as tolerance for standing to increase ability to tolerate ADLs and IADLs.
Dynamic standing task with reaching out of base of support to put away snack items in kitchen with Min-Mod A	15 min	#2	*Occupations and Activities:* Dynamic standing balance will increase ADL performance and decrease fall risk.

SOAP note: 12/3/—, 2:00 pm–2:55 pm

S: Client noted “I can’t go for much longer than this” after standing for 3 minutes.

O: Client participated in skilled OT services at outpatient OT clinic for 55 minutes to address strength, endurance, balance, pain, and ROM. Client is oriented ×4 with pain complaints in shoulders at night after sleeping in one position for too long. He also complains of pain in the shoulders during ADL tasks at 5/10 on a pain scale. OTA performed prolonged stretch to B shoulders and use of ultrasound for 1.5 W/cm^2 for 10 minutes with 2/10 pain noted after, and an increase from 90 degrees to 100 degrees shoulder flexion on the right and 70 degrees to 75 degrees on the left noted. Client stood in kitchen for 4 × 3 min during snack preparation with Min A for balance and endurance, and 2-min rest breaks between tasks. He was able to demonstrate dynamic standing while moving items in the kitchen with Mod A.

A: Client demonstrated improvement in PROM and a decrease in pain in bilateral shoulders during stretching and ultrasound by OTA. He was able to stand for 1-min longer each time and with 1-min shorter rest periods than previous sessions, showing increased activity tolerance. Client is a good rehab candidate due to improvements in PROM and pain and tolerance of endurance tasks. Client would benefit from continued OT to address functional task performance in static and dynamic standing.

P: Client will be seen for 3 weeks, 60-minute sessions, 2×/week to address ROM, pain management, balance, strength, and endurance. OT will continue to work through contracture and pain for increasing ROM for daily PROM and ADL performance. Client will be educated on SROM strategies during next session.

Yolanda Peters, COTA/L, 12/3/—, 3:00 pm

TREATMENT SESSION 2

What could you do next with this client?

TREATMENT SESSION 3

What could you do next with this client?

REFERENCES

1. Guillain-Barré syndrome fact sheet. (2011). National Institute of Neurological Disorders and Stroke. Retrieved from http://www.ninds.nih.gov/disorders/gbs/detail_gbs.htm
2. Guillain-Barré syndrome or GBS disease. (n.d.). Retrieved from http://www.physiotherapy-treatment.com/gbs-disease.html.
3. Guillain Barré syndrome. (2016). Retrieved from http://www.mayoclinic.org/diseases-conditions/guillain-barre-syndrome/basics/definition/con-20025832
4. Van Den Berg, B., Walgaard, C., Drenthen, J., Fokke, C., Jacobs, B. C., & Van Doorn, P. A. (2014). Guillain-Barré syndrome: Pathogenesis, diagnosis, treatment and prognosis. *Nature Reviews Neurology, 10*(8), 469–482. http://dx.doi.org/10.1038/nrneurol.2014.121
5. Guillain Barré syndrome. (n.d.). Retrieved from http://www.gbsnz.org.nz/guillain_barre_syndrome
6. NINDS Chronic Inflammatory Demyelinating Polyneuropathy (CIDP) information page. (2016). Retrieved from http://www.ninds.nih.gov/disorders/cidp/cidp.htm
7. About myasthenia gravis. (2016). Retrieved from https://www.mda.org/disease/myasthenia-gravis
8. Myasthenia gravis fact sheet. (2010). National Institute of Neurological Disorders and Stroke. Retrieved from http://www.ninds.nih.gov/disorders/myasthenia_gravis/detail_myasthenia_gravis.htm
9. Test and diagnostic methods. (2015). Myasthenia Gravis Foundation of America, Inc. Retrieved from http://www.myasthenia.org/WhatisMG/TestDiagnosticmethods.aspx
10. What makes MG worse? (2016). Retrieved from http://www.myastheniagravis.org/about-mg/
11. Poliomyelitis. (2016). Retrieved from http://www.who.int/mediacentre/factsheets/fs114/en/

12. A polio free U.S. thanks to vaccine efforts. (2016). Retrieved from http://www.cdc.gov/features/poliofacts/
13. What is polio? (2014). Retrieved from http://www.cdc.gov/polio/about/
14. Recognizing the symptoms of polio. (n.d.). Retrieved from http://www.healthline.com/health/poliomyelitis#Symptoms4
15. Post-polio syndrome fact sheet. (2012). National Institute of Neurological Disorders and Stroke. Retrieved from http://www.ninds.nih.gov/disorders/post_polio/detail_post_polio.htm
16. DMD gene. (2016). Genetics home reference. Retrieved from http://ghr.nlm.nih.gov/gene/DMD
17. Flanigan, K. M. (2014). Duchenne and Becker muscular dystrophies. *Neurological Clinician, 32,* 671–688.
18. Pangalila, R. F., van den Bos, G. A., Bartels, B., Bergen, M., Stam, H. J., & Roebroeck, M. E. (2015). Prevalence of fatigue, pain, and affective disorders in adults with Duchenne muscular dystrophy and their associations with quality of life. *Archives of Physical Medicine and Rehabilitation,96*(7), 1242–1247.
19. Care for Duchenne. (2016). Retrieved from http://www.parentprojectmd.org
20. Emflaza (deflazacort) for the treatment of Duchenne muscular dystrophy. (2017). Retrieved from http://www.drugdevelopment-technology.com/projects/emflaza-deflazacort-for-the-treatment-of-duchenne-muscular-dystrophy/
21. Duchenne muscular dystrophy. (2016). Retrieved from https://www.mda.org/disease/duchenne-muscular-dystrophy/
22. Yiu, E. M. & Kornberg, A. J. (2015). Duchenne muscular dystrophy. *Journal of Paediatrics and Child Health, 51*(8), 759–764.
23. Becker muscular dystrophy—Medical management. (2016). Retrieved from https://www.mda.org/disease/becker-muscular-dystrophy/medical-management
24. Berthelsen, M. P., Husu, E., Christensen, S. B., Prahm, K. P., Vissing, J., & Jensen, B. R. (2014). Anti-gravity training improves walking capacity and postural balance in patients with muscular dystrophy. *Neuromuscular Disorders, 24*(6), 492–498.
25. Sveen, M. L., Andersen, S. P., Ingelsrud, L. H., Blichter, S., Olsen, N. E., Jonck, S., ... & Vissing, J. (2013). Resistance training in patients with limb-girdle and becker muscular dystrophy. *Muscle and Nerve, 47*(2), 163–169.
26. Charcot-Marie-Tooth disease. (2016). Retrieved from https://www.mda.org/disease/charcot-marie-tooth
27. What is CMT? (n.d.). Retrieved from http://www.cmtausa.org/index.php?option=com_content&view=article&id=70&Itemid=28
28. Treatment and management of CMT. (n.d.). Retrieved from http://www.cmtausa.org/resource-center/treatment-management/
29. Sman, A. D., Hackett, D., Fiatarone Singh, M., Fornusek, C., Menezes, M. P., & Burns, J. (2015), Systematic review of exercise for Charcot-Marie-Tooth disease. *Journal of the Peripheral Nervous System, 20,* 347–362.
30. Therapeutic approaches. (2014). Retrieved from http://www.curesma.org/research/our-strategy/drug-discovery/therapeutic-approaches/
31. Myotonic muscular dystrophy—Types of myotonic MD. (2016). Retrieved from https://www.mda.org/disease/myotonic-muscular-dystrophy/types
32. Managing DM. (n.d.). Myotonic Dystrophy Foundation. Retrieved from http://www.myotonic.org/living-dm/managing-dm
33. Myotonic muscular dystrophy. (n.d.). Retrieved from www.mda.org.au
34. Wahl, M. (2012). MMD research: Seeking to free proteins from a toxic web. Retrieved from https://www.mda.org/quest/article/mmd-research-seeking-to-free-proteins-from-a-toxic-web
35. Lindeman, E., Leffers, P., Spaans, P., Drukker, J., Reulen, J., Kerckhoffs, M., & Koke, A. (1995). Strength training in patients with myotonic dystrophy and hereditary motor and sensory neuropathy: A randomized clinical trial. *Archives of Physical Medicine and Rehabilitation, 76,* 7.
36. Kierkegaard, M., Harms-Ringdahl, K., Edström, L., Widén Holmqvist, L., & Tollbäck, A. (2011). Feasibility and effects of a physical exercise programme in adults with myotonic dystrophy type 1: A randomized controlled pilot study. *Journal of Rehabilitation Medicine, 43*(8), 695–702.
37. Limb girdle muscular dystrophy. (2016). Retrieved from https://www.mda.org/disease/limb-girdle-muscular-dystrophy/
38. Narayanaswami, P., Weiss, M., Selcen, D., David, W., Raynor, E., Carter, G., ... & Amato, A. A. (2014). Evidence-based guideline summary: Diagnosis and treatment of limb-girdle and distal dystrophies. *Neurology, 83,* 1453–1463.
39. Limb girdle muscular dystrophy. (2016). Genetics Home Reference. Retrieved from http://ghr.nlm.nih.gov/condition/limb-girdle-muscular-dystrophy
40. What is FSH? (2010). Friends of FSH research. Retrieved from http://www.fshfriends.org/fsh/
41. Facioscapulohumeral muscular dystrophy. (2016). Retrieved from https://www.mda.org/disease/facioscapulohumeral-muscular-dystrophy/signs-and-symptoms
42. Padua, L., Aprile, I., Frusciante, R., Iannaccone, E., Rossi, M., Renna, R., ... & Ricci E. (2009). Quality of life and pain in patients with facioscapulohumeral muscular dystrophy. *Muscle Nerve, 40,* 200.
43. van der Kooi, E. L., Lindeman, E., & Riphagen, I. (2005). Strength training and aerobic exercise training for muscle disease. *Cochrane Database of Systematic Reviews,* 1, CD003907.
44. Craig, M., & McDonald, M. D. (2010). Physical activity and exercise in FSHD: A physician's and a patient's perspectives. Retrieved from: https://www.fshsociety.org/assets/pdf/FSHSocietyPatientIPRN2010_McDonald.pdf
45. What is SMA? (n.d.). Retrieved from www.fightsma.org/what-sma
46. MDA celebrates FDA approval of Spinraza for treatment of spinal muscular atrophy. (2016). Retrieved from www.mdausa.org
47. Physical/occupational therapy. (n.d.). Spinal Muscular Atrophy Clinical Research Center. Retrieved from http://columbiasma.org/pt-ot.html
48. Hansen, M., & Garcia, S. (n.d.). Guillian-Barré syndrome, CIDP and variants: Guidelines for the physical and occupational therapist. Retrieved from https://www.gbs-cidp.org/wp-content/uploads/2012/01/PTOTGuidelines.pdf
49. All about GBS. (2016). Retrieved from http://www.gbs-cidp.org/gbs/all-about-gbs/
50. Matsuda, P. N., Verrall, A. M., Finlayson, M. L., Molton, I. R., & Jensen, M. P. (2015). Falls among adults aging with disability. *Archives of Physical Medicine and Rehabilitation, 96*(3), 464–471.
51. Bendixen, R. M., Lott, D. J., Senesac, C., Mathur, S., & Vandenborne, K. (2014). Participation in daily life activities and its relationship to strength and functional measures in boys with Duchenne muscular dystrophy. *Disability Rehabilitation, 36*(22), 1918–1923.
52. Smith, A. E., Molton, I. R., & Jensen, M. P. (2016). Self-reported incidence and age of onset of chronic comorbid medical conditions in adults aging with long-term physical disability. *Disability and Health Journal,9*(3), 533–538.
53. Cook, K. F., Molton, I. R., & Jensen, M. P. (2011). Fatigue and aging with a disability. *Archives of Physical Medicine and Rehabilitation, 92*(7), 1126–1133. doi:10.1016/j.apmr.2011.02.017
54. Larsson, L. M., & Lexell, J. (2010). A positive turning point in life—How persons with late effects of polio experience the influence of an interdisciplinary rehabilitation programme. *Journal of Rehabilitation Medicine, 42*(6), 559–565.

Chapter 32

Degenerative Diseases of the Central Nervous System: Understanding and Management

Amber L. Ward, MS, OTR/L, BCPR, ATP/SMS and Megan McDermond Shein, OTR/L

LEARNING OUTCOMES

After studying this chapter, the student or practitioner will be able to:

32.1 Describe common degenerative diseases and specific characteristics of each

32.2 Identify applicable occupational therapy treatment interventions associated with common degenerative diseases

32.3 Describe common assistive technology and adaptations for management of occupational performance for clients with a degenerative disease

32.4 Identify the classification systems and scales associated with dementia and what they mean for occupational performance

32.5 Discuss the burden a degenerative disease takes on the client, caregiver, and support system

KEY TERMS

Bradykinesia
Bilevel positive airway pressure (BiPAP)
Chorea
Dementia
Dyskinesias
Dyspnea
Dystonia
Dyspraxia
Fasciculations
Frontotemporal dementia
Hypermetabolic
Orthopnea
Pseudobulbar affect
Rigidity
Sundowning
Wandering

Clients with progressive disorders present with a special set of needs and a constantly changing set of skills and strengths throughout the course of the disease. The occupational therapy assistant (OTA) has a role in working with individuals with these disorders in maintaining function, independence, and quality of life (QoL) for as long as possible. Although each of the diseases covered in this chapter has significant differences, each can be life-limiting and have a significant impact on the lives of the client and family as well as the OTA caring for them. Some clients/families will deal with this adversity by seeing it as a challenge, and others will have significant psychosocial issues in dealing with the stress, limitations, and progressive changes that accompany diseases of this sort. Also, OTAs who work with clients with life-limiting diseases must also practice self-care and monitor their own feelings of grief and loss for the struggles of their clients.

This chapter will focus on diseases that affect the central nervous system (CNS), including amyotrophic lateral sclerosis (ALS) and its variants, multiple sclerosis (MS), Huntington's disease (HD), Parkinson's disease (PD), and other movement disorders and dementias, including Alzheimer's disease (AD).

AMYOTROPHIC LATERAL SCLEROSIS

Amyotrophic lateral sclerosis (ALS), also known as Lou Gehrig's disease in the United States and motor neuron disease in many other countries, affects motor neurons in the brain and spinal cord, and affects all voluntary muscle control including breathing and swallowing.[1] Motor neurons send impulses that control the muscles from the brain to the brainstem and spinal cord and from there to the specific muscles. ALS is often a quickly progressive disorder, and clients with ALS will have significant adaptation and equipment needs as their weakness increases. In order to receive a diagnosis of ALS, many other diseases must first be ruled out, and since no definitive test for ALS currently exists, the diagnostic process can be challenging. A firm diagnosis requires both upper and lower motor neuron signs; upper motor signs include increased reflexes and increased muscle tone (observable when the information from the brain to the spinal cord is disrupted), and lower motor signs include atrophy, weakness, and decreased reflexes (observable when the information from the spinal cord to the muscles is disrupted). Both signs must be exhibited for an ALS diagnosis, all other differential diagnoses must be ruled out, and an electromyography (EMG) is performed as well. Blood tests must rule out heavy metal toxicity or other conditions such as Lyme disease. Unfortunately, a client may initially seek out a primary care physician or orthopedist due to a weakness in the hand or ankle, and can be misdiagnosed with carpal tunnel syndrome, back/disc problems, or cervical issues as the cause of the weakness. These conditions may actually exist but are erroneously considered the root cause of the symptoms, and clients do not improve after spinal or carpal tunnel surgeries as they should. The delayed diagnosis is often due to a delayed referral to a neurologist.[2] By the time a client is sent to a neurologist or an ALS specialist, it can often be 1 or 2 years later, after numerous other visits to specialists while trying to find an accurate diagnosis.

Presentation

Clients can experience their first ALS symptom with any combination of symptoms: in an arm or leg, all in one side or on both sides, proximally or distally, in the bulbar regions of speech and swallowing, or in the respiratory system. Many clients have cramping and **fasciculations** (muscle twitching), especially when the muscle is overtired or overworked. If the client presents with primarily upper motor neuron signs at the time of diagnosis, the condition can be called primary lateral sclerosis (which is slower progressing) or upper motor predominant ALS. These clients have increased tone and spasticity, increased reflexes, and decreased balance/movement as their first symptoms. When a client has primarily lower motor neuron signs at the time of diagnosis, it is called progressive muscular atrophy or lower motor predominant ALS. These clients have weakness, low tone, atrophy, and decreased reflexes in all affected muscle groups. When a client has speech and swallowing deficits initially, it is called progressive bulbar palsy or bulbar predominant ALS. Sensation is not affected in persons with ALS, nor is hearing, sphincter muscle control, or gastrointestinal function. Vision and visual muscles can be affected in the very late stages of the disease as the eye muscles weaken. Cognition and behavior can be affected in approximately 50% of persons with ALS, especially with executive functioning, behavior and personality.[3] **Pseudobulbar affect,** or uncontrollable emotionality out of proportion to the situation, with laughing and/or crying, can be common. Some clients will experience depression and have difficulty with coping. A **frontotemporal dementia** (cognitive, behavioral, language changes) is associated with ALS and affects about 20% of clients.[3] Respiratory functioning, diaphragm functioning, and speech and swallowing are eventually affected in most people. ALS does not generally cause pain as a primary symptom, but rather secondarily by cramping, decreased ROM or stiffness, frozen shoulder, and pain from immobility.[4]

PROGRESSION AND LIFE EXPECTANCY

The life expectancy for most persons with ALS is on average 2 to 5 years from symptom onset, but some live less time and many survive much longer. Certainly, those with respiratory or swallowing symptoms early on will have more difficulty in a shorter period than clients with hand weakness as a first symptom. It generally is a rapidly progressing disease, but not in all cases, and typically the pace of change over time seen initially continues through the course of the disease. ALS is considered a fatal disease. Attendance at a quarterly multidisciplinary clinic has been proven in research to increase life expectancy, potentially due to the proactive care and aggressive symptom management.[5] The weakness from ALS is progressive, and eventually the client can only move his or her eyes. Ultimately, the eye muscles stop working, and the client is "locked in" where they have no ability to communicate or move, though their thinking and awareness may be intact.

Clients with respiratory weakness initially use **bilevel positive airway pressure (BiPAP),** volume ventilation (BiPAP-like settings on a ventilator) with a mask (Fig. 32-1) or nasal pillows (interface that covers only the nostrils), and some later in the progression also choose to get a ventilator with tracheostomy (a surgically created hole in the trachea with a tube connecting it to a ventilator to provide an alternate method for breathing). BiPAP differs from a continuous positive airway pressure (CPAP) machine used for sleep apnea in that the BiPAP device not only "pushes" the air, but "pulls" it as well. Many clients will receive a volume ventilator instead of BiPAP that has settings for use with a mask, and can easily transition with the same machine to full ventilation with tracheostomy as well. If chosen, ventilation with tracheostomy would be generally used 24 hours a day, and the client may or may not be able to speak or swallow once receiving it. Persons with ALS have diaphragm weakness, not an oxygen exchange issue, and so typically do not require supplemental oxygen unless they have an underlying chronic obstructive pulmonary disease (COPD) or other respiratory issue. They may have difficulty with **dyspnea** (shortness of breath) or **orthopnea** (shortness of breath with lying flat), which will require the use of respiratory support to sleep and eventually to use full time as well.

Decreased safe swallowing means a feeding tube will be recommended for most clients at some point. Initially, clients will have difficulty with dry or crunchy type food consistencies as well as thin liquids. Safe swallowing

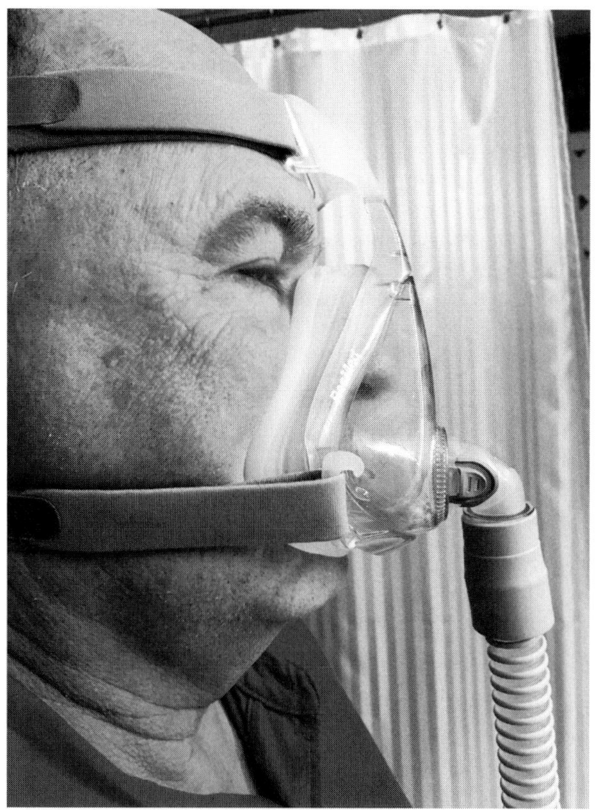

FIGURE 32-1. A client wearing a BiPAP mask for breathing.

strategies include a chin tuck, small bites and sips, thickening liquids, and avoiding problem foods that cause choking (see Chapter 12 for details). Many clients must change diet/liquid consistencies to softer foods and thicker liquids to minimize the risk for choking and aspiration. Most clients can have small tastes of food for pleasure even after getting the feeding tube. These amounts of food are so small that the person is tasting and smelling the food more than swallowing it. Proactive care means placing the feeding tube before the person loses excessive weight, is struggling to eat/drink, or is compromised in respiratory status. Many surgeons will not perform the feeding tube procedure when breathing status is too low, unless performing the tracheostomy at the same time, as there is a risk for difficulty with removal from surgical ventilator support. This means that some clients will get the feeding tube when respiration is beginning to change, but swallowing may not yet be compromised, especially because ALS has a known course. ALS is known to be **hypermetabolic** (increased metabolism and speed of processing food) in most people, and so maintaining a high-calorie diet can be important as well.[6] When combined with decreased ability to self-feed due to arm or hand weakness and slow or poor swallow, it can be difficult to consume enough calories; clients often lose weight quickly.

Due to progressive weakness, most clients with ALS will end up using a wheelchair of some sort. With leg/trunk weakness, the progression of equipment is typically from a cane to a rollator style walker to a power wheelchair, along with a manual or transport wheelchair as a backup. Other necessary equipment may include ankle-foot orthoses, hospital bed, patient lifter with sling, bathing and toileting equipment, and many other types of adaptive equipment and adaptations. Whichever power wheelchair is chosen must have significant long-term flexibility as the client's ability to control the chair will certainly change over time. A specialty seating clinic will have resources and knowledge to assist the client in choosing the appropriate equipment. See Chapter 15 for further details.

RESEARCH, MEDICAL TREATMENT, AND EXERCISE

Currently there are only two Food and Drug Administration (FDA)-approved drugs that affect the rate of progression of ALS, Rilutek® (riluzole) and Radicava® (edaravone), but many other drugs are in testing. Both medications are expensive and may be difficult to have covered by insurances. Neudexta® (dextromethorphan and quinidine combo) is a drug for pseudobulbar affect symptoms. Other medications are used for symptom management, such as depression, anxiety, pain, constipation, and cramping. Research is ongoing to find the cause and reason behind ALS as well as to decrease the rate of progression. Many research projects for persons with ALS are beginning to have a "fast track" with the FDA to test new ALS drugs more quickly. As per the FDA, "Fast track is a process designed to facilitate the development, and expedite the review of drugs to treat serious

TECHNOLOGY AND TRENDS

The Kinova® Jaco robotic arm is an amazing device that attaches to the client's power wheelchair and is controlled by the wheelchair joystick and two switches. It has movements in all planes, multiple joints, and three fingers for a three-jaw chuck grasp and release. It also has memory functions that allow the user to save steps for repetitive tasks such as self-feeding. Whichever way the client controls the wheelchair, be it hand, head array, foot joystick, or sip-and-puff control, he or she can control the robotic arm in the same manner. Therefore, the client is not limited in control over the robotic arm as long as he or she has some means to control the chair. Clients have used it for self-feeding, drinking, opening cupboards and the refrigerator, playing tug with the family dog, and grasp/release/reach of all sorts. Although it may be too costly for many clients, it may be achievable through fund raising, some private insurances, VA benefits, and vocational rehabilitation.

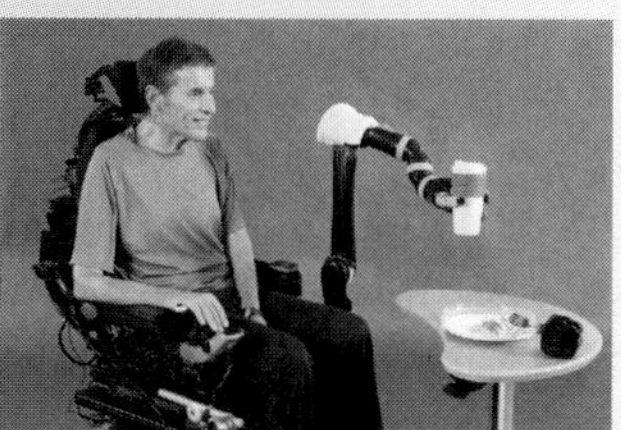

Client using robotic arm to drink and self-feed.

conditions and fill an unmet medical need."[7] Some drugs being tested for ALS also have "orphan" status, including "drugs which are defined as those intended for the safe and effective treatment, diagnosis or prevention of rare diseases/disorders that affect fewer than 200,000 people in the U.S., or that affect more than 200,000 persons but are not expected to recover the costs of developing and marketing a treatment drug."[7] These designations assist with getting drugs to testing and market faster.

Exercise studies, particularly related to the correct amount of exercise that clients with ALS should perform at the various stages of weakness, are ongoing. The current exercise standard at most ALS clinics is that exercise is acceptable when the muscle group is at least a 3+/5; the focus is on endurance, balance, and light resistance, instead of the "feel the burn" expected with maximal effort.[8]

Occupational Therapy Intervention

The occupational therapy (OT) practitioner is the multidisciplinary team member (with ALS teams worldwide, the term multidisciplinary is used instead of interdisciplinary) with much to offer the client with ALS. Many times, a client will not have a need for long-term ongoing therapy, but simply a short round of education and training, adaptation, safety, range of motion (ROM) exercises, and functional management for occupational performance. The client with ALS will not generally benefit from traditional strengthening exercises to build muscle, but may be able to maintain strength longer with careful exercise. OT goals may focus on increasing ROM to avoid pain and contractures, using adaptive equipment, or educating the client and family how to perform safe transfers. As a client who ambulates with a walker progresses in weakness to needing a power wheelchair, many other tasks can change as well. These may include transfers to the tub and toilet, getting safely in and out of bed and bed positioning, donning lower extremity (LE) clothing. The safe use of a power wheelchair in the home and community is also a consideration for these clients. A client with significant dominant hand/thumb weakness will have difficulty with writing, keyboarding, using the phone, self-feeding, cutting food, buttoning, shoe tying, key turning, bottom wiping, opening water bottles and jars, and many other tasks (see Chapter 14 on adaptive equipment). A client with one-sided UE and LE weakness will require hemi-dressing techniques and other equipment and adaptations similar to someone with one-sided weakness such as caused by a cerebrovascular accident (CVA) (see Chapter 33). Clients with fatigue and breathing difficulties will require energy conservation and work simplification as well as a mobility device to avoid further shortness of breath and fatigue. This same client may use a communication device and respiratory support as well. A client with significant shoulder weakness may require support in standing/bed/wheelchair, ROM education, techniques and equipment to avoid painful reaching, dressing adaptations, and adapted bathing and toilet hygiene.

For clients with less active movement, ROM, positioning in the bed, recliner, and wheelchair, as well as skin integrity are important. If clients cannot roll themselves in bed, a caregiver may need to assist. Some clients with a weak diaphragm will not lie flat or tilt back in the wheelchair for pressure relief because they have shortness of breath in that position. These clients may choose to sleep in a recliner or sleep with numerous pillows propping them up so they can stay somewhat upright while sleeping. Clients may also not tilt/recline back fully in the power wheelchair for pressure relief for the same reason. Because of the combination of sitting all day/night on their tailbone without good relief, pressure relief and skin management becomes even more critical due to an inability to off-load tissues, as well as potentially decreased nutrition from self-feeding, eating, and swallowing difficulties. Even though clients with ALS have intact sensation, they are at high risk for skin breakdown and pressure injuries from the combination of these issues.

So much of the OT treatment for clients with ALS depends on what sort of weakness the client has and how it is affecting him or her functionally. At an ALS clinic, traditionally the OT practitioner sees the client with ALS every 3 months for solving new problems and challenges, and so that OT practitioner may refer the client to home health or

OT Practitioner's Viewpoint

As an OT practitioner who works primarily with clients with progressive disorders, I have a unique and sometimes difficult job. Many other OT practitioners have asked how I can handle a job in which people die and no one "gets better." While the job has its daily challenges and I grieve for each life lost, I focus on the amazing ways I can help my clients. I find that OT treatment with these progressive diagnoses is very focused on function. I have options, tools, tricks, and ideas for nearly every problem clients and caregivers throw my way, and I keep them functioning at the highest level possible. Many times, clients will think they have to give up a cherished task or role, only to find out I have an adaptation. I had a gentleman who could not use his arms and needed to use his TV remote with his big toe. Having tried the large TV remotes without success, he came to me with the problem of tiny remote buttons and a large big toe. Together, we created the "Toetroller," a toe splint that attaches with Velcro® on his big toe, and has a downward pointer that can hit the individual buttons. Problem solved, all with scrap splinting material and Velcro®. It changed his life, and I was glad to assist. ~ Amber L. Ward, MS, OTR/L, BCPR, ATP/SMS

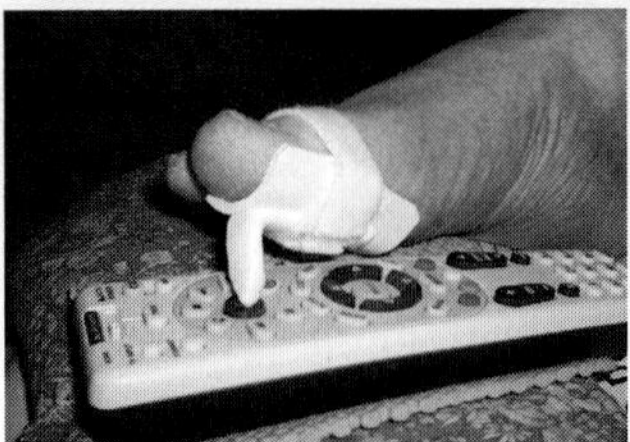

The Toetroller.

outpatient OT for further education and training. The home health OTA working with the client with ALS may focus on home safety, tub/shower and toilet transfers and equipment, positioning and bed mobility, activities of daily living (ADL) and instrumental activities of daily living (IADL) adaptation and performance, and ROM. A client with ALS might go to an outpatient setting to work on decreasing pain and increasing ROM in a sore shoulder as well.

A general guideline for exercise early in the disease process would include performing only submaximal resistive exercise, with a focus on lighter weights, versus heavy weights. Aerobic exercise, such as swimming, walking, or biking, can be good choices to maintain heart health, general fitness, and ROM. Generally, aerobic exercise is to tolerance. The exercise should not tire clients to the point where functionality or balance is compromised or they risk a fall due to fatigue. Fatigue can be a major problem for clients with ALS, and many have difficulty changing routines for fatigue management and energy conservation. A focus on maintaining full ROM is important, especially because as the muscles weaken, the active range also decreases.[8]

Many ALS Association (ALSA) and Muscular Dystrophy Association (MDA) clinics have access to a loan closet, which can assist the OTA from any setting (not necessarily associated with the clinic) to provide equipment, such as a bedside commode or shower seat, as required for a client with ALS. The OTA should also refer the client to a seating clinic for a specialized power wheelchair with flexibility in features that will meet the client's long-term needs.

MULTIPLE SCLEROSIS

Multiple sclerosis (MS) is a disorder of the central nervous system that affects the myelin coating around nerve fibers and causes plaques to form in the brain and spinal cord.[9] The location of the damage in the brain and/or spinal cord determines the type and severity of the symptoms. MS is more common in Caucasians of Northern European ancestry, in women, and those with low levels of vitamin D. Smoking also increases the risk for developing MS.[10]

In order for the physician to make a diagnosis of MS, the client must meet all of the following criteria:

- Have evidence of damage in at least two separate areas of the CNS, which includes the brain, spinal cord, and optic nerves on magnetic resonance imaging (MRI) with contrast
- Have evidence that the damages occurred at least 1 month apart
- Must have ruled out all other possible diagnoses through MRI, blood tests, and clinical testing[11]

Progression, Life Expectancy, and Symptoms

In general, MS is not considered a fatal disease, and most people with MS have a normal or near-normal life expectancy. In fairly rare cases, complications of MS such as pneumonia can shorten life, though many complications are preventable or manageable. In very rare instances of rapid-onset, MS can be fatal. Because MS lesions may appear in any area of the brain or spinal cord, MS symptoms can vary widely in location and severity. MS can affect every system including muscle dysfunction, sensory changes, visual changes, cognitive and behavioral symptoms, gastrointestinal and sexual effects, and many more. See Table 32-1 for a listing of MS symptoms and treatments. MS is separated into four types, and clients may move between types as the disease progresses over the years (Table 32-2). Stress, heat, and emotional or physical trauma can exacerbate the disease and cause relapses. These relapses, also known as exacerbations or flare-ups, are periods of new or worsening symptoms that generally last a few days to weeks or months. For some clients, the remissions (improvement) mean they go back to their prior level, and others do not regain full function. While pregnant, most women with MS have fewer relapses, even though most MS medications are not safe to take during pregnancy. After

TABLE 32-1 Multiple Sclerosis Symptoms and Treatment

MORE COMMON SYMPTOMS	OT TREATMENT
Fatigue	Education and training for energy conservation, work simplification, sitting to cook, and sitting to complete dressing and grooming
Weakness	Encourage submaximal strengthening exercises if in an exacerbation/remission cycle; encourage use of adaptive equipment and compensatory techniques.
Numbness/tingling	Teach safety considerations for hot/sharp items.
Dizziness/vertigo	Teach safety awareness when dizzy.
Sexual problems	Help explore options for safe and fulfilling sexual experiences.
Emotional changes	Suggest counseling and/or support group; encourage staying active.
Visual changes	Suggest working with a neuro-ophthalmologist for vision or OT practitioner specializing in vision rehabilitation; adapt for changes in acuity (e.g., with magnifiers).
Pain	Suggest relaxation techniques and ways to work through pain.

Continued

TABLE 32-1 Multiple Sclerosis Symptoms and Treatment (continued)

MORE COMMON SYMPTOMS	OT TREATMENT
Walking difficulties	Teach about safety and balance awareness, working on making the home safer, and wheelchair or walker use.
Bladder dysfunction	Encourage discussion with physician or urologist for medications and treatments.
Spasticity	Encourage ROM, stretching, AROM, weight-bearing, and use of medications.
Bowel problems	Medications; teach bowel program to help avoid accidents.
Cognitive changes	Teach about modification of home environment and safety considerations, alarms, medication reminders, phone use, calendars, and memory strategies. Refer for driving evaluation as needed.
Depression	Encourage being active and seeking psychological assistance and volunteer or group activities.
LESS COMMON SYMPTOMS	
Speech problems	Refer to speech language pathologist for communication options, use iPad® text to speech; write down words.
Tremors	Encourage use of Liftware Steady™ for self-feeding and modifications of ADLs.
Seizures	Encourage medication management, safety, and no driving.
Swallowing problems	Refer to speech language pathologist; use chin tuck, thickened liquids; may need modified barium swallow test for safe swallowing; avoid certain textures.
Itching	Medication, relaxation
Hearing loss	Refer to audiologist.
Breathing problems	Refer to respiratory therapist or pulmonologist; teach about energy conservation, work simplification techniques, management of shortness of breath with pursed-lip breathing, and taking rest breaks.
Headaches	Medication, relaxation, massage

TABLE 32-2 Multiple Sclerosis Types[10,11]

Relapsing-remitting MS • The most common disease course • Characterized by clearly defined relapses/exacerbations of worsening neurological function that are followed by partial or complete recovery periods (remissions), during which symptoms improve partially or completely • Approximately 85% of people with MS are initially diagnosed with relapsing-remitting MS.	Secondary-progressive MS • Follows after the relapsing-remitting course • Most people who are initially diagnosed with relapsing-remitting MS will eventually transition to secondary progressive, which means that the disease will begin to progress more steadily (although not necessarily more quickly), with or without relapses.
Primary-progressive MS (PPMS) • Characterized by steadily worsening neurological function from the beginning • Although the rate of progression may vary over time with occasional plateaus and temporary, minor improvements, there are no distinct relapses or remissions. • About 10% of people with MS are diagnosed with PPMS.	Progressive-relapsing MS • Least common of the four disease courses • Characterized by steadily progressing disease from the beginning and occasional exacerbations along the way • May or may not experience some recovery after these attacks; the disease continues to progress without remissions.

giving birth, relapse rates tend to rise in the first 3 to 6 months, and the risk for relapse is estimated to be 20% to 40%.[12]

Research, Medical Treatment, and Exercise

Numerous drugs are available to slow the progression of MS, prevent or reduce the severity of relapses, and decrease the severity of its symptoms. However, currently no drug exists that can cure MS. In addition to the MS drugs taken orally, by injection or intravenously, physicians often prescribe intravenous steroids for serious relapses, followed by oral steroids.[13] Clients may also take medications to manage specific symptoms, such as depression, spasticity, pain, and bladder dysfunction.

Studies of people living with MS have shown that exercise can help combat fatigue and depression, improve strength, and result in increased participation in social activities.[14] Many people receive occupational and physical therapy to regain strength after an exacerbation with relapsing/remitting MS.[14] Despite the often unpredictable course of MS, exercise programs designed to increase cardiorespiratory fitness, muscle strength, and mobility provide benefits that improve a client's quality of life while reducing the risk for secondary disorders such as pain and balance issues.[15] Most studies recommend close supervision from the physician or practitioner and subsequent modification of any exercise program to address concerns with overheating, fatigue, balance, and other medical management.[15] Many clients with MS are sensitive to overheating and require a cooling vest or other ways to stay cool in the heat, as heat can cause an exacerbation or relapse (Fig. 32-2). Some clients with MS simply avoid going outside in the heat, which may limit participation in valued occupations, or some chose to move to cooler climates.

Occupational Therapy Treatment

OT is often prescribed by the physician to improve a client's level of function after an MS exacerbation or due to a problem caused by a progression, and this may typically occur through inpatient rehabilitation, outpatient rehabilitation, or home health therapy. Treatment will depend on the specific symptoms seen, but often focuses on adapting ADL and IADL for performance skills, accommodating for strength, balance, pain, and safety issues, as well as cognitive/visual management, all resulting from the relapse or progression. Precautions for any program are to avoid overheating, which can occur both indoors and outdoors, as it can lead to further exacerbation or worsening of symptoms. Another precaution includes performing only submaximal resistive exercise, with a focus on lighter weights, versus heavy weights. Generally, aerobic exercise is to tolerance. Fatigue can be a major problem as well for persons with MS, and when first diagnosed, many have difficulty changing their routines to manage fatigue and conserve energy.

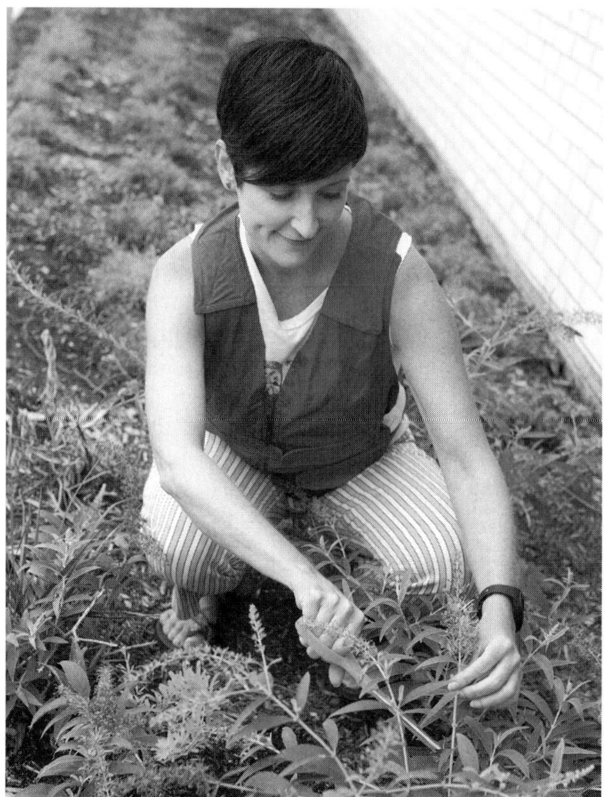

FIGURE 32-2. A person with multiple sclerosis wearing a cooling vest to enable outside leisure pursuits during hot weather.

Adaptive equipment and techniques may be required to increase a client's independence for desired occupational performance. Techniques and equipment, such as sitting to don pants using a reacher or dressing stick when leg weakness or stiffness is present, or using large-handled utensils for self-feeding when hand weakness is present, may be offered. Sitting on a stool can assist with balance and fatigue management in the kitchen and bathroom during functional tasks. A shower seat may be needed for fatigue management earlier than for impaired balance, and clients with MS should avoid long, hot showers due to the effects of overheating. Visual and cognitive strategies are important to address as well, such as managing double vision or placing a call list on a phone for clients with a memory issue. Many clients with MS want to continue working and may need assistance with an alternative mouse/keyboard at work or a driving evaluation for adaptive options. OT services can also be recommended for a wheelchair seating or mobility equipment evaluation, home modification recommendations, and self-feeding/swallowing performance. OT services prescribed are often for management of changes in occupational performance skills due to a progression of the disease. In these cases, the treatment is generally short in duration and focuses on adaptive equipment and techniques as well as ROM/stretching, pain management, safety, and accommodation. Examples might be treatment by the OTA for management of shoulder pain and ROM caused by weakness, use of a bottom wiper for toilet hygiene due to hand and arm weakness, or a home safety assessment to advise about eliminating throw rugs, having appropriate lighting, and installing grab bars in the bathroom. At times with relapsing/remitting MS, the client can improve after the relapse to close to the prior level of functioning, and the OT practitioner may use a biomechanical model instead of focusing on strictly compensatory methods. Generally with primary and secondary progressive MS, once the strength is lost due to steady disease progression, it cannot be regained.

The client with MS may initially require mobility equipment, such as a cane, walker, or wheelchair, for fatigue management, energy conservation, and mobility, and later may use a manual wheelchair or scooter for longer distances. Eventually, many clients will use a power wheelchair full time for all mobility, pressure relief,

THE OLDER ADULT

About 4.6% to 9.4% of adults with MS who are diagnosed after 55 years of age tend to have a more progressive course with more motor impairments and a poorer prognosis overall.[16] The average age of onset of ALS is between 40 and 70 years of age.[17] The peak incidence rates of PD are between 70 and 79 years of age.[18] Dementia is more common in those older than 65 years of age.[19] These statistics are noteworthy, as many progressive diseases affect the older adult, and many times symptoms are attributed to the effects of aging instead of to a specific disorder. If an older adult has balance difficulties or memory problems, the first thought of the primary care physician may not be PD or AD, therefore, diagnosis and treatment may be delayed. For example, a client may go to the primary care doctor for back pain and leg weakness, who then refers the client to an orthopedic physician. This doctor orders a Computerized tomography (CT) of the spine, and finds spinal disc degeneration. Surgery is performed, and after a period of recovery, the client's condition does not improve. The orthopedic surgeon then refers the client to a neurologist who diagnoses ALS. This scenario is all too common, and some clients may have unnecessary surgeries, procedures, and treatments from inaccurate diagnoses. Clients who are older may have numerous chronic conditions that interfere with the diagnostic process, and may wait longer to be diagnosed based on their complexity. Older adults also tend to react differently to medications than their younger peers, and may take more medications overall, increasing the likelihood of drug interactions. Some older adults have fewer personal and financial resources to manage their progressive disease process, and when they live alone, may face difficulty staying home as the disease progresses. Many times the OT practitioner can assist to keep clients in their homes as long as possible by adapting for occupational performance and addressing safety and functional mobility.

and positioning. Since many insurances require 5-7 years from the purchased mobility device, the OTA should refer the client to a seating clinic for full evaluation and management.

HUNTINGTON'S DISEASE

Huntington's disease (HD) is a neurodegenerative genetic disease which causes the death of brain cells. Symptoms generally begin to appear from 30 to 50 years of age, but the disease may affect those as young as 2 years of age and as old as 80 years of age.[20] Complications such as pneumonia, heart disease, and physical injury from falls reduce life expectancy to around 20 years from the point when symptoms begin.[20] Suicide accounts for about 9% of deaths.[20] HD currently has no cure, with only symptom management at this time.

Progression, Life Expectancy, and Symptoms

HD is generally broken down into three stages: an early stage with subtle changes in mood, movement, and cognition; a midstage with numerous ADL/IADL difficulties, jerky and uncoordinated movement, cognitive, and behavioral changes; and a late stage in which the client requires 24/7 total care. Clients with HD may experience varying degrees of difficulty in the various stages, including:

- Cognitive: Planning abilities, insight, judgment/reasoning, memory, creative thinking, and diminished orientation
- Psychological: Denial about the disorder, anger and grief about changes, behavioral problems, such as attention seeking, and psychotic and abusive behavior
- Physical: Poor coordination, poor balance, ataxia (lack of coordination), **chorea** (rapid, jerky, forceful movements), decreased stamina and endurance, and **dyspraxia** (inability to link thought to movement)

Initial symptoms may include involuntary movements, alterations in quality of voluntary movement, difficulty with concentration, or changes in behavior (Table 32-3).[21] Onset and progression varies widely from person to person. Serious loss of weight can accompany the movement disorder portions of the disease due to constant movement, and getting enough nutrition can be challenging due to difficult self-feeding with chorea and decreased muscle control.[21] Up to 98% of clients may exhibit neuropsychiatric symptoms during the disease course, the most common being dysphoria (general dissatisfaction with life), agitation, irritability, apathy, and anxiety.[22] A small percentage exhibit more significant symptoms such as those similar to paranoid schizophrenia, as well as delusions, obsessions and compulsions, and hallucinations.[23]

For HD, genetic testing can be performed if there is a family history of the disease before symptoms appear and can confirm whether a person or embryo has the genes that cause the disease. Diagnosis can be made following the appearance of symptoms consistent with HD, and genetic testing can confirm a diagnosis in a person with no family history (either none available or a new mutation in a gene). Autosomal dominant mutation (50% of children will inherit the disease) of a gene called *HTT* causes an abnormally long version of the protein *Huntingtin*, which gradually damages the brain, although the reasons are not fully understood.[24] HD usually runs its fully fatal course in 10 to 30 years with an average of 20 years.[25] It has been observed that the earlier in life the symptoms of HD appear, the faster the disease progresses. A client who is bedridden during the final stages of Huntington's disease often dies from complications such as heart failure or pneumonia.[26]

RESEARCH, MEDICAL TREATMENT, AND EXERCISE

Medical care for those with HD is typically symptom management, and medication management for psychotic and mental health symptoms as well as for the movement disorder. Medications are available to suppress involuntary movements, but they produce side effects, and typically,

TABLE 32-3 Huntington's Disease[21,26]

PROBLEMS WITH HUNTINGTON'S	SYMPTOMS	OT TREATMENT	TREATMENT RATIONALE
Involuntary movements	• Chorea (jerking or twitching movements) • Akathisia (motor restlessness or need for constant movement) • Dystonia (sustained posturing of a body part)	Stabilize proximally to offer some distal control. Offer safe ways to move and be restless.	Proximal or near stability allows the distal limb to have potentially increased control, such as placing the elbow on the table for more stability during meals. Safe movements may be in bed or on a mat on the floor when restless, so there is nothing hard to kick or be injured by.
Voluntary movement problems	• Akinesia (delayed initiation or reaction) • Bradykinesia (slowness of movement) • Hand-eye coordination • Difficulty with smaller movements • Impairment in modulation of force of movement • Incoordination of movement • Alteration of rhythmical/ repetitive movements	Give extra time to initiate; give cues as needed. Adaptations for fine motor control difficulties; use buttonhook, Oelastic shoelaces, zipper pull. Use plastic ware for eating (less hard and less breakable).	Extra time may be as much as 90 extra seconds, and extra cues may assist as well. Adaptive equipment may assist with fine motor control problems. Note that decreased cognition may also affect learning of new equipment. Plastic plates and cups can survive being dropped and are lighter and safer.
Cognitive symptoms	• Difficulty controlling impulses • Difficulty with concentration, attention, and multitasking • Perseveration (repeating the same thought), decreased initiation (beginning or ending activities), irritability, and outbursts • Short-term memory with new learning	Memory: Strategies such as lists, phone reminders and alarms, and calendars Attention: Perform difficult tasks in quiet setting without distraction.	Memory strategies can mean the difference in being able to stay home alone and manage things such as medications and turning off a stove appropriately. Decreasing distraction will increase the potential for concentration and success.
Psychiatric symptoms	• Anxiety, depression • Blunted affect (reduced display of emotions), aggression • Egocentrism • Compulsive behavior • Addictions like gambling and alcoholism, hypersexuality • Psychiatric disorders	Refer for medication management, counseling	Psychiatrists can offer medication management, and psychologists or social workers can offer counseling. These are generally out of the OT realm, except for basic empathetic understanding and holistic care during functional task management.
Other symptoms	• Muscle atrophy • Cardiac failure • Diabetes • Osteoporosis • Testicular atrophy	Accommodation for muscle weakness and atrophy with adaptive equipment and techniques	Adaptive equipment and techniques can assist with progressive weakness/ atrophy and are the clear focus for the OTA. Education on safe ADL/IADL performance for clients with diabetes, osteoporosis, and cardiac issues will be important.

clients with HD are less bothered by the involuntary movements as they are by the side effects. Tetrabenazine (Xenazine®) is approved by the FDA to treat chorea associated with HD but may increase the risk for depression and suicidal thoughts or behavior.[26] Exciting studies are ongoing that involve testing drugs that reduce the amount of the huntingtin protein, and which may slow disease progression.

Exercise is considered a possibility for the client with HD in the early stages, as long as balance is functional enough to avoid falls, the client does not "overdo it," and potential cardiac issues are monitored. Therapy and exercise are typically to prevent loss of function for as long as possible and to learn to compensate for changes in strength, balance and coordination. Research on rehabilitation for the person with HD is ongoing; for example, Norwegian scientists observed that rehabilitation and exercise lead to improvements in balance, walking ability, and physical quality of life in clients with HD.[27] The results of a number of these studies support the idea that a sustained program of regular exercise and rehabilitative therapy are of benefit to clients with HD.[27]

Occupational Therapy Treatment

Treatment by the OTA will vary, depending on the client's needs and goals, the severity of the symptoms, and the client's stage as below. Many of the symptoms begin in a mild fashion such as minor involuntary movements or slightly slurred speech, and progress to more significant deficits such as complete lack of voluntary control, and limited speech and swallowing.

EARLY STAGE

With motor movement, clients with HD in the early stage will display involuntary twitching in their fingers, toes, and face, and decreased coordination during occupational performance.[29] Clients need a consistent daily routine incorporating the use of lists, calendars, and notes to assist with organization. The client may have difficulty coping with changes to routine, low motivation, difficulty organizing daily tasks, and impaired decision making. Depression, irritability, and disinhibition are common, and some clients experience hypersexuality, which can cause relationship problems.[29,30]

The OTA may teach the caregiver to break tasks down into simple steps, ask questions with yes/no or a list of choices, and label items around the house with their names and functions. Clients who are still working will need to reduce outside stimuli in the office or working environment to concentrate. Home safety is also a priority due to balance and tripping concerns with rugs and clutter. Clients with HD may need to be assessed for safety during cooking and lawn care, for example. An exercise routine can be established that focuses on safe ways to move and stay as fit as possible within the balance and cardiac restrictions. At this stage, the speed of processing may be slower, and speech may begin to be slurred. Cues and choices for decision making may assist clients with early cognitive deficits. Clients will have difficulty learning and retaining motor memories, therefore retraining a client to perform a safe transfer technique or bathing program may not be retained without cues.[29]

MID STAGE

In the mid stage, clients will have difficulty driving (motor as well as cognitive) and managing work and household tasks. Clients with HD often lack initiation, therefore, a caregiver who is helping a client with HD during the midstage of the disease may suggest a task or activity and offer help to get started, as well as make lists for daily hygiene tasks. The caregiver may want to pair items, such as a shirt and pants that match, for easier dressing and grooming. The client must build in rest periods for fatigue management, and use items such as a shower mitt, electric razor, or built-up toothbrush handle, for managing fine motor control problems. Self-feeding and eating is especially difficult for clients at this stage due to motor control challenges such as ataxia and chorea as well as swallowing. The OTA can suggest using a sturdy chair that will not tip; clients can wrap their legs around chair legs and keep their elbows on the table for proximal stability and to decrease extra movements while self-feeding (Fig. 32-3). Adaptive equipment for toileting and bathing safety will be required due to balance and uncontrollable movements. Items such as a Toilevator® to raise the height of the toilet in a stable way, or a tub bench with suction cup feet will make these tasks safer. The early stage behavioral concerns continue such as disinhibition and irritability, and some clients show increased

EVIDENCE-BASED PRACTICE

An article published in 2015 noted the effect of multidisciplinary treatment for 9 months on the brain structure and cognition of clients with HD. These clients received weekly in-clinic physical therapy exercise program consisting of supervised aerobic and resistance exercises for 1 hour each week, a home-based exercise program involving self-directed muscle strengthening and fine motor exercises to be done for 1 hour, three times per week, and OT, which consisted of a variety of paper-and-pencil, verbal planning, memory, and problem-solving exercises designed to enhance cognition and executive function.[28] The researchers found evidence of increased gray matter volume in the right caudate and bilaterally in the dorsolateral prefrontal cortex, as well as an improvement in verbal learning and memory after 9 months of multidisciplinary rehabilitation.[28] These findings "collectively indicate that neuroplasticity may still be present in HD and amenable to multidisciplinary rehabilitation."[28] Many clients and caregivers may feel that there is nothing to be done for the relentless progression of HD. It has been proven in this exciting research and others that positive changes can occur, which may preserve functional occupational performance in these clients for longer.

Cruickshank, T. M., Thompson, J. A., Domínguez, D. J. F., Reyes, A. P., Bynevelt, M., Georgiou-Karistianis, N., ... & Ziman, M. R. (2015). The effect of multidisciplinary rehabilitation on brain structure and cognition in Huntington's disease: An exploratory study. Brain and Behavior, *5(2), e00312. http://doi.org/10.1002/brb3.312*

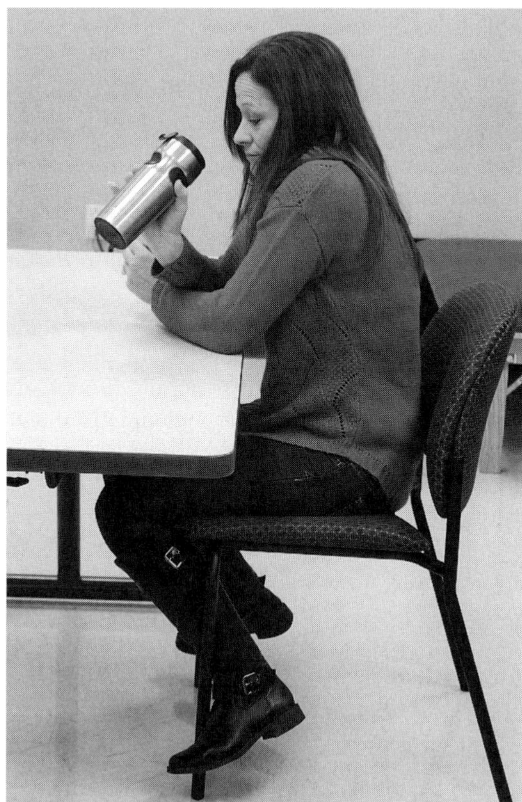

FIGURE 32-3. Person prepares for self-feeding using techniques that give her extra stability. She has her legs hooked around the chair and her arms stabilized on the table so that she can drink.

apathy as the disease continues, losing interest in previously desired activities.[30]

LATE STAGE

The client in the late stage can no longer manage basic ADL tasks, and requires assistance for most tasks. Motor symptoms are severe. By this point, choreatic movements have usually stopped, although some clients continue to experience severe chorea.[30] Instead, clients generally have the greatest difficulty with voluntary movements, and often experience **rigidity** (tightness of muscles on both sides of the joint), **dystonia** (muscle contractions that cause slow repetitive movements or abnormal postures), and **bradykinesia** (slowness of movement).[30] One goal is to avoid skin breakdown by padding body parts in both the wheelchair and in the bed. Specialized wheelchair seating will be required for the client through a seating clinic. Bed positioning will also be important for contracture management as well as comfort and the avoidance of skin issues including pressure injuries. The OTA may fabricate orthotics and perform PROM to avoid contractures, as well as education and training for the caregivers to perform PROM. The orthoses will need to be padded to maintain ROM without compromising skin integrity. Cognitive impairments can be a significant issue, but most clients with HD will understand speech and recognize loved ones.[30] Between "4% to 11% of clients will experience psychosis with auditory and visual hallucinations in this stage."[30] Many clients have difficulty thinking and communicating clearly, so decisions about end-of-life care often fall to physicians and caregivers unless there are specific advanced directives already established. Advanced directives are legal documents that note who is in charge of medical decision making if the client is unable (medical power of attorney) as well as what treatments are desired at the end of life (living will).

PARKINSON'S DISEASE

As many as 1 million people in the United States live with Parkinson's disease (PD), which is more than the combined number of people diagnosed with ALS, MS, and muscular dystrophies.[31] Approximately 60,000 Americans are diagnosed with PD each year, and this number does not reflect the thousands of cases that go undetected. Men are one and a half times more likely to have PD than women.[31] The root cause of PD is currently unknown, and many experts think it is caused by a combination of genetic and environmental factors, which may vary from person to person. In some people, genetic factors may play a primary role; in others, illness, an increase in certain proteins, an environmental toxin, or another event may contribute to PD.[31] Scientists know there is neuron death associated with PD, especially in the substantia nigra (part of the basal ganglia in the midbrain), but are unsure of the trigger that starts the cell death process.[32]

To diagnose PD, the physician takes a thorough neurological history and performs a physical examination. Because no standard diagnostic tests for PD exist, the diagnosis rests on the clinical information provided by the person with PD and the findings of the neurological examination.[31] Other diagnoses can also cause some of the symptoms of PD, such as essential tremor (tremors in hands, head, arms, voice, legs), multisystem atrophy (tremor, rigidity, loss of coordination, speech problems), corticobasal ganglionic degeneration (rigidity, poor balance, dystonia, dysphasia), progressive supranuclear palsy (apathy, masklike face, decreased balance, slowed movements, decreased cognition), and medication/toxic causes.[31,32]

Progression, Life Expectancy, and Symptoms

PD has a generally normal life expectancy, is slowly progressive, and is not considered a fatal disease. The progression of PD symptoms can take 20 years or even longer, but the rate of progression varies from person to person. Clinically, the disease process is broken up into five stages that can assist with understanding its progression.[33] To give clients an idea about how far their disease has progressed, many physicians use the five-stage Hoehn and Yahr scale for the staging of PD, which is broken down into the following stages:

- **Stage one:** Symptoms affect only one side of the body.
- **Stage two:** Symptoms begin affecting both sides of the body, but balance is still intact.

- **Stage three:** Symptoms are mild to moderate and balance is impaired, but the person can still function independently.
- **Stage four:** Symptoms cause severe disability, but clients can still walk or stand without assistance.
- **Stage five:** Symptoms cause the client to become wheelchair-bound or bedridden, unless assisted.[34]

The Unified Parkinson's Disease Rating Scale (UPDRS) is more complicated than the Hoehn and Yahr scale and takes into account the client's cognitive and other nonmotor symptoms.[35] Other scales separate the symptoms into mild, moderate, and severe, and each stage can last many years.[31]

Mild PD is characterized by the following:

- Movement symptoms may be inconvenient, but do not affect daily activities
- Movement symptoms, often tremor, occur on one side of the body.
- Friends may notice changes in a person's posture, walking ability, or facial expression.
- PD medications suppress movement symptoms effectively.
- Regular exercise improves and maintains mobility, flexibility, ROM, and balance, and also reduces depression and constipation.

Moderate PD is characterized by the following:

- Movement symptoms occur on both sides of the body.
- The body moves more slowly.
- Trouble with balance and coordination may develop.
- "Freezing" episodes—when the feet feel stuck to the ground—may occur.
- PD medications may "wear off" between doses.
- PD medications may cause side effects, including **dyskinesias** (involuntary movements).
- Regular exercise continues to be important for good mobility and balance.
- OT practitioners may provide strategies for maintaining independence.

Advanced PD is characterized by the following:

- Client has great difficulty walking; in wheelchair or bed most of the day.
- Client is unable to live alone.
- Client needs assistance with all daily activities.
- Cognitive problems may be prominent, including hallucinations and delusions.
- Balancing the benefits of medications with their side effects becomes more challenging.[31]

The life expectancy for PD is not shortened by the disease itself, but certain symptoms can lead to death, including serious falls, pneumonia from aspiration and immobility, and choking from decreased swallowing. The four hallmark symptoms seen with PD include the following:

- Tremor of the hands, arms, legs, jaw, or face
- Bradykinesia or slowness of movement
- Rigidity or stiffness of the limbs and trunk
- Postural instability or impaired balance and coordination; may fall backward, or sideways when turning

The tremors are generally seen at rest or when relaxed, although certainly intention tremors (purposeful movement toward a target) and postural tremors (when holding a position against gravity) can also be seen in the PD population. Table 32-4 presents other common motor and nonmotor symptoms of PD. Many researchers believe that nonmotor symptoms may precede motor symptoms—and a Parkinson's diagnosis—by years.[36] The most recognizable early nonmotor symptoms include loss of sense of smell, constipation, rapid eye movement (REM) behavior disorder (a sleep disorder), mood disorders, urinary urgency, and orthostatic hypotension (low blood pressure when standing up). Some or all of these may be present before the hallmark signs of PD are exhibited. In 10%-65% of persons with PD, a lack of norepinephrine can cause a neurogenic orthostatic hypotension (nOH), with feeling faint and dizzy after standing short periods. Most clients have a forward and stooped posture, and some clients may exhibit pseudobulbar affect as well.[31]

RESEARCH, MEDICAL TREATMENT, AND EXERCISE

Aggregates, or clusters of specific substances within brain cells called Lewy bodies, are microscopic markers of PD.[36] Researchers believe that Lewy bodies hold an important clue to the cause of PD. Although many substances are found within Lewy bodies, scientists are most concerned with the protein alpha-synuclein because it is found in clumps within all Lewy bodies, and the cells cannot break it down. This is currently an important focus among PD researchers.[36] Other areas of emerging research include stem cell implantation as a treatment technique, which are in clinical trials in humans with PD, and gene-modifying therapy. Gene-modifying therapy has three approaches: to increase dopamine production, to adjust the excitatory or inhibitory pathways of the brain, and to use growth hormones to slow progression or even reverse the disease process.[39] To date, "gene therapy for Parkinson's disease has been administered by drilling a hole in each side of the skull and then injecting the selected dose of the viral vector (a virus containing the gene) into the desired brain region (either putamen or subthalamic nucleus) using image-guided surgical techniques."[39] While it is emerging as a potential future treatment option, stem cell therapy and related research have a long way to go.

An increasing number of medications can assist with management of some PD symptoms, but those can lose effectiveness over time or have an increased risk for side effects as the amount of medication required increases. Some medications also have significant side effects, such as additional movement and coordination problems, which increase as the medication amounts increase. Three surgical procedures that may be performed on clients with PD are thalamotomy, pallidotomy, and deep brain stimulation.

TABLE 32-4 Common Motor and Nonmotor Symptoms in Parkinson's Disease[31,37,38]

MOTOR SYMPTOMS	NON-MOTOR SYMPTOMS
Freezing (temporary inability to move)	Sleep disturbances
Masklike facial expression	Constipation
Festination—Short, accelerating steps, often on tiptoe when walking	Bladder problems
Dystonia—Sustained muscle contractions cause twisting and repetitive movements or abnormal postures	Excessive saliva
Impaired gross motor coordination	Weight loss or gain
Akathisia (a state of agitation, distress, and restlessness)	Vision and dental problems
Difficulty swallowing	Fatigue and loss of energy
Cramping	Depression, fear, and anxiety
Micrographia—Small handwriting	Skin problems (oily, flaking, dry, excessive sweating)
Unwanted acceleration of gait or voice	Cognitive issues (memory, slowed thinking, dementia in some cases)
Stooped posture with a tendency to lean forward, especially over a walker	Impulsive behaviors
Impaired fine motor dexterity and motor coordination	Sexual problems (ejaculation, erection, orgasm)
Poverty of movement (e.g., decreased arm swing during ambulation)	
Speech problems—Softness of voice or slurred speech caused by lack of muscle control; may talk quickly as well; generally speak in a monotone voice	
Sexual dysfunction—Weakness, poor control	
Drooling—Due to decreased oral-motor control	

In thalamotomy, the goal of the surgery is to permanently end tremors or other involuntary movement by placing a small lesion in the thalamus. Clients who receive the most benefit from thalamotomy are usually younger adults with PD with tremors predominantly, and one-sided (or mainly one-sided) symptoms. However, the effects of thalamotomy on the other main symptoms of PD are much less predictable and may in some cases cause worsening of bradykinesia.[40]

In pallidotomy, the goal is to "abolish drug-induced dyskinesias, tremor, rigidity, and bradykinesia by placing a lesion in the ventral posterior globus pallidus."[40] Only clients with treatment-resistant PD that has clearly responded to dopamine replacement therapy in the past would be considered candidates for pallidotomy.

Deep brain stimulation (DBS) is a surgical procedure in which electrodes are inserted into the specific spots in the brain that are involved in motor function. A device called an impulse generator (IPG), which is similar to a pacemaker, is implanted under the client's collarbone to provide electrical impulses to the electrodes[31] (Fig. 32-4). For many people, DBS can dramatically relieve some symptoms and improve quality of life. It is most effective in clients with tremors for whom medication is having side effects. Studies show benefits lasting at least 5 years.[31] Although all three surgeries can have dramatic results, they are not appropriate for every person with PD, and the disease still continues to progress despite the treatment.

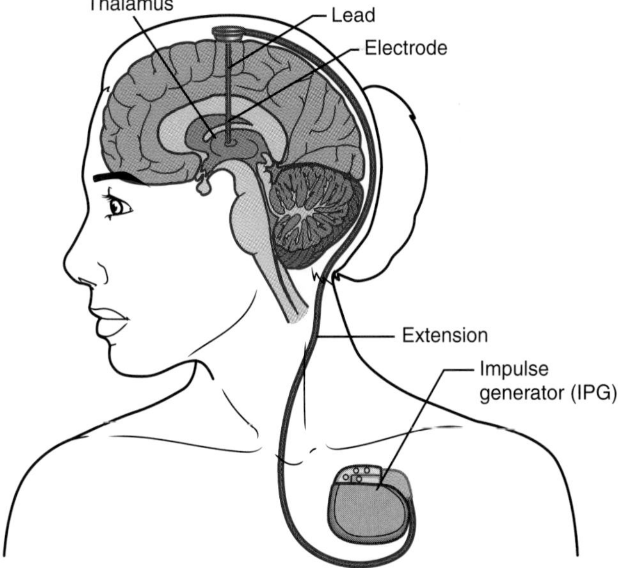

FIGURE 32-4. Deep brain stimulation sends electrical impulses to areas of the brain thought to be causing the movement problems.

For clients with PD, exercising may increase muscle strength, flexibility, and balance. Exercise can also improve well-being and reduce depression or anxiety. Exercises such as walking, swimming, dancing, water aerobics, or stretching may be beneficial.[36] For example, numerous studies have noted that clients have shown improvements following the initiation of dance therapy. These improvements from the dancing were seen in balance—especially moving backward, position and awareness of self in space, rising from a chair, 6-minute walk test, and other formalized tests.[41] A precaution during all exercise activities would be to account for balance deficits to keep the client safe.

Occupational Therapy Treatment

Certainly, treatment the OTA provides will vary depending on the individual needs of the client and caregivers, the severity and types of symptoms, the functional effect of symptoms on the client, and the present stage of the disease.

MILD PARKINSON'S TREATMENT

For clients with mild PD, regular exercise improves and maintains mobility, flexibility, ROM, and balance, and can assist with maintaining the ability to perform functional tasks. Most people do not need or seek OT in this stage. However, programs called LSVT BIG® and LSVT LOUD® exist that work to increase clients' motor control, fluidity, and strength with both movement and speech. Clients with PD tend to make smaller and smaller movements with walking and writing, as well as quieter/faster sounds with less mouth movement when speaking. BIG® focuses on making larger movements, as well as balance and motor control, and is often run by OT practitioners or physical therapists (Fig. 32-5). LOUD® focuses on speaking loudly, clearly, and more slowly and is facilitated by speech language pathologists (SLPs). Clients are educated and trained in the techniques and then expected to add the exercises to their daily routines.

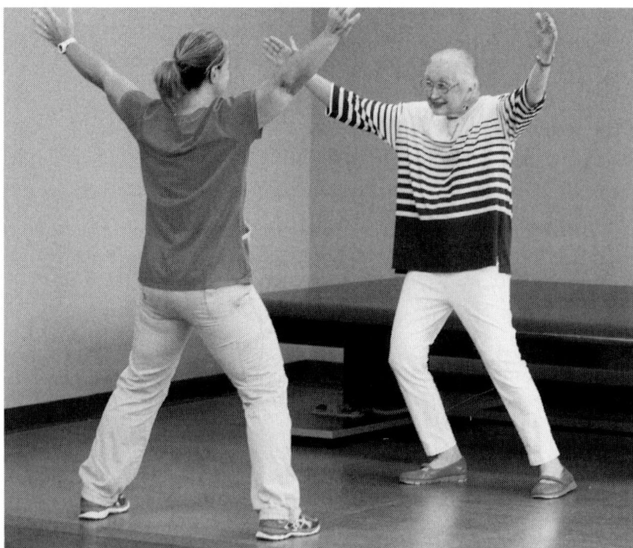

FIGURE 32-5. A client with PD learning the LSVT BIG® program.

Adaptive equipment, including a shower seat or tub bench, may assist clients who have mild balance challenges during bathing; the client may need to sit while donning pants. A large-handled utensil may keep the spoon or fork more securely in the hand during self-feeding, and a straw and lid will help keep a drink from spilling due to movement challenges. Precise tasks such as putting on makeup or pulling only one pill from a container may also require adaptations such as larger brushes and foam for the makeup brushes and weekly preloaded pill boxes.

> **COMMUNICATION**
>
> Nothing is more difficult than learning one has a life-limiting and potentially serious disorder. After receiving such news, clients go through the stages of grief for life as they knew it, and often require counseling or medications to battle depression and anxiety. The OTA can assist clients to create a "new normal" by providing them with the tools needed to remain independent for as long as possible. The OTA may not treat clients with a progressive disorder for a long duration, but may see them every 6 months to 1 year for a "tune-up" and with a refocus on the new problems and concerns that have developed since their last session. When independence is no longer an option, the focus of OT can shift to quality of life and keeping it as high as possible. When quality of life deteriorates and symptom management is exhausted, then hospice or palliative care can assist the client and family.

MODERATE PARKINSON'S TREATMENT

Issues around balance, coordination, tremors, and involuntary movements can affect functional performance of clients with moderate PD. Tremor may affect ability to perform self-feeding and grooming tasks, and other ADL and IADL tasks may become frustrating. OT practitioners can offer adaptive equipment and adaptive techniques for those tasks. Examples might be a reacher to don pants, a zipper pull to grasp a small zipper, a pen with an alternate shape, or weighted utensils or wrist weights to trial for self-feeding. The Liftware Steady™ spoon/fork has a gyroscope built into the handle that decreases spillage from tremors. Balance challenges will require equipment for safe bathing and toileting as well as mobility. A transfer tub bench or higher toilet will assist. A U-Step brand walker or cane has a laser light that shines on the ground to give the client who frequently "freezes" something to step over to restart ambulation. This walker type also has the brakes always locked, and the client squeezes the brakes to make the walker intentionally move. This is safer than standard rollator walkers, because the combination of small steps and stooped posture means that the rollator or rolling walker can get away from the client.

Adaptation for cognitive and memory tasks is often needed such as lists, medication reminders, and a call bell. Home safety and home and community mobility are paramount, with a walker, manual wheelchair, or power wheelchair to get around more safely. A seating clinic can assist with determining the correct manual or power wheelchair to meet the needs at the time of evaluation and for the future.

ADVANCED PARKINSON'S TREATMENT

For clients with advanced PD, positioning in bed and the wheelchair are important as the body grows more rigid and less control is evident. Padding pressure points is important to avoid pressure injuries, and ROM and stretching are needed daily as well. Caregiver education and training is often required so he or she can manage to safely care for the dependent loved one. Tasks performed by caregivers, such as transfers, safe ambulation, performance of daily ROM, assistance with ADL and IADL tasks, and bed mobility and positioning will require education and training by an OT practitioner. For example, learning proper ways to manage their own body mechanics and the positioning of their loved one during transfers will be paramount for caregivers.

Wheelchair management can be complex for positioning in the advanced stage, and should be addressed by a seating clinic. Often the wheelchair of choice is a manual wheelchair with tilt and recline as well as positioning components or an "attendant" joystick in the back of the power wheelchair for caregiver control. Typically, this is because clients with PD in the advanced stage cannot safely control a power wheelchair due to rigidity and decreased initiation. Tilt is used for pressure relief and to prevent some of the stooped posture and forward head position by providing a mechanical advantage. Recline is used to perform clothing management, to use a urinal, and to stretch out the back and hips for repositioning and comfort. The OTA may also address equipment management in bed/bathing/toileting, patient lifters, hospital beds, and safe handling and transfers.

DEMENTIA AND RELATED DISEASES

In population studies, 13.9% of persons 71 years of age and older in the United States have some type of dementia, and that number is expected to increase.[42] By 2050 the number of persons 65 years of age and older with AD, the most common type of dementia, may triple, from 5.2 million to a projected 11 to 16 million as the baby boomer generation ages.[42] **Dementia** is a term describing a variety of diseases and conditions that develop when nerve cells in the brain die or no longer function normally, and cause changes in a person's memory, behavior, and ability to think clearly.[42] Dementia in all forms is an irreversible, progressive brain disease that slowly destroys memory and thinking skills, and eventually even the ability to carry out the simplest tasks. In most people with AD specifically, symptoms first appear when people are in their mid-60s.[43] With other dementias, the appearance of symptoms depends on the course of the disease or root cause for the age at onset and course/duration of the dementia.

Dementia is an umbrella term for a category of diseases; underneath the umbrella are over 100 different "spokes." Some of the most common include: AD, vascular dementia, chronic traumatic encephalopathy, Lewy body dementia (LBD), frontotemporal lobar dementia, alcohol- or drug-related dementias, white matter diseases, and many other types of dementia.[43] The comparison of words like *dementia* and *cancer* can make it easier to understand the terminology. For example, breast cancer is different from skin cancer, but both diseases are cancer. Similarly, AD, the most common type of dementia, is different from vascular dementia, but both diseases are dementia.

For clients showing symptoms of dementia, it is critical to get an accurate assessment from a physician in order to determine whether the client's symptoms are from a dementia or another cause, such as a CVA, tumor, sleep disturbances, side effects of medications, or other conditions that may be treatable and possibly reversible. Assessment should include a comprehensive history and physical, neurological examination, CT scan or MRI of the brain, laboratory tests, as well as a family interview.[43]

The impact of all types of dementia reaches beyond the client with the diagnosis, causing a ripple effect of challenges for professionals and family members providing care for the client with dementia. The cost to care for persons with dementia in the United States was estimated to be $236 billion in 2016, but the cost for family caregivers is unaccounted and substantial.[44] OT practitioners in a variety of settings support clients with dementia and their families, whether or not the diagnosis is the primary reason for referral. Approximately 25% of all hospitalized clients older than 75 years of age have a secondary diagnosis of dementia.[45] It is estimated that in long-term care, 60% to 80% of clients have some type of dementia.[46] As part of a broad range of behavioral and environmental intervention strategies, training caregivers in specific communication and management skills has been identified as an important need, and one that OT practitioners are best qualified to address.[19] These communication and management skills are addressed in the next section, along with numerous tips and techniques for the OTA to manage the client with dementia.

Progression, Life Expectancy, and Symptoms

Many dementias have differing symptoms and can progress very differently. The classic symptom often associated with dementia is memory changes, but many clients can have motor, visual, and other changes, as noted in Table 32-5. In AD, abnormal deposits of proteins form amyloid plaques and tau tangles throughout the brain, and once-healthy neurons begin to work less efficiently.[47] Over time, neurons lose their ability to function and communicate with each other, and eventually they die.[47] As the functions the neurons were responsible for in each specific area of the brain can no longer be performed (such as integrating complex thoughts or laying down new memories), the client has new symptoms.[47] In LBD, abnormal deposits develop in brain cells, and the development of plaques and tangles in the brain is also possible.[48] In many of the dementias, the diagnosis is clinical and symptom-based, and the definitive diagnosis is made via autopsy after the person's death. AD

TABLE 32-5 Dementia Types and Characteristics

DEMENTIA TYPES/CAUSES	DEMENTIA CHARACTERISTICS[44]
Alzheimer's disease	• Difficulty remembering recent conversations, names; early memory loss • Apathy and depression, withdrawal from work and social activities • Trouble understanding visual images and spatial relationships • Impaired communication • Disorientation, confusion • Poor judgment • Behavioral changes: anxiety, agitation, sleep disturbances • Ultimately, difficulty speaking, swallowing, and walking
Vascular dementia	• Impaired judgment or impaired ability to make decisions, plan, or organize • Decreased motor function, especially slow gait and poor balance
Dementia with Lewy bodies	• Many of Alzheimer's symptoms with less significant memory impairment • Sleep disturbances • Well-formed visual hallucinations • Slowness, gait imbalance, or other Parkinsonian movement features • Early visuospatial impairment
Mixed dementia	• Characterized by the hallmark abnormalities of more than one cause of dementia
Frontotemporal lobar dementia	• Marked changes in personality and behavior • Difficulty with producing or comprehending language • Memory is typically spared in the early stages of disease
Creutzfeldt-Jakob disease	• Rapidly fatal disorder • Memory impairment • Coordination problems • Behavioral changes
Normal pressure hydrocephalus	• Difficulty walking • Memory loss • Inability to control urination
Wernicke-Korsakoff syndrome (low thiamine often caused by alcohol abuse)	• Severe memory deficits • Other thinking and social skills often spared
Posterior cortical atrophy	• Difficulty processing visual information • Difficulties with visual tasks such as reading a line of text, judging distances • Trouble distinguishing between moving objects and stationary objects • Inability to perceive more than one object at a time • Disorientation • Difficulty maneuvering, identifying, and using tools or common objects • Hallucinations • Difficulty performing mathematical calculations or spelling • Anxiety
Chronic traumatic encephalopathy—Repeated blows to the head/concussions as with many sports	• Memory loss • Confusion • Personality changes (including depression and suicidal thoughts) • Erratic behavior (including aggression) • Problems paying attention and organizing thoughts • Difficulty with balance and motor skills

is the sixth leading cause of death in the United States.[44] Those with AD live an average of 8 years after their symptoms become noticeable to others, but survival can range from 4 to 20 years, depending on age and other health conditions.[44] Typically, the life expectancy following a diagnosis of dementia is about 10 years, and many clients with dementia die of lung or kidney infections caused by immobility (muscles no longer move effectively or functionally, client may be confined to a wheelchair or bed) rather than the dementia itself.[49] Underreporting of dementia may also occur, as a client may have died with a diagnosis of dementia, but from pneumonia or malnutrition on the death certificate. Dementias are also associated with effects such as poor balance with falls, unsafe behavior, difficulty with self-feeding and swallowing, pneumonia, and immobility, which can all cause mortality. How quickly the dementia progresses, depends on the type and the area of the brain that is affected. It is certainly possible for a client to have more than one type of dementia, and all of the dementias have slightly different symptoms and progressions (Table 32-5).

A common effect from the symptoms that occur in the mid to late stages of dementia is called **sundowning**, characterized by increased anxiety, agitation, confusion, disorientation, and pacing, and is generally seen later in the day.[50] Studies show that as many as 66% of clients with AD can experience sundowning.[50] It has been found to not be as much about the sun going down, but is more about brain fatigue. The client with dementia struggles all day with the stresses of performing functional tasks as well as navigating the environment and making sense of confusing concepts. As the day progresses, the client seems to exhibit a decreased tolerance to stimuli, until he or she finally has a "meltdown." Sundowning symptoms may worsen with the absence of an established routine (such as on vacation), variances in diet/liquid intake, lack of sleep, a stressed caregiver, and physical fatigue.[50]

Wandering is another effect of the symptoms of dementia, and is caused by confusion and disorientation.[44] Whereas the walking about or wandering may seem aimless, generally most clients have a purpose and an intended destination. Tracking the episodes of wandering may assist the caregiver to determine the root cause such as hunger/thirst, pain, boredom, anxiety, stress, or confusion about the time. Sixty percent of clients with AD will wander, and it can be seen at any stage of the disease.[44] Clients who may be at higher risk for wandering are those who appear lost in a new or changed environment, or those who return late from regular walks or drives.

SCREENING AND ASSESSMENT TOOLS

Dementia is often considered in stages of progression, and many screening and assessment tools can be used to identify the client's current stage of dementia. Some examples include a screening tool such as the Mini Mental State Examination (MMSE),[51] and descriptive assessments such as the Global Deterioration Scale (GDS),[52] the Allen Cognitive Level Scale (ACL),[53] and Teepa Snow's Senior Gems.[54]

The MMSE is a 30-question tool often used to determine cognitive impairment both in the medical setting for diagnostic use and in the research setting. It takes about 10 minutes to administer, and assesses the areas of orientation, immediate memory, short-term memory, as well as language functioning.[51]

The GDS can be utilized as an assessment tool to determine the severity and progression of both cognitive and functional abilities.[52] It is based on behavioral observation of the client, and is used for clients with a dementia diagnosis. The ACL scale may be used in assessment/intervention with any diagnosis that affects level of cognitive function.[53] The levels utilize functional activity performance as a basis for evaluation of cognitive processing. The seven stages in the GDS matched with the similar levels of the ACL include:[52,53]

GDS Stage 1: No Cognitive Decline/ACL Level 6: Planned Actions: No memory deficits

GDS Stage 2: Very Mild Cognitive Decline/ACL Level 5: Exploratory Action level: Client may have subjective statements of "I am getting more forgetful," however deficits are not noted by others or identified under testing situations.

GDS Stage 3: Mild Cognitive Decline/ACL Level 5: Exploratory Action level: May be referred to as Mild Cognitive Impairment (MCI). Earliest clear-cut deficits seen with intensive interview and family members or coworkers start noticing deficits, especially in cognitively demanding occupations. The client may start to forget important appointments, perform poorly on concentration and calculation tests, start to misplace valuable items such as financial documents, and be slower to learn new information.

GDS Stage 4: Moderate Cognitive Decline/ACL Level 4: Goal Directed Activity: These clients function best in a familiar environment, and continue to need autonomy and control.

Behaviors: The client may begin to withdraw from challenging situations or activities in general, and tends to be anxious, angry, depressed, and in denial. He or she may perceive others as the problem, still desire autonomy, and tend to refuse new ideas.

Physical Mobility: The client may walk a bit slower than normal.

ADLs: Clients can still perform basic ADLs as they are goal directed and familiar. The client will understand the beginning, middle, and end of an activity, and may benefit from structure and setup. There will be difficulties with performance of IADLs, and most clients are no longer safe drivers.

Communication: The client appears socially appropriate and functional but may be focused on themselves more than others. He or she is able to make needs known and participate in conversation. The client may have difficulty naming objects, people, and places, and have limited reading comprehension. Cues may be required for word finding.

GDS Stage 5: Moderately Severe Cognitive Decline/ACL Level 3: Manual Action Level: These clients may still look normal with jewelry and makeup (if this was their routine before decline). Clients typically cannot manage at home alone without assistance and are often admitted to a skilled nursing facility due to cognitive deficits. They are often not oriented to reality, and a delusion may be their perception of reality, such as an older woman who expresses the anxious need to check on the turkey for Thanksgiving dinner while in the facility. They are not goal directed and may wander. Clients at this level may exhibit sexual acting out, and they may be impatient, paranoid, or suspicious.

Physical Abilities: Clients can still use their hands to manipulate and explore and may use different grasps for different objects. Clients may feel physically cold, may take longer for body temperature to adjust, and are able to sustain actions for at least 1 minute.

Vision: Tunnel vision is approximately 14 inches in front of the body. It can be startling when approaching from the back or from their sides, as their peripheral vision becomes much more compromised, causing a startled response. This startle may cause the client potentially to reach out to hit. Because the client has effectively lost depth perception and peripheral vision at this level, balance, walking, and all ADL tasks will be affected.

ADLs: Begin to decline, and the client benefits from visual, verbal, and tactile cues. There is still independence in toileting, although the client has decreased ability to choose clothing. There is still a sense of completion of a task when materials are used up such as at the end of a meal.

Communication: Clients often repeat themselves, may have difficulty being understood, and complex language is hard for them to understand. The client may not be able to answer detailed questions, but can still name familiar objects.

OT practitioner/Caregiver approaches: The client at this level needs 24-hour care, with additional time to perform tasks (2 to 3 times). When possible, provide functional and rote activities to perform.

GDS Stage 6: Severe Cognitive Decline/ACL Level 2: Postural Changes: These clients do not like to change clothes, and will remove and misplace items such as dentures, glasses, and hearing aids.

Behaviors: The client at this level will be found wandering for self-stimulation (without a verbalized agenda). They may display obsessive symptoms from the past such as a homemaker who focuses on dusting, an electrician who tries to remove outlet covers, or a mailman attempting to deliver mail. Clients may be sensitive to environmental stimuli, which can prompt behaviors of agitation. They will act on what they think, feel, hear, sense, and taste in the moment without thought. There can be high resistance to an unfamiliar caregiver, and clients may fear being alone. Many clients like to "go shopping" and put items in and out of a bag or cupboard. They typically have no boundaries and will take items from other clients and staff. Clients can display anxiety, agitation, and violent episodes based on negative stimulation, and sometimes being physically cold or experiencing discomfort can facilitate hostility.

Physical Mobility: Many clients at this level will exhibit a shuffling gait, stooped posture, loss of trunk rotation, and loss of righting reactions, which can lead to an increased risk for falls. Most clients respond to music and repetitive rhythmical movements and may like to dance.

Vision Changes: Loss of peripheral vision can occur, and the client may startle if not approached from the front.

ADLs: The client may not recognize everyday objects and may not be able to sequence through rote activities such as toileting, dressing, grooming, and oral hygiene. The client may display loss of fine motor skills, including difficulty with buttoning and fastening items. Self-feeding is generally intact, but the OTA or caregivers may start noticing difficulties with holding and using the utensil appropriately or eating very quickly or very slowly. Motor apraxia (difficulty with motor planning) and agnosia (inability to interpret sensory information leading to inability to recognize objects) becomes evident in this stage. Clients may become incontinent and can get their days and nights mixed up.

Communication: Responses may be limited to one or a few words; clients may revert to languages acquired earlier in life and may have a decreased ability to communicate wants and needs. Clients can be completely aphasic, although they may be able to respond to simple "yes" or "no" questions with regard to comfort. They may only respond to those directly in front of them and in the line of sight.

GDS Stage 7: Late Dementia/ACL Level 1: Automatic Action: These clients have poor ability to sit up and will rely on a wheelchair most of the time. They will display difficulty holding their head up or effectively swallowing at times, and may pocket food in their mouth. They often will finger and manipulate buttons, strings, zippers, and keys securely sewn to an apron or cloth for hours. At this level, clients are totally dependent on others for survival, and are unable to manage physical needs. They are completely incontinent, and dependent for all ADLs including self-feeding. Client may have end-of-life dysphagia issues and weight loss as well as malabsorption.

Physical mobility: Clients at this level have a loss of basic mobility and are dependent on manual wheelchair mobility, with decreased ability to stand, sit up, or hold up their head. They are at a high risk for pressure injuries, contractures, and loss of swallowing.

Communication: In most clients at this level, the basic verbal abilities are lost, although they may yell or grunt to express themselves, respond with facial grimacing, or use repetitive words. Most clients will respond to touch and may turn their head to track someone but will have difficulty establishing eye contact.

In another less commonly used scale, occupational therapist Teepa Snow developed a measurement tool, The Living Gems™, based on the Allen Cognitive Scale levels.[54] The Living Gems™ scale uses gemstones instead of numbers as a way to consider a client, which may be easier for some clients or caregivers to understand. Departing from the numeric system allows changes between levels to be more fluid, not constant or in one direction.[54] For example, a client may present skills and abilities of an emerald in the daytime when feeling rested and engaged, but change to an amber when tired or sick. Even a healthy person can appreciate that the brain is operating at the sapphire level on most days, but under stress, a healthy person will slip to diamond and have more difficulty dealing with change or controlling emotions only to return to sapphire when the stress subsides. The gems include:

Sapphire—Normal aging, or "true blue"

Diamond—"Rigid and sharp." The first signs of cognitive decline

Emerald—"On the go." This includes word finding and comprehension difficulties; clients think they are in another place and time, they "have to get home," and there is a decline in personal care, often wearing the same soiled clothing for days.

Amber—"Softest, most changeable." These clients are all about being in the moment, all about sensation, and there is no safety awareness.

Ruby—Stop. There is a great risk for falls in this stage with decreased fine motor control. Clients still have large, big movements, with increased walking and increased sleeping.

Pearl—Clients are tightly hidden within themselves, much like that of an oyster shell, with increasing contractures and deteriorating sensory and motor abilities.[54]

OT practitioners are well prepared to provide interventions that focus on safety and independence during desired occupations for clients with a variety of conditions and in a variety of settings.[54] OT practitioners' focus on client factors and the performance skills of a particular client means that OT practitioners understand the needs of the clients they treat. The benefit of staging a client is that it reduces trial and error, avoids learned dependency, sets up accurate expectations, guides treatment, and increases accountability to manage expenses.[52,53] Too often, practitioners will discharge clients prematurely from skilled intervention due to the client not making sufficient progress or reaching maximum potential. There are opportunities, however, where the OT practitioner could be setting up a plan of care based on the cognitive stage the client is exhibiting, and modifying interventions to meet the needs of the client now and for the future.

RESEARCH, MEDICAL TREATMENT, AND EXERCISE

Medications are currently available to treat dementia. These drugs work by regulating neurotransmitters, the chemicals that transmit messages among neurons and may help clients maintain thinking, memory, and speaking skills, as well as with certain behavioral problems, such as agitation.[51] However, none of the currently available drugs change the underlying disease process, their effectiveness varies from person to person, and they may only be beneficial for a limited time. Many of the drugs also have serious side effects, such as nausea, vomiting, loss of appetite, headache, dizziness, confusion, and increased frequency of bowel movements.[50,51]

In addition to medication, other medical treatment for dementia can include symptom management for conditions such as constipation, depression, and pain from immobility. A rapidly growing amount of literature strongly suggests that exercise, specifically aerobic exercise, may slow or improve cognitive impairment and reduce dementia risk for the general population.[55] Among patients with dementia or mild cognitive impairment, randomized controlled trials documented better cognitive scores after 6 to 12 months of exercise compared with controls who did not exercise.[55] OTAs who work with clients with dementia can assist with general exercise through tasks such as balloon volleyball, walks, and recumbent biking to tolerance and observing safety issues such as balance (Fig. 32-6).

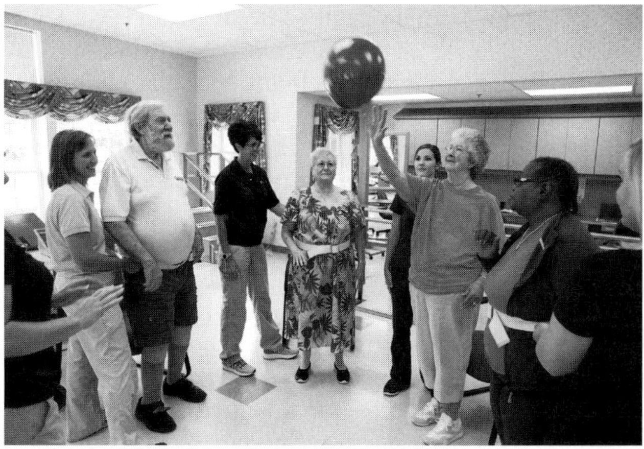

FIGURE 32-6. Balloon volleyball game with day program for clients with dementia.

OCCUPATIONAL THERAPY TREATMENT IN THE STAGES

Dementia-specific interventions have two common pitfalls. First, the focus may be only on what is lost or impaired without the understanding of what the client with dementia can still do at each stage of the disease. Second, the intervention may be too narrowly focused on the single client, the person with dementia. A more effective plan is to engage the caregiver team in using person-centered strategies that work for this client and make participating easier for both the client with dementia and the caregiver(s). Many interventions will focus on the OTA sharing strategies and techniques, as well as training with caregivers until they have adapted routines for each stage of the disease.

Many family caregivers and professionals may be more familiar with the memory changes associated with dementia, but dementia is also a language disorder.[44] Many caregivers recognize that giving a person verbal instruction is often ineffective, but may not have considered another approach to sharing information—specifically, showing a person what one wants them to do. Imagine speaking to a person who is not proficient in English. In such an interaction, one may automatically use fewer words, move one's body and gesture more, and pick up a prop to indicate an action. This combination of cues is also a better strategy for giving information to clients with dementia.[44]

Stages with Treatment: The following are treatment and caregiver strategies that OT practitioners can implement for each dementia stage as defined earlier. Typically, the evaluating occupational therapist or SLP will be the primary clinicians responsible for staging a client based on objective and subjective clinical testing, as well as skilled observation. The stages should be documented on the initial evaluation and discussed with other treating practitioners as well as all caregivers involved in the care of the client.

GDS Stage 1: No Cognitive Decline/ACL Level 6: Planned Actions: No memory deficits, no OT treatment

GDS Stage 2: Very Mild Cognitive Decline/ACL Level 5: Exploratory Action level—Generally no OT treatment.

GDS Stage 3: Mild Cognitive Decline/ACL Level 5: Exploratory Action level: Strategies the OTA might utilize are using tools to assist with forgetfulness such as phone note pad, calendars, and making lists. Concentration can be enhanced with a quieter space with fewer distractions. New information may need to be written down or rehearsed to put into long-term memory. A GPS may assist with getting to the desired location while walking or driving.

GDS Stage 4: Moderate Cognitive Decline/ACL Level 4: Goal-Directed Activity: Giving choices can assist the OTA and caregiver by gaining increased cooperation, as can strategies to decrease anxiety by keeping outings to familiar places. The OTA can schedule the client at the same time each day or week, and assist caregivers in setting up a schedule. The OTA may need to tap into automatic or rote activities, such as handing clients a toothbrush instead of asking them to brush their teeth. The client will have difficulties with performance of IADLs, and are no longer a safe driver. The OTA and any new caregiver staff should take the time to develop a rapport, to be reassuring so as not to increase anxiety. Be aware that this is the last opportunity to introduce a new assistive device if they have not previously used one such as a cane, walker, reacher, dressing stick, or sock aid. A collaboration with physical therapy, as well as the rest of the care team and family, may be appropriate to determine any necessary mobility devices and education. In this stage, it is important to ensure that the client knows how to safely use an assistive device such as a walker or cane. This is even more critical if the client has never used an assistive device.

GDS Stage 5: Moderately Severe Cognitive Decline/ACL Level 3: Manual Action Level: The OTA should approach clients directly in front of them due to tunnel vision, extend the hand as though to shake their hand, while saying their name in a cheerful tone of voice. As ADLs begin to decline, the client benefits from visual, verbal, and tactile cues. The OTA should eliminate excessive verbiage and use simple statements versus complex stories. The OTA should give increased time for answering simple, one-step questions—up to 90 seconds. The client at this level needs 24-hour care, with additional time to perform tasks (2 to 3 times as much). When possible, provide functional and rote activities to perform. Tasks such as brushing hair, wiping down a table, folding towels, or sorting socks are potential options. Instruction necessary for caregivers in this stage is on how to set up tasks for client successful completion. The OTA can provide techniques such as having all clothing and showering items ready to go with the bathroom already warm, and bathing at a familiar time or when already taking off clothing to change.

GDS Stage 6: Severe Cognitive Decline/ACL Level 2: Postural Changes: Self-feeding is generally intact, but the OTA or caregivers may start noticing difficulties with holding and using the utensil appropriately or self-feeding and eating very quickly or very slowly. The tone of voice and body language can be the key to communication at this level, and the OTA can connect with these clients through touch. The OTA should encourage the caregiver and facility to provide consistency in staff assignments as much as possible and try to anticipate needs such as pain and toileting. Simplify ADL tasks such as grooming, dressing, and bathing, and place only items necessary for task completion in direct line of sight in sequential order. For this level, use tactile, visual, and modeling to cue the client, and try to avoid frustration and a negative tone as the client can still sense this.

GDS Stage 7: Late Dementia/ACL Level 1: Automatic Action: Most clients at this level will respond to touch and may turn their head to track the OTA. The client at this level requires total care with a focus on comfort. The OTA and caregivers can provide sensory stimulation such as music, soft cloth to touch, or movement in their chair. Other focuses will be skin management, contracture management, and fall prevention. The OTA can also monitor swallowing and self-feeding skills while the nurse or caregiver also notes weight changes and hydration.[52,53]

SUNDOWNING TREATMENT

The following are some sundowning strategies to make life easier for both the client and caregiver for the afternoon/evening hours:[56]

1. Encourage healthy, enjoyable (not exhausting) exercise during the day to get endorphins and blood flowing. This will promote a relaxing and low-key evening to help switch the body end-of-day focus (Fig. 32-7).

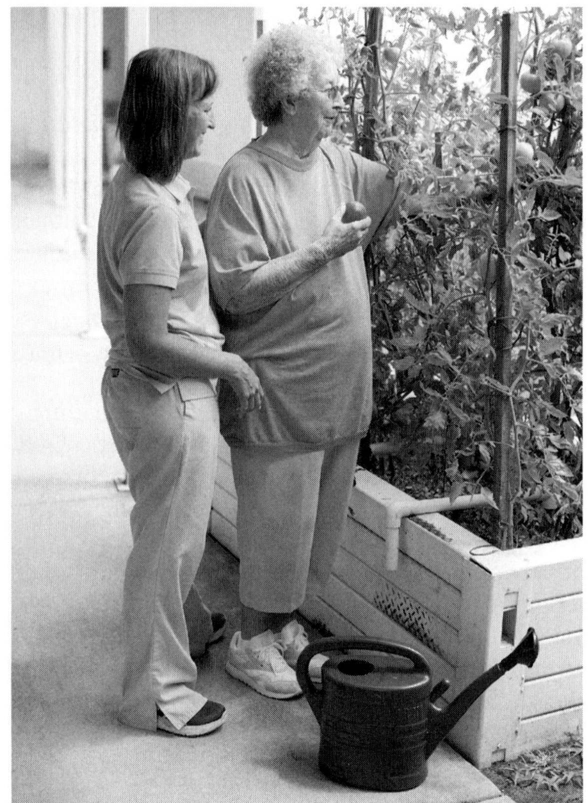

FIGURE 32-7. Resident working with an OTA in the garden.

2. Turn on lights in the rooms that will be occupied during the evening.
3. Try to keep the client engaged in a meaningful task, such as looking at pictures, playing a game, or sorting and folding laundry.
4. Select one or more of the rooms to become a "quiet place" where there is bright light and soothing music.
5. If this time marks a particular trend in the client's life, try to mimic what they may have done at that time in the past. It may include setting the table, picking up children from school, or reading the newspaper, and these "normal" activities may be comforting.
6. Only allow brief naps during the day of 20 minutes or less. Hours of sleeping can confuse the body's circadian rhythms and keep clients awake at night.
7. If pacing is involved, make sure the path is clear to increase safety.
8. If increased frustration or agitation seems to be happening, hold the client's hand, or put a hand on his or her back or knee. Sometimes a soothing massage can be comforting and decrease tension that may be building.
9. Promote evenings of positive interactions and memories.
10. Maintain a comfortable temperature in the home.

Often, healthcare providers need to search further to see what is triggering the negative behavior. Is the client cold or hungry? Offer a snack or a glass of water. Is there a need to use the restroom, or is the diaper soiled? Offer them a hand, and take them to the toilet.[56]

TREATMENT FOR WANDERING

Wandering is a huge concern for families, caregivers, and clients with dementia. Clients may get bored, frightened, and upset or confused about time and place. They may think they are late for work and walk out the door, or get confused trying to find the bathroom and go out the wrong door. The best way to prevent wandering is to keep the individual engaged and active. One idea that may help keep the client safe is to make the environment secure by putting deadbolts on the door high and out of reach. Put a stop sign on the door that clients attempt to exit from. Put a familiar restroom sign on the bathroom door, and leave the light on so that the client can locate the bathroom. If the problem is extensive, consider alarm mats or alarmed doors or windows. Look for patterns and triggers. Clients may wander off in the morning because they think it is time to go to work. Consider telling the caregiver to register the individual with the National Alzheimer's Association wandering prevention program called Medic Alert/Safe Return.[57]

General Strategies

It is important for the OTA to get to know the client with dementia and know what types of activities are calming to them and those that are exciting. Be mindful of the verbal and nonverbal communication as well as that of other caregivers; when verbal language decreases, the client may rely on nonverbal cues more often. Very often, clients become agitated because they cannot tell the OT practitioner or caregiver that they are cold or incontinent. Clients in moderate to advanced stages of dementia cannot autoregulate body temperatures, so make sure they are wearing multiple layers of clothing, such as a thermal undershirt, shirt, and sweater to maintain body heat. Pay attention to temperature, noise level, and lighting in the environment. Very often, clients are "parked" in front of a nursing station for observation, yet these areas tend to be the busiest and noisiest locations on the units. Consider an alternative place to relocate the client where there is safety and supervision that is less stimulating. Lighting is an important element to consider as well. Bright light from time in the sun or internal lighting is effective in the treatment of seasonal affective disorder; some benefits were reported for restlessness, but a particular beneficial effect has been found for sleep disturbances with dementia.[58]

Aromatherapy may also be very beneficial; however, it is important to be aware of what scents clients preferred or disliked earlier in their life. Aromatherapy seems to be safe and effective and may have an important role in managing behavioral problems in clients with dementia.[58] Scents with a strong citrus smell can help to calm the limbic system. The OT practitioner can further their knowledge of aromatherapy through continuing education. In addition to the sense of smell, the sense of touch should be considered, also. Individuals may accept a weighted baby doll, stuffed animal, or a fidget quilt (a quilt with items sewn on for touching such as buttons, keys, or ribbons), and the OTA may find that signs of restlessness or agitation decrease with these objects.

Inappropriate remarks and touching can be a difficult behavior to manage with those with dementia. Be aware of how the OTA is presenting to the client; the OTA's attire should be professional and conservative. Avoid low necklines, and make sure that the shirt does not rise up when assisting clients. If inappropriate remarks occur, in a kind but firm demeanor, either redirect attention to another task, calmly state that the behavior is not appropriate, or leave the room and return at another time. Some clients have fewer behaviors with a caregiver of a certain age or gender. The OT practitioner can also mention to the client's family or friends who visit that the client may benefit from simply holding someone's hand or from a warm embrace from family, because these are human needs that may not be fulfilled for this population. If no family members visit the client who is in a long term care facility, the OT practitioner may discuss the need with the social worker, who may be able to arrange for a volunteer to visit. OT practitioners frequently modify the demands of an activity in order for a client to reach his or her goals. Activity demands are the aspects of an activity, which include the objects, space, social demands, sequencing or timing, required actions, and required underlying body functions and body structure needed to carry out the activity.[59] Modifications to activities may include changing the materials used, varying the space in which the activity is carried out, and providing social interaction in the form of verbal cues. Other modifications may include resequencing the required steps or actions of an activity, and/or altering the position of the person completing the activity.[59]

Remember that clients can fluctuate between the dementia stages due to stress, illness, acute medical conditions such as a urinary tract infection, sepsis (blood infection), depression, and many other reasons. Minor fluctuations can occur in all individuals due to fatigue and stress. Occupational performance is composed of emotional, physical, and cognitive factors and must also be considered when determining the stage of dementia. A client may be able to cognitively engage in a chosen activity, however may not demonstrate interaction due to depression, hearing loss, or disinterest in the task. This is why it is also important to recognize the client's social and leisure interests, in order to identify and implement the most relevant and purposeful occupation for the client. Table 32-6 provides some ideas to engage clients with dementia into meaningful activity.

Group treatments are a potential option for dementia management as well. It is important to consider the composition of the group members to try to match persons at a similar stage or level, as possible, to increase the success of the group. Selection of those clients with fewer behavioral challenges may also make the group run more smoothly. Tasks for a higher-level group might include making a snack such as peanut butter on crackers or a smoothie, an exercise group in standing, or a craft activity. A mid-level group might perform seated exercise movements to music and sing along, or play bingo. A lower-level group might catch or hit a balloon, fold towels, or color pictures. Many times, the lower the level of the participants, the smaller the number of participants possible due to the increased amount of assistance each group member requires. At times a group member may be having an off day, and will have a behavioral disruption in the group. If it is safe, letting the client leave may be appropriate, or asking another staff

TABLE 32-6 Dementia ADL Treatments, Level, and Precautions

OT ADL TREATMENTS	DEMENTIA LEVEL	PRECAUTIONS AND CONTRAINDICATIONS
Offer finger foods; place directly in line of vision.	5, 6, 7	Make sure the client's hands are washed before self-feeding. Watch pace of bites and chewing.
Limit the number of utensils offered.	5, 6	Make sure the client can manipulate utensil being offered. Be aware if the utensil could be used as an object to throw if agitated. Metal utensils increase sensory input over plastic ones due to weight.
Limit the number of food choices presented.	5, 6	Too much food presented on a plate can actually overwhelm and diminish appetite.
Provide highly contrasting tableware.	5, 6	Increases visual awareness of plate or utensils (such as a red plate, utensils, and cup). Avoid white plates on white tablecloth so plate can be easily seen.
Give full assist first bite; try to fade out amount of assist with subsequent bites as automatic movements take over.	5, 6	Be aware of any diet restrictions such as modified liquids or mechanical soft/puree diets.
Limit the number of choices of objects on the bathroom counter.	5, 6	Keep protective ointments for the body away from toothpaste.
Eliminate "visual pollution," which is distracting in the room and for ADLs.	4, 5, 6	Too many visual cues posted are distracting and ignored. Difficult with figure ground issues
Provide brightly colored visual cues on personal tools or on shelves of medicine cabinet.	4, 5, 6	Try to keep to minimum. May benefit from visual cues such as pictures of recognizable objects like comb, toothbrush if word recognition is a concern
Identify via observation or from family member interview, which article of clothing does client don/doff first, second, and third.	4, 5, 6	Keep to same routine that the client is used to doing.
Set up manicure stations, wash hands in warm soapy water, rinse fingers, dry, and apply lotion (make sure lotion is not noxious smelling to client).	3, 4, 5, 6	Wash hands pre- and post-activity. Make sure fingers do not go in the client's mouth.

member to assist may be necessary. Even with mixed functional levels, a group may be possible. An exercise group may be run for example, with the higher-level participant following closely what the leader is doing and assisting to lead exercises, and others participating with extra physical or verbal cues (Table 32-7). Sometimes individual treatment can be done by the OTA within a group activity setting that is led by the activity director or recreation staff.

The development of a functional maintenance program (FMP) is critical to help maintain the highest functional level for the individual. This is a program that focuses on strategies, tools, and techniques for management of the client's behavior and skills as they relate to functional tasks as the dementia progresses. It is critical as well to observe the caregiver's follow-through with recommended strategies and interventions before discharge and the client's response to the FMP so that any changes can be made.

QUALITY OF LIFE, IMPACT ON CLIENT AND FAMILY, AND CAREGIVER BURDEN

These neurodegenerative diseases have commonalities in that they are progressive and have a high impact on the client and family. Studies have shown that a lower physical

TABLE 32-7 Dementia UE Therapeutic Exercises

OT IADL AND LEISURE TREATMENTS	DEMENTIA LEVEL	PRECAUTIONS AND CONTRAINDICATIONS
Rolling pin with cookie dough or play dough	4, 5	Be observant that client does not use rolling pin as a weapon.
Use a feather duster to dust high and low; can be graded to remain in base of support or to grade to outside of base of support in sitting or standing.	3, 4, 5	Use a gait belt if balance is a concern.
Hang laundry on a clothes line.	3, 4, 5	Use a gait belt if balance is a concern.
Wash windows.	3, 4, 5	Make sure window cleaner is not placed in mouth or sprayed in eyes. Use a gait belt if balance is a concern.
Sort clothing, and place in varying dresser drawer heights.	3, 4, 5	Use gait belt if standing and if balance is a concern.
Place coins in a piggy bank.	3, 4, 5, 6	Make sure coins are not placed in mouth.
Use orange plastic netting found on construction sites (which can be purchased at a hardware store), and weave various different textures throughout the plastic.	3, 4, 5	Make sure items are not placed in mouth.
Color in a coloring book.	3, 4, 5	Make sure crayons are not placed in mouth.
Use finger paint.	3, 4, 5, 6	Wash hands pre- and post-activity. Make sure fingers do not go in mouth.
Apply peanut butter to pine cones and then roll in bird seed; hang from a tree using piece of yarn.	3, 4, 5	Wash hands pre- and post-activity. Make sure fingers do not go in mouth. Use gait belt for balance.
Paint clay pots, and then plant a flower or herb in it; water daily with watering can.	3, 4, 5	Wash hands pre- and post-activity. Make sure fingers do not go in mouth. Use gait belt for balance.
Set up two basins, one with warm water, and have client wring out a washcloth from one basin to the other.	3, 4, 5	Wash hands pre- and post-activity. Make sure fingers do not go in mouth. Use gait belt for balance. Wipe up any spills to avoid slipping.
Blow bubbles, and have the client try to reach for the bubbles.	3, 4, 5	Wash hands pre- and post-activity. Make sure fingers do not go in mouth. Use gait belt for balance. Wipe up any spills to avoid slipping.
Make beaded jewelry.	3, 4, 5	Wash hands pre- and post-activity. Make sure beads do not go in mouth.

Continued

TABLE 32-7 Dementia UE Therapeutic Exercises (continued)

OT IADL AND LEISURE TREATMENTS	DEMENTIA LEVEL	PRECAUTIONS AND CONTRAINDICATIONS
Sand a simple project such as a bird house.	3, 4, 5	Make sure items do not go in mouth.
Bat a balloon with a hand, or use a badminton racquet.	3, 4, 5	Use gait belt for balance. Make sure client does not use racquet as a weapon.
Throw and catch a ball.	3, 4, 5	Use gait belt for balance.
Play putt-putt golf.	3, 4	Use gait belt for balance. Make sure client does not use club as a weapon.
Pick flowers or tomatoes from a bush, and carry back to clinic in a basket; pick blossoms or autumn leaves from trees overhead.	3, 4, 5	Use gait belt for balance if performing activity in standing.
Sort clothing; fold laundry.	3, 4, 5, 6	Use gait belt for balance if performing activity in standing.
Water outside plants; can vary the amount of water inside the can to add resistance.	3, 4, 5	Use gait belt for balance if performing activity in standing. Watch for spills, which could cause slips.
Vacuum and sweep.	3, 4, 5	Use gait belt for balance if performing activity in standing.
Put canned food items away at varying heights.	3, 4, 5	Use gait belt for balance if performing activity in standing. Make sure client does not use cans as a weapon. May need assist for grip.
Throw beanbags, or play shuffleboard.	3, 4, 5	Use gait belt for balance if performing activity in standing.
Go for a walk on different terrain.	3, 4, 5	Use gait belt for balance. Watch for elopement risk if out of the secure area.
Set a table, wipe off the table, and clear the table.	3, 4, 5	Use gait belt for balance if performing activity in standing. Wash hands pre- and post-activity. Use plastic plates, if possible, to avoid breakage.
Deliver newspaper or mail to the other clients.	3, 4, 5	Use gait belt for balance if performing activity in standing.
Dance to familiar music.	3, 4, 5	Use gait belt for balance if performing activity in standing. Pick familiar or preferred music.
Use a small parachute to lift arms up and down (with others).	3, 4, 5	Use gait belt for balance if performing activity in standing.

level of functioning in many diseases does not necessarily have an impact on QoL on clients, and that QoL can remain high through the course of the disease.[60] Most of these diseases however, place an astounding burden on the caregiver as it relates to finances, disability, providing care, and having personal resources to manage keeping the person with a progressive disorder in the home. Generally, at some point in the progression of the disease, the client cannot work, and a caregiver may also have to stop working to care for the client. The result of not working often means that finances may be difficult. Many clients choose to go on disability from the federal government, which means they are legally unable to work or be retrained to work. Determination of disability through the Social Security Administration in the United States can be difficult to obtain due to the burden of proof required and the extended period of time it can take to receive. Clients with ALS have a 6-month to disability "fast track," but others have to wait at least 2 years for disability determination and benefits. Clients with a determined disability status receive Medicare benefits, even though they are not 65 years of age.

Respite and caregiving assistance may be needed to keep clients in the home, especially as they become more dependent. Some disease-specific organizations have support groups, equipment loan closets, and financial support available for members with the specific diagnosis. Some clients and families will hire paid caregivers to assist, or the client may have to move into a facility for increased care needs. If the client requires a tracheostomy with a ventilator, he or she may live at home with 24-hour support; alternatively, here are a few facilities in each state or region that will accept those clients. Therefore, clients may have to live far from home and supportive resources (family, friends, etc.) if they need a skilled nursing facility and choose mechanical ventilation.

Sexual Activity

When diseases have an onset in adulthood, many times adults will be in stable relationships and be sexually active with their partners. Progressive diseases can affect sexuality and intimacy in many ways. Fatigue and depression can be factors affecting interest and energy level, and medications can have side effects that impact performance or desire.

Certainly, physical weaknesses can impact the ability to not only have intercourse, but to reach out to hug or show intimacy. Difficulty with muscle control, tremors, or ataxia might mean that when the client reaches out to caress a partner, that touch hits out or becomes noxious instead. Many times, caregivers are tired and stressed from their caregiving duties, leaving them with few energy reserves, and a view of their family member as a "patient," not a sexual partner. For many clients, however, sexual desire does not decrease with age or immobility. The disconnect between the ability to perform certain movements and communicate effectively and what can be imparted to the partner is difficult to overcome. For example, clients who cannot move their arms or facial muscles and use a communication device to speak "I love you" in a synthesized voice, may not impart the same feelings as a strong hug, a smile, and an endearment in the client's own voice as before the weakness.

The OTA can assist in many aspects of sexuality management, and should initiate conversations with clients about this important ADL. OT practitioners can assist with advice on physical tools and techniques to accommodate for weakness such as a wedge or extra pillows, having the client in side-lying or on the bottom for sexual activity, and vibrator and dildo modification for easier holding with weak grasp. The OTA may also encourage open communication between partners about needs and desires, offer handouts and information, and encourage counseling or respite if indicated.

SUMMARY

Clients with the significant and progressive disorders noted in this chapter have many varied symptoms that can impact occupational performance. The physical, sensory, visual, behavioral, and cognitive symptoms can evolve and change over days, weeks, months, or years, causing an inability to maintain roles and can impact client factors and performance skills. The OTA's role is to identify strengths and deficits, modify tasks for maximum independence, and promote dignity with a sense of value. While typically not getting stronger or making classic improvements in therapy, each client with a progressive disorder has a need for intervention by the OTA at various times through the disease course.

REVIEW QUESTIONS

1. A client with dementia presents as a GDS stage 5. During the day program, this client may demonstrate which of the following characteristics?
   a. They still desire autonomy and tend to refuse new ideas.
   b. They are goal directed.
   c. They may use different grasps for different objects.
   d. They exhibit a shuffled gait and stooped posture.
2. A client with ALS is beginning to have difficulty with fine motor tasks on his dominant side. Which types of functional tasks would be difficult to complete?
   a. Zippers only
   b. Opening sugar packets, nail clipping, shoe tying, buttons
   c. Opening the microwave and oven
   d. Donning pants and shoes
3. When introducing adaptive equipment or devices to a client with dementia, it is *best* to introduce it them no later than:
   a. GDS Stage 3
   b. GDS Stage 4
   c. GDS Stage 5
   d. GDS Stage 6
4. A client with PD has slow and deliberate movements when the OTA observes him grooming and self-feeding. Which symptom is he displaying?
   a. Tremors
   b. Cognitive changes
   c. Balance challenges
   d. Bradykinesia
5. A caregiver of a client with HD is asking the OTA what types of therapy interventions the client would participate in during outpatient OT to increase strength and functional abilities for daily tasks. How should the OTA respond?
   a. Exercise with low reps and low exertion only
   b. Upper extremity exercises, balance tasks, and therapy in the pool
   c. Exercise with maximum repetitions and maximum weights only
   d. Exercise is not indicated with this population.
6. A 55-year-old client with primary progressive MS would be appropriate for which three of the following types of OT services?
   a. Strengthening exercises to regain function
   b. Adaptive techniques for ADL tasks
   c. Balance and mobility safety during kitchen tasks
   d. Cognitive retraining to return to work
   e. Memory adaptations
   f. Liftware Steady™ for tremor management during self-feeding
7. Clients who present as a GDS stage 6 may demonstrate which of the following characteristics?
   a. They wander for self-stimulation.
   b. They lose basic verbal abilities.
   c. Delusion is a part of their reality.
   d. They can still use their hands to manipulate and explore.
8. Any client with a degenerative disease must think proactively and look forward to the future for their needs for adaptive equipment and accessible options. The OTA is responsible for advising a client with ALS when to start the power wheelchair evaluation process and would do so when which of the following is apparent?
   a. When they can ambulate 2 miles while walking the dog without difficulty
   b. When they have been to the emergency room two times with broken bones from falling over the past 6 months
   c. When they are able to safely control it
   d. When ambulating with the walker is becoming less safe and distances are less functional
9. The OTA is working on a memory care unit at an adult day program. He or she sees a client having word-finding and comprehension difficulties during a craft activity and has noticed a decline in the client's personal care over the past few months. The OTA knows that this client has now entered which stage of dementia?
   a. Pearl
   b. Emerald
   c. Ruby
   d. Sapphire

10. A client with tremors, stiffness of movement, and micrographia from PD would note which three of the following issues when paying bills?
    a. Checks would be potentially illegible if written out.
    b. Online bill paying with an adapted keyboard and mouse may be easier.
    c. The client would not be able to pay the bills.
    d. The client would not be able to remember when to pay the bills due to decreased memory.
    e. There would not be an issue with paying the bills with these symptoms.
    f. A wrist weight and arm support may assist.

CASE STUDY

A 30-year-old man with ALS named Randy lives alone in a one-level apartment with two steps, and is estranged from his parents. He works in an office setting and is often on the computer and phone. He has an extensive friend network, but will not talk about his diagnosis or the changes his friends see in him. He enjoys Nascar, watching and listening to country music, eating out, and playing tennis. He has a 5-year-old daughter whom he sees two weekends a month, but was never married. Randy has right leg and right arm weakness and is right-handed. He is also slightly dysarthric. He wears a right ankle AFO due to foot drop, and uses a cane for balance when out of the home. His strength in his RUE is 3+/5 shoulder, 3/5 elbow, 3/5 wrist, 3/5 finger extension, and 3/5 finger flexion. He drives as he needs to, to and from work and for shopping, and says he is fine to drive because he "raises his leg instead of moving his ankle on the brake and gas."

1. What are some of Randy's immediate needs for adaptive equipment and techniques for the following occupations?
   - Bathing in his tub/shower combo
   - Toileting and hygiene
   - Dressing and grooming
   - Self-feeding, including cutting food
   - Driving
   - Work tasks
   - Leisure
   - Child care
2. What will soon become some of the issues as Randy's disease progresses, and what will he have to think about long term?

PUTTING IT ALL TOGETHER — Sample Treatment Session and Documentation

Setting	Memory support unit at assisted living facility, 24-hour caregiver support
Client profile	Clara, an 88-year-old, widowed client with a medical history of dementia, unspecified hemorrhage of GI tract, hx of closed fx unspecified part neck of femur, dysphagia, osteoporosis, degenerative joint disease, hypertension
History	A pleasant 88-year-old, frail client, Clara, who has lived on the memory care unit for the past 2 years. She presents in a manual wheelchair. Her daughter stated she had an episode with sciatica nerve pain and has been in a wheelchair since then, approximately 2 years ago. She was an elementary school teacher for 43 years. She has three children, but was not able to recall that. Per her daughter's report, the client liked to work in the yard, liked to dig in the dirt, was an avid "walker," never was a napper, and enjoyed cooking. She now presents in a manual wheelchair and demonstrates inappropriate behaviors when she becomes agitated. She would benefit from skilled OT to address and identify more appropriate activities and then train the caregivers on these activities.
Insurance	Humana—State Health Plan, must call for preauthorization after the initial evaluation is completed; once this was done, authorized for 8 visits.
Psychological	Client was referred to skilled OT intervention due to inappropriate behaviors such as "digging into her pants" and smearing feces on the wall and around her room, as well as demonstrating destructive behaviors in her room. She also has a habit of "spitting" on the table and the floor and attempting to spit on another client's plate.
Social	She is a widowed female with no interaction noticed with other clients on the unit. She appears to be sensory deprived or seeking sensory interaction.
Cognitive	GDS Stage 6, decreased safety awareness, judgment, and insight. Attempts to communicate with staff verbally, however, speech is unintelligible most of the time. She can follow one-step commands with increased time to process (requires approx. 90 seconds)
Motor and Manual Muscle Testing (MMT)	Not able to follow MMT due to cognition, however both LE and UE AROM and PROM appear WFL. Strength in BUE's appears grossly 3+/5, and BLE appears grossly 3/5 to 3+/5. Client is right-hand dominant. Her static sitting balance is fair, dynamic sitting Fair, static standing Fair –, and dynamic standing Fair –. Fall predictors are: age older than 80, arthritis, balance impairment, female gender, gait impairment, impaired ADL, impaired cognition, impaired strength, and five or more medications, including pain pill, which puts her at a greater than 78% risk for falls. Skin intact, denies pain, demonstrated coordination with a mild impairment

PUTTING IT ALL TOGETHER Sample Treatment Session and Documentation (continued)

ADL	Independent with pureed diet; staff gives client a plastic spoon as they report she has thrown the stainless spoon across the room. She can grasp a glass and bring to her mouth and drink from it. Noticed is an increased "hacking" noise as well as spitting after eating. Personal hygiene is Mod A, oral hygiene is Mod A, bathing and dressing Max A, toileting Max A, transfers Mod A.
IADL	Dependent for all IADLs
Goals	Short-term goals (within 15 days): 1. Client will respond to specific sensory activities and behavioral approaches that will be determined to reduce manipulation of feces and smearing it on the wall by 75%. 2. Client will show increased tolerance by 50% of caregiver follow-through with toileting in the morning during ADL routine, and then after every meal and before bedtime. 3. Client will "rummage" through individually selected sensory containers to reduce inappropriate behaviors to less than 50% of the time. Long-term goals (within 30 days): 1. Client will perform toileting routine in bathroom with Min A with Mod verbal and gestural cues. 2. Client will increase tolerance of caregiver follow-through with FMP by 75% in order to maximize self-care performance.

OT TREATMENT SESSION 1

THERAPEUTIC ACTIVITY	TIME	GOAL(S) ADDRESSED	OTA RATIONALE
Educate family on OT plan of care. Request that they bring in some green beans to fidget with/snap; also requested that they bring in a weighted baby doll. Also request a trial ordering of a one-piece outfit that snaps/buttons in the back. Suggest that they bring in lemon popsicles or fruit ices, and lotions or oils with a strong lavender or citrus scent for nursing staff to apply to the client during morning routine.	30 min	#1 and #3	*Education and Training:* Instructed and educated family in OT plan of care. Requested green beans as client previously loved to dig in the dirt, and loved to snap beans. A trial of this activity will be completed to determine whether it would decrease anxiety and inappropriate behaviors. Weighted baby doll would provide a calming sensory object as well as give the client something to care for as she was a very devoted mother per family report, and a schoolteacher of 43 years. Lemon-flavored food would assist with cleansing the palette. Current pureed diet has low sensory texture; client most likely feels she has phlegm in her mouth and is spitting to get rid of it; eating an Italian ice with a metal spoon would provide more sensory stimulation. One-piece outfits that fasten in the back may decrease client access to buttocks. Also instructed caregivers to layer with undershirt or sweater, to help client stay warm.
Educate caregivers on the importance of a toileting schedule.	25 min	#2	*Education and Training:* Educated and instructed caregivers on the importance of providing Min A with toilet transfer and then staying in the bathroom with the client in order to reduce the risk for falls. Instructed caregivers that client may need to sit a little longer than usual in order to have a bowel movement. Discussed with nurse supervisor that client may "sense" constipation, therefore will try to "dig" it out. Suggested that nurse supervisor talk with physician and determine whether a review of medications could be completed. Client may benefit from changing out pain medications (which can be constipating).

Continued

PUTTING IT ALL TOGETHER Sample Treatment Session and Documentation (continued)

SOAP note: 3/5/—, 2:00 pm–2:50 pm

S: Client said "Come sit down here with me," when she saw the OTA enter the room.

O: Client participated in therapeutic activities on the memory care unit to determine what type of strategies would be beneficial to decrease negative behaviors such as playing in her feces and spitting on the floor. The client was orally and tactile oriented. Identified sensory activities such as snapping green beans needs done with close supervision due to client attempting to eat them. Required 1:1 close supervision and was able to sustain attention to task approximately 5 min. Presented a weighted baby doll, which client kept on her lap for the remainder of the session. It was also noted that other clients would attempt to come up to the client and socialize with her about the "baby." Client was presented with a metal spoon and fruit ice, and was able to self-feed appropriately from cup with metal utensil, with approximately 75% reduction in spitting behaviors at the end of the session.

A: Client smiling and engaging with other clients while she was holding the baby doll. Further instruction to caregivers is recommended to offer a metal spoon versus a plastic spoon in order to provide more sensory input to this client. Caregivers will need further instruction in which sensory activities have been effective in reducing negative behaviors.

P: Continue to see client for OT services 1X/day for 60 min for 2 weeks. Caregiver instruction on regular toileting schedule, how to present one-step verbal cues, gestural cues, and to eliminate excessive verbal jargon. Educate caregivers about the characteristics of clients with this stage of dementia.

Rebecca Jones, COTA/L, 3/5/—, 4:30 pm

TREATMENT SESSION 2

What could you do next with this client?

TREATMENT SESSION 3

What could you do next with this client?

REFERENCES

1. Amyotrophic lateral sclerosis (ALS) Fact Sheet, NINDS. (2015). Retrieved from http://www.ninds.nih.gov/disorders/amyotrophiclateralsclerosis/detail_ALS.htm
2. Nzwalo, H., Abreu, D., Swash, M., Pinto, S., & de Carvalhoaf, M. (2016). Delayed diagnosis in ALS: The problem continues. *Journal of the Neurological Sciences, 43*(1–2), 173–175.
3. Strong, M., Grace, G. M., Freedman, M., Lomen-Hoerth, C., Woolley, S., Goldstein, L. H., ... & Figlewicz, D. (2010). Consensus criteria for the diagnosis of frontotemporal cognitive and behavioral syndromes in amyotrophic lateral sclerosis. *Amyotrophic Lateral Sclerosis, 10*(3), 131–146.
4. Handy, C. R., Krudy, C., Boulis, N., & Federici, T. (2011). Pain in amyotrophic lateral sclerosis: A neglected aspect of disease. *Neurology Research International,* vol. 2011. doi:10.1155/2011/403808
5. Rooney J., Byrne S., Heverin M., Tobin K., Dick A., Donaghy C., & Hardiman, O. (2015). A multidisciplinary clinic approach improves survival in ALS: A comparative study of ALS in Ireland and Northern Ireland. *Journal of Neurology and Neurosurgery Psychiatry, 86*(5), 496–501.
6. Bouteloup C., Desport J. C., Clavelou P., Guy N., Derumeaux-Burel H., Ferrier A., & Couratier P. (2009). Hypermetabolism in ALS patients: An early and persistent phenomenon. *Journal of Neurology, 256*(8), 1236–1242.
7. Fast track, breakthrough therapy, accelerated approval, priority review. (2015). Retrieved from www.fda.gov
8. Lui, A. J., & Byl N. N. (2009). A systematic review of the effect of moderate intensity exercise on function and disease progression in amyotrophic lateral sclerosis. *Journal of Neurologic Physical Therapy, 33,* 68–87.
9. McDonald W. I., Compston A., & Edan G. (2001). Recommended diagnostic criteria for multiple sclerosis: Guidelines from the International Panel on the diagnosis of multiple sclerosis. *Annals of Neurology,* 50(1), 121–127.
10. Multiple sclerosis FAQs. (n.d.). Retrieved from http://www.nationalmssociety.org/What-is-MS/MS-FAQ-s
11. Diagnosing MS. (n.d.). Retrieved from http://www.nationalmssociety.org/Symptoms-Diagnosis/Diagnosing-MS
12. Pregnancy and reproductive issues. (n.d.). National Multiple Sclerosis Society. Retrieved from www.nationalmssociety.org
13. Treating multiple sclerosis. (n.d.). Retrieved from http://www.hopkinsmedicine.org/neurology_neurosurgery/centers_clinics/multiple_sclerosis/conditions/multiple_sclerosis_treatments.html
14. Rietberg M. B., Brooks D., Uitdehaag B. M., & Kwakkel G. (2011). Exercise therapy for multiple sclerosis: A review. *The Cochrane collaboration.* Chichester, United Kingdom: John Wiley & Sons.
15. White L. J., & Dressendorfer R. H. (2004). Exercise and multiple sclerosis. *Sports Medicine, 34*(15), 1077–1100.
16. Bermel, R. A., Rae-Grant, A. D., & Fox, R. J. (2010). Diagnosing multiple sclerosis at a later age: More than just progressive myelopathy. *Multiple Sclerosis, 16*(11), 1335–1340.
17. Who Gets ALS? (2016). Retrieved from www.alsa.org
18. Hirsch, L., Jette, N., Frolkis, A., Steeves, T., & Pringsheim, T. (2016). The incidence of Parkinson's disease: A systematic review and meta-analysis. *Neuroepidemiology, 46,* 292–300.
19. Gitlin L. N., Corcoran M., Winter L., Boyce A., & Hauck W. W. (2001). A randomized, controlled trial of a home environmental intervention: Effect on efficacy and upset in caregivers and on daily function of persons with dementia. *Gerontologist, 41*(1), 4–14.
20. What is Huntington's disease? (2016). Retrieved from http://hdsa.org/what-is-hd/
21. Imbriglio, S. (2010). Physical and occupational therapy family guide series. Huntington's Disease Society of America.
22. Paulsen, J., Ready, R., Hamilton, J., Mega, M., & Cummings, J. (2001). Neuropsychiatric aspects of Huntington's disease. *Journal of Neurology, Neurosurgery, and Psychiatry, 71*(3), 310–314. http://doi.org/10.1136/jnnp.71.3.310
23. Scher, L. M., & Kocsis, B. J. (2012). How to target psychiatric symptoms of Huntington's disease. *Current Psychiatry, 11*(9), 34–39.
24. Walker F. O. (2007). Huntington's disease. *Lancet, 369*(9557), 218–228. doi:10.1016/S0140-6736(07)60111-1. PMID 17240289
25. Pringsheim, T., Wiltshire, K., Day, L., Dykeman, J., Steeves, T., & Jette, N. (2012). The incidence and prevalence of Huntington's disease: A systematic review and meta-analysis. *Movement Disorders, 27*(9), 1083–1091. doi:10.1002/mds.25075
26. Swierzewski, S. J. (2015). Huntington's disease symptoms, prognosis. Retrieved from http://www.healthcommunities.com/huntingtons-disease/treatment.shtml
27. Maiuri, T. (2013). More evidence points to Huntington's disease exercise benefit. Retrieved from http://en.hdbuzz.net/151

28. Cruickshank, T. M., Thompson, J. A., Domínguez D, J. F., Reyes, A. P., Bynevelt, M., Georgiou-Karistianis, N., ... & Ziman M. R. (2015). The effect of multidisciplinary rehabilitation on brain structure and cognition in Huntington's disease: An exploratory study. *Brain and Behavior, 5*(2), e00312. http://doi.org/10.1002/brb3.312
29. Lios, S. (2010). The cognitive symptoms of Huntington's disease. Retrieved from http://web.stanford.edu/group/hopes/cgi-bin/hopes_test/the-cognitive-symptoms-of-huntingtons-disease/
30. Reddy, R. (2011). Stages of Huntington's disease. Retrieved from http://web.stanford.edu/group/hopes/cgi-bin/hopes_test/stages-of-huntingtons-disease/
31. What is Parkinson's Disease? (n.d.). Retrieved from www.pdf.org
32. What causes Parkinson's disease? (n.d.). Retrieved from http://nihseniorhealth.gov/parkinsonsdisease/whatcausesparkinsonsdisease/01.html
33. Roos, R. A. C., Jongen, J. C. F., & Van Der Velde, E. A. (1996). Clinical course of patients with idiopathic Parkinson's disease. *Movement Disorders, 11*, 236–242. doi:10.1002/mds.870110304
34. McCoy, K. (n.d.). Recognizing the progression of Parkinson's disease symptoms. Retrieved from http://www.everydayhealth.com/parkinsons-disease/parkinsons-disease-progression.aspx
35. The unified Parkinson's disease rating scale (UPDRS): Status and recommendations. (2003). *Movement Disorders, 18*, 738–750. doi:10.1002/mds.10473
36. Causes of Parkinson's disease. (n.d.). Retrieved from http://www.mayoclinic.org/diseases-conditions/parkinsons-disease/basics/causes/con-20028488
37. Chaudhuri, K. R., & Schapira, A. H. V. (2009). Non-motor symptoms of Parkinson's disease: Dopaminergic pathophysiology and treatment. *The Lancet Neurology, 8*(5), 464–474.
38. Khoo, T. K., Yarnall, A. J., Duncan, G. W., Coleman, S., O'Brien, J. T., Brooks, D. J., Barker, R. A., & Burn, D. J. (2013). The spectrum of nonmotor symptoms in early Parkinson disease. *Neurology, 80*(3), 276–281. doi:10.1212/WNL.0b013e31827deb74
39. Gene therapy for PD. (n.d.) Retrieved from http://pdcenter.neurology.ucsf.edu/professionals-guide/gene-therapy-pd
40. Cosgrove, G. R., & Eskandar, E. (n.d.). Thalamotomy and pallidotomy. Retrieved from http://neurosurgery.mgh.harvard.edu/functional/pallidt.htm
41. Earhart, G. M. (2009). Dance as therapy for individuals with Parkinson disease. *European Journal of Physical Rehabilitation Medicine, 45*(2), 231–238.
42. Alzheimer's disease facts and figures. (2012). Retrieved from http://www.alz.org/downloads/facts_figures_2012.pdf
43. About Alzheimer's disease: Alzheimer's basics. (n.d.). Retrieved from https://www.nia.nih.gov/alzheimers/topics/alzheimers-basics
44. 2016 Alzheimer's disease facts and figures. (2016). Retrieved from www.alz.org
45. Cerejeira, J., Lagarto, L., & Mukaetova-Ladinska, E. B. (2012). Behavioral and psychological symptoms of dementia. *Front Neurology, 3*, 73.
46. Wilkins, C. H., Moylan, K. C., & Carr, D. B. (2005). Diagnosis and management of dementia in long-term care. *Annals of Long Term Care, 16*(12).
47. Alzheimer's disease fact sheet. (2015). Retrieved from https://www.nia.nih.gov/alzheimers/publication/alzheimers-disease-fact-sheet
48. Lewy body dementia symptoms. (n.d.). Retrieved from https://www.lbda.org/content/symptoms
49. The later stages of dementia. (2012). Retrieved from https://www.alzheimers.org.uk/site/scripts/documents_info.php?documentID=101
50. Cramer, L. (n.d.). Taking a fresher look at sundowning. Alzheimer's Association Caregiver Tips and Tools. Number 36.
51. Tombaugh, T. N. & McIntyre, N. J. (1992). The mini-mental state examination: A comprehensive review. *Journal of the American Geriatrics Society, 40*(9), 922–935.
52. Reisberg, B., Ferris, S. H., de Leon, M. J., & Crook, T. (1982). The global deterioration scale for assessment of primary degenerative dementia. *American Journal of Psychiatry, 139*, 1136–1139.
53. Velligan, D. I., Bow-Thomas, C., Mahurin, R., Miller, A., Dassori, A., & Erdely, F. (1998). Concurrent and predictive validity of the Allen cognitive levels assessment. *Psychiatry Research, 80*(3), 287–298.
54. Snow, T. (2016). The GEMS brain change model. Retrieved from http://teepasnow.com/events/teepas-gems/
55. Ahlskog, J. E., Geda, Y. E., Graff-Radford, N. R., & Petersen, R. C. (2011). Physical exercise as a preventive or disease-modifying treatment of dementia and brain aging. *Mayo Clinic Proceedings, 86*(9), 876–884.
56. Larsen, D. (2012). 11 tips for dealing with sundowning and dementia. Retrieved from www.aplaceformom.com
57. National Alzheimer's Association. (n.d.). Retrieved from http://www.alz.org/care/dementia-medic-alert-safe-return.asp
58. Fu, C.-Y., Moyle, W., & Cooke, M. (2013). A randomized controlled trial of the use of aromatherapy and hand massage to reduce disruptive behavior in people with dementia. *BMC Complementary and Alternative Medicine, 13*, 165.
59. American Occupational Therapy Association. (2014). Occupational therapy practice framework: Domain and process (3rd ed.). *American Journal of Occupational Therapy, 68*(Suppl 1), S1–S48.
60. Bromberg, M. B. (2008). Quality of life in amyotrophic lateral sclerosis. *Physical Medicine Rehabilitation Clinical North America, 19*(3), 591–605.

ACKNOWLEDGMENTS

I would like to thank Genesis Rehab Services for promoting education to their employees on treating residents who have dementia, as well providing numerous resources to their clinicians. Most of all, I would like to remember and honor my mother, Audrey J. McDermond, who had dementia. Mom always taught me to "go out and be a voice for those who cannot speak up for themselves." ~ Megan McDermond Shein, OTR/L

Chapter 33

Cerebrovascular Accident: Critical Aspects and Components of Care

Melinda Cozzolino, OTD, OTR/L, MS, CRC, BCN

LEARNING OUTCOMES

After studying this chapter, the student or practitioner will be able to:

33.1 Describe the physiological mechanisms that cause the various types of cerebrovascular accident

33.2 Explain the effects of cerebrovascular accident based on location in the brain

33.3 Determine the various resulting physical and psychosocial effects of cerebrovascular accident

33.4 Discuss the functional impact of a cerebrovascular accident on a client

33.5 Develop treatment intervention plans for clients experiencing various effects of cerebrovascular accident

33.6 Use current evidence based research to develop treatment plans

KEY TERMS

Cerebrovascular accident (CVA)
Compensatory movements
Contraversive pushing
Feedback
Flaccidity
Flat affect
Hemianesthesia
Hemiparesis
Hemiplegia
Hemorrhagic stroke
Hypertonicity
Ideational apraxia
Ideomotor apraxia
Ischemic stroke
Neuroplasticity
Stroke
Synergy pattern
Transient ischemic attack (TIA)
Unilateral neglect
Venous thromboembolism (VTE)

According to the American Stroke Association,[1] a stroke occurs every 40 seconds and is the fifth leading cause of death in the United States as of 2016. A **cerebrovascular accident (CVA),** also known as a **stroke,** occurs when blood flow to the brain is interrupted, resulting in oxygen not being able to reach parts of the brain. Where the brain lacks enough oxygen, damage to that neural tissue occurs, resulting in many types of symptoms.

The interruption of blood flow can occur for a short period, as is the case of a **transient ischemic attack (TIA).** This results in symptoms being present for usually less than 24 hours.[2] Despite the short duration of symptoms with a TIA, it is a serious condition and can be a warning sign of a future, more permanent and significant stroke to come. The cost of stroke, including the cost of health care and missed days of work, is estimated to be $34 billion each year in the United States.[3] Stroke is the leading cause of disability in the United States,[1] and the lasting effects experienced by clients are commonly treated in occupational therapy (OT).

RISK FACTORS

Stroke has associated modifiable and nonmodifiable risk factors. Modifiable, or preventive, risk factors are those a person can change and/or control. They include hypertension (high blood pressure), smoking, coronary heart disease, hyperlipidemia (high cholesterol), obesity, diabetes, and drug abuse. Hypertension has been cited as a leading cause of stroke, with nearly 70% of people who have a stroke being hypertensive.[4] Cigarette smoking has long been linked to both the incidence of stroke and coronary heart disease.[5] Coronary heart disease alone is the leading cause of death in the United States and a contributing factor to stroke.[6] High cholesterol has been linked to the incidence of stroke,[7] and obesity (having a high body mass index [BMI]) has long been discussed as a risk factor for stroke. New research points to the accumulation of visceral adipose tissue (VAT), also known as "fatty tissue" as having a correlation with increased stroke risk.[8] Diabetes has also been cited as a risk factor for stroke. Most recently, the length of time a person has diabetes has been independently linked to stroke with risk increasing 3% each year, thus an individual who has diabetes for greater than 10 years has a threefold risk for stroke compared with individuals who have newer onset diabetes.[9] Substance abuse is being increasingly cited as a source of stroke.[10]

Nonmodifiable risk factors are those beyond a person's control, such as gender, race, and age. A woman's risk for having a stroke between the ages of 55 and 75 years is 21%, which is higher than a man's risk of 14%–17% at the same age .[11] The risk of first-time stroke is twice as high in African Americans than in other races.[12] The risk of having a stroke doubles with every decade of age over the age of 55 years.[12] Recent evidence has shown, however, that there is a shift in this commonly cited age risk factor, with reported incidence of 45% of people who had a stroke under the age of 65 years out of a sample of 7740 people.[13] During the first year following a stroke, the risk of recurrent stroke is one in four, and that risk is 18% at 4 years after the stroke.[14]

Quickly identifying the signs of a stroke is important for early, potentially life-saving medical treatment. The early warning signs can be remembered as FAST, standing for **F**ace, **A**rm, **S**peech, **T**ime.[15]

- Face: **F**—Ask the person to smile. Does one side of the face droop?
- Arm: **A**—Ask the person to raise both arms. Does one arm drift downward?
- Speech: **S**—Ask the person to repeat a simple phrase. Is the speech slurred or odd?
- Time: **T**—Time is of the essence. If any of these signs are present, call 911.

TYPES OF STROKE

As previously described, stroke is a disease of blood flow in the brain. When blood flow is disrupted, brain cells are deprived of oxygen, and this ultimately results in cell death. The two primary types of stroke are ischemic and hemorrhagic. An **ischemic stroke** is the most common type of stroke and occurs when there is some type of blockage of blood flow. Common causes of ischemic stroke are blood clots, which are typically from cardiac sources. An embolic stroke is another type of ischemic stroke that occurs when a clot breaks free and travels through a vessel before causing a blockage. This traveling clot, called an *embolus*, may originate from vascular plaques or deep vein thrombosis (DVT). Forty percent of the time, the cause of an ischemic stroke is unknown.[16] A thrombotic stroke occurs as a result of buildup inside of the blood vessel, usually through atherosclerotic disease. This buildup occludes (blocks) the artery. A **hemorrhagic stroke** occurs when a blood vessel ruptures or leaks, most commonly because of hypertension bleeds, malformed blood vessels or veins, aneurysms (blood vessel weakness), or it may be spontaneous.[16,17] Hemorrhagic stroke causes the excess blood to come in contact with other brain tissue. This contact is often an irritant and results in more secondary complications for the affected individual. These strokes can also cause the skull to fill up with ruptured blood, squeezing brain tissues and causing significant pressure increases and damage. For hemorrhagic strokes, medical treatment often includes an endovascular procedure or other more invasive surgery. To treat a hemorrhagic stroke caused by an aneurysm or arteriovenous malformation (AVM), the surgeon performs the endovascular procedure by threading a tube from an artery in the groin up to the affected area in the brain. The tube houses a small wire stent, which can be inserted into the artery to prevent rupture.[18] Surgery is sometimes required to stop the bleeding. One type of surgery is to cut open the skull and place a clip at the aneurysm to stop the bleeding. Another surgery is to repair or remove the AVM.[19]

TECHNOLOGY AND TRENDS

Optimal medical treatment for an ischemic stroke depends on timing. Quick identification of the symptoms of a stroke (FAST) help to get the client emergency medical attention. The "gold standard" of stroke care has been tissue plasminogen activator (tPA, also known as intravenous line [IV] rtPA, given through an IV in the arm). The medication travels through the bloodstream and works to quickly dissolve the clot that is blocking the normal passage of blood in the brain. The medication can be given within the first 3 hours of the initial onset (up to 4.5 in some clients).[18] However, the tPA is not always effective, and some people do not get medical attention fast enough to even qualify for the drug.[20]

Another type of treatment is an endovascular procedure, in which the physician inserts a catheter with a stent (wire cage) device into an artery in the groin and threads it up through the arterial pathways to the location of the clot in the brain. The physician guides the stent to "grab" the clot, pulls it into the catheter, and pulls it back out through the artery.[18] Other times, the stent fills/repairs the spot of the hemorrhagic bleed, and is left in that spot as support.

Sometimes, individuals who have experienced a stroke are medically treated with both tPA and the endovascular procedure. In fact, the endovascular procedure can be more effective because it physically removes the clot rather than waiting for medication to dissolve the clot.[20] In a Canadian research study, 53% of clients who had both treatments were functionally independent 3 months after the stroke versus just 29% of clients who were given only the tPA. Furthermore, the study found that 91% of clients were alive 3 months after the stroke versus 81% of the tPA only group.[20]

EFFECTS OF STROKE

The early signs of stroke directly correlate with the function of the part of the brain that has lost blood flow and oxygen. In general, certain areas of the brain are responsible for certain types of functions (Table 33-1 and Fig. 33-1). The common impairments following a stroke that impede occupational participation can be broken down into these major categories: neuromuscular and movement-related functions, sensory-perceptual functions, mental-cognitive functions, and other bodily functions.[21]

Neuromuscular and Movement-Related Functions

Clients who have experienced a stroke present with a variety of neuromuscular and movement-related symptoms, including loss of control of voluntary movement and coordination. Many of the terms in the following sections have been

TABLE 33-1 Common Arteries and Symptoms

ARTERY	SYMPTOMS/PROBLEMS
Internal carotid	Hemianopsia, aphasia, hemiparesis
Anterior cerebral	Hemiparesis, especially in contralateral legs
Middle cerebral	Contralateral hemiplegia, aphasia, homonymous hemianopsia, neglect, anosognosia,
Posterior cerebral	Ataxia, dizziness, diplopia, hemiparesis, hemianopsia, dysphasia, dysarthria
Basilar	Breathing difficulties, sensory/balance disorders, ataxia, nystagmus, tremors, vomiting
Cerebellar	Sensory, headaches, fever, vomiting, balance changes, dizziness, coordination

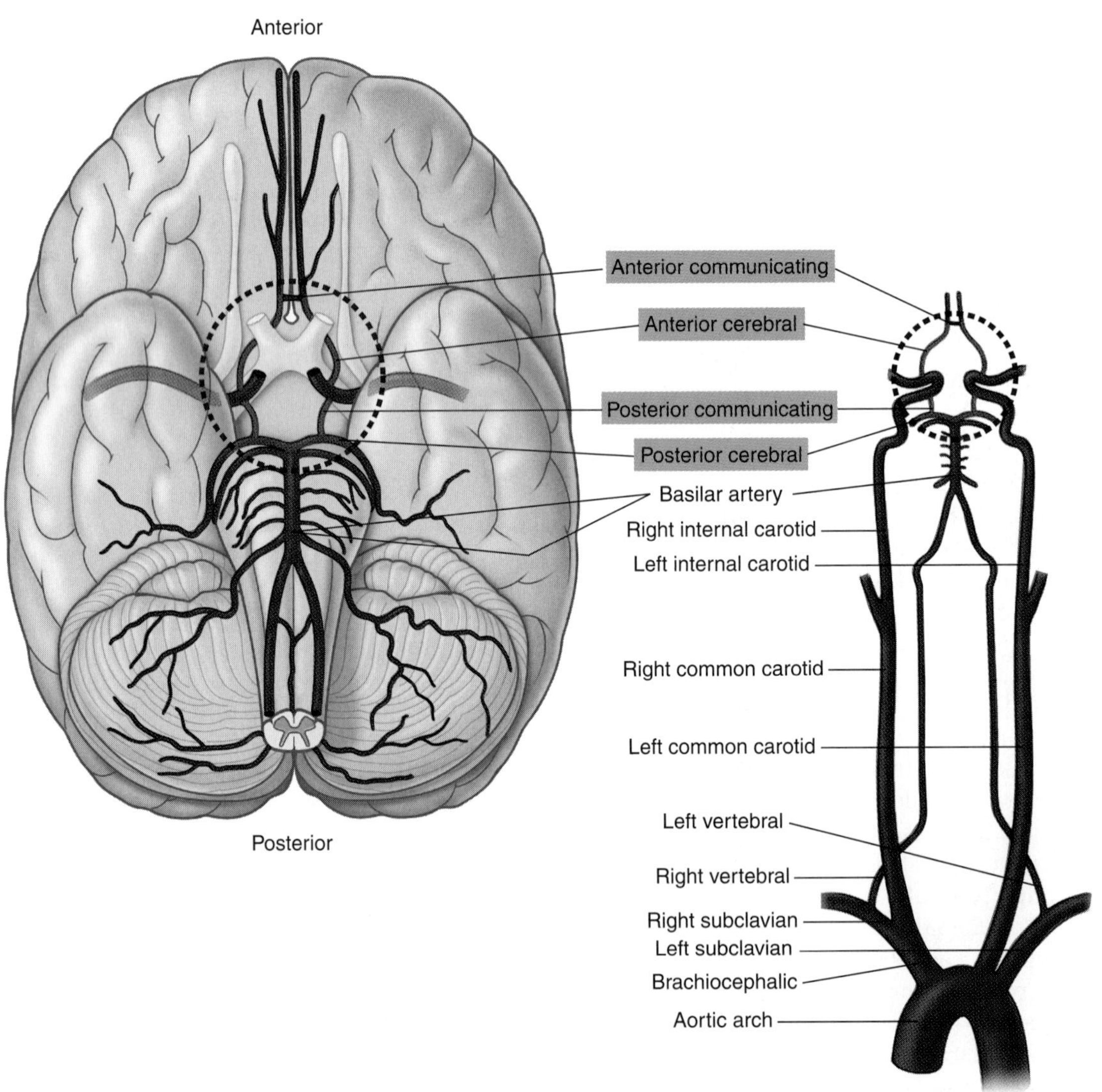

FIGURE 33-1. Arteries and locations in the brain.

defined thoroughly in earlier chapters, so there will only be a short review in this chapter.

Clients may have hemiplegia or hemiparesis as well as flaccidity or spasticity. **Hemiplegia** is a significant weakness or paralysis that affects one side of the body, whereas **hemiparesis** is a milder weakness that affects one side of the body. **Hypertonicity,** or *spasticity,* refers to an abnormally strong skeletal muscle that is resistant to stretch and is velocity dependent. In **flaccidity,** the opposite of spasticity, a person has no muscle tone or resistance to passive stretch; the limb appears floppy. Many times clients will have flaccidity initially and then progress to spasticity with a synergy pattern as the brain begins to recover. Clients who have had a stroke may present with a stereotypical flexor or extensor **synergy pattern** of the upper extremity (UE) (Fig. 33-2). Both are considered abnormal synergies that prevent clients from performing independent functional activities. There is significant variety in both client presentation as well as references and resources with regards to the patterns. Flexor synergy is the most common, and the pattern presents as:

- Scapula adducted
- Shoulder externally rotated and abducted
- Elbow in flexed position
- Forearm supinated
- Wrist flexed
- Fingers flexed

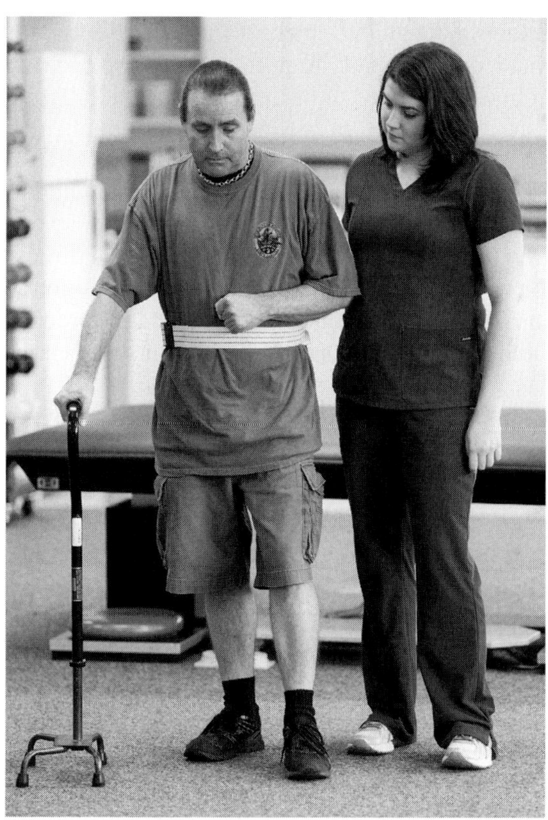

FIGURE 33-2. Common flexor synergy pattern of upper extremity after a stroke.

Extensor synergy pattern presents as:

- Scapula abducted
- Shoulder internally rotated and adducted
- Elbow in extended position
- Forearm pronated
- Wrist extended or flexed
- Fingers variable[22]

Clients who have had a stroke may also experience abnormal movements. These may include *ataxia,* which refers to abnormal voluntary movements that are of normal strength but are jerky and inaccurate and interfere with achieving the goal of specific movement and, in some cases, prevent independent performance of occupations. All of the problems with voluntary movement, coordination, and involuntary movements may result in decreased joint range of motion (ROM), which results in the inability to move a body part through the arc of desired motion. **Shoulder subluxation** may also occur, and this is the misalignment of the humeral head in the glenoid fossa, causing the humerus to be positioned outside of the joint cavity. Its causes include weak/flaccid rotator cuff and other shoulder musculature, and nonalignment of the scapula on the rib cage.[23] The subluxation is typically inferior, when the head of the humerus hangs downward from the joint cavity, but subluxations can be anterior (forward) and posterior (backward) as well, generally from abnormal tone or imbalanced musculature at the shoulder. The occupational therapy assistant (OTA) should be aware of and try to prevent a weak or flaccid affected arm from hanging without support. The amount of subluxation is often measured informally as "one-finger" and "two-finger," referring to distance out of the joint. Later in the chapter, specific positioning methods will be discussed.

Sensory-Perceptual Function

Clients who have had a stroke may experience residual effects related to sensory-perceptual areas of function. These symptoms may include problems with the visual system, as loss in specific areas of the visual field (field cut) occurs frequently. *Hemianopsia* (one sided field cut) and *diplopia,* or double vision, are types of visual problems people may experience following a stroke. See Chapter 10 for specific details.

Sensory problems following a stroke also include the way the body is able to feel. **Hemianesthesia** is the loss of feeling in one side of the body, usually the same side that has movement changes. Loss of the ability to feel touch, temperature, and loss of proprioception (being aware of where a limb is located) are safety concerns and also impact occupational performance.

Mental-Cognitive Functions

Following a stroke many people have cognitive symptoms. These individuals may have problems with their ability to pay attention, remember things, problem-solve, organize, and prioritize tasks (executive functioning). They may appear to not recognize or "ignore" half their body or items in the space opposite the side where their stroke occurred. This phenomenon is called *unilateral neglect.* They may also deny or not notice that they are having any problems at all, this is known as *anosognosia.*

After a stroke, individuals may have difficulty recognizing the appropriate use of an object. They may try to comb their hair with their toothbrush or eat their soup with a knife. They may not be able to visually recognize a common object but can describe its use. These types of cognitive symptoms are known as *agnosia. Apraxia* is another type of cognitive symptom that affects a person's ability to complete a known sequence of movements. Individuals with apraxia will have intact strength, sensation, and movement ability, but they cannot complete the task. They may place the cheese on top of a sandwich instead of between the slices of bread, don their bra over their shirt, or pour cream on top of their eggs instead of in their coffee. There are specific types of apraxia named for the difficulties a person is having, such as dressing apraxia and constructional apraxia. See Chapter 11 for further information on cognition.

Emotional/Behavior Functions

Emotional and behavioral effects fall under the large category of mental-cognitive symptoms. A person who has had a stroke may experience frustration, anxiety, or depression. These may occur as a result of knowing that he or she has acquired a chronic illness or as a result of neurological changes in the brain.[12] Neurological changes in the brain may also result in a person presenting with a flat affect. A **flat affect** is seen when a person does not display any emotional expressions and body gestures. He or she appears to have a stony expression, with little reaction to things around them. The opposite of a flat affect is *emotional lability,* which is seen when a person is unable to control any emotional expression. He or she may cry at something benign that never would have caused them to cry before or laugh at inappropriate times. The emotional/behavioral symptoms of a stroke are often undiagnosed, untreated, and very frustrating for the individual and his or her family members. These symptoms may or may not improve over time.

Other Effects

Other residual effects commonly occurring following a stroke include problems with language. *Wernicke's aphasia* is an impairment of the ability to understand language. People with Wernicke's aphasia have intact hearing; they simply cannot understand what is being said to them or what is written. It is described as *receptive aphasia. Expressive aphasia* (Broca's aphasia) is when a person cannot talk or express himself or herself using language or writing. The individual can often understand what is being said but cannot respond in a timely or appropriate manner. Another type of language problem is *dysarthria.* Dysarthria is similar to other motor problems in that it involves weakness, spasticity, or incoordination of the muscles needed for speaking, and the speech sounds garbled. See Chapter 12 for further information on communication issues.

In addition to the effects of stroke relating to a specific area of the brain, effects can differ, depending on which side of the brain is impacted, the right or left hemisphere. The myth of "right brain versus left brain" has been debunked by the scientific community. Nonetheless, hemispheric differences do exist. Of the people who are right handed, 95% to 99% have their language centers in the left hemisphere of the brain. Seventy percent of left-handed people also have their language centers in the left hemisphere of the brain. It has also been noted that vision and attention are more dominantly represented in the right hemisphere of the brain.[24] These differences, along with what is known about how the motor and sensory systems work, allow for some educated guesses when someone has had a stroke. It must be remembered that each person is different and that brains are shaped by experiences, so these impairments may not always appear in everyone. Refer to Table 33-2 for a list of neurological functional areas, but also keep in mind these general "rules of thumb" are based on the side of the brain where a stroke may occur; these represent the most common type of stroke (middle cerebral artery).

COMMON LONG-TERM MEDICAL COMPLICATIONS FOLLOWING A STROKE

A stroke is a life-changing event that can affect many aspects of a clients' ability to participate in the occupations they choose and need to participate in. In addition to the wide array of symptoms defined previously, clients who have had a stroke and their caregivers will also need to contend with, and work to prevent, a number of conditions that may arise after a stroke. Working with clients and their families to address the following areas are of the utmost importance for OT practitioners. In each of the following sections, there is information on how the OT practitioner can address, or advocate for, care in that specific area.

TABLE 33-2 Neurological Functional Areas

A STROKE ON THE RIGHT SIDE OF THE BRAIN OFTEN RESULTS IN:	A STROKE ON THE LEFT SIDE OF THE BRAIN OFTEN RESULTS IN:
Left-sided hemiparesis or hemiplegia	Right-sided hemiparesis or hemiplegia
Left-sided proprioceptive and sensory impairments	Right-sided proprioceptive and sensory impairments
Visual hemianopsia	Visual hemianopsia
Left-body and visual neglect	Aphasia
Left-sided motor apraxia	Bilateral motor apraxia
Lack of insight into deficits	Problems with managing food in the mouth
Problems with swallowing	

Contractures

Clients who have had a stroke are prone to developing *contractures*, which are ROM impairments that occur as a result of decreased elasticity of the tissue around a joint. Such tissues include muscles, tendons, and ligaments; the tissue loses its elasticity as a result of a number of symptoms, including decreased active movement, incoordination, spasticity, and abnormal synergistic movement patterns. Contractures are prevented through passive range of motion (PROM), active-assistive range of motion (AAROM), and active range of motion (AROM) and by maintaining a prolonged stretch of the area through the use of positioning and orthoses.[16] Treating the spasticity itself can also be helpful. Some medicines given orally, via an injection, or internal pump have been used successfully, such as Botox™ and baclofen. In extreme cases, surgery is performed to "release" the shortened, contracted tissues.

Osteoporosis

Bone is a living tissue that is constantly cycling through a process of shedding and replacement of cells. Osteoporosis occurs when the bone sheds cells faster than they can be replaced, and this causes the bone to become brittle, weak, and more prone to fractures.[25] Since clients who have had a stroke often have hemiparesis, this results in unequal weight-bearing through one half of the body. Lack of normal movement and inconsistent weight-bearing can lead to osteoporosis. As a result of balance challenges as well as osteoporosis, these clients may be more prone to falls and fractures. Prevention of osteoporosis is achieved through active weight-bearing exercise, active motion, strengthening, and medical management.

Seizures

Clients who have had a stroke are more prone to experiencing a seizure similar to that caused by epilepsy. The National Stroke Association places the incidence at around 5% in the early stages following a stroke,[26] and some other sources place this at a higher rate (3%–38%).[16] Later-onset seizures can occur as well, with a reported incidence of 6% to 18%.[16] Seizures are best managed through use of pharmaceutical agents, as well as education on necessary actions to take if they occur (see Chapter 4).

Deconditioning

Following a stroke, individuals can become easily and quickly deconditioned, particularly as a result of bedrest immediately following the stroke and the subsequent immobility that can occur in association with the effects of the stroke. Hemiparesis/hemiplegia, visual-perceptual symptoms, and cognitive symptoms all can play a role in a person's ability to seek and maintain physical fitness. Chronic deconditioning can exacerbate other symptoms, such as weakness, fatigue, and muscle atrophy, and also can affect cardiovascular health and have a negative impact on urinary function. Treatment for deconditioning is early and aggressive mobility and exercise.

Urinary Tract Dysfunction

It is common to experience urinary incontinence following a stroke, with an early incidence rate of 37% to 79% and with one third of those individuals still having a problem with incontinence 1 year after the stroke.[27] Urinary incontinence is thought to be caused by weak or hypertonic urinary sphincter muscles and as a result of inattention and immobility. Treatment of urinary incontinence includes establishing a scheduled voiding routine, managing the diet, pelvic floor exercises, and proper hygiene; an indwelling or condom catheter is sometimes required to decrease other negative effects, such as skin breakdown and infections.

Skin Breakdown and Sores

Pressure injuries are a common problem for any person who is immobilized. Following a stroke, clients are at risk of skin breakdown and sores because of the effects of the stroke, such as decreased sensation, decreased movement, spasticity, and contractures. Cognitive and perceptual problems may impact a person's ability to either change body positions frequently or recognize the importance of doing so. Swallowing and feeding problems may lead to malnutrition that could hasten skin breakdown. The OTA plays an important role in the prevention of pressure injuries by initiating a positioning schedule and educating and training the client, his or her family, and other healthcare practitioners to follow program the correctly and frequently. Maintaining proper nutrition and keeping skin clean and dry are other ways to prevent pressure injuries. The use of a pressure relief mattress and pressure-relieving chair cushions will also help in preventing pressure injuries and skin breakdown. See Chapter 8 for more detailed information on wounds and their prevention and treatment.

Dysphagia

Dysphagia (difficulty swallowing) following a stroke has a reported incidence of 37% to 45%.[28] Swallowing problems can lead to malnutrition, aspiration, and pneumonia. The OT practitioner has a role in assisting clients with swallowing and feeding. OT practitioners work with speech language pathologists (SLPs) and dietitians to determine the most proper course of treatment for the client with dysphagia. Treatment can include positioning, exercises, stimulation, modified swallowing techniques, and modified diets. See Chapter 12 for more details on swallowing.

Deep Vein Thrombosis

DVT is the formation of blood clots in the venous system. A **venous thromboembolism (VTE)** occurs when the blood clot dislodges and moves within the circulatory system, ultimately causing a blockage that can be fatal. The incidence rate of DVT following a stroke is 23% to 75%, with a mortality rate of 10%.[16] Factors for developing a DVT are the same as the risk factors for stroke, such as cardiac disease and obesity, and other factors directly related to the effects of the stroke, such as immobility. Treatment of DVT is prevention; most commonly, people are placed on a low dose of heparin, an anticoagulant. Early mobility programs are also important for the prevention of DVT. Once a DVT is discovered, medications are administered intravenously, and the client is placed on bedrest until the DVT has been cleared. Therapy should continue bedside; the OT practitioner and the client should avoid moving the limb with the DVT.

Psychological Factors

Numerous psychological factors are associated with a stroke. Typical emotional reactions tend to follow a life-threatening illness and subsequent hospitalization. Clients feel overwhelmed and anxious and experience a sense of loss of control. Social isolation and depression are common during the early stages of post-stroke recovery. Role changes and dependence on others will often result in a feeling of loss of self-worth. Grief, guilt, anger, fear, and shame are all common and appropriate reactions to illness and disability. The rate of diagnosable depression following a stroke is around 30%, but this condition is often undertreated.[29] The rate of poststroke anxiety is reported at 28%.[30] Treatment of the psychological factors related to a stroke should be incorporated into all aspects of intervention. The OT practitioner should address coping strategies and role changes with the client. Setting realistic, achievable goals will increase a person's sense of self-worth. Providing clients with activities or modifications that can provide them with a sense of control is also helpful. Support groups, peer support, and counseling are beneficial. Pharmaceutical management is often warranted, and a psychiatrist should be consulted.

Falls

Individuals who have experienced a stroke are at a great risk for falling. Stroke-related symptoms, such as hemiparesis/hemiplegia, decreased sensation, and changes in cognition and visual-perceptual abilities all increase the risk for a fall. Falls can occur at all stages of recovery. During the inpatient stage, between 10.5% and 47% of clients will experience a fall. Among clients dwelling in the community, the prevalence of falls ranges from 40% to 73% 3 months after the stroke, and 43% to 70% at 1 year follow-up.[31] Older adults who have experienced a stroke are at a greater risk for fractures following a fall because of the presence of osteoporosis, as mentioned earlier. Fall prevention is crucial following a stroke, and many communities have established educational and prevention programs for older adults and individuals who have experienced a stroke. Prevention, which involves the entire team of healthcare providers, should include medical management (some medications could increase dizziness or confusion), balance and strength training, cognitive training, environmental modifications, and mobility aid training.[32]

STROKE REHABILITATION: OVERVIEW

The effects of stroke vary widely, as explained thus far, yet some common issues are seen in motor, process, and social skills throughout the phases of stroke rehabilitation. The remaining sections of this chapter are dedicated to providing evidence-based treatment interventions. To assist the reader, Table 33-3 offers as an overview of the most

TABLE 33-3 Commonalities and Occupational Therapy Intervention Strategies for Phases of Stroke Rehabilitation

PHASE OF INTERVENTION	WHAT CLIENT MAY BE EXPERIENCING IN THIS SETTING/PHASE	PROBABLE INTERVENTION FOCUS	ADDITIONAL CONSIDERATIONS
Acute care (average of 4 days after stroke, can be up to 30 days for LTAC)[33] Hospital setting or LTAC	<u>Motor:</u> Flaccid hemiplegia Apraxia Swallowing/feeding issues Max A to dependent assistance for bed mobility and transfers Max A to dependent assistance for self-care <u>Process Skills:</u> Hemianopsia Disorientation Decreased alertness/arousal level <u>Social Interaction:</u> Aphasia (left brain lesion)	1. Positioning • Bed • Support for flaccid limb • Educate team members and family on how to position limb 2. Early mobilization • Bed mobility • Transfers to wheelchair • Transfers to commode 3. Work with team for bedside feeding in upright position 4. Set up room to allow participation if neglect is present (call bell/phone positioned to the unaffected side) 5. Bedside bathing and grooming, oral care	Primary goal is medical stabilization Work to increase out of bed endurance to ready for transfer to rehabilitation program

TABLE 33-3 Commonalities and Occupational Therapy Intervention Strategies for Phases of Stroke Rehabilitation (continued)

PHASE OF INTERVENTION	WHAT CLIENT MAY BE EXPERIENCING IN THIS SETTING/PHASE	PROBABLE INTERVENTION FOCUS	ADDITIONAL CONSIDERATIONS
Inpatient rehabilitation setting (approximately 9–22 days depending on mild, moderate, or severe)[34]	Motor: Hemiplegia with tone changes Arm may have higher tone Synergy patterns may be present Apraxia Dysphagia/self-feeding deficits could be improving Min-Mod A for functional mobility Min-Mod A for self-care More energy, but needs structured rest periods Process: More alert and oriented Cognitive/perceptual deficits more noticeable with increased activity Social: Aphasia Impulsivity/behavioral issues	1. Motor learning principles/task oriented functional activities to improve upper extremity function. • Use: Mirror therapy, bilateral UE training, action observation, mental practice, weight-bearing techniques, functional electrical stimulation, sensory reeducation • Positioning needs continue • Think about orthotics 2. Activities of daily living (ADLs) training in context with own clothing. Teach hemi-dressing techniques 3. Self-feeding training or groups 4. Insight training and remediation/compensation for visual-perceptual deficits 5. Behavioral interventions, as needed, with interdisciplinary team 6. Functional mobility training incorporating transfers to many different surfaces (bed, toilet, chairs, tub bench, car, etc.) 7. Light instrumental activities of daily living (IADLs) (snack or light meal prep)	Restore or compensate for performance skill deficits Prepare for discharge to home Home evaluation Home modification recommendations Secure adaptive equipment and durable medical equipment (DME) Caregiver training
Community (outpatient or home health)	Motor: Hemiparesis Tone/synergy with some volitional movement More energy, but still needs scheduled down times Has improved but deficits remain Apraxia mostly resolved Supervision—Min A for functional mobility Supervision—Min A for self-care IADLs require assistance Process: Alert and oriented May develop insight into cognitive/perceptual deficits Social: Aphasia improved but be may present Impulsivity improved but still requires some support for safety Psychosocial: Depression/anger may be present	1. Motor learning principles/task oriented functional activities to improve UE function. • Setup and monitor home programs to include: CIMT • Mirror therapy • Bilateral UE training • Action observation • Mental practice • Weight-bearing techniques • Functional electrical stimulation • Sensory reeducation 2. ADLs • Adaptive equipment and techniques to increase independence 3. IADLs • Adaptive equipment, meal preparation, house work, computer, money management 4. Return to work or volunteer work 5. Return to driving, if possible	Community reentry Secure adaptive equipment and DME Caregiver training Transportation must be addressed to gain access to community Accessible public transportation Leisure access Return to work or retraining, if possible Caregiver support

Continued

TABLE 33-3 Commonalities and Occupational Therapy Intervention Strategies for Phases of Stroke Rehabilitation (continued)

PHASE OF INTERVENTION	WHAT CLIENT MAY BE EXPERIENCING IN THIS SETTING/PHASE	PROBABLE INTERVENTION FOCUS	ADDITIONAL CONSIDERATIONS
Skilled nursing facility or long-term care (May be short-term rehabilitation or long-term/lifetime)	Motor: Hemiparesis or hemiplegia with tone changes Arm may have higher tone Synergy patterns present Pain syndromes may be present, most likely in the shoulder Mod–Max A is required for ADLs and IADLs Process: Visual-perceptual deficits (neglect) are often present Social: Language deficits may persist (aphasia) Impulsivity Psychosocial: Anger/Depression common in first 6 months	1. Positioning in bed, chair and during transfers is important to provide support and minimize pain • Lap or arm trays support arm in wheelchair • Taping, orthotics with soft covers (prevent skin breakdown) may also help • Slow, prolonged stretching to UE to maintain range and inhibit contractures • Modalities to decrease pain 2. Modify the room to enhance participation in ADLs, IADLs, and mobility. • Call bell/phone/TV remote in reach and accessible. • Items set up on the right side if left neglect is present 3. Active engagement and social participation through facility activities program and group leisure pursuits 4. ADL—provide adaptive equipment and training to facilitate maximum potential	Staff and caregiver training Meaningful participation Social connections Provide activity program or work with activity director to engage client

common concerns and basic OT interventions by phase. The table is meant to be a general guide to increase overall understanding of stroke rehabilitation; it is *not* a treatment plan because every client has specific and unique needs. Additionally, clients may not progress through rehabilitation in the exact order presented in the table, as indicated in Figure 33-3, which shows the various pathways of OT care following a stroke.

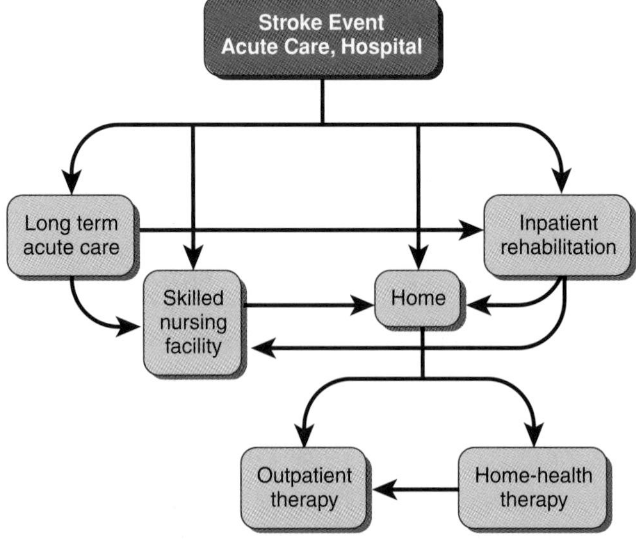

FIGURE 33-3. Pathways of care.

Importance of the Interprofessional Team in Stroke Rehabilitation

The residual effects of a stroke are vast and affect many areas of function. To adequately treat and rehabilitate a person following a stroke requires an interprofessional team of medical professionals, including OT practitioners. The term *interprofessional* means learning and working with others and being better for that learning; it is "purposeful and has to be fit for that purpose."[35] Numerous studies have documented the relationships among interprofessional team members resulting in better outcomes for clients who have experienced a stroke. One Canadian study completed with community-dwelling home care clients included an interprofessional team comprising a care coordinator, a registered nurse, a physiotherapist/physical therapist and a physical therapist assistant (PTA), an occupational therapist and an OTA, a SLP, a registered dietitian, a social worker, a personal support worker/social worker, family members, and the client. The team of professionals upheld the standards of interprofessional teamwork by working with and learning from one another, having open and frequent communication, and working toward a common purpose. The outcome of this work was improved scores for the client on a number of measures compared with clients who received treatment as usual.[36] Other team members, not included in this study but often seen, are the physician/physiatrist, recreational therapist, nurse assistant, psychologist/psychiatrist, equipment supplier, and chaplain. All of these professions contribute to the rehabilitation of a person who has had a stroke, and by working in an interprofessional manner, they improve the outcomes of that client's rehabilitation.

INTERVENTIONS FOR MOTOR IMPAIRMENTS

As previously mentioned, many people experience motor impairments following a stroke. This section will discuss the best practice for providing interventions for the common areas of motor impairments, specifically the UE, and for dysphagia.

Intervention and Management of Upper Extremity Impairments

Somewhat of a paradigm shift has occurred in recent years in the treatment of UE functional impairments following a stroke. Current evidence and advancements in neuroscience have provided support for certain types of interventions while negating others. Accreditation standards that guide OT education require knowledge of both evidence as well as current practice. Researchers performed a survey of current practice in relation to neurological treatment.[37] They found that of the 167 responding clinicians, most reported that the techniques that fell under the "task-oriented approach" were the most widely used. This was followed, in order of responses, by neurodevelopmental treatment (NDT), proprioceptive neuromuscular facilitation (PNF), Brunnstrom, constraint-induced movement therapy (CIMT) (which will be classified as a form of the task-oriented approach in this chapter), and Rood. NDT, PNF, Brunnstrom, and Rood are older frames of reference (FORs) for stroke intervention and are considered more traditional and hierarchical. Although current understanding of neurophysiology does not match the original premise for many of these FORs, they all have some clinical relevance and are still utilized clinically. To that end, each FOR will be discussed briefly here (a review from Chapter 8), with additional detail provided for the more current models of practice that are supported by evidence, such as the motor-learning techniques that guide the task-oriented approach.

NEURODEVELOPMENTAL TREATMENT

NDT was originally developed in the 1940s as a means to address abnormal movement in adults who had experienced a stroke and in children with cerebral palsy. This view of motor control revolved around feeling and learning the correct way to perform a movement. A person must *feel* normal movement to learn and later perform it. Abnormal movement patterns (spasticity and synergies) perpetuate and reinforce abnormal movement patterns and need to be inhibited. Once these abnormal patterns are inhibited, then normal patterns can be relearned. Inhibition of abnormal movements and facilitation of normal movements occur through the skilled OT practitioner performing learned *handling* techniques through a motor developmental sequence.[38] Once a client has learned a normal movement, it is repeated and eventually incorporated into functional tasks. The goal is to have voluntary control over normal movements while inhibiting abnormal movements. Using abnormal movements to complete a task is discouraged under the NDT approach. Although using an all-inclusive NDT approach has not been supported by evidence,[39,40] elements are useful to incorporate into other more contemporary approaches. Using the key points of control (proximal: pelvis, shoulders, trunk; distal: wrist, feet) during transfers and positioning is a good way to facilitate proper movement and positioning. Using some abnormal tone (spasticity) reduction techniques can be helpful before initiating ADLs. Reflex-inhibiting postures/patterns (RIPs) are another piece of NDT that can be incorporated into more contemporary models. RIPs are those positions and patterns of movement that are essentially opposite of the client's abnormal position. For example, if a client has the elbow in a flexed position at rest, the RIP that will be helpful and place muscles on stretch is to provide ROM and positioning into elbow extension. Here is the sequence an OT practitioner can perform to inhibit spasticity in a hemiparetic arm by using RIPs.

- Have the client in a comfortable, supported sitting position.
- Use proximal (trunk, pelvis, shoulder girdle) to distal (elbow, wrist) key points of control as places to provide input/control movement using the hands.
- Begin with the shoulder, and provide physical input to correct the adduction and internal rotation the humerus will most likely be in. Correct by slowly moving the humerus into slight abduction and external rotation to have it in a neutral position.
- Keep the humerus in this neutral position, and slowly and firmly provide pressure to the top of the forearm (elbow will most likely be flexed), and stretch into extension.
- Once the OTA feels the biceps relax a bit, move the hand slowly from the client's forearm to the wrist, and move the wrist into a neutral position because the wrist will be in a flexed position. Leave the fingers flexed at this point.
- When the OTA feels the client's wrist begin to relax into this neutral position, slowly and gently extend the fingers.
- Be careful not to overextend the wrist or fingers as damage to tendons and ligaments can occur. Carpal bones may be dislocated.

Once the OT practitioner has taken the time to obtain this position, participation in ADLs and weight-bearing activities are much more feasible for the client.

PROPRIOCEPTIVE NEUROMUSCULAR FACILITATION

PNF is defined as "a method of promoting or hastening the response of the neuromuscular mechanism through stimulation of the proprioceptor."[38] In the late 1930s, Herman Kabat found that when the distal segments were stimulated, the more proximal segments were also stimulated. PNF uses the body's proprioceptive system as a way to facilitate and/or inhibit muscle contraction.

PNF uses early motor learning theory as a basis for some of its stimulation. It proposes that using the stronger muscle groups will facilitate the weaker muscle groups (irradiation). Reciprocal innervation uses active movement to inhibit unwanted reflexes.[38] PNF considers multiple sensory stimulation beneficial with the OT practitioner using visual, physical, and verbal prompts. Additionally, PNF proposes the use of diagonal patterns, which can be easily incorporated into, and form the basis of, many functional tasks as a means to promoting motor recovery. For example, the D1 shoulder flexion pattern begins with shoulder flexion, adduction and external rotation, forearm supination, wrist radial deviation, and finger flexion. The arm is raised and across the midline of the trunk. The ending position for D1 flexion is shoulder extension, abduction, external rotation, forearm pronation, wrist ulnar deviation and finger extension. The arm comes diagonally across the body in a downward and outward pattern. D2 flexion begins with shoulder flexion, abduction and external rotation, forearm supination, wrist radial deviation and finger extension. The arm is raised away from the body and is brought down and across the trunk, ending with shoulder extension, adduction, internal rotation, pronation, wrist ulnar deviation, and finger flexion.[41] Incorporating these patterns (through physical and verbal prompts) into therapy and functional tasks is thought to enhance motor recovery. Many ADLs and IADLs are naturally suited for PNF. Placing a laundry basket to one side and at knee height will force the client to use diagonal patterns when hanging laundry on the clothesline. Placing a grocery bag in a specific position will promote the use of diagonal patterns while putting groceries into the cabinet or refrigerator. Having the ironing board positioned at a slight vertical angle can enhance the motor recovery of the limb through the activity of ironing. Thoughtful rearrangement of items used in everyday tasks can be a means to use PNF concepts to promote motor recovery.

BRUNNSTROM APPROACH

Signe Brunnstrom, a Swedish physical therapist, developed the theory of movement therapy in the 1950s. Similar to the other traditional theorists, Brunnstrom believed that movement was produced through lower-level reflexes being integrated or controlled by higher centers (cortical).[42] However, the neuroscience behind Brunnstrom's theory does not match current thinking about neuromuscular control. Brunnstrom documented many clinical observations of people's UE and lower extremity (LE) movement patterns after a stroke. Brunnstrom believed that after a stroke, a person's limb will move through seven stages of recovery, with each stage demonstrating different levels of abnormal tone or synergy patterns. These stages are explained in Chapter 8. While acknowledging the existence and debilitating effects of abnormal synergistic movement patterns, the Brunnstrom theory deviates from NDT in that it advocates the use of the primitive reflexive patterns to accomplish tasks, if possible, whereas NDT advocates inhibition of reflex patterns and promotion of normal movement. The Brunnstrom therapy follows a developmental sequence, facilitates movement through sensory stimulation to facilitate or inhibit synergies until they are under voluntary control. Although some of the Brunnstrom theory of treatment is outdated, some of the stages of motor recovery are still relevant. The Fugl-Meyer Assessment of Motor Recovery after a stroke is a popular and well-utilized assessment that is based on the Brunnstrom stages of motor recovery. Treatment interventions using this approach are dependent on the client's current stage. Interventions should follow a proximal-to-distal sequence. In stages I and II, the client's arm is either flaccid or just beginning to show reflex patterns. Here, the OT practitioner would facilitate reflex development. The OTA would use associated reactions by resisting elbow flexion on the less affected side to promote a biceps contraction on the affected side and use sensory techniques, such as tapping and vibration over groups, to facilitate the reflexive synergy pattern. Once the client moves into stage III (has synergy), and stage IV (some active movement outside of synergy), the OT practitioner would place the client's arm into a position, such as elbow extension, and have the client hold that position. Once the client is able to hold the position, the OT practitioner would have him or her begin to work on movement outside of the synergy pattern more independently. The OT practitioner can also provide resistance to movements (stage V), such as incorporating reaching tasks to provide a target for elbow extension, wiping tables, or putting dishes away with active guidance from the OT practitioner, as needed. The client could complete homework to use the newly acquired movement patterns multiple times a day. The Brunnstrom approach also uses weight-bearing techniques once the client has more control of the limb outside of synergy patterns.

ROOD APPROACH

The Rood approach is named after Margaret Rood, a clinician who was both an occupational therapist and a physical therapist. Rood's thinking was in line with other traditional theories at the time (1950s)—that voluntary control of movement emerged from reflexes that were present at birth.[38] Rood believed that appropriate sensory stimulation can elicit a motor response to either facilitate movement in a weak or flaccid muscle or inhibit abnormal tone. She incorporated icing, brushing, vibration, tapping, stroking, proprioceptive stimuli, joint compression, and quick stretches applied by the OT practitioner to facilitate movement. To inhibit abnormal tone (spasticity), Rood used sensory stimulation, such as neutral warmth, slow rhythmic rocking, and maintaining a sustained muscle stretch. As with the other early motor approaches, the motor/reflex/sensory systems, as Rood understood them at the time, have been disproven. The clinical significance of her therapeutic techniques remains, however, and is applied to other more current theories. For example, an OTA may provide slow sustained muscle stretch to inhibit the tone of a limb as a preparatory measure before movements, such as rolling out pizza dough, as a functional task under the task-oriented model of practice.

NEUROPLASTICITY

Neuroplasticity is the ability of the nervous system to change; it occurs at the cellular level. Neurons (nerve cells) can change their functions, the types of neurotransmitters they manufacture and transmit, and their genetic material; they can also develop more synapses, build more dendrites, and regrow after damage.[43] Neuroplasticity is a permanent change in the cellular structure and the way these cells communicate. It is necessary for learning and memory, task mastery, and recovery after injury. Although the term neuroplasticity was originally coined in the late 1800s, it was not until the 1990s that the nervous system's capacity to change could be fully understood with the ability to better image and see the cells of the nervous system in action with functional magnetic resonance imaging (fMRI) and positron emission tomography (PET).[44] Once this concept was understood, therapeutic interventions and animal experiments were developed and tested to determine what could enhance these changes.[45] The concept of neuroplasticity facilitating a permanent structural change in the nervous system following damage informs current therapeutic techniques and aligns with the principles of motor learning.

MOTOR LEARNING

Motor learning refers to how a person acquires or changes motor skills. How a person practices a skill and the feedback received during this practice are core concepts of motor learning theory.[46] OT practitioners need to pay close attention to how they are structuring practice sessions and providing feedback to their clients. Employing the techniques of motor learning across the continuum of care could improve the functional outcomes of individuals with motor impairments. Researchers summarize the structure and definitions of practice as follows:[47,48]

1. *Massed practice versus distributed practice*—Massed practice is continuous practice with few rest breaks. Distributed practice is when rest breaks occur in between practice trials. Massed practice has been shown to be more effective for motor learning. Individuals following a stroke are most likely to be quite fatigued, making true massed practice difficult. OT practitioners should remember this principle but use their client's abilities as a guideline.
2. *Variable practice versus constant practice*—Variable practice is when one piece of the practice is altered in some way. Using different size cups to drink from to practice grasp and release is an example of variable practice. Constant practice is practicing the same thing in the same way. Variable practice is thought to be better for motor learning. Through different types of practice the motor system is forced to problem-solve in new ways and thus adapts more readily to newly learned ways of completing a movement.
3. *Whole-task practice versus part-task practice*—Whole-task practice is when a client practices the whole task in its entirety. Part-task practice is when the task is broken down into smaller parts and those individual parts are practiced. Whole-task practice is thought to be better for motor learning. Whole-task practice, similar to variable practice, enhances motor problem-solving.
4. *Blocked practice versus random practice*—Blocked practice is when the same skill is practiced over and over until an improvement is seen. An example of this is a drill on a sports team. Practicing kicking a soccer ball with the inside of the foot over and over until a person can perform that single task well. Random practice, in contrast, is when the skill is practiced at different times in a different order. Kicking the soccer ball with the inside of the foot is practiced alongside dribbling the ball. Blocked practice shows immediate improvement in the discrete task, but random practice is thought to be better for long-term learning.

Feedback is another concept important for motor learning and involves information about a client's performance of a task, used as a basis for improvement. How an OT practitioner provides feedback, both the timing and content/type of feedback, has been shown to have an impact on recovery of a motor skill.[46] The two types of feedback are intrinsic—that which can be felt within and how one interacts with the environment—and extrinsic—the feedback provided by others. Extrinsic feedback is what an OT practitioner or coach provides, and it is meant to provide insight into and supplement a person's intrinsic feedback. Extrinsic feedback is subdivided into knowledge of results and knowledge of performance. Knowledge of results describes the outcome and the goal of the action and its success or failure. Saying "That was a terrific throw!" is an example of knowledge of results because it offers no feedback provided on the actual movements. Conversely, saying, "Try straightening the elbow more during the throw" is an example of knowledge of performance because it provides feedback related to the actual movements.

The timing of feedback is also important. Feedback should not be given while a person is performing a task but, instead, be delayed for about 5 seconds; this allows the person to first think about his or her performance. Feedback should be varied, not be provided each time, and be offered in a question/answer type of format, such as "How do you think that went?" Feedback should be faded over time—that is, more feedback is given during the beginning of learning and less is given over time.[48,49]

TASK-ORIENTED APPROACH

The OT task-oriented approach closely aligns with motor learning theories and has been supported by evidence.[50-52] It is based on a systems model of motor control. This means that occupational performance comes from the interaction between the individual and the environment. The principles of motor learning are applied by using the concepts of practice and feedback previously discussed. Learning comes out of a client's practice and interaction with the environment. Facilitating experimentation with different strategies leads to solving motor problems. The approach is client based and client driven—that is, the client chooses what he or she would like to work on and is an active participant in goal setting. Most importantly, the OT task-oriented approach is occupation-based. It uses functional tasks as a mode of therapeutic intervention. Intervention will change on the basis of the client's needs and the environment in which the task is being practiced.[53]

Newer therapeutic techniques, such as CIMT and bilateral training use the task-oriented approach as a model of intervention. Other newer interventions use cognitive strategies as ways to enhance task-oriented modes of therapy. These include mirror therapy, action observation (AO), mental practice, and virtual reality, and will be described later.

CONSTRAINT-INDUCED MOVEMENT THERAPY

CIMT involves restraining the less impaired arm in an oven mitt, cast, hand restraint, or sling. Clients wear the restraint for a minimum of 6 hours and up to 90% of their day. While wearing the restraint, clients participate in massed practice with functional tasks, which forces the more impaired arm to complete the functional tasks unassisted (Fig. 33-4). Research supports the use of CIMT for enhancing neuroplastic changes in the nervous system and improving UE function.[54-56] Modified CIMT (mCIMT) programs have also been found to be effective. They require less therapy time (1-hour sessions three times a week) and the use of restraint for 5 hours daily.[57] CIMT has been shown to be most effective in clients who have met the following criteria:

- A minimum of 10 degrees active wrist extension
- 10 degrees of active thumb abduction and extension
- 10 degrees of active abduction and extension in two or more digits.
- At least 3 months poststroke[58]

Client fatigue, client compliance, caregiver support, and cost are all factors to consider before implementing a CIMT program. Nonetheless, it is the most evidence-supported, task-oriented UE rehabilitation program available at this time.

BILATERAL TRAINING

Bilateral training uses both UEs to complete functional tasks simultaneously. The less affected limb assists the affected limb in massed practice task completion. Using both limbs simultaneously is thought to engage both hemispheres of the brain

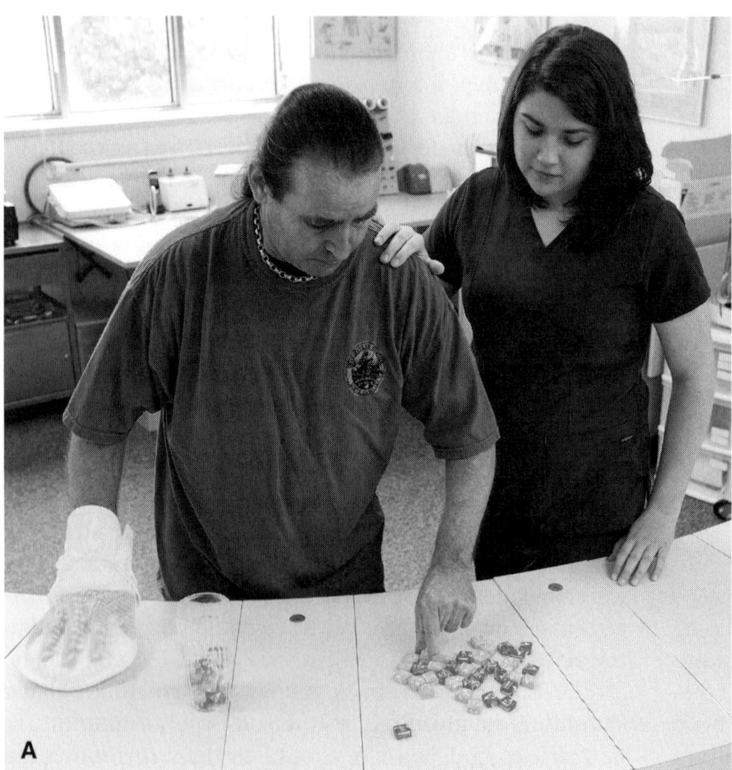

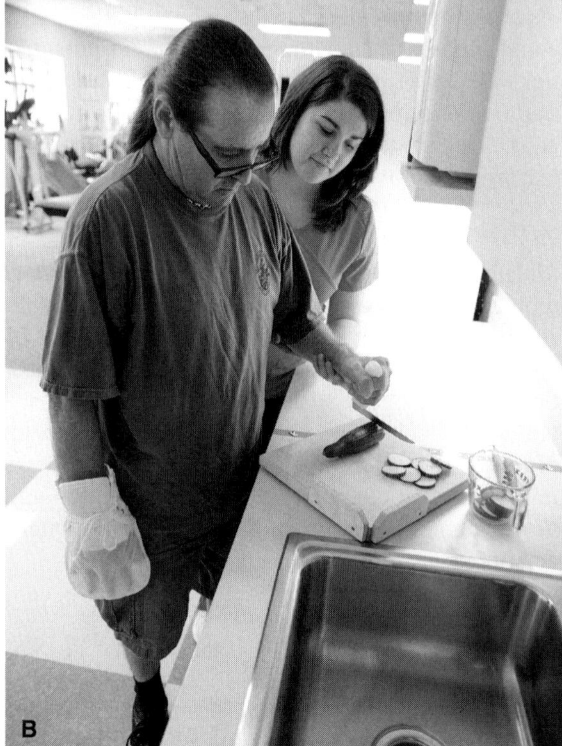

FIGURE 33-4. Constraint-induced movement therapy. **A.** Fine motor task. **B.** Gross motor task.

OT Practitioner's Viewpoint

The hospital-based outpatient clinic where I worked offered a traditional, 2-week CIMT program for several years. I was fortunate to have the opportunity to work with clients who were at various poststroke stages—from 3 months to several years—and were seeking the next level of functional gains. I am pleased to share that all who met the criteria for the program made functional gains during their 2 weeks, and some reported continued progress afterward as well.

Working with clients in the CIMT program was simultaneously challenging and rewarding. As the OTA, I was responsible for developing the treatment activities for clients, which was a demanding job because the protocol requires the client to perform tasks repeatedly in 20-minute intervals, with each task focusing on a specific skill or movement. I sought to provide activities that were intrinsically or extrinsically meaningful to each client to help them engage in the long therapy sessions and have optimal functional outcomes. I used my activity analysis skills constantly to develop and adjust the activities for the clients in the program; some activities were completed in 20 minutes, whereas others were multiday projects worked on in 20-minute increments. A few of the clients' favorite activities were scooping fresh melon balls, whisking pudding, making a toy car for a grandchild (sanding, painting, and assembling), designing tile mosaic patterns, hammering, and playing active games. Any activity that involved a food product became a same day reward for clients to eat at lunch, which was very motivating. Lunchtime was also therapeutic; clients brought their lunches or prepared them onsite, all while wearing the mitt on the unaffected UE and doing all tasks with the affected UE. By the end of the program, one client who was right hand dominant, left side affected stated, "I feel as though I am left-handed now."

With client permission, I took pictures and videos throughout the 2 weeks. At times of low confidence or discouragement, I directed the client's attention to view the earlier videos for increased self-awareness of progress attained. Clients were typically reenergized to keep working hard. At the end of the 2 weeks, clients received copies of the videos.

At the end of the 2-week program, in addition to physical assessments to measure progress, we also assessed the client's perceptions of their progress and their overall experience. One man who was the most dedicated, hardworking client I have ever worked with stated that he struggled to complete his 2 hours of daily HEP after the 4-hour session in the clinic because he did not have the same accountability and assistance/feedback and was also fatigued. He also mentioned that involving his spouse early on in the therapy sessions would have been beneficial because she would have better understood the demands of the program and could have assisted him at home to encourage him to complete his HEP. He actually continued to make progress after the CIMT and was able to return to a very physically demanding job in a competitive industry.

CIMT and mCIMT are evidence-based interventions with positive outcomes for the clients who meet the inclusion criteria. Many CIMT programs have moved to the mCIMT model due to insurance reimbursement issues and the time and staff resources required to hold a traditional program. Therefore, in providing the mCIMT program, OT practitioners should carefully design activities and methods of accountability for optimal client outcomes. ~ Amy J. Mahle, MHA, COTA/L

and increase the chances of neuroplasticity occurring. One study that compared bilateral massed practice training with equal hours of a CIMT program found that clients in both groups showed improvements.[56] Bilateral training is sometimes paired with an adjunctive type of intervention. Electromyography (EMG)–triggered neuromuscular stimulation and bilateral arm training with rhythmic auditory cueing (BATRC) have both been found to produce positive results[59,60] in improving UE function. The rhythmic auditory cuing simply is sound (cues) synchronized to movement. Motor areas are found to be active when clients listen to musical rhythms, and rhythm may be a means to improve efficiency in movement relearning.[61] A research study examined clients who completed bilateral training with BATRC and compared them with a group of clients who completed the same bilateral therapy but did not use BATRC.[59] The study used both UE assessments and an fMRI machine to look at cortical changes. Both groups showed improvement, but the results of the BATRC group on the fMRI machine looked different, causing the researchers to speculate about the different impacts these two types of intervention have on the cortex.

WEIGHT-BEARING

Weight-bearing through the more affected limb has been a therapeutic staple for many years. As understanding of neuroscience increases, so does the rationale for why there may be therapeutic benefits to having clients weight-bear through their more affected limb. A recent hypothesis identifies increased excitability in the motor cortex[62] during weight-bearing activities. Weight-bearing is important to prevent osteoporosis, facilitate proper postural alignment, and maintain soft tissue lengthening. Weight-bearing is best completed in conjunction with functional task performance. Using the more affected limb to hold a piece of paper in place during writing and placing the limb on the counter as a postural support when unloading a dishwasher are good examples of functional weight-bearing tasks. During a weight-bearing task, the less affected limb should be performing functional tasks. By performing functional tasks with guidance from the OT practitioner, clients will use proper weight-shifting, resulting in trunk engagement. Weight-bearing must be performed with proper alignment, or damage may occur to joints and tissues (Fig. 33-5). Proper positioning of the more affected UE is as follows:

- Palm arches of the hand must be maintained (hand should not be completely flat).

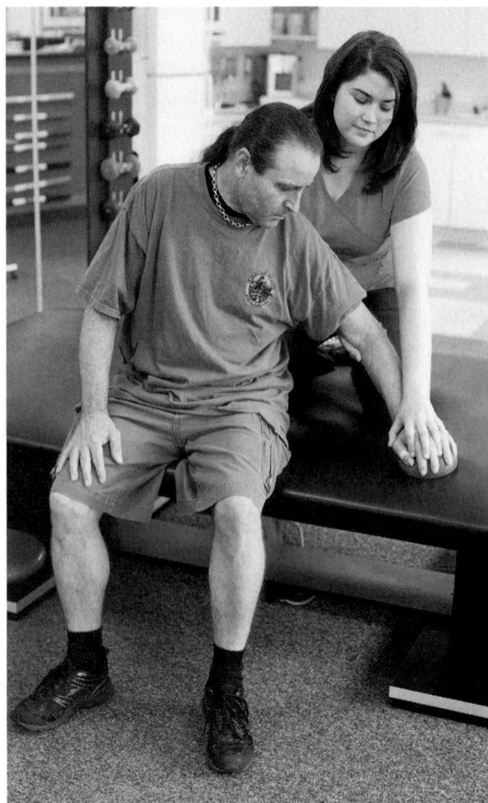

FIGURE 33-5. The OTA is assisting the client to obtain proper alignment for weight-bearing before initiating a functional task with non-affected UE.

- Thenar eminence, hypothenar eminence, metacarpal heads, and the palmar surfaces of the fingers should be touching the surface. The OT practitioner should be able to slide a finger between the web space and the first metacarpal head under the hand until it touches the hypothenar eminence.[63]
- Extreme shoulder internal rotation, forced elbow extension, and an inactive trunk should be avoided.[63]
- Weight-bearing through the forearm is also recommended.

STRENGTHENING

In the past, strengthening was an area where OT practitioners were tentative to engage for fear of increasing a client's spasticity. It is now known that although spasticity will appear to increase during active exertion, the effects are short lived. The benefits of strength training far outweigh any disadvantages. Ample evidence supports the use of general strengthening programs to increase UE function.[64,65] *Strengthening* is defined as any intervention that attempts an effortful, repetitive muscle contraction. The OTA must be thoughtful about how the client can be engaged in strengthening. Having a client place and hold the affected limb in different gravity-eliminated planes, with and without assistance, is a good way to strengthen. For example, the client should lie supine on a mat, and then the arm should be positioned at 90 degrees of shoulder flexion, with elbow extended. The client is cued to "hold" this position, while the OT practitioner provides support, as needed. This position has the scapula in a supported position and removes the pressure of gravity, so the client can strengthen the shoulder complex without fear of harming the delicate joint. Another reaching position that is safe for the client is to have him or her bend forward at the waist in a seated position to reach for items on the floor. This position has the shoulder at 90 degrees of flexion, also on a gravity-eliminated plane. Having the client reach for and grasp different functional objects is in line with motor learning theory. The classic activity of having the client "dust the table" is another early strengthening task that serves to eliminate gravity. The client should be in either the seated or standing position with the affected arm on a cloth placed on a table. He or she should then move the arm forward, back, and side to side. Incorporating the affected limb into as many functional tasks as possible will also serve to strengthen the arm. The OT practitioner should distinguish himself of herself from the physical therapy (PT) team members by incorporating functional, occupation-focused tasks into the strengthening program.

As the arm strengthens, other treatments in this category may include muscle reeducation, progressive resistance exercises (Chapter 9), electrical stimulation (see below and Chapter 18), and mental practice (see below).

COGNITIVE STRATEGIES USING A TASK-ORIENTED APPROACH

Some of the common concerns with regard to the rehabilitation of clients who have had a stroke is the decreased length of stay in rehabilitation and declining reimbursement for outpatient therapies. The average length of stay following a stroke is 8.9, 13.9, and 22.2 days for mild, moderate, and severely impaired individuals, respectively.[34] A 10-year study reported a 24% decrease in the length of stay for the period 1989 to 2009.[66] The general rule of thumb for inpatient therapy settings is that a client receives a minimum of 3 hours of therapy a day for 6 days a week. The cognitive strategies used as an adjunct to regular therapy can provide a safe and productive means for clients to participate in their recovery process.

Mirror Therapy: *Mirror therapy* is a technique in which the more affected forearm, wrist, and hand are placed behind a freestanding mirror or a table mirror, with the reflection of the less affected limb visible to the client. The more affected limb is hidden from view. The client is instructed to complete active movements and simple functional tasks with the less affected limb while looking in the mirror. The mirror image provides the illusion that the more affected limb is actually moving simultaneously with the less affected limb (Fig. 33-6). This illusion triggers neurons in the motor cortex, as if the more affected limb were actually performing the movements. The theory is that cortical stimulation will lead to neuroplasticity and

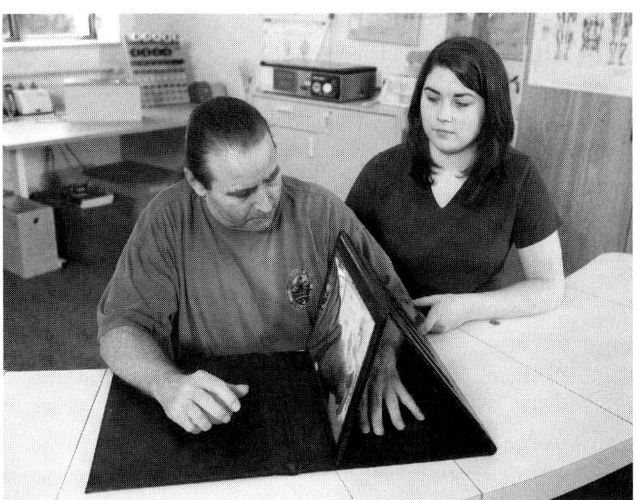

FIGURE 33-6. Mirror therapy.

regrowth of damaged neurons. Evidence supports the use of mirror therapy,[67,68] both in the clinical setting and in an independent home program.[69] The "how to" of mirror therapy differs among the available resources. One leading study recommends a frequency of two times a week in the clinic and four times a week at home for 150 repetitions of movement for each session.[70] Rotation of activities is helpful. Some activities used by the clients in this study included drinking from a cup, turning a key, and picking up coins (Table 33-4).

TABLE 33-4 Mirror Therapy Protocol[70]

Box	Begin with a flexible, shatter proof mirror, not warped or magnified Keep vertical Minimum size 15 inch height × 18 inch length
Hands	Need to be kept identical Remove jewelry, accessories Cover birthmarks and tattoos
Positioning	Client sits comfortably at a table Involved hand is inside the box, out of view Other hand rests in front of the mirror Client looks into mirror to view image
Stage 1	Initial observation Perform basic finger movements of uninvolved hand
Stage 2	Attempt bilateral movements Move from gentle to more intense Incorporate wrist and forearm movements
Stage 3	Incorporate tools and objects Use functional tasks as much as possible Follow the ideas of the task-oriented approach, where tasks are client driven and meaningful Find the "just right challenge"

Action Observation: In AO, the client watches another person perform a functional task, and the client will then attempt to perform the task. Watching a person perform a task stimulates the motor neurons in the cortex, and this is thought to promote neuroplasticity. A recent study compared two groups of individuals with hemiparesis following a stroke.[71] One group watched videos of people performing a motor task five times and then were asked to complete this task five times. The OT practitioner chose the motor tasks, which were specific to each client's needs. Examples of the tasks were picking up coins, taking a drink, and flipping cards. This group was compared with another group of subjects who did not watch the task being performed but read a written text of directions explaining how to perform the task. The last group received and completed their typical therapy. The AO video group showed positive results, with the clients in this group having better scores at the end of the study compared with the other groups. This one study demonstrated the simplicity of AO and its potential benefits when used as an adjunct to other therapies.

Clients can safely and independently perform AO. OT practitioners should begin developing a motor video library to be used in home programs or during the multiple hours of the day or week when the client is not in therapy (Box 33-1).

Mental Practice: Mental practice is a cognitive strategy in which a client mentally rehearses a motor task before attempting to complete it. The reason behind the effectiveness of this theory is similar to that of other cognitive strategies discussed—facilitation of the motor cortex to promote neuroplasticity. The client listens to an audio recording that includes contextual and motor imagery. Many studies have shown that mental practice may improve ADL function and UE function when used alongside physical performance of a task.[72,73] Recommended protocols are not available yet, and the amount of time a client should listen to audio description of the mental imagery differs among studies. One study suggested that a 60-minute mental practice session was best when used after each 30-minute traditional OT session, three times a week.[73] Mental practice is a safe technique that the client can participate in independently outside of scheduled therapy sessions.

BOX 33-1
Guidelines for Action Observation

Demonstrate a task before asking a client to perform it.
Video of task should be no longer than 5 minutes.
Video should include tasks within the client's ability and interest.
Have the client complete repetitions of the viewed motor task (5 minutes).
Time frame is five to six 30-minute sessions per week.

DEVICES USED WITH THE TASK-ORIENTED APPROACH

Functional electrical stimulation (FES) is a treatment modality that uses electrical pulses to specific muscles to elicit a muscle contraction. The stimulation of the sensory system is also thought to promote neuroplastic changes in the cortex. Once muscle contraction occurs, the client attempts to perform a functional task. Grasping and releasing objects is a good example of a functional task that can be performed with an electrically stimulated muscle contraction. Different types of electrical stimulation units are available, all with the same purpose. More information can be found in Chapter 18 on electrical stimulation. There is evidence to support an increase in UE function[74] and decrease in spasticity.[75] However, these improvements in muscle function do not always translate to improvements in activity performance.

Ample evidence exists to support the use of FES as a preparatory method intervention. Bioness H200 is an example of a FES unit that contains preprogrammed sessions that an OT practitioner can choose from, making it easy to program and use it in therapy[76] (Fig. 33-7). Clients and their caregivers can be taught to don/doff units and perform home exercise programs independently.

MANAGING THE UPPER EXTREMITY AFTER THE STROKE

An understanding of the complexity of the shoulder joint is important to be able to provide appropriate treatment and educate clients and caregivers. See Chapter 23 for further details on the shoulder. The human shoulder is the most mobile joint in the body. This wide ROM also makes the shoulder joint inherently unstable. This instability is compensated for by rotator cuff muscles, tendons, ligaments, and the glenoid labrum. It is important to keep in mind that along with the shoulder, the scapula is also moving simultaneously into scapular protraction, retraction, elevation, and depression. The simultaneous movements of the scapula and the shoulder are called *coupled movements.* When the arm is moving into a certain position, the scapula is moving into a related position. The role of the scapula is to provide stability to the glenohumeral joint so that the arm can move into desired, interdependent positions, which include the following:[77]

GLENOHUMERAL JOINT MOVEMENT/POSITION	SCAPULAR MOVEMENT/POSITION
Flexion	Depression
Extension	Elevation
Abduction	Upward rotation
Adduction	Downward rotation
Internal rotation	Protraction
External rotation	Retraction

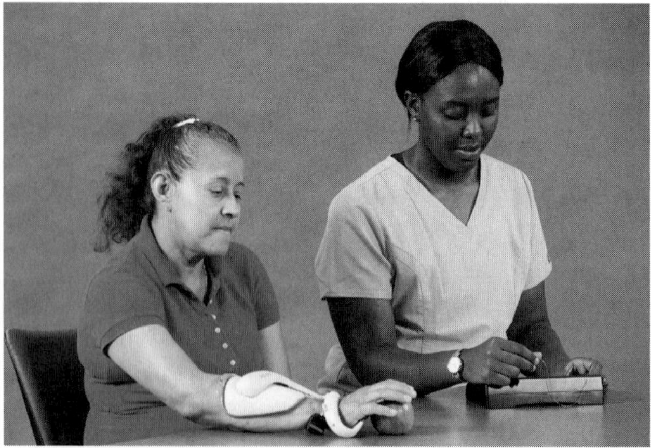

FIGURE 33-7. Client using the Bioness neuromuscular functional electrostimulation unit while performing a functional task.

The effects of a stroke often prevent the arm and shoulder from working together as they are meant to. Spasticity, weakness, and poor positioning, including glenohumeral subluxation, can all contribute to this problem. When the arm and scapula are not moving together as they are meant to, tendons, bursa, and ligaments can become impinged (pinched), causing pain and inflammation. Moving the arm through PROM without the scapula also moving can cause harm to the soft tissue. Prevention is imperative and is discussed further in this chapter.

After a stroke, the affected UE will go through stages of motor recovery. The Brunnstrom stages are the most widely referred to staging of the motor recovery after a stroke. Many assessments of motor recovery and interventions refer to these stages (Fugel-Meyer Stroke Assessment Scale, Chedoke McMaster Stroke Assessment Scale). An individual may not move through each stage and can become stuck in any one or a combination of two stages, although the stages have a predictive pattern of movement.

When considering the Brunnstrom stages, two concepts, in particular, are notable—spasticity and synergy. Both these conditions can lead to further UE and shoulder complications resulting from tissue shortening and cause contractures, misalignment of joints, improper positioning, and, at times, pain. The presence of UE pain is a limiting factor in recovery and occurs in 48% to 84% of individuals after a stroke.[78] In addition to spasticity and synergy, pain can be caused by trauma to the shoulder complex as a result of improper positioning and handling (tendonitis, bursitis, rotator cuff tears) or adhesive capsulitis (frozen shoulder). Here, we will examine the techniques used to protect the UE from damage and prevent the onset of pain.

Positioning: Proper positioning to support the UE, decrease the chance of subluxation, and maintain soft tissue length should be an OT practitioner's top priority in every stage of the client's recovery. When a client is first seen in the acute care setting in the 24 hours after a stroke, the OT practitioner should initiate a bed positioning program. Clients will require repositioning approximately every 2 hours.

Bed positioning can reduce contractures and pain, the risk of pressure injuries, edema, and spastic and synergistic positions. Bed positioning is important throughout recovery as up to two thirds of individuals who have had a stroke also have sleep disordered breathing.[79] Some symptoms seen because of the sleep disorders include snoring, fatigue, insomnia, irritability, shortness of breath, and depression. These individuals should mention their symptoms to their physician because other sources of treatment could be available (Table 33-5).

OT practitioners should educate and train caregivers and other members of the interprofessional team on proper positioning. Pictures of positions are sometimes helpful to caregivers.

Proper positioning for sitting is important to support the UE. In the seated position, the UE should be positioned with support under the elbow to prevent subluxation at the shoulder caused by the weight of the arm hanging. The elbow and the forearm can be supported with pillows, a table stand, or a lap tray if the client is in a wheelchair. It is best to limit the amount of internal rotation of the shoulder—that is, the arm should be kept away from the person's lap or trunk (Fig. 33-8).

Proper positioning for standing can be a complex task, which often requires collaboration with the PT and nursing

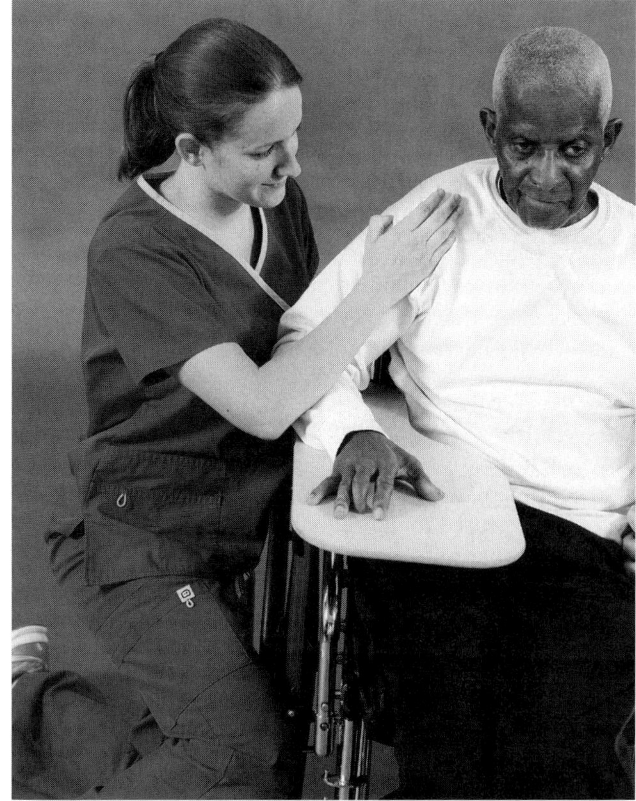

FIGURE 33-8. Proper wheelchair position to support the upper extremity.

TABLE 33-5 Bed Positioning Recommendations

Supine	Head supported on a flat pillow (slight flexion) Shoulder blade (scapula) pulled slightly forward, resting on a pillow Shoulder should be slightly away from the body (abducted) Shoulder should be placed in neutral or externally rotated Elbow should be straight Forearm should be neutral Wrist and fingers straight Entire arm should be supported by pillows
Side-lying on unaffected side	Affected arm should be supported on pillows or cushions so scapula is protracted and shoulder is in approximately 70 degrees shoulder flexion Elbow, wrist, fingers straight Hip flexed, knee flexed and supported by pillows or cushions on affected side
Side-lying on affected side	Shoulder blade should be pulled forward (protracted) to prevent a lot of weight through the shoulder joint Shoulder in some external rotation Elbow is straight or bent slightly Forearm is supinated Wrist and fingers straight Affected leg has knees flexed and supported by pillows or cushions, and nonaffected as desired

Note: Trunk should always be in alignment with all positions

staff. Supporting the arm to prevent shoulder damage while the limb is initially flaccid should be a top priority. When the client is in the standing position, the shoulder is susceptible to traction injury or subluxation. Many OT practitioners are quick to turn to the use of a sling as the answer to this problem. Before choosing to use a sling, the OT practitioner should carefully consider the pros and cons and the goals in prescribing one. A generic sling cannot be used to correct subluxation because there is no commercially available standard sling that can properly position the UE to prevent subluxation.[74] The typical sling holds the limb opposite the recommended positions. Most slings hold the UE in shoulder internal rotation and elbow flexion. Maintaining this position could increase the rate of contracture. According to Gillen, the cons of prescribing a sling outweigh the pros. The only instance for prescribing a sling, as supported by evidence, is when the client is in the flaccid stage,[62] for transfers and initial gait training, and never while in bed or sitting. One study reports that the GivMohr® sling can reduce subluxation in shoulders after a stroke.[80] The GivMohr® sling attaches to the trunk and provides some weight-bearing and support through the limb, at the hand. If the client uses a walker, the affected limb can be supported on that to an extent but assistance may be required to maintain grasp. The OT practitioner may fabricate a supportive orthosis or use Velcro® strapping to assist to maintain hand positioning. Standing is a good opportunity for shoulder management and weight-bearing through the affected side as well. This will not only protect the shoulder from the arm hanging but also involves the affected side in such tasks as grooming at the sink or putting away dishes.

Taping: Taping has been used as an adjunct to support the shoulder after a stroke. Adhesive rigid taping has been shown to decrease pain but not to increase ROM or function.[81] Kinesio® taping is gaining popularity, but there is lack of evidence to support its use in clients after a CVA. There are many anecdotal reports of pain relief (Fig. 33-9). The premise is that the tape provides support to the joint or muscle while decreasing inflammation.

Orthotics: Another type of intervention that falls under the category of UE support and prevention of abnormalities and pain is the use of orthotics. See Chapter 19 for a discussion on orthosis application and fabrication procedures. Orthotics are used to maintain soft tissue length, decrease edema and spasticity, and protect joint integrity. They can also be used to enhance function and movement, as with a wrist extension orthotic or a dynamic extension orthotic.

Range of Motion: Facilitating ROM is another common therapeutic technique that OT practitioners employ as a means of maintaining joint integrity and preventing pain and deformities. A review of the foundational information on ROM presented in Chapter 7 is as follows:

- *AROM*—Client moves his or her own limb
- *AAROM*—OT practitioner and client move limb together

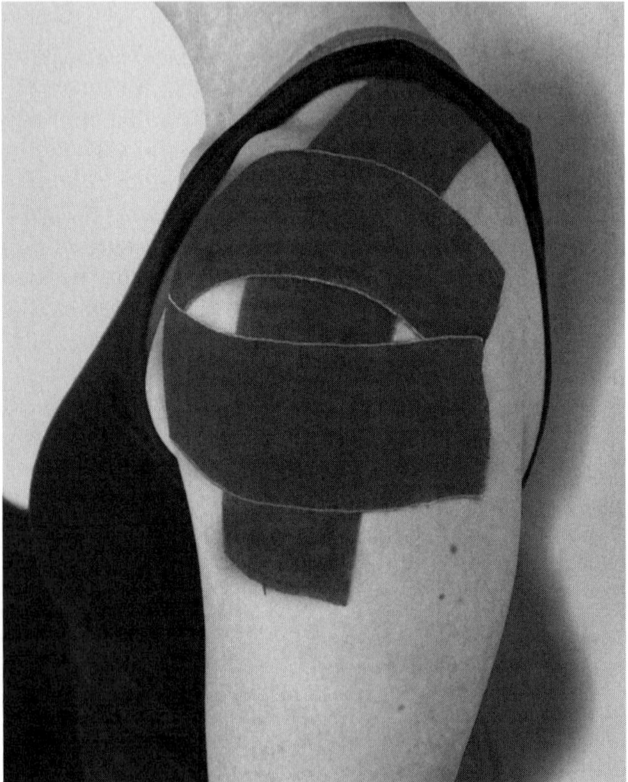

FIGURE 33-9. Kinesio® taping of shoulder.

- *PROM*—OT practitioner moves arm for client
- *Self-ROM*—Client moves weaker limb with stronger one

A systematic review found that stretching had little lasting impact on spasticity, activity, or most importantly, pain.[82] Aggressive ROM activities, such as using an overhead pulley or pushing through significant spasticity, have been found to increase the incidence of shoulder pain and injury.[83] Evidence supports gentle ROM within a person's pain tolerance. It is imperative during performance of ROM exercises that the OTA ensure that the scapula is in proper position and is moving along with the shoulder. The OT practitioner should perform scapular mobilizations if there is increased muscle tone in the muscles around the scapula before ranging the shoulder. Scapular mobilizations involve the OT practitioner having the client positioned in the sitting or side-lying position so that the practitioner can place his or her hand on the client's affected scapula. Here, the OTA places the palm of his or her hand on the flat part of the client's scapula and attempts to slowly and firmly move it in the direction of elevation, depression, protraction, retraction, upward, and downward rotation.[84] For certain movements, it may be helpful to position the inferior borders of the client's scapula in the web of the OTA's hand between the thumb and the index finger. The OTA will place his or her other hand lateral to the client's sternum and below the clavicle to provide support of the joint complex. Following scapular mobilizations, ROM of the shoulder should be performed with the OT practitioner passively facilitating scapular movements coupled with arm movements. If the OTA is unable to achieve scapular movements, he or she should not perform shoulder ROM above 90 degrees of flexion or abduction. This is because for these movements, the glenohumeral joint only moves through part of the full ROM, and the other part of the ROM is the movement of the scapula in a 2:1 ratio. If the muscles around the scapula are tight or weak, excessive motion will occur at the glenohumeral joint with attempts at full ROM.

Clients should be encouraged to perform gentle and pain-free ROM on their own in whatever capacity they can. Actively engaging the more affected limb increases sensory feedback, decreases perceptual/neglect syndromes, and provides the client with some sense of control. Clients should be well instructed and informed to go slowly and gently and not move if they feel pain, and *not stretch their shoulder past 90 degrees of flexion or abduction.* When the shoulder is pushed above this range, damage and impingement of shoulder tissues can occur, causing pain syndromes. "Rocking the baby" movement and pushing a towel on a table are good ROM activities for clients to perform in a safe way.

Compensatory Movements: The student or novice OTA may have concerns about how to provide the proper level of support and assistance as clients are recovering from a stroke. The OTA may be tempted to provide support to the point that the client is not really working, in an attempt to make the client feel good, make it easier for both the client and OTA, and to avoid frustration. As a helping professional, it may be uncomfortable to let the client struggle; there is a delicate balance between too much assistance and not enough. With too much support, clients will not make the desired improvements as quickly as they should, and with too little support, the clients will become frustrated and often will use abnormal compensatory movement to perform the desired task. They may also work so hard that they overfatigue the muscle, which would result in pain or temporary increased weakness.

Compensatory movements are strategies the client may use to replace weaker or less functional muscles when attempting to move. Examples would be trunk lean or rotation along with shoulder/scapular elevation when trying to reach up or out or shoulder abduction when attempting to grasp or pick up an item.

While working with the client who is beginning to have UE muscle return, careful attention is required to provide the "just right challenge." For instance, if the client is straining and using compensatory movements to reach up for an item on a shelf, the OTA could either bring the item down to a more manageable level or provide increased assistance for the reaching task. The OTA may place one hand or arm on the client to block the abnormal movement at the trunk or shoulder while cuing to move with a more normal movement pattern and assist the client through the AAROM required to reach with the other hand. The OTA may find that the first time or two through a task, such as opening the fingers to fit around a cup, the client may be providing a certain percentage of the power to move the limb while the OTA provides the rest in the assist. As the client tires, his or her ability to assist will go down. The OTA can experiment with his or her hand or arm placement on the client for most effective support and control as well as the type of task and movement required for the activity. Even clients who have very little active movement may find it motivating to see the arm move toward a desired item as the OTA encourages them to reach. Some clients may be able to move the arm without assist but may perform the movement in an abnormal way, which does not help strengthen the weakest muscles. In these cases, the OTA may provide cuing and some assist for the client to perform the movement without compensation.

Overview of Upper Extremity Interventions

- Focus treatment on functional task retraining by choosing meaningful tasks.
- Use motor learning principles of massed practice, whole task practice, variable practice, and delayed thoughtful feedback.
- Make the client an active participant in the therapy process.
- Incorporate strengthening and resistive exercise.
- Use CIMT (when appropriate).
- Use bilateral training and weight-bearing during functional tasks.
- Use cognitive strategies as an addition to therapy time.
- Use mirror therapy, action observation, and mental imagery as home programs, and hold the client accountable for completing it.
- Provide education and training in proper positioning.
- Train the client to perform self-ROM exercises, and have him or her perform it gently and slowly and *never* beyond 90 degrees of shoulder flexion or abduction.
- Use slings sparingly.
- Consider using an orthotic as an aid to enhance function.
- Encourage use of the affected UE in all daily tasks.

Self-Feeding, Eating, and Swallowing

Self-feeding, eating, and swallowing are complex tasks requiring coordination between the nervous, motor, sensory, physiological systems, as well as the context in which the task is being performed. The acts of self-feeding, eating, and swallowing are also steeped in cultural meaning and significance. Feeding, eating, and swallowing are an important part of one's social life and the culture in which a person was raised and lives. See Chapter 12, for a thorough review of the factors involved in self-feeding, eating, and swallowing.

Self-feeding, eating, and swallowing are within the domain of practice for occupational therapists and OTAs.[84] It is an OTA's ethical responsibility to seek supervision and continuing education to advance his or her skill level and knowledge.

An assessment of self-feeding and swallowing should be incorporated into all initial evaluations in the acute care setting. OT practitioners should work with SLPs, dietitians, respiratory therapists, physicians, and nursing staff to assess the need for intervention, as appropriate. An OT practitioner should first perform oral motor assessments, observe and adjust positioning, and perform gross observations for visual perceptual difficulties, such as a left neglect or apraxia. Then, the OT practitioner should observe the mealtime and initiate an evaluation by using foods that are easier to swallow, such as thick pureed substances. OT practitioners should follow the physician's orders in the chart as well as the national dysphagia diet recommendations for progression of a food trial. To review the information in Chapter 12, the levels are pureed/spoon-thick liquids, mechanically altered/honey liquids, soft foods/nectar liquids, and regular/thin liquids.

Intervention for Self-Feeding, Eating, and Swallowing

Interventions for dysphagia after a stroke include positioning, self-feeding, modified diets, incorporating posture and techniques, exercises and strengthening, and use of adaptive equipment. Dysphagia after a stroke carries a threefold increased mortality risk and a sixfold to sevenfold increased risk of aspiration pneumonia.[85]

POSITIONING

Positioning interventions include obtaining an upright seated position. This position enhances alertness, provides the best mechanical position for feeding and swallowing, and is a more natural context for a person to eat in. The client should be moved to a chair or wheelchair and sit at a table for best positioning. If the client is unable to move to a chair, then an attempt should be made to have the bed in the most upright position possible. It is best to have clients feed themselves, if at all possible; this allows the system ample time to prepare itself to receive the food. If a client has left unilateral neglect, items may need to be placed toward the right hand side in the field of vision initially.

SELF-FEEDING

Feeding interventions include help with UE coordination and increasing awareness of food approaching the mouth (visually and olfactory); manual guiding and alternating food textures may help if a client has apraxia. Use of CIMT may be helpful to increase UE coordination on the affected side while feeding.

POSTURES AND TECHNIQUES

Use of postures and techniques have been shown to be of some use in working with clients who have dysphagia. Different head and body positions known to influence pharyngeal dimensions, movement of the food bolus, and structural movements during swallowing have been documented.

1. Chin tuck: Is used to initiate a swallow and assist to potentially protect the airway by constricting it. It is thought that a chin tuck position may decrease aspiration in some, but should not be recommended to the exclusion of further testing.
2. Head turn: Head rotated toward the weaker side in conjunction with a chin tuck can also decrease aspiration.
3. Mendelsohn maneuver: Involves cueing a client to push tongue into hard palate while swallowing which helps by opening the pathway for a swallow[85]

There is significant disagreement with each of these strategies as far as when to employ and with which type of weakness. For example, if a chin tuck alone is recommended for a client with silent aspiration who takes larger bites, it will almost certainly be ineffective. More SLPs are recommending a neutral position to start, with a modified barium swallow study for further information to guide treatment options.

EXERCISES AND STRENGTHENING

Exercises and strengthening interventions can also be incorporated into treating eating and swallowing deficits. Examples include ROM exercises of the jaw, tongue, and cheek, and oral motor tasks, such as blowing air into a balloon and sucking through a straw. Lip and tongue exercises have proven useful with clients after a stroke to increase strength and coordination.

ADAPTIVE EQUIPMENT

The OT practitioner can recommend many types of adaptive equipment that are available for the client experiencing difficulty feeding, eating, and swallowing. Modified plates (scoop dish, guards) assist the person to use one hand for getting food onto the utensil. Many types of modified utensils are available, some coated with rubber (to protect teeth), some with large handles (for weak grasp), and some weighted (for tremors). A self-leveling utensil is the Liftware Level™ that allows the client to self-feed by keeping the food level, no matter how the client's UE moves. Modified cups and complex power feeders are also available. The OTA may need to guide/support the client with weakness through scooping food and taking the hand to the mouth and back to the plate, providing the "just right challenge." OT practitioners are encouraged to review Chapters 12 and 14 for discussions on further options for adaptive equipment and periodically review supply catalogs and websites for any new ideas; they should have an array of items on hand to provide to the client during trials.

INTERVENTIONS FOR SOMATOSENSORY IMPAIRMENTS

The human sensory system allows for interaction with, and interpretation of, the world. Through vision, hearing, tasting, sense of smell, and sense of touch, individuals perceive and integrate the information from the environment. This section will focus on only one system of sensation, the somatosensory system. The term *somatosensory* refers to sensation coming from skin, joints, and muscles,[86] and includes sensations such as vibration, firm and light touch, pressure, texture, stereognosis (manipulation and identifying an object in the hand without vision), proprioception (feeling where body parts are in space without vision), temperature sensation, and pain.[87] Deficits of these sensations appear to be common after stroke, with prevalence rates ranging from 11% to 85%.[86] A systematic review found that somatosensory deficits had a negative impact on functional recovery after a stroke.[86] Most people will have impaired sensation on the contralateral side of the body—that is, the arm, trunk, and leg on the side opposite the hemisphere that is damaged.

The principles that guide intervention in sensory modalities are the same as those that guide motor interventions—neuroplasticity-promoting cortical reorganization and application of motor learning methods. In fact, the motor and somatosensory systems are completely intertwined and reliant on one another for optimal performance. It makes sense that if the motor system is impaired because of a CVA, so, too, is the sensory system. It also stands to reason that the same principles could be used to guide intervention for both systems.

Interventions for sensory retraining have little evidence to support them. One of the earliest methods of sensory retraining involved passive stimulation and bombardment.[87] This type of training involves the OT practitioners passively providing stimulation to limbs via different textures or electrical stimulation. Although not harmful, this passive type of intervention is not recommended because there is no true active engagement on the part of the client and therefore will have little carry over into functional tasks.[87]

Researchers have developed a transfer-enhanced training approach, the SENSe program. The SENSe program incorporates seven principles based on the concepts of neuroplasticity and motor learning principles (use of feedback, variable practice, and massed practice).[88] The SENSe principles of training have been identified and are guided by these three core principles:

"1. Use of goal-directed attentive exploration and anticipation trials to enhance sensory thresholds and processing,
2. Calibration of the client's impaired touch sensation internally by reference to more normal touch sensation experienced through the unaffected hand and via vision, and
3. Graded progression of training across a matrix of somatosensory tasks that vary in degree of difficulty and sensory attribute training."[87]

In the SENSe program, clients perform sensory tasks by using objects and textures that are carefully selected and are meaningful to them. Empirical evidence supports the effectiveness of this program.[88] OT practitioners should incorporate sensory tasks into their interventions for individuals who have had a stroke.

INTERVENTIONS FOR COGNITIVE IMPAIRMENTS

The arena of cognitive rehabilitation after a stroke is changing. In the past, interventions focused on domain specific areas. There were and still are interventions specifically for attention span impairments, memory problems, and executive functioning disorders. It was often assumed in the past that working in one area would translate to improved function overall. For example, the assumption was that if an OT practitioner worked to improve a person's attention span through pencil-and-paper activities in the clinic, the person would be better able to perform work tasks as well. Each domain area of cognition was and still is treated as its own subspecialty area. The earlier discussion on the advancements of neuroscience also applies to the area of cognitive rehabilitation. We now know that all of the cognitive processes are interconnected; they all work with and are dependent on one another for proper functioning. For example, a person cannot use his or her executive functioning skills to plan for a weekend camping trip if he or she lacks the attention span to write a grocery list. If a person has the attention span to write a grocery list but has executive functioning difficulties, he or she would not have the initiation to write the list or even know that writing a list is the best place to start. Advancements in neuroimaging techniques have confirmed what many OT practitioners have known for a long time—that one simply cannot treat the areas of cognition as different units. In addition to overlapping cognitive areas, all cognitive abilities are further influenced by an individual's behavioral, emotional, and physical abilities, as well as the environment and context in which these tasks are performed.

Cognitive interventions should assist clients in achieving a more accurate understanding of their own strengths and limitations. Goals of cognitive rehabilitation after stroke should include improving cognitive and behavioral skills and compensating for limitations. Goals should also involve assisting a client to understand and teach ways to manage their emotional reactions to make changes in their functional ability. Cognitive interventions after a stroke should be eclectic, functional, and relate to the goals and needs of clients and their families. Here, more than in many other areas, OT practitioners must rely on caregivers to support the intervention plan and provide follow-up "treatment." The caregiver *must* be an active member of the team.

A thorough overview of all cognitive deficits and cognitive rehabilitation strategies is provided in Chapter 11. Intervention strategies for problems faced by individuals who have had a stroke are discussed below.

Attention Impairments

Interventions for attention impairments can be divided into two main categories: (1) interventions that focus on improving or remediating the underlying attentional deficits, and (2) interventions that improve skills or provide compensatory strategies for performance of ADLs and IADLs. The first, which is improving or remediating the underlying deficits, is often based on laboratory and clinical methods. A direct and strong link to improvements in an individual's everyday functioning has yet to be made. Researchers have found that there is limited to no evidence to support interventions focused on a specific attention domain having any positive effect on occupational performance.[21]

The second area of intervention for individuals with attention deficits focuses on improving daily living skills and increasing participation in occupations despite the presence of attention problems. This approach would be considered a compensatory approach. It utilizes self-management strategies, environmental supports, and external aids.

The three types of self-management strategies are as follows:[89]

1. Orienting procedures: Encourages clients to monitor their activities in a purposeful, conscious way to avoid attention drifting. Clients are taught to ask themselves questions to provide reorientation, such as "What am I doing?" "What comes next?" These questions are asked after being cued by some type of external reminder, such as an alarm on a phone or watch.
2. Pacing: After neurological damage has occurred, fatigue is often a concern. Teaching pacing strategies can be helpful. Scheduling uninterrupted work times, scheduling breaks, setting realistic goals, and

self-monitoring of progress and fatigue are examples of self-pacing.

3. Key ideas log: Individuals who have had a stroke often complain of having difficulty switching between tasks because they lose their train of thought and cannot resume the original task. By writing down, verbally recording on a smartphone or audio recorder, or entering a note in a smartphone, clients can quickly note key ideas or questions so that they can address them later without interrupting their current attention.[89]

To utilize any strategy, a client must be provided with multiple types of practice. Use of the principles of motor learning may provide practice and enhance learning of the strategy. Individuals must overpractice the strategy so that it becomes a habit. The OTA must work with caregivers to train them on how to reinforce strategies for forming habits.

Environmental supports must be employed in conjunction with self-management strategy training. It is important to assess the environment and task to be completed and modify to manage attention accordingly. Box 33-2 summarizes the findings on many types of strategies for clinicians and caregivers.[90]

Other research has suggested the client use a "do not disturb" sign as a helpful tool to maintain attention in a situation where the client may be interrupted multiple times. Another recommendation is for the client to get sufficient exercise as a means to enhance thinking skills.[89]

Memory Impairments

Memory is a complex process involving many different aspects and areas of the brain and the ability of these areas to effectively communicate with one another. Many different techniques have been employed in an effort to improve a person's memory after a stroke. A systematic review found strong evidence to support the use of specific memory interventions, including internal and external memory strategy training, errorless learning, and remediation, compensatory and self-help approaches, encoding techniques, and training in cognitive assistive technology (CAT).[91] (See Chapter 11 for details of these interventions.) Although this review noted many positive results, it also pointed out that many of the studies do not focus on occupational performance as an outcome measure. The lack of improved performance of ADLs as an outcome measure in many studies led the review to conclude that evidence to support interventions that improve memory is limited.[21] OT practitioners should have improved occupational performance as the main goal in any and all rehabilitation efforts.

Some general suggestions when working with individuals with memory impairments include the following:

- Make instructions short and to the point.
- For training, use functional tasks that have meaning to the client.
- Avoid talking too quickly.
- Break down a large task into smaller parts, have the client overlearn each part, and then put it all back to form a whole task (part-whole learning).
- Incorporate extra practice and rehearsal.
- Teach rehearsal strategies.[90]
- Incorporate pictures, which may be better remembered.
- Strategically place environmental cues.
- Use errorless learning techniques.
- Provide education and training to family members and caregivers; it is crucial for them to learn and incorporate strategies.[92]
- Consider creating short videos, using the client or caregiver's smartphone or other device, if available.

A combination of internal and external strategies would be best to improve functional performance in an individual with memory deficits. All strategies should be rehearsed and overlearned in a client's natural settings. In devising a functional memory book and providing training in the use of it, the best practice is to individualize the strategy and overteach it, and its use should be reinforced by all staff and caregivers. Some sections of the functional memory book that are recommended include an orientation section, calendar, memory log, to-do lists, names of relevant people and their contact information, and task-specific sections, related to the individual needs.[93]

The following is a list of environmental adaptations and cues, which can be easily incorporated into a client's life:[92]

- Color-code keys with matching colors on locks.
- Keep a central location for a family communication board, keys, phone, wallet, and so on.
- Use 7-day pill box.
- Label doors with pictures of what is inside the room. Label drawers, cabinets, and so on.
- Place important items, such as wallets, where they cannot be missed (e.g., by the entryway).

BOX 33-2

Environmental Supports as Attention Strategies

Avoid overstimulating/distracting environments.
Face away from visual distractors during tasks.
Wear earplugs.
Shop or go to restaurants at off-peak times
Label cupboards and drawers.
Reduce clutter and visual distractors.
Use self-instruction strategies.
Learn self-pacing strategies.
Control the rate of incoming information.
Self-manage effort and emotional responses during tasks.
Learn monitoring or shared attentional resources when multitasking.
Manage the home environment to decrease stimuli (turn off phones, TV, radios).
Close doors and curtains.
Keep surfaces, cabinets, closets, and refrigerators organized and uncluttered.
Use daily checklists for work, self-care, and IADLs.[90]

- Place a reminder list on the back of the entry door (e.g., what to take along, safety checklist before leaving the house).

Another study provided a list of electronic assistive technology for individuals with memory loss after a stroke:[90]

- Electronic pill box
- Microwave with preset times
- Adaptive stove controls to turn off an electric stove after a certain period or when the heat becomes excessive
- A phone with programmable memory buttons
- A phone that is programmed to speak the name of the person being called
- A locator attachment to keys and on cell phone
- Recorders used to cue a behavioral sequence, such as morning care
- Timers set for turning on/off the lights or the stove
- Automatic shut-off for appliances, such as irons and televisions

Executive Functioning Impairments

Executive functions are considered the highest order of cognitive functions. They are defined as "those functions that enable a person to engage successfully in independent, purposive, self-serving behavior."[90] Executive functioning is covered in depth in Chapter 11; in addition, the literature identifies the following list of 20 areas that are executive functioning deficits: poor abstract thinking ability, impulsivity, confabulation, planning deficits, euphoria, poor temporal sequencing, lack of insight, apathy, disinhibition, variable motivation, shallow affect, aggression, lack of concern, perseveration, restlessness, decreased response inhibition, know–do dissociation, distractibility, poor decision making, and lack of concern for social rules.[90] Prospective memory is often included as a component of executive functioning. *Prospective memory* refers to one's ability to remember something that has to be completed in the future, such as stopping to buy dog food on the way home after work. Most often, individuals with impaired executive functioning abilities demonstrate the most difficulty when presented with new and novel situations. Within the clinic, impaired executive functioning ability has been linked to poor IADL performance and to depression.[94]

Much of the research and writing about executive functioning impairment has been done on individuals who had experienced traumatic brain injury (TBI), not on stroke. There are differences in the presentation of these two types of conditions, and therefore applying intervention strategies designed for individuals with TBI to those who had a stroke may not be the best practice. A systematic review involving only studies on individuals who had a stroke[95] found only 12 studies that met their criteria and no studies that addressed the acute stage of recovery. Although only a small number of studies were included, those researchers found some encouraging results for both remedial (computer-based training of working memory and dual tasking) and compensatory interventions (cognitive strategy use and paging system). Some of the studies reported generalization of skills to real-life situations as an outcome, showing promise for enhanced function.

Four broad categories of interventions for those living with impairments of executive functions are (1) environmental modifications, (2) compensatory strategies, (3) task-specific training, and (4) training in metacognitive strategies.[90] Many of the interventions overlap and are also applicable to other areas, such as memory and attention concerns. Interventions in similar categories include environmental management, which is further divided into organization of physical space and manipulation of physiological factors; teaching task-specific routines; training on the selection and execution of cognitive plans; and providing metacognitive strategies/self-instructional training.[89]

ENVIRONMENTAL MANAGEMENT

Environmental management strategies involve organizing the client's physical space to provide the support needed for successful and safe task completion. Completing an assessment of the client's living space is crucial to recommending the most meaningful strategies. Environmental management is a joint effort among the client, his or her caregivers, and OT practitioners. Some examples are given in Box 33-3.[89]

BOX 33-3
Environmental Management Strategies

Labeling cupboard contents
Bulletin boards with separate labeled sections for different types of information
Rearranging the refrigerator with specific food on specific shelves
Designating a place for clutter
Establishing clutter free work space zones
Setting up bill paying systems
Using large family planning calendars
Placing a family message center on fridge
The use of Post-Prompt® or strategically placed cues can assist in compensating for deficits. Some examples of Post-Prompts® include:
- Leaving what is needed to take to school by front door (keys, lunch, bag...)
- Morning ADL/Grooming routine checklist in bathroom
- Menus for specific meals posted on fridge

Going to bed or leaving house routine posted (lights out, door locked, iron off, take medication, set alarm...)
- Operating procedures for laundry, dishwasher, computer, etc. posted near item
- Conversation prompts, such as photo albums or books, placed in strategic locations
- Schedules to assist with time management, placed wherever necessary.

MANIPULATION OF PHYSIOLOGICAL FACTORS

Manipulation of physiological factors is another area related to environmental management and includes the following:

- **Nutrition**: Eating healthy and avoiding mind altering substances such as caffeine, alcohol, and sugar
- **Sleep hygiene**: Relaxation training and a fixed schedule for sleep/wake times
- **Activity level**: Over-/understimulation may be more difficult to manage after a stroke. Helping individuals set up a schedule and providing training in self-pacing strategies, with prescribed rest periods built in, will be helpful.
- **Medication monitoring**: Often an issue for individuals who have a neurological deficit. Teaching individuals to track their medications and how they may affect behaviors is important. Use of external aids, such as pill boxes, post prompts, and calendars, can help manage the schedule.[89]
- **Teaching task-specific routines:** Involves teaching a client behaviors and strategies for a specific setting or problem. The process is similar to teaching other compensatory strategies. The first step is writing a task analysis, in which the routine is broken into single, logical, sequenced steps; developing and implementing a checklist that makes each of the steps very clear; providing sufficient practice for each step using errorless learning techniques; and, last, making sure that reinforcement and motivation to succeed at the task are embedded into the training.[89]

TRAINING IN THE SELECTION OF COGNITIVE PLANS

The selection of cognitive plans is another area OT practitioners can use to work with individuals with executive functioning difficulties. The activities chosen are designed to manage impairments in initiation, prospective memory, and impulsivity. These activities are unique in that they focus on generalization to natural environments. Some examples include having the client complete various planning scenarios, beginning with hypothetical events (discussing what sorts of movies might be shown nearby) and moving toward actual event planning (looking up actual times/location for a specific movie). The objectives of the strategies and activities are to increase accuracy in listing the essential steps involved in a multicomponent task, increase the accuracy of sequencing, and improve organization or efficiency in planning.[89] Examples of planning tasks include planning meals, parties, fundraising projects; planning and ordering therapy sessions; and arranging a surprise date.

Another type of activity that falls into this category is errand completion. Errand completion tasks are arranged to address planning, sequencing, initiation, and execution. They incorporate compensatory strategies. They should progress from concrete activities to abstract activities. Some examples are as follows:

1. A concrete hospital-based activity: Going to the hospital gift shop to determine hours, going to the cafeteria to look at the menu or get a bottle of water from the vending machine.
2. A concrete community-based activity: Finding the way to a store by using the bus schedule, buying stamps, or determining the price of a particular item on a menu.

The last category of tasks for training in the selection and execution of cognitive plans includes time management tasks and prospective memory tasks. Examples of time management tasks are to have the client keep track of a specific number of minutes and inform the practitioner when that time has passed. Clients should develop their own schedules and adhere to them, with decreasing cues from others.

METACOGNITIVE STRATEGIES

The last approach to helping people manage executive function impairments is utilizing metacognitive strategies and self-instructional training techniques. Clients are taught to ask questions about the task demand, provide answers to the questions via cognitive rehearsal and planning, talk to themselves about steps in the process (verbal self-talk), use overt verbalizations (whispering inner talk), and self-reinforcement upon task completion.[89] One common self-management strategy is goal management training. Goal management training involves selecting goals, partitioning the task into sub-goals, remembering the steps of the task during performance of it, and monitoring the task outcome. The steps taught to clients are as follows:

1. Asking themselves, "What am I doing?" (STOP)
2. Defining the "main task" and selecting the main goal (DEFINE)
3. Listing the steps (LIST)
4. Asking themselves whether they know the steps and rehearsing the steps (LEARN)
5. Executing the task (DO IT)
6. Asking themselves, "Am I doing what I planned to do?" (CHECK)[90]

Self-Awareness and Insight Impairments

The reported frequency of *anosognosia* (denial of weakness or impairments) ranges from 28% to 85% in clients who have sustained damage to the right hemisphere of the brain after a stroke, and up to 17% in clients with damage to the left hemisphere of the brain, indicating that right hemisphere damage is more associated with anosognosia.[96] Clients may be aware of the hemiplegia, but not of their cognitive/perceptual impairments (e.g., neglect). Lack of awareness or insight into impairments, regardless of subtype, has been associated with decreased scores on the functional independence measure (FIM™) at discharge, decreased motivation, difficulty with strategy/compensatory use, decreased safety, lack of appropriate goal setting, decreased error detection, less sustained attention capacity, decreased vocational and employability outcomes, and decreased overall sense of well-being.[90] It has also been associated with enhanced caregiver distress.[97]

Research evidence is limited with regard to any interventions used to work with individuals who have awareness or insight problems after a stroke. Three types of interventions that are often employed simultaneously or at varying times during the rehabilitation process are (1) individual awareness-enhancing program, (2) caregiver training, and (3) education.[89]

INDIVIDUAL AWARENESS-ENHANCING PROGRAM

This program focuses on the client and has two approaches: the educational approach and the experiential approach. The goal of an education approach is providing clients with information that they currently lack and can internalize. Examples of interventions strategies using an educational approach include the following:[90]

- Providing clients with information about their injury through print materials, videos and audiotapes, whichever method can accommodate their current status
- Having clients view videos and share what does and does not match their current function
- Reviewing medical records with clients
- Developing a personalized stroke education notebook with clients
- Having caregivers and the client assess the client's status and then compare the ratings
- Reviewing the scores of assessments and discussing their meaning
- Video recording client performance and reviewing it
- Role play reversal—OT practitioner or a caregiver performs a task and makes errors, and the client works to identify them
- Always working to present information in a way that does not incite a defensive reaction

EXPERIENTIAL EXERCISES

Experiential exercises are another way to enhance an individual's self-awareness. The goal of experiential exercises is to have clients experience changes in their ability and recognize the changes. Some examples of experiential exercise include the following:

- Comparing predicted performance and actual performance
- Performance tracking through use of self-monitoring logs or behavioral logs
- Incorporating the client into the goal setting process, which must be understood by the client[89]

CAREGIVER EDUCATION AND TRAINING

Education and training of the caregiver is an important factor in the success of the client. The approaches listed above can also be applied to the caregiver. In addition to the client's anosognosia, caregivers can experience a type of unawareness of their loved one's deficits because of stress, emotions, and lack of education. It is important to assess the caregiver's expectations, as not all clients will improve and get "back to normal." The caregiver may be well aware of the deficits but may merely want their loved one to "admit" that he or she has a problem or deficit. This need for admission is often counterproductive to the therapeutic process.

FUNCTIONAL TASKS FOR SELF-AWARENESS

Functional tasks can be used as a means to enhance client self-awareness. Many of the previously described concepts can be applied using functional occupations as the mode of delivery. The following examples are recommended:[90]

- Encourage the client to describe his or her anticipated difficulties before beginning the task.
- Plan out how the client would handle new situations.
- Ask the client to evaluate and describe his or her performance upon completion of the task.
- Ask the client if he or she could improve performance and how.
- Provide feedback about observed difficulty.
- Provide practice opportunities.
- Use video feedback.

Gillen further recommends use of specific prompting procedures during functional task performance as means to enhance awareness. Asking questions, such as "How do you know this is correct?" or saying, "This is not correct because..."; "Try this way"; "Try this (explain strategy, out loud, slowly).[90]

Other suggestions for improving a client's self-awareness and insight after a stroke would be to provide opportunities for group sessions. Group sessions have proven helpful to increase self-awareness.[98] Receiving peer feedback is often accepted better than receiving feedback from an authority figure, such as a physician or an OT practitioner.

Individuals With Aphasia

Aphasia is defined as an acquired communication disorder resulting from brain damage and is characterized by impairment of language modalities—speaking, listening, reading, and writing. It is not a deficit of sensory, motor, intellectual, or psychiatric functioning.[99] The National Aphasia Association reports that about a third of all strokes result in aphasia.[100] People with aphasia have a lower quality of life (QoL) and report that they participate in fewer activities compared with people who have had a stroke who do not have subsequent aphasia.[101] Many types of aphasia/communication disorders are found in the literature and are discussed fully in Chapter 12. Here, we will discuss the types most commonly seen following a stroke: Broca's aphasia (expressive, nonfluent) and Wernicke's aphasia (receptive, fluent).

Broca's aphasia results in clients having difficulty with speech production. They often present as alert and oriented and can utter a few automatic responses, such as "Yes" or a swear word. Their speech is awkward and labored, with difficulty initiating words. Their sentences are shortened and choppy. It is important to remember that clients with Broca's aphasia also have some limitations in understanding language. They have great difficulty understanding spoken number words. Reading and writing are also impaired. A person with Broca's aphasia may say things like: Sky... b...b...bird... b...b....black... f...f...f...feed... bad" to indicate that a crow ate all of the bird seed in the feeder. The speech is substantive, just not fluent.

Wernicke's aphasia (fluent aphasia, receptive) is a triad of characteristics of difficulties with processing the meaning of written and spoken language, which includes fluent but paraphasic speech (wrong word substitution), reduced speech comprehension, and anosognosia (lack of awareness of erroneous speech output).[99] The speech of clients with Wernicke's aphasia contains a mix of normal words and neologisms (made-up words) and does not usually have any recognizable meaning. The language has intact flow and intonation but does not make sense to the communication partner. It may present as something like this: "Birdabirda a bird, stupid... seechippy (made-up word for sunflower seed), mean, stupid. It is outside. Goolupies (made up word to indicate smaller birds?) are gone" to indicate that crows ate all of the bird seed in the feeder. People with Wernicke's aphasia may not recognize that they have a language deficit and become frustrated when others do not understand what they are trying to communicate. These individuals have problems with both the expressive and receptive aspects of speech. Comprehension of written words and writing is also impaired. Writing usually reflects spoken language, lacking in meaningful content.

OT practitioners work side by side with SLPs to assist people with aphasia to recover from the effects of stroke. Although the SLP directly addresses language deficits, OT practitioners can employ techniques to assist clients with aphasia with language comprehension and language production. Some general suggestions for enhancement of communication after a stroke are provided in Table 33-6.

In their synthesis of evidence on outcome measures for people with aphasia presented at the Annual Conference of the American Occupational Therapy Association (AOTA), Berger and Escher described six key principles, as presented in Table 33-7.[103]

Individuals With Apraxia

Apraxia is the deficit associated with praxis skills, which are skills that help a person to store skilled movement patterns in memory and interact in the environment and with the objects in it. Praxis has two steps that allow an individual to perform functional, purposeful, skilled movement. The first step is *ideation* (development of a concept)—what to do, what objects are in front of a person, and how should the client use them to perform the desired task. The second step is *production*, which refers to knowing how to perform a task and completing the movement sequence.[90] This skill set is not limited to one particular region of the brain; rather, it is believed that it involves more than one cerebral lobe and the white matter that connects them. Apraxia refers to lack of these skills.

Apraxia is defined as a disorder of purposeful skilled movement, which is not the result of sensory or motor deficits (weakness, abnormal muscle tone, decreased proprioceptive sense, etc.) or deficits in comprehension.[90,104] The prevalence of apraxia has been reported to be 28% to 57% in individuals who have had a left brain stroke and 0% to 34% in individuals with damage to their right brain. Recently, researchers found that apraxia is associated with decreased function at admission and discharge, but they did

TABLE 33-6 Enhancement of Communication[102]

TO ENHANCE EXPRESSION:	TO ENHANCE COMPREHENSION:
Use the phrase "I know you know____" to show that the OTA understands the problem is with expression, not knowledge.	Identify if there is a hearing loss.
Acknowledge breakdown in communication and encourage the client to repair.	Slow the rate of your speech, but maintain normal intonation.
Accept and encourage use of gestures and facial expressions.	Reduce distractions from the environment.
Engage their friends and family in providing topics.	Use face-to-face communication.
Provide clear choices.	Signal topic shifts "on another topic...."
Talk about personally relevant topics and shared experiences.	Use simple direct sentences.
Give client the time to talk.	Use short phrases interspersed with appropriate pauses.
Tolerate the client's silence, but encourage them to take part in conversation.	Identify communication breakdowns and use repair strategies (rephrasing, simpler words, slow rate...).
	Use visual props.
	Write down important words.
	Emphasis important words.
	Have only one person talk at a time (if co-treating, choose which therapist will talk for that session).[99]

TABLE 33-7 Key Principles for Clients With Aphasia[103]

Principle 1: Use pictures.	Photographs are preferred over cartoons/clipart. Use pictures made for adults (not childish). Use pictures that show meaning not just for decoration. Use captions and link writing with pictures.
Principle 2: Provide choices.	Give one message at a time. Use Likert scale 1–5 versus 1–10. Use close ended questions: Yes, no, maybe.
Principle 3: Use simple vocabulary and syntax.	Use Grade 5 reading level. Use active voice with common words. Write while talking. Use short sentences (five or fewer words).
Principle 4: Use clear presentation.	Use large font (18–24) and san serif font (Arial and Calibri). Use plenty of white space around text. Only capitalize first letter of sentence. Use bold font for important information. (Do not underline or use capitals.) Use headings to organize information.
Principle 5: Provide supported conversation.	Provide scaled levels of support based on client's needs (e.g., repeat question, simplify and restate, combine yes/no questions). Spoken support—slower pace, natural tone of voice Gestural support—body orientation, symbolic gestures Verification—ensure client understands question, and vice versa. Teach-back technique ensures the client understands you.
Principle 6: Provide "positive" environment.	Plan for face to face interviews/treatment. Decrease background noise. Decrease visual distractions. Ensure physical comfort (seating, bathroom, temperature, hunger, etc.). Allow enough time.

not find any difference related to lesions sites in the right brain or the left brain.[105]

Many types of apraxia are named in the literature; however, this section will focus on ideational apraxia and ideomotor apraxia. Although these can occur together or separately, it is important to attempt to determine which type is more prevalent because the therapy strategies differ. **Ideational apraxia** is a deficit in the knowledge of what needs to be done in a task. For example, knowledge of using a tool correctly may be impaired (toothpaste smeared on sink, using a knife to eat soup), or the sequence of the task may be off (mustard on top of sandwich, not inside). **Ideomotor apraxia** (motor apraxia) is a disorder in the production of purposeful movement. The person understands what needs to occur to complete the task but cannot physically perform it despite not having any physical or sensory deficits. It is as though the stored motor pattern in the person's memory is gone. Individuals with ideomotor apraxia display clumsy movements that appear inflexible or static, and the timing and speed of movements are off. They have difficulty performing movements that involve crossing the midline or require multiple joints.[90] A diagnostic screening method often used to detect ideomotor apraxia involves having the individual pantomime the use of an object with their body ("Show me how to blow out a match" or "Show me how you would comb your hair").

As with many therapeutic interventions, treatment for apraxia falls into two broad categories, described as restorative or adaptive.[92] Restorative methods attempt to decrease the impairment itself, and adaptive interventions focus on improving activity performance despite the presence of apraxia.[90] Evidence from research does not support the restorative approach.[90]

A study has provided data that further support and demonstrate the transferability of strategy training.[106] Strategy training is an intervention method created by OT practitioners and teaches clients strategies to compensate for apraxia. The treatment focuses on specific training of tasks chosen by the client. The OT practitioner categorizes specific errors observed during task performance and provides instructions or education, depending on which category of error was observed. The three types of errors identified are as follows:

1. Initiation (developing a plan and selecting appropriate objects)
2. Execution (task performance)
3. Control (control and correcting activities to ensure end results)[107]

Clients with deficits in initiation were given specific instructions. Instructions were provided in this order: verbal, auditory, tactile, gesturing, pointing, handing objects, and beginning the task together.[90] Problems in execution were treated with assistance, ranging from verbal assistance (naming of steps of activity) to physical assistance, such as guiding movements. Areas of control were treated with feedback. Feedback included knowledge of results (describing the results of the action "good throw") to taking control of the task and not allowing errors (errorless learning).[90]

The following is a list of potential interventions for those living with functional limitations related to apraxia:[108]

- Use functional tasks that are familiar to clients.
- Use their already formed habits and routines.

- Collaborate with clients and their caregivers to choose the tasks to focus on.
- Practice these activities in the appropriate environment and context (dressing in the bathroom in the morning).
- Use strategy training interventions to develop internal or external compensations during task performance.
- Focus interventions based on the type of errors made.
- Practice functional activities with vanishing cues.
- Provide graded assistance via graded instructions, assistance, or feedback during task performance.
- Practice functional activities using errorless learning techniques.

Strategies to Promote Generalization of Treatment

Generalization is the ultimate goal of cognitive rehabilitation. Taking what was learned and accomplished in therapy and applying it to a real-life experience should be the goal of therapy. Generalization should be explicit, planned for, and taught. Strategies to assist this process are as follows:[89]

- Provide explicit instructions during training, but try a variety of target skills, and have clients overpractice.
- Practice in a variety of natural settings.
- Change the environment to support new skills and behaviors.
- Enlist assistance from significant others and OT colleagues, as required.
- Identify barriers to maintenance, and plan for high-risk situations.
- Plan for setbacks.
- Plan booster sessions; for example, schedule a follow-up appointment for 3 months later.

INTERVENTIONS FOR VISUAL-SPATIAL/ PERCEPTUAL IMPAIRMENTS

The visual system is complex, involving six pairs of ocular muscles, four cranial nerves (optic, oculomotor, trochlear, and abducens), the thalamus, all four lobes of the cerebral cortex, and many connecting pathways in between. See Chapter 10 for visual anatomy, deficits, and details. It is not hard to imagine that after a stroke, individuals would have some form of difficulty with regard to vision or visual/perceptual ability. The incidence is reported to be 50% to 70% in right hemisphere damage and 30% to 50% in left hemisphere damage.[109] People who have visual impairments following neurological damage have difficulties with ADLs, are at a higher risk for falls, and have poor rehabilitation outcomes.[110]

Individuals With Visual Field Deficits

The location of the neurological damage dictates the location and type of visual field deficit. Chapter 10 provides a review of the locations of damage and the implications. Individuals can have loss of their upper field of vision, lower field of vision, or, most commonly (30%), loss of one side of their visual field. This is known as *hemianopsia* (or *hemianopia* or *hemiopia*). A person with damage to the right hemisphere may lose the ability to see items on the left side when looking forward. With the loss of one half of the visual field comes other difficulties, such as inaccurate saccades (the ability to look from one object to another, quickly and accurately) and difficulty with visual scanning, causing the person to take a longer time searching the environment, as when trying to locate an object on a shelf or a chair in a room.[111]

Individuals With Diplopia

Diplopia, or double vision, is a common problem that occurs after a neurological injury such as a CVA. Eyes become misaligned, and as a result, an image is not seen in its entirety. The goal of intervention is to produce singular vision. To this end, OT practitioners may work to strengthen muscles through visual therapy or teach compensatory methods with adaptive techniques and equipment (see Chapter 10 for details).

Individuals With Visual-Spatial Deficits

The presence of visual-spatial problems after a stroke has been associated with an increase in falls,[112] and a lower QoL.[113] The incidence of visual-spatial impairments following a stroke is reported to be as high as 38%.[108] Individuals with these impairments have reported feeling unsafe, having difficulty interacting with their environment and difficulty with car transfers and wheelchair maneuverability, and feeling that familiar objects are now feeling unfamiliar.[114] The presence of visual-spatial problems impacts ADL and IADL performance.

The functional approach is now thought to be the best type of intervention for these disorders. Focusing on task-specific activities (dressing, car transfers), teaching strategies, and modifying the environment are appropriate interventions. In general, OT practitioners should use less directional language (over, under, right/left); provide less visual cues and more auditory and tactile cues; utilize audio recordings of strategies for independent practice times; use tactile feedback, when possible (slide hand on counter or desk to reach for an object); and encourage the client to work slowly. The environment should also be modified (Box 33-4).

Individuals With Unilateral Neglect

Unilateral neglect has been defined as "the failure to report, respond, or orient to novel or meaningful stimuli presented to the side opposite a brain lesion when this failure cannot be attributed to either sensory or motor defects."[90] Although unilateral neglect can occur in individuals with right brain damage and in those with left brain damage, it is the most common clinical presentation with right hemisphere damage (left hemiparesis or hemiplegia). The incidence

BOX 33-4

Environmental Modifications for Visual-Spatial Problems

Decrease clutter.
Minimize items in drawers.
Organize and label items.
Color code.
Place items in the same place.
Use contrasting colors (orange toothbrush on white counter).
Use colored duct tape on handles and switches.
Place bright tape on counter edges, stairs and shelves.

rate of neglect has been reported in a literature review to be 12% to 100% in individuals with right brain damage and 0% to 76% in those with left brain damage.[115,116] Neglect is thought to be a lateralized attention disorder and is often seen in conjunction with hemianopsia, but it is not a visual issue of itself. Clients with neglect can have extrapersonal or unilateral spatial neglect. Extrapersonal neglect, also called peripersonal or near extrapersonal neglect, occurs when a person neglects items within arm's reach. Far extrapersonal neglect occurs when a person neglects items farther away from the body. In peripersonal or near extrapersonal neglect, a person will not be able to locate items on the left side of the meal tray or find the call bell on the left side. A client with far extrapersonal neglect will not be able to see the OT practitioner on the left side or the picture on the wall. The individual will also have difficulty watching television or reading. With unilateral body/personal neglect, the person does not respond to or orient to the neglected side (most often the left) of the body. Personal neglect is most clearly seen during ADL tasks, and the individual does not wash or dress the neglected side of the body. Interestingly, these clients often lack awareness of their neglect. When asked if he or she is ready to leave their room, the individual will respond by saying yes, although he or she has only one arm in the sleeve of the shirt and one leg in the pants. The severity of an individual's neglect has been associated with decreased FIM™ scores, increased length of hospital stay, and decreased functional outcomes for reading and writing.[117]

Many of the interventions discussed earlier in this chapter can also be applied when working with individuals with neglect. Awareness training techniques have been useful for individuals with neglect.[90] Using meaningful tasks, predicting performance and comparing performance with actual results, discussing compensatory strategies, using mirrors, and video recording performance can all be useful when applied in a supportive way.

As neglect is believed to be a result of attention deficits, the interventions discussed previously in relation to attention would also be beneficial in this case. Training individuals to use self-alerting strategies as a means for increasing their attention has been shown to reduce unilateral neglect.[118] An example would be a person having a timer go off at various times to cue the individual to scan to the left and find a predetermined anchor (watch on hand, clock on wall).

Scanning training has been a positive intervention for individuals with neglect. As previously discussed, training in scanning patterns, both large (full room, larger environment) and small (table top, reading, games), can be useful to those with neglect.[90] The lighthouse strategy is another method of scanning that has been documented as being helpful to individuals with neglect.[119] (See Chapter 10 for a description of scanning training in more detail.)

Limb activation or spatiomotor cueing is based on the concept of neuroplasticity, with the idea that stimulating or moving the neglected limb or limbs may stimulate activity in the damaged region of the brain, leading to neuroplastic changes. The client is encouraged to locate the neglected limb and engage it in the task, either actively or as an assist. Locating the affected limb may also serve as an "anchor" for the client, having him or her scan to that side of the body before participating in a functional task. A literature review on limb activation after a stroke reported many positive results from past work.[120] At the conclusion of the study, the researchers put forth a new hypothesis that limb activation works as an arousing agent to orient individuals toward their neglected side.

Mental practice/imagery is a newer technique being used for individuals with neglect. Many people with neglect also have hemiparesis/hemiplegia, which makes it difficult to actively engage the arm. Mental practice/imagery is a technique in which clients are instructed to visualize performing a motor task. A case-series study demonstrated cortical/neuroplastic changes after use of mental imagery.[121] The study noted, however, that although cortical changes were evident, no functional improvements in limb function were noted. Previous research has reported positive results with the use of mental imagery as an adjunct to traditional therapies.[90] Mirror therapy, which has been discussed earlier in this chapter, is another type of therapy that may assist individuals with neglect.

Safety is a concern for individuals who have neglect. When outside of a therapeutic environment, where the OTA will be stimulating and drawing attention to the affected side, environmental adaptations can serve as means to increase safety and allow clients to more fully engage in their surroundings. While the client is in the hospital, the call bell should always be placed on the unaffected side for safety. Phone and light switches should also be placed on the unaffected side. Closets and cabinets should be organized such that most needed items are toward the nonaffected side. Bright colored tape can be placed on doorways and signage placed to help individuals navigate more safely and independently.

Individuals With Contraversive Pushing

Contraversive pushing is a newer term used to describe the phenomenon that Davis coined in 1985 as "pusher syndrome." Contraversive pushing is when a person who has had a stroke pushes away from the less affected side. The client literally pushes toward the hemiparetic side, which obviously would cause many safety concerns. Contraversive pushing occurs in about 10% of all individuals who have had strokes and is present with both right and left brain lesions.[122] It is now believed that contraversive pushing occurs as a result of a damage to the ventral posterior lateral nuclei of the thalamus. Individuals with contraversive pushing will orient their body tilted toward their affected side in the sitting or standing position. They will actively push themselves further toward the affected side and resist correction by anyone who attempts to "straighten" them, seemingly pushing into them. Clients feel that they are sitting or standing straight when they are, in fact, tilted approximately 18 degrees toward the affected side when their eyes are open. When in complete darkness, they are able to correctly identify when they are in an upright, straight position according to research.[122] This finding demonstrates that individuals who have these symptoms have a mismatch between their visual and vestibular systems in relation to how gravity is perceived. They feel they are erect even when they can see that the body is tilted. Contraversive pushing often resolves after 6 months, but rehabilitation efforts take on average 3.6 weeks longer for individuals with it to achieve the same results as peers without it.[123]

As contraversive pushing is now known to be a disorder of a person's perception of gravity when in the sitting or standing position, therapy should occur with the client in that position. The visual system is generally intact and can therefore be utilized in treatment. Individuals are unable to spontaneously correct their deficits but can be trained to use their visual system to take in information from their surroundings and make corrections with practice. Clients need to be retrained about what upright and straight is and feels like. This training can be provided with visual aids, such as sitting upright in front of a mirror that has a vertical line down the middle (Fig. 33-10). Once clients can see that they are correctly aligned, they are less likely to do the actual pushing. With practice, clients will gain confidence with feeling upright, push less, and feel more secure with the OT practitioner's physical cues and assistance. The following sequential order is recommended for treatment:[122]

1. Have clients realize their disturbed perception of erect body position.
2. Have clients visually explore the surroundings and the body's relation to the surroundings.
3. Ensure that the clients sees that they are oriented upright, use visual aids (mirrors, doors, windows, etc.).
4. Ensure that clients learn the movements necessary to reach and obtain an upright body position.
5. Have clients maintain the upright position while performing functional tasks.[122]

To be ensure client safety during transfers and sitting on the side of the bed, the OTA may initially have the client use the stronger hand to hold the more affected hand, to decrease the ability to "push." Once the client has begun to compensate, both arms may assist with balance and transfers as able.

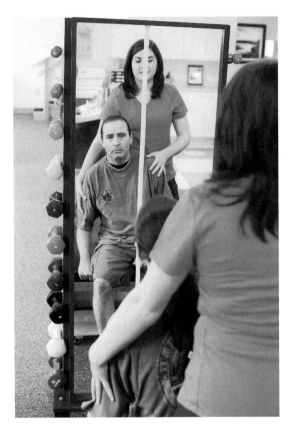

FIGURE 33-10. Intervention to address midline awareness.

Individuals With Agnosia

Agnosia is an umbrella term that means the inability to recognize sensory information in absence of any sensory impairment. An example would be a client with auditory agnosia (with normal hearing) who could not recognize a ringing phone by the sound alone. The damage is to the cortical regions that interpret that sensation. Treatment of agnosia in a client post-CVA is primarily compensatory in nature. Compensatory strategies and education include training the client to use other sensory modalities instead of the one that has been lost. For example, one strategy is to instruct a person with visual agnosia to use tactile information to find a pen on the table or a person with auditory agnosia to use visual cues to find a barking dog.

PSYCHOSOCIAL IMPACT OF STROKE

The psychosocial impact of a stroke can be significant as clients come to terms with their new reality. Clients may experience confusion, loss of control, role reversals, fear, anxiety, and a sense of isolation. They often experience a loss of dignity and feelings of guilt associated with suddenly being dependent on others. They could also be sad as a result of being separated from their homes, their families, their gardens, or their pets. All of this contributes to an initial emotional reaction that OT practitioners need to acknowledge, be patient with, and open to discussing, as needed. Depression, anxiety, and anger are all common mood disorders seen in individuals after a stroke.

Interventions That Address Psychological Impairments

Poststroke depression (PSD) is common, with a prevalence rate of 33% to 66%.[124] Clients with PSD have more functional disability, poorer rehabilitation outcomes, reduced QoL,[125] and increased mortality (three times the rate of those without PSD) compared to peers. PSD is characterized by "unrelenting feelings of sadness, anhedonia (inability to feel pleasure), helplessness, worthlessness, and/or hopelessness; loss of pleasure or interest in all activities; change in appetite, weight, or sleep pattern; psychomotor retardation or agitation; loss of energy; loss of concentration; or suicidal ideation."[126]

Poststroke anxiety is defined as an overwhelming sense of worry or fear. It may involve physical manifestations, such as decreased energy and concentration, fast heart rate, muscle tension, headaches, and shortness of breath.[124] Depression and anxiety tend to occur together. The prevalence of poststroke anxiety is thought to be 11% to 28%.[124] Individuals with anxiety are more likely to refuse therapy and are at times fearful to participate fully. Additionally, posttraumatic stress disorder (PTSD) is being recognized in stroke survivors with an estimated prevalence rate of 13% to 23%.[127]

Anger, although rarely discussed or researched, is often seen in individuals who have had a stroke. Anger may manifest as "explosive outbursts, decreased impulse control, increased irritability, hostility, insult, derogatory remarks, and reactive aggression."[124] The prevalence rate of anger after a stroke is estimated at 15%.[128] Anger can become a hurdle during the rehabilitation process, often causing stress among team members and between caregivers and clients and may lead to the client refusing to participate in therapy.

The presence of depression, anxiety, and anger can all negatively impact the rehabilitation process and affect outcomes. Once detected, actions and interventions can be initiated to help the client. Referral to a psychiatrist should be made by the team, and psychopharmaceutical medications may be administered. Medication should be administered in conjunction with other therapies that offer treatment and compensatory strategies. A model for using a modified cognitive behavioral therapy administered by a psychologist and an OT practitioner is available for individuals facing mood disorders after a stroke.[129] The core principle of cognitive behavioral therapy is that thoughts—not external factors, such as people or situations—drive feelings and behaviors. Although promising, this protocol has yet to be tested for its clinical efficacy.

Social support and promotion of active participation has also been noted to assist people with mood disorders after a stroke.[126] Involving clients in volunteering and leisure activities can often get them socially involved and connected. A client who had many roles and responsibilities at a former job may feel worthless now; a new role helping others learn to read or learn to use computers might improve mood and life purpose. A workaholic may have had few leisure pursuits formally and after the stroke has been sitting alone watching television all day. The OTA can introduce new or modified leisure options, either sedentary or more active and those that involve others. Educating and training on problem-solving techniques can assist with improving coping strategies. Some clients feel trapped in the home, and although they may not be able to do gardening on a giant plot as in the past, large pots of tomatoes or flowers on the porch will get them outside and digging in the dirt. The psychosocial impact of stroke can be devastating for many, and OT practitioners have the skills and training to help such individuals.

INTERVENTIONS FOR ACTIVITY OF DAILY LIVING AND INSTRUMENTAL ACTIVITY OF DAILY LIVING IMPAIRMENTS

Return to desired independence in performing ADLs and IADLs for people who have had a stroke should be a goal in OT throughout all levels of the rehabilitation process. Goals should be developed at each level of recovery in conjunction with the client and his or her caregiver/family. OT practitioners should keep the conversation regarding ADL/IADL goals open at all times, taking into account that the goals will and should change as the client moves along the recovery process and develops a deeper awareness of his or her abilities. It is the role of the OT practitioner to assist the client in problem-solving ways to compensate for residual deficits so that he or she can be more independent.

A review of the literature found that 1 year after discharge, 83% of the subjects followed up on still had cognitive dysfunction and that 20% were dependent in performing ADLs.[130] One year after the stroke, few had returned to work, with only 20% working, mostly on a part-time basis, 3 years after stroke. For individuals who had neglect and/or aphasia, the outcomes were worse, with only 11% having returned to work compared to 44% of clients without these deficits working 3 years after stroke. Cognitive and visual-spatial deficits appear to have a greater impact on ADL and IADL independence after a stroke.

A large systematic review was conducted to examine the role of OT and ADLs with individuals who had had a stroke.[131] The review concluded with a strong supportive statement: "Occupational therapy after stroke 'works' in that it improves outcome in terms of ability in personal ADLs." The following section will provide tips on some basic ADLs and IADLs.

Activities of Daily Living

Before beginning any basic ADL interventions, the OT practitioner should examine the environment for safety. Can the client navigate the environment where the ADLs will be performed in a safe way? Is there ample room for him or her to move? Is the bed/chair stable? Can the client reach needed items? In a bedroom, for example, all extra items should be removed. Box 33-5 notes environmental modifications to enhance performance.

Browsing websites or catalogs for adaptive equipment along with the client can serve to educate, assist with goal setting, and as a prop for problem-solving. It is good practice to keep some assistive devices in the clinic for clients to try out before purchasing. Many communities have loan closets available, and clients can borrow equipment from there. In addition to specialized medical supply companies, many mainstream store chains are stocking assistive devices and DME. See Chapter 14 for further information on equipment and adaptations in all sections below.

PERSONAL HYGIENE AND GROOMING

Personal hygiene and grooming most often can be performed more efficiently and independently with the use of adaptive equipment, assistive devices, and alternative/compensatory strategies. Oral hygiene can be performed with an electric toothbrush and automatic toothpaste dispenser, or the affected side can stabilize the toothpaste tube while opening and applying on a brush. Applying deodorant using the unaffected side can be easier with a spray, and adaptations for the spray nozzle on aerosol cans are available. Hairstyling is easiest with short hair that can be air-dried. Hands-free hair dryer holders that attach to the wall or sit on the counter are also commercially available and may be helpful. Grooming tools can be modified with cylindrical foam, Velcro®, or splinting material. Some clients find it helpful to set up a grooming station on the kitchen table so that they can sit with arms supported fully on the table. A self-standing mirror, basin, cup with water, and all grooming supplies can be placed on the table for easier access than using a wheelchair or standing at the sink.

> **BOX 33-5**
> **Environmental Modifications for Enhancing ADL/IADL Performance**
>
> There should be no unnecessary items on the bed stand or dresser.
> Place needed items within reach.
> Lower clothes hanger racks in closet.
> Replace knobs on dresser drawers, or use shelves.
> Rearrange furniture so that the client can transfer to nonaffected side more often.
> Remove throw rugs.
> Enhance lighting.
> Room temperature should be warm (cold increases unwanted high tone).

TOILETING AND TOILET HYGIENE

Remote switches for lamps or motion activated lights can illuminate the path to the bathroom for safer trips to the toilet at night. The toilet paper should be placed within reach and mounted on the unaffected side. Flushable wipes are recommended because they cause less friction and require less strength for cleaning the body. Paper or wipes can be used with a toilet aid for easier reaching. A bidet seat can be installed on any toilet to ensure hygiene; the bidet provides a warm water wash and air-drying. Grab bars should be placed where the client is most likely to reach for support (consider placement for assistance with stand-to-sit and sit-to-stand). If the bathroom is too far away, a bedside commode should be made available near the bed or external catheters (for men) for the nighttime. Various shapes of urinals for men and for women can be used to increase safety during independent urination.

BATHING AND SHOWERING

Bathing and showering environments often have many extrinsic factors that can cause falls (e.g., slippery surfaces, poorly designed tubs, bathroom fixtures, lack of grab bars, or clutter), making them potentially dangerous.[132] Nonslip mats should be used inside and outside the tub or shower. A tub bench helps avoid stepping over the tub onto the weaker leg. Use of a handheld shower is recommended, as it allows the individual to control the temperature and water flow while seated. Grab bars should be installed where the client is most likely to need them to be, and this is determined through practice and observation. See Chapter 14 for grab bar installation and other home modifications. Necessary items for bathing are placed within easy reach. For one-handed bathing, long-handled sponges, wash mitts, bath brushes, and liquid soap in a pump container are all useful. A flexible or bendable sponge can be bent to the correct angle to wash the unaffected limb, which is often a challenge.[133] During drying, for energy conservation, a large terry cloth towel, chamois, or robe can be used to absorb much of the water in a safe manner. To wash while seated by a sink, the arm and axilla of the affected limb is placed into the sink basin.[133] A wet/soaped washcloth is placed over the edge of the sink and the client can wash the less affected limb over this cloth, and once washing is completed, the client can use that arm to bath the rest of the body. A long-handled sponge (with a bendable handle) is helpful here as well.

DRESSING

Dressing is best accomplished by opting to wear loose-fitting clothing with fewer buttons and fasteners. Clients need to be in a safe/supported position, and the OT practitioner should be able to provide assistance for the "just right challenge," as needed. The client should be in a stable chair with arms (edge of bed for a challenge), clothing placed within reach, and feet touching the floor for stability (a stool is

COMMUNICATION

Communication is often a challenging area when a client is recovering and healing after a stroke. The client, during the various stages of recovery over time, may be at different locations, including acute care, long-term acute care, skilled nursing facility, inpatient rehabilitation, outpatient, home health, or home. Each location will have different staff with different methods of performing therapy, a variety of skill levels and years of experience, and clients will have different needs as they progress. The communication between facilities may be poor even within the same hospital system, not to mention across regions or between competitors. The OTA in a home health providing OT services for a client may see that there is a transfer tub bench sitting in a spare room while the client and caregiver struggle with a lawn chair in the shower. After gathering more information, the OTA learns that the inpatient rehabilitation OTA ordered a tub bench because the client mentioned the availability of the tub. Unfortunately, no one explained to the client and the caregiver that the glass door should be removed, that the bench works best with a hand held shower, or that the client would have to have the back toward the water controls to get the legs moved around the toilet in the small bathroom.

Similarly, an OTA with 20 years of experience in an outpatient facility may attempt to use FES to stimulate wrist extension in the affected side, not realizing that the inpatient practitioner already tried it; with poor results as the client could not tolerate it. If possible, OTAs should send along contact information for themselves and any pertinent information about status, current and future needs, and equipment used or ordered for the client to give to the next OT practitioner. Improved communication between settings will help the client and the caregiver navigate the confusing world of health care and enhance continuity of care over all practice settings.

used, if needed). The OT practitioner should allow the client to take rest breaks and provide simple, clear instructions because dressing has inherent cognitive, motor, and visual-spatial challenges. Individuals who have use of one hand will benefit from zipper pulls and Velcro® in place of buttons or a buttonhook, where possible. Bras should be modified to have Velcro® in place of hooks, or a pullover sports bra or a lined camisole may be easier to manage.

The sequence of dressing may need to be changed to conserve energy, for example, donning shirt–resting–donning pants sequence; sitting to don pants instead of standing; or donning underwear/pants together and standing only once to pull them up. Donning socks before pants eliminates the challenge of managing the bottom of the pant leg while donning the sock. Alternatively, the client may don a sock and then the pant leg on the same side and then do the same on the other side.

Clients should be given directions for alternative dressing techniques, as listed in the following sections[133] (Fig. 33-11).

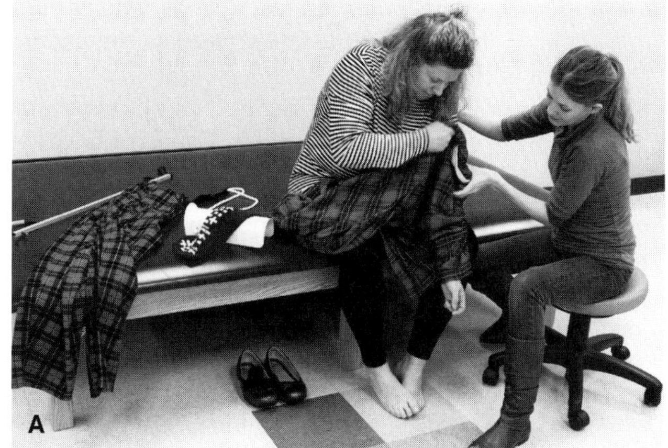

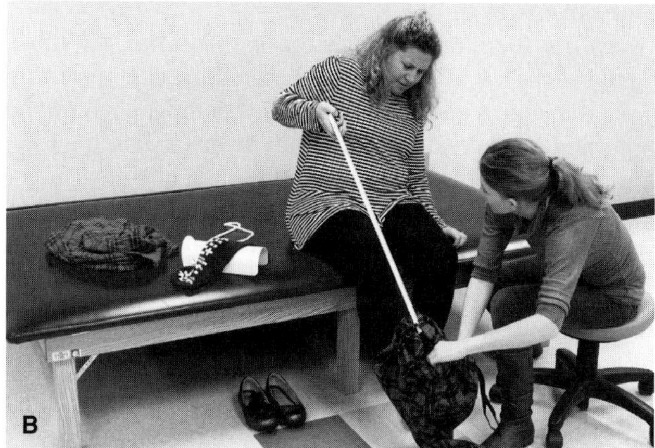

FIGURE 33-11. Hemi-dressing techniques. **A.** Upper body. **B.** Lower body.

Upper Extremity (Seated): Teach the client to:

- Always dress the affected arm first, pull clothing up to the shoulder. Start with the affected arm placed on the lap. Bunch up the sleeve, and place over the affected hand and wrist. It may be helpful to lean slightly forward with the affected arm reaching toward floor, between the knees, while bringing the sleeve up over the arm. This helps manage spasticity in a gravity-reduced position. Be sure to bring the sleeve up over the elbow to the shoulder. Clients who have poor sitting balance should take extra caution.
- Place the unaffected limb inside the shirt, and pull the shirt up to the shoulder.
- Put the head and neck inside the shirt (if a pullover shirt)
- Straighten the sleeve by rubbing the arm along the leg.
- Pull the shirt down over the torso (use dressing stick to assist, if needed).

Lower Extremity (Seated):

- Cross the affected leg over the other knee or ankle, if possible.
- Place the correct pant leg over the foot (using reacher or dressing stick, as needed) and then straighten the leg into the pant leg.
- Dress the less affected leg next.

- Pull up the pants (and/or underwear as well) as high as they will go while in the seated position, shifting the weight back and forth.
- Stand to pull up underwear/pants; it may be necessary to lean on a wall or the walker for support or have assistance to maintain balance.

A dressing stick and or reacher may be helpful for both upper and lower body dressing. The dressing stick can push up a bra strap, push the shirt down the back, pull on a pant loop to pull pants onto the leg, or help doff clothing. The reacher can grab the waistband of the pants to extend the reach to the foot and assist with maintaining balance in the sitting position to avoid reaching too far forward.

Donning Socks:

- Cross the affected leg over the opposite knee, if possible.
- Use the less affected hand to open the sock by inserting the fingers and thumb into the opening, opening the fingers to create a space, pull the sock onto the toes, and spread it all the way to heel.
- Pull the sock over the heel.
- A stool is sometimes helpful to don socks in the sitting position.

Donning Shoes:

- Similar to donning a sock, cross the affected limb over the opposite knee, if possible.
- Open the shoe as wide as possible, and place the toes into it.
- Pull the shoe on over the heel; use a step stool or the floor to push the foot inside the shoe.
- A long-handled shoehorn may be helpful to get the heel to slide into the shoe without the back of the shoe buckling.
- Use Velcro® fasteners, magnetic closures (available in various magnetic forces), or elastic shoelaces, which are easier to manage than shoelaces that need to be tied. One-handed shoelace tying is an option, and a number of resources describing this technique are available on the Internet. The benefit is that this technique does not involve any new purchases; however, getting the shoelaces pulled tight enough can be difficult.

Alternative techniques may be required for clients with an ankle-foot orthosis (AFO). Typically, clients wear a knee-high sock with an AFO, so donning this sock can be challenging. The orthotic starts underneath the foot, spans the dorsal LE ending just below the knee, and may have a rigid or hinged joint at the ankle. It is held on with Velcro® straps at the ankle and just below the knee. For donning while seated, a small stool may be helpful, or the use of a special device, the Original AFO Assist® (see Fig. 33-12) may be considered. The Original AFO Assist® provides the option of an angled or straight surface that holds the AFO in place while it is donned. After donning of the AFO, the additional bulk of the AFO at the ankle and the flat, rigid foot support make donning shoes traditionally much more difficult.

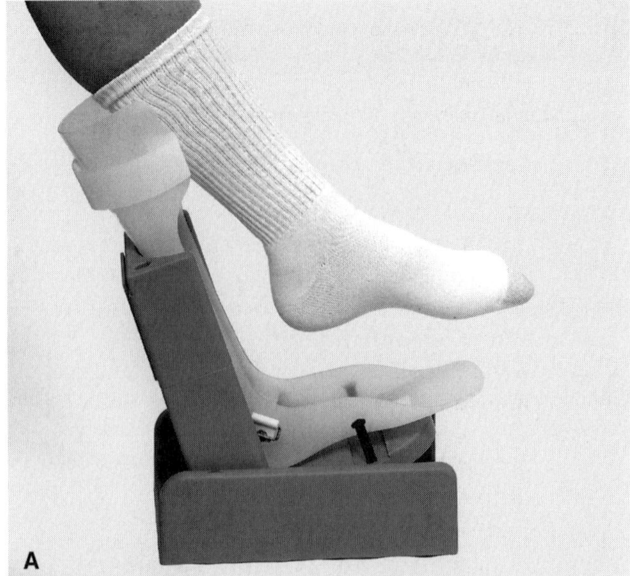

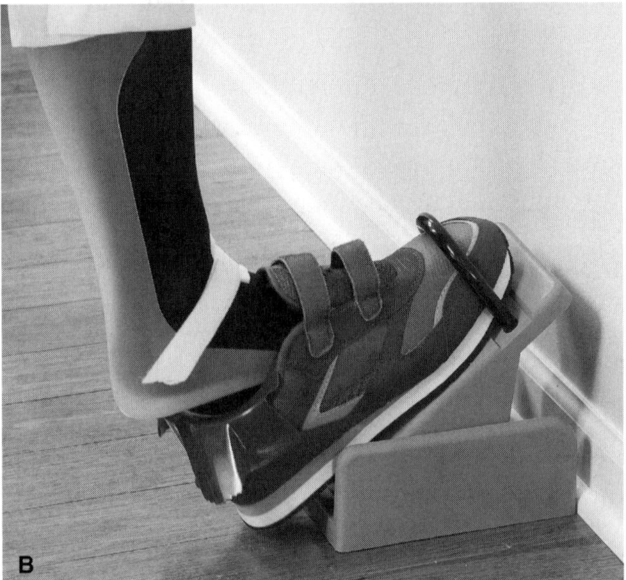

FIGURE 33-12. **A.** An AFO is difficult to don for some clients, and the angled support, such as provided by the Original AFO Assist®, can help. **B.** The Original AFO Assist® also assists with donning the shoe while wearing the bulky AFO.

Clients may use the Original AFO Assist® to don the AFO while sitting in a chair or long sitting on a mat or bed. Clients can use a the specially designed shoe portion on the Original AFO Assist® or a small stool to push against to safely don a shoe while seated, and a long shoehorn may assist.

SEXUAL ACTIVITY

Decreased libido, impaired erectile and ejaculatory functions, decreased vaginal lubrication, impaired ego and self-esteem, and depression are noted effects of stroke on sexual function.[135] The side effects that often accompany stroke, such as motor, sensory, cognitive, communicative, and visual-spatial impairments, can also impact the ability to participate in sexual activities. Other medical complications,

EVIDENCE-BASED PRACTICE

In an article published in the *American Journal of Occupational Therapy,*[134] the authors reported on a study looking at how motor functioning after a stroke affected the client's ability to complete dressing tasks independently. The research noted that balance was strongly associated with the independence level in dressing and that certain values on the Berg Balance Scale (BBS) could be a cut-off point to note dressing independence versus the need for supervision or assistance. Their results suggested that "balance is a more important function influencing dressing independence than motor and cognitive functions." The BSS assesses balance in older adults, and the highest score possible is 56. In this study, a BBS score of 44 points was the cut-off value for independence in dressing, and a BBS score of 32 points was the cut-off value to show at least a supervision level of dressing functionality. OT practitioners could potentially use these values as the criteria for determining the level of assistance required by a client for dressing, thus achieving accurate goal setting and treatment expectations.

The authors of the study did note that the values only assess balance, and certainly functional abilities in the trunk, upper extremities, and cognition must also be considered. They found that clients with a BSS score under 44 could still potentially be independent with dressing if they have a strong trunk, less affected UE function, and good cognition. Similarly, clients may require assistance to dress even with a BSS of greater than 32, if they have poor cognitive functioning. A misjudgment based on these scenarios could lead to a fall, so all factors should be taken into account when working with the client on dressing and for determining the client's level of functioning.

Fujita, T., Sato, A., Yamamoto, Y., Otsuki, K., Tsuchiya, K., & Tozato, F. (2016). Motor function cutoff values for independent dressing in stroke patients. American Journal of Occupational Therapy, 70, 3.

such as diabetes, hypertension, and cardiac conditions, bring their own problems and concerns in relation to sexual functioning. Societal attitudes regarding sex and caregiver stress and fatigue further complicate sexual rehabilitation and options. Following a stroke, dependence in the performance of ADLs has been shown as a strong predictor of decreased sexual activity after a stroke.[136] At times, the OT practitioner may not bring up the subject of sexual activity as the population of clients who have had a stroke is composed primarily of older adults. This form of ageism, with its own prejudice and discrimination, assumes that the older adult will not be interested in sex or is not sexually active. OT practitioners not only have the knowledge to address issues related to sexual activity after a stroke,[137] but they also have the responsibility to do so.

Jack Annon proposed the acronym PLISSIT for the levels of intervention that should be applied with regard to the client's sexuality.[135] The levels are as follows:

- Permission: Is simply reassuring the client that having sexual feelings or concerns related to sexuality is normal and acceptable to talk about. The OT practitioner should be proactive and bring up the subject of sexuality early (during evaluation when talking about ADLs) in the process to bring a sense of normalcy around discussion of the topic. All OT practitioners can and should function at this level, being sure to not project their own personal beliefs.
- Limited information: Is the next level of intervention. Here, the OT practitioner provides information to dispel myths or fears. Education groups, pamphlets, handouts, and Internet links may all be helpful. The OT practitioner can also refer the client to other personnel who can provide information. For example, the client could have fear that sex will cause him or her to have another stroke. It may be helpful in this case to have the client consult the physician. The OT practitioner can function as a liaison in this case. For the OT practitioner who is uncomfortable with initiating the discussion on sexual activity, a handout may be a way to begin the conversation.
- Specific suggestions: Suggestions include the OT practitioner gathering full information regarding the specific problem. The OTA will need to have knowledge of various sexual activities to address the concerns the client may be describing. The OT practitioner may or may not be able to provide direct intervention but can refer the client, as needed. An example of suggestions in this step of the model would be positional changes. Often, individuals will not be able to participate in sexual activity the same way as before the stroke because of the effects of stroke. Taking the bottom position, lying on the hemiparetic side, or sitting in a chair with the partner on top of the client are some of the positional suggestions the OT practitioner can offer. Having the client focus less on the sexual act itself and more on affection, touch, and intimacy may also be appropriate.
- Intensive therapy: In this step, formal training in sex therapy is required, and since this is beyond the scope of OT practice, the client should be referred appropriately to a practitioner specializing in this area.

Mobility/Transfers During Activities of Daily Living

Many occupations require moving from one place to another, and mobility may be vital for functional performance. Chapter 13 provides details regarding many types of transfers, and Chapter 15 addresses types of mobility, including wheelchair use. A client who has had a stroke presents unique challenges in relation to transfers. Visual-perceptual deficits require that the OTA allow the client to take time for visual recognition of the environment before moving. Attention, language, and motor planning deficits may be compensated for with the use of tactile cues and visual demonstration by the OTA. An OT practitioner should use key points of control (shoulder girdle and pelvis) and client momentum to assist with transfers. When the client is in the seated position, the OT practitioner should have the client "scoot forward" or "butt walk" by using lateral shifting of the pelvis and trunk from side to side. This not only accomplishes the forward movement but also assists with increasing trunk strength and awareness of body position. A forward trunk lean is also important here to avoid premature LE extension resulting from higher extensor tone tendencies of the legs. Once the client has scooted forward and has the feet flat on the floor, he or she should be instructed to rock forward by putting weight through both LEs and shifting weight forward. The flaccid or synergistic affected arm should be cradled in front of the client by either the client or the OT practitioner so that it is protected, and the arm with some movement should be involved in assisting to push the client forward and off the seated surface. Repeating this motion of rocking forward can prepare the client to stand incorporating both sides of the body. Asymmetry during transfers has been associated with an increased risk for falls; therefore, spending time to teach and train clients to ensure symmetry during the sit-to-stand process is beneficial.[138] The OT practitioner's hands are positioned on the client's shoulder girdle and pelvis, with a gait belt and assistance, as needed. Momentum can be used by the client to rock forward and move into the standing position, with the OT practitioner providing additional support to the affected knee to prevent it from "buckling" as it accepts weight. The OT practitioner can place his or her legs on both sides of the client's weaker knee and gently squeeze to provide support there, or use his or her knees on the outside of both knees of the client. Once the client is in the standing position, the OT practitioner can use tactile cues and physical support, as mentioned above, to assist the client with proper weight-shifting to pivot to the desired surface. The OT practitioner must recognize that moving into a seated position requires more motor control than coming to the standing position. The client will require physical cues and assistance to maintain trunk flexion and slowly lower the body onto the desired surface. Verbal cues should be kept to a minimum for clients with aphasia. Practicing sit-to-stand transfers and performing functional tasks in the sitting and standing positions, which require weight shift and reaching, will assist with increasing strength and balance, ultimately leading to improved ability to complete desired occupations safely.

Clients who are ambulatory may use a cane or a walker. With their PT teammates, the OT practitioner should encourage the use of a mobility device as appropriate for weight-bearing through the more affected arm during ambulation. The rollator style walker also has brakes and a built-in seat, which may be helpful when a rest break is required or for sitting on while grooming at the sink. At times, the OTA may work with the physical therapist or the PTA in a co-treatment situation if the more dependent client has to stand during a functional task. Clients may use a wheelchair for some or all of their mobility. A client may propel a manual wheelchair at a "hemi-height," which is lower to the ground to allow for one arm, one leg (stronger side) propulsion without sliding out of the chair. Some clients will use a one-arm-drive manual wheelchair, which has an extra wheel rim on the strong side to control both wheels from one side. Clients who are improving in ambulation may rent a lightweight manual wheelchair for a few months as a backup for moving over long distances and to avoid fatigue. Some clients will be safer and more efficient with power mobility because it can facilitate mobility and help with pressure relief and repositioning. The OTA can collaborate with PT teammates and the clinic staff helping with wheelchair seating for a consistent, safe, and appropriate approach with transfers and mobility.

Instrumental Activities of Daily Living

IADLs include a wide range of practices, as mentioned earlier. Here, it is important to set goals with the client and his or her caregiver to determine the need for, and the feasibility of, the client returning to previous roles and responsibilities.

KITCHEN TASKS, MEAL PREPARATION, AND SHOPPING

One area that almost everyone will have to participate in at some point is preparing food/snacks and cleaning the kitchen. After a stroke, individuals can often manage kitchen tasks safely, with properly placed items, pacing of work, and use of adaptive devices. The following is a list of strategies for the kitchen:

- Use already prepared food, when possible; many grocery stores now sell precut vegetables and marinated meat.
- Incorporate rest breaks, and avoid overly complicated recipes.
- Rotating shelf ("Lazy Susan") inserts, peg boards, and magnetic knife holders allow for easy access to items.
- Use nonstick cooking utensils and pans, and use smaller-sized and lighter weight pans.
- Retrieve items from oven shelves by standing to the side (instead of in front) in case of balance challenges.
- Move heavy and hot pots from the stovetop to the sink by placing them on a towel or large pot holder, and pulling them along the counter surface to transport.
- Invest in a rolling cart for transporting hot items, taking dishes to set the table, or transporting items when both hands have to be kept on the walker for balance.

A number of commercially available devices that serve to stabilize items for one-handed control include the following: a one-handed cutting board with vertical edge to hold bread during spreading, nonskid pads and/or Dycem®, bowls with nonskid bottoms, use of a stand-up mixer while baking, a countertop or wall-mounted jar opener, an electric one-handed can opener, and a holder to secure pots on the stove for secure stirring. Meal preparation tasks, such as chopping vegetables, can be performed sitting at the table, and stirring a pot on the stove can be less fatiguing and safer when done seated on a stool or walker seat.

Shopping for food can be difficult because of transportation challenges, poor balance or endurance, difficulty reaching high or low, or cognitive changes. A reacher can assist with items on higher shelves or staff at the store may be asked to assist. The OTA can recommend a service that delivers groceries to the home or ordering online for home delivery or store pick-up. Friends, family, neighbors, or members of a faith community may assist with getting groceries. Some communities have Meals on Wheels programs, in which a free meal is delivered daily to the client's home.

HOUSEHOLD MANAGEMENT

The management of household tasks and roles can be difficult for the client who has had a stroke. The client may prefer a certain level of cleanliness that the spouse may not be able to maintain. Some families hire someone to assist with cleaning tasks, or friends and family may take turns to provide assistance. For dishwashing, a suction bottle brush can be used to clean glasses and other dishes in the sink, and heavy rubber or vinyl gloves may increase the client's ability to hold onto a slippery plate. Use a dishwasher for all items that are dishwasher-safe. For cleaning and dusting surfaces, long-handled brooms, dustpans, and brushes may be used. Swiffer® dusters are lightweight and easy to use. The client should be aware of balance challenges when reaching high, squatting, or using a heavy vacuum cleaner. Consider using a robot or lightweight vacuum. A dressing stick or reacher can assist with laundry transfer from the washer to the dryer and then to the basket. The rolling cart, as mentioned earlier, can help transport the basket to another room.

DRIVING AND COMMUNITY MOBILITY

Interventions in this area focus on safety and the interests and concerns of the client and his or her caregivers and these issues along with the role of the OT practitioner are discussed thoroughly in Chapter 16. Driving is often a goal for individuals recovering from stroke and has an impact on a person's sense of independence. After a stroke, a client may have sensory, motor, cognitive, and visual-spatial impairments, which will impede safe driving. The generalist OT practitioner is trained to assess the client in all of these areas and provide useful information to the rehabilitation team's conversation about whether a client can safely resume driving. Each state and country has different requirements for obtaining and maintaining a driver's license and reporting laws. It is imperative that OT practitioners know the laws of the area in which they are working.

As discussed in this chapter, it is evident that many individuals have visual-spatial and visual field cuts (neglect and hemianopsia), hemiplegia/hemiparesis, spasticity, communication limitations, impulsivity, or poor insight into their deficits and memory concerns, rendering them incapable of returning to safe driving. The OTA can assist with specific assessments that are part of the driving evaluation. It is the OT practitioner's role to perform a solid evaluation; report the findings to the team, the client, and his or her caregivers; and refer the client to a driving specialist, as appropriate.

Leisure

Tapping into leisure interests can serve to motivate the client and be used during strength and balance training. After a stroke, many individuals have residual impairments that result in activity limitations, and researchers have found that occupational gaps are reported in 87% of the population studied 1 year after the stroke.[139] Those authors reported that dependency in self-care and performance of IADLs and previous leisure activities had a negative effect on life satisfaction. Clients experience many barriers related to leisure participation, such as "internal barriers, lack of knowledge, decreased skills, decreased opportunities, environmental barriers, attitudes, architectural, transportation, rules and regulations, barriers of omission, economic, communication barriers, social skills, ability to speak and ability to listen."[108] The OTA addressing issues related to leisure must begin with conversations with the client and his or her caregivers/family members to prioritize the client's interests and determine the feasibility of engaging in leisure pursuits. Therapy should then address the client's limitations, provide adaptive equipment, and problem-solve adaptive techniques for leisure participation. For example, a client who loves to play golf may think that this leisure pursuit is gone from their lives. An OTA can recommend adaptations to the clubs for grip and balance options that can be attached to the golf cart if playing; or other related activities, such as riding along with friends in the cart, keeping score, playing Wii® golf or miniature golf, or even explaining the game rules to a grandchild while watching golf on TV together. As with ADLs and IADLs, many modifications to leisure activities are available and can be purchased or fabricated. Education regarding community resources should also be provided. Many communities have alternative transportation programs, independence centers, and adaptive leisure activities. For example, many ski resorts have adaptive ski programs, and most larger cities have adapted sports of all types. Adapted travel resources for clients with disabilities can be found for every destination. It is the duty of the OTA to be knowledgeable about these resources.

Rest and Sleep

Rest and sleep are listed as occupations in the *Occupational Therapy Practice Framework, 3rd edition* (OTPF-3)[140] and are defined as "activities related to obtaining restorative rest and sleep to support healthy, active engagement in other occupations." Rest and sleep include the actual act of sleeping as well as the activities around sleep, such as brushing teeth, putting on pajamas, setting the alarm, or other things that may be part of the sleeping preparation ritual. It is believed that after a stroke, 50% of individuals have difficulty sleeping.[141] Insomnia, sleep-related breathing disorders, and sleep–wake cycle disorders are common. In addition to those sleep disorders, pain, lack of exercise, and impaired mobility can further exacerbate sleep problems. Having proper sleep is imperative for an individual to fully function in the rehabilitation process as well as for helping the brain and body heal. OT practitioners can assist in this occupation through recommending proper positioning and by training caregivers in repositioning schedules. Refer to the section on positioning for more information about proper positioning. On average, a person should reposition himself or herself or be repositioned by a caregiver every 2 hours. A person may only require a pillow for re-adjustment or may require a complete turn performed by a caregiver. Pillows, wedges, towel rolls, and hospital beds are all equipment that could be used to assist in enhancing comfort for sleeping.

If the client has been diagnosed with insomnia, medication could be helpful, and the OT practitioner or client/family should speak to the physician about this. Sleep-related breathing disorders can be addressed through the use of a continuous positive airway pressure (CPAP) machine, which is prescribed by a physician and managed by a respiratory therapist.

Researchers have found that after providing clients in the intensive care unit with education and providing simple over-the-counter sleep remedies (e.g., eye mask, ear plugs, white noise machine, etc.), clients self-reported improvements in fatigue, sleep disturbance, wake performance, and perceived disturbances in physical function.[142] Recommended education for the client and his or her caregiver includes the following instructions:

- Keep the bedroom dark and at a comfortable temperature.
- Prevent and avoid noises that might cause wakefulness.
- Increase movement and exercise during the day.
- Have exposure to light during the day.
- Follow a regular sleep schedule. Go to bed and wake up the same time every day.
- Have a bedtime routine. For example, take a warm bath before bedtime. Listen to calming music, or read a book.
- Use the bedroom only for sleep or sex. Do not eat food or watch TV in bed.
- Certain foods and drinks can lead to sleep problems. Consume foods and drinks that are caffeine-free. Avoid coffee, tea, certain soft drinks, and chocolate after the late afternoon or evening.
- Plan to have dinner at least 3 hours before bedtime.
- Make sure that the stomach is neither too full nor empty before bedtime.
- Avoid eating heavy meals that can cause poor sleep.
- Stop consuming drinks 2 hours before bedtime. Drinking fluids at night can lead to frequent trips to the bathroom.
- Avoid alcoholic drinks at night. Alcohol may help with falling asleep, but sleep is then often restless.[143]
- Limit the use of electronic devices before bedtime or use night shift/change color tone of electronics to warm tones versus blue tones a few hours before bedtime.

Work

The prevalence rate of stroke is increasing among younger individuals. Researchers found that over half the clients in one large study (N = 7740) treated at a large medical center were of working age.[13] This, coupled with the fact that aging Americans are choosing to work longer, makes return to work (RTW) an important factor for OT practitioners to consider when treating adults with stroke. See Chapter 17 for details about work. Best practices for OT practitioners related to RTW for clients with a stroke were developed on the basis of findings from a qualitative study by experts in the field, and include the following:

1. When important to the client, address RTW early after a stroke and emphasize RTW as an end goal.
2. Conduct comprehensive, occupation-centered evaluations and assessments.
3. Integrate coping and metacognitive strategies (awareness/understanding of thoughts) into interventions.
4. Address the readiness and capability of the employer and work environment to receive the employee after a stroke.
5. Advocate for support services as needed.[144]

THE YOUNGER ADULT

Strokes in young adults are relatively uncommon, with the incidence at 10% to 15% of all strokes, although there is a disproportionately large economic impact because of disability before an adult's most productive years.[145] Both young and older adults have the same modifiable risk factors; however, the prevalence of these risk factors is not the same in these two age groups. Hypertension, heart disease, and diabetes are the most common risk factors among older adults.[146] In contrast, in the case of young clients with stroke, the most common risk factors are dyslipidemia (high cholesterol), smoking, and hypertension.[147] The incidence of ischemic stroke in younger adults is also increasing, although the reasons have not been fully determined.[148] The OTA can assist with community health efforts to decrease smoking, increase exercise and activity, and promote healthy eating and regular checkups. The young client may have concerns about study, work, active leisure pursuits, the future, and caring for a family with children at home. Young adults may also have different priorities with regard to therapeutic goals, preferences for treatment, leisure activities, and use of technology compared with their older counterparts.

The world of work is vast, and it is virtually impossible for an OT to have knowledge of all occupations. An OT practitioner is skilled, however, at activity analysis and can apply this analysis to the job a client desires to return to. The OT practitioner will need to understand the job's demands and the skills, ability, and knowledge to perform that job. The OTA can use publicly available resources, such as O*NET (Occupational Information Network), published electronically by the US Department of Labor. O*NET provides a good start for the OTA to understand a job's demands, as well as the knowledge and skills required to perform that job well.[149] The OTA must also consider the environment (e.g., temperature, noise, lighting, smell, surface, etc.), tools and equipment used, and coworker support in the environment. The OTA can, with permission from the client, speak directly to the employer to gain insight into the specifics of the job duties and the culture of the work environment. In addition to learning the specifics about a particular job, OT practitioners will need to develop knowledge in work regulations and laws. The Family Leave Act, Social Security Disability, and the Americans with Disability Act are examples of laws and regulations that an OT practitioner should be knowledgeable about. If it is deemed that the client is unable to return to his or her former occupation, a referral can be made to the state's Vocational Rehabilitation Services for a more formal evaluation and financial support to pursue other options, such as education or training.

Work can give an individual a sense of identity, habit, routine, confidence, meaning, and self-worth. Often, one of the first things asked when meeting someone new is "What do you do?" A stroke greatly impacts a person's ability to RTW, thus impacting their sense of place in the world. With increasing numbers of individuals of work age having strokes, the OT profession needs to incorporate more RTW education and intervention into its everyday practice. If RTW is not possible, the client may want to consider volunteering options.

Religious/Spiritual Activities and Expression

To many clients, their faith and belief systems are important in their daily lives. The OTA should be aware of cultural differences, which may mean that the client does no work (therapy) on a certain day of rest in the week or has dietary preferences associated with beliefs. Turning the pages of the Bible or the Koran may require a book holder or support and a finger cot (rubber finger) for turning pages. Many religious texts are also available online, as audiobooks/CDs, or as an app with audio options. Clients may miss the social and spiritual aspects of a study group, and the group may be able to meet in the client's home instead of at the church, synagogue, or temple. Some organizations have transportation options for helping members get to services when they have difficulty driving or if car transfers are a problem. OT practitioners should inquire about assisting with this important occupation and be aware of their own biases toward others' religious or spiritual practices. The OT practitioner may also inquire about using the virtual context to join study groups or participate in religious services.

MILD STROKES

Many students and new graduates assume, on the basis of what they have read about stroke and the stages of recovery, that every client with a stroke has significant disabilities with flaccidity and/or hemiplegia. This, however, is not the case, especially with the improvements and timing of medical treatments for stroke, such as with tissue plasminogen activator (tPA) and endovascular medical procedures, which can reduce the effects of strokes. Not all clients in the acute setting experience flaccidity; some clients have hemiparesis, with some movement in the arm and the leg from the onset. They may have mild weakness throughout the arm and/or the leg or exhibit distal weakness with relative proximal strength. These clients may go home directly from the initial hospitalization, with a prescription for either outpatient or home health therapy, instead of going through intensive rehabilitation. The changes in functionality can however, be significant, because even slight weakness can make some occupations, roles, and tasks challenging and frustrating. The OTA may provide skilled therapy to these clients at home or in the clinic, with a focus on adaptive equipment and techniques, safety, and strengthening. Some clients may be out of work on short-term disability, and some may have longer-term impairments that affect function.

CAREGIVER AND FINANCIAL CONCERNS

The focus after a stroke is often on the individual who sustained the stroke and his or her needs for recovery. However, the literature on caregiving notes that caring for someone with a chronic condition can have significant effects on the physical and emotional health of the caregiver.[150] Some clients and their caregivers have a large support network with ample resources to assist, whereas some others may have a limited number of friends/family, with one caregiver providing all the care. Some caregivers may have to not only provide dependent care but also give up working to do so, which imposes a financial burden on them as well. The client's home may require costly modifications, and there may be additional costs for long-term medications, DME, and many other health-related expenses. Clients may be eligible for disability payments (income), but that process can take 2 to 3 years, and finances may become tight while waiting for the approval.

Some clients may be virtually immobile when in bed, requiring assistance to change positioning every few hours and for toileting overnight. This may result in lack of sleep for busy caregivers, adding to the stress and physical toll of lifting, moving, and caring for the client. The client and the caregiver may disagree on how tasks in the home should be performed, and this may cause extra tension. The client may desire to perform transfers in the standing position instead of using the patient lift, but this method may hurt the caregiver's back while assisting. With regard to all goals, therapy sessions, and practice locations, the OTA should consider not only the needs of the client but also those of the caregiver. For instance, a client may refuse to have an external/paid caregiver come into the home to assist with care; however, that refusal may mean that the caregiver never gets a break. The OTA and the client can make a list of tasks for which the client would be willing to have assistance and create a plan that begins with an aide or friend providing company and light housekeeping a few hours a week while the caregiver takes a break. The OTA could also train friends and family (besides the main caregiver) in some tasks, such as performing ROM, and help create a daily calendar for the person responsible for assisting with ROM.

Caregiver burden has been investigated in the study area of stroke, and it has been found that caregivers use a wide variety of coping strategies to avoid burnout. In one study, the most common coping strategies used by caregivers were active problem-solving, positive distraction with enjoyable tasks, seeking social support, identifying solutions to problems faced, and having strong faith.[151]. The OTA may be able to refer a caregiver to a support group or offer problem-solving strategies to make performance of ADL tasks easier.

WHEN THEY DON'T GET BETTER

Certainly, most clients who have had a stroke make some recovery in the months and years after the stroke. The recovery may not, however, be enough to resume desired occupational pursuits and, in some cases, even to go home at all. It may be sad and frustrating to the client and the caregiver as well as to the OTA that despite everyone's best efforts, the recovery has stopped or is limited. The occupational therapist and the OTA, as well as the rest of the team, will need to discuss how long therapy should be continued, when there is no or very limited improvement. The client who was hoping to go home from inpatient rehabilitation may have to go to a skilled nursing facility for care when the spouse or the family simply cannot provide adequate care at home. These cases can be challenging, but the OTA can be a resource for clients and the caregivers to continue to perform ROM, stimulate and engage the weakened limbs, perform/assist with any ADL tasks as abilities allow, and enjoy leisure pursuits as they are able.

SUMMARY

A CVA is a fairly common medical condition that an OT practitioner will likely encounter multiples times in his or her career and may provide primary intervention for the residual effects of a stroke or secondary intervention when treating other challenges faced by their clients. Although the symptoms of clients vary in severity, it is important that the causes, complications, and residual functional abilities be thoroughly understood. The wide variety of symptoms, although discussed separately in the chapter, are not seen in isolation clinically. OTAs must use clinical reasoning to integrate all of the client's symptoms into treatment sessions. For example, the task demands of dressing are not only related to motor skills but will also contain challenges to vision, attention, executive functioning, sensation, and others. The OTA generally works as part of a team caring for clients who have had a stroke, and good communication with all team members is vital to provide quality care to the client and to avoid duplication of efforts or missed opportunities. This chapter reviewed recent evidence for providing interventions for individuals who have had a stroke. Specific strategies for intervention were provided on the basis of the most recent evidence available. The evidence is, however, constantly changing, and if the OTA finds working with clients after a stroke a desired practice area, then he or she has the responsibility to stay current on research findings and techniques through lifelong learning.

REVIEW QUESTIONS

1. A client has UE spasticity after a stroke. The shoulder will *most likely* be in which of the following fixed positions?
   a. Flexion and abduction
   b. Extension and adduction
   c. External rotation and abduction
   d. Internal rotation and adduction
2. During an OT intervention session, a client who has had a right CVA demonstrates a tendency to ignore items on the left side. When documenting this behavior, what should the OTA report?
   a. Agnosia
   b. Unilateral inattention
   c. Poor right/left discrimination
   d. Poor visual scanning
3. When teaching self-ROM exercises to a client who has had a CVA, it is important that the OT practitioner instruct the client to *not*:
   a. Perform them more than three times in a day
   b. Stretch the shoulder beyond 90 degrees of flexion
   c. Stretch shoulder into external rotation
   d. Bend elbow too slowly
4. Which three of the following should the OTA remember when speaking to a client with aphasia?
   a. Give the person the time to talk.
   b. Slow the rate of speech but maintain normal intonation.
   c. Accept and encourage use of gestures and facial expressions.
   d. Attempt to guess what the person is saying.
   e. Have the client write it down.
   f. Use a family member as an interpreter.
5. A client with left unilateral neglect would benefit from being educated in which of the following strategies?
   a. Transfers to the left side
   b. Placing the call bell on the left side
   c. Lighthouse strategy
   d. Reading out loud

6. Mrs. Willard is 72 years old, married, and was in very good health before she experienced a ischemic stroke during the night while asleep, and subsequently, was not able to receive tPA. The effects of the stroke have been significant for her and rehabilitation progress is expected to be very slow. Which of the following psychosocial concerns would she be *most likely* to have?
   a. Hallucinations
   b. Depression
   c. Memory loss
   d. Combative behaviors
7. An OT practitioner is conducting a chart review in an acute care setting. The client had a large left hemisphere stroke. Which of the following symptoms would the OT practitioner *most likely* see upon first meeting the client?
   a. Diplopia
   b. Aphasia
   c. Unilateral neglect
   d. Left-sided hemiparesis
8. When using the principles of motor learning while working with a client who has had a stroke, an OT practitioner will do which of the following?
   a. Provide PROM.
   b. Provide opportunities for varied practice.
   c. Use a mirror in therapy.
   d. Provide a splint for wrist support.
9. Which three of the following are cognitive strategies used to enhance motor function?
   a. Mirror therapy
   b. Mental practice
   c. Action observation
   d. Weight-bearing through affected limb
   e. Playing Uno®
   f. Writing a journal
10. A client who has had a right CVA displays limited movement in the left wrist extensors. Using the Rood approach, which technique is considered effective to facilitate left wrist extension?
   a. Maintaining firm pressure over the wrist extensor muscles
   b. Slow stroking of the wrist extensor muscles
   c. Quick stretching of the wrist flexor muscles
   d. Fast brushing over the wrist extensor muscles

CASE STUDY

Lucy is a 62-year-old retired nurse. One year ago, she experienced a right carotid artery CVA. She spent 13 days in acute care, 30 days in a renowned rehabilitation center, and 5 weeks in a subacute rehabilitation center. Lucy lived with her daughter and son-in-law for 6 months and received home-health care assistance, and she required 24-hour supervision. She currently resides in a skilled nursing facility and attends an interdisciplinary community reentry program 3 days a week. She has expressed dissatisfaction with her current living arrangement and lack of independence.

Medical History

Remarkable for a left-shoulder replacement (status post 2 years ago); gastric bypass surgery (14 years post), and a history of depression.

Evaluation Results

Self-care ADLs:

Feeding—Following setup, Lucy can self-feed with right UE

Grooming—Following setup, Lucy can comb hair, brush teeth, and wash face. She is able to wash hands but requires assistance to wash right side.

Dressing—Lucy requires maximal assistance to dress her upper body. Maximal assistance is required to dress LEs and don socks and shoes.

Bathing—Lucy requires maximal assistance for all bathing and washing hair.

Toileting—Maximal assistance is required for clothing management and hygiene

Functional Mobility/Transfers:

Lucy's primary mode of mobility is a manual wheelchair. She has a Roho® cushion in her chair to prevent skin breakdown. She is dependent for propelling and steering of the chair.

Bed mobility requires minimal assistance to reposition in the bed. Maximal assistance is required for supine-to-sit and sit-to-stand transfers. Her dynamic sitting and standing are both poor, requiring maximal assistance to be maintained. She requires maximal assistance to perform a stand–pivot transfer (to toilet, chair, bed, and car). She is able to walk a few steps with use of a hemi-walker and maximal assistance. Her endurance is poor, and she fatigues easily during functional mobility activities.

Process Skills:

Cognition—Scores of the Mini-Mental State Examination did not detect any cognitive deficits. Speech intelligibility is within normal limits, with Lucy being articulate and quick witted. She is appropriate during social interaction, although at times interruptive and tangential. She is able to maintain a steady flow of conversation with no detectable receptive deficits.

Visual screening—Lucy demonstrates decreased visual attention, has left sided hemianopsia, and left neglect is noted with Lucy requiring cues to scan to the left or to bring her left UE into view or in a supported position. She is unable to read without anchors and assistance. Some depth perception issues were noted during a cutting task and during observation during feeding. The Motor-Free Visual Perception Test (MVPT) was administered to gather more information regarding her visual perceptual areas of functioning. She demonstrated significant deficits with this assessment. She had difficulty with form constancy, visual closure, and visual short-term memory. She required continuous cueing to scan to the left during this assessment. She became increasingly frustrated and discontinued this standardized assessment halfway through. It is evident that Lucy has many visual-perceptual deficits, which greatly impact her function and safety.

Psychosocial—Lucy was administered the Becks Depression Scale, and her scores indicated moderate depression. She scored in the "somewhat bad" range on a Global Quality of Life scale. These scores indicate that she is unhappy with her current level of functioning and does not feel as though she has adequate supports.

Insight—Lucy's level of insight into her deficits or functional level is questionable. Although not formally assessed, she makes frequent comments on how she cannot wait to "walk again" to get back to her home and live independently. She mentions that she does not have difficulties in areas where she requires a great deal of assistance.

Leisure:

Lucy's past leisure pursuits included quilting, reading, and gardening. Current leisure interests include socializing at meals, going out to eat, visiting with family, and TV viewing.

Motor Skills:

Active AROM—Right UE is WFL; left UE has no AROM

Passive PROM—Right UE is WFL Left UE—WFL

Joint integrity and tone—Left UE has a noted two-finger glenohumeral subluxation. Lucy's left arm fluctuates between a flexor synergy pattern and an extensor synergy pattern. At rest, her arm is supported on a pillow, and her hand is in a tight fisted position. She wears a soft splint on her hand.

Sensation—Left UE and LE touch sensation is impaired. Lucy reports that she has minimal sensation on her left side and it feels numb.

Coordination—Left UE, unable. Right UE coordination is mildly impaired because of visual-perceptual problems.

Pain—Lucy reports significant pain in her left shoulder and hand and her left hip and knee.

Goals

1. Lucy will increase attendance to her left arm with 80% accuracy during a variety of structured and unstructured activities within 8 weeks.
2. Lucy will attend to stimuli placed within her left visual field during structured activity 80% of the time within 8 weeks.
3. Lucy will increase use of left UE by using it as a gross assist while making a sandwich with no more than two verbal cues within 6 weeks.
4. Lucy will demonstrate three techniques to complete AAROM and self-ROM of left UE, with no cues for safety, within 3 weeks.
5. Lucy will complete bathing following setup and no more than three verbal cues within 8 weeks.

Case Study Questions

1. Lucy has many areas and goals that require attention. How does the OT practitioner prioritize which area to focus on?
2. How does the OT practitioner address/approach her lack of insight into her deficits?
3. Design a treatment plan that will address three of her goals simultaneously.

PUTTING IT ALL TOGETHER Sample Treatment Session and Documentation

Setting	Outpatient rehabilitation, referred from inpatient rehabilitation, where client spent 2 weeks
Client Profile	Mrs. R, 62 y/o, experienced a L CVA 3 weeks ago, resulting in R hemiplegia
Work History	Employed as an administrative assistant in the public school system for 26 years, but is currently on disability leave
Insurance	State Employee Health Insurance, limited to 30 visits for OT/PT combined
Psychological	Depression s/p CVA
Social	Married. Client typically enjoys preparing meals for husband and self. Adult daughter, Carrie, lives nearby and is expecting a baby in a few months—the very first grandchild—and client is hoping to be able to assist Carrie the first few weeks after the baby arrives.
Cognitive	Short-term memory affected
Motor & Manual Muscle Testing (MMT)	Client presents with moderate spasticity and flexor synergy in her RUE. The RUE testing includes: 100 degrees AROM shoulder flexion (PROM 120 degrees) Lacks 10 degrees (or 170 degrees) AROM elbow extension (PROM 180 degrees) 5 degrees AROM wrist extension (PROM 25 degrees) 0 degrees AROM finger extension (PROM normal) AROM LUE WNL MMT RUE: NT due to spasticity MMT LUE: 4+ throughout Ambulates with quad cane
ADL	Mod A bathing, Min A LB dressing, Min A UB dressing
IADL	Max A cooking due to memory loss and limited use of RUE
Goals	Within 4 weeks: 1. Client will be Mod I for bathing and dressing with the use of appropriate AE and techniques. 2. Client will increase AROM by 10 degrees for shoulder and 5 degrees for wrist extension to improve functional ADL & IADL tasks. 3. Client will grasp ADL objects, such as cup or brush, and use functionally at a Min A level. 4. Client will demonstrate adapted techniques for diapering and bottle-feeding a baby with Min A.

OT TREATMENT SESSION 1

THERAPEUTIC ACTIVITY	TIME	GOAL(S) ADDRESSED	OTA RATIONALE
Moist heat applied to R shoulder with passive stretch to increase ROM. Client side-lying on nonaffected side, giving OTA access to R shoulder.	15 min	#2, and indirectly #1, #3, and #4	*Preparatory Method:* PAM (moist heat) can help to decrease spasticity, relaxing the muscles to allow for greater PROM and to increase AROM. Using passive stretch during heating for better outcomes allows practitioner to bill for skilled therapeutic intervention.

PUTTING IT ALL TOGETHER Sample Treatment Session and Documentation (continued)

THERAPEUTIC ACTIVITY	TIME	GOAL(S) ADDRESSED	OTA RATIONALE
Followed by education for client and husband and training in weight-bearing on RUE while seated edge of mat.	3 min	#2	*Preparatory Method; Education and Training:* Weight-bearing temporarily decreases spasticity and assists to normalize tone while providing proprioceptive input. Used directly before AROM to help facilitate voluntary movement of RUE.
Teach shoulder AROM exercises for RUE, in supine and side-lying on mat. Give client HEP handout, make sure client can perform return demonstration. Shoulder flexion, shoulder abduction, protraction/retraction, & elevation.	20 min	#2	*Preparatory Task and Training:* Performed directly after the moist heat, PROM & weight-bearing to carryover controlled AROM and build shoulder strength. Trained in HEP for carryover at home. Will follow up next visit to assess compliance with HEP and check with husband.
Functional NEMS applied to R wrist extensors. Client to grasp a thick plastic cup during "on" phase, then used with hairbrush. Client's RUE supported on an incline wedge, with wrist positioned off the edge to allow for unrestricted ROM.	20 min	#2 and #3	*Preparatory Method:* Using NEMS to deliver electric impulse to stimulate the wrist extensors for muscle reeducation. Performed with functional objects due to evidence-based research best practices.

SOAP note: 7/3/—, 2:00 pm–2:58 pm

S: Client states, "I hope I can still help my daughter when the baby arrives," and "Will I ever get back the use of my R arm?" Husband present for treatment session.

O: Client participated in OP therapy session to address R shoulder & wrist ROM and neuromuscular reeducation. No c/o pain, only stiff RUE. Moist heat applied to client's R shoulder in sidelying while OTA performed passive stretch shoulder flexion to approximately 125 degrees. Weight-bearing on RUE, seated on edge of mat, to decrease spasticity in preparation for AROM & exercises. Client supine & sidelying for RUE AROM & exercises x 10 reps within available range (shoulder flexion, shoulder abduction, protraction/retraction, elevation). Client provided HEP handout of exercises, able to return demo HEP with 1 correction for technique. Functional NEMS to R wrist extensors, client performed grasp/release with thick plastic cup placed midline (NEMS settings:10 pps, 220 mS, 5 sec on, 10 sec off, synchronous), able to grasp cup 11/15 attempts when in visual field.

A: Moist heat & passive stretch were successful to increase PROM R shoulder flexion by 5 degrees. Client NEMS greater than 75% effective for functional grasp/release with wrist extension. Client will benefit from continued NEMS program & support from husband for HEP due to short term memory issues.

P: Next visit, continue to work on PROM/AROM RUE, functional use of RUE, focus on adapted bathing & dressing techniques, & follow up on HEP. Discuss possible NEMS home program with OT.

Jane Brooker, COTA/L, 7/3/—, 5:15 pm

OT TREATMENT SESSION 2

What could you do next with this client?

OT TREATMENT SESSION 3

What could you do next with this client?

REFERENCES

1. Mozaffarian, D., Benjamin, E. J., Go, A. S., Arnett, D. K., Blaha, M. J., Cushman, M., ... & Turner, M. B. (2016). Heart disease and stroke statistics—2016 update: A report from the American Heart Association [published online ahead of print December 16, 2015]. *Circulation, 133*(4), e38–e360. doi:10.1161/CIR.0000000000000350
2. National Stroke Association. (2011). What is TIA? Retrieved from http://www.stroke.org/understand-stroke/what-stroke/what-tia
3. Centers for Disease Control and Prevention. (2015). Stroke facts. Retrieved from http://www.cdc.gov/stroke/facts.htm
4. Abdulhamid, K. (2009). Hypertension and stroke. *International Journal of Cardiology, 137*(Suppl 1), S23. doi:10.1016/j.ijcard.2009.09
5. Wolf, P., D'Agostino, R., Kannel, W., Bonita, R., & Belanger, A. (1988). Cigarette smoking as a risk factor for stroke: The Framingham study. *JAMA, 259*, 1025.
6. Powers, B. J., Danus, S., Grubber, J. M., Olsen, M. K., Oddone, E. Z., & Bosworth, H. B. (2011). The effectiveness of personalized coronary heart disease and stroke risk communication. *The American Heart Journal, 161*(4), 673–680. http://dx.doi.org.ezproxy.ithaca.edu:2048/10.1016/j.ahj.2010.12.021

7. Zhang, Y., Tuomilehto, J., Jousilahti, P., Wang, Y., Antikainen, R., & Hu, G. (2012). Total and high-density lipoprotein cholesterol and stroke risk. *Stroke, 43,* 1768–1774. doi:10.1161/STROKEAHA.111.646778
8. Obesity and Diabetes Week. (2015). New obesity and diabetes findings from University of Kuopio Hospital outlined [Increased visceral adipose tissue as a potential risk factor in patients with embolic stroke of undetermined source (ESUS)]. *Obesity & Diabetes Week* 13. *General OneFile.* Retrieved from: http://go.galegroup.com/ps/i.do?id=GALE%7CA416671461&v=2.1&u=nysl_sc_ithaca&it=r&p=ITOF&sw=w&asid=d4156bcc7511fda2326d3a74aed314e1
9. Banerjee, C., Moon, Y., Paik, M., Rundek, T., Mora-McLaughlin, C., Vieira, J., ... & Elkind, M. (2012). Duration of diabetes and risk of ischemic stroke: The Northern Manhattan study. *Stroke, 43,* 1212–1217. doi:10.1161/STROKEAHA.111.641381
10. Esse, K., Fossati-Bellani, M., Traylor, A., & Martin-Schild, S. (2011). Epidemic of illicit drug use, mechanisms of action/addiction and stroke as a health hazard. *Brain and Behavior, 1,* 44–54. http://dx.doi.org/10.1002/brb3.7
11. Seshadri, S., Beiser, S., Kelly-Hayes, M., Kas, C. S., Au, R., Kannel, W. B., & Wolf, P. A. (2006). The lifetime risk of stroke: Estimates from the Framingham study. *Stroke, 37,* 345–350. http://dx.doi.rg/10.1161/01.STR.0000199613.38911.b2
12. American Stroke Association. (2016). Stroke risk factors. Retrieved from http://www.strokeassociation.org/STROKEORG/AboutStroke/UnderstandingRisk/Understanding-Stroke-Risk_UCM_308539_SubHomePage.jsp
13. Wolf, T., Baum, C., & Connor, L. T. (2009). Changing face of stroke: Implications for occupational therapy practice. *American Journal of Occupational Therapy, 63,* 621–625.
14. Jeffrey, S. (2010). Risk for recurrent stroke, death high in hospitalized stroke patients. *Medscape.* Retrieved from http://www.medscape.com/viewarticle/717586
15. National Stroke Association. (2017). Act FAST. Retrieved from http://www.stroke.org/understand-stroke/recognizing-stroke/act-fast
16. Bartels, M. (2011). Pathophysiology, medical management, and acute rehabilitation of stroke survivors. In G. Gillen (Ed.), *Stroke rehabilitation* (pp. 1–48). St. Louis, MO: Elsevier.
17. Perna, R., & Temple, J. (2015). Rehabilitation outcomes: Ischemic versus hemorrhagic strokes. *Behavioural Neurology,* Epub 2015 Jul 12. http://dx.doi.org/10.1155/2015/891651
18. American Heart Association. (2013). Stroke treatments. Retrieved from http://www.strokeassociation.org/STROKEORG/AboutStroke/Treatment/Stroke-Treatments_UCM_310892_Article.jsp#.WI0CxLGZORs
19. National Heart, Blood, and Lung Institute. (2017). How is a stroke treated? Retrieved from https://www.nhlbi.nih.gov/health/health-topics/topics/stroke/treatment
20. American Heart Association News. (2015). Clot-removing devices provide better outcomes for stroke survivors. Retrieved from http://news.heart.org/clot-removing-devices-provide-better-outcomes-stroke-survivors/
21. Wolf, T., & Nilsen, D. (2015). *Occupational therapy practice guidelines for adults with stroke.* Bethesda, MD: AOTA Press.
22. Saebo. (2017). Important facts about stage 2 of stroke recovery. Retrieved from https://www.saebo.com/important-facts-stage-2-stroke-recovery/
23. Ada, L., Foongchomcheay, A., & Canning, C. G. (2009). Supportive devices for preventing and treating subluxation of the shoulder after stroke. *Cochrane Database Systematic Review, 1,* 1–25.
24. Corballis, M. (2014). Left brain, right brain: Facts and fantasies. *Biology, 12*(1), e1001767. http://dx.doi.org/10.1371%2Fjournal.pbio.1001767
25. Mayo Foundation for Education and Research. (2016). Osteoporosis. Retrieved from http://www.mayoclinic.org/diseases-conditions/osteoporosis/basics/definition/con-20019924
26. National Stroke Association. (2016). Seizures following a stroke. Retrieved from http://www.stroke.org/we-can-help/survivors/stroke-recovery/post-stroke-conditions/physical/seizures-and-epilepsy
27. Dumoulin, C., Korner-Bitensky, N., & Tannenbaum, C. (2007). Urinary incontinence after stroke: Identification, assessment, and intervention by rehabilitation professionals in Canada. *Stroke, 38,* 2745–2751. doi:10.1161/STROKEAHA.107.486035
28. Martino, R., Foley, N., Bhogal, S., Diamant, N., Speechley, M., & Teasell, R. (2005). Dysphagia after stroke: Incidence, diagnosis, and pulmonary complications. *Stroke, 36,* 2756–2763, doi:10.1161/01.STR.0000190056.76543.eb
29. Paolucci, S. (2008). Epidemiology and treatment of post-stroke depression. *Neuropsychiatric Disease and Treatment, 4*(1), 145–154.
30. Åström, M. (1996). Generalized anxiety disorder in stroke patients: A 3-year longitudinal study. *Stroke, 27,* 270–275. doi:10.1161/01.STR.27.2.270
31. Weerdesteyn, V., de Niet, M., van Duijnhoven, H., & Geurts, A. (2008). Falls in individuals with stroke. *The Journal of Rehabilitation Research and Development, 45*(8), 1195–213. doi:10.1682/JRRD.2007.09.0145
32. Fall Prevention Center for Excellence. (2016). Basics of fall prevention. Retrieved from http://stopfalls.org/what-is-fall-prevention/fp-basics/
33. Winstein, C. J., Stein, J., Arena, R., Bates, B., Cherney, L. R., Cramer, S. C., ... & Zorowitz, R. D. (2016). Guidelines for adult stroke rehabilitation and recovery: A guideline for healthcare professionals from the American Heart Association/American Stroke Association. *Stroke, 47*(6), e98–e169.
34. Camicia, M., Wang, H., DiVita, M., Mix, J., & Niewczyk, P. (2016). Length of stay at inpatient rehabilitation facility and stroke patient outcomes. *Rehabilitation Nursing, 41*(2), 78–90.
35. Hammick, M., Freeth, D., Cooperman, J., & Goodsman, D. (2009). *Being interprofessional.* Malden, MA: Polity Press.
36. Markle-Reid, M., Orridge, C., Weir, R., Browne, G., Gafni, A., Lewis, M., ... & Thabane, L. (2011). Interprofessional stroke rehabilitation for stroke survivors using home care. *The Canadian Journal of Neurological Sciences, 38*(2), 317–334.
37. Schriner, M., Thome, J., & Carrier, M. (2014). Rehabilitation of the upper extremity after stroke: Current practice as a guide for curriculum. *The Open Journal of Occupational Therapy, 2,* 1. http://dx.doi.org/10.15453/2168-6408.1056
38. Kielhofner, G. (2009). *Conceptual foundations of occupational therapy practice* (4th ed.). Philadelphia, PA: F. A. Davis Company.
39. Hafsteinsdttir, T. B., Algra, A., Kapelle, L. J., & Gypdonock, M. H. F. (2005). Neurodevelopmental treatment after stroke: A comparative study. *Journal of Neurology and Neurosurgery in Psychiatry, 76,* 788–792. doi:10.1136/jnnp.2004.042267
40. Hiraoka, K. (2001). Rehabilitation effort to improve upper extremity function in post-stroke patients: A meta-analysis. *Journal of Physical Therapy Science, 13,* 5–9.
41. Burton, L., & Brigham, H. (2013). Proprioceptive neuromuscular facilitation: The foundation of functional training. *FMS* screening. Retrieved from http://www.functionalmovement.com/articles/screening/2013-07-04_proprioceptive_neuromuscular_facilitation_the_foundation_of_functional_training
42. Chattergee, S. (2015). Brunnstrom concept. Retrieved from http://www.slideshare.net/Drsubhasishchatterje/brunnstrom
43. Lundy-Ekman, L. (2013). *Neuroscience: Fundamentals for rehabilitation* (4th ed.). St. Louis, MO: Elsevier.
44. Fuchs, E., & Flügge, G. (2014). Adult neuroplasticity: More than 40 years of research. *Neural Plasticity, 2014,* 541870. doi:10.1155/2014/541870DOI: 10.1017/S0317167100011537
45. Corbetta, D., Sirtori, V., Moja, L., & Gatti, R. (2010). Constraint induced movement therapy in stroke patients: Systematic review and meta-analysis. *European Journal of Physical and Rehabilitation Medicine, 46,* 537–544.
46. Schumway-Cook, A., & Woollacott, M. H. (2012). *Motor control: Translating research into clinical practice* (4th ed.). Philadelphia, PA: Lippincott Williams & Wilkins.
47. Birkenmeier, R. (2015). Core concept in motor recovery and rehabilitation after stroke. In T. J. Wolf & G. M. Giles (Eds.), *Stroke: Interventions to support occupational performance* (pp. 119–144). Bethesda, MD: AOTA Press.

48. Giuffrida, C., & Maitra, K. (2011). *Motor learning and motor control: Contemporary approaches.* Philadelphia, PA: AOTA Press.
49. SPS Bulletin. (2016). Using feedback during student practice. Retrieved from http://www.mr-pbet.com/Downloads/SPSB-Feedback.pdf
50. Michelsen, S. M., Dannenbaum, R., & Levin, M. F. (2006). Task-specific training with trunk restraint on arm recovery in stroke: Randomized control trial. *Stroke, 37,* 186–192.
51. Woodbury, M. L., Howland, D. R., McGuirk, T. E., Davis, S. B., Senesac, C. R., Kautz, S., & Richards, L. G. (2009). Effects of trunk restraint combined with intensive task practice on poststroke upper extremity reach and function: A pilot study. *Neurorehabilitation and Neural Repair, 23,* 78–91. http://dx.doi.org/10.1177/15459683083318836
52. Bayona, N. A., Bitensky, J., Salter, K., & Teasell, R. (2005). The role of task-specific training in rehabilitation therapies. *Topics in Stroke Rehabilitation, 12*(3), 58–65.
53. Mathiowetz, V. (2011). Task-oriented approach to stroke rehabilitation. In G. Gillen (Ed.), *Stroke rehabilitation* (pp. 80–99). St. Louis, MO: Elsevier.
54. Azab, M., Al-Jarrah, M., Nazzal, M., Maaah, M., Sammour, M. A., & Jamous, M. (2009). Effectiveness of constraint-induced movement therapy (CIMT) as home-based therapy on Barthel Index in patients with chronic stroke. *Topics in Stroke Rehabilitation, 16*(3), 207–211.
55. Shi, Y. X., Tian, J. H., Yang, K. H., & Zhao, Y. (2011). Modified constraint induced movement therapy versus traditional rehabilitation in patients with upper extremity dysfunction after stroke: A systematic review and meta-analysis. *Archives of Physical Medicine and Rehabilitation, 92,* 972–982. http://dx.diu.org/10.1016/j.apmr.2010.12.036
56. Hayner, K., Gibson, G., & Giles, G. M. (2010). Comparison of constraint induced movement therapy and bilateral treatment of equal intensity in people with chronic upper extremity dysfunction after cerebrovascular accident. *American Journal of Occupational Therapy, 64,* 528–539.
57. Page, S. J., Sisto, S. A., & Levine, P. (2002). Modified constraint-induced movement therapy in chronic stroke. *American Journal of Physical Medicine and Rehabilitation, 81,* 870–875.
58. Wolf, S. L., Winstein, C. J., Miller, J. P., Taub, E., Uswatte, G., Morris, D., ... & Nichols-Larsen, D. (2006). Effect of constraint-induced movement therapy on upper extremity function 3 to 9 months after stroke: The EXCITE randomized clinical trial. *JAMA, 296,* 2095–2104. http://dx.doi.org/10.1001/jama.296.17.2095
59. Whitall, J., Waller, S. M., Sorkin, J. D., Forrester, L. W., Macko, R. F., Hanley, D. F., Goldberg, A., & Luft, A. (2011). Bilateral and unilateral arm training improve motor function through differing neuroplastic mechanisms: A single-blinded randomized controlled trial. *Neurorehabilitation and Neural Repair, 25,* 118–129. http://dx.doi.org/10.1177/1545968310380685
60. Cauraugh, J. H., Lodha, N., Naik, S. K., & Summers, J. J. (2010). Bilateral movement training and stroke motor recovery progress: A structured review and meta-analysis. *Human Movement Science, 29,* 853–870. http://dx.doi.org/10.1016/.j.humov.2009.09.004
61. Chen, J. L., Penhune, V. B., & Zatorre, R. J. (2008). Listening to musical rhythms recruits motor regions of the brain. *Cerebral Cortex, 18,* 2844–2854. doi:10.1093/cercor/bhn042
62. Schaechter, J. (2004). Motor rehabilitation and brain plasticity after hemiparetic stroke. *Progress in Neurobiology, 73,* 61–72. doi:10.1016/j.pneurobio.2004.04.001
63. Gillen, G. (2011). Upper extremity function and management. In G. Gillen (Ed.), *Stroke rehabilitation* (pp. 218–279). St. Louis, MO: Elsevier.
64. Harris, J. E. & Eng, J. J. (2010). Strength training improves upper-limb function in individuals with stroke: A meta-analysis. *Stroke, 41,* 136–140.
65. Ada, K., Dorsch, S., & Canning, C.G. (2006). Strengthening interventions increase strength and improve activity after stroke: A systematic review. *Australian Journal of Physiotherapy, 52,* 241–248. http://dx.doi.org/10.1016/S0004-9514(06)70003-465
66. Hall, M., Levant, S., & DeFrances, C. (2012). Hospitalization for stroke in U.S. hospitals, 1989–2009. NCHS data brief. Retrieved from http://www.cdc.gov/nchs/products/databriefs/db95.htm
67. Thieme, H., Mehrholz, J., Pohl, M., Behes, J., & Dohl, C. (2012). Mirror therapy for improving motor function after stroke. *Cochrane Database of Systematic Reviews, 3,* CD008449. http://dx.doi.org/10.1002/14651858.CD008449.pub2
68. Bondac, S., Booth, J., Budde, G. A., Caruso, K., DeRosa, M., Earl, B., ... & Humphreys, J. (2015). Mirror therapy and task oriented training to improve UE function after stroke: A case series. *Archives of Physical Medicine and Rehabilitation, 96*(10), e113. http://dx.doi.org/10.1016/j.apmr.2015.08.378
69. Nilsen, D. M., & DiRusso, T. (2014). Brief report—Using mirror therapy in the home environment: A case report. *American Journal of Occupational Therapy, 68,* e84–e89. http://dx.doi.org.ezproxy.ithaca.edu:2048/10.5014/ajot.2014.010389
70. Bondac, S., Budde, G., Caruso, K., & Earl, B. (2016). *Combining mirror therapy and occupation-based, task-oriented approach to improve upper extremity function in chronic stroke.* Chicago, IL: AOTA Press.
71. Dettmers, C., Nedelko, V., Hassa, T., Starrost, K., & Schoenfeld, M. A. (2014). "Video therapy": Promoting hand function after stroke by action observation training—A pilot randomized controlled trial. *International Journal of Physical Medicine and Rehabilitation, 2,* 189. doi:10.4172/2329-9096.1000189
72. Nilsen, D. M., Gillen, G., & Gordon, A. M. (2010). Use of mental practice to improve upper-limb recovery after stroke: A systematic review. *American Journal of Occupational Therapy, 64*(5), 695–708.
73. Page, S. J., Dunning, K., Hermann, V., Leonard, A., & Levine, P. (2011). Longer versus shorter mental practice sessions for affected upper extremity movement after stroke: A randomized controlled trial. *Clinical Rehabilitation, 25,* 627–637. http://dx.doi.org/10.1177/0269215510395793
74. Alon, G., Levitt, A. F., & McCarthy, P. A. (2007). Functional electrical stimulation enhancement of upper extremity functional recovery during stroke rehabilitation: A pilot study. *Neurorehabilitation and neural repair, 21,* 207–215. http://dx.doi.org/10.1177/1545968306297871
75. Marconi, B., Filippi, G. M., Koch, G., Giacobbe, V., Pechioli, C., Versace, V., ... & Calagirone, C. (2011). Long-term effects on cortical excitability and motor recovery induced by repeated muscle vibration in chronic stroke patients. *Neurorehabilitation and Neural Repair, 25,* 48–60. http://dx.doi.org/10.1177/1545968310376757
76. Bioness H200. Retrieved from http://www.bioness.com/Products/H200_for_Hand_Paralysis.php
77. Chai, H. M. (2004). The shoulder complex. Retrieved from www.pt.ntu.edu.tw/hmchai/kines04/kinupper/shoulder.htm
78. Swati, M., Teasell, R., & Foley, N. (2013). Evidenced based review of stroke rehabilitation. Retrieved from http://www.ebrsr.com/sites/default/files/chapter11_hemiplegicshoulder_final__16ed.pdf
79. National Stroke Association. (2010). Recovery after stroke: Sleep disturbances. Retrieved from https://www.stroke.org/sites/default/files/resources/NSAFactSheet_SleepDisorders_2014.pdf
80. Dieruf, K., Poole, J. L., Gregory, C., Rodriguez, E. J., & Spizman, C. (2005). Comparative effectiveness of the GivMohr sling in subjects with flaccid upper limbs on subluxation through radiologic analysis. *Archives of Physical Medicine and Rehabilitation, 86,* 2324–2329.
81. Grampurohit, N., Pradhan, S., & Kartin, D. (2015). Efficacy of adhesive taping as an adjunct to physical rehabilitation to influence outcomes post-stroke: A systematic review. *Topics in Stroke Rehabilitation, 22*(1), 72.
82. Katalinic, O. M., Harvey, L. A., Herbert, R. D., Moseley, A. M., Lannin, N. A., & Schurr, K. (2010). Stretch for the treatment and prevention of contractures. *Cochrane Database of Systematic Reviews, 9,* CD007455. http://dx.doi.org/10.1002/14651858.CD007455.pub2
83. Kumar, R., Metter, E. J., Mehta, A. J., & Chew, T. (1990). Shoulder pain in hemiplegia: The role of exercise. *American Journal of Physical Medicine and Rehabilitation, 69*(4), 205–208.
84. Hall, C., & Thein Brody, L. (2005). *Therapeutic exercise: Moving toward function* (2nd ed.). Philadelphia, PA: Lippincott Williams & Wilkins.
85. Singh, S., & Hamdy, S. (2006). Dysphagia in stroke patients. *Postgraduate Medical Journal, 82*(968), 383–391.
86. Meyer, S., Karttunen, A. H., Thijs, V., Feys, H., & Verheyden, G. (2014). How do somatosensory deficits in the arm and hand relate to upper limb impairment, activity, and participation problems after stroke? A systematic review. *Physical Therapy, 94*(9), 1220—1231.

87. Carey, L. (2015). Core concepts in sensory impairment and recovery after stroke. In T. Wolf & G. Giles (Eds.), *Stroke: Interventions to promote occupational performance* (pp. 95–118). Bethesda, MD: AOTA Press.
88. Carey, L., Macdonell, R., & Matyas, T. A. (2011). SENSe: Study of the effectiveness of neurorehabilitation on sensation: A randomized controlled trial. *Neurorehabilitation and Neural Repair, 25*(4), 304–313. doi:10.1177/1545968310397705
89. Sohlberg, M., & Mateer, C. (2001). *Cognitive rehabilitation.* New York, NY: Guilford Press.
90. Gillen, G. (2009). *Cognitive and perceptual rehabilitation: Optimizing function.* St. Louis, MO: Elsevier.
91. Radomski, M. V., Anheluk, M., Bartzen, M. P., & Zola, J. (2016). Effectiveness of interventions to address cognitive impairments and improve occupational performance after traumatic brain injury: A systematic review. *American Journal of Occupational Therapy, 70,* 7003180050. http://dx.doi.org.ezproxy.ithaca.edu:2048/10.5014/ajot.2016.020776
92. Zoltan, B. (2007). *Vision, perception, and cognition: A manual for the evaluation and treatment of the adult with acquired brain injury* (4th ed.). Thorofare, NJ: Slack.
93. Sohlberg, M. M., & Mateer, C. A. (1989). Training use of compensatory memory books: A three stage behavioral approach. *Journal of Clinical Experimental Neuropsychology, 11*(6), 871–891.
94. Pohjasvaara, T., Leskela, M., Vataja, R., Kalska, H., Ylikoski, R., Hietanen, M., ... & Erkinjuntti, T. (2002). Post-stroke depression, executive dysfunction and functional outcome. *European Journal of Neurology, 9*(3), 269–275. doi:10.1046/j.1468-1331.2002.00396.x
95. Poulin, V. (2012). Efficacy of executive function interventions after stroke: A systematic review. *Topics in Stroke Rehabilitation, 19*(2), 158. doi:10.1310/tsr1902-158
96. Jehkonen, M., Laihosalo, M., & Kettunen, J. (2006). Anosognosia after stroke: Assessment, occurrence, subtypes and impact on functional outcome reviewed. *Acta Neurologica Scandinavica, 114*(5), 293–306. doi:10.1111/j.1600-0404.2006.00723.x
97. Prigatano, G. P., Borgaro, S., Baker, J., & Wethe, J. (2005). Awareness and distress after traumatic brain injury: A relative's perspective. *Journal of Head Trauma Rehabilitation, 20*(4), 359–367.
98. Lundqvist, A., Linnros, H., Orlenius, H., & Samuelsson, K. (2010). Improved self-awareness and coping strategies for patients with acquired brain injury—A group therapy programme. *Brain Injury, 24*(6), 823–832. doi:10.3109/02699051003724986
99. Stewart, C., & Riedel, K. (2011). Managing speech and language deficits after stroke. In G. Gillen (Ed.), *Stroke rehabilitation: A function-based approach* (pp. 534–552). St. Louis, MO: Elsevier.
100. National Aphasia Foundation. (2016). Aphasia fact sheet. Retrieved from http://www.aphasia.org/aphasia-resources/aphasia-factsheet/
101. Hillari, K. (2011). The impact of stroke: Are people with aphasia different to those without? *Disability and Rehabilitation, 33*(3), 211–218.
102. Stewart, C. & Riedel, K. (2016). Managing speech and language deficits after stroke. In G. Gillen (Ed.), *Stroke rehabilitation: A function-based approach* (pp. 673–689). St. Louis: Elsevier.
103. Berger, S., & Escher, A. (2016). *Outcome measures for people with aphasia.* Presented at the American Occupational Therapy Association National Conference, Chicago, IL. Chicago, IL: AOTA Press.
104. Gillen, G., & Brockmann-Rubio, K. (2011). Treatment of cognitive-perceptual deficits: A function-based approach. In G. Gillen (Ed.), *Stroke rehabilitation: A function-based approach* (pp. 501–533). St. Louis, MO: Elsevier.
105. Civelek, G. M., Atalay, A., & Turhan, N. (2015). Association of ideomotor apraxia with lesion site, etiology, neglect, and functional independence in patients with first ever stroke. *Topics in Stroke Rehabilitation, 22*(2), 94–101.
106. Geusgens, C. V., Van Heugten, C. M., Cooijmans, J. J., Jolles, J., & Van Den Heuvel, W. A. (2007). Transfer effects of a cognitive strategy training for stroke patients with apraxia. *Journal of Clinical & Experimental Neuropsychology, 29*(8), 831–841. doi:10.1080/13803390601125971
107. van Heugten, C., Dekkar, J., Deelman, B. G., van Dijk, A. J., Stehmann-Saris, J. C., & Kinebanian, A. (1998). Outcome of strategy training in stroke patients with apraxia: A phase II study. *Clinical Rehabilitation, 12*(4), 294–303. http://dx.doi.org.ezproxy.ithaca.edu:2048/10.1191/026921598674468328
108. Gillen, G. (2011). Managing visual and visuospatial impairments to optimize function. In G. Gillen (Ed.), *Stroke rehabilitation: A function-based approach* (pp. 417–437). St. Louis, MO: Elsevier.
109. Funk, J., Finke, K., Reinhart, S., Kardinal, M., Utz, K. S., Rosenthal, A., ... & Kerkhoff, G. (2013). Effects of feedback-based visual line-orientation discrimination training for visuospatial disorders after stroke. *Neurorehabilitation and Neural Repair, 27*(2), 142–152.
110. Jones, S., & Shinton, R. (2006). Improving outcome in stroke patients with visual problems. *Age Ageing, 35*(6), 560–565. doi:10.1093/ageing/afl074
111. Zihl, J. (1995). Visual scanning behavior in patients with homonymous hemianopia. *Neuropsychologia, 33*(3), 287–303. http://dx.doi.org.ezproxy.ithaca.edu:2048/10.1016/0028-3932%2894%2900119-A
112. Teasell, R. (2002). The incidence and consequences of falls in stroke patients during inpatient rehabilitation: Factors associated with high risk. *Archives of Physical Medicine and Rehabilitation, 83*(3), 329–333. doi:10.1053/apmr.2002.29623
113. Cumming, T., Brodtmanna, A., Darby, D., & Bernhardta, J. (2014). The importance of cognition to quality of life after stroke. *Journal of Psychosomatic Research, 77*(5), 374–377. doi:10.1016/j.jpsychores.2014.08.009
114. Lampinin, J., & Tham, K. (2003). Interaction with the physical environment in everyday occupation after stroke: A phenomenological study of persons with visuospatial agnosia. *Scandinavian Journal of Occupational Therapy, 10*(4), 147–156. doi:10.1080/11038120310016580
115. Bowen, A., Mckenna, K., & Tallis, R. (1999). Reasons for variability in the reported rate of occurrence of unilateral spatial neglect after stroke. *Stroke, 30,* 1196–1202. doi:10.1161/01.STR.30.6.1196
116. Bowen, A., & Lincoln, N. B. (2008). Cognitive rehabilitation for special neglect following stroke. *Cochrane Database of Systematic Reviews, 7,* CD003586. http://dx.doe.org/10.1002/14651858.CD003586.pub2
117. Cherney, L. R., Halper, A. S., Kwasnica, C. M., Harvey, R. L., & Zhang, M. (1999). Recovery of functional status after right hemisphere stroke: Relationship with unilateral neglect. *Archives of Physical Medicine and Rehabilitation, 82*(3), 322–328. doi:10.1053/apmr.2001.21511
118. Robertson, I. H., Tegner, R., Tham, K., Lo, A., & Nimmo-Smith, I. (1995). Sustained attention training for unilateral neglect: Theoretical and rehabilitation implications. *Journal of Clinical and Experimental Neuropsychology, 17,* 416–430.
119. Niemeier, J. P. (2002). Visual imagery training for patients with visual perceptual deficits following right hemisphere cerebrovascular accidents: A case study presenting the lighthouse strategy. *Rehabilitation Psychology, 47*(4), 426–437. http://dx.doi.org.ezproxy.ithaca.edu:2048/10.1037/0090-5550.47.4.426
120. Butler, B. C., & Eskes, G. (2014). Effect of limb movements on orienting of attention in right-hemisphere stroke. *Experimental Brain Research. 232*(1), 89–101. doi:10.1007/s00221-013-3722-y
121. Butler, A., & Page, S. (2006). Mental practice with motor imagery: Evidence for motor recovery and cortical reorganization after stroke. *Archives of Physical Medicine and Rehabilitation, 12*(Suppl2), S2–S11. http://dx.doi.org/10.1016/j.apmr.2006.08.326
122. Karnath, H. O., & Boetz, D. (2003). Understanding and treating "pusher syndrome." *Physical Therapy, 83,* 1119–1125.
123. Bassile, C., & Hayes, S. (2011). Gait awareness. In G. Gillen (Ed.), *Stroke rehabilitation: A function-based approach* (pp. 389–416). St. Louis, MO: Elsevier.
124. Muneshwar Babulal, G., & Tabor O'Connor, L. (2015). Core concepts in emotional regulation and psychosocial issues after stroke. In T. Wolf & G. Giles (Eds.), *Stroke: Interventions to support occupational performance* (pp. 187–209). Bethesda, MD: AOTA Press.

125. Hermann, N., Seitz, D., Fischer, H., Saposnik, G., Calzavara, A., Anderson, G., & Rochon, P. (2011). Detection and treatment of post stroke depression: Results from the registry of the Canadian stroke network. *International Journal of Geriatric Psychiatry, 26*(11), 1195–1200. doi:10.1002/gps.2663
126. Falk-Kessler, J. (2011). Psychological aspects of stroke rehabilitation. In G. Gillen (Ed.), *Stroke rehabilitation: A function-based approach* (pp. 49–65). St. Louis, MO: Elsevier.
127. Edmondson, D., Richardson, S., Fausett, J. K., Falzon, L., Howard, V. J., & Kronish, I. M. (2013). Prevalence of PTSD in survivors of stroke and transient ischemic attack: A meta-analytic review. *PLoS ONE, 8*(6), e66435. http://doi.org/10.1371/journal.pone.0066435
128. Choi-Kwon, S., Han, K., Cho, K., Choi, S., Suh, M., Nah, H., & Kim, J. S. (2013). Factors associated with post-stroke anger proneness in ischaemic stroke patients. *European Journal of Neurology, 20*(9), 1305–1310. doi:10.1111/ene.12199
129. Kootker, J. A., Rasquin, S. M. C., Smits, P., Geurts, A. C., van Heugten, C. M., & Fasotti, L. (2015). An augmented cognitive behavioral therapy for treating post-stroke depression: Description of a treatment protocol. *Clinical Rehabilitation, 29*(9), 833–843. http://dx.doi.org.ezproxy.ithaca.edu:2048/10.1177/0269215514559987
130. Hofgren, C., Bjorkdahl, A., Esbjornsson, E., & Stibrant Sunnerhagen, K. (2009). Recovery after stroke: Cognition, ADL-function and return to work. *Journal of the Neurological Sciences, 283*(1-2), 316. doi:10.1016/j.jns.2009.02.287
131. Legg, L., Drummond, A., Leonardi-Bee, J., Gladman, J. R. F., Corr, S., Donkervoort, M., ... & Langhorne, P. (2007). Occupational therapy for patients with problems in personal activities of daily living after stroke: Systematic review of randomized trials. *British Medical Journal, 335*(7626), 922–925. doi:10.1136/bmj.39343.466863.55
132. Pynos, J., Steinman, B., Quyen Do Nguyen, A., & Bressette, M. (2012). Assessing and adapting the home environment to reduce falls and meet the changing capacity of older adults. *Journal of Housing for the Elderly, 26*, 137–155. doi:10.1080/02763893.2012.673382
133. Ryan, P., & Sullivan, J. (2011). Activities of daily living adaptations: Managing the environment with one-handed techniques. In G. Gillen (Ed.), *Stroke rehabilitation: A function-based approach* (pp. 716–734). St. Louis, MO: Elsevier.
134. Fujita, T., Sato, A., Yamamoto, Y., Otsuki, K., Tsuchiya, K., & Tozato, F. (2016). Motor function cutoff values for independent dressing in stroke patients. *American Journal of Occupational Therapy, 70*, 3.
135. Farman, J., & Dicker Friedman, J. (2011). Sexual function and intimacy. In G. Gillen (Ed.), *Stroke rehabilitation: A function-based approach* (pp. 648–664). St. Louis, MO: Elsevier.
136. Kimura, M., Murata, Y., Shimoda, K., & Robinson, R. (2001). Sexual dysfunction following stroke. *Comprehensive Psychiatry. 42*(3), 217–222. doi:10.1053/comp.2001.23141
137. MacRae, N. (2010). Sexuality and aging. In R. H. Robnett & W. C. Chop (Eds.), *Gerontology for the health care professional* (pp. 235–258). Sudbury, MA: Jones and Bartlett.
138. Cheng, P. T., Wu, S. H., Liaw, M. Y., Wong, A. M., & Tang, F. T. (2001). Symmetrical body-weight distribution training in stroke patients and its effect on fall prevention. *Archives of Physical Medicine and Rehabilitation, 82*(12), 1650–1654.
139. Eriksson, G., Aasnes, M., Tistad, M., Guidetti, S., & von Koch, L. (2012). Occupational gaps in everyday life one year after stroke and the association with life satisfaction and impact of stroke. *Topics in Stroke Rehabilitation, 19*(3), 244–255.
140. American Occupational Therapy Association. (2014). Occupational therapy practice framework: Domain and process (3rd ed.). *American Journal of Occupational Therapy, 68*(Suppl.1), S1–S48. http://dx.doi.org/10.501/ajot.2014.682006
141. National Stroke Association. (2016). Sleep after stroke. Retrieved from http://www.stroke.org/we-can-help/survivors/stroke-recovery/post-stroke-conditions/physical/sleep
142. Heidt, S., Scott, J. R., Clore, K., David, C., Johnson, M., Gappy, B., ... & Farrehi, P. (2016). Sleep-enhancing education intervention effect on patient-reported outcomes in hospitalized adults. *American Journal of Occupational Therapy, 70*(4_Supplement_1), 7011510216p1. doi:10.5014/ajot.2016.70S1-PO4122.
143. The National Stroke Association. (2016). Tips to manage sleep problems at home. Retrieved from http://www.stroke.org/we-can-help/survivors/stroke-recovery/post-stroke-conditions/physical/sleep
144. Bondoc, S., & Scott, S. (2016). Supporting return to work for persons with stroke: A survey of occupational therapy practice patterns. *American Journal of Occupational Therapy, 70*(4_Supplement_1), 7011510190p1. doi:10.5014/ajot.2016.70S1-PO1102.
145. Smajlović, D. (2015). Strokes in young adults: Epidemiology and prevention. *Vascular Health and Risk Management, 11*, 157–164.
146. Smajlović, D. Ž., Salihović, D., Ibrahimagić, O.Ć., & Sinanović, O. (2013). Characteristics of stroke in young adults in Tuzla Canton, Bosnia and Herzegovina. *College Anthropology, 37*, 515–519.
147. Putaala, J., Metso, A. J., Metso, T. M., Konkola, N., Kraemer, Y., Haapeniemi, E., ... & Tatlisumak, T. (2009). Analysis of 1008 consecutive patients aged 15 to 49 with first-ever ischemic stroke: The Helsinki Young Stroke Registry. *Stroke, 40*, 1195–1203.
148. Mackey, J. (2014). Evaluation and management of stroke in young adults. *Continuum (Minneapolis, Minnesota), 4*(20), 352–369.
149. National Center for O*NET Development. (2017). O*NET online help: OnLine overview. *O*NET OnLine*. Retrieved from https://www.onetonline.org/help/online/
150. Kamel A. A., Bond A. E., & Sivarajan Froelicher, E. (2012). Depression and caregiver burden experienced by caregivers of Jordanian patients with stroke. *International Journal of Nursing Practice, 18*, 147–154.
151. Kumar, R., Kaur, S., & Redemma, K. (2015). Burden and coping strategies in caregivers of stroke survivors. *Journal of Neurology and Neuroscience, Special Issue*, S1.

ACKNOWLEDGMENTS

The author would like to thank Christa Gallie-Weiss, MS, OTR/L, CAPS, RYT 200, CA, for her shared wisdom and editorial efforts.

Chapter 34

Traumatic and Acquired Brain Injury: Management and Treatment

Heidi A. Van Keulen, OTR/L, CBIS

LEARNING OUTCOMES

After studying this chapter, the student or practitioner will be able to:

34.1 Distinguish between traumatic brain injury and acquired brain injury

34.2 Describe the levels of the Rancho Level of Cognitive Functioning Scale

34.3 Describe occupational therapy interventions for the symptoms associated with the different stages of brain injury

34.4 Explain the role of the occupational therapy practitioner in educating family members and caregivers involved in assisting a client with a brain injury

KEY TERMS

Acquired brain injury (ABI)
Anoxic brain injury
Closed head injury (CHI)
Comorbidity
Confabulate
Diffuse axonal injury (DAI)
Open head injury (OHI)
Traumatic brain injury (TBI)
Vegetative state

Working with individuals who have a brain injury and their families is one of the most challenging and rewarding areas of occupational therapy (OT) practice. Damage to the brain, whether mild or severe, can have a profound impact on an individual's life and on the lives of his or her loved ones. Every aspect of life may be affected, including the individual's physical health, emotional well-being, vocation, relationships, leisure, and the ability to complete daily occupations.

A conflict exists within the brain injury community about the definitions of **traumatic brain injury (TBI)** versus **acquired brain injury (ABI).** TBI is generally defined as an insult to the brain from an external source, and the Brain Injury Network in its definition of ABI includes TBI, cerebrovascular accident (CVA), brain illness/infection, and any other brain injury acquired after birth.[1] Other sites and organizations still separate TBI from ABI and consider ABI to take place on the cellular level throughout the brain and TBI to affect just a specific area following trauma. In 2011, the American Academy of Neurology updated its definition of TBI to say that TBI is a form of ABI. Generally, a TBI has trauma as the cause of the injury but still is an acquired injury. This chapter will separate ABI and TBI simply to give structure to the chapter as traumatic and anoxic/nontraumatic.

A brain injury can be classified at a minimum as mild loss of consciousness and/or confusion and disorientation for a period less than 30 minutes. A mild TBI may also be referred to as a *concussion.* A moderate TBI is characterized by loss of consciousness lasting 30 minutes to 24 hours and may include skull fracture. A severe TBI is associated with loss of consciousness for more than 24 hours and memory loss after the injury for more than 24 hours.[2] Even with mild brain injury, the consequences to a person's life can be dramatic and life changing. The effects of a brain injury can be profound, and a severe injury may leave a client in a permanently unresponsive or **vegetative state** (full absence of awareness and responsiveness).

Considerable data have been reported more for TBI than for ABI, but as of 2014, TBI was the leading cause of death in the United States for persons age 1 to 44 years, and every year, approximately 52,000 deaths occur from TBI. An estimated 2.4 million children and adults in the United States sustain a TBI, and another 795,000 individuals sustain an ABI from nontraumatic causes each year.[3,4] Currently, more than 5.3 million children and adults live with disabilities as a result of a TBI and another 4.7 million from disability caused by CVA.[5]

HEALTHCARE TEAM MEMBERS AND ROLE OF OCCUPATIONAL THERAPY

The members of the multidisciplinary or interdisciplinary team can be extensive, depending on the client's location, whether in the intensive care unit (ICU), acute care, inpatient rehabilitation, outpatient, home health, skilled nursing facility, or home. The team includes doctors, including a neurologist and a physiatrist (rehabilitation doctor), neuropsychologist, nurses, and certified nursing assistants (CNAs) and may include a social worker who will work with the client and family on insurance/disability issues, setting up home care or outpatient service, and counseling. The speech language pathologist (SLP) will generally work on speech, swallowing, and cognitive issues. The respiratory therapist manages respiratory health, including oxygen, ventilator support, cough assist, high-frequency chest wall oscillation (often called a VEST), continuous positive airway pressure or bilevel positive airway pressure machines (CPAP/BiPAP), and breathing. The nutritionist or dietitian assesses the client's caloric intake and output, diet and diet consistencies, and energy consumption. The physical therapist and physical therapist assistant (PTA) addresses balance, mobility, and strength as well as transfers and ambulation. Last, the occupational therapist and occupational therapy assistant (OTA) bring the healthcare team together with a holistic focus on function. The OT practitioner uses the information from the SLP about the client's swallowing test and assists the client with the process of self-feeding and eating and drinking to meet the nutritional needs. The OT practitioner uses mobility information from the physical therapist to determine safe methods for bathing, toileting, and standing to transfer after dressing. In addition, the OT practitioner works in conjunction with the neuropsychologist to address the impact of cognitive, behavioral, and/or emotional challenges for day-to-day function. The OT practitioner may also work with vocational rehabilitation practitioners on skills needed for returning to work in the future. Because the client with a TBI/ABI can have a variety of symptoms, the occupational therapist and OTA will address each one affecting the client's performance of functional tasks. After the occupational therapist completes the client evaluation, the OTA will perform many of the day-to-day treatments and education and training with the client and his or her family.

FROM THE INTENSIVE CARE UNIT TO THE HOME AND COMMUNITY

Generally, clients with severe brain injuries arrive at the emergency department, and after stabilization, many end up in surgery or the ICU, depending on symptoms and severity of injury. Often, many ancillary injuries are involved in addition to the brain injury, including fractures, lung collapse or puncture, burns, and other injuries or comorbidities that the team must attend to. A **comorbidity** is an injury or health condition that occurs in addition to the primary injury and affects the overall plan of care. For example, someone who has a TBI may also have diabetes and/or additional injuries sustained in the accident that caused the TBI. Most clients with a severe brain injury remain in a coma state in the ICU from 1 to 3 weeks while they are medically stabilized (Fig. 34-1). OT begins in the ICU as soon as the client is medically stable for movement; this might include passive range of motion (PROM) and bed mobility and positioning. Family education and training begins early in these areas. The OTA can begin to teach the client's family members in PROM exercises and positioning, both of which are important for preserving joint mobility and preventing contracture when a client is in a coma (Figs. 34-2 and 34-3).

In the case of clients who are medically able to tolerate movement, positions are typically changed from supine to side-lying on both sides on a schedule of every 2 hours to prevent pressure injuries. Different types of specialty beds and/or mattresses may be used to assist with positioning and skin management. Some examples are beds with air mattresses, beds that can bring the client to the standing position, and beds that can turn the client 360 degrees. Whatever the position, particular care is paid to the bony prominences, including heels, ankles, knees, hips, head, and elbows. Special soft orthoses or high-top tennis shoes may be used to prevent foot drop, which occurs when gravity

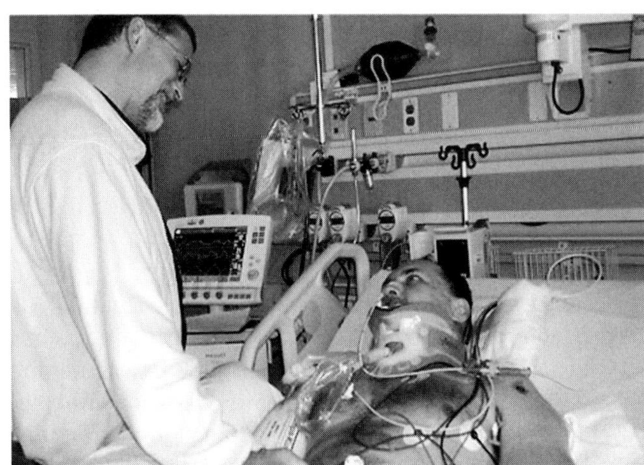

FIGURE 34-1. A client early in recovery from a brain injury, when the focus of care is meeting medical needs.

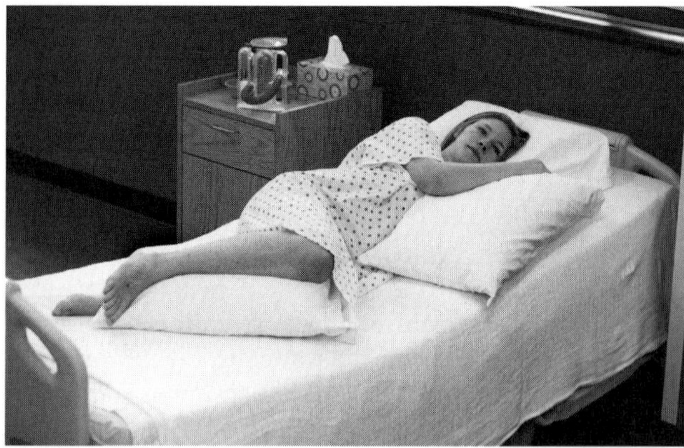

FIGURE 34-2. A client positioned in side-lying position. Pillows are used to provide support and keep pressure away from bony prominences, such as knees and ankles.

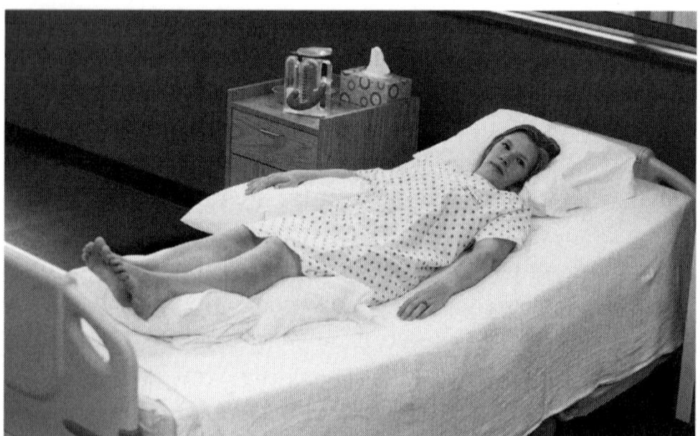

FIGURE 34-3. Placing pillows under the affected arm, knee(s) and ankle(s), helps to prevent pressure for a client positioned supine.

and/or muscle tone pull the foot into plantar flexion (toes pointed). If the ankles become contracted, the client would have difficulty standing and walking later on. Some clients after a brain injury and/or spasticity/immobility develop neurogenic heterotopic ossification, which is a pathological bone formation in the joint(s) (see Chapter 35 for details).

Once stable, many clients transition either to an inpatient rehabilitation center or a skilled nursing facility (subacute rehabilitation) to begin more intensive therapy. The rehabilitation period can be 3 to 6 weeks, and it is here that the client relearns many skills and receives education and training about management of his or her condition. During rehabilitation, the focus of skilled OT intervention is to assist the client to reach maximal levels of independence in all areas of ADLs and potentially other areas of occupation as well. In addition to the services of the physiatrist, other services during this period typically include OT, physical therapy (PT), the services of the SLP, therapeutic recreation, nursing, psychology, and social work. From rehabilitation, the transition can be home or to a skilled nursing facility (SNF), depending on the family's ability to care for the individual. If the client goes home, home care is often set up, and the client receives home health services that may include nursing, OT, PT, SLP and those of the social worker, as needed. If appropriate, transition to an outpatient brain injury program may be possible to continue the client's work toward being fully functional and independent. A client with a brain injury may experience positive changes even years after the injury, and the therapy process is never really completed.

Glasgow Coma Scale and Rancho Level of Cognitive Functioning Scale

The two common scales that are used to track the recovery progress in clients with brain injuries are the Glasgow Coma Scale (GCS) and the Rancho Level of Cognitive Functioning Scale (LCFS). The GCS is a measure that is frequently used early in the recovery process. It measures three parameters—eye movements, verbal responses, and motor responses; overall scores can range from 3 to 15. Lower scores indicate a more severe brain injury[6] (Table 34-1). The LCFS was developed in 1972 at the Rancho Los Amigos Neurorehabilitation Center, revised in November 1974 by Malkmus and Stenderup, and revised again by Hagen, one of its original developers, in 1997 to include 10 levels. However, the original eight-level scale is still often used because more research was done using it. The scale was developed to help plan treatment, track recovery, and classify outcome levels.[7] (Table 34-2). The treatment strategies discussed in this chapter are organized according to the original eight levels of the LCFS, which is most commonly used throughout rehabilitation settings. The levels of the LCFS look straightforward, but in reality, not all clients move smoothly through each level. A client with a brain injury may move from level 2 to level 4 and never show any true level 3 activity. They may go back and forth between levels and seem to reverse for a time, which may result from fatigue, medications, or other factors. A client may reach level 3 and never progress beyond that point. The pace at which a client proceeds through the levels or even if he or she will proceed is difficult to predict. Even if a person reaches level 8, it does not necessarily mean that the individual is exactly as he or she once was because the person may exhibit changes in personality, behavior, or functional abilities. Also, the level the OTA sees in the morning with grooming may be very different from the one the physician sees later in the morning after multiple therapy sessions due to fatigue throughout the day.

Expectations for Recovery

TBI and ABI can cause a variety of symptoms and problems that can range from slight headache to severe damage with brain swelling and coma or a vegetative state. *Coma* is defined as complete loss of arousal, with no sleep–wake cycles present.[9] A *vegetative state* is a "condition of wakeful unconsciousness" with spontaneous eye opening, but no purposeful, behavioral responses to stimulation.[9] The term *persistent vegetative state* refers to a vegetative state that lasts at least 1 month.[9] Recovery from brain injury symptoms can also vary and be difficult to predict. Many clients make

TABLE 34-1 Glasgow Coma Scale[6]

Eye Opening
4—Spontaneous
3—Eye opening to verbal command
2—Eye opening to pain
1—No eye opening
Verbal Response
5-Oriented to person, place, month, and year
4—Confused
3—Inappropriate words
2—Sounds, but words not understandable
1—No verbal response
Motor Response
6-Obeys commands
5—Localizes pain
4—Withdraws to pain
3—Abnormal flexion to pain
2—Abnormal extension to pain
1—No motor response
GCS = Eye + Verbal + Motor

TABLE 34-2 Rancho Level of Cognitive Functioning Scale (LCFS), Also Known as Rancho Los Amigos Scale[8]

Level I—*No response*
Level II—*Generalized response*
Level III—*Localized response*
Level IV—*Confused, agitated response*
Level V—*Confused, inappropriate, non-agitated response*
Level VI—*Confused, appropriate response*
Level VII—*Automatic, appropriate response*
Level VIII—*Purposeful, appropriate response*

an amazing recovery from their time in the ICU through to rehabilitation, going from a comatose state to walking and talking, but most persons with a brain injury require supervision and some assistance when they return home. Some clients are left with significant weakness and residual effects of the brain insult, depending on the area of the brain impacted. Some people remain in a persistent vegetative state for months, years, or the remainder of their lives. Every brain injury is different, and the recovery is impacted by many factors, including overall health, the location(s) of the brain impacted, the mechanism of injury, substance abuse history, age, socioeconomic status, support systems, education level, nutritional status, work history, spiritual beliefs, and smoking.[10] Recovery is inherently unpredictable, making it difficult to determine what level of function a client may achieve. This unpredictability may be a source of frustration for clients and their families. Being a supportive advocate of the client and his or her family is an important role of the OT practitioner throughout the recovery process.

TRAUMATIC BRAIN INJURY

A TBI is defined by an external force impacting the head and therefore the brain inside the skull. Very often, the TBI is caused by a car or motorcycle accident, sports injury, gunshot wound, fall, or getting hit by something, and symptoms can be from a mild concussion to a skull fracture with severe brain injury, swelling, and bleeding. Mild TBI may cause a temporary dysfunction of thinking, balance, memory, and orientation. A more severe TBI can result in brain bruising, torn brain tissues, bleeding within the skull, and other physical damage to the brain that can cause long-term complications or even death.[11]

Types of Injuries and Areas of Injury

Open head injury (OHI) occurs when the skull is penetrated, such as by a bullet, and typically involves focal damage (confined to a small part of the brain). A **closed head injury (CHI)** does not involve penetration of the skull but results in both focal and broad diffuse damage (occurring throughout the brain).[12] Because a CHI may involve swelling, it often presents with primary damage from the injury, followed by secondary damage as the brain swells within the skull. Increased intracranial pressure occurs because there is a limited amount of space within the skull. Think about what happens if a person sprains his ankle while wearing boots. As the ankle swells because of the injury, the swelling increases beyond the limit of the boot, and the person feels the pressure when there is no more room in the boot. The same thing happens if the brain swells from an injury. Often, surgery is required to manage the pressure within the skull, and sometimes a piece of the skull is removed and saved to be replaced after the swelling goes down (Fig. 34-4) These clients will often wear a padded helmet to protect the area when balance is poor and risk of further damage is high. Certainly, the areas of the brain that are injured will influence the ultimate symptoms the client experiences as well as the severity of the injury. When a TBI is the result of a car accident or other external force to one side of the head, a "coup-contra-coup" (front-to-back or side-to-side) effect can occur—that is, bouncing back and forth within the skull injures the area of the brain opposite the initial injury.[2]

Diffuse Axonal Injury

Diffuse axonal injury (DAI) occurs in about half of all severe head traumas, making it one of the most common TBIs.[13] Instead of occurring in a certain focal area, it occurs over a more widespread area and is one of the leading causes of death in people with TBI.[13] It is not caused by a blow or impact to the head, but by the brain moving with acceleration and deceleration as well as compression and stretching inside the skull, often causing injuries to many parts of the brain. The axons, which are parts of the neurons that move messages between the nerve cells, get broken and stretched in many places. This shearing injury, or tissue sliding over tissue, causes damage, resulting in the death of brain cells,

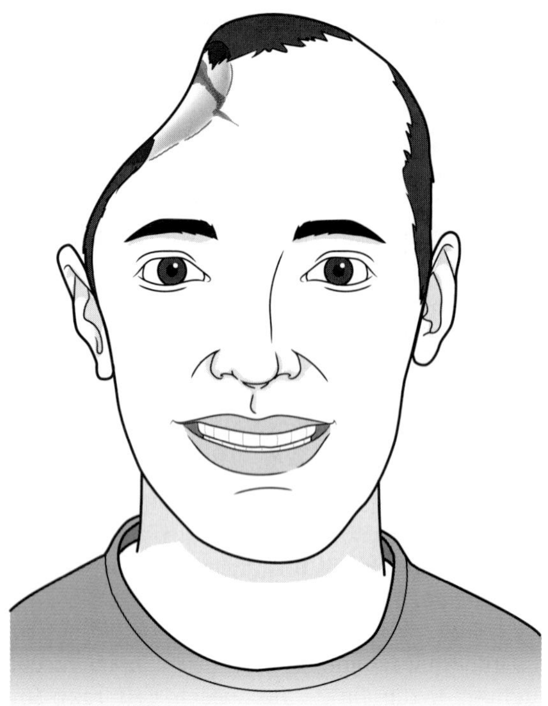

FIGURE 34-4. This client had a piece of bone removed from the skull to accommodate swelling of the brain.

which also causes swelling.[13] Once those nerve cells are disrupted and the links between them are broken, the signal process cannot occur, and such functions as movement, speech, and even those that support life cannot occur.[14]

ACQUIRED BRAIN INJURY

ABI was traditionally not thought to be caused by an impact, but from other causes of brain insult, including lack of oxygen as a result of drowning or choking, drug and alcohol overdose or abuse, and chemical toxicity or abuse. Now the term ABI is more overarching to include TBI. ABI can be caused by a CVA, infection, or brain aneurysm and, by definition, occurs after birth. There can be a multitude of reasons for the insult, but many of the results and symptoms of ABI and CVA, such as memory loss, confusion, balance deficits, and motor difficulties, are similar. The symptoms of any ABI vary, depending on the areas of the brain affected. Progressive and degenerative diseases, such as Alzheimer's disease, and brain injuries present at birth, such as cerebral palsy, are not considered ABIs.[3] See Chapter 33 for comprehensive information on CVA.

Anoxia and Other Nontraumatic Acquired Brain Injuries

Anoxic brain injury can also be called *cerebral hypoxia* or *hypoxic–anoxic injury* and is a serious and life-threatening insult to the brain. After 4 minutes of significantly low oxygen levels, brain cells begin to die, and after 5 minutes, permanent anoxic brain injury can result. The greater the lack of oxygen, the more widespread and serious the injury will be.[13] The lack of oxygen can result from a physical means, such as choking; toxic or metabolic anoxia, which causes the body's oxygen to not be used effectively, such as with side effects of drugs; carbon monoxide poisoning; or anemic anoxia, such as when the lungs cannot process the oxygen efficiently because of chronic obstructive pulmonary disease (COPD) or pneumonia. Tumors can grow and invade spaces of the brain and cause direct damage as well as damage resulting from increased pressure around the tumor. Viruses and bacteria can cause brain damage via encephalopathy or meningitis. Anoxic brain injury can occur in the event of a cardiac arrest and the resulting lack of oxygen. Near-drowning is another cause of anoxic or hypoxic brain injury. In anoxic brain injury, the brain is completely deprived of oxygen, and in hypoxic brain injury, the brain receives insufficient oxygen.

BRAIN ANATOMY

It has to be kept in mind that a brain injury can affect any part or parts of the brain. To review the anatomy of the brain, the left side of the brain controls movement of the right side of the body, as well as mathematical skills, reasoning, writing, and speaking. The right side of the brain controls the left side of the body as well as insight, musical ability, imagination, creativity, and awareness of three dimensions. Each side of the brain is further subdivided into lobes (Fig. 34-5). The parietal lobes control movement, sensation, and sense of space. The cortical motor homunculus is a pictorial representation of the motor cortex and the body parts it controls (see Chapter 8, Fig. 8-3). The frontal lobes control movement, judgment, behavior, executive function skills, personality, and memory. The occipital lobes control and interpret what we see. The temporal lobes are involved in memory, language, and emotional regulation. The cerebellum coordinates balance, timing, and movement. The brainstem connects the spinal cord to the brain and controls automatic functions, such as breathing, blood pressure, and arousal. If the brainstem is even minimally damaged, it can cause coma or a minimally conscious state.[15]

SYMPTOMS AND TREATMENT BY LEVEL

The OT plan of care is always individualized on the basis of the symptoms the client is experiencing, his or her life roles, and the needs of the client and the family. Symptoms of a brain injury vary, depending on the area of the brain affected, the extent of the brain injury, and the mechanism of injury.

Symptoms may include the following:

- Dysphagia (difficulty swallowing)
- Hemiparesis/hemiplegia (one-sided weakness)
- Visual impairment
- Vestibular difficulties, such as with balance, or dizziness
- Sensory impairments (numbness, difficulty with temperature sensation)

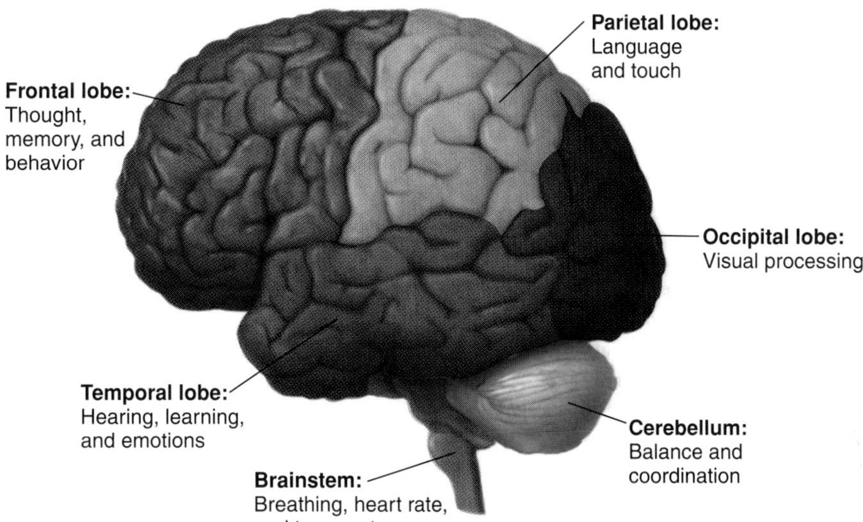

FIGURE 34-5. The location of the lobes of the brain.

- Ataxia (decreased coordination and motor planning)
- Cognitive deficits—memory, judgment, attention, insight, executive functions
- Apraxia (difficulty with skilled movements)
- Aphasia (lack of speech or language processing)
- Decreased level of consciousness
- Motor and muscle weakness
- Personality changes and behavioral disorders
- Perceptual deficits (sense of position in space)[16]

Some symptoms may not be apparent early during the client's recovery process. For example, difficulties with speech, including aphasia, may not be observed in a client who is still on the ventilator or has not yet regained consciousness. It must be kept in mind that if the brain injury is the result of trauma, such as a fall or a car accident, the client may have additional injuries, including fractures or internal injuries.

Rancho Level I—No Response

The client who is classified as being at LCFS level I is not responding to external stimulation and is likely still in the acute care hospital and possibly the ICU. Clients at level I do not open their eyes and do not respond to painful stimuli, such as sternal rubbing or any other stimulation. If the client is medically able to tolerate therapeutic intervention, OT services are focused on positioning and PROM, but the primary focus of the client's care is management of the medical condition. Positioning is crucial to prevent pressure injuries, by minimizing pressure on bony prominences, such as heels, tailbone, elbows, and the base of skull. Positioning is also helpful in minimizing stress to the joints that may be affected by increased or decreased muscle tone by supporting the joints in a safe position in the case of decreased tone or by minimizing increased tone, when possible. In clients with increased tone, the OTA would observe what impact each position has on tone. For example, placing a client in the side-lying position with slight hip flexion may decrease tone in the extensor muscles. If a client's medical condition allows, positions may be changed from supine to side-lying every 2 hours. PROM is important to maintain joint mobility and to prevent contractures. If appropriate, on the basis of the client's medical condition, family members may be instructed and trained on a PROM program. The OT practitioner may fabricate hand orthotics to maintain a functional hand position and monitor the fit as well as the client's ability to tolerate the orthotic.

At this stage, the OT practitioner may administer an assessment, such as the *JFK Coma Recovery Scale-Revised* (CRS-R), which was designed "to assist with differential diagnosis, prognostic assessment, and treatment planning in patients with disorders of consciousness."[16] The CRS-R is an instrument that can be utilized by providers in multiple disciplines, including physicians, SLPs, and OT practitioners, to objectively measure an individual's responses to specific stimuli over time. The CRS-R assesses the client's ability to respond to auditory, visual, and tactile stimulations. The scale also looks at the client's ability to follow commands and communicate. The results of the CRS-R can be used by the OTA to determine what type of stimulation the client is responding to, if any. Clients who are functioning at Level I are dependent for all occupations.

Rancho Level II—Generalized Response

An individual who is functioning at Level II of the LCFS reacts to stimulation inconsistently in a nonspecific, nonpurposeful manner and is considered to be in a vegetative state. The client may not respond to all stimulations, and the responses may not be specific to the stimulus. For example, the client may respond to auditory stimulation with changes in the respiratory rate or depth or heart rate. The person with a brain injury at this level may be in an acute care hospital or inpatient rehabilitation facility. The OT plan of care at this level focuses on positioning; PROM; use of orthotics, as needed; sensory stimulation; and family education. The goal of using orthotics is to preserve a functional hand position, so the OTA may fabricate a resting hand orthosis or an antispasticity orthosis. Colored thermoplastic material or straps can be used to enhance the client's awareness of the affected extremity, and the color may also prevent loss within the sheets when bedding is changed.

Treatment interventions with sensory stimulation focus on providing specific sensory input and observing the client's responses. For example, the OTA might use a penlight or brightly colored object for visual tracking. Pictures of loved ones and familiar objects are useful in eliciting responses and can be an effective way to include the client's valued occupations into treatment. The OTA may use pictures of the client's children, or with a client who plays the drums, the drumsticks may be used to incorporate IADLs and leisure or work. The OTA may also observe how the client responds to movement, such as PROM exercises, rolling, or changes in position. A mechanical lift may be used for vestibular stimulation with clients who are medically stable. When the client is no longer on a ventilator and the tracheostomy has been capped, the OTA may begin using scents, such as peppermint or orange, for stimulation. Lavender is a soothing scent that promotes relaxation and sleep. The OTA should check for allergies, negative associations, or irritants (vinegar, ammonia) before using certain scents. Garlic or mustard are safer noxious odor choices to trial. Clients who have a tracheostomy will not be able to smell because they are not breathing through their noses. Some scents should be non–food-related ones because the client is most likely not eating by mouth. Some examples of non-food scents are eucalyptus, pine, or florals. Scents may be presented one at a time and then client responses observed and documented by the OTA. At this level, responses to stimulation may be delayed, and the OTA may need to wait 10 to 20 seconds before presenting the next scent. The OTA may use familiar toiletry items for bathing or dress the client in his or her own clothing that has been washed with the familiar laundry detergent. A washcloth with a scent on it may be left within 12 inches of the client's nose to allow for a delayed response but should be removed after a period (15–30 minutes) to prevent overstimulation.

Management of the level of environmental stimulation is an important topic in family education and training. The OTA may educate family members in communicating in simple terms with the client. For example, directions and verbal cues should comprise one or two words. Pictures paired with a single word written on a piece of paper, such as "sit." Education on quiet time for the client to rest is also important. Some of the stimulation is unavoidable, such as the noise of a ventilator, alarms on medical monitoring devices, and bright overhead lighting needed to allow nurses and physicians to provide necessary medical care. Lighting is also important in providing environmental cues for time of day. For example, opening the blinds during the day to allow natural light into the room signals daytime and turning off the lights at night provides the cue to go to sleep. Family members can be educated in minimizing conversation in the client's presence, particularly on topics that might be upsetting. Conversation around the client may be overstimulating, but it can also lead to paranoia if the client is understanding only some of what is being said. Whispering around the client can add to the client's paranoia. Encounters with the client should always begin with a simple introduction, such as "Hi, John. I'm Heidi from occupational therapy," and the OTA can educate family members on beginning their visits in a similar fashion. Closure is also important, and family members should be taught to tell the client, "I'm going to get lunch, but I'll be back tonight."

Additionally, if the individual is medically able to tolerate it, the OTA may begin working on head control and balance while sitting at the edge of the bed or sitting up in the wheelchair. With sitting at the edge of the bed, the OTA would provide assistance for balance and facilitate reaching for familiar items. With transfers or sitting without support at this level, the OTA would likely need assistance from a rehabilitation aide or technician for safety because the client may not be able to provide assistance. In some cases, the use of a patient lifter may be the safest method for transfers. At this level, co-treatments with the physical therapist may be provided. For example, the physical therapist may assist the client to sit at the edge of the bed while the OTA works on grooming tasks or helps with donning of the shirt. Even though the client who is functioning at a Level II of the LCFS is not yet following commands, the OTA should communicate in simple terms with the client. For example, before repositioning the client in sitting at the edge of the bed, the OTA should tell the client what is being done using simple phrases, such as "I'm going to help you sit up now."

Rancho Level III—Localized Response

Level III of the LCFS is characterized by localized responses. The client responds in a specific manner to stimuli, but responses may be delayed and inconsistent. The client may be in an acute care hospital or may have transitioned to an inpatient rehabilitation facility. At this point, the client is considered to be in a minimally conscious state and OT is focused on sensory stimulation and family education. Documentation of the client's responses is important for showing progress over time, such as number of times per trials that the client visually tracked or followed a command (visual tracking 2/4 trials 30 degrees past midline to both sides). Some clients at this level have increased tone (hypertonicity or spasticity), and OT will include positioning and possibly orthoses for management of increased tone. For example, the client's position may impact muscle tone, whether from contact between body parts and the surface of the bed, or gravity acting on feet/ankles encouraging plantar flexion. Side-lying with slight hip flexion may decrease extensor tone, potentially preventing some foot drop. The OT practitioner, PT practitioner, or physician may perform the Modified Ashworth Scale, which assesses hypertonicity in various muscles on a zero to four point scale.[17] See Table 8-7 for further details.

Range of motion (ROM) is important for the prevention of contractures, and family members can be educated to carry out PROM exercises on a daily basis (Fig. 34-6). The OTA may begin active assistive range of motion (AAROM) in an attempt to have the client try to assist with moving while the OTA primarily moves the limb. Management of the environment

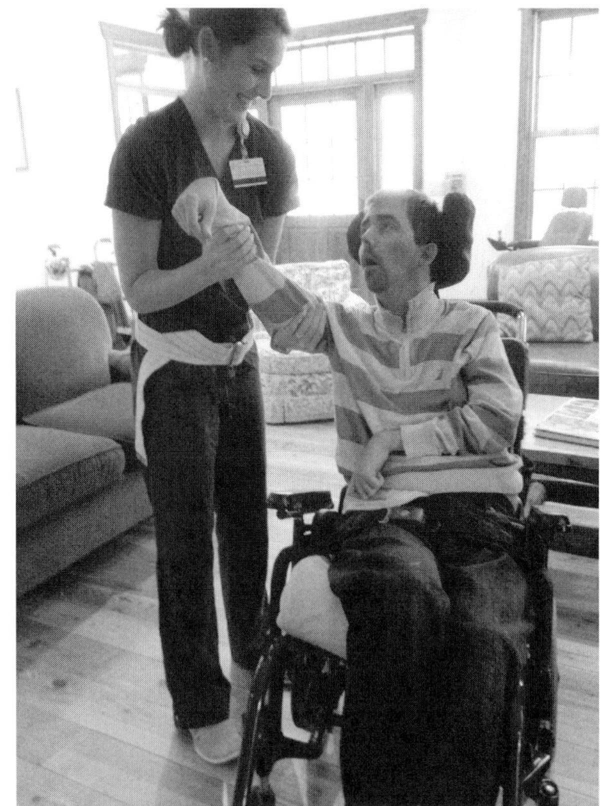

FIGURE 34-6. The client and the OTA are working on active assisted range of motion (AAROM).

is crucial because the client is not able to process multiple sensory inputs simultaneously. Because the client has difficulty with attention and processing sensory input, it is difficult for them to determine what to attend to and what to ignore. For example, if a sock is wrinkled within someone's shoe and causing that person discomfort while he or she is driving, that person will ignore it because driving requires the attention. An individual who is functioning at this Rancho Level is unable to separate relevant details from irrelevant, and may fixate on or react out of proportion to ones within the environment.

SENSORY STIMULATION—OLFACTORY

The olfactory cortex, as well as the amygdala and hippocampus, is part of the limbic system, which regulates emotion. Because of the connection between the olfactory cortex and the hippocampus, memories associated with smells typically have a strong emotional component.[18] Olfactory stimulation can be used to facilitate increased level of arousal. One way is to use familiar toiletry items, such as soap, for grooming/hygiene tasks and the client's own clothing laundered with familiar detergents, keeping in mind that clients with a tracheostomy will not be able to smell unless the tracheostomy is capped. The OTA may observe how a client responds to both pleasant and noxious scents. Different scents are better presented one at a time and may include spices, floral or botanical scents, or food scents. Using familiar scents, such as the client's usual aftershave, is a way to incorporate ADL occupations into the intervention.

SENSORY STIMULATION—GUSTATORY

Clients who are currently functioning at a Rancho Level III may not yet be eating by mouth because of swallowing dysfunction, cognitive deficits, and/or a tracheostomy. Gustatory stimulation can be performed by using a lemon swab, but the client's swallowing abilities should be discussed ahead of time with the SLP or the physician. Temperature can be incorporated by using lemon swabs stored in the freezer. The cold in addition to the lemon flavor will increase awareness of the stimulation and overall alertness. "Toothettes," which are disposable mouth swabs made of spongy material, come in different flavors, such as mint, and may also be used for gustatory stimulation. The OT practitioner must be aware that some clients may reflexively bite down on the toothette, so it must be kept outside of the teeth if possible. The OTA may educate the family to assist the client with oral care, incorporating gustatory stimulation by using mouthwash on a toothette or toothbrush with a minty flavor. A suction toothbrush can be used to prevent aspiration during oral care by pulling the excess liquid and saliva out of the mouth. The sense of taste is dependent on the olfactory sense, and clients who are unable to smell have a diminished sense of taste.[18]

SENSORY STIMULATION—AUDITORY

Excess noise in the environment can be distracting and should be minimized as much as possible. When several people are present, only one person should speak at a time. The OT practitioner should keep directions simple and clear and allow the client time, as long as 15 seconds, to respond. Family members and other staff may need education and training about minimizing auditory distractions, keeping directions simple, and allowing the client enough time to respond. Familiar music, including current favorite tunes, old favorites, and singing, can be used for stimulation in an otherwise low-stimulation environment. With excessive stimulation, the client may "shut down" and stop responding to stimulation. Using familiar music is another way to incorporate occupation into intervention at this level.

SENSORY STIMULATION—VISUAL

Keeping the environment free of clutter and other visual distractions is beneficial to facilitate attention. Overhead fluorescent lighting may be overstimulating, and it is helpful for therapy sessions to take place in a room where lighting can be modulated. Photographs of family members, friends, and pets are useful during therapy but should be displayed in such a way that they can be removed from view when the individual is resting. Depending on the location of the brain injury, the client may demonstrate less attention to one side, so stimuli should be presented on both sides. The OT practitioner should educate family members to encourage the client to look to both sides.

The client may be experiencing vision difficulties, such as difficulty processing visual input, *diplopia* (double vision), difficulty visually focusing, or *homonymous hemianopsia*, which is a visual field cut or loss of vision on one side (see

Chapter 10 for in-depth vision information). A group of symptoms known as posttrauma vision syndrome (PTVS) may occur after a brain injury and may include occasional blurriness (words on a page seen as running together) and stationary objects appearing to move. Clients may also have difficulties with balance and spatial orientation, especially in crowded environments.

SENSORY STIMULATION—VESTIBULAR

The vestibular system is responsible for maintenance of equilibrium and balance and has a role in coordinating head and eye movements. Because of the relationship between the reticular activating system and the vestibular system, changes in the client's position may affect his or her level of alertness. Clients often are more alert when upright in the sitting position rather than in the reclined or supine position.[18] The client's medical condition should be considered at all times and vital signs monitored closely during vestibular stimulation. *Orthostatic hypotension* refers to drop in blood pressure related to a change in position from supine to sitting or sitting to standing, and it may occur in individuals who have been not been standing or walking for some time. Orthostatic hypotension causes dizziness and possibly loss of consciousness, if severe. If a client is experiencing orthostatic hypotension, positioning in the sitting or supine position, with the lower extremities (LEs) elevated, can help alleviate symptoms. Slow transitioning from supine to sitting is achieved by raising the head of the bed first, allowing the client time to adjust to the new position before raising the head of the bed higher, and then ultimately getting the client into the sitting position. The physician may also order compression stockings and/or wrapping the LEs with elastic bandages to assist with circulation of blood back to the heart. The physical therapist may be addressing the client's tolerance for upright positioning by using a tilt table, which is a piece of equipment that provides full-body support and moves the client from supine to standing upright gradually. Clients may experience dizziness or vertigo because of disturbances in the vestibular system related to the TBI. Vestibular treatment is a specialized intervention that advanced practitioners use for clients with disturbances to the vestibular system.

Rancho Level IV—Confused, Agitated Response

When a client is functioning at Rancho Level IV, his or her behavior may be bizarre and inappropriate, with poor attention and short-term memory. The client may demonstrate impulsivity, balance deficits, poor safety awareness, and agitation; he or she may be in an inpatient rehabilitation facility unless the medical condition requires a higher level of care. The client is also likely exhibiting poor insight into the deficits resulting from the brain injury. Managing the amount of sensory stimulation continues to be important, as the client may be easily overstimulated, and this may lead to agitation and lack of participation and/or cooperation with therapeutic intervention.

OT Practitioner's Viewpoint

In the multiple years that I have been treating clients with brain injuries in an inpatient rehabilitation setting, I have found that compassion and therapeutic use of self are the tools that I use the most and that have the greatest impact on my clients in treatment sessions. Many individuals with ABI are confused or have aphasia. Cognitive and language deficits make everyday interactions very difficult and possibly even disturbing or frightening for the client, and that can result in agitation or difficult behavior. In my experience, some of the behavior that a client may exhibit makes sense when you consider that the client does not consistently recall his or her location or situation. The medical care that is required can be frightening, and the client's responses often "make sense" if you try to put yourself in his or her shoes. In my opinion, it is especially important to not take client's behavior personally and to remember that as difficult as it may be to provide the care that the client needs, it is far more difficult to be confused and vulnerable. I have found that if I keep in mind that every client is loved by someone and treat each one the way that I would want my family to be treated, I am able to be kind and compassionate in the face of difficult client behaviors. I have also observed that when I engage therapeutic use of self by modulating the volume of my voice and my facial expression with individuals who are agitated, my therapy sessions are more successful. The reverse is also true—if I am struggling to be patient and positive, my clients sense it and my sessions do not go as well as they should. One strategy that is helpful is to model deep breathing and/or sighing with clients who may be anxious or agitated. I have found that taking that pause also helps me calm myself and put the treatment session back on track. ~ Heidi A. Van Keulen, OTR/L, CBIS

Clients who are mobile and are functioning at Level III or IV on the LCFS may require restraints because of their poor safety awareness. Restraints may include the use of wrist restraints or mitts that restrict movement to prevent the client from pulling out intravenous lines, feeding tubes, or tracheostomy/ventilator tubing. Placing all four bed rails up is considered a restraint because it restricts a client's ability to get out of bed. As clients become more mobile and impulsive, a netbed or veil bed may be used to prevent them from falling because some clients will climb up and over the rails (Fig. 34-7). Some facilities place the mattress on the floor and/or provide one-on-one supervision 24 hours a day for clients who are at risk of falling. When clients are out of bed in wheelchairs, restraints, such as a utility belt that prevents the client from getting out of the wheelchair without assistance, may be used (Fig. 34-8). The need for restraints must have a physician's order and must be documented on a daily basis. Restraints are utilized only as long as they are necessary for client safety.

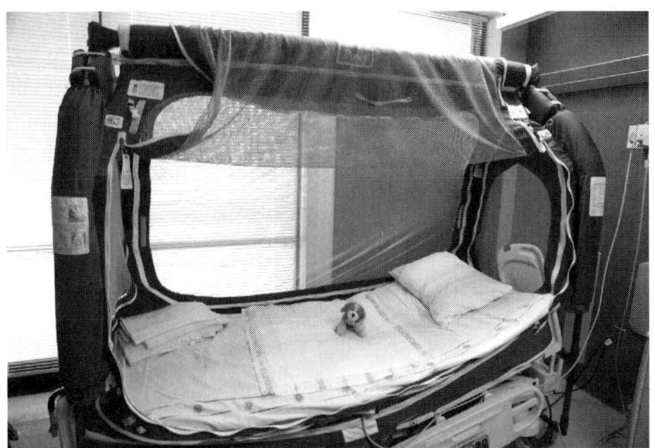

FIGURE 34-7. A netbed is a restraint used to prevent a client who is able to move but is confused. The client may try to get out of bed putting him or her at risk for falls. The netting zips and unzips from the outside.

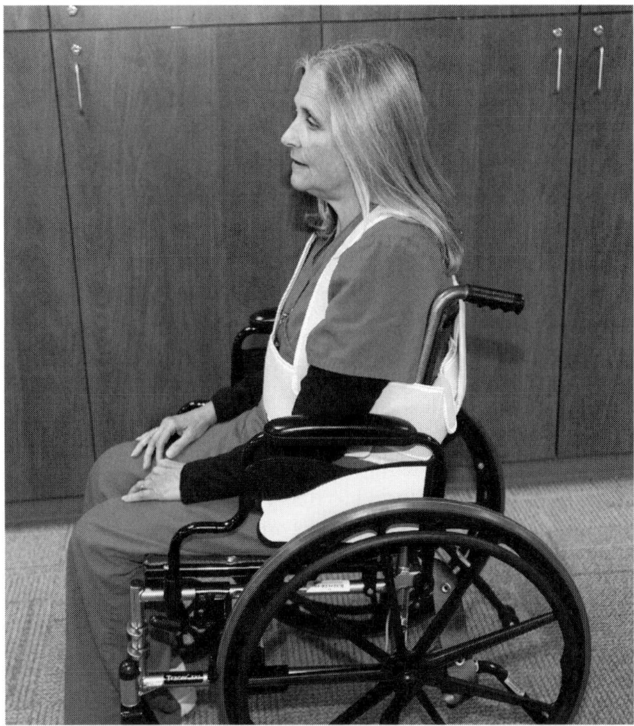

FIGURE 34-8. The utility belt is a restraint used to prevent falls in a client who is impulsive and has poor balance.

The OT plan of care is focused on attention, safety awareness, behavior management, and ADLs/IADLs. Familiar occupations are included in a safe manner. For example, for a client who works in food service or enjoys cooking for family, simple food preparation tasks may be included in a way that ensures safety, such as making instant pudding. Therapy sessions should take place in a low stimulation environment, and the OTA should keep instructions simple. Therapeutic use of self is crucial, as the demeanor and tone of voice used by the OT practitioner can affect the client's behavior. For example, if the OTA is using a confrontational tone of voice in correcting or providing feedback to a client who is confused, the client at Level IV will likely become frustrated and agitated. However, if the client is becoming increasingly frustrated, and the OTA responds in a quiet, soothing tone of voice, the client may calm down or at least not escalate further. Many facilities require specific training of their staff in the management of agitation and violent behavior, such as Crisis Prevention Institute's *Nonviolent Crisis Intervention®*, which emphasizes early use of nonphysical techniques for preventing and managing disruptive behavior as well as appropriate use of physical intervention to manage aggressive behavior in the least restrictive, safest manner.[19] Education of family members continues to be important during this stage, as many people struggle with the uncharacteristic and often inappropriate behavior of their loved one. The OT practitioner is in a position to model behavior management techniques and appropriate levels of stimulation for family members. It is also important that the OTA look for signs of increasing agitation in clients at this level. For example, if a client is showing increased motor restlessness, vocal outbursts, or frustration, a change in activity or a break from stimulation might be necessary. The OTA must also avoid taking the client's behavior personally, even though the client may be insulting because of a lack of social awareness. Responding to the client who is confused, agitated, and or inappropriate can be a challenge for the new practitioner. Use clinical judgment for deciding when to go along, redirect, reorient, confront, or ignore incorrect client behaviors and reactions. For example, a client who is in a netbed says, "Let me out of jail!" repeatedly. The OTA might have to decide which of their own actions would facilitate a calmer demeanor in the client. Another example is the client who keeps asking for his or her mother (who died in the same car accident). The OTA could remind the client his or her mother is deceased, could distract the client to another topic or activity, or could ignore the client and keep talking. Each of these actions may have a different response (crying, agitation/anger). The OTA should discuss cases or clients with the supervising occupational therapist, nursing staff, or other teammates for management advice.

The OT plan of care also continues to address balance, motor control, fine motor coordination, safety awareness, functional mobility, and cognitive skills needed for completing ADLs/IADLs, in addition to attention, safety awareness, and behavior. Therapy sessions should include activities that are functional as well as meaningful to the client. The OTA should discuss the client's hobbies, interests, and responsibilities with the family. ADLs/IADLs can be used as treatment activities. Standing balance can be worked on while standing at the sink for brushing teeth or combing hair. Sitting balance can be addressed by having the client sit edge of bed with feet supported to don a shirt. Using the client's own toiletries and completing tasks in context is helpful for individuals who are confused. For example, working on dressing in the morning following bathing is more meaningful for learning than working on components of dressing in the therapy gym in the afternoon because the activity is occurring in its natural environment and within the client's typical routine. Balance can also be addressed by having the client reach for items in the kitchen cabinets, clean a mirror, or make a bed.

Motor control and fine motor skills can be addressed with games, crafts, and technology depending on client interests. Playing checkers or dominoes challenges reaching, grasp/release, and coordination as well as problem-solving and attention. Putting together a small wooden birdhouse addresses problem-solving, sequencing, strength, attention, and fine motor coordination.

For many clients who are functioning at a Level IV of the LCFS, cognitive impairments may be limiting function more than any other deficit (see Chapter 11 for details on cognition). Sometimes, simply following one-step directions and participating in a functional task, such as face washing, may be an accomplishment for a treatment session. Attention can be addressed with a simple, familiar task, such as folding or sorting laundry, if that is a meaningful IADL for the client. OT sessions may also include orientation activities with the use of a calendar or memory activities, such as having the client identify loved ones in pictures. Working in a quiet, low-stimulation environment facilitates attention better than a busy environment. Decreasing the visual clutter by removing unneeded items from view and increasing contrast is also helpful. For example, if the OTA is working on visual scanning by having the client locate specific playing cards on the table, placing the cards on a dark surface facilitates attention better than a light-colored surface because the background of the cards is white. A client at this level may be able to identify common objects, such as coins or keys, verbally or by pointing. All tasks must be carefully graded to avoid frustration and subsequent agitation.

Because clients functioning at Level IV of the LCFS may have poor awareness of their deficits, they may not be motivated to participate in therapy sessions, and that presents a challenge for the OTA. Flexibility and creativity are key because the client may not be willing to participate in the interventions that were planned but may participate in some other activities. In that case, it is up to the OTA to find a way to make the activities therapeutic. For example, if a client refuses to go to the therapy gym to work on cognitive skills, the OTA could offer to take a walk with the client. While walking around the facility, the OTA could ask the client to locate specific items, such as exit signs, restrooms, specific numbers, or the elevator, to work on attention and visual scanning.

A structured schedule that includes quiet time for rest without stimulation is helpful to people who are confused. In the inpatient rehabilitation setting, a client might begin the day by completing a shower and getting dressed with the OTA, followed by breakfast with the SLP to work on swallowing. After a 30- to 60-minute break, the client might work on ambulation with PT. The rest of the day would typically include more therapy as well as time for rest breaks between sessions.

When the mechanism of injury is an accident or fall, the client may have multiple injuries including fractures. Depending on how much time has passed since the injury and the severity of the fracture, the client may have a cast or air-splint and be restricted from putting weight on the extremity to allow the bone to heal. For clients who are functioning at Levels IV, V, or VI, confusion and memory difficulties may affect their ability to comply with weight-bearing precautions, affecting clinical decision making related to techniques utilized for transfers and ADLs. For example, a transfer board may be the safest transfer technique to prevent the client from weight-bearing on an LE with a fracture, even though the individual is physically capable of performing a stand–pivot transfer on one leg. This is especially true if the client is not capable of recalling the weight-bearing precautions in the course of the transfer. Consultation with the physical therapist or the PTA is important for the OTA to carry over transfer techniques as well as the use of appropriate ambulatory devices for mobility, such as a walker, wheelchair, or cane. The OTA should provide education and training to the family on toilet and shower transfer techniques specific to the client and communicate with nursing staff for carryover of techniques.

Rancho Level V—Confused, Inappropriate, Non-agitated Response

Level V is characterized by confusion and inappropriate responses, but the individual is no longer as agitated. Memory and attention continue to be impaired, and the client is not able to retain new information. Poor insight may still to be an issue because the client may not recognize his or her own limitations or may not have the ability to complete tasks safely. At this point, the client may still be in an inpatient rehabilitation facility or subacute rehabilitation facility or may have transitioned to his or her home with 24-hour supervision and home health or outpatient OT services. The cognitive, sensorimotor, and behavioral issues related to brain injury can impact how the individual functions in society for the rest of his or her life.[20] The OT plan of care addresses cognition, functional mobility, social awareness, motor control, balance, ADLs/IADLs, and fine motor coordination, incorporating occupations that are meaningful to the client. The OTA should begin treatment sessions by introducing himself or herself and orienting the client to the date and purpose of the session. For example, the OTA might say, "My name is Anna, and I'm with occupational therapy. Today is Monday, March 25, 2018. We are going to work on dressing." To address balance, the OTA may work with the client seated on a mat and engaged in reaching for clothing to place in a laundry basket. Standing balance can be addressed by performing standing activities in the kitchen (reaching for items in cabinets or washing dishes at the sink) or playing a simple game in standing at a table. Cognition can be addressed by performing functional tasks, such as counting change, making a sandwich, creating a grocery list, or writing appointments on a calendar. Kitchen activities are a good way to address

COMMUNICATION

Communicating with the client who has a brain injury can be challenging, especially if the client has slow processing, motor planning deficits, or receptive aphasia. The OTA should provide directions and verbal cues in clear, simple language and give the client time to respond. If a client does not respond right away, it is very tempting to repeat or rephrase the direction. Unfortunately, if the OTA provides verbal cues and repeats or rephrases while the client is still processing the direction initially given, then the OTA may actually make things more difficult by overstimulating the client.

Collaboration with the SLP is crucial for determining communication strategies that enable the client to be successful. Knowing a client's cognitive strengths and challenges, as well as his or her communication issues, will assist the OTA in providing effective treatment. For example, a client who has dysarthria, motor planning issues related to speaking, or expressive aphasia will have difficulty communicating his or her wants and needs, but the understanding of directions may not be affected. The approach to communication will be different in this case from the approach for a client who has receptive aphasia or severe cognitive deficits. A client with severe cognitive deficits benefits from simple phrases and additional time for processing. A client who has receptive aphasia benefits from simple phrases and gestures or possibly a picture communication board. A client who has dysarthria and motor difficulties with producing speech does not have difficulty with understanding what the OTA is communicating to him or her and may become frustrated or even insulted if the OTA is speaking in simple phrases but may benefit from a communication board. A client who has expressive aphasia has an issue with producing the language to communicate and is not able to write to communicate either. Clients who have expressive aphasia may repeat phrases in response to questions or may be able to sing.

problem-solving, attention, sequencing, and safety awareness, such as while making a cup of coffee. The client must work on the multiple steps of making coffee, kitchen safety, and problem-solving when there is no sugar for the coffee.

ADLs are often a staple of treatment sessions because they can be used in a variety of ways and because of their importance in overall independence. An ADL session may address carryover of adaptive techniques, such as using a sock aid to don socks or one-handed dressing techniques for donning a shirt. The OTA may work on balance by having the client brush hair, or perform oral care standing at the sink. Sequencing can be addressed by having the client place in order pictures of the steps in getting dressed. Problem-solving can be addressed by having the client choose clothing, with the OTA providing verbal cues, as needed, for matching colors, or choosing clothing appropriate for the weather and the situation.

IADLs should be discussed with the client and the family to determine what activities are meaningful to the client. If the client enjoys cooking, then the OTA could include working on a simple recipe to address sequencing, problem-solving, memory, and safety awareness. Does the client remember each step, or does he or she have to refer to the recipe multiple times for each step? Does the individual remember to turn the stove off or use an oven mitt to handle hot items? If the client is hoping to return to driving in the future, the OTA could address cognition and balance by having the client use a map of a building to locate specific areas, such as the cafeteria, elevators, restrooms, or a given room number. For clients who enjoy gardening, the OTA may incorporate planting a container garden to work on upper extremity (UE) strength or balance if working while standing.

Because the client is not able to retain new information consistently, therapy activities should include familiar tasks that are meaningful to the client and are functional as well. Throughout the rehabilitation process, involvement of the family is important because it gives them the opportunity to provide care and increases their comfort level before the client is discharged home.

At this level, the person with a brain injury continues to be confused and have difficulty with memory. OT sessions may include orientation activities using calendars, clocks, and other environmental cues. In all rehabilitation settings, a written daily schedule may be used to assist with orientation. Attention is typically impaired at this level, and this affects the client's ability to complete even basic tasks. Treatment sessions in a quiet environment helps with attention, and so does reducing visual clutter. For example, a client in inpatient rehabilitation will receive his or her dinner on a tray with a drink, dessert, utensils, and condiments. Placing only the plate on the table with the utensils facilitates attention to the plate, feeding, and eating. Providing instructions in simple language, one step at a time, and allowing the client enough time to respond before providing additional verbal cues is helpful. Documentation of activities in which the client maintains sustained and focused attention is important, along with the amount of time he or she was able to engage to show progress.

Rancho Level VI—Confused, Appropriate Response

The client who is functioning at Level VI of the LCFS continues to demonstrate difficulties with recent memory but is able to use external cues for direction. For example, the client may not be oriented to the date but may be able to determine that he or she can look to the calendar for a cue. Responses are typically appropriate in the context of the situation. The client may demonstrate emerging insight into his or her deficits, but it is likely inconsistent. Clients at this level may **confabulate,** or describe events that did not happen but which they believe did happen. For example, the individual may relate a story about going to the store the previous evening, even though he or she is still in the inpatient rehabilitation facility. Twenty-four-hour supervision is likely still required because of memory

THE OLDER ADULT

Adults over 75 years of age have the highest rates of TBI hospitalizations and are more likely to die of their injuries.[5] The leading cause of TBI in older adults is falls.[5] Treatment of the older adult with TBI may be complicated by comorbidities, making it important for the OTA to be aware of the client's history and prior level of functioning. For example, some older adults may have decreased ROM related to osteoarthritis. Even older adults who are living alone may have assistance from family members for managing finances or medication management. Preexisting conditions, such as dementia or Parkinson's disease, may put the client at risk for a fall that could lead to a brain injury. The older adult may have age-related hearing loss or vision issues that increase their risk of falls. As with any client, occupational history is important for working with the older adult. Compensatory strategies to assist with memory deficits may be different from those used with a young adult. For example, an older adult may not be as comfortable with technology and may prefer to use a paper calendar or datebook rather than a smartphone calendar app. Home safety and accessibility may be factors, and a home health OTA may make suggestions to improve safety and accessibility in the kitchen and bathrooms.

deficits, and the client may be in a rehabilitation facility or at home with home health or outpatient services, depending on the client's medical status and the families' ability to provide care.

A structured environment is helpful because clients are able to use external cues for direction, and the OTA may need to provide education and training to the family in incorporating structure into daily life. Assisting the client to keep a daily schedule and a calendar is helpful for orientation, incorporating structure, and self-advocacy by directing the client to external cues and giving him or her the opportunity to take responsibility for following the schedule. Using a daily schedule also helps transition the client to being an active participant in his or her daily life, rather than having others direct all the activities. The client may use a traditional calendar/planner, the calendar function on a smartphone/tablet, or a computer-based schedule/calendar. The OT plan of care addresses safety awareness, balance, motor control, fine motor coordination, and cognition during all occupations.

Balance activities continue to be addressed through dynamic activities in the sitting and standing positions, as well as functional mobility with whatever ambulation device is being used by the client. The OTA may have the client reaching for items in the upper and lower cabinets in the kitchen or carrying items from the refrigerator to the counter for food preparation tasks. Safety awareness can be addressed with the use of cards with pictures of household and community activities and having the client identify safe and unsafe behaviors. The OTA may also want to engage the client in hands-on activities because some clients are able to identify unsafe behaviors in pictures but may not demonstrate awareness of their own unsafe behaviors or be able to generalize.

For clients with physical impairments related to the brain injury, the OTA may need to introduce adaptive equipment, such as a reacher, elastic shoelaces, sock aid, or long-handled sponge, for increased independence with ADLs. Carryover of adaptive techniques will still be challenging for the client because of memory deficits, so practice and repetition are important. Some clients may benefit from visual cues, such as a picture showing how to use a sock aid. Adaptive equipment may only be used for a short time, depending on the client's physical progress. For example, a client may need a reacher, dressing stick, and/or sock aid because he or she is wearing a thoracic-lumbar-sacral-orthosis (TLSO) after a fractured vertebrae. The TLSO limits trunk mobility, making it difficult for the client to reach the feet. Once the fracture has healed, the adaptive equipment use can be faded out. The OTA may also address IADLs, such as washing clothes, washing dishes, and simple food preparation. Memory deficits may be limiting, and the client may forget important steps, such as turning off the oven. Difficulty with sequencing may make it difficult for the client to follow the steps of a simple recipe or steps required to wash a load of laundry.

Motor control can be addressed through performance of bilateral tasks, such as the upper body ergometer or resistance band exercise program. Exercise programs, in general, can be used to address motor control along with memory for following a written exercise program, keeping in mind that not all clients enjoy exercise. Folding laundry or using a rolling pin to roll out cookie dough are also ways to address bilateral motor control for clients who enjoy those activities. Many clients who have a brain injury may be debilitated and weaker overall because of prolonged hospitalization and will benefit from an exercise program for increased activity tolerance as well. Strengthening, for both proximal and distal muscle groups, can be helpful in addressing fine motor coordination, especially in preparation for fine motor tasks. Meaningful tasks can be helpful in addressing fine motor coordination, such as craft activities, handwriting, or playing checkers, by working on grasp of the checkers or holding a pen or paintbrush.

Therapy sessions may also begin to include dual task practice, which involves challenging two skills simultaneously. For example, playing a card or board game while standing at the table addresses balance and cognitive skills at the same time. Building a model or small birdhouse from written directions challenges fine motor coordination along with cognition. Another example is asking a client to name items in a particular category, such as animals or fruit, while playing catch to challenge cognition along with motor skills. For all clients, the OTA should be including occupations that fit the context of their life roles, whatever they may be.

Games, in general, are effective for challenging functional cognition. Recalling the rules of a familiar game challenges long-term memory. The sequence of turn-taking requires that a client read social cues and figuring out a strategy for game play involves problem-solving skills. Incorporating games into OT sessions can also provide a means to educate family members in ways to interact with their loved one and assist in continued progress at home. Computer games can be beneficial, especially because computers provide the client with consistent auditory or visual responses, which people rarely do.

Some clients may have difficulty with initiation—that is, they may not engage in an activity without being prompted.[20] Other issues that clients may face include difficulty evaluating what is important in the environment or a situation, difficulty understanding cause and effect (how their actions affect others), difficulty adapting to changes in routine, and difficulty with empathy (being able to see things from someone else's point of view).[20] Part of the OTA's role is to provide ongoing feedback and verbal cues to the client in the course of treatment sessions. Communication with the SLP is helpful for consistency in addressing issues with the client. For example, if the client continues talking in spite of nonverbal cues that the listener is losing interest, the OTA may provide a verbal cue ("It looks like Dr. Smith may need to go see other patients."). As the client improves, the OTA may work with the client and the SLP to find a subtle cue, such as a touch on the hand or the shoulder to let the client know he or she is talking too much. For clients who have decreased initiation, the OTA may need to provide verbal or tactile cues to prompt the client to begin a task. As the client makes progress, visual cues, such as a schedule, or auditory cues, such as an alarm clock or kitchen timer, may be used to remind the client to begin a task. For example, a client who has difficulty with initiation may have a hard time getting started on a task, such as showering. Termination of an activity may be an issue, in which case the client may continue washing the same body part over and over, rather than moving on to the next body part.

Rancho Level VII—Automatic, Appropriate Response

At this level, the client's behavior is becoming more appropriate in familiar settings and carryover of new learning is beginning to be evident, although at a slower rate than before the TBI. Although the client is able to perform his or her daily routines and initiate social interaction, overall judgment continues to be impaired. Insight may continue to be limited. For this reason and many others, the client may not be able to live alone without some degree of supervision. At this point, the client is likely receiving OT services in an outpatient or home health setting, and vocational rehabilitation services may be involved to address skills needed to return to work.

At this level, the focus of the OT plan of care is shifting to a greater emphasis on IADLs specific to the life roles the client will return to (Fig. 34-9). However, some clients may

TECHNOLOGY AND TRENDS

The use of technology presents many opportunities for increasing independence in clients with TBI. The OTA may use various websites and software products for the computer that are available as treatment modalities to address memory, problem-solving, and visual perceptual skills. They include activities that challenge visual memory, scanning, recall, reaction time, and problem-solving through games. Playing Solitaire® on the computer, for example, is a way to address scanning, matching, sequencing, and problem-solving strategy. The computer also provides consistent verbal and visual feedback to the client. Examples of other devices that may assist clients include a medical alert device that helps a client who is unsupervised for some or most of the day to notify emergency services in the event of a fall. A door alarm may be used to alert a family member to the possibility of an individual with memory deficits wandering off or other potential safety hazards that could be encountered outside the home. Some pill boxes can be programmed with customizable reminders to assist with medication compliance and reduce the amount of supervision that may be necessary. Smartphone apps can be used for medication reminders. The OTA's role is to assist the client and his or her family to determine how the technology that is in place can be customized to assist in day-to-day living and to make recommendations for other products and services that may be helpful.

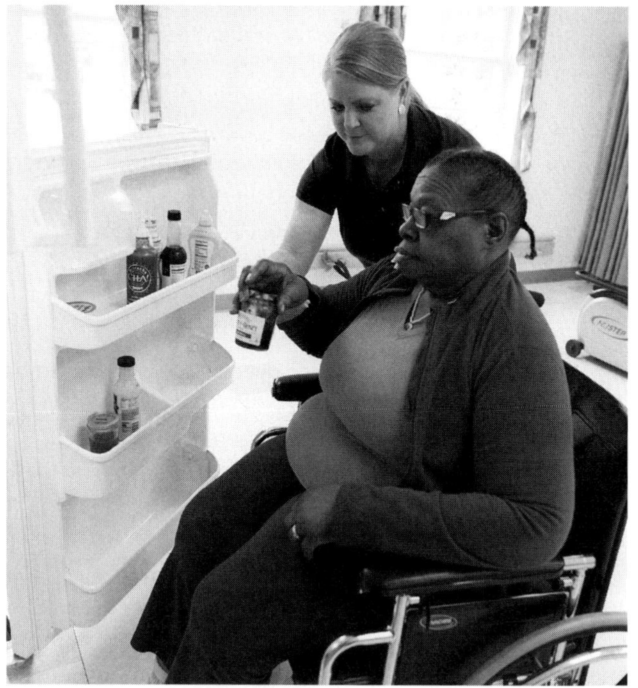

FIGURE 34-9. The OTA is working on food preparation, which is an IADL, with this client, who needs to be able to prepare meals to live alone safely.

still be recovering from other physical injuries that may be affecting their level of independence for basic ADLs. OT sessions would then continue to address adaptive techniques to increase the client's independence and safety, including adaptive equipment, as needed. For example, if the client has hemiparesis, the OTA would teach one-handed techniques for donning a shirt. The OTA may also teach the client how to use a reacher for threading pants over the feet or a sock aid for donning socks.

IADL treatment may focus on money management, including using money in a community setting, such as a restaurant or a shop. The OTA could simulate the activity with a sales flyer from the newspaper or a menu. Is the client able to select a meal and calculate a tip? Can the client make a shopping list, given a certain amount of money and a recipe? Medication management is an important skill the OTA may practice with the client, including setting up a pill box, as needed. During an OT session, medication management could be simulated with a list of prescriptions and bottles filled with empty capsules, jelly beans, or pieces of cereal to use in setting up a weekly pill box.

The OTA as well as the rest of the team will be providing direction to the family on the level of supervision that the client requires for safety. The Supervision Rating Scale (SRS) is a helpful tool that was designed to measure the amount of supervision a client receives from caregivers (Table 34-3).[21] While the ratings are based on the level of supervision received, not on the amount recommended,[21] the language used to describe supervision in the SRS can be useful for making recommendations to family members.

At this point, the plan of care should also include some strategies to assist the client in managing ongoing cognitive deficits, and technology may be helpful. OT practitioners can teach a client to use a digital watch or smartphone to set reminders to take medication as scheduled. Some pharmacies will provide medications in a "blister pack" with a client's morning and evening medications appropriately packaged to minimize medication errors. Calendar

TABLE 34-3 Supervision Rating Scale (SRS)[21]

Level 1: INDEPENDENT	
1	The patient lives alone or independently. Other persons can live with the patient but cannot take responsibility for supervision (e.g., a child or elderly person).
2	The patient is unsupervised overnight. The patient lives with one or more persons who *could* be responsible for supervision, but they are *all* sometimes absent.
Level 2: OVERNIGHT SUPERVISION	
3	The patient is only supervised overnight. One or more supervising persons are always present overnight but are *all* sometimes absent for the rest of the day.
Level 3: PART-TIME SUPERVISION	
4	The patient is supervised overnight and part time during waking hours but is allowed on independent outings. One or more supervising persons are always present overnight and are also present during part of waking hours every day. However, the patient is sometimes allowed to leave the residence without being accompanied by someone who is responsible for supervision.
5	The patient is supervised overnight and part time during waking hours but is unsupervised during working hours. Supervising persons are *all* sometimes absent for enough time for them to work full-time outside the home.
6	The patient is supervised overnight and during most waking hours. Supervising persons are *all* sometimes absent for periods longer than 1 hour but less than the time needed to hold a full-time job.
7	The patient is supervised overnight and during almost all waking hours. Supervising persons are *all* sometimes absent for periods shorter than 1 hour.
Level 4: FULL-TIME INDIRECT SUPERVISION	
8	The patient is under full-time indirect supervision. At least one supervising person is *always* present but does not check on the patient more than once every 30 minutes.
9	Same as #8 plus requires overnight safety precautions (e.g., a deadbolt on outside door).
Level 5: FULL-TIME DIRECT SUPERVISION	
10	The patient is under full-time direct supervision. At least one supervising person is always present, and the supervising person checks on the patient more than once every 30 minutes.
11	The patient lives in a setting in which the exits are physically controlled by others (e.g., a locked ward).
12	Same as #11 plus a supervising person is designated to provide full-time line-of-sight supervision (e.g., an escape watch or suicide watch).
13	The patient is in physical restraints.

applications on a smartphone or tablet can be shared between the client and family members to help the client to be more independent while still having the supervision he or she needs.

Therapy sessions may also include some community outings so that the client can put new skills to use in a natural setting (Fig. 34-10). An outing to a coffee shop gives the client the opportunity to practice social skills and money management when ordering and paying for a drink. Community outings may be done in a group setting with several clients and/or as a co-treatment with the SLP, physical therapist, or recreational therapist. For clients who have more physical disabilities and may be using a wheelchair or assistive device for walking, an outing with the OTA and the caregiver can be an opportunity to practice toilet transfers in a public restroom.

Groups are also an opportunity to address social skills. The OTA and the SLP may work together with a group of clients. Activities may include role playing different scenarios to increase clients' awareness of body language, facial expressions, and other social cues that they may have difficulty interpreting. Group sessions also provide the opportunity for the OTA and the clients to review their performance in community outings and social interactions to facilitate increased insight.

OT groups may be used to address the skills required for community integration and independent living. Community outings are often featured. For example, the OTA may work on planning a meal on the first day with a group of clients to work on organization of a task, negotiation with a group, and money skills/budgeting. The OTA and a rehabilitation aide may take the group to the grocery store and the next day using public transportation. Each client is assigned several items to locate and purchase in the store to work on social skills (asking for assistance), money management (to pay for the items), and using environmental cues (signs in the store to locate items.) After returning to the clinic, the clients put the items away, thus working on organization skills. For the third session, the OTA works with the clients on preparing a meal to address kitchen safety, following directions/recipe, planning, and organization of tasks.

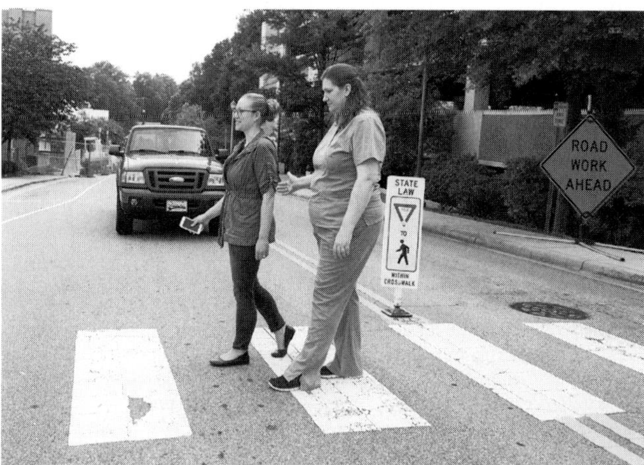

FIGURE 34-10. The OTA is addressing community reintegration skills, such as functional mobility and safety awareness.

Group sessions provide an opportunity to address social skills. Following community outings, the OTA may facilitate discussion with clients to reflect on their performance on tasks and social interactions. The OTA may not only provide feedback but also facilitate the clients evaluating their own performance and others' performance; the OTA may also help clients with providing feedback in a socially appropriate way. Role playing challenging social situations is also a useful tool to assist the clients in reading social cues, such as facial expression, tone of voice, and body language.

Rancho Level VIII—Purposeful, Appropriate Response

Level VIII of the LCFS is characterized by appropriate responses to the environment. The client is oriented but continues to demonstrate impaired abstract reasoning (the ability to use logic and creativity in problem-solving and to make predictions) compared with his or her level of function before the injury. At this level, clients will typically be receiving services in an outpatient or home health setting or possibly as part of a day program. The focus of rehabilitation continues to be maximization of the skills needed for the client to be as independent as possible and may include vocational rehabilitation and/or a driving evaluation. Vocational rehabilitation services assist the client in developing the skills needed to return to a previous job or a different job.

Driving evaluations are a specialized service provided by some occupational therapists in an outpatient setting (see Chapter 16 for details). Driving simulations can be performed with computer-based equipment to evaluate the skills needed for driving, such as vision, reaction time, and coordination. The physician may require a client to have a driving evaluation to be cleared to return to driving. If a client is not yet ready to return to driving, the OT plan of care may address the skills needed to access public transportation, such as reading a bus schedule, purchasing a bus pass, or using a taxi.

The OT plan of care at Level VIII is focused on higher-level cognitive skills, including medication management, money management, community integration, and home management. The OTA may now begin addressing the skills needed for returning to work. To address money management, the OTA may use paper and pencil tasks to address the functional math skills needed for paying bills, banking, and setting a budget. The OTA may also work on the client's use of a computer for accessing a bank account or paying bills or the use of a calculator to aid math calculations. For clients who continue to have difficulty with money management, technology can be a useful adaptive strategy. For example, the client may be able to set up an alert through the bank's website or through an app that will send a text message or email when the account balance reaches a set level to avoid overdrawing. When addressing medication management skills, the OTA may work on reading medication labels for safety interactions, strategies for taking medications correctly, and what to do to avoid running out of prescription medications. In addressing home management skills, the OTA may work on menu planning, home safety, or pet care, depending on the client's needs. For example, the OTA may set up the kitchen in the clinic with staged safety hazards and have the client locate the safety issues. Picture cards depicting safety issues can also be used, although they are not as powerful as the actual environment.

For clients who are no longer able to engage in their preferred leisure activities, the OT professional may provide help with exploring new leisure interests or adaptive techniques to allow participation. Some clients may also continue to work on balance and fine motor skills. OT sessions provide an opportunity for clients to try activities they may not have participated in previously. The OTA can facilitate exploring those activities by talking to clients about preferences and activities that they may like to try and include these into the treatment sessions. The OTA may also adapt and grade those activities to challenge balance and/or fine motor skills. For example, balance could be addressed while the client is playing air hockey or a video game standing on a balance board. In addition to rehabilitating needed skills, the OTA should also assist the client and family in developing adaptive strategies to compensate for deficit areas. Adaptive strategies may be high-tech, such as smartphone apps that could be used to remind the client to take their medication, or low-tech, such as a day planner or 7-day pill box. A work simulation unit with tasks needed for return to work, such as the Valpar unit, can be beneficial for addressing work-related skills. See Chapter 17 for more details on work.

PSYCHOSOCIAL IMPACT

Brain injury has a significant impact on the psychosocial aspects of an individual's life. Memory deficits, communication issues, personality changes, and difficulty reading social cues affect personal relationships with family, friends, and significant others. The dynamics of the relationship with a romantic partner may be changed by a shift in roles because of the partner's taking on the role of caregiver. An individual with a brain injury may not be able to return to a prior job or leisure activities for some time, if ever, which may result in grieving for what has been lost. Many people derive a large amount of self-esteem from job success or role as a parent. Day-to-day activities that used to be automatic

EVIDENCE-BASED PRACTICE

The American Occupational Therapy Association (AOTA) website has a number of resources, including practice guidelines, for OT professionals treating clients who have TBI. Critically appraised topics and papers are available through AOTA's *Evidence-Based Literature Review Project.* The AOTA also published six systematic reviews as part of this initiative. The reviews cover visual and visual perceptual performance, motor function, sensory stimulation in disorders of consciousness, social participation, cognitive impairments, and occupational performance, as well as psychosocial, behavioral, and emotional impairments.

- For visual and visual-perceptual deficits in adults with TBI, the evidence shows preliminary support for scanning training with visual field deficits, the use of adaptive strategies, and cognitive retraining approach, along with the use of meaningful occupations for carryover into daily living.[22] Vision is a complex function that requires continued study and review of the evidence for effective treatment interventions.
- For motor impairments related to TBI, the evidence suggests that exercise programs may be beneficial.[23] The available research data on the effects of multidisciplinary rehabilitation programs and computer-based interventions on motor function are limited.[23] Motor function provides a basis for many other skills and also may be affected by other deficits, including cognition, vision, and sensory function.[23]
- The evidence supports the use of bimodal (directed at two senses) or multimodal (directed at all five senses) sensory stimulation for clients with disorders of consciousness.[24]
- Strong evidence supports the use of dual-task practice, compensatory strategies, and assistive technology for clients with cognitive deficits following brain injury.[25]

Working with clients who have brain injuries is challenging because every brain and every injury is different. Combining the available evidence with good clinical reasoning is the best way to provide effective OT interventions.

Berger, S., Kaldenberg, J., & Carlo, S. (2016). Effectiveness of interventions to address visual and visual perceptual impairments to improve occupational performance in adults with traumatic brain injury: A systematic review. American Journal of Occupational Therapy, 70, *7003180010.*

Chang, P. F. J., Baxter, M.F., & Risskey, J. (2016). Effectiveness of interventions within the scope of occupational therapy practice to improve motor function of people with traumatic brain injury: A systematic review. American Journal of Occupational Therapy. 70, *7003180020.*

Padilla, R., & Domina, A. (2016). Effectiveness of sensory stimulation to improve arousal and alertness of people in a coma or persistent vegetative state after traumatic brain injury: A systematic review. American Journal of Occupational Therapy, 70, *7003180030.*

Radomski, M.V., Anheluk, M.P., & Zola, J. (2016). Effectiveness of interventions to address cognitive impairments and improve occupational performance after traumatic brain injury: A systematic review. American Journal of Occupational Therapy, 70, *7003180050.*

may require more thought and effort following a brain injury, resulting in increased fatigue just from navigating daily life. In addition to this, many individuals may merely seem unchanged after a brain injury, and this may lead the people in their lives to have unrealistic expectations of their abilities. Depression and anxiety can be a part of the psychosocial impact of the brain injury as the client grieves for losses and adjusts to new ways of living.

CLIENT AND FAMILY EDUCATION AND TRAINING

A comprehensive program for treatment of the client with a brain injury will include education provided by all disciplines. The OT professional provides education and training to assist the client and family with adapting to life with a brain injury. Depending on client needs, education and training may focus on safety, cognitive issues, balance deficits, functional mobility, and/or motor issues that affect ADLs and IADLs. Social awareness and behavior management may be addressed by a team comprising the OTA, the SLP, the social worker, and the psychologist. After demonstrating safe techniques for assisting the client with ADLs, transfers, and functional mobility, which is also an ADL according to the *Occupational Therapy Practice Framework: Domain & Process, 3rd edition* (OTPF-3), the OTA would have family members practice providing assistance.[26] The OTA could then provide feedback on body mechanics for transfers and other safety considerations. Teaching family members strategies to allow the individual with the brain injury to be as independent and as safe as possible is crucial. Family members often help the client more than they need to because of trying to be helpful. The OTA can educate them on how to provide assistance while allowing the client to be as independent as he or she is able. Because of the holistic nature of OT and the role it plays in occupations, the OT professional is also in a unique position to provide on-the-spot education in the context of functional tasks. For example, performing a cooking task is an opportunity to reinforce education about the client's nutritional needs that the dietitian or nurse may have addressed previously. Reeducation is also important because of the memory deficits that often accompany brain injury. Reinforcement of education to caregivers is important because stress and fatigue may affect their ability to retain new information.

The family of the individual with the brain injury may require education on safety considerations for the home. In some cases, modifications to the home for accessibility may be necessary. For example, grab bars in the bathroom may be needed for safety in toileting or bathing. A ramp may be needed to make the home accessible for a client who is using a wheelchair at discharge. If the home has two levels and it is not safe for the client to use the stairs, then he or she may have to remain on the first floor initially. The OT professional may provide education on safety related to memory deficits, such as the risk of the oven being left on or the water left running. Family members may need to remind the client to eat or take medication in a timely manner. For clients who continue to demonstrate memory deficits and poor insight, education should include securing items that are important, such as credit cards, or items that may pose a safety risk, such as car keys or firearms which may be present in the home.

Although many clients and family members believe that the client will function better once he or she is at home in a familiar environment, this is not always the case. While the client is continuing to make progress, he or she may not have good insight into personal deficits, and that can lead to frustration after discharge home. If a client has poor insight, he or she is less likely to use adaptive strategies and may be resistant to supervision by family members. Many individuals with a brain injury do not recognize that they have deficits and, therefore, do not see the need for adaptive strategies or supervision. Some clients also have difficulty with initiation following a brain injury. Some clients who go home sit around playing video games or watching TV all day and resist the efforts of caregivers to engage them. The caregivers may need assistance from the OTA in creating a supportive, engaging environment, where the client can take on specific responsibilities. This can be especially challenging with regard to reemerging roles of a parent of a 24-year-old now living back at home and needing supervision, or a client who wants to return to the role of a working spouse but is frustratingly unable to do so.

Alcohol abuse may also be an issue because as many as two thirds of individuals with TBI have a prior history of alcohol abuse.[26,27] Sometimes, when clients return home, familiar behaviors, friends, and patterns reemerge for the client, some of which may have led to the brain injury in the first place. Alcohol and/or drug use or abuse delay the healing process and can interfere with therapy. It can also be a reason for the client being discharged from an outpatient brain injury therapeutic group. Clients and their families may benefit from brain injury support groups in the community.

SEXUAL ACTIVITY

Sexual activity is an ADL and falls within the domain of OT practice.[26,28] The client with a brain injury may experience changes in their sexuality—increased or decreased desire as well as changes in arousal.[28] The client may also experience changes in his or her relationships due to a spouse taking on a caregiver role, the possibility of self-esteem issues related to the disability, and physical challenges to sexual functioning and intimacy. The OTA plays a role in educating the client with brain injury and his or her partner in sexuality related to brain injury. Some issues may be related to or helped by medications prescribed by the physician and the client may have other health issues that affect sexual functioning. For example, the OTA may educate the client on options for positions to assist with physical deficits related to his or her injuries, such as placing pillows to provide support that might be needed. The OTA would also educate the client and family about socially and sexually appropriate behavior. Some clients continue to have difficulty reading social cues and/or recognizing when something is not appropriate to say in a given situation. Role playing different social situations/interactions is a helpful strategy for teaching the client how to read social cues, such as tone of voice, facial expression, and body language, as well as what impression he or she may be giving to others based on their social cues. The OTA might also use pictures, asking the client to identify what the person in the picture is feeling as indicated by the presented facial expression. Educating family members on the difficulties that the client may be having with interpreting social cues as well as awareness of the impact of his or her own behavior is an important part of the OTA's role. Some clients who have decreased inhibition will make sexually or socially inappropriate remarks, and some clients with a brain injury may be hypersexual. The hypersexuality can manifest as constant and obsessive desire for sex and can lead to unsafe behaviors. Even more common is decreased libido after a brain injury; either scenario can put a significant strain on partner relationships. Some caregivers note that it is difficult to consider a spouse that they assist with toileting and bathing, or one that is impulsive, irrational, or childish behavior, as a sexual partner.

SUMMARY

Every brain injury is unique and life changing, and no two brain injuries are alike. The impact on an individual and every member of his or her network is enormous. The OTA's holistic view and focus on function for each individual is an important part of the rehabilitation process, from the ICU to home health or outpatient settings. OTAs working at every level of the rehabilitation continuum address occupations to assist the client in regaining the highest level of function possible. Whether the goal is to help the client return to work or to educate the family to provide care in the home, the OTA is an important member of the team working toward the ultimate goal. The person-centered focus of OT places practitioners in the position to change the lives of the clients they serve in a positive way, through the use of occupations that are meaningful to the client.

REVIEW QUESTIONS

1. Gladys had a TBI 4 weeks ago and is now at home and receiving outpatient OT services. She has difficulty with recent memory and new learning. She is oriented to time by using a calendar and clock for direction. Gladys is still demonstrating some confusion. At what level of the LCFS is Gladys functioning?
   a. Level VII—Automatic, appropriate response
   b. Level IV—Confused, agitated response
   c. Level V—Confused, inappropriate, non-agitated response
   d. Level VI—Confused, appropriate response
2. Fred is a 60-year-old man who has a TBI as a result of a motorcycle accident. He also sustained a pelvic fracture, so the physician ordered no weight-bearing on the right lower extremity. Fred is currently functioning at Level IV of the LCFS, with poor memory, poor safety awareness, and balance deficits. What challenges would the OT practitioner expect to have in working on ADLs with Fred?
   a. ADLs would not be a problem because they are automatic, familiar tasks.
   b. Following weight-bearing precautions with toilet transfers
   c. Carrying over adaptive techniques for ADL and transfers
   d. Walking from the bed to closet for clothing retrieval
3. Cheryl is a 20-year-old college student with a diagnosis of an anoxic brain injury from a near-drowning following a boating accident. She was recently evaluated in an acute rehabilitation facility and found to have poor balance, memory deficits, poor attention, difficulties with problem-solving, and poor impulse control. At this point, Cheryl requires steadying assistance for bathing, dressing, toileting, and transfers, and is functioning at Level V of the LCFS. Her goal is to return to school when she is able. What would the OTA working with Cheryl focus on?
   a. Handwriting and study skills working toward returning to school
   b. Problem-solving for IADLs
   c. Attention and standing balance for increased safety with ADLs and transfers
   d. Memory strategies, such as using a smartphone for medication reminders and keeping a calendar
4. George is a new client in an outpatient clinic. He is a 35-year-old man who had a TBI after falling from a ladder 6 months ago. George lives with his wife and 7-year-old son and is only interested in outpatient therapy to work on his goals to return to driving and his job as a manager of the service department of a car dealership. The OT evaluation showed deficits in problem-solving, sequencing, abstract reasoning, mild fine motor deficits in the left hand, and mild memory deficits. How would the OT practitioner address George's goal of returning to work?
   a. Give him a crate of equipment to sort and organize on a shelf to simulate a task that he might do at work to encourage participation in therapy sessions.
   b. Educate the client that returning to work at this time is not realistic.
   c. Ask the doctor to refer George for a driving evaluation since he will need to drive to return to work.
   d. Give him a TheraPutty® exercise program to address his fine motor deficits.
5. Betty is a 67-year-old woman who had an anoxic brain injury following a cardiac arrest 3 months ago. She demonstrates mild balance deficits, mild memory deficits, and problem-solving deficits. She has been living alone since her husband passed away, and she has a daughter who lives nearby. Betty has been staying with her daughter after being discharged from the hospital but wants to return to her home. Where would the OT practitioner focus treatment during outpatient sessions with Betty?
   a. Safety awareness, medication management, and fine motor coordination
   b. Balance, safety awareness, and food preparation
   c. Fine motor coordination, home management, strengthening, and balance
   d. Adaptive strategies for home management, balance, medication management, and getting around the kitchen with her walker

6. Angie had a TBI when thrown from the passenger seat during a motor vehicle accident 7 weeks ago. She is currently in an inpatient rehabilitation facility and currently functioning at a Level V on the LCFS. Which of the following would be the *most* appropriate treatment?
   a. Applying favorite scented lotion
   b. Simply looking at photos of family and pets
   c. ADLs of bathing, dressing, and grooming in her room
   d. Afternoon exercise session in the busy therapy gym
7. Which three of the following would be part of the OT plan of care for a client who is functioning at Level II of the LCFS?
   a. ADLs
   b. Sensory stimulation
   c. Memory strategies
   d. Education of family members in overstimulation
   e. Money management tasks
   f. ROM and positioning
8. The OT practitioner is working with a client who has left hemiparesis and is functioning at Level VII of the LCFS. Which of the following strategies would be appropriate for working on upper body dressing?
   a. Just dress the client, because he is not capable of new learning.
   b. Teach hemi-dressing techniques in the context of dressing. Practice often because more time is required for carry-over of new learning.
   c. Explain and demonstrate hemi-dressing techniques on a doll.
   d. Explain hemi-dressing techniques in detail, using photographs of the steps of donning a shirt.
9. The OTA sees a client in the acute hospital 2 days after he was thrown from his motorcycle. He sustained a TBI, left tibial fracture, and is in a medically induced coma state. Which of the following areas would be a good place to begin with OT education and training with his family members?
   a. Sexuality
   b. Behavior and overstimulation
   c. ADLs and transfers
   d. PROM UE exercises
10. Which three of the following technologies may be used to increase a client's independence and safety in the home setting in the context of mild cognitive deficits?
   a. Using the reminder function on a smartphone for taking medication
   b. Environmental control unit
   c. Reacher
   d. Elastic shoelaces
   e. Daily calendar or planner for scheduling
   f. Medications filled in blister packs by the pharmacy

CASE STUDY

Marty, a 27-year-old man, was involved in a motor vehicle collision. He was not wearing a seatbelt and was ejected from the vehicle he was driving. Marty's injuries included a TBI with diffuse axonal injury, right clavicle fracture, right tibia fracture, and vertebral fractures at C4 and C5. He was intubated at the scene and had an initial GCS score of 3. Marty underwent a craniectomy, with the bone flap removed to manage intracranial pressure. A tracheostomy was placed, and Marty was dependent on the ventilator for 4 weeks. A gastrostomy tube was placed for nutrition and medication. Marty had a cervical collar to stabilize his spine and a temporary brace to immobilize his right leg. OT consultation was sought 2 weeks after the admission, when Marty was in the neurology ICU. The occupational therapist evaluated Marty and developed a plan of care that focused on positioning and ROM. The orthopedist wrote an order restricting ROM of the right shoulder and ankle. The OTA carried out the plan of care and also began education of Marty's parents in issues related to brain injury. Some of the sessions were deferred by the nurse or the physician because of abnormalities in his vital signs.

After 4 weeks in the ICU, Marty was breathing without the ventilator and began to respond to tactile stimulation. He was inconsistently following commands. OT treatment focused on managing the level of environmental stimulation, sitting balance, head control, visually tracking objects and people in the environment, and following commands. The OTA also educated his family regarding overstimulation and trained them to perform PROM exercises.

After Marty moved to an inpatient rehabilitation facility, he was evaluated by the occupational therapist. He was dependent for bathing, dressing, toileting, and all transfers. Marty still had the tracheostomy in place and was receiving all his nutrition and hydration through the gastrostomy tube. He was not allowed to put weight on his right UE or the right LE, and he was wearing the cervical collar to stabilize his vertebral fractures. Transitional movements were more difficult because of Marty's non–weight-bearing status and difficulty with new learning for adaptive movement and transfer techniques. Simple, direct commands of one to two steps increased his understanding, but Marty was not able to read written commands because of difficulties with his vision. Marty was also required to wear a helmet when out of bed because of the craniectomy. OT sessions focused on ADLs, balance, safety awareness, attention, memory, and family education/training. The OTA taught the family on providing assistance with ADLs and dependent transfers and on providing verbal cues and directions without overstimulating Marty. The OTA also educated the family on managing Marty's behaviors. He was agitated for several days, but changes in medication along with reducing stimulation in the environment improved the agitation. During the 3 weeks he spent at inpatient rehabilitation, Marty was able to have the tracheostomy removed, and he began to self-feed and drink by mouth. He went back to the hospital for surgery to replace the bone flap in his skull and was discharged home from there.

Marty was discharged to his parents' home and began receiving outpatient OT services. His parents and other family members provided 24-hour supervision and assisted Marty with taking showers and with transfers. He was able to put weight on his right arm to assist with transfers, but he still had a cast on his leg and the cervical collar in place. Marty's safety awareness improved with routine and familiar ADLs, such as upper and lower body dressing, and he was able to carry over new learning, including sequencing the steps for adaptive techniques for transitional movements with the cast in place. Outpatient OT focused on memory strategies, problem-solving, IADLs, and strengthening of the right UE.

About 6 months after his injury, Marty was still staying with his parents but was doing well with intermittent supervision, with his parents being able to leave him for up to 2 to 3 hours at a time during the day. His physician referred him for a driving evaluation, due to his instance on driving, and he was receiving vocational rehabilitation services in addition to outpatient OT and speech therapy. Marty began volunteering at a local food bank for 10 hours a week to develop the skills needed to return to his former job in a grocery store. Marty worked with his OTA on using his smartphone for medication reminders, using public transportation to get to his volunteer site and therapy appointments, and using a planner to keep to a schedule. They also worked on simple cooking skills and shopping for food to meet Marty's goal of moving out of his parents' home when he was able to return to work. The OTA started with simple cold food preparation, such as making a sandwich, and then moved on to using the microwave for heating frozen dinners, and finally to simple cooking on the stove, such as scrambled eggs.

OT was an essential part of the team approach that facilitated Marty's return to independence after his brain injury.

1. After Marty was admitted to the inpatient rehabilitation hospital, what possible methods would the OTA use for safely transferring him from the wheelchair to the toilet without putting weight on the right upper and lower extremities?
2. What are some strategies that the OTA could teach Marty in outpatient therapy sessions to help him compensate for his memory deficits?
3. What other IADLs would the OTA work on with Marty (in addition to the ones listed in the case study) to make it possible for him to move out of his parents' home and live independently?

PUTTING IT ALL TOGETHER Sample Treatment and Documentation

Setting	Inpatient rehabilitation
Client Profile	Cathy is a 67-year-old female with a diagnosis of TBI following a fall from a step stool. She has a history of R knee osteoarthritis and high blood pressure.
Work History	Cathy is retired, but works part time as a hostess in a restaurant.
Insurance	Medicare Part A and B
Psychological	She has a history of anxiety.
Social	Cathy lives with her husband. They have a dog and a cat. She has a daughter and grandson who live nearby.
Cognitive	She is oriented to person, place, and time, but she tends to become confused at the end of the day. She is impulsive and has difficulty with moderate to complex problem-solving. Safety awareness and memory for recent events are impaired.
Motor & Manual Muscle Testing (MMT)	Sitting balance is good, but Cathy has difficulties with standing balance. She typically requires Min A for standing balance. Her strength is 5/5 for BUEs, and grossly 4/5 in BLEs.
ADL	Cathy feeds herself, completes grooming, and dons a shirt and bra with supervision for problem-solving. She requires Min A for bathing, shower transfers, toileting, and toilet transfers. She requires Min A for donning underwear, pants, socks, and shoes.
IADL	Cathy requires Min A for balance with kitchen tasks and pet care. She requires Min A for complex money tasks like balancing her checkbook.
Goals	Within two weeks: 1. Client will perform LE dressing with Mod I using adaptive equipment, as needed. 2. Client will perform bathing and shower transfers with Mod I using a shower chair. 3. Client will perform simple food prep with supervision using a rolling walker for balance.

OT TREATMENT SESSION 1

THERAPEUTIC ACTIVITY	TIME	GOAL(S) ADDRESSED	OTA RATIONALE
Shower on a shower seat	30 min	#2	*Preparatory Method; Occupations:* Practice in context of natural environment; trained client in the use a long-handled sponge.
Dressing edge of bed with adaptive equipment	15 min	#1	*Occupations:* Seated LB dressing edge of bed. Practice in context of natural environment
Education on use of sock aid	10 min	#2	*Occupations; Education and Training:* Compensatory strategies for dressing. Trained client in use of sock aid.

SOAP note: 12/2/—, 8:00 am–8:55 am

S: "I really want to wash my hair."

O: Client participated in skilled OT session in room and bathroom for ADL program. No complaints of pain. Client washed LEs with education and training for use of long-handled sponge. After skilled instruction, client transferred from wheelchair to shower chair with Min A. Client required supervision because of balance deficits and min cues for use of grab bars. Client washed all body parts with use of long-handled sponge. OTA instructed client in threading pants and underwear on feet seated at edge of bed because of standing balance deficits. Client required Min A to don pants and underwear safely, and steadying

PUTTING IT ALL TOGETHER Sample Treatment and Documentation (continued)

assistance with standing to pull up pants. OTA demonstrated use of sock aid for donning socks. Client was able to don socks with Min A and verbal cues provided for recall of techniques.

A: Client demonstrated increased independence with bathing and LE dressing with use of adaptive equipment. Client will require further education and practice with techniques to reach goals.

P: Continue further practice of dressing and bathing techniques to assess carryover. Continue plan of care.

Amanda Adams, OTA/L, 12/2/—, 1:00 pm

TREATMENT SESSION 2

What could you do next with this client?

TREATMENT SESSION 3

What could you do next with this client?

REFERENCES

1. Public policy of brain injury network. (2008). Retrieved from www.braininjurynetwork.org
2. Savage, R. (2009). Understanding the brain and brain injury. In *The Essential Brain Injury Guide* (4th ed., pp. 38–53). Vienna, VA: Brain Injury Association of America.
3. About TBI. (2015). Retrieved from www.biausa.org
4. TBI: Get the facts. (2016). Retrieved from www.cdc.gov/traumaticbraininjury
5. Ficker-Terrill, C., Flippo, K., Antoinette, T., & Braunling McMorrow, D. (2009). Overview of brain injury. In *The Essential Brain Injury Guide* (4th ed., pp. 4–5). Vienna, VA: Brain Injury Association of America.
6. Teasdale, G., & Jennett, B. (1974). Assessment of coma and impaired consciousness: A practical scale. *Lancet, 2,* 81–84.
7. Sander, A. (2002). The level of cognitive functioning scale. *The Center for Outcome Management in Brain Injury.* Retrieved from http://tbims.org/combi/lcfs
8. Hagen, C., Malkmus, D., & Durham, P. (1972). *Levels of cognitive functioning.* Downey, CA: Rancho Los Amigos Hospital.
9. Giacino, J. T., Fins, J. J., Laureys, S., & Schiff, N. D. (2014). Disorders of consciousness after acquired brain injury: The state of the science. *Nature Reviews Neurology, 10*(2), 99–114.
10. Page, T. (2009). Health, medications, and medical management. In *The Essential Brain Injury Guide* (4th ed., pp. 57–80). Vienna, VA: Brain Injury Association of America.
11. Traumatic brain injury: Definition. (2014). Retrieved from www.mayoclinic.org
12. Definitions related to TBI. (n.d.). Retrieved from www.traumaticbraininjury.com
13. Diffuse axonal injury. (2016). Retrieved from www.brainandspinalcord.org
14. Brain injury: How the brain functions. (2011). Retrieved from www.braininjuryinstitute.org
15. Anatomy of the brain: The basics. (2016). Retrieved from www.braininjury101.org/details/anatomy
16. Giacino, J., & Kalmar, K. (2006). Coma recovery scale—Revised. The Center for Outcome Management in Brain Injury. Retrieved from http://www.tbims.org/combi/crs
17. Bohannon, R., & Smith, M. (1987). Interrater reliability of a modified Ashworth scale of muscle spasticity. *Physical Therapy, 67*(2), 206.
18. Gutman, S. A. (2008). *Neuroscience for rehabilitation professionals: The essential neurologic principles underlying rehabilitation practice* (2nd ed.). Thorofare, NJ: Slack.
19. Caraulia, A. P., & Steiger, L. K. (1997). *Nonviolent crisis intervention: Learning to defuse explosive behavior.* Dubai, UAE: CPI Publishing.
20. Antoinette, T., Strauss, D., & Trudel, T. (2009). Understanding & treating functional impacts of brain injury. In: *The Essential Brain Injury Guide* (4th ed., pp. 82–105). Vienna, VA: Brain Injury Association of America.
21. Boake, C. (2001). The supervision rating scale. The Center for Outcome Measurement in Brain Injury. Retrieved from http://www.tbims.org/combi/srs
22. Berger, S., Kaldenberg, J., & Carlo, S. (2016). Effectiveness of interventions to address visual and visual perceptual impairments to improve occupational performance in adults with traumatic brain injury: A systematic review. *American Journal of Occupational Therapy, 70,* 7003180010.
23. Chang, P. F. J., Baxter, M. F., & Risskey, J. (2016). Effectiveness of interventions within the scope of occupational therapy practice to improve motor function of people with traumatic brain injury: A systematic review. *American Journal of Occupational Therapy, 70,* 7003180020.
24. Padilla, R., & Domina, A. (2016). Effectiveness of sensory stimulation to improve arousal and alertness of people in a coma or persistent vegetative state after traumatic brain injury: A systematic review. *American Journal of Occupational Therapy, 70,* 7003180030.
25. Radomski, M. V., Anheluk, M. P., & Zola, J. (2016). Effectiveness of interventions to address cognitive impairments and improve occupational performance after traumatic brain injury: A systematic review. *American Journal of Occupational Therapy, 70,* 7003180050.
26. American Occupational Therapy Association. (2014). Occupational therapy practice framework: Domain and process (3rd ed.). *American Journal of Occupational Therapy, 68*(Suppl. 1), S1–S48. http://dx.doi.org/10.5014/ajot.2014.682006
27. Bombardier, C. H., & Turner, A. (2009). Alcohol and traumatic disability. In R. Frank & T. Elliott (Eds.), *The Handbook of Rehabilitation Psychology* (2nd ed., pp. 241–258). Washington, DC: American Psychological Association Press.
28. Sander, A. M., & Maestas, K. L. (2014). Sexuality after traumatic brain injury. *Archives of Physical Medicine and Rehabilitation, 95,* 801–802.

Chapter 35

Spinal Cord Injury and Disease: Factors and Essential Care

Raheleh G. Tschoepe MS, OT/L

LEARNING OUTCOMES

After studying this chapter, the student or practitioner will be able to:

35.1 Describe the physiological mechanisms that cause the various types of spinal cord injury/disease

35.2 Explain the impacts of complete versus incomplete spinal cord injury/disease.

35.3 Determine the various resulting physical and psychosocial ramifications of spinal cord injury/disease

35.4 Describe the functional impact of spinal cord injury/disease on the client, family, friends, and community

35.5 Identify intervention plan priorities for clients with various levels of spinal cord injury/disease

KEY TERMS

Anterior cord syndrome	Orthostatic hypotension
Atelectasis	Paralysis
Autonomic dysfunction	Paraparesis
Autonomic dysreflexia (AD)	Paraplegia
Bradycardia	Radicular pain
Central pain	Scapulohumeral rhythm
Complete spinal cord injury (SCI)	Sepsis
Dermatome	Septicemia
Hypoxia	Somatosensation
Incomplete spinal cord injury/disease (SCI/D)	Spina bifida
Intrathecal	Spinal cord disease
Mechanical pain	Stenosis
Myotome	Tenodesis
Nontraumatic SCI/D	Tetraplegia
Neurogenic heterotopic ossification (nHO)	Transverse myelitis
	Traumatic SCI
	Zone of partial preservation

One in 11,000 people in the United States will have a spinal cord injury (SCI). Support networks of family, friends, caregivers, healthcare providers, and community members must be prepared to assist these individuals.[1] Occupational therapy assistants (OTAs) play a critical role in facilitating participation in meaningful activities, education and training about spinal cord injury and disease (SCI/D), and empowerment. Living well with SCI/D requires a lifelong commitment to maintaining healthy routines and fully being able to engage in desired occupations. OT practitioners specialize in enabling clients with SCI/D to explore and practice desired activities in safe and supportive environments so clients can maximize their ability to achieve goals and live life to its fullest.[2]

This chapter begins by providing an overview of SCI/D, including its causes, classifications, and medical interventions. It next paints broad strokes about the health implications of spinal cord injury (SCI) and how OT supports the quality of life (QoL) of people living with SCI/D. It then goes on to explore functional outcomes at each level of injury and target areas of OT intervention with a focus on occupation and activity; preparatory methods and tasks; and advocacy and groups. The final section of the chapter describes the continuum of care along which clients with SCI/D, their support networks, and OTAs work together to maximize independence, promote wellness and empowerment, and improve QoL.

SPINAL CORD INJURY AND DISEASE

Spinal cord injury (SCI) results from injury to the spine that fractures and dislocates the vertebrae, causing damage to spinal cord tissue.[3] Additional damage from the traumatic injury usually occurs over days or weeks because of bleeding, swelling, inflammation, and fluid accumulation in and around the spinal cord.[4] **Nontraumatic SCI** or **spinal cord disease** includes tumors, infections, inflammation, and autoimmune or degenerative processes that damage spinal cord tissue.[5] In the past, all spinal cord damage was known as SCI, but the more current and correct term is SCI/D. SCI/D can cause sudden, dramatic, and pervasive trauma to an individual's physical, physiological, emotional, and psychosocial state. SCI/D survivors must first confront the immediate, life-altering impact directly after their injury. SCI/D has the potential to affect QoL, role fulfillment, participation in meaningful and purposeful activities, financial well-being, family and community dynamics, body image, and relationships (Box 35-1 and Fig. 35-1).

Etiology

The etiology (causes) of SCI/D illustrated by the three individuals in Box 35-1 are each different. Suzanna's complete paraplegia was caused by a *traumatic* SCI. **Paraplegia** is caused by injury to the thoracic, lumbar, or sacral spinal cord and results in lower extremity (LE) weakness or paralysis.[6] **Paralysis** is the complete loss of muscle function in an area of the body[5]. The OTA may also hear the term **paraparesis,** which is a partial loss of function or strength in the lower limbs. José experienced injury to his spinal cord as a result of a *nontraumatic* pathological process with resulting incomplete tetraplegia. **Tetraplegia** is caused by injury to the cervical spinal cord and results in UE and LE weakness or paralysis in all four extremities.[6] Quadriplegia is a term used in the past for the same region of damage, but tetraplegia is now the accepted term. Carol lives with incomplete paraplegia from a nontraumatic spinal cord disease. The impact on all their lives, however, is undoubtedly significant. Suzanna, José, Carol, and their support networks will work with OT practitioners throughout the continuum of care who will help them navigate strategies and resources as they live their lives with SCI/D.

Incidence and Prevalence

There are 12,500 new cases of SCI each year in the United States, and there were 276,000 persons living with SCI in 2014.[7] The leading causes of SCI include vehicle crashes, followed by falls, acts of violence (mainly gunshot wounds), and sports.[7] After 45 years of age, falls are the leading cause of SCI.[8] The average age at injury since 2010 has been 42, an increase since the 1970s, when the average age of someone with an SCI was

BOX 35-1
Three Examples of SCI/D

Traumatic spinal cord injury: Suzanna was on a spring break trip in Central America and, while driving a moped, was involved in a collision with a car and ejected from the moped. She was immediately unable to move and feel her legs. She was flown and admitted to the nearest trauma hospital, where she underwent a thoracic laminectomy and fusion. She had a traumatic T4 complete SCI.

Nontraumatic spinal cord injury: José was a 70-year-old contractor who over a period of 3 months felt he was declining in his upper body strength to lay drywall, complained of tingling and numbness in his feet, and found it increasingly difficult to urinate after feeling the urge. Jose's family depends on his income, so despite his symptoms, he was unable to take time off from work to address these medical issues. One day while hanging drywall, Jose's lower body weakness progressed to the point that he was unable to stand. He was transported by ambulance to the hospital, evaluated by a physician, and admitted for an emergent decompression of his cervical spine. The physician diagnosed Jose with cervical spinal stenosis, or narrowing of his spinal canal, caused by aging and degenerative changes, resulting in compression of his spinal cord. He now lives with nontraumatic C5 incomplete tetraplegia.

Nontraumatic spinal cord injury: Carol is a 60-year-old health care professional, wife, and grandmother of 11 grandchildren. She was diagnosed with cancer originating in her spine. As a result of the compression from the growing tumor on her thoracic spinal cord, she experiences debilitating pain throughout her chest and back and has muscle weakness in her LEs that renders her unable to sit or stand for more than 30 minutes at a time. As a result of this spinal cord disease, she has T4-T7 incomplete paraplegia.

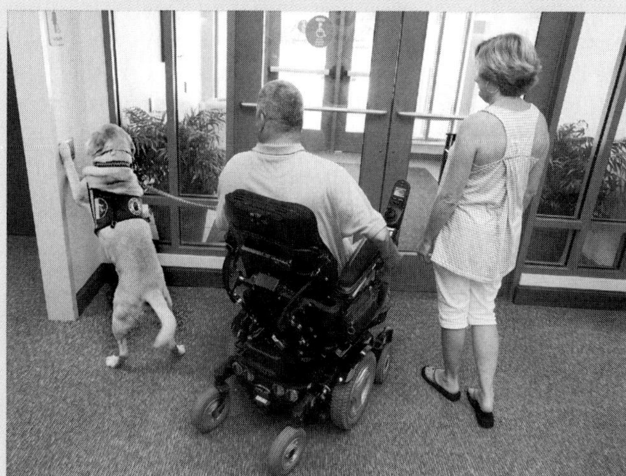

FIGURE 35-1. Jose with incomplete C5 SCI, his wife, and service dog.

29 years of age. The average age is increasing with an aging, yet active population. This aging population is at risk for falls, and therefore the percentage of SCI due to falls is increasing.[9] From 1997 to 2000, 28% of SCIs were associated with falls in older adults 65 years of age and older. This average increased to 66% from 2010 to 2012 in individuals 65 years of age and older.[1]

Cause of Death

According to the World Health Organization (WHO), mortality risk for a person with SCI/D is highest in the first year after injury and remains high compared with the general population. Mortality risk increases with injury level and severity and is strongly influenced by availability of timely, quality medical care.[9]

The leading causes of death in individuals with SCI/D are pneumonia and septicemia.[7] Pneumonia is an infection that inflames the air sacs in one or both lungs.[10] Clients with SCI/D are particularly vulnerable to pneumonia because if their diaphragm, abdominal, and accessory breathing muscles are affected by their level of SCI/D, it will make coughing and taking deep breaths difficult. This makes clearing their lungs of dangerous bacteria difficult. **Sepsis** is a potentially life-threatening complication of an infection that can spread into the bloodstream, causing rampant infection known as **septicemia**.[11] Clients with SCI/D may become septic when they have an existing condition, such as a bladder infection, kidney stone, or bowel impaction, for example. They may not realize or feel they have a problem until the condition is advanced. Clients with SCI/D also experience a higher incidence of secondary complications such as pressure injuries and bladder infections that put them at higher risk for life-threatening septicemia.

Occupational Therapy

A study of QoL 5 years post–medical discharge after traumatic SCI found that participation was the mediating factor between level of impairment and QoL.[12] In other words, the level of SCI/D was not as predictive of QoL as the clients' ability to participate meaningfully in their life. If clients could continue to do the things that were important to them, this mitigated the impact of their SCI/D. OT practitioners guide clients with SCI/D in relearning activities of daily living (ADL) and instrumental activities of daily living (IADL), as well as all other occupations. Use of activities grounded in purposeful and meaningful occupation are also used to build strength, improve endurance and coordination, and promote full engagement. By assessing and understanding the supports and barriers within occupations, client factors, performance skills, and performance patterns, the OT practitioners and client create goals that are congruent with the client's context and environment. Interactions between these domains impact the client's occupational identity, well-being, and participation in life.[13]

NEUROLOGIC CLASSIFICATION OF SPINAL CORD INJURY/DISEASE

An insult to the spinal cord affects the efferent (motor) pathways from the brain to the UEs and LEs as well as the afferent (sensory) pathways from the body to the brain. Think of the spinal cord as an interstate connecting the brain (the capital city) to the states, cities, and small towns, north and south, all along the highway. In this analogy, cars can be used to symbolize neurological signals traveling up and down this highway to deliver information from town to town, city to city, and state to state.

Information traveling north to the capitol carries sensory information. This provides the brain information to process regarding what the body is sensing. Information traveling south from the brain carries motor information. This provides the body with direction to move in a volitional, coordinated, safe, and purposeful movement pattern. When there is an interruption along the highway due to bad weather, traffic congestion, construction, or an accident, cars are slowed down or cannot get through at all. The analogy is similar for SCI/D. If trauma or disease causes an interruption in the flow of information between the brain and the spinal cord, sensory and motor signals cannot reach their destinations. As a result, someone with SCI/D experiences varied degrees of paralysis, loss of somatosensation, and autonomic dysfunction. **Somatosensation** is the body's ability to process information about pain, temperature, touch, and proprioception. The autonomic nervous system controls the body's most basic functions including heart rate, blood pressure, breathing rate, and digestion, and SCI/D can cause **autonomic dysfunction** in many cases.

Complete Versus Incomplete Spinal Cord Injury and Disease

The extent to which the spinal cord is damaged determines the overall physiological impact and function on the individual. A **complete SCI/D** means there is total lack of sensory and motor function preserved in the S4-S5 sacral segments.[14] An **incomplete SCI/D** means there is sensory function and/or partial motor below the level of injury, and includes the S4-S5 sacral segment (anal sensation or voluntary external sphincter motor control).[14] It is now more common for clients to have an incomplete injury of their spinal cord due to advances in emergency and acute management.[15]

Of all individuals with SCI/D, 20% have complete tetraplegia, 32% have incomplete tetraplegia, 27% have complete paraplegia, and 21% have incomplete paraplegia.[16] It is important to remember that clients with SCI/D experience a diverse spectrum of symptoms impacting their lives, and the chapter will address both the symptoms and potential treatment.

The spinal cord is separated into cervical, thoracic, lumbar, and sacral zones. Each section of the cord has control over various muscles and areas of sensation. Figure 35-2 shows the separations and basic functions.

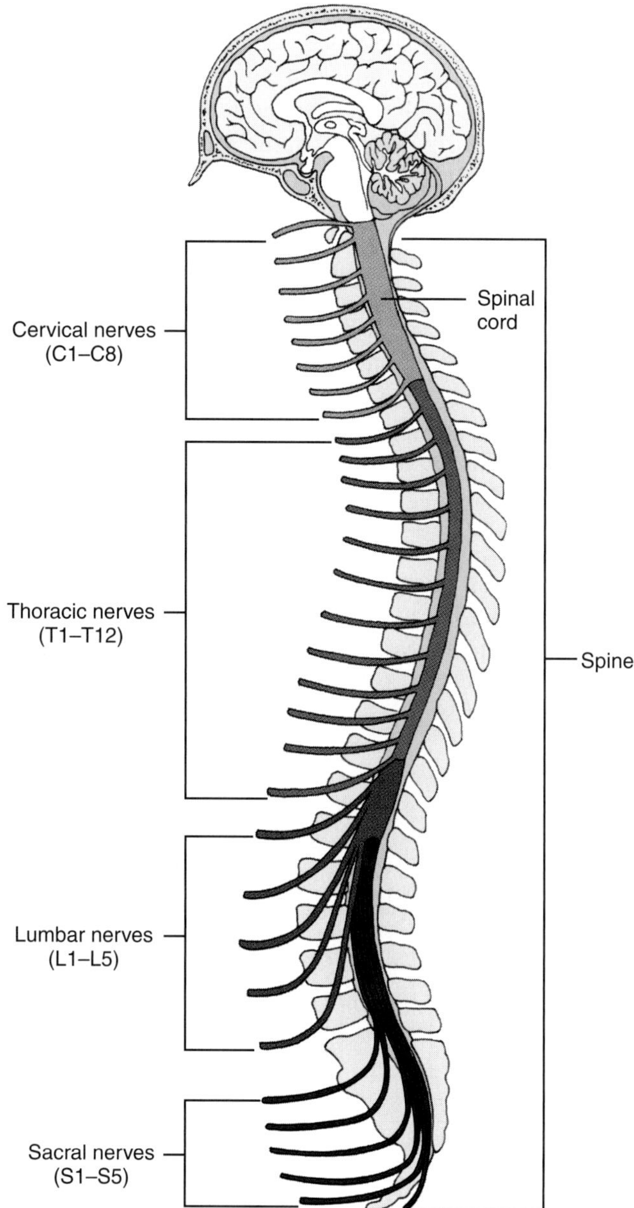

FIGURE 35-2. Spinal cord levels.

The American Spinal Injury Association Impairment Scale

The American Spinal Injury Association (ASIA) has developed a system used to classify SCI/D as complete (ASIA Impairment Scale A) or incomplete (ASIA Impairment Scale B, C, D, or E) (Fig. 35-3). The assessment, the ASIA Impairment Scale (AIS), is based on a test of muscle strength and somatosensation and is used to define two motor, two sensory, and one neurological level.[16] The OTA may hear other healthcare professionals refer to the classification as ASIA A or ASIA B, which is actually incorrect terminology as each component is determined for the right and left side of the body. The motor component of the AIS tests the strength of 10 key muscles in the myotomes between spinal levels C5 and T1, and L2 and S1. A **myotome** is a group of muscles innervated by a single spinal nerve.[17] For example, the C5 myotome includes the biceps and deltoid muscle groups that allow the shoulder and elbow to flex. So, the C5 myotome is tested by assessing bicep strength. The somatosensory component of the AIS tests touch and pin-prick sensation in 28 key dermatomes. A **dermatome** is the area of skin supplied with afferent nerve fibers by a single posterior spinal root. The C5 dermatome is tested in the areas of the medial anterior upper arm over the biceps area, for example. The motor and sensory components of the AIS are then used to derive one overall neurological level for each side.[16]

The assessment is performed by a clinician such as a physician or a physical or occupational therapist. Training in the use of the AIS is mandatory for those completing the assessment.[18]

COMPLETE SPINAL INJURY—ASIA IMPAIRMENT SCALE A

This level (AIS A) of SCI/D indicates there is no motor or sensory function in the S4-S5 segments of the spinal cord, and there is no volitional movement or somatosensation below the level of injury. For example, an individual who has a C5 AIS A SCI/D has voluntary movement of elbow and shoulder flexors and sensation in only the C1-C5 dermatomes. The **zone of partial preservation** is a term used with complete, AIS A individuals who have some level of sparing below the level of injury and above S5.[19,20] For example, a client may have intact motor or sensory from T1-T3, indicating some intact fiber pathways. While highly unlikely, it is not impossible that a client with AIS A would ambulate with long leg braces and assistance; in a review by Morganti and colleagues, 3 out of 117 clients were able to do so.[19] It is more likely that the zone of partial preservation is to a limited sparing such as pin-prick sensation at C7.

INCOMPLETE SPINAL INJURY—ASIA IMPAIRMENT SCALE B, C, D, AND E

Incomplete SCI/D indicates varying levels of motor and sensory function below the level of injury. Figure 35-3 provides specific definitions of each of the AIS levels B, C, D, and E. AIS B indicates the presence of sensation below the level of injury, with AIS C and D indicating sensory and motor function below the level of injury. AIS E indicates normal sensory and motor function.

INCOMPLETE SYNDROMES

Incomplete spinal cord syndromes describe patterns of motor and sensory function with incomplete SCI/D (Table 35-1). OT practitioners must be able to educate clients and their support systems on the functional implications of these patterns. Since patterns of motor and somatosensory function vary among these types of incomplete injuries, they will affect clients' capacities in different ways.

MEDICAL INTERVENTION

Most treatment options for acute traumatic SCI/D are directed at minimizing progression of the initial injury and preventing secondary injury.[22] The ABCDE algorithm of advanced trauma life support includes ensuring stability of airway, breathing, and circulation and minimizing disability and exposure. Cervical collars and backboards are used for spine immobilization in prehospitalization stages. Surgery to stabilize the spine is undertaken after life-threatening injuries have been assessed and treated. Intensive care unit (ICU) admission is considered for all clients with a cervical-level SCI/D or the inability to regulate their blood pressure and heart rate, as well as those with other injuries that independently warrant ICU admission. Avoidance of hypotension (low blood pressure) and **hypoxia** (lack of oxygen) may minimize secondary neurological injury. The use of intravenous steroids to reduce inflammation throughout the body is controversial, but is thought to positively impact overall neurological recovery. Clients with cervical-level SCI/D have compromised respiratory systems because muscles that help them breathe, such as the diaphragm and abdominal muscles, are not fully innervated. Tracheostomy soon after the injury, especially in these clients with injuries above C5, may reduce the number of ventilator days and the incidence of ventilator-associated pneumonia. Devices such as a Cough Assist work to mobilize secretions in the lungs during mechanical ventilation. These devices serve as respiratory assists and exaggerate inhalation and exhalation, creating a rapid change in air pressure that makes coughing more powerful in order to break up mucus in the lungs.[22]

Research suggests that early consultation of an interdisciplinary team to begin mobilization with the client streamlines care and may improve long-term outcomes.[22] The interdisciplinary team involved in a client's early mobilization often includes, but is not limited to, the occupational therapist, OTA, physical therapist, physical therapist assistant, recreational therapist, respiratory therapist, dietitian, and nursing staff. Early mobilization includes facilitating movement in bed through passive range of motion (PROM) and active range of motion (AROM) exercises, training to roll side to side for pressure relief, bed-level ADLs, elevating the head of the bed to accomplish these activities, as well as beginning to work on upright positioning tolerance and transferring to a

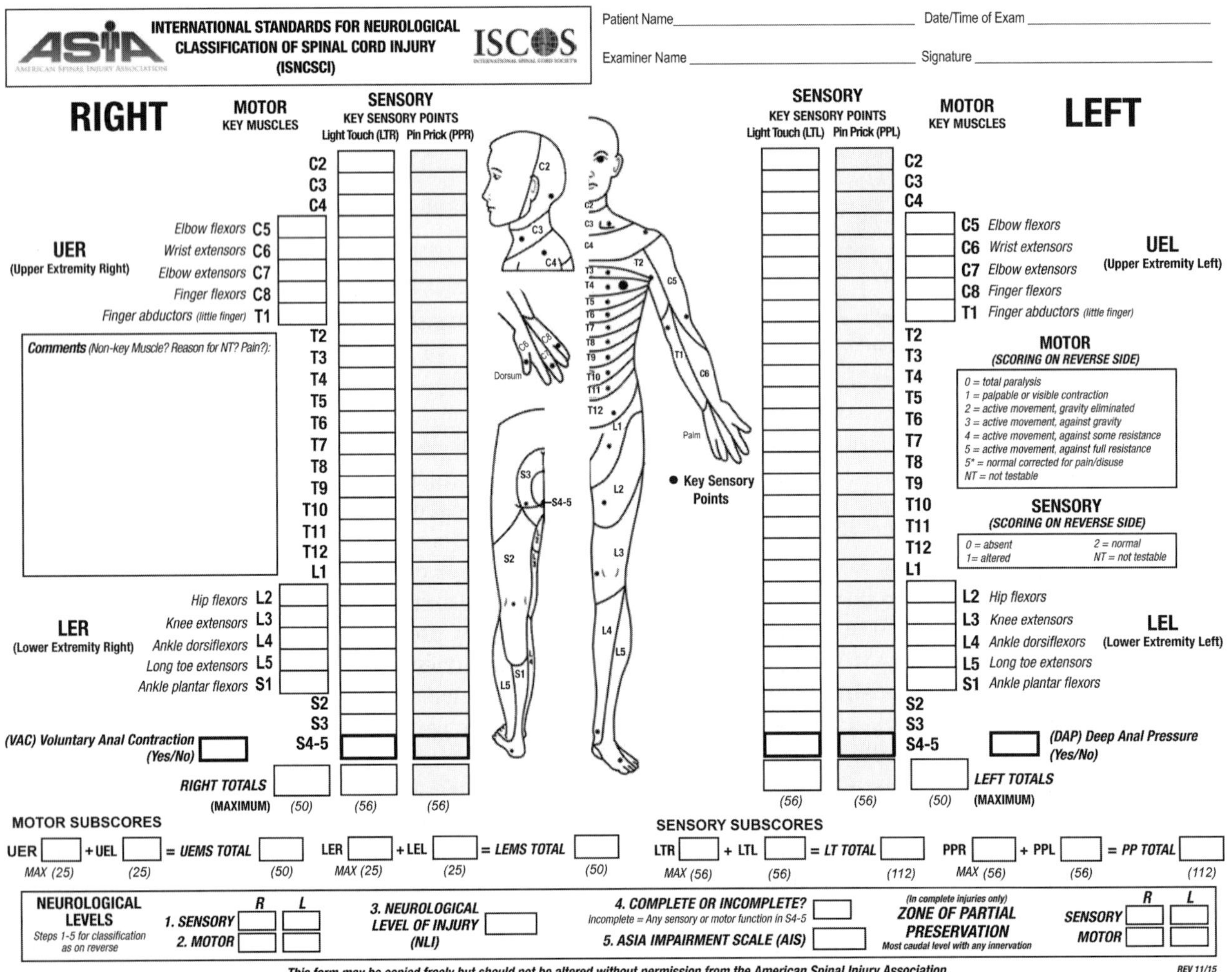
ASIA — AMERICAN SPINAL INJURY ASSOCIATION
INTERNATIONAL STANDARDS FOR NEUROLOGICAL CLASSIFICATION OF SPINAL CORD INJURY (ISNCSCI)
ISCOS — INTERNATIONAL SPINAL CORD SOCIETY

Patient Name______ Date/Time of Exam______
Examiner Name______ Signature______

RIGHT

MOTOR — KEY MUSCLES
SENSORY — KEY SENSORY POINTS — Light Touch (LTR) Pin Prick (PPR)

C2, C3, C4

UER (Upper Extremity Right)
Elbow flexors C5
Wrist extensors C6
Elbow extensors C7
Finger flexors C8
Finger abductors (little finger) T1

Comments (Non-key Muscle? Reason for NT? Pain?):

T2, T3, T4, T5, T6, T7, T8, T9, T10, T11, T12, L1

LER (Lower Extremity Right)
Hip flexors L2
Knee extensors L3
Ankle dorsiflexors L4
Long toe extensors L5
Ankle plantar flexors S1

S2, S3, S4-5

(VAC) Voluntary Anal Contraction (Yes/No)

RIGHT TOTALS (MAXIMUM) (50) (56) (56)

LEFT

SENSORY — KEY SENSORY POINTS — Light Touch (LTL) Pin Prick (PPL)
MOTOR — KEY MUSCLES

C2, C3, C4

UEL (Upper Extremity Left)
C5 Elbow flexors
C6 Wrist extensors
C7 Elbow extensors
C8 Finger flexors
T1 Finger abductors (little finger)

T2, T3, T4, T5, T6, T7, T8, T9, T10, T11, T12, L1

MOTOR (SCORING ON REVERSE SIDE)
0 = total paralysis
1 = palpable or visible contraction
2 = active movement, gravity eliminated
3 = active movement, against gravity
4 = active movement, against some resistance
5 = active movement, against full resistance
5* = normal corrected for pain/disuse
NT = not testable

SENSORY (SCORING ON REVERSE SIDE)
0 = absent 2 = normal
1= altered NT = not testable

LEL (Lower Extremity Left)
L2 Hip flexors
L3 Knee extensors
L4 Ankle dorsiflexors
L5 Long toe extensors
S1 Ankle plantar flexors

S2, S3, S4-5

(DAP) Deep Anal Pressure (Yes/No)

LEFT TOTALS (MAXIMUM) (56) (56) (50)

MOTOR SUBSCORES
UER ☐ + UEL ☐ = UEMS TOTAL ☐ LER ☐ + LEL ☐ = LEMS TOTAL ☐
MAX (25) (25) (50) MAX (25) (25) (50)

SENSORY SUBSCORES
LTR ☐ + LTL ☐ = LT TOTAL ☐ PPR ☐ + PPL ☐ = PP TOTAL ☐
MAX (56) (56) (112) MAX (56) (56) (112)

NEUROLOGICAL LEVELS (Steps 1-5 for classification as on reverse) — R L
1. SENSORY ☐ ☐
2. MOTOR ☐ ☐

3. NEUROLOGICAL LEVEL OF INJURY (NLI) ☐

4. COMPLETE OR INCOMPLETE? ☐
Incomplete = Any sensory or motor function in S4-5
5. ASIA IMPAIRMENT SCALE (AIS) ☐

(In complete injuries only) ZONE OF PARTIAL PRESERVATION — Most caudal level with any innervation — R L
SENSORY ☐ ☐
MOTOR ☐ ☐

This form may be copied freely but should not be altered without permission from the American Spinal Injury Association.

REV 11/15

FIGURE 35-3. The ASIA Assessment.

Muscle Function Grading

0 = total paralysis

1 = palpable or visible contraction

2 = active movement, full range of motion (ROM) with gravity eliminated

3 = active movement, full ROM against gravity

4 = active movement, full ROM against gravity and moderate resistance in a muscle specific position

5 = (normal) active movement, full ROM against gravity and full resistance in a functional muscle position expected from an otherwise unimpaired person

5* = (normal) active movement, full ROM against gravity and sufficient resistance to be considered normal if identified inhibiting factors (i.e. pain, disuse) were not present

NT = not testable (i.e. due to immobilization, severe pain such that the patient cannot be graded, amputation of limb, or contracture of > 50% of the normal ROM)

Sensory Grading

0 = Absent

1 = Altered, either decreased/impaired sensation or hypersensitivity

2 = Normal

NT = Not testable

When to Test Non-Key Muscles:

In a patient with an apparent AIS B classification, non-key muscle functions more than 3 levels below the motor level on each side should be tested to most accurately classify the injury (differentiate between AIS B and C).

Movement	Root level
Shoulder: Flexion, extension, abduction, adduction, internal and external rotation **Elbow:** Supination	C5
Elbow: Pronation **Wrist:** Flexion	C6
Finger: Flexion at proximal joint, extension. **Thumb:** Flexion, extension and abduction in plane of thumb	C7
Finger: Flexion at MCP joint **Thumb:** Opposition, adduction and abduction perpendicular to palm	C8
Finger: Abduction of the index finger	T1
Hip: Adduction	L2
Hip: External rotation	L3
Hip: Extension, abduction, internal rotation **Knee:** Flexion **Ankle:** Inversion and eversion **Toe:** MP and IP extension	L4
Hallux and Toe: DIP and PIP flexion and abduction	L5
Hallux: Adduction	S1

ASIA Impairment Scale (AIS)

A = Complete. No sensory or motor function is preserved in the sacral segments S4-5.

B = Sensory Incomplete. Sensory but not motor function is preserved below the neurological level and includes the sacral segments S4-5 (light touch or pin prick at S4-5 or deep anal pressure) AND no motor function is preserved more than three levels below the motor level on either side of the body.

C = Motor Incomplete. Motor function is preserved at the most caudal sacral segments for voluntary anal contraction (VAC) OR the patient meets the criteria for sensory incomplete status (sensory function preserved at the most caudal sacral segments (S4-S5) by LT, PP or DAP), and has some sparing of motor function more than three levels below the ipsilateral motor level on either side of the body.
(This includes key or non-key muscle functions to determine motor incomplete status.) For AIS C – less than half of key muscle functions below the single NLI have a muscle grade ≥ 3.

D = Motor Incomplete. Motor incomplete status as defined above, with at least half (half or more) of key muscle functions below the single NLI having a muscle grade ≥ 3.

E = Normal. If sensation and motor function as tested with the ISNCSCI are graded as normal in all segments, and the patient had prior deficits, then the AIS grade is E. Someone without an initial SCI does not receive an AIS grade.

Using ND: To document the sensory, motor and NLI levels, the ASIA Impairment Scale grade, and/or the zone of partial preservation (ZPP) when they are unable to be determined based on the examination results.

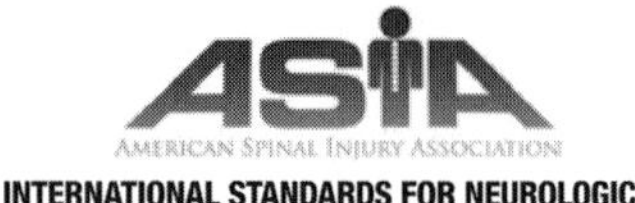

INTERNATIONAL STANDARDS FOR NEUROLOGICAL CLASSIFICATION OF SPINAL CORD INJURY

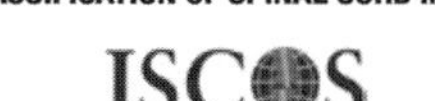

Steps in Classification

The following order is recommended for determining the classification of individuals with SCI.

1. Determine sensory levels for right and left sides.
The sensory level is the most caudal, intact dermatome for both pin prick and light touch sensation.

2. Determine motor levels for right and left sides.
Defined by the lowest key muscle function that has a grade of at least 3 (on supine testing), providing the key muscle functions represented by segments above that level are judged to be intact (graded as a 5).
Note: in regions where there is no myotome to test, the motor level is presumed to be the same as the sensory level, if testable motor function above that level is also normal.

3. Determine the neurological level of injury (NLI)
This refers to the most caudal segment of the cord with intact sensation and antigravity (3 or more) muscle function strength, provided that there is normal (intact) sensory and motor function rostrally respectively.
The NLI is the most cephalad of the sensory and motor levels determined in steps 1 and 2.

4. Determine whether the injury is Complete or Incomplete.
(i.e. absence or presence of sacral sparing)
If voluntary anal contraction = ***No*** *AND all S4-5 sensory scores =* ***0***
AND deep anal pressure = ***No,*** *then injury is* ***Complete.***
Otherwise, injury is ***Incomplete.***

5. Determine ASIA Impairment Scale (AIS) Grade:

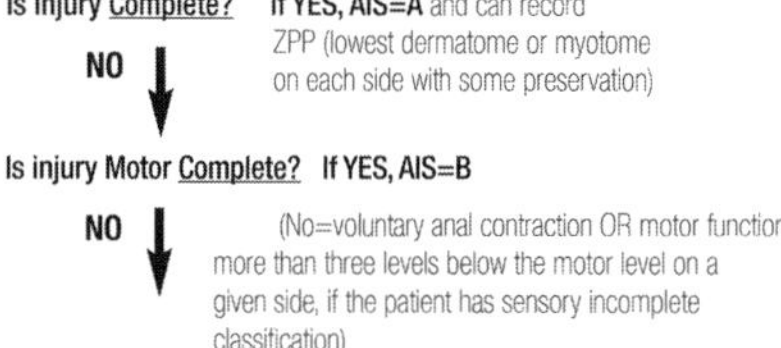

Is injury Complete? **If YES, AIS=A** and can record ZPP (lowest dermatome or myotome on each side with some preservation)

NO ↓

Is injury Motor Complete? **If YES, AIS=B**

NO ↓ (No=voluntary anal contraction OR motor function more than three levels below the motor level on a given side, if the patient has sensory incomplete classification)

Are at least half (half or more) of the key muscles below the neurological level of injury graded 3 or better?

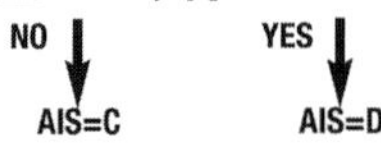

NO ↓ **AIS=C** **YES** ↓ **AIS=D**

If sensation and motor function is normal in all segments, AIS=E
Note: AIS E is used in follow-up testing when an individual with a documented SCI has recovered normal function. If at initial testing no deficits are found, the individual is neurologically intact; the ASIA Impairment Scale does not apply.

FIGURE 35-3.—continued

wheelchair, with a lift or transfer board. It is critical for team members to have clearance from the client's physician before beginning mobilization and to understand and be prepared to address symptoms from autonomic instability/dysfunction (specifically addressed later).

An example of early mobilization is Brooke, a 18-year-old girl who sustained a T2 incomplete SCI/D after a tumor removed from her spinal cord left her temporarily unable to feel or move her legs or to sit without assistance. The occupational therapist evaluates Brooke in the step-down unit, and after confirming with her medical team determines it is appropriate for Brooke and her family to begin progressively elevating the head of her bed. The occupational therapist also recommends performing PROM exercises on her legs, performing AROM in her upper body, and completing functional tasks. The ability to be active and begin taking care of herself will mean a lot to Brooke, including grooming and using her smartphone to communicate with friends, which can be done with the head of the bed elevated. The OTA has demonstrated competence in this area of early SCI/D mobilization and works with Brooke and her family to help them understand the importance of and techniques for early mobilization strategies, all while communicating progress back to the interdisciplinary team as they work with Brooke toward similar goals.

External Fixators and Orthotics

Some clients with SCI/D will require an external fixator called a halo instead of surgery to repair a cervical fracture. A halo is composed of a ring of metal drilled into the skull with screws, and attached down-posts that hook to a rigid, lightweight fleece-lined vest that straps to the torso (Fig. 35-4) Typically clients wear the halo for 12 weeks with weekly checkups if home, and daily care if in the hospital or rehabilitation center. About 60% of clients will experience pin loosening that requires the physician to tighten, and 10% to 20% of clients will develop pin site infections.[23] Some clients are able to ambulate with the halo, although balance may be affected for a short period. Clients cannot drive with the halo, and should not get any portion of the vest wet to avoid localized skin issues. Clients and caregivers will be taught care for the pin sites and how to care for skin under the vest, typically by nursing staff.

Some clients will have a thoracolumbosacral orthosis (TLSO), which is a rigid spinal orthosis that spans the thoracic, lumbar, and sacral spine, and is used to provide post-traumatic

TABLE 35-1 Incomplete Spinal Cord Syndromes

NAME	SYMPTOMS	FUNCTIONAL ISSUES
Anterior cord syndrome: Damage to front of spinal cord	Loss/decrease pain, temperature below injury level, touch, vibration, proprioception relatively spared	Essentially this client presents as an AIS B (sensory incomplete). They tend to progress a little quicker with therapy goals because proprioception and light touch are intact.
Central cord syndrome: Damage to middle of spinal cord	Loss of arm function, some leg function may be preserved as well as bowel/bladder	Generally, this client has significantly more impairment in the UEs than the LEs. The degree of impairment varies. Spasticity is often an issue. Many of these clients do better with lower body ADLs than upper body ADLs because they have the balance to lean forward and reach down, but UE weakness limits upward reaching. Bladder function is often impaired but has the potential for recovery.
Posterior cord syndrome: Damage to back of spinal cord	Good muscle power, pain and temperature, decreased muscle coordination	Functional performance for all ADLs can be impacted due to poor motor control.
Brown-Séquard syndrome: Damage to one side of spinal cord	Loss/decrease of muscle power with intact pain/temperature on one side, opposite on the other side	In many ways this client appears to have hemiplegia, but sensory awareness on each side of the body is different. Level of injury is going to affect specific impairments. Safety education is critical since the side with active movement most likely has minimal pain/temperature awareness.
Cauda equina syndrome: Damage to cauda equina	Partial to complete loss of movement/sensation below level of injury	This client will typically progress quickly with seated-level ADLs, but will have difficulty with dynamic standing balance, standing-level ADLs, and IADLs.[21]

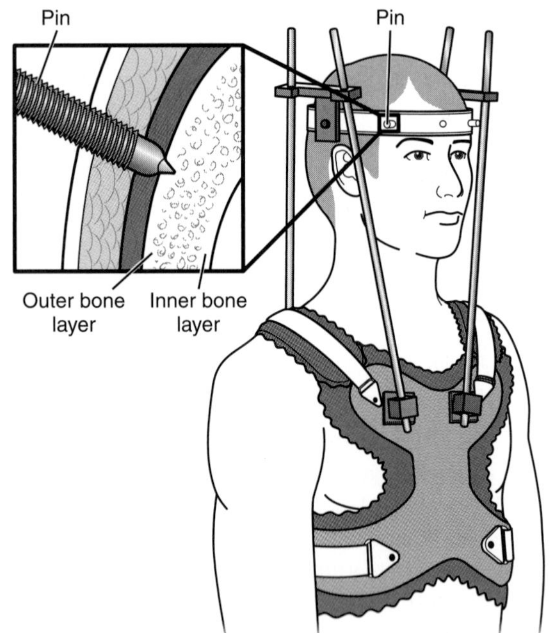

FIGURE 35-4. Halo external fixator and vest.

and post-surgical stabilization.[24] It generally stabilizes from T5-L4 (may stabilize to S5), is custom made into two pieces like a clamshell, and has a soft inner lining. The TLSO is often used to provide nonoperative management of more complex or multilevel fractures.[24] The duration of wear is typically up to 3 months. The client is not allowed out of bed without the TLSO, and must log-roll without twisting or bending the spine to be moved or move in the bed.

Clients may also be required to wear a restrictive and supportive cervical collar for cervical immobilization. The wearing schedule may be 24/7 or only worn when out of bed. The most frequently prescribed rigid collars are the Aspen®, Malibu, Miami J, and Philadelphia® collars, and all these can be used with additional chest and head extension pieces to increase stability.[25] In general, most collars do not provide a significant amount of restriction of motion and can show variability depending on fit and consistency of use.

IMPACT OF SPINAL CORD INJURY AND DISEASE ON BODY FUNCTIONS

OT practitioners provide skilled intervention to address the multitude of lifelong secondary complications and conditions resulting from SCI/D. This next section summarizes the health implications of SCI/D and how OT supports the QoL of people living with SCI/D. Complications resulting from SCI/D impact body functions. It is important for OTAs to understand the functional implications of these changes and integrate this understanding into clinical reasoning. This section also focuses on the education and training areas of intervention because this is a keystone of SCI/D rehabilitation.

Mental Functions

Mental health includes a client's psychological and emotional well-being as well as social and cognitive function. When a client's mental well-being is compromised, challenges occur and put the body at risk.

DEPRESSION AND MOTIVATION

A higher prevalence of psychological comorbidity (departure from a state of well-being) occurs in individuals with SCI/D compared with the general population.[26] This psychological comorbidity has been studied in the acute and rehabilitation phases as well as in the chronic stages when clients have returned to their communities. It has been suggested that levels of depression, anxiety, and/or stress remain substantially higher in people with chronic SCI/D than in the general population,[27] and that both personal and injury factors play a role.[28] One study found that people who had a history of depression or substance abuse or who had more permanent neurological impairment were at higher risk for depression after their SCI/D.[28] Factors that have been associated with post-SCI/D depression include past coping mechanisms, premorbid personality, social situations, degree of paralysis, age, education level, substance abuse, perceived level of social support, and locus of control.[16,28]

Psychological and emotional distress affects clients' capacity to engage in the rehabilitation process, retain SCI/D education and training, and envision outcomes that will positively impact their ability to function in daily activities in a meaningful and purposeful way post-rehabilitation. OT practitioners work with clients and family members to facilitate meaningful participation as a way of fostering mental health. If research demonstrates that QoL and mental health are related to participation, it would follow that bridging the gap between disability and function through adapted participation is the expertise of the OT practitioner. As OT practitioners teach and train clients to participate again in meaningful activities as well as develop roles and routines around these activities, the result is encouraging positive mental health.

OT practitioners must also communicate and collaborate closely with mental health specialists to promote clients' coping skills. Access to mental health providers will vary depending on the setting. OT practitioners naturally fit with rehabilitation counselors, neuropsychologists, pastoral staff, and social workers regarding goals for coping mechanisms and helping to paint a future of mental, emotional, physical, and spiritual health and success. In the inpatient rehabilitation setting, it is relatively easy to communicate in a team atmosphere in which the client and family are actively engaged with the interdisciplinary team on a daily or weekly basis. As clients move into community settings along the continuum of care, this collaboration can be more challenging. It will take initiative by and commitment from the OT practitioner and mental health providers to address a client's ongoing mental health and wellness issues.

The *Occupational Therapy Practice Framework: Domain and Process, 3rd edition* (OTPF-3) defines emotional well-being as regulation and range of emotions; appropriateness and lability of emotions.[7] Clients may turn to a range of healthy and unhealthy coping mechanisms. "The individual with the SCI as well as their friends, family, and community members all struggle to find coping mechanisms as they go through the grieving process. They may experience anger, grief, despondency, denial, depression, and apathy. The incidence of ongoing depression appears to be strongly linked to restrictions in participation."[16] It is important that OT practitioners do not mistake a client who is struggling to adapt for a client who is "unmotivated" or lacks determination for rehabilitation.[16] In fact, OT practitioners can be clients' strongest advocates in communicating the impact of psychosocial stressors on the rehabilitation course.

SCI/D and occupational science research also demonstrate that the context, environment, and personal factors that shape clients' lives will impact their rehabilitation course and ultimately their QoL. Clients with SCI/D identify positive thinking (e.g., optimism, hope, and positive attitude), perseverance and determination, and social support from friends and family as important contributors to their ability to adapt in spite of experiencing traumatic events that resulted in SCI.[29] OT practitioners can educate and engage clients' social support network throughout the therapy process to create a shared vision of participation and wellness.

FATIGUE

Physiological, psychological, and environmental factors affect an individual's perceptions of energy level. Acutely, persistent pain, antispasmodic medications, constant waking for turning and vital checks, demanding therapy sessions, and psychosocial adjustment contribute to fatigue early on. As clients return to the community, pain and medications may continue to contribute to fatigue, and reintegration into daily activities and routines contributes to psychosocial and physiological fatigue. Activities that once were second nature now consume more energy. OT practitioners play an important role in education and training before discharge into the community and upon reintegration into the community.

COGNITION: DUAL DIAGNOSIS WITH TRAUMATIC BRAIN INJURY

Up to 40% to 50% of individuals with SCI/D also have a concomitant brain injury.[6] This may impact the client's ability to achieve his or her maximal levels of function due to barriers with higher-level cognitive functions, attention, memory, and sequencing of complex movements.[7] Often, OT practitioners may be the first to notice a difficulty in retaining and transferring information from one therapy session to another and along the rehabilitation course in general. It is the practitioner's responsibility to notify the physician and rehabilitation team of a suspected issue. A comorbid brain injury often means close collaboration with other team members and family to ensure the education is being carried over and reinforced by a variety of methods including in verbal, visual, demonstration, and written forms.

One longitudinal study found that individuals who experienced a comorbid traumatic brain injury actually had similar outcomes to matched comparison groups with either only SCI or only traumatic brain injury.[30] They

OT Practitioner's Viewpoint

Often, working with a client with SCI/D means constant reassessment of goals and priorities, especially during inpatient rehabilitation when client factors, performance skills, and performance patterns are so dynamic. As an example, Damion was shot in the neck during an altercation in his neighborhood, resulting in a C6 AIS D SCI/D. He had severe pain and weakness throughout the right (dominant) side of his body, and increasing strength and sensation in the left side of his body. His trunk control was poor, and he struggled with spasticity that was relatively controlled on oral antispasmodics. He had neurogenic bowel and bladder and required intermittent self-catheterization and a nightly bowel program. In the first half of Damion's stay on inpatient rehabilitation, his goal was to move out of state to his father-in-law's home where he would have the physical assistance of his father-in-law and also continue outpatient rehabilitation. At this time, Damion's wife was unable to provide physical lifting assistance due to a medical condition. Our goals were on course with this discharge plan for him to be able to transfer with assistance from his power wheelchair to a transfer tub bench (TTB) to bathe. His father-in-law practiced these transfers and the bathing process from bed level to TTB on a weekly basis with OT. As Damion's discharge approached, he, his wife, and the rehabilitation team determined that traveling out of state at this point in his recovery was not recommended. Discharge to Damion's mother's home was the next best option. Damion's relationship with his mother had always been strained, and during family training he struggled with trusting his mother to safely transfer him as well as to perform such intimate tasks as bathing and bowel program when his wife was unavailable. After in-depth discussion with Damion and the rehabilitation team, I revised Damion's goals such that he would be performing bathing at the bed level, where he could safely bathe himself. This would be his strategy until he grew strong enough to transfer into the shower without requiring physical assistance. Initially, this transition felt to me as if we were regressing in terms of functional goals, however, this new goal reflected Damion's need to feel secure and independent in a potentially turbulent home environment.

Damion's story illustrates the point that intervention plans are dynamic and reflect the ever-changing experiences of our clients. We must be prepared to meet our clients where they are. When contexts, environments, and activity demands change, so too must our plan of care. ~ Raheleh G. Tschoepe, MS, OT/L

attributed this unexpected outcome to the fact that individuals in their study who had dual diagnoses were afforded longer rehabilitation stays. These stays may have provided them the opportunity to learn adaptations to participation resulting in better outcomes on measures such as the Functional Independence Measure (FIM).

It is critical, therefore, that OT practitioners are aware of the impact of concomitant traumatic brain injury on short- and long-term SCI rehabilitation since the client's ability to follow directions, attend, and remember are critical cognitive functions in learning new and adaptive skills. See Chapter 11 for further information and treatment for cognitive challenges, and Chapter 34 on brain injury.

Sensory and Skin Functions

The integumentary system serves to protect the body and act as the initial point of contact of sensory information of touch, pressure, temperature, and pain, and also is responsible for producing sweat to cool the body. When the skin's functions are compromised, challenges occur and put the body at risk.

SKIN INTEGRITY

Think about sitting at a dining room table, desk, car seat, plane seat, and movie theater seat. How long can a person sit in one place before feeling the need to reposition an arm, foot, or leg, or change the posture? The body's ability to sense discomfort and communicate it to the brain is a vital capacity that people with SCI/D often lose, placing them at high risk for inability to feel pain and adjust accordingly. Without active movement, these clients often have compromised circulation throughout their bodies, leaving them prone to pressure injuries. Skin breakdown is the number one reason for hospital readmission in individuals with SCI/D. Skin is the body's largest organ and is what protects the body from infection. The Consortium of Spinal Cord Medicine Pressure Ulcer Prevention and Treatment Clinical Practice Guidelines notes that individuals with SCI/D have a reduced blood supply and reduced blood flow below the level of injury.[31] Also, clients with cervical levels of injury can have cardiovascular insufficiency, placing them at an especially high risk for pressure injuries.

The combination of poor sensation, muscle weakness, and decreased circulation make susceptibility to skin breakdown highly likely. Addressing skin integrity is a critical interdisciplinary effort, and OT practitioners are skilled in addressing this topic from the perspective of habits, routines, rituals, and roles. OT practitioners teach pressure relief strategies, provide critical skin care education, and integrate pressure relief schedules into an individual's activities and routines. This process of habit formation and routine building begins during the inpatient rehabilitation stay and continues as the client reintegrates and works to find a new normal. Skin care habits and routines will change as clients' contexts change over time and as they age. Including this education in anticipation of such change over time is an important part of SCI/D education and training between the OT practitioner and their clients and families.

Bony areas such as (but not limited to) the ischial tuberosities, sacrum, hips, heels, skull, and ankles are especially susceptible to breakdown because they lack adipose tissue protection. Also, people with SCI/D typically lie in bed and sit in wheelchairs, which means these body parts are in constant contact with unforgiving surfaces. Teaching pressure relief is a vital role for OT practitioners to help clients avoid pressure injuries, infection, and potentially death. Throughout this book, the older terms of "pressure sores" and "pressure ulcers" have been changed to the updated term "pressure injuries".

Education about how functional mobility affects skin care includes providing a general understanding of the physiological responses to prolonged sitting or lying and applying pressure relief strategies across mobility contexts including during seated and lying activities as well as when transferring from one surface to another. Applying pressure relief strategies will include:

- Power and manual wheelchair use with use of power seat functions, including tilt, recline, and elevating center mount leg platform
- Use and protection of upper extremities (UEs) for performing pressure relief
- Understanding how to move, roll, and transition from supine to sitting and sitting to supine
- Understanding how to move body parts across various surfaces correctly such as when in a hospital or standard bed, on the commode, transferring to a sofa, dining room chair, booth in a restaurant or in/out of a car

Establishing hygiene habits such as ensuring cleanliness after self-catheterization, bowel program, sexual activity, and physical activity to ensure dry and intact skin versus wet or soiled skin, which tends to break down quickly, will be vital. It is important to teach clients to move their body parts to access areas that may be difficult to see in plain view and to use skin inspection mirrors as well as to direct family and care staff about thorough and frequent skin inspection.

It is important for clients with SCI/D to develop a routine that includes skin check habits and pressure relief options. It may be especially effective for OT practitioners to instill these habits early on during ADL retraining, when clients can learn how to streamline their routines to maximize endurance and minimize effort. This can be done while simultaneously learning to integrate their skin care routine and minimize external forces that may put their skin at risk during these ADL routines.

PAIN

Pain is unfortunately very common in the aftermath of SCI/D. It may be acute and temporary or chronic, lasting more than 6 months to 1 year. It is a barrier with which the client must cope on a daily basis.[32] The three common types of pain post SCI/D include mechanical pain, radicular pain, and central pain. **Mechanical pain** is local soft-tissue pain associated with the injury; it is common in traumatic cases in which bones and soft tissue were compromised. It is also common when the SCI/D has caused weakness in a muscle group, leading to dysfunction of an extremity. Mechanical pain is common in the shoulders of clients with tetraplegia because disruption of the **scapulohumeral rhythm** (coordination between the scapula and humerus). This can develop because of overuse, impingement, propelling a manual wheelchair, weight-bearing for transfers or pressure relief, and/or hooking an arm over the wheelchair handle for stability, leading to imbalance and pain with movement. **Radicular pain** is often described as a shooting or burning sensation that often follows the distribution of the nerve. **Central pain** (also called neurogenic or neuropathic pain) originates in the spinal cord and is thought to be the result of misdirected neural sprouting after the injury.

Pain continues to be a complication for most clients after SCI/D with implications for occupational performance, emotional well-being, and QoL. Pain becomes chronic after 6 months when it is unresponsive to any intervention, and may evolve into a barrier and pervade the client's life.[6] Pain negatively impacts perceived cognitive, emotional, and physical functioning and QoL after SCI/D.[33]

The importance of pain management lies in understanding that there are many different causes of pain as well as pharmacological and nonpharmacological strategies to address them. It is important to be aware that psychosocial and environmental factors contribute to the perception and experience of pain. These factors include, among others, mood, cognition, relationships, and job satisfaction.[34] OT practitioners observe contexts in which pain is a barrier to participation and work with clients and their support networks to mitigate these contributing factors.

Researchers have demonstrated approaches that individuals with physical disabilities can use to manage anticipated and unexpected pain, specifically by occupation prioritization through energy conservation and work simplification strategies.[34] OTAs can apply this evidence to interventions with clients with SCI/D. Education and training on preventing pain as much as possible includes employing an exercise regimen of stretching, strengthening or cardio workouts, maintaining a healthy routine of exercise, diet, and sleep, and avoiding stress. In addition, OTAs can teach clients with SCI/D how to prioritize their daily activities including planned rest times and opportunities for physical, emotional, and mental restoration.[34]

Wheelchair seating and positioning is another area of opportunity for addressing pain management. If the client uses wheeled mobility full time or even part time, OT and PT seating specialists are experts in assessing whether the seating and positioning components such as the wheelchair cushion, back support, headrest, and other components are contributing to or could relieve pain symptoms, and clients should be referred for seating evaluations as appropriate (see Chapter 15 for further details). Similar characteristics can be assessed with bed positioning, bathing and toileting equipment, and leisure and recreation equipment. For example, some beds are semielectric with standard mattresses, yet others have low air-loss mattresses for increased pressure relief. The rehabilitation team should assess which is most appropriate functionally and medically as well as identify the insurance coverage criteria for various options. OT practitioners should also apply clinical reasoning to selection of bathing and toileting equipment, taking into account characteristics between equipment that minimizes pain and maximizes function and safety. Rolling shower commodes that tilt, have padded surfaces, swing-away arms and legrests, and a cutout for the bowel program provide very different support for pressure relief than standard plastic bedside commodes.

Observation of daily activity and applying principles of ergonomics, work simplification, and energy conservation to these particular activities and to daily routines can make a significant impact on the contributing factors of pain. Observing the number of times and the manner in which someone with paraplegia transfers from bed to wheelchair during a morning dressing routine will provide the OT practitioner insight into a potential risk for a painful upper extremity (UE) repetitive strain injury. Similarly, analyzing a meal preparation process for a client with a C7 SCI/D may lead the OTA to provide recommendations for ergonomic setup of his or her kitchen and cooking tools to improve environmental access and task efficiencies.

Interventions that strengthen the client's belief in his or her own abilities to manage pain are an important component of therapy.[34] OT practitioners have the skill set to empower clients with these tools for a greater sense of control and efficacy in managing their pain.

SENSITIVITY TO TEMPERATURE

Often clients with SCI/D have difficulty regulating body temperature due to poor blood circulation and autonomic dysfunction causing decreased ability to manage body temperature via sweating and shivering. Clients with SCI/D typically do not sweat or shiver below the level of injury, and some clients with high level tetraplegia do not sweat above the injury either. This leaves them prone to hypothermia or overheating. In addition, clients are prone to frostbite and sunburn due to compromised somatosensation. OT education should emphasize strategies to maintain neutral body temperatures and prevent harm to the skin from extreme temperature environments. Having awareness of the outside and inside temperature and humidity will be important. OTAs educate clients on layering clothing in cold climates and being vigilantly aware of where insensate areas of their body may come into contact with hot surfaces in warmer climates.

Muscle Functions

The normal function of muscles is interrupted by SCI/D due to the interruption of the neuronal pathways. Muscles may not receive the message to contract (flaccid muscles), or may receive repeated messages with no information returning to the brain, resulting in abnormally high muscle tone (spasticity or spasms).

SPASTICITY

Spasticity, also called spastic hypertonia, can be defined as disordered sensorimotor control, resulting from an upper motor neuron (UMN) lesion, presenting as intermittent or sustained

THE OLDER ADULT

WHAT CAUSES SCI/D IN OLDER ADULTS?

SCI/D is typically associated with younger adult populations. The same mechanisms of injury that cause spinal injury in younger populations also affect older adults. However, older adults more often experience SCI/D related to degenerative aging processes leading to cervical spinal stenosis and as a result of falling and injuring their necks.

HOW DOES SCI/D PRESENT DIFFERENTLY IN OLDER ADULTS THAN IN YOUNGER ADULTS?

Because of the mechanisms of spinal injury, older adults are especially prone to the central cord syndrome type of incomplete SCI. Central cord syndrome is caused by injury to the central part of the spinal cord, and because of the way the spinal tracts are organized, causes weakness disproportionately in the UEs and trunk more than the LEs. Strength also typically returns in the LEs before the UEs. The resulting pattern of functional return is that older adults are often walking before they regain the ability to use their UEs, which limits their ability to care for themselves and to resume caregiving roles.

HOW IS REHABILITATION FROM SCI/D UNIQUE FOR OLDER ADULTS?

Older adults experience sensory, motor, cardiovascular, respiratory, digestive, genitourinary, and mental function changes associated with aging. Some of these changes include a decline in vision, hearing, muscle and bone strength, joint flexibility, and cognition. These age-related declines in body functions impact motor and process skills, and the capacity for rehabilitation. Taking into account their preexisting chronic conditions within the complexities of acute SCI/D creates a picture of a complex path to rehabilitation and return to previous performance patterns and meaningful occupation. Rehabilitation is often a longer course for older adults that extends from the acute inpatient hospital setting to long-term care settings. The client's health insurance guidelines dictate the extent and length of time therapy services are provided in these settings. Case managers help clients and their caregivers navigate these complex issues.

HOW DO CONTEXT AND ENVIRONMENT IMPACT OLDER ADULTS LIVING WITH SCI/D?

Older adult partners often assume the role of caregiver as they and their loved ones age. As caregivers, they are an invaluable part of the care recipient's context and social environment. This can be a gradual process as partners age and benefit from increasing assistance in all areas of occupation. Changes resulting from SCI/D however typically occur as a sudden, dramatic change. The resulting functional challenges require a significant shift and increase in the type and level of caregiving responsibilities. The aging partner may not themselves have the physical, cognitive, and emotional capacity to fulfill this new level of caregiving duty. In yet another scenario, the caregiving partner may experience SCI/D and now both the caregiver and the care recipient are in a difficult predicament. The interdisciplinary team's role in all scenarios is to work with the older adult client and their support network to examine the available resources in planning the way ahead.

THE OLDER ADULT (continued)

CONSIDERATIONS FOR OCCUPATIONAL THERAPY

Rehabilitation from the impact of SCI/D can be a long and challenging road. The SCI/D OT intervention illustrated throughout this chapter also applies to older adults experiencing SCI/D, however OT practitioners should be sensitive to the implications of experiencing such traumatic change late in life. At a time when there may already be limited physiological and cognitive reserve, older adults benefit from dialogue and relationship throughout the rehabilitation continuum. Focus must be on providing understanding of the process and on providing continual hope and support during the treatment planning process. OTAs can encourage reflection of meaning in the older client's previous life experiences and to also find purpose in their current and future experiences living with SCI/D. Occupational therapists and OTAs will likely set OT goals and scaffold interventions more conservatively than for a younger client.

OTAs work closely with the interdisciplinary team as they also provide education and training to the older caregiving partners of clients with SCI/D. The team must take into account the caregiver's capacities and the caregiving context and environment and include relevant supports and resources for the discharge plan. For instance, it would be safer for both a 75-year-old client with a C6 AIS C SCI/D and her 77-year-old spouse to use a lift for transfers in and out of the power wheelchair. If the client, her spouse, and the rehabilitation team decided it was safe to plan for discharge home, the OTA and other team members would heavily emphasize mobility training and education using the lift in preparation for going home.

A NEW MEMBER OF THE REHABILITATION TEAM

In addition to the team members listed in the "Meet the Team" box, the client's **geriatrician** will be a key member of the team, especially as the client transitions from the acute hospital to the outpatient setting. A geriatrician is a physician who specializes in the medical care of older adults. They collaborate with the interdisciplinary rehabilitation team providing expertise in aging-related considerations.

involuntary activation of muscle.[35] Typically, the spinal cord is in spinal shock with no reflexes or increased tone for the first few weeks to months, then reflex activity returns. About 65% to 78% of clients with SCI/D will experience spasticity to varying degrees, and the length of time symptoms last can be weeks to months or for a lifetime. The spasticity can manifest with these clients as sudden involuntary movements in muscles, hyperactive reflexes, and involuntary muscle tightness (spasms).[36] Most clients with SCI/D will have spasticity, although those with cervical or incomplete injuries are more likely than those with paraplegia or with complete injuries.[37] Spasticity is primarily managed by medication and positioning for the SCI/D population. Medications include those that act on the central nervous system and those that act at the level of the muscle itself or neuromuscular junction peripherally. Physicians may recommend **intrathecal** spasticity medication, which is delivered directly to the spinal cord via a pump, in cases of severe spasticity that inhibits function, jeopardizes safety, and causes significant pain.

OT intervention for spasticity is complex and requires client-centered, interdisciplinary care and clinical reasoning.[38] OT practitioners may use bracing, orthotics, and casting to passively lengthen the spastic muscle and its tendons. Functional electrical stimulation has also shown effectiveness when combined with functional practice and bracing in some clients with UE spasticity.[6] Research has shown the benefits of this combined modality therapy in clients with UE spasticity as a result of neurological deficit. OTAs employ these spasticity management strategies and teach clients and their caregivers the most effective combinations. Strategies may include using rhythmic passive movements, consistent passive muscle stretch, and active exercise. Spasticity may also respond to various physical agent modalities for which they are indicated. These modalities include moist heat, ice, and electrical stimulation (see Chapter 18). OT's educational role in nonpharmacological spasticity management is important because spasticity can lead to contracture, pain, and skin breakdown. It also can make volitional movement, care provider–assisted movement, and self-care difficult. Clients may have LE spasticity that may make transfers less safe, make it difficult to sleep, and make wheelchair mobility difficult; some clients have reported being nearly knocked out of their manual wheelchairs by spasms. Some clients do, however, use their spasticity functionally for transfers, dressing, and to increase circulation.[37] The OT practitioner will teach the client to manage spasticity during ADL, IADL, and mobility tasks. As mentioned earlier, an intrathecal Baclofen pump can be surgically placed to manage spasticity with direct application of Baclofen to the spine without the side effects of the oral medication. Clients should be educated on how to note changes in their spasticity type or frequency and inform their physician, because it may herald an infection or pressure injury.[37] Competence in spasticity management includes a holistic understanding of the client, empowering the client in the decision-making process, and recognizing the complexity and diversity of clients living with spasticity.[38]

Musculoskeletal and Movement-Related Functions

Clients with SCI/D are at risk for UE pain and injury because there is an increased reliance on the shoulders, elbows, wrists, and hands with LE paralysis. The Consortium for Spinal Cord Medicine recommends beginning education and training about risks and ways to prevent problems in the acute phase of recovery as UE pain and injury can lead to pervasive challenges with self-care, functional mobility, and all areas of IADLs.[39]

OT practitioners should emphasize strategies for preservation of UE structures and function through all facets of intervention. These strategies include the ergonomics of transfers and wheelchair-propulsion techniques; equipment selection, training, and environmental adaptations; and exercise.[39]

Ergonomic strategies for preventing UE pain and injury include minimizing the force and frequency of UE tasks as well as minimizing extreme joint positions during functional mobility and activities.[39] OTAs educate and train their clients to find comfortable positions in their wheelchairs during rest and sleep that avoid direct pressure on shoulders and distribute support. Education and training of the support network is necessary to avoid pulling on the client's arms when providing physical assistance. OTAs observe their clients using mobility equipment and provide recommendations for performing activities, adapting equipment, and modifying the environment in ways to put less strain and pressure on UE joints. This might include a power wheelchair or power assist wheels on a manual wheelchair for longer distances, or a tub bench instead of a shower seat for a less intense transfer. Attention to the client's access of the physical environment can be important, such as ramps being less steep at one inch of rise for every foot of length or the front door on the home requiring a low amount of force to open. Clients benefit from strategies to avoid UE pain and strain during transfer training. The Consortium recommends that all clients who can transfer themselves use a transfer-assist device such as a transfer board to decrease strain through the UEs. Finally, OTAs can work with physical therapy (PT) colleagues to incorporate ROM and strengthening exercises and activities into daily routines to improve clients' UE flexibility and strength.[39]

NEUROGENIC HETEROTOPIC OSSIFICATION

Neurogenic heterotopic ossification (nHO) is pathological bone formation in joints caused by central nervous system damage or insult and has an incidence of greater than 50% of people with SCI/D.[40] The OTA may also hear the term heterotopic ossification (HO), which is the term generally used for the bone formation with traumatic damage such as with burns or accidents. nHO is mostly seen in the affected joints at or below the level of injury for people with SCI/D and most often in the hip, knees, elbows, and shoulder joints. It involves bone material building in the connective tissue around the joint which then causes limited ROM and contracture. Onset of nHO usually occurs within 1 month to several months' post-injury.[32] Risk factors for nHO include prolonged immobilization, muscle spasticity, and long hospital length of stay.[32] Symptoms include fever, increase in spasticity, warm and swollen extremity, and/or ROM limitations. Some of these signs are similar to symptoms of deep vein thrombosis (DVT) and fracture. Diagnosis is made by ultrasound, CT scan, and/or blood tests. The etiology of nHO is uncertain, however in animal studies it has been shown to develop after repeated and aggressive passive movements of immobilized joints. It is prudent, therefore, for clients, their caregivers, and family members to employ gentle stretching into the home program and for the OT practitioner to educate them to be aware of signs or symptoms that stretching is overly aggressive.

Typically, nHO is managed with pharmacological measures and in extreme cases with surgery. Surgery can be risky, creating complications, and is thought to exacerbate the condition. It is only undergone when the condition is thought to have stabilized after 1 to 2 years of onset and when function and QoL are negatively impacted.[6] It is important that OTAs are aware of nHO symptoms as therapy practitioners are often the first providers to recognize this condition when it is adversely affecting functional performance. Also, OT practitioners are experts in providing adaptive ways of coping with the limitations brought about by decreased ROM and resulting challenges in functional mobility and self-care activities.

OT and PT practitioners have significant roles in nHO management.[27] While the nHO is medically managed, OT practitioners can provide recommendations for positioning to minimize pain and discomfort. Clients with nHO also benefit from adaptive equipment training when limited LE or UE ROM inhibits positioning and reach. OT practitioners in a specialty seating clinic can reassess for wheelchair positioning and seating options. Other interventions should include education on indications or contraindications to stretching, depending on the stage of nHO progression and on the methods of medical management such as medication management within the setting of clients' daily routines. Clients who have undergone surgical and medical management for nHO often undergo extensive rehabilitation as they learn to adapt, function, and receive education and training on possible strategies for nHO recurrence.[40]

PERFORMING OCCUPATIONS WITH FIXATORS AND ORTHOTICS

Clients with a halo fixator will require numerous adaptations by the OT practitioner. Clothing will need to have a button/zip front to go around the brace, and an undershirt split at the top seams that can go under the vest. Hair washing is typically a dry-rub shampoo, although some clients use a handheld shower or water pitcher and numerous towels to wash the hair. Showers are typically contraindicated until the halo is removed and the pin sites heal, unless the client can carefully use a handheld shower to avoid getting the vest wet. Clients must lie on their side while a caregiver unfastens the vest and assists with washing the trunk. The vest is closed, and the process is repeated on the other side. Sleeping can be challenging, and a hospital bed is useful to assist with positioning along with numerous pillows. Getting out of bed should be accomplished by rolling to the side, moving legs off the side, and then sitting up. Once the halo is removed, the head will feel heavy and wobbly, and generally a rigid cervical collar is prescribed.

The TLSO can be challenging for clients to don independently. Most clients prefer a T-shirt between the skin and the TLSO. The brace is donned in the bed with the client in the supine position. Generally, to don the brace, the client log-rolls to the side, and the back portion is pushed under as far as possible. The client log-rolls to supine, the back shell is straightened, and the straps are located. The top is then placed on the body, and the straps fastened. A similar method is used to apply a cervical collar before getting out of bed. See Figure 20-3a for a picture of donning the TLSO.

STANDING FRAMES AND TILT TABLES

Clients with SCI/D have the obvious symptoms of weakness and sensory changes, but there are also numerous secondary complications exacerbated by prolonged sitting. Those can be osteoporosis, spasticity, pressure injuries, bone demineralization, renal calculi (kidney stones), and contractures.[41] Because clients with SCI/D who sit and have an altered pattern of loading of the LEs, a loss of 50% to 60% of their bone mineral density can occur over time.[42] This loss occurs the most during the first year of injury, but continues through the client's life. The most beneficial method of pressure injury prevention is complete offloading of the pressure points, which can be obtained by standing.[42] A regular standing program for those with SCI/D, initiated early on can be valuable for health as well as improvement in sleep, QoL, and well-being.[43]

Numerous options exist for reaching a standing position. Clients who have high-level tetraplegia and less head/trunk control may require a tilt table for standing. The motorized tilt table starts flat, the client is in supine, and then once the client is strapped in, the whole table can be tilted to any degree to fully standing. This also allows the client to progress slowly at first to avoid orthostatic hypotension (dizziness, fainting from low blood pressure). Clients who have head and upper trunk control can use a standing frame. Typically, there is a seat or harness, and a block for the knees and chest. The client is raised to a standing position with a hydraulic crank as either the harness is pulled forward or the seat is raised. Standing frames can be either for static standing or have a dynamic component where the foot supports move forward and backward with bilateral arm movement on poles. The dynamic standing does allow the client to get exercise and weight-bearing at the same time, but typically use is limited to a client with an SCI/D at C7 or lower. Manual and power wheelchairs can have standing options as well, but this feature is difficult to procure through most insurances (see Chapter 15 for details). Some clients note orthostatic complaints such as dizziness, headache, and fatigue, although these improve with use of an abdominal binder and LE compression stockings as well as repetition of standing.[43] The recommendations generally are for 30 to 60 minutes, three or more times per week.[44]

Cardiovascular System Functions

When first thinking about an individual with SCI/D, one would not naturally tend to think that cardiovascular functions could be compromised. The following sections, however, impart crucial information for client safety.

ORTHOSTATIC HYPOTENSION

Cardiovascular dysfunction is another frequent cause of morbidity and mortality in people with SCI/D.[45] Disrupted autonomic pathways as a result of SCI/D lead to unstable cardiovascular systems, which then lead to significant fluctuations in blood pressure, blood flow deregulation, and low resting blood pressure.[45] Physical inactivity, impaired blood sugar control, widespread inflammation, and lipid abnormalities also contribute to this cardiovascular dysfunction. This autonomic dysfunction accelerates age-related health issues and can cause cardiac impairment, cerebrovascular accident (CVA), cognitive deficits, and impairments to rehabilitation.[45]

Blood pressure regulation is one of the most difficult challenges post-SCI/D and another reason that early mobilization is an important aspect of rehabilitation. **Orthostatic hypotension** is a sudden drop in blood pressure due to insufficient venous return to the brain.[6] This is also commonly known as postural hypotension because when someone changes position quickly (supine to sitting, sitting to standing), blood pressure drops dramatically. The Consensus Committee of the American Autonomic Society and the American Academy of Neurology defines orthostatic hypotension as a decrease in systolic blood pressure of 20 mmHg or more, or in diastolic blood pressure of 10 mmHg or more, upon the assumption of an upright posture from a supine position, regardless of whether symptoms occur. It is also possible in other types of clients who have prolonged bedrest during their hospital stay or who spend long periods of time in bed at home due to medical or psychosocial issues.[6] The blood pools in the LEs which, due to paralysis in SCI/D, likely do not have adequate muscle strength to pump the blood back up to the brain or abdomen.[45] Symptoms of orthostatic hypotension include feeling faint, seeing spots, temporarily losing hearing or having tinnitus (ringing of the ears), temporary loss of vision, loss of color in the face, and nausea. It is important to understand that clients with SCI/D tend to have healthy blood pressures, which might be considered low for their able-bodied peers.

As clients with SCI/D begin the adjustment process, it is important to gradually introduce upright positions using tools in the physical environment such as elevating the head of the bed during and between therapy sessions, practicing sitting at the edge of the bed with assistance from the OTA, and using mobility equipment such as tilt tables, tilt-in-space manual wheelchairs, and power wheelchairs that assist accommodation to being upright. It is also important to continually monitor and document the client's vital signs both to receive a baseline for comparison and to track progress for activity tolerance over time.

Prevention is the mainstay of intervention for cardiovascular dysfunction, with a focus on educating the client, family, and care providers.[45] Prevention of orthostatic hypotension involves maintaining hydration (within fluid restriction guidelines if applicable), avoiding large meals, and avoiding heat stress. Clients can be encouraged to elevate the head of the bed 10° to 20° in a semi-upright position for short periods to allow the body to accommodate to an upright position over time. Practitioners also employ external modalities such as abdominal binders, LE compression stockings, and gradient elastic bandage wrapping of bilateral LEs to prevent orthostatic hypotension. OTAs educate and train clients and their support networks on how to incorporate these modalities into client routines. Often these modalities must be grouped with the therapeutic strategies previously mentioned and pharmacological intervention. The eventual goal is to decrease reliance on these over time as the client is exposed to being upright over longer and more consistent periods of time.[45]

AUTONOMIC DYSREFLEXIA

Autonomic dysreflexia (AD) is an exaggerated, reflexive sympathetic response, generally in an individual with a complete SCI/D at T6 or above. This response causes a very high blood pressure and potentially life threatening symptoms that happen due to stimuli such as pain, irritation, constipation, or a full bladder, which would not be an issue for an individual without an SCI/D. There is loss of supraspinal sympathetic nervous system control that can occur at any time after neurogenic spinal shock has resolved.[6] Typically, the resting blood pressure of clients with SCI/D is lower than before SCI/D, being between 90 and 110 mmHg for the systolic number. A sudden increase in systolic blood pressure of more than 20 mmHg is one symptom of AD.[6] This points to a critical area of education for OT practitioners. Clients and their support system should know their baseline blood pressure so that if there is a deviance from that, they can inform general health care providers who may not see a systolic blood pressure of 150 mmHg for example, as aberrant. Other signs of AD include severe headache, **bradycardia** (slowness of heart rate), goosebumps, flushing, and sweating above the level of their injury.[46]

Because AD is a medical emergency, when someone with a SCI/D is in AD, the OTA first calls for medical assistance while looking for the cause to resolve the noxious issue. Next, the OTA works to lower the blood pressure by removing any constricting clothing or items from the client's body, then sitting him or her up as much as possible to orthostatically drop the blood pressure. Medical management of chronic AD includes a variety of methods including Botox injections, oral medications, and surgical intervention.[46]

AD has numerous triggers; the three most common causes include problems with bowel, bladder, and skin function. Problems with bowel dysfunction may include stool impaction or pressure and pain from a hemorrhoid. Noxious stimuli from the urinary system may include kidney stones, urinary tract infection (UTI), or a kinked indwelling catheter. Numerous skin function issues triggering AD include pressure injuries, ingrown toenails, unknowingly sitting or lying on an object, and tightly fitting or impinging clothing. Other causes reported by physicians for AD included skeletal fractures, sexual intercourse, gall bladder dysfunction, sunburn, pregnancy, and childbirth.[46] AD is considered a medical emergency and can cause CVA, retinal detachment, heart attack, seizures, or death.[46]

Prevention of AD, like orthostatic hypotension, is the primary method of intervention by OT practitioners. It involves educating the individual, family, and care providers on causes of AD. OT practitioners who work with clients with SCI/D must be knowledgeable of the signs and symptoms of AD, how to prevent AD, and how to manage it. They must also educate and train their client and client's support system to do the same.

An illustration of a case of AD when the client is at home would be the following example: Fatima's husband Abdul had a C5 AIS A SCI. As part of his daily stretching routine, Fatima stretched her husband's hip into abduction while he was lying in bed, and they both noted that he suddenly broke out into an unusual sweat and complained of feelings of uneasiness and severe headache. Because of his level of injury, Abdul could not feel this pain per say, but he did recognize these odd symptoms as his body's way of communicating discomfort associated with stretching, and noted the AD. They both recalled the training on AD they had received by their OTA, and moved quickly. They ceased stretching in that moment; Fatima raised the head of Abdul's bed, and noted that the covers were wadded up behind him. Once she found this problem, the AD resolved quickly, and the next time they stretched, Fatima proceeded more carefully to smooth the blankets before starting. They did not have a recurrence of the AD symptoms.

DEEP VEIN THROMBOSIS

Deep vein thrombosis (DVT) is the formation of a blood clot in a vein due to compromised circulation. All individuals living with SCI/D are at risk,[6] and DVTs are a significant cause of morbidity and mortality in the population living with SCI/D.[39] They are most commonly formed in the LEs, abdomen, or pelvic areas. A DVT may dislodge from the venous wall, forming an embolus (unattached clot); travel from the point of origin in the vein; and enter the circulatory system. It may then enter and occlude the pulmonary circulatory system, possibly causing a pulmonary embolism (PE). OT practitioners' skills in observation and familiarity with the client are important to note if there is asymmetry in the LEs, abdomen, or pelvic areas with change in color, temperature, and/or size. A DVT is diagnosed by a physician usually with peripheral vascular imaging. If the imaging is positive (there is a DVT), bedrest and anticoagulation medication for the client will likely be prescribed to prevent embolus formation, which can be life threatening. Filters can be surgically placed in the inferior vena cava (IVC filters) to capture emboli that have dislodged before they do damage; IVC filters are used more often in clients who cannot tolerate anticoagulants or who have had more than one DVT.[47] OT practitioners also play an important role in educating clients and their caregivers about DVT prevention, signs and symptoms of DVT, and DVT management related to physical activity levels. Research shows that DVT can be most prevented by physical activity and following the anticoagulation plan set forth by the physician. DVT prevention is one of the most important reasons for OTAs to encourage and train regarding physical activity for clients with SCI/D from early mobilization in the acute hospitalization phase to adaptive leisure and sports in the community reintegration phase.[6]

Respiratory System Functions

Breathing is often compromised in clients with SCI/D. The phrenic nerve that innervates the diaphragm may be compromised or completely paralyzed in clients with spinal injury above the C4 level, requiring the client to have ventilation support. In lower cervical and thoracic injuries, the abdominal, intercostal, and latissimus dorsi muscle strength that supports breathing is weak or absent. Respiratory system compromise pervasively impacts and changes the capacity for clients with SCI/D to participate in therapy. Impaired muscles of inhalation prevent deep breaths, leading to **atelectasis** (collapse or closure of a lung) and related gas-exchange and lung-compliance abnormalities.[48] Clients' decreased or lack of ability to cough leads to significant risk for pulmonary infection or persistent infection.[49] It causes decreased ability to clear secretions. Respiratory therapists and PT practitioners may incorporate pulmonary exercises to the daily routine to prevent lung mucous buildup. Clients with high cervical spinal injuries and those who are sedentary are especially susceptible to secondary complications from respiratory compromise.

OT practitioners support prevention of secondary respiratory complications by working with clients and their support networks to incorporate respiratory hygiene strategies into their routines. OT/PT practitioners and caregivers may perform assisted coughs (sometimes called an assisted cough). This is an effective tool for assistance in clearing secretions (Fig. 35-5). This is especially important for clients with injury above C5 who lack innervation to the motor neurons responsible for inspiration and expiration.[31] The assisted cough is performed if the client requests it, is trying to cough, is short of breath, or if the OTA hears congestion in the throat or chest. The procedure for an assisted cough includes:[50]

- Place the client on his or her back, if possible. If he or she is sitting, make sure the wheelchair is locked. If the client has a reclining wheelchair, recline the chair back and lock it.
- Place the thumb of each hand together and spread the fingers wide apart, forming what looks like a butterfly. Next, put butterfly hands on top of the client's stomach area. Do not put them on top of the ribs or bony areas.
- Ask the client to take 3 to 5 deep breaths. On the last breath, the OTA will help the client breathe out by pushing in and up, using a firm, steady pressure. Use smooth motion. At the same time as the pushing, ask the client to try to cough as hard as possible.
- Repeat this as needed. The client may wish to rest between coughs.

OTAs should encourage clients and their friends, family members, and caregivers to frequently wash their hands, avoid smoking, and prevent the client's exposure to illness. In addition, OTAs promote physical activity and identify strategies and resources to promote clients to be physically active. Establishing these new habits and ingraining these lifestyle modifications is important to pulmonary health.

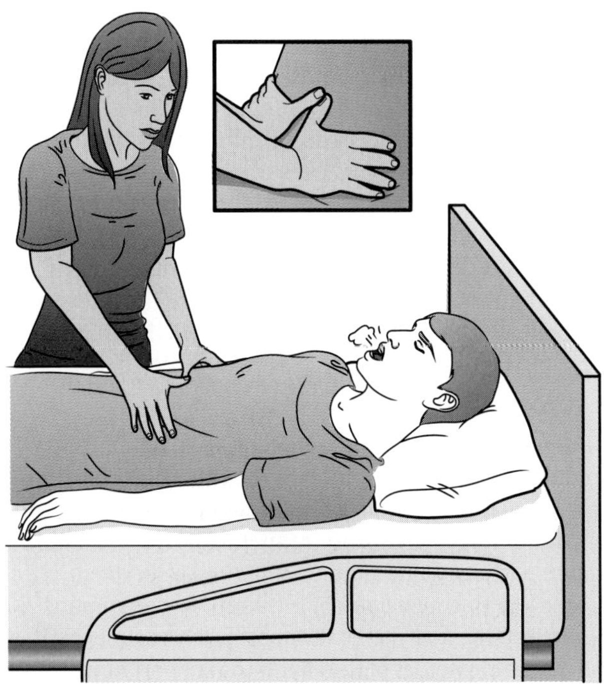

FIGURE 35-5. Closely observe hand placement for the assisted cough procedure.

Neurogenic Bladder

After SCI/D, the transmission of information via motor information from the brain to the bladder and via sensory signals from the bladder to the brain is impaired. As a review, UMNs are part of the central nervous system and are housed within the brain and spine. Lower motor neurons (LMNs) are part of the peripheral nervous system and connect the spinal cord to the muscles. Clients with SCI/D affecting UMN function will experience more spasticity of the bowels and bladder, while those who have SCI/D affecting LMN function will experience flaccid symptoms because there is a loss of spinal cord–mediated reflexes.[6] Whether the injury involves UMN or LMN lesions has implications for bowel and bladder management.

If the injury is above the conus medullaris (the most distal portion of the spinal cord below the L2 vertebral level), the injury leads to spastic paralysis of the bladder (bladder will not empty without assistance). Injury below the conus medullaris directly impacts the bladder and results in flaccidity with urine leakage.

After SCI/D, clients must manage their bladder to prevent bladder, urinary tract, and renal dysfunction. There are different ways clients with SCI/D manage their bladder function, including types of catheterization or surgical options.

INTERMITTENT CATHETERIZATION

Intermittent catheterization is the most common type of strategy and involves introducing a sterile catheter into the bladder every 4 to 6 hours to drain it manually. This strategy is the most effective and least likely to cause UTI compared with the use of indwelling catheters, which stay in longer periods. Intermittent catheterization is effective for men and women, however women with SCI/D often meet with more barriers, due to anatomical differences. Women without sensation in the S2-S3 dermatome of the vaginal area have a marked increase in difficulty, as they are unable to feel the orifice through which the catheter enters. For instance, it is not uncommon to unintentionally insert the catheter into the vagina. For both genders with SCI/D, body habitus (body build), preexisting medical conditions involving the bladder, and level of SCI/D may complicate intermittent catheterization. Self-catheterization for someone with tetraplegia is more challenging due to compromised hand function than for someone with paraplegia whose hand function is intact.

INDWELLING CATHETERIZATION

An alternative to intermittent catheterization is the placement of an indwelling catheter of which there are different types. It remains in the bladder, and urine drains into a bag attached to the client's leg or wheelchair. The indwelling catheter is changed generally every 2 to 4 weeks in most cases, and has an air- or saline-filled balloon to maintain its placement in the bladder. The physiatrist and urologist will help the client determine which is the most effective bladder management system (Fig. 35-6).

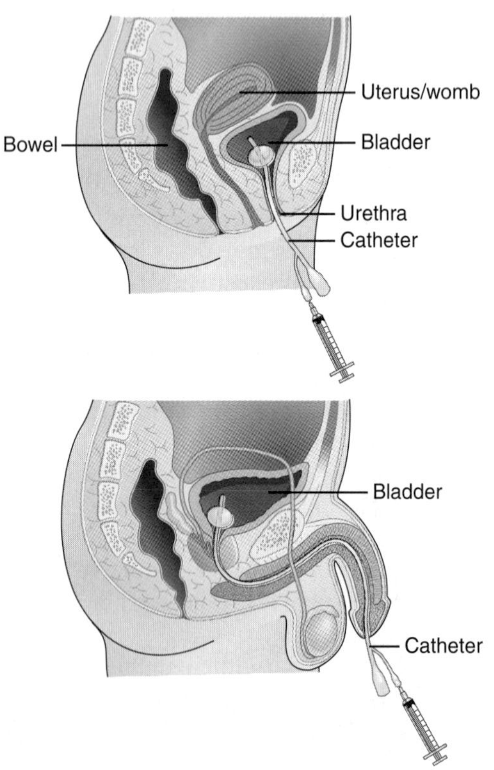

FIGURE 35-6. Indwelling catheters: Female and male.

SURGICAL OPTIONS

Urologists work with clients with SCI/D to determine whether surgical options of bladder diversion (such as suprapubic catheter) are appropriate. These surgical options often improve independence in bladder management for clients who have limited UE function and who lack access to caregivers. For clients in these situations, intermittent and indwelling catheterization is often not practical or safe. The urologist works with the client and support network to negotiate the risks and benefits of surgical intervention.

The OT practitioner plays a key role in educating clients on bladder management strategies and incorporating them into the daily routine. OT practitioners analyze the client's capabilities and assess the activity demands to determine how the client can have the most independence and safety with bladder management. OTAs work closely with their clients and their support networks to adapt the physical environment so that clients learn to perform intermittent catheterization from the bed, from the wheelchair, or over the commode. OTAs provide adaptive equipment options such as thigh spreaders to place on the legs, adaptive clamps to hold catheters, and mirrors that improve independence with intermittent self-catheterization, especially for women. OTAs adapt all parts of the bladder management routine, which improves function and safety, and embed these adaptations into routine. OT collaboration with clients, their support network, and their medical team is crucial.

Research demonstrates that there is a paternalistic model in the decision-making process about how people with SCI/D empty their bladders, causing a mismatch in roles between how people prefer to make decisions and how they are actually involved in the process.[51] OT practitioners have a valuable role on the interdisciplinary team, advocating for the client at the head of that team, and constructing a picture for the client about the impact of bladder management medical decisions on daily life and QoL. Evidence illustrates that a three-way decision may be most effectively made among the client, caregivers, and physician about an intervention that is likely to be carried out in the home. The OT practitioner has a role in explaining the implications of each decision on daily life as well as training the client post–medical intervention on how to integrate the intervention at home, work, school, and other areas of the community.

Neurogenic Bowel

Neurogenic bowel management after spinal injury is a predictor of QoL.[52] The inability to maintain control over bowel function negatively affects every aspect of daily function including community reintegration, vocational and leisure participation, relationships, and self-esteem.

The key to bowel control is a routine that emphasizes a balance of the most medically appropriate regimen with the functional capacities of the client, the support network, and QoL considerations. OTAs educate clients on the importance of establishing a consistent routine including physical activity, diet and hydration, bowel medication, and stool evacuation, which is pivotal in bowel program success.

Traditionally the bowel program is performed once a day every day or every other day and takes 30 to 45 minutes to complete. Bowel management can be a challenging process physically, emotionally, and mentally as clients and their support networks wrap their minds around learning how to manage this function in a new way. It requires understanding their bodily functions differently and more intimately. Clients who require assistance for bowel management should also be prepared and empowered to direct their bowel care.

Because bowel function patterns can be unpredictable and difficult to regulate for clients with incomplete spinal cord injury, effective management involves close orchestration with the client, support network, OT practitioner, physician, and dietitian.

Similar to bladder function, location of spinal cord involvement affects the pattern of neurogenic bowel management. For complete injuries above the conus medullaris (UMN involvement), parasympathetic nervous system–mediated spinal reflexes are intact, causing the anal sphincter to have increased tone (be spastic). When the injury is below the conus (LMN involvement), the spinal cord–mediated reflexes are inhibited and the result is a flaccid anal sphincter.

Generally speaking, the bowel program for a client with UMN involvement is more predictable than that for a client with LMN involvement or an incomplete spinal cord injury. Clients with spastic bowels require the balance of oral and/or rectal medication as well as **digital stimulation** of the anus via a gloved finger or tool to evacuate stool (Fig. 35-7). The technique is generally to move the finger or tool gently in a circular motion.

The regimen for someone with a flaccid bowel is more difficult to manage and can hinge on balancing fiber intake and hydration. There is more chance for an accidental evacuation of the bowels with a flaccid bowel, and clients are often afraid to leave the home for fear of an episode of incontinence.

Bowel programs can be conducted in bed, on a standard toilet (with or without cushioning depending on the client's ability to perform effective pressure relief), or using durable medical equipment (DME). DME options include an array of bedside commodes ranging from standard three-in-one commodes with fixed arms and hard, plastic seats or those with drop-down arms and padded seats to more complex tilt-in-space commodes that provide pressure relief and blood pressure management. Bedside commodes may be free-standing, placed over the toilet, or even placed in the shower (see Chapter 14 for options). Clients with levels of complete injury at and below C6 can more likely tolerate performing their bowel program on a padded three-in-one commode over the toilet because they have the capacity to relieve pressure adequately and routinely. Using DME over the toilet offers a raised commode surface for increased safety and ease of transfer. It also provides space between the 3-in-1 commode and the toilet for the client or caregiver to perform digital stimulation, and has a safety frame for additional balance support. If clients are able, learning to perform the bowel program on a standard toilet, however, provides flexibility within the community and during travel where DME may not be available. Placing grab bars around a standard toilet can provide the addition of security for balance. Due to lack of manual dexterity and hand strength in clients with a cervical spinal injury, OT practitioners can provide education about use of digital stimulators or "dil sticks" meant to provide safe anal stimulation for evacuation (Fig. 35-8). They can also educate on suppository inserters as effective tools for suppository insertion and stool evacuation. As with other adaptive equipment, OTAs educate the client

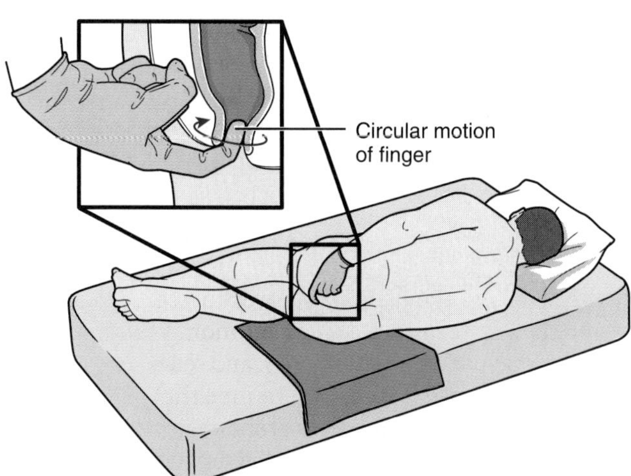

FIGURE 35-7. Anal stimulation performed in the bed for bowel program.

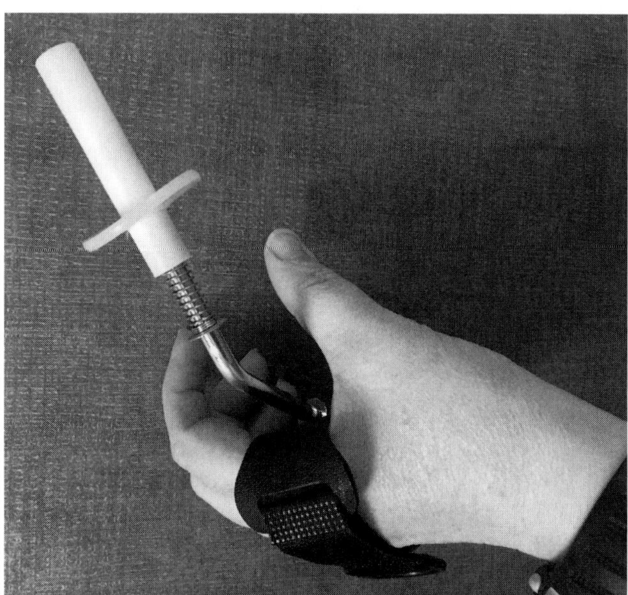

FIGURE 35-8. Bowel stimulator (dil stick) suppository inserter with cuff.

and caregivers on the purpose and usefulness of these tools, training the client and caregivers how to incorporate them as part of the program. The OTA may need to create an adaptive device to hold the stimulator more securely to the weak hand for some clients.

Bowel programs for clients with complete injuries above C6 may be performed on more supportive reclining or tilt-in-space shower/commode chairs with tall backs, with wheels and headrests for head, neck, and trunk support. These commodes also often have swing-away armrests for transfer ease and legrests for LE support. The advantage to this rolling chair is that both the bladder/bowel program and the shower with cleanup can be performed in the same chair without additional transfers, which conserves energy and time.

The OTA can work with nursing staff in the inpatient setting to ensure daily carryover of bowel program DME and adaptive equipment. This interdisciplinary work encourages problem solving and optimizing preparation for returning to the community.

Clients with high levels of cervical spinal injury, those with secondary complications such as pressure injuries or blood pressures that fluctuate, or those who do not have the resources to purchase DME may choose to perform the bowel program from the bed (Box 35-2). Often a caregiver would assist with this process.[52] Clients would lie on their side to encourage bowel evacuation.[53]

PARALYTIC ILEUS

Autonomic dysfunction as a result of SCI/D may cause **paralytic ileus** during the spinal shock phase of recovery, when there is temporary loss or depression of all or most reflex activity below the level of the SCI/D in the period after injury.[53] This may last from 48 to 72 hours post–injury.[54] Due to the ileus, clients are unable to digest food, and the result is nausea, vomiting, severe abdominal distension, and gastrointestinal blockage. This issue is medically managed by emptying the bowel contents via a tube and providing nutrition via nasogastric tube and hydration intravenously.

Reproductive Functions: Sexual Activity

A client's sexuality is affected by all of the SCI/D sequelae discussed in this chapter. Sexuality encompasses identity, role, and self-esteem, in addition to the physical aspects of intimacy. Sexuality is a complex integration of biological, cultural, spiritual, social, relational, and psychological factors.[55] Sexual expression is not only what occurs in the privacy of one's home but goes to the core of how individuals relate to other people and how they feel about themselves.[56] It is important that clients can rely on their rehabilitation team for care, concern, accurate information, referral, and follow-up when needed. Professional support can ensure that lives are full and enriched, as well as long and healthy.[57]

BOX 35-2
Bladder/Bowel Scenarios

LMN NEUROGENIC BOWEL AND BLADDER MANAGEMENT

Martha had a tumor in her lumbar spine at the cauda equina, the bundle of nerve roots that exit the spinal cord at the L2 vertebral level, resulting in LMN damage. As a result of nerve compression, she had decreased motor function in both LEs and bowel and bladder dysfunction resulting from a flaccid bowel and bladder. She was unable to control either function voluntarily as she continually leaked urine and stool, causing emotional distress. As part of neurogenic bowel and bladder education and training, Martha's OTA taught her how to manage her indwelling urinary catheter when dressing and how to perform perineal hygiene during bathing. The OTA also worked with the nutritionist and physiatrist to educate Martha on the importance of a bowel routine to prevent bowel incontinence.

UMN NEUROGENIC BOWEL AND BLADDER MANAGEMENT

Travis had a T4 complete SCI after a dirt bike accident, damaging the UMNs at the thoracic spinal cord level. Travis had resulting paralysis and spasticity of his core, back, and LE muscles as well as spastic neurogenic bowel and bladder. Travis' OTA taught him how to perform intermittent self-catheterizations from the bed and from his wheelchair as well as how to perform a bowel program with digital stimulation on a padded commode.

NEUROGENIC BLADDER

Pamela has incomplete tetraplegia as a result of a continually growing syrinx (fluid-filled sac) in her spinal cord, creating pressure to the cord and resulting in progressive worsening of her tetraplegia. She, her physiatrist, and her urologist are aware that her tetraplegia will likely continue to progress due to her medical issues. As a result, the urologist finds it most functionally and medically beneficial to insert a suprapubic tube in her bladder rather than continuing to attempt intermittent self-catheterization, which Pamela reports is becoming more difficult by the day. Latoya's fall off her skateboard resulted in a sacral SCI and she now lives with an indwelling urinary catheter. Her outpatient OTA organizes an outing to her school where she, Latoya, and the school nurse, work to assess how best to empty her collection bag while at her high school during the day. Bernard, a 70-year-old man with a C5 complete SCI is unable to self-catheterize due to a long history of osteoarthritis in both hands before SCI. The OTA at the skilled nursing facility where Bernard is receiving therapy works with him and his wife every day to teach his wife how to intermittently catheterize him from the bed and power wheelchair so she is comfortable catheterizing him whether they are at home or visiting family members.

After SCI/D, sexual activity for men and women can be impacted by urinary and bowel incontinence, urinary tract infection, autonomic dysreflexia, pain, and spasticity.[56] Although much of the current research around SCI/D lies in the area of fertility, because fertility is often not negatively affected by SCI/D, research efforts instead should be focused on areas such as urinary incontinence.[54,58] Addressing sexual activity in OT intervention is important because having positive sexual experiences after SCI/D is linked with higher QoL and better psychological well-being.[59] Women may have difficulties with lubrication and positioning, and men often have difficulty initiating and maintaining an erection, ejaculation, and positioning.

For men with SCI/D, some are able to achieve erections quite easily, others can achieve erections only occasionally, and some are unable to achieve erections at all. The ability to achieve an erection does not necessarily depend on the level of injury. Three basic kinds of erections are possible. They are psychogenic erections, which occur as a result of having sexy thoughts or by looking at erotic pictures, reflexogenic erections that occur as a result of direct physical stimulation of the penis, surrounding area, or even a LE (e.g., when dressing), and spontaneous erections, which could occur from a full bladder.[56] At T11 and above, reflexogenic erections are generally possible, psychogenic are not, and less than 10% of men can have ejaculations.[60]At T11 and below complete injury, psychogenic erections are generally possible, reflexogenic are not, and if sacral nerve injury is involved, ejaculations are not generally possible.[60] For women, they may have decreased lubrication, decreased sensation or muscle control, more difficulty achieving an orgasm, and it may feel different. Women below T6 injury may find use of a vibrator helpful.

Men with SCI/D may be able to initiate and maintain erections with the assistance of various prescription medications via pill or a shot in the penis as well as devices such as constriction rings, vacuum suction, or a surgically implanted penile prosthesis.[61] Fertility is often preserved in women, although they must be carefully monitored.[49] Both men and women should have regular gynecological/prostate examinations, respectively.

It is important for OT practitioners to understand the impact of sexual dysfunction on habits, routines, and roles. Sexual activity is an ADL, and OT practitioners can use the Ex-PLISSIT model to facilitate a discussion about sexuality in a sensitive, holistic manner with clients and their partners, which has been described in detail in Chapter 33.[62] The "Ex" prefix focuses on giving clients an opportunity to express initial or later concerns. It is helpful for OT practitioners to use this framework as research demonstrates that sexuality is one area of intervention many feel disinclined to address due to a number of reasons including perceived inadequate knowledge.[63] Sexuality and sexual activity should be recognized and approached as any other ADL, benefiting from relearning and reframing.

Topics appropriate for intervention by OT practitioners include positioning to maximize safety, comfort, and performance in contexts in which intimacy may occur. For example, OT practitioners can discuss safety, comfort, and performance in bed, from the wheelchair, and on a padded floor in the room of a house. Guidelines also encourage OT practitioners to consider a variety of possibilities for intimate activities that may include use of other bodily senses when sense of touch is impaired or absent.[57] For example, OTAs can educate clients on the use of aromatic massage oils, incorporating mirrors for visual feedback, and wearing adaptive clothing that allows increased independence with clothing management resulting in a greater sense of autonomy and sensuality. OT interventions for sexuality also include discussions about safety related to skin care. OTAs provide education about skin checks and thorough hygiene after intimate activity; bowel and bladder management before and after activity to prevent episodes of incontinence and autonomic dysreflexia; and the use of positioning strategies and tools to maximize skin protection and overall comfort with functional performance. For example, the OT practitioner may recommend positioning for spasticity management, self-catheterization technique before sexual activity, and modification of adaptive devices for a client with tetraplegia. The OT practitioner can create handouts with information for men and women at the various SCI/D levels to have available for clients and as a conversation starter.

OT intervention also includes psychosocial support, where the individual is taught and encouraged to resume pre-injury roles that reconnect them with their individual identities. This is also promoted as they relearn or learn to direct the meaningful, purposeful, and necessary activities of their daily lives. In learning to maximize their functional capacities in other areas of ADLs and IADLs, OT practitioners can educate and empower clients to apply these same strategies to their intimate lives.

FUNCTIONAL OUTCOMES AFTER COMPLETE SPINAL CORD INJURY: GOALS AND AREAS OF INTERVENTION

It can be helpful to have a general understanding of the expected functional outcomes clients with SCI/D may ultimately achieve. This section describes functional outcomes at each level of injury and target areas of OT intervention with a focus on occupation and activity; preparatory methods and tasks; and advocacy and groups. It includes a brief summary of a few key levels of SCI/D and reasonable goals and outcomes at each level of function, as well as more information in Table 35-2. (Note that this table of levels and functionality will at times be difficult to follow regarding clients with incomplete SCI/D as they are written for the complete injury, and clients may not fit into a specific category, or may be different levels on each side of the body.) It is equally important to understand that goal attainment and functional outcome levels will be

COMMUNICATION

A common phrase is "It takes a village..." in reference to the idea that multiple people, working in unity to accomplish a goal, do more good than one person in isolation. This is especially true for intervention with the individual with SCI/D throughout the continuum of care. Medical treatment, case management, counseling, physical therapy, OT, speech language pathology, and nursing care are not provided in isolation of one another.

The interdisciplinary team is integral to successful outcomes for both the client and his or her family and care providers. To accomplish interdisciplinary care, intervention should be individualized to the client and family; be client-driven; and be a goal-oriented process. This means that plans of care are carried out with input to and from and attention to all aspects of the client's rehabilitation. As part of this interdisciplinary team, OTAs communicate with other members of the team to address barriers and maximize supports. The benefit is to the client and also to the team members who learn from one another through the process.

OT's specialized contribution—OT practitioners have unique contributions to the interdisciplinary team. OT practitioners are skilled observers and analyzers; seeing clients as occupational beings who desire returning to what is meaningful and purposeful in their lives. The team consists of the client, family, support network, and often the following providers:

Physiatrist (rehabilitation physician)
Primary care physician
Urologist
Neuropsychologist
Mental health and rehabilitation counselor
Occupational therapist
Occupational therapy assistant
Physical therapist
Physical therapist assistant
Speech language pathologist
Recreational therapist
Case manager or social worker
Nurse
Certified nursing assistant
Personal care assistant

impacted by individual client characteristics; the course of medical events; psychosocial and environmental supports or lack thereof; and cognitive abilities. For instance, older age and obesity are characteristics that could drastically affect outcomes.[64] Secondary medical complications such as urinary tract infections, pressure injuries, fractures, chronic pain, and depressive symptoms are potential consequences of SCI/D that can cause functional limitations.[65] These complications can exacerbate the experience of living with SCI/D and affect long-term health, productivity, dignity, mobility, and overall independence.[65] As OTAs learn what to expect in terms of facilitating outcomes for clients with SCI/D at various levels, they must keep in perspective a holistic view of the characteristics of clients and their situations and how these might affect their outcomes.

A common goal for clients with higher cervical levels of injury is independence with direction of their care, including ADLs and IADLs. Foundational to independent direction of ADLs and IADLs is the ability to direct skin inspection, body positioning, assisted cough, and prevention and management of autonomic dysreflexia and orthostatic hypotension.

Long-Term Goals by Neurological Level

The following discusses long-term goals for clients based on the neurological level of their SCI/D.

CERVICAL TETRAPLEGIA: C2-C4

Strength and Somatosensation: Clients with this level of injury have no strength in or control of their arms, trunk, or legs. Due to paralysis or weakness of the diaphragm, clients with C3 and above complete SCI/D require constant breathing assistance from an external ventilator, a pneumatic electric machine that forces room air into the lungs (inspiration) and the client passively exhales (expiration).[32] Some ventilators are set to provide constant and steady assistance, and others are set to trigger when the client initiates a breath. Many ventilators do not let the lungs fully exhale to avoid atelectasis and other lung collapses. Not all clients with a C4 tetraplegia are ventilator dependent, although some are, especially at night. Occupational therapists and OTAs work with clients and their caregivers to understand how to safely carry out self-care and IADL tasks considering the ventilator and its components. Portable ventilators can also be attached to power wheelchairs, promoting community mobility and participation. The respiratory therapist can be a resource for the OTA to learn to feel comfortable with the ventilator and its various beeps and alarms.

Adaptive Equipment and Functional Mobility: OT practitioners educate, train, and empower these clients to direct their self-care and determine types of equipment they desire in their day-to-day living. They may have neck movement, head control, and potentially shoulder shrug. Traditionally, many clients use mouth sticks, a head mouse, or voice activation to participate in activities such as artwork, keyboarding, and turning pages of a book (Fig. 35-9). Technologic advances offer clients with tetraplegia opportunities to engage with and control their environment with greater levels of independence. For example, electronic ADLs (EADLs) (formerly known as environmental control units) as well as smartphone and smart-home technologies allow hands-free ability to operate lights, televisions, and appliances and to open doors. Low- and high-tech adaptations are highly individualized and require time to learn and integrate into routines. High-tech options also tend to be cost-prohibitive, and OT

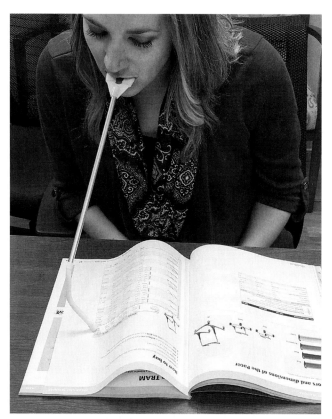

FIGURE 35-9. A person with tetraplegia using a mouth stick to turn pages.

practitioners play an important role in connecting clients with available resources. In addition to adaptive strategies for environmental control, clients usually drive power wheelchairs with alternative drive controls such as pneumatic "sip and puff" control, chin mini joystick control, or head control.

Activities of Daily Living Goals: Teaching clients to independently direct their own care is paramount. OT practitioners offer valuable skills in activity analysis, including the time needed to accomplish tasks, and can assist clients plan and prioritize tasks that can be delegated to formal and informal care providers. They can also help clients outline the components and time commitments of a daily and weekly routine as well as to create scripts on how to most clearly verbalize directions to caregivers.

CERVICAL TETRAPLEGIA: C5

Strength and Somatosensation: Clients with this level of injury have limited UE strength and arm function. They have no strength in or control of their trunk or LEs. They have neck strength and can shrug their shoulders. The hallmark of the C5 SCI/D level is C5 spinal nerve innervation to the anterior deltoid and biceps muscle groups, enabling elbow flexion and some shoulder control, which opens up a significant level of movement and functionality. Clients with this level of spinal cord injury do not have strength in their triceps for elbow extension or active control in their wrists or hands.

TECHNOLOGY AND TRENDS

OT practitioners introduce and educate clients with tetraplegia and the inability to engage the world with their hands to assistive technologies that promote participation using other body functions. Even as this chapter is read, more advanced technologies are being developed and marketed to promote participation for clients with SCI/D and other conditions who have limited use of their arms. Eye gaze or tracking technology is an effective and evolving area of assistive technology that provides independence for individuals with high levels of SCI/D who cannot use their UEs to communicate, control their environment, and participate in meaningful and purposeful tasks that typically involve use of their hands. Eye gaze technology works by allowing users to scan computer screens with their eyes then dwell on the item they desire to click on. When their eyes dwell on the item, this serves like a switch to select and activate the item. Eye gaze software technology provides opportunity for efficient and fluid computer access. The *New Mobility* article, "The Eyes Have It," references a few of many eye gaze technologies on the market.[66] The Grid software is another example, and allows people to create custom screens and keyboards for adapted access.[67] OT practitioners can work with clients who benefit from this assistive technology to evaluate for and educate and instruct clients and their support systems in its use and integration into their goals and routines. Currently the Centers for Medicare and Medicaid Services and private insurers consider this type of technology medically necessary if it is used as a speech-generating device. It is not considered medically necessary and therefore not funded for uses other than speech generation. OT practitioners can work with clients and their support systems to find alternative funding sources for other uses of this technology since clients with SCI/D typically benefit from this technology for access and connection purposes rather than for speech generation. OT practitioners should also continue to advocate to their legislators on behalf of their clients for the medical necessity of these devices and more importantly educate their clients and support systems on how to self-advocate for these devices and the impact on their QoL.

Another example of an assistive technology option is the Tecla. This technology allows a client to use external switches or the client's power wheelchair controller to access iOS and Android phones, tablets, and PC and Mac computers. Clients with tetraplegia can access the external switches with any part of their body that can voluntarily make contact with the switch or through their power wheelchair drive control. This way they can use the Tecla to send and receive emails, surf the Internet, read, access environmental controls, make phone calls, and use smart phone or tablet apps.[68]

Rehabilitation practitioners, clients with SCI/D, and their support systems should advocate for changes in health care policy and health insurance reimbursement to support the rapid evolution of assistive technology designed to provide independence and QoL for clients. Eye gaze and other assistive technologies like the Tecla are examples of avenues through which clients can return to work, school, and to participate in activities that allow them to feel productive, connected, fulfilled, and whole.

(Text continued on page 942)

TABLE 35-2 SCI/D Levels

LEVEL	MOVEMENTS GAINED/ SPARED	AREA OF OCCUPATION	FUNCTIONAL GOALS—CLIENT CAN:	OCCUPATIONS AND ACTIVITIES
C1-C4	Some neck/ head control, more at C3-C4 cervical levels C4 will have shoulder shrug from trapezius and levator scapulae and some diaphragm control, but unable to cough	ADLs	• Independently direct self-care • Independently drive power wheelchair with alternative drive control(s) • Perform pressure relief every 30 minutes while in power wheelchair	• Practices talking through dressing routine with caregiver • Uses chin-controlled joystick to drive power wheelchair in bedroom, bathroom, and living area
C1-C4		IADLs	• Independently or with setup use technology integrated into power wheelchair to control a tablet	• Creates and edits emails to family using voice-control software
C1-C4		Rest/sleep	• Independently direct positioning for comfort and schedule for pressure relief during sleep routines	<u>Activities</u> • Selects sleep clothes and pillows to minimize areas of discomfort and pressure when in bed • Directs caregiver to set an alarm to wake and change position every 2 hours
C1-C4		Education/ work/leisure	• Independently participate in online continuing education	<u>Occupations</u> • Writes a term paper using voice-dictation software. (Applies to C4 off vent)
C5	Head, neck, shoulder, gain biceps brachii for elbow flexion, supination	ADLs	• Independently direct bathing and dressing activities • Independently drive power wheelchair with joystick or alternative drive control(s) • Use mobile arm support and bilateral wrist orthotics to feed self	• Practices bringing fork and spoon to mouth using mobile arm support • Drives power wheelchair with joystick to school bus stop to pick up daughter

PREPARATORY METHODS AND TASKS	EDUCATION AND TRAINING	ADVOCACY AND SELF ADVOCACY	GROUP INTERVENTIONS
<u>Tasks</u> • OTA performs PROM of UEs and LEs through full ROM twice a day <u>Modalities</u> • OTA administers heat to bicep to improve PROM for upper body dressing <u>Orthotics</u> • OTA fabricates and issues antideformity orthotic to prevent hand contracture, decrease pain <u>Assistive Technology & Environmental Modifications</u> • OTA educates client on home modifications for a ceiling lift to transfer to a power wheelchair <u>Wheeled mobility</u> • OTA recommends setting a pressure-relief timer on client's smartphone	<u>Education</u> • OTA educates caregivers on causes for and strategies to prevent autonomic dysreflexic episodes • OTA educates client and caregivers on role of HEP for maintaining PROM for range necessary in dressing and bathing <u>Training</u> • OTA instructs formal care provider on performing UE and LE PROM • OTA trains caregivers on performing assisted cough for respiratory health	• Calls insurance company to ask for increased nursing hours	• Joins support group at inpatient rehab center with other clients at this level
<u>Modalities</u> • OTA performs neck ROM and strengthening exercises <u>Assistive Technology and Environmental Modification</u> • OTA sets up chin control and tablet on power wheelchair with ergonomic considerations for varied tilt and recline seating positions	<u>Education</u> • OTA educates caregiver on selecting switches based on client's current strengths and abilities <u>Training</u> • OTA instructs client on sequence of switch activation to compose an email	• Advocates for insurance reimbursement of technology through power wheelchair	• Joins SCI peer group to discuss the benefits of creating an assistive technology loan closet
<u>Preparatory Tasks</u> • Client employs breathing techniques to promote rest and relaxation	<u>Education</u> • OTA educates caregiver on the role of ROM exercises before and when waking from sleep <u>Training</u> • OTA instructs caregiver on supine and side-lying positions for pressure relief of bony prominences	• Fights insurance company for a specialty lateral rotation bed so caregivers do not have to get up every 2 hours to turn	
<u>Preparatory methods</u> • OTA recommends ergonomic workstation setup from power wheelchair	<u>Training</u> • OTA instructs client on how to use voice-dictation software	<u>Self-Advocacy</u> • Educates teacher and classmates about condition and needs	• Joins online computer gaming group; controls computer with eye gaze or head mouse
<u>Tasks</u> • Client performs shoulder, scapular, and bicep strengthening exercises using modified equipment <u>Modalities</u> • OTA provides massage to bilateral UEs to reduce dependent edema and	<u>Education</u> • OTA educates caregiver on use of power seating for intermittent catheterization from the wheelchair <u>Training</u> • OTA instructs formal care provider on performing bowel	• Is proactive in planning schedule to stay on time with intermittent catheterization and bowel program times in order to prevent autonomic dysreflexia or other medical issues	• Participates in a lunch group with others using a mobile arm support and other adaptations

Continued

TABLE 35-2 SCI/D Levels (continued)

LEVEL	MOVEMENTS GAINED/ SPARED	AREA OF OCCUPATION	FUNCTIONAL GOALS—CLIENT CAN:	OCCUPATIONS AND ACTIVITIES
C5, *continued*			from power wheelchair with Min A from caregiver	
C5		IADLs	• Independently operate a smartphone and tablet with a stylus and lap tray	• Signs up to read to daughter's elementary school class using Web-based scheduling tool • Builds sitting endurance for activities outside of home
C5		Rest/sleep	• Independently direct neurogenic bowel and bladder routine before sleep to prevent incontinence and autonomic dysreflexic episodes	<u>Activities</u> • Practices use of powered leg bag emptier in preparation for sleep
C5		Education/ work/leisure	• Participate in volunteer activities in daughter's elementary school classroom	<u>Occupations</u> • Reads to daughter's class from power wheelchair using a tablet
C6	Gain latissimus dorsi, serratus anterior, wrist extensors, pronation	ADLs	• Groom and self-feed seated in wheelchair with Mod I • Dress with Mod I to Min A from bed • Bathe with Mod I to Min A sitting on padded TTB or commode chair. May still prefer rolling shower wheelchair for comfort and energy conservation • Perform intermittent self-catheterization with Mod I to Mod A • Perform bowel program with Min A to Mod A seated on padded commode • Independently transfer between bed and power wheelchair with transfer board • Independently drive power wheelchair with joystick	• Practices using toothbrush and hairbrush with built-up handle and tenodesis • Practices applying universal cuff to various self-feeding and grooming tools • Practices intermittent self-catheterization from power wheelchair (more likely with males than females) • Dresses from bed using circle and long sitting positions and using tenodesis for clothing management • Practices sponge bathing from bed, learning to lift and manipulate LEs with UEs and

PREPARATORY METHODS AND TASKS	EDUCATION AND TRAINING	ADVOCACY AND SELF ADVOCACY	GROUP INTERVENTIONS
improve AROM/PROM for feeding • OTA applies therapeutic taping to shoulders for support and pain management Orthotics • OTA identifies and issues wrist orthotic with universal cuff for tool use • OTA obtains elbow stabilization orthotic for nighttime wear to prevent elbow flexion contractures	program from tilt-in-space commode		
Modalities • OTA performs stretching to bilateral wrists before donning wrist orthotics Assistive Technology and Environmental Modification • OTA modifies lap tray for smartphone use	Education • OTA educates caregiver on setup of power wheelchair lap tray and smartphone Training • OTA instructs client and caregiver on optimal UE positioning to prevent pain and fatigue during activity	• Asks caregiver to assist with meal setup in a certain preferred way	• Communicates in an online blog about pet care with SCI
Assistive Technology • OTA recommends a ceiling lift to transfer from power wheelchair to bed	Education • OTA educates on creating a routine to minimize client/caregiver disruption during sleep Training • OTA instructs caregiver on supine and side-lying positions for pressure relief of bony prominences		
Preparatory methods • OTA modifies stylus for tablet use	Training • OTA instructs client in how to use stylus to navigate book application on tablet	• Speaks to the teacher in daughter's classroom about best ways to be involved	• Explores options with local adapted sports club such as waterskiing in supportive equipment
Tasks • Client performs shoulder, bicep, and wrist strengthening exercises using wrist weights and modified equipment • OTA performs stretching to tight hamstring and hip internal rotators in preparation for dressing in circle sit • OTA modifies pants for increased independence with dressing and intermittent catheterization • Client practices transitioning between supine, side-lying, prone, long sit, circle sit,	Education: • OTA instructs client and caregivers on home exercise and stretching program • OTA educates on importance of preserving tenodesis grasp when stretching, transferring, or using UEs to support self in sitting • OTA educates client on importance of incorporating skin inspection into daily ADL routine	• Tells partner alternative options to try for sexual stimulation	• Participates in a wheelchair Zumba class for strength and endurance training as well as social interaction

Continued

TABLE 35-2 SCI/D Levels (continued)

LEVEL	MOVEMENTS GAINED/ SPARED	AREA OF OCCUPATION	FUNCTIONAL GOALS—CLIENT CAN:	OCCUPATIONS AND ACTIVITIES
C6, *continued*			• Independently verbalize positioning considerations for sexual activity	using tenodesis, in preparation to bathe in shower • Practices using modified suppository inserter with tenodesis while sitting on padded commode • Performs pressure relief every 20 minutes while seated on padded commode during 45-minute bowel program • Drives power wheelchair from college dorm to classrooms across campus using power seat functions to safely navigate grades and uneven terrain
C6		IADLs	• Independently navigate public transportation with power wheelchair (some use manual wheelchair) • Independently prepare breakfast and lunch in college dorm • Independently load self and power wheelchair into adapted van and drive safely with adaptations	• Accesses city bus from campus to urban downtown location • Practices opening and closing condiment containers and food packaging using tools and tenodesis grasp • Practices using adapted meal preparation tools and tenodesis grasp • Orders groceries online for pickup
C6		Rest/sleep	• Independently direct neurogenic bowel and bladder routine before sleep to prevent incontinence and autonomic dysreflexic episodes • Independently position self in bed to promote comfort and prevent pressure injury	Activities • Lists areas for and schedule of assistance with neurogenic bowel and bladder programs in preparation for sleep • Modifies dorm room bed with wedges and pillows necessary for positioning at night • Sets a recurring alarm to wake him every 2 hours to change sleep positions
C6		Education/ work/leisure	• Maintain a full-time student course load • Maintain a part-time to full-time office job	Activities • Practices packing and unpacking his backpack • Practices preparing breakfast • Selects the most direct route to classes • Uses touch screen on his laptop to take notes

PREPARATORY METHODS AND TASKS	EDUCATION AND TRAINING	ADVOCACY AND SELF ADVOCACY	GROUP INTERVENTIONS
and short sit positions in preparation for ADLs • OTA provides activities to train dynamic sitting balance Modalities • OTA provides FES to wrist extensors to strengthen radial wrist extension and train tenodesis grasp/release patterns Orthotics • OTA identifies and issues universal cuff and/or foam grips for tool use			
Preparatory Tasks • OTA provides scapular stabilization exercises to build proximal upper body strength and stabilization for distal mobility • Client performs regular exercise routine to build physical endurance Assistive Technology and Environmental Modification • OTA recommends environmental modifications in the dorm room and bathroom for safety and efficiency of function	Education • OTA educates caregiver on setup of power wheelchair lap tray and smartphone • OTA educates on process to procure an adapted van Training • OTA instructs client and caregiver on optimal UE positioning to prevent pain and fatigue during activity • OTA educates client on kitchen safety from wheelchair level	• Uses computer to research financing options for new versus used adapted vans	
Tasks • OTA recommends stretching in prone as part of home exercise program to promote sleeping in this position; to achieve stretching of muscles in the anterior shoulders and hips; and to achieve pressure relief from posterior bony prominences	Education • OTA educates on creating a routine to minimize client/caregiver disruption during sleep Training • OTA instructs client on the importance of undisrupted sleep to promote healthy sleep/wake cycles and active participation	• Speaks with physician about options to help with management of spasms that disrupt sleep	
Preparatory methods • OTA modifies zippers and closures on client's backpack Assistive Technology • OTA recommends interfacing smartphone technology with power wheelchair	Training • OTA educates on ways to carry course materials on wheelchair safely	• Meets with disability services counselor on campus to arrange for a note-taker in certain classes	• Joins organization on campus that goes to local high schools to talk about risks of drinking and driving and violence

Continued

TABLE 35-2 SCI/D Levels (continued)

LEVEL	MOVEMENTS GAINED/ SPARED	AREA OF OCCUPATION	FUNCTIONAL GOALS—CLIENT CAN:	OCCUPATIONS AND ACTIVITIES
C7	Wrist flexors, triceps	ADLs	• Groom and self-feed seated in wheelchair with Mod I • Dress with Mod I from bed or wheelchair • Bathe with Mod I sitting on padded TTB or commode chair • Perform intermittent self-catheterization with Mod I • Perform bowel program with Mod I seated on padded commode • Independently transfer between bed and power wheelchair with transfer board or press-over transfer • Independently drive power wheelchair with joystick or propel manual wheelchair with UEs • Independently verbalize positioning considerations for sexual activity	• Practices using toothbrush and hairbrush with built-up handle or modified grip • Practices applying modified grip for various self-feeding and grooming tools • Practices intermittent self-catheterization from bed, wheelchair, and/or toilet • Dresses from bed using circle and long sitting positions or from wheelchair with modified grasp and engaging triceps for clothing management • Practices sponge bathing from bed, learning to lift and manipulate LEs with UEs and engaging triceps, in preparation to bathe in shower • Practices using modified bowel stimulator while sitting on padded commode • Propels manual wheelchair with power assist from downtown office to bus stop
C7		IADLs	• Perform household tasks such as washing dishes and laundry with Mod I • Prepare healthy meals and clean up with Mod I • Grocery shop with Mod I	• Loads dishwasher with lightweight, plastic dishes • Transfers laundry from washer to dryer; may use dressing stick for reach • Coordinates propelling manual wheelchair while pushing a grocery cart • Loads trunk of car with grocery bags
C7		Rest/sleep	• Transfer from wheelchair to high bed surfaces when traveling with Mod I to Min A	<u>Activities</u> • Practices transferring from wheelchair to high surface using transfer board • Uses standing frame for 45 minutes per day to promote better sleep
C7		Education/ work/leisure	• Join and play on a quad rugby team	<u>Occupations</u> • Participates in weekly quad rugby practices

PREPARATORY METHODS AND TASKS	EDUCATION AND TRAINING	ADVOCACY AND SELF ADVOCACY	GROUP INTERVENTIONS
Tasks • Client performs shoulder, bicep, triceps, and wrist strengthening exercises using wrist weights and modified equipment • OTA provides dynamic sitting balance activities in preparation for dressing from wheelchair and reaching for bowel program • Client practices activities reaching outside of and returning to base of support in preparation for IADL at wheelchair level Modalities • OTA provides FES to scapular stabilizers to facilitate strengthening and stabilization	Education • OTA educates client and caregiver on causes of and strategies to prevent autonomic dysreflexia • OTA educates client and caregiver on wheelchair seating and positioning components that protect UE integrity • OTA educates on importance of padded bathroom equipment for skin integrity Training • OTA instructs client on how to break down and reassemble a manual wheelchair • Training on manual wheelchair propulsion in community, ramps, and so on • OTA demonstrates and teaches technique for using skin inspection mirror to perform daily skin check	• Requests reasonable accommodations for workplace restroom	• Joins a group of women with SCI that meets monthly through a local chapter of United Spinal Association for exchange of information/ resources specific to women's health after SCI/D
Modalities • OTA ace wraps client's LEs to prevent orthostatic hypotension when sitting upright. • Client practices balancing while scooted to the edge of the seat in wheelchair in order to reach for items in kitchen and laundry room Assistive Technology and Environmental Modification • OTA modifies office workstation setup with ergonomic considerations for UE preservation	Education • OTA recommends modification to household appliances: front-loading washer and dryer Training • OTA instructs client on coordinating wheelchair propulsion while participating in activities such as cooking, shopping, and doing laundry	Self-Advocacy • Requests assistance in loading trunk of car with groceries • Uses insurance money from accident to purchase an adapted van	• OTA facilitates a cooking group and includes a peer mentor who demonstrates adapted kitchen utensils
Assistive Technology • OTA recommends use of transfer board for unleveled transfers when traveling	Education • OTA educates on creating a routine to minimize client disruption during sleep Training • OTA instructs client on consistent routine formation around sleep	Self-Advocacy • Contacts hotel before travel to inquire if beds in wheelchair-accessible rooms are the correct height for transfers	
Preparatory Tasks • Client carries out regular strengthening, stretching, and endurance-building exercise program	Education • OTA provides resources on local adaptive sports organizations and ideas for fund-raising for adapted sports equipment	Self-Advocacy • Applies for a grant to get a rugby chair	• Travels with quad rugby team to a tournament against other teams

Continued

TABLE 35-2 SCI/D Levels (continued)

LEVEL	MOVEMENTS GAINED/ SPARED	AREA OF OCCUPATION	FUNCTIONAL GOALS—CLIENT CAN:	OCCUPATIONS AND ACTIVITIES
C8-T1	C8— Add strength and precision of fingers, gain finger flexors T1—Add intrinsics in hand	ADLs	• Groom seated in wheelchair with Mod I • Dress with Mod I from bed or wheelchair • Bathe with Mod I sitting on padded TTB or commode chair • Perform intermittent self-catheterization with Mod I • Perform bowel program with Mod I seated on padded commode • Independently transfer between car driver seat to wheelchair with transfer board	• Practices curling hair with curling iron while seated at vanity in manual wheelchair • Practices inserting suppository in bed before transfer to toilet for bowel program • Performs intermittent self-catheterization in public restroom • Practices transfers from wheelchair to padded commode and padded TTB • Tries on clothing in store dressing room from manual wheelchair
C8-T1		IADLs	• Babysit grandchildren with Mod I • Drive with hand controls with Mod I • Maintain flower garden with Mod I	• Prepares meals for grandchildren • Picks up grandchildren from after-school program twice per week • Weeds garden, and plants new shrubs • Practices balancing while scooted to the edge of the seat in wheelchair in order to reach items in dishwasher
C8-T1		Education/ work/leisure	• Return to work with Mod I • Engage in health maintenance by swimming at a local recreation center	Occupations • Returns to working a job with flexibility to telecommute • Attends open swim time at recreation center three times per week
T2-T12	Increasing trunk/back and core strength, more with each lower level	ADLs	• Groom seated in a wheelchair with independence • Dress with Mod I from bed or wheelchair • Bathe with Mod I sitting on padded TTB or commode chair • Perform intermittent self-catheterization with Mod I • Perform bowel program with Mod I seated on padded commode • Independently transfer between car driver seat to wheelchair	• Performs intermittent self-catheterization in public restroom • Uses standing frame 60 minutes per day to calm spasticity, which interferes with ADLs
T2-T12		IADLs	• Be able to sit on the floor to change son's diaper • T2-T8 injury: Stand using bilateral knee-ankle-foot orthoses (KAFOs) along with a walker or crutches for meal prep task in kitchen • T10-T12 injury: walk household distances independently with KAFOs and assistive devices	Activities • Practices uneven level transfers with progression to floor transfers • Performs reaching tasks while standing for progressing lengths of time in preparation for meal task

PREPARATORY METHODS AND TASKS	EDUCATION AND TRAINING	ADVOCACY AND SELF ADVOCACY	GROUP INTERVENTIONS
Tasks • Client practices bed mobility skills needed to position in side-lying for suppository insertion • OTA instructs client on clothing adaptations that may increase ease of self-catheterization from wheelchair • OTA educates on prone exercise program for scapular strengthening	Education • OTA educates client on benefits of regular physical activity for prevention of chronic conditions after SCI • OTA educates client and caregiver on protecting UE integrity during community mobility and community transfers Training • OTA instructs client on impact of water buoyancy on blood pressure	• Advocates for more accessible bathroom at work for self-catheterization	
Assistive Technology and Environmental Modification • OTA modifies car keys for improved grasp • OTA modifies garden with raised beds	Education • OTA recommends Certified Driving Rehabilitation Specialist for hand-control training	• Asks children to pick up and wash clothing to assist around the house	• Takes a cooking class at the local community college • Takes young dog to obedience classes to cut down on pulling behaviors during walks (manual wheelchair level)
Preparatory Methods • OTA provides aquatic exercises designed to build endurance and strength • Client practices transferring from manual wheelchair to pool lift chair	Training • OTA instructs client on how to transport work-related items while propelling wheelchair to minimize shoulder strain	• Speaks with manager and human resources about accommodations required	• Although has the ability to work from home, attends weekly team meetings • Signs up for an adaptive scuba diving class
Tasks • Client practices LE management skills while in wheelchair to increase independence with dressing • Client practices clothed transfers to TTB in preparation for more difficult unclothed transfers during bathing	Education • OTA educates client on benefits of regular physical activity for prevention of chronic conditions after SCI • OTA educates client and caregiver on protecting UE integrity during community mobility and community transfers Training • OTA trains client on balance tasks to increase compensation for weakness and strengthen available muscles	• Advocates for ADA bathroom at work, even though it is a small company and it is not required • Contacts restaurant before going out to ensure it is accessible and will be a positive experience	• OTA takes multiple clients on an outing to a local restaurant while they are still in the inpatient rehab setting to prepare them for community reentry
Assistive Technology and Environmental Modification • Train with a crutch, walker, or cane to be able to carry things, open doors, and so on	Education • OTA educates on problem solving and using tools in the environment to assist with floor transfers • OTA recommends Certified Driving Rehabilitation specialist for hand- control training	• Requests that Vocational Rehabilitation Services pay for a wheelchair that allows standing for job duties, such as to reach supplies and interact with customers at eye level	• Participates in a wheelchair skills group

Continued

TABLE 35-2 SCI/D Levels (continued)

LEVEL	MOVEMENTS GAINED/ SPARED	AREA OF OCCUPATION	FUNCTIONAL GOALS—CLIENT CAN:	OCCUPATIONS AND ACTIVITIES
T2-T12, *continued*				
T2-T12		Rest/sleep	• Transfer from wheelchair to high bed surfaces when traveling with Mod I	Activities • Practices transferring from wheelchair to high surface
T2-T12		Education/ work/leisure	• Return to work in an office with Mod I	Occupations • Returns to full-time desk job Activities • Joins an adapted gym to increase strength and provide stress relief
L1 and below	L2 hip flexion, L3 knee extension, L4 ankle dorsiflexion, L5 great toe extension, S1 ankle plantar flexion	ADLs	• Groom with independence • Dress with Mod I to independent from bed or wheelchair • Bathe with Mod I sitting on padded TTB or commode chair • Perform intermittent self-catheterization with Mod I • Perform bowel program with Mod I seated on padded commode • Use sexual enhancements for maintaining erection with Mod I	• Performs sit-to-stand transition training to allow client to manage clothing while standing • Performs static and dynamic standing balance training for ADLs and IADLs
L1 and below	Ambulation best below L3	IADLs	• Independently drive by using a car adapted with hand controls • Transfer to car driver seat with Mod I • Mod I with household and community ambulation for IADLs, with or without use of braces and assistive devices (KAFOs and ankle-foot orthoses [AFOs])	• Practices disassembling wheelchair to place into car
L1 and below		Rest/sleep	• Independently perform LE stretching before bed to decrease leg spasms at night	Activities • OTA practices use of leg lifter as needed to get legs into standard bed
L1 and below		Education/ work/leisure	• Return to work at independent level if desk/office job (may need job retraining for more active job)	Activities • Stands intermittently at work to decrease leg spasms throughout day

PREPARATORY METHODS AND TASKS	EDUCATION AND TRAINING	ADVOCACY AND SELF ADVOCACY	GROUP INTERVENTIONS
	• Advanced wheelchair training: uneven surfaces, rough terrain, ramps, curbs, "wheelies" and transfers from floor to wheelchair		
Assistive Technology • May prefer adjustable bed to standard bed	Education • OTA educates on using a small laundry detergent bottle with a lid to perform self-catheterization into at night to prevent spills		
Assistive Technology and Environmental Modification • Client volunteers at local men's shelter to serve meals with a portable ramp for the step	Training • Drives independently using an adapted van or a car adapted with hand controls	Self-Advocacy • Applies to Vocational Rehabilitation Services since he cannot return to employment as a plumber	• Meets another person with SCI, who recommends a hand cycle to trial for road biking
Tasks • Use of functional electrical stimulation (FES) to perform some functional tasks while standing or with ambulation	Education • OTA educates on options for bowel management via timing of caffeine, fiber, and water	• Discusses with his primary care physician the need for referral to a counselor specializing in sexuality issues	• Meets a group of men from an adapted tennis team for coffee and breakfast
Assistive Technology and Environmental Modification • Use an adaptable-height table in kitchen for meal preparation ease whether sitting or standing	Education • OTA educates on importance of skin inspection after doffing braces to prevent skin breakdown Training • Floor transfer training in order to allow client to continue with interest in mechanical work on his car	• Discusses with spouse the need for a new washer and dryer for ease of access whether sitting in a wheelchair or standing	• Queries a group of friends over lunch about the best lightweight vacuum
Environmental Modifications • Client removes box spring from bed to lower the height of the mattress for easier transfers	Education • OTA educates on importance of elevating heels when sleeping to prevent pressure injuries	• Discusses the "handicapped" room received at a hotel during a trip, which was not accessible with a large chair next to a very high bed	
Environmental Modifications • Client asks for and uses a stool at a party for energy conservation Assistive Technology • Client invests in a specialized wheelchair basketball chair	Training • Use of a manual wheelchair for energy conservation and some functional mobility	Self-Advocacy • Discusses the need for a handicapped parking sticker to not ambulate/propel wheelchair as far • Discusses the need to get a special key to use college-restricted elevators	• Participates in an adapted sports program for exercise and social interaction

Adaptive Equipment and Functional Mobility: Because of this lack of wrist and hand strength, clients can use a dorsal wrist support with a universal cuff attachment for increased independence with self-feeding and grooming activities. This dorsal wrist support keeps the wrist in a neutral or slightly extended position while the universal cuff holds the utensil or tool. This adaptive equipment can also assist with other desired activities such as operating a keyboard or tablet using a stylus (Fig. 35-10). Even with wrist stabilization, clients with C5 spinal injuries in the early stages may benefit from a mobile arm support that attaches to a wheelchair or table. The mobile arm support provides shoulder, elbow, and wrist support and aids in active assisted ROM to support UE use for tasks such as self-feeding and grooming. (See Figure 12-2.)

Activities of Daily Living Goals: Clients with a C5 level of injury require maximum or total assistance with their ADLs, although some may gain minimal independence with certain tasks. However, with dorsal wrist support and universal cuff attachment, clients can learn to groom and self-feed with setup to moderate assistance. Some clients can don a large T-shirt with practice and some assist, but most other dressing requires total assist. Bathing transfers will generally be dependent, but with a supportive seat, the client should be able to use a wash mitt and liquid soap to reach the arms, chest, groin, and possibly upper legs. Toileting tasks usually require total assistance. Clients with a C5 level of injury can independently drive a power wheelchair with a joystick or alternative drive control that is modified and programmable according to the client's capacities. EADLs can assist at this level as well as with computer, work, phone, and home access. Clients at this level may drive a specially modified and adapted van. It is important for OT practitioners to employ clinical reasoning and engage with the client to determine what activities are important to carry out as independently as possible and what can be delegated. UE preservation and energy conservation strategies are critical quality-of life considerations when prioritizing ADL and IADL goals.

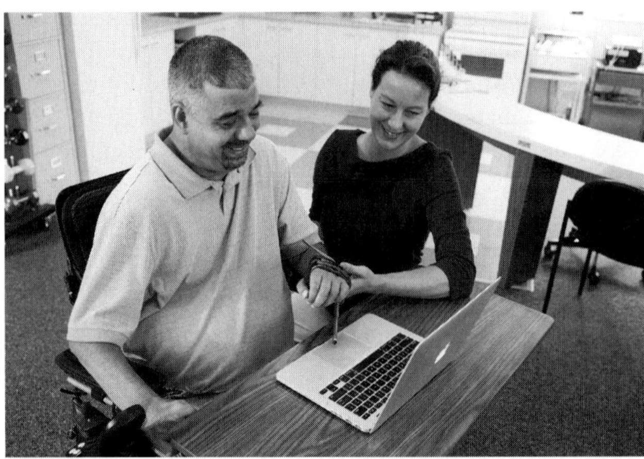

FIGURE 35-10. A person with C5 tetraplegia using stylus in a wrist support to use a tablet.

CERVICAL TETRAPLEGIA: C6

Strength and Somatosensation: Clients with this level of SCI/D have strength in their wrist extensor muscles. With this additional muscle group, they are able to use their UEs more functionally for ADLs and IADLs as well as for functional mobility and wheelchair propulsion. With wrist extension, they have the mechanism called **tenodesis,** which allows passive grasp between the index finger and thumb or a gross grasp in the palm of the hand.[6] With tenodesis, as the wrist extends, the fingers flex and the thumb adducts, and as the wrist flexes (performed at this level by relaxing the wrist extensors, since there is no active wrist flexion), the fingers extend and the thumb abducts (Fig. 35-11). This allows for functional grasp and release and some lateral pinch with the thumb and index finger.

It is critical that clients with this level of injury/disease avoid inadvertently stretching out the finger flexors and thumb by stretching incorrectly. Clients and their caregivers should be instructed and trained to flex the wrist in order to extend the fingers and to flex the fingers when extending the wrist. This preserves the natural mechanism that occurs when the wrist is extended and the fingers flex. When clients unknowingly extend or stretch their fingers out while their wrist is extended, they may lose the grasping mechanism of flexed fingers with an extended wrist. Even more important is that the thumb does not get overstretched. When the wrist extends and the fingers flex, the thumb passively adducts as well for a pinch movement. If the thumb gets overstretched into abduction, it may no longer reach the index finger for a functional pinch. See Figure 35-12 for an example of a product called the ThumDuction™ Strap to protect the thumb into adduction. Many OT practitioners do not actually stretch the thumb of clients at this SCI/D level, since a slightly tighter pinch may be more functional.

Adaptive Equipment and Functional Mobility: Orthotics and bracing may be used to preserve tenodesis in the event of hypertonicity, via a resting hand orthosis. A tenodesis brace may also be worn externally to strengthen the tenodesis grasp, however these braces are bulky, heavy, and difficult to function in meaningful tasks outside of isolated hand function exercise purposes. Generally, they are not used in most rehabilitative centers any longer.

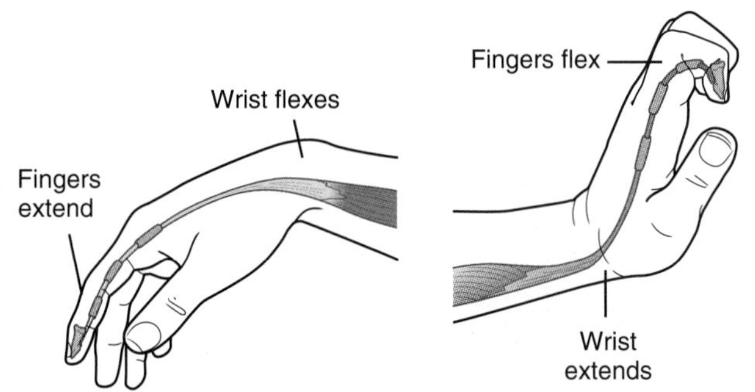

FIGURE 35-11. Tenodesis.

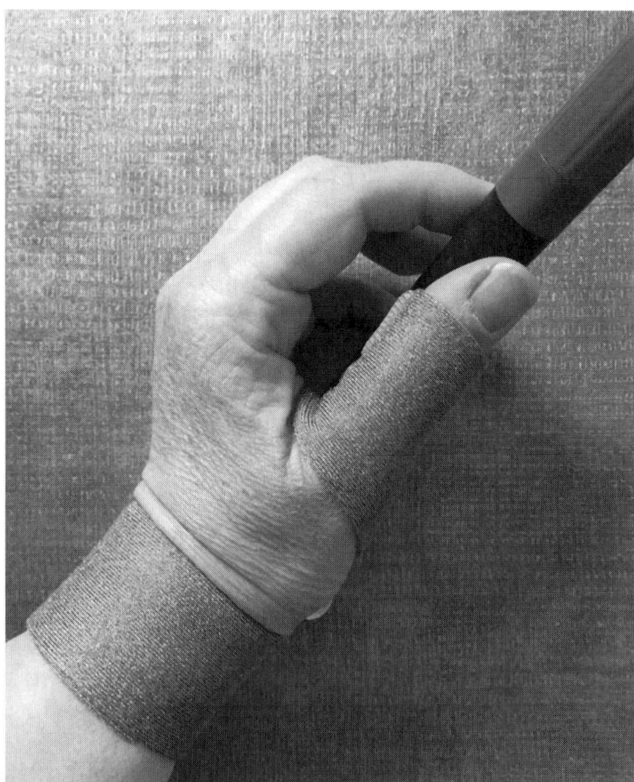

FIGURE 35-12. ThumDuction™ Strap to support the thumb in tenodesis grasp and avoid excessive abduction.

With a tenodesis grasp, clients may benefit from objects with lightweight, built-up or extended handles to maximize their grasp and reach at the wheelchair level. Lightweight foam tubing can help manage items such as toothbrushes, utensils for self-feeding, writing, and art tools, or a client may use a universal cuff to hold the item. Tasks requiring force when using tenodesis, such as hair brushing and tooth brushing, can be difficult, as tenodesis does not generally have a forceful grip. A cuff made from a spare loop of Velcro® could be attached to items for a stronger force as the client performs the task. Lightweight electric toothbrushes and razors are simple solutions for ADL independence (Fig. 35-13).

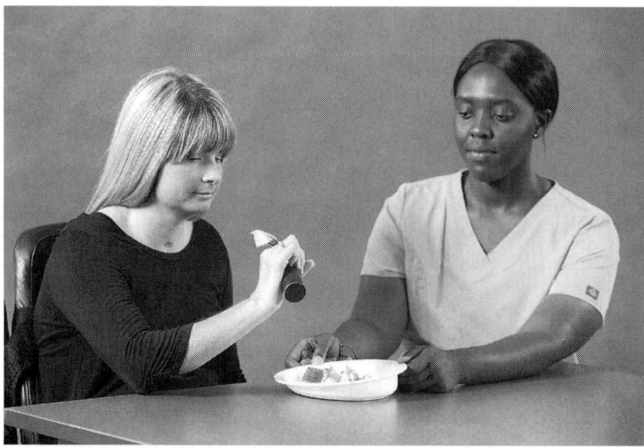

FIGURE 35-13. Using tenodesis to lift a large-handled fork.

Bathroom and shower equipment should be chosen and integrated into the client's routine with careful attention. Some clients with this level of injury benefit from more complex rehab commode/shower wheelchairs that tilt in space for blood pressure and pressure relief management. Others do not require this complexity and function well with upright tub transfer benches (TTBs), commodes, and shower chairs. Factors such as skin integrity risks, blood pressure stability, availability of caregiver assistance, and time since injury are all factors involved in the clinical reasoning process when an OTA is helping to decide which DME is most appropriate for the client and caregivers.

Clients with a C6 level of injury may propel a manual or power wheelchair, and this decision is made initially and in subsequent evaluations by an OT or PT at a seating clinic in a team effort with the client and caregivers or family members. The OTA may be involved in training with use of the mobility device in daily activities and also reinforcing the UE strengthening regimen for protection of their UEs. Sometimes a power wheelchair is recommended depending on the individual characteristics of the client. Some examples for power wheelchair indication at C6 include older age, heavier body build, history of or risk for repetitive shoulder strain injuries, and poor pulmonary status.

Activities of Daily Living Goals: Most clients with C6 levels of SCI/D benefit from at least a minimal level of assistance with many ADLs, but may progress to achieving higher levels of independence over time with practice and task and environmental modifications. Clients with C6 SCI/D can often perform grooming tasks and self-feed meals with modified independence or supervision/set-up using a universal cuff, using tools with built-up handles, or by holding tools in a modified manner. Some clients use tenodesis, and others find success by weaving or threading tools such as pens and forks between their fingers, using tightness in their finger flexors to their advantage.

Clients can generally perform upper body dressing and assist with lower body dressing. Many can perform bladder and bowel management with adaptive equipment and techniques. Bathing can be performed with a nylon mesh body scrubber or washcloth held with tenodesis grasp, liquid soap, pump bottles, and at times a long sponge. Since energy conservation and UE preservation are important considerations in daily routine, some people benefit from assistance for ADLs and choose to have more independence around IADLs.

ADLs, such as dressing, can be accomplished at the bed or wheelchair level, and OTAs should collaborate with clients and caregivers to assess the impact of the physical environment on independence, safety, and energy. For instance, many clients begin toileting, dressing, and bathing routines in bed as they improve strength, balance, endurance, and confidence and gradually progress to bathing in the shower, performing their bowel program over the toilet, and self-catheterizing from the wheelchair, while they continue to dress in bed.

CERVICAL TETRAPLEGIA: C7

Strength and Somatosensation: Clients with this level of injury typically are considerably more independent than the previous levels because at the C7 level they have innervation of triceps, wrist flexors, and finger extensors.[6] While they do not have innervation of finger flexors, they can use a tenodesis grasp for grasp and release of objects and have the additional ability to actively extend their fingers. Triceps strength responsible for active elbow extension is helpful during transfers because the extended elbow facilitates a co-contraction on both sides of the joint during transfers for increased support and balance. Clients with this level of function can rely on their UEs for transfer assistance as they prop in sitting and move across the transfer board or perform a press-over transfer. Of course, triceps strength also plays an important role in other activities such as reaching for a grab bar during bathing, retrieving an object from the floor or overhead cabinet, or propelling a manual wheelchair.[6]

Clients with this level of injury also have strength in the pectoralis, serratus anterior, and latissimus dorsi muscles.[6] These muscles allow improved strength and stability in the scapulae and UEs for wheelchair propulsion and transfers, rolling in bed, and self-care activities.[6]

Adaptive Equipment and Functional Mobility: Adaptive equipment that is helpful for clients with C6 SCI/D are often also helpful for clients with C7 SCI/D. Built-up handles and modified grasp techniques may be useful because grasp is weak although active release is present at this level.

OT practitioners work with clients and their caregivers to assess for the most appropriate and medically necessary power or manual wheelchair. Clients, OT practitioners, and complex rehabilitation equipment suppliers may be successful in seeking and leveraging resources to acquire both a power and manual wheelchair for disparate purposes. For instance, a young woman with C7 tetraplegia who attends a large university on a hilly campus may choose to use a power wheelchair while driving around campus for energy conservation and shoulder preservation purposes but use a manual wheelchair in her dorm where space is limited. Attention must be drawn to UE protection and preservation as well as energy conservation and safety.

DME, such as TTBs, shower chairs, and shower/commode combination chairs, allow for independence for many with bathing and/or bowel program completion and related clothing management, together with handheld shower heads and grab bars.

Activities of Daily Living Goals: Clients with a C7 level of spinal cord injury can perform ADLs with modified independence by using modified techniques or adaptive equipment. Generally, lower body dressing is easier from the bed with rolling, but may also be performed from the chair. They often benefit from modified strategies and techniques for fine motor coordination and weak grasp, such as identifying ways to maximize finger extension functionally, but do not usually depend on a significant amount of adaptive equipment for self-feeding and grooming. At this level of function, men and women may be able to self-catheterize from bed, wheelchair, or toilet with modified grasp and use of mirrors for visual guidance (Box 35-3).

CERVICAL TETRAPLEGIA: C8

Strength and Somatosensation: Clients with C8 complete tetraplegia have the additional capacity of innervation to their thumb and finger flexors.[6] Because of this strength, they need not fully rely on a tenodesis grasp or adaptive equipment as they have greater fine motor strength and control. They also have greater strength in their triceps and shoulder muscles, which allows more functional independence.[6]

Adaptive Equipment and Functional Mobility: Due to continued paralysis of their trunk and LE muscles, clients with C8 SCI/D benefit from specialty bathing and toileting

BOX 35-3
Tendon Transfers

A surgery that has been available for over 40 years, but is still relatively uncommon is tendon transfer for clients with tetraplegia. It is estimated that 65% to 75% of clients with C5-C7-level tetraplegia could benefit from UE surgery to move tendons from muscles with movement to assist movement in other areas, but only about 14% get the surgery.[69] Some of the proposed reasons for the low numbers may be lack of communication and cross-specialty collaboration, poor access to care, and lack of knowledge.[69] Common surgical options are to move posterior deltoid or part of the biceps to triceps, and brachioradialis to the wrist or thumb. Increased triceps movement would increase independence with reaching overhead, weight shifting, and transfers, while increased hand function could allow pinch and/or grasp and release for self-catheterization and ADLs.[69] Most tendon transfers are done at 1 year or more post-injury.

Another procedure that is gaining popularity is a nerve transfer, either alone or in combination with tendon transfer(s). Generally, this level of surgery is appropriate for clients with C6-C7 tetraplegia. A peripheral nerve from a muscle (brachialis for instance) above the level of injury is moved to a muscle without current nerve innervation due to the SCI/D.[70] Once a connection is established, clients undergo extensive therapy to train the brain to recognize the new nerve signals.[70] Since the nerve regenerates at about a millimeter per day or about 1 inch per month, the process can take 6 to 24 months to see a functional pinch with the thumb and index finger.

DME. It is also very individualized whether power or manual wheelchair use is recommended. Either type of wheelchair is a possibility and is determined by a combination of body function, contextual considerations, and environmental considerations.

Activities of Daily Living Goals: Clients with C8 SCI/D can achieve independence with all ADLs and transfers. Shoulder and scapular stability and strength proximally combined with distal triceps, forearm, wrist, and relative intrinsic hand muscle strength provide greater UE function and overall independence with self-care and mobility.

THORACIC TETRAPLEGIA: T1

Strength and Somatosensation: Clients with T1 complete paraplegia have very functional hand use. They continue to have some weakness in their intrinsic hand muscles affecting the finesse of very fine motor activities.[6]

Adaptive Equipment and Functional Mobility: The capacity for stronger proximal and distal UEs means more independence, stability, and fluidity of performance. Fully functional UEs also allow for some compensation because clients with this level of injury have continued weakness of trunk muscles. OT practitioners recommend and teach clients how to use specialty bathing and toileting DME. As for clients with C7 and C8 SCI/D, either a power or manual wheelchair may be functionally and medically appropriate.

Activities of Daily Living Goals: With T1 tetraplegia, clients can independently perform all self-care and mobility tasks. As is the case with clients with a higher level of tetraplegia, self-care training and education often begin in bed, but because of increased strength in their UEs enabling improved function and balance, they may more quickly transition to showering, dressing from the wheelchair, and managing bowel and bladder functions over the toilet.

THORACIC PARAPLEGIA T2-T12

Clients with thoracic paraplegia between the levels of T2 and T12 have full UE strength and varying degrees of trunk strength. Clients with more caudal (lower) levels of injury have more innervation of trunk muscles and thus greater strength, balance, control, and capacity for controlled, volitional movement.[6] Depending on factors intrinsic and extrinsic to the client, these clients can propel a manual wheelchair and use upright shower and commode equipment without tilt or recline features. They benefit from commode and shower seats that are padded and have cutouts to protect their skin and provide access for self-catheterization and their bowel program.

LUMBAR AND SACRAL PARAPLEGIA L1-S5

Clients with lumbar and sacral paraplegia do not have injuries that are classified as complete.[6] They have varying abilities to ambulate and therefore, different degrees of reliance on manual wheelchairs. While these are all considered LMN injuries, clients will have varying functional abilities because the lumbar and sacral spinal cord innervate different myotomes and dermatomes. For example, the lumbar spinal cord innervates most LE muscles, so an injury in this area will likely impact walking ability. An injury in the sacral spinal cord may not affect walking to as great an extent. Spinal involvement in the lumbar or sacral spine does not impact UE or trunk strength and somatosensation. Clients are independent with self-care tasks and functional mobility and may have bowel and bladder involvement. As discussed in the neurogenic bowel and bladder section of this chapter, LMN injuries often lead to complex bowel and bladder management issues. While clients with this level of injury theoretically have the UE gross and fine motor physical capacity to perform bowel and bladder management functions, they (as with all SCI/D levels) may benefit from assistance of a caregiver due to challenges coping emotionally.

Occupational Therapy Areas of Intervention

This section discusses OT areas of intervention to develop short- and long-term goals with the client.

OCCUPATIONS AND ACTIVITIES

The OT practitioner and client work together to develop a vision of the client's short- and long-term goals and through the therapeutic use of occupations and activities, work toward these goals. When OT practitioners and clients have a mutual understanding of meaningful goals, OTAs identify functional activities that contribute to accomplishing these goals. Activities include components of occupations that hold meaning, relevance, and perceived utility for clients.[7] Occupation- and activity-based interventions facilitating ADL and IADL relearning are powerful because they reflect the client's motivations, desires, and purposes.

For example, a client with a T4 SCI/D may have a goal for showering daily before a college class. Because of the T4 SCI/D and resulting trunk and LE paralysis, he will benefit from bathing seated on a TTB. The OT practitioner grades this ADL by beginning the first day with sponge bathing at the bed level. This activity teaches the client to manage his legs with his arms; to understand what it feels like to balance and control his trunk with head, neck, and UE; to build endurance for an activity that will soon be accomplished in the shower; to establish patterns of energy conservation for a taxing activity; to perform regular skin checks; and to observe and continually monitor ROM. The OTA is able to grade the activity with dressing and bathing as the client's activity tolerance and confidence builds.

Clients with SCI/D are at risk for the secondary complications discussed in the body functions section of this chapter. Prevention of secondary complications such as pressure injuries, urinary tract infections, fecal impaction, orthostatic hypotension, autonomic dysreflexia, DVTs, and contractures is paramount. OTAs educate and train clients and their support systems about how incorporating activities such as skin checks, bowel and bladder programs, and regular physical activity consistently promotes their desired occupations. The college student with a T4 SCI/D might work with an OTA to outline how these health and wellness activities can be integrated into his daily routine and support his occupation of student.

PREPARATORY METHODS

Preparatory methods are activities that the OT practitioner uses to prepare the client for or during the performance of occupations. A preparatory method may also be something the OT practitioner gives to the client to use in the home environment, such as an orthotic, which will support the client's ability to perform occupations. The focus of the preparatory method is on what the OT practitioner does.[13]

Wheeled Mobility: OT practitioners work together with the client, the client's family, and the seating specialist to narrow down the best wheelchair seating and positioning fit for the client. The client is afforded opportunity to trial various types of medically and functionally appropriate wheelchairs and through this process, identifies the wheelchair with the seating clinic specialist that best facilitates the client's lifestyle and goals.

ADL and IADL training at the wheelchair level is graded according to level of injury and activity and occupational demands. As with all OT intervention related to SCI/D, this involves close collaboration between the OT practitioner and the client. Understanding the environment to which the client will be discharging is instrumental in planning and preparation.[32] With the advantage of technology today, clients and their families may take photos and video and share this media with their therapy team to facilitate successful wheelchair mobility training before discharge. When discharge to the client's home environment is not possible, acquiring as much information about the environment to which the client is discharging will facilitate success and will help the client and OT practitioner anticipate barriers that can be at least in part addressed through wheelchair mobility training. OT provides a valuable perspective when these clients and their families prepare for discharge to the community.

For clients with complete SCI/D levels between C6 and L2, wheelchair mobility training includes learning to transfer safely and efficiently between a wheelchair and various surfaces throughout the day. These surfaces may include the toilet or bedside commode, shower chair or TTB, bed, sofa, recliner, dining chairs, and the floor. Transferring onto a high, standard bed with a soft mattress would be different from transferring onto an adjustable hospital bed. Car transfers are also important for the OTA and PT staff to fully train the client and caregiver on, including both the transfer and loading mobility equipment (Fig. 35-14). See Chapter 13 on transfers for details.

For clients with complete injury above C6, mobility training often consists of building tolerance toward getting safely in and out bed with mobility equipment and the assistance of one or more people. This equipment may include a transfer board or lift. One of the most important goals for these clients is to be able to independently direct their mobility.

For clients with complete SCI/D at L2 and below, the possibility of assisted ambulation and/or standing is greater, and the OTA works with clients to integrate standing, ambulation, or combined wheelchair use and functional ambulation in daily living skills.

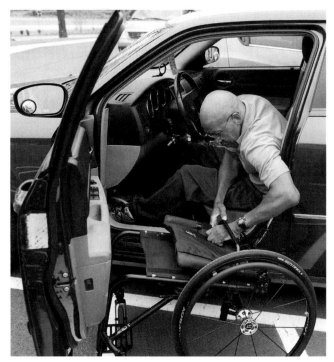

FIGURE 35-14. Car transfer with loading of manual wheelchair. Note how this client, with a cervical SCI (and no trunk control) has learned techniques for bracing against the car frame and his left leg to maintain balance during the loading.

Assistive Technology and Environmental Modifications: When SCI/D leads to tetraplegia and the client has UE impairment, OT practitioners recommend adaptive equipment and assistive technology to maximize clients' ability to participate to their fullest ability. Once it is assessed that the equipment is a best fit between the client and the task, the OTA and client work to generalize its use across environmental variables including settings, times of day, and task variations.

OT practitioners are highly skilled in assessing the physical and environmental contexts in which their clients live. The inpatient rehab phase is a valuable time to work with clients and their support teams to begin making decisions about home modifications. The priorities may include a ramp for entrance into the home; widened doorways or removal of doors into bathrooms and bedrooms; clearing space throughout the home to allow wheelchair access; rearranging commonly accessed items to be at shoulder level for UE preservation, assessing flooring options, and so on. Other priorities for modifications may include vehicle access by power or manual wheelchair. The Consortium for Spinal Cord Medicine recommends the Americans with Disabilities Act (ADA) guidelines for minimum environmental modification guidelines.

Orthotic Fabrication: For clients with tetraplegia, orthotics can be important for functional hand use. Hand function increases independence even when LE function is lost or compromised. Fabrication of orthoses often begins in the acute phase, continues with more intensity in the inpatient rehabilitation phase, and is then refined in the post–inpatient rehabilitation phase.

C4 and Above: Clients with complete SCI/D at these levels do not have hand function, and so orthosis use is aimed at preventing painful and harmful contractures.[6] Positioning the hand in a sustained resting position over prolonged periods is recommended.[6] The preferred position for someone with no hand function or who may gain tenodesis function is in the intrinsic plus position with the hand metacarpophalangeal (MCP) joints in flexion and interphalangeal (IP) joints in extension (Fig. 35-15).

C5 Tetraplegia: Clients with function at the C5 level often have the ability to bend at the elbow using their elbow flexors and even anterior deltoid compensation, and can bring their hand to their face with these muscles.[6] With lack of wrist extension, however, it is difficult and puts clients at a mechanical disadvantage to attempt to bend their elbow and lift their hand against gravity. Orthotics that support the wrist in a comfortable and safe neutral position while also supporting function in the hands can help clients with SCI/D to grossly manage objects between the forearms or wrists. The addition of a universal cuff in conjunction with a wrist supportive orthosis allows for use of utensils, writing tools, a stylus, and grooming items. In these cases, OT practitioners teach clients to use their arms in such a way as to prevent overuse in maladaptive patterns that may contribute to shoulder pain from torquing their shoulder in an adaptive abduction or "chicken wing" position, proximally, to gain distal advantage of the task. OT practitioners often also fabricate orthotics to maintain these clients' elbows in extension overnight to prevent elbow flexion contractures.

C6 Tetraplegia: The hallmark of a client with C6 tetraplegia is the presence of wrist extension. With active wrist extension, one can achieve passive finger flexion if the flexor tendons are not elongated by inappropriate stretching. This lever system of combined wrist extension and finger flexion provides the client with a modified grasp. The client can use passive thumb adduction and finger flexion to grasp objects and opposing passive extension of the same fingers to release objects. In order to preserve this action of tenodesis, the hand is held in the intrinsic plus position with the orthotic (Fig. 35-15). This is considered to be the more conservative approach to encourage and maintain tenodesis.[6] In cases in which there is increased flexibility in finger and thumb flexors, the best way to increase the effectiveness of the tenodesis grasp is to induce shortening of the extrinsic thumb and finger flexors.[6] More aggressive orthotic strategies in this case involve flexing the MCP and proximal IP joints with the thumb positioned against the side of the second digit.[6] The wrist is held in extension with the orthotic.[6] This type of orthotic fabrication should be done under close supervision of an occupational therapist. IP ROM should be regularly maintained to prevent flexion contractures and the client should also be made aware of the long-term results.[6]

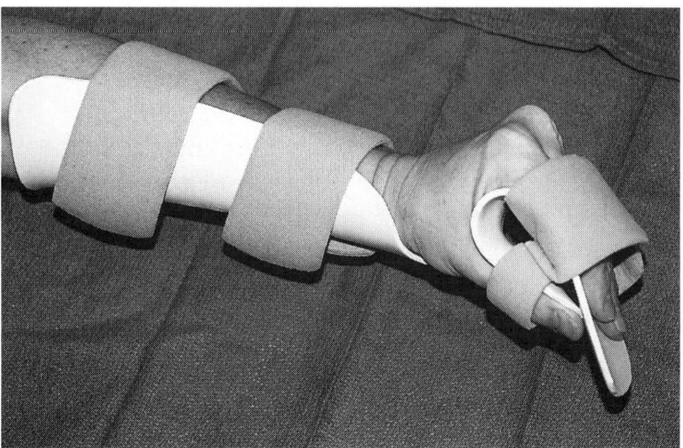

FIGURE 35-15. Intrinsic plus hand position orthotic.

PREPARATORY TASKS

Preparatory tasks are activities that the client performs that "target specific client factors or performance skills."[13] The activities may simulate actual occupations or parts of an occupation, and may not be as meaningful to the client as actually performing the occupation.[13]

Positioning: OTAs will educate and train their clients and caregivers on positioning their bodies during activity and when resting in ways that will prevent pressure injuries, contractures, and pain, and promote stability, movement, and circulation. Care should always be taken to prevent pressure on bony prominences and to limit time spent in one position. OTAs should teach clients and their support networks that when the client is in a wheelchair, he or she should shift weight off of the pelvis, spine, heels, and other bony areas. This process of shifting weight is called pressure relief. In other words, someone with limited UE use who uses a power wheelchair should use the power seating options (tilt, recline, elevating leg rests) available to them to relieve pressure every 30 minutes for 2 minutes. This relieves pressure from and increases circulation in areas prone to pressure injuries such as the sacrum, ischial tuberosities, and greater trochanters. OTAs train manual wheelchair users how to perform lateral shifts and forward leans every 20 minutes (Fig. 35-16). Clients and their caregivers should also establish a consistent pressure relief schedule during rest and sleep times. This means turning in bed every 2 hours to change positions between left and right side-lying, prone, and supine positions. Technology can assist, as smartphones can remind clients to perform their pressure relief until it becomes a habit.

Clients and their caregivers should also be aware that positioning to encourage flexibility and mobility is critical for wellness. OTAs encourage shoulder preservation with positioning the shoulders in abduction and external rotation using pillows when in bed and the use of wheelchair seating to maintain upper and lower body alignment, neutral pelvic positioning, and symmetry in all planes of motion.

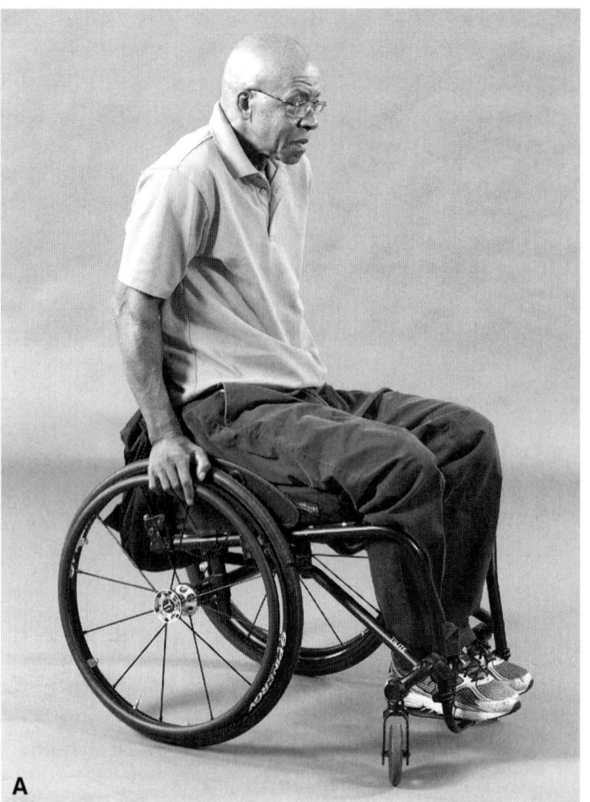

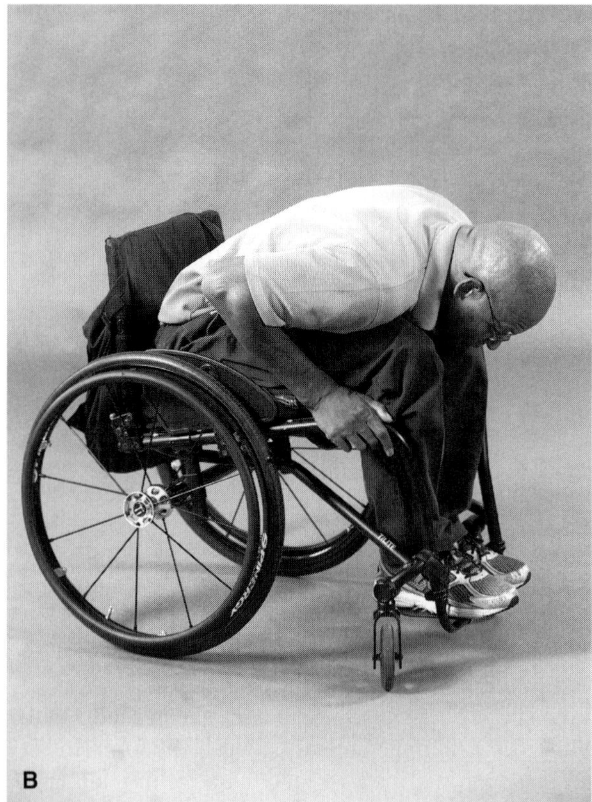

FIGURE 35-16. Pressure relief strategies. **A.** Press up. **B.** Lean forward.

Therapeutic Exercise: After SCI/D, stretching and building physical endurance for activity is an integral part of daily routine that prepares and continues to provide clients the capacity for passive and active movement and meaningful participation. OT practitioners and PT practitioners collaborate to create a regimen of exercises that varies in intensity and purpose over the course of the continuum of care and lifespan. The components of the fitness program reflect clients' level of injury and their overarching goals. Educating clients and their support network is key to any exercise program so that they understand the purpose of daily stretching, ROM, and strengthening to promote wellness and functional activity. While PT practitioners instruct clients on particular exercises, OTAs work to integrate these exercises into daily routines and in a manner that will promote healthy and sustainable habits. Limited flexibility in passive knee extension may be a barrier to a client being able to put on pants, for example. When OTAs notice this during a session focused on dressing, they can collaborate with PT practitioners on a hamstring stretching routine to promote independence and safety with dressing. OTAs also collaborate with clients to identify ways of participation in functional leisure activities that promote physical fitness and psychosocial well-being. These activities may include wheelchair sports, weight lifting, or aquatics.

Promoting flexibility, strength, endurance, and overall fitness is an interdisciplinary effort along the continuum of care and across the lifespan of the client with SCI/D. Early after injury, OTAs may perform and teach family members to range the client's shoulders on a regular schedule to prevent contractures in positions of immobility. Protecting the weakened shoulder while providing ROM for clients with higher levels of injury is important to avoid pain and nerve impingement. All ROM should be gentle, with awareness of both client and OTA/family positioning. The arm should be fully supported with the thumb or palm up to assist with slight external rotation and avoid impingement. The shoulder should not be passively moved beyond 90 degrees of flexion and abduction unless the scapula moves through full upward rotation. To perform full shoulder ROM, the OTA may need to assist the scapula to move into rotation. See Chapter 7 for more information on safe ROM. The family who assists with this program will appreciate feeling they have a helping role.

OTAs and recreational therapists often work together with clients with SCI/D in inpatient rehabilitation to identify meaningful adapted leisure activities promoting health and wellness. When clients return to their communities, OT practitioners connect them with community resources for adapted leisure and networks of peer groups who can encourage return to or explore new options for leisure and recreation.

Advocacy and Groups: Self-advocacy and advocacy is an important part of being empowered to stand up for rights, to advance policy, and to build awareness about what it means to live a healthy life with SCI. Teaching, training, and encouraging self-advocacy is a therapeutic intervention and a valuable skill that OTAs impart to clients. Healthcare policies may dictate the type of wheelchair and wheelchair components for which clients qualify with which diagnosis. As healthcare costs rise, options for complex rehabilitation technologies are narrowing, and OTAs should encourage clients to be vocal about their needs and rights. OTAs can also empower clients with SCI/D to self-advocate within their communities, educating their healthcare networks, community associations, family, and friends about what it means to live well with SCI/D.

Often, OT practitioners use group intervention to educate about advocacy and self-advocacy. Groups provide opportunities for clients with SCI/D to connect with peers and share their journeys, strategies, resources, and ideas with others. Adapted sports programs exist in many communities for competitive and noncompetitive activities such as cycling, water and snow skiing, basketball, rugby, golf, tennis, and many others.

Education and Training: An abundance of education and training after SCI/D for clients and their caregivers is necessary as clients are literally relearning everything from how to accomplish basic daily tasks to fulfilling roles and reintegrating into their communities. This education and training begins from the moments after SCI/D through the life course. Much of the education and training provided revolves around the body functions described in this chapter, and as clients with SCI/D transition through various roles and stages in life, they may benefit from ongoing education and reinforcement of this information. OTAs may encounter opportunities for education with clients in the outpatient or home health OT setting or in innovative community-based settings.

THE CONTINUUM OF OCCUPATIONAL THERAPY ACROSS THE LIFESPAN

After SCI, clients may wonder about their life's trajectory, their purpose, and their identity. Are they the same person after their injury? Will they be able to do the same things that were meaningful for them and to others? How much assistance and care will they need, and for how long? Can they restore their strength, endurance, and coordination? Will they walk again? What about sex? Can they have families? Can they take care of their families? Can they return to school or work? Will their families and friends treat them differently? They question how they will reestablish their roles, routines, rituals, and habits.

OTAs work with clients with SCI/D in a variety of settings to help address these and other concerns. Clients receive OT after injury or with recurrence of SCI/D-related complications in acute hospitals, inpatient rehabilitation facilities, and skilled nursing facilities; 90% of clients transition from inpatient rehabilitation settings to private homes.[71] Clients may continue OT services with home health or in outpatient clinics. Of those who do not return to home settings, most are discharged to skilled nursing facilities or assisted living centers. Gains in rehabilitation can be seen for years after onset of injury, however the most gains are achieved in the first year. Therefore, research suggests that this time be focused on aggressive rehabilitation.[72]

Rehabilitation after SCI/D is an interdisciplinary effort. To be an effective member of the team, OT practitioners must be additionally skilled in communication, teamwork, and team problem-solving to maximize the benefit for their client. Depending on the setting and services offered, intervention may be provided individually, in groups, or both. The opportunity to provide OT in one-on-one and group models and with a diverse team of professionals affords a multitude of client-centered strategies for intervention.

While the focus of OT intervention in each practice setting may differ slightly, what remains consistent is occupation as the medium for change and return to daily living as the goal. OT practitioners facilitate restoration of meaning and discovering novel meaning through occupation-centered practice. Clients relearn basic self-care skills, learn new ways to fulfill valued roles, and reintegrate into their communities.

Occupational Therapy in Acute Care

In the first days and weeks after SCI/D when the focus is on life-saving measures and medical stability, OT approaches to intervention focus mainly around preparatory methods and tasks; education; and advocacy. The cornerstone of all of these is education and training as the client and caregivers are receiving copious amounts of medical information. The acute hospital environment sets the stage for inpatient or subacute rehabilitation, and skillful integration of rehabilitation approaches helps to prepare for that transition.

In addition to education and training, occupational therapists and OTAs in acute settings prepare clients with SCI/D physically and mentally for gradual upright activity. With careful consideration of the level of SCI/D and related complexities, physiological tolerance, medical indications, and physician orders, it may be appropriate for OTAs to begin easing clients into upright and out-of-bed functional activities. Clients benefit from performing familiar grooming and self-feeding tasks with the head of the bed elevated, sitting at the edge of the bed with support, or in chairs—all with constant and close supervision and monitoring from the OT practitioner and other members of the interdisciplinary team.

OT practitioners can introduce adaptive equipment in this stage to provide independence and control over the hospital room environment where clients often feel the most restricted. For clients with limited UE function, OTAs can provide and teach clients how to use an adapted call bell. They can also provide and teach clients how to use a universal cuff to push buttons on the hospital bed or television remote, manage their meals, and brush their teeth.

OTAs should also work with the team to begin a regimen of ROM, positioning for pressure relief, and education regarding the importance of activity in the acute stages for body function health.

Inpatient Rehabilitation and Skilled Nursing Facility Rehabilitation

Inpatient rehab is an important time to begin to build on skills from acute care and develop habits and routines around self-care and functional mobility. The rehabilitation team is there to educate, train, problem-solve with, encourage, and empower the client and family to envision a life with SCI/D outside of the hospital walls. OTAs work with clients and caregivers to establish healthy performance patterns around body functions such as skin care, bowel and bladder management, respiratory function, physical fitness, and endurance for meaningful activity at the wheelchair level (Fig. 35-17). OTAs teach clients to embed care for their body functions in sustainable and consistent routines. Inpatient rehabilitation affords the opportunity to work with clients in simulating these routines every day as they prepare to return to their natural environments.

Skilled nursing facilities can have rehabilitation options for clients who intend to return home but need extra time to progress, and it is generally less intensive than inpatient rehabilitation. Many of the same types of tasks and training are performed as in the inpatient setting, and more and more insurance companies are choosing this type of site instead of the potentially more costly inpatient rehabilitation. Some clients, despite additional time, are not able to return home, and then would transition to a long-term type of care in this setting.

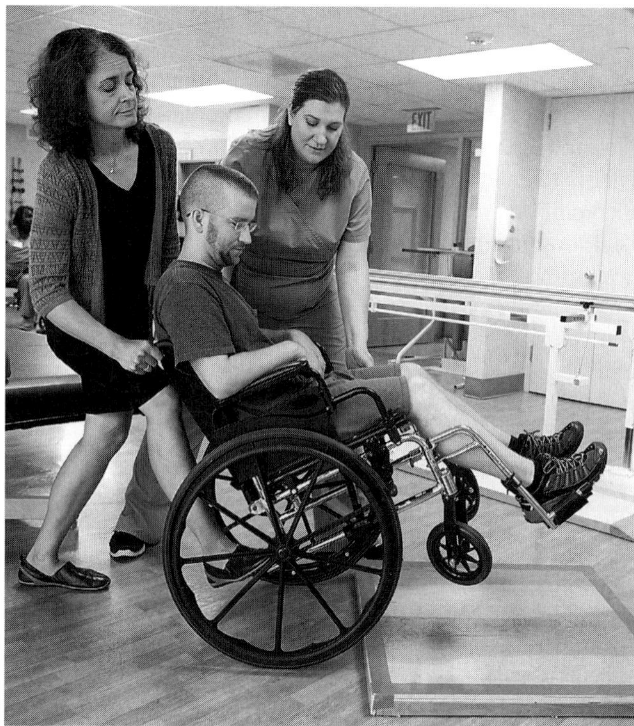

FIGURE 35-17. OTA working with client and spouse as they prepare to go home.

Post-Inpatient Rehabilitation

The role of the OT practitioner in home health, outpatient, and community-based rehabilitation settings is critical to reinforce and progress clients' goals. As the acute and inpatient rehabilitation phases are an intense time of medical stabilization and learning, it is not uncommon that clients and their family members have difficulty after discharge remembering

EVIDENCE-BASED PRACTICE

Pettersson and colleagues conducted qualitative research of power mobility device (PMD) users and found that assessment of both home environment and clients' perceptions of their autonomy is an important part of integrating the PMD into their lives.[73] Researchers also found that environmental barriers at entrances to homes might create challenges to outdoor autonomy. Finally, the investigators concluded that practitioners involved in PMD provision should be aware of the negative impacts presented by environmental barriers on autonomy to prevent accessibility problems and encourage mobility and participation in their clients.[73]

As this evidence suggests, clients with SCI/D who use PMD for functional mobility must have an environment that supports integration of the PMD in meaningful indoor and outdoor activities, or these clients are at risk for participation restrictions. OTAs educate and train clients in the use of their PMD through occupation. As the PMD becomes the essential component of their functional mobility, it also becomes an integral vessel for participation. OTAs identify their client's meaningful performance patterns and strategize solutions to indoor and outdoor environmental barriers to participation. They work with the client and client's support network to also connect with community resources around environmental modification. OTAs also facilitate their client learning how to perform daily activities from the PMD in the inpatient rehabilitation, outpatient clinic, home, and community contexts.

Pettersson, C., Brandt, A., Mansson Lexell, E., & Iwarsson, S. (2015). Autonomy and housing accessibility among powered mobility device users. American Journal of Occupational Therapy, 69, *6905290030. http://dx.doi.org/10.5014/ajot.2015.015347*

and integrating the education and skills learned in the hospital. OT practitioners in the community reinforce SCI/D education and ADL/IADL skills, reevaluate goals, and work with clients through their transition back home and into their communities. OTAs also work with clients to progress and refine daily living and functional mobility skills.

Incomplete Spinal Cord Injury

It is challenging to predict the functional goals for clients with incomplete levels of injury. Much depends on the mechanism and extent of injury, the client's characteristics, and psychosocial and environmental supports.[6] OT practitioners use their clinical reasoning, observation skills, and interdisciplinary, collaborative, client-centered approach to determine goals and intervention ideas. These ideas are often fluid, and as the client surpasses the expected functional returns or has not improved to the SCI level expected, the OT plan of care reflects this fluidity.

SPINA BIFIDA

Spina bifida is a condition occurring in the womb where the spinal column does not close all the way, potentially causing spinal nerve damage.[74] Clients may have no symptoms up to severe symptoms that present with severe muscle weakness and sensory difficulties. Some clients with spina bifida can walk with an assisted device such as forearm crutches, and some use manual or power wheelchairs. Usually, as adults, clients with spina bifida are well used to managing functionally, and may see the OT practitioner only after a shoulder surgery or at a seating clinic for a new wheelchair.

TRANSVERSE MYELITIS

Transverse myelitis is an autoimmune system disorder of unknown cause that attacks the spinal cord causing inflammation, and has a rapid onset that occurs over hours to weeks. The nerves, as a result of the inflammation and subsequent loss of myelin sheaths, are unable to conduct signals between the brain and parts of the body. The level at which the damage occurs will determine the functionality of the client, although most have thoracic damage with weakness, bowel/bladder changes, pain and sensory changes below that level. Some clients recover with little to no residual effects within 3-6 months, and others will have lifelong issues with weakness, spasticity, and pain.[75] Most clients with transverse myelitis do go through inpatient rehabilitation, and the OTA will certainly be part of the treatment team there and in the community.

SUMMARY

SCI/D impacts people's lives in dramatic ways. OT practitioners have a lens through which they envision possibility, participation, and purpose for their clients and their caregivers. With this lens, therapy is occupation-based and client-centered, collaborative, team-based, and empowering. Because clients with SCI/D may have significant challenges in performing many occupations, OT practitioners are powerful contributors to the interdisciplinary team, facilitating clients at every level of injury and their families and caregivers to engage in meaningful occupations through adaptive methods and equipment, strategies, orthotic fabrication, DME recommendations, driving and mobility options, environmental modifications, and so on. Clients with SCI/D must develop new habits and routines that help them to maintain healthy and meaningful lives. OTAs partner with clients and caregivers to achieve the new vision of a productive and fulfilling life.

REVIEW QUESTIONS

1. Jon has a T4 AIS A SCI/D. As a result of this condition, where would you suggest he check for water temperature when bathing?
   a. His feet
   b. His hands
   c. His thighs
   d. His stomach
2. Mrs. Caldwell fell while descending a flight of stairs, resulting in a C6 incomplete SCI/D. She can stand and is regaining movement in her arms and wrists, so she can bring her hands to her mouth with control of her wrist. However, she does not have strength in her hands to hold utensils. What piece of adaptive equipment would the OTA recommend next?
   a. Mobile arm support
   b. Mouth stick
   c. Universal cuff
   d. Universal cuff with wrist support
3. Jake experienced a T4 complete AIS A SCI/D after a motorcycle accident, and during an OT session feels a sudden, intense headache; has goose bumps above his level of injury; and he is sweating. The OTA checks his blood pressure, and it is 20 mmHg above his baseline blood pressure of 95/60. What is the *first* thing the OTA should suspect?
   a. Orthostatic hypotension
   b. Neurogenic heterotopic ossification
   c. The flu
   d. Autonomic dysreflexia
4. Anna has a T10 AIS B SCI/D. Which three of the following would the OTA expect to be preserved based on this level of classification?
   a. Sensation in her legs
   b. Strength in her thighs
   c. The ability to walk
   d. Normal bladder function
   e. Sensation in her feet
   f. Independent breathing
5. Brad has a C6 AIS C SCI/D as a result of a gunshot wound to the neck. His 25-year-old daughter would like to assist with stretching her father's UEs and LEs during evenings and weekends. What mechanism would the OTA emphasize protecting during stretching?
   a. Tenodesis: Flexing the wrist while extending the fingers
   b. Tenodesis: Extending the wrist while extending the fingers
   c. Tenodesis: Flexing the wrist while flexing the fingers
   d. Tenodesis: Extending the wrist while ignoring the fingers

6. Juanita has a T12 AIS A SCI/D and has concerns about sexuality post-injury. The OTA gives what sort of information to her to assist?
   a. Recommendations to focus on intimacy
   b. Recommendations on specific types of birth control
   c. Instruction on a routine to incorporate self-catheterization before sexual activity
   d. Recommendations to perform skin integrity checks before sexual activity
7. Jon has a C7 AIS D SCI/D and is regaining "gross strength" in his right hand and fine motor strength in his left hand. Which is the *most* accurate example of how he can use his right hand?
   a. Hold a water bottle with his right hand
   b. Type an email with both hands
   c. Pick up a pill with the right hand
   d. Tie his shoes using both hands
8. Miriam has a C5 AIS A SCI/D and will be going home with her husband, mother, and sister who will rotate care provision. Her family seeks information on expected independence levels upon discharge to home. Which three of the following expectations should the OTA educate the family on?
   a. She can expect to brush her teeth with some assistance from family.
   b. She can expect to dress herself independently.
   c. She can expect to shift positions in the bed and wheelchair with some assistance from family.
   d. She can expect to drive her power wheelchair independently with alternative controls.
   e. She can expect to empty her bowel and bladder independently.
   f. She can expect to perform pressure relief independently with use of tilt/recline on her power wheelchair.
9. During a transfer from bed to tilt-in-space shower chair, Ben complains of sudden dizziness, nausea, lightheadedness and ringing in his ears. The OTA should suspect that Ben is experiencing which of the following?
   a. Autonomic dysreflexia
   b. Orthostatic hypotension
   c. A spasm
   d. Spinal shock
10. Marguerite has a T4 AIS B SCI/D and is learning to put makeup on seated at the sink in her wheelchair. During an episode when Marguerite complains of feeling suddenly faint, the OTA encourages:
   a. Continued participation in the activity until the feeling subsides
   b. Returning to bed for the rest of the day
   c. Tilting back in her wheelchair until the feeling subsides, and then resuming activity
   d. Loosening all tight clothing, as this is likely an autonomic dysreflexia episode

CASE STUDY

Candace is a 20-year-old college student living at home with her parents. She is in nursing school and a personal trainer at her local gym. She is a weight lifter and exercise enthusiast. During a girls' night out, Candace and three of her friends were in a motor vehicle collision (MVC). Candace was the restrained driver. During the scene of the accident, it was determined that Candace required specialized medical care, and she was emergently flown to the nearest trauma hospital, 2 hours from her home and the scene of the accident. At the hospital, physicians determined Candace's injuries resulted in a T5 complete SCI.

Candace's parents work full time to support their family and remain at her side during her entire acute stay and alternate time staying overnight during her inpatient rehabilitation stay.

During her 4 weeks on the inpatient rehabilitation unit, she works with OT and PT 3 hours or more per day to relearn all aspects of her daily living in preparation for discharge back home. These activities are graded with the assistance of the OT practitioner such that Candace experiences and practices them at the bed level initially and then progresses to the wheelchair level. The activities include use of an ultra-lightweight wheelchair for independent mobility and ADL/IADL accomplishment; grooming; dressing from bed and her wheelchair; bathing and performing her bowel program on a specialized commode chair in the shower; intermittent self-catheterization; completing laundry and cooking tasks; carrying a backpack and necessary supplies; and transferring on and off exercise equipment for continued strength training. The OT practitioner also works consistently with her family including her parents and grandparents in preparation for going home. These preparations include SCI/D education and training; connection with resources; recommendations for adaptive equipment, and home modifications. Perhaps one of the most poignant preparatory strategies the OT practitioner offered was the creation of a shared vision with Candace and her family of her long-term goals of returning to school and personal training.

After discharge from inpatient rehabilitation, Candace received outpatient OT services where her skills were refined and intervention focused on higher-level daily skills in preparation for return to school and work.

1. How would an OT practitioner begin to prioritize an intervention plan for Candace at the (a) acute care, (b) inpatient rehabilitation, and (c) outpatient phases of her SCI rehab?
2. Considering her level and type of injury, what body structures and functions warrant particular attention when working toward ADL and mobility training? What body functions might Candace not have at the T5 level in her trunk, for instance?
3. Considering Candace's age and stage in development, who might the OTA encourage Candace to invite to participate in her OT sessions before discharge?
4. What referral sources might the OTA consider providing Candace considering her level of injury, age, and stage in development?

PUTTING IT ALL TOGETHER Sample Treatment Session and Documentation

Setting	Acute inpatient rehabilitation after 5 days in acute care
Client profile	Mr. C is a 50 y/o male with new-onset transverse myelitis (TM). He awoke one morning with sudden loss of bladder control and pain and weakness in his legs. He attempted to walk to his car to drive himself to his primary care physician when his legs collapsed. His wife drove him to the emergency department, where neurology diagnosed the TM. He lives with his wife and works full time in information technology at a local firm in his town. His wife works full time as a museum curator in a town 10 miles from their home. They live in a one-story, narrow, ranch home built in the 1970s with three steps to enter. Mr. C has one daughter who attends college full-time, 30 miles away. He reports not having much leisure time outside of work but that he does like to play golf and go out for meals with his wife.
Work history	Has been working for his IT firm for 15 years and before that was a stay-at-home father
Insurance	Aetna: Approved for 3 weeks
Psychological	Currently notes feelings of depression, anxiety, and being out of control of this situation and its management
Social	He is a highly social person and hosts many gatherings at his home. He considers his colleagues to be his social support system. Considers himself an extrovert with a type A personality, however admits he struggles with interpersonal conflict at times.
Cognitive	Intact; alert and oriented to person, place, date, and situation
Sensation, Motor, and Manual Muscle Testing	T4 AIS A SCI/D 4/5 strength BUE 0/5 strength at and below T4 Light touch and pin prick intact C3-T3, bilaterally Light touch and pin prick absent T4 and below, bilaterally Noted intermittent but predictable spasms throughout BLE which occur during position changes (supine to and from sitting) Modified Ashworth Scale: 1+/4 In supine, PROM of BLE is normal Unable to sit without back support for any period of time Sits in ultra-lightweight manual wheelchair with tall, hard back with constant assist for balance
ADL	From supine in bed, requires: Setup assistance with upper-body bathing, dressing, and grooming; Max A to dependent assistance with LE bathing and dressing; dependent assistance for bowel program and intermittent catheterization From wheelchair level, requires: Max assistance for UE bathing and dressing; supervision for grooming; dependent assist for LE bathing and dressing; dependent assistance for bowel program and intermittent catheterization
IADL	Requires: Mod A for light meal preparation Max A for light housekeeping Min A for work-related (laptop, phone) tasks at the wheelchair level
Goals	Within 3 weeks, client will demonstrate: 1. Supervision for bathing seated on TTB with AE. 2. Mod I with dressing from the bed 3. Mod A with LE dressing from the wheelchair and Mod I with UE dressing from the wheelchair. 4. Mod I with grooming at the wheelchair level 5. Mod I with intermittent self-catheterization at wheelchair level every 6 hours 6. Mod I with bowel program on raised toilet surface 7. Independent verbalization of signs and symptoms of a UTI as well as strategies to prevent and manage a UTI 8. Mod I light meal preparation at the wheelchair level, demonstrating safety and adapted techniques for managing sharp and hot kitchen items 9. Mod I light housekeeping tasks such as bed making and laundry at the wheelchair level, relevant to his role at home 10. Mod I performance of work-related computer tasks at the wheelchair level, verbalizing strategies for energy conservation in the workplace throughout the day.

Continued

PUTTING IT ALL TOGETHER Sample Treatment Session and Documentation (continued)

OT TREATMENT SESSION 1

THERAPEUTIC ACTIVITY	TIME	GOAL(S) ADDRESSED	OTA RATIONALE
Verbal bowel and bladder management education	30 min	#5, #6, #7, and indirectly #10	*Education; Self-Advocacy:* Necessary to build a foundation of understanding for purpose of bowel and bladder programs and to feel empowered to advocate when he feels something is not functioning well.
Supply setup, education, and self-catheterization training with sterile kit.	30 min	#5 and #7	*Education and Training; Occupation and Activities:* Present basic information on purpose of various aspects of catheters and be able to compare/contrast their benefits to make educated decision with the rehab team. Progress training beginning at the bed level to build understanding and confidence before a more challenging, wheelchair level of performance. Training begins in the bed also to eliminate more difficult performance skills such as balance, endurance, and wheeled mobility.
Transfer training to raised toilet surface with grab bars and transfer board; clothing management training	20 min	#3, #6, and indirectly, #10	*Occupation and Activities; Preparatory Methods:* Begin mobility training to toilet where bowel program will happen at home. Begin to build strength, endurance, and balance necessary to perform this independently and daily. Provide exposure to modification possibilities in context to demonstrate support to activity.
Education and written information provided for bathroom modifications	30 min	#1, #3, and #6	*Education and Training:* Provide written and video education on modifications so client may share with his wife and contractor to begin making decisions in preparation for discharge to home.

SOAP note: 10/5/—, 1:45 pm-2:50 pm

S: Client states, "I never thought I would have to control my urine and stool this way. But if it's what I have to, I will do it. I just don't want my wife to have to help me."

O: Client participated in OT ADL session focused on bowel and bladder management strategies and mobility related to bowel and bladder management. OTA provided verbal, written, and video instruction on bowel and bladder management strategies to prevent, identify, and manage complications. Client return verbalized three strategies to prevent urinary tract infection and bowel incontinence. OTA presented and educated client on the two options for intermittent self-catheterization including the straight catheter and the closed catheter kit. After skilled instruction, the client selected training on the closed catheter kit, and with one verbal cue, demonstrated ability to properly lay out supplies while maintaining a sterile environment. Since this was the first training session, client self-catheterized from bed, where he had more balance and room to work. OTA instructed client on clothing management before and after self-catheterization. Client performed with one-step verbal cues with Mod A overall. After a rest break, client transferred to wheelchair and raised toilet surface with assist of grab bars—Mod A with transfer board. He doffed and donned pants prior and after transfer with Max A. After exploring the modification options available through practice, the OTA provided client with written and video information on home modifications focusing on the toilet and shower in preparation for discussion next session.

A: Client made progress toward goals today. He will benefit from continued practice and reinforcement of these activities within a daily routine. He will benefit from continued therapeutic activity to refine motor control and to build strength and endurance for these physically demanding tasks. He will also benefit from a referral to rehab psychology counseling to cope with the psychosocial challenges of these activities.

P: Next ADL session, progress to self-catheterization training at the wheelchair level, continue transfer training to toilet, and begin discussion of bowel program training on the raised toilet. Discuss preparedness to self-catheterize independent of nursing assistance q6 hours.

Carolyn Johnson, COTA/L 10/5/—, 5:30 pm

TREATMENT SESSION 2

What could you do next with this client?

TREATMENT SESSION 3

What could you do next with this client?

REFERENCES

1. Jain, N. B., Nitin, B., Ayers, G. D., Peterson, E. N., Harris, M. B., Morse, L., ... & Garshick, E. (2015). Traumatic spinal cord injury in the United States, 1993-2012. *Journal of the American Medical Association, 313*(22), 2236–2243.
2. American Occupational Therapy Association (AOTA). (n.d.). Occupational therapy: Improving function while controlling costs. Retrieved from http://www.aota.org/About-Occupational-Therapy/Professionals.aspx
3. Spinal cord injury information page: Definition. National Institute of Neurological Disorders and Stroke. (2017). Retrieved from https://www.ninds.nih.gov/disorders/all-disorders/spinal-cord-injury-information-page
4. Spinal cord injury. (2015). Mayo Clinic. Retrieved from www.mayoclinic.org/spinalcordinjury
5. U.S. National Library of Medicine. Spinal cord diseases. (2017). Retrieved from: https://medlineplus.gov/spinalcorddiseases.html
6. Harvey, L. (2008). *Management of spinal cord injuries: A guide for physiotherapists*. Edinburgh, United Kingdom: Churchill Livingstone Elsevier.
7. National Spinal Cord Injury Statistical Center. (2015). Facts and figures at a glance. Birmingham, AL: University of Alabama at Birmingham.
8. Van den Berg, M. E., Castellote, J. M., Mahillo-Fernandez, I., & de Pedro-Cuesta, J. (2010). Incidence of spinal cord injury worldwide: A systematic review. *Neuroepidemiology, 34*, 184–192.
9. DeVivo, M. J. (2012). Epidemiology of traumatic spinal cord injury: Trends and future implications. *Spinal Cord, 50*, 365–372.
10. Spinal cord injury. (n.d.). World Health Organization. Retrieved from http://www.who.int/mediacentre/factsheets/fs384/en/
11. Sepsis. (n.d.). Mayo Clinic. Retrieved from http://www.mayoclinic.org/diseases-conditions/sepsis/home/ovc-20169784
12. Erosa, N. A., Berry, J. W., Elliott, T. R., Underhill, A. T., & Fine, P. R. (2014). Predicting quality of life 5 years after medical discharge for traumatic spinal cord injury. *British Journal of Health Psychology, 19*(4), 688–700.
13. American Occupational Therapy Association. (2014). Occupational therapy practice framework: Domain and process (3rd ed.). *American Journal of Occupational Therapy, 68*(Suppl. 1), S1–S48.
14. What is a complete vs. incomplete injury? (2016). Retrieved from https://www.christopherreeve.org/living-with-paralysis/newly-paralyzed/how-is-an-sci-defined-and-what-is-a-complete-vs-incomplete-injury
15. Ginis, K. M., Latimer, A. E., Hicks, A., & Craven, B. C. (2005). Development and evaluation of an activity measure for people with spinal cord injury. *Medicine and Science in Sports and Exercise, 37*(7), 1099–1111.
16. Pneumonia. (n.d.). Mayo Clinic. Retrieved from http://www.mayoclinic.org/diseases-conditions/pneumonia/basics/definition/con-20020032
17. Neurological examination. (2009). Retrieved from www.neurosurgical.com
18. The AIS. Spinal cord injury research evidence. (n.d.). Retrieved from https://www.scireproject.com/outcome-measures-new/american-spinal-injury-association-impairment-scale-ais-international-standards#
19. Morganti, B., Scivoletto, G., Ditunno, P., Ditunno, J. F., & Molinari, M. (2005). Walking index for spinal cord injury (WISCI): Criterion validation. *Spinal Cord, 43*(1), 27-33. http://dx.doi.org/10.1038/sj.sc.3101658
20. Institute of Medicine. (2005). Spinal cord injury: Progress, promise and priorities (p. 35). Washington, DC: The National Academies Press.
21. Incomplete spinal cord injury. (2017). Retrieved from http://www.spinal-injury.net/incomplete-spinal-cord-injury.htm
22. Markandaya, M., Stein, D. M., & Menaker, J. (2012). Acute treatment options for spinal cord injury. *Current Treatment Options in Neurology, 14*, 175–187.
23. Traynelis, V., & Waziri, A. (2016). Cervical spine bracing options: halo ring, crowns, or vest. Retrieved from www.spineuniverse.com
24. Thoracolumbosacral orthosis (TLSO). (2017). Retrieved from http://www.cascadeorthotics.com/thoracolumbosacral-orthosis-tlso-cascade-orthotics/
25. Khadir, S. A., Neubourg, S., & Lowe, R. (n.d.). Cervical collar. Retrieved from www.physio-pedia.com
26. Craig, A., Tran, Y., & Middleton, J. (2009) Psychological morbidity and spinal cord injury: A systematic review. *Spinal Cord, 47*, 108–114.
27. Migliorini, C., Sinclair, A., Brown, D., Tonge, B., & New, P. (2105). Prevalence of mood disturbance in Australian adults with chronic spinal cord injury. *Internal Medicine Journal, 45*, 1014–1019.
28. Dryden, D. M., Saunders, L. D., Rowe, B. H., May, L. A., Yinnakoulias, N., Svenson, L. W., ... & Voaklander, D. C. (2005). Depression following traumatic brain injury. *Neuroepidemiology, 25*, 55–61.
29. Monden, K. R., Trost, D., Catalano, D., Garner, A. N., Symcox, J., Driver, S., Hamilton, R. G., & Warren, A. M. (2014). Resilience following spinal cord injury—A phenomenological review. *Spinal Cord, 52*, 197–201.
30. Nott, M. T., Baguley, I. J., Heriseanu, R., Weber, G., Middleton, J. W., Meares, S., ... & Chilko, S. (2014). Effects of concomitant spinal cord injury and brain injury on medical and functional outcomes and community participation. *Topics in Spinal Cord Injury Rehabilitation, 20*(3), 225–235.
31. Consortium for Spinal Cord Medicine Clinical Practice Guidelines. (2014). *Pressure Ulcer Prevention and Treatment following Injury: A clinical practice guideline for health-care practitioners* (2nd ed.). Paralyzed Veterans of America. Retrieved from http://www.pva.org/media/pdf/CPG_Pressure%20Ulcer.pdf
32. Trombly Latham, C. A., & Radomski, M. V. (2013). *Occupational Therapy for Physical Dysfunction.* (7th ed.). Philadelphia, PA: Lippincott Williams & Williams.
33. Murray, R. F. (2007). Impact of spinal cord injury on self-perceived pre- and postmorbid cognitive, emotional, and physical functioning. *Spinal Cord, 45*(6), 1099–1111.
34. Dudgeon, B. J., Tyler, E. J., Rhodes, L. A., & Jensen, M. P. (2006). Managing usual and unexpected pain with physical disability: A qualitative analysis. *American Journal of Occupational Therapy, 60*, 92–103.
35. Spasticity. (n.d.) Retrieved from: https://www.scireproject.com/book/export/html/1417
36. Villines, Z. (2016). Understanding spasticity after a spinal cord injury. Retrieved from https://www.spinalcord.com/blog/understanding-spasticity-after-a-spinal-cord-injury
37. What is spasticity? (2017). Retrieved from https://www.christopherreeve.org/living-with-paralysis/health/secondary-conditions/spasticity
38. Colclough, S., Copley, J., Turpin, M., Justins, E., & De Monte, R. (2015). Occupational therapists' perceptions of requirements for competent upper limb hypertonicity practice. *Disability and Rehabilitation, 37*(16), 1416–1423.
39. Do, J. G., Kim du H., & Sung, D. H. (2013). Incidence of DVT after spinal cord injury in Korean patients at acute rehabilitation unit. *Journal of Korean Medicine Spinal Cord Injury, 28*(9), 1382–1387.
40. Gil, J. A., Waryasz, G. R., Klyce, W., & Daniels, A. H. (2015). Heterotopic ossification in neurorehabilitation, *Rhode Island Medical Journal, December*, 32–34.
41. Doolin-Carver, A. J. (2012). Standing tall post-injury. Rehab management. Retrieved from www.rehabpub.com
42. Dionyssiotis, Y., Lyritis, G. P., Mavrogenis, A. F., & Papagelopoulos, P. J. (2011). Factors influencing bone loss in paraplegia. *Hippokratia, 15*, 54–59.
43. Walicka-Cupry_, K., Bejer, A., & Domka-Jopek, E. (2007). Significant effects of prolonged standing in spinal cord injury survivors. *Fizjoterapia, 15*(3), 18–22.
44. Clinical guideline for standing adults following spinal cord injury. (2013). Retrieved from http://www.mascip.co.uk/wp-content/uploads/2015/05/Clinical-Guidelines-for-Standing-Adults-Following-Spinal-Cord-Injury.pdf
45. Phillips, A. A., & Krassioukov, A.V. (2015). Contemporary cardiovascular concerns after spinal cord injury: Mechanisms, maladaptations, and management. *Journal of Neurotrauma, 32*, 1927–1942.

46. Caruso, D. (2015). Prevention of recurrent autonomic dysreflexia: A survey of current practice. *Clinical Autonomic Research, 25*(5), 293–300.
47. Peña, C. (2016). Inferior vena cava (IVC) filter placement and removal. Retrieved from https://www.radiologyinfo.org/en/info.cfm?pg=venacavafilter
48. Atelectasis. (n.d.). Mayo Clinic. Retrieved from http://www.mayoclinic.org/diseases-conditions/atelectasis/basics/definition/con-20034847
49. Brown R., DiMarco A. F., Hoit J. D., & Garshick, E. (2006). Respiratory dysfunction and management in SCI. *Respiratory Care, 51*(8), 853–868; discussion 869–870.
50. Assist cough. (2017). Retrieved from http://www.myshepherdconnection.org/respiratory/assist-cough
51. Engkasan, J. P., Ng, C. J., & Low, W. Y. (2014). Factors influencing bladder management in male patients with spinal cord injury: A qualitative study. *Spinal Cord, 52*, 157–162.
52. Burns, A. S., St. Germain, D., Connolly, M., Delparte, J. J., Guindon, A., Hitzig, S. L., & Craven, B. C. (2015). Phenomenological study of neurogenic bowel from the perspective of individuals living with spinal cord injury. *Archives of Physical Medicine and Rehabilitation, 96*, 49–55.
53. Consortium for Spinal Cord Medicine Clinical Practice Guidelines. (1998). Neurogenic Bowel Management in Adults with Spinal Cord Injury.
54. Pryor, J., Fisher, M., & Middleton, J. (2014). Management of the neurogenic bowel for adults with spinal cord injuries. Retrieved from https://www.aci.health.nsw.gov.au/__data/assets/pdf_file/0019/155215/Management-Neurogenic-Bowel.pdf
55. Sexual health. (n.d.). The World Health Organization. Retrieved from: http://www.who.int/topics/sexual_health/en/.
56. Bodner, D. (2010). Sexuality and reproductive health in adults with spinal cord injury: A clinical practice guideline for health-care professionals. *The Journal of Spinal Cord Medicine, 33*(3), 281–336.
57. Bodner, D. (2011). What you know and what you should know: Sex and spinal cord injury. *Journal of Spinal Cord Medicine, 34*(4), 349.
58. Cramp, J. D., Courtois, F. J., & Ditor, D. S. (2015). Sexuality for women with spinal cord injury, *Journal of Sex & Marital Therapy, 41*(3), 238–253. doi:10.1080/0092623X.2013.869777
59. Fritz, H. A., Dillaway, H., & Lysack, C. L. (2015). "Don't think paralysis takes away your womanhood": Sexual intimacy after spinal cord injury. *American Journal of Occupational Therapy, 69*, 6902260030. http://dx.doi.org/10.5014/ajot.2015.015040
60. Sexual functioning for men after a spinal cord injury. (2015). Retrieved from https://craighospital.org/resources/sexual-function-for-men-after-a-spinal-cord-injury
61. Sexuality and sexual function after spinal cord injury. (2015). The Model Systems Knowledge Translation Center. Retrieved from http://www.msktc.org/lib/docs/Factsheets/SCI_Sexuality.pdf
62. Taylor, B., & Davis, S. (2007). The extended PLISSIT model for addressing the sexual wellbeing of individuals with an acquired disability or chronic illness. *Sex Disability, 25*, 135–139.
63. Summerville, P., & McKenna, K. (1998). Sexuality education and counseling for individuals with SCI: Implications for occupational therapy. *British Journal of Occupational Therapy, 61*(6), 275–279.
64. Consortium for Spinal Cord Medicine. (2000). Outcomes following spinal cord injury: Clinical practice guidelines for healthcare professionals. *Journal of Spinal Cord Medicine, 23*(4), 289–316.
65. Munce, S., Webster, F., Fehlings, M. G., Straus, S. E., Jang, E., & Jaglall, S. B. (2014). Perceived facilitators and barriers to self-management in individuals with traumatic spinal cord injury: a qualitative descriptive study. *BMC Neurology, 14*, 48.
66. Boatman, M. (2013). New technology: The eyes have it. *New Mobility, 26*.
67. Software. Thinksmartbox. (2016). Retrieved from https://thinksmartbox.com/our-software
68. Assistive technology hands-free. Tecla. (2016). Retrieved from https://gettecla.com
69. Bednar, M. S. (2016). Tendon transfers for tetraplegia. *Hand Clinics, 32*(3), 389–396.
70. Fox, I. K., Davidge, K. M., Novak, C. B., Hoben, G., Kahn, L. C., Juknis, N., ... & Mackinnon, S. E. (2015). Use of peripheral nerve transfers in tetraplegia: Evaluation of feasibility and morbidity. *Hand (New York, N.Y.), 10*(1), 60–67.
71. Wallace, M. A., & Kendall, M. B. (2014). Transitional rehabilitation goals for people with spinal cord injury: Looking beyond the hospital walls. *Disability Rehabilitation, 36*(8), 642–650.
72. Grant, R. A., Quon, J. L., & Abbed, K. M. (2015). Management of acute traumatic spinal cord injury. *Current Treatment Options Neurology, 17*(2), 334.
73. Pettersson, C., Brandt, A., Mansson Lexell, E., & Iwarsson, S. (2015). Autonomy and housing accessibility among powered mobility device users. *American Journal of Occupational Therapy, 69*, 6905290030. http://dx.doi.org/10.5014/ajot.2015.015347
74. What is spina bifida? (2015). Spina Bifida Association. Retrieved from http://spinabifidaassociation.org/project/what-is-spina-bifida/
75. Transverse myelitis fact sheet. (n.d.). Retrieved from https://www.ninds.nih.gov/Disorders/Patient-Caregiver-Education/Fact-Sheets/Transverse-Myelitis-Fact-Sheet

ACKNOWLEDGMENTS

For their contributions to this chapter, immeasurable thanks to Jenny Womack, OT, FAOTA, for her ceaseless encouragement, mentorship, and support; to Amy Mahle, OTA and Amber Ward, OT, for their leadership and guidance in this incredible project; to Kara Cantoni, OT, for offering her clinical expertise and clarity in chapter revisions; to Dr. Heather Walker for her SCI mentorship and teachings; to Courtney Matrunick, PT, and other colleagues in SCI for the "real world" teamwork that inspired much of this chapter's content; and the deepest gratitude to my clients with SCI and their support systems for the priceless gift of allowing me to partner with them through their journeys living with SCI.

Chapter 36

Polytrauma and Complex Multiple Conditions

Melissa D. Brawley, MS, OTR/L

LEARNING OUTCOMES

After studying this chapter the student or practitioner will be able to:

36.1 Define polytrauma and describe common medical diagnoses involved in the complex client

36.2 Explain the clinical presentation of clients with polytrauma, including the physical and psychosocial impacts

36.3 Describe common lines, tubes, and drains, as well as safe and effective management during the delivery of occupational therapy services

36.3 Explain the role of the occupational therapy practitioner with this population and the research supporting early occupational therapy intervention for the client who has complex medical conditions

36.4 Develop treatment intervention based on performance and the client's place within the continuum of care

36.5 Determine the appropriate time to initiate, modify, or terminate occupational therapy intervention based on the client's response to treatment

KEY TERMS

Activity
Comorbidity
Critical illness myopathy (CIM)
Critical illness polyneuropathy (CIP)
Mechanism of injury (MOI)
Mechanical ventilation
Premorbid
Polytrauma

It is a late Friday night, which has quickly changed to early Saturday morning, around 2:00 am, and Josh is with a small group of friends. The alcohol consumption started after dinner and continued at a party for several hours. Josh separated from the group and headed to his dorm. Staggering across the street, he entered the building and stumbled up the stairwell to the third floor. Josh made his way down the hall, shook his head after remembering his room was on the second floor and in the co-ed dorm; the third floor housed only girls. He hurriedly made his way back to the stairwell, took two steps down, tripped, and fell down eight steps until he hit the wall at the landing. Josh vomited, choked, and became unconscious. The next morning around 8:00 a.m. a student found Josh, and 10 minutes later the emergency services arrived.

TRAUMA, MULTIPLE CONDITIONS, AND CRITICAL ILLNESS

A situation can completely change in the blink of an eye, and most often, that is the scenario in polytrauma cases. According to the Department of Veterans Affairs, **polytrauma** is defined as "two or more injuries to physical regions or organ systems, one of which may be life threatening, resulting in physical, cognitive, psychological, or psychosocial impairments and functional disability."[1] It could be the result of a single car accident caused by the mother who dropped her cell phone and reached down to get it, triggering her car to run off of the road directly into a tree. It could be the result of the construction worker who slipped off of his 25-foot ladder while doing his last painting job of the day and realized that when he caught his breath, he could not move or feel below the waist. Whatever may be the circumstances or risk factors surrounding a traumatic situation, clients who experience polytrauma undergo total disruption of their lives (Fig. 36-1).

Activity, External Cause of Injury, and Mechanism of Injury

Activity is the term used to describe what the injured person was doing when a potentially life-threatening injury occurred.[2] The World Health Organization (WHO) categorizes

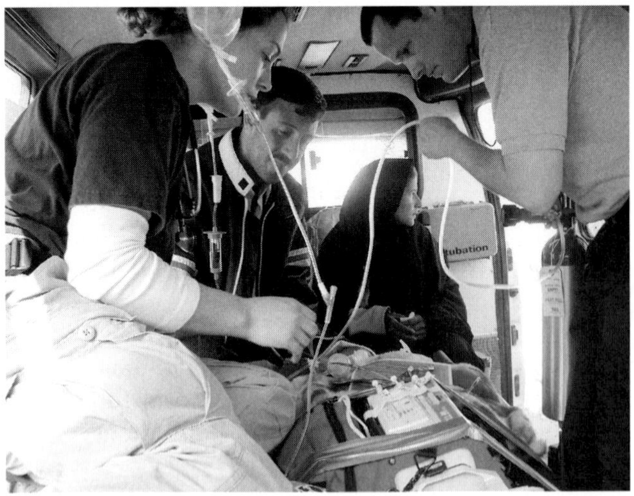

FIGURE 36-1. Polytrauma often begins with a life-threatening event, such as a car accident, fall, or act of violence. *(FEMA/Marty Bahamonde.)*

such activities as either leisure activities, sports and exercise, working at house or yard, working at paid job, driving or riding in a motor vehicle, and other.[2] Of these categories, 25% of all injury episodes have been reported as occurring during leisure activities.[2] The causal primary activity for injured clients varies by age. Research has shown that children under the age of 15 years are most often injured when participating in a leisure-related activity, whereas sports were the leading activity among injured youth 15 to 24 years of age.[2] In the case of adults 25 to 64 years of age, the leading activity when injured is reported as working at a paid job, and the leading activity for older adults over the age of 65 years is categorized under "other" activities.[2] The "other" category includes housework, shopping, volunteer work, sleeping, resting, eating, drinking, cooking, receiving hands-on care from another person, and specified activities.[2]

The terms *occupation* and *activity* are used on a daily basis by occupational therapy (OT) practitioners because each is highly valued and recognized for its influence on health and well-being. Occupations and activities are encompassed within the domain of OT and are used to "describe participation in daily life pursuits."[3] Although their meanings are distinct, both occupations and activities are involved before, during, and after an injury. All of the activities occurring at the time of a client's potentially life-threatening injury, as mentioned above, represent various occupations. The activity occurring at time of the client's injury is relevant to the OT practitioner as a means of understanding and establishing the client's dynamic occupational profile.

Although it is important for the OT practitioner to understand the activity occurring at the time of injury, there are other factors that are essential to truly understanding the performance skills and client factors after injury. The term *external cause of injury* is used to categorize the circumstances of the injury. This includes two axes—the mechanism or cause (e.g., fall, motor vehicle) and the manner or intent (e.g., accidental, self-inflicted, assault).[2]

The **mechanism of injury (MOI)** was historically used as a component of triage for the trauma client and later evolved into an indicator of major trauma as well as an indicator for transport to a major trauma center.[4] For injuries resulting in hospitalization subsequent to emergency department (ED) treatment or injuries resulting in an ED visit followed by release (without hospitalization or other transfer), MOI is defined as the precipitating cause or the cause that started the chain of events that led to the injury.[2]

Several other characteristics are also used to describe the MOI. Energy, or the force behind the mechanism, is generally applied in characteristic patterns. The various types of energy include mechanical, gravitational, thermal, chemical, electrical, and radiant. Mechanical energy is the energy associated with the motion and position of an object, such as a car, traveling in the direction of another object. Gravitational energy is stored in the height of the object. An example of this is the energy behind the tree limb that falls down on the logger. Thermal energy is energy that comes from heat, whereas chemical energy is derived from the bonding of chemical compounds and often is released in the form of heat. Electrical energy is produced by electrical charges that can subsequently produce other forms of energy, including thermal and light energy. Lightning is an example of electrical energy. Radiant energy is energy transmitted from electromagnetic waves, as in the case of microwaves or ultraviolet (UV) waves. Thermal, chemical, electrical, and radiant forms of energy can all produce a burn mechanism. The majority of traumatic injuries occur as a result of mechanical or gravitational forces.[5]

The means by which a specific type of energy is transferred to the tissues of the body include blunt force, penetrating force, crush, burn, or blast. Blunt mechanisms of injury primarily seen in the client with the multiple trauma include motor vehicle collisions (MVCs), automobile versus pedestrian incidents, falls, and being struck by or against an object.[5]

Within every MVC, four collisions occur. These include vehicle collision, body collision, internal organ collision, and secondary impacts. During a collision, parts of the vehicle, such as the bumper, hood, and frame, come in contact with an external site, which commonly include trees, other vehicles, guardrails, and so on. The body collides with safety devices, including seat belts and air bags, or the steering wheel, dashboard, or windshield. The internal organs impacted generally include the brain, aorta, lungs, heart, and abdominal organs. Secondary impacts include flying objects and other passengers.[5] Over half the MVCs are frontal impacts; however, rear impacts, lateral impacts, or rollover collisions can result in devastating injuries. The mortality rate is fourfold higher among clients who are ejected from the vehicle compared with the rates among those who remain in the vehicle.[5]

In addition to MVCs, other mechanisms can result in multiple trauma injuries. Automobile versus pedestrian injuries are also very common among those who experience multiple trauma. In this biomechanical situation, a significant amount of mass is transmitted to the pedestrian, with very little going to the vehicle. The location of the client's injuries will depend primarily on the points of contact with the vehicle. The injuries resulting from automobile versus moped or automobile versus cyclist are similar. Falls involve the same laws of physics, with every second of falling resulting in significant acceleration.[5] A fall with a drop height of approximately 13 feet will result in impact at 20 miles per hour, a fall from a two-story building with a drop height of 20.5 feet will result in impact at 25 miles per hour, and a fall with a drop height of 30 feet will result in impact at approximately 30 miles per hour (the acceleration is not constant).[5] When an individual has been struck by or against an object, he or she has experienced a blow. An example of this type of injury is a logger injured on the job with blunt force after being struck by a large tree branch. The force of the blow is equal to the mass of the object times its velocity squared.[5]

Although blunt injury is the most common form of injury, other injury mechanisms include penetrating injuries caused by firearms, stabs/slashes, impalement, crushing, burns, and blasts. Burns are the only type of injury that does not involve mechanical or gravitational force. The energy source for burns is thermal, chemical, electrical, or radiant.[5]

The manner or intent of injury is assigned by trained hospital staff on the basis of information obtained from the client's medical record. The categories include unintentional, assault–other, assault–sexual, legal intervention, and self-harm. *Unintentional injuries* are those that are "not deliberately inflicted, including any such injury described as an 'accident,' regardless of whether inflicted by oneself or by another person."[2] *Assault injuries* are nonfatal injuries that result as "acts of violence where physical force by one or more persons is used with the intent of causing harm, injury, or death to another person."[5] *Legal intervention injuries* are those injuries sustained as a result of police or law enforcement intervention in the course of official duties. *Self-harm injuries* result from deliberate or self-directed violence. Injuries sustained by military personnel may vary and potentially include many of the categories noted above.

The intent and the mechanism of injury are described within the client's medical record and allow OT practitioners to more fully understand the course of treatment and sequence of events during the client's subsequent hospitalization and rehabilitation path.

Diagnoses

The definitions of the term *polytrauma*, or multiple trauma, have proven to be inconsistent over time and a clear and valid definition across academia and clinical practice is still lacking.[6] An accepted definition across research articles identifies polytrauma as at least two or more injuries, of which at least one is life threatening, with an injury severity score (ISS) score of 16 or greater. The ISS is an internationally validated and accepted trauma score, which allows for direct comparison of polytrauma injuries.[7] The ISS has been shown to be a reliable predictor of survival and mortality.[7] Each of the six body regions (head/neck, face, chest, abdomen, extremities, external) is given a score between one to six points (the Abbreviated Injury Scale score), including minor, moderate, serious, severe, critical, and maximal (untreatable), respectively. The scores of the most severely injured regions are tallied for a score. If any single score is a maximal of 6, the individual is automatically rated the highest ISS score.[8] Figure 36-2 presents ISS definition categories. More detailed definitions describe polytrauma as complex multiple injuries on both lower extremities (LEs), a combination of one upper extremity (UE) and one LE injury, or complex pelvis/acetabulum fractures.[9]

Polytrauma-related diagnoses include fractures of the skull, neck and trunk, UEs and LEs, as well as dislocations, sprains, and strains of joints and associated muscles. Common fractures include those of the skull base, femur, tibia and fibula, acetabulum, ribs, sternum, humerus, scapula, clavicle, radius, and ulna. Fractures have been recognized as the primary type of injury in all age groups—from children to young adults and older adults.[2] LE injuries in general are recognized as the most common; however, the most common fractures resulting from falls are those of the pelvis, hip, humerus, and wrist.[10]

Intracranial injuries include concussions; cerebral lacerations and contusions; and subarachnoid, subdural, extradural (between inner skull and outer dura layers), and intracranial hemorrhages. Traumatic brain injury (TBI) is common in polytrauma and can vary dramatically in severity.[11] The term *traumatic brain injury* encompasses all intracranial injuries because they relate to brain damage as a result of external mechanical force. The classic presentation of TBI includes loss of consciousness, posttraumatic amnesia, and the presence of skull fracture or objective neurological and radiological findings.[2] See chapter 34 for more specific information on TBI.

Internal injury diagnoses include traumatic pneumothorax and/or hemothorax, with or without open wound into the thorax. *Pneumothorax* refers to a collapsed lung, which usually occurs as a result of air leaking into the space between the lungs and the chest wall. In many cases, individuals with multiple trauma present with an additional chest

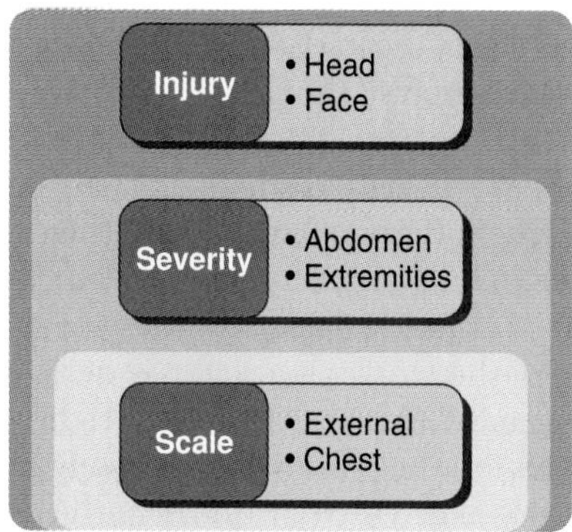

FIGURE 36-2. ISS definition categories. The scale is used to quickly assess the severity of injuries in six body regions.

injury, including hemothorax, rib fracture, lung contusion, or contusion of the chest wall.[12] Hemothorax is the collection of blood in the pleural space between the lungs and the chest wall. *Traumatic pneumohemothorax* is a combination of these two and is an associated polytrauma injury that can occur with or without an open wound into the thorax.

Chest injury is one of the most common multiple trauma–related injuries with over one third of individuals experiencing a complication related to chest contusion or trauma.[13] Related internal injuries include those that involve the heart, lung(s), diaphragm, esophagus, or bronchus.

When the heart is punctured, pronounced bleeding into the chest cavity may result. If the pericardium (the membrane around the heart) is significantly torn, *pericardial tamponade,* which refers to the entrapment of blood within the pericardium, may occur. The result is increased pressure between the pericardium and the heart; the pressure compresses the heart and interferes with efficient circulation. Cardiac tamponade is a critical condition and requires immediate attention to prevent vital organs from going without oxygenated blood.

With chest contusion and multiple trauma, clients are at an increased risk for experiencing lung contusion and acute lung injury.[14] In fact, one out of five individuals who experience polytrauma face a pulmonary contusion diagnosis and will likely require mechanical ventilation for at least the first 48 hours of hospitalization.[15] **Mechanical ventilation** is defined as the use of an external device for gas exchange within the lungs and is often required to sustain pulmonary function in the setting of respiratory distress. These clients are at risk for the development of acute respiratory distress syndrome (ARDS), pneumonia, and long-term respiratory insufficiency. ARDS is characterized by the rapid onset of respiratory failure. Certain criteria must be met for a diagnosis of ARDS, including onset within 1 week of a known clinical insult, demonstration on chest radiography, respiratory failure not explained by cardiac failure or fluid overload, and certain oxygenation requirements.[16]

Liver and splenic injuries are common in individuals who experience polytrauma when there is blunt or penetrating abdominal trauma. Because of the anatomical location of the liver and spleen within the abdominal cavity in highly vascularized areas, both organs are prone to injury.[17] The grade of the liver or splenic laceration is often found during a review of the client's chart. Liver injury is classified on the basis of the severity of the injury and ranges from grade I, with a small-surface hematoma, to grade VI, in which there is disruption of the vascular supply to the organ and hepatic avulsion or the actual tearing away of the organ.[18] Spleen injuries are also classified on the basis of the worsening severity of the injury and range from grade I, with a small-surface hematoma, to grade V, in which the spleen is completely shattered or when there is a hilar vascular injury of the spleen at the point of insertion of the splenic artery and the splenic vein. Kidney, bladder, ureter, gall bladder, peritoneum, and retroperitoneum injuries may also be associated with polytrauma.

Superficial injuries, as well as open wounds, contusions, and abrasions, may present at various locations on the body. These are common in pedestrian accidents, motorsport collisions, or injuries as a result of ejection. Burns to or foreign body penetration of a particular area or orifice may present with multiple other severe injuries in polytrauma. Multiple injuries only occur in approximately 5% of burns cases.[19] Orthopedic injuries are the most common, followed by soft tissue injuries, and head injuries.[19] A burn injury often complicates the diagnosis and treatment of the individual who has experienced polytrauma, by increasing the risk of sepsis and multisystem organ failure. See chapter 28 for more detailed information on burns.

Injuries to the nerves include those impacting the spinal cord as well as those to the nerve roots and spinal plexus. Spinal cord injury (SCI) occurs when there is an insult to the spinal cord resulting in motor, sensory, and/or autonomic changes. Traumatic SCI can be categorized into primary and secondary injuries. Primary injury occurs as a result of flexion, rotation, extension, compression, contusion, and shearing, as well as fracture-dislocation, ligamentous tears or disruption, and/or herniation of intervertebral disks. These primary injury events occur at the time of trauma and result in a series of secondary mechanisms similar to those found in TBI. Secondary injury includes spinal ischemia (lack of blood or oxygen) and spinal inflammation or edema. With the leading cause of SCI in the United States being motor vehicle accidents (MVAs)[20], it is not surprising that a high percentage of these individuals present with multiple injuries.[21,22] See chapter 35 for detailed information on SCI.

An example of a spinal plexus injury would be a brachial plexus injury. The brachial plexus is comprised of nerves that originate in the neck region. This network of nerves branches off to form other nerves that control movement and sensation in the UEs. The radial, median, and ulnar nerves originate in the brachial plexus. Brachial plexus injuries in adults have been identified in more than 1% of polytrauma clients cases in a single-institution study.[23] Minor brachial plexus injuries occur with stretching or compression, with more severe injuries resulting when there is tear or rupture of the nerves. The most severe form of brachial plexus injury is avulsion, which occurs when the nerve root is torn from the spinal cord. The prognosis for functional recovery after a brachial plexus injury depends on the severity of the injury. In less severe cases, where the nerves are only stretched, recovery can occur without treatment. In severe cases, however, surgery may be required, with adequate recovery occurring if the surgery is performed within 6 to 7 months of the initial injury. After this time frame, the chances of the muscle recovering function after surgical nerve repair are low.

Unspecified injuries and systemic injuries are often a result of the body's response to injury. System-wide injuries are those that affect the entire body, rather than a single body region. Poisoning and various types of toxicity account for most system-wide injuries.[2] The most pronounced system-wide injury affecting this client population, as observed clinically, is sepsis, also referred to as *septic shock*.

Sepsis occurs when an infection results in the formation of toxins, which are released into the bloodstream and cause a system-wide inflammatory response. Sepsis remains the most common cause of ARDS, with 46% of the cases triggered by a pulmonary source.[14,16] Sepsis is a critical condition and will most likely result in hemodynamic instability, which can progress to the level of septic shock marked by severe hypotension. Other forms of shock as a result of trauma include cardiogenic, neurogenic, and hypovolemic shock, also known as hemorrhagic shock. These types of severe system-wide injuries may result in multisystem organ failure (MSOF) because of their impact at the cellular level.

Nontrauma Critical Illness

Some individuals experience critical illness in a different form, where there is no isolated traumatic event or mechanism of injury. Their illness progresses to a severe medical situation, for example, a tooth abscess resulting in sepsis or serious pneumonia necessitating prolonged mechanical ventilation. Wound infections, cellulitis (tissue inflammation), necrotic tissue (dead tissue), urinary tract infections, and pneumonia are clinically observed as common medical issues that may become complicated in the setting of increased severity and certain premorbid or preexisting conditions in the individual. These medical conditions may then develop into sepsis, as described above, or systemic inflammatory response syndrome (SIRS). SIRS is an inflammatory state affecting the whole body, resulting in increased heart rate (HR) and respiratory rate (RR), increased white blood cell count, and fever. SIRS is exclusive of sepsis in that it is nonspecific and may not be caused by an infection.

Other examples of complications that may result from medical conditions include **critical illness polyneuropathy (CIP)** and **critical illness myopathy (CIM).** These complications arise as a result of prolonged mechanical ventilation, prolonged intensive care unit (ICU) stay, and prolonged used of sedation medications. *Critical illness polyneuropathy* is defined as an acute disorder primarily affecting motor and sensory axons, causing severe limb and respiratory muscle weakness.[24] *Critical illness myopathy* has a similar definition; however, it is an acute disorder of the muscle, with flaccid presentation and symmetrical weakness.[24] Both CIP and CIM result in prolonged ventilator assistance, increased hospital length of stay, and longer rehabilitation periods. Improvement may take weeks in mild cases and as long as months in more severe cases. Recovery and rehabilitation involve progressive reinnervation of muscles as well as restoration of sensory function. Over 50% of clients achieve full recovery; however, for the remaining population, recovery may be incomplete, resulting in a change in the client's level of functional independence or, sadly, death in some.[24]

RISK FACTORS

Traumatic injury places a significant burden on society with an estimated combined cost of $671 billion in medical treatment and lost productivity related to all death and physical injuries over the course of a single year (2013) in the United States alone.[25,26] The risk of hospitalization related to a traumatic injury varies by age and gender, and it is important to identify at-risk populations for injuries that require more than minimal medical attention. Understanding individuals who are more likely to be injured seriously enough to require hospitalization will facilitate the prevention of unintentional injuries.

Gender, age, behaviors, and lifestyle are all identifiable risk factors when considering those more likely to experience polytrauma. Just over two out of every three individuals experiencing major trauma are males, with the highest rate of injury found in the age group of 15- to 24-year-olds.[2,5] This is not surprising given the general interest in sports and high-risk activities, such as motorsports, including those involving all-terrain vehicles and motorcycles, in this population. Risky behaviors and lifestyle choices increase the likelihood of trauma. This includes association with gangs and violence, living in areas with high crime rates, and alcohol and/or drug abuse.

COMORBIDITIES AND COMPLICATIONS

The term **comorbidity** refers to the presence of one or more conditions that exist along with a primary disease or disorder. These can be medical conditions that exist independent of each other or medical conditions that are related. In clients in both the acute and subacute phases of rehabilitation after polytrauma, it is very likely that their injuries or diagnoses are related.

The Neurological System

Injuries of the brain, spinal cord, and peripheral nervous system can have varying impacts both within and across multiple medical conditions. These conditions often affect functional mobility, fine motor skills, skin and joint sensation or proprioception, behavior and emotional regulation, bowel and bladder functions, communication, visual-perceptual skills, cognition, and even the client's level of consciousness. Although many neurological conditions, such as TBI, improve or can be managed with treatment, some injuries result in chronic functional deficits.

Several different comorbidities and complications are related to a neurological insult, such as abnormal tone, seizures/epilepsy, hydrocephalus (collection of fluid within the brain), and migraine headaches. The presence of hypertonic spasticity, which is an abnormal increase in involuntary muscle tone, is responsible for shortening of soft tissue over time. Spasticity can lead to the development of joint contracture, which can only be corrected with orthopedic surgery. Contractures can lead to musculoskeletal conditions, as described in the next section.

In approximately 5% of clients with TBI, seizures may occur.[27] Early posttraumatic seizures are an associated complication occurring within the first week of the initial injury, and late posttraumatic seizures occur after the first week, with an 80% chance of recurrence.[27] A seizure is a serious event and requires immediate medical attention. Clinically, altered mental status or an altered level of consciousness can be seen in the period after an epileptic seizure. This is referred to as the *postictal state,* which can also consist of significant fatigue or weakness.

Hydrocephalus is categorized as communicating or noncommunicating, depending on the cause of the obstruction. Noncommunicating hydrocephalus occurs secondary to an obstruction in the ventricular system before the point at which cerebrospinal fluid (CSF) exits the fourth ventricle. Communicating hydrocephalus is the most common form after TBI and occurs when the obstruction is in the subarachnoid space.[28] Clients with hydrocephalus are often treated with surgical placement of a drainage system referred to as a *shunt*. The system diverts CSF from the central nervous system (CNS) and the brain region to another area of the body, where it is then absorbed as part of the normal circulation process.

Interestingly, most TBI survivors experience fewer postinjury comorbidities compared with those with orthopedic injuries and those who have experienced a cerebrovascular accident (CVA). The most frequently reported postinjury conditions include hypertension, musculoskeletal conditions, ear-nose-throat issues, and psychiatric/behavioral disturbances.[29]

The Musculoskeletal System

Abnormal tone as a result of neurological changes can cause hypertonicity, spasticity, and eventually joint contractures. Contractures begin with shortening of the muscles, which causes tight tendon cords. As time goes on, the surrounding nerves, skin, and joint capsules can also become tight. Exercise in the form of passive range of motion (PROM) or active assisted range of motion (AAROM) can help prevent contracture. However, when tightness has impacted the joint capsule, the contracture will require surgical intervention.

Heterotopic ossification (HO) refers to the abnormal presence of bone in soft tissue where bone normally does not exist.[30] This musculoskeletal complication is most often precipitated by trauma, such as with a fracture, but can also have a neurogenic cause, as with TBI or SCI (then called neurogenic heterotopic ossification [nHO]).[30] Symptoms of HO/nHO include localized swelling, pain, warmth, and loss of ROM. See Chapter 35 for more information on both types.

Compartment syndrome is an acute complication of injury or trauma to the musculoskeletal system and can lead to irreversible tissue damage. It is a critical condition in which the pressure within the closed segments of a person's limbs, consisting of fascia and bone (also known as *osseofascial compartment*), rises to a level that affects the delivery of blood across tissues. This poor perfusion leads to cellular anoxia, muscle ischemia, and tissue death, also called necrosis. Tissue death can then lead to a systemic inflammatory response or septic event, which can be fatal. Many different trauma-related injuries or conditions may precipitate acute compartment syndrome, including fractures, contusions, bleeding disorders, burns, and gunshot wounds.[31]

Complex injuries that involve both skeletal injury and vascular injury may result in limb amputation if salvaging efforts are unsuccessful. This happens with severe trauma resulting in disruption of arterial supply and loss of distal pulses. Amputation is a complication of complex injury but may be necessary to preserve the remainder of the limb or as a lifesaving measure. This is often the case in the event of muscle necrosis (tissue death) and wound contamination. In the instance of vascular damage and orthopedic fracture, revascularization through repair takes priority over orthopedic fracture stabilization because of the risk involved. See Chapter 24 for further information on amputations.

The development of fat embolism syndrome is another complication related to musculoskeletal trauma. This occurs when bone marrow fat from the fracture site embolizes (clots) and enters the pulmonary blood vessel network. The series of events that follow can result in acute hypoxemia (low oxygenation of blood) and other pulmonary compromise, as well as change in mental status. The incidence of fat embolism syndrome increases from 2% in single long-bone fractures to nearly 15% in polytrauma with pelvic and/or LE fractures.[32]

The Cardiopulmonary System

The hallmark risk related to polytrauma is pulmonary compromise.[33] Two common complications related to cardiopulmonary function after trauma are deep vein thrombosis (DVT) and pulmonary embolism (PE). These two complications can adversely affect client outcomes and have been reported to occur more often in cases of polytrauma than in isolated injuries.[34] DVT is the formation of a blood clot in the deep veins primarily in the LEs; however, it may also be observed in the UEs. PE can be life-threatening and is caused by the detachment of a clot, which then travels to the lungs. Signs and symptoms of acute PE include shortness of breath, sharp chest pain, increased HR, increased respiratory rate (RR), and the production of pink or bloody mucus. In individuals who have experienced polytrauma, significant measures are taken for prophylaxis of DVT because it is a major thromboembolic complication. If the occupational therapy assistant (OTA) suspects a client to have DVT or PE, the OTA should return the client to the bed and immediately seek the attention of a nurse or physician. If the medical team is testing the client for possible DVT or PE, OT treatment should be withheld until the test result is confirmed negative; and in case of a positive result, treatment should be withheld until the client has received appropriate medical treatment. In the early stages of HO/nHO, the symptoms can mimic those associated with DVT. Radiological findings and other further testing are used to distinguish the two.

Development of ARDS is a complication of polytrauma and may present initially or postoperatively. ARDS is characterized by hypoxemia that cannot be corrected by administration of extra oxygen and by demonstration of chest infiltration on radiology reports or scans. The prevalence of ARDS increases with severity of injury and with the occurrence of injuries in multiple anatomical regions.[35] Clinically, it is indicated by the need for mechanical ventilation for greater than 48 hours. The need for prolonged mechanical ventilation can lead to other complications, including ventilator-associated pneumonia and delirium resulting from a protracted ICU stay. If the medical team determines that mechanical ventilation has to continue well into the client's course, a tracheostomy tube may be placed. A tracheostomy tube is a plastic tube inserted through a surgical opening in the windpipe and provides a means of ventilation for clients with ARDS and other pulmonary injuries. Table 36-1 provides a brief description of ventilator terms and modes. Tracheostomy allows for a more secure airway and more gradual options during ventilator weaning. Weaning from the ventilator is generally determined by the pulmonologist and respiratory therapist and allows the client to rely less and less on the ventilator to eventually breathing on his or her own. The longer the client has been on the ventilator, the more difficult is the weaning process; it can be impacted by other health issues and can occur over minutes to days.

The Endocrine, Integumentary, and Gastrointestinal Systems

Approximately 30% to 50% of clients with TBI experience endocrine complications, such as diabetes insipidus, anterior hypopituitarism, antidiuretic hormone imbalance causing hyponatremia, cerebral salt wasting, and primary adrenal insufficiency.[36] Diabetes insipidus is characterized by intense thirst despite intake of fluids and causes the production of large amounts of urine. In hypopituitarism, a disorder of the pituitary gland, the gland either fails to produce one or more of its hormones or does not produce enough of them. This can impact the body's functions, including growth, reproduction, and blood pressure (BP) regulation. Hyponatremia is an electrolyte condition in which the level of sodium in blood is too low. Similarly, cerebral salt wasting syndrome results in hyponatremia caused by brain trauma or the presence of brain lesions. Complex medical management of polytrauma often results in prolonged periods of bedrest. Evidence suggests that within 3 days of bedrest, there is an increase in insulin resistance caused by impaired glucose delivery and uptake. This results in changes related to regulation of energy storage, regulation of protein metabolism, and potential insulin insufficiency.[37-39]).

In polytrauma cases, another major complication related to prolonged bedrest or limited mobilization impacts the integumentary system. Clients with spinal cord injuries, those

TABLE 36-1 Snapshot of Ventilator Settings

MODE	DEFINITION
IMV: Intermittent mandatory ventilation	Client receives a preset tidal volume and RR but it allows the client to breathe spontaneously between predetermined ventilator breaths
SIMV: Synchronized intermittent mandatory ventilation	RR and tidal volume are set. Similar to IMV but prevents "stacking" of inspiratory tidal volume (V_t = amount of gas inhaled during a normal cycle)
PRVC: Pressure regulated volume control	Vent controls both pressure and volume, every breath is a machine breath however the client can trigger breaths above the set rate. Volume is based on body weight.
PCV: Pressure control ventilation	Delivers a set airway pressure at prescribed rate, tidal volume is variable. Client can trigger breaths above the set rate but will be given a machine breath.
Volume Support	Client-initiated breath mode that targets tidal volume based on the client's inspiratory effort.
PSV: Pressure support ventilation	Commonly used as a weaning mode. Considered a spontaneous breathing mode, delivering a set pressure to overcome airway resistance and support the patient's efforts. Client regulates RR and tidal volumes with support from the ventilator. V_t set by lung compliance. Lowest pressure support is usually 5 mm H_2O to overcome resistance of tubing system.
CPAP: Continuous Positive Airway Pressure	Positive pressure is maintained throughout the respiratory cycle, providing essentially positive end expiratory pressure (PEEP) with increased fraction of inspired oxygen (FIO_2). Indicated during vent weaning and intended to decrease the work of breathing in clients who are spontaneously breathing.

with poor nutritional status, and some frail or very old clients have compromised skin integrity, and the propensity for developing pressure-related injuries increases significantly. A pressure injury, formerly called a decubitus ulcer, results from remaining in a given position over prolonged periods when circulation is compromised, particularly over a bony prominence, such as the sacrum. Such injuries can result in infection, significant pain, or the need for surgical intervention. See chapter 8 for more information.

Gastrointestinal complications in the polytrauma population include stress ulcers, dysphagia, bowel diarrhea or incontinence, constipation, and elevated levels on liver function tests. Bowel obstructions are clinically observed and are present when there is a blockage of the small or large intestine. Medication and toileting procedures are used to improve the motility of the gastrointestinal tract. Because of the effects of narcotic pain medication on the gastrointestinal system (typically constipation), bowel regimens are generally initiated early on during hospitalization.

Dysphagia, or difficulty swallowing, may present as a primary result of the brain damage or as a result of other medical conditions, such as respiratory compromise and ventilator use. Dysphagia often requires an alternate means of nourishment to maintain adequate caloric intake, especially during the rehabilitative process. This may be provided via a nasogastric (NG) tube (through the nose to the stomach) or a percutaneous endoscopic gastrostomy (PEG) tube (through the stomach wall to the stomach) or intravenously.

Premorbid Conditions and Risks

A client's **premorbid** status, or medical condition before the disease occurrence, can be an indicator and ultimately a potential risk factor for complications and other related conditions. Such conditions that have been observed clinically include older age, obesity, tobacco abuse, chronic obstructive pulmonary disease (COPD), alcohol abuse, and dementia.

Age as a risk factor has been evaluated. Older clients who have experienced trauma have a higher mortality rate compared with younger clients,[33,40] whereas, the opposite is true for developing complications after trauma.[23] A possible explanation is that the higher mortality in older adults may actually reduce the chances of complications developing in this group.[33]

It is widely known that obesity is an independent risk factor for various morbidities. The influence of excess body mass has been studied to understand its impact on those who are critically ill. Obesity has been revealed as the highest risk factor for development of MSOF because of altered inflammatory reaction; however, it does not have a significant influence on mortality.[41]

MEDICAL TREATMENT

The medical management of the client with complex polytrauma generally is performed at a level I trauma center. As described in Table 36-2, trauma hospitals are designated by range in level of care from I to IV. The phases of trauma care can be categorized as the prehospital phase, the hospital phase (including acute, primary, secondary and tertiary periods), and the rehabilitative phase.

THE OLDER ADULT

The treatment of geriatric polytrauma clients (age greater than 64 years) is known to be associated with both higher mortality and morbidity. However, geriatric trauma clients treated at centers that are more experienced and manage a higher proportion of older clients have demonstrated improved outcomes. Older clients who presented for care at medical facilities that treat more than 50% geriatric clients have been shown to be 33% more likely to survive than those presenting for care at medical facilities that treat a low (10%) proportion of geriatric clients. This evidence supports the prospective benefit of treating older trauma clients at centers specializing in their condition and expanding the availability of specialty facilities across the nation.[42,43]

TABLE 36-2 Levels of Trauma Care

HOSPITALS	LEVEL I	LEVEL II	LEVEL III	LEVEL IV
Ability to Manage Polytrauma Care	Full range of specialists and equipment available 24 hours per day	24-hour availability for all essential specialties, staff, and equipment	Resources for emergency resuscitation, surgery, and intensive care of most trauma patients	Initial evaluation, stabilization, diagnostic capabilities with transfer agreements to higher level centers
Trauma Management	Ongoing research, leader in trauma education and injury prevention, referral source for nearby regions	Comprehensive trauma care	Transfer agreements with level I or level II trauma centers that provide backup resources	Trauma trained nurse is immediately available, physicians are available on call

During the prehospital phase, paramedics focus on life support protocols and maintain communication with hospital personnel regarding the client's history, if available, and the mechanism, time, and circumstances of the injury. Often, clients who have experienced polytrauma arrive at the hospital on life support, and also may have spine immobilization, which involves use of a backboard and/or rigid cervical collar to maintain optimal positioning of the cervical spine. Hemorrhage is managed with direct pressure, prefabricated orthoses are utilized for immobilization, and open wounds are covered in sterile bandage.[32]

The acute hospital phase involves a fast, yet systematic, approach to evaluation and management. Vitals and radiographic findings are performed and assessed. During this phase, the client's airway, breathing/ventilation, circulation, disability, and exposure/environmental control are evaluated. Rapid resuscitation and orthopedic intervention occur during this phase, as indicated. Resuscitation intervention includes placement of all venous access, blood transfusion, and fluid solutions as indicated to increase mean arterial pressure. BP and HR are indicators of adequate resuscitation, and when necessary, central venous pressure or pulmonary capillary wedge pressure (via sensor inserted into pulmonary artery branch) may be warranted as a more accurate measure of hemodynamic stability.[32]

Surgical Intervention

Surgical intervention during the hospital phase may be emergent or scheduled. Hemorrhage and other vascular compromise, such as occlusion related to trauma, are managed as emergent events. Angiography (blood vessel imaging), completion arteriography (vessel imaging using dye), embolization (selective occlusion of blood vessels), exploration and vascular ligation (surgical tying of veins), patch angioplasty (repair by patch of a vessel wall), and bypass graft (replacement of vein or artery segment) are surgical management options for vascular repair. Fasciotomy is the emergent operative procedure to treat compartment syndrome, and it involves cutting the fascia to relieve increased pressure. The goal with all of the above vascular interventions is to preserve tissue or muscle perfusion. This is crucial to the tissue oxygenation cascade to ensure viability of the region, organ, and system.

Intracranial, subdural, subarachnoid, and intraventricular hemorrhages involve immediate consultation of a neurosurgeon to determine the need for operative or non-operative management. Surgical procedures related to head trauma include craniotomy with hemorrhage evacuation or craniectomy for bone flap removal to relieve increased intracranial pressure. Neurosurgeons make decisions regarding surgical intervention on the basis of the client's neurological presentation and radiology findings. Repeat scans are usually taken over the first 24 to 48 hours to determine whether a client is neurologically stable in the event of non-operative or operative management.

Orthopedic injuries are managed by the trauma team or the orthopedic consultative service. Non-operative management is an option with orthopedic injuries and is clinically observed with rib fractures, scapular fractures, sternal fractures, and some facial or clavicle fractures. Conversely, open reduction and internal fixation (ORIF) is a method of surgically repairing a bone fracture. Open reduction means opening the fracture area via incision allowing the surgeon to reconstruct the broken bone with hardware. ORIF involves the use of an intramedullary nail or rod to stabilize bone. It may also involve the use of plates and screws. In some instances, an external fixator ("ex-fix") is used to treat open fractures or as a temporary solution (Fig. 36-3). In this type of surgery, holes are drilled into uninjured areas of bone around the fracture, with placement of pins into the holes. Externally, a metal

COMMUNICATION

With clients who have experienced complex multiple trauma or who are critically ill, the best outcomes occur when there is effective communication and collaboration among members of the medical team. An interdisciplinary approach is the best practice and essential to service delivery. The medical record gives an idea of the overall plan, but in-person verbal communication gives the most up-to-date information specific to that clinician's area of practice.

The respiratory therapist is an example of a teammate who is a source of information regarding the client's ventilator weaning and overall pulmonary status. Verbal communication between the OTA and the respiratory therapist may include the client's respiratory response to activity and OT intervention on a given vent setting, what to change next time, information regarding respiratory reserve, secretions, physical recovery compared with respiratory recovery, and need for portable ventilator use when the client is showering.

Daily rounds or unit-based "huddles" are great avenues of interdisciplinary communication in the acute care setting. The term "rounds" typically indicates the presence of a physician or midlevel provider such as a nurse practitioner or physician assistant. Other disciplines are often invited and speak on different aspects of the client's care and hospital course, depending on the intent of the rounds. "Huddles" are more department/unit specific and typically are focused on workflows, for example, OT or PT practitioners or SLPs needing help with their workload or nurses reporting on which clients are being discharged that day. Nursing staff "huddles" are a great way for the OTA to present any changes or barriers to the client's discharge plan because the clinical case manager is often present. Handoff from the occupational therapist to the OTA is commonly used in the case of complex polytrauma client. This interaction allows the evaluating occupational therapist to give the OTA firsthand information that may not be directly available on the medical record. It allows for collaboration on treatment strategies or family dynamics that will set the OTA up for success.

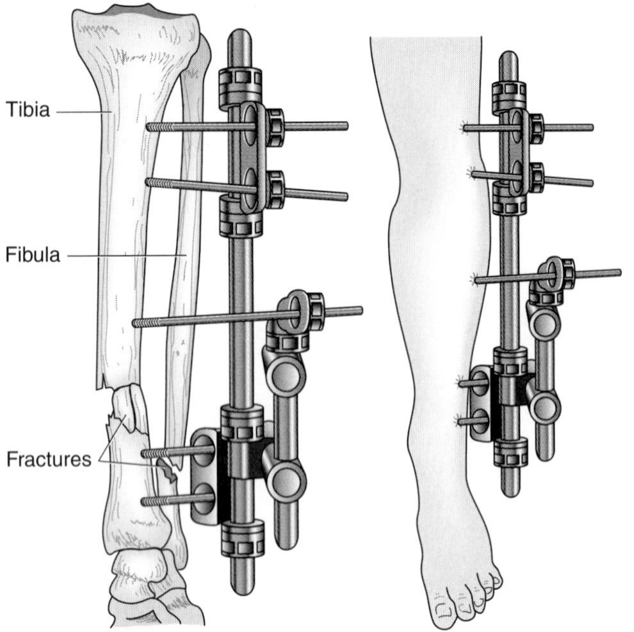

FIGURE 36-3. External fixator (ex-fix).

rod with a particular framework of clamps creates a rigid support. The ex-fix is used to keep the bones stabilized and in alignment. It is typically worn anywhere from a few weeks to several months, with the orthopedic surgeon determining the time frame.

Spinal fractures are usually managed by the neurosurgery service as a consultation when the client is admitted to the hospital. Based on the injury to the spine, recommendations are made for operative or non-operative treatment. Minor stable fractures of the spinous or transverse process are generally treated non-operatively based on clinical findings. Ligamentous injuries from trauma may be caused by subluxation or dislocation of the vertebrae and are likely to be treated conservatively. The presence of a stable spinal fracture indicates that there is no identifiable threat to the spinal cord. Unstable vertebral body fractures, compression fractures, or any trauma resulting in cord compromise, require neurosurgical intervention. The goal of surgery is to stabilize the spinal column, prevent spinal deformity, and improve the neurological presentation. Spinal stabilization surgery involves decompression of the spinal cord, possible fusion of vertebrae, or corpectomy (removal of vertebrae).

Other surgical procedures are performed as a means of opening a space in a particular body region to manage trauma and determine the treatment course. Laparotomy is a surgical procedure in which the abdomen is opened. This may be to repair, remove, or wash out a region or organ within the abdominal cavity. Clinically, this is common with gunshot wounds or stab wounds. The small bowel is the most commonly injured structure when there is penetrating trauma.[5] Problems associated with a bowel injury include infection or peritonitis, edema, or fluid loss. In severe trauma cases, where life-saving surgical intervention is required on unstable clients, the abdomen is packed and left open, with definitive closing deferred until the client is more stable and out of a state of shock. The presence of edema may also prevent abdominal closure. In this event, a patch is placed and gradually tightened during a series of return trips to the operating room.

Some clients may have experienced blunt trauma and sustained spleen or liver injuries. Spleen injuries can be managed non-operatively, and proper discharge education is provided to prevent the risk of rupture. Operative management includes splenectomy (removal), splenorrhaphy (repair), or angioembolization (minimally invasive procedure to stop bleeding).[5] Liver injuries, however, are managed more aggressively compared with spleen injuries, given that hepatectomy (liver removal) is not an option. If surgical intervention is indicated, it typically occurs as a means of packing or repairing specific structures.[5] Thoracotomy is a surgical procedure in which the chest is opened to treat an injury or to remove blood, infection, or fluid. Video-assisted thoracoscopic surgery (VATS) is a less invasive alternative to thoracotomy and is used for the same indications.

Lines, Tubes, and Drains

Other surgical interventions for serious injuries found in clients who have experienced complex polytrauma include placement of drains and tubes. See Appendix A for location, purpose, and rehabilitation considerations for common lines, tubes, and drains by system.

Medication

Clients who have multiple serious injuries related to trauma or critical illness will likely receive many different medications as pharmacological treatment during the course of their

TECHNOLOGY AND TRENDS

It is clearly the focus of the trauma team and the team in the ICU to keep the client who has experienced polytrauma stable and alive. A study by Vieira and colleagues showed that skeletal muscle deteriorates rapidly in traumatically injured and mechanically ventilated clients, especially in the first 5 days.[44] One of the newest techniques being studied is to use neuromuscular electrical stimulation (NMES) on muscles to preserve their size and strength while the client is ventilated and sedated. One benefit to NMES is that it does not require the client's participation in any way, as the muscle is electrically stimulated to contract with electrodes on the muscle belly. In another study by Vieira and colleagues in 2016, it was shown that with NMES, the studied quadriceps muscle of the clients was 23.7 percent less thick in the controls, whereas the NMES group, the size did not change.[45] The authors of the article noted that because they only studied one muscle for 5 days, the next steps are to study multiple muscles for longer periods as well as functionally. A population that typically ends up so significantly weak after weeks in the ICU may have a chance of maintaining some strength with future options.

recovery. The main groups of medication that the OTA must be familiar with are those used to manage pain, anxiety/agitation, BP, and arrhythmias (irregular heartbeats).

Sedative medications modulate signals within the client's CNS and serve to calm and to increase comfort. These medications may be in the form of continuous fast-acting infusions that can be turned off with limited effects after just minutes. Other sedative medications are used for conscious sedation during procedures or for more long-term sedation in the critical care environment. OT treatment times must be carefully planned around the use of sedative medication because clients may be too lethargic to participate in OT. In the case of stronger sedative medications, such as Versed®, treatment may not be appropriate within hours after administration or at any time that day, depending on the use and medical plan. Propofol, however, is a medication that will allow for client participation if given in a small dose or if its administration has been recently stopped. See Table 36-3 for the most commonly used sedative medications in the ICU.

Analgesics are used to manage pain and may be administered orally or given intravenously for faster results. Common analgesics used to treat clients who have experienced polytrauma fall within the opioid drug class and include oxycodone, hydrocodone, hydromorphone, codeine, morphine, and tramadol. Pain medications have a number of side effects, including dizziness, nausea, vomiting, constipation, abdominal pain, skin rash, and heartburn. Clients with severe injuries and multiple fractures will usually be prescribed scheduled pain medication with an "as needed," or PRN, option as well while the client is in the hospital setting. The goal is pain management leading to an overall decrease in pain during the client's acute and subacute phases of recovery.

Vasopressors are used to manage low BP. Clients requiring the use of these medications may continue to be hemodynamically unstable. Antiarrhythmics and antihypertensives are other cardiac medications that can cause hypotension, drowsiness, and nausea. Close collaboration with nursing staff and the whole medical team is required to determine whether the medication is being tapered off (not increased in the past 2 hours) and if BP is stable.

Many other medications are used in the acute and subacute environments following polytrauma. Cognitive stimulants are often used in the case of CVA and TBI; diuretics are commonly used to treat edema, which may result after fluid resuscitation; and an array of antibiotics are used to treat infection. Thorough review of the client's medical record and close communication with the medical team will provide insight into the medications used and their potential effects related to OT interventions. This often requires assessment during every treatment session, depending on the setting.

FUNCTIONAL IMPAIRMENT

Depending on the nature of the injury and the severity of the trauma, the client may experience minor to major impairments. The following sections discuss both physical and psychosocial impairments that should be considered in the OT practitioner's intervention plan.

Physical Presentation: Motor and Praxis

Clients who have experienced complex polytrauma may present with motor control and strength deficits, depending on the injury and the overall course. The client's initial evaluation or reevaluation will provide information regarding strength, motor control, ideation, motor planning, and execution. In the acute phase of rehabilitation, clients may present with significant weakness associated with their injury, edema caused by resuscitation efforts, and an overall deconditioned state. It is not uncommon for OTAs to treat clients with multiple injuries and conditions and who have trace or only gravity-eliminated strength at the acute phase. Across the continuum of care, it is important for the OTA to focus on the client's further development of functional strength and functional movement patterns to develop that strength.

Observation of the client during the initial moments of the session will provide insight into the individual's performance related to motor skills and praxis on that day. Spilled food on the client's bed, gown, or food tray is an indicator of possible motor control deficits. This could also be an indicator, however, of proximal weakness resulting in distal coordination deficits. The client's response to nonfunctional motor commands such as manual muscle testing will provide, at a minimum, information regarding generalized strength. However, asking the client to perform a

TABLE 36-3 Sedation Medications

MEDICATION	EFFECTS	ONSET IN MINUTES	HALF-LIFE IN HOURS	ADVERSE REACTIONS
Versed®	Sedation	2-5	3-12	Delirium, hypotension
Ativan®	Sedation Analgesia	5-20	10-20	Delirium, metabolic acidosis
Propofol®	Sedation	1-2	1.5-12.4	Hypotension
Precedex®	Sedation Analgesia	5-10	2	Bradycardia, hypotension

functional task such as using objects as targets across the midline, with a functional end goal, will lead to identification of any problems related to praxis. An example of this would be the grooming task of brushing teeth, in which the items are placed to the left side of the sink for a client who is right-hand dominant. The client's regard, reach, and grasp of the items, as well as management of the toothpaste on the toothbrush and reaching to turn on the water, require a high level of motor planning and motor coordination.

Functional motor skills may be impaired in the presence of fractures, wounds, or neurological injury. ROM can be limited in the presence of a fracture and, depending on the operative or non-operative plan, it may be encouraged aggressively or contraindicated. Physician orders regarding weight-bearing and ROM should be considered first when anticipating the physical motor performance a client may demonstrate.

With clients who have a brain injury and are at a low performance level, motor skills may be assessed by giving basic commands and paying close attention to differentiate intentional or purposeful motor movement from reflexive movement. The client's cognitive abilities may limit the potential for demonstration of motor skills. Placement of common objects, such as a ball or television remote, over the client's hands on the dorsal aspect will allow the OTA to potentially elicit a functional grasp upon command while eliminating the possibility of reflexive movement. Close attention should be paid to any purposeful or nonpurposeful movement patterns in the population at the low performance level. Simple observation before treatment intervention may allow the practitioner to understand motor skills and patterns the client is demonstrating at rest as well.

Physical Presentation: Sensory and Perceptual

With regard to the client's loss of or change in sensation, the condition may improve or worsen throughout the rehabilitation phase and should be continuously monitored. Recovery from CIP is characterized by progressive reinnervation of muscle and restoration of sensory function that may take anywhere from weeks to months.[24] A traumatic neurological injury, such as SCI or TBI, can leave clients with significant sensory changes. Neurogenic pain, which is pain from a central cause versus a wound or injury, may develop and cause significant limitations with shoulder and scapular function in clients with SCI. Clients who have experienced polytrauma presenting after a traumatic limb amputation may experience phantom limb sensation and/or phantom limb pain. Sensory changes or loss can be devastating to an already traumatized client.

Perceptual skills are those skills required to take in, organize, and interpret one's current environment. Visual changes may result from trauma to the face and orbital regions or from TBI. These changes often present in the form of blurry or double vision. Cognitive deficits combined with visual deficits make the client's perception of the situation especially challenging.

Delirium as a result of a prolonged ICU stay may be an additional contributor to perceptual skill changes. Delirium is characterized by a disturbance of consciousness, with cognitive changes resulting in short-term memory impairment, attention deficits, and disorientation. It generally develops acutely and presents with a fluctuating course.

Physical Presentation: Balance and Posture

The client who has experienced polytrauma is likely to present with impairments related to functional balance and posture as a result of an array of contributing factors. Pain in sitting or standing, changes in the ability to bear weight through an extremity, muscle weakness, and cognitive impairment are all indicators that a client is likely to have balance and postural control deficits. Consider the client who had arthritis and chronic pain before the trauma, is cognitively impaired after an acute TBI, and also presents with an acute right distal radius fracture and fractures of the left tibia and fibula with an external fixator in place. This client is likely to present with challenges to balance in the sitting position because of the inability to prop himself with his right UE, pain from the premorbid arthritis in BUEs, pain at fracture or injury sites, and confusion in orientation to situation or location.

Overall weakness in the extremities is an indicator of core muscle weakness, especially following critical illness. Core weakness related to deconditioning or a neurological injury, such as TBI, will result in challenges to completion of activities of daily living (ADLs) in unsupported sitting. Often, clients will present with functional challenges even in a supported sitting posture. Postural changes may occur after a prolonged ICU stay or hospitalization. Clinically, this has been observed by clients presenting with posterior pelvic tilt, shoulders that are rounded and internally rotated, and a flexed trunk. The exception to this typical postural presentation in critical illness is seen in clients who have experienced abdominal injuries and surgeries. These clients typically position themselves in extension because of abdominal pain and the fear of moving that may cause increased pain in that area. From the edge of the bed, it is not uncommon for this client to present in significant trunk extension, often requiring the assistance of a second person to maintain the client's balance.

Psychosocial Presentation: Cognition

Cognitive changes as a result of polytrauma may range from presentation in a comatose state to emergence from a comatose state to impulsivity and high distractibility with multistep ADL routines. Various assessment tools are available for use by OT practitioners to determine a client's cognitive abilities in a subjective or objective manner. In the acute care setting, common tools include the Glasgow Coma Scale, the Rancho Los Amigos Level of Cognitive Function Scale, and the JFK Coma Recovery Scale. Understanding the client's ability to follow simple or complex commands, respond to various stimulus, interact with the environment, and problem-solve are foundational to planning treatment intervention. See Chapter 11 on cognition or Chapter 34 on TBI for more information.

Polytrauma often causes short- and long-term effects on the client's psychological and emotional well-being. Once clients are aware of the situation and the degree of their injury, they may experience posttraumatic stress disorder (PTSD). The client who is able to recall the traumatic incident that caused the injury may have flashbacks or panic attacks. On clinical observation, clients who become aware of their cognitive deficits may mask them out of fear or embarrassment. In other instances, clients may be unaware of their cognitive deficits because of the nature of the injury. This may cause a direct change in the client's performance skills, and this ultimately impacts the client's performance patterns. Clients may experience depression as a result of their changing roles, and this places significant stress on both the clients and the new caregivers.

Psychosocial Presentation: Communication

Communication changes in the client who has experienced complex trauma may result from placement of an artificial airway, such as an endotracheal tube (ETT) (into the windpipe through the mouth) or a tracheostomy tube. The inability to effectively communicate is often a significant source of fear and anxiety in clients who are ventilated. In some instances, speech language pathologists (SLPs) or respiratory therapists have issued a Passy Muir® valve (PMV) for use in clients who have a tracheostomy tube in place and can tolerate valve use (the valve can make it harder to breathe, since it replaces ventilator tubing). It is a one-way valve placed over the end of the tracheostomy tube (without the ventilator) and is often the first opportunity for both the client and his or her loved ones to hear the client's voice after prolonged hospitalization. The client must be able to produce sufficient expiratory air flow through the vocal cords to produce speech. This may take practice for retraining the upper airway but is a great opportunity for clients to let their voices be heard. Some clients, however, may not be able to tolerate increased activity level with the valve in place because of a feeling of not being able to catch the breath, coughing, intolerance to the one-way valve, or the need for increased ventilation and oxygen. Close monitoring of oxygenation saturations and RR is indicated.

Motor and cognitive skills guide practitioners in understanding the client's ability to handwrite or point to a communication board as a form of effective communication. Appropriate and effective modifications should be considered, such as a basic or complex picture or letter board that the client points to with either hands or a mouth stick. An adapted call bell is often required for clients who are unable to demonstrate adequate fine motor skills for calling the nursing station in the acute care environment. Adapted call bell options consist of a bulb or pancake mechanism that either requires a gross grasp or gross motor movement pattern of the UE or even the head (Fig. 36-4). Another option is a sip-and-puff call bell that requires the client to move air across a small tube that is placed close to their mouth. Collaboration with the SLP and the rest of the client's care team will maintain consistency among providers when helping the client be successful in expressive communication.

Psychosocial Presentation: Emotional Regulation

Traumatic circumstances and significant life changes caused by injury can be a major challenge in this specific client population. This can occur as a result of the injury, as in the case of a client presenting for rehabilitation after a frontal brain injury. This client may be easily angered and agitated by simple requests. This same frustration and agitation can also be seen in a client coping with the long-term implications of his or her traumatic injury, such as a complete SCI. Establishing and building rapport, as well as allowing for continuity among OT practitioners, is beneficial

EVIDENCE-BASED PRACTICE

Much of the literature on rehabilitation of clients with critical illnesses captures the long-term effects on the client's physical, social, and psychological well-being. Early mobility and skilled therapy intervention at the level of the ICU has been explored and shown to be effective in decreasing hospital length of stay, and research studies have attempted to demonstrate significant functional outcomes. Research exploring any positive effects of these early interventions on the client's quality of life after the rehabilitation process is limited. With this client population at risk for depression and posttraumatic stress disorder, it does not capture the implementation of effective and holistic psychosocial services.

Recently, however, there has been a shift, and researchers are looking at the impact of peer support in ICU rehabilitation. Peer support allows for direct engagement with other clients who have experienced, or are currently experiencing, the same health care service trajectory. This can be in the form of support groups or one-on-one peer visitation. Research has demonstrated the effectiveness of support groups in recovery in the case of clients who have cancer, burns, or diabetes.[46] There is a small body of qualitative evidence showing that clients in the ICU have benefited from peer support. Future research should be aimed at integrating this into holistic ICU rehabilitation service delivery and exploring the effectiveness in quality of life outcomes after critical illness and polytrauma.[46]

McPeake J., & Quasim, T. (2016). The role of peer support in ICU rehab. Intensive and Critical Care Nursing, *37, 1-3.*

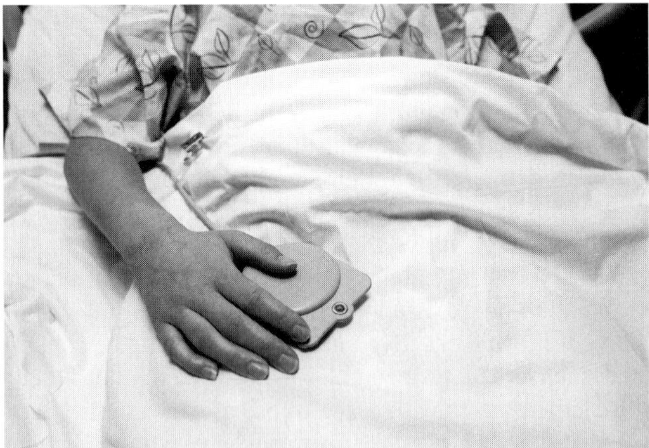

FIGURE 36-4. Adaptive pancake call bell for hospital bed. The client presses anywhere on the call bell to activate the signal.

to those clients with complex polytrauma and emotional challenges. Family members can also present with an assortment of emotions because of stress and changing roles.

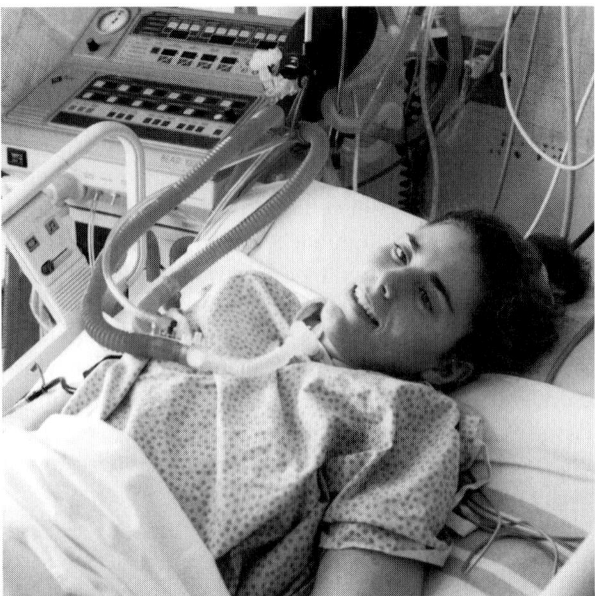

FIGURE 36-5. Client in the ICU.

TREATMENT AND INTERVENTION

OT treatment and intervention specific to polytrauma involves taking a look at all of the factors preventing the person from completing his or her valued occupations. Understanding specific factors will allow the OTA to develop appropriate treatment strategies to decrease the burden of impairment while also building skills needed to participate in, or complete, daily routines.

Role of the Occupational Therapy Assistant

The role of the OTA is to provide rehabilitative services to clients who have experienced polytrauma (Fig. 36-5). The goal is to improve the client's overall quality of life in all aspects, including cognitive, physical, and emotional. The OTA collaborates closely with the occupational therapist because these cases can be complex. Supervision is provided by occupational therapists with regard to the plan of care and appropriate frequency and intensity of services, given the injuries.

ACUTE CARE GOALS

Acute care OT goals focus on maximizing independence and promoting increased function with basic ADLs. The goal of the OTA is to help clients get to the next level of care outside of the acute trauma center environment. This could be inpatient rehabilitation, subacute rehabilitation, home health, outpatient therapy, or home with supervision and assistance from family. The process involves intervention centered on the client's goals, home environment, and support after discharge. The OT process is unique in that it challenges OT practitioners to promote optimal independence, decrease pain, and increase overall safety with ADLs and instrumental activities of daily living (IADLs).

Acute care OT often starts at the level of the ICU and may involve monitoring a client's response to treatment in terms of activity tolerance or providing basic education to family on appropriate ways to position their loved one. Often, acute care OT intervention includes training the client in foundational skills needed to progress to basic ADL performance. These foundational skills include safe transition from supine to sitting at the edge of the bed, sustained grasp on an ADL object, or following two-step commands. These foundational skills may be written as short-term, 2-week, acute care goals with the level of independence or accuracy gradually increased to reflect the client's progress.

SUBACUTE CARE GOALS

OT goals beyond the acute care setting are directed toward completion of actual ADL routines and capture those areas necessary for a safe discharge home or to the community setting. Subacute focuses less on the foundational skills and more on dimensions of independence. This includes shower transfers, bathing, dressing, and bowel management to list a few, but it also encompasses cognitive skills, such as comprehension, problem-solving, and health management. Long-term goals that are addressed in the subacute setting include family- or caregiver-directed tasks, as taught and demonstrated by the OTA. Education goals are centered on delivery of all necessary information to promote client and caregiver success in the home or community.

Gaining Competence in Polytrauma

Early OT intervention for clients who have experienced complex polytrauma involves critical thinking and experience beyond the entry level for the OT practitioner. ICU and step-down ICU levels of care require supervision and mentoring (potentially an OT Fellowship), along with skills-based competencies. Practitioner orientation and higher level competencies are site specific and are usually necessary for OT practitioners to gain confidence in skills for treating clients with lower-level TBI or those with acute SCI.

EVIDENCE-BASED RESEARCH

The importance of OT in the ICU setting for clients who are critically ill has been determined, as well as the use of early activity and therapy to prevent or treat the neuromuscular complications of critical illness.[14,47] Earlier OT intervention has been linked to lower median doses of sedatives, improved delirium status, improved functional mobility status, and decreased ICU stay, as well as hospital length of stay.[48] Delivery of OT services in the critical care environment involves an interdisciplinary approach, where there is frequent communication and collaboration among team members. The team consists of the client, the client's family, physicians (gastroenterologist, pulmonologist, or other specialties), a nurse, respiratory therapist, SLP, dietitian, occupational therapist, OTA, physical therapist, physical therapist assistant (PTA), social worker, and clinical case manager.

EFFECTS OF PROLONGED BEDREST

Clients who have experienced prolonged bedrest or immobility are at risk for physical, psychological, and physiological complications and adverse events. Research has demonstrated that immobility may lead to a decreased metabolic rate, negative nitrogen balance, tissue atrophy, bone demineralization, electrolyte and fluid imbalance, change in body temperature with increased perspiration, loss of fluids, and insulin resistance even in clients without diabetes.[49] Gastrointestinal complications related to prolonged bedrest include disruption of peristalsis (the muscle contractions that move food through the digestive tract), hypomobility, constipation, and impaction. Clients are also at risk for urinary issues, including urinary stasis (urine accumulation), urinary tract infection (UTI), kidney stones, and incontinence.[49] Slowed RR, increased risk of hypoxemia, and overall decreased respiratory movement resulting in stasis of secretions, have been reported to be complications of prolonged bedrest. The cardiovascular impact of a slowed and static system results in the potential development of orthostatic hypotension (rapid drop in BP with movements such as sitting up or standing), DVT, or hypovolemia (decreased blood volume).[49]

Behavioral and Emotional Considerations

The client's behavioral and emotional response to the trauma they experienced may manifest in anger, tearfulness, denial, or a withdrawn affect. These behavioral or emotional changes arise as clients begin to process their injuries and the changes they are experiencing. Therapeutic use of self and establishing rapport with clients will allow them to feel comfortable sharing their emotions while collaborating with the OTA to achieve desirable goals.

Client Safety

Safety always comes first when providing OT interventions across settings. Ensuring client safety during treatment involves gathering all necessary information related to the client's condition as well as preparing the environment for the treatment session. Close monitoring of the client and the client's response to treatment is always indicated, especially with clients who are in the acute phase of polytrauma. Anticipating adverse events will allow OTAs to maintain safety for clients and for themselves. The use of proper equipment, including a gait belt, rolling walker, or wheelchair, as appropriate, as well as the help of a therapy technician, will increase safety when performing functional mobility. Adherence to all precautions, including spinal, weight-bearing, and ROM, must be ensured. This can prove to be challenging with clients who have experienced a TBI or delirium, for example, and they may not remember their precautions. Clients who present for treatment after craniectomy (removal of part of the skull) generally require use of a helmet during functional mobility because of lack of a protective bone flap. Compliance with all necessary bracing, helmeting, and protective orthotics must be maintained during OT unless the requirements have been lifted by physician orders.

WHEN TO START

Before initiating treatment with the client who has experienced polytrauma, it is imperative to perform a thorough review of the individual's medical record. This is especially true when providing treatment in the acute care setting because the client's condition can change frequently. Any modifications to precautions, including weight-bearing status, activity orders, or ROM orders, should be noted. Laboratory values within normal limits or consistent across time should be observed. While reviewing the client's chart, the OTA should take note of any critical events and precautions or indications for treatment. If a client has had a change in status, or major surgery beyond placement of a line or tube, the evaluating or supervising occupational therapist should be notified. Clearance with the nurse is best practice when working with complex cases, as nurses may have up-to-date information not yet available within the medical chart. Communication with the nursing staff will assist the OT practitioner in determining the best time for treatment, depending on procedures, testing, and medication.

Before treatment, all OT practitioners should take note of the lines, tubes, drains, and airway in place. Visually scanning the environment and writing down information about the lines and tubes on a small piece of paper is good practice to ensure that all are noted while in the room and later during documentation. For the OTA to gain an understanding of how much support the client requires, ventilator settings and use of supplemental oxygen should be noted. Baseline vitals should be recorded if the client is being monitored through an ICU monitoring system or if the client is on basic telemetry. This will provide information regarding the client's resting state and allow for close monitoring of the client's response to treatment, as mentioned above. Continual assessment for nonverbal signs and symptoms of pain should occur, as well as any client changes, such as diaphoresis (sweating), pallor, change in mental status, and significant change in vital signs. See Table 36-4 for normal resting vital signs.

WHEN TO MODIFY

OT intervention should be modified if the client requires increased rest for recovery of vital signs, including oxygen saturation and RR. A normal response to activity and intervention would be an appropriate increase in HR, RR, and BP. An increase in HR from 1 to 49 beats per minute (bpm) is generally expected with exertion. A RR increase to the 20s and 30s may require rest breaks for recovery. A change in BP with a decrease of more than 20 mmHg from the initial assessment of vitals may require further investigation to determine whether the client is symptomatic with hypotension or orthostatic hypotension. If the client is symptomatic, the nurse should be made aware and can assist with determining whether treatment may be continued, if modified. Mean arterial pressure (MAP) is utilized to determine tissue perfusion, and normally, it should range from 80 to 100 mmHg. A MAP of less than 60 mmHg may signal inadequate tissue perfusion, and a MAP of less than 65 to 80 mmHg should involve modification of treatment. Change in peripheral oxygen saturation (SpO_2), with a decrease greater than 10% of the client's baseline, requires modification of the intervention. This may involve communication with the client's nurse or the respiratory therapist to increase the amount of oxygen being delivered. Rest breaks and cueing for pursed-lip breathing will generally allow for increased oxygen saturations.

WHEN TO STOP

The OTA should consider stopping treatment when there are significant changes in vital signs for no apparent reason; see Table 36-5 for basic guidelines.[48] Ventilator dyssynchrony, or a mismatch between the client's breaths and the ventilator breaths, is a situation in which treatment should be stopped or modified, and the respiratory therapist should be notified.[48] Client distress, as observed by nonverbal cues or gestures, as well as unsafe combativeness, are scenarios when OT intervention should be discontinued and nursing staff notified. New-onset arrhythmia, onset of myocardial infarction, concern for airway device integrity, endotracheal tube removal, and the client falling are also scenarios in which treatment should stop so that the client's medical needs are met.

When modification of treatment does not result in stable vitals or desirable client presentation, treatment should be discontinued. An example of this would be a client's HR being 100 bpm at the start of the therapy session, reaching 135 bpm with activity, and staying between 130 and 140 bpm despite a 5-minute seated rest break. The OTA would expect to see a decrease to a resting HR of 100 bpm. In the acute care setting, the nurse must be made aware of those situations when OT intervention is modified or discontinued.

TABLE 36-4 Normal Vital Signs

VITAL SIGN	NORMAL RESTING RANGE
Heart rate (HR)	60–100 bpm (beats per minute)
Respiratory rate (RR)	12–20 breaths per minute
Blood pressure (BP)	110–119 mmHg systolic BP 60–79 mmHg diastolic BP
Mean arterial pressure (MAP)	80–100 mmHg
Oxygen saturation	95%–100%

TABLE 36-5 Basic Guidelines for Stopping Treatment

VITAL SIGN	PRESENTATION
Mean arterial pressure (MAP)	<65 mmHg
Heart rate (HR)	<40 or >130 beats per minute
Respiratory rate (RR)	<5 or >40 breaths per minute
Oxygenation (SpO_2)	<88% saturation

MANAGEMENT OF LINES AND TUBES

After taking initial inventory of the client's lines, tubes, and drains, the OTA must consider the projected path or plan for the client to take during the treatment session. Bed level ADL activity or exercises rarely demand positioning or repositioning of lines and tubes. Awareness of the placement of lines, tubes, and drains in relation to the client and his or her extremities is generally all the OTA must maintain. If functional mobility is performed, more critical thinking is involved.

The first question to ask oneself when preparing to perform functional mobility with a client who has multiple lines, tubes, and drains is "What is connected that cannot be moved?" If the client is supported by a ventilator, this will determine in which direction he or she must mobilize. Unless it is a portable home ventilator in the inpatient rehabilitation or home setting, the ventilator restricts the space in which the client can move. There is, however, the option in the acute care setting to place the client on a portable ventilator for treatment beyond the reach of the standard bedside ventilator. This must be performed by the respiratory therapist, as ordered by the physician.

Other tubing that may limit the distance or direction in which a client can move includes those drains connected to the wall or to a monitoring system. Clients with drains or tubes that lead to wall suction and a canister for emptying of the contents may be restricted to move in a certain direction unless the nurse assists in making the suction unit portable. More invasive lines that are secured with electrical monitoring, such as central venous pressure (CVP) lines and arterial lines, must also be considered first. With a physician's order, these lines may be adapted or unhooked by the nurse before treatment. CNS drains, such as ventriculostomy and lumbar drains, must be clamped, which also involves a physician's order and management by the nurse before initiating activity or treatment.

All other tubes or drains are made portable by pinning or taping them to the client's clothing or by moving them via the intravenous (IV) pole to which they are connected. More than likely, the nurse is able to adapt a peripheral IV line, which does not involve continuous infusion, for brief periods during OT intervention. It is necessary to anticipate the direction of the lines and tubes and how much assistance will be needed to manage them during any treatment. If more than one hand is needed to manage the lines and tubes, and more than one hand is needed to safely assist the client, the assistance of a rehabilitation technician is indicated.

Once lines, tubes, and drains have been organized before OT intervention, the OTA must ensure that the path is free of clutter or objects that may be a safety hazard. Drains that can be secured to the client's clothing must be secured with a clip or pin before mobilization. In the instance that a tube or drain gets pulled, the OTA must make sure the client is seated or supine while applying pressure to the site with sterile gauze. The OTA should assess the client's pain level and provide all necessary information to the bedside nurse if treating in the acute care setting.

Treatment Approaches

Treatment approaches will differ, depending on the environment the client is currently in, his or her medical status, and the nature and severity of the injuries. Goals will change and be adapted as the client regains strength and function and on the basis of the discharge location and amount of assistance or supervision available.

THE CONTINUUM OF CARE AND TREATMENT SETTINGS

The initial phase of rehabilitation for clients who have experienced polytrauma occurs in the acute care setting, usually while the client is receiving care in the ICU or the step-down ICU. At this point, the occupational therapist would have evaluated the client and established short-term goals, usually for 2-week periods. These goals may range from increasing the client's awareness of self and environment to completing a two-step ADL task with minimal cueing for sequence. Acute care goals address the foundational skills needed for participation in basic ADLs, such as grooming, dressing, bathing, and toileting. The emphasis is on increasing ROM, strength, cognitive skills, visual-perceptual skills, safety awareness, balance, and coordination to a level at which simple ADL routines can be performed. Other acute care level goals include education and training to the client and his or her family, positioning, orthotics, functional bed mobility retraining, and development of increased activity tolerance. Depending on the injury, clients may be introduced to compensatory techniques or temporary ways of completing ADLs and functional mobility until weight-bearing precautions or bracing restrictions are lifted. This may involve recommendations for durable medical equipment (DME) or training in the use of adaptive equipment to increase overall safety and independence.

Acute care OTAs work closely with caregivers, social workers, and case managers to determine the best place for the client after discharge from the acute care setting. This involves understanding the client's home environment, social support system, and availability of assistance after discharge. Most clients who have experienced polytrauma with multiple injuries and prolonged hospitalizations require additional rehabilitation after discharge from the hospital. These clients are likely to be discharged to inpatient rehabilitation hospitals or subacute rehabilitation centers.

Inpatient rehabilitation meets the client's rehabilitation needs in an environment where there is less emphasis on the medical complexity of the client's condition and more emphasis on preparing for the home environment. Inpatient rehabilitation hospitals serve clients who have experienced polytrauma and have TBIs, multiple fractures, and spinal cord injuries. These clients receive a minimum of 3 hours of scheduled therapy time, which is usually split among physical therapy (PT), OT, and speech language pathology. At this level of rehabilitation, goals are specific to a functional outcome measure, such as the functional independence measure. Inpatient rehabilitation aims to increase the client's ADL performance while preparing the client's family for the transition back into the home and the community. At this point in the continuum of care, clients further develop ROM, strength, balance, cognitive skills, visual-perceptual skills, and coordination beyond the level of foundational skills. Clients work to take the level of independence that they have achieved and apply that to the home and community environments. On the basis of the client's progress and needs, recommendations are made for specialized mobility devices and cushions, adaptive equipment, and all necessary DME.

Subacute rehabilitation is also a level of rehabilitation beyond the acute hospital setting, and it establishes more home and community goals for clients. Subacute rehabilitation may be affiliated with a skilled nursing facility; however, it is usually a place for a short-term stay until the client is independent enough to return to his or her previous home environment. Subacute rehabilitation generally has a slower pace compared with inpatient rehabilitation and may be indicated for clients who have multiple fractures (three or more extremities affected). This level of rehabilitation is appropriate when clients are unable to demonstrate tolerance for approximately 3 hours of therapy per day but could likely tolerate 2 hours. Often, clients who have experienced polytrauma, are discharged to a subacute rehabilitation facility until these precautions are lifted and they can fully participate in inpatient rehabilitation.

In some instances, however, clients with three or more extremities under non–weight-bearing precautions are discharged home, with adequate assistance and equipment in place.

Both acute and subacute rehabilitation facilities aim to increase the client's level of function for feeding, dressing, showering/bathing, item retrieval, grooming, toileting, completing functional transfers, and safe mobility during occupations. OT practitioners make recommendations for modification of the home environment, if needed, and family members carry out these recommendations if resources are available. IADLs are incorporated into the client's treatment, as appropriate. The goal is to increase client independence and medical management following polytrauma. Continual assessment is performed in the rehabilitation setting to determine the client's need for home health OT or outpatient OT.

Home health OT services are established when the client continues to require skilled OT intervention within the home environment. Clients are generally eligible when their condition is expected to improve within a reasonable period, when an OT practitioner is needed to safely and effectively perform skilled therapy, including modifying the home environment for safe and effective performance of ADLs and IADLs, or to teach a maintenance program for the specific condition.

Outpatient OT services, community reintegration services, and return-to-work (RTW) services are all rehabilitation options that clients may be offered after multiple traumatic injuries or a critical illness. These settings establish higher-level goals related to fine motor skills, dexterity, higher-level cognition and processing skills, IADLs, work hardening, ergonomics, and injury prevention training. OT services at this level promote continued health, well-being, and prevention of complications. Clients will have reached a level of independence, self-awareness, and reintegration far beyond what they first experienced when their journey began in the acute care environment.

DETERMINING HOW TO PLAN A TREATMENT SESSION

OT sessions vary significantly across settings and are highly client specific. Treatment planning depends on the client's clinical picture as well as the client's overall level of functioning and amount of assistance available at discharge. Considerations include the extent of injuries, medical stability, the precautions in place, the client's readiness to participate, how effectively pain is being managed, and the personal goals communicated.

PREPARATORY TASKS AND METHODS

Therapeutic exercise is commonly used in OT practice as a method for ensuring joint integrity, tone management, and the progression of strength. Therapeutic exercise includes PROM, AAROM, active range of motion (AROM), resistive therapeutic exercise, and exercise to build muscle endurance. Performance and education related to therapeutic exercise are integral throughout the continuum of care because it allows for improved occupational participation.

Design, fabrication, application, and fitting of orthotics are skills required of OTAs for clients with multiple trauma conditions. This may involve fabricating static orthoses for positioning after severe brain injury or fabricating a dynamic orthotic after tendon repair following a laceration. Braces and collars are orthotics that generally must be applied before the initiation of functional mobility or functional ADL routines. The use of prosthetic devices is an essential part of the OT intervention provided after traumatic amputation and usually occurs at the inpatient rehabilitation or outpatient phase of recovery.

Environmental modification is often used to promote overall success of a particular ADL or IADL within a specific environment. At the level of the ICU, OT practitioners are able to modify the environment to promote adequate sleep–wake cycles and encourage client participation. Encouraging family members to bring in familiar items from home, such as framed photos or a blanket, usually leads to positive outcomes related to engaging the client in the environment. Turning lights on during waking hours and allowing an appropriate amount of noise will also serve to alert clients to be involved with the environments. Another example of environmental modification includes reducing the amount of clutter or items within a space when asking a client to perform a focused task. This will reduce the likelihood of a client with TBI becoming distracted.

Physical agent modalities (PAMs) and techniques to enhance a client's sensory, motor, perceptual, and cognitive processing are all treatment strategies with this client population. Heat or ultrasound may be needed to manage pain or increase ROM. Stimulation of a client in a low-level coma, also known as a (persistent) vegetative state, aims to elicit a sensory response for emergence out of the vegetative state. This includes providing tactile stimulation, such a brushing motion of bristles over the extremities, rubbing with a soft sponge or washcloth, or providing a brief pinch using the thumb and the index finger.

Manual therapy techniques to enhance performance skills include promoting improved balance and posture at the edge of the bed and eliciting head and neck control, as well as scapular stabilization, for example, in preparation for a grooming task. Manual therapy intervention techniques also include the use of retrograde massage and Kinesio® taping for edema, as well as shoulder subluxation. Kinesio® taping is a treatment method used to support and stabilize muscles and joints while still allowing for ROM. The properties of the tape can also create a bond to help lift the epidermis and allow edema to more freely move versus pooling within the interstitial space. Tone inhibition, as well as weight-bearing techniques, in the situation of neurological involvement, are provided manually as a means of allowing for improved function in the affected extremity.

Training in techniques to enhance functional mobility begins with the client's ability to roll side to side, sit at the edge of the bed, and progress to a bedside commode transfer.

From there, clients progress to development of the preparatory skills needed to transfer in and out of the bathroom for ADL routines. For critically ill clients, functional mobility–related preparatory treatment consists of core strength development, manual development of bed mobility skills, progression from sitting to standing, and weight shifting.

ACTIVITIES

An assortment of meaningful and relevant activities provide clients with the challenge needed to advance independence and safety following critical illness or polytrauma. Reaching in the closet to select a shirt, monetary problem-solving, and gathering ADL items needed for a bathing routine are all activities that require cognitive abilities after brain injury or ICU delirium. While using critical thinking, OTAs should be guided by a common principle of sequential progression of activity based on individual client tolerance.[28]

OCCUPATION-BASED INTERVENTION

ADLs involve creativity and working around multiple lines and tubes with clients who have experienced polytrauma. Tooth brushing may be a challenge because of dysphagia and the presence of a tracheostomy tube, so the use of a suction toothbrush with mouthwash may be more appropriate for oral hygiene. The suction machine with the toothbrush attachment pulls all saliva and mouthwash out, decreasing the risk for aspiration. Shampoo caps lined with no-wash shampoo are a great way to incorporate bilateral UE use and coordination while completing a task that is a meaningful occupation. If cleared by a physician, showering can be performed in the ICU setting, even with clients on a tracheostomy collar (oxygen support) or ventilator support. Showering with a tracheostomy collar necessitates the use of a portable oxygen tank and a handheld shower nozzle. Precautions include ensuring that the client does not spray water from the shower nozzle directly at the tracheostomy site. Taping plastic or cloth to the neck above the tracheostomy will assist to prevent water from running in it from hair washing. In the acute environment, showering with a ventilator involves collaboration with the respiratory therapist to place the client on a portable ventilator and programming all the necessary settings. Since the ventilator is a closed tubing system attached to the tracheostomy collar, the only precaution is to spot-check the client's vital signs and to keep the ventilator dry on the other side of the shower curtain. This may involve placing the ventilator on a higher level so water does not run down the tubing to the machine. Clients who progress to showering with a tracheostomy collar or ventilator have usually been hospitalized for a significant amount of time. This milestone becomes the highlight of their rehabilitation experience and allows them to feel like a "real person" again.

Occupations may require temporary or long-term use of adaptive equipment and/or DME. Allowing clients to try out the equipment with daily routines in the acute care or inpatient rehabilitation setting, before determining whether they will truly utilize it in the home environment, is something OTAs should strive to do if the resources are available. Examples of such adaptive equipment include a reacher, long-handled sponge, sock aid, toilet aid, universal cuff, built up utensil handles, skin inspection mirror, and dressing stick. See Chapter 14 for further information on adaptive equipment.

EDUCATION AND TRAINING

Education is an ongoing part of providing OT intervention. Clients who have experienced polytrauma and their family members often require a significant amount of education and training with repetition to understand changes. With new weight-bearing precautions, equipment recommendations, and safety modifications, clients and their families rely on the expertise of the OTA to guide them on how to carry out their daily routines safely once they return home. In this instance, the changes are temporary and will last until precautions are lifted after follow-up with the orthopedic physician. However, in many cases, the changes are long term. In the instance of clients with SCI, education on positioning, skin checks, pressure relief, ROM exercises, bowel and bladder programs, and the orthotic wear schedule is an ongoing process. In fact, this education and training likely occurs through the continuum of care in both the acute care hospital and inpatient rehabilitation phases. Verbal and visual demonstration, handouts, and return demonstration are all strategies used by OTAs when providing client or caregiver education and training.

OT Practitioner's Viewpoint

A favorite activity that a client of mine found both purposeful and meaningful required him to recall the ingredients of his homemade banana pudding recipe. This client was involved in a head-on motor vehicle collision, which resulted in a TBI, right proximal humerus fracture, left distal radius fracture, lung contusion, and abdominal surgery for small bowel obstruction as a medical complication. Not only did the client engage in listing out the banana pudding ingredients, he then used fine motor skills and bilateral integration after the injury to slice a banana. The banana he sliced was used to garnish the pudding made by the OT practitioner who used the recipe provided by the client despite his memory deficits related to the brain injury. Another meaningful situation came up after a client was feeling a significant sense of loss of independence from sustaining a traumatic C6 SCI following a MVC. The client was an artist by trade, his favorite medium being acrylic and oil paint. Multiple sessions were spent building his upper extremity strength and coordination with use of bilateral wrist drop orthoses. The orthoses were modified to hold paintbrushes. In one of his acute care OT treatment sessions, the client was able to participate in a painting activity using the orthoses seated in a tilt-in-space wheelchair while still on the ventilator. By the end of his hospitalization, the client was able to voice his appreciation for the therapy intervention focusing on what was most important to him. ~ Melissa D. Brawley, MS, OTR/L

Clients with TBI have a very different appearance from how they were before their injury, and their presentation may continue to fluctuate during physical and/or cognitive recovery. Many family members need help coping with this change. Education is focused on teaching the family ways to maintain a necessary sleep–wake cycle, such as keeping lights off at night and on during the day, bringing in natural light, and providing appropriate simulation during day time while avoiding constant noxious stimuli. Handouts are helpful to describe ways the family should appropriately interact with the client along with reasons and explanations.

Clients with orthopedic injuries may need to wear bracings, slings, or orthotics. The frequency or wear schedule, method of maintenance, and keys to incorporating the orthotic into daily routines are all topics of client education. When spinal fractures are managed non-operatively, clients generally must adhere to spinal precautions and may be required to wear a back brace when upright or out of bed.

Regardless of the education being provided, the OTA must remember to assess the client's and his or her family members' comfort levels following all education and training so that follow-up can occur, as needed. Checking for understanding, carryover, and readiness will build rapport and allow the family to express concerns even if they are afraid to ask. It is important during the treatment of clients who have experienced polytrauma and multiple conditions to remind the family and loved ones to care for themselves as well. Caregivers should be directed to available resources for support so that their own needs are also met during such a difficult journey.

SUMMARY

Although polytrauma can be complicated and slightly intimidating because of the multiple systems involved, the OTA has an array of options to offer the client with this type of injury. These clients and their caregivers look to OT practitioners to provide them with the opportunities to reengage, participate, and succeed in even the most basic activities that are meaningful to them. For the client who has experienced polytrauma and has been through a life-threatening situation, OT focuses on ensuring the highest quality of life in each moment. Every stage of the recovery process presents new and different opportunities for the OTA to provide the appropriate interventions to these clients within an interdisciplinary team structure. Providing OT to this population demands both critical and creative thinking and involves many psychosocial considerations.

REVIEW QUESTIONS

1. The client is receiving maintenance IV fluids and needs to practice a shower transfer before discharge. Which of the following is the *best* method?
   a. Simulate the shower transfer because IV tubing is too short.
   b. Hold the shower transfer until the physician discontinues the IV.
   c. Ask the nurse to adapt the line briefly for the shower transfer.
   d. Ask the family to demonstrate management of the IV pole with the transfer.
2. The newest client on the unit was admitted after a motorcycle accident that caused an intracranial hemorrhage, pneumothorax, damage to the liver, and multiple fractures. Which three of the following are tasks the OTA should do *before* treatment of this client?
   a. Determine weight-bearing status and allowed ROM of limbs with fractures.
   b. See if there is IV-line delivery of analgesics.
   c. Ask the family for a status report from overnight.
   d. Check if the client is scheduled for surgery to drain cerebrospinal fluid from the brain ventricles.
   e. Check the chart for oxygen saturation, heart rate, or other precautions to monitor.
   f. Ask the nurse what level of cognitive functioning and awareness the client has been exhibiting.
3. A 35-year-old client is referred for OT after a car accident where she sustained numerous cuts and contusions, a mild concussion, stage 2 and 3 burns over 10% of her body, and a right pelvic fracture (non–weight-bearing status). She was the driver in the accident, and her two daughters were killed in the accident. Which of the following is the *best* treatment for this client?
   a. Observation of the client to see if she exhibits PTSD and depression
   b. Establishment of rapport as the OTA helps her perform tooth brushing and hair brushing
   c. Passive range of motion and family education
   d. Education and training on wound dressing and management
4. What should the OTA do if the client's heart rate is 40 bpm while bathing in the standing position?
   a. Modify treatment
   b. Continue treatment
   c. Stop treatment
   d. Grade treatment
5. A client with a traumatic brain injury presents as a Rancho Level II with no command-following or eye-opening. He is withdrawing his extremities to deep pain stimuli and is hypotonic. The OTA is seeing the client two times per week, and the client's family is willing to help in his recovery. Which of the following would be the *most* appropriate handout to provide to the family?
   a. Facts about mild brain injury
   b. Tips for decreasing agitation in a client with TBI
   c. An educational tool for sympathetic storming
   d. A coma stimulation program for the family
6. Which three of the following are the appropriate reasons why the OTA should plan to defer treatment immediately after the client's PEG procedure?
   a. The client will be very sore at the site with any movement after the procedure.
   b. The client now has a tube; OT intervention is contraindicated.
   c. The client will remain sedated and/or very drowsy after the procedure.
   d. The client will now have tube feedings instead of food by mouth.
   e. The client may have difficulty participating immediately after the procedure.
   f. The client is too critically ill.
7. Which of the following has been identified as the highest risk factor for multisystem organ failure (MSOF) after sepsis or an acute inflammatory response?
   a. Age
   b. Gender
   c. Obesity
   d. Mechanism of injury

8. The OTA arrives to treat a client who sustained a low-level TBI, has multiple fractures, and is wearing a cervical collar. His eyes are closed, and he is not alert or interactive. What is the *best* course of action?
   a. Notify the nurse that the client is nonresponsive.
   b. Defer treatment because the client is sleeping.
   c. Modify the environment and provide various forms of stimulation.
   d. Perform passive range of motion and allow the client to rest.
9. Which of the following is the safest and most therapeutic bedside commode transfer situation for a polytrauma client with lower extremity injuries and non–weight-bearing in bilateral lower extremities precautions?
   a. None, a bedpan must be used.
   b. The use of a transfer board to drop-arm bedside commode, with OTA and therapy technician assist for safety
   c. Stand pivot on the right leg because the fracture site has been stabilized
   d. Hoyer lift to the bedside commode with nursing staff present
10. While standing at the sink for OT, the polytrauma client with tracheostomy complains of increasing dizziness and presents with diaphoresis, including a change to pale skin color. What is the *best* course of immediate action?
   a. Modify the grooming tasks from two to one, and encourage the client to continue.
   b. Stop treatment, assist the client to sitting, and call the nurse and stay to monitor the client until the nurse's arrival.
   c. Stop treatment, assist the client back to bed, and leave him or her with the call bell if symptoms do not improve.
   d. Leave the client standing at the sink, and retrieve a vitals machine to assess.

CASE STUDY

Jasmine is an 18-year-old female status post car accident as an unrestrained driver, resulting in subarachnoid hemorrhage, intracranial hemorrhage, rib fractures, pulmonary contusion, acute respiratory failure, right distal radius fracture, and right femur fracture. Jasmine underwent a left craniotomy, tracheostomy placement, right distal radius repair, and right femur intramedullary (IM) nail placement. She is on restrictions for non–weight-bearing (NWB) through her right UE and weight-bearing as tolerated (WBAT) through her right LE. She is beginning to follow simple commands 75% of the time, tolerate tracheostomy collar trials off the ventilator, and move her extremities purposefully. Jasmine has been cleared for progressive mobility by both neurosurgery and trauma physicians.

Jasmine is in her first semester at college, where she was living in the dorms on the first floor with elevator access. She has a very supportive family and an older brother who is also attending the same college. Jasmine enjoys music, spending time with her friends, and volunteering with the Humane Society.

The focus of the initial OT intervention in this case should be to increase Jasmine's awareness of self and environment through increased alertness and consistent command following as she has experienced a TBI. Education would include a family program and ensuring an environment that promotes sleep and wake periods as tolerated by Jasmine. Upright sitting in the bed, at the edge of the bed, or out of the bed should increase levels of alertness because of the reticular activating system in the brain, which senses changes in position and environment. Jasmine should be provided with simple one-step commands with increased time to process them and carry them out (approximately 10 seconds). Basic ADL objects may be placed near her hand to check for purposeful grasp and functional use of familiar objects to command. An example would be presentation of a warm, soapy, wet washcloth with the simple command, "Wash your face."

With functional mobility retraining, a second person will be needed to assist with safety and management of lines and tubes. Once at the edge of the bed, Jasmine will likely need verbal cues or reminders for maintaining her NWB precaution to right UE, such as not to push with that arm on the mattress for increased balance. With progression to out-of-bed sitting, Jasmine may have significant pain, and the inability to tolerate placing weight through her right leg for a pivot transfer on the left LE. When working toward this transfer, a gait belt should be used, given Jasmine's weakness and cognitive status. The chair or bedside commode should be placed to the left, which is the direction in which the transfer will go because this is her stronger, less involved side.

Collaboration with the team members would involve PT practitioners to know the client's progress with functional mobility, including success, barriers, and approaches. Collaboration with nursing staff would involve pain medication scheduling as well as any procedures for the day that may interfere with OT delivery. Respiratory therapy practitioners will provide information regarding Jasmine's ventilation weaning progress and whether Jasmine should mobilize on increased ventilator support. SLPs will have information regarding her cognitive skills for comparison as well as progress toward use of a PMV and advancing toward taking food and drink by mouth. The case manager will communicate discharge plans—likely to inpatient rehabilitation, where her OT goals will expand to ADL routines, higher-level cognitive skills, and reintegration into the community.

Given Jasmine's love for volunteering for animal services, pet therapy may be incorporated into treatment by presenting a dog as a familiar visual stimulus. Other sensory input could be applied in this treatment scenario because the OTA may provide verbal cues and manual assist to facilitate visual attention and reach to the dog for petting as a purposeful movement. The OTA may also instruct Jasmine's family to bring in a few photos of Jasmine's friends and family members or her favorite blanket to make the environment more personal and visually appealing.

1. What performance skills will the OTA need to address to improve Jasmine's function?
2. As Jasmine progresses through the rehabilitation continuum of care, what might one expect to see as a client-centered community integration goal?
3. Describe the psychosocial deficits that may be present in Jasmine after her polytrauma.

PUTTING IT ALL TOGETHER Sample Treatment and Documentation

Setting	Acute, hospital admission to level I trauma center
Client Profile	48 y/o female unrestrained driver s/p MVC with C4 incomplete SCI, T8 and T9 compression fractures, pneumothorax, acute respiratory failure, L distal radius fracture. Surgeries: cervical spinal fusion, tracheostomy, and PEG placement Precautions: Spinal, Aspen® (cervical) collar on at all times, thoracic lumbar sacral orthotic (TLSO) with head of bed greater than 45 degrees, invasive lines, skin integrity, compression stockings for BP control, aspiration
Work History	Worked at a convenience store part time
Insurance	Self pay with process started to obtain Medicaid
Psychological	History of depression, polysubstance abuse; positive for cocaine, benzodiazepines, and ETOH (alcohol) on arrival
Social	Lives alone in a 2nd floor apartment with 6 y/o son. Separated from husband, disclosed to social worker there is a history of physical and emotional abuse. Supportive retired parents live an hour away in a one-story ranch.
Cognitive	No deficits
Motor & Manual Muscle Testing (MMT)	R handed RUE: 0/5 digits, 0/5 wrist, 2-/5 pronation/supination, 3/5 elbow flexion, 2+/5 elbow extension, 3-/5 shoulder flexion and scapular elevation 4/5 shrug. LUE: 0/5 digits, unable to assess wrist or pronation/supination due to short arm cast, 0/5 elbow flexion, elbow extension, 1/5 shoulder flexion and scapular elevation, 4/5 shrug
ADL	Grooming: Dependent Bathing: Dependent Upper Body Dressing: Dependent Lower Body Dressing: Dependent Feeding: Dependent (NPO) Toileting: Dependent
IADL	Dependent
Goals	Within 2 weeks: 1. Client will direct in bed and out of bed pressure relief schedule with Mod I 2. Client will direct RUE orthotic wear schedule with Mod I 3. Client will complete simple oral hygiene with Mod A, use of RUE orthotic as needed 4. Client will complete simple feeding task for ice chip/spoon to mouth with Min A, use of RUE orthotic, as needed 5. Client's family will complete BUE therapeutic exercises with Mod I with handout, as needed.

OT TREATMENT SESSION 1

THERAPEUTIC ACTIVITY	TIME	GOAL(S) ADDRESSED	OTA RATIONALE
Orthotic need: R wrist drop orthosis to improve function, improve positioning. Review with OT given injury is incomplete. Obtain order from trauma midlevel provider. Call orthotics company to order prefabricated orthotic once client's palm measured and size determined. Once orthotic is delivered, educate client on purpose and positioning, demonstrate technique to apply, educate on wear schedule, post information in visible area within client's room, and perform skin check after 1 hour of wear. Make adjustments, as needed. Educate nursing staff on orthotic wear schedule and purpose.	34 min	#2 and indirectly #3 and #4	*Preparatory Methods:* A dorsal wrist drop orthosis will support the client's weak wrist in her dominant extremity where there is proximal strength. Orthotic training and education can be billed for services provided.

PUTTING IT ALL TOGETHER Sample Treatment and Documentation (continued)

THERAPEUTIC ACTIVITY	TIME	GOAL(S) ADDRESSED	OTA RATIONALE
ADL: Placement of hospital bed in semireclined position. Oral hygiene grooming task with suction toothbrush in R wrist drop orthosis. Suction toothbrush utilized due to client with tracheostomy in place and failed swallow evaluations by SLP (aspiration precautions).	10 min	#3	*Occupations:* Engaging in the actual grooming task promotes functional movement patterns to build strength and muscle endurance. Allows for neuro-reeducation to elicit muscle memory during a familiar and routine task.

SOAP note: 10/1/—, 10:00 am–10:44 am

S: Client supine in bed, RN cleared session. Client's parents present, mom stated, "I wish she would be able to use her arms."

O: Client participated in acute OT session to address orthotic need for R wrist positioning and improved function in preparation for ADL performance. Trauma telephone order obtained for orthotic. Client's palm width measured at 3" with size small orthotic required. Orthotic applied, fit well with no immediate signs of skin irritation. Orthotic check performed after 1 hour with no signs of redness or client complaints. Issued handout with photo of orthotic, wear schedule, and purpose. All education and training provided to client and family, with parents able to return at Mod I with use of handout. Client performed oral hygiene grooming task with use of R wrist drop orthosis. Dependent for setup with verbal and Max A for functional movement pattern for toothbrush to mouth. Pt performed with Max A proximally to achieve accuracy for toothbrush to mouth. Verbal cues throughout for shoulder movement pattern for brushing motion. Overall client completed task with Max A.

A: Client receptive to R wrist drop orthosis for positioning and improved function. Orthosis with good fit and client's family able to verbalize rationale and wear schedule. Client improved from dependent to Max A for oral hygiene with use of orthosis. Client will continue to benefit from acute OT services to progress functional independence related to weakness s/p SCI.

P: Continue OT plan of care at 5×/week frequency to address RUE function, progress LUE as able and provide client education and training in preparation for client directed care and ADL participation s/p SCI and polytrauma.

Miriam Stein, COTA/L; 10/1/—, 12:35 pm

TREATMENT SESSION 2

What could you do next with this client?

TREATMENT SESSION 3

What could you do next with this client?

REFERENCES

1. Pohlman, M. C., Schweickert, W. D., Pohlman, A. S., Nigos, C., Pawlik, A. J., Esbrook, C. L., ... & Kress, J. P. (2010). Feasibility of physical and occupational therapy beginning from the initiation of mechanical ventilation. *Critical Care Medicine, 38*(11), 2089–2094.
2. Bergen, G., Chen, L. H., Warner, M., & Fingerhunt, L. A. (2008). *Injury in the United States: 2007 chartbook.* Hyattsville, MD: National Center for Health Statistics.
3. Occupational therapy practice framework: Domain and process, 3rd edition. (2014). *American Journal of Occupational Therapy, 68,* S1–S48.
4. Boyle, M. J. (2007). Is mechanism of injury alone in the prehospital setting a predictor of major trauma—A review of the literature. *Journal of Trauma Management and Outcomes, 1*(1). doi:10.1186/1752-2897-1-4
5. Criddle, L. M. (2012). *Trauma care after resuscitation.* Scappoose, OR: The Laurelwood Group.
6. Butcher, N. E., & Balogh, Z. J. (2014). Update on the definition of polytrauma. *European Journal of Trauma and Emergency Surgery, 40,* 107–111.
7. Baker, S. P., O'Neill, B., Haddon, Jr. W., & Long, W. B. (1974). The injury severity score: A method for describing patients with multiple injuries and evaluating emergency care. *The Journal of Trauma, 14*(3), 187–196.
8. Brohi, K. (2007). Injury severity score. Retrieved from http://www.trauma.org/index.php/main/article/383/
9. Kosar, S., Seelen, H. A. M., Hemmen, B., Evers, S. M. A. A., & Brink, P. R. G. (2009). Cost-effectiveness of an integrated 'fast track' rehabilitation service for polytrauma patients involving dedicated early rehabilitation intervention programs: Design of a prospective, multi-centre, non-randomised clinical trial. *Journal of Trauma Management & Outcomes, 3,* 1–9. doi:10.1186/1752-2897-3-1
10. Rothstein, J., Roy, S., & Wolf, S. (1997). *The rehabilitation specialist's handbook.* Philadelphia, PA: F. A. Davis.
11. Thurman, D. J., Sniezek, J., Johnson, D., Greenspan, A., & Smith, S. (1995). *Guidelines for Surveillance of Central Nervous System Injury.* Atlanta, GA: Centers for Disease Control and Prevention.
12. Zhang, M., Liu, Z. H., Yang, J. X., Gan, J. X., Xu, S. W., You, X. D., & Jiang, G. Y. (2006). Rapid detection of pneumothorax by ultrasonography in patients with multiple trauma. *Critical Care, 10*(4), R112. doi:10.1186/cc5004
13. Michalska, A., Jurczyk, A. P., Machała, W., Szram, S., & Berent, J. (2009). Pulmonary contusion and acute respiratory distress syndrome (ARDS) as complications of blunt chest trauma. *Archiwum Medycyny Sadowej Kryminologii, 59,* 148–154.
14. Rubenfeld, G. D., Caldwell, E., Peabody, E., Weaver, J., Martin, D. P., Neff, M., Stern, E. J., & Hudson, L. D. (2005). Incidence and outcomes of acute lung injury. *New England Journal of Medicine, 353*(16), 1685–1693.
15. Hamrick, M. C., Duhn, R. D., & Ochsner, M. G. (2009). Critical evaluation of pulmonary contusion in the early post-traumatic period: Risk of assisted ventilation. *The American Surgeon, 75*(11), 1054–1058.
16. Modrykamien, A. M., & Gupta, P. (2015). The acute respiratory distress syndrome. *Proceedings (Baylor University. Medical Center), 28*(2), 163–171.

17. Cirocchi, R., Boselli, C., Corsi, A., Farinella, E., Listorti, C., Trastulli, S. ... & Fingerhut, A. (2013). Is non-operative management safe and effective for all splenic blunt trauma? A systematic review. *Critical Care, 17*(5), R185. doi:10.1186/cc12868
18. Ahmed, N. & Vernick, J. J. (2011). Management of liver trauma in adults. *Journal of Emergencies, Trauma and Shock, 4*(1), 114–119. doi:10.4103/0974-2700.76846
19. Purdue, G. F., Hunt, J. L. (1989). Multiple trauma and the burn patient. *The American Journal of Surgery, 158*, 536–539.
20. National Spinal Cord Injury Statistical Center. (2014). Spinal cord injury facts and figures at a glance. Birmingham, AL: University of Alabama at Birmingham.
21. Lieutaud, T., Ndiaye, A., Frost, F., & Chiron, M. (2010). Registry group: A 10-year population survey of spinal trauma and spinal cord injuries after road accidents in the Rhone area. *Journal of Neurotrauma, 27*, 1101–1107.
22. Herbert, J. S. & Burnham, R. S. (2000). The effect of polytrauma in persons with traumatic spine injury: A prospective database of spine fractures. *Spine, 25*, 55–60.
23. Midha, R. (1997). Epidemiology of brachial plexus injuries in a multitrauma population. *Neurosurgery, 40*, 1182–1189.
24. Hermans, G., Jonghe, B. D., Bruyninckx, F., & Van den Berghe, G. (2008). Clinical review: Critical illness polyneuropathy and myopathy. *Critical Care, 12*(6), 238.
25. Florence, C., Haegerich, T., Simon, T., Zhou, C., & Luo, F. (2015). Estimated lifetime medical and work loss costs of emergency department treated nonfatal injuries, United States 2013. *MMWR Morbidity and Mortality Weekly Report, 64*(38), 1078–1082.
26. Florence, C., Simon, T., Haegerich, T., Luo, F., & Zhou, C. (2015). Estimated lifetime medical and work loss costs of fatal injuries, United States 2013. MMWR *Morbidity and Mortality Weekly Report, 64*(38), 1074–1077.
27. Englander, J., Cifu, D. X., & Diaz-Arrastia, R. (2010). *Seizures after traumatic brain injury*. Seattle, WA: University of Washington Model Systems Knowledge Translation Center.
28. Parcell, D. L., Ponsford, J. L., Rajaratnam, S. M., & Redman, J. R. (2006). Self-reported changes to nighttime sleep after traumatic brain injury. *Archives of Physical Medicine and Rehabilitation, 87*(2), 278–285.
29. Holcomb, E. M., Millis, S. R., & Hanks, R. A. (2012). Comorbid disease in persons with traumatic brain injury: Descriptive findings using the modified cumulative illness rating scale. *Archives of Physical Medicine and Rehabilitation, 93*(8), 1338–1342. doi:10.1016/j.apmr.2012.04.029
30. Shehab, D., Elgazzar, A. H., & Collier, B. D. (2002). Heterotopic ossification. *Journal of Nuclear Medicine, 43*(3), 346–353.
31. Olson, S. A., & Glasgow, R. R. (2005). Acute compartment syndrome in lower extremity musculoskeletal trauma. *Journal of the American Academy of Orthopaedic Surgeons, 13*(7), 436–444.
32. Turen, C. H., Dube, M. A., & LeCroy, M. C. (1999). Approach to the polytraumatized patient with musculoskeletal injuries. *Journal of the American Academy of Orthopaedic Surgeons, 7*(3), 154–165.
33. Mondello, S., Centrell, A., Italiano, D., Fodale, V., Mondello, P., & Ang D. (2014). Complications of trauma patients admitted to the ICU in level I academic trauma centers in the United States. *BioMedical Research International, 2014*, 473419. doi:10.1155/2014/473419
34. Boone, L. B., Johnson, K. D., Weigelt, J., & Scheinberg, B. (1989). Early versus delayed stabilization of femoral fractures: A prospective randomized study. *Journal of Bone and Joint Surgery of America, 71*, 336-340.
35. White, T. O., Jenkins, P. J., Smith, R. D., Cartlidge, C. W., & Robinson, C. M. (2004). The epidemiology of posttraumatic adult respiratory distress syndrome. *Journal of Bone and Joint Surgery, 86*(11), 2366–2376.
36. Klein, M. J. (2014). Post head injury endocrine complications clinical presentation. Retrieved from http://emedicine.medscape.com/article/326123-clinical#a0217
37. Saunders, C. B. (2015). Preventing secondary complications in trauma patients with implementation of a multidisciplinary mobilization team. *Journal of Trauma Nursing, 22*(3), 170–175. doi:10.1097/JTN.0000000000000127
38. Stuart, C. A., Shangraw, R. E., Prince, M. J., Peters, E. J., & Wolfe, R. R. (1988). Bedrest-induced insulin resistance occurs primarily in muscle. *Metabolism, 37*(8), 802–806.
39. Hamburg, N. M., McMackin, C. J., Huang, A. L., Shenouda, S. M., Widlansky, M. E., Schulz, E., ... & Vita, J. A. (2007). Physical inactivity rapidly induces insulin resistance and microvascular dysfunction in healthy volunteers. *Arteriosclerosis Thrombosis Vascular Biology, 27*, 2650–2656.
40. Taylor, M. D., Tracy, J. K., Meyer, K., Pasquale, M., & Napolitano, L. M. (2002). Trauma in the elderly: Intensive care unit resource use and outcome. *Journal of Trauma—Injury, Infection and Critical Care, 53*(3), 407–414.
41. Andruszkow, H., Veh, J., Mommsen, P., Zeckey, C., Hildebrand, F., & Frink, M. (2013). Impact of the body mass on complications and outcome in multiple trauma patients. *Mediators of Inflammation, 2013*, 345702. doi:10.1155/2013/345702
42. Zafar, S. N., Obirieze A., Schneider, E. B., Hashmi, Z. G., Scott, V. K., Greene, W. R., ... & Haider, A. H. (2015). Outcomes of trauma care at centers treating a higher proportion of older patients: The care for geriatric trauma centers. *The Journal of Trauma and Acute Care Surgery, 78*(4), 852–859.
43. Zafar, S. N., Shah, A. A., Zogg, C. K., Hashmi, Z. G., Greene, W. R., Haut, E. R., ... & Haider, A. H. (2016). Morbidity or mortality? Variations in trauma centres in the rescue of older injured patients. *Injury, 47*(5), 1091–1097.
44. Vieira, L., Melo, P., Maldaner, V., Santana, L. V., Nobrega, O. T., Durigan, J., ... & Cipriano, G. (2016). Early neuromuscular electrical stimulation preserves skeletal muscle size and echogenicity in mechanically ventilated polytrauma patients. *American Journal of Respiratory Critical Care Medicine, 193*, A4518.
45. Vieira, L., Melo, P., Maldaner, V., Xavier, A., Souza, V. C., Silva, P. E., ... & Cipriano, G. (2016). Skeletal muscle atrophy occurs early and rapidly in the first 5 days after emergency admission in mechanically ventilated polytrauma patients. *American Journal of Respiratory Critical Care Medicine, 193*, A4517.
46. McPeake, J., & Quasim, T. (2016). The role of peer support in ICU rehab. *Intensive and Critical Care Nursing, 37*, 1–3.
47. Morris, P. E., Griffin, L., Berry, M., Thompson, C., Hite, R. D., Winkelman, C., ... & Haponik, E. (2011). Receiving early mobility during an intensive care unit admission is a predictor of improved outcomes in acute respiratory failure. *American Journal of Medical Science, 341*(5), 373–377.
48. Needham, D. M., Korupolu, R., Zanni, J. M., Pradhan, P., Colantuoni, E., Palmer, J. B., ... & Fan, E. (2010). Early physical medicine and rehabilitation for patients with acute respiratory failure: A quality improvement project. *Archives of Physical Medicine and Rehabilitation, 91*, 536–542.
49. Dean, E. (1993). Bedrest and deconditioning. *Neurology Report, 17*(1), 6–9.

Chapter 37

The Pediatric Client—All Grown Up

Denise K. Donica, DHSc, OTR/L, BCP, FAOTA and Jamie Bittner, MS, OTR/L

LEARNING OUTCOMES

After studying this chapter the student or practitioner will be able to:

37.1 Explain various health impairments that are diagnosed in childhood but continue to affect individuals as they transition from childhood to adulthood

37.2 Identify legislation that impacts adults with disabilities and their occupational performance

37.3 Describe how sensory processing may impact occupational performance

37.4 Review contexts where intervention may occur for adults with disabilities

37.5 Explain the occupations of activities of daily living, instrumental activities of daily living, work, and education that the occupational therapy assistant can address when working with adults with disabilities

KEY TERMS

Nonprogressive condition
Progressive condition
Sensory processing
Stereotypic behaviors
Transition

With the discovery of many of the foundational skills for occupational therapy (OT) practice with adults who have physical impairments, it is important to recognize that entering the world of OT is a journey (Fig. 37-1). Treating each client will take the OT practitioner down a different path even when the diagnoses are the same. As an occupational therapy assistant (OTA), it is important to understand what causes the turns in the path, the unexpected events, and how to handle these situations.

The individual clients that OTAs treat are often identified by the presence of one or more health conditions or diagnoses. When learning about these impairments and learning about OT practice, it is easy to separate the diagnoses into pediatric and adult impairments. However, in reality, not all diagnoses are purely pediatric or purely adult. Some conditions are considered pediatric because the individual becomes symptomatic during infancy or childhood, whereas with other conditions, the individual becomes symptomatic in adulthood. However, many of the health impairments typically viewed as pediatric in nature are not conditions that diminish their effects as the individual grows into adulthood. As a result of advancements in health care as well as the nature of a specific impairment, many individuals with what are typically known as "pediatric" conditions grow into adulthood and continue to have limitations on occupational performance. This chapter intends to explore how OTAs can enhance occupational performance with the individual who has grown up from a pediatric client to an adult client.

PACKING FOR THE TRIP—KNOWING THE CONDITIONS

The first thing to be done before beginning the journey with a client is to make sure that all the necessary items are packed for the trip. The OTA will need to pack the knowledge of common health impairments that are diagnosed in childhood but continue to impact an individual into adulthood. As clients progress through life, leaving the role of student in the traditional elementary and secondary education context, he or she enters a world with diminishing support and increasing responsibility.

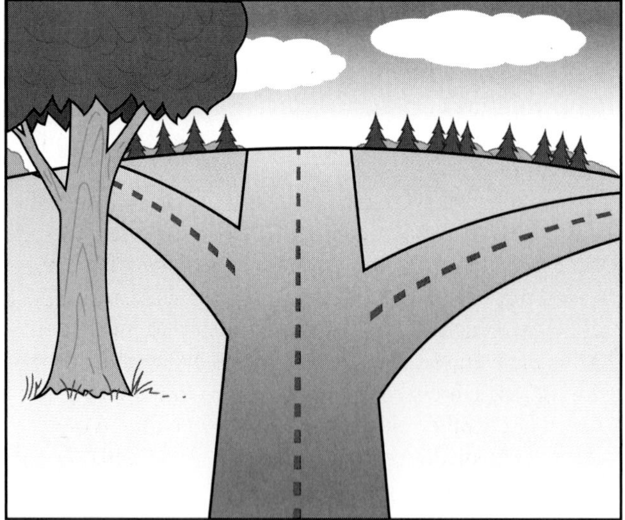

FIGURE 37-1. Occupational therapy practice is a journey.

OT Practitioner's Viewpoint

OT practitioners often identify with a certain population in which they work. However, it is important to remember that all are OT practitioners, not a "pediatric" practitioner or one who "works with adults." There are many important considerations when working with individuals across the lifespan to improve occupational performance. The pediatric client all grown up reminds the OT practitioner that there are important components to integrate into practice with those transitioning into adulthood and in adulthood, such as sensory processing knowledge. It is also important to recognize that a condition that is primarily known as "pediatric" may affect individuals differently in adulthood, and knowledge and understanding about those contributors to occupational performance are critical to maximizing quality of care. ~ Denise K. Donica, DHSc, OTR/L, BCP, FAOTA

Although the journey to treat individuals with developmental disabilities is not a new one for OT practitioners, working with adults who have transitioned from childhood with a variety of different conditions is still relatively new. In fact, a 2001 qualitative study on this **transition** (from childhood to adulthood) reported that those young adults viewed themselves as the first generation with disabilities surviving into adulthood, as well as residing within the community.[1] The following section provides a brief description of some of the most common conditions frequently diagnosed in a client in childhood and how they might impact that same individual as an adult (Fig. 37-2).

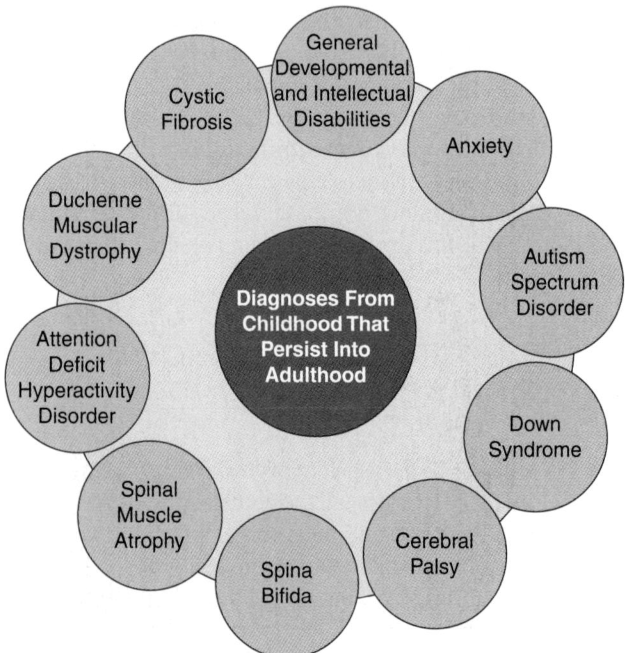

FIGURE 37-2. Common health impairments diagnosed in childhood that continue to impact individuals into adulthood.

Anxiety

The first diagnosis to explore is anxiety, a common impairment in both adulthood and childhood. A variety of anxiety diagnoses that currently exist have evolved over time because of changes to the *Diagnostic and Statistical Manual.* The current *Diagnostic and Statistical Manual of Mental Disorders, Fifth edition* (DSM–5),[2] a publication of the American Psychiatric Association, classifies mental disorders on the basis of diagnostic criteria. The DSM-5 includes the following anxiety disorders: separation anxiety disorder, selective mutism, specific phobia, social anxiety disorder, panic disorder, agoraphobia, generalized anxiety disorder, and substance/medication-induced anxiety disorder. The differences in the disorders relate to what causes the anxiety as well as the age at which the symptoms appear. Typically, the anxiety must persist over 6 months to meet the criteria for a diagnosis of an anxiety disorder.[2] A common characteristic of all of these disorders is that they share some element of fear that induces the anxiety in an individual, causing muscle tension and the fight-or-flight responses. Anxiety disorders may be diagnosed in childhood, and certain diagnoses predispose themselves to different anxiety disorders in adulthood.[3] Diagnosis of an anxiety disorder occurs in 11% to 30% of individuals in middle childhood or adolescence.[3-5]

Some anxiety disorders may be found in childhood but not in adulthood (e.g., separation anxiety disorder), whereas other anxiety disorders may develop in adulthood but are rare in childhood (e.g., agoraphobia and panic disorder).[3] However, diagnosis of an anxiety disorder in childhood may be a predictor of another anxiety disorder or depression in adulthood, and those with a childhood diagnosis tend to have poorer outcomes as adults.[2-4]

Understanding the role that anxiety plays in daily function is critical when treating an adult who may have anxiety.

Copeland et al.[3] identified some adult outcomes related to a childhood diagnosis of anxiety. All participants in this study who had received an anxiety diagnosis at some point during childhood demonstrated impairments in at least one area of function (health, financial, or interpersonal) as an adult and some had impairments in multiple areas of function.[3] A childhood diagnosis of anxiety also negatively impacts self-esteem in the adult. Although self-esteem increases during adolescence and into adulthood for both nonaffected and affected populations, those having an anxiety diagnosis during childhood have consistently much lower self-esteem across the lifespan.[5] Research findings indicate that there is an increased prevalence of anxiety disorders in females, as well as an increased risk for negative outcomes for females in adulthood. Other factors that may impact the effects of anxiety in adulthood include the number of experienced life stressors, personality characteristics, and comorbidities.[4] Anxiety may be coupled with a physical impairment or other psychosocial impairment; thus, it is important for the OTA to be aware of this common condition because it may impact any or all areas of occupation.

Autism Spectrum Disorder

Continuing to pack for the journey, the OTA next comes to information about autism spectrum disorder (ASD), a common childhood neurodevelopmental disorder. Although diagnosis of ASD may occur at any time during the lifespan, symptoms must be present during childhood to meet the diagnostic criteria.[2] An ASD diagnosis must include two important criteria: (1) deficits in both social communication and social interaction that are present across contexts, and (2) repetitive behavior patterns. These criteria must cause impairments in various occupations and cannot be explained by another condition.[2] It is important for the OTA to recognize that although ASD is the current diagnosis listed in the DSM-5, former editions of this manual have included additional diagnoses on this spectrum, such as Asperger's syndrome and pervasive developmental disorder–not otherwise specified (PDD-NOS). The OTA may work with clients who are identified to have these conditions diagnosed during childhood. In addition to the DSM-5 criteria, individuals with autism are often noted to have deficits in sensory processing.

One research study indicates that the ASD symptom severity tends to decrease as the individual matures from childhood to early adulthood,[6] but studies overall have had mixed results with regard to symptoms of ASD and the debate on whether the symptoms decrease with age or not continues.[7] Therefore, no assumption can be made for an adult with ASD.

The public school system in the United States often provides support for individuals with ASD as well as other disabilities through 21 years of age. At this point, individuals typically leave this system with less independence compared with their peers, thus depending more on family members or other caregivers.[8] Individuals with ASD have difficulty generalizing skills from one context to another as well as recognizing others' perceptions.[7] As individuals with ASD transition to adulthood, the nature of the impairments in communication and social skills can impact their ability to assume new roles, such as employee, college student, or roommate.

Data collected between 2000 and 2011 indicated that less than 20% of adults with ASD are living independently or semi-independently[6] (Fig. 37-3). One of the difficulties in transitioning to independent living is the shift in responsibility for self-management.[7] The ability to complete activities of daily living (ADLs) and instrumental activities of daily living (IADLs), including medication management, can be difficult for individuals with ASD, especially when the amount of medications increases with aging.[6] This dependence on family members may lead to increased stress and strain on the family unit. In fact, Graetz determined that 77% of families in her study felt that their relatives with ASD would not have an opportunity to live outside of their homes, thus always requiring some level of caregiving.[8]

Likewise, this study showed that 58% of the adults with ASD required some level of assistance for ADLs, and 84% required some level of assistance for IADLs. As the OT practitioner is well aware, the management of life tasks, such as ADLs and IADLs, requires more than just the person's ability to perform individual activities.[7]

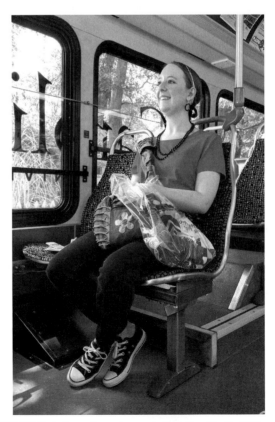

FIGURE 37-3. Independence is a goal of adults with disabilities, but unfortunately less than 20% of adults with ASD live independently or semi-independently.

Further data collected show that adults with ASD tend to be unmarried and unemployed.[6] Also, only 25% had one or more friends, and only 14% were reported to be married or in a long-term relationship.[6] **Stereotypic behaviors** (repetitive movements of self or objects) negatively impact the development of meaningful relationships as well as successful employment opportunities.[6] Inflexibility and limited language development also limit employment opportunities.[6,7] In fact, in a survey of individuals with a family member who had ASD, 80% reported that the family member with ASD had expressive language skills that were somewhat or greatly affected, and 82% reported that their family member had receptive language skills that were somewhat or greatly affected. During 2000 to 2011, approximately 49% of adults with ASD were either in some kind of employment, including paid, sheltered, or voluntary work, or in an educational program. Many of these jobs were poorly paid and required a low level of skill.[6] Adults with ASD who had an intellectual impairment were also less likely to be employed for pay or as a volunteer. Of the total surveyed, only 13% had an employment opportunity that allowed them to work daily, or almost daily, and only 8% worked once a week.[8]

Because of the difficulties that exist with behavior management in adults with ASD coupled with communication and social deficits, working with these clients can be challenging and stressful. For example, a client's maladaptive behaviors may have become habitual, limiting his or her residential options and opportunities to engage in social occupations, and this may lead to poorer occupational outcomes.[9]

ASD is common among children, and because of its high prevalence rate in childhood, as these children age, the prevalence rate among adults is increasing as well. It is important for the OTA to have a basic understanding of the social, communication, and sensory deficits that impact an individual with autism because common occupations, such as living skills, education, and work, may all be impacted by these characteristics. OT is the profession from which understanding of sensory processing developed and will be discussed later in the journey preparation.

Attention Deficit Hyperactivity Disorder

Attention deficit-hyperactivity disorder (ADHD) is another condition commonly diagnosed during childhood and continues to affect these individuals as adults. ADHD is a condition that includes a consistent presentation of inattentive tendencies and/or hyperactive and impulsive tendencies that impact a person's functioning across multiple contexts. To meet the diagnostic criteria, the symptoms of ADHD have to be present before age 12 years, but actual diagnosis may not occur in childhood. In fact, it has been reported that many adults have ADHD and remain undiagnosed and/or untreated.[10,11] Research indicates that there is a significant genetic component to ADHD.[2,12,13]

ADHD is categorized into three subtypes—inattentive, hyperactive/impulsive, and combined—differentiated by the symptoms present. The inattentive subtype is behavioral in nature and characteristic of at least six symptoms for at least 6 months (only five are necessary for diagnosis at age 17 years or older). Symptoms may include limited attention to detail, difficulty with prolonged attention, avoidance of tasks requiring much mental effort, difficulty organizing, and distractibility and forgetfulness. The hyperactive/impulsive type is motor in nature; diagnostic criteria require the individual to have at least six symptoms for 6 months (only five are necessary for a diagnosis at age 17 years or older). These symptoms include persistent fidgeting or movement, excessive talking, inability to engage in activities quietly, impulsive speech and tendency to interrupt others, and/or difficulty taking turns. ADHD can occur as one of these two subtypes primarily, or it can exist as a combined presentation that includes both the inattentive and the hyperactive/impulsive qualities.[2] This combined type typically manifests as doing without thinking. It is critical that the symptoms appear consistently and in multiple contexts for the criteria for diagnosis to be met.

The presentation of ADHD does appear to change as children mature into adulthood.[12] First, ADHD has a very high rate of comorbidity with certain conditions, such as learning disabilities, depression, conduct disorder, intermittent explosive disorder, and personality disorders, resulting in increased healthcare expenses.[2,13,14] Therefore, this condition has not only a direct impact on the individual and his or her family but also on society in general. Research indicates that as these individuals age, the motor-based symptoms seem to become less prevalent, but restlessness, poor planning, excessive talking, and inattention persist.[11,12] Societal expectations of an individual to assume increased responsibility and autonomy after adolescence cause the individual to struggle as deficits related to these areas (e.g., education, work, and IADLs) become more prevalent in daily life.

Second, literature indicates that adults with ADHD have less education than the typical population and have more difficulties with employment and productivity.[12,15] Compounding these challenges are difficulties with social relationships and personal relationships, including marriage. Those who manage to be employed typically have lower incomes, increased risk for substance use and abuse, and more documented accidents related to driving.[11,12,16]

The diagnosis of ADHD in an adult is associated with negative life events, whether the ADHD is of the inattentive type or the hyperactive type.[16] However, because adults with ADHD struggle with these inherent challenges, they are often viewed as lazy or unmotivated by others.[13]

Attachment to others and limited independence in performing tasks are noted difficulties for adults with ADHD. These adults tend to have insecure attachment styles, characterized by fear, or they may be preoccupied with certain tendencies.[17] This may result in the individual's difficulty with taking on more responsibility with age and developing independence from direct support from others. Limited independence can be a strain on family support systems.

Adults with ADHD also report that they have limited self-awareness skills; however, they are more aware of the needs of others,[17] impacting interpersonal relationships in all settings. These deficits could impact work effectiveness as well as productivity. Conversely, as the support from family begins to diminish as the individual grows older, new deficits may emerge or become more problematic.[11]

Decision-making skills are affected in adults with ADHD. It has been noted that impulsivity is a common characteristic. With impulsivity, decisions are made before considering the consequences of a choice. It should not be a surprise that individuals with ADHD are more likely to participate in activities that are risky, which is likely a result of this tendency toward impulsive decision making.[18]

On the positive side, it is important for OTAs to also know the strengths of individuals with various health impairments because this knowledge may impact treatment planning and recommendations. Adults with ADHD have reported feeling that their diagnosis had promoted creativity, which can, in fact, enhance productivity and relationships.[11]

A study by Lensing et al. performed on adults ages 50 years or older living with a diagnosis of ADHD reported that there is reduced life satisfaction in these individuals compared with those without ADHD. Individuals with ADHD also lived alone more compared with the non-ADHD group and experienced more unemployment. This study's findings supported other research indicating that difficulties with employment early in life may persist throughout the course of the individual's life.[19]

Cerebral Palsy

Cerebral palsy (CP) is the term for a collection of conditions that are characterized by impairments in motor functioning that may or may not include cognitive impairments. CP is the result of neurological damage that occurs around the time of birth (before, during, or soon after), and those with CP typically present with altered muscle tone, differences in posture, difficulty in coordination, and weakness.[20] The type and level of impairment depends on the area of the brain where the injury occurred. Because this condition is often diagnosed very soon after birth, it is common for supports to be in place for children with CP and their families during the early years. Pediatricians are familiar with the condition, and the educational system offers many resources. However, once a child becomes an older adolescent and transitions from pediatric care to adult care, many changes occur in the provision of care for individuals with CP.[21-23]

At the time that this challenging transition occurs from pediatric medical care to adult medical care, it is common that the new adult-focused healthcare provider spends less time with the client with CP and has less knowledge of the disorder and its impact on occupational performance and daily life skills. In fact, research indicates that few physicians discuss the transition that would occur in healthcare management—from the physician's standpoint, from an insurance perspective, or with regard to changes in responsibility for the individual with CP.[21-23] Another primary concern is the lack of coordination between the pediatric care provider and the adult care provider.[22] Not only is there a perceived lack of communication during this time of transition, the actual amount and frequency of services that the individual with CP is eligible to receive decrease abruptly.[22] This lack of support is critical because transition to adulthood is the time when the individual with CP is potentially taking over responsibility for his or her own medical decisions, and yet the individual gets less support from healthcare providers, affecting his or her ability to be successful in this new role.[23] This transition may also leave the individual with feelings of sadness and abandonment.[22] Because of the psychosocial impacts that occur during this time of transition, it is important for the OTA to be aware of the client's mental health and consider providing coping strategies and other resources to meet the client's needs that may not be physical in nature. In addition, the OTA needs to be aware of this change and prepare the individual and the family for the new responsibilities as well as the imminent decrease in support from the healthcare system for people with CP. It is recommended that this medical transition planning occur during the individual's teenage years.[23]

Cerebral palsy is a **nonprogressive condition** (a static disorder which does not get worse). However, it is typical that daily function is impacted later in life, not as a direct result of cerebral palsy but because of a secondary condition.[21,24] Common symptoms found in adults with CP include weakness, contractures, depression, social isolation, and pain, which all impact an individual's ability to complete ADLs and IADLs. These symptoms can also impact the individual's ability to form social relationships and maintain employment.[21] Pain itself is a primary symptom that has negative impacts on quality of life for those with CP in adulthood.[21] It is not uncommon for an adult with CP to have complaints of new symptoms, which are often mistaken by physicians as symptoms of CP when, in fact, they may result from secondary conditions. These secondary conditions may cause additional symptoms, such as foot deformities, hip dysplasia, pain, arthritis, and contractures. These secondary conditions are often causes of functional declines for those with CP.[24]

Some adults with CP have difficulties with ADLs, learning, and education, as well as communication.[21] All of these areas of difficulty may impact the individual's ability to live alone once adulthood is reached. Many families continue to care for an adult with CP because of the physical impairments the individual has to contend with. Often, the individual with CP requires home modifications to increase independence with self-care tasks and decrease the responsibilities of caregivers or family. Home modifications may include installing helpful adaptations in the bathroom and the bedroom.[25] See Chapter 14 for adaptations and home modification information.

Weight-bearing is important throughout the lifespan of an individual with CP because it is necessary to have increased functional mobility within the home. For example, transfers may require less physical assistance if the client can bear weight on the legs, thus protecting the caregiver, and this may allow for an individual's increased independence with bathroom tasks. Proper footwear and foot position are critical for weight-bearing.[24] The physical dependency is often viewed as the most demanding aspect of care by family and caregivers.[25] This continued level of dependence on family or caregivers may impact the social relationships of the client and family throughout the life of the individual with CP.[25]

When looking at employment rates, severity of motor dysfunction impacts the person's likelihood of receiving further education or being employed. A review of the literature indicates that only about 10% to 65% of individuals with CP are employed, with most of the studies indicating less than 40% are employed.[23]

Adolescence is a critical time to make positive impacts on functional skills, which may also influence future success and independence. Practice of self-care tasks and either performing or directing IADL tasks is important for the client with CP to eventually live with less assistance. Participation in physical and social activities during adolescence is a predictor of future involvement in these activities and adult independence.[21,23] Limited social activities may impact the ability to form healthy social relationships, friendships, and dating opportunities.[23]

The significant advances in technology in recent years have opened doors for adults with CP (Fig. 37-4). Many assistive technologies are available to meet the needs of these individuals, such as smartphone "apps," home automation, and a variety of computer access methods. Although technology has opened the door to enhanced social opportunities for those with physical disabilities through social communities online,[23] many of the other technologies that increase mobility and independence may be prohibitively expensive.[23]

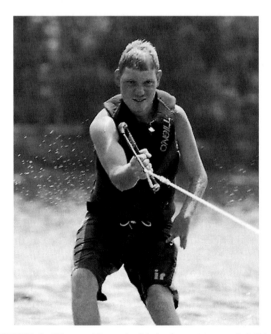

FIGURE 37-4. Clients with cerebral palsy have a range of abilities that allow them to participate in meaningful leisure occupations in adulthood.

Although CP results in a range of impairments that may impact an individual across his or her lifespan, it is important to realize that CP is a spectrum of conditions and that not all individuals spiral into a pattern of increased disability during adulthood. Blackman and Conaway's research findings support that childhood services may have a positive impact on the skill development of those with CP.[21] In fact, research has found that as children with CP grow up, the level of caregiver assistance does decrease, whereas the functional independence of the individual with CP increases. However, the level of severity of motor dysfunction is the best predictor of ability for self-care, mobility, and social function. Those with minimal severity tended to have the highest function in all areas.[26] Working with adults who have CP may involve working on many aspects of OT described in *Occupational Therapy Practice Framework, 3rd edition* (OTPF-3),[27] ranging from basic self-care tasks to community mobility and financial skills to employment-related tasks.[23] The CP may also be a secondary disorder to the condition the OT practitioner is treating the client for, such as a hip fracture from a fall or to improve range of motion (ROM), strength, and hand function after carpal tunnel surgery.

THE OLDER ADULT

This chapter focuses on important considerations in working with adults who have diagnoses that were established when the clients were children. Many conditions that are diagnosed early in life continue to impact individuals into adulthood. It is not uncommon to see clients as older adults with these conditions as well. Looking at the evidence will help highlight why it is important to recognize that the aging process may be different for an individual with a disability compared with one without.

Research has been conducted to explore executive function and memory changes in adults who were diagnosed with ASD (primarily high-functioning individuals). It has been determined that older adults (ages 51–83 years) with ASD tend to have impairments that mirror those in children with ASD, including sustained attention, working memory, and verbal letter fluency. Interestingly, children with ASD are commonly identified as having difficulty with cognitive flexibility, which is not present in older adults, suggesting that this deficit may disappear with age. Compared with older adults without ASD, aging individuals tend to show a faster decrease in performance of verbal letter fluency while adults with ASD experience a decrease in visual memory skills more quickly. Further research is necessary, but this research does suggest that the aging process is different for those with ASD than those without.[28]

Continued

Another example of differences in the aging process occurs with those who have CP. As CP is typically classified as a physical condition, it is expected that physical declines may be different during the aging process for these individuals than those without CP. A systematic review identified that, when looking at ambulatory adults with CP, at least 25% of them experience declines in gait earlier than adults without CP. In addition, those with higher levels of pain, fatigue, and bilateral motor impairment are at higher risk of gait decline.[29] Therefore, it is important for the OTA to recognize how this may impact an individual's functional mobility, transfers, and safety with ADLs and IADLs as the individual becomes an older adult.

It is also important to recognize that although CP may have physical impacts during the aging process, psychosocial impacts may also occur. For example, individuals with CP have been found to experience more loneliness than adults without disability. Adults with CP who were independent communicators reported more loneliness than those who used augmentative and alternative communication (AAC). Research suggests that although these differences were not significant, those who use AAC may feel less lonely because they often had someone they could talk to as part of the AAC. The study suggested loneliness may be impacted by inappropriate placement of the adults with CP in group homes, separation from family and friends in residential settings, decreased leisure and social opportunities, and limited experiences in competitive work as an adult.[30] Therefore, the OTA needs to recognize loneliness may be a factor for adults with CP and opportunities for social relationships must be explored as living situations change over time. These are just a few examples of how aging with a disability may impact someone differently from the typical aging process.

Cystic Fibrosis

Cystic fibrosis (CF) is an autosomal recessive condition that is most common in the Caucasian population. It is marked by multisystem dysfunction but primarily impacts the respiratory and digestive systems. This condition is typically diagnosed through a newborn screening or through a sweat test to determine whether there is dysfunction caused by a mutation of the CF transmembrane conductance regulator (CFTR) protein. CF causes the body to produce very thick and sticky mucus found in the organs, especially the lungs. Historically, CF has been viewed as a pediatric diagnosis because it was often diagnosed early in life and life expectancy of those diagnosed with CF was so poor that these individuals did not survive into adulthood. However, with advances in medical care, the life expectancy has been improved significantly, and it is common for individuals with CF to live into their 30s and 40s and possibly even reach retirement age. Because of this newly extended life expectancy, treatment of individuals with CF as adults is a relatively new concept.[31,32]

CF has many variations and levels of presentation; therefore, building rapport with the client to determine the specific presentation for that individual will be important for the OTA. It is essential to examine the ways respiratory function and digestion affect individuals with CF. They may have very specific nutritional requirements due to their individual digestive concerns. Because of the effects of CF on the pancreas, it is common that food is not absorbed correctly.[32,33] As a result, the adult with CF may follow a specific diet and/or medical regimen that is an important ADL. Independent management of these routines will be critical. Another common concern for individuals with CF who are age 25 years and older is acquiring CF-related diabetes mellitus; this may affect survival rates as well as nutritional factors and pulmonary exacerbations.[32]

Awareness of pulmonary dysfunction, the classic symptom of CF, is vital for OTAs. Clients also typically have chronic lung infections and airway obstruction, with respiratory disease being a common cause of death.[31,33] Another factor found to be associated with poor lung function is methicillin-resistant *Staphylococcus aureus* (MRSA). Approximately one fifth of individuals with CF have been found to carry MRSA in their lungs.[32] The lung obstruction is so critical that it often requires daily treatments to enhance lung function.[33]

In addition to the pulmonary and digestive impacts, CF may also affect an individual's reproductive system. Typically, males with CF are infertile, whereas females with CF are fertile and even able to carry a pregnancy to full term.[32,33] It is important for the OTA to be aware of these reproductive impacts on adults with CF so that the topic of sexuality can be addressed, as appropriate. As individuals move into adulthood, it is also common that they develop other comorbidities not discussed above.[33]

Treatment that individuals with CF receive is very time intensive and occurs across the lifespan. Individuals with CF receive frequent antibiotic treatments for the chronic lung infections and experience many pulmonary exacerbations.[32] During these exacerbations, lung function is compromised, as is the ability to complete daily life tasks, including ADLs, IADLs, work, and education.

A variety of methods are used for airway clearance. They range from positive end expiratory pressure (PEEP) devices, chest drainage techniques, to high-frequency chest wall oscillation vests to help break up the mucus in the lungs[31,32] (Fig. 37-5). Research has not found any one method to be more effective than the others. Typically, it depends on the personal preference of the client or the physician. As the disease process continues, it is possible that lung transplantation may be a required medical treatment for end-stage lung disease.[32]

As individuals with CF transition into adulthood, transition of medical care from pediatric care providers to adult care providers is an important aspect. Research has shown that decline in pulmonary function can be reduced when the individual transitions to adult care instead of remaining with pediatric providers. The Cystic Fibrosis Foundation offers resources to help with this transition and to support clients with CF.[34]

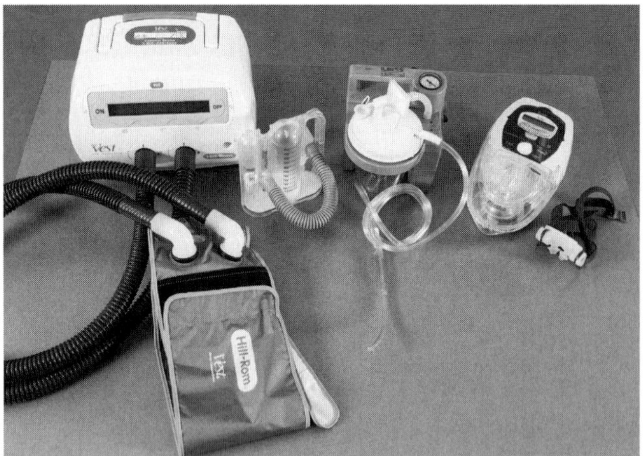

FIGURE 37-5. Equipment used for individuals with cystic fibrosis. *From left*: High Frequency Chest Wall Oscillation (VEST), incentive spirometer, suction machine, continuous positive airway pressure (CPAP) machine, and nasal option (instead of mask) for CPAP.

CF impacts many areas of occupation for an individual. First, ADLs and IADLs include some important activities related to self-management. The severity of an individual's condition impacts the range of unique activities that must be included as ADLs and IADLs.[33] One research study indicated that 89% of clients with CF required daily treatments for airway obstruction.[35] Fatigue can be a factor as well as decreased endurance; many clients are sedentary as activity can cause shortness of breath. Learning pacing and self-management techniques is important for the client, but so is asking for assistance when techniques cannot be completed independently.[33] Although the lifespan of an individual with CF has increased, CF is still a **progressive condition,** (changing and worsening over time) which will result in increased healthcare costs and potentially more caregiving as the individual ages. Complex medical care is often required because of comorbidities that are more common in older individuals. Medication management is a complicated task for a client with CF because it involves dealing with many types and various forms of medications. Often, family members or other caregivers are needed to help with IADLs, such as shopping, cooking, and gardening. Support is often provided by the parents of the individual, even if the adult with CF is married. It is important to keep in mind that as the adult with CF is aging, so are the parents of that person, who might also need to manage complications related to their own aging process. Loss of parental support is often correlated with a decrease in health for the individual with CF. Often, home-based medical services allow for daily activity management so that the client can continue to participate in other important occupations, such as education and leisure.[33]

Because individuals with CF are living longer, postsecondary education and work opportunities are now important considerations. Many factors, including nutrition, pulmonary sufficiency, susceptibility to illnesses, and amount of time required for treatments, may determine whether or not an individual with CF is able to have a job. Individuals with CF often have limited employment opportunities, but many of them do work at least on a part-time basis or volunteer. One important predictor of employment status is the completion of some postsecondary education. Therefore, it is important to encourage education after high school and provide recommendations for modifications that might help facilitate success for these students to assist with future employment opportunities. Reduction in work hours can be a way to maintain employment when complications occur as the disease process progresses.[35] Sick days are commonly utilized for undergoing part of the course of antibiotic treatment, which may last 15 days.

Although CF is primarily known as a physical disability, its psychosocial impacts must be considered by the OTA. Having a progressive condition, such as CF, can greatly impact the mental health and quality of life of the client. It is important to note that although increased symptoms of anxiety and depression may be seen in adolescents with CF, these rates are significantly higher in the parents of adolescents with CF. Therefore, the mental health of parents as well as that of clients with CF must be addressed by healthcare professionals. Screening for mental health concerns and quality of life changes is an important consideration.[36,37]

Down Syndrome

Down syndrome (DS) is a genetic impairment caused by an extra chromosome 21 in all or some of the cells. Intellectual disability is one of the most significant effects of DS. In fact, intellectual disability is caused more by DS than any other genetic condition. As with many other conditions described in this chapter, life expectancy for individuals with DS has greatly increased in the recent years and now may extend into the 60s. In addition to the intellectual disabilities that accompany DS, multiple other health-related issues and comorbidities can occur, [38,39] and may include congenital heart disease, hearing loss, and ophthalmological problems,[39] cancer, infectious diseases, digestive system disorders, orthopedic disorders, and gynecological issues.[40,41] It is also common for individuals with DS to become obese. Diet is an important consideration because of concerns related to obesity, potential for diabetes, and metabolic issues.[39] Because of comorbidities, especially cardiovascular disease, it is expected that adults with DS will experience increasing health-related problems as they age.[40] Another classic symptom of DS is the tendency for the individual to avoid cognitively challenging activities. This characteristic can be problematic when the OTA is trying to teach the client a new skill, and it impacts the client's ability to learn.[38,39] Individuals with DS also have difficulty with working memory, which also impacts their ability to learn.[38,41] As adults with DS age, they have an increased risk for developing early-onset Alzheimer's disease.[38]

An important precaution for the OTA to be aware of when working with a client of any age who has DS is the potential for atlantoaxial instability. This disorder results in excessive mobility at the cervical end of the spine where the C1 and C2 vertebrae meet. Often, individuals with DS do not have symptoms related to the instability, but it is possible for the spinal cord to become compressed here.[39] In addition to this instability, motor milestones are delayed, with low muscle tone generally seen.[38,41] Difficulty in motor skills can result in gross motor coordination and fine motor control challenges as well, although many skills can be learned with repetition.[38] (Fig. 37-6).

Individuals with DS typically have difficulty with expressive language, and it impacts them through childhood and adulthood. However, they tend to have stronger receptive language than expressive language. Despite communication challenges, social skills are typically a strength of individuals with DS because they make good eye contact and are empathetic. In fact, they use these strengths as a tool to avoid performing the challenging tasks described above. However, social involvement has been found to decrease as the individual ages.[41]

In addition to learning difficulties, individuals with DS can have challenges with self-regulation. It is difficult for them to control their desires as well as their automatic responses to others. However, individuals with DS have strengths in visual perceptual skills.[38] Because of the perceptual strengths, individuals with DS tend to enjoy arts and crafts as well as the performing arts, such as dancing and singing.[38]

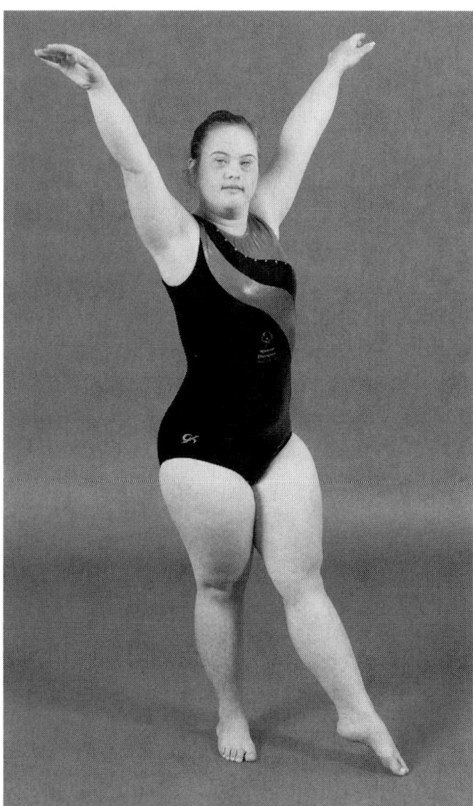

FIGURE 37-6. Although individuals with Down syndrome are not commonly involved in sports, this woman is very active in many sports and was a gold medalist in the North Carolina Special Olympics.

Individuals with DS may have some challenges regarding sexuality and reproduction. As with CF, it is common for women with DS to be fertile and able to bear children, whereas men have reduced sperm counts and are often infertile.[39] However, because of the intellectual disability, it is important that individuals with DS have sexual education to support them in making informed decisions related to sexuality and reproduction. Women with DS often demonstrate behavior related to premenstrual syndrome and are documented to have difficulty with menstrual hygiene. They also have earlier onset of menopause compared with individuals with intellectual disabilities alone.[39,41]

Research has indicated that sometimes the OT practitioner on the team is less likely to provide the diagnosis and focus instead on the characteristics of the condition to communicate how the intervention being provided relates specifically to that client.[38] As with many conditions discussed in this chapter, there is limited information available in the literature on the care of the individual with the given diagnosis in adulthood.[40] It is common for the person with DS to live with family members. Sometimes, the caregiver may end up being an older sibling who is also a caregiver for aging parents.[41] Some clients transition to a group home or skilled nursing facility when parents pass away due to lack of other caregivers.

When looking at the occupational performance of adults with DS, participation in IADLs is a relative strength. Research has found that individuals with DS complete household management tasks, meal preparation and cleanup, and personal care with greater independence and success compared with those with other developmental disabilities.[41] In addition, one third to two thirds of adults with DS complete ADLs, including feeding, toileting, bathing, and dressing, independently.[41] However, it is important to note that safety is a concern when working with an individual of any age with DS.[38] It is typical for independence in ADLs and IADLs to increase throughout adolescence and into young adulthood. Unfortunately, it is common to see declines in these skills beginning around age 40 to 45 years.[41] The level of cognitive function best predicts the level of independence for an individual with DS.[41] Likewise, the higher the level of functional independence with ADLs, the better are the chances of the individual with DS obtaining employment.[42] If individuals are involved in decision making throughout the transition process occurring within education, they are more likely to be involved in open employment opportunities (the same employment available to a regular worker, and with a regular wage).[42] Studies have shown trends in employment among individuals with DS. Employment is often part time as opposed to full time. Positions typically held by those with DS include retail, food service, and custodial or stocking jobs.[41] Volunteer opportunities may be another fulfilling possibility for clients with DS. It is important for the OTA to advocate for the individual with DS throughout his or her lifespan and help facilitate the young adult to assume roles as a worker, whether paid or not.

Duchenne Muscular Dystrophy

Duchenne muscular dystrophy (DMD), a neuromuscular impairment in males, is characterized by progressive muscle weakness. Typically, the disease progresses such that the individual is unable to walk independently and often is using a wheelchair for mobility by the time he reaches early adolescence. As he advances in age, further complications, such as respiratory problems, swallowing challenges, and severe arm and leg weakness tends to occur, and the individual may require more support from family members, especially parents. Along with these changes, weakness in the muscles necessary for sufficient respiration requires the individual to decide if he wants to endure mechanical ventilation. If not, his lifespan is shortened.[43-45] The choice to use mechanical ventilation becomes a decision of the individual with DMD once the individual reaches adulthood. Having to make this decision, as well as other medical-related decisions, results from a shift in responsibility during the time of transition. Unfortunately, it is not uncommon for individuals to feel as though others do not think they are "worth" the cost and amount of medical care required because of their limited life expectancies.[43] It is important for the OTA to be aware of this progression and anticipate the cycle of emotions and frustrations that the client may go through. Advocacy and support are critical roles of the OT practitioner.

Individuals with DMD face another issue that is common to many pediatric clients who enter adulthood—resources for their care becoming scarce after they complete high school. Early adolescence is often a time filled with worry and fear of what is to come for the individual with DMD, especially in relation to health concerns, ability to go to college, and long term independence.[43,46] However, research shows that psychosocial adjustment may actually improve as the individual ages.[46] Unfortunately, it is not uncommon for individuals with DMD to complete their education and then be at home without employment or other meaningful activities to engage in during the day.

Many individuals with DMD do not move out to live on their own due to lack of care, or limited financial options. There is a societal expectation for this to occur after secondary education is finished, but this is the time when their dependence on others is nearly complete. Many individuals with DMD feel that they could move out with the correct supports in place, but they still fear doing it and therefore often remain at home.[46] It is very important for the young adult with DMD to be involved in the planning for his own care. See Chapter 31 for further information on adults with DMD.

Spina Bifida

Spina bifida is a neurological condition that develops prenatally when the neural tube does not close completely, thus requiring surgery to close the spine within 48 hours after birth. Individuals with spina bifida often demonstrate leg weakness and possibly paralysis, loss of sensory function, problems with bowel and bladder function, and various contractures and deformities.[47,48] It is important for OTAs to recognize the latex sensitivities and allergies that are common in this population. Spina bifida is more common in females than in males.[47] Because of the complexities of this condition, it is important to ensure a cohesive transition from pediatric medical care to adult care.[48] Over the years, medical interventions have improved, resulting in greater life expectancy for those with spina bifida.[47] However, general health and quality of life in individuals with spina bifida decline during adolescence and early adulthood.[49,50] Quality of life was found to be correlated not only with age but also with the level of the spinal cord lesion.[50] In addition, decreased mobility in adolescents and adults with spina bifida is correlated with increased depression symptomology,[51] and decreased physical mobility is a primary symptom which affects occupations that the OT practitioner can address to increase independence (Fig. 37-7). OT can be an important contributor to enhancing not only improved mobility, but to increasing quality of life through improved independence with daily life skills.

Adolescents and adults with spina bifida struggle for independence, although many live alone as adults. Self-management of complications caused by spina bifida can be challenging. Urinary issues impact independence, so some individuals with spina bifida use self-catheterization to increase independence.[52] Lower extremity weakness can cause a reliance on forearm crutches or a manual wheelchair, which can lead to significant shoulder pain as an adult. Adults with spina bifida are less likely to have a driver's license, which is one factor that limits their ability to be involved in social activities and to maintain employment.[49,52] The OT practitioner can refer to a driving evaluation program or a driving rehabilitation specialist to have clients assessed for alternatives, such as hand controls, and vocational rehabilitation.

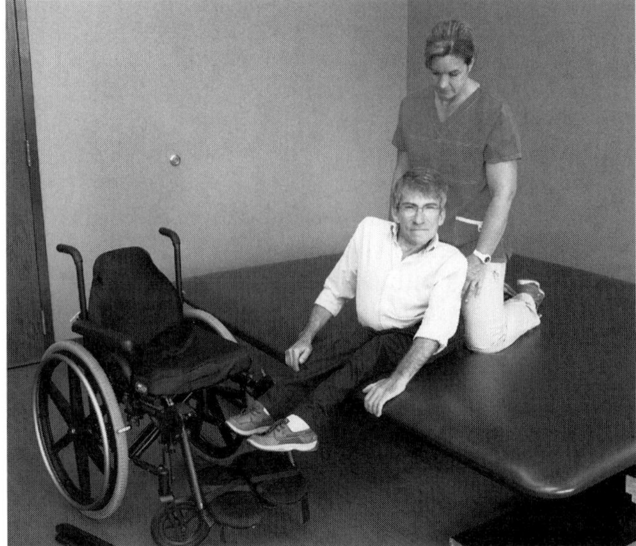

FIGURE 37-7. Functional mobility helps to maintain psychological well-being and promote independence.

Another medical complication in adults with spina bifida is lymphedema, especially in those with lesions at the thoracic level and those that use powered mobility.[53] This complication is caused by decreased sensation in the limbs as well as muscle weakness, which limits lymphatic drainage.[53] Among adults with spina bifida, there is increased prevalence of hypertension and obesity, so they should continue to be monitored for hydrocephalus (abnormal build-up of fluid in the brain) and shunt (a drain which moves extra fluid from the brain to another place in the body where it can be absorbed) malfunctions, urological issues, and changes in mobility and ability to complete daily occupations.[47,48,53] A focus on healthy eating, wellness, and physical activity to tolerance is important.

Sexual function is affected in individuals with spina bifida, although little is known about this in adolescents and young adults.[54] Research has shown that adolescents receive the typical sexual education information in school but may receive limited additional personalized information in relation to spina bifida from physicians. Urinary incontinence is a barrier to sexual activity, as may be the lack of sensation in the genitals and achieve an erection/ejaculation. The OTA may offer specific positions or adaptive techniques as needed to facilitate this ADL, or refer to further counseling by a therapist specializing in sexual issues, as necessary.

Spinal Muscle Atrophy

The last condition for which information is needed in preparation for the journey is one mentioned in Chapter 31. Spinal muscle atrophy (SMA) is a genetic, progressive disorder that is autosomal recessive. An individual with SMA experiences degeneration of spinal alpha motor neurons, and this results in progressive skeletal muscle weakness and paralysis. There are currently four primary types of SMA. Type 1 is the most severe, presents with severe weakness, and, generally, will result in death by age 2 to 5 years. Type 2 is diagnosed at 6–18 months. Typically, these children can sit but not walk and are in a power wheelchair from a very early age. Type 3 has an onset of adolescence to early adulthood, and type 4 has an onset in adulthood. Each type of SMA has its own issues, but there can certainly be secondary concerns as a client ages with pain, pressure injuries, obesity from immobility, osteoporosis from decreased weight-bearing, lower extremity swelling and edema with decreased circulation, scoliosis, progressive voluntary muscle weakness with potential contractures in all body regions, and increasing difficulty with all desired occupations.[55] It is rare for a client with SMA to have cognitive symptoms, so most of the support an OT practitioner will give is adaptations for changes due to physical progression.

Because of the physical care which may be required and a potential dependence on parents as caregivers, young adults with SMA 2 and 3 may have difficulty with dating, socialization, and intimacy/sexuality. Other issues for clients may revolve around attending college, finding a job and living on their own. See Chapter 31 for more information on SMA.

General Developmental and Intellectual Disabilities

The common developmental and intellectual disabilities that are diagnosed in childhood and are seen in individuals as they mature into adulthood have been described previously. However, the OTA may also see individuals with both types of disabilities not already discussed. When caring for a client with unfamiliar conditions, OTAs have the responsibility of seeking specific resources to learn about the symptoms of and expectations for those conditions.

Working with individuals with intellectual disabilities and cognitive delays may require the use of techniques for skill development that are based in psychology. For example, individuals with severe intellectual disabilities were found to improve in their abilities to complete multistep IADL tasks through a process called *simultaneous prompting*. Here, the individual was provided with a task and received verbal praise immediately following correct completion of the step. If there was an error, verbal prompts, physical cueing, or gestures were provided to help the individual complete the task correctly. A tangible reinforcer, such as a reward, was provided at the end of the session.[56] This technique or other behavior modification techniques might be used with any of the tasks within an occupation to increase an individual's success and increase independence for those with cognitive challenges. While there can be differences with an adult who acquires a cognitive disability due to an injury or disease process from an individual with a congenital cognitive disability, many useful cognitive treatment strategies may be similar to those found in Chapter 11.

Psychosocial Impact

The conditions presented above that the OT practitioner must consider when packing for his or her journey comprise both physical and psychosocial diagnoses. It is important for the OTA to recognize that although it is clear that psychosocial diagnoses may impact the individuals' own and their families' mental health, individuals with physical conditions may also have signs of psychosocial challenges. The OTA should always be alert to identify signs of anxiety, depression, and stress when working with clients and families. Refer to the earlier discussions in this chapter for specific risks related to specific conditions.

The remainder of the chapter will discuss resources and services for adults with disabilities. These sections are not diagnosis specific but, rather, are organized by topic. Now that the OTA is finished packing for the journey, the next need is to look at the map of resources.

LOOKING AT THE MAP—NAVIGATING THE RESOURCES

Going on a journey is always more fun with friends. Who is joining practitioners for this journey? In the client's childhood, typically there are two primary care-providing teams—medical-based services and/or education-based services. The pediatric medical-based team may extend into adulthood for the client, whereas the education-based team crosses into the client's adulthood but, as alluded to earlier, typically ends before the individual reaches age 22 years. This section will first explore the team for medical-based services. After these teams are considered, legislation that potentially impacts these clients will be discussed.

Medical Team

The medical team may include individuals from various disciplines, depending on the setting or context in which services are delivered. These contexts will be discussed in the next section. However, it is not uncommon to see any combination of the following professionals on the team, depending on both the diagnosis and the context. A medical physician is typically the head of the team and makes the ultimate decisions regarding the client's care, such as deciding if the client should be referred to OT services. The medical team also includes nursing staff, dietitian, social worker, speech language pathologist (SLP), audiologist, physical therapy (PT) practitioners, recreational therapist, ophthalmologist or optometrist, specialty medical provider (e.g., cardiologist or orthopedic specialist), and OT practitioners. As the individual moves from childhood to adulthood, many of these team members may change to different providers or may include other specialists. In fact, the client's care may change to a different physical location as well. This time of transition can be difficult for the family and the client, as mentioned earlier in the chapter.

Education Team

Throughout school, students with disabilities are supported by an education team, which is referred to as the Individualized Education Plan (IEP) team. This team includes the parents of the student, at least one regular education teacher (if the student participates in regular education), at least one special education teacher, a representative of the local education agency who is responsible for supervising the provisions of the specially designed instruction, an individual who can interpret evaluation results (e.g., school psychologist), and others who have knowledge about the student, including related service providers, such as occupational therapists, OTAs, physical therapists, or SLPs. Typically, students are not invited to IEP meetings until it is time to discuss transition planning for life after high school. This transition planning is required to occur when the student turns 16 years of age but may occur when the student reaches age 14 years. It is important that this transition process includes the student's interests and preferences.[57] Involvement in the team meeting is a great way for the student to start practicing self-advocacy skills.

As students with disabilities grow into young adults, it is important for them to understand their rights and the laws that support their individual needs. This "transition" is a delicate process because it can introduce a wide variety of emotions and questions regarding the disability that can impact performance at school, at home, and in the community. Whenever the student is going to be attending a meeting that involves decision making, it is important that three things occur: (1) The student needs to be prepared for the meeting beforehand and given time to ask questions; (2) the other attendees should be prepared regarding the topics to be discussed, how to best communicate with the student, and what issues should be discussed at a different time if they surface; and (3) a statement should be made at the beginning of the meeting that clearly identifies the student's role in the meeting.[58] The goal is to make the meeting a positive experience wherein the student realizes that the people sitting around the table are there to support his or her goals and future dreams. After the meeting, it is important to review what occurred during the meeting and what decisions were made.[58] The IEP is used to guide the day-to-day education of the student over the coming year. All team members are involved as goals are monitored and progress is noted throughout the year. (56[59]).

COMMUNICATION

As the pediatric client grows into adulthood, some important changes in communication occur as part of the OT process. The client becomes an advocate for his or her own needs when moving into adulthood. However, this role change is not necessarily a natural process, and often the client needs to be educated on what this advocacy role means. This education should happen early in adolescence, but it does not always occur.

When working with a child, the parent or caregiver has authority over the decisions that are made. However, when these children become legal adults, a shift in responsibility occurs. Likewise, communication changes. The OTA should understand the family's culture through the therapeutic use of self within the therapeutic relationship. Culture may have an impact on how the family adjusts to this significant role change. Although family members may continue to be important members of the team, it is important for the OTA to communicate with the adult client, promote self-advocacy for him or her, and include him or her in discussions related to OT services. The input from the family should not be discredited. The family often knows more about the client than anyone else involved. However, this shift can be a very delicate issue for families.

Often, parents and caregivers have had many years of control over the decisions. If the adult with the disability has a differing opinion, this can create a stressful situation for all involved. It will be important to know who has legal authority for decision making. If the OTA senses disagreement between the adult with a disability and the family, it is recommended that the OTA be an active listener and report the details of the situation to the supervising occupational therapist. This will facilitate a healthy discussion between the occupational therapist and OTA to determine what the source of disagreement is and problem-solve options for resolution.

The individuals on the education team may change from year to year, but the team will remain involved in the student's educational experience as long as the student is in the primary or secondary education system, which can continue until the student reaches the age of 21. At that time, decisions will be made regarding opportunities for further education or other occupations to engage in after high school. Many adults with disabilities may receive assistance from Vocational Rehabilitation, a federal and state funded service in the United States, which provides support for further education, adaptations, and employment exploration and training.

A Brief History of Legislation for People With Disabilities

It is always important to know where one is coming from and where one is going when planning a trip. There are specific rights and laws that prohibit discrimination against individuals with disabilities, and these rights and laws ensure that people with disabilities have the same rights as everyone else in the United States. The primary laws that impact individuals with disabilities that are important to know along the journey will be reviewed here.

AMERICANS WITH DISABILITIES ACT OF 1990

One of the most important laws the OT practitioners must be familiar with is the Americans with Disabilities Act (ADA) (P.L. 101–336), which was signed by President George H. W. Bush on July 26, 1990. This civil rights law prohibits discrimination on the basis of disability in a variety of public sectors. These include employment situations, state and local government programs, and public accommodations, such as access to buildings, commercial facilities, public transportation options, and telephone services. This equal opportunity law was modeled after the Civil Rights Act of 1964 as well as on Section 504 of the Rehabilitation Act of 1973, which prohibits discrimination on the basis of race, color, gender, religion, or origin. The ADA Amendments Act (P.L. 110–325) was passed in 2008 and included revisions to the accessibility design, impacting state and local governments and public accommodations.[60]

To be protected under the ADA, the individual must have a disability defined in a specific way for this law. An individual with a disability, according to the ADA, has an impairment that can be physical or mental. The identified impairment must significantly limit at least one major life activity. If not, the person must have a history of having an impairment that does this or be perceived by others as having an impairment that meets these criteria. In general, all people who have disabilities that meet the ADA definition of a disability are covered. A specific list of disabilities, by name, has not been provided by the ADA.[60]

INDIVIDUALS WITH DISABILITIES EDUCATION IMPROVEMENT ACT OF 2004

Another important law that the OT practitioner must be familiar with when working with students with disabilities who are transitioning into adulthood is the Individuals with Disabilities Education Act (IDEA) (P.L. 108–446). This law governs state and public agencies throughout the nation with regard to early intervention, special education, and related services.[61] The purpose of IDEA is to ensure that all students with disabilities receive free and appropriate public education (FAPE) in the least restrictive environment, based on their individual needs. Care providers from outside agencies, such as vocational rehabilitation agencies, are often involved during this time. This is part of the transition services section that includes postsecondary goals in the areas of education, employment, and independent living. Specific documentation requirements also exist regarding students who have IEPs.[62]

REHABILITATION ACT OF 1973—SECTION 504

The Rehabilitation Act of 1973 (P.L. 93–112) prohibits discrimination based on the presence of a disability. This protection covers federal programs that receive federal monies, programs that are federally conducted, and federal employment.[60] What does this mean? It can be simply stated as the national law that protects qualified individuals from discrimination based on their disability.[62]

Who is covered under this law? An individual with a disability is defined by this law as a person "with a physical or mental impairment which substantially limits one or more major life activities."[63] Such individuals should not be denied benefits or excluded from or discriminated against in any program or activity that is funded with federal financial assistance. This protection includes organizations and employers in which each agency is responsible for enforcing its own regulations.

With regard to employment, qualified individuals with disabilities should be able to perform the essential functions of the job, given reasonable accommodations, in which they had been hired to perform. This is the area in which OT services can be beneficial to an individual with a disability. As a profession, OT practitioners excel in understanding how to modify or provide an accommodation to a person who otherwise would have difficulties completing a job task. For example, consider a 19-year-old young adult with autism who is entering the workforce for the first time. In school, this individual has an IEP and is working on community integration goals to gain more independence and skills in preparation for life after high school. An OTA can be involved in many areas in this situation and provide expert assistance to this individual. According to the American Occupational Therapy Association (AOTA) Member Data Survey (2016), 19.9% of occupational therapists and 15.2% of OTAs work in schools, but working with the adolescent population is a small percentage of those practitioners' caseloads.[64] Furthermore, of the occupational therapists who reported working in the high school setting, less than 10% reported spending their time providing transition services.[65] OT practitioners should expand their thinking to be more inclusive of the adolescents and young adults going through times of transition.

IDEA emphasizes the delivery of transition services in major performance areas that are typically addressed by OT practitioners.[66] These areas include work, education, independent living, play and leisure, and social participation.

Thus, the skill set required for OT practice has changed, but it should not be reduced as the student client transitions from high school, and beyond.

With regard to the earlier example of the student entering the workforce, the student is protected under IDEA and Section 504 of the Rehabilitation Act. The role of OT in this example is to work as a liaison between the employer and the student and to provide assistance with how the student can perform the job tasks expected of him provided reasonable accommodations and/or modifications. OT practitioners can support individuals with disabilities in unique and unparalleled ways. The process of activity analysis and synthesis is most useful to break down cognitive and psychosocial skills into component parts.[67] These parts can be addressed separately until all steps can be integrated in the correct sequence and functional performance of the job description is attained.

Section 504 ensures that all students with medical or other disabilities have equal access to education via accommodations and modifications for qualifying students. Unfortunately, the 504 plan does not generally transition to college with students, although many colleges and universities will assist with accommodations, as required.

HIGHER EDUCATION OPPORTUNITY ACT OF 2008

The reauthorization of the Higher Education Act of 1965 brought about the Higher Education Opportunity Act (HEOA) of 2008 (P.L. 110–315). This legislation requires that federal financial assistance be made available to individuals with intellectual disabilities.[62] If they meet the criteria for the diagnosis of "intellectual disability" and are attending an approved transition program, they are eligible for work study and federal grants without having a high school diploma; however, they are ineligible for student loans. In addition, transition and postsecondary programs for students with intellectual disabilities exist in 23 states and provide individualized support for students in college. They add a focus on not only academics, but also work experiences, IADLs, and independent living, as well as social experiences.[68]

ASSISTIVE TECHNOLOGY ACT OF 2004

Millions of Americans with disabilities work, play, go to school, and are contributing members of their communities each day. For many of these individuals, assistive technology devices are a valuable tool to improve their lives and facilitate independence. *Assistive technology* is defined as any type of item that is used to improve the ability of an individual with a disability to function. This could be a piece of equipment that has been modified or something purchased commercially.[61] The Assistive Technology Act of 1998 (P.L. 105–394) was amended in 2004 (P.L. 108–364) to provide states with federal funding from the U. S. Department of Education.[69] The effort of this public law is to "improve the provision of assistive technology to individuals with disabilities through comprehensive statewide programs of technology-related assistance, for individuals with disabilities of all ages."[69] This law is not limited to school-aged persons. With regard to the adult population, assistive technology could be used to support postsecondary options, vocational rehabilitation, and community living activities.

LEGAL INDEPENDENCE

During the transition from childhood to adulthood, young adults are developing the skill of self-determination, which involves many components that facilitate the individual's ability to make decisions and advocate for himself or herself. These components include self-esteem, self-advocacy, independence in life tasks, and self-efficacy.[57,70] Young adults with disabilities participate in intervention planning and goal writing. Self-determination initially revolves around school performance and goals but then expands to include life skills, such as ADLS, IADLs, and, potentially, employment.[62]

When an individual reaches 18 years of age, parents are no longer the guardians of the individual, which means that the individual is now legally responsible to make decisions and sign consents regarding care. The parent(s) may apply for guardianship to maintain this right, but two criteria must be fulfilled. It must be clear that the individual is incompetent with regard to a major life area, and there must be a need for guardianship. It is important for families to plan ahead because a process must occur for guardianship to be granted to another individual and if it is not completed before the 18th birthday, guardianship goes to the individual.[62]

CONTEXT OF OCCUPATIONAL THERAPY SERVICES

OT services are provided in a variety of settings during clients' adulthood. Settings may be within the community, educationally based, work related, or medically based.

Community Settings

Community-based services are usually designed on the basis of a needs assessment to determine what needs exist for individuals within the given community. These programs may be developed in collaboration with universities, or a grant proposal may be written to provide funding to pay for the program designed and the involvement of OT practitioners.

One example of a local, community-based program is the Bridge Program, which was designed by OT practitioners to assist adults with psychiatric disabilities develop needed life skills. The program includes the development of social skills, such as public speaking, stress management, and professional behaviors. It also includes work-related skills, such as time management, computer and Internet skills, reading skills, basic math skills, and applying for jobs. Individuals in the program also develop education-related skills, such as study skills, library skills, completing financial aid forms, exploring available programs, studying for placement tests, and completing school applications. As a collaborative effort between OT practitioners and OT students, this program has been shown to be effective in improving skills of the participants.[67]

The above program is a description of just one type of community-based services. Community-based services are likely to occur in group settings; therefore, it will be important for the OTA to refer back to what was learned during his or her training on group process and effective management of OT groups to have a full understanding of how to work with these adults.

Postsecondary Education

OTAs may have a role in working with clients in postsecondary settings because of the unique skills of OT practitioners to help problem-solve appropriate accommodations that promote improved occupational performance of these adults with disabilities. The AOTA identifies multiple roles for OT practitioners working with this population. OT practitioners may help students understand their rights; work with the student, family, and Disability Support Services to determine adaptations that may facilitate success in academic tasks and tasks related to postsecondary education; and coach students with education-related skills, such as time management, mobility, personal device care. These services may be provided through community or government agencies or through the disability support services offices located at postsecondary institutions.[71]

Employment

Although it is not as uncommon for employers to hire adults with disabilities, some challenges still exist. These challenges include not knowing how to offer adaptations and accommodations and how to communicate about a position to an individual with a disability. Individuals with disabilities often face limited opportunities for advancement in some of the positions that companies are required to provide. Many misperceptions about people with disabilities in the workplace still persist, including limited confidence in their abilities.[72]

Adults with disabilities who maintain positions in the workforce identify some important benefits of having a job. First, socialization within the workplace is meaningful. Second, society places value on the ability of a person to work. Therefore, when an adult with a disability has a job, this individual feels that he or she is contributing to society.[72] Culturally, individuals are often defined by the work that they do. Often, when one individual meets another, they introduce themselves by their names and their work. Therefore, many individuals desire to have some job and thus a place in society.

Many research studies have been performed on work trends related to various disabilities. One study found that 53% of participants with CP who volunteered went on to obtain competitive employment, which is an increase from past studies. In addition, 33% of the participants were financially independent as a result of having jobs.[73] Different types of work opportunities include competitive work, semicompetitive work, sheltered employment, volunteer work, and homemaking. Competitive work involves an individual with a disability having a job, where pay is commensurate with skills. Semicompetitive work is when an individual with a disability has significant modifications and earns less than minimum wage for the work done. Sheltered employment is a setting for individuals with disabilities that is separate from that for able-bodied peers. Volunteering and homemaking tasks are unpaid and are very broadly defined.[73,74]

Acute Care

Even though an OTA may not work in a unit designed specifically for adults who have had disabilities from childhood, an individual who has one of the aforementioned diagnoses may be a client at a variety of different settings. As noted previously, many of these conditions have comorbidities or additional concerns that increase as the individual ages. For example, an individual with DMD may be dropped during a transfer and break a leg, thus requiring acute orthopedic care. If the OTA is assigned to this client, the OTA must be aware of the orthopedic concerns involving the broken leg, the healing process, treatment precautions, and so on. In addition, the preexisting diagnosis of DMD is critical to understanding how this may impact the functioning of the client, premorbid functioning, expectations, appropriate equipment, and handling techniques.

Physical as well as psychological disabilities may coexist with acute conditions. If an individual is diagnosed with anxiety or ASD and is hospitalized for an infection that has caused severe debility, it will be important for the OTA to know how those conditions impact an individual to be able to interpret the client's behaviors and responses. Having a premorbid disability often complicates both medical care and the aging process.[6,24,41]

Outpatient and Home Health Services

Outpatient and home health OT services are typically recommended after an initial hospital stay. If OTAs are working in adult settings, it is important for the OTA to be prepared for this therapeutic journey with the client. As in the acute care setting, if the client has a comorbid condition that was present before the reason for current medical services, the OTA must understand what this symptomatology includes and how it may impact the client's participation and occupational performance in the clinic or at home.

"HOW'S THE WEATHER?" UNDERSTANDING SENSORY PROCESSING

When planning a journey, it is always important to look at the weather report. The weather impacts how one prepares for the journey and helps one anticipate changes that may need to be made. Just as weather impacts people differently, so does **sensory processing**. When preparing for a journey through OT, it is important to understand how sensory input, and the way it is processed, impacts an individual. To explore this idea of sensory processing, Winnie Dunn's model of sensory processing, now known as the *Sensory Processing Framework*, will be described here.[75,76]

Each individual's neurological system impacts the way sensory information is interpreted. At some level of habituation, the individual stops being aware of sensory inputs. For example, when a person is sitting in a classroom and a projector is turned on, he or she hears the sound it makes. However, over time sitting in that classroom, the body tunes out that sound or becomes habituated to it. If this does not happen, it is very difficult to concentrate on new information being provided or the task at hand. Likewise, if a person is unable to habituate to the feeling of a tag in a shirt, that can limit the individual's functional performance of a task.[62,63] In contrast, if the fire alarm goes off while someone is sitting in the classroom, that person quickly jumps out of his or her seat and runs to the hallway. People have been sensitized to this sound (and possibly smell, if smoke is present as well), and they make a quick decision about responding to it. This recognition of stimuli is called *sensitization*. Sensory input is interpreted by the body along a continuum that ranges from sensitization to habituation. The way this input is interpreted may depend on the sense being stimulated.[75,76]

At the same time that the body's neurological system is interpreting sensory input, behavioral responses also occur. When the sensory input is detected, the individual determines how to respond to this input. The way in which one responds is called *self-regulation*, which occurs either in an active way or in a passive way. For example, responding to a fire alarm would be an active response to the stimulus of sound. An example of a passive response to sound is saying a person's name to get his or her attention and the individual does not seem to acknowledge that anything was said.[76] Active and passive responses may vary, depending on the type of sensory input, and follows a continuum.

Because of the interaction between the neurological system and the behavioral system, an individual's sensory processing can be characterized in four different ways: registration/bystander, sensitivity/sensor, seeking/seeker, and avoiding/avoider. Although the original model was constructed around young children, it has been recognized that sensory processing also impacts adolescents and adults.[75,76] Therefore, it is important to have a general understanding of these systems and sensory processing approaches when working with adults. For example, an adult with ASD may not want to perform a certain work task because he or she does not like the texture and feel of the uniform. If the OT practitioner does not have a good understanding of how sensory processing may impact function, it may remain undiscovered. It is also important to understand that an individual may belong to any of the different categories with regard to different types of sensory inputs, or it may change depending on context. The four areas are described in Table 37-1.

TABLE 37-1 Sensory Processing Preferences

SENSORY PROCESSING PREFERENCES	DESCRIPTION/TENDENCIES	EXAMPLES
Registration/Bystanders	Likely to miss sensory input (not hearing one's own name) Need lots of sensory input to notice it because they habituate so quickly Passive in their responses because they do not typically notice input	Name may need to be said multiple times or in a louder or different tone of voice to be noticed These individuals are usually very easy going but interaction with them may be frustrating because they may appear like they do not care or are ignoring stimuli when really their neurological system is not registering the input.[75,76]
Sensitivity/Sensors	Passive approach to self-regulation but sensitive to sensory input	Notice stimuli quickly and may see details that others may miss Would likely cover his/her ears when the fire alarm went off or may ask others to be quiet if the environment is too loud[75,76]
Seeking/Seekers	Habituate quickly to sensory input so it takes more input than most people for the individual to sense the input Have an active self-regulation strategy	Seek out additional sensory input May require extra movement to stay alert In a classroom setting, they may be the ones wiggling in their chairs, kicking their desks, or chewing on pencils. This may be distracting to a teacher or employer who may think the individual is being obstinate or not paying attention.[75,76] Adults with ADHD have been identified as sensory seeking.[12]

TABLE 37-1 Sensory Processing Preferences (continued)

SENSORY PROCESSING PREFERENCES	DESCRIPTION/TENDENCIES	EXAMPLES
Avoiding/Avoiders	Sensitive to sensory input, so they detect very small changes in the environment Active in their behavioral response	They often leave the context if they become overwhelmed by sensory input, or they may refuse to go certain places in anticipation of the sensory input. For example, an individual may have developed a friendship but avoids social situations with the person because of the intensity of sensory stimuli in that context. Thus, the relationship remains limited. However, these individuals may demonstrate strengths in creating organization and structure as to minimize unexpected sensory input.[75,76]

Sensory processing impacts individuals in different ways. It is known that individuals with a variety of diagnoses, including learning disabilities, display difficulties with sensory processing.[9] Understanding that this may be a factor in the behavior and decisions made by a person is critical for the OT practitioner to understand on the journey so that he or she may enhance the occupational performance of the pediatric clients who have now grown up.

THE GOAL OF THE JOURNEY—ENABLING OCCUPATION

Transition from childhood to adulthood can be a very challenging time for the client and for the client's family. In fact, families and clients have reported that after high school, most services end. This leaves them feeling abandoned and alone in the battle to develop necessary skills that are often delayed.[1] By bridging the gap in support for the client, OTAs can truly enhance the journey of the client.

OT practitioners typically use one (or more) of the five primary approaches to OT when designing an intervention. These approaches include creating, establishing or restoring, maintaining, modifying, or preventing.[27] The primary approaches that will be discussed throughout the remainder of this chapter will be restoring, maintaining, and modifying; however, preventing further disability is also important as the individual continues to age.

Before providing OT services to an adult with a disability, it is important to recognize the role of that individual in the treatment planning process. This process should be client-centered, and the individual should be empowered to be involved in decision making and goal setting.[58] When looking at intervention strategies specifically, physical

EVIDENCE-BASED PRACTICE

Sensory processing challenges have been studied in children with both ASD and ADHD, but little research has been done on adults with ASD and ADHD. A recent study by Clince et al. was conducted to explore and compare sensory processing patterns of adult students in postsecondary education who have ASD and ADHD to inform OT practice and review functional implications of these patterns.[77] In this study, 28 students with ADHD and 27 students with ASD participated by completing the Adolescent/Adult Sensory Profile.[78] In addition, a subset of the students completed semistructured interviews. As a result, the students with ASD were similar to most people in all sensory processing preferences, except Sensation Seeking, where 63% scored less compared with most people. The adults with ADHD did not show consistency in results, but 71.4% scored more compared with most people for low registration and 60.7% scored similar to most people for sensation avoiding. Those with ADHD were significantly higher in sensation seeking than the ASD participants.[77]

With regard to the implications of these sensory processing patterns on daily life as a postsecondary student, the responses tended to revolve around the importance of appropriate sensory input in the study and examination environments, impact of sensory processing on choice of leisure activities, and impacts of sensory processing on social life. This study is important to highlight to the OTA how sensory processing continues to impact individuals into adulthood and the implications this may have on an individual's daily life.

Clince, M., Connolly, L., & Nolan, C. (2016). Comparing and exploring the sensory processing patterns of higher education students with attention deficit hyperactivity disorder and autism spectrum disorder. American Journal of Occupational Therapy, 70, *7002250010.*

Brown, C., & Dunn, W. (2002). Adolescent/adult sensory profile: User's manual. *San Antonio, TX: Pearson.*

adaptations may be similar to strategies discussed elsewhere in this text and can be used for a variety of conditions that traditionally have onset in adulthood. However, the approaches used and the behavior management strategies for adult clients who have intellectual and developmental disabilities may be very different. Likewise, the role that sensory processing plays in an individual's behavior and occupation is critical to consider.

Occupations will be discussed in a manner consistent with the OTPF-3.[27] Considerations will be discussed by occupation, taking into account not only the physical assistance or adaptations that might be addressed but also how sensory processing may affect performance of that task.

Activities of Daily Living

As an individual transitions from childhood to adulthood, the level of responsibility may change. Within society, it is expected that young adults be independent in the performance of ADLs. However, disability may impact that level of independence. However, if an OTA is working with an adult who is not independent in these tasks, facilitating performance of these tasks will likely become a primary priority. Cognitive, physical, psychological, and sensory impairments may impact intervention in these areas. With the goal of enabling occupations, important things to consider within each of the identified occupations will be discussed.

DRESSING

Dressing skills include the cognitive skills of planning and sequencing the dressing tasks as well as the physical capability to manipulate clothes and place them correctly. In fact, it is common that older individuals who have cognitive difficulties are unable to complete dressing tasks independently.[79] The OTA may work with the client on sequencing the tasks to dress while also working with the caregiver on how to cue the client to increase independence with dressing tasks.

Individuals with decreased sensation and decreased fine motor skills may have difficulty with fasteners and tying shoelaces. When considering shoelace tying, it is important to recognize the individual's orthopedic needs for specific supports in the shoes. Many types of shoes that can accommodate different motor needs are now available, but the availability may be limited, depending on the type of support needed. Sitting while dressing is a recommendation that can help increase safety and independence with dressing tasks.[79] Difficulty with the ability to dress is highly correlated with the ability to complete other ADLs and IADLs. Therefore, it is important for the OTA to recognize that someone who has difficulty with dressing is probably going to struggle with other ADLs and/or IADLs.[79]

A significant number of adaptive devices and equipment have been developed to increase independence with dressing. Of the commonly used devices, those assisting with lower body dressing, including socks and shoes, are the most commonly owned and used. Other commonly owned and used devices include button hooks and dressing sticks.[79] However, equipment may be owned but not used in some cases. It is important for the OTA to ensure that equipment that is recommended for purchase is usable by the client, its purpose is understood, and the client finds it meaningful so that the client and/or family is not making an unnecessary purchase.

Sensory processing may impact dressing as well. The client may avoid certain colors of clothing or some textures that are not comfortable. Different fabric textures within the clothing or the presence of tags may also be bothersome. However, many clothing companies are now offering "tagless" options for shirts, pants, and even undergarments. Therefore, such items are much easier to find, and there are many more options than there used to be. This tactile sensitivity in the client is important to keep in mind when preparing the individual for employment. Some adults with disabilities may not be able to communicate these sensory difficulties and instead may show their responses through behaviors. Some individuals may avoid a certain job because of the way the uniform feels. Because of motor skill challenges or sensory processing difficulties, any occupation that has specific dress requirements may also impact an individual's ability to participate. However, if participating in the occupation is a desire of the client, this is an area that the OTA should address.

BATHING

Bathing and showering are important activities to help an individual remain clean as well as healthy.[80] If an individual has limited mobility, the process of bathing or showering can be physically challenging and may require the assistance of another person and/or some equipment. The OTA may work to train caregivers on proper bathing techniques and transfers in and out of the bathtub or shower. The OTA may also recommend adaptive equipment to decrease the strain on the caregiver or to increase the independence and safety of the individual. It is important to teach proper sequencing of steps for safety reasons. For example, if the individual has limited balance, it may be safer to dry the individual while he or she is seated. Transferring a dry person is safer than transferring a wet one. It is important for the OTA to be aware of current equipment available as well as its cost and the resources available to the individual. In some areas, there may be equipment loan programs, where equipment can be tested with the client before purchase. However, properly placed grab bars and nonslip surfaces are frequently recommended by OT practitioners and are important for safety.[81] OT practitioners are urged to promote safe environments and provide education to prevent falls of adults dwelling in the community-. The presence of safety equipment does not guarantee understanding or competence in its use.[82]

Those with disabilities have been found to take longer time in the shower and may skip steps in the bathing process. Decreased motor function, challenges sequencing steps, or perseveration on a step may all contribute to the decreased efficiency.[80] If motor skills are a challenge, adapting the specific tasks within bathing may be necessary for improved success and efficiency. For example, using a wash mitt may help an individual who has limited grasp. If cognitive skills are impaired, then providing a picture sequencing chart or marking the shower knob position for the appropriate water temperature may be helpful strategies.

When considering sensory processing and bathing, multiple sensory inputs should be considered. First, the individual may be averse to certain soap smells. In addition, the individual may have very sensitive skin that limits the options of products that can be used in this occupation. Textures of towels and washcloths may be a factor, as well as the feel of the water hitting the skin. Some individuals may not like a light spray of the shower but may tolerate a more forceful massaging spray. Change of environment may also impact functional performance.

PERSONAL HYGIENE AND GROOMING

Hygiene and grooming tasks often require the use of small objects, such as toothbrush and toothpaste, fingernail file and clippers, brush and comb, makeup and lip gloss, razor and shaving cream, deodorant, perfume or cologne, among other items. Personal hygiene and grooming tasks often involve the opening and closing of small containers through twisting, flipping, or squeezing and thus require the use of one hand to stabilize while the other hand does the work. Individuals with weakness, poor endurance, or tremors may have difficulty performing these types of tasks. Individuals who have difficulty coordinating both sides of the body to work together may have difficulty with the fine motor and coordination skills as well. Many adaptive devices are available to help make these tasks easier if the motor skills is a challenge for the individual. Often, adaptive devices can be made from everyday items as well. These adaptations are only limited by the creativity of the OTA.

Cognitive skills may also impact the ability to complete hygiene and grooming tasks independently. Not understanding the purpose or when to do a task can be problematic. Teaching the steps of a task with visual cues as well as verbal cues can be a beneficial way to practice something that should become routine (See the "Technology and Trends" box for a description of an iPad® application designed for this purpose).

Many different sensations are experienced during grooming and hygiene activities. Products used have various smells, and many have a perfume-type scent. Some of the activities require tolerance of various tactile inputs. For example, shaving tasks for males or females often require the use of shaving cream. Some individuals seek out the sensation of the shaving cream on skin while others cannot tolerate it. As technologies to facilitate everyday life tasks advance, more options may become available in regular stores. For example, there are disposable razors that have shaving gel included with the blade. Such razors do not require the use of shaving cream. Fingernail clipping is

TECHNOLOGY AND TRENDS

Over the last few years, the use of electronic devices, such as tablets, iPads®, and smartphones, has become commonplace for a multitude of functions. Along with the development of these tablets, individual fee-based or free apps have been created for download on a device. When updates or changes are made to the application, or "app," the user of the app is notified through the device and can choose to update the app. Many apps have become tools used in intervention by OT practitioners. When considering adults with disabilities, three types of apps in particular may be helpful for the OTA to use in intervention and to help train the individual and/or the family in specific ADLs or IADLs.

ADL and IADL Training—Sequencing:

Apps are available on the iPad® to help OTAs train clients who are having difficulty sequencing ADLs. For example, "Sequencing Tasks" has four different bundle "apps" that help teach the client appropriate steps by combining multiple sensory inputs for three-step tasks: (1) A real-time video is shown demonstrating the task while each step is stated orally; (2) a still photo of each step is displayed with a one-line written direction and auditory cue; and (3) the client is asked to order the steps involved in the activity. The steps are stated verbally when touching the photo. Tasks included are ADLs, such as brushing teeth, eating, putting on shoes, donning a shirt, and grooming tasks. IADLs include sweeping, purchasing an item, riding in a car, stapling papers, putting on an adhesive bandage, making a sandwich, doing laundry, and making food. The leisure activity of painting a picture is also available.

Other sequencing apps on iPad® include more steps for a more complete and thorough task completion, such as "iDo Hygiene" and "iDo Dressing." These apps include the ability to record one's own video and would be very useful to clients who have difficulty generalizing skills or who are motivated by watching their own successful task completion. These apps also have activities where the client can match the step to a photo and order the steps into a correct sequence. These apps also include a game that the client may play with the OTA or caregiver and answer questions or complete tasks related to the ADLs being addressed in the app.

OTAs are recommended to search and explore apps related to sequencing and ADL and IADL tasks. These apps do cost money, and the OTA will want to ensure that he or she is purchasing or suggesting the best fit for the client's needs.

IADL—Medication Management:

"CareZone" is a free app for the iPad® or android tablet or smartphone designed for medication management that includes many features for both clients and caregivers. CareZone allows the individual to input data on all medications by taking photos of the labels. This app will track all prescriptions and can also include over-the-counter medications and supplements. Alerts can be set for when to take medications as well as when to refill a prescription. In addition, the medication list can be emailed or printed for communication with caregivers and/or medical professionals. A contact section includes the prescribing

Continued

physicians and the pharmacies where the prescriptions are maintained. Photos of insurance cards and other relevant items can be stored and notes and checklists can be created for personal use. The OTA could train the client and caregiver as appropriate on use of this app to assist in medication management and potential increase independence in this task for a client with a disability.

IADL—Money Management and Budgeting:

A budgeting and money management app, "Bills for iPad®" and "Bills Organizer" for android both have a free and a paid version. These apps are designed to help an individual track his or her monthly spending. A dollar amount available to spend each month is established, and then monthly bills and expenses are tracked. A calendar is included where the due dates for bills can be listed for reminders. A color coding system is used on the calendar to identify bills overdue, bills planned for payment, and expenses paid. Visual cues notify the user if too much money has been spent. Bills can be sorted into a variety of categories, including cell phone, credit cards, house repair, insurance, loans, taxes, and other. Other features may be available, such as adding income to the calendar, for more complex money management tasks. Bills for iPad® includes a feature where the individual's bills can by synced together with loved ones for assistance with oversight of spending. Reports can be exported to Excel as well. A password can be set on the app for privacy. One of these apps or something similar may be used by the OTA to help train the client to plan for bill payment and to budget money. Family members can use it to help oversee client spending or to manage the tasks for which the client continues to need supervision.

another task that can elicit a behavioral response because of the sensation experienced during the task. In addition, hair washing, cutting, and brushing could evoke avoidance responses from those with sensory processing difficulties.

In addition to the olfactory and tactile inputs from grooming and hygiene tasks, sound can also be problematic. Hair dryers and electric razors are two primary examples. If the sounds produced by these are problematic, the OTA may want to explore with the client and the family alternative means to meet the grooming needs of the individual. For example, bathing at a different time of day when hair can be air-dried may eliminate the need to use a hairdryer.

PERSONAL DEVICE CARE

A variety of personal assistive devices might be required for daily functioning of an individual with disabilities. It is important to recognize that the use of personal assistive devices is likely to increase with age for those with progressive as well as nonprogressive conditions. For example, vision will deteriorate over time. Even if the individual does not require visual correction at the time of transition into adulthood, visual correction needs will occur later in life because of the normal aging process. Visual correction may require glasses or contact lenses or other specialized devices that have more durability or made for another purpose. Hearing aids are another common device that may be required. Changing the batteries and placing the aid appropriately are necessary tasks. Care of any of these hearing aid devices may require the ability to modulate pressure for success, and the inability to modulate pressure may be very costly.

Additional devices used by individuals may include devices for mobility, such as canes, walkers, and wheelchairs. All of these have their own required maintenance and repair. They may also include prosthetics or orthotic devices. Assistive technology or any of the specialized adaptive devices listed in the other sections as options are also personal assistive devices. It is important to make sure that when a specific device is recommended and/or issued to a client, the client and/or caregivers are educated on not only how to use the device but also on the required care and maintenance. It is possible that the device may facilitate independence for the adult with disabilities; however, that individual may require assistance in the care of the device.

TOILETING AND TOILET HYGIENE

Managing toileting needs and hygiene is an activity that occurs multiple times throughout the day. Physical, cognitive, and sensory processing needs can all have impacts on these very important and frequent ADL needs. When considering toileting and toilet hygiene from a physical standpoint, the client must have sufficient strength, endurance, and balance to complete a transfer from a surface to the standard toilet. Often, a raised toilet seat and grab bars are recommended if there is difficulty with any of these physical components. If a caregiver is involved in a transfer because of the client's limited mobility, it is important for the OTA to be aware of proper body mechanics and transfer techniques that must be taught, if necessary. See Chapter 13 on transfers for further information about these techniques. Toilet hygiene from a physical approach also requires sitting balance, strength, and ROM. Grab bars are important to assist with sitting balance to allow for proper hygiene.

When considering toileting and toilet hygiene with someone who has cognitive difficulties, consistency in teaching and training is very important. Repetition is required for developing routines with ADL tasks, although some clients may never demonstrate awareness or concern about toileting or hygiene issues.

Sensory processing challenges can have a significant impact on toileting and toilet hygiene. In fact, toilet training for those with ASD is a laborious process. Sensitivities may include sitting on a cold seat, the texture of the toilet paper, the sound of the toilet flushing, accidental splash of water, and the smell in the bathroom. These individuals may also have difficulty with using a public bathroom.[83] It is important for the OTA to be aware of such sensitivities to help determine possible alternatives to increase independence and success with toileting.

In addition, when females become adults, toilet hygiene becomes more complicated with the addition of menstrual hygiene needs. It is recommended that management of menstrual needs for individuals with DS and other disorders include family training, behavior management approach, and potential medical interventions, such as hormone treatment. The OTA may notice behavioral symptoms related to menstruation and premenstrual syndrome that impact occupational performance of the client.[39] Understanding additional needs during the medical process for health and wellness is also important.[41]

FEEDING AND EATING

Feeding and eating are considered two distinct processes in OT. *Feeding* involves the process of getting the food to the mouth. *Eating* involves oral motor and sensory skills to physically manipulate the food in the mouth and then coordinate swallowing. It is important for the OTA to recognize that any intervention in this area first requires a complete evaluation of feeding and eating skills by an occupational therapist. It is also important to note that age-related changes occur in oral motor skills, as well as sensory changes in touch, vision, taste, and so on, which may impact the feeding and eating experience.[84]

Motor skills are a primary factor in feeding abilities. Often, weakness or incoordination make the feeding task challenging. Posture in preparation for the feeding and eating tasks is important. For example, customized seating may be important for adults with CP because of scoliosis, which is common in these individuals. Positioning is critical for adults to increase occupational performance and to minimize further medical complications resulting from scoliosis and poor seating.[24] Feeding utensils must be considered with regard to the individual's motor abilities, as well as availability and client preference. The OTA may engage in preparatory activities to help improve skills for feeding, but these activities should always have a direct correlation with the occupation. It is also important for the client to understand the purpose of the activity. Contrived feeding activities should be used sparingly if the client does not understand the link between the activity and function.

In addition to feeding modifications and techniques, an OTA may be involved in interventions for eating and swallowing. This chapter does not provide information regarding training for the OTA on eating interventions, and the OTA should refer to Chapter 12 for more information, and also seek other texts or continuing education opportunities to learn these specific skills. Intervention may include preparatory oral motor exercises, where to place the food in the mouth, positioning of the head and neck for swallowing, and environmental modifications, to name a few.[84] In addition to continuing education opportunities, OTAs who are interested in advancement of their knowledge in this area may choose to pursue specialty certification through the AOTA in Feeding, Eating, and Swallowing (SCFES-A)

SEXUAL ACTIVITY

As individuals grow from childhood into adulthood, it is important to recognize that education about sexual development and sexuality is just as important for those with disabilities as it is for those without. Many professionals avoid this topic in their discussions with individuals with disabilities, and therefore many clients lack any education on it.[62,85] In fact, less value is often placed on this important ADL than on other activities, such as bathing, dressing, and toileting.[86] However, OT practitioners can and should address all aspects of ADLs.

First of all, any practitioner who is educating a client and his or her family about the intimate topic of sexuality should first be aware of his or her own beliefs, values, and biases that could impact the therapeutic relationship. Next, the OTA should be aware of the impact the client's specific disability has on sexual development and function.[85] For example, males who have CF or DS are typically infertile, whereas females with these two conditions are fertile.[32,33,39] The OTA should also be aware of the cultural and social contexts of the individual's family when addressing this issue.[85] Last, the OTA may be responsible for collaborating with the client and his or her family to determine an approach to sharing this information with the client in a way that is understandable if the individual has cognitive or processing deficits.[85,87] As the individual ages, the OTA may also play a role in providing suggestions for positioning because of the physical challenges faced by the individual or in providing social skills training related to relationship development and interpreting social cues.

The specific impairment that an individual is facing may also directly impact the individual's sexual expression. For example, individuals with ASD who have difficulty with communication, socialization, and interpreting social cues may display inappropriate sexual behaviors as adults.[85,87] In the past, it was believed that individuals with ASD had no desire for intimacy, but more recent studies have indicated that this may not be the case.[87] Because of this need, various programs have been developed specifically to provide sex education to individuals with ASD.[87,88] It is important that the approach is developmentally appropriate for the client. Topics that should be addressed include relationship development, understanding social cues and communication related to sexuality, and how and when to become involved in sexual activities. Because individuals with developmental disabilities often have limited understanding of sexuality, they are easily exploited.[85] The OTA may be a great resource to help locate and/or provide such information for the individual's parents and/or caregivers or to identify a referral source and communicate this information to the supervising occupational therapist.

Instrumental Activities of Daily Living

When individuals with disabilities become adults, different arrangements may be made for their living situation. Some individuals may live independently in their own homes. However, many do live with family members. In addition to these two options, residential settings where individuals may reside with a group of individuals with disabilities are available.[62] Various supports are available for many of the IADLs that will be discussed in this section. The OTA should be aware of what supports are available to a client, what skills the client must have to be able to reside in or maintain the desired living situation, and in what skills the clients wants to become more independent.

COMMUNICATION MANAGEMENT

With the advancements in technology, communication management is not limited to only verbal communication but now includes use of a variety of systems and devices, such as smartphones, computers, and tablets, to communicate needs. It may also include specialized communication devices for clients who have hearing or visual impairments as well as other disabilities.[27] Therefore, the OTA may be involved in helping the client use a familiar device in a new context, occupation, or role. The OTA may also need to teach the client how to use a new device within a given occupation to increase functional performance.

DRIVING AND COMMUNITY MOBILITY

Preparing for the possibility of driving and other means of community mobility begins in high school. This is an important area that OT should address because driving and community mobility impact access to various occupations. Although the occupational therapist will be evaluating the client to determine the needs related to driving and community mobility as well as fitness to drive, the OTA can be involved in intervention for the various aspects of this IADL.

One important skill to address is the ability to transfer in and out of a car independently and load the wheelchair, if one is used. If the client cannot do these two things independently, then another individual will always need to be present to aid in these preparatory tasks even if the client has the skills to drive. Another important skill that a client must have is the ability to find his or her way from point A to point B. The OTA may address the client's problem-solving skills to see if he or she can read a map, such as in a shopping mall or store. This is a critical preparatory skill not only for driving but also for independence in community mobility.[89]

In terms of sensory processing, the client must be able to tolerate sitting in the front seat of a car. This may not be a familiar experience for the client. The client must not only be able to process the sensory input from this position but also be able to follow simple driving-related tasks, such as calling out important street signs and giving directions to a destination.[89] In addition to the items listed above, specific client factors, such as ROM, strength, coordination, visual perception, reflex integration, and ability to disassociate head movements from body movements (to turn the head to look without the whole body moving) are all possible areas to address.[89]

In a survey of 143 individuals who have an adult family member with ASD, it was determined that 49% of those with ASD had never had access to public transportation.[8] This lack of community mobility negatively impacts the individual's ability to engage in social occupations or employment opportunities. Research also shows that individuals with ADHD are more likely to be involved in accidents, but their performance improves with the use of long-acting methylphenidate.[90]

Therefore, the role of OT practitioners includes working on the client's predriving skills, such as coordination, reaction time, social interaction, and handling emergencies. In addition, demonstrating confidence, managing impulsivity, and being able to regulate sensory input are also important skills that clients must have. Although driving may not be a possible IADL for everyone, community mobility skills such as map reading and using the Global Positioning Service (GPS), as well as use of public transportation, should be addressed, as appropriate.[89-91] OTAs who have a specific interest in driving and community mobility may work to obtain the specialty certification in driving and community mobility (SCDCM-A) through the AOTA.

Many of the above skills can be addressed by occupational therapists and OTAs who are general practitioners. When they see that the intervention requires more specialized knowledge in the area of driving rehabilitation, it is important for the client to be referred to a driving rehabilitation specialist for further training specific to driving as well as for possible adaptations or limitations that may impact driving abilities. See Chapter 16 for further driving information.

FINANCIAL MANAGEMENT

Managing and budgeting money is a skill that is required for complete independence as an adult. However, independence with money management is not essential for living independently. When working in this area, it will be important for the OTA to understand both the client and the client's family's past roles and desires for future involvement in money management. The OTA must understand the client's source of income and required expenses and be aware of spending money available. Once the background information has been obtained and goals determined, it will be important to identify what skills need to be addressed. Some skills related to financial management may include simple math skills, use of a calculator, writing a check, using online banking and bill payment options, use of an automated teller machine, credit card and bank card use, and how to handle an issue with a bill.

HEALTH MANAGEMENT AND MAINTENANCE

The client's role in health management and maintenance are part of health and wellness promotion. The OTA may be involved in helping the client make good decisions on health-related behaviors and nutrition. Routines related to physical fitness and medication may also be included.[27] Role-playing anticipated situations may be one way to help promote independence in this area.

HOME ESTABLISHMENT AND MANAGEMENT

Many skills are required in maintaining a home. Some of these skills may still be necessary, even if the client does not live independently or in a single-family residence. Physical, cognitive, and sensory limitations may limit an individual's ability to maintain a vehicle, the yard, the house, appliances, and so on. In addition, the client needs to know who to contact for help, if necessary.[27] Therefore, the OTA may address physical limitations to performing a task and may explore appropriate modifications or accommodations to increase success. It may also be important to prioritize the most important IADLs for the individual because many of the IADLs may cause significant stress and energy expenditure. It may not be feasible to participate in all of the possible roles that may be necessary. The client thus needs to learn to balance activities for energy conservation.

Sensory processing needs may impact the individual's desire and willingness to participate in home establishment and management tasks. For example, the client may not tolerate the sound of the vacuum cleaner, or the smell of household cleaners may be overwhelming to a client. Therefore, the OTA may need to find alternatives, if necessary (e.g., unscented dish detergent).

MEAL PREPARATION AND CLEANUP

Depending on the individual's living situation, the client may or may not be directly involved in planning, preparing, and serving meals.[27] It is possible that the client is guided to complete specific steps within this process and is taught through repetition of tasks. This would require the ability to physically complete the components of the task as well as the ability to learn a specific sequence. To be independent in performing the occupation as a whole, planning and problem-solving are also necessary abilities. This is also an important skill that can lead to success in a specific setting where the client may work as a volunteer or for pay.

Although there are many sensory components to meal preparation and cleanup, if this is completed in the client's own home, then the sensory input can be predictable, and this makes it easier to work through the IADL with a client. If meal preparation and cleanup are performed in a work context, knowing what sensory inputs may occur would be important to address these potential situations with the client.

SHOPPING

Shopping includes grocery shopping, shopping for household goods, and online shopping. It includes the ability to physically maneuver oneself within the store setting around aisles and rows, have the endurance to complete the task, and be able to complete the monetary transaction required to purchase items. Shopping may also include the ability to locate and select items in a digital environment and complete a monetary transaction in the virtual context.[27]

Because of the complexity of the shopping occupation, many areas need to be addressed by OT. First, the physical ability to get around in the store or use the online device to be able to locate items of interest is important. Skill development or adaptation to various components of shopping tasks may be required. Cognitively, determining an appropriate shopping list, selecting appropriate items for purchase, sequencing steps involved in the shopping process, and problem-solving in getting an item that is out of reach or unavailable are all skills that may be addressed. Last, it is important to consider how sensory processing may affect the shopping process. Shopping in a large department store or mall can result in an overwhelming amount of sensory input—from the florescent lights and visual movement, the use of an elevator or escalator, the competing smells from stores and restaurants, the unexpected touch of passersby, or the unanticipated sounds. It is important for the OTA to be aware of the client's sensory processing and how it may impact the shopping experience in an unpredictable setting.

SAFETY AND EMERGENCY MAINTENANCE

In any context, especially if the client is alone, it is important for the individual to understand safety issues, be able to recognize how to prevent dangerous situations and identify when they occur, and be able to notify appropriate individuals of an emergency.[27] Safety awareness is critical if the client is expected to be alone for any amount of time during the course of a day. Once the client's safety awareness is determined, then the OT practitioner may be required to establish proper emergency responses and make adaptations to allow for independence with these tasks. Any safety measures for clients home alone, such as automatic door openers or emergency assist lines, should also be considered for how access will occur when the power goes out.

RELIGIOUS AND SPIRITUAL ACTIVITIES AND EXPRESSION

The occupation of involvement in religious and spiritual activities may include organized religion, or it may be a connectedness with nature or the common good.[27] Ensuring that a client is able to meet his or her goals in terms of religious and spiritual participation requires the OTA to have an established rapport with the client and the supervising occupational therapist to be aware of what activities are important to the client related to this occupation. Views of religion and spirituality are not always addressed upon evaluation or as openly as part of the therapeutic relationship. OT may address access to the activities, physical roles of participation, or how sensory processing challenges impact performance in this area.

Education

For young adults who are transitioning out of the K-12 education setting, there are various postsecondary education options available. The traditional settings are universities and community colleges. However, on-the-job training or specialized coursework may also be options. Most colleges or universities have an office for disability support services (DSS). Unlike the public K-12 system, at the postsecondary level, it is the responsibility of the individual to report their disability to DSS to be considered for accommodation of specific needs. These reasonable accommodations, such as audio books, sign language interpreter, and note taker, are required to be provided through Section 504 of the Rehabilitation Act of 1973 if the institution receives federal funding.[62,92]

The OT practitioner's role becomes more of a guided support service to promote independence in the student. One of the most difficult transitions for students is to go from a structured, nurturing environment, such as a high school, to a more independent, self-supporting role in higher education. Self-advocacy skills are most important during this transition because support services are not "seeking out" the students in need; the student must initiate them. The U. S. Department of Education provides vocational rehabilitation state grants for the state to provide vocational rehabilitation services. These services must give priority by significance in disability if not all eligible individuals can be served. These services are designed to help individuals with either physical or mental impairments prepare for employment, obtain employment, be successful and maintain their employment, or regain employment, if necessary.[93] Such services can include counseling, training, transportation, job placement, education, and assistive technology.

As the student seeks postsecondary educational opportunities, it is his or her responsibility to follow-up with vocational rehabilitation services to request assistance. Once vocational rehabilitation services are established, they are provided for life as long as the person continues to qualify as a person with a disability. If there is a change in life events, such as a person no longer needs educational supports but now requires job placement assistance, he or she is responsible to make the contact with the agency. The OTA can be most useful by providing services to young adults in self-advocacy skills and communication skills that are necessary for this to occur.

FORMAL EDUCATION PREPARATION

The *US News* reported that about 3% of teens who have been diagnosed with a learning disability struggle so much in their classes in high school that they give up on their hopes to go to college and pursue their lifelong dreams of a career.[94] Although the graduation rate hit its highest level (81%) in 2012 to 2013,[95] the graduation rate for students with disabilities generally remains very low (around 60%).[96] OT practitioners value the prospect of individuals with disabilities getting into a career based on their strengths, interests, needs, and personal preferences. It is the job of OT practitioners to work diligently with clients to achieve this goal.

OCCUPATIONAL THERAPY'S ROLE IN THE TRANSITION OF HIGH SCHOOL STUDENTS

The role of OT in the transition process for high school students is to help them grow and learn to be as independent as possible.[66] Occupational therapists and OTAs can be part of the transition team because they have specialized knowledge and skills to support the following areas related to transition:

- Developing and sustaining positive work habits and skills
- Preparing the student and his or her family for changes in roles and routines related to independent living
- Teaching strategies for successful community living
- Determining supports for employment through role assessment and activity and work analysis
- Supporting self-determination and self-advocacy skills in school and through community integration
- Recommending modifications and equipment for community mobility
- Collaborating with transition team members and school staff
- Exploring behavioral, psychosocial, and sensory needs of clients
- Facilitating daily living skills and independent living skills
- Fostering development of functional skills such as time management, organization, and safety
- Working with clients to identify leisure and recreation activities

The role of OT during the student's transition is critical for the individual with a disability to ensure a smooth transition to life after high school is related to the client's postsecondary goals. As can be imagined, if occupational therapists and OTAs were able to provide these transition-related services to students with disabilities while they were still in high school, how much better prepared for their "trip" would these students be?

POSTSECONDARY OPTIONS

Many postsecondary options exist for students who complete high school, whether they have disabilities or not. Being adequately prepared for postsecondary education can make their journey a success.[97] OT practitioners can assist with the process of career and college exploration as well as the actual steps of applying to the programs. Students with disabilities may select any program in which they are qualified but are strongly urged to research their options, review documentation, and understand program requirements to make sure it is a good fit for them.

A campus visit would be a great way for a student to get a feel for the campus environment, visit the disabilities service office, and meet with an academic advisor. It is not unusual for a student to change his or her mind after visiting a campus or enrolling in a program. Understanding the reasoning behind their decisions can sometimes be the most useful tool to discovering what is best for them.

College includes 2- and 4-year institutions. Four-year colleges help students earn their bachelor's degree and/or graduate degree. They have specific requirements for application, such as minimal GPA (grade point average) standards, SAT (Scholastic Aptitude/Assessment Test) or ACT (American College Testing) scores, essays, and interviews, depending on the school. College campuses vary in size and location. OT practitioners can facilitate conversations with students on what would be the best college environment for them to attend. For example, should the college campus be located on a bus line? Are there hills that would be difficult for manual wheelchair propulsion? Does it need to be close to home? Do the students need to participate in a work-study program? Would they prefer for their class size to be small, or can they handle a large group of students in a lecture class? All of these questions and many others can assist students with disabilities in choosing the right school for them based on their strengths, preferences, and needs.

Students who attend 2-year colleges can earn their associate degree or technical certifications, and these courses include programs such as Automotive, Childcare Development, Cosmetology, Computer Programming, Agriculture, and many more. These types of career and technical education programs focus on career training and include technical training, employability skills, work ethics, industry certification, and/or direct links to career paths.

An apprenticeship is another great option for students with disabilities interested in paid on-the-job training with an employer.[97] Students can receive classroom instruction directly related to the trade or industry in which they are interested in working.

Work

Individuals with disabilities often enter the workforce later in life than those without disabilities. It is common for individuals without disabilities to have paid employment during their high school years, but this is generally where exploring employment interests and abilities occurs for those with disabilities.[62]

EMPLOYMENT INTERESTS

Individuals with disabilities should begin exploring interests related to potential employment while they are still in high school. This movement toward paid employment is a required component in the student's IEP as part of transition planning.[62] For students in the high school setting, the goal of employment exploration is to learn more about themselves. For example, does the student like working outside compared with working inside? Does the student prefer working with people or the general public? What kind of schedule would suit the student? Is the student a morning person or need a job that requires working primarily at night? All of these questions need to be further explored for students with different types of disabilities.

OT practitioners can assist with the evaluation of the students' strengths, skills, personal preferences, and needs. It is best when a variety of work environments can be observed and tried by the student to get real-life experience with what the day-to-day job may look and feel like. Students can discover that a job is not for them. For example, if a student thought he wanted to work outside in a landscaping job and discovers later on that he does not like to get his hands dirty and dislikes being in the heat all day, it is a good thing. Students with disabilities need to discover for themselves what their preferences are with this type of job exploration.

Vocational Rehabilitation Services are a great resource for students and families with disabilities when it comes to job exploration and employment. Students, parents, teachers, counselors, social workers, nurses, OT practitioners, or any other person related to the transition team can all make referrals. Vocational Rehabilitation counselors will assist students and their families with completing applications and then will develop individualized plans for employment.

EMPLOYMENT SEEKING

Looking for a job is an exciting, yet challenging, experience for anyone. For people with disabilities, it is important to remember that the regulations of the ADA are in place to ensure that they have an equal opportunity to work.[98] Work options for individuals with disabilities include competitive employment or noncompetitive employment options.[62] OT practitioners can assist individuals with disabilities in identifying job opportunities they are interested in.[66] This includes preemployment skills, such as completing, submitting, and reviewing application materials; preparing for interviews; working on a resume and cover letter; and discussing job benefits. OTAs can use their clinical reasoning skills to determine the relationship between the individual client factors and how that could affect job performance.

JOB PERFORMANCE

The OTPF-3 describes job performance as an area of occupation, including "work skills and patterns; time management; relationships with coworkers, managers, and customers; leadership and supervision; creation, production, and distribution of products and services; initiation, sustainment, and completion of work; and compliance with work norms and procedures."[27] The company will have certain job expectations from the new employee. These include hard skills, such as the teachable, specific abilities of a job, as well as soft skills, which are harder to quantify and are more subjective. OTAs can work with clients on both sets of skills. For example, hard skills, such as computer programming skills or the ability to change the oil in a car, are often listed on a resume. Soft skills relate more to how a person can interact with people. Examples of soft skills include communication, teamwork, enthusiasm, dependability, flexibility, and motivation. Soft skills are more difficult to teach but are very effective in obtaining employment and keeping it.

OT practitioners facilitate intervention strategies throughout their engagement with clients. For example, in high school, a student may be having difficulties with turning in an English paper on time. Instead of not turning it in at all and just receiving a zero on the paper, the student could learn communication strategies and self-advocacy skills to explain to the teacher what modifications to the task would help him complete the assignment independently and in a timely manner. By learning both hard skills and soft skills while still in school, individuals with disabilities will have an easier time transferring those skills to the work environment.

EXPLORATION OF VOLUNTEERING OPPORTUNITIES

Volunteering is an excellent way to gain experience and on-the-job training while improving a person's quality of life. For example, a young adult loves animals and wants to have a career one day working as a veterinarian technician. This is a career that requires a certificate from a community college or certified program. While in high school, the student may decide to volunteer at a local animal rescue group or walk dogs in his or her neighborhood to gain experience. Exploring volunteering opportunities allows the individual the opportunity to participate in unpaid "work" as it relates to their personal skills, interests, location, and available time.[27]

Leisure and Social Participation

In OT, engagement in occupation, while supporting health and participation in life, is the overarching outcome of the intervention process.[27] OT practitioners believe that "active engagement in occupation promotes, facilitates, supports, and maintains health and participation."[27] Participation in leisure and social activities is intrinsically motivating to the individual and does not require commitment to obligatory time, such as with work, self-care, or sleep. Participation in such activities facilitates balance and self-esteem and can reduce stress. Many communities have adapted sports and leisure programs that support clients with disabilities.

KNOWING YOUR CO-PILOT—COLLABORATION WITH THE OCCUPATIONAL THERAPIST

A team member of primary importance, whatever the context of services, is the supervising occupational therapist. The occupational therapist performs evaluation of the client, writes up the treatment plan, and establishes goals. Although the OTA may be the primary individual providing OT services, it is important that the OTA not pursue the journey alone. Regular communication with the occupational therapist about the client's progress, the family's involvement, and the client's successes and challenges along the way are important.

REFLECTING ON THE JOURNEY—PUTTING IT ALL TOGETHER

The trip, with all its planning, is finally ready to begin! It is the OT practitioner's privilege to be involved with young adults and adults with disabilities as they transition from the familiarity of life routines and services in their childhood to the new challenges of adulthood, and it is an exciting journey for an OTA. While on this journey, it is important to remember the things discussed in this chapter. First, the OTA must pack for the journey—that is, have knowledge of the condition(s) that the client has because these conditions can impact the client's ability to engage in meaningful occupations. Second, the OTA must navigate through the resources to know what support and rights apply to the client. Third, the OTA must anticipate and understand the individual's difficulties and needs. These factors impact functioning differently in different contexts and may be something no other professional has picked up on. Last, the OTA should work collaboratively with the client and his or her family and the supervising occupational therapist to achieve the overarching goal of OT—enabling the client's occupational performance. As the OTA travels along this journey, he or she will continue to explore new resources available to enhance skills and knowledge of occupational performance. Good luck on the journey!

REVIEW QUESTIONS

1. A 23-year-old adult who uses a wheelchair for mobility is going to have lunch at the cafeteria, which is in the oldest building on campus. When the student gets to the building, she notices an updated entrance that has an automatic door. This entrance allows her to enter the building independently. Which law was *most likely* the basis of this entrance being installed?
   a. Individuals with Disabilities Education Act
   b. Rehabilitation Act—Section 504
   c. Americans with Disabilities Act
   d. Higher Education Opportunity Act
2. A client is in a work setting where the required task is to press a button when the bell rings. The client is taught this task and is responding well initially. However, after a few minutes, the client stops pressing the button when the bell rings. The supervisor is puzzled because the client does not appear distressed and has not moved from the work area. What is the *most likely* explanation that the OTA can provide for this behavior on the basis of a sensory processing framework?
   a. The client is an auditory avoider and needs to get away from the stimulus.
   b. The client is an auditory bystander and has habituated to the stimulus.
   c. The client is an auditory seeker and needs more rings to respond.
   d. The client is an auditory sensor and needs the stimulus to be minimized.
3. An OTA is working with a client with DMD who has legal independence. The family does not agree with the decision the client is making regarding areas of importance for OT treatment. What is the *best* approach that the OTA can take in this situation?
   a. The client is independent and can make his own choices; the OTA should act in accordance with the client's decisions.
   b. The family has an important role in the client's life and should be allowed to overrule the client's decision.
   c. The OTA should hear from both the family and the client and make a decision based on the best argument.
   d. The OTA should take the concerns back to the supervising occupational therapist and discuss the options and legal issues.
4. A student who has DS and is in high school, receives special education services and has an established IEP. At what age is transition planning first required to occur and the student invited to be involved in team meetings and planning for future after high school?
   a. 14 years
   b. 16 years
   c. 18 years
   d. 21 years

5. A 26-year-old adult with ASD is expressing interest in learning to drive. Within OT, the OTA attempts some activities that would be important for driving and community mobility preparation. Which three of the following activities would be the *most* appropriate for the OTA to do for the client?
   a. Conducting visual perceptual and visual motor assessments to evaluate if these skills are adequate for driving
   b. Having the client follow a map in the local shopping mall to see if the client can locate requested stores in the mall
   c. Allowing the client to drive in an empty parking lot to look for appropriate sequencing of driving tasks
   d. Referring the client to a driving rehabilitation specialist to address any intervention related to driving
   e. Working with the client on identifying different road signs related to driving and safety
   f. Teaching the client to read a public bus schedule and plan for travel between points of interest
6. Anxiety is a common diagnosis across the lifespan of individuals with disabilities. Why is it important for an OTA to be aware of its presence when treating a client with a musculoskeletal condition?
   a. Anxiety is often coupled with physical health impairments.
   b. Anxiety causes physical pain that must be considered.
   c. Anxiety may limit an individual's willingness to take pain medications.
   d. Anxiety decreases a client's muscle strength and endurance.
7. The diagnosis of ASD must include deficits in social communication and interaction and what other component?
   a. Sensory processing difficulties
   b. Repetitive behaviors
   c. Learning disability
   d. Fine motor coordination challenges
8. A young adult with ADHD of the hyperactive/impulsive type is working with an OTA on vocational tasks to prepare to work in a fast food restaurant setting. Which three of the following situations should the OTA expect might be issues based on the diagnosis?
   a. Starting a task before directions are given
   b. Not recalling multiple step directions
   c. Excessive talking at inappropriate times
   d. Difficulty organizing necessary tasks
   e. Not consistently completing activities
   f. Fidgeting with nearby items
9. A client with CF mentions concerns regarding sexual intimacy with a partner. What must the OTA determine *first* when approaching this topic with the client?
   a. What positions are optimal for someone with decreased lung capacity
   b. What strategies have been ineffective for the client
   c. What adaptive equipment is available and affordable
   d. What the client and family's cultural beliefs are
10. The OTA is working with a young adult who wants to be more involved socially with peers. The OTA is aware that this individual is an avoider. Keeping this in mind, what is the *most likely* reason the OTA will consider for the individual not getting out of the car to join a pool party with peers?
   a. Poor self-image regarding swim attire
   b. Limited understanding of social cues
   c. Overwhelming sounds from the event
   d. Discomfort with own swimming abilities

CASE STUDY

OTAs learn that every client they work with hold a special place in their hearts and teach memorable lessons along the way. One of my most memorable clients is Mckenzie. Mckenzie has autism, a mild cognitive impairment, and low muscle tone in her upper extremities.

Mckenzie is a sweet, hard-working student and is always eager to please. She has a number of friends at her current high school and has become an individual who demonstrates independence and confidence. When Mckenzie first started her 10th grade year, there were a number of areas that required OT intervention.

Biomechanical:

When the intervention began, Mckenzie required assistance from OT for completing basic work tasks related to her body position in space and body awareness, crossing the midline, sequencing, strength, endurance, and speed. Functionally, Mckenzie was unable to sweep with a broom; wipe a table from one end to the other effectively; or complete classroom tasks, such as using a three-hole punch or opening and closing her binders without requiring physical assistance. She had difficulty sequencing the steps of a task or understanding how to move her body appropriately to complete the task. Currently, Mckenzie is independently completing all of the school-based activities required of her. She is able to use tools to complete jobs and has become a role model for other students. This is because Mckenzie has had enough training and repetition in each area for her body to learn and understand how to move and function. The biomechanical piece of completing a functional task is only one part of a complex process.

Student Role/Social/Communication:

Mckenzie is a student who always wants to please her teachers and peers and works very hard to assist them when she can. Mckenzie has been working on self-determination skills, confidence in making decisions, communicating her wants and needs, and asking for help when needed. She has a nice group of friends, eats with them during lunch, and tells a good joke now and then. She is a pleasure to be around. Although Mckenzie needs to continue working on her social and communication-related skills, she has made tremendous progress. She makes independent suggestions during class, volunteers to help others without needing to be asked, and expresses her opinions. She is becoming her own person and a self-advocate for what she needs and wants.

Graphic Communication:

Mckenzie's handwriting lacks legibility, and she requires additional time to complete hand-written assignments. At school, Mckenzie has been able to work with her teachers on completing assignments. She works with peers to copy models and examples and uses the computer as much as possible. Using basic computer skills and computer programs has become a major focus with Mckenzie this past year and has become her preference. She is making progress but continues to require assistance to complete her work.

Work:

Mckenzie demonstrates confidence, pride, and accomplishment, which are the most important qualities for work. She is a loved member of the student body in her high school. As part of the Occupational Course of Study Program, Mckenzie continues to put in her school-based and community-based hours to earn her high school diploma. She has just recently demonstrated independence with school-based jobs, but the same tasks are much more difficult for her to do in a new environment. She requires one-to-one assistance from an adult for each step of a multistep task during community outings with her class. Learning how to complete a task, with practice and expectations, is easier than developing the confidence and pride.

Postsecondary Options:

The Transition Plan in Mckenzie's IEP takes into consideration that Mckenzie wants to go to college, live with a roommate, and work as a receptionist in a pediatrician's office. To help Mckenzie learn work skills that would be useful in an office, she is assisting the business manager in the front office of her school with answering the school phone, taking messages, making photocopies, greeting visitors, and completing some basic filing. In her life skills course, Mckenzie works closely with her teacher and the OT practitioner on financial management skills, meal preparation and cooking, housekeeping, and transportation options. She has been referred to a vocational rehabilitation agency and will be starting on career exploration soon. Mckenzie is currently completing her 11th grade year and is looking forward to the 12th grade.

1. Identify two interventions that may have been used to address Mckenzie's skill deficits in the biomechanical area.
2. Identify three additional skills not mentioned in the case described above that would be important for Mckenzie to demonstrate to be successful in the career she would like to pursue.
3. On the basis of the information presented in this chapter, what unforeseen hurdles may Mckenzie face as she transitions from high school into the work setting?

PUTTING IT ALL TOGETHER Sample Treatment and Documentation

Setting	Inpatient rehabilitation center
Client Profile	49 y/o male with a L femur fracture at the joint with hip replacement surgery due to a fall. Past history of Cerebral Palsy with use of walker for stability. Client was reaching to pick up an item off the floor and fell. In acute hospital for 2 days, then sent to rehab. Precautions: Full hip precautions with non-weight-bearing in LLE
Work History	Owns an insurance company with 3 employees. Works full time in the office.
Insurance	Private insurance
Psychological	History of anxiety, controlled with minimal medication taken regularly
Social	Lives with wife and two sons in a ranch home with zero entry. Enjoys going to son's sporting events as well as professional sporting events
Cognitive	No deficits
Motor & Manual Muscle Testing (MMT)	R handed RUE: 5/5 throughout LUE: 5/5 throughout, mild increased tone during mobility tasks RLE: 5/5 with slightly internally rotated at hip with ambulation LLE: NT
ADL	Grooming: Independent Bathing: Mod A shower seat Upper Body Dressing: Independent Lower Body Dressing: Mod A Feeding: Independent Toileting: Mod A Toilet Transfers: Mod A
IADL	Shares chores with spouse, riding lawnmower for yard, sits on walker seat for some cooking
Goals	Within 2 weeks: 1. Client will be Mod I with all ADLs while following hip precautions. 2. Client will be Mod I with all transfers and mobility during ADL and IADL tasks. 3. Client will demonstrate safety awareness during ADL and IADL tasks with Mod I and use of adaptive equipment for fall prevention.

OT TREATMENT SESSION 1

THERAPEUTIC ACTIVITY	TIME	GOAL(S) ADDRESSED	OTA RATIONALE
Bed mobility and transfer to wheelchair while following hip precautions, and training on the same.	10 min	#2, #3	*Education and Training; Occupations:* Engaging in the actual bed mobility and transfer will increase carryover for safety and hip precautions. OTA will assess the client as he rolls and moves for recall and performance in functional tasks.
Client to perform morning ADL program, including toileting, bathing, grooming and dressing. Focus on following hip precautions and safety awareness during all tasks.	45 min	#1, #2, #3	*Education and Training; Occupations:* Engaging in the actual tasks will increase carryover for safety and hip precautions. OTA will assess the client's recall and performance in functional tasks.

PUTTING IT ALL TOGETHER Sample Treatment and Documentation (continued)

SOAP note: 11/24/—, 7:00 am–7:55 am

S: Client supine in bed, client noted he was tired, but ready to learn enough to go home.

O: Client participated in OT session in room to address bed mobility, transfers, and ADL performance while adhering to hip precautions and safety. He was able to roll in bed with Min A and Min cues to fully follow hip precautions. He noted pain at 4/10 with movement, but had just received pain medications from nursing staff. Supine to sit with Min A, and transfer to wheelchair with Mod A to keep weight fully off of LLE. Client performed toilet transfer to higher commode with Mod A, and Min cues to maintain hip precautions during toilet hygiene. Client able to complete grooming without assistance, and sponge bathe at sink from wheelchair with Min A and use of long sponge and reacher to manage towel for drying. Client donned UB clothing independently, LB clothing with Min A, Min cues and use of reacher, dressing stick, sock aid, long shoehorn, and slip-on shoes for completion.

A: Client receptive to adaptive equipment for improved function. He did require cues for hip precautions, and OTA will put up reminders near bed and in bathroom of the precautions. Client does require cues for all steps of ADL and mobility process including non-weight-bearing for safety awareness. Client will continue to benefit from OT services to progress functional independence related to all goals.

P: Continue OT plan of care daily to address ADL/IADL performance, safety and hip precautions, and continue to provide client education and training in to ensure ability to return home.

Emily Rheinbolt, COTA/L, 11/24/—, 12:35 pm

TREATMENT SESSION 2

What could you do next with this client?

TREATMENT SESSION 3

What could you do next with this client?

REFERENCES

1. Stewart, D. A., Law, M. C., Rosenbaum, P., & Williams, D. G. (2001). A qualitative study of the transition to adulthood for youth with physical disabilities. *Physical & Occupational Therapy in Pediatrics, 21*, 3–21.
2. American Psychiatric Association. (2013). *Diagnostic and statistical manual of mental disorders* (5th ed.). Washington, DC: Author.
3. Copeland, W. E., Angold, A., Shanahan, L., & Costello, E. J. (2014). Longitudinal patterns of anxiety from childhood to adulthood: The great smoky mountains study. *Journal of the American Academy of Child & Adolescent Psychiatry, 53*(1), 21–33.
4. Asselmann, E., & Beesdo-Baum, K. (2015). Predictors of the course of anxiety disorders in adolescents and young adults. *Current Psychiatry Report, 17*(7), 1–8. doi:10.1007/s11920-014-0543-z
5. Maldonado, L., Huang, Y., Chen, R., Kasen, S., Cohen, P., & Chen, H. (2013). Impact of early adolescent anxiety disorders on self-esteem development from adolescence to young adulthood. *Journal of Adolescent Health, 53*, 287–292. doi:10.1016/j.jadohealth.2013.02.025
6. Howlin, P., & Moss, P., (2012). Adults with autism spectrum disorders. *The Canadian Journal of Psychiatry, 57*(5), 275–283.
7. Kao, Y. C., Kramer, J. M., Liljenquist, K., & Coster, W. J. (2014). Association between impairment, function, and daily life task management in children and adolescents with autism. *Developmental Medicine & Child Neurology, 57*, 68–74. doi:10.1111/dmcn.12562
8. Graetz, J. E. (2010). Autism grows up: Opportunities for adults with autism. *Disability & Society, 25*(1), 33–47. doi:10.1080/09687590903363324
9. Manente, C. J., Maraventano, J. C., LaRue, R. H., Delmolino, L., & Sloan, D. (2010). Effective behavioral intervention for adults on the autism spectrum: Best practices in functional assessment and treatment development. *The Behavior Analyst Today, 11*, 36–48.
10. Kessler, R. C., Berglund, P. A., Demler, O., Jin, R., & Walters, E. E. (2005). Lifetime prevalence and age-of-onset distributions of DSM-IV disorders in the National Comorbidity Survey Replication. *Archives of General Psychiatry, 62*(6), 593–602.
11. Asherson, P., Akehurst, R., Kooij, J. J. S., Huss, M., Beusterien, K., Sasane, R., ... & Hodgkins, P. (2012). Under diagnosis of adult ADHD: Cultural influences and societal burden. *Journal of Attention Disorders, Supplement 16*(5), 20S–38S. doi:10.1177/1087054711435360
12. Weiss, N. (2011). Assessment and treatment of ADHD in adults. *Psychiatric Annals, 41*(1), 23–31.
13. Valentine, S., & Kennedy, B. L. (2012). Recognizing and treating adult ADHD. *The Nurse Practitioner, 37*(3), 41–46.
14. Ryden, E., Thase, M. E., Straht, D., Adberg-Wistedt, A., Bejerot, S., & Landen, M. (2009). A history of childhood attention-deficit hyperactivity disorder (ADHD) impacts clinical outcome in adult bipolar patients regardless of current ADHD. *Acta Psychiatrica Scandinavica, 120*, 239–246.
15. Gjervan, B., Torgersen, T., Nordahl, H. M., & Rasmussen, K. (2012). Functional impairment and occupational outcome in adults with ADHD. *Journal of Attention Disorders, 16*(7), 544–552. doi:10.1177/1087054711413074
16. Garcia, C. R., Bau, C. H. D., Silva, K. L., Callegari-Jacques, S. M., Salgado, C. A. I., Fischer, A. G., ... & Grevet, E. H. (2012). The burdened life of adults with ADHD: Impairment beyond comorbidity. *European Psychiatry, 27*, 309–313.
17. Koemans, R. G., van Vroenhoven, S., Karreman, A., & Bekker, M. H. J. (2015). Attachment with autonomy problems in adults with ADHD. *Journal of Attention Disorders, 19*(5), 435–446. doi:10.1177/1087054712453170
18. Mäntlylä, T., Still, J., Gullberg, S., & Del Missier, F. (2012). Decision making in adults with ADHD. *Journal of Attention Disorders, 16*(2), 164–173. doi:10.1177/1087054709360494
19. Lensing, M. B., Zeiner, P., Sandvik, L., & Opjordsmoen, S. (2015). Quality of life in adults aged 50+ with ADHD. *Journal of Attention Disorders 19*(5), 405–413. doi:10.1177/1087054713480035
20. Koman, L. A. (2004). Cerebral palsy. *The Lancet, 363*, 1619–1631.
21. Blackman, J. A., & Conaway, M. R. (2014). Adolescents with cerebral palsy: Transitioning to adult health care services. *Clinical Pediatrics, 53*(4), 356–363. doi:10.1177/0009922813510203
22. Lariviere-Bastien, D. L., Bell, E., Majnemer, A., Shevell, M., & Racine, E. (2013). Perspectives of young adults with cerebral palsy on

transitioning from pediatric to adult healthcare systems. *Seminars in Pediatric Neurology, 20*(2), 154–159. doi:10.1016/j.spen.2013.06.009

23. Frisch, D., & Msall, M. E. (2013). Health, functioning, and participation of adolescents and adults with cerebral palsy: A review of outcomes research. *Developmental Disabilities Research Reviews, 18,* 84–94.
24. Murphy, K. P. (2010). The adult with cerebral palsy. *Orthopedic Clinics of North America, 41,* 595–605. doi:10.1016/j.ocl.2010.06.007
25. Pimm, P. L. (1996). Some of the implications of caring for a child or adult with cerebral palsy. *British Journal of Occupational Therapy, 59*(7), 335–341.
26. Phipps, S., & Roberts, P. (2012). Predicting the effects of cerebral palsy severity on self-care, mobility, and social function. *The American Journal of Occupational Therapy, 66*(4), 422–429. doi:10.5014/ajot.2012.003921
27. American Occupational Therapy Association. (2014). Occupational therapy practice framework: Domain & process (3rd ed.). *American Journal of Occupational Therapy, 68,* S1–S48. doi:10.5014/ajot.2014.682006
28. Geurts, H. M., & Vissers, M. E. (2012). Elderly with autism: Executive functions and memory. *Journal of Autism and Developmental Disorders, 42,* 665–675.
29. Morgan, P., & McGinley, J. (2014). Gait function and decline in adults with cerebral palsy: A systematic review. *Disability and Rehabilitation, 36*(1), 1–9.
30. Balandin, S., Berg, N., & Waller, A. (2006). Assessing the loneliness of older people with cerebral palsy. *Disability and Rehabilitation, 28*(8), 469–479.
31. Hurt, K., & Bilton, D. (2012). Cystic fibrosis. *Medicine, 40,* 273–276.
32. O'Sullivan, B. P., & Freedman, S. D. (2009). Cystic fibrosis. *The Lancet, 373,* 1891–1904. doi:10.1016/S0140-6736(09)60327-5
33. Edwards, J., Clarke, A., & Greenop, D. (2013). Adults with cystic fibrosis—Responding to a new ageing population. *Chronic Illness, 9,* 312–319. doi:10.1177/1742395313479982
34. Tuchman, L., & Schwartz, M. (2013). Health outcomes associated with transition from pediatric to adult cystic fibrosis care. *Pediatrics, 132,* 847–853. doi:10.1542/peds.2013-1463
35. Laborde-Casterot, H., Donnay, C., Chapron, J., Burgel, P. R., Kanaan, R., Honore, I., ... & Hubert, D. (2012). Employment and work disability in adults with cystic fibrosis. *Journal of Cystic Fibrosis, 11,* 137–143. doi:10.1016/j.jcf.2011.10.008
36. Besier, T., & Goldbeck, L. (2011). Anxiety and depression in adolescents with CF and their caregivers. *Journal of Cystic Fibrosis, 10,* 435–442. doi:10.1016/j.jcf.2011.06.012
37. Schmitz, T.G., Henrich, G., & Goldbeck, L. (2006). Quality of life with cystic fibrosis—Aspects of age and gender. *Klinische Padiatrie, 218* (1), 7–12.
38. Daunhauer, L. A., & Fidler, D. J. (2011). The Down syndrome behavioral phenotype: Implications for practice and research in occupational therapy. *Occupational Therapy in Health Care, 25,* 7–25. doi:10.3109/07380577.2010.535601
39. Roizen, N. J., & Patterson, D. (2003). Down's syndrome. *The Lancet, 361,* 1281–1289.
40. Ross, W. T., & Olsen, M. (2014). Care of the adult patient with Down syndrome. *Southern Medical Journal, 107,* 715–721.
41. Steingass, K. J., Chicoine, B., McGuire, D., & Roizen, N. J. (2011). Developmental disabilities grown up: Down syndrome. *Journal of Developmental & Behavioral Pediatrics, 32,* 548–558.
42. Foley, K. R., Jacoby, P., Girdler, S., Bourke, J., Pikora, T., Lennox, N., ... & Leonard, H. (2013). Functioning and post-school transition outcomes for young people with Down syndrome. *Child: Care, Health and Development, 39,* 789–800. doi:10.1111/cch.12019
43. Abbott, D., & Carpenter, J. (2014). "Wasting precious time": Young men with Duchenne muscular dystrophy negotiate the transition to adulthood. *Disability & Society, 29,* 1192–1205. doi:10.1080/09687599.2014.916607
44. Spies, S., Schipper, K., Nollet, F., & Abma, T. A. (2010). A patient's journey: Duchenne muscular dystrophy. *British Medical Journal, 341,* 1101–1103. doi:10.1136/bmj.c4364
45. Hamdani, Y., Mistry, B., & Gibson, B. E. (2014). Transitioning to adulthood with a progressive condition: Best practice assumptions and individual experiences of young men with Duchenne muscular dystrophy. *Disability and Rehabilitation, Early Online,* 1–8. doi:10.3109/09638288.2014.956187
46. Usark, D., King, E., Cripe, L., Spicer, R., Sage, J. Kinnet, K., ... & Varni, J. W. (2012). Health-related quality of life in children and adolescents with Duchenne muscular dystrophy. *Pediatrics, 130,* e1559–e1566. doi:10.1542/peds.2012-0858
47. Mitchell, L. E., Adzick, N. S., Melchionne, J., Pasquariello, P. S., Sutton, L N., & Whitehead, A. S. (2004). Spina bifida. *The Lancet, 364,* 1885–1895.
48. Liu, J. S., Greiman, A., Casey, J. T., Mukherjee, S., & Kielb, S. (2016). A snapshot of the adult spina bifida patient—High incidence of urologic procedures. *Central European Journal of Urology, 69,* 72–77. doi:10.5173/ceju.2016.596
49. Liptak, G. S., Kennedy, J. A., & Dosa, N. P. (2010). Youth with spina bifida and transitions: Health and social participation in a nationally represented sample. *The Journal of Pediatrics, 157*(4), 584–588. doi:10.1016/j.peds.2010.04.004
50. Young, N. L., Sheridan, K., Burke, T. A., Mukherjee, S., & McCormick, A. (2013). Health outcomes among youths and adults with spina bifida. *The Journal of Pediatrics, 162*(5), 993–998.
51. Dicianno, B. E., Kinback, N., Chaikind, L., Holmbeck, G. N., Donlan, R. M., Bellin, M. H., ... & Collins, D. M. (2015). Depressive symptoms in adults with spina bifida. *Rehabilitation Psychology, 60*(3), 246–253. doi:10.1037/rep0000044
52. Ridosh, M., Braun, P., Roux, G., Bellin, M., & Sawin, K. (2011). Transition in young adults with spina bifida: A qualitative study. *Child: Care, Health and Development, 37*(6), 866–874. doi:10.1111/j.1365-2214.2011.01329.x
53. Garcia, A. M., & Dicianno, B. E. (2011). The frequency of lymphedema in an adult spina bifida population. *American Journal of Physical Medicine & Rehabilitation, 90*(2), 89–96.
54. Cardenas, D. D., Topolski, T. D., White, C. J., McLaughlin, J. F., & Walker, W. O. (2008). Sexual functioning in adolescents and young adults with spina bifida. *Archives of Physical Medicine and Rehabilitation, 89,* 31–35.
55. Noritz, G. (2017). Medical management of adults with SMA. Retrieved from http://www.curesma.org/documents/support—care-documents/2017-conference-presentation.pdf
56. Dollar, C. A., Fredrick, L. D., Alberto, P. A., & Luke, J. K. (2012). Using simultaneous prompting to teach independent living and leisure skills to adults with severe intellectual disabilities. *Research in Developmental Disabilities, 33,* 189–195.
57. Juan, H. G., & Swinth, Y. (2010). As students become adults: The role of occupational therapy in the transition process. *Journal of Occupational Therapy, Schools, & Early Intervention, 3,* 255–267. doi: 10.1080/19411243.2010.520249
58. Lotan, G., & Ells, C. (2010). Adults with intellectual and developmental disabilities and participation in decision making: Ethical considerations for professional-client practice. *Intellectual and Developmental Disabilities, 48,* 112–125. doi:10.1352/1934-9556-48.2.112
59. Jackson, L. (2007). *Occupational therapy services for children and youth under IDEA.* (3rd ed.). Bethesda, MD: AOTA Press.
60. United States Department of Justice, Civil Rights Division. (2009). Information and technical assistance on the Americans with Disabilities Act. Retrieved from http://www.ada.gov
61. U. S. Department of Education. (n.d.). Building the legacy: IDEA 2004. Retrieved from http://idea.ed.gov/explore/home
62. Dosa, N. P., White, P. H., & Schuyler, V. (2013). Future expectations: Transition from adolescence to adulthood. In M. L. Batshaw, N. J. Roizen, & G. R. Lotrecchiano (Eds.), *Children with disabilities* (7th ed.). Baltimore, MD: Paul H. Brookes Publishing.
63. U. S. Department of Health and Human Services, Office for Civil Rights (2006). Your rights under section 504 of the Rehabilitation Act (fact sheet). Retrieved from http://www.hhs.gov/ocr/civilrights/resources/factsheets/504.pdf

64. American Occupational Therapy Association. (2016). Work setting trends for occupational therapy: How to choose a setting. Retrieved from http://www.aota.org/education-careers/advance-career/salary-workforce-survey/work-setting-trends-how-to-pick-choose.aspx
65. Arnold, K. (2000). *The occupational therapist's role in the high school.* Durham, NH: University of New Hampshire.
66. American Occupational Therapy Association. (2008). Transitions for children and youth how occupational therapy can help (fact sheet). Retrieved from https://www.aota.org/-/media/Corporate/Files/AboutOT/Professionals/WhatIsOT/CY/Fact-Sheets/Transitions.pdf
67. Gutman, S. A., Kerner, R., Zombek, I., Dulek, J., & Ramsey, C. A. (2009). Supported education for adults with psychiatric disabilities: Effectiveness of an occupational therapy program. *American Journal of Occupational Therapy, 63,* 245–254.
68. University of Massachusetts Boston (2015). Think college! College options for people with intellectual disabilities. Retrieved from http://www.thinkcollege.net/topics/opportunity-act
69. Association of Assistive Technology Act Programs. (n.d.). Assistive Technology Act of 1998, as amended Public Law 10-364. Retrieved from http://www.ataporg.org/summaryact.html
70. Swinth, Y. (2000). The development of self-determination by students with disabilities: What is the role of occupational therapy? *School System Special Interest Section Quarterly, 7,* 1–4.
71. American Occupational Therapy Association. (2013). Students with disabilities in post-secondary education settings: How occupational therapy can help (fact sheet). Retrieved from http://www.aota.org/-/media/Corporate/Files/AboutOT/Professionals/WhatIsOT/CY/Fact-Sheets/Post-secondary-Education.pdf
72. Toldra, R. C., & Santos, M. C. (2013). People with disabilities in the labor market: Facilitators and barriers. *Work, 45,* 553–563. doi:10.3233/WOR-131641
73. Murphy, K. P., Molnar, G. E., & Lankasky, K. (2000). Employment and social issues in adults with cerebral palsy. *Archives of Physical Medicine and Rehabilitation, 81,* 807–811.
74. USA Social Security Administration. (2012). Services for sheltered workshops (RS 02101.270). Retrieved from http://policy.ssa.gov/poms.nsf/lnx/0302101270
75. Dunn, W. (1997). The impact of sensory processing abilities on the daily lives of young children and their families: A conceptual model. *Infants and Young Children, 9*(4), 23–35.
76. Dunn, W. (2014). *Sensory profile 2: User's manual.* Bloomington, MN: PsychCorp.
77. Clince, M., Connolly, L., & Nolan, C. (2016). Comparing and exploring the sensory processing patterns of higher education students with attention deficit hyperactivity disorder and autism spectrum disorder. *American Journal of Occupational Therapy, 70,* 7002250010.
78. Brown, C., & Dunn, W. (2002). *Adolescent/adult sensory profile: User's manual.* San Antonio, TX: Pearson.
79. Mann, W. C., Kimble, C., Justiss, M. D., Casson, E., Tomita, M., & Wu, S. S. (2005). Problems with dressing in the frail elderly. *American Journal of Occupational Therapy, 59,* 398–408.
80. Reistetter, T. A., Chang, P. F. J., & Abreu, B. C. (2009). Showering habits: Time, steps, and products used after brain injury. *American Journal of Occupational Therapy, 63,* 641–645.
81. Clemson, L., Mackenzie, L., Ballinger, C., Close, J. C. T., & Cumming, R. G. (2008). Environmental interventions to prevent falls in community-dwelling older people: A meta-analysis of randomized trials. *Journal of Aging and Health, 20,* 954–971. doi:10.1177/0898264308324672
82. Korp, K. E., Taylor, J. M., & Nelson, D. L. (2012). Bathing area safety and lower extremity function in community-dwelling older adults. *OTJR: Occupation, Participation and Health, 32,* 22–29. doi:10.3928/15394492-20110805-01
83. LaVesser, P., & Hilton, C. L. (2010). Self-care skills for children with an autism spectrum disorder. In H. M. Kuhaneck & R. Watling (Eds.), *Autism: A Comprehensive Occupational Therapy Approach* (3rd ed). Bethesda, MD: AOTA Press.
84. Boczko, F. & Feightner, K. (2007). Dysphagia in the older adult: The roles of speech-language pathologists and occupational therapists. *Topics in Geriatric Rehabilitation, 23,* 220–227.
85. D'Amico, M., & Cahill, S. M. (2015). Addressing sexuality with individuals with developmental disabilities and their families across the lifespan. *Developmental Disabilities Special Interest Section Quarterly, 38,* 1–3.
86. Hattjar, B., Parker, J. A., & Lappa, C. L. (2008). Addressing sexuality with adult clients with chronic disabilities: Occupational therapy's role. *OT Practice, 13*(11), CE-1–CE-8.
87. Sullivan, A., & Caterino, L. C. (2008). Addressing the sexuality and sex education of individuals with autism spectrum disorders. *Education and Treatment of Children, 31,* 381–394. doi:10.1353/etc.0.0001
88. Koller, R. (2000). Sexuality and adolescents with autism. *Sexuality and Disability, 18,* 125–135.
89. Strzelecki, M. V. (2011). Green light go: Helping teens with disabilities take the wheel. *OT Practice, 16,* 8–19.
90. Cox, D. J., Madaan, V., & Cox, B. S. (2011). Adult attention-deficit/hyperactivity disorder and driving: Why and how to manage it. *Current Psychiatry Reports, 13,* 345–350. doi:10.1007/s11920-011-0216-0
91. American Occupational Therapy Association. (2012). The occupational therapy role in driving and community mobility across the lifespan (fact sheet). Retrieved from http://www.aota.org/-/media/Corporate/Files/AboutOT/Professionals/WhatIsOT/CY/Fact-Sheets/Driving.pdf
92. U. S. Department of Education, Office for Civil Rights. (2011). *Students with disabilities preparing for post-secondary education.* Retrieved from http://www2.ed.gov/about/offices/list/ocr/transition.html
93. U. S. Department of Education. (2014). Programs: Vocational rehabilitation state grants. Received from http://www2.ed.gov/programs/rsabvrs/index.html
94. Clark, K. (2010). 8 steps for learning disabled students who want to go to college. Retrieved from http://www.usnews.com/education/articles/2010/12/02/8-steps-for-learning-disabled-students-who-want-to-go-to-college
95. U. S. Department of Education. (2015). U.S. high school graduation rate hits new record high. Retrieved from http://www.ed.gov/news/press-releases/us-high-school-graduation-rate-hits-new-record-high
96. U. S. Department of Education, Institute of Education Sciences, National Center for Education Statistics. (2015). Retrieved from https://nces.ed.gov/
97. Project 10: Transition Education Network. (2015). Identifying post-secondary options. Retrieved from http://project10.info/DetailPage.php?MainPageID=196&PageCategory=Post-secondary%20Education&PageSubCategory=
98. United States Department of Labor. (n.d.). Disability resources: Americans with disabilities act. Retrieved from http://www.dol.gov/dol/topic/disability/ada.htm

ACKNOWLEDGMENTS

The authors would like to thank Megan Inman, MLIS, Research Assistant Professor at East Carolina University, for her assistance and expertise in locating relevant research articles used in the development of this chapter.

Lines, Leads, and Tubes

Melissa D. Brawley, MS, OTR/L

Lines, Leads, Tubes: Vascular

	LOCATION	PURPOSE	REHABILITATION PRECAUTIONS
Arterial Line (A-line)	• Radial or femoral placement • Accurate reading when level with the right atrium of the heart	• Used for constant monitoring of systolic and diastolic blood pressure	• Monitor waveform, avoid decreased amplitude with changes in position, ROM • If dislodged, hold strong pressure over site with sterile gauze, notify nurse
Central Venous Catheter	• Subclavian, jugular, or femoral vein placement and travels directly to the heart • Tip is 2 cm above the right atrium	• Used to monitor central venous pressure (CVP); administer drugs, fluids, and blood; and obtain venous blood	• Do not kink catheter. • Routine range of motion (ROM) can be performed without restriction. • If dislodged, hold pressure over site with sterile gauze, notify nurse
IV Tubing and Pumps	• Central or peripheral insertion sites	• Used to deliver medications, IV nutrition, blood, or fluids at a prescribed rate	• Ensure adequate slack for ROM and mobility. • Notify nurse of alarm
Patient Controlled Analgesia (PCA)	• Placed with peripheral IV or epidural catheter	• IV pain pump used by the client to assist with pain management	• Clients with epidural catheters may have decreased strength and sensation in lower extremities; assess appropriately.
Permacath or Mediport	• Large external catheter that is inserted into a large central vein of the chest or arm	• Provides long-term vascular access for dialysis or chemotherapy	• Do not break or dislodge.
Peripherally Inserted Central Catheter (PICC)	• Inserted into the brachial vein and travels through the axillary vein • Empties into the superior vena cava	• Used for long-term administration of antibiotics and/or total parenteral nutrition (TPN)	• Make sure sterile dressing over insertion site remains dry and intact. • Avoid taking blood pressure in the extremity with the line present.
Pulmonary Artery Catheter (Swan-Ganz or PA Catheter)	• Commonly inserted into the subclavian or internal jugular veins then through the heart to the pulmonary artery • Has plastic sheath around catheter and is usually colored	• Calculates a variety of pressures and volumes including pulmonary artery pressure • Small balloon at end of catheter may be temporarily inflated to measure cardiac output and fluid balance	• Assure PA catheter is not in wedge or balloon-inflated position; do not dislodge • Monitor waveform before and during therapy treatment • Routine ROM, mobility, and positioning may be performed without restriction.

Lines, Leads, Tubes: Cardiopulmonary (Pulmonary)

	LOCATION	PURPOSE	REHABILITATION PRECAUTIONS
Chest Tube	• Commonly placed for removal of air: second, third, or fourth intercostal space • Commonly placed for removal of fluid: sixth, seventh, or eighth intercostal space	• Used for treatment of pneumothorax, hemothorax, pleural effusion, empyema, bronchopleural fistula, and mediastinal fluid • Used for removal of fluid or blood in the pleural or mediastinal space	• Keep chamber below insertion site to prevent backflow • Avoid pulling, disconnecting, or kinking. • If dislodged, stop activity, notify nurse, and apply pressure over site with sterile gauze; monitor vital signs.
Pumpless Extracorporeal Lung Assist/ Extracorporeal Membrane Oxygenation (pECLA, ECMO)	• Venovenous or arteriovenous access ports	• Indicated for clients with reversible cardiac or pulmonary failure • Oxygenates the blood and removes carbon dioxide outside of the body; may assist heart in circulating blood	• Need physician clearance for ROM in extremity with access ports • Use extreme care not to dislodge cannula. • Monitor vital signs and laboratory results.
Pigtail Catheter	• Usually pericardial • May drain into a chamber, Foley, or ostomy bag	• Similar to a chest tube, smaller lumen • Used to drain fluid over a longer period of time	• Keep chamber below insertion site to prevent backflow • Avoid pulling, disconnecting, or kinking.

Lines, Leads, Tubes: Cardiopulmonary (Cardiac)

	LOCATION	PURPOSE	REHABILITATION PRECAUTIONS
Ventricular Assist Device (VAD)	• Interabdominal or intraabdominal pump • Valve inserted into the left ventricle and outflows to the ascending aorta (HeartMate™ product)	• Indicated to assist function of the right, left, or both ventricles to circulate blood for clients who are awaiting a heart transplant, in refractory cardiogenic shock, persistent ventricular failure with an alternative to heart transplant	• Specialized education and skills competency required before treating clients with a VAD • Monitor vital signs and output rates of device • Monitor device line at all times. • Always check battery power before treatment.
Temporary Pacemaker	• Threaded through the internal jugular or femoral artery to the heart, where electrodes are placed directly on the heart muscle	• Indicated for clients who require temporary pacing of heart rate	• Client on bedrest if pacemaker is located in the femoral artery • Wires can pull out easily; avoid tension and kinking. • ROM of limb or cervical spine is generally restricted. • Client on bedrest for 3 hours after wires are pulled to assure absence of cardiac tamponade

Lines, Leads, Tubes: Genitourinary

	LOCATION	PURPOSE	REHABILITATION PRECAUTIONS
Gastrostomy Tube/ Percutaneous Endoscopic Gastrostomy Tube (G-Tube, PEG Tube)	• Percutaneous endoscopic gastrostomy (PEG) tube is most commonly used and inserted endoscopically to the stomach	• Provides enteral feeding, supplemental nutrition; administers medications and fluid • Can be used for drainage of gastric contents	• Tube feeds may be disconnected by nurse for therapy; must be reconnected • Apply abdominal binder loosely to prevent accidental dislodging of tube. • If dislodged, find nursing staff to reinsert immediately—hole starts to close quickly; if at home, insert new tube in stoma if possible or reinsert/ tape old one in stoma temporarily

Continued

Lines, Leads, Tubes: Genitourinary (continued)

	LOCATION	PURPOSE	REHABILITATION PRECAUTIONS
Jejunostomy Tube (J-Tube)	• Enters the jejunum instead of the stomach	• Provides enteral feeding, administration of medications and fluid, or drainage	• Same as above
Orogastric Tube or Nasogastric Tube (OGT, NGT)	• Orogastric tube enters through the mouth and reaches to the stomach • Nasogastric tube enters through the nose to the stomach	• Used to administer nutrition, fluid, or medications • Large-bore tubes allow for drainage of gastric contents either to gravity or suction	• Can be disconnected with nurse approval • Secure tubing to prevent dislodging. • Tube feeds should be held when head of the bed is less than 30 degrees to prevent aspiration
Dobhoff Tube (DHT)	• Enters through the nose to the stomach	• Small-bore feeding tube used to administer nutrition, fluid, or medications • Preferred due to the low risk for developing sinusitis and tissue breakdown of the nares	• Same as above • May require flushing by the nurse to prevent clogging after being disconnected
Duval or Abdominal Drain	• Usually placed in the pancreatic bed	• Used for fluid drainage following abdominal surgery	• Avoid tugging on tubing. • Keep drainage bag below the level of insertion.
Ostomy Components	• Colostomy bag is located over the stoma site at the large intestine or colon • Ileostomy bag is located over the stoma site at the small intestine or ileum	• Used for stool collection	• Consider asking the nurse to empty contents of the bag before activity to prevent detachment or leakage.
Rectal Catheter	• Placed in the rectum	• Used for drainage and collection of stool	• Avoid dislodging during activity.

Lines, Leads, Tubes: Integumentary

	LOCATION	PURPOSE	REHABILITATION PRECAUTIONS
Hemovac	• Near surgical incision site	• Used postoperatively to collect drainage • Spring-activated chamber provides low-pressure suction for active drainage	• Avoid tugging. • Clip to clothing or gown with activity
Jackson-Pratt Drain (JP Drain)	• Near surgical incision site	• Used for drainage collection • When compressed, the chamber creates low-pressure suction for active drainage.	• Avoid tension and tugging. • Secure collection bag to gown, or place in a telemetry pouch for easy management during activity
Wound Vac Dressing/ System	• Over a deep, extensive wound or graft/flap site • Black sponge in wound, sealed by clear plastic with suction tubing attached	• Negative pressure system is used to provide an optimal wound-healing environment.	• Suction unit may be unplugged from wall outlet and operate off of battery power for short periods during activity.

Lines, Leads, Tubes: Dialysis Access

	LOCATION	PURPOSE	REHABILITATION PRECAUTIONS
Arteriovenous Fistula or Graft	• Common sites include forearm (radial artery to cephalic vein) and leg (posterior tibial artery to long saphenous vein)	• Used as a vascular access site for long-term hemodialysis management	• Do not take blood pressure on this extremity. • If dialysis is ongoing, specific physician orders are needed for activity.
Continuous Arteriovenous or Venovenous Hemodialysis	• Vas cath or permacath site • Subclavian, jugular, or femoral veins are common locations for ports	• Used for continuous renal replacement therapy • Hemofilter and dialyzer serve as an artificial kidney. • Used for clients who are critically ill to manage fluid and electrolyte imbalances	• ROM usually limited to 90 degrees shoulder flexion and abduction for clients with axillary access • Monitor vital signs and respiratory status. • Need physician order for functional mobility with ongoing dialysis
Peritoneal Dialysis	• Flexible catheter tube is placed in the abdomen	• Used for home dialysis treatment • Dialysis is manually instilled and drained into the peritoneum.	• Monitor respiratory status, as there is direct pressure placed on the diaphragm.

Lines, Leads, Tubes: Neurological

	LOCATION	PURPOSE	REHABILITATION PRECAUTIONS
Intracranial Pressure Monitor	• Subarachnoid or subdural space for bolt or screw • Epidural sensory may be used as is located in the epidural space • Camio bolt is placed in subdural, subarachnoid, intraventricular, or intraparenchymal location.	• Measures intracranial pressure (ICP), allows for fluid removal or medication administration • Pressure is equal to the pressure exerted by the brain matter, blood, and cerebrospinal fluid (CSF) against the skull. • Normal ICP is 0–15 mmHg.	• Do not pull, kink, or put pressure on the device. • Hold or stop treatment if ICPs rise greater than 20 mmHg or different value communicated by the physician or nurse • Client will likely be on bedrest
Ventriculostomy or Intraventricular Catheter	• Placed in the anterior horn of lateral ventricle of the nondominant hemisphere • Connects to transducer and to drainage bag for CSF collection	• System is either open and draining or clamped and works on a pressure gradient so that when there is an increase in pressure from CSF, it can drain.	• Must clamp for activity or any change in position • Clamping the drain changes the amount of drainage and must be a physician order; nurse will perform clamping
Lumbar Drain	• Placed at L3-4 or L4-5 in most cases • May be inserted during a lumbar puncture procedure	• Used to drain CSF	• Do not pull or kink. • Must be clamped by nurse
Cisternal or Subdural Drains	• Cisternal drain is located at the base of the skull. • Subdural drain is located within the subdural space.	• Used to drain blood or CSF	• Do not pull or kink. • Must be clamped by nurse

Lines, Leads, Tubes: Respiratory

	LOCATION	PURPOSE	REHABILITATION PRECAUTIONS
Nasal Cannula	• Oxygen tubing in the nares	• Provides oxygen • Used for 1–6 liters of O_2	• Manage tubing away from client's feet to prevent falls • Watch kinks and pulling. • Use O_2 carrier and tank for distance longer than tubing attached to the wall
Nonrebreather Mask	• Oxygen mask located over the client's nose and mouth	• Gives 60%–100% oxygen • Allows for no rebreathing of expired air	• Generally an indication of respiratory distress • Check with nurse before treating as the client likely has no reserve for activity.
Endotracheal Tube (ETT) or Nasotracheal Tube (NTT)	• Artificial airway is placed into the client's trachea via the mouth or nose, respectively, which terminates approximately 2 cm from the carina.	• Process of placing the ETT is called *intubation* • Process of removing the ETT is called *extubation* • Provides mechanical ventilation through ventilator support	• Make sure ETT is not accidentally pulled as the cuff that holds it in place could damage the vocal cords. • Safe to complete all activity to client tolerance • Monitor vital signs.
Tracheostomy Tube	• Tracheal stoma site is placed surgically. • Tracheostomy tube is placed within the stoma to bypass the upper airway (nose and mouth).	• To easily and safely provide increased ventilation and deliver oxygen to the lungs • To bypass an obstructed upper airway • To clear out secretions	• Make sure tube remains secure during treatment • Monitor secretions coughed out of the tube, and report to nurse as appropriate.
Trach Collar	• Collar is placed over the client's tracheostomy tube.	• To provide humidified oxygenation	• Make sure collar remains over the tracheostomy tube and does not become disconnected from the wall or water-collection bag
Venturi	• Tracheal stoma site is placed surgically. • Tracheostomy tube is placed within the stoma to bypass the upper airway (nose and mouth).	• To easily and safely provide increased ventilation and deliver oxygen to the lungs • To bypass an obstructed upper airway • To clear out secretions	• Make sure tube remains secure during treatment • Monitor secretions coughed out of the tube, and report to nurse as appropriate.

Answers to Review Questions

CHAPTER 1

1. B, D, E
2. D
3. B
4. B
5. C
6. A
7. A, B, F
8. C
9. B
10. D

CHAPTER 2

1. B
2. D
3. B, D, E
4. A
5. B, C, F
6. A
7. A
8. D
9. D
10. B

CHAPTER 3

1. C
2. A
3. B
4. B
5. B, E, F
6. B
7. A
8. D
9. D
10. A, C, D

CHAPTER 4

1. B, E, F
2. B
3. A, D, E
4. A
5. D
6. A, B, D
7. C
8. D
9. B
10. C

CHAPTER 5

1. A, B, E
2. C
3. A, C, E
4. C
5. A
6. C
7. B
8. A
9. D
10. C

CHAPTER 6

1. A
2. B
3. C, E, F
4. B, E, F
5. C
6. C
7. B
8. A
9. D
10. C

CHAPTER 7

1. C
2. B
3. B
4. C
5. B
6. B, C, E
7. A
8. A, E, F
9. A
10. D

CHAPTER 8

1. C
2. D
3. B
4. C
5. B, C, E
6. A
7. A, B, E
8. B
9. B, D, E
10. A

CHAPTER 9

1. A, C, F
2. C
3. B
4. D
5. A, C, D
6. B
7. B
8. B
9. C
10. C

CHAPTER 10

1. A, B, D
2. A
3. C
4. D
5. A, C, F
6. B
7. C
8. B
9. B
10. A

CHAPTER 11

1. B
2. D
3. C
4. D
5. A
6. B, C, E
7. A
8. B
9. A, B, E
10. A

CHAPTER 12

1. A
2. C
3. B
4. C
5. C
6. A
7. B
8. A, D, E
9. C
10. B, C, F

CHAPTER 13

1. C
2. B
3. D
4. B
5. A
6. C
7. B
8. D
9. A, C, F
10. B, E, F

CHAPTER 14

1. A
2. A, C, D
3. C, D, E
4. B
5. D
6. B
7. D
8. A
9. C
10. C

CHAPTER 15

1. A
2. C
3. C
4. A
5. C
6. B
7. B, C, D

8. B
9. C
10. A, D, E

8. C
9. B
10. C

8. A
9. C
10. D

8. B
9. A, B, E
10. A, B, C

CHAPTER 16

1. C
2. B, D, E
3. B, E, F
4. B
5. B, E, F
6. A
7. B
8. D
9. C
10. C

CHAPTER 17

1. B, C, E
2. A
3. A, D, E
4. B
5. D
6. C
7. D
8. A, B, D
9. B
10. B

CHAPTER 18

1. C
2. C
3. C
4. C
5. C
6. C
7. B
8. A, B, D
9. A
10. C

CHAPTER 19

1. A
2. B, C, D
3. C
4. D
5. A
6. C
7. A
8. B
9. C
10. B, D. E

CHAPTER 20

1. B, C, F
2. C
3. C, E, F
4. C
5. B
6. A, C, D
7. D

CHAPTER 21

1. A, C, F
2. B, C, D
3. A, E, F
4. A
5. D
6. A
7. B
8. B
9. C
10. C

CHAPTER 22

1. B, C, E
2. C
3. B
4. B, C, E
5. A
6. A
7. B
8. A
9. D
10. A

CHAPTER 23

1. A
2. C
3. C
4. A, B, F
5. B
6. A
7. A, C, D
8. C
9. A
10. A

CHAPTER 24

1. C
2. D
3. B
4. B, C, F
5. B
6. C
7. A
8. B, C, F
9. A
10. B

CHAPTER 25

1. A
2. B, C, E
3. D
4. C
5. A
6. A, D, F
7. B

CHAPTER 26

1. A
2. A, D, E.
3. C
4. B, E, F
5. C
6. B
7. A
8. D
9. A
10. B

CHAPTER 27

1. A
2. B
3. B, D, E
4. A
5. B, C, E
6. A, C, F
7. D
8. B
9. C
10. D

CHAPTER 28

1. B
2. D
3. B
4. A, B, D
5. C
6. D
7. B
8. A
9. C
10. B, C, F

CHAPTER 29

1. C
2. A, D, F
3. A,C, D
4. D
5. B
6. B
7. A
8. B
9. B
10. A, B, E

CHAPTER 30

1. C
2. C
3. A, E, F
4. C
5. D
6. D
7. D

CHAPTER 31

1. B
2. B
3. C
4. D
5. A
6. C
7. A
8. C, E, F
9. A, B, D
10. B

CHAPTER 32

1. C
2. B
3. B
4. D
5. B
6. B, C, E
7. A
8. D
9. B
10. A, B, F

CHAPTER 33

1. C
2. B
3. B
4. A, B, C
5. C
6. B
7. B
8. B
9. A, B, C
10. D

CHAPTER 34

1. D
2. B
3. C
4. A
5. D
6. C
7. B, D, F
8. B
9. D
10. A, E, F

CHAPTER 35

1. B
2. C
3. D
4. A, E, F
5. A
6. C
7. A

8. A, D, F
9. B
10. C

CHAPTER 36

1. C
2. A, E, F
3. B
4. C
5. D
6. A, C, E
7. C
8. C
9. B
10. B

CHAPTER 37

1. C
2. B
3. D
4. B
5. B, E, F
6. A
7. B
8. A, C, F
9. D
10. C

glossary

A

Acalculia Impaired ability to calculate numbers

Accommodation Making changes so an individual has the same access to work, school, and housing as individuals without a disability experience

Acquired brain injury (ABI) Traumatic brain injury, cerebrovascular accident, brain illness, or any other brain injury acquired after birth

Acquired immunodeficiency syndrome (AIDS) The medical diagnosis assigned at the final stages of the HIV infection, when symptoms, infections, and diseases become clinically apparent (with additional indicators, such as an extremely low CD4 cell count) and as the complexity of symptoms increases to include the presence of opportunistic infections and disease(s)

Active assistive range of motion (AAROM) Joint movement that occurs when the movement of the body or any of its parts occurs partially through the individual's own efforts (or attempts at movement) and is accompanied by the aid of an individual (typically, a member of the healthcare team or a caregiver) or some device, such as an exercise machine

Active expiration A breathing technique in which clients contract the abdominal muscles while they exhale to relieve shortness of breath and improve the effectiveness of the lungs for breathing

Active range of motion (AROM) Joint movement that occurs when muscles act on the joint and cause voluntary movement such as bending the wrist up and down without any assistance from external forces; a product of muscle strength

Activities of daily living (ADLs) Tasks that one performs to take care of oneself, (e.g., bathing, toileting, grooming, dressing)

Activity analysis An ongoing part of the OT process that allows practitioners to understand and address the skills and external components needed for the performance of any given activity

Activity and occupational demands The components of activities and occupations that occupational therapy practitioners consider during the clinical reasoning process

Activity limitation A person is unable to perform a meaningful task or action (e.g., unable to bend over to tie one's shoes)

Activity (Activities) The term used to describe what the injured person was doing when the injury occurred (as in Chapter 17); a class of culturally accepted actions people perform on a daily basis (general definition); or carefully selected components of intervention to help clients achieve occupational performance (throughout text)

Acute settings A setting in which an individual requires daily monitoring from a physician and round-the-clock care (e.g., hospital)

Adapting Offering an alternative way to perform a task, modifying or substituting objects used in performing the activity

Adaptive equipment (AE) Devices that are used to enhance occupational performance, such as a device to assist with buttons or a larger-handled fork

Adherence The ability of material to bond to itself

Advocacy Seeking the best for another individual or group and often communicating on their behalf

Against gravity Movements that occur in a vertical plane (e.g., away from the floor or toward the ceiling)

Agnosia The inability to recognize an object by sight despite adequate cognition, normal language skills, normal visual acuity, and intact visual fields

Agonist A muscle or muscle group that causes the motion and is sometimes referred to as the *prime mover*

Agraphia Impaired ability to write

Air speed In fluidotherapy, the rate that the cellulose particles are moving, which can be adjusted to the appropriate level for the client to tolerate

Airway obstruction A blocking of the airway as a result of choking on foods, which impedes normal breathing

Alexia without agraphia Inability to read letters, words, or sentences, yet ability to write

Allograft (homograft) Cadaver skin used as a temporary wound coverage

Alternating attention The ability to shift focus between two tasks or activities, each requiring thought

Alternating current (AC) The type of current used in neuromuscular electrical stimulation

Alternative transportation Any other form of transport besides driving, such as biking or public transportation

Amplitude The maximum amount of current delivered in one pulse

Amputation The loss of parts of a limb, a whole limb, or multiple limbs

Angina pectoris A condition characterized by chest pain or tightness that results from reduced blood flow in coronary arteries, most commonly as a result of coronary artery disease

Anosognosia Denial of impairments

Anoxic brain injury A serious and life-threatening insult to the brain due to lack of oxygen

Antagonist A muscle that performs the opposite motion of the agonist

Anterior cord syndrome A medical condition in which the anterior spinal artery, the primary blood supply to the front of the spinal cord, is interrupted, causing ischemia or infarction of the spinal cord

Anterograde amnesia The inability to make new memories after a neurological event

Anticipatory awareness A high level of awareness in which the client is able to anticipate the effects of his or her impairment before it occurs (for example, a memory-impaired client writes out a grocery list)

Antiretroviral therapy (ART) A medication regimen comprising several different medications selected from over 25 potential medications in accordance with U.S. Department of Health and Human Services (DHHS) guidelines to reduce the amount of HIV within a person's body

Aphasia A communication impairment affecting receptive and/or expressive language abilities

Applicator The ultrasound tool that delivers the ultrasonic energy or sound waves

Apraxia A motor speech disorder caused by damage to the area of the brain that is responsible for coordinated and controlled muscle movement

Aquatic therapy Water-based therapy for clients who have difficulty with muscle strength, muscle tone, weight-bearing, joint pain, joint flexibility, balance, healing, and/or sensory perception

Arthrodesis Joint fusion surgery

Arthroplasty Rebuilding of a joint (commonly referred to as *joint replacement*)

Arthroscopy A minimally invasive procedure that involves making small incisions around a joint; the incisions allow passage of a scope (miniature camera) and miniaturized surgical instruments

Artificial disk replacement A surgical procedure for relieving low back pain in which the intervertebral disk in the spine is replaced with a mechanical device

Aspiration The passage of any substance into the airway or trachea, which can lead to pneumonia

Assistive devices Items that can help compensate for client weakness, disability, and/or increased distance or height difference between surfaces (e.g., mobility devices and durable medical equipment)

Assistive technology (AT) An umbrella term that includes assistive, adaptive, and rehabilitative devices for persons with disabilities and also includes the process used in selecting, locating, and using them

Atelectasis Collapse or closure of a lung

Attention Process Training (APT) An attention training method for those with neurological impairment (based on a hierarchical model developed by Sohlberg and Mateer)

Augmentative and alternative communication (AAC) A term for all forms of communication—other than speaking—used to communicate wants, needs, and ideas

Autograft A graft of the client's own skin

Autoimmune disease An immune system disorder in which the immune system triggers a response that actively destroys healthy cells. The trigger is not an external source, such as a virus, but an abnormal response as the body begins to attack itself

Autonomic dysfunction A condition in which there is damage to the nerves of the autonomic nervous system of the body

Autonomic dysreflexia (AD) An exaggerated, reflexive sympathetic response, generally in an individual with a complete T6 or above SCI/D

Axis (axes) of the body Imaginary longitudinal lines through the body, around which movement occurs in planes

Axonotmesis A severe nerve injury that may be the result of a crush or traction injury. Motor loss is expected, and although there is the potential for recovery, it may take a long time

B

Baby Boomers The generation born between 1945 and 1964

Back precautions A list of movements that should or should not be done, provided to clients after back surgery, such as: no bending, no twisting, and specific limits on how much they can lift

Backward chaining A technique in which the practitioner provides significant (or total) assistance in all steps of the sequence except the last step of the task, which the client performs. The practitioner lends less assistance in the step before the last step as the client becomes proficient

Bariatric A branch of medicine that deals with all stages of obesity—from its cause to its treatment

Basal ganglia disorders Syndromes and movement disorders thought to arise from abnormalities or disturbances in the basal ganglia

Beam nonuniformity ratio (BNR) An indicator of the variability of the intensity delivered through the ultrasound (specifically, the ratio of the highest intensity of the beam to the average intensity of the beam delivery)

Benign tumor A noncancerous growth of tissue

Bilevel positive airway pressure (BiPAP) A device used by clients with respiratory problems, generally caused by diaphragmatic weakness or lung air exchange issues; BiPAP not only "pushes" the air, but "pulls" it as well

Biologics A class of disease-modifying antirheumatic drugs (DMARDs), called *biological response modifiers*, that target the parts of the immune system that cause inflammation and damage to joints and tissues

Body mass index (BMI) An assessment and screening tool to monitor for overweight and obesity; it is a value derived from the mass (weight) and height of an individual

Body mechanics A term that conveys the concept of how to best position the body in space to avoid injury and has foundational principles in anatomy and kinesiology

Bolus An assemblage of solids and liquids that will be swallowed and is created as one chews this mixture of materials into a cohesive unit

Bouchard's nodes Hard, bony growths seen in clients with osteoarthritis on the proximal interphalangeal joints of the fingers

Boutonnière deformity A hyperextension deformity of a finger, which is bent toward the palm at the joint nearest the knuckle and bent back away from the palm at the joint farthest from the knuckle

Bradycardia A heart rate that is slower than normal

Bradykinesia Slowness of movement

Bruxism The grinding of teeth

Burn A type of injury to the skin caused by heat, chemicals, electricity, friction, or radiation, resulting in a wound

Burnout A psychological syndrome as a result of chronic workplace stress and is often associated with compassion fatigue

Bursa Fluid-filled sacs that surround and protect the shoulder and other places where bone meets bone (e.g., elbow, knee)

Bursitis An inflammation of the bursa

C

Canadian Model of Occupational Performance and Engagement (CMOP-E) A model that depicts the client at the center, with spirituality as the core motivating principle, which is foundational for the cognitive, affective (behavioral), and physical aspects. Surrounding this core is the individual's occupations, followed by the outermost layer, the environment

Canadian Occupational Performance Measure (COPM) A semistructured interview that measure a client's self-perception of barriers that impact occupational performance in everyday living, and explores self-care, productivity, and leisure issues on a scale of 1 to 10, with the goal of increasing performance satisfaction

Cancer Disease in which there is rapid, uncontrolled growth and spread of abnormal cells, most often forming a tumor

Cancer-related fatigue (CRF) A debilitating impairment of cancer patients characterized by a chronic, subjective feeling of overwhelming exhaustion from which one cannot recover

Cancer rehabilitation A process that assists the client with cancer to obtain maximum physical, social, psychological, and vocational functioning within the limits created by the disease and its resulting treatment

Capsuloligamentous complex A series of connective tissue that surrounds and supports the glenohumeral joint to provide stability by limiting the amount of translation (movement) and rotation of the humeral head away from the glenoid fossa

Cardiomyopathy A disease of the heart muscle; three common types of cardiomyopathy are dilated, hypertrophic, and restrictive

Casting motion to mobilize stiffness (CMMS) A technique in which casting is used to immobilize some joints while encouraging a specific motion to regain motion in the stiff hand

Central pain Neurogenic pain that originates in the spinal cord and is thought to be the result of misdirected neural sprouting after the injury

Central vision The acute and clear vision of the center of the visual field. Central vision is necessary for reading, facial identification, and object identification

Cerebellum (cerebellar) disorders Involving the cerebellum in which a client's movements may appear jerky, segmented, awkward, and uncontrolled

Cerebral akinetopsia An inability to perceive movement of objects, such as a ball in motion

Cerebrovascular accident (CVA) An event that occurs when blood flow to the brain is interrupted, resulting in oxygen not being able to reach parts of the brain; also called a *stroke*

Certification National or state regulation that exists to maintain the integrity of the profession and protect the public. To work as an OTA in the United States, one must pass a national certification examination, which is followed by licensure in the state of work. OTAs in Canada may attend a community college or gain skills through on-the-job training, and they do not have to take a national certification examination

Chaining technique A tool for breaking down functional tasks into steps, then chaining them together one by one as the client learns each step

Charge In neuromuscular electrical stimulation, the total amount of electricity being delivered to the client during each pulse

Chemotherapy-induced peripheral neuropathy (CIPN) A disabling side effect of cancer treatment in which the chemotherapy agents used to treat cancer also damage the peripheral nerves

Chemotherapy-related cognitive dysfunction A possible side effect of chemotherapy drugs that impairs cognitive function and may present during or after treatment

Chorea Rapid, jerky, forceful movements

Chronic disease A persistent or lifelong condition that can be controlled and self-managed over time but is not curable

Chronic disease self-management The client's active participation in the healthcare process, self-monitoring of symptoms, symptom management, making informed decisions about their health, adhering to medical recommendations, and managing the impact of the condition on their daily lives

Chronic fatigue syndrome (CFS) A condition characterized by long-term, extreme fatigue that does not improve with rest and may actually worsen with activity

Chronic inflammatory demyelinating polyneuropathy (CIDP) CIDP is closely related to Guillain Barré syndrome in symptoms, and is often considered its chronic counterpart

Chronic obstructive pulmonary disease (COPD) An irreversible lung disease in which individuals progressively experience difficulty breathing when air flow in the lungs is disrupted by damage to the alveolar walls and/or thickening of the airways

Chunking Breaking down information into small pieces as a memory technique

Closed head injury (CHI) A head injury that does not involve penetration of the skull but results in both focal and broad diffuse damage (occurring throughout the brain)

Cognitive rehabilitation therapy (CRT) A systematic, therapeutic intervention to retrain individuals with any type of cognitive impairment who have difficulty carrying out daily activities that were once automatic

Comorbidity An injury or health condition that occurs in addition to the primary injury and affects the overall plan of care

Compassion fatigue A psychological state resulting from the prolonged care of individuals who are suffering. It is a direct result of ignoring the symptoms of stress and inattention to personal emotions over time

Compassion satisfaction Feelings of gratification of caregiving that can be enhanced by practitioners who effectively use coping strategies to reduce stress and increase opportunities for relaxation

Compensatory movements Abnormal motions the client may use to replace weaker or less functional muscles when attempting to move

Compensatory strategies Techniques and behavior modifications that are used to compensate for a deficit or injury. In clients with visual field deficits, a compensatory strategy might be having the client turn his or her head toward the impaired visual field to bring missing areas into view

Complete SCI/D A total lack of sensory and motor function below the level of spinal cord injury or disease

Complex regional pain syndrome (CRPS) A chronic pain syndrome that develops either in the upper or lower extremity and is characterized by swelling; stiffness; burning pain; hypersensitivity to cold; changes in skin color, hair growth, and nail growth; and a loss of functional use of the extremity (formerly called *reflex sympathetic dystrophy*)

Complex rehabilitation technology (CRT) Products and associated services, including devices that require a specialty process (evaluation, fitting, programming, and training), designed to meet the specific needs of clients with congenital, progressive, or degenerative neuromuscular disorders

Comprehensive driving evaluation An assessment of a client's driving skills, abilities, and rehabilitation potential to return to driving by a healthcare professional that includes a complete clinical assessment of physical, cognitive, vision, and/or perception abilities

Concentric contraction A contraction that occurs when the muscles shorten and the muscle attachments (origin and insertion) move toward each other when there is joint movement

Confabulate In clients with certain types of memory impairment, clients may fabricate descriptions of events that did not happen but which the client believes did happen

Congestive heart failure (CHF) A chronic and progressive condition in which the heart loses its ability to pump effectively to meet the body's need for blood and oxygen

Constructional apraxia Difficulty or inability to perform the act of building, assembling, or drawing objects

Continuous passive motion machine (CPM) A device used in rehabilitation following a soft tissue trauma that provides early protected motion to healing soft tissues. The CPM is commonly used for treating elbows, shoulders, and knees for contractures or mobilization after surgery to enhance connective tissue strength, facilitate ROM, and evacuate joint hemarthrosis

Continuum of care A concept involving a system that guides and tracks clients over time through a comprehensive array of health services spanning all levels and intensity of care

Contraindication A specific condition that indicates a particular technique or device should not be used, such as the use of a physical agent modality or device for a client

Contrast In vision, contrast refers to the ability to distinguish between similar shades of light and dark or between an object and its background

Contraversive pushing A term used to describe the phenomenon in which a person who has had a stroke pushes away from the less affected side

Controlled motion Active motion of an involved joint or previously immobilized structure

Convergence In vision, moving the eyes symmetrically and inward toward the midline to focus on a single point

Coronary artery bypass graft (CABG) A procedure to replace occluded coronary arteries with grafts of arteries or veins from other parts of the body

Cortical blindness The total or partial loss of vision in a normal-appearing eye caused by damage to the brain's occipital cortex

Corticosteroids Steroid medications (cortisone, prednisone, hydrocortisone) that mimic the effects of hormones that are naturally produced in the body, but exceed the body's normal levels. This helps to decrease inflammation and suppress the body's immune system, which is why it is used in inflammatory and autoimmune conditions such as arthritis

Cranial nerve palsy Damage to cranial nerves III, IV, or VI that leads to weakness or paralysis of the eye muscles

Critical illness myopathy (CIM) An acute disorder of the muscle, with flaccid presentation and symmetrical weakness

Critical illness polyneuropathy (CIP) An acute disorder primarily affecting motor and sensory axons, causing severe limb and respiratory muscle weakness

Cryotherapy The local use of low and freezing temperatures to control pain and inflammation

Custom fabricated (C/F) An orthosis that has components that are molded or fabricated for one specific client. The orthosis may be fabricated based on clinically derived castings, tracings, measurements, or images such as x-rays of a given body part. Fabrication requires substantial work and cost

Cystic fibrosis (CF) A genetic condition characterized by increased production of very thick mucus that blocks airways needed for breathing

D

Deep partial-thickness burn Burn involving the entire epidermis and going deeper into the dermis

DeLorme's method of progressive resistive exercise (PRE) An exercise procedure in which small loads are used initially and increased gradually after each set of 10 repetitions

Dementia A group of diseases and conditions that develop when nerve cells in the brain die or no longer function normally and cause changes in a person's memory, behavior, and ability to think clearly

Dermatome The area of skin supplied with afferent nerve fibers by a single posterior spinal root

Desensitization A program for hypersensitivity of the upper extremity that involves exposure to stimulation in order to normalize sensory input and to decrease pain. Because the goal of desensitization is to decrease pain and improve hand function, the client should be slowly introduced to more uncomfortable textures, immersion particles, and vibration, eventually desensitizing the hypersensitive extremity

Diabetes A group of diseases characterized by the presence of elevated blood sugar, or hyperglycemia

Diaphragmatic breathing A strategy used to promote increased use of the diaphragm muscle and reduce overuse of the accessory muscles for breathing

Diathermy An application of electrically induced heat or high-frequency electromagnetic currents used to increase blood flow and heat fibrous tissues

Diffuse axonal injury (DAI) A traumatic brain injury in which damage occurs in the form of extensive lesions over a wide area and is one of the leading causes of death in persons with a TBI

Diplopia Double vision caused by the two eyes not working together because of muscle or nerve weakness

Direct current (DC) A continuous flow of unidirectional electrons between the anode (positive) electrode and the cathode (negative) electrode. This type of current accumulates a charge as a result of the unidirectional flow of uninterrupted current

Disability A broad term encompassing three areas: impairments, activity limitations, and participation restrictions

Disarticulation Amputation at a joint line (between bones)

Discectomy Surgery to remove herniated disc material that is pressing on a nerve root or the spinal cord

Disease-modifying antirheumatic drugs (DMARDs) Medications that help to slow the progression of the rheumatoid arthritis disease process

Divided attention The ability to simultaneously attend to multiple stimuli

Documentation Up-to-date records that assist professionals and caretakers with appropriate decision-making in regard to the treatment and care of the client; often written as an evaluation or treatment note and considered a legal record

Drape The ability of the thermoplastic material to conform to structures (when heated) without too much handling

Drive lockout A safety feature of some power wheelchairs that prevents the chair from moving if the chair is tilted or reclined too much for safe driving

Driver rehabilitation specialist (DRS) A diverse group of providers (e.g., engineers, driving instructors, healthcare professionals) who specialize in driving rehabilitation

Duty cycle The period that ultrasound is being delivered during the treatment time

Dynamic (orthosis) An orthosis that has movable or elastic parts and is used to improve motion, provide controlled motion, or compensate for loss of motion

Dynamometer A device used to objectively assess gross grip strength

Dysarthria A motor speech impairment caused by damage to the brain

Dyskinesias Involuntary movements

Dysphagia An impairment in the ability to swallow

Dyspnea Shortness of breath

Dyspraxia Inability to link thought to movement

Dystonia Muscle contractions that cause slow repetitive movements or abnormal postures

E

Early protected motion Active or passive range of motion that is performed to the uninvolved structures surrounding an injury or immobilized joint

Eccentric contraction A contraction that occurs when there is joint motion but the muscle appears to lengthen; that is the muscle attachments (origin and insertion) move away from each other

Effective radiating area (ERA) The circular area on the sound head from which ultrasound energy radiates

Electromyography (EMG) An electrical test of nerve and muscle function

Electronic aids to daily living (EADL) Environmental control options that allow a client to interact with and manipulate electronic items and devices from a wheelchair, mobile phone, computer, tablet, or remote

Emergent awareness A type of awareness in which a client is able to identify an impairment as it is occurring

Energy conservation An intervention in which clients are taught strategies to minimize muscle fatigue, joint stress, and pain by using the body efficiently and doing things to save energy

Episodic memory Type of memory responsible for storing information about events that were experienced

Ergonomics The design of tools, systems, environments, or tasks to maximize a client's occupational performance, prevent injury, and promote safety and health

Errorless learning technique A tool for presenting important information to a client in a way that eliminates trial and error and guesswork

Eschar Dead tissue

Escharotomy A surgical incision made through the eschar (dead tissue) within the burn wound to release the pressure of the swollen tissues and restore blood flow

Evidence-based practice (EBP) A blend of quality research, clinical knowledge, and input from clients regarding their values and beliefs used as a clinical decision-making framework

Evidence-based treatment Using evidence-based practice (EBP) to incorporate research and clinical expertise in a client-centered manner

Executive functions Cognitive processes carried out in the frontal lobes of the brain that are necessary for control of behavior and that help individuals to be organized, make decisions, problem solve, and regulate behavior in a way that allows for independence and safety in managing daily activities

Explicit/declarative memory The memory of facts and events, which can be consciously recalled

Expressive communication Conveying a message—thoughts, questions, ideas, and concerns—to an intended recipient. Speaking, writing, and gesturing, or any combination of the three, are forms of expressive communication

External fixator A device that has long screws that are inserted into the bones on each side and connected to a frame outside the body to stabilize the bones

F

Fasciculations Small, involuntary twitching, generally in a muscle

Fasciotomy A procedure in which the fascia (connective tissue) is cut through to relieve tension/pressure

Feedback A concept important for motor learning that involves information about a client's performance of a task, used as a basis for improvement

Feeding The action of getting the food or drink and bringing it to the mouth; also called *self-feeding*

Fibromyalgia A chronic condition characterized by widespread pain

Fitness to drive The ability of the driver to drive safely despite a physical impairment, meeting all necessary mental or physical requirements

Flaccidity The absence of muscle tone

Flat affect A phenomenon seen when a person does not display any emotional expressions and body gestures. The person appears to have a stony expression, with little reaction to things around him or her

Focused attention The type of attention that allows for the identification of specific sensory information. For example, it is focused attention that allows a person to orient to sounds, smells, and tactile stimuli

Foraminotomy A decompression surgery that is performed to enlarge the foramen (passageway where a spinal nerve root exits the spinal canal)

Forward chaining A technique in which a task is performed from the very beginning, step by step, adding steps as the practitioner progresses the client in the acquisition of skills. The practitioner provides necessary assistance for step one, with the goal of less and less assistance on each successive attempt

Frame of reference A multifaceted perspective that helps the practitioner to focus on addressing the underlying causes that limit occupations, whether due to activity limitation, impairment, or restriction, in order to assist a client to meet his or her desired goals

Frontotemporal dementia A dementia associated with amyotrophic lateral sclerosis and other conditions that is characterized by specific cognitive, behavioral, and language changes

Fulcrum The axis (center) of a goniometer

Full-thickness burn A burn that involves both layers of skin (epidermis and dermis) and extends to the hypodermis, or subcutaneous fat. Characteristics include a surface that is firm, dry, and leathery and a variety of possible colors, depending on the cause of the burn, that may range from charred (black), pale white, yellow, or nonblanching red

Functional capacity evaluation (FCE) A systematic process of identifying a client's real abilities and/or limitations to perform sustained work

Functional capacity report (FCR) A definitive statement written by an occupational therapy practitioner of what the employer can reasonably expect from the client in terms of his or her ability to sit, stand, stoop, squat, bend, walk, climb (both ladders and stairs), lift and carry, push and pull, and work in a variety of postures and positions within his or her pain tolerance

Functional electrical stimulation (FES) The electrical stimulation of targeted muscles during a functional task. The stimulation period is coordinated with performing a functional task

Functional range of motion (functional ROM) The minimum movement required from a specific joint for the performance of activities of daily living or for any client-specific task (not necessarily full range of motion)

Fusiform swelling A condition that occurs in rheumatoid arthritis in which an entire finger or one joint swells and loses the definition of the individual phalanges

G

Generalization The ability to apply learned skills and techniques learned under one set of circumstances to both predictable and unpredictable environments

Global amnesia Almost total disruption in memory

Goniometer The tool used to measure the arc of motion of a joint

Goniometry The measurement of the arc of motion of a joint using a goniometer

Graded motor imagery A technique to treat chronic pain in the upper extremity that uses three steps to influence the sensorimotor cortex in the brain: laterality training, imagined hand movements, and mirror visual feedback

Graded stimuli The process, for example, of starting with softer textures and then progressing to rougher textures

Grading Adjusting the complexity of a task by altering the demands of the task or the environment or assisting the client to change in order to enable or enhance functional abilities; providing the "just-right" challenge to a client

Gravity The force that attracts an item to the center of the earth, occurring naturally in the environment and exerting a form of resistance to muscle power

Gravity-minimized (-eliminated, -lessened, -reduced) Alternative terms for the horizontal plane position used when testing weaker muscles to reduce the resistance of gravity on muscle power

Guillain-Barré syndrome (GBS) An acute and life-threatening motor neuron disease that rapidly causes severe muscle weakness, including the muscles of speech, swallowing, and respiration

H

Health literacy The client's ability to obtain, process, communicate, and understand medical language or health information so that he or she can manage a health condition and make informed, educated healthcare choices (also incorporates cultural and social nuances concerning health)

Health management and maintenance An instrumental activity of daily living that involves the development of a health-promotion regimen for the client

Health promotion Initiatives to have a population reach a state of complete physical, mental, and social well-being (e.g., the national initiative *Healthy People 2020*)

Health-related quality of life (HRQOL) A multidimensional concept that focuses on the impact of health status on quality of life and includes domains related to physical, mental, emotional, and social functioning

Heberden's nodes Hard, bony growths seen in clients with osteoarthritis on the distal interphalangeal joints of the fingers and toes

Hemianesthesia A sensory problem following a cerebrovascular accident (stroke) or other brain insult, specifically the loss of feeling on one side of the body, usually the same side that has movement changes

Hemianopsia Vision loss in one-half of the visual field in one eye

Hemiarthroplasty A hip surgery used to treat a fractured hip that involves replacing half of the hip—the ball portion and not the socket portion (*hemi* means half, and *arthroplasty* means joint replacement)

Hemi-inattention Decreased awareness of one side of the body and/or the environment

Hemi-neglect A severe form of hemi-inattention that refers to no awareness of the left side of the body and/or environment; also called *unilateral neglect*

Hemiparesis A mild weakness that affects one side of the body

Hemiplegia A significant weakness or paralysis that affects one side of the body

Hemorrhagic stroke A cerebrovascular accident (stroke) that occurs when a blood vessel ruptures or leaks, most commonly because of hypertension bleeds, malformed blood vessels or veins, aneurysms (blood vessel weakness), or it may be spontaneous

Heterotrophic ossification (HO) An abnormal calcification process occurring in and around damaged joints, most often in the elbow or shoulder, severely limiting joint movement and interfering with the ability to perform everyday tasks

Hip movement precautions Postsurgical movement instructions for clients who have undergone hip surgery

Home exercise program (HEP) A customized passive and active range of motion daily exercise routine

Homunculus A representation of the human body, with distortions to show how the various areas of the body are represented in the brain. Those areas with large representation have more sensory receptors in the brain compared with those with smaller representation

Hospice care End-of life care that strives to ease the difficulties during the last stages of terminal illnesses

Human immunodeficiency virus (HIV) A virus that targets the CD4 T lymphocytes, also called *CD4 cells* or *T cells,* and in the process, continues to replicate itself

Hypermetabolic Characterized by increased metabolism and speed of processing food

Hypersensitivity Occurs when the client has an extreme physical response to a stimulus or condition; often perceived as exaggerated response to the stimulus as compared to other individuals

Hypertension A condition in which there is an excessive amount of force being exerted against the walls of arteries as blood is pumped throughout the body by the heart (high blood pressure)

Hypertonicity An abnormally strong skeletal muscle that is resistant to stretch and is velocity dependent; the involuntary contraction can occur when the muscle is not actively working

Hypertrophic scar A scar characterized by its dark red–purple "angry" color; it is thick, firm to the touch, and itchy; it results from the complex processes that are required to heal a large (burn) wound. Instead of forming neatly, the scar tissue forms randomly and creates the rough texture

Hyposensitivity Occurs when a stimulus is applied and the client does not feel it or perceives it with less intensity as compared to other individuals

Hypotonicity Decreased muscle tone

Hypoxia Lack of oxygen

I

Ideational apraxia A deficit in the knowledge of what needs to be done in a task.

Identification The process of helping the client realize that the tasks used in therapy are tied to individual client goals and have great personal value to them to achieve a desired outcome

Ideomotor apraxia A disorder in the production of purposeful movement. The client understands what needs to occur to complete the task but cannot physically perform it despite not having any physical or sensory deficits

Idiopathic pulmonary fibrosis A progressive lung condition of unknown cause in which the lungs become fibrotic, scarred, and stiff over time

Immobilization The process of holding a joint in place with an orthotic, cast, or brace

Impingement syndrome A clinical syndrome in which rotator cuff tendons and bursa become irritated, trapped, or compressed by movements at the shoulder

Impairment Difficulty with a body part(s) or the way the body functions

Implicit/procedural memory Remembering how to perform tasks, such as riding a bicycle or playing the piano; it is automatic

Inclusion Involving a person with a disability in all aspects of society, despite the person's disability

Incomplete spinal cord injury/disease (SCI/D) A partial motor and/or sensory function below the level of injury, including the lowest sacral segment (anal sensation or voluntary external sphincter motor control)

Initiation The internal ability to begin a task

Injury prevention The strategies to keep injuries from ever occurring

Instrumental activities of daily living (IADLs) Tasks that are performed just beyond the scope of caring for one's own body and are more complex (e.g., cooking, medication management, light housework, driving)

Integration The process in which the individual personally values the goals, and the goals become part of his or her internal drive

Intellectual awareness The most basic level of awareness, in which a client is able to identify that impairments do exist. When asked, clients would be able to verbalize some or all of their impairments

Interactive driving simulator A computer-controlled environment that represents selected aspects of the driving experience considered to be representational of real-world driving and allows objective measurements of clients' responses to designated driving tasks and scenarios and how the responses influence subsequent events within the limits of the parameters of the simulation program through accelerator, brake, and steering components

Interdisciplinary team Involves a variety of healthcare professionals from different disciplines who work interdependently on common goals for the client

Interferential current (IFC) A treatment modality that consists of two separate channels delivering different frequencies of electrical stimulation simultaneously. The channels are set up so that their paths cross, literally interfering with each other

Interlaminar implant A *U*-shaped implant that fits between the spinous processes located in the lumbar region of the spine. The implant is designed to maintain a fixed distance between the spinous processes to support and stabilize without a reduction in the range of movement and motion

Intrathecal Administered directly into the spinal theca

Iontophoresis The delivery of transdermal drugs or chemicals into the tissue via low-amplitude DC current; a physical agent modality

Ischemic stroke The most common type of cerebrovascular accident (stroke), occurring when there is some type of blockage of blood flow (typically a blood clot)

Isokinetic exercise Exercises that provide a changing resistance with a constant velocity that allows for maximal force throughout the full range of motion

Isometric exercise Exercises performed when the muscle contracts but the joint does not move

Isometric muscle contraction A static contraction that occurs when tension is developed in the muscle but no movement occurs and muscle length does not change

Isotonic exercise Exercises performed with weights or elastic bands and provide a constant amount of resistance throughout the full range of motion

Isotonic muscle contraction A muscle contraction that occurs when the muscle length and the joint angle change when a muscle contracts

J

Joint laxity The relative instability of a joint; the freedom of movement within a joint

Joint preservation or **joint protection** A set of principles in managing arthritic conditions with the goal of reducing joint stress, decreasing pain, and preserving joint structure

Joystick throw How far the joystick must be pushed before a power wheelchair responds with movement

K

Keloid scar A scar in which there is overgrowth of tissue beyond the original wound; such scars can be firm or rubbery and can vary in color

Kinematics The study of motion

Knee resurfacing Minimally invasive knee surgery performed only on the damaged or arthritic parts of the knee. Jagged bone edges or spurs are trimmed and removed. Only the inner side or outer compartment of the knee joint is replaced with an implant

Kyphoplasty A procedure that creates space in a compressed or collapsed vertebra with a balloon-type device and injection of a special cement to restore the damaged vertebrae height to relieve pain

L

Laminectomy A decompression surgery that enlarges the spinal canal to relieve pressure on the spinal cord or nerves

Legal blindness A term used by the government to determine whether a client qualifies for government services and benefits. Legal blindness means that the acuity is no better than 20/200 with best correction in the better-seeing eye (glasses or after surgery) or only 20 degrees of total visual field or less in the better-seeing eye

Length of stay (LOS) The number of days a client will receive care in a given setting

Licensure Regulation by national or state board to maintain the integrity of the profession and protect the public. State licensures vary, but most states require annual licensure renewal, which entails proof and documentation of a specific number of hours of continuing education, plus a license renewal fee. In Canada, only occupational therapists are licensed, and not all have to pass a national certification examination to gain licensure; it varies province by province

Lifelong learning Developing a natural desire to seek and discover opportunities for continual self-improvement as a practitioner and to incorporate new learning into practice

Lifestyle modification Building new, health-supporting routines in clients to address potential risk factors for chronic diseases

Lipedema A bilateral, symmetrical increase in stored fat, generally of the lower extremities

Long-term memory The virtually unlimited capacity to store (and retrieve) information and memories over a long period of time

Lymphedema A condition of localized fluid retention and tissue swelling caused by a mechanical dysfunction within the lymphatic system—a system that helps protect the body from disease and is responsible for moving interstitial fluid back into the bloodstream. It may present as swelling in the lower part of the arms and legs, but can encompass the entire extremity

M

Maceration Skin breakdown caused by excessive moisture in contact with the skin

Manual edema mobilization (MEM) A technique used for decreasing edema in the orthopedic population. MEM differs from manual lymph drainage, as it is used in an acute condition to decrease edema in an intact lymph system.

Manual muscle testing (MMT) A means of assessing muscle strength that measures the maximal contraction of a muscle or a muscle group

Manual wheelchair Self-propelled or caregiver-propelled wheelchair. A multitude of types, features, and support systems for positioning and pressure relief as well as weight are available

Maximum medical improvement (MMI) The state in which an injured employee's healing process has plateaued and additional medical interventions or traditional therapy interventions are no longer of benefit to the client

Mechanical pain Local soft tissue pain associated with spinal cord injury; it is common in traumatic cases in which bones and soft tissue were compromised

Mechanical ventilation The use of an external device for gas/air exchange, often required to sustain pulmonary function in the setting of respiratory distress

Mechanism of injury (MOI) The precipitating cause or the cause that started the chain of events that led to the injury

Medically at-risk drivers Clients who have medical conditions that could affect driving performance; typically, assessment is required

Megahertz (MHz) The unit of measure that expresses 1 million vibrations per second for the ultrasound wave frequency

Memory How the mind stores and remembers information. See also *episodic, explicit/declarative, implicit/procedural, long-term, semantic, sensory, short-term, and working*

Memory orthotics The ability of the thermoplastic material to return to its original shape once reheated

Metastasis Cancerous cells from the tumor that break away and travel to other parts of the body, where they may continue to grow and form more tumors

Mirror therapy (MT) A treatment for phantom limb pain in which a client sits parallel to a mirror that blocks the view of the affected limb and creates an illusion that tricks the brain into thinking that the limb is intact

Mirror visual feedback (MVF) The use of a mirror to assist the client with visualizing sensory input while watching the uninvolved hand

Mobility-related activities of daily living (MRADLs) Any activity of daily living (ADL) for which a mobility device would be used in the completion

Modalities Therapeutic methods or agents, such as deep heat and cryotherapy

Model of Human Occupation (MOHO) A model developed by Gary Kielhofner that focuses intervention on a client's volition (willingness to do something) and the client's habituation (how the client does things), which leads to improved competence, identity, and occupational adaptation

Model of practice A way of viewing the relationship of the person, environment, occupation, and desired outcomes, and can serve to help test theories

Morbidly obese One hundred pounds or more overweight

Motivational interviewing A client-centered communication style targeted at obtaining pertinent information from a client, including demonstrating empathy and compassion, while eliciting their story and working toward enhancing the client's self-efficacy. Used to facilitate behavior change in individuals who may be ambivalent, hesitant, or resistant to change

Motor neuron A cell body located in the spinal cord or brain which controls muscle

Movable arm The movable part of the goniometer that rotates on the circular disc

Multidisciplinary team A team consisting of various professionals from different disciplines who each provide their own healthcare service to the client

Muscle coordination The smooth rhythmic interaction of muscle function without the presence of tremors or ataxia

Muscle endurance The ability of a muscle or a muscle group to perform repeated contractions against a resistance or to maintain an isometric contraction over time

Muscle grade Score assigned during manual muscle testing that depends on the clinical judgment, knowledge, and experience of the OT practitioner, and is based on whether a muscle can move the body part against gravity

Muscle strength The maximal amount of tension or force that a muscle or muscle group can voluntarily exert in one maximal effort, when type of muscle contraction, limb velocity, and joint angle are specified

Muscular dystrophy A group of rare diseases that cause progressive muscle weakness and loss of muscle mass. In muscular dystrophy, gene mutations interfere with production of the proteins necessary to form healthy muscle

Myasthenia gravis (MG) An autoimmune disease that occurs when the immune system attacks the body's own tissues; that attack interrupts the connection between nerve and muscle

Myelin A coating, or sheath, on axons that insulates and nourishes them

Myocardial infarction (MI) A condition in which a portion of the heart muscle has reduced blood flow that is sustained for an extended period. This reduction in blood flow limits oxygen that is necessary for heart functioning and leads to damage and necrosis, or death, of cardiac tissues; also known as a *heart attack*

Myotome A group of muscles innervated by a single spinal nerve

Myotonia The inability to relax a muscle at will

N

National Highway Traffic Safety Administration (NHTSA) An agency under the U.S. Department of Transportation. In its mission to save lives and reduce crashes, it has collaborated with the American Occupational Therapy Association to expand driver rehabilitation service programs, policies, and strategies

Neurogenic heterotopic ossification (nHO) Pathological bone formation in joints caused by central nervous system damage or insult

Neuromuscular electrical stimulation (NMES) The electrical stimulation of muscles to improve muscle strength and function

Neuromuscular junction The connection between nerve and muscle

Neuroplasticity The ability of the nervous system to change at the cellular level

Neuropraxia (Neurapraxia) A peripheral nerve injury that is usually the result of nerve compression or repetitive stress. With neuropraxia, sensory changes may occur, but recovery is expected

Neurotmesis A nerve injury in which the nerve has either been lacerated or transected and will require surgery in order to improve

Nonprogressive condition A condition in which the disorder itself does not cause further or ongoing changes in medical, physical, or cognitive health

Nonsteroidal anti-inflammatory drugs (NSAIDs) Medications that reduce inflammation (swelling) and pain (analgesic)

Nontraumatic spinal cord injury or disease Tumors, infections, inflammation, and autoimmune or degenerative processes that damage spinal cord tissue

Nosocomial Hospital-acquired (generally infections)

O

Obese Over 20% higher-than-expected weight

Obesity A condition characterized by an atypical measure of fat content that has the potential to negatively impact one's health

Object permanence The ability to recognize that an object is available and present despite it being outside of the visual field

Occupational alienation A sense of isolation or frustration from the removal of an occupation or from participating in activities that do not satisfy or support an individual's needs

Occupational deprivation The loss of choice or diversity beyond an individual's control

Occupational dysfunction A condition in which an individual incurs a disruption caused by an important life event, an environmental change, or a temporary illness or injury that has not been resolved; occupational performance deficits; or a lengthy state of occupational deprivation

Occupational imbalance A disproportion among work, rest, and play that occurs when an individual's occupational engagement fails to meet physical, social, mental, and rest needs, which can have the outcome of boredom or burnout

Occupational injustice Individuals or a group of people that experience a lack of meaningful occupation. This may manifest as the risk factors of occupational deprivation, occupational alienation, occupational imbalance, and occupational marginalization

Occupational marginalization An individual's inability to apply daily choices and use decision-making while engaging in occupations

Occupational performance The client's ability to desire, recall, plan, and carry out occupations based on internal desire or external stimuli and demands

Occupational profile The summary of information about the client, which includes occupational history and daily life tasks, interests, and values

Occupational risk factors The loss of the balance between lifestyle and environment that affect an individual's health and well-being

Oculomotor control The ability to control eye movements

Off the shelf (OTS) Orthotics or equipment that is prefabricated and requires minimal self-adjustment for use and does not require expertise in fitting, trimming, or bending; some assembly may be required

Older drivers Drivers who are 65 years of age or older. Advanced age combined with functional impairments associated with medical conditions put older drivers at risk for crashes and life-threatening injuries

Oncology The branch of medicine concerned with the diagnosis and treatment of cancer

Open head injury (OHI) A head injury that occurs when the skull is penetrated, such as by a bullet, and typically involves largely focal damage (confined to a small part of the brain)

Open-reduction internal fixation (ORIF) A procedure in which a hip or other fracture is reduced or put back in place, and an internal fixation device (such as a metal plate) is placed on the bone to hold the broken bone together

Opportunistic infections Infections caused by pathogens (e.g., viruses, protozoa) that take advantage of an opportunity not normally available, such as a human host with a weakened immune system

Orthopnea Shortness of breath that occurs with lying flat

Orthosis (orthoses, *pl*) A brace or other device used as a treatment intervention to treat a variety of diagnoses to assist clients in the return to engagement in occupation. Orthoses are used for protection, positioning, and improving range of motion

Orthostatic hypotension A form of low blood pressure that occurs when standing up from sitting or lying down.

Orthostatic hypotension is common in clients who have been bedbound primarily in the supine position for extended periods

Osteoarthritis (OA) Degenerative joint disease or degenerative arthritis; chronic condition affecting the joints, occurring when the cartilage on the ends of bones wears down or is destroyed

Osteotomy A procedure in which the surgeon corrects a bone defect by cutting it and then repositioning the bone

P

Palliative care A multidisciplinary approach that focuses on alleviating suffering and improving the quality of life for clients with advanced illnesses

Panniculus The excessive adipose (fat) tissue in the lower abdominal region that hangs down, creating an increased "pull" against the client's lower back

Paralinguistic communication The nonverbal parts of communication, such as gasps, sighs, and/or facial expressions

Paralysis The complete loss of muscle function in an area of the body

Paraparesis A partial loss of function or strength in the lower limbs

Paraplegia Lower extremity weakness or paralysis caused by injury or disease to the thoracic, lumbar, or sacral spinal cord

Partial knee replacement Minimally invasive knee surgery performed only on the damaged or arthritic parts of the knee. Jagged bone edges or spurs are trimmed and removed. Then only the inner side or outer compartment of the knee joint is replaced with an implant

Partial-thickness burn A burn that extends through the epidermis and into the dermis; also called *second-degree burn*

Participation restriction A person cannot be involved in a specific life situation (e.g., an individual who uses a wheelchair would not be able to perform the typical job of a police officer on patrol)

Passive range of motion (PROM) Joint movement caused only by an external force, such as an individual or a device, and typically having a higher degree of ROM than active movement

Penetration During swallowing, the passage of materials into the laryngeal region but not past the vocal folds into the trachea

Perceptual completion The phenomenon in which the brain "fills in" blind spots in the field of vision with what it thinks should be there

Performance skill The small, observable, goal-directed actions the client uses to perform daily activities, which are learned and developed over time

Peripheral vision Commonly called *side vision;* it also includes upper and lower vision and enables the effective navigation of the environment and anticipation of surrounding objects

Person-Environment-Occupation-Performance (PEOP) A model that explains the interaction between the person, environment, occupation, and performance of those occupations in five dimensions (psychological, neurological, spiritual, physiological, and motor factors) to understand how these dimensions interact with one another to promote well-being and quality of life; formerly the PEO model

Phantom limb pain Pain perceived to be coming from an amputated body part

Phantom limb sensation Sensations (e.g., itching, touch) in a specific part of, or throughout, the whole limb that was amputated

Phasic alertness The momentary, rapidly occurring (within milliseconds) readiness to respond, such as to a reaction time test or when woken abruptly (e.g., the sound of a baby crying)

Phasic bite An ineffective chewing pattern in which the jaws move up and down with no lateral movement

Phonophoresis The use of ultrasound to enhance the delivery of topically applied drugs; a physical agent modality

Physiatrist A physician specializing in rehabilitation medicine

Physical agent modalities (PAMs) Procedures and interventions that are applied to alter specific client factors, such as body functions related to pain and neuromusculoskeletal, skin, or movement-related functions

Physical job description A written document that identifies the physical requirements necessary to perform a job's essential functions. When these physical requirements are identified in measurable terms, simulated work tasks can be designed for the rehabilitation process

Pinch gauge A device used to assess pinch strength

Pitting edema Soft, swollen area that leaves an indentation after gentle pressure (such as with a finger) is applied and released

Plasmapheresis A method by which whole blood is removed from the body and processed so that the red and white blood cells are separated from the plasma, or liquid portion of the blood

Polytrauma Two or more injuries, at least one of which is life threatening, with an Injury Severity Score (ISS) of 16 or greater

Post-acute setting A setting in which an individual requires intermittent monitoring by a physician, and is generally after an acute hospitalization (e.g., inpatient rehabilitation [IPR] facilities and long-term acute care [LTAC] facilities)

Post-polio syndrome A condition that affects polio survivors 15 to 40 years after recovery from an initial attack of the poliomyelitis virus. Most often, polio survivors start to experience gradual new weakening in muscles that were previously affected by the polio infection

Post-traumatic amnesia The period of confusion immediately after a traumatic brain injury when the individual is unable to make new memories

Power wheelchair An electric motor–powered mobility device

Pragmatic communication The verbal and nonverbal skills that govern social communication. These skills include the use of language for different purposes, such as greeting, informing, and requesting. Pragmatics also involve modifying language to meet the needs of the communication partner

Praxis Motor planning

Prefabricated (P/F) Orthotics that are non–custom fabricated and require minimal self-adjustment for use and do not require expertise in fitting, trimming, or bending; also called *off the shelf (OTS)*

Premorbid A medical condition already present before a disease or injury occurrence

Presbyphagia Characteristic age-related changes in the swallowing mechanism of otherwise healthy older adults

Pressure injuries Wounds caused by compression or direct application of force (e.g., pressure on skin over a bony prominence)

Pressure Compression or direct application of force (e.g., pressure on skin over a bony prominence)

Primary literature Actual research studies conducted with research participants

Primitive reflex A reflex action present in newborns that integrates into normal movements in neurologically sound adults; may reappear in cases of brain insult or damage

Professional self-care Engaging in behaviors and activities that increase energy, lower stress, and contribute to health and well-being

Progressive condition A condition in which the disorder itself causes ongoing injuries and deterioration in medical, physical, or cognitive health

Proportional control In amputation, the proportional relationship of the elicited strength of the selected muscle contraction to the speed and grip force of the terminal device; alternatively, in power mobility devices, the way a wheelchair joystick moves, where increased deflection of the joystick in any direction causes a corresponding increase in speed in that direction

Prosthesis/Prosthetic device An artificial device designed to replace a missing part of the body

Prosthetic socks Material that fills the space between a socket and the residual limb. Unlike typical socks, prosthetic socks are shaped similar to the residual limb and are sometimes cut to best accommodate the limb and the socket

Prosthetist A medical professional who is trained to fabricate and fit a prosthetic

Provocative testing Testing to provoke symptoms to clarify the site of injury and rule out other diagnoses

Pseudobulbar affect Uncontrollable emotionality, with laughing and/or crying, often not matching the stimulus in content or degree of response

Pulse duration The amount of time that the electrical current stimulus has to be on a body part to generate a motor response, in microseconds

Pulse frequency The number of pulses or periods that the ultrasound is being delivered, expressed in milliseconds

Pulsed current With modulations, meaning the current is turned on and off for brief intervals in short periods

Purposeful activity An activity that the client wants to do and that has meaning for him or her

Pursed-lip breathing (PLB) A technique of exhaling through tightly pressed (pursed) lips and inhaling through the nose with the mouth closed; this technique is used by clients with pulmonary conditions to control and maintain breathing when experiencing shortness of breath

Q

Qualitative Research that aims to find answers to subjective questions, such as experiences and personal stories, which cannot be replicated

Quality of life (QoL) The client's general well-being

Quantitative Research that deals with numbers, logic, objectivity, and finding a cause and effect, which is easily associated with a measurable, objective number. Should be able to be accurately and precisely replicated, and the goal is for the results to be generalized, or applied to other similar situations

R

Radicular pain A shooting or burning sensation that often follows the distribution of the nerve

Radiculopathy A compression of the nerve root in the foraminal opening, which can occur due to bone spurs, herniated or degenerated discs, arthritis, fractures, or facet joint problems, causing pain and possible neurological symptoms to radiate along the path of the nerve

Ramp time The amount of change in pulse intensity or duration from start time to peak intensity in electrical modalities

Range of motion (ROM) The available movement of a joint, whether active or passive, measured within a specific plane

Readmission An admission back to the hospital after being discharged from care

Receptive communication The ability to understand language; the ability to receive, process, and comprehend information to effectively communicate with a partner

Reimbursement The payment of a healthcare provider for a service

Repair and remodeling phase A phase in wound healing in which tissue regeneration and repair of the injured muscle takes place

Resilience The interaction of risk factors and protective resources that produces individual variations in response to stressors

Resistance The load that must be overcome for motion to occur (e.g., the weight of the body part being moved, the pull of gravity on that body part, or an external weight)

Response inhibition The ability to inhibit the inclination to direct attention toward something distracting

Resting hand orthosis A support used to immobilize or position the wrist, fingers, and thumb in a functional position

Retrograde amnesia The loss of memory of events and information that occurred before the brain injury or condition

Reverse total shoulder arthroplasty A surgical procedure in which the ball-and-socket prosthesis construction is reversed, wherein the ball is fitted on the glenoid side, and the cup is situated on the humeral side

Revision surgery In hip revision surgery, a procedure performed to repair an artificial hip joint that has been damaged due to infection, dislocation, or normal wear and tear of the prosthetic hip

Rigid braces An orthotic, such as the thoracolumbar sacral orthosis (TLSO), that is a form-fitting thermoplastic material limiting most movement

Rigidity In muscles, the inability of the muscles to relax normally; alternatively, in orthotics, the strength of the orthotic material when exposed to repeated stress

Rotator cuff disease Damage to the rotator cuff that results in pain and can be due to trauma, overuse, repetitive motion, inflammation, or degeneration

Rotator cuff (muscles) Four muscles (the supraspinatus, infraspinatus, teres minor, and subscapularis) that stabilize the shoulder and hold the head of the humerus into the glenoid cavity to maintain the principal shoulder joint

S

Safe-patient-handling (SPH) equipment designed to reduce work-related injuries. Examples include manual and electric portable lifts, overhead track lifts, and standing-aid lifts

Scapulohumeral rhythm Coordinated movement between the scapula and humerus

Scar contracture A complication of a burn injury in which skin tissue is replaced with scar tissue that is shorter and less extensible. The result is loss of range of motion in the affected area

Scar maturation The latter stages of wound healing, the synthesis and remodeling phase, in which the wound is closed and scar remodeling is progressing. This process of scar remodeling toward scar maturation continues for 12 to 18 months during which time the texture, height, and color of the scar is changing and can be influenced by therapeutic interventions to achieve the best movement and appearance possible

Scooter An electric motor–powered mobility device that turns with a tiller (central post in front of the seat for turning)

Scotoma The central blind spot that occurs with age-related macular degeneration

Screening Using an informal assessment tool to evaluate a client's abilities

Secondary literature Research that evaluates and sorts numerous primary research studies to identify the best overall evidence for a topic and includes systematic reviews, meta-analyses, evidence-based practice guidelines, and critically appraised topics

Secondary traumatic stress The natural, unpreventable stress incurred from the knowledge of a traumatic event of another and the desire to provide assistance to that person

Selective attention The ability to focus on one item while mentally identifying and distinguishing nonrelevant information. This skill gives the ability to filter out extraneous information coming into a person's sensory system

Self range of motion (SROM) Passive range of motion performed by the client alone, generally a nonaffected limb will assist an affected one

Self-efficacy An individual's self-perceptions and beliefs (and judgments) about his or her own capabilities, which have a direct effect on the individual's actions

Self-management The client's ability to take responsibility for managing his or her chronic disease, including maintaining knowledge of the condition and developing problem-solving skills to recognize and navigate lifestyle changes

Self-management support Healthcare professionals aim to increase a clients' skills and confidence in their care, and provide ongoing assessment of progress, goal setting, and problem-solving

Self-monitoring A method of self-observation that requires clients to actively analyze one's actions, thoughts, and feelings with the goal of achieving desired health outcomes

Semantic memory A type of memory that is responsible for storing information about the world, including knowledge about the meaning of words, as well as general knowledge

Sensation Sensory input from objects and others in the environment, as well as from an individual's body, that is received by nuclei in the thalamus, which then relays it to the appropriate area in the cerebral hemispheres for interpretation; a physical feeling experienced by sensory receptors in the skin and joints that provides awareness of the body's contact with objects and temperatures in the immediate environment

Sensory memory A form of unconscious memory in which constant sensory information is taken in, stored for less than 1 second, and then is gone. Sensory memory allows an individual the ability to look at something for a split second and then describe it

Sensory processing Term that refers to how an individual's neurological system impacts the way sensory information is interpreted. At some level of habituation, the individual stops being aware of sensory inputs

Sensory reeducation A process of retraining the brain to correctly interpret and to learn to distinguish various sensory inputs

Sepsis A potentially life-threatening complication of an infection that can spread into the bloodstream, causing rampant infection called *septicemia*

Septicemia A rampant, serious infection that occurs when a bacterial infection elsewhere in the body enters the bloodstream

Serial casting A casting process used in both neuro-rehabilitation and orthopedic settings to improve passive range of motion; it involves applying, removing, and reapplying a series of lightweight casts

Shear (Shearing) forces Internal force generated by the motion of bone and subcutaneous tissue relative to skin, which is restrained from moving because of frictional forces (e.g., when a seated client slides down a chair, when a client slides across a transfer board, or when the head of a bed is raised by more than 30 degrees)

Short-term disability A disability lasting 6 months or less

Short-term memory The brain's ability to retain about seven items for about 10 seconds to 1 minute. It can be thought of as the ability to remember and process at the same time

Shoulder instability The degree of shoulder subluxation, which can range from mild slipping out of the fossa to complete dislocation

Shoulder subluxation The misalignment of the humeral head in the glenoid fossa, causing the humerus to be positioned outside of the joint cavity

Shrinker An elastic socklike garment used to control edema after an amputation

Sialorrhea Drooling

Side-scoot transfer A type of transfer typically used for a client who has greater weakness of the lower extremities and involves the client using the stronger upper extremities in an extension/depression pattern while leaning the trunk anteriorly, lifting the buttocks off of the surface, bearing weight on the knees and feet, and performing a small sideways motion toward the new surface

Skin substitutes Temporary coverage for a severe burn when skin is unavailable. A skin substitute initially "tricks" the wound into thinking that the coverage is skin

Socket The piece of a prosthesis that fits around the residual limb to attach the residual limb to the rest of the prosthesis

Somatosensation Denoting sensation of the body—tactile (touch) and proprioceptive senses that contribute to perception of body position and limb movement, including sensations of pressure, warmth, and vibrations

Sound head Part of the handheld applicator that transmits the ultrasonic energy or sound waves through the coupling agent (gel or water) to the tissue

Spaced retrieval technique Similar to errorless learning; however, in spaced retrieval the client is asked to remember the information for increasingly longer periods of time

Spasticity An involuntary increase in muscle tone with increased velocity of movement

Spina bifida A condition occurring in the womb in which the spinal column does not close all the way, potentially causing spinal nerve damage

Spinal cord disease The nontraumatic tumors, infections, inflammation, and autoimmune or degenerative processes that damage spinal cord tissue

Spinal fusion Surgery to join, or fuse, two or more vertebrae so there is no movement between them

Squat-pivot transfer A transfer that is typically used with a client who needs greater-than-minimal assistance to transfer from a wheelchair or is unable to come to a standing position

Standing lift Durable medical equipment specifically designed to safely secure, lift, and transfer clients from a seated position to a standing position

Stand-pivot transfer A transfer that is primarily used with a client who needs less assistance but is unable to step with the lower extremities when in a standing position

Stand-step transfer A transfer that is used with a client who requires less assistance and is able to step with the lower extremities when in a standing position

Static progressive An orthosis that uses inelastic parts to position a joint at the available end ROM with the intent of improving passive range of motion by manually adjusting tension

Static (orthosis) An orthosis that does not have movable parts and is usually designed to protect, restrict motion, and provide proper positioning

Stationary arm The part of the goniometer that does not move

Stemmer's sign A clinical test for lymphedema. It may be positive if the thick fold of skin of the forefoot cannot be pinched and lifted

Stenosis The abnormal narrowing of a body channel. In spinal cord disease, stenosis means a narrowing of the bony spinal channel

Stereotypic behaviors Repetitive behaviors (such as body rocking) that tend to be harmless but nevertheless interfere with adjustment and participation

Stroke A cerebrovascular accident (CVA), which occurs when blood flow to the brain is interrupted, resulting in oxygen not being able to reach parts of the brain. Where the brain lacks enough oxygen, damage to that neural tissue occurs, resulting in many types of symptoms

Substitutions Movements that result from a muscle's attempt to compensate for the function of a weaker muscle

Sundowning Neuropsychiatric symptoms that occur in the mid to late stages of dementia, characterized by increased anxiety, agitation, confusion, disorientation, and pacing, and generally seen later in the day

Super obese The weight status of an individual with a BMI of 50.0 to 59.9

Superficial burn A burn that involves only the epidermis and appears like simple sunburn. Characteristics include pain upon touch, redness, and possibly edema; also called *first-degree burn*

Superficial partial-thickness burn Burn involving the entire epidermis and the top part of the dermis

Survivorship Care for clients living with, through, and beyond cancer. The goal of survivorship is to decrease the risk for recurrence and prevent new cancers, optimize health by reducing the consequences of cancer and cancer treatments, facilitate recovery, and nurture resiliency and well-being; may be used with other disorders, such as burns

Suspension The way the socket is held onto the residual limb

Sustained attention The ability to remain focused and on task for an extended period of time

Swallowing A complex process involving the mouth, pharynx, larynx, and esophagus. These systems work together to form the swallowing mechanism and are responsible for transporting foods and liquids from the mouth into the stomach for digestion

Swan neck deformity A permanent deformity of the finger in which the joint closest to the fingertip is bent toward the palm while the joint nearest to the palm is bent away from it

Symptom magnification A phenomenon in which clients magnify their pain behaviors, either consciously or unconsciously, for secondary gain

Synergy pattern Stereotypical movements of the extremities following a brain insult or injury

Synovectomy A procedure that removes diseased synovium when rheumatoid arthritis causes the synovial tissue in a joint to become severely inflamed

Synovial joints Three joints separated by synovial fluid and cartilage and encapsulated by a synovial membrane, specifically the glenohumeral, acromioclavicular, and sternoclavicular joints

T

Targeted muscle reinnervation (TMR) A procedure that uses the residual nerves from the amputated limb and transfers them to remaining muscles that have not been biomechanically functional since the amputation

Tendinitis Inflammation of the tendon resulting from microtears and typically due to overuse or repetitive strain

Tendinopathy Disease of the tendon; clinical presentation includes tenderness on palpation and pain, often when exercising or with movement

Tendinosis Tendon degeneration that occurs when the rate of damage exceeds the rate of healing

Tenodesis The synergistic movement between the wrist and fingers; when the wrist is passively or actively flexed, the fingers extend, and when the wrist is passively or actively extended, the fingers flex

Terminal device (TD) The most distal component of the prosthesis that acts as the hand

Tetraplegia Upper-extremity and lower extremity weakness or paralysis in all four extremities caused by injury to the cervical spinal cord; formerly called *quadriplegia*

Theory A broad method used to understand how something works. Theories define the relationship between concepts to help direct and guide the understanding of practitioners, and they are the foundation of models of practice

Therapeutic use of self How the practitioner uses herself or himself as a therapeutic tool throughout the intervention process in words and actions in order to build a therapeutic relationship with the client that enables the client to achieve goals; considered a type of intervention by the *Occupational Therapy Practice Framework, 3rd edition.*

Thermoplastic material A heat-moldable material used for orthotic fabrication

Thumb spica orthosis An orthosis used to immobilize the thumb in a protected or functional position. Clients who have been diagnosed with arthritis, de Quervain's tenosynovitis, scaphoid fractures, and traumatic injuries, such as an ulnar collateral ligament injury to the thumb, can benefit from the use of a thumb spica orthosis

Tilt-in-space manual wheelchair A dependent manual wheelchair that features manual tilt (the whole seat tips backward on the base) typically controlled by the caregiver

Tissue necrosis Death of body tissue

Tone The continuous state of muscle contraction

Tongue thrust A chewing pattern often referred to as *reverse swallow*, in which the tongue pushes forward during the attempt to chew and swallow

Topographical orientation A mental map as to where things are located in both public and personal spaces, assisting in interpreting landmarks to find the way

Total body surface area (TBSA) An evaluation tool used to estimate the "size" of a burn as a percentage of body surface area, using the "rule of nines" in adults

Total hip replacement or **arthroplasty (THR)** A procedure that involves surgically removing the entire hip joint (acetabulum and femoral head and neck) and replacing it with an artificial joint (prosthesis)

Total knee arthroplasty or replacement (TKR) A procedure in which a surgeon removes damaged cartilage and bone and reshapes the bony surfaces to fit the prosthesis, or artificial joint. The surgeon cements the prosthetic components into place, including a metal femoral shell, a metal and plastic tibial component, and a plastic patellar component

Traction A procedure that involves using the mechanical force of weight and pulleys set up on a bed frame to put tension on displaced bone to put it back in position and keep it stable

Transcutaneous electrical nerve stimulation (TENS) A unit that utilizes electrodes to deliver pulsed current to stimulate nerves for relieving pain

Transdisciplinary team A type of interdisciplinary team in which members often blur professional lines, believing that one professional can fill the roles of others on the team when necessary

Transfemoral amputation An above the knee amputation (through the femur bone)

Transfer Movement of the body from one site to another

Transfer belts Beltlike devices that help decrease the risk for falls or injury during a transfer. Transfer belts should be positioned low on the client's waist (just above the iliac crests) and snug to prevent slipping along the abdomen and trunk

Transfer boards Assistive devices used to increase the safety of transfers. Transfer boards are flat, smooth boards and vary in length, weight-bearing capacity, weight, shape, and function; sometimes called *slide boards*

Transhumeral amputation An above the elbow amputation (through the humerus bone)

Transient ischemic attack (TIA) A brief, event accompanied by symptoms (generally one-sided weakness or difficulty communicating) that last from minutes to less than 24 hours. Despite the short duration of symptoms with a TIA, it is a serious condition and can be a warning sign of a future, more permanent and significant cerebrovascular accident to come

Transition The complex process of moving from one life stage to another (e.g., from adolescence to adulthood); alternatively, the height difference between one floor surface and the doorway or another type of flooring

Transradial amputation An amputation below the elbow (through the radius and ulna bones)

Transtheoretical Model of Behavior Change (TTM) An evidenced-based model that describe the five intentional stages a person often goes through when making a behavior change

Transtibial amputation An amputation below the knee (through the tibia and fibula bones)

Transverse myelitis An autoimmune system attack on the body's spinal cord that occurs over hours to weeks. The nerves are unable to conduct signals between the brain and the body

Traumatic brain injury (TBI) An injury to the brain that by definition has trauma as the cause of the injury but still is an acquired injury

Traumatic spinal cord injury (SCI) A sudden, traumatic blow to the spine that causes injury to the thoracic, lumbar, or sacral spinal cord and often results in weakness or sensory changes

Tremor dampening An advanced power wheelchair programming feature that can be used for clients with a tremor or less controlled movements because it keeps the chair moving straight despite extraneous movements

Tumor A mass of cells that has no function in the body

U

Ulnar drift A deformity of the hand in which swelling of the metacarpophalangeal joints causes the fingers to become displaced, tending to move toward the little finger

Ultrasound intensity The ultrasonic power that is delivered to the client per area, expressed in watts per square centimeter (W/cm^2)

Ultrasound power The intensity measure by which the ultrasound is delivered to the client, expressed in watts (W), over the course of a treatment

Unilateral neglect A poststroke phenomenon in which the person appears to "neglect," or not recognize, half of his or her body or items in the space opposite the side where the cerebrovascular accident occurred, and is not related to visual deficits

Universal design (UD) The design of tools or environments to improve accessibility and usability for persons of all ages and abilities, to enhance safety, and to prevent injury

V

Vascular dementia The second leading cause of dementia, caused by a stroke, a series of strokes, or other vascular changes

Vasocompression units Devices used to reduce swelling, including the extremities, after surgery or for treating chronic conditions such as lymphedema; commonly referred to as *intermittent compression units*

Vegetative state A condition seen in clients after a brain injury or cerebrovascular accident in which there is wakefulness but no awareness or consciousness; spontaneous eye opening may occur, but no purposeful, behavioral responses to stimulation

Vehicle modifications Adaptations or structural changes to a passenger car, van, or other motor vehicle that allow a client with a disability to safely drive or ride as a passenger

Venous thromboembolism (VTE) A condition in which blood clots form in the venous system and dislodge and move within the circulatory system, ultimately causing a blockage that can be fatal

Vicarious trauma A natural, unpreventable impact that repeated emotional contact with trauma survivors has on a caregiver that can interfere with the person's sense of meaning and worldview

Viscosity A term that refers to a liquid's thickness or resistance to flow

Visual attention The ability of the visual system to attend to visual information in the environment, as well as to determine what information is relevant and irrelevant to a situation

Visual field deficit A blind spot in a portion of the visual field, which may occur based on the location of an injury in the brain

Visual fields Total area where objects can be seen by one or both eyes

Visual scanning The ability to move the eyes to obtain information. The normal scanning pattern is left to right, top to bottom

Volar wrist orthosis An orthosis used to immobilize the wrist in a protected or functional position

W

Wandering An effect of the symptoms of dementia caused by confusion and disorientation. Although the walking about of wandering may seem aimless, most clients have a purpose and an intended destination

Waveform A visual illustration of the pulse waveform, much like the wave patterns on an electrocardiogram (ECG) for the heart

Weight-bearing In orthopedics, how much weight the client is allowed to place on a healing fracture or post-surgery; alternatively, a treatment method used after a brain injury or cerebrovascular accident to normalize muscle tone and increase sensory awareness in a limb

Wheeled mobility Any type of device with wheels that facilitates movement (e.g., manual wheelchair, power wheelchair, scooter, motor vehicle)

Within normal limits (WNL) Within normal, acceptable guidelines

Work capacity evaluation (WCE) A comprehensive evaluation that precedes the work conditioning program or the work hardening program. This assessment not only covers the client's musculoskeletal abilities but also includes the ability to perform work-related functions

Work conditioning A program designed to focus on specific physiological issues (flexibility, strength, and endurance) that prohibit the client from participating in more work-related activities

Work hardening A program designed to use the client's participation in real work activities to improve his or her functional improvement

Work simplification An intervention in which clients with chronic diseases are taught strategies to minimize fatigue and pain by modifying work tasks and employing strategies to save energy

Working memory The temporary storage and manipulation of information in the mind. This information will quickly disappear if not consciously retained by rehearsing it, associating it with other information already in long-term memory, or by giving it meaning

World Health Organization (WHO) An agency of the United Nations that is concerned about international public health and initiation of global health responses

X

Xenograft A tissue graft from another species

Y

Z

Zone of partial preservation A term used with complete (AIS A) individuals who have some level of sparing below the level of injury and above S5

index

Note: Page numbers followed by *f* refer to figures; page numbers followed by *t* refer to tables; page numbers followed by *b* refer to boxes.

D

E

I

N

O

P

Q

R

S

T

U

V

W

X

Y

Z